PDR® 2010 EDITION NURSE'S DRUG HANDBOOK

THE INFORMATION STANDARD FOR PRESCRIPTION DRUGS AND NURSING CONSIDERATIONS

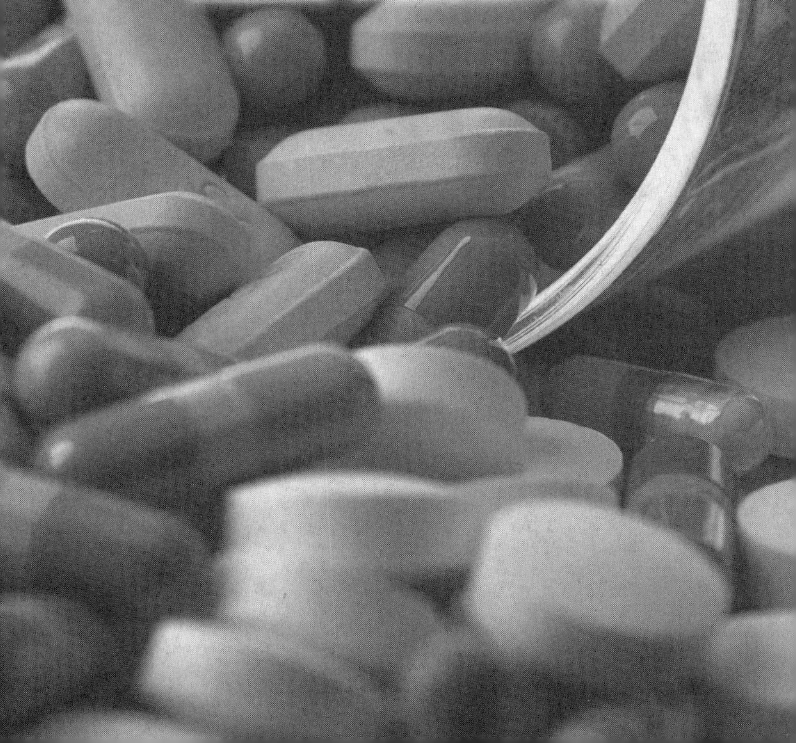

PDR® Nurse's Drug Handbook

2010 EDITION
Senior Director, Editorial & Publishing: Bette Kennedy
Director, Clinical Services: Sylvia Nashed, PharmD
Manager, Clinical Services: Nermin Shenouda, PharmD
Drug Information Specialists: Anila Patel, PharmD; Christine Sunwoo, PharmD; Greg Tallis, RPh
Manager, Editorial Services: Lori Murray
Associate Editor: Jennifer Reed
Contributing Clinical Editors: Pamela Hsieh, PharmD; Shalini Shah, PharmD
Senior Director, Client Services: Stephanie Struble
Project Manager: Gary Lew
Manager, Production Purchasing: Thomas Westburgh
Manager, Art Department: Livio Udina
Electronic Publishing Designer: Carrie Spinelli Faeth

Senior Director, Copy Sales: Bill Gaffney
Senior Product Manager: Richard Buchwald

PHYSICIANS' DESK REFERENCE
Executive Vice President, PDR: Thomas Rice
Vice President, Product Management: Cy Caine
Vice President, Publishing & Operations: Valerie Berger
Vice President, Clinical Relations: Mukesh Mehta, RPh
Vice President, Strategy & Business Development: Ray Zoeller
Vice President, Finance: Donna Santarpia

ISBN: 978-156363-746-9

Printed in the United States

CONTENTS

FOREWORD . . . vii

HOW TO USE THIS BOOK . . . ix

DRUG MONOGRAPH KEY . . . xi

CONCISE DRUG MONOGRAPHS . . 1-1190

BRAND/GENERIC INDEX . . . I-1-I-24

THERAPEUTIC CLASS INDEX . . . I-25-I-52

VISUAL IDENTIFICATION GUIDE . . . V1-V8

APPENDIX: REFERENCE TABLES

Abbreviations, Measurements, and Calculations

Abbreviations, Acronyms, and Symbols . A1
Calculations and Formulas . . . A7
Tables for Pharmacy Calculations . . . A15

Professional Organizations, Boards, and Other Information Centers

Drug Information Centers . . . A17
Poison Control Centers . . . A23
Certification Programs for Nurses . . . A29
Professional Associations for Nurses . . A31
Nurse Practitioner Programs by State . . A33
Professional Associations for NPs . . . A37

OTC Drug Comparison Charts

Central Nervous System
Antipyretic Products . . . A39
Headache/Migraine Products . . . A43
Insomnia Products . . . A49
Smoking Cessation Products . . . A51
Weight Management Products . . . A53

Dermatology
Acne Products . . . A59
Antifungal Products . . . A63
Contact Dermatitis Products . . . A65
Dandruff Products . . . A67
Diaper Rash Products . . . A69
Dry Skin Products . . . A71
Psoriasis Products . . . A83
Wound Care Products . . . A85

Gastrointestinal
Antacid and Heartburn Products . . . A87
Antidiarrheal Products . . . A91
Antiflatulant Products . . . A93
Hemorrhoidal Products . . . A95
Laxative Products . . . A97

Ophthalmic
Artificial Tear Products . . . A101
Ophthalmic Decongestant/ Antihistamine Products . . . A103

Respiratory
Allergic Rhinitis Products . . . A105
Is it a Cold, the Flu, or an Allergy? . . . A109
Cough-Cold-Flu Products . . . A110
Nasal Decongestant/ Moisturizing Products . . . A125

Miscellaneous
Analgesic Products . . . A129
Canker and Cold Sore Products . . . A135

Rx Drug Comparison Charts

Cardiology
ACE Inhibitors . . . A137
Antiarrhythmic Agents . . . A138
Angiotensin II Receptor Blockers (ARBs) and Combinations . . . A145
Beta-Blockers . . . A147
Calcium Channel Blockers . . . A151
Cholesterol-Lowering Agents . . . A153
Coagulation Modifiers . . . A155
Diuretics . . . A161
Lipid Management . . . A163

Dermatology
Acne Management: Systemic Therapies . . . A165
Acne Management: Topical Therapies . . . A167
Psoriasis Management: Systemic Therapies . . . A169
Psoriasis Management: Topical Therapies . . . A171
Topical Corticosteroids . . . A173

Endocrinology
Insulin Formulations . . . A175
Oral Antidiabetic Agents . . . A177

Gastroenterology
Antiemetics . . . A179
H_2 Antagonists and Proton Pump Inhibitors (PPIs) Comparison . . . A185

Infectious Disease
Antibiotic Sensitivity Chart
Aminoglycosides . . . A186
Carbapenems/Monobactams . . . A190
Cephalosporins . . . A194

Fluoroquinolones A199
Macrolides and Clindamycin A203
Penicillins. A207
Sulfonamides A211
Tetracyclines A211
Miscellaneous A215
Drug Treatments for Common STDs . .A219
Flu Vaccines A223
HIV/AIDS Pharmacotherapy A225
HIV/AIDS Complications Therapy. . . .A229
Management of Hepatitis B and Hepatitis C A231
Oral Antibiotics A235
Systemic Antibiotics A237
Systemic Antifungals A269

Musculoskeletal
Ankylosing Spondylitis Agents. A273
Bone Mineral Density Classification/Tests. A275
Dietary Calcium Intake A277
Gout Agents A279
Osteoarthritis Agents A281
Osteoporosis Agents A283
Rheumatoid Arthritis Agents A287

Obstetrics and Gynecology
Gynecological Anti-Infectives. A289
Hormone Therapy A291
Oral Contraceptives A293

Oncology
Breast Cancer Treatment Options. . . .A295
Breast Cancer Risk Factors A301
Chemotherapy Regimens. A303
Colorectal Cancer Treatment Options. .A307

Ophthalmology
Administration Guidelines for Eye Drops & Ointment A309
Glaucoma Agents. A311

Neurology and Pain Management
ADHD Agents A313
Alzheimer's Disease Agents A317
Antiparkinson's Agents A318
Opioid Products A322
Oral Anticonvulsants A327
Oral Narcotic Analgesics A329
Triptans for Acute Migraine A331

Psychiatry
Antidepressants A333
Antipsychotic Agents A335
Bipolar Disorder Pharmacotherapy . . .A337

Pulmonology
Administration Guidelines for Dry Powder Inhalers. A341
Administration Guidelines for Metered-Dose Inhalers A343
Asthma Management. A345
Asthma Treatment Plan A347

Urology
Urological Therapies A349

Immunization Charts
Recommended Immunization Schedule for Persons Aged 0-6 Years A351
Recommended Immunization Schedule for Persons Aged 7-18 Years A353
Catch-up Immunization Schedule for Persons Aged 4 Months–18 Years Who Start Late or Who Are More Than 1 Month Behind A355
Recommended Adult Immunization Schedule, by Vaccine and Age Group A357
Vaccines That Might Be Indicated for Adults Based on Medical and Other Indications. A361

Miscellaneous
Alcohol-Free Products A365
Common Laboratory Test Values A369
Cytochrome P450 Enzymes: Substrates, Inducers, and Inhibitors. .A373
Drugs Excreted in Breast Milk A383
Drugs That May Cause Photosensitivity A385
Drugs That May Cause QT Prolongation. A389
Drugs That May Cause Stevens-Johnson Syndrome and Toxic Epidermal Necrolysis (TEN) . .A391
Drugs That Should Not Be Crushed . .A393
Generic Availability Guide. A399
Lactose- and Galactose-Free Drugs . .A405
Poison Antidote Chart A407
Sugar-Free Products A413
Sulfite-Containing Products A419
Use-in-Pregnancy Ratings A421
Vitamin Comparison Table A428

FOREWORD

Nurses play a crucial role in healthcare delivery. Paramount in this role is the safe administration of medications and expertise in educating patients about their medication therapy. Given today's fast-paced healthcare system, the continual introduction of new medications, and the ongoing release of new information about established medications, nurses need a reference that presents up-to-date information accurately and in a reader-friendly format. The *PDR® Nurse's Drug Handbook, 2010 Edition* is this reference.

Physicians' Desk Reference® is a well-known and trusted resource for medication information—and *PDR Nurse's Drug Handbook* follows in this tradition. This important reference is specifically designed for nurses and presents sections concisely detailing the therapeutic class, indications, dosage, how the medication is supplied, relevant warnings and precautions, key adverse reactions, interactions, pregnancy category, mechanisms of action, pharmacokinetics, and nursing considerations for each entry. Nursing considerations include content specific to assessing, monitoring, and counseling patients, and administering medications.

The *PDR Nurse's Drug Handbook* is organized to foster rapid identification of vital drug information. Medications can be identified by both their generic and brand names and their therapeutic class. Special sections provide important considerations when caring for women who are pregnant or breastfeeding, children, and older adults. Other useful resources include more than 100 charts and tables about medications for specific chronic problems such as hypertension, headache, HIV, and diabetes; immunizations; generic availability; poison antidotes; lactose-, galactose-, and sugar-free product lists; and a full-color visual identification guide. New for 2010 are tables providing detailed information about metered-dose and dry powder inhalers for asthma, medications for glaucoma, hepatitis management, flu vaccines, drugs that affect cytochrome P450 enzymes, and much more.

The *PDR® Nurse's Drug Handbook, 2010 Edition* provides easily accessible, critical information that informs nursing practice and patient education efforts. With its convenient size and clear layout, nurses have swift access to concise, authoritative information. This book is a useful and trusted source for medication information among nurses.

Ivy M. Alexander, PhD, C-ANP
Associate Professor
Director–Adult, Family, Gerontological, and
Women's Health Primary Care Specialty
Yale University School of Nursing

How to Use This Book

The *PDR® Nurse's Drug Handbook, 2010 Edition* allows you to quickly locate important drug information so you can care for patients with confidence. The guide includes over 1,100 monographs providing current, organized information for more than 1,500 of the most commonly used drugs. This handy reference is the perfect companion for practicing nurses, nursing students, and other healthcare professionals.

This compact guide is divided into four discrete sections. The **first section** consists of **concise drug monographs** based on FDA-regulated prescribing information. These monographs are organized alphabetically by brand name. When a brand is no longer available, the generic name is used. Monographs may include:

- Brand Name
- Generic Name
- Manufacturer
- FDA/DEA Schedule
- Black Box Warnings
- Therapeutic Class
- Indications
- Dosage (adults, pediatrics, special populations)
- How Supplied (dosage form/strength)
- Contraindications
- Warnings/Precautions
- Adverse Reactions
- Interactions
- Pregnancy Category/Breastfeeding Precautions
- Mechanism of Action
- Pharmacokinetics
- Nursing Considerations
    - —Assessment
    - —Monitoring
    - —Patient Counseling
    - —Administration and Storage

The **second section** comprises an extensive collection of **tables and key references** to help nurses assess drug therapy and patient safety. Tables provided include Rx and OTC drug comparisons; the most common abbreviations, acronyms, and symbols used by healthcare professionals; and professional associations for nurses. Within the drug comparison tables, drugs are organized alphabetically and by class for easy lookups. These tables and references may include, but are not limited to:

- Brand/Generic Name
- How Supplied (dosage form/strength)
- Indications
- Initial and Max Dosages
- Usual Dosage Range
- Most Common Side Effects

The **third section** of the *PDR® Nurse's Drug Handbook, 2010 Edition* contains two **indices**—one with drugs indexed by brand and generic name and the other organized by therapeutic class.

The **final section** contains a **Visual Identification Guide** featuring product images listed by brand name. This section helps you quickly verify the identity of a capsule, tablet, or other solid oral medication. Each product image contains both the generic and brand name, strength, and the name of its supplier. Other strengths and dosage forms may be available; please check the full prescribing information for a complete listing of all strengths and dosage forms.

Important Information About Product Labeling

Entries in the *PDR® Nurse's Drug Handbook, 2010 Edition* are drawn from FDA-regulated product labeling as published in *Physicians' Desk Reference®* or supplied by the manufacturer. The entries are compiled and updated on a regular basis by a staff of experienced pharmacists. While diligent efforts have been made to ensure the accuracy of each entry, it is essential to bear in mind that the information presented here is merely a synopsis of key points in the official labeling, and that the complete labeling contains additional precautionary information that may be of significance in specific cases. Similarly, please remember that only common and dangerous adverse reactions and interactions are included here, and that numerous less-prevalent adverse effects may be reported in the complete labeling. If an entry leaves any question unanswered, be sure to consult *Physicians' Desk Reference* or the manufacturer for additional information.

The function of the publisher is the compilation, organization, and distribution of this information. In organizing and presenting the material in the *PDR® Nurse's Drug Handbook, 2010 Edition*, the publisher does not warrant or guarantee any of the products described, or perform any independent analysis in connection with any of the product information contained herein.

The *PDR® Nurse's Drug Handbook, 2010 Edition* assumes no obligation to obtain and include any information in these entries other than that provided by the manufacturer. The publisher does not warrant, guarantee, or advocate the use of any product described herein. The publisher and editors do not assume, and expressly disclaim, any liability for error, omissions, or typographical errors in the information contained herein or for misuse of any of the products listed.

DRUG MONOGRAPH KEY[1, 2]

BRAND NAME FDA/DEA Class*

generic (Manufacturer)

Black Box Warning: A brief description of the black box warning(s) that appear in the beginning of the official FDA-approved labeling for the drug.

OTHER BRAND NAMES: Brand name drugs that have the same generic components as the monograph drug.

THERAPEUTIC CLASS: Based on the active ingredients and their mechanism of action.

INDICATIONS: Only includes FDA-approved indications.

DOSAGE: Dosages for adults, pediatrics, and/or special populations as indicated in the official FDA-approved labeling.

HOW SUPPLIED: Product description including strength, formulation, [package size], and scored tablet information.

CONTRAINDICATIONS: Details harmful conditions related to the use of the drug and disease states or patient populations in which use of the monograph drug should be avoided.

WARNINGS/PRECAUTIONS: Details harmful conditions related to the use of the drug and disease states or patient populations where caution is dictated.

ADVERSE REACTIONS: Denotes side effects and adverse reactions listed in the official FDA-approved labeling as occurring with greater frequency (generally at a rate of ≥3%) or deemed significant based on the clinical judgment of the editors. Other side effects may be included if deemed serious or life-threatening. For a complete list of adverse reactions, please refer to the official FDA-approved labeling.

INTERACTIONS: Includes the effects and implications of other drugs and food on the monograph drug based on official FDA-approved labeling.

PREGNANCY: Indicated pregnancy and breastfeeding precautions and, when available, the FDA pregnancy rating system category.†

MECHANISM OF ACTION: Includes pharmacologic drug class and a brief description, or proposed mechanism, of how the drug produces its therapeutic effect.

PHARMACOKINETICS: Brief description of the important parameters described in the FDA-approved labeling related to the absorption, distribution, metabolism, and elimination of the drug. The majority of parameters included are an average or the approximate values provided in the FDA-approved labeling. Only a select group of parameters are included. Refer to the full prescribing information for more detailed pharmacokinetics information.

- **Absorption:** The process by which the drug enters the bloodstream and becomes bioavailable. Absorption parameters may include time to peak plasma concentration (T_{max}), area under the curve (AUC), peak plasma concentration (C_{max}), and absolute bioavailability.
- **Distribution:** Parameters related to the dispersion and dissemination of the monograph drug through bodily fluids and tissues. Distribution parameters may include plasma protein binding and volume of distribution (V_d).
- **Metabolism:** Summary of the biotransformation or detoxification of the parent compound into metabolites. Associated enzymes and active metabolites are included if applicable.
- **Elimination:** The parameters associated with the removal of the drug from the body. Elimination parameters may include elimination/terminal half-life ($T_{1/2}$) and percentage eliminated through urine or feces.

NURSING CONSIDERATIONS

Assessment: Contains specific parameters and laboratory tests that the patient must be assessed for or undergo prior to starting treatment with the drug.

Monitoring: Information used for monitoring patients currently treated with the drug. Monitoring points may include specific lab tests and drug-related or condition-specific information.

Patient Counseling: A compilation of important treatment information to discuss with the patient.

Administration: Guidelines for preparing the monograph drug for administration, rate of administration, proper administration technique, and/or compatibility. Please see the Dosage section. For more details on the step-by-step administration process, refer to the full prescribing information for the drug. **Storage:** Instructions for safe storage and disposal of the monograph drug.

[1] Drug monographs contain concise information. Not all fields described in the Drug Monograph Key are included in every monograph. For more detailed information, please see the full FDA-approved labeling information for the drug.

[2] To identify abbreviated terms used within monographs, refer to the Abbreviations, Acronyms, and Symbols table in the appendix on page A1.

*FDA/DEA CLASS

OTC:	Available over-the-counter.
RX:	Requires a prescription.
CII:	Controlled substance; high potential for abuse.
CIII:	Controlled substance; some potential for abuse.
CIV:	Controlled substance; low potential for abuse.
CV:	Controlled substance; subject to state and local regulation.

†FDA USE-IN-PREGNANCY RATINGS

The FDA use-in-pregnancy rating system weighs the degree to which available information has ruled out risk to the fetus against the drug's potential benefit to the patient. The ratings, and the interpretation, are as follows:

CATEGORY	INTERPRETATION
A	**CONTROLLED STUDIES SHOW NO RISK.** Adequate, well-controlled studies in pregnant women have failed to demonstrate a risk to the fetus in any trimester of pregnancy.
B	**NO EVIDENCE OF RISK IN HUMANS.** Adequate, well-controlled studies in pregnant women have not shown increased risk of fetal abnormalities despite adverse findings in animals, or, in the absence of adequate human studies, animal studies show no fetal risk. The chance of fetal harm is remote, but remains a possibility.
C	**RISK CANNOT BE RULED OUT.** Adequate, well-controlled human studies are lacking, and animal studies have shown a risk to the fetus or are lacking as well. There is a chance of fetal harm if the drug is administered during pregnancy; but the potential benefits may outweigh the potential risk.
D	**POSITIVE EVIDENCE OF RISK.** Studies in humans, or investigational or post-marketing data, have demonstrated fetal risk. Nevertheless, potential benefits from the use of the drug may outweigh the potential risk. For example, the drug may be acceptable if needed in a life-threatening situation or serious disease for which safer drugs cannot be used or are ineffective.
X	**CONTRAINDICATED IN PREGNANCY.** Studies in animals or humans, or investigational or post-marketing reports, have demonstrated positive evidence of fetal abnormalities or risk which clearly outweighs any possible benefit to the patient.

Concise Drug Monographs

ABBOKINASE
RX

urokinase (Abbott)

THERAPEUTIC CLASS: Thrombolytic agent

INDICATIONS: Lysis of acute massive pulmonary emboli (PE) and PE accompanied by unstable hemodynamics.

DOSAGE: *Adults:* LD: 4400 IU/kg IV at 90mL/hr over 10 min. Maint: 4400 IU/kg/hr IV at 15mL/hr for 12 hrs. Flush line after each cycle. For IV use only.

HOW SUPPLIED: Inj: 250,000 IU

CONTRAINDICATIONS: Active internal bleeding, intracranial neoplasm, arteriovenous malformation, aneurysm, bleeding diathesis, severe uncontrolled arterial HTN. Recent (within 2 months) CVA, intracranial or intraspinal surgery, trauma including resuscitation.

WARNINGS/PRECAUTIONS: Prior to use obtain Hct, platelet count, and aPTT. Increased risk of bleeding; fatalities due to hemorrhage, including intracranial and retroperitoneal, reported. Avoid IM injections, nonessential patient handling, frequent venipunctures. Use upper extremity vessels when performing arterial punctures. Increased risk of bleeding with recent (within 10 days) major surgery, obstetrical delivery, organ biopsy, previous puncture of noncompressible vessels, serious GI bleeding, high likelihood of left heart thrombus, subacute bacterial endocarditis, hemostatic defects including those secondary to severe hepatic or renal disease, pregnancy, cerebrovascular disease, diabetic hemorrhagic retinopathy, and any other condition in which bleeding may be a significant hazard or difficult to manage. May carry risk of transmitting infectious agents.

ADVERSE REACTIONS: Bleeding, fatal hemorrhage, anaphylaxis, allergic-type or infusion reactions.

INTERACTIONS: Increased risk of serious bleeding with other thrombolytic agents, anticoagulants, or agents inhibiting platelet function (eg, ASA, other NSAIDs, dipyridamole, GP IIb/IIIa inhibitors).

PREGNANCY: Category B, caution in nursing.

MECHANISM OF ACTION: Thrombolytic agent; acts on the endogenous fibrinolytic system. Converts plasminogen to the enzyme plasmin. Plasmin degrades fibrin clots, fibrinogen, and some plasma proteins.

PHARMACOKINETICS: Distribution: V_d=11.5L. **Metabolism:** Liver. **Elimination:** Bile, urine; $T_{1/2}$=12.6 min.

NURSING CONSIDERATIONS

Assessment: Assess for active internal bleeding, recent (within 2 months) cerebrovascular accident or intracranial or intraspinal surgery; recent trauma (eg, cardiopulmonary resuscitation), intracranial neoplasm, arteriovenous malfunction, aneurysms, bleeding diathesis, and severe uncontrolled arterial HTN. Assess use in patients who had recent (within 10 days) major surgery, obstetrical delivery, organ biopsy, or previous puncture of non-compressing vessels. Assess use in patients with recent (eg, within 10 days) GI bleeding, patients at risk for left heart thrombus, presence of subacute bacterial endocarditis, hemostatic defects (eg, secondary to severe hepatic or renal disease), pregnancy, cerebrovascular disease, diabetic hemorrhagic retinopathy, and any condition in which bleeding might constitute a significant hazard. Assess for drug interactions. Obtain baseline hematocrit, platelet count, and an activated partial thromboplastin time (aPTT).

Monitoring: Monitor for signs/symptoms of bleeding (eg, intracranial hemorrhage, retroperitoneal bleeding), anaphylaxis, and other infusion reactions (eg, fever, hypoxia, cyanosis, dyspnea, hypotension), cholesterol embolization (eg, livedo reticularis, "purple toe" syndrome, acute renal failure, cerebral infarction), and transmission of infectious disease. Monitor for clinical response, vital signs (BP), Hct, platelet count, and aPTT.

Patient Counseling: Instruct to contact physician immediately if allergic reactions (eg, anaphylaxis, bronchospasm, orolingual edema, urticaria, skin rash, and pruritus) or bleeding occur. Counsel about the risk of viral transmission from medication.

Administration: IV route. Do not reconstitute until immediately before use. Discard any unused portion. 1) Reconstitute. Aseptically add 5 mL of SWFI, without preservatives to vial. Do not use bacteriostatic water. 2) After reconstituting, visually inspect vial for discoloration or presence of particulate matter. Solution should be pale and straw-colored. 3) Further dilute using 0.9% NS or D5W, USP. **Storage:** Refrigerate at 2-8°C (36-46°F).

ABELCET

amphotericin B lipid complex (Enzon) **RX**

THERAPEUTIC CLASS: Polyene antifungal

INDICATIONS: Treatment of invasive fungal infections in patients refractory to or intolerant of conventional amphotericin B therapy.

DOSAGE: *Adults:* 5mg/kg IV at 2.5mg/kg/hr.
Pediatrics: ≥16 yrs: 5mg/kg IV at 2.5mg/kg/hr.

HOW SUPPLIED: Inj: 5mg/mL

WARNINGS/PRECAUTIONS: Anaphylaxis reported. D/C if respiratory distress occurs. Monitor SCr, LFTs, serum electrolytes, CBC during therapy.

ADVERSE REACTIONS: Chills, fever, increased SCr, multi-organ failure, NV, hypotension, respiratory failure, dyspnea, sepsis, diarrhea, headache, heart arrest, HTN, hypokalemia, infection, kidney failure, pain, thrombocytopenia.

INTERACTIONS: Antineoplastics may potentiate renal toxicity, bronchospasm, hypotension. Corticosteroids and corticotropin may potentiate hypokalemia, predisposing patients to cardiac dysfunction. May potentiate digitalis toxicity. Increased risk of flucytosine toxicity. Acute pulmonary toxicity reported with leukocyte transfusions. Nephrotoxic drugs (eg, aminoglycosides, pentamidine) enhance potential for renal toxicity. Cyclosporine within several days of bone marrow ablation associated with nephrotoxicity. Hypokalemia effect may enhance curariform effect of skeletal muscle relaxants. May cause increased myelotoxicity and nephrotoxicity with concomitant zidovudine.

PREGNANCY: Category B, not for use in nursing.

MECHANISM OF ACTION: Acts by binding to sterols in cell membrane of susceptible fungi, with resultant change in membrane permeability.

PHARMACOKINETICS: Absorption: C_{max}=1.7mcg/mL, AUC=14mcg•h/mL. **Distribution:** V_d=131L/kg. **Elimination:** $T_{1/2}$=173.4 hrs.

NURSING CONSIDERATIONS

Assessment: Assess for hepatic/renal impairment and possible drug interactions.

Monitoring: Monitor for anaphylatic reaction, hypotension, bronchospasm or respiratory distress, arrhythmias, shock, chills, and fever. Frequently monitor creatinine, LFTs, serum electrolytes (Mg, K^+) and CBC.

Patient Counseling: Inform about risks/benefits.

Administration: IV infusion. Do not dilute with saline solution or mix with other drugs or electrolytes. **Storage:** 2-8°C (36-46°F); admixture stable for 48 hrs at 2-8°C (36-46°F) and additional 6 hrs at room temperature. Avoid light exposure and freezing.

ABILIFY

RX

aripiprazole (Bristol-Myers Squibb/Otsuka America)

Elderly patients with dementia-related psychosis treated with atypical antipsychotic drugs are at an increased risk of death; most appeared to be cardiovascular (eg, heart failure, sudden death) or infectious (eg, pneumonia) in nature. Aripiprazole is not approved for the treatment of patients with dementia-related psychosis. Children, adolescents, and young adults taking antidepressants for major depressive disorder and other psychiatric disorders are at increased risk of suicidal thinking and behavior.

OTHER BRAND NAMES: Abilify Discmelt (Bristol-Myers Squibb/Otsuka America)

THERAPEUTIC CLASS: Partial D_2/$5HT_{1A}$ agonist/$5HT_{2A}$ antagonist

INDICATIONS: (PO) Acute and maintenance treatment of schizophrenia in adults and adolescents aged 13-17 yrs. Acute and maintenance treatment of manic and mixed episodes associated with bipolar I disorder with or without psychotic features in adults and pediatrics aged 10-17 yrs. Adjunctive therapy to antidepressants for acute treatment of major depressive disorder (MDD) in adults. Adjunctive therapy to either lithium or valproate for the acute treatment of manic and mixed episodes associated with bipolar I disorder with or without psychotic features in adults and pediatrics aged 10-17 yrs. (Inj) Acute treatment of agitation associated with schizophrenia or bipolar disorder, manic or mixed, in adults.

DOSAGE: *Adults:* (PO) Schizophrenia: Initial/Target: 10-15mg qd. Titrate: Should not increase before 2 weeks. Max: 30mg/day. Bipolar Disorder (Monotherapy or Adjunct): Initial/Target: 15mg/day. Max: 30mg/day. MDD: Initial: 2-5mg/day. Titrate: May adjust dose at increments of ≤5mg/day at intervals ≥1 week. Range: 2-15mg/day. Max: 15mg/day. Periodically reassess need for maintenance therapy. Oral sol can be given on mg-per-mg basis up to 25mg. Patients receiving 30mg tabs should receive 25mg of oral sol. (Inj) Agitation: 9.75mg IM. Range: 5.25-15mg IM. Max: 30mg/day; initiate PO therapy as soon as possible. Concomitant Strong CYP3A4 Inhibitors (eg, ketoconazole, clarithromycin): Reduce usual aripiprazole dose by 50%. Concomitant CYP2D6 Inhibitors (eg, quinidine, fluoxetine, paroxetine): Reduce usual aripiprazole dose by 50%. Concomitant CYP3A4 Inducers (eg, carbamazepine): Double aripiprazole dose.

Pediatrics: Schizophrenia (13-17 yrs)/Bipolar Disorder (Monotherapy or Adjunct) (10-17 yrs): Initial: 2mg/day. Titrate: 5mg after 2 days. May adjust dose in 5mg/day increments. Recommended: 10mg/day. Max: 30mg/day. Periodically reassess need for maintenance therapy. Oral sol can be given on mg-per-mg basis up to 25mg. Patients receiving 30mg tabs should receive 25mg of oral sol. Concomitant Strong CYP3A4 Inhibitors (eg, ketoconazole, clarithromycin): Reduce usual aripiprazole dose by 50%. Concomitant CYP2D6 Inhibitors (eg, quinidine, fluoxetine, paroxetine): Reduce usual aripiprazole dose by 50%. Concomitant CYP3A4 Inducers (eg, carbamazepine): Double aripiprazole dose.

HOW SUPPLIED: Tab, Orally Disintegrating: (Discmelt) 10mg, 15mg; Tab: 2mg, 5mg, 10mg, 15mg, 20mg, 30mg; Sol: 1mg/mL [150mL]; Inj: 7.5mg/mL

WARNINGS/PRECAUTIONS: May develop tardive dyskinesia, NMS. Monitor for hyperglycemia, worsening of glucose control with DM, FBG levels with diabetes risk. Increased incidence of cerebrovascular adverse events (stroke) in elderly dementia patients. Orthostatic hypotension reported; caution with cardiovascular disease, conditions predisposed to hypotension (eg, dehydration, hypovolemia). May lower seizure threshold. Potential for cognitive and motor impairment. May disrupt body's temperature regulation. Possible esophageal dysmotility and aspiration; caution in patients at risk for aspiration pneumonia. Observe vigilance in treating psychosis associated with Alzheimer's.

ADVERSE REACTIONS: Headache, asthenia, rash, blurred vision, rhinitis, cough, tremor, anxiety, insomnia, nausea, vomiting, lightheadedness, somnolence, constipation, akathisia, extrapyramidal disorder, somnolence, oropharyngeal spasm, grand mal seizure, jaundice, nasopharyngitis, dizziness.

INTERACTIONS: May potentiate effect of antihypertensives. Caution with anticholinergic agents, other centrally acting drugs. Avoid alcohol. CYP3A4 inducers (eg, carbamazepine) may lower blood levels. CYP3A4 inhibitors (eg, ketoconazole, itraconazole) or 2D6 inhibitors (eg, quinidine, fluoxetine, paroxetine) can increase blood levels.

PREGNANCY: Category C, not for use in nursing.

MECHANISM OF ACTION: Psychotropic agent; mechanism not established. Proposed that efficacy is mediated through a combination of partial agonist activity at D_2 and 5-HT_{1A} receptors and antagonist activity at 5-HT_{2A} receptors.

PHARMACOKINETICS: Absorption: Absolute bioavailability 87% (PO), 100% (IM); T_{max}=3-5 hrs (PO), 1-3 hrs (IM). **Distribution:** V_d=404L or 4.9L/kg (PO); plasma protein binding 99% (PO). **Metabolism:** Hepatic via dehydrogenation, hydroxylation, and N-dealkylation. Dehydro-aripiprazole (active metabolite) CYP3A4 and 2D6 enzymes (PO). Not systemically evaluated (IM). **Elimination:** Urine (25%), feces (55%); $T_{1/2}$=75-146 hrs.

NURSING CONSIDERATIONS

Assessment: Assess for dementia-related psychosis, risk of suicidal behavior in children or adolescents/young adults, clinical diagnosis of bipolar disorder, use of drug in patients who have a history of cardiovascular or cerebrovascular disease or history of seizures, and risk of aspiration pneumonia. Assess baseline fasting blood glucose levels in patients at risk for hyperglycemia.

Monitoring: If patient remains on therapy for longer than 6 weeks, perform periodic clinical evaluations to determine treatment responsiveness. Monitor for unusal changes in behavior, signs of worsening depression, risk of suicidality, signs/symptoms of NMS, TD, and hyperglycemia, hypotension, and for dysphagia, dystonia, and extrapyramidal symptoms while on therapy. Measure fasting blood glucose levels if symptoms develop. Periodically evaluate serum glucose levels in patients at risk for DM.

Patient Counseling: Counsel family members or caregivers to contact physician if signs of agitation, irritability, changes in behavior, or suicidal ideation occur. Counsel about cognitive/motor impairment; use caution when operating machinery/driving. Avoid alcohol consumption. Medication may affect body's ability to lower body temperature; instruct to take appropriate measures (eg, adequate hydration when performing strenuous activities, exposed to extreme heat, on concomitant medications with anticholinergic activity). Inform that medication can be taken with/without food. Instruct that disintegrating tab is to be placed on tongue; can be taken without liquid. Do not split tablet.

Administration: Oral route and IM administration. **Storage:** 25°C (77°F); excursions permitted to 15-30°C (59-86°F). Opened bottles of oral solution may be used for up to 6 months after opening, not beyond expiration date. Store injections in original container, protect from light.

ABRAXANE — RX

paclitaxel protein-bound particles (Abraxis)

> **Do not administer to patients with metastatic breast cancer who have baseline neutrophil counts of less than 1,500 cells/mm³. Perform peripheral blood cell counts on all patients to monitor occurrence of bone marrow suppression, primarily neutropenia. Should only be administered under the supervision of a physician experienced in the use of cancer chemotherapeutic agents. Do not substitute for or with other paclitaxel formulations.**

THERAPEUTIC CLASS: Antimicrotubule agent

INDICATIONS: Treatment of breast cancer after failure of combination chemotherapy for metastatic disease or relapse within 6 months of adjuvant chemotherapy. Prior therapy should have included an anthracyline unless clinically contraindicated.

DOSAGE: *Adults:* 260mg/m² IV over 30 min every 3 weeks. Severe neutropenia (neutrophil <500 cells/mm³ for week or longer) or severe sensory neuropathy (Grade 3 or 4): Hold dose until neutrophil >1500 cells/mm³ or sensory neuropathy resolves to Grade 1 or 2. Reduce subsequent courses to 220mg/m², if recurrence reduce subsequent courses to 180mg/m².

HOW SUPPLIED: Inj: 100mg

CONTRAINDICATIONS: Patients with baseline neutrophil counts of < 1,500 cells/mm³.

WARNINGS/PRECAUTIONS: Perform frequent blood counts to monitor for bone marrow suppression. Men should be advised to not father a child while receiving treatment. Remote risk for transmission of viral diseases; theoretical risk for transmission of Creutzfeldt-Jacob disease. Sensory neuropathy occurs frequently. Reports of injection site reactions.

ADVERSE REACTIONS: Neutropenia, infectious episodes, anemia, hypotension, ECG abnormalities, dyspnea, cough, sensory neuropathy, ocular/visual disturbances, arthralgia, myalgia, NV, asthenia, abnormal liver function test.

PREGNANCY: Category D, not for use in nursing.

MECHANISM OF ACTION: Antimicrotubule agent; promotes assembly of microtubules from tubulin dimers and stabilizes microtubules by preventing depolymerization. This stability results in inhibition of the normal dynamic reorganization of the microtubule network that is essential for vital interphase and mitotic cellular functions.

PHARMACOKINETICS: Absorption: C_{max}=18,741ng/mL. **Distribution:** V_d=632L/m², plasma protein binding (89-98%). **Metabolism:** Liver via CYP2C8 (6α, 3'-p-dihydroxypaclitaxel, major metabolite). **Elimination:** Urine (4% unchanged, ≤1% metabolite), feces (approximately 20%).

NURSING CONSIDERATIONS

Assessment: Assess baseline neutrophil counts ≤1,500 cells/mm³ and history of heart disease.

Monitoring: Perform frequent peripheral blood cell counts to monitor occurrence of bone marrow suppression, primarily neutropenia, which may be severe and result in infection. Closely monitor infusion site for possible infiltration during drug administration.

Patient Counseling: Advise women of childbearing potential to avoid becoming pregnant while on drug. Immediately report any signs of fever or other sign of infection. Avoid contact with skin. If contact occurs wash skin immediately and thoroughly with soap and water.

Administration: IV. 1) Reconstitute each vial by injecting 20mL of 0.9% NaCl. 2) Slowly inject 20mL of 0.9% NaCl over a minimum of 1 min, using sterile syringe to direct solution flow onto the inside wall of the vial. 3) Once injection is complete, allow vial to sit for a minimum of 5 min. 4) Gently swirl or invert vial. Avoid generation of foam. Visually inspect parenteral drug products for particulate matter and discoloration prior to administration. **Storage:** Store vials in original cartons at 20-25°C (68-77°F). Retain in original package to protect from light.

ACANYA RX

clindamycin phosphate - benzoyl peroxide (Arcutis)

THERAPEUTIC CLASS: Antibacterial/keratolytic

INDICATIONS: Topical treatment of acne vulgaris in patients ≥12 yrs.

DOSAGE: *Adults:* Apply pea-sized amount to face qd. Not for oral, ophthalmic, or intravaginal use.
Pediatrics: ≥12 yrs: Apply pea-sized amount to face qd. Not for oral, ophthalmic, or intravaginal use.

HOW SUPPLIED: Gel: (Clindamycin-Benzoyl Peroxide) 1.2%-2.5% [50g]

CONTRAINDICATIONS: History of regional enteritis, ulcerative colitis, or antibiotic-associated colitis.

WARNINGS/PRECAUTIONS: Diarrhea, bloody diarrhea, and colitis (eg, pseudomembranous colitis) reported; d/c if significant diarrhea occurs. Antiperistaltic agents (eg, opiates, diphenoxylate with atropine) may prolong and/or worsen severe colitis, and may result in death. Minimize exposure to natural and artificial sunlight after application.

ADVERSE REACTIONS: Erythema, scaling, itching, burning, and stinging.

INTERACTIONS: Avoid with topical or oral erythromycin. Caution with concomitant topical acne therapy (eg, peeling, desquamating, or abrasive agents). May potentiate neuromuscular blockers.

PREGNANCY: Category C, not for use in nursing.

MECHANISM OF ACTION: Clindamycin: Binds to 50S ribosomal subunits of susceptible bacteria and prevents elongation of peptide chains, thereby suppressing bacterial protein synthesis. Benzoyl peroxide: Oxidizing agent with bacteriocidal and keratolytic effects.

NURSING CONSIDERATIONS

Assessment: Assess for history of regional enteritis, ulcerative colitis, or antibiotic-associated colitis, diarrhea, bloody diarrhea, and active colitis, possible drug interactions, and pregnancy/nursing status.

Monitoring: Monitor for erythema, scaling, itching, burning, and stinging.

Patient Counseling: Instruct to apply medication as directed and avoid direct contact with mouth, eyes, vagina, or lips. Avoid applying on cuts or open wounds and washing of face more than 3 times a day. Instruct to wash hands with soap and water after application. Advise not use more than the recommended amount and not to apply more often than once daily. Instruct to notify physician if any signs or symptoms of local skin irritation, pregnant or intend to be pregnant. Advise to minimize exposure to natural and avoid artificial sunlight; to minimize exposure to sunlight wear a wide-brimmed hat or other protective clothing and use a sunscreen with SPF 15 rating or higher during treatment.

Administration: Topical route. See PI for admixing instructions. **Storage:** Store at room temperature up to 25°C (77°F). Do not freeze. Keep jar tightly closed.

ACCOLATE

zafirlukast (AstraZeneca) **RX**

THERAPEUTIC CLASS: Leukotriene receptor antagonist

INDICATIONS: Prophylaxis and chronic treatment of asthma.

DOSAGE: *Adults:* 20mg bid. Administer 1 hr ac or 2 hrs pc.
Pediatrics: ≥12 yrs: 20mg bid. 5-11 yrs: 10mg bid. Administer 1 hr ac or 2 hrs pc.

HOW SUPPLIED: Tab: 10mg, 20mg

WARNINGS/PRECAUTIONS: Cases of life-threatening hepatic failure reported; if suspected, d/c therapy. Not for treatment of acute asthma attacks. Bioavailability decreases with food. Hepatic dysfunction and systemic eosinophilia reported.

ADVERSE REACTIONS: Headache, infection, nausea, diarrhea, hypersensitivity reactions including angioedema.

INTERACTIONS: Coadministration with warfarin increases PT time; monitor closely. Caution with drugs metabolized by CYP2C9 (eg, tolbutamide, phenytoin, carbamazepine) or CYP3A4 (eg, dihydropyridine CCBs, cyclosporine, cisapride, astemizole). Increased levels with ASA. Decreased levels with erythromycin, theophylline. May increase theophylline levels.

PREGNANCY: Category B, not for use in nursing.

MECHANISM OF ACTION: Leukotriene receptor antagonist (LTRA); selective and competitive receptor antagonist of leukotriene D_4 and E_4 (LTD_4 and LTE_4), components of slow-reacting substance of anaphylaxis (SRSA); inhibits bronchoconstriction.

PHARMACOKINETICS: Absorption: Rapid. (Adult) C_{max}=326ng/mL; T_{max}=2 hrs; AUC=1137ng•h/mL. (7-11 yrs) C_{max}=601ng/mL; T_{max}=2.5 hrs; AUC=2027ng•h/mL. (5-6 yrs) C_{max}=756ng/mL; T_{max}=2.1 hrs; AUC=2458ng•h/mL. **Distribution:**

V_d=approximately 70L; plasma protein binding (>99%). **Metabolism:** Liver, hydroxylation via CYP2C9. **Elimination:** $T_{1/2}$=10 hrs.

NURSING CONSIDERATIONS

Assessment: Assess for hepatic dysfunction, bronchospasm (status asthmaticus), nursing status, and possible drug interactions. Obtain baseline LFTs.

Monitoring: Monitor LFTs and for PT, signs/symptoms of hepatotoxicity, eosinophilia, vasculitic rash, worsening pulmonary symptoms, cardiac complications, neuropathy, and hypersensitivity reactions (eg, urticaria, angioedema, rash).

Patient Counseling: Counsel to take drug at least 1 hr before or 2 hrs after meals. Do not decrease dose or stop taking other anti-asthma medications unless instructed by physician. Do not use if nursing. Advise to seek medical attention if experience symptoms of liver dysfunction (eg, right upper quadrant abdominal pain, nausea, fatigue, lethargy, pruritus, jaundice, flulike symptoms, anorexia), eosinophilia, vasculitic rash, worsening pulmonary symptoms, cardiac complications, neuropathy, and hypersensitivity reactions (eg, urticaria, angioedema, rash).

Administration: Oral route. **Storage:** 20-25°C (68-77°F). Protect from light and moisture. Dispense in original air-tight container.

AccuNeb

albuterol sulfate (Dey)

RX

THERAPEUTIC CLASS: Beta$_2$-agonist

INDICATIONS: Relief of bronchospasm with asthma.

DOSAGE: *Pediatrics:* 2-12 yrs: Initial: 0.63mg or 1.25mg tid-qid via nebulizer. 6-12 yrs with severe asthma, >40kg or 11-12 yrs: Initial: 1.25mg tid-qid.

HOW SUPPLIED: Sol, Inhalation: 1.25mg/3mL, 0.63mg/3mL [3mL, 25[s]]

WARNINGS/PRECAUTIONS: Hypersensitivity reactions reported. Fatalities reported with excessive use. Caution with cardiovascular disorders, especially coronary insufficiency, arrhythmias and HTN. May need concomitant anti-inflammatory agents. Can produce paradoxical bronchospasm. Caution with DM. May cause hypokalemia.

ADVERSE REACTIONS: Asthma exacerbation, otitis media, allergic reaction, gastroenteritis, cold symptoms.

INTERACTIONS: Avoid other short-acting sympathomimetic bronchodilators and epinephrine. Extreme caution within 2 weeks of MAOI or TCA use. Monitor digoxin. ECG changes and/or hypokalemia with non-K^+-sparing diuretics may worsen. May be antagonized by β-blockers.

PREGNANCY: Category C, not for use in nursing.

MECHANISM OF ACTION: β_2 adrenergic agonist; stimulates adenyl cyclase, enzyme that catalyzes formation of ATP.

PHARMACOKINETICS: Absorption: (3mg): C_{max}=2.1ng/mL, T_{max}=0.5 hrs. **Elimination:** (4 mg): $T_{1/2}$=5-6 hrs.

NURSING CONSIDERATIONS

Assessment: Assess for CVD (coronary insufficiency, cardiac arrhythmias, HTN), hyperthyroidism, DM, and possible drug interactions.

Monitoring: Monitor for signs/symptoms of cardiovascular effects (eg, increased BP, palpitations), worsening of symptoms, paradoxical bronchospasm, destabilization of asthma, and hypersensitivity reactions (eg, anaphylactic, urticaria, angioedema, rash, bronchospasm, oropharyngeal edema).

Patient Counseling: Instruct not for relief of acute respiratory symptoms. Seek medical attention if symptoms worsen, therapy becomes less effective, need more inhalation from short-acting β_2-agonist than usual, or if experience destabilization of asthma, paradoxical bronchospams, and hypersensitivity (eg, anaphylactic, urticaria, angioedema, rash, bronchospasm, oropharyngeal edema).

Administration: Inhalation route. **Storage:** Between 2-25°C (36-77°F). Protect from light and excessive heat. Store vials in protective foil pouch at all times. Once removed, use within 1 week. Discard if solution not colorless.

ACCUPRIL

quinapril HCl (Parke-Davis) **RX**

ACE inhibitors can cause death/injury to developing fetus during 2nd and 3rd trimesters. Stop therapy if pregnancy detected.

THERAPEUTIC CLASS: ACE inhibitor

INDICATIONS: Treatment of hypertension. Adjunct therapy in heart failure with diuretics and/or digitalis.

DOSAGE: *Adults:* HTN: If possible, d/c diuretic 2-3 days prior to therapy. Initial: 10-20mg qd; 5mg qd with concomitant diuretic. Titrate at intervals of at least 2 weeks. Usual: 20-80mg/day given qd-bid. CrCl >60mL/min: Initial: 10mg/day. CrCl 30-60mL/min: Initial: 5mg/day. CrCl 10-30mL/min: Initial: 2.5mg/day. Heart Failure: Initial: 5mg bid. Titrate at weekly intervals. Usual: 10-20mg bid. CrCl >30mL/min: Initial: 5mg/day. CrCl 10-30mL/min: Initial: 2.5mg/day.

HOW SUPPLIED: Tab: 5mg*, 10mg, 20mg, 40mg *scored

CONTRAINDICATIONS: History of ACE inhibitor-associated angioedema.

WARNINGS/PRECAUTIONS: D/C if angioedema, jaundice, or if marked LFT elevation occurs. Risk of hyperkalemia with DM, renal dysfunction. Persistent nonproductive cough reported. Monitor WBCs in renal or collagen vascular disease. Anaphylactoid reactions reported. Fetal/neonatal morbidity and death reported. Monitor for hypotension in high-risk patients (heart failure, surgery/anesthesia, hyponatremia, high-dose diuretic therapy, recent intensive diuresis, dialysis, or severe volume and/or salt depletion, etc). Caution with CHF, renal dysfunction, and renal artery stenosis. Less effective on BP in blacks and more reports of angioedema than nonblacks.

ADVERSE REACTIONS: Fatigue, headache, dizziness, cough, NV, hypotension, chest pain.

INTERACTIONS: Decreases tetracycline absorption (possibly due to magnesium content in quinapril); consider interaction with drugs that interact with magnesium. May increase lithium levels. Hypotension risk with diuretics. Increased risk of hyperkalemia with K^+-sparing diuretics, K^+ supplements, or K^+-containing salt substitutes.

PREGNANCY: Category C (1st trimester) and D (2nd and 3rd trimesters), not for use in nursing.

MECHANISM OF ACTION: Angiotensin-converting enzyme inhibitor; inhibits ACE activity, reducing angiotensin II formation.

PHARMACOKINETICS: Absorption: T_{max}=1hr. (Quinaprilat) T_{max}=2 hrs. **Distribution:** Plasma protein binding (97%). **Metabolism:** De-esterification. Quinaprilat (active metabolite). **Elimination:** (Quinaprilat) Renal; $T_{1/2}$=2hrs.

NURSING CONSIDERATIONS

Assessment: Assess for pregnancy status, volume/salt depletion, collagen vascular disease (systemic lupus erythematosus [SLE], scleroderma), CHF, DM, possible drug interactions, ischemic heart disease, cerebrovascular disease, and renal impairment.

Monitoring: Monitor renal function for 1st few weeks; WBC in patients with collagen vascular disease periodically. Monitor for signs/symptoms of hypotension, anaphylactoid or hypersensitivity reactions, head/neck and intestinal angioedema, agranulocytosis, hyperkalemia, and renal dysfunction.

Patient Counseling: Inform of pregnancy risks. Instruct inadequate fluid intake or fluid loss may lead to drop in BP resulting in lightheadedness or syncope; avoid K^+ supplements or salt substitutes. Advise to seek medical attention if symptoms of hypotension (syncope), anaphylactoid or hypersensitivity reactions, angioedema (head/neck; abdominal pain with/without NV), infection (sore throat, fever), or hyperkalemia occur.

Administration: Oral route. **Storage:** 15-30°C (59-86°F). Protect from light.

ACCURETIC

RX

quinapril HCl - hydrochlorothiazide (Parke-Davis)

ACE inhibitors can cause death/injury to developing fetus during 2nd and 3rd trimesters. Stop therapy if pregnancy detected.

THERAPEUTIC CLASS: ACE inhibitor/thiazide diuretic

INDICATIONS: Treatment of hypertension. Not for initial therapy.

DOSAGE: *Adults:* Initial (if not controlled on quinapril monotherapy): 10mg-12.5mg or 20mg-12.5mg tab qd. Titrate: May increase after 2-3 weeks. Initial (if controlled on HCTZ 25mg/day but significant K^+ loss): 10mg-12.5mg or 20mg-12.5mg tab qd. If previously treated with 20mg quinapril and 25mg HCTZ, may switch to 20mg-25mg tab qd.

HOW SUPPLIED: Tab: (Quinapril-HCTZ) 10mg-12.5mg*, 20mg-12.5mg*, 20mg-25mg* *scored

CONTRAINDICATIONS: History of ACE inhibitor-associated angioedema, anuria, sulfonamide hypersensitivity.

WARNINGS/PRECAUTIONS: D/C if angioedema, jaundice, or marked LFT elevation occurs. Risk of hyperkalemia with DM, renal dysfunction. Persistent nonproductive cough reported. Monitor WBCs in renal or collagen vascular disease. Anaphylactoid reactions reported. Fetal/neonatal morbidity and death reported. Monitor for hypotension in high-risk patients (heart failure, surgery/anesthesia, hyponatremia, severe volume/salt depletion, etc). Caution with CHF, renal or hepatic dysfunction, and renal artery stenosis. Less effective on BP in blacks and more reports of angioedema than nonblacks. May exacerbate or activate SLE. Monitor serum electrolytes. Avoid if CrCl ≤30mL/min/1.73m². May increase cholesterol, TG, and uric acid levels and decrease glucose tolerance.

ADVERSE REACTIONS: Dizziness, headache, cough, myalgia.

INTERACTIONS: Decreases tetracycline absorption (possibly due to magnesium content in quinapril); consider interaction with drugs that interact with magnesium. Increase risk of hyperkalemia with K^+-sparing diuretics, K^+ supplements, or K^+-containing salt substitutes. Potentiates orthostatic hypotension with alcohol, barbiturates, and narcotics. Adjust insulin and antidiabetic drugs. Impaired absorption with cholestyramine, colestipol. Corticosteroids and ACTH deplete electrolytes. May decrease response to pressor amines. Potentiates other antihypertensives. May increase responsiveness to skeletal muscle relaxants. Risk of lithium toxicity. NSAIDs decrease diuretic effects.

PREGNANCY: Category C (1st trimester) and D (2nd and 3rd trimesters), not for use in nursing.

MECHANISM OF ACTION: Quinapril: Angiotensin-converting enzyme inhibitor; inhibits ACE activity reducing angiotensin II formation. HCTZ: Thiazide diuretic; affects renal tubular mechanism of electrolyte reabsorption directly increasing excretion of Na^+ and Cl^-, and indirectly reducing plasma volume.

PHARMACOKINETICS: Absorption: Quinapril: T_{max}=1 hr. (Quinaprilat) T_{max}=2 hrs. **Distribution:** Quinapril: Plasma protein binding (97%). HCTZ: V_d=3.6-7.8L/kg; plasma protein binding (67.9%); crosses placenta. **Metabolism:** Quinapril: De-esterification. Quinaprilat (metabolite). **Elimination:** Quinaprilat: Renal; $T_{1/2}$=2 hrs. HCTZ: Kidney (61%); $T_{1/2}$=4-15 hrs.

NURSING CONSIDERATIONS

Assessment: Assess for pregnancy status, possible drug interactions, volume/salt depletion, collagen vascular disease (systemic lupus erythematosus [SLE], scleroderma), CHF, DM, ischemic heart disease, cerebrovascular disease, anuria, sulfonamide hypersensitivity, renal/hepatic impairment.

Monitoring: Monitor renal function for 1st few weeks; WBC in patients with collagen vascular disease periodically. Monitor for signs/symptoms of hypotension, anaphylactoid or hypersensitivity reactions, head/neck and intestinal angioedema, agranulocytosis, hyperkalemia, electrolyte imbalance, exacerbation or activation of SLE, precipitation of gout, hyperglycemia, renal/hepatic dysfunction.

Patient Counseling: Inform of pregnancy risks. Advise that inadequate fluid intake or loss of fluids may lead to drop in BP resulting in lightheadedness or syncope. Advise to seek medical attention if symptoms of angioedema (head/neck; abdominal pain with/without NV), infection (sore throat, fever), hypotension (syncope), hypersensitivity reactions, hyperkalemia, or electrolyte imbalance (dry mouth, thirst, weakness) occurs.

Administration: Oral route. **Storage:** 20-25°C (68-77°F).

ACCUTANE — RX

isotretinoin (Roche Labs)

Not for use by females who are or may become pregnant, or if breastfeeding. Birth defects have been documented. Increased risk of spontaneous abortion, and premature births reported. Approved for marketing only under special restricted distribution program called iPLEDGE™. Must have 2 negative pregnancy tests. Repeat pregnancy test monthly. Use 2 forms of contraception at least 1 month prior, during, and 1 month following discontinuation. Must fill written prescriptions within 7 days; refills require new prescriptions. May dispense maximum of 1 month supply. Prescriber, dispensing pharmacy, and patient must be registered with iPLEDGE.

OTHER BRAND NAMES: Sotret (Ranbaxy) - Claravis (Barr) - Amnesteem (Genpharm)

THERAPEUTIC CLASS: Retinoid

INDICATIONS: Severe recalcitrant nodular acne unresponsive to conventional therapy, including systemic antibiotics.

DOSAGE: *Adults:* Initial/Usual: 0.5-1mg/kg/day given bid for 15-20 weeks. Max: 2mg/kg/day (for very serious cases). Adjust for side effects and disease response. May discontinue if nodule count reduced by >70% prior to completion. Repeat only if necessary after 2 months off drug. Take with food. *Pediatrics:* ≥12 yrs: Initial/Usual: 0.5-1mg/kg/day given bid for 15-20 weeks. Max: 2mg/kg/day (for very serious cases). Adjust for side effects and disease response. May discontinue if nodule count reduced by >70% prior to completion. Repeat only if necessary after 2 months off drug. Take with food.

HOW SUPPLIED: Cap: 10mg, 20mg, 40mg

CONTRAINDICATIONS: Pregnancy, paraben sensitivity (preservative in gelatin cap).

WARNINGS/PRECAUTIONS: Acute pancreatitis, impaired hearing, anaphylactic reactions, inflammatory bowel disease, elevated TG and LFTs, hepatotoxicity, premature epiphyseal closure, and hyperostosis reported. May cause depression, psychosis, aggressive and/or violent behaviors, rarely suicidal ideation/attempts and suicide; may need further evaluation after discontinuation. May cause decreased night vision, and corneal opacities. Associated with pseudotumor cerebri. Check lipids before therapy, and then at intervals until response established (within 4 weeks). D/C if significant decrease in WBC, hearing or visual impairment, abdominal pain, rectal bleeding, or severe diarrhea occurs. Monitor LFTs before therapy, weekly or biweekly until response established. May develop musculoskeletal symptoms. Avoid prolonged UV rays or sunlight, and donating blood up to 1 month after discontinuing therapy. Caution with genetic predisposition for age-related osteoporosis, history of childhood osteoporosis, osteomalacia, other bone metabolism disorders (eg, anorexia nervosa). Spontaneous osteoporosis, osteopenia, bone fractures, and delayed fracture healing reported; caution in sports with repetitive impact. Use 2 forms of effective contraception for 1 month. Female patients of childbearing potential must fill and pick up the prescription within 7 days of the date of specimen collection for the pregnancy test. Must only be dispensed in no more than 30-day supply and with a Medication Guide.

ADVERSE REACTIONS: Cheilitis, dry skin and mucous membranes, conjunctivitis, blood dyscrasias, epistaxis, decreased HDL, elevated cholesterol and TG, elevated blood sugar, arthralgias, back pain, hearing/vision impairment, rash, photosensitivity reactions, psychiatric disorders, abnormal menses, cardiovascular disorders.

INTERACTIONS: Avoid vitamin A. Limit alcohol consumption. Avoid use with tetracyclines; increased incidence of pseudotumor cerebri. Pregnancy reported with oral and injectable/implantable contraceptives. Avoid St. John's wort; may cause breakthrough bleeding with oral contraceptives. Caution with drugs that cause drug-induced osteoporosis/osteomalacia and affect vitamin D metabolism (eg, corticosteroids, phenytoin).

PREGNANCY: Category X, not for use in nursing.

MECHANISM OF ACTION: Retinoid; not established. Suspected to inhibit sebaceous gland function and keratinization.

PHARMACOKINETICS: Absorption: C_{max}=862ng/mL (fed), 301ng/mL (fasted); T_{max}=5.3 hrs (fed), 3.2 hrs (fasted); AUC=10,004ng•hr/mL (fed), 3703ng•hr/mL (fasted). **Distribution:** Plasma protein binding (99.9%). **Metabolism:** Liver via CYP2C8, 2C9, 3A4, and 2B6; 4-*oxo*-isotretinoin, retinoic acid, and 4-*oxo*-retinoic acid (active metabolites). **Elimination:** Urine, feces; $T_{1/2}$=21 hrs (isotretinoin), 24 hrs (4-*oxo*-isotretinoin).

NURSING CONSIDERATIONS

Assessment: Assess that females have had 2 negative pregnancy tests separated by at least 19 days, and are on 2 forms of effective contraception: A primary form (eg, tubal sterilization, partner's vasectomy, intrauterine device, or hormonal) and a secondary form (barrier, vaginal sponge) for at least 1 month prior to administration. Assess that females are not nursing. Assess for hypersensitivity to parabens, history of psychiatric disorder, risk of hyperlipidemia (eg, DM, obesity, increased alcohol intake, lipid metabolism disorder or family history of such disorder). Obtain lipid levels profile and LFTs. Assess for possible drug interactions.

Monitoring: Monitor for signs/symptoms of psychiatric disorders (eg, depression, mood disturbances, psychosis, aggression, suicidal ideation), pseudotumor cerebri (eg, papilledema, headache, NV, visual disturbances), hyperlipidemias (eg, elevated serum TG), acute pancreatitis, hearing impairment, hepatotoxicity, inflammatory bowel disease (regional ileitis), decreased bone mineral density, hyperostosis, premature epiphyseal closure, musculoskeletal symptoms (eg, arthralgia), neutropenia, agranulocytosis, hypersensitivity reactions, visual impairments, corneal opacities, and decreased night vision. Monitor lipid levels and LFTs, glucose levels, and CPK levels until response to drug is established. Monitor that females remain on 2 forms of contraception during therapy and for 1 month following discontinuation.

Patient Counseling: Instruct to read the guidelines and sign the Patient Information/Informed Consent form. For females of childbearing potential, instruct that 2 forms of contraception are required starting 1 month prior to initiation, during treatment, and for 1 month following discontinuation. Inform that monthly pregnancy tests are required before new prescription is issued. Counsel not to share drug with anyone and not to donate blood during therapy and 1 month following discontinuation. Instruct to take with a meal and swallow capsule with a full glass of liquid. Inform that transient flare of acne may occur when initiating treatment. Counsel to notify physician if signs of depression, mood disturbances, psychosis, or aggression occur. Instruct to avoid wax epilation and skin resurfacing procedures during therapy and for 6 months following. Counsel to avoid prolonged exposure to UV rays or sunlight. Inform that decreased tolerance to contact lenses during and after therapy may occur.

Administration: Oral route. **Storage:** 15-30°C (59-86°F). Protect from light.

ACEON

perindopril erbumine (Solvay) RX

ACE inhibitors can cause death/injury to developing fetus during 2nd and 3rd trimesters. Stop therapy if pregnancy detected.

THERAPEUTIC CLASS: ACE inhibitor

INDICATIONS: Treatment of hypertension (HTN). Risk reduction of cardiovascular mortality or nonfatal myocardial infarction in patients with stable coronary artery disease (CAD).

DOSAGE: *Adults:* HTN: If possible, d/c diuretic 2-3 days prior to therapy. Initial: 4mg qd; 2-4mg/day given qd-bid with concomitant diuretic. Maint: 4-8mg/day given qd-bid. Resume diuretic if BP not controlled. Max: 16mg/day. Elderly (>65 yrs): Initial: 4mg/day given qd-bid. Max (usual): 8mg/day. Renal Impairment: CrCl >30mL/min: Initial: 2mg/day. Max: 8mg/day. CAD: Initial: 4mg qd for 2 weeks. Maint: 8mg qd. Elderly (>70 yrs): Initial: 2mg qd for 1 week. Titrate: 4mg qd for Week 2. Maint: 8mg qd.

HOW SUPPLIED: Tab: 2mg*, 4mg*, 8mg* *scored

CONTRAINDICATIONS: History of ACE inhibitor-associated angioedema.

WARNINGS/PRECAUTIONS: D/C if angioedema, jaundice, or if marked LFT elevation occurs. Risk of hyperkalemia with DM, renal dysfunction. Persistent nonproductive cough reported. Monitor WBCs in renal and collagen vascular disease. Anaphylactoid reactions reported. Fetal/neonatal morbidity and death reported. Monitor for hypotension in high-risk patients (heart failure, surgery/anesthesia, hyponatremia, prolonged diuretic therapy, or volume and/or salt depletion). Caution with CHF, renal dysfunction, and renal artery stenosis. Less effective on BP in blacks and more reports of angioedema than nonblacks. Avoid if CrCl <30mL/min.

ADVERSE REACTIONS: Cough, headache, asthenia, dizziness, diarrhea, edema, respiratory infection, lower extremity pain.

INTERACTIONS: May increase lithium levels. Hypotension risk with diuretics. Increased risk of hyperkalemia with K^+-sparing diuretics, drugs that increase serum K^+, or K^+ supplements. Caution with gentamicin.

PREGNANCY: Category D, caution in nursing.

MECHANISM OF ACTION: Angiotensin-converting enzyme inhibitor; inhibits ACE activity, decreasing plasma angiotensin II, decreasing vasoconstriction, increasing plasma renin activity, and decreasing aldosterone secretion.

PHARMACOKINETICS: Absorption: Rapid; absolute bioavailability (75%); T_{max}=1 hr. Perindoprilat: Absolute bioavailability (25%); T_{max}=3-7 hrs. **Distribution:** Plasma protein binding (60%). Perindoprilat: Plasma protein binding (10-20%). **Metabolism:** Hepatic esterases (hydrolysis), glucuronidation, cyclization. Perindoprilat (active metabolite). **Elimination:** Urine (4-12%); $T_{1/2}$=0.8-1 hr. Perindoprilat: $T_{1/2}$=3-10 hrs.

NURSING CONSIDERATIONS

Assessment: Assess for pregnancy status, volume/salt depletion, collagen vascular disease (systemic lupus erythematosus [SLE], scleroderma), CHF, DM, possible drug interactions, ischemic heart disease, cerebrovascular disease, renal/hepatic impairment.

Monitoring: Monitor renal function for 1st few weeks; WBC in patients with collagen vascular disease periodically. Monitor for signs/symptoms of hypotension, anaphylactoid or hypersensitivity reactions, head/neck and intestinal angioedema, agranulocytosis, hyperkalemia, renal/hepatic dysfunction.

Patient Counseling: Inform of pregnancy risks. Instruct that inadequate fluid intake or loss of fluids may lead to drop in BP resulting in lightheadedness or syncope; avoid K+ supplements or salt substitutes. Advise to seek medical attention if symptoms of hypotension (syncope), anaphylactoid or hypersensitivity reactions, angioedema (head/neck; abdominal pain with/without NV), infection (sore throat, fever), hyperkalemia or hepatic dysfunction occur.

Administration: Oral route. **Storage:** 20-25°C (68-77°F). Protect from moisture.

ACETAZOLAMIDE — RX
acetazolamide (Various)

OTHER BRAND NAMES: Diamox Sequels (Duramed)

THERAPEUTIC CLASS: Carbonic anhydrase inhibitor

INDICATIONS: Adjunctive treatment for: (Cap, Extended-Release/Inj/Tab) chronic simple (open-angle) glaucoma, secondary glaucoma and preoperatively in acute angle-closure glaucoma where delay of surgery is desired in order to lower IOP; edema due to CHF and drug-induced edema; centrencephalic epilepsies (petit mal, unlocalized seizures). (Cap, Extended-Release/Tab) Prevention or amelioration of symptoms associated with acute mountain sickness in climbers attempting rapid ascent and in those who are very susceptible to acute mountain sickness despite gradual ascent.

DOSAGE: *Adults:* (Cap, Extended-Release) Glaucoma: 500mg bid. (Cap, Extended-Release/Tab) Acute Mountain Sickness: 500mg-1g/day in divided doses; 1g for rapid ascent. Initiate 24-48 hrs before ascent and continue for 48 hrs while at high altitude or longer as needed. (Inj/Tab) Open-Angle Glaucoma: Usual: 250mg-1g IV/PO qd in divided doses. Secondary Glaucoma/Pre-op Treatment of Closed-Angle Glaucoma: (IV/PO) 250mg q4h or 250 mg bid if on short term therapy or 500mg followed by 125mg or 250mg q4h in severe cases. Epilepsy: Monotherapy: 8-30mg/kg/day in divided doses. Usual: 375mg-1g/day. Combination Therapy: Initial: 250mg qd. Titrate: If needed up to 1g/day. CHF/Drug-Induced Edema: Initial: 250-375mg qam for 1-2 days. Maint: After initial edema fluid loss, give on alternating days, or for 2 days alternating with day of rest.

HOW SUPPLIED: Cap, Extended-Release: 500mg; Inj: 500mg; Tab: 125mg*, 250mg* *scored

CONTRAINDICATIONS: In sodium- or potassium-depleted patients, marked hepatic or kidney impairment, cirrhosis, suprarenal gland failure, hyperchloremic acidosis, (with long-term therapy) chronic noncongestive angle-closure glaucoma.

WARNINGS/PRECAUTIONS: Rare reports of fatal sulfonamide hypersensitivity reactions (eg, Stevens-Johnson syndrome, toxic epidermal necrolysis, fulminant hepatic necrosis, anaphylaxis, agranulocytosis, aplastic anemia, other blood dyscrasias) have occurred. D/C drug if this occurs. Sensitizations may recur when a sulfonamide is readministered irrespective of the route of administration. Dose increase does not increase diuresis and may result in decreased diuresis and increased drowsiness. Use with caution if patient predisposed to acid/base imbalances (elderly with renal impairment), DM, or impaired alveolar ventilation. Monitor serum electrolytes. Obtain CBC and platelet count before therapy and at regular intervals during therapy.

ADVERSE REACTIONS: Paresthesia, hearing dysfunction, tinnitus, loss of appetite, taste alteration, GI disturbances, polyuria, drowsiness, confusion, metabolic acidosis, electrolyte imbalance, transient myopia.

INTERACTIONS: Caution with high-dose ASA. May increase phenytoin levels; may increase occurrence of osteomalacia. May decrease levels of primidone, lithium. May increase effects of other carbonic anhydrase inhibitors, folic acid antagonists, quinidine, amphetamine. May prevent urinary antiseptic effect of methenamine. Increased risk of renal calculus formation with sodium bicarbonate. May increase levels of cyclosporine.

PREGNANCY: Category C, not for use in nursing.

MECHANISM OF ACTION: Carbonic anhydrase inhibitor. In eye: Decreases secretion of aqueous humor, reducing IOP. In CNS: Appears to retard abnormal, paroxysmal excessive discharge from CNS neurons. Diuretic effect is due to action in kidney, which produces reversible reaction involving hydration of carbon dioxide and dehydration of carbonic acid.

PHARMACOKINETICS: Absorption: T_{max} = 3-6 hrs (Sequels); 1-4 hrs (Tab)

NURSING CONSIDERATIONS

Assessment: Assess for sulfonamide allergy, depressed sodium and/or K^+ blood serum levels, hepatic/renal disease/dysfunction, suprarenal gland failure, hyperchloremic acidosis, and cirrhosis. With long-term therapy, assess for chronic non-congestive angle-closure glaucoma. Assess use with impaired glucose tolerance or DM, pulmonary obstruction or emphysema, and in pregnant/nursing females. Assess baseline levels of CBC and platelet counts. Assess for possible drug interactions.

Monitoring: Monitor for signs/symptoms of severe sulfonamide reaction (eg, Stevens-Johnson syndrome, toxic epidermal necrolysis, fulminant hepatic necrosis, anaphylaxis, agranulocytosis, aplastic anemia, and other blood dyscrasias). Monitor with concomitant high-dose ASA therapy for signs/symptoms of anorexia, tachypnea, lethargy, metabolic acidosis, and coma. Monitor for decrease in diuresis and increase in drowsiness when dose is increased. Perform periodic monitoring of CBC, platelet counts, and serum electrolytes.

Patient Counseling: Inform about potential manifestations of severe sulfonamide reaction (eg, anaphylaxis, fever, rash, Stevens-Johnson syndrome, toxic epidermal necrolysis, crystalluria, bone marrow depression, thrombocytopenic purpura, leukopenia, agranulocytosis). Instruct to notify physician of all drugs being taken while on medication (eg, ASA). Advise medication may cause drowsiness and myopia; may impair ability to operate machinery/drive. Advise if using medication for acute mountain sickness that gradual ascent should be taken. If rapid ascent undertaken, drug does not obviate need for prompt descent if severe forms of high-altitude sickness occur.

Administration: Oral route; intravenous route. **Storage:** Oral: (Sequels/Tab) 20-25°C (68-77°F); Inj: (Vial) 15-30°C (59-86°F); (Reconstituted) 2-8°C (36-46°F); use within 12 hrs of reconstitution.

ACETYLCYSTEINE — RX

acetylcysteine (Various)

THERAPEUTIC CLASS: Acetaminophen antidote/Mucolytic

INDICATIONS: Adjunctive mucolytic therapy in acute and chronic bronchopulmonary disease; pulmonary complications of cystic fibrosis and surgery; tracheostomy care; during anesthesia; post-traumatic chest conditions; atelectasis; diagnostic bronchial studies. Antidote for acute acetaminophen (APAP) toxicity.

DOSAGE: *Adults:* Antidote: Empty stomach by lavage or emesis before administration. Administer immediately, regardless of quantity, if APAP ingestion ≤24hrs. LD: 140mg/kg PO then 70mg/kg PO q4h for 17 doses starting 4 hrs after LD. D/C if predetoxification APAP level is in nontoxic range and overdose occurred at least 4 hrs before assay. Obtain 2nd plasma level if range is nontoxic and time of ingestion is unknown or <4 hrs. Mucolytic: Nebulization (face mask, mouth piece, tracheostomy): 1-10mL of 20% or 2-10mL of 10% q2-6h. Usual: 3-5mL of 20% or 6-10mL of 10% 3-4 times/day. Closed Tent or Croupette: Up to 300mL of 10% or 20%. Direct Instillation: 1-2 mL of 10% or 20% q1-4h. Percutaneous Intratracheal Catheter: 1-2mL of 20% or 2-4mL of 10% q1-4h. Diagnostic Bronchograms: Give before procedure. 2-3 doses of 1-2mL of 20% or 2-4mL of 10%.

Pediatrics: Antidote: Empty stomach by lavage or emesis before administration. Administer immediately, regardless of quantity, if APAP ingestion ≤24hrs. LD: 140mg/kg PO then 70mg/kg PO q4h for 17 doses starting 4 hours after LD. D/C if predetoxification APAP level is in nontoxic range and overdose occurred at least 4 hrs before assay. Obtain 2nd plasma level if range is nontoxic and time of ingestion is unknown or <4 hrs. Mucolytic: Nebulization (face mask, mouth piece, tracheostomy): 1-10mL of 20% or 2-10mL of 10% q2-6h. Usual: 3-5mL of 20% or 6-10mL of 10% 3-4 times/day. Closed Tent or Croupette: Up to 300mL of 10% or 20%. Direct Instillation: 1-2 mL of 10% or 20% q1-4h. Percutaneous Intratracheal Catheter: 1-2mL of 20% or 2-4mL of 10% q1-4h. Diagnostic Procedures: Give before procedure. 2-3 doses of 1-2mL of 20% or 2-4mL of 10%.

HOW SUPPLIED: Sol: 10%, 20%

WARNINGS/PRECAUTIONS: (Oral) D/C if generalized urticaria or encephalopathy due to hepatic failure develops. May aggravate vomiting; evaluate with risk of gastric hemorrhage. (Inhalation) Monitor asthmatics. D/C if bronchospasm progresses.

ADVERSE REACTIONS: (Oral) N/V, other GI symptoms. (Inhalation) Stomatitis, NV, fever, rhinorrhea, drowsiness, clamminess, chest tightness, bronchoconstriction.

PREGNANCY: Category B, caution in nursing.

MECHANISM OF ACTION: N-acetyl derivative. Mucolytic: Opens disulfide linkages in mucus, thereby lowering viscosity. Antidote: Protects liver by maintaining or restoring glutathione levels, or by acting as alternate substrate for conjugation with, and thus detoxification of reactive metabolites, reducing extent of liver injury.

PHARMACOKINETICS: Metabolism: Deacetylation, oxidation.

NURSING CONSIDERATIONS

Assessment: Assess for possible drug interactions, asthma, esophageal varices, and peptic ulcers.

Monitoring: Monitor for signs/symptoms of bronchospasm, encephalopathy, gastric hemorrhage, and hypersensitivity reactions.

Patient Counseling: Advise to seek medical attention if symptoms of bronchospasm, encephalopathy, gastric hemorrhage, or hypersensitivity reactions (urticaria) occur.

Administration: Mucolytic: Inhalation route. Antidote: Oral route. Dilute 20% solution with NS for injection or sterile water for inhalation. Refer to full PI for administration techniques. **Storage:** 20-25°C (68-77°F), or 2-8°C (36-46°F) after opening; stable for 96 hrs.

ACIPHEX RX

rabeprazole sodium (Eisai/PRICARA)

THERAPEUTIC CLASS: Proton pump inhibitor

INDICATIONS: Short-term treatment in the healing and symptomatic relief of erosive or ulcerative gastroesophageal reflux disease (GERD). Maintenance of healing and reduction in relapse rates of heartburn symptoms in patients with erosive or ulcerative GERD. Treatment of daytime and nighttime heartburn and other symptoms associated with GERD. Short-term treatment in the healing and symptomatic relief of duodenal ulcers (DU). In combination with amoxicillin and clarithromycin as a 3-drug regimen for the treatment of patients with *H.pylori* infection and DU disease (active or history within the past 5 yrs) to eradicate *H.pylori* and reduce the risk of DU recurrence. Long-term treatment of pathological hypersecretory conditions, including Zollinger-Ellison syndrome.

DOSAGE: *Adults:* Erosive/Ulcerative GERD: Healing: 20mg qd for 4-8 weeks. May repeat for 8 weeks if needed. Maint: 20mg qd. Symptomatic GERD: 20mg qd for 4 weeks. May repeat for 4 weeks if needed. DU: 20mg qd after morning meal for up to 4 weeks. May need additional therapy. *H.pylori* Triple Therapy: 20mg + clarithromycin 500mg + amoxicillin 1g, all bid (qam and qpm) with food for 7 days. Pathological Hypersecretory Conditions: Initial: 60mg qd. Titrate: Adjust according to need. Maint: Up to 100mg qd or 60mg bid. May treat up to 1 yr. Swallow tabs whole; do not chew, crush, or split.
Pediatrics: ≥12 yrs: Symptomatic GERD: 20mg qd for up to 8 weeks.

HOW SUPPLIED: Tab, Delayed-Release: 20mg

WARNINGS/PRECAUTIONS: Symptomatic response does not preclude the presence of gastric malignancy. Caution with severe hepatic impairment.

ADVERSE REACTIONS: Headache, diarrhea, nausea, vomiting, abdominal pain, and taste perversion with triple therapy.

INTERACTIONS: May alter absorption of pH-dependent drugs (eg, ketoconazole, digoxin). May inhibit cyclosporine metabolism. May increase digoxin plasma levels and decrease ketoconazole levels. Concomitant use with warfarin increases the INR and PT time; monitor PT/INR. Increased rabeprazole and clarithromycin levels with triple therapy.

PREGNANCY: Category B, not for use in nursing.

MECHANISM OF ACTION: Proton pump inhibitor; suppresses gastric acid secretion by inhibiting the gastric (H^+, K^+)-ATPase enzyme at the secretory surface of the gastric parietal cell. Blocks the final step of gastric acid secretion.

PHARMACOKINETICS: Absorption: T_{max}=2-5 hrs; absolute bioavailability (52%). **Distribution:** Plasma protein binding (96.3%). **Metabolism:** Extensive. Liver via CYP3A4 to sulphone (primary metabolite) and CYP2C19 to desmethyl rabeprazole (primary metabolite). **Elimination:** Urine (90%), feces; $T_{1/2}$=1-2 hrs.

NURSING CONSIDERATIONS

Assessment: Assess for hypersensitivity to other proton pump inhibitors, presence of gastric malignancy, severe hepatic impairment, pregnancy/nursing status, and possible drug interactions.

Monitoring: Monitor for allergic reactions, clinical improvement, and pathological changes in gastric mucosa. If on concomitant therapy with antibacterial agents, monitor for signs/symptoms of *C. difficile*.

Patient Counseling: Instruct to swallow tablet whole with water; do not chew, crush, or split tablet. May take with/without food. Inform if dose is missed, take drug as soon as possible. If almost time for the next dose, skip missed dose and go back to normal schedule; do not take 2 doses at same time. Instruct to contact physician if signs of hypersensitivity reaction (hives, swelling of face, eyelids, lips, tongue, or throat) occur.

Administration: Oral route. **Storage:** 15-30°C (59-86°F); store in dry place, out of reach of children.

ACLOVATE RX

alclometasone dipropionate (GlaxoSmithKline)

THERAPEUTIC CLASS: Corticosteroid

INDICATIONS: Relief of the inflammatory and pruritic manifestations of corticosteroid-responsive dermatoses.

DOSAGE: *Adults:* Apply bid-tid. Reassess if no improvement after 2 weeks. *Pediatrics:* ≥1 yr: Apply bid-tid. Reassess if no improvement after 2 weeks.

HOW SUPPLIED: Cre, Oint: 0.05% [15g, 45g, 60g]

WARNINGS/PRECAUTIONS: May produce reversible HPA axis suppression, manifestations of Cushing's syndrome, hyperglycemia, and glucosuria. Use appropriate antifungal or antibacterial agent with dermatological infections. Peds may be more susceptible to systemic toxicity. Avoid occlusive dressings. Avoid diaper area. Not for use in diaper dermatitis. D/C if irritation occurs. Caution in peds.

ADVERSE REACTIONS: Itching, burning, erythema, dryness, irritation, papular rash, folliculitis, acneiform eruptions, hypopigmentation, perioral dermatitis, allergic contact dermatitis, secondary infection, skin atrophy, striae.

PREGNANCY: Category C, caution in nursing.

MECHANISM OF ACTION: Corticosteroid; has anti-inflammatory, antipruritic, and vasoconstrictive properties. Anti-inflammatory mechanism not established. Suspected to act by the induction of phospholipase A_2 inhibitory proteins (lipocortins), which may control the biosynthesis of potent mediators of inflammation (eg, prostaglandins, leukotrienes) by inhibiting the release of their common precursor, arachidonic acid. Arachidonic acid is released from membrane phospholipids by phospholipase A_2.

PHARMACOKINETICS: Distribution: Systemically administered corticosteroids are found in breast milk.

NURSING CONSIDERATIONS

Assessment: Assess use in pregnant/nursing females.

Monitoring: Monitor for occurrence of HPA axis suppression through periodic monitoring of ACTH stimulation, a.m. plasma cortisol, and urinary-free cortisol tests. Monitor for manifestations of Cushing's syndrome, hyperglycemia, and glucosuria while on therapy. Monitor for development of skin irritation. If present, d/c medication. Monitor for signs of allergic contact dermatitis (eg, failure to heal) and signs of concomitant skin infections. In pediatric patients, monitor for HPA axis suppression, Cushing's syndrome, linear growth retardation, delayed weight gain, and intracranial HTN.

Patient Counseling: Instruct to use externally and as directed. Counsel to avoid contact with eyes and that treated skin area should not be bandaged. Instruct not to use medication on face, underarms, or groin areas unless directed by a physician. Counsel to notify physician if any signs of improvement do not occur within 2 weeks of starting medication.

Administration: Apply topically. **Storage**: 2-30°C (36-86°F).

ACTIGALL RX

ursodiol (Watson)

THERAPEUTIC CLASS: Bile acid

INDICATIONS: Treatment of radiolucent, noncalcified gallbladder stones <20mm in diameter in patients unable to undergo cholecystectomy. Prevention of gallstone formation in obese patients experiencing rapid weight loss.

DOSAGE: *Adults:* Treatment: 8-10mg/kg/day given bid-tid. Obtain ultrasound at 6 month intervals for 1 yr. Continue therapy after stones have dissolved and confirm with repeat ultrasound within 1-3 months. Prevention: 300mg bid.

HOW SUPPLIED: Cap: 300mg

CONTRAINDICATIONS: Calcified cholesterol stones, radiopaque stones, radiolucent bile pigment stones, unremitting acute cholecystitis, cholangitis, biliary obstruction, gallstone pancreatitis, biliary-gastrointestinal fistula, bile-acid hypersensitivity.

WARNINGS/PRECAUTIONS: Therapy is not associated with liver damage. Monitor LFTs at the initiation of therapy and periodically thereafter. Caution in elderly.

ADVERSE REACTIONS: Abdominal pain, constipation, diarrhea, dyspepsia, flatulence, NV, arthralgia, coughing, viral infection, bronchitis, pharyngitis, back pain, myalgia, headache, sinusitis, upper respiratory tract infection.

INTERACTIONS: Decreased absorption with bile acid sequestrants and aluminum based antacids. Estrogens, oral contraceptives, and clofibrate encourage gallstone formation.

PREGNANCY: Category B, caution in nursing.

MECHANISM OF ACTION: Bile acid; suppresses hepatic synthesis, cholesterol secretion, and inhibits intestinal cholesterol absorption; actions combine to change bile from cholesterol-precipitating to solubilizing, resulting in bile conducive to cholesterol stone dissolution.

PHARMACOKINETICS: Absorption: Small bowel (90%). **Metabolism:** Liver (1st pass, conjugation). **Elimination:** Feces.

NURSING CONSIDERATIONS

Assessment: Assess for type of bile pigment stones (calcified cholesterol, radiopaque, radiolucent), unremitting acute cholecystitis, cholangitis, biliary obstruction, gallstone pancreatitis, biliary GI fistula, and possible drug interactions. Obtain baseline SGOT (AST) and SGPT (ALT).

Monitoring: Ultrasound should be taken in 6-month intervals for first year. If appear dissolved, continue therapy and confirm on repeat ultrasound within 1-3 months. If partial dissolution not seen by 12 months, success is greatly reduced. Monitor SGOT (AST) and SGPT (ALT) periodically. Signs/symptoms of hypersensitivity reactions.

Patient Counseling: Seek medical attention if symptoms of hypersensitivity or allergic reactions occur.

Administration: Oral route. **Storage:** Store at 25°C (77°F); excursions permitted to 15-30°C (59-86°F). Dispense in tight container.

ACTIQ CII
fentanyl citrate (Cephalon)

May cause life-threatening hypoventilation in opioid non-tolerant patients. Only for cancer pain in opioid tolerant patients with malignancies. Keep out of reach of children and discard properly. Concomitant use with moderate and strong CYP3A4 inhibitors may cause fatal respiratory depression.

THERAPEUTIC CLASS: Opioid analgesic

INDICATIONS: Management of breakthrough cancer pain in patients with malignancies who are already receiving and are tolerant to opioid therapy.

DOSAGE: *Adults:* Initial: 0.2mg (consume over 15 min). Titrate: Redose 15 min after previous dose is completed. No more than 2 units per breakthrough pain episode. May increase to next highest available strength if several breakthrough episodes (1-2 days) require more than 1 unit per pain episode. Repeat titration for each new dose. Max: 4 units/day. Prescribe 6 units with each new titration. The lozenge should be sucked, not chewed, and consumed over 15 min.
Pediatrics: ≥16 yrs: Initial: 0.2mg (consume over 15 min). Titrate: Redose 15 min after previous dose is completed. No more than 2 units per breakthrough pain episode. May increase to next highest available strength if several breakthrough episodes (1-2 days) require more than 1 unit per pain episode. Repeat titration for each new dose. Max: 4 units/day. Prescribe 6 units with each new titration. The lozenge should be sucked, not chewed, and consumed over 15 min.

HOW SUPPLIED: Loz: 0.2mg, 0.4mg, 0.6mg, 0.8mg, 1.2mg, 1.6mg

CONTRAINDICATIONS: Opioid non-tolerant patients and management of acute or postoperative pain.

WARNINGS/PRECAUTIONS: Caution with COPD, hepatic or renal dysfunction. Risk of clinically significant hypoventilation. Extreme caution with evidence of increased ICP or impaired consciousness. Can produce morphine-like dependence. Increased risk of dental decay; ensure proper oral hygiene. Caution with bradyarrhythmias, liver or kidney dysfunction. Patients on concomitant CNS depressants must be monitored for a change in opioid effects. May impair mental and/or physical status.

ADVERSE REACTIONS: Respiratory depression, circulatory depression, headache, hypotension, shock, N/V, constipation, dizziness, dyspnea, anxiety, somnolence.

INTERACTIONS: Concomitant use with other CNS depressants, including opioids, sedatives, hypnotics, general anesthetics, phenothiazines, tranquilizers, skeletal muscle relaxants, sedating antihistamines, potent inhibitors of CYP3A4 (eg, erythromycin, ketoconazole, itraconazole, ritonavir, troleandomycin, clarithromycin, nelfinavir and nefazodone) or moderate inhibitors (eg, amprenavir, aprepitant, diltiazem, erythromycin, fluconazole, fosamprenavir, and verapamil) and alcohol may result in increased plasma concentrations. Avoid grapefruit juice. Avoid within 14 days of MAOIs.

PREGNANCY: Category C, not for use in nursing.

MECHANISM OF ACTION: Narcotic agonist analgesic: Principle therapeutic effect is analgesia. Not established. A μ-opioid receptor agonist. Specific CNS opioid receptors for endogenous compounds have been identified throughout brain and spinal cord and play a role in analgesic effects.

PHARMACOKINETICS: Absorption: Rapidly absorbed from buccal mucosa; slow absorption of swallowed fentanyl from GI tract. Absolute bioavailability

(50%); C_{max}= 0.39-2.51ng/mL; T_{max}=20-40 min. **Distribution:** V_d=4L/kg; plasma protein binding (80-85%). Rapidly distributed to brain, heart, lungs, kidneys, spleen; slowly to muscles and fat. Readily crosses placenta; found in breast milk. **Metabolism:** Liver, via CYP3A4; intestinal mucosa; norfentanyl (metabolite). **Elimination**: Urine (major), feces; $T_{1/2}$=7 hrs.

NURSING CONSIDERATIONS

Assessment: Assess for risk of drug misuse, abuse, or diversion; acute/chronic post-op pain; opioid intolerance; COPD; increased ICP or impaired consciousness; pregnancy/nursing status; hepatic/renal function; and drug interactions.

Monitoring: Monitor for signs/symptoms of respiratory and CNS depression, bradycardia, circulatory depression, hypotension, shock, impaired mental/physical abilities, abuse/addiction, dental decay, and hypersensitivity reactions (eg, anaphylaxis). Monitor glucose levels with DM.

Patient Counseling: Inform that medication must be kept out of reach of children; may be fatal to child. Seek immediate help if child accidentally consumes medication. Instruct to properly discard partially used units. Inform that use may impair mental/physical abilities and to use caution if performing hazardous tasks (eg, operating machinery/driving). Notify physician of all concurrently used medications or before taking any other medications. Avoid consumption of grapefruit juice and alcohol. Instruct to maintain proper dental hygiene during therapy and consult dentist to ensure proper dental care. Advise diabetics that medication contains approximately 2g sugar/unit. Advise to contact physician for any signs of respiratory depression (eg, difficulty breathing, extreme drowsiness with slowed breathing, slow shallow breathing, faintness, dizziness, confusion). Instruct to avoid abrupt withdrawal. Patient may drink water prior to use, but should not eat or drink anything during use. Advise that if dizziness, nausea, or sleepiness develops before medication is completely dissolved, to remove medication from mouth. Notify physician if have 4 episodes of breakthrough pain.

Administration: Oral route. 1) Do not open blister package until ready to use. 2) Place in mouth between cheeks and gums and actively suck on medication. 3) Move around in mouth, especially along cheeks. Twirl handle often. 4) Finish completely in 15 min to get most relief. Do not bite or chew. 5) Dispose of immediately or put in temporary storage bottle following use. **Storage:** 20-25°C (68-77°F); excursions permitted between 15-30°C (59-86°F). Protect from freezing and moisture. Do not use if blister package has been opened.

ACTIVASE

RX

alteplase (Genentech)

THERAPEUTIC CLASS: Thrombolytic agent

INDICATIONS: To improve ventricular function, reduce incidence of congestive heart failure, and reduce mortality with acute myocardial infarction (AMI). Management of acute ischemic stroke and acute massive pulmonary embolism (PE).

DOSAGE: *Adults:* AMI: Accelerated Infusion: >67kg: 15mg IV bolus, then 50mg over next 30 min, and then 35mg over next 60 min. ≤67kg: 15mg IV bolus, then 0.75mg/kg (max 50mg) over next 30 min, then 0.50mg/kg (max 35mg) over next 60 min. Max: 100mg total dose. 3-Hr Infusion: ≥65kg: 60mg in 1st hr (give 6-10mg as IV bolus), then 20mg over 2nd hr, then 20mg over 3rd hr. <65kg: 1.25mg/kg over 3 hrs as described above. Stroke: 0.9mg/kg IV over 1 hr (max 90mg total dose). Administer 10% of total dose as IV bolus over 1 min. PE: 100mg IV over 2 hrs. Start heparin at end or immediately after infusion when PTT or PT ≤2x normal.

HOW SUPPLIED: Inj: 50mg, 100mg

CONTRAINDICATIONS: (AMI, PE) Active internal bleeding, history of cerebrovascular accident (CVA), recent intracranial/intraspinal surgery or trauma, intracranial neoplasm, arteriovenous (AV) malformation, aneurysm, bleeding diathesis, severe uncontrolled HTN. (Stroke) Active internal bleeding, AV malformation, intracranial neoplasm or hemorrhage, aneurysm, bleeding diathesis, uncontrolled HTN, subarachnoid hemorrhage, seizure at stroke onset. Recent intracranial or intraspinal surgery, serious head trauma, previous stroke.

WARNINGS/PRECAUTIONS: Weigh benefits/risks with recent major surgery, cerebrovascular disease, recent GI or GU bleeding, recent trauma, HTN, left heart thrombus, acute pericarditis, subacute bacterial endocarditis, hemostatic defects, severe hepatic dysfunction, pregnancy, diabetic hemorrhagic retinopathy or other hemorrhagic ophthalmic conditions, septic thrombophlebitis or occluded AV cannula at a seriously infected site, elderly, any other bleeding condition that is difficult to manage. For stroke, also weigh benefits/risks with severe neurological deficit or major early infarct signs on CT. Cholesterol embolism and internal/superficial bleeding reported. Arrhythmias may occur with reperfusion. Avoid IM injection, noncompressible arterial puncture, and internal jugular or subclavian venous puncture. Caution with readministration.

ADVERSE REACTIONS: Bleeding.

INTERACTIONS: Increased risk of bleeding with heparin, vitamin K antagonists, drugs that alter platelets (eg, ASA, dipyridamole, abciximab) given before, during, or after alteplase therapy.

PREGNANCY: Category C, caution in nursing.

MECHANISM OF ACTION: Tissue plasminogen activator; has property of fibrin-enhanced conversion of plasminogen to plasmin. Produces limited conversion of plasminogen in absence of fibrin. Binds to fibrin in thrombus and converts entrapped plasminogen to plasmin. Initiates local fibrinolysis with limited systemic proteolysis.

PHARMACOKINETICS: Metabolism: Liver. **Elimination:** $T_{1/2}$=5 min (initial).

NURSING CONSIDERATIONS

Assessment: In patients with acute MI or PE, assess for presence of active internal bleeding, history of cerebrovascular accident, trauma, aneurysm, known bleeding diathesis, and severe uncontrolled HTN. In patients with acute ischemic stroke, assess for presence or history of hemorrhage, surgery, serious head trauma, previous stroke, uncontrolled HTN, and possible drug interactions.

Monitoring: Monitor for signs/symptoms of bleeding (eg, internal, superficial, surface bleeding), cholesterol embolism (eg, livedo reticularis, "purple toe" syndrome, acute renal failure, gangrenous digits), and for allergic reactions (eg, anaphylactoid reaction, laryngeal edema, orolingual angioedema, rash, urticaria). Monitor BP frequently and arrhythmias with acute MI.

Patient Counseling: Inform about risk of bleeding with medication. Instruct to notify physician if any type of allergic reaction develops during therapy.

Administration: IV route. Reconstitute using appropriate volume of SWFI (without preservatives) to vial. Do not use Bacteriostatic Water for Inj, USP. Reconstitute to a final concentration of 1mg/mL. Reconstitute just prior to use. May further dilute using an equal volume of 0.9% NS or D5W to yield concentration of 0.5mg/mL. Do not add any other medication to infusion solutions containing drug. Discard any unused infusion solution. **Storage:** Lyophilized: Controlled room temperature not to exceed 30°C (86°F), or under refrigeration 2-8° (36-46°F). Protect from excessive exposure to light. Reconstituted: 2-30° (36-86°F); use within 8 hrs.

ACTIVELLA RX

norethindrone - estradiol (Novo Nordisk)

Estrogens and progestins should not be used for the prevention of cardiovascular disease or dementia. Increased risks of MI, stroke, invasive breast cancer, PE, and DVT in postmenopausal women (50-79 yrs of age) reported. Increased risk of developing probable dementia in postmenopausal women ≥65 yrs of age reported.

THERAPEUTIC CLASS: Estrogen/progestogen combination

INDICATIONS: For women with intact uterus, treatment of moderate to severe vasomotor symptoms associated with menopause, vulvar/vaginal atrophy and prevention of postmenopausal osteoporosis.

DOSAGE: *Adults:* 1 tab qd.

HOW SUPPLIED: Tab: (Estradiol-Norethindrone) 1mg-0.5mg, 0.5mg-1mg

CONTRAINDICATIONS: Pregnancy, breast cancer, abnormal genital bleeding, estrogen-dependent neoplasia, DVT, thromboembolic disorders, stroke, liver dysfunction or disease.

WARNINGS/PRECAUTIONS: Risk of gallbladder disease, endometrial and breast cancer, fetal congenital reproductive tract disorder, elevated BP, and hypercalcemia with breast cancer or bone metastases. Possible risk of cardiovascular disease. Increased risk of DVT, stroke, and PE; increased risk of endometrial, breast, and ovarian cancer with prolonged use. Risk of probable dementia-unknown risk in postmenopausal women under 65 years of age. Monitor for fluid retention with asthma, epilepsy, migraine, and cardiac/renal dysfunction. Avoid in post-menopausal women without a uterus. D/C if vision disturbances or thrombotic disorders occur. Caution with depression, DM, severe hypocalcemia. Acceleration of PT, PTT. Hypercoagulability effects. Impaired glucose tolerance. Increased triglycerides, fibrin/fibrinogen, and plasmin/plasminogen activity.

ADVERSE REACTIONS: Back pain, headache, nasopharyngitis, sinusitis, insomnia, upper respiratory tract infection, breast pain, postmenopausal bleeding/vaginal hemorrhage, endometrial thickening, uterine fibroid, pain in extremities, nausea, and diarrhea.

INTERACTIONS: CYP3A4 inducers (eg, St. John's wort, phenobarbital, carbamazepine, rifampin) may reduce estrogen levels. CYP3A4 inhibitors (eg, erythromycin, clarithromycin, ketoconazole, itraconazole, ritonavir, grapefruit juice) may increase estrogen levels.

PREGNANCY: Category X, caution in nursing.

MECHANISM OF ACTION: Estrogen/progestogen combination. Estradiol: Binds to nuclear receptors in estrogen-responsive tissues and modulating pituitary secretion of gonadotropins, luteinizing hormone (LH) and follicle-stimulating hormone (FSH), through negative-feedback mechanism. Norethindrone: Exerts effect in target cells by binding to specific progesterone receptors that interact with progesterone-response elements in target genes. Enhances cellular differentiation and opposing actions of estrogens by decreasing estrogen receptor levels, increasing local metabolism of estrogens to less active metabolites, and inducing gene products that blunt cellular responses to estrogen.

PHARMACOKINETICS: Absorption: Estradiol (E_2): Well-absorbed, T_{max}=5-8 hrs. Norethindrone (NET): Rapid. **Distribution:** Estrogens found in breast milk. E_2: Sex-hormone-binding globulin (37%); albumin (61%); unbound (1-2%). NET: Sex-hormone-binding globulin (36%); albumin (61%). **Metabolism:** E_2: Liver to estrone, E_1 (metabolite); estriol (major urinary metabolite); enterohepatic recirculation via sulfate and glucuronide conjugation; biliary secretion of conjugates into the intestine, and hydrolysis in intestine; CYP3A4 (partial). NET: 5α-dihydro-norethindrone and tetrahydro-norethindrone (metabolites). **Elimination:** E_2: Urine; $T_{1/2}$=12-14 hrs. E_1: Urine; $T_{1/2}$=12-14 hrs. NET: $T_{1/2}$=8-11 hrs.

NURSING CONSIDERATIONS

Assessment: Assess for abnormal genital bleeding, presence or history of breast cancer, estrogen-dependent neoplasias, DVT, PE, active or recent (within past yr) arterial thromboembolic disease (eg, stroke, MI), liver dysfunction/disease, and known/suspected pregnancy. Assess use in patients undergoing surgery associated with increased risk of thromboembolism, under prolonged immobilization, and with history of hypertriglyceridemia, hypothyroidism, renal dysfunction, or presence of severe hypocalcemia. Assess use in women ≥65 yrs old, nursing patients, and those with DM, asthma, epilepsy, migraines or porphyria, SLE, and hepatic hemangiomas. Assess for possible drug and lab test interactions.

Monitoring: Monitor for signs/symptoms of cardiovascular disorders (eg, MI, stroke, venous thrombosis, PE), malignant neoplasms (eg, breast, endometrial, ovarian cancer), dementia, gallbladder disease, hypercalcemia, visual abnormalities (eg, retinal vascular thrombosis), increased BP, hypertriglyceridemia, hypothyroidism, fluid retention, cholestatic jaundice, exacerbation of endometriosis and other conditions (eg, asthma, DM, epilepsy, migraine, porphyria, SLE, and hepatic hemangiomas). Perform annual mammography and periodic monitoring of BP. Monitor thyroid function if patient on thyroid hormone replacement therapy. In cases of undiagnosed, persistent, or recurrent vaginal bleeding in women with uterus, perform adequate diagnostic measures (eg, endometrial sampling) to rule out malignancies.

Patient Counseling: Inform that estrogens may increase risk for uterine and breast cancer, heart attack, stroke, blood clots, and dementia. Report any unusual vaginal bleeding, breast lumps, dizziness or faintness, changes in speech, severe headaches, chest pain, SOB, leg pain, changes in vision, or vomiting. Advise to perform monthly self breast exam, and have annual gynecologic exam (breast exam, mammography).

Administration: Oral route. **Storage:** Store in dry place; protect from light. Store at room temperature, 25°C (77°F), excursions permitted to 15-30°C (59-86°F).

ACTONEL

risedronate sodium (Procter & Gamble)

RX

THERAPEUTIC CLASS: Bisphosphonate

INDICATIONS: Prevention and treatment of osteoporosis in postmenopausal women, glucocorticoid-induced osteoporosis in men and women. Increase bone mass in men with osteoporosis. Treatment of Paget's disease in men and women.

DOSAGE: *Adults:* Paget's Disease: 30mg qd for 2 months. May retreat after 2 months. Postmenopausal Osteoporosis Prevention/Treatment: 5mg qd or 35mg once weekly or 75mg on 2 consecutive days each month or 150mg once a month. Glucocorticoid-Induced Osteoporosis: 5mg qd. Increase Bone Mass in Men with Osteoporosis: 35mg once weekly. Take at least 30 min before 1st food or drink of day other than water. Swallow tab in upright position with 6-8 oz plain water. Do not lie down for 30 min after dose.

HOW SUPPLIED: Tab: 5mg, 30mg, 35mg, 75mg, 150mg

CONTRAINDICATIONS: Hypocalcemia; inability to stand or sit upright for at least 30 min.

WARNINGS/PRECAUTIONS: May cause upper GI disorders (eg, dysphagia, esophagitis, esophageal or gastric ulcer). Treat hypocalcemia and other disturbances of bone and mineral metabolism before therapy. Give supplemental calcium and vitamin D if dietary intake is inadequate. Avoid with severe renal impairment (CrCl <30mL/min). Osteonecrosis, primarily in the jaw, has been reported. Postmarketing reports of severe and occasionally incapacitating bone, joint, and/or muscle pain, has been reported.

ADVERSE REACTIONS: Asthenia, diarrhea, abdominal pain, nausea, constipation, peripheral edema, arthralgia, leg cramps, headache, dizziness, sinusitis, rash, tinnitus.

INTERACTIONS: Calcium supplements and calcium-, aluminum-, and magnesium-containing agents may interfere with absorption; space doses.

PREGNANCY: Category C, not for use in nursing.

MECHANISM OF ACTION: Bisphosphonate; has an affinity for hydroxyapatite crystals in bone and acts as an antiresorptive agent. Inhibits osteoclast-mediated bone resorption and modulates bone metabolism.

PHARMACOKINETICS: Absorption: Relatively rapid; T_{max}=1 hr; (30mg) absolute bioavailability (0.63%). **Distribution**: V_d=6.3L/kg, plasma protein binding (24%). **Elimination**: Urine, feces (unabsorbed dose); $T_{1/2}$=480 hrs.

NURSING CONSIDERATIONS

Assessment: Assess for hypocalcemia and other bone disturbances or problems with mineral metabolism; treat appropriately. Assess for ability to stand or sit upright for 30 min, severe renal impairment (CrCl <30mL/min), risk of osteonecrosis, pregnancy/nursing status, and possible drug interactions. Assess hormonal status if treatment is for glucocorticoid-induced osteoporosis; consider appropriate replacement therapy.

Monitoring: Monitor for signs/symptoms of upper GI disorders (eg, dysphagia, esophagitis, esophageal or gastric ulcers), jaw osteonecrosis, and musculoskeletal pain.

Patient Counseling: Counsel to take as directed. Take 30 min before first food or drink of day other than water. Take while in an upright position (eg, sitting or standing) with a full glass of plain water (eg, 6-8oz). Instruct to avoid laying down for 30 min following administration. Advise to avoid chewing or sucking tablet. Contact physician if develop symptoms of esophageal disease (eg, difficulty or pain with swallowing, retrosternal pain, worsening heartburn) before continuing medication. Instruct that if taking 35mg once weekly dosing, and miss dose, 1 tablet should be taken on the morning after remembering dose was missed; return to originally scheduled day of once-weekly dosing. Take supplemental calcium and vitamin D if dietary intake is inadequate; take with food at separate time from medication. Advise to consider weight-bearing exercises as well as modification of behavioral factors (eg, excessive cigarette smoking, alcohol consumption).

Administration: Oral route. **Storage**: 20-25°C (68-77°F).

ACTONEL WITH CALCIUM — RX

risedronate sodium - calcium carbonate (Procter & Gamble)

THERAPEUTIC CLASS: Bisphosphonate

INDICATIONS: Treatment and prevention of postmenopausal osteoporosis.

DOSAGE: *Adults:* Risedronate: 35mg once weekly (Day 1 of 7-day treatment cycle). Take at least 30 min before 1st food or drink of day other than water. Swallow tab in upright position with 6-8oz of plain water. Do not lie down for 30 min after dose. Calcium: 1250mg qd with food on each of remaining 6 days (Days 2-7 of the 7-day treatment cycle).

HOW SUPPLIED: Tab: (Risedronate Sodium) 35mg; Tab: (Calcium Carbonate) 1250mg

CONTRAINDICATIONS: (Risedronate) Hypocalcemia; inability to stand or sit upright for at least 30 min. (Calcium) Hypercalcemia from any cause (eg, hyperparathyroidism, hypercalcemia of malignancy, sarcoidosis).

WARNINGS/PRECAUTIONS: (Risedronate) May cause upper GI disorders (eg, dysphagia, esophagitis, esophageal or gastric ulcer). Treat hypocalcemia and other disturbances of bone and mineral metabolism before therapy. May cause osteonecrosis, primarily in jaw. Avoid with severe renal impairment (CrCl <30mL/min). (Calcium) Should not be used to treat hypocalcemia. Daily intake above 2000mg has been associated with increased risk of adverse effects, including hypercalcemia and kidney stones. Patients with achlorhydria may have decreased absorption of calcium. Severe and occasionally incapacitating bone, joint, and/or muscle pain in patient taking bisphosphonates reported.

ADVERSE REACTIONS: Risedronate: Infection, pain, flu syndrome, abdominal pain, headache, asthenia, HTN, constipation, dyspepsia, nausea, arthralgia, nausea, diarrhea, dizziness, myalgia. Calcium: Constipation, flatulence, nausea, abdominal pain, and bloating.

INTERACTIONS: Risedronate: Calcium supplements, and calcium-, aluminum-, and magnesium-containing agents may interfere with absorption; space doses. Calcium: May reduce absorption of levothyroxine, fluoroquinolones, tetracycline. Calcium absorption reduced when taken with systemic glucocorticoids. Reduced urinary excretion of calcium with use of thiazide diuretics. Absorption of calcium increased with use of vitamin D and analogues. May interfere with absorption of iron. Take iron and calcium at different times of the day.

PREGNANCY: Category C, not for use in nursing.

MECHANISM OF ACTION: Risedronate: Bisphosphonate; inhibits osteoclast-mediated bone resorption and modulates bone metabolism. Calcium: Major substrate for mineralization; has antiresorptive effect on bone. Suppresses PTH secretion and decreases bone turnover.

PHARMACOKINETICS: Absorption: Risedronate: Relatively rapid. T_{max}=1 hr; absolute bioavailability (30mg): (0.63%). **Distribution**: Risedronate: V_d=6.3L/kg, plasma protein binding (24%). Calcium: Plasma protein binding (40%). **Elimination**: Risedronate: Urine, feces (unabsorbed dose); $T_{1/2}$=480 hrs. Calcium: Renal, feces (unabsorbed dose).

NURSING CONSIDERATIONS

Assessment: Assess for hypocalcemia and other bone disturbances; treat appropriately prior to therapy. Assess for hypercalcemia from any cause (eg, hyperparathyroidism, hypercalcemia of malignancy, sarcoidosis), inability to stand or sit upright for 30 min, severe renal impairment (CrCl <30mL/min), risk of osteonecrosis, history of kidney stones or hypercalciuria, achlorhydria, pregnancy/nursing status, and possible drug interactions.

Monitoring: Monitor for signs/symptoms of GI disorders (eg, dysphagia, esophagitis, esophageal or gastric ulcers), osteonecrosis, musculoskeletal pain, and kidney stone formation. Perform periodic monitoring of urinary calcium excretion in patients with kidney stones.

Patient Counseling: Actonel: Advise to take as directed. Take at least 30 min before first food or drink of day other than water. Take in an upright position (eg, sitting or standing) with a full glass of plain water and avoid lying down for 30 min after administration. Avoid chewing or sucking medication. Contact physician if develop symptoms of esophageal disease (eg, difficulty or pain swallowing, worsening heartburn). If patient misses one 35mg dose taken once weekly, instruct to take 1 tablet the morning after remembering and return to taking 1 tab once a week on originally scheduled day; avoid taking 2 tabs in one day. Advise to take supplemental calcium and vitamin D if dietary intake is inadequate. Counsel to consider weight-bearing exercises and modification of certain behavioral factors (eg, excessive cigarette smoking, alcohol consumption). Calcium: Instruct to take with food.

Administration: Oral route. **Storage**: 20-25°C (68-77°F); excursions permitted to 15-30°C (59-86°F).

ACTOPLUS MET — RX

pioglitazone HCl - metformin HCl (Takeda)

Thiazolidinediones may cause or exacerbate CHF in some patients. Actoplus Met is not recommended in patients with symptomatic heart failure.

THERAPEUTIC CLASS: Thiazolidinedione/biguanide

INDICATIONS: Adjunct to diet and exercise to improve glycemic control in type 2 diabetes mellitus in patients already treated with a combination of pioglitazone and metformin or whose diabetes is not adequately controlled with metformin alone, or for those patients who have initially responded to pioglitazone alone and require additional glycemic control.

DOSAGE: *Adults:* Individualize dose. Prior Pioglitazone/Metformin: Base on current regimen. Prior Metformin Monotherapy or Pioglitazone Monotherapy: Initial: 15mg-500mg or 15mg-850mg qd-bid. Titrate: Gradually increase after assessing adequacy of therapeutic response. Max: (Pioglitazone) 45mg, (Metformin) 2550mg. Elderly/Debilitated/Malnourished: Conservative dosing; do not titrate to max dose.

HOW SUPPLIED: Tab: (Pioglitazone-Metformin) 15mg-500mg, 15mg-850mg

CONTRAINDICATIONS: Established NYHA Class III or IV heart failure, renal disease or dysfunction (eg, SrCr ≥1.5mg/dL [males], ≥1.4mg/dL [females], or abnormal CrCl) and metabolic acidosis, including diabetic ketoacidosis. Temporarily d/c in patients undergoing radiologic studies involving intravascular iodinated contrast materials.

WARNINGS/PRECAUTIONS: (Metformin) Lactic acidosis reported (rare); increased risk with renal dysfunction, increased age, DM, CHF, and other conditions with risk of hypoperfusion and hypoxemia. Avoid in patients ≥80 yrs unless normal renal function. Monitor renal function and for ketoacidosis and metabolic acidosis. Avoid in renal/hepatic impairment. D/C in hypoxic states (eg, CHF, shock, acute MI), loss of blood glucose control due to stress (give insulin), acidosis, dehydration, sepsis. Temporarily d/c prior to surgery (due to restricted food intake) and procedures requiring IV iodinated contrast materials. May decrease serum B_{12} levels. Increased risk of hypoglycemia in elderly, debilitated/malnourished, adrenal or pituitary insufficiency, or alcohol intoxication. Alcohol known to potentiate effect of metformin on lactate metabolism. (Pioglitazone) May cause fluid retention and exacerbation/initiation of heart failure; d/c if cardiac status deteriorates. Avoid if NYHA Class III or IV cardiac status. Use lowest approved dose if systolic heart failure (NYHA Class II). Not for use in type 1 diabetes or for diabetic ketoacidosis treatment. Caution with edema. Dose-related wt gain reported. Ovulation in premenopausal anovulatory patients may occur; risk of pregnancy with inadequate contraception. May decrease Hgb and Hct. Avoid with active liver disease, if ALT levels >2.5x ULN. D/C if jaundice occurs or ALT >3x ULN on therapy. Macular edema reported.

ADVERSE REACTIONS: Upper respiratory tract infection, diarrhea, nausea, edema, headache, UTI, sinusitis, dizziness, weight increase, new onset or worsening diabetic macular edema.

INTERACTIONS: (Pioglitazone) Possible loss of contraception with ethinyl estradiol and norethindrone; caution when coadministering. Ketoconazole may inhibit pioglitazone metabolism; evaluate glycemic control more frequently. Risk for hypoglycemia with insulin or oral hypoglycemic agents. May cause reduction of midazolam levels. (Metformin) Furosemide, nifedipine, cimetidine, cationic drugs (eg, digoxin, amiloride, procainamide, quinidine, quinine, ranitidine, trimethoprim, vancomycin, triamterene, morphine) may increase metformin levels. Thiazides, other diuretics, corticosteroids, phenothiazines, thyroid products, estrogens, oral contraceptives, phenytoin, nicotinic acid, sympathomimetics, CCBs, or isoniazid may cause hyperglycemia. Risk of hypoglycemia with alcohol. Excess alcohol may increase potential for lactic acidosis. May decrease furosemide levels. An enzyme inhibitor of CYP2C8 (eg, gemfibrozil) may significantly increase AUC of pioglitazone and an enzyme inducer of CYP2C8 (eg, rifampin) may significantly decrease AUC of pioglitazone.

PREGNANCY: Category C, not for use in nursing.

MECHANISM OF ACTION: Pioglitazone: Thiazolidinedione; insulin sensitizing agent, enhances peripheral glucose utilization. Metformin: Biguanide; decreases endogenous hepatic glucose production.

PHARMACOKINETICS: Absorption: Pioglitazone: T_{max}=2-4 hrs. Metformin: Absolute bioavailability (50-60%), C_{max}=5µg/mL. **Distribution:** Pioglitazone: V_d =0.63L/kg, plasma protein binding (99%). Metformin: V_d =654L. **Metabolism:** Pioglitazone: Hydroxylation and oxidation (extensive); CYP450 2C8 and 3A4. Metformin: No hepatic metabolism. **Elimination:** Pioglitazone: Bile (unchanged), feces (metabolites), $T_{1/2}$=3-7 hrs (pioglitazone), 16-24 hrs (total pioglitazone). Metformin: Urine (unchanged), $T_{1/2}$=6.2 hrs.

NURSING CONSIDERATIONS

Assessment: Obtain baseline LFTs, renal function, CBC. Assess for lactic acidosis, CHF, macular edema, type 1 DM, diabetic ketoacidosis, pregnancy status, and possible drug interactions. Assess history of hepatic insufficiency, renal impairment, and abnormal CrCl.

Monitoring: Monitor FPG and HbA_{1c} periodically for glycemic control and therapeutic response. Perform LFTs, hematologic parameters, renal function, and eye exams periodically. Monitor for signs/symptoms of heart failure, edema, lactic acidosis, diabetic ketoacidosis, fractures.

Patient Counseling: Inform to d/c with unexplained hyperventilation, myalgia, malaise, unusual somnolence symptoms. Counsel to report unexplained GI symptoms, rapid increase in weight or edema, SOB, NV, abdominal pain, fatigue, anorexia, or dark urine. Inform to avoid excessive alcohol intake. Counsel females about use of reliable contraception. Advise on importance of regular follow-up visits.

Administration: Oral route. **Storage:** 25°C (77°F); excursions permitted to 15°C (59-86°F). Keep container tightly closed. Protect from moisture and humidity.

ACTOS RX
pioglitazone HCl (Takeda)

Thiazolidinediones may cause or exacerbate CHF in some patients. Pioglitazone is not recommended in patients with symptomatic heart failure.

THERAPEUTIC CLASS: Thiazolidinedione

INDICATIONS: Adjunct to diet and exercise, to improve glycemic control in type 2 diabetes mellitus.

DOSAGE: *Adults:* Monotherapy: Initial: 15-30mg qd. Max: 45mg/day. Combination Therapy: Initial: 15-30mg qd. Max: 30mg/day. Decrease insulin dose by 10-25% if hypoglycemia occurs or if plasma glucose is <100mg/dL. Decrease sulfonylurea dose with hypoglycemia also.

HOW SUPPLIED: Tab: 15mg, 30mg, 45mg

CONTRAINDICATIONS: Established NYHA Class III or IV heart failure.

WARNINGS/PRECAUTIONS: May cause fluid retention and exacerbation/initiation of heart failure; d/c if cardiac status deteriorates. Avoid if NYHA Class III or IV cardiac status. Use lowest approved dose if systolic heart failure (NYHA Class II). Not for use in type 1 diabetes or for diabetic ketoacidosis treatment. Caution with edema. Dose-related wt gain reported. Ovulation in premenopausal anovulatory patients may occur; risk of pregnancy with inadequate contraception. May decrease Hgb and Hct. Avoid with active liver disease, if ALT levels >2.5x ULN. Check LFTs before therapy, every 2 months for 1 yr, and periodically thereafter, or if hepatic dysfunction symptoms occur. D/C if jaundice occurs or ALT >3x ULN on therapy. Macular edema reported. Increased incidence of bone fracture was noted in female patients.

ADVERSE REACTIONS: Upper respiratory tract infection, myalgia, tooth disorder, headache, sinusitis, pharyngitis, transient CPK level elevations, CHF, weight gain, aggravated DM, edema, dyspnea, new onset or worsening of diabetic macular edema.

INTERACTIONS: Possible loss of contraception with ethinyl estradiol and norethindrone; caution when co-administering. Ketoconazole may inhibit pioglitazone metabolism; evaluate glycemic control more frequently. Risk for hypoglycemia with insulin or oral hypoglycemic agents. May cause reduction of midazolam levels. An enzyme inhibitor of CYP2C8 (such as gemfibrozil) may significantly increase the AUC of pioglitazone and an enzyme inducer of CYP2C8 (such as rifampin) may significantly decrease the AUC of pioglitazone.

PREGNANCY: Category C, not for use in nursing.

MECHANISM OF ACTION: Thiazolidinedione; decreases insulin resistance in the periphery and liver resulting in increased insulin-dependent glucose disposal and decreased hepatic glucose output.

PHARMACOKINETICS: Absorption: T_{max}=within 2 hrs (fasting), 3-4 hrs (with food). **Distribution:** V_d=0.63±0.41 L/kg; plasma protein binding (>99%). **Metabolism:** Hydroxylation and oxidation; active metabolites: M-II and M-IV (hydroxy derivatives), M-III (keto derivative); CYP450 enzymes: 2C8, 3A4. **Elimination:** Urine (15-30%), bile (unchanged), feces (metabolites); $T_{1/2}$=3-7 hrs (pioglitazone), 16-24 hrs (total pioglitazone).

NURSING CONSIDERATIONS

Assessment: Assess for history of insulin-induced hypoglycemia, serum ALT, HbA_{1c}, active liver disease, class III or IV symptomatic heart failure, and other drug interactions. After initiation and dose increases, observe carefully for signs/symptoms of heart failure, including excessive and rapid weight gain, dyspnea, and/or edema.

Monitoring: Perform FPG and HbA_{1c} measurements periodically to monitor glycemic control and therapeutic response. Monitor for signs/symptoms of heart failure, liver function tests (serum ALT), and hematological parameters (Hgb/Hct). Monitor adverse events related to fluid retention after initiation and with dose increases.

Patient Counseling: Advise to adhere to dietary instructions and to regularly test blood glucose and glycosylated hemoglobin. Drug can be taken with/without meals once daily; if dose is missed, do not double dose the following day. Instruct to report SOB, rapid increase in weight or edema, unexplained NV, anorexia, fatigue, and dark urine immediately.

Administration: Oral route. **Storage:** 25°C (77°F); excursions permitted to 15-30°C (59-86°F). Keep container tightly closed. Protect from moisture and humidity.

ACULAR

RX

ketorolac tromethamine (Allergan)

THERAPEUTIC CLASS: NSAID

INDICATIONS: Ocular itching due to seasonal allergic conjunctivitis. Postoperative inflammation in cataract extraction.

DOSAGE: *Adults:* 1 drop qid. Post-op Inflammation: Begin 24 hrs post-op and continue for 2 weeks.
Pediatrics: ≥3 yrs: 1 drop qid. Post-op Inflammation: Begin 24 hrs post-op and continue for 2 weeks.

HOW SUPPLIED: Sol: 0.5% [3mL, 5mL, 10mL]

WARNINGS/PRECAUTIONS: May increase ocular tissue bleeding in conjunction with ocular surgery. Avoid use with contact lenses. D/C if corneal epithelium breakdown occurs. Caution in known bleeding tendencies, complicated ocular surgeries, corneal denervation, corneal epithelial defects, DM, ocular surface diseases (eg, dry eye syndrome), rheumatoid arthritis, or repeat ocular surgeries within a short period of time. Caution if used >24 hrs prior to surgery and use beyond 14 days post-surgery.

ADVERSE REACTIONS: Transient stinging/burning, superficial keratitis or infections, allergic reactions, ocular inflammation, corneal edema, iritis.

INTERACTIONS: Potential for cross-sensitivity to acetylsalicylic acid, phenylacetic acid derivatives, and other NSAIDs. Caution with agents that may prolong bleeding time. Increased potential for healing problems with topical steroids.

PREGNANCY: Category C, caution in nursing.

MECHANISM OF ACTION: NSAID; inhibits prostaglandin biosynthesis.

PHARMACOKINETICS: Absorption: C_{max}=95ng/mL; T_{max}=12hrs.

NURSING CONSIDERATIONS

Assessment: Assess for drug hypersensitivity, cross-sensitivity reactions, bleeding tendencies, complicated ocular surgeries, corneal denervation, corneal epithelial defects, DM, ocular surface disease (dry eye syndrome), rheumatoid arthritis, possible drug interactions.

Monitoring: Monitor for bleeding of ocular tissues (hyphema), healing problems, keratitis, epithelial breakdown, corneal thinning/erosion/ulceration/perforation.

Patient Counseling: Advise not to use while wearing contact lenses. Caution during nursing/late pregnancy.

Administration: Intraocular route. **Storage:** 15-25°C (59-77°F), protect from light.

ADALAT CC
nifedipine (Schering)

RX

OTHER BRAND NAMES: Afeditab CR (Watson)

THERAPEUTIC CLASS: Calcium channel blocker (dihydropyridine)

INDICATIONS: Treatment of hypertension.

DOSAGE: *Adults:* Initial: 30mg qd. Titrate over 7-14 days. Usual: 30-60mg qd. Max: 90mg/day. Take on empty stomach. Swallow tab whole.

HOW SUPPLIED: Tab, Extended-Release: (Adalat CC, Afeditab CR) 30mg, 60mg, (Adalat CC) 90mg

WARNINGS/PRECAUTIONS: May cause hypotension; monitor BP initially or with titration. May exacerbate angina from β-blocker withdrawal. CHF risk, especially with aortic stenosis or β-blockers. Peripheral edema reported. May increase angina or MI with severe obstructive CAD. Caution in elderly.

ADVERSE REACTIONS: Headache, flushing, heat sensation, dizziness, peripheral edema, fatigue, asthenia.

INTERACTIONS: β-blockers may increase risk of CHF, severe hypotension, or angina exacerbation. Possible hypotension with fentanyl. Monitor digoxin, quinidine, and coumarin levels. CYP3A4 inhibitors (eg, ketoconazole, erythromycin, protease inhibitors) may increase levels. Avoid grapefruit juice. Cimetidine may increase levels. CYP3A4 inducers (eg, phenytoin, St. John's wort) may decrease levels.

PREGNANCY: Category C, not for use in nursing.

MECHANISM OF ACTION: Calcium channel blocker; involved in peripheral arterial vasodilatation and consequently reduction in peripheral vascular resistance.

PHARMACOKINETICS: Absorption: Complete; absolute bioavailability (84-89%); C_{max}=115ng/mL; T_{max}=2.5-5 hrs. **Distribution:** Plasma protein binding (92-98%); found in breast milk. **Metabolism:** Liver (extensive). **Elimination:** Urine (60-80% as metabolite/unchanged), feces (metabolite); $T_{1/2}$=7 hrs.

NURSING CONSIDERATIONS

Assessment: Assess for hypotension, CHD, aortic stenosis, hepatic/renal impairment, pregnancy/nursing status, and possible drug interactions.

Monitoring: Carefully monitor BP and HR during initial administration and titration. Monitor for signs/symptoms of CHF, hypotension, cholestasis with/without jaundice, peripheral edema, angina, MI, lab tests (eg, elevations in alkaline phosphatase, CPK, LDH, SGOT, and SGPT), decrease in platelet aggregation, increased bleeding time, positive direct Coombs' test with/without hemolytic anemia, and reversible elevation in BUN and serum creatinine.

Patient Counseling: Instruct to swallow whole; do not chew, divide, or crush. Take on empty stomach. Do not take with grapefruit juice. Inform about potential benefits/risks and to report any adverse reactions to physician. Notify if pregnant/nursing.

Administration: Oral route. **Storage:** Below 30°C (86°F); in tight, light-resistant container. Avoid moisture.

ADDERALL
amphetamine salt combo (Shire)

CII

High potential for abuse; avoid prolonged use. Misuse of amphetamine may cause sudden death and serious cardiovascular adverse events.

THERAPEUTIC CLASS: Sympathomimetic amine

INDICATIONS: Treatment of attention deficit disorder with hyperactivity (ADHD) and narcolepsy.

DOSAGE: *Adults:* Narcolepsy: Initial: 10mg/day. Titrate: May increase by 10mg/day every week. Usual: 5-60mg/day. Give 1st dose upon awakening, and additional doses q4-6h.
Pediatrics: ADHD: 3-5 yrs: Initial: 2.5mg qd. Titrate: May increase by 2.5mg weekly. ≥6 yrs: 5mg qd-bid. May increase by 5mg weekly. Max (usual): 40mg/day. Narcolepsy: 6-12 yrs: Initial: 5mg/day. May increase by 5mg weekly. ≥12 yrs: Initial: 10mg/day. Titrate: May increase by 10mg/day every week. Usual: 5-60mg/day. Give 1st dose upon awakening, and additional doses q4-6h.

HOW SUPPLIED: Tab: 5mg*, 7.5mg*, 10mg*, 12.5mg*, 15mg*, 20mg*, 30mg* *scored

CONTRAINDICATIONS: Advanced arteriosclerosis, symptomatic cardiovascular disease, moderate to severe HTN, hyperthyroidism, glaucoma, agitated states, history of drug abuse, during or within 14 days of MAOI use.

WARNINGS/PRECAUTIONS: May exacerbate symptoms of behavior disturbance and thought disorder in psychotic patients. Caution when using stimulants to treat patients with comorbid bipolar disorder because of concern for possible induction of mixed/manic episode in such patients. Stimulants at usual doses can cause treatment emergent psychotic or manic symptoms (eg, hallucinations, delusional thinking, mania) in children and adolescents without prior history of psychotic illness. Aggressive behavior or hostility reported in clinical trials and the postmarketing experience of some medications indicated for the treatment of ADHD. Monitor growth in children. May lower convulsive threshold; d/c in presence of seizures. Visual disturbances reported with stimulant treatment. May exacerbate Tourette's syndrome and phonic or motor tics. Caution with HTN and monitor BP. Interrupt occasionally to determine if patient requires continued therapy. Sudden death reported in children with structural cardiac abnormalities; avoid use in children or adults with structural cardiac abnormalities.

ADVERSE REACTIONS: HTN, tachycardia, palpitations, CNS overstimulation, dry mouth, GI disorders, anorexia, impotence, urticaria, rash, angioedema, anaphylaxis, Stevens-Johnson syndrome.

INTERACTIONS: GI acidifying agents (guanethidine, reserpine, glutamic acid, etc) and urinary acidifying agents (ammonium chloride, etc) decrease efficacy. MAOIs may cause hypertensive crisis. Potentiated by GI and urinary alkalinizers, propoxyphene overdose. Potentiated effects of both agents with TCAs. May delay absorption of phenytoin, ethosuximide, phenobarbital. Potentiates meperidine, norepinephrine, phenobarbital, phenytoin. Antagonized by haloperidol, chlorpromazine, lithium. Antagonizes adrenergic blockers, antihistamines, antihypertensives, veratrum alkaloids (antihypertensive). Avoid co-administration with alkalinizing agents (eg, antacids).

PREGNANCY: Category C, not for use in nursing.

MECHANISM OF ACTION: CNS stimulant; thought to block reuptake of norepinephrine and dopamine into presynaptic neuron and increase release of these monoamines into extraneuronal space.

PHARMACOKINETICS: Absorption: T_{max}=approximately 3 hrs (fasted). **Metabolism**: CYP2D6 (oxidation): 4-hydroxy-amphetamine and norephedrine. **Elimination**: Urine, $T_{1/2}$=9.77-11 hrs (d-amphetamine), 11.5-13.8 hrs (l-amphetamine).

NURSING CONSIDERATIONS

Assessment: Assess for agitation, glaucoma, tics, family history of Tourette's syndrome, cardiovascular conditions (eg, severe HTN, angina pectoris, cardiac abnormalities, arrhythmias, heart failure, recent MI), hyperthyroidism or thyrotoxicosis, bipolar illness, history of drug dependence or alcoholism.

Monitoring: Monitor for cardiac abnormalities, exacerbations of behavior disturbances and thought disorder, bipolar illness, aggression, seizures, and visual disturbances. Periodic monitoring of CBC, differential and platelet count, LFTs. Monitor height and weight in children.

Patient Counseling: Inform about risks of treatment, appropriate use, drug abuse/dependence. Caution while operating machinery/driving.

Administration: Oral route. **Storage**: 20-25°C (68-77°F).

ADDERALL XR

amphetamine salt combo (Shire)

CII

High potential for abuse; avoid prolonged use. Misuse of amphetamine may cause sudden death and serious cardiovascular adverse events.

THERAPEUTIC CLASS: Sympathomimetic amine

INDICATIONS: Treatment of attention deficit hyperactivity disorder (ADHD).

DOSAGE: *Adults:* Initial: 20mg qam. Currently Using Adderall: Switch to Adderall XR at the same total daily dose, taken once daily. Titrate at weekly intervals as needed. Swallow cap whole or open cap and sprinkle contents on applesauce; do not chew beads.
Pediatrics: ≥6 yrs: Initial: 10mg qam. Titrate: May increase weekly by 5-10mg/day. Max: 30mg/day. 13 to 17 yrs: Initial: 10mg/day. Titrate: May increase to 20mg/day after one week. Currently Using Adderall: Switch to Adderall XR at the same total daily dose, taken once daily. Titrate at weekly intervals as needed. Swallow cap whole or open cap and sprinkle contents on applesauce; do not chew beads.

HOW SUPPLIED: Cap, Extended-Release: 5mg, 10mg, 15mg, 20mg, 25mg, 30mg

CONTRAINDICATIONS: Advanced arteriosclerosis, symptomatic cardiovascular disease, moderate to severe HTN, hyperthyroidism, glaucoma, agitated states, history of drug abuse, during or within 14 days of MAOI use.

WARNINGS/PRECAUTIONS: May exacerbate symptoms of behavior disturbance and thought disorder in psychotic patients. Caution when using stimulants to treat patients with comorbid bipolar disorder because of concern for possible induction of mixed/manic episode in such patients. Stimulants at usual doses can cause treatment emergent psychotic or manic symptoms (eg, hallucinations, delusional thinking, mania) in children and adolescents without prior history of psychotic illness. Aggressive behavior or hostility reported in clinical trials and postmarketing experience of some medications indicated for the treatment of ADHD. Monitor growth in children. May lower convulsive threshold; d/c in presence of seizures. Visual disturbances reported with stimulant treatment. May exacerbate Tourette's syndrome and phonic or motor tics. Caution with HTN and monitor BP. Interrupt occasionally to determine if patient requires continued therapy. Sudden death reported in children with structural cardiac abnormalities; avoid use in children or adults with structural cardiac abnormalities. May decrease appetite.

ADVERSE REACTIONS: Abdominal pain, asthenia, fever, infection, viral infection, loss of appetite, diarrhea, NV, emotional lability, insomnia, nervousness, weight loss, dry mouth, headache, urticaria, anaphylaxis.

INTERACTIONS: GI acidifying agents (guanethidine, reserpine, glutamic acid, etc) and urinary acidifying agents (ammonium chloride, etc) decrease efficacy. MAOIs may cause hypertensive crisis. Potentiated by GI and urinary alkalinizers, propoxyphene overdose. Potentiated effects of both agents with TCAs. May delay absorption of phenytoin, ethosuximide, phenobarbital. Potentiates meperidine, norepinephrine, phenobarbital, phenytoin. Antagonized by haloperidol, chlorpromazine, lithium. Antagonizes adrenergic blockers, antihistamines, antihypertensives, veratrum alkaloids (antihypertensive). Avoid coadministration of alkalinizing agents (eg, antacid).

PREGNANCY: Category C, not for use in nursing.

MECHANISM OF ACTION: CNS stimulant; thought to block reuptake of norepinephrine and dopamine into presynaptic neuron and increase release of these monoamines into extraneuronal space.

PHARMACOKINETICS: Absorption: T_{max}=7 hrs. **Metabolism**: CYP2D6 (oxidation): 4-hydroxy-amphetamine and norepinephrine (metabolites). **Elimination**:

Urine (30-40%). D-amphetamine: $T_{1/2}$=10 hrs (adults), 11 hrs (adolescents aged 13-17 years), 9 hrs (6-12 years). l-amphetamine: $T_{1/2}$=13 hrs (adults), 13-14 hrs (adolescents aged 13-17), 11 hrs (6-12 yrs).

NURSING CONSIDERATIONS

Assessment: Assess for agitation, glaucoma, tics, family history of Tourette's syndrome, cardiovascular conditions (eg, severe HTN, angina pectoris, cardiac abnormalities, arrhythmias, heart failure, recent MI), hyperthyroidism or thyrotoxicosis, bipolar illness, history of drug dependence or alcoholism.

Monitoring: Monitor for cardiac abnormalities, exacerbations of behavior disturbances and thought disorder, bipolar illness, aggression, seizures, and visual disturbances. Periodic monitoring of CBC, differential and platelet count, LFTs. Monitor height and weight in children.

Patient Counseling: Inform about risk of treatment, appropriate use, drug abuse/dependence. Caution while operating machinery/driving.

Administration: Oral route. **Storage**: 15-30°C (59-86°F).

ADVAIR

RX

salmeterol xinafoate - fluticasone propionate (GlaxoSmithKline)

Long-acting β_2-adrenergic agonists, such as salmeterol, may increase risk of asthma-related deaths. Use of diskus should be reserved for patients not adequately controlled on other medications or whose disease severity warrants initiation with 2 maintenance therapies.

THERAPEUTIC CLASS: Corticosteroid/beta$_2$ agonist

INDICATIONS: Long-term, maintenance treatment of asthma in patients ≥4 yrs. (250/50 only): Maintenance treatment of airflow obstruction in patients with COPD, including chronic bronchitis and/or emphysema; to reduce exacerbations of COPD in patients with history of exacerbations.

DOSAGE: *Adults:* Asthma: 1 inh q12h. Without Prior Inhaled Corticosteroid (CS) Therapy/Inadequate Control on Current Inhaled CS: Initial: 100/50 or 250/50 bid. Max: 500/50 bid. If no response within 2 weeks, may increase to higher strength. COPD: (250/50 only): 1 inh q12h. Rinse mouth after use. *Pediatrics:* ≥12 yrs: Asthma: 1 inh q12h. Without Prior Inhaled Corticosteroid (CS) Therapy/Inadequate Control on Current Inhaled CS: Initial: 100/50 or 250/50 bid. Max: 500/50 bid. If no response within 2 weeks, may increase to higher strength. (100/50 only): 4-11 yrs: Symptomatic on Inhaled CS: 1 inh q12h. Rinse mouth after use.

HOW SUPPLIED: Disk (Inhalation): (Fluticasone-Salmeterol) (100/50) 0.1mg-0.05mg/inh, (250/50) 0.25mg-0.05mg/inh, (500/50) 0.5mg-0.05mg/inh [60 blisters]

CONTRAINDICATIONS: Status asthmaticus, other acute asthma or COPD episodes, and hypersensitivity to milk proteins.

WARNINGS/PRECAUTIONS: Deaths due to adrenal insufficiency have occurred with transfer from systemic corticosteroids to inhaled corticosteroids. Resume oral corticosteroids during stress or severe asthma attack. Observe for adrenal insufficiency, systemic corticosteroid withdrawal effects, hypercorticism, reduction in growth velocity (pediatrics). More susceptible to infection. Not for acute bronchospasm. D/C if bronchospasm occurs after dosing. Caution with TB; untreated systemic fungal, bacterial, viral, or parasitic infections; or ocular herpes simplex. *Candida* infection of mouth and pharynx, glaucoma, hypersensitivity reactions, increased IOP, cataracts reported. Monitor for increasing use of β_2-agonists. QTc interval prolongation reported with large doses. D/C if paradoxical bronchospasm occurs. Caution with cardiovascular or CNS disorders, convulsive disorders, thyrotoxicosis, DM, and ketoacidosis. May produce hypokalemia, hyperglycemia, and eosinophilic conditions.

ADVERSE REACTIONS: Upper respiratory tract inflammation, pharyngitis, sinusitis, cough, hoarseness, headaches, GI effects, musculoskeletal pain, palpitations.

INTERACTIONS: Extreme caution with TCAs or MAOIs during or within 14 days of use. Antagonized by β-blockers. Caution with non-K^+-sparing diuretics; ECG changes, hypokalemia may develop. Concomitant use with strong CYP3A4 inhibitors (eg, ritonavir, atazanavir, indinavir, ketoconazole) is not recommended.

PREGNANCY: Category C, caution in nursing.

MECHANISM OF ACTION: Fluticasone: Corticosteroid with anti-inflammatory activity; inhibits multiple cell types (eg, mast cells, eosinophils, neutrophils, macrophages, lymphocytes) and mediators (eg, histamine, eicosanoids, leukotrienes and cytokines) involved in inflammation and asthmatic response. Salmeterol: Long-acting β_2-adrenergic agonist; stimulates intracellular adenyl cyclase, which catalyzes conversion of ATP to cAMP, producing relaxation of bronchial smooth muscle and inhibition of release of immediate hypersensitivity mediators from cells (eg, mast cells).

PHARMACOKINETICS: Absorption: Fluticasone: (Asthma, 500 bid) C_{max}=110pg/mL, (COPD, 250 bid) 53pg/mL. Salmeterol: C_{max}=167pg/mL, T_{max}=20 min. **Distribution:** Fluticasone: V_d=4.2L/kg; plasma protein binding (91%). Salmeterol: Plasma protein binding (96%). **Metabolism:** Fluticasone: Liver via CYP3A4. Salmeterol: Liver, via CYP3A4 to α-hydroxysalmeterol (metabolite). **Elimination:** Urine, feces; Fluticasone: $T_{1/2}$=7.8 hrs. Salmeterol: $T_{1/2}$=5.5 hrs.

NURSING CONSIDERATIONS

Assessment: Assess if asthma is controlled by inhaled corticosteroids and occassional use of short-acting β_2-agonists. Assess for risk factors for decreased bone mineral content (eg, tobacco use, advanced age, sedentary lifestyle, family history of osteoporosis, drugs that decrease bone mass), CVD (eg, coronary insufficiency, cardiac arrhythmia, HTN), convulsive disorder, thyrotoxicosis, DM, history of increased IOP, glaucoma, cataracts, concomitant diseases like status asthmaticus, active or quiescent pulmonary TB, ocular herpes simplex, untreated systemic fungal, bacterial, parasitic or viral infections, and possible drug interactions. Obtain baseline bone mineral density, eye exam, and lung function prior to therapy.

Monitoring: Monitor bone mineral density and lung function periodically. Perform periodic eye exams. Monitor for localized oral infections with *Candida albicans*, decreased bone mass, upper airway symptoms (laryngeal spasm, irritation, swelling), worsening or acutely deteriorating asthma (increased use of inhaled β_2-agonist, decreased lung function), asthma instability (serial objective measures of airflow), body height in children, development of glaucoma, increased IOP, posterior subcapsular cataracts, adrenal insufficiency (eg, fatigue, weakness, NV, hypotension), paradoxical bronchospasm, eosinophilic conditions, pneumonia, and hypersensitivity reactions.

Patient Counseling: Inform not to d/c therapy unless directed by physician. Instruct to never exhale into diskus, never attempt to take diskus apart. Activate and use in a level, horizontal position, never wash mouthpiece or any part, keep dry. Inform not to use for sudden symptoms of SOB or acute bronchospasm. Advise to rinse mouth after inhalation. Inform may cause reduction in growth velocity (pediatric) and may also unmask allergies (eg, rhinitis, conjunctivitis, eczema). Warn to avoid exposure to chickenpox or measles. Seek medical attention if exposed to chickenpox or measles, worsening of existing TB, infections or ocular herpes simplex, symptoms do not improve or worsen during periods of stress or severe asthmatic attack, adrenal insufficiency (eg, fatigue, weakness, NV, hypotension), paradoxical bronchospasm or hypersensitivity reactions occur.

Administration: Oral inhalation. 1) Hold with 1 hand and put thumb of other hand on thumbgrip. Push thumb away from self until mouthpiece appears and snaps into position. 2) Hold in level, flat position with mouthpiece towards self. Slide lever away from self until it clicks. 3) Exhale fully, then put mouthpiece in lips and breath in quickly and deeply. Hold breath for 10 seconds or as long as comfortable. Breath out slowly. **Storage:** 20-25°C (68-77°F). Keep away from heat and sunlight. Discard 1 month after removal from pouch or when indicator reads "0", whichever comes first.

ADVAIR HFA

RX

salmeterol xinafoate - fluticasone propionate (GlaxoSmithKline)

Long-acting β_2-adrenergic agonists, such as salmeterol, may increase risk of asthma-related deaths.

THERAPEUTIC CLASS: Corticosteroid/beta$_2$ agonist

INDICATIONS: For long-term, maintenance treatment of asthma.

DOSAGE: *Adults:* Asthma: 2 inh q12h. Without Prior Inhaled Corticosteroid (CS): Initial: 2 inh of 45/21 bid or 1 inh of 115/21 bid. Max: 2 inh of 230/21 bid. Current Inhaled CS: Beclomethasone: ≤160mcg/day use 2 inh of 45/21 bid, 320mcg/day use 2 inh of 115/21 bid, 640mcg/day use 2 inh of 230/21 bid. Budesonide: ≤400mcg/day use 2 inh of 45/21 bid, 800-1200mcg/day use 2 inh of 115/21 bid, 1600mcg/day use 2 inh of 230/21 bid. Flunisolide: ≤1000mcg/day use 2 inh of 45/21 bid, 1250-2000mcg/day use 2 inh of 115/21 bid. Flunisolide HFA: ≤320mcg/day use 2 inh of 45/21 bid, 640mcg/day use 2 inh of 115/21 bid. Fluticasone Aerosol: ≤176mcg/day use 2 inh of 45/21 bid, 440mcg/day use 2 inh of 115/21 bid, 660-880mcg/day use 2 inh of 230/21 bid. Fluticasone Powder: ≤200mcg/day use 2 inh of 45/21 bid, 500mcg/day use 2 inh of 115/21 bid, 1000mcg/day use 2 inh of 230/21 bid. Mometasone Powder: 220mcg/day use 2 inh of 45/21 bid, 440mcg/day use 2 inh of 115/21 bid, 880mcg/day use 2 inh of 230/21 bid. Triamcinolone: ≤1000mcg/day use 2 inh of 45/21 bid, 1100-1600mcg/day use 2 inh of 115/21 bid. If no response within 2 weeks, increase to higher strength.
Pediatrics: ≥12 yrs: Asthma: 2 inh q12h. Without Prior Inhaled Corticosteroid (CS): Initial: 2 inh of 45/21 bid or 1 inh of 115/21 bid. Max: 2 inh of 230-21 bid. Current Inhaled CS: Beclomethasone: ≤160mcg/day use 2 inh of 45/21 bid, 320mcg/day use 2 inh of 115/21 bid, 640mcg/day use 2 inh of 230/21 bid. Budesonide: ≤400mcg/day use 2 inh of 45/21 bid, 800-1200mcg/day use 2 inh of 115/21 bid, 1600mcg/day use 2 inh of 230/21 bid. Flunisolide: ≤1000mcg/day use 2 inh of 45/21 bid, 1250-2000mcg/day use 2 inh of 115/21 bid. Flunisolide HFA: ≤320mcg/day use 2 inh of 45/21 bid, 640mcg/day use 2 inh of 115/21 bid. Fluticasone Aerosol: ≤176mcg/day use 2 inh of 45/21 bid, 440mcg/day use 2 inh of 115/21 bid, 660-880mcg/day use 2 inh of 230/21 bid. Fluticasone Powder: ≤200mcg/day use 2 inh of 45/21 bid, 500mcg/day use 2 inh of 115/21 bid, 1000mcg/day use 2 inh of 230/21 bid. Mometasone powder: 220mcg/day use 2 inh of 45/21 bid, 440mcg/day use 2 inh of 115/21 bid, 880mcg/day use 2 inh of 230/21 bid. Triamcinolone: ≤1000mcg/day use 2 inh of 45/21 bid, 1100-1600mcg/day use 2 inh of 115/21 bid. If no response within 2 weeks, increase to higher strength.

HOW SUPPLIED: MDI: (Fluticasone-Salmeterol) (45/21) 0.045mg-0.021mg/inh, (115/21) 0.115mg-0.021mg/inh, (230/21) 0.230mg-0.021mg/inh [120 inhalations]

CONTRAINDICATIONS: Status asthmaticus or other acute asthma.

WARNINGS/PRECAUTIONS: May increase the risk of asthma-related death. Should only be given to patients not adequately controlled by other asthma-controller medications (eg, low- or medium-dose inhaled corticosteroids) or when disease severity requires need to start 2 maintenance therapies. Not to be given to patients with rapidly deteriorating or potentially life-threatening episodes of asthma. Avoid to treat acute symptoms. Should not be used for transferring patients from systemic corticosteroid therapy. Should not be coadministered with inhaled, long-acting β_2-agonist and strong CYP3A4 inhibitors (eg, ketoconazole, ritonavir). Should not exceed recommended dosage. Life-threatening paradoxical bronchospasm reported; d/c therapy immediately; start alternative therapy. Immediate hypersensitivity reactions (eg, urticaria, angioedema, rash, and bronchospasm) may occur. Upper airway symptoms (eg, laryngeal spasm, irritation, or swelling, stridor and choking) and lower respiratory tract infections (eg, pneumonia) reported. Caution in CVD, convulsive disorders, thyrotoxicosis, active or quiescent TB, untreated systemic fungal, bacterial, viral, or parasitic infection, and ocular herpes simplex. Prolonged use may affect normal bone metabolism and bone mineral density. *Candida* infection of mouth and pharynx, glaucoma, hypersensitivity reactions, increased IOP, cataracts reported. Cases of eosinophilic conditions reported. Caution in elderly.

ADVERSE REACTIONS: Upper respiratory tract infection, throat irritation, upper respiratory tract inflammation, headaches, dysphonia, nausea, vomiting, musculoskeletal pain, menstruation symptoms.

INTERACTIONS: Extreme caution with TCAs or MAOIs during or within 14 days of use. Antagonized by β-blockers. Caution with non-potassium sparing diuretics; ECG changes, hypokalemia may develop. Potentiated by ketoconazole, ritonavir, erythromycin, other CYP3A4 inhibitors.

PREGNANCY: Category C, caution in nursing.

MECHANISM OF ACTION: Fluticasone: Corticosteroid with anti-inflammatory activity; inhibits multiple cell types (eg, mast cells, eosinophils, neutrophils, macrophages, lymphocytes) and mediators (eg, histamine, eicosanoids, leukotrienes and cytokines) involved in inflammation and asthmatic response. Salmeterol: β_2-adrenergic agonist; stimulates intracellular adenyl cyclase, which catalyzes conversion of ATP to cAMP, producing relaxation of bronchial smooth muscle and inhibition of release of immediate hypersensitivity mediators from cells (eg, mast cells).

PHARMACOKINETICS: Absorption: Fluticasone: Absolute Bioavailability (5.3%); Salmeterol: C_{max}=150pg/mL; T_{max}=5-10 mins. **Distribution:** Fluticasone: V_d=4.2L/kg; plasma protein binding (99%). Salmeterol: Plasma protein binding (96%). **Metabolism:** Fluticasone: Liver, via CYP3A4. Salmeterol: Extensive by hydroxylation. **Elimination:** Fluticasone: Feces (major), urine (<5%); $T_{1/2}$=7.8 hrs. Salmeterol: Feces (60%), urine (25%); $T_{1/2}$=5.5 hrs.

NURSING CONSIDERATIONS

Assessment: Assess if asthma is controlled by inhaled corticosteroids and occasional use of short-acting β_2-agonists. Assess for risk factors for decreased bone mineral content (eg, tobacco use, advanced age, sedentary lifestyle, family history of osteoporosis, drugs that decrease bone mass), CVD (eg, coronary insufficiency, cardiac arrhythmia, HTN), convulsive disorder, thyrotoxicosis, DM, history of increased IOP, glaucoma, cataracts, concomitant diseases like status asthmaticus, active or quiescent pulmonary TB, ocular herpes simplex, untreated systemic fungal, bacterial, parasitic or viral infections, and possible drug interactions, and pregnancy/nursing status. Obtain baseline bone mineral density, eye exam, and lung function prior to therapy.

Monitoring: Monitor bone mineral density and lung function periodically. Perform periodic eye exams. Monitor for localized oral infections with *Candida albicans*, decreased bone mass, upper airway symptoms (laryngeal spasm, irritation, swelling), worsening or acutely deteriorating asthma (increased use of inhaled β_2-agonist, decreased lung function), asthma instability (serial objective measures of airflow), body height in children, development of glaucoma, increased IOP, cataracts, adrenal insufficiency (eg, fatigue, weakness, NV, hypotension), paradoxical bronchospasm, eosinophilic conditions, pneumonia, and hypersensitivity reactions. Closely monitor patients with hepatic disease.

Patient Counseling: Counsel that Advair HFA is not used to relieve acute asthma symptoms. Instruct to seek physician if signs of seriously worsening asthma occur. Inform not to d/c therapy unless directed by physician. Counsel about β_2-agonists common adverse reactions (eg, palpitations, chest pain, rapid HR, tremor, or nervousness) during therapy. Instruct regular eye examinations in long-term therapy. Inform not to use for sudden symptoms of SOB or acute bronchospasm. Counsel on appropriate use: priming inhaler before use, rinsing mouth after inhalation, not to swallow, to clean inhaler once a week, and to never immerse in water. Inform may cause reduction in growth rate (pediatrics), may unmask allergies (eg, rhinitis, conjunctivitis, eczema). Warm to avoid exposure to chickenpox or measles. Seek medical attention if exposed to chickenpox or measles, worsening of existing TB, infections, or ocular herpes simplex, symptoms do not improve or worsen, during periods of stress or severe asthmatic attack, fatigue, weakness, NV and hypotension, paradoxical bronchospasm, or hypersensitivity reactions occur.

Administration: Oral inhalation. Prime inhaler by releasing 4 test sprays into air, away from face, shaking well for 5 seconds before each spray. If not used for 4 weeks or dropped, reprime by releasing 2 test sprays into air, shaking well before each spray. **Storage:** 25°C (77°F); excursions permitted to 15-30°C (59-86°F). Store with mouthpiece down. Do not puncture, store, or use near heat or open flame.

ADVICOR

RX

lovastatin - niacin (Abbott)

THERAPEUTIC CLASS: B-complex vitamin/HMG-CoA reductase inhibitor

INDICATIONS: Treatment of hypercholesterolemia when use of both Niaspan (niacin ER) and lovastatin is appropriate. (Niacin ER) Treatment of primary hypercholesterolemia and mixed dyslipidemia, hypertriglyceridemia, and secondary prevention of cardiovascular events. (Lovastatin) Treatment of primary hypercholesterolemia, primary and secondary prevention of cardiovascular events. See individual labeling for further details.

DOSAGE: *Adults:* ≥18 yrs: Initial: 500mg-20mg qhs. Titrate: Increase by no more than 500mg of niacin every 4 weeks. Max: 2000mg-40mg. Concomitant Cyclosporine/Danazol: Max Lovastatin: 20mg/day. Concomitant Amiodarone/Verapamil: Max Lovastatin: 40mg/day. Swallow tab whole. Take with low-fat snack. Pretreat 30 min prior with ASA to reduce flushing.

HOW SUPPLIED: Tab: (Extended-Release Niacin-Lovastatin) 500mg-20mg, 750mg-20mg, 1000mg-20mg, 1000mg-40mg

CONTRAINDICATIONS: Active liver disease, unexplained persistent elevations in serum transaminases, active PUD, arterial bleeding, pregnancy, nursing mothers.

WARNINGS/PRECAUTIONS: Do not substitute for equivalent dose of immediate-release niacin. Myopathy, rhabdomyolysis, severe hepatotoxicity reported. Caution with history of liver disease or jaundice, heavy alcohol use, hepatobiliary disease, peptic ulcer, diabetes, unstable angina, acute phase of MI, gout, renal dysfunction. Monitor LFTs prior to therapy, every 6-12 weeks for 1st 6 months, and periodically thereafter. May elevate PT, uric acid levels. D/C if AST or ALT ≥3x ULN persists, if myopathy diagnosed or suspected, and a few days before surgery. May reduce phosphorous levels. May disrupt therapy during a course of treatment with systemic antifungal azole, a macrolide antibiotic or ketolide antibiotic.

ADVERSE REACTIONS: Flushing, asthenia, flu syndrome, headache, infection, pain, GI effects, hyperglycemia, myalgia, pruritus, rash.

INTERACTIONS: May potentiate ganglionic blockers, vasoactive drugs. Decreased niacin clearance with ASA. Separate bile acid sequestrants by 4-6 hrs. Avoid concomitant alcohol and hot drinks; may increase flushing and pruritus. Antidiabetic agents may need adjustment. Caution with niacin-containing nutritional supplements. Increased risk of skeletal muscle disorders with CYP3A4 inhibitors (eg, cyclosporine, itraconazole, ketoconazole, erythromycin, clarithromycin, telithromycin, protease inhibitors, nefazodone, >1 quart/day of grapefruit juice), verapamil, fibrates (eg, gemfibrozil). Monitor warfarin. Caution with drugs that diminish levels or activity of steroid hormones (eg, ketoconazole, spironolactone, cimetidine). Caution with acute MI and nitrates, CCBs, and adrenergic blockers.

PREGNANCY: Category X, not for use in nursing.

MECHANISM OF ACTION: Niacin: Vitamin B complex; not completely understood and may include various actions, including partial inhibition of free fatty acids from adipose tissue and increased lipoprotein lipase activity. Decreases hepatic synthesis rate of VLDL-C and LDL-C. Lovastatin: Inhibits HMG-CoA reductase enzyme, which is needed for conversion of HMG-CoA to mevalonate. Has LDL-lowering effect by involving both reduction of VLDL-C concentration and induction of the LDL receptor, leading to reduction of production and/or increased catabolism of LDL-C.

PHARMACOKINETICS: Absorption: Niacin: C_{max}=18mcg/mL, T_{max}=5 hrs. Lovastatin: Incomplete, C_{max}=11ng/mL, T_{max}=2 hrs. **Distribution:** Niacin: Serum protein binding (20%), found in breast milk. Lovastatin: Plasma protein binding (95%), crosses blood-brain/placental barrier. **Metabolism:** Niacin: Rapid and extensive. Through conjugation pathway. Lovastatin: Liver (extensive) via CYP3A4. Lovastatin acid, 6'-hydroxy (active metabolites). **Elimination:** Niacin: Urine (60%); $T_{1/2}$=20-48 min. Lovastatin: Urine (10%), feces (83%), bile; $T_{1/2}$=4.5 hrs.

NURSING CONSIDERATIONS

Assessment: Assess for active liver disease or unexplained persistent serum transaminase elevations, active peptic ulcer disease or arterial bleeding, pregnancy/nursing status, alcohol intake, DM, upcoming surgery, unstable angina, acute phase of MI, gout, and possible drug interactions. Perform LFTs prior to therapy. Control dyslipidemia with appropriate diet, exercise, and weight reduction in obese patients and treat other underlying medical problems before instituting therapy.

Monitoring: Monitor for signs/symptoms of myopathy, rhabdomyolysis (eg, pain, tenderness, or weakness), acute renal failure, endocrine dysfunction, flushing, CNS toxicity (eg, optic nerve degeneration), CNS vascular lesions (eg, hemorrhage, edema), false elevations of urinary/plasma catecholamines and false-positive reactions in urine glucose test. Periodic monitoring of LFTs, CK, blood glucose, phosphorus levels, platelets, and uric acid.

Patient Counseling: Inform about risks/benefits and report promptly any signs of unexplained muscle pain, tenderness, or weakness to physician. Avoid alcohol and hot drinks around time of drug administration. Notify physician if pregnant/nursing or if dizziness occurs. Take as prescribed. Inform that flushing is a common side effect of drug and taking aspirin or NSAIDs 30 min before administration of drug may decrease it.

Administration: Oral route. Take drug whole at bedtime; do not crush or chew. Do not take on empty stomach or with grapefruit juice. **Storage:** 20-25°C (68-77°F).

AEROBID

flunisolide (Forest)

RX

OTHER BRAND NAMES: Aerobid-M (with menthol) (Forest)

THERAPEUTIC CLASS: Corticosteroid

INDICATIONS: Maintenance treatment of asthma as prophylactic therapy in patients ≥6 years and to reduce or eliminate the need for oral systemic corticosteroidal therapy.

DOSAGE: *Adults:* Initial: 2 inh bid. Max: 4 inh bid. Rinse mouth after use. *Pediatrics:* 6-15 yrs: 2 inh bid. Rinse mouth after use.

HOW SUPPLIED: MDI: 0.25mg/inh [7g]

CONTRAINDICATIONS: Primary treatment of status asthmaticus or other acute asthma attacks.

WARNINGS/PRECAUTIONS: Deaths due to adrenal insufficiency have occurred with transfer from systemic corticosteroids to inhaled corticosteroids. Resume oral corticosteroids during stress or severe asthma attack. Observe for adrenal insufficiency, systemic corticosteroid withdrawal effects, and growth suppression (children). More susceptible to infections. Not for acute bronchospasm. D/C if bronchospasm occurs after dosing. Caution with tuberculosis of the respiratory tract; untreated systemic fungal, bacterial, viral, or parasitic infections; or ocular herpes simplex. *Candida* infection of the mouth and pharynx reported.

ADVERSE REACTIONS: Upper respiratory infection, diarrhea, stomach upset, cold symptoms, nasal congestion, headache, nausea, vomiting, sore throat, unpleasant taste.

PREGNANCY: Category C, caution with nursing.

MECHANISM OF ACTION: Corticosteroid; demonstrated marked anti-inflammatory and anti-allergic activity in test systems.

PHARMACOKINETICS: Metabolism: Liver (1st pass). Metabolite (6β-OH). **Elimination:** $T_{1/2}$=1.8 hrs.

NURSING CONSIDERATIONS

Assessment: Assess for concomitant diseases such as status asthmaticus, active or quiescent pulmonary TB, untreated systemic fungal, bacterial or parasitic or viral infections, and possible drug interactions.

Monitoring: Monitor for localized oral infections with *Candida albicans*, body height in children, adrenal insufficiency, paradoxical bronchospasm, pulmonary infiltrates with eosinophilia, and hypersensitivity reactions.

Patient Counseling: Inform that medication is not for relief of acute bronchospasm. Inform that therapy may unmask allergies (eg, rhinitis, conjunctivitis, eczema). Warn to avoid exposure to chickenpox or measles. Advise to seek medical attention if exposed to chickenpox or measles, symptoms worsen or do not improve, during periods of stress or severe asthmatic attack, adrenal insufficiency, paradoxical bronchospasm or hypersensitivity reactions occur.

Administration: Oral inhalation. **Storage:** Do not puncture. Do not use or store near heat or open flame. Exposure to temperatures above 49°C (120°F) may cause container to explode. Never throw container into fire or incinerator. Keep out of reach of children.

AGGRASTAT — RX

tirofiban HCl (Medicure)

THERAPEUTIC CLASS: Glycoprotein IIb/IIIa inhibitor

INDICATIONS: In combination with heparin, for treatment of acute coronary syndrome, in patients being medically managed or undergoing PTCA or atherectomy.

DOSAGE: *Adults:* Initial: 0.4mcg/kg/min IV for 30 min. Maint: 0.1mcg/kg/min IV. Continue through angiography and for 12-24 hrs after angioplasty or atherectomy. CrCl <30mL/min: Administer at half of usual rate of infusion.

HOW SUPPLIED: Inj: 0.05mg/mL, 0.25mg/mL

CONTRAINDICATIONS: Active internal bleeding, acute pericarditis, severe HTN, concomitant parenteral GP IIb/IIIa inhibitor, hemorrhagic stroke, aortic dissection, thrombocytopenia with prior exposure. Bleeding diathesis, stroke, major surgical procedure, or severe physical trauma within past 30 days. History of intracranial hemorrhage or neoplasm, arteriovenous malformation, aneurysm.

WARNINGS/PRECAUTIONS: Bleeding reported. Monitor platelets, Hgb, Hct before treatment, within 6 hrs after loading infusion, and daily during therapy. Monitor platelets earlier if previous GP IIb/IIIa inhibitor use. Determine APTT before and during therapy with heparin. Caution with platelets <150,000/mm^3, hemorrhagic retinopathy, chronic hemodialysis patients, femoral access site in percutaneous coronary intervention. Minimize vascular and other trauma. D/C if thrombocytopenia confirmed or if bleeding cannot be controlled by pressure.

ADVERSE REACTIONS: Bleeding, nausea, fever, headache, edema, anaphylaxis.

INTERACTIONS: Avoid other parenteral GP IIb/IIIa inhibitors. Increased bleeding with heparin and ASA. Caution with other drugs that affect hemostasis (eg, warfarin). Increased clearance with levothyroxine, omeprazole.

PREGNANCY: Category B, not for use in nursing.

MECHANISM OF ACTION: Glycoprotein IIB/IIIa inhibitor; reversible antagonist of fibrinogen binding to the GP IIb/IIIa receptor, the major platelet surface receptor involved in platelet aggregation. Inhibits platelet aggregation.

PHARMACOKINETICS: Absorption: C_{max}=0.01-25mcg/mL. **Distribution:** V_d=22-43L; plasma protein binding (35%). **Metabolism:** Limited. **Elimination:** Urine (65%), feces (25%); $T_{1/2}$=2 hrs.

NURSING CONSIDERATIONS

Assessment: Assess for presence or history (within previous 30 days) of internal bleeding; history of intracranial hemorrhage, intracranial neoplasm, arteriovenous malformation, or aneurysm; history of thrombocytopenia following previous exposure to the medication; history of any stroke; major recent surgical procedure or severe trauma; history, symptoms, or findings of aortic dissection; severe HTN; concomitant use of another parenteral GP IIb/IIIa inhibitor; and acute pericarditis. Assess use in patients with platelet counts <150,000/mm³, presence of hemorrhagic retinopathy, and those in chronic hemodialysis. Assess for drug interactions. Obtain baseline platelet counts, Hgb, and Hct.

Monitoring: Monitor for signs/symptoms of bleeding, allergic reactions (eg, anaphylaxis), and thrombocytopenia. Monitor platelet counts, Hgb, and Hct within 6 hours of loading infusion, and at least daily thereafter.

Patient Counseling: Counsel to notify physician if allergic reaction (eg, anaphylaxis) or bleeding occurs.

Administration: IV route. Dilute. 1) If using 500mL of 0.9% NS or D5W, withdraw and discard 100mL from bag and replace this volume with 100mL of drug injection from two 50mL vials. 2) If using 250mL of 0.9% NS or D5W, withdraw and discard 50mL from bag and replace this volume with 50mL of drug injection from one 50mL vial. Mix well prior to administration. **Storage:** 25°C (77°F) with excursions permitted between 15-30°C (59-86°F). Protect from light. Do not freeze.

AGGRENOX

dipyridamole - aspirin (Boehringer Ingelheim)

RX

THERAPEUTIC CLASS: Platelet aggregation inhibitor

INDICATIONS: Reduce risk of stroke in patients with transient brain ischemia or complete ischemic stroke due to thrombosis.

DOSAGE: *Adults:* 1 cap bid (am and pm).

HOW SUPPLIED: Cap: (Dipyridamole Extended-Release/ASA) 200mg-25mg

CONTRAINDICATIONS: NSAID allergy, children or teenagers with viral infections, syndrome of asthma, rhinitis, nasal polyps.

WARNINGS/PRECAUTIONS: Increased risk of bleeding with chronic, heavy alcohol use. Caution with inherited or acquired bleeding disorders, severe CAD, and hypotension. Monitor for signs of GI ulcers and bleeding. Avoid with history of peptic ulcer disease, severe renal failure (CrCl <10mL/min). Risk of hepatic dysfunction. Not interchangeable with individual components of ASA and Persantine tabs. Avoid in 3rd trimester of pregnancy.

ADVERSE REACTIONS: Headache, dyspepsia, abdominal pain, NV, diarrhea, fatigue, arthralgia, pain, hemorrhage.

INTERACTIONS: May decrease effects of ACE inhibitors, cholinesterase inhibitors, phenytoin, β-blockers. Potentiates adenosine, acetazolamide, methotrexate, oral hypoglycemics, valproic acid. Anticoagulants increase risk of bleeding. Decreased effects of diuretics in renal or cardiovascular disease. NSAIDs may increase risk of bleeding and decrease renal function. May antagonize uricosuric agents.

PREGNANCY: Category D, caution in nursing.

MECHANISM OF ACTION: Dipyridamole: Platelet aggregation inhibitor. Inhibits uptake of adenosine into platelets, endothelial cells, and erythrocytes. Leads to increase in adenosine, which acts on platelet A_2-receptor to stimulate platelet adenylate cyclase and increase platelet cyclic-3',5'-adenosine monophosphate (cAMP) levels. Platelet aggregation is then inhibited in response to stimuli such as platelet activation factor (PAF), collagen, and adenosine diphosphate (ADP). Also responsible for inhibiting phosphodiesterase (PDE). Weakly inhibits cAMP-PDE. Therapeutic levels of dipyridamole inhibit cyclic-3',5'-guanosine monophosphate-PDE (cGMP-PDE), which helps to augment the increases in cGMP that are produced by endothelium-derived relaxing factor (EDRF). ASA: Platelet aggregation inhibitor. Irreversibly inhibits platelet cyclooxygenase. Leads to inhibition in the generation of thromboxane A_2, a powerful inducer of platelet aggregation and vasoconstriction.

PHARMACOKINETICS: Absorption: Dipyridamole: C_{max}=1.98mcg/mL; T_{max}=2 hrs. ASA: C_{max}=319ng/mL; T_{max}=0.63 hrs. **Distribution:** Dipyridamole/ASA found in breast milk. Dipyridamole: V_d=92L; plasma protein binding (99%). ASA: V_d=10 L; plasma protein binding (poor); salicylic acid (ASA metabolite): highly protein bound (concentration dependent). **Metabolism:** Dipyridamole: Liver (conjugation); monoglucuronide (metabolite) (low activity). ASA: Liver (conjugation); salicylic acid (metabolite). **Elimination:** Dipyridamole: Feces (95%), urine (low); $T_{1/2}$=15.5 hrs. ASA: Urine; $T_{1/2}$=0.33 hrs, $T_{1/2}$=1.71 hrs (metabolite).

NURSING CONSIDERATIONS

Assessment: Assess for hypersensitivity to NSAIDs, asthma, rhinitis, nasal polyps, severe renal failure, and severe hepatic dysfunction. Assess use in presence of inherited or acquired bleeding disorders (eg, liver disease, vitamin K deficiency), pregnancy/nursing, history of active peptic ulcer disease, presence of severe coronary artery disease (eg, unstable angina or recently sustained MI), and hypotension. Assess for drug interactions.

Monitoring: Monitor for signs/symptoms of allergic reactions (eg, urticaria, angioedema, bronchospasm), coagulation abnormalities (including bleeding time), GI effects (eg, stomach pain, heartburn, NV), elevated hepatic enzymes (hepatic failure), bleeding (eg, GI, intracranial hemorrhage), increased BUN, increased serum creatinine, hyperkalemia, and proteinuria. If used in pediatrics, monitor for Reye's syndrome.

Patient Counseling: Inform patients who consume ≥3 alcoholic drinks every day are at increased risk for bleeding. Advise to contact physician if any signs of abnormal bleeding or allergic reactions occur. Instruct to swallow medication whole, with/without food. If intolerable headaches occur during initial treatment, advise to switch to 1 capsule at bedtime and low-dose aspirin in the morning. Advise to return to normal treatment regimen as soon as possible, usually within 1 week.

AGRYLIN

RX

anagrelide HCl (Shire)

THERAPEUTIC CLASS: Platelet-reducing agent

INDICATIONS: Treatment of thrombocythemia secondary to myeloproliferative disorders.

DOSAGE: *Adults:* Initial: 0.5mg qid or 1mg bid for at least 1 week. Moderate Hepatic Impairment: Initial: 0.5mg qd for at least 1 week. Titrate: Increase by no more than 0.5mg/day per week. Max: 10mg/day or 2.5mg/dose. Adjust lowest effective dose to reduce and maintain platelets <600,000/mcL. Monitor platelets every 2 days during first week, then weekly thereafter until reach maintenance dose.
Pediatrics: Initial: 0.5mg qd. Titrate: Increase by no more than 0.5mg/day per week. Max: 10mg/day or 2.5mg/dose. Adjust to lowest effective dose to reduce and maintain platelets <600,000/mcL. Monitor platelets every 2 days during first week, then weekly thereafter until reach maintenance dose.

HOW SUPPLIED: Cap: 0.5mg, 1mg

CONTRAINDICATIONS: Severe hepatic impairment.

WARNINGS/PRECAUTIONS: Caution with heart disease, renal or hepatic dysfunction. Perform pre-treatment cardiovascular exam and monitor during treatment; may cause cardiovascular effects (eg, vasodilation, tachycardia, palpitations, CHF). Monitor closely for renal toxicity if creatinine ≥2mg/dL or hepatic toxicity if bilirubin, SGOT, or LFTs >1.5x ULN. Monitor blood counts, renal and hepatic function while platelets are lowered. Increase in platelets after therapy interruption. Reduce dose in moderate hepatic impairment.

ADVERSE REACTIONS: Headache, palpitations, asthenia, edema, GI effects, dizziness, pain, dyspnea, fever, chest pain, rash, tachycardia, malaise, pharyngitis, cough, paresthesia.

INTERACTIONS: Sucralfate may interfere with absorption. Exacerbated effects of products that inhibit cyclic AMP PDE III (inotropes: milrinone, enoximone, amrinone, olprinone, cilostazol).

PREGNANCY: Category C, not for use in nursing.

MECHANISM OF ACTION: Platelet-reducing agent; not established. Suspected to reduce platelet production resulting from a decrease in megakaryocyte hypermaturation. Inhibits cyclic AMP phosphodiesterase III (PDEIII). PDEIII inhibitors can also inhibit platelet aggregation.

PHARMACOKINETICS: Metabolism: Liver, CYP1A2 (partial). RL603 and 3-hydroxy anagrelide (major metabolites). **Elimination**: Urine; $T_{1/2}$=1.3 hrs.

NURSING CONSIDERATIONS

Assessment: Assess for severe hepatic impairment, pregnancy/nursing status, and drug interactions. Assess use in presence of known or suspected heart disease; perform pretreatment CV exam. Assess use in presence of moderate hepatic impairment and renal insufficiencies.

Monitoring: Monitor platelet counts every 2 days during first week of treatment and at least weekly thereafter until maintenance dose is reached. Perform periodic monitoring of blood counts (hemoglobin, white blood cells), liver function (SGOT, SGPT), and renal function (serum creatinine, BUN). Monitor for signs/symptoms of CV effects (eg, palpitations, vasodilation, tachycardia, and congestive heart failure), thrombocytopenia, and renal impairment.

Patient Counseling: Advise to notify physician if CV effects (eg, palpitations) occur. Advise periodic laboratory tests while on medication. Counsel that platelet counts usually rise within 7-14 days of therapy at the proper dosage.

Administration: Oral route. **Storage:** 25°C (77°F); excursions permitted to 15-30°C (59-86°F). Store in light-resistant container.

ALAMAST RX

pemirolast potassium (Vistakon)

THERAPEUTIC CLASS: Mast cell stabilizer

INDICATIONS: Prevention of ocular itching due to allergic conjunctivitis.

DOSAGE: *Adults:* 1-2 drops in affected eye qid.
Pediatrics: ≥3 yrs: 1-2 drops in affected eye qid.

HOW SUPPLIED: Sol: 0.1% [10mL]

WARNINGS/PRECAUTIONS: May reinsert soft contact lens after 10 min, if eyes are not red. Contains lauralkonium chloride; may be absorbed by soft contact lens.

ADVERSE REACTIONS: Headache, rhinitis, cold/flu symptoms, ocular burning/discomfort, dry eye, foreign body sensation.

PREGNANCY: Category C, caution in nursing.

MECHANISM OF ACTION: Mast cell stabilizer; inhibits type I immediate hypersensitivity reaction, antigen-induced release of inflammatory mediators (eg, histamine, leukotriene C_4, D_4, E_4) from human mast cell; also inhibits the chemotaxis of eosinophils into ocular tissue, blocks the release of mediators from human eosinophils, and prevents calcium influx into mast cells upon antigen stimulation (not established).

PHARMACOKINETICS: Absorption: C_{max}=4.7ng/mL, T_{max}=0.42 hrs. **Elimination:** Urine (10-15% unchanged); $T_{1/2}$=4.5 hrs.

NURSING CONSIDERATIONS

Assessment: Assess for known drug hypersensitivity.

Monitoring: Monitor for anaphylaxis and adverse reactions.

Patient Counseling: Counsel not to touch dropper tip to eyelid or surrounding areas and not to wear contact lenses if eye is red.

Administration: Intraocular route. **Storage:** 15-25°C (59-77°F).

ALBENZA
RX

albendazole (GlaxoSmithKline)

THERAPEUTIC CLASS: Broad-spectrum anthelmintic

INDICATIONS: Treatment of parenchymal neurocysticercosis and cystic hydatid disease of the liver, lung, and peritoneum.

DOSAGE: *Adults:* Hydatid Disease: ≥60kg: 400mg bid. <60kg: 7.5mg/kg bid up to 800mg/day. Take with meals for 28 days, then 14 days drug-free, repeat for a total of 3 cycles. Neurocysticercosis: Same dose as Hydatid disease. Treat for 8-30 days.
Pediatrics: ≥6 yrs: Hydatid Disease: ≥60kg: 400mg bid. <60kg: 7.5mg/kg bid up to 800mg/day. Take with meals for 28 days, then 14 days drug-free, repeat for a total of 3 cycles. Neurocysticercosis: Same dose as Hydatid disease. Treat for 8-30 days.

HOW SUPPLIED: Tab: 200mg

WARNINGS/PRECAUTIONS: Monitor blood counts at the beginning of each 28-day cycle, and every 2 weeks during therapy; bone marrow suppression, aplastic anemia, and agranulocytosis have been reported. May continue if total WBC and absolute neutrophil count decrease are modest and do not progress. Not for use in pregnancy unless no other therapy is appropriate. Avoid pregnancy at least 1 month after discontinuing therapy. D/C immediately if become pregnant. Treatment for neurocysticercosis should include anticonvulsants and steroids. Examine for retinal lesions before therapy. Elevated LFTs reported. Can cause bone marrow suppression, aplastic anemia, and agranulocytosis in patients with and without underlying hepatic dysfunction.

ADVERSE REACTIONS: Abnormal LFTs, abdominal pain, NV, headache.

INTERACTIONS: Monitor theophylline levels during and after therapy. Increased levels with dexamethasone, praziquantel, and cimetidine.

PREGNANCY: Category C, caution in nursing.

MECHANISM OF ACTION: Broad-spectrum anthelmintic; exerts action by inhibitory effect on tubulin polymerization, which results in loss of cytoplasmic microtubules.

PHARMACOKINETICS: Absorption: GI tract (poorly absorbed); C_{max}=1.31mcg/mL; T_{max}=2-5 hrs. **Distribution:** Plasma protein binding (70%). **Metabolism:** Liver; metabolite: Albendazole sulfoxide (major metabolite). **Elimination:** Bile, urine (<1%); $T_{1/2}$=8-12 hrs.

NURSING CONSIDERATIONS

Assessment: Assess CBC with platelet count and differential, LFTs, renal function, retinal lesions in cases of neurocysticercosis, pregnancy status, and for possible drug interactions.

Monitoring: Monitor CBC with platelet count and differential, LFTs, renal function, hypersensitivity reactions.

Patient Counseling: Instruct that tab may be crushed or chewed; swallow with water. Take with food. Caution females of childbearing age against becoming pregnant during and 1 month following treatment. Counsel about side effects. Inform about need for regular monitoring of blood counts and LFTs.

Administration: Oral route. **Storage:** 20-25°C (68-77°F).

ALBUTEROL
RX

albuterol sulfate (Various)

THERAPEUTIC CLASS: $Beta_2$-agonist

INDICATIONS: (Aerosol) Prevention and treatment of bronchospasm with reversible obstructive airway disease. Prevention of Exercise-Induced Bronchospasm (EIB). (Sol) Relief of bronchospasm with reversible obstructive airway disease and acute attacks of bronchospasm in patients ≥12 yrs. (Tab; Tab, Extended-Release) Relief of bronchospasm with reversible obstructive airway disease in patients ≥6 yrs. (Syrup) Relief of bronchospasm in patients ≥2 yrs with reversible obstructive airway disease.

DOSAGE: *Adults:* Bronchospasm: (Aerosol) 2 inh q4-6h or 1 inh q4h. (Repetabs) Initial: 4-8mg q12h. Max: 32mg/day. (Sol) 2.5mg tid-qid by nebulizer. (Syrup, Tabs) 2-4mg tid-qid. Max: 32mg/day (8mg qid). Elderly/β-Adrenergic Sensitivity: (Syrup, Tabs) Initial: 2mg tid-qid. Max: (Tabs) 8mg tid-qid. EIB: (Aerosol) 2 inh 15 min before activity.
Pediatrics: Bronchospasm: >14 yrs: (Syrup) Initial: 2-4mg tid-qid. Max: 8mg qid. ≥12 yrs: (Aerosol) 2 inh q4-6h or 1 inh q4h. (Sol) 2.5mg tid-qid by nebulizer. (Tabs) Initial: 2-4mg tid-qid. Max: 8mg qid. >12 yrs: (Repetabs) Initial: 4-8mg q12h. Max: 32mg/day. 6-14 yrs: (Syrup) Initial: 2mg tid-qid. Max: 24mg/day. 6-12 yrs: (Repetabs) Initial: 4mg q12h. Max: 24mg/day. (Tabs) Initial: 2mg tid-qid. Max: 24mg/day. 2-5 yrs: (Syrup) Initial: 0.1mg/kg tid (not to exceed 2mg tid). Titrate: May increase to 0.2mg/kg/day. Max: 4mg tid. EIB: ≥12 yrs: (Aerosol) 2 inh 15 min before activity.

HOW SUPPLIED: MDI: 0.09mg/inh [17g]; Sol (neb): 0.083% [3mL, 25ˢ], 0.5% [20mL]; Syrup: 2mg/5mL; Tab: 2mg*, 4mg*; Tab, Extended-Release (Repetabs): 4mg *scored

WARNINGS/PRECAUTIONS: Hypersensitivity reactions reported. Monitor for worsening asthma. Fatalities reported with excessive use. Caution with cardiovascular disorders, especially coronary insufficiency, arrhythmias and HTN. May need concomitant corticosteroids. Can produce paradoxical bronchospasm. Caution with DM, hyperthyroidism, seizures. May cause transient hypokalemia.

ADVERSE REACTIONS: Tachycardia, increased BP, tremor, nervousness, dizziness, nausea/vomiting, palpitations, paradoxical bronchospasm, heartburn, rhinitis, respiratory tract infection.

INTERACTIONS: Avoid other sympathomimetic agents. Extreme caution with MAOIs and TCAs. Monitor digoxin. May worsen ECG changes and/or hypokalemia with non-K^+-sparing diuretics. Antagonized by β-blockers.

PREGNANCY: Category C, not for use in nursing.

MECHANISM OF ACTION: β_2-adrenergic agonist; stimulates intracellular adenyl cyclase, which catalyzes conversion of ATP to cAMP to produce relaxation of bronchial smooth muscle and inhibition of release of mediators of immediate hypersensitivity from cells (mast cells).

PHARMACOKINETICS: Absorption: (Aerosol) T_{max}=2-4 hrs. (Syrup, Tab) Rapid. C_{max}=18ng/mL; T_{max}=2 hrs. **Elimination:** (Aerosol) Urine (28%); $T_{1/2}$=3.8 hrs. (Syrup, Tab) $T_{1/2}$=5 hrs.

NURSING CONSIDERATIONS

Assessment: Assess for CVD (coronary insufficiency, cardiac arrhythmias, HTN), convulsive disorder, hyperthyroidism, DM, and possible drug interactions.

Monitoring: Monitor for signs/symptoms of CV effects (increased BP, palpitations), worsening of symptoms, destabilization of asthma, paradoxical bronchospasm, and hypersensitivity reactions (anaphylactic, urticaria, angioedema, rash, bronchospasm).

Patient Counseling: Seek medical attention if worsening of symptoms, therapy becomes less effective, need more inhalation from short-acting β_2-agonist than usual, paradoxical bronchospams, and hypersensitivity (anaphylactic, urticaria, angioedema, rash, bronchospasm) occur.

Administration: Oral inhalation, oral route. (Aerosol) 1) Shake well. 2) Breathe out fully through mouth. 3) While breathing in deeply and slowly through mouth, depress the top of metal canister. 4) Hold breath as long as possible. 5) Cleanse inhaler thoroughly and frequently. 6) Recommend "test spray" into air before using for first time. **Storage:** (Inhalation) 2-25°C (36-

77°F). Protect from light. Store in pouch until time of use. (Aerosol) 15-30°C (59-86°F). Shake well before using. (Tab) 20-25°C (36-77°F). Protect from light. Dispense in tight, light-resistant container. (Syrup) 15-30°C (59-86°F). Dispense in tight, light-resistant container.

ALCORTIN

RX

iodoquinol - hydrocortisone (Primus)

THERAPEUTIC CLASS: Corticosteroid/Anti-infective

INDICATIONS: "Possibly" Effective: Contact or atopic dermatitis, impetiginized eczema, nummular eczema, endogenous chronic infectious dermatitis, stasis dermatitis, pyoderma, nuchal eczema and chronic eczematoid otitis externa, acne urticata, localized or disseminated neurodermatitis, lichen simplex chronicus, anogenital pruritus (vulvae, scroti, ani), folliculitis, bacterial dermatoses, mycotic dermatoses such as tinea (capitis, cruris, corporis, pedis), monliasis, intertrigo.

DOSAGE: *Adults:* Apply to affected area(s) tid-qid.
Pediatrics: ≥12 yrs: Apply to affected area(s) tid-qid.

HOW SUPPLIED: Gel: (Hydrocortisone-Iodoquinol) 2%-1% [2g]

WARNINGS/PRECAUTIONS: For external use only. Avoid eyes. D/C if irritation develops. May stain skin, hair, or fabrics. Risk of systemic absorption with treatment of extensive areas or use of occlusive dressings. Increased risk of systemic absorption in children. Iodoquinol may interfere with thyroid tests. False-positive phenylketonuria test reported. Prolonged use may result in overgrowth of nonsusceptible organisms.

ADVERSE REACTIONS: Burning, itching, irritation, dryness, folliculitis, hypertrichosis, acneiform eruptions, hypopigmentation, perioral dermatitis, allergic dermatitis, skin maceration, secondary infection, skin atrophy, striae, miliaria.

PREGNANCY: Category C, caution in nursing.

MECHANISM OF ACTION: Corticosteroid/Anti-infective. Hydrocortisone: Corticosteroid; possesses anti-inflammatory, antipruritic, and vasoconstrictive properties. Anti-inflammatory effect unclear; however, there is a recognizable correlation between vasoconstrictor potency and therapeutic efficacy. Iodoquinol: Anti-infective; possesses both antifungal and antibacterial properties.

PHARMACOKINETICS: Absorption: Hydrocortisone: Absorbed from normal intact skin. Inflammation of skin increases absorption. **Metabolism:** Hydrocortisone: Liver and most body tissues. Tetrahydrocortisone and tetrahydrocortisol (metabolites). **Elimination:** Hydrocortisone: Urine (unchanged and glucuronides). Iodoquinol: Urine (3-5% glucuronide).

NURSING CONSIDERATIONS

Assessment: Assess for known hypersensitivity to aloe vera, glycine, histidine, lysine, or palmitic acid. Assess use in pregnant/nursing females.

Monitoring: Monitor for development of systemic toxicity in children if large areas of body are treated or if occlusive dressings used (eg, diapers, plastic pants) on treated areas. With prolonged therapy, monitor for occurrence of overgrowth of non-susceptible bacteria. Monitor for lab test interactions (eg, thyroid function tests, ferric chloride tests for phenylketonuria [PKU]). If necessary, perform thyroid function tests 1 month after therapy end.

Patient Counseling: Instruct parents of pediatric patients not to use tight-fitting diapers or plastic pants on child being treated in diaper area. Counsel to keep medication away from eyes. If contact occurs and irritation develops, counsel to d/c medication and apply appropriate therapy. Inform that medication may cause staining of skin, hair, or fabrics and burning, itching, irritation, or dryness.

Administration: Topical route; external use only. **Storage:** Store at room temperature, 15-30°C (59-86°F). Keep out of reach of children. Keep tightly closed.

ALDACTAZIDE

hydrochlorothiazide - spironolactone (Pharmacia & Upjohn) **RX**

Tumorigenic in chronic toxicity animal studies; avoid unnecessary use. Not for initial therapy.

THERAPEUTIC CLASS: K^+-sparing diuretic/thiazide diuretic

INDICATIONS: Management of edematous conditions (CHF, hepatic cirrhosis with edema/ascites, nephrotic syndrome) and hypertension.

DOSAGE: *Adults:* Edema: 100mg/day per component qd or in divided doses. Maint: 25-200mg/day per component. HTN: 50-100mg/day per component qd or in divided doses.

HOW SUPPLIED: Tab: (Spironolactone-HCTZ) 25mg-25mg, 50mg-50mg* *scored

CONTRAINDICATIONS: Acute renal impairment, significantly impaired renal excretory function, hyperkalemia, acute or severe hepatic dysfunction, anuria, sulfonamide hypersensitivity.

WARNINGS/PRECAUTIONS: Monitor for fluid/electrolyte imbalance. Caution with renal and hepatic dysfunction. Hyperchloremic metabolic acidosis reported with decompensated hepatic cirrhosis. Mild acidosis, gynecomastia, transient BUN elevation, hypercalcemia, hyperglycemia, hyperuricemia, hypomagnesemia, and sensitivity reactions may occur. D/C if hyperkalemia occurs. Risk of dilutional hyponatremia. Enhanced effects in post-sympathetectomy patient. May increase cholesterol and TG levels. May manifest latent DM.

ADVERSE REACTIONS: Gastric bleeding, ulceration, gynecomastia, impotence, agranulocytosis, fever, urticaria, confusion, ataxia, renal dysfunction, blood dyscrasias, electrolyte disturbances, weakness, irregular menses, amenorrhea.

INTERACTIONS: Risk of hyperkalemia with K^+-sparing diuretics, K^+ supplements, NSAIDs, ACE inhibitors. Alcohol, barbiturates, or narcotics potentiate orthostatic hypotension. Corticosteroids, ACTH may intensify electrolyte depletion. Reduced vascular response to norepinephrine. Increased response to nondepolarizing skeletal muscle relaxants. Risk of digoxin, lithium toxicity. NSAIDs may reduce effects. Antidiabetic agents may need adjustment.

PREGNANCY: Category C, not for use in nursing.

MECHANISM OF ACTION: Spironolactone: Aldosterone antagonist; competitively binds to receptors at aldosterone-dependent sodium-potassium exchange site. HCTZ: Thiazide diuretic; promotes excretion of sodium and water by inhibiting reabsorption.

PHARMACOKINETICS: Absorption: Spironolactone: C_{max}=80ng/mL; T_{max}=2.6 hrs. HCTZ: Rapid; T_{max}=1-2 hrs. **Distribution:** Spironolactone: Plasma protein binding (90%). **Elimination:** Spironolactone: Urine (major), bile (minor). HCTZ: Urine.

NURSING CONSIDERATIONS

Assessment: Assess for renal impairment (insufficiency, anuria, impairment of excretion), hepatic impairment (failure), hyperkalemia, pregnancy status, possible drug interactions, systemic lupus erythematosus, DM, sulfonamide hypersensitivity, history of allergy or bronchial asthma.

Monitoring: Monitor serum electrolytes, serum K^+, and renal function periodically. Monitor for signs/symptoms of electrolyte imbalance, hyperkalemia, gynecomastia, hyperglycemia, exacerbation or activation of SLE, hyperuricemia or precipitation of gout, hypersensitivity reactions, hepatic/renal impairment.

Patient Counseling: Instruct to avoid K^+ supplements and foods containing high levels of K^+. Inform of pregnancy risks. Advise to seek medical attention if symptoms of electrolyte imbalance (dry mouth, thirst, weakness), hyperkalemia (paresthesia, fatigue, muscle weakness), or hypersensitivity reactions occur.

Administration: Oral route. **Storage:** Below 25°C (77°F).

ALDACTONE

RX

spironolactone (Pharmacia & Upjohn)

Tumorigenic in chronic toxicity animal studies; avoid unnecessary use.

THERAPEUTIC CLASS: K^+-sparing diuretic

INDICATIONS: Management of primary hyperaldosteronism (diagnosis, short-term preoperative, and long-term maintenance treatment); edematous conditions (CHF, hepatic cirrhosis with edema/ascites, nephrotic syndrome); hypertension. Treatment and prophylaxis of hypokalemia.

DOSAGE: *Adults:* Hyperaldosteronism: (Diagnostic) 400mg/day for 3-4 weeks or 400mg/day for 4 days. (Preoperative) 100-400mg/day. Maint: Lowest effective dose. Edema: Initial: 100mg/day given qd or in divided doses for at least 5 days. Maint: 25-200mg/day given qd-bid. HTN: Initial: 50-100mg/day given qd or in divided doses. Titrate: Adjust at 2-week intervals. Hypokalemia: 25-100mg/day.

HOW SUPPLIED: Tab: 25mg, 50mg*, 100mg* *scored

CONTRAINDICATIONS: Anuria, acute renal insufficiency, significantly impaired renal excretory function, hyperkalemia.

WARNINGS/PRECAUTIONS: Monitor for fluid/electrolyte imbalance. Caution with renal and hepatic dysfunction. Hyperchloremic metabolic acidosis reported with decompensated hepatic cirrhosis. Mild acidosis, gynecomastia, transient BUN elevation may occur. D/C and monitor ECG if hyperkalemia occurs. Risk of dilutional hyponatremia.

ADVERSE REACTIONS: Gastric bleeding, ulceration, gynecomastia, impotence, agranulocytosis, fever, urticaria, confusion, ataxia, renal dysfunction, irregular menses, amenorrhea.

INTERACTIONS: Risk of hyperkalemia with K^+-sparing diuretics, K^+ supplements, NSAIDs, ACE inhibitors. Alcohol, barbiturates, or narcotics potentiate orthostatic hypotension. Corticosteroids, ACTH may intensify electrolyte depletion. Reduced vascular response to norepinephrine. Increased response to nondepolarizing skeletal muscle relaxants. Risk of digoxin, lithium toxicity. NSAIDs may reduce effects.

PREGNANCY: Category C, not for use in nursing.

MECHANISM OF ACTION: Aldosterone antagonist; competitively binds to receptors at aldosterone-dependent Na^+-K^+ exchange site in distal convoluted renal tubule, causing increased Na^+ and water excretion and K^+ retention.

PHARMACOKINETICS: Absorption: C_{max}=80ng/mL; T_{max}=2.6 hrs. **Distribution:** Plasma protein binding (>90%). **Elimination:** Urine (major), bile (minor).

NURSING CONSIDERATIONS

Assessment: Assess for renal impairment (insufficiency, anuria, impairment of excretion), hepatic impairment, hyperkalemia, pregnancy status, and possible drug interactions.

Monitoring: Monitor serum K^+, electrolytes, and renal function periodically. Monitor for signs/symptoms of electrolyte imbalance, hyperkalemia, gynecomastia, hypersensitivity reactions, renal/hepatic dysfunction.

Patient Counseling: Instruct to avoid K^+ supplements and foods containing high levels of K^+, including salt substitutes. Advise to seek medical attention if symptoms of electrolyte imbalance (dry mouth, thirst, weakness), hyperkalemia (paresthesia, fatigue, muscle weakness), or hypersensitivity reactions occur.

Administration: Oral route. **Storage:** Below 25°C (77°F).

ALDARA

RX

imiquimod (Graceway)

THERAPEUTIC CLASS: Immune response modifier

INDICATIONS: Actinic keratoses on face or scalp in immunocompetent adults. External genital and perianal warts/condyloma acuminata. Biopsy-confirmed, primary superficial basal cell carcinoma (sBCC) in immunocompetent adults, with a maximum tumor diameter of 2cm, located on trunk (excluding anogenital skin), neck, or extremities (excluding hands and feet), only when surgical methods are medically less appropriate and follow-up can be assured.

DOSAGE: *Adults:* Use before bedtime. Actinic Keratosis: Usual: Apply 2x/week to defined area on face or scalp (but not both concurrently). Wash off after 8 hrs with soap and water. Max: 16 weeks. External Genital and Perianal Warts/ Condyloma: Usual: Apply 3x/week. Wash off after 6-10 hrs with soap and water. Use until warts are clear. Max: 16 weeks. May suspend use for several days to manage local reactions. Do not occlude treatment area. sBCC: Apply 5x/ week for 6 weeks. If tumor diameter is 0.5 to <1cm, use 4mm (10mg) of cream. If tumor is ≥1 to <1.5cm, use 5mm (25mg) of cream. If tumor is ≥1.5 to 2cm, use 7mm (40mg) of cream. Max diameter of tumor: ≤2cm. Treatment area should include a 1cm margin of skin around the tumor. Wash off after 8 hrs with soap and water.

Pediatrics: ≥12 yrs: External Genital and Perianal Warts/Condyloma: Usual: Apply 3x/week before bedtime. Wash off after 6-10 hrs with soap and water. Use until warts are clear. Max: 16 weeks. May suspend use for several days to manage local reactions. Do not occlude treatment area.

HOW SUPPLIED: Cre: 5% [12 pkts]

WARNINGS/PRECAUTIONS: Not for urethral, intra-vaginal, cervical, rectal, or intra-anal human papilloma viral disease. Avoid sexual contact while cream is on skin. May weaken condoms and diaphragms; avoid concurrent use. Avoid or minimize exposure to sunlight. May exacerbate inflammatory skin conditions. Avoid contact with eyes, lips, nostrils. Avoid after surgery or with sunburn until tissue is healed.

ADVERSE REACTIONS: Wart (erythema, erosion, flaking, edema) and application site reactions (bleeding, burning, itching, pain), flu-like symptoms, headache.

INTERACTIONS: Avoid topical drugs immediately after treatment of warts.

PREGNANCY: Category C, safety in nursing not known.

MECHANISM OF ACTION: Immune response modifier; not established. In basal cell carcinoma, suspected to increase infiltration of lymphocytes, dendritic cells, and macrophages in the tumor lesion. In external genital warts, suspected to induce mRNA encoding cytokines, including interferon-α at the treatment site.

PHARMACOKINETICS: Absorption: C_{max}=0.1ng/mL (12.5mg, face), 0.2ng/mL (25mg, scalp), 3.5ng/mL (75mg, hands/arms). **Distribution:** Excreted in breast milk. **Elimination:** Urine: Male (0.11%), female (2.41%).

NURSING CONSIDERATIONS

Assessment: Assess use with pre-existing autoimmune conditions, immunosuppression, basal cell nevus syndrome or xeroderma pigmentosum. For treatment of superficial basal cell carcinoma, assess proper diagnosis (eg, biopsy). Assess use in inherent sensitivity to sunlight, current sunburn, and in pregnancy/nursing. Assess for possible drug interactions.

Monitoring: Monitor for signs/symptoms of local inflammatory reactions (eg, weeping or erosion) and for systemic reactions (eg, flu-like symptoms: malaise, fever, nausea, myalgias). Monitor for clinical signs of improvement.

Patient Counseling: Inform to wash hands before and after applying cream. Before applying, wash treatment area with mild soap and water and allow area to dry thoroughly (at least 10 min). Avoid contact with eyes, lips, and nostrils. Warn to avoid exposure to sunlight (including sunlamps) and to use protective clothing (eg, hat) or sunscreen when using medication. Advise patients with sunburns not to use the cream until fully recovered. Advise female patients to take special care when applying the cream at the vaginal opening because of local skin reactions on the delicate moist surfaces, which may result in pain or swelling and may cause difficulty in passing urine. When using for the treatment of actinic keratosis or superficial basal cell carcinoma, wash the treatment area with mild soap and water 8 hrs following application of the cream.

When using for the treatment of external genital warts, wash treatment area with mild soap and water 6-10 hrs following application of cream.

Administration: Topical application. **Storage:** Store at 4-25°C (39-77°F). Do not freeze.

ALESSE RX

ethinyl estradiol - levonorgestrel (Wyeth)

OTHER BRAND NAMES: Lessina (Barr) - Aviane (Duramed)

THERAPEUTIC CLASS: Estrogen/progestogen combination

INDICATIONS: Prevention of pregnancy.

DOSAGE: *Adults:* 1 tab qd for 28 days, then repeat. Start 1st Sunday after menses begin or 1st day of menses.

HOW SUPPLIED: Tab: (Ethinyl Estradiol-Levonorgestrel) 0.02mg-0.1mg

CONTRAINDICATIONS: Thrombophlebitis, DVT or thromboembolic disorders, pregnancy, cerebrovascular or coronary artery disease, undiagnosed abnormal genital bleeding, cholestatic jaundice of pregnancy or jaundice with prior pill use, hepatic adenomas or carcinomas, active liver disease (as long as liver function has not returned to normal), breast cancer or other estrogen-dependent neoplasia, thrombogenic valvulopathies, thrombogenic rhythm disorders, diabetes with vascular involvement, uncontrolled HTN.

WARNINGS/PRECAUTIONS: Cigarette smoking increases risk of serious cardiovascular side effects; risk increases with age (especially >35 yrs) and heavy smoking. Increased risk of MI, vascular disease, thromboembolism, stroke and gallbladder disease. Retinal thrombosis, hepatic neoplasia, carcinoma of breast and reproductive organs reported. May cause glucose intolerance. May increase BP, elevate LDL levels or cause other lipid changes, fluid retention, breakthrough bleeding, and spotting. May cause or exacerbate migraine. May develop visual changes with contact lens. Diarrhea and/or vomiting may reduce absorption. Increased risk of MI with HTN, hyperlipidemia, obesity, and diabetes. D/C if jaundice, significant depression or ophthalmic irregularities develop. Perform annual physical exam. Use before menarche is not indicated. May affect certain endocrine, LFTs and blood components.

ADVERSE REACTIONS: NV, breakthrough bleeding, spotting, amenorrhea, migraine, depression, vaginal candidiasis, edema, weight changes.

INTERACTIONS: Reduced effects, increased breakthrough bleeding, and menstrual irregularities with rifampin, barbiturates, phenylbutazone, phenytoin, griseofulvin, topiramate, some protease inhibitors, modafinil, ampicillin, tetracyclines, and possibly with St. John's wort. Troleandomycin may increase risk of intrahepatic cholestasis. Ascorbic acid, APAP, CYP3A4 inhibitors (eg, indinavir, fluconazole, troleandomycin), atorvastatin may increase plasma levels. Increased plasma levels of cyclosporine, theophylline, and corticosteroids.

PREGNANCY: Category X, not for use in nursing.

MECHANISM OF ACTION: Oral contraceptive: Inhibits ovulation by suppression of gonadotropins. Causes changes in cervical mucus (increases difficulty of sperm entry into uterus) and in endometrium (reduces likelihood of implantation).

PHARMACOKINETICS: Absorption: Levonorgestrel: Rapid and complete, bioavailability (100%), C_{max}=2.8ng/mL (single dose), 6.0ng/mL (multiple doses), T_{max}=1.6 hrs (single dose), 1.5 hrs (multiple doses); Ethinyl Estradiol: Rapid, bioavailability; (38-48%); C_{max}=62 pg/mL (single dose), 77pg/mL (multiple doses), T_{max}=1.5 hrs (single dose), 1.3 hrs (multiple doses). **Distribution:** Levonorgestrel: Primarily bound to SHBG. Ethinyl estradiol: Plasma protein binding (97%). **Metabolism:** Levonorgestrel: Reduction, hydroxylation, and conjugation. Ethinyl Estradiol: Hepatic, via CYP3A4 (hydroxylation), methylation, and glucuronidation. **Elimination:** Levonorgestrel: Urine (40-68%), feces (16-48%); $T_{1/2}$=36 hrs. Ethinyl Estradiol: $T_{1/2}$=18 hrs.

NURSING CONSIDERATIONS

Assessment: Assess for thromboembophlebitis or thromboembolic disorder, past history of DVT, CVD, CAD, uncontrolled HTN, thrombogenic valvulopathies, thrombogenic rhythm disorders, major surgery with prolonged immobilization, DM, headache with focal neurological symptoms, known/suspected or history of carcinoma (of breast, endometrium) or known/suspected estrogen-dependent neoplasia, undiagnosed abnormal genital bleeding, cholestatic jaundice of pregnancy or jaundice with prior pill use, hepatic adenomas or carcinomas, active liver disease, and known/suspected pregnancy. Assess use in patients who are >35 years and heavy smokers (≥15 cigarettes/day). Assess use with HTN, hyperlipidemias, obesity, DM, or in patients at increased risk for thrombosis. Assess for possible drug interactions.

Monitoring: Monitor for venous and arterial thrombotic and thromboembolic events (eg, MI, thromboembolism, and stroke), hepatic neoplasia, gallbladder disease, ocular lesions, HTN, bleeding irregularities, onset or exacerbation of headaches or migraines, and ectopic pregnancy. Monitor fasting blood glucose levels in DM and prediabetic patients, BP with history of HTN, lipid levels with a history of hyperlipidemia. Monitor for signs of liver dysfunction (eg, jaundice) and signs of depression with previous history. Refer patients with contact lenses to an ophthalmologist if visual changes occur. Perform annual history and physical exam.

Patient Counseling: Inform that drug does not protect against HIV infection and other STDs. Instruct women who are initiating therapy to use additional method of protection during first 7 days of use. Take exactly as directed and at intervals not exceeding 24 hrs. Advise that if pill missed, take as soon as remembered; take next dose at regularly scheduled time. Inform may experience spotting, light bleeding, or stomach upset during first 1-3 packs of pills. Instruct to continue using therapy and to contact physician if symptoms persist. Counsel to avoid smoking while on medication.

Administration: Oral route. **Storage:** Store at controlled room temperature 20-25°C (68-77°F).

ALIMTA

pemetrexed disodium (Lilly) **RX**

THERAPEUTIC CLASS: Antifolate

INDICATIONS: In combination with cisplatin for the treatment of patients with unresectable malignant pleural mesothelioma who are not candidates for curative surgery. Monotherapy for the treatment of patients with locally advanced or metastatic non-small cell lung cancer (NSCLC) after prior chemotherapy. In combination with cisplatin for the initial treatment of locally advanced or metastatic NSCLC.

DOSAGE: *Adults:* Premedication: Dexamethasone: 4mg PO bid day before, day of, and day after pemetrexed. Folic Acid: At least 5 daily doses (350-1000mcg) during 7 days prior to pemetrexed. Continue for 21 days after last pemetrexed dose. Vitamin B_{12}: 1000mcg IM once during week preceding first pemetrexed dose and every 3 cycles thereafter. Treatment: Mesothelioma/NSCLC: 500mg/m^2 IV over 10 min on Day 1 of each 21-day cycle with cisplatin 75mg/m^2 infused over 2 hrs beginning 30 min after pemetrexed. NSCLC/Single Agent: 500mg/m^2 IV over 10 minutes on day 1 of each 21-day cycle. Refer to PI for dose adjustments for hematologic, nonhematologic and neurotoxicities.

HOW SUPPLIED: Inj: 100mg, 500mg

WARNINGS/PRECAUTIONS: Avoid use if CrCl <45mL/min. May suppress bone marrow function. With pleural effusions, ascites, consider draining prior to therapy. Monitor CBCs, for nadir and recovery before each dose and on Days 8 and 15 of each cycle. Do not begin new cycle unless ANC ≥1500 cells/mm^3, platelets ≥100,000 cells/mm^3, CrCl ≥45mL/min.

ADVERSE REACTIONS: N/V, fatigue, dyspnea, hematologic effects, constipation, chest pain, anorexia, fever, infection, stomatitis, pharyngitis, rash/desquamation.

INTERACTIONS: Delayed clearance with nephrotoxic or tubularly secreted drugs (eg, probenecid). Reduced clearance with ibuprofen; caution with CrCl <80mL/min. In mild-moderate renal insufficiency, avoid NSAIDs with short elimination half-lives from 2 days prior to 2 days following therapy. Interrupt dosing of NSAID with longer half-lives from at least 5 days before to 2 days following therapy.

PREGNANCY: Category D, not for use in nursing.

MECHANISM OF ACTION: Antifolate agent; disrupts folate-dependent metabolic processes essential for cell replication. Inhibits thymidylate synthase, dihydrofolate reductase, glycinamide ribonucleotide formyltransferase, and folate-dependent enzymes involved in the *de novo* biosynthesis of thymidine and purine nucleotides.

PHARMACOKINETICS: Distribution: Steady-state V_d=16.1L. Plasma protein binding (81%). **Elimination:** Urine (70-90%); $T_{1/2}$=3.5 hrs.

NURSING CONSIDERATIONS

Assessment: Assess for renal/hepatic impairment, pregnancy status, CBC with differential and platelet count.

Monitoring: CBC with differential, platelet count, LFTs, creatinine clearance, hypersensitivity reactions.

Patient Counseling: Instruct to wear gloves. Advise if solution comes in contact with skin, wash skin with soap and water immediately; if contact is with mucous membranes, flush thoroughly with water. Instruct to take folic acid and vitamin B_{12} as prophylactic measure to reduce toxicity.

Administration: IV infusion after reconstitution with 0.9% sodium chloride.
Storage: 25°C (77°F); excursions permitted to 15-30°C (59-86°F).

ALINIA — RX

nitazoxanide (Romark)

THERAPEUTIC CLASS: Antiprotozoal agent

INDICATIONS: Treatment of diarrhea caused by *Cryptosporidium parvum* and *Giardia lamblia.*

DOSAGE: *Adults:* ≥12 yrs: *G.lamblia* Diarrhea: 500mg q12h for 3 days. Take with food.
Pediatrics: C.parvum/G.lamblia Diarrhea: 1-3 yrs: 100mg (5mL) q12h for 3 days. 4-11yrs: 200mg (10mL) q12h for 3 days. *G.lamblia* Diarrhea: ≥12 yrs: 500mg (1 tab or 25mL) q12h for 3 days. Take with food.

HOW SUPPLIED: Sus: 100mg/5mL [60mL]; Tab: 500mg [60[s], 3-Day Therapy Packs, 6[s]]

WARNINGS/PRECAUTIONS: Caution with hepatic and biliary disease, renal disease. Contains 1.48g sucrose/5mL. Safety and effectiveness have not been established in HIV positive or immunodeficient patients.

ADVERSE REACTIONS: Abdominal pain, diarrhea, headache, nausea.

INTERACTIONS: Highly protein bound; caution with other highly plasma protein-bound drugs with narrow therapeutic indices.

PREGNANCY: Category B; caution in nursing.

MECHANISM OF ACTION: Antiprotozoal agent; interferes with the pyruvate, ferredoxin oxidoreductase enzyme-dependent electron transfer reaction, which is essential to anaerobic energy metabolism.

PHARMACOKINETICS: Absorption: Tizoxanide: (Tab, 500mg) 12-17 yrs: C_{max}=9.1mcg/mL, T_{max}=4 hrs, AUC=39.5mcg•hr/mL; ≥18 yrs: C_{max}=10.6mcg/mL, T_{max}=3 hrs, AUC=41.9mcg•hr/mL. (Sus, 100mg) 1-3 yrs: C_{max}=3.11mcg/mL, T_{max}=3.5 hrs, AUC=11.7mcg•hr/mL; 4-11 yrs: C_{max}=3mcg/mL, T_{max}=2 hrs, AUC=13.5mcg•hr/mL. **Distribution**: Tizoxanide: Plasma protein binding (>99%). **Metabolism**: Hydrolysis, glucuronidation: Tizoxanide and tizoxanide glucuronide (active). **Elimination**: Urine (33%), bile and feces (66%). Refer to PI for complete kinetics information.

NURSING CONSIDERATIONS

Assessment: Assess for hepatic, renal/biliary impairment, HIV infection, DM, possible drug interactions.

Monitoring: Monitor for abdominal pain, diarrhea, nausea, LFTs, and CBC.

Patient Counseling: Counsel to take exactly as directed. Shake well prior to administration. Report lack of response or adverse effects.

Administration: Oral route, should be taken with food. Reconstitute with 48mL of water and keep tightly closed. Sus may be stored for 7 days. **Storage:** 25°C (77°F); excursions permitted to 15-30°C (59-86°F).

ALLEGRA — RX

fexofenadine HCl (Sanofi-Aventis)

THERAPEUTIC CLASS: H_1-antagonist

INDICATIONS: (ODT) 6-11 yrs; (Sus) 2-11 yrs: Relief of symptoms associated with seasonal allergic rhinitis in children. (ODT) 6-11 yrs; (Sus) 6 months-11 yrs: Treatment of uncomplicated skin manifestations of chronic idiopathic urticaria in children. (Tab) Relief of symptoms associated with seasonal allergic rhinitis and treatment of uncomplicated skin manifestations of chronic idiopathic urticaria in adults and children ≥6 yrs.

DOSAGE: *Adults:* Tab: Rhinitis/Urticaria: 60mg bid or 180mg qd. Renal Dysfunction: Initial: 60mg qd.
Pediatrics: Tab: ≥12 yrs: Rhinitis/Urticaria: 60mg bid or 180mg qd. Renal Dysfunction: Initial: 60mg qd. 6-11 yrs: Rhinitis/Urticaria: 30mg bid. Renal Dysfunction: Initial: 30mg qd. ODT: Rhinitis/Urticaria: 6-11 yrs: 30mg bid. Renal Dysfunction: 30mg qd. Sus: Rhinitis: 2-11 yrs: 30mg (5mL) bid. Renal Dysfunction: 30mg (5mL) qd. Urticaria: 2-11 yrs: 30mg (5mL) bid. Renal Dysfunction: 30mg (5mL) qd. 6 months to <2 yrs: 15mg (2.5mL) bid. Renal Dysfunction: 15mg (2.5mL) qd.

HOW SUPPLIED: Tab: 30mg, 60mg, 180mg; Tab, Orally Disintegrating: 30mg; Sus: 30mg/5mL

ADVERSE REACTIONS: Headache, cough, upper respiratory tract infection, back pain, fever, pain, otitis media, vomiting, diarrhea.

INTERACTIONS: Increased plasma levels with erythromycin or ketoconazole. Avoid concomitant aluminum- and magnesium-containing antacids. Fruit juices (eg, grapefruit, orange, and apple) may decrease levels.

PREGNANCY: Category C, caution in nursing.

MECHANISM OF ACTION: Antihistamine with selective peripheral H_1-receptor antagonist activity; prevents antigen-induced bronchospasm and histamine release from peritoneal mast cells.

PHARMACOKINETICS: Absorption: Rapid; (Cap, 120mg) T_{max}=2.6 hrs; (Cap, 60mg) C_{max}=131ng/mL; (Tab, 60mg) C_{max}=142ng/mL; (Tab, 180mg) C_{max}=494ng/mL; (Sus, 30mg) C_{max}=118.0ng/mL, T_{max}=1.0 hrs. **Distribution:** Plasma protein binding (60-70%). **Metabolism:** Liver (5%). **Elimination:** Urine (80%), feces (11%); $T_{1/2}$=14.4 hrs.

NURSING CONSIDERATIONS

Assessment: Assess for hepatic/renal impairment, pregnancy/nursing status, and possible drug interactions.

Monitoring: Monitor for side effects and treatment efficacy.

Patient Counseling: Advise to take as prescribed and not to exceed recommended dose. D/C and consult physician if adverse effects occur.

Administration: Oral route. Take with water. Shake suspension bottle before use. **Storage:** 20-25°C (68-77°F); cool, dry place.

ALLEGRA-D RX

fexofenadine HCl - pseudoephedrine HCl (Sanofi-Aventis)

THERAPEUTIC CLASS: H_1-antagonist/sympathomimetic amine

INDICATIONS: Relief of symptoms of seasonal allergic rhinitis.

DOSAGE: *Adults:* 60mg-120mg tab bid or 180mg-240mg tab qd without food. Renal Dysfunction: Initial: 60mg-120mg tab qd; avoid 180mg-240mg tab. Do not crush or chew.
Pediatrics: ≥12 yrs: 60mg-120mg tab bid or 180mg-240mg tab qd without food. Renal Dysfunction: Initial: 60mg-120mg tab qd; avoid 180mg-240mg tab. Do not crush or chew.

HOW SUPPLIED: Tab, Extended-Release: (Fexofenadine-Pseudoephedrine) (12-Hour) 60mg-120mg, (24-Hour) 180mg-240mg

CONTRAINDICATIONS: Narrow-angle glaucoma, urinary retention, severe HTN, severe CAD, within 14 days of MAOI therapy.

WARNINGS/PRECAUTIONS: Caution with HTN, DM, ischemic heart disease, increased IOP, hyperthyroidism, renal impairment, or prostatic hypertrophy. May produce CNS stimulation with convulsions or cardiovascular collapse with hypotension.

ADVERSE REACTIONS: Headache, insomnia, nausea, dry mouth, dyspepsia, throat irritation.

INTERACTIONS: Increased plasma levels with erythromycin or ketoconazole. Avoid MAOIs. Increased ectopic pacemaker activity can occur with digitalis. Caution with other sympathomimetic amines. Reduced effects of antihypertensive drugs which interfere with sympathetic activity (eg, methyldopa, mecamylamine, reserpine).

PREGNANCY: Category C, caution with nursing.

MECHANISM OF ACTION: H_1-receptor antagonist/sympathomimetic amine. Fexofenadine: Selective peripheral H_1-receptor antagonist; inhibits antigen-induced bronchospasm and histamine release from peritoneal mast cells. Pseudoephedrine: Exerts a decongestant action on the nasal mucosa.

PHARMACOKINETICS: Absorption: Fexofenadine: Rapidly absorbed; C_{max}=634ng/mL (single dose), 674ng/mL (multiple doses); T_{max}=1.8-2 hrs. Pseudoephedrine: C_{max}=394ng/mL (single dose), 495ng/mL (multiple doses); T_{max}=12 hrs. **Distribution:** Fexofenadine: Plasma protein binding (60-70%). Pseudoephedrine: V_d=2.6-3.5L/kg. **Metabolism:** Fexofenadine and pseudoephedrine: Hepatic (5% of fexofenadine; <1% of pseudoephedrine). **Elimination:** Fexofenadine: Feces (80%), urine (11%); $T_{1/2}$=14.6 hrs. Pseudoephedrine: $T_{1/2}$=7 hrs.

NURSING CONSIDERATIONS

Assessment: Assess for narrow-angle glaucoma, urinary retention, MAOI therapy presently or within past 14 days, severe HTN, and severe CAD. Assess for idiosyncrasies to adrenergic agents or other drugs of similiar chemical structure. Assess use in patients with HTN, DM, ischemic heart disease, increased IOP, hyperthyroidism, renal impairment, prostatic hypertrophy, and in pregnant/nursing females. Assess for drug interactions.

Monitoring: Monitor for signs/symptoms of CNS stimulation with convulsions and for cardiovascular collapse with accompanying hypotension.

Patient Counseling: Instruct to take on empty stomach with water; swallow tab whole, do not break or chew. Instruct not to exceed recommended dose. Counsel to d/c and contact physician if nervousness, dizziness, or sleeplessness occur. Avoid concurrent use with OTC antihistamines and decongestants.

Administration: Oral route. **Storage:** 20-25°C (68-77°F). Store in tightly-closed container in a cool, dry place, away from children.

ALOPRIM RX

allopurinol sodium (Nabi)

THERAPEUTIC CLASS: Xanthine oxidase inhibitor

INDICATIONS: Management of elevated serum and urinary uric acid levels in patients with leukemia, lymphoma, and solid tumor malignancies receiving cancer therapy when oral therapy is not tolerated.

DOSAGE: *Adults:* Initial: 200-400mg/m²/day IV as qd or in divided doses every 6, 8, or 12 hrs. Max: 600mg/day. CrCl 10-20mL/min: 200mg/day. CrCl 3-10mL/min: 100mg/day. CrCl <3mL/min: 100mg/day at extended intervals.
Pediatrics: Initial: 200mg/m²/day IV as qd or in divided doses every 6, 8, or 12 hrs.

HOW SUPPLIED: Inj: 500mg

CONTRAINDICATIONS: Previous severe reaction to therapy.

WARNINGS/PRECAUTIONS: D/C at first appearance of hypersensitivity; increased risk in decreased renal function. Monitor LFTs during early stages of therapy in liver disease. Monitor renal function and uric acid levels; adjust dose if needed. Maintain sufficient fluid intake to yield a daily urinary output ≥2L. Drowsiness, hepatotoxicity, bone marrow suppression reported.

ADVERSE REACTIONS: Skin rash, eosinophilia, local injection site reaction, NV, diarrhea, renal failure/insufficiency.

INTERACTIONS: Decrease mercaptopurine and azathioprine dose to 1/3-1/4 of usual dose. Increased risk of skin rash with ampicillin, amoxicillin. Increased toxicity and risk of hypersensitivity with thiazide diuretics; monitor renal function. Caution with anticoagulants. Hypoglycemia reported with chlorpropamide. Enhanced myelosuppressive effects of cyclophosphamide, other cytotoxic agents. Increased cyclosporine levels. Increased urinary excretion of uric acid with uricosuric agents. Monitor PT with dicumarol.

PREGNANCY: Category C, caution in nursing.

MECHANISM OF ACTION: Xanthine oxidase inhibitor; reduces production of uric acid by inhibiting the biochemical reactions immediately preceding its formation.

PHARMACOKINETICS: Absorption: Absolute bioavailability (100%); C_{max}=1.58µg/mL (100mg), 5.12µg/mL (300mg); T_{max}=0.5 hrs; AUC=1.99 hr•µg/mL (100mg), 7.1 hr•µg/mL (300mg). **Metabolism:** Oxidative; oxypurinol (active metabolite). **Elimination:** Urine (12% unchanged); $T_{1/2}$=1 hr (parent), 24.1 hrs (oxypurinol).

NURSING CONSIDERATIONS

Assessment: Assess for prior history of severe reaction to drug (eg, skin rash, Stevens-Johnson syndrome). Obtain serum uric acid to provide correct dosage and schedule.

Monitoring: Monitor for allergic reactions, severe hypersensitivity reactions (eg, exfoliative, urticarial, and purpuric lesions, Stevens-Johnson syndrome), generalized vasculitis, hepatotoxicity, serum uric acid, LFTs, BUN, SrCr, and PT.

Patient Counseling: Advise to report any adverse events to physician.

Administration: IV route. Contents of each 30mL vial should be dissolved with 25mL of sterile water for injection. **Storage:** 25°C (77°F); excursions permitted to 15-30°C (59-86°F).

ALOXI RX

palonosetron HCl (Eisai)

THERAPEUTIC CLASS: 5-HT_3 receptor antagonist

INDICATIONS: (Cap) Prevention of nausea and vomiting with moderately emetogenic cancer chemotherapy associated with initial and repeat courses. (Inj) Prevention of acute nausea and vomiting associated with initial and repeat courses of moderately and highly emetogenic cancer chemotherapy. Prevention of postoperative nausea and vomiting (PONV) for up to 24 hrs following surgery.

DOSAGE: (Cap) Chemo-Induced N/V: 0.5mg 1 hr prior to chemotherapy with or without food. (Inj) Chemo-Induced N/V: 0.25mg IV single dose 30 min before start of chemo. Repeated dosing within 7 day interval not recommended. PONV: 0.075mg IV single dose 10 sec before induction of anesthesia.

HOW SUPPLIED: Cap: 0.5mg; Inj: 0.25mg/5mL, 0.075mg/1.5mL

WARNINGS/PRECAUTIONS: Hypersensitivity reaction may occur.

ADVERSE REACTIONS: (Cap/Inj) Headache, constipation; (Inj) diarrhea, dizziness.

PREGNANCY: Category B, not for use in nursing.

MECHANISM OF ACTION: 5-HT_3 receptor antagonist with antiemetic and antinausea properties.

PHARMACOKINETICS: Absorption: (Cap) Absolute bioavailability (97%); C_{max} = 0.81ng/mL, T_{max} = 5.1 hrs, AUC= 38.2 ng•h/mL; (Inj) C_{max}=5.6ng/mL, AUC=35.8ng•hr/mL. **Distribution:** (Cap/Inj) V_d=8.3L/kg; plasma protein binding (62%). **Metabolism:** (Cap/Inj) 50% metabolized via CYP2D6; N-oxide-palonosetron and 6-S-hydroxy-palonosetron (primary metabolites). **Elimination:** (Cap) urine (85-93%), feces (5-8%); $T_{1/2}$=37 hrs; (Inj) urine (40%); $T_{1/2}$=40 hrs.

NURSING CONSIDERATIONS

Assessment: Assess for pre-existing cardiac impairment, hypokalemia or hypomagnesemia, congenital QT syndrome, and possible drug interactions.

Monitoring: ECG monitoring of prolongation of QT interval.

Patient Counseling: Advise to report all medical conditions (eg, heart problems), if taking diuretics, anti-arrhythmics, or anthracyclines, and any pain, redness, or swelling around infusion site. Instruct to read patient insert.

Administration: IV route. **Storage:** 20-25°C (68-77°F); excursions permitted to 15-30°C (59-86°F); avoid light exposure and freezing.

ALPHAGAN P — RX

brimonidine tartrate (Allergan)

THERAPEUTIC CLASS: Selective $alpha_2$ agonist

INDICATIONS: Treatment of open-angle glaucoma and ocular hypertension.

DOSAGE: *Adults:* 1 drop tid, give q8h. Space dosing of other topical products that lower IOP by 5 min.
Pediatrics: ≥2 yrs: 1 drop tid, give q8h. Space dosing of other topical products that lower IOP by 5 min.

HOW SUPPLIED: Sol: 0.1% [5mL, 10mL, 15mL], 0.15% [5mL, 10mL, 15mL] (contains Purite)

CONTRAINDICATIONS: Concomitant MAOI therapy.

WARNINGS/PRECAUTIONS: Caution with severe CV disease, hepatic or renal dysfunction, depression, cerebral or coronary insufficiency, Raynaud's phenomenon, orthostatic hypotension, thromboangiitis obliterans. Wait 15 min before reinserting contacts with 0.2% solution. Monitor IOP.

ADVERSE REACTIONS: Oral dryness, ocular hyperemia, ocular pruritus, burning, stinging, ocular allergic reaction, blurred vision, foreign body sensation, fatigue, drowsiness, headache, conjunctival follicles.

INTERACTIONS: See Contraindications. May potentiate CNS depressants. May reduce BP; caution with β-blockers, antihypertensives, cardiac glycosides. Caution with TCAs. May be given with other topical products to lower IOP.

PREGNANCY: Category B, not for use in nursing.

MECHANISM OF ACTION: An α-2-adrenergic receptor agonist; reduces aqueous humor production and increases uveoscleral outflow.

PHARMACOKINETICS: Absorption: T_{max}=0.5-2.5 hrs. **Metabolism:** Liver (extensive). **Elimination:** Urine (74%).

NURSING CONSIDERATIONS

Assessment: Assess for depression, cerebral or coronary insufficiency, Raynaud's phenomenon, orthostatic hypotension, or thromboangiitis obliterans. Assess renal/hepatic function prior to therapy, for MAO inhibitor therapy, other drug interactions, and use in nursing females.

Monitoring: Perform routine monitoring of IOP while on therapy. Monitor for signs of decreased pulse rate and BP levels while on medication.

Patient Counseling: Advise drug may cause fatigue; use caution during hazardous activities that require mental alertness.

Administration: Ocular route. May be used concomitantly with other topical ophthalmic products to lower IOP; should be administered at least 5 min apart. **Storage:** 15-25°C (59-77°F).

ALREX — RX

loteprednol etabonate (Bausch & Lomb)

THERAPEUTIC CLASS: Corticosteroid

INDICATIONS: Relief of signs and symptoms of seasonal allergic conjunctivitis.

DOSAGE: *Adults:* 1 drop qid.

HOW SUPPLIED: Sus: 0.2% [5mL, 10mL]

CONTRAINDICATIONS: Viral diseases of the cornea and conjunctiva, including epithelial herpes simplex keratitis, vaccinia, and varicella. Mycobacterial infection and fungal diseases of the eye.

WARNINGS/PRECAUTIONS: Caution with glaucoma, herpes simplex, diseases causing thinning of cornea/sclera and other ocular viral infections. Prolonged use can cause glaucoma or secondary ocular infections (eg, fungal). Monitor IOP beyond 10 days of therapy. Wait 10 min after instillation before inserting soft contact lenses. Re-evaluate if no response after 2 days.

ADVERSE REACTIONS: Elevated IOP, foreign body sensation, itching, chemosis, epiphora, blurred vision, burning on instillation, discharge, dry eyes, photophobia.

PREGNANCY: Category C, caution in nursing.

MECHANISM OF ACTION: Corticosteroid; anti-inflammatory agent, not established. Inhibits edema, fibrin deposition, capillary dilation, leukocyte migration, fibroblast proliferation, deposition of collagen, and scar formation associated with inflammation by induction of phospholipase A_2 inhibitory protein lipocortin.

PHARMACOKINETICS: Absorption: C_{max}<1ng/mL.

NURSING CONSIDERATIONS

Assessment: Assess for viral diseases of the cornea and conjunctiva (eg, epithelial herpes simplex, keratitis (dendritic keratitis), vaccinia and varicella, mycobacterial infection of the eye and fungal diseases of ocular structure, known hypersensitivity to drug components, glaucoma, and possible drug interactions.

Monitoring: Monitor for secondary ocular infections, fungal infections, masking or enhancement of existing infections, thinning of the cornea or sclera, perforation, glaucoma, damage to optic nerve, defects in visual acuity, and posterior subcapsular cataract formation.

Patient Counseling: Avoid touching dropper tip to eyes, fingers, or any surface. Notify physician if symptoms persist or worsen. Do not wear contact lenses if eyes are red or irritated.

Administration: Intraocular route. **Storage:** 15-25°C (59-77°F). Do not freeze.

ALTABAX — RX
retapamulin (GlaxoSmithKline)

THERAPEUTIC CLASS: Pleuromutilin antibacterial

INDICATIONS: Topical treatment of impetigo caused by susceptible strains of microorganisms, in patients ≥9 months.

DOSAGE: *Adults*: Apply thin layer (up to 100 cm^2 in total area) bid for 5 days. May cover with sterile bandage or gauze.
Pediatrics: ≥9 months: Apply thin layer (up to 2% total BSA) bid for 5 days. May cover with sterile bandage or gauze.

HOW SUPPLIED: Oint: 1% [5g, 10g, 15g]

WARNINGS/PRECAUTIONS: D/C if sensitization or irritation occurs. Not intended for oral, intranasal, ophthalmic or intravaginal use. May cause super-infection during therapy.

ADVERSE REACTIONS: Application site reactions.

INTERACTIONS: Coadministration with ketoconazole may increase levels.

PREGNANCY: Category B, caution in nursing.

MECHANISM OF ACTION: Pleuromutilin antibacterial; selectively inhibits bacterial protein synthesis by interacting at a site on the 50S subunit of the bacterial ribosome. The binding site involves ribosomal protein L3 and is in the region of the ribosomal P site and peptidyl transferase center. By binding to this site, peptidyl transfer is inhibited, P-site interactions are blocked, and the formation of normal active 50S ribosomal subunits is prevented.

PHARMACOKINETICS: Absorption: Low systemic exposure. Following application to 800cm^2 of intact skin: C_{max}=3.5ng/mL (multiple doses). Following application to 200cm^2 of abraded skin: C_{max}=11.7ng/mL (single dose), 9.0ng/mL (multiple doses). **Distribution:** Plasma protein binding (94%). **Metabolism:** Liver via CYP3A4 (mono-oxygenation, N-demethylation). **Elimination:** Not investigated.

NURSING CONSIDERATIONS

Assessment: Assess for proper diagnosis of bacterial organisms, use in nursing females, and possible drug interactions.

Monitoring: Monitor for signs/symptoms of sensitization reactions or severe local irritation, and for the development of overgrowth of nonsusceptible organisms (superinfection).

Patient Counseling: Counsel drug is for external use only; avoid contact with eyes, mouth, inside of nose, or inside of female genital area. May use sterile bandage or gauze dressing after applying ointment. Wash hands following application (if hands are not the treatment area). Take the medication for full recommended time; notify physician if symptoms do not improve within 3-4 days after starting treatment or if irritation, redness, itching, burning, blistering, oozing at treatment site develops.

Administration: Topical route. **Storage**: Store at 25°C (77°F); excursions permitted to 15-30°C (59-86°F).

ALTACE — RX
ramipril (King)

ACE inhibitors can cause death/injury to developing fetus during 2nd and 3rd trimesters. Stop therapy if pregnancy detected.

THERAPEUTIC CLASS: ACE inhibitor

INDICATIONS: Hypertension, alone or with thiazide diuretics. To decrease hospitalization and mortality in stable post-MI patients that show signs of congestive heart failure. To reduce risk of MI, stroke, and cardiovascular (CV) death in patients ≥55 yrs who are at risk due to history of coronary artery disease, stroke, peripheral vascular disease, or diabetes with at least one other CV risk factor.

DOSAGE: *Adults:* HTN: Initial: 2.5mg qd. Maint: 2.5-20mg/day given qd or bid. Add diuretic if BP not controlled. CrCl <40mL/min: Initial: 1.25mg qd. Titrate/ Max: 5mg/day. CHF Post-MI: Initial: 2.5mg bid, 1.25mg bid if hypotensive. Titrate: Increase to 5mg bid. CrCl <40mL/min: Initial: 1.25mg qd. Titrate: May increase to 1.25mg bid. Max: 2.5mg bid. Risk Reduction of MI, Stroke, Death (≥55 yrs): Initial: 2.5mg qd for 1 week. Increase to 5mg qd for next 3 weeks. Maint: 10mg qd. Reduce or d/c diuretic if possible. With Volume Depletion/ Renal Artery Stenosis: Initial: 1.25mg qd.

HOW SUPPLIED: Cap: 1.25mg, 2.5mg, 5mg, 10mg

CONTRAINDICATIONS: History of ACE inhibitor-associated angioedema.

WARNINGS/PRECAUTIONS: D/C if angioedema, jaundice, or if marked LFT elevation occurs. Risk of hyperkalemia with DM, renal dysfunction. Persistent nonproductive cough and anaphylactoid reactions reported. Monitor WBCs in renal and collagen vascular disease. Fetal/neonatal morbidity and death reported. Monitor for hypotension in high-risk patients (heart failure, surgery/ anesthesia, hyponatremia, high-dose diuretic therapy, recent intensive diuresis, dialysis, or severe volume and/or salt depletion, etc). Caution with CHF, renal dysfunction, severe liver cirrhosis and/or ascites, and renal artery stenosis. Less effective on BP in blacks and more reports of angioedema than nonblacks. May reduce RBCs, Hgb, WBCs, or platelets. May cause agranulocytosis, pancytopenia, and bone marrow depression.

ADVERSE REACTIONS: Hypotension, cough, dizziness, fatigue, angina, impotence, Stevens-Johnson syndrome.

INTERACTIONS: May increase lithium levels. Hypotension risk with diuretics. Increased risk of hyperkalemia with K^+-sparing diuretics, K^+ supplements, or K^+-containing salt substitutes. NSAIDs may worsen renal failure and increase serum potassium.

PREGNANCY: Category C (1st trimester) and D (2nd and 3rd trimesters), not for use in nursing.

NURSING CONSIDERATIONS

Assessment: Assess for pregnancy status, possible drug interactions, volume/ salt depletion, DM, collagen vascular disease, CHF, hepatic/renal impairment. Obtain baseline BP, renal function and WBC with differential (impaired renal function).

Monitoring: Monitor renal function periodically; BP in first 2 weeks and at dosage change. If impaired renal function, monitor WBC with differential before therapy, at 2-week intervals for 3 months, and then periodically during therapy. Monitor for signs/symptoms of hypotension, anaphylactoid or hypersensitivity reactions, head/neck and intestinal angioedema, infection, and neutropenia/agranulocytosis.

Patient Counseling: Inform of pregnancy risks. Instruct that inadequate fluid intake or loss of fluids may lead to drop in BP resulting in lightheadedness or syncope; avoid K^+ or salt substitutes. Advise to seek medical attention if symptoms of angioedema (head/neck; intestinal/abdominal pain with/without NV), infection (sore throat, fever), syncope, or hypersensitivity reactions occur.

Administration: Oral route. **Storage:** 59-86°F.

ALTOPREV — RX

lovastatin (Sciele)

THERAPEUTIC CLASS: HMG-CoA reductase inhibitor

INDICATIONS: Adjunct to diet, to slow progression of coronary atherosclerosis in coronary heart disease. Adjunct to diet, for reduction of elevated total cholesterol (total-C), LDL-C, Apo B, and TG, and to increase HDL-C in patients with primary hypercholesterolemia (heterozygous familial and non-familial) and mixed dyslipidemia (Fredrickson types IIa and IIb). To reduce risk of MI, unstable angina and coronary revascularization procedures in patients with asymptomatic cardiovascular disease, average to moderately elevated Total-C and LDL-C, and below average HDL-C.

DOSAGE: *Adults:* Initial: 20, 40, or 60mg qhs. Consider immediate-release lovastatin in patients requiring smaller reductions. May adjust at intervals of ≥4 weeks. Concomitant Fibrates/Niacin (≥1g/day): Try to avoid. Max: 20mg/day. Concomitant Amiodarone/Verapamil: Max: 20mg/day. CrCl <30mL/min: Consider dose increase of >20mg/day carefully and implement cautiously. Swallow whole; do not chew or crush.

HOW SUPPLIED: Tab: Extended-Release: 20mg, 40mg, 60mg

CONTRAINDICATIONS: Active liver disease, unexplained persistent elevations of serum transaminases, pregnancy, nursing mothers.

WARNINGS/PRECAUTIONS: May increase serum transaminases and CPK levels; consider in differential diagnosis of chest pain. D/C if AST or ALT ≥3x ULN persists, if myopathy diagnosed or suspected, and a few days before major surgery. Monitor LFTs prior to therapy, at 6 weeks, 12 weeks, then periodically or with dose elevation. Caution with heavy alcohol use and/or history of hepatic disease. Caution with dose escalation in renal insufficiency. Lovastatin immediate-release found to be less effective with homozygous familial hypercholesterolemia. Rhabdomyolysis (rare), myopathy reported.

ADVERSE REACTIONS: Nausea, abdominal pain, insomnia, dyspepsia, headache, asthenia, myalgia.

INTERACTIONS: Due to increased risk of myopathy: suspend lovastatin if itraconazole, ketoconazole, erythromycin, or clarithromycin must be used; avoid other CYP3A4 inhibitors (protease inhibitors, nefazodone, >1 quart/day of grapefruit juice); avoid gemfibrozil (reduce max lovastatin dose if must be used); reduce max lovastatin dose with amiodarone, verapamil, if must be used; caution with other fibrates, ≥1g/day of niacin. Avoid use with cyclosporine. Monitor warfarin. May blunt adrenal and/or gonadal steroid production; caution with steroid hormone suppressive drugs (eg, ketoconazole, spironolactone, cimetidine).

PREGNANCY: Category X, not for use in nursing.

MECHANISM OF ACTION: HMG-CoA reductase inhibitor; reduces LDL-C and total-C.

PHARMACOKINETICS: Absorption: Lovastatin: C_{max}=5.5ng/mL, T_{max}=14.2 hrs, AUC=77ng•h/mL. Lovastatin acid: C_{max}=5.8ng/mL, T_{max}=14.2 hr, AUC=87ng•h/mL. **Distribution:** Plasma protein binding (>95%). Crosses blood brain/placental barriers. **Metabolism:** Liver (extensive), β-hydroxy acid (active inhibitor). **Elimination:** Urine, bile.

NURSING CONSIDERATIONS

Assessment: Assess for active liver disease, pregnancy/nursing status, DM, alcohol intake, homozygous familial hypercholesterolemia, and possible drug interactions. Perform LFTs prior to therapy.

Monitoring: Monitor for signs/symptoms of myopathy/rhabdomyolysis (eg, pain, tenderness, or weakness), CNS toxicity (eg, optic nerve degeneration), and CNS vascular lesions (eg, hemorrhage and edema). Monitor CK levels, LFTs, and endocrine function.

Patient Counseling: Inform about risks/benefits; promptly report signs of myopathy (eg, unexplained muscular pain, tenderness, or weakness).

Administration: Oral route. Take drug whole; do not crush or chew. **Storage:** 20-25°C (68-77°F). Avoid excessive heat and humidity.

ALVESCO

RX

ciclesonide (Sepracor)

THERAPEUTIC CLASS: Non-halogenated glucocorticoid

INDICATIONS: Maintenance treatment of asthma as prophylactic therapy in adults and adolescents ≥12 yrs.

DOSAGE: *Adults:* Previous Bronchodilator Alone: Initial: 80mcg bid. Max: 160mcg bid. Previous Inhaled Corticosteroid Therapy: Initial: 80mcg bid. Max: 320mcg bid. Previous Oral Corticosteroid Therapy: Initial: 320mcg bid. Max: 320mcg bid.
Pediatrics: ≥12 yrs: Previous Bronchodilator Alone: Initial: 80mcg bid. Max: 160mcg bid. Previous Inhaled Corticosteroid Therapy: Initial: 80mcg bid. Max: 320mcg bid. Previous Oral Corticosteroid Therapy: Initial: 320mcg bid. Max: 320mcg bid.

HOW SUPPLIED: MDI: 80mcg/actuation [60 actuations], 160mcg/actuation [60 or 120 actuations]

CONTRAINDICATIONS: Status asthmaticus or other acute episodes of asthma.

WARNINGS/PRECAUTIONS: *Candida albicans* infections of mouth and pharynx may occur; examine periodically and treat accordingly. Advise to rinse mouth after inhalation. Caution with active or quiescent TB infections, untreated local/systemic bacterial/fungal infections, systemic viral or parasitic infections, or ocular herpes simplex. Risk for more severe/fatal course of infections (eg, chickenpox, measles); avoid exposure in patients who have not had the disease or been properly immunized. Risk of adrenal insufficiency and withdrawal symptoms when replacing oral corticosteroids with inhaled corticosteroids; monitor closely. Taper dose if symptoms of hypercorticism and adrenal suppression occur. May cause reduced growth velocity in pediatrics. May decrease bone mineral density (BMD) with prolonged treatment; monitor and treat accordingly. Caution with history of glaucoma, increased IOP, and cataracts; monitor closely. Acute asthma episodes or bronchospasm may occur; d/c use and institute alternative treatment if occur.

ADVERSE REACTIONS: Headache, nasopharyngitis, sinusitis, pharyngolaryngeal pain, upper respiratory infection, arthralgia, nasal congestion, pain in extremity, back pain.

INTERACTIONS: Ketoconazole may increase levels of the pharmacologically active metabolite des-ciclesonide; co-administer with caution.

PREGNANCY: Category C, caution in nursing.

MECHANISM OF ACTION: Corticosteroid: exerts anti-inflammatory actions with affinity to glucocorticoid receptor that inhibits activities of multiple cell types (mast cells, eosinophils,basophils, lymphocytes, macrophages, and neutrophils) and mediators (histamine, eicosanoids, leukotrienes, and cytokines) involved in asthmatic response.

PHARMACOKINETICS: Absorption: Ciclesonide: Absolute bioavailability: 22%. Des-ciclesonide (active metabolite): 63%; C_{max}=1.02ng/mL in asthmatic patient. **Distribution:** Ciclesonide: V_d=2.9L/kg. Des-ciclesonide: V_d=12.1L/kg. **Metabolism:** Liver, via CYP3A4, CYP2D6 (hydrolysis); des-ciclesonide (active metabolite). **Elimination:** Feces (60%), urine (≤20%), and bile. $T_{1/2}$=ciclesonide (0.71 hrs), des-ciclesonide (6-7 hrs).

NURSING CONSIDERATIONS

Assessment: Assess for risk of impaired adrenal function, presence of status asthmaticus or other acute episodes of asthma and potential worsening of current infection (TB, ocular herpes simplex), history of increased IOP, glaucoma, and/or cataracts, under systemic corticosteroid therapy, and hypersensitivity to drug.

Monitoring: Monitor for signs of adverse effects in oral cavity, change of vision, growth velocity measurement (stadiometry) especially for pediatrics, BMD, corticosteroid effects of hypercorticism and adrenal suppression, and urinary cortisol level.

Patient Counseling: Advise that drug is not a bronchodilator and not intended to provide rapid relief of breathing difficulties during asthmatic attack. Instruct that medication must be taken at regular intervals as recommended, and not as emergency measure. Caution to not inhale more often than what is advised. Instruct that it may take 4 weeks or longer to feel full benefit. Instruct to report if symptoms do not improve in that time frame or if condition worsens at any point during treatment. Instruct to not stop treatment even if feeling better unless told to do so. Inform that if dose is missed, wait and take regularly scheduled next dose. Advise to test spray inhaler on 1st use or if it has not been used for more than 10 days.

Administration: Inhalation route. Inhaler is fitted with dose indicator which shows how much medication is left during use. Dose indicator display will move every 10th time puff is taken. Dose indicator display window will turn red when there are only 20 puffs remaining; this means that inhaler must be replaced soon. Inhalation Steps: 1) Close lips around mouthpiece, keeping tongue below it. 2) While breathing in deeply and slowly, press down on center of dose. Fully depress canister until it stops moving in adapter while delivering dose. When finished breathing in, hold breath for about 10 sec, or for as long as is comfortable. Breathe out gently. 3) After taking dose, rinse mouth with water and spit out; do not swallow. Do not wash inhaler in water. **Storage:** Store at room temperature. Keep out of reach of children. Contents under pressure. Do not puncture. Temperature above 120°F (49°C) may cause bursting. Never throw into fire.

AMARYL

RX

glimepiride (Sanofi-Aventis)

THERAPEUTIC CLASS: Sulfonylurea (2nd generation)

INDICATIONS: Adjunct to diet and exercise, to improve glycemic control in type 2 diabetes mellitus. May use in combination with metformin or insulin.

DOSAGE: *Adults:* Initial: 1-2mg qd with breakfast or 1st main meal. Titrate: After 2mg, may increase by up to 2mg every 1-2 weeks. Maint: 1-4mg qd. Max: 8mg qd. Amaryl/Metformin: Add Metformin to 8mg qd for better glucose control. Amaryl/Insulin Therapy: If FBG >150mg/dL on 8mg qd, add low-dose insulin; increase insulin weekly as needed. Renal Insufficiency: Initial: 1mg qd. Elderly/Debilitated/Malnourished/Hepatic Insufficiency: Dose conservatively to avoid hypoglycemia.

HOW SUPPLIED: Tab: 1mg*, 2mg*, 4mg* *scored

CONTRAINDICATIONS: Diabetic ketoacidosis.

WARNINGS/PRECAUTIONS: Increased cardiovascular mortality. Hypoglycemia risk if debilitated, malnourished, or with adrenal, pituitary, renal or hepatic insufficiency. Hypoglycemia may be masked in elderly. May lose blood glucose control with stress. Secondary failure may occur. D/C if skin reactions persist or worsen.

ADVERSE REACTIONS: Dizziness, nausea, asthenia, headache, hypoglycemia.

INTERACTIONS: Potentiated hypoglycemia with alcohol, NSAIDs, highly protein-bound drugs, such as salicylates, sulfonamides, chloramphenicol, coumarins, probenecid, MAOIs, miconazole, and β-blockers. Risk of hyperglycemia with diuretics, corticosteroids, phenothiazines, thyroid products, estrogens, oral contraceptives, phenytoin, nicotinic acid, sympathomimetics, and isoniazid. Monitor for hypoglycemia when switching from long-acting sulfonylurea, and with combination therapy with insulin and metformin. Hypoglycemia may be masked with β-blockers/sympatholytic agents.

PREGNANCY: Category C, not for use in nursing.

MECHANISM OF ACTION: Sulfonylurea; lowers blood glucose by stimulating insulin release from functioning pancreatic beta cells.

PHARMACOKINETICS: Absorption: Complete (GI tract); T_{max}=2-3 hrs; (4mg PO) C_{max}=308ng/mL. **Distribution:** (IV) V_d=8.8L, (PO) 21.8L; plasma protein binding (99.5%). **Metabolism:** Complete (liver); CYP2C9; major metabolites: M1 & M2. **Elimination:** Urine (60%), feces (40%); $T_{1/2}$=5.3 hrs.

NURSING CONSIDERATIONS

Assessment: Assess for signs/symptoms of hypoglycemia, loss of control (fever, trauma, infection), risk of cardiovascular mortality, hepatic porphyria, hyponatremia, allergic reactions, thrombocytopenia, leukopenia, agranulocytosis, and hepatitis (cholestasis, jaundice), and potential drug interactions.

Monitoring: Monitor fasting blood glucose and glycosylated hemoglobin (every 3-6 months) to determine response to therapy and glycemic control.

Patient Counseling: Instruct to have a proper diet and exercise and regularly test blood glucose. Inform about risks of hypoglycemia (symptoms, treatment) and conditions that predispose to development.

Administration: Oral route. **Storage:** 15-30°C (59-86°F). Dispense in well-closed containers.

AMBIEN CIV

zolpidem tartrate (Sanofi-Aventis)

THERAPEUTIC CLASS: Imidazopyridine hypnotic

INDICATIONS: Short-term treatment of insomnia characterized by difficulties with sleep initiation.

DOSAGE: *Adults:* Tab: Usual: 10mg qhs. Elderly/Debilitated/Hepatic Insufficiency: Initial: 5mg. Decrease dose with other CNS depressants. Max: 10mg qd. Reevaluate if insomnia persists after 7-10 days.

HOW SUPPLIED: Tab: 5mg, 10mg

WARNINGS/PRECAUTIONS: Severe anaphylactic/anaphylactoid reactions reported. Abnormal thinking, behavior changes and complex behaviors (eg, sleep driving) reported. Worsening of depression or suicidal thinking may occur; use lowest feasible amount to avoid intentional overdose. Withdrawal symptoms may occur with rapid dose reduction or discontinuation. Potential impairment of activities requiring complete mental alertness (eg, operating machinery) after ingestion and following day. Avoid with alcohol. Monitor elderly and debilitated patients for impaired motor performance. Caution with hepatic impairment, mild to moderate COPD or sleep apnea, impaired drug metabolism or hemodynamic responses. Avoid if you cannot get a full night's sleep.

ADVERSE REACTIONS: Drowsiness, dizziness, headache, nausea, diarrhea, drugged feeling, dyspepsia, myalgia, lethargy, memory loss, anxiety, abnormal thoughts and behavior, tongue or throat swelling.

INTERACTIONS: Decreased alertness with imipramine. Impaired alertness and psychomotor performance with chlorpromazine. Additive psychomotor impairment with alcohol and other CNS depressants. Rifampin may decrease effects. Flumazenil may reverse effect.

PREGNANCY: Category B, not for use in nursing.

MECHANISM OF ACTION: Imidazopyridine, a non-benzodiazepine hypnotic; binds to $GABA_A$ receptor complex at the α-subunit/benzodiazepine receptor, the major modulatory site. GABA receptor complex modulation is hypothesized to be responsible for the sedative, anticonvulsant, anxiolytic, myorelaxant properties.

PHARMACOKINETICS: Absorption: Rapid. C_{max}=59ng/mL (5mg), 121ng/mL (10mg). T_{max}=1.6 (5mg, 10mg). **Distribution:** Plasma protein binding (92.5%). **Metabolism**: CYP450. **Elimination**: Renal; $T_{1/2}$=2.6 hrs (5mg), 2.5 hrs (10mg).

NURSING CONSIDERATIONS

Assessment: Carefully assess for primary psychiatric and/or medical illness or depression prior to initiation. Assess for presence of pre-existing respiratory impairment (eg, myasthenia gravis, sleep apnea syndrome, COPD), hepatic/renal impairment, possible drug interaction, and history of addiction or abuse of drugs or alcohol.

Monitoring: Monitor for anaphylactic/anaphylactoid reactions, insomnia, abnormal thinking, behavioral changes, complex behaviors (eg, sleep driving, suicidal thinking), visual and auditory hallucinations. Monitor patients with hepatic/renal impairment, and for drug abuse/dependence with long-term treatment.

Patient Counseling: Counsel to take immediately before bedtime and not with or right after meals. Inform about benefits/risks with long-term use. Caution needed when performing hazardous tasks (eg, operating machinery/driving). Counsel on tolerance, dependence, and withdrawal signs/symptoms. Do not take with alcohol.

Administration: Oral route. **Storage:** 20-25°C (68-77°F).

AMBIEN CR — CIV

zolpidem tartrate (Sanofi-Aventis)

THERAPEUTIC CLASS: Imidazopyridine hypnotic

INDICATIONS: Treatment of insomnia, characterized by difficulties with sleep onset and/or sleep maintenance.

DOSAGE: *Adults:* 12.5mg qhs. Elderly/Debilitated/Hepatic Insufficiency: 6.25mg qhs. Swallow whole; do not divide, crush, or chew.

HOW SUPPLIED: Tab, Extended-Release: 6.25mg, 12.5mg

WARNINGS/PRECAUTIONS: Use smallest possible effective dose, especially in elderly. Abnormal thinking and behavior changes reported with use of sedative/hypnotics. Caution with depression and conditions that could affect metabolism or hemodynamic responses. Signs and symptoms of withdrawal reported with abrupt discontinuation of sedative/hypnotics. Monitor elderly and debilitated patients for impaired motor and/or cognitive performance.

ADVERSE REACTIONS: Headache, somnolence, dizziness, nausea, hallucinations, back pain, myalgia, fatigue.

INTERACTIONS: Increased effect with alcohol and other CNS depressants. Rifampin may decrease effects. Flumazenil reverses effect.

PREGNANCY: Category C, not for use in nursing.

MECHANISM OF ACTION: Imidazopyridine, non-benzodiazepine hypnotic; binds to $GABA_A$ receptor complex at the α-subunit/benzodiazepine receptor, the major modulatory site. GABA receptor complex modulation is hypothesized to be responsible for the sedative, anticonvulsant, anxiolytic, myorelaxant properties.

PHARMACOKINETICS: Absorption: Rapid; 12mg: C_{max}=134ng/mL, T_{max}=1.5 hrs, AUC=740ng•hr/mL. **Distribution:** Plasma protein binding (92.5%). **Metabolism**: CYP450. **Elimination:** Urine; $T_{1/2}$=2.8 hrs.

NURSING CONSIDERATIONS

Assessment: Assess for primary psychiatric illness or depression, pre-existing respiratory impairment (eg, COPD, sleep apnea syndrome), hypersensitivity reactions, hepatic/renal impairment, possible drug interactions, and history of alcohol abuse.

Monitoring: Monitor for anaphylactic/anaphylactoid reactions, abnormal thinking, behavioral changes, complex behavior (eg, sleep driving, hallucinations). Monitor patients with hepatic/renal impairment, and those on long-term treatment for drug abuse/dependence.

Patient Counseling: Counsel to take just before bedtime without food; do not crush, divide, or chew, and do not take when drinking alcohol. Caution against hazardous tasks (eg, driving/operating machines). Inform about risks/benefits of use.

Administration: Oral route. **Storage:** 15-25°C (59-77°F).

AMBISOME — RX

amphotericin B (Astellas)

THERAPEUTIC CLASS: Polyene antifungal

INDICATIONS: Empirical therapy for presumed fungal infection in febrile, neutropenic patients. Treatment of *Aspergillus, Candida,* or *Cryptococcus* infections refractory to amphotericin B deoxycholate or where renal impairment or unacceptable toxicity precludes its use. Treatment of cryptococcal meningitis in HIV-infected patients. Treatment of visceral leishmaniasis.

DOSAGE: *Adults:* Empiric Therapy: 3mg/kg/day IV. Systemic Infections (*Aspergillus, Candida, Cryptococcus*): 3-5mg/kg/day IV. Cryptococcal Meningitis in HIV: 6mg/kg/day IV. Visceral Leishmaniasis: Immunocompetent: 3mg/kg/day IV on Days 1-5, 14, 21. May repeat course if needed. Immunocompromised: 4mg/kg/day IV on Days 1-5, 10, 17, 24, 31, 38. *Pediatrics:* 1 month-16 yrs: Empirical Therapy: 3mg/kg/day IV. Systemic Infections (*Aspergillus, Candida, Cryptococcus*): 3-5mg/kg/day IV. Cryptococcal Meningitis in HIV: 6mg/kg/day IV. Visceral Leishmaniasis: Immunocompetent: 3mg/kg/day IV on Days 1-5, 14, 21. May repeat course if needed. Immunocompromised: 4mg/kg/day IV on Days 1-5, 10, 17, 24, 31, 38.

HOW SUPPLIED: Inj: 50mg

WARNINGS/PRECAUTIONS: If anaphylaxis occurs, d/c all further infusions. Significantly less toxic than amphotericin B deoxycholate. Monitor renal, hepatic, hematopoietic function and electrolytes (especially K^+, Mg^{++}).

ADVERSE REACTIONS: Chills, asthenia, back pain, pain, infection, chest pain, HTN, hypotension, tachycardia, GI hemorrhage, diarrhea, NV, hyperglycemia, hypokalemia, dyspnea.

INTERACTIONS: Concurrent use of antineoplastic agents may potentiate renal toxicity, bronchospasm, hypotension. Corticosteroids and corticotropin may potentiate hypokalemia. May potentiate digitalis toxicity. May increase flucytosine toxicity. Acute pulmonary toxicity with leukocyte transfusions reported. Nephrotoxic drugs enhance potential for renal toxicity. May enhance curariform effect of skeletal muscle relaxants due to hypokalemia. Imidazoles (eg, ketoconazole, miconazole, clotrimazole, fluconazole) may induce fungal resistance; caution with combination therapy, especially in immunocompromised patients.

PREGNANCY: Category B, not for use in nursing.

MECHANISM OF ACTION: Antifungal agent; acts by binding to the sterol component of the cell membrane, which leads to changes in cell permeability and cell death in susceptible fungi. Also binds to the cholesterol component of the mammalian cell, leading to cytotoxicity.

PHARMACOKINETICS: Absorption: IV administration of variable doses resulted from different parameters. **Metabolism:** Not known.

NURSING CONSIDERATIONS

Assessment: Assess cultures, renal function, and possible drug interactions.

Monitoring: Monitor for acute infusion reactions (eg, chills, hypotension, hypoxia, rash), renal, hepatic and hematopoietic function, and serum electrolytes (particularly Mg^+ and K^+).

Patient Counseling: Seek medical attention if symptoms of acute reaction occur (eg, fevers, chills, respiratory symptoms). May receive pretreatment medication to help prevent acute infusion reactions. Infusion time may be reduced to approximately 60 min if treatment is well tolerated.

Administration: IV infusion. Reconstitute. 1) Add 12mL of Sterile Water For Inj, USP to vial. 2) Shake vial until all solids are completely dispersed. 3) Further dilute using 5% Dextrose. Must be diluted to a final concentration of 1.0-2.0 mg/mL in adults, (0.2-0.5mg/mL may be appropriate for infants and children). Discard partially used vials. Infuse over a period of 120 min. If using an existing IV line, must flush with 5% Dextrose prior to infusion. Otherwise, another IV line must be used. **Storage:** Unopened vials: 25°C (77°F). Reconstituted: 2-8°C (36-46°F) stored for 24 hrs. Diluted Product: Injection should commence within 6 hrs of dilution with 5% Dextrose Injection.

AMERGE **RX**

naratriptan HCl (GlaxoSmithKline)

THERAPEUTIC CLASS: 5-$HT_{1B/1D}$ agonist

INDICATIONS: Acute treatment of migraine with or without aura.

DOSAGE: *Adults:* ≥18 yrs: 1mg or 2.5mg taken with fluids; may repeat dose once after 4 hrs. Max: 5mg/24 hrs. Mild-Moderate Renal/Hepatic Impairment: Initial: Lower dose. Max: 2.5mg/24 hrs. Safety of treating >4 headaches/30 days not known.

HOW SUPPLIED: Tab: 1mg, 2.5mg

CONTRAINDICATIONS: Uncontrolled HTN, ischemic cardiac disease, cerebrovascular or peripheral vascular syndromes, other significant CVD, severe renal or hepatic impairment, basilar or hemiplegic migraine, within 24 hrs of another 5-HT_1 agonist, ergotamine-containing or ergot-type drugs (eg, dihydroergotamine, methysergide).

WARNINGS/PRECAUTIONS: Confirm diagnosis. Supervise 1st dose and monitor cardiac function in those at risk of CAD (eg, HTN, hypercholesterolemia, smoker, obesity, diabetes, CAD family history, postmenopausal women, males >40 yrs). Monitor cardiovascular function with long-term intermittent use. May cause vasospastic reactions or cerebrovascular events. Serotonin syndrome may occur; symptoms may include mental status changes, autonomic instability, neuromuscular aberrations, and GIT symptoms. Caution with renal or hepatic dysfunction. Avoid in elderly.

ADVERSE REACTIONS: Paresthesias, dizziness, drowsiness, malaise/fatigue, throat and neck symptoms (eg, pain/pressure sensation).

INTERACTIONS: Ergotamine-containing and ergot-type drugs (eg, dihydroergotamine, methysergide) drugs may cause prolonged vasospastic reactions. Avoid other 5-HT_1 agonist drugs within 24-hr period due to additive effects. Serotonin syndrome reported with combined use of an SSRI or SNRI.

PREGNANCY: Category C, caution in nursing.

MECHANISM OF ACTION: Selective 5-HT_1 receptor agonist; binds with high affinity to 5-$HT_{1D/1B}$ receptors; two theories explain its efficacy in migraine. One theory suggests that activation of 5-$HT_{1D/1B}$ receptors located on intracranial blood vessels, including those on arteriovenous anastomoses, leads to vasoconstriction that correlates with relief of migraine. Another suggests that activation of 5-$HT_{1D/1B}$ receptors in the trigeminal system results in inhibition of pro-inflammatory neuropeptide release.

PHARMACOKINETICS: Absorption: Well-absorbed; bioavailability (70%); T_{max}=2-3 hrs. **Metabolism:** Via CYP450 isoenzymes. **Distribution:** V_d=170L, plasma protein binding (28-31%); found in breast milk. **Elimination:** Urine (50% unchanged, 30% metabolites); $T_{1/2}$=6 hrs.

NURSING CONSIDERATIONS

Assessment: Confirm diagnosis of migraine before therapy. Assess for IHD (eg, angina pectoris, Prinzmetal's variant angina, MI or documented silent MI), HTN, hemiplegic/basilar migraine, presence of risk factors (eg, hypercholesterolemia, smoking, obesity, DM, strong family history of CAD, female with surgical/physiological menopause, or male >49 yrs), ECG changes, hepatic/renal impairment, pregnancy/nursing status, and possible drug interactions.

Monitoring: Administration of 1st dose should be in physician's office or medically staffed and equipped facility as cardiac ischemia may occur in absence of clinical symptoms; ECG should be obtained immediately during interval in those with risk factors. Monitor for signs/symptoms of cardiac events (eg, coronary vasospasm, acute MI, arrhythmia, ECG changes, follow-up coronary angiography), cerebrovascular events (eg, hemorrhage, stroke, TIAs), peripheral vascular ischemia, colonic ischemia with bloody diarrhea and abdominal pain, serotonin syndrome (eg, mental status changes, autonomic instability, neuromuscular aberrations and/or GI symptoms), ophthalmic effects, increased BP, and anaphylaxis/anaphylactoid reactions.

Patient Counseling: Inform about potential risks of therapy (eg, symptoms of serotonin syndrome such as confusion, hallucinations, fast heartbeat, fever, sweating, muscle spasms, and diarrhea), especially if taken with SSRIs or SNRIs. Instruct to report adverse reactions to physician. Advise to take exactly as directed. Instruct to notify if pregnant/nursing or planning to become pregnant.

Administration: Oral route. **Storage:** 20-25°C (68-77°F).

AMEVIVE
alefacept (Astellas) **RX**

THERAPEUTIC CLASS: Immunosuppressive agent

INDICATIONS: Treatment of moderate to severe chronic plaque psoriasis for candidates of systemic therapy or phototherapy.

DOSAGE: *Adults:* 7.5mg IV bolus or 15mg IM once weekly for 12 weeks. May initiate retreatment with an additional 12-week course if CD4+ T-lymphocyte counts are within normal range and a 12-week minimum interval has passed since the previous course of treatment. CD4+ T-Lymphocyte Counts <250 cells/mL: Withhold dose. D/C if counts remain below 250 cells/mL for 1 month.

HOW SUPPLIED: Inj: (IV) 7.5mg, (IM) 15mg

CONTRAINDICATIONS: HIV.

WARNINGS/PRECAUTIONS: Do not initiate with CD4+ T-lymphocyte counts below normal; monitor every 2 weeks. May increase risk of malignancies; do not administer to patients with history of systemic malignancy. May increase risk of infection or reactivate latent, chronic infections; avoid with clinically important infections, caution with chronic or history of recurrent infections; d/c if serious infection develops. D/C if serious hypersensitivity reactions occur. Caution in elderly. Avoid concurrent phototherapy.

ADVERSE REACTIONS: Pharyngitis, dizziness, increased cough, nausea, pruritus, myalgia, chills, injection-site pain/inflammation, lymphopenia, malignancies, serious infections, hypersensitivity reactions.

INTERACTIONS: Avoid with other immunosuppressive agents.

PREGNANCY: Category B, not for use in nursing.

MECHANISM OF ACTION: Immunosuppressive agent; interferes with lymphocyte activation by specifically binding to the lymphocyte antigen CD2, and inhibiting LFA-2/CD2 interaction. Causes reduction in subsets of CD2+ T lymphocytes (primarily CD45RO+), presumably by bridging between CD2 on target lymphocytes and immunoglobulin Fc receptors on cytotoxic cells, such as natural killer cells, which results in reduction of circulating total CD4+ and CD8+ T-lymphocyte counts.

PHARMACOKINETICS: Distribution: V_d=94mL/kg. **Elimination:** $T_{1/2}$=270 hrs.

NURSING CONSIDERATIONS

Assessment: Assess for HIV infection, history of systemic malignancy or risk of malignancy, chronic infections or a history of recurrent infection, immunosuppressants or phototherapy, immunization status, hepatic impairment, pregnancy/nursing status, and possible drug interaction or alcohol intake. Prior to initiation or subsequent course of therapy, patient should have normal CD4+ T lymphocytes.

Monitoring: Requires monitoring of CD4+ T lymphocyte counts every 2 weeks throughout the course of the 12-week dosing regimen. Monitor for signs/symptoms of infection during or after a course of therapy. Monitor for new infections, malignancies, hypersensitivity reactions (urticaria, angioedema, anaphylactic reactions, or serious allergic reaction), signs/symptoms of hepatic injury, and WBCs.

Patient Counseling: Inform about potential risks/benefits of therapy and to report any signs/symptoms of infections, malignancy, or liver injury to physician. Notify physician if pregnant/nursing or planning to become pregnant.

Administration: IV and IM routes. Use only under supervision of a physician. **Storage:** 2-8°C (36-46°F). Protect from light, retain in carton or drug/diluent pack until time of use.

AMICAR

RX

aminocaproic acid (Xanodyne)

THERAPEUTIC CLASS: Monoamino carboxylic acid anti-fibrinolytic

INDICATIONS: To enhance hemostasis when fibrinolysis contributes to bleeding.

DOSAGE: *Adults:* IV: 16-20mL (4-5g) in 250mL diluent during 1st hr, then 4mL/hr (1g) in 50mL of diluent. PO: 5g during 1st hr, then 5mL (syr) or 1g (tabs) per hr. Continue therapy for 8 hrs or until bleeding is controlled.

HOW SUPPLIED: Inj: 250mg/mL [20mL]; Syrup: 1.25g/5mL; Tab: 500mg*, 1000mg* *scored

CONTRAINDICATIONS: Active intravascular clotting process, disseminated intravascular coagulation without concomitant heparin.

WARNINGS/PRECAUTIONS: Avoid in hematuria of upper urinary tract origin due to risk of intrarenal obstruction from glomerular capillary thrombosis or clots in renal pelvis and ureters. Skeletal muscle weakness with necrosis of muscle fibers reported after prolonged therapy. Consider cardiac muscle damage with skeletal myopathy. Avoid rapid IV infusion. Thrombophlebitis may occur. Contains benzyl alcohol; do not administer to neonates due to risk of fatal "gasping syndrome." Do not administer without a definite diagnosis of hyperfibrinolysis.

ADVERSE REACTIONS: Edema, headache, anaphylactoid reactions, injection site reactions, pain, bradycardia, hypotension, abdominal pain, diarrhea, nausea, vomiting, agranulocytosis, increased CPK, confusion, dyspnea, pruritus, tinnitus.

INTERACTIONS: Increased risk of thrombosis with Factor IX Complex concentrates, Anti-Inhibitor Coagulant concentrates.

PREGNANCY: Category C, caution in nursing.

MECHANISM OF ACTION: Monoamino carboxylic acid anti-fibrinolytic; fibrinolysis inhibitory effects are exerted principally by inhibition of plasminogen activators and, to a lesser extent, through antiplasmin activity.

PHARMACOKINETICS: Absorption: (PO) C_{max}=164mcg/mL; T_{max}=1.2 hrs. **Distribution:** (PO) V_d=23.1L; (IV) V_d=30L. **Metabolism:** Adipic acid (metabolite). **Elimination:** Renal: Urine (65% unchanged), (11% metabolite); $T_{1/2}$=2 hrs.

NURSING CONSIDERATIONS

Assessment: Assess for evidence of active intravascular clotting, proper diagnosis of hyperfibrinolysis (hyperplasminemia), pregnancy/nursing status, and possible drug interactions. Assess use in presence of hematuria of the upper urinary tract origin.

Monitoring: Monitor for signs/symptoms of subendocardial hemorrhages, fatty degeneration of the myocardium, skeletal muscle weakness with necrosis of muscle fibers (rhabdomyolysis, myoglobinuria, acute renal failure), cardiac muscle damage, thrombophlebitis, and neurological deficits (eg, hydrocephalus, cerebral ischemia, cerebral vasospasm). In patients with upper urinary tract bleeding, monitor for signs/symptoms of intrarenal obstruction (eg, glomerular capillary thrombosis, clots in renal pelvis and ureters). If used in pediatrics, monitor for "gasping syndrome" in neonates. Monitor CPK levels in patients on long-term therapy. Perform periodic monitoring to determine amount of fibrinolysis present.

Patient Counseling: Advise not to administer without definite diagnosis (laboratory finding indicative of hyperfibrinolysis). Instruct to contact physician if unusual muscle weakness or pain develops.

Administration: IV or Oral routes. IV: Use compatible intravenous vehicles (eg, Sterile Water for Injection, Sodium Chloride for Injection, 5% Dextrose or Ringer's Injection). Rapid IV administration may induce hypotension, bradycardia, and/or arrhythmias. **Storage:** 15-30°C (59-86°F).

AMIKACIN RX

amikacin sulfate (Various)

Potential for ototoxicity and nephrotoxicity. Neuromuscular blockade, respiratory blockade reported. Avoid potent diuretics and other neurotoxic, nephrotoxic, and ototoxic drugs.

THERAPEUTIC CLASS: Aminoglycoside

INDICATIONS: Short-term treatment of serious infections due to susceptible strains of gram-negative bacteria. Shown to be effective in bacterial septicemia; respiratory tract, bone/joint, CNS (including meningitis), skin and soft tissue, and intra-abdominal infections; burns and postoperative infections; complicated and recurrent urinary tract infections (UTI) due to susceptible strains of microorganisms.

DOSAGE: *Adults:* (IM/IV) 15mg/kg/day given q8h or q12h. Max: 15mg/kg/day. Heavier Wt Patients: Max: 1.5g/day. Recurrent Uncomplicated UTI: 250mg bid. Usual Duration: 7-10 days. D/C therapy if no response after 3-5 days. D/C if azotemia increases or if progressive decrease in urinary output occurs. Renal Impairment: Reduce dose.

Pediatrics: 15mg/kg/day given q8h or q12h. Newborns: LD: 10mg/kg. Maint: 7.5mg/kg q12h. Usual Duration: 7-10 days. D/C therapy if no response after 3-5 days. D/C if azotemia increases or if progressive decrease in urinary output occurs. Renal Impairment: Reduce dose.

HOW SUPPLIED: Inj: 50mg/mL, 250mg/mL

CONTRAINDICATIONS: History of serious toxic reactions to aminoglycosides.

WARNINGS/PRECAUTIONS: May aggravate muscle weakness; caution with muscular disorders (eg, myasthenia gravis, parkinsonism). May cause fetal harm in pregnancy. Contains sodium metabisulfite, allergic reactions may occur especially in asthmatics. Maintain adequate hydration. Assess kidney function before therapy, then daily.

ADVERSE REACTIONS: Ototoxicity, neuromuscular blockage, nephrotoxicity, skin rash, drug fever, headache, paresthesia, tremor, nausea, arthralgia, anemia, hypotension.

INTERACTIONS: Increased nephrotoxicity with cephalosporins. Significant mutual inactivation may occur with β-lactams (eg, penicillin, cephalosporins). Cross-allergenicity between aminoglycosides. Avoid potent diuretics (eg, ethacrynic acid, furosemide), bacitracin, cisplatin, amphotericin B, paromomycin, polymyxin B, colistin, vancomycin, other aminoglycosides, and other neurotoxic, nephrotoxic and ototoxic drugs. Increased risk of neuromuscular blockade and respiratory paralysis with anesthetics, neuromuscular blockers, or massive transfusions of citrate-anticoagulated blood.

PREGNANCY: Category D, not for use in nursing.

MECHANISM OF ACTION: Semi-synthetic aminoglycoside antibiotic derived from kanamycin.

PHARMACOKINETICS: Absorption: Rapidly absorbed after IM administration. (IV) C_{max}=38mcg/mL. **Distribution**: V_d=24L; plasma protein binding (0-11%); crosses placenta. **Elimination**: Urine; $T_{1/2}$ ≥2 hr; (IM) 91.9% at 8 hrs, 98.2% at 24 hrs; (IV) 84% at 9 hrs, 94% at 24 hrs.

NURSING CONSIDERATIONS

Assessment: Assess for pregnancy/nursing status, renal impairment, muscular disorders (eg, myasthenia gravis, parkinsonism) and for possible drug interactions. Assess renal function tests prior to and throughout therapy.

Monitoring: Periodic monitoring of urea, creatinine, CrCl, audiometric testing changes, 8th nerve function, serum concentrations of the drug and urine (specific gravity, proteins, presence of cells/casts). Monitor for signs/symptoms of nephrotoxicity, neurotoxicity (vestibular and permanent bilateral auditory ototoxicity, vertigo, numbness, skin tingling, muscle twitches, and convulsions), cochlear damage, neuromuscular blockade, respiratory paralysis, and CDAD.

Patient Counseling: Inform about potential risks/benefits of therapy and to report signs of ototoxicity (eg, dizziness, vertigo, tinnitus, roaring in the ears, and hearing loss). Notify physician if pregnant/nursing or planning to become pregnant. Inform that drug treats bacterial infections only. Take as prescribed.

Administration: IV, IM route. Obtain pretreatment body weight to calculate correct dosage. **Storage**: 20-25°C (68-77°F).

AMILORIDE
amiloride HCl (Various)

RX

THERAPEUTIC CLASS: K^+-sparing diuretic

INDICATIONS: Adjunct therapy in CHF or hypertension to help restore normal serum K^+ levels and to prevent hypokalemia.

DOSAGE: *Adults:* Initial: 5mg qd. Titrate: Increase to 10mg/day. If hyperkalemia persists, may increase to 15mg/day then to 20mg/day with careful monitoring. Take with food.

HOW SUPPLIED: Tab: 5mg

CONTRAINDICATIONS: Hyperkalemia, anuria, acute or chronic renal insufficiency, diabetic neuropathy, K^+-sparing agents (eg, diuretics), and K^+ supplements, K^+ salt substitutes, K^+-rich diet (except with severe hypokalemia).

WARNINGS/PRECAUTIONS: Risk of hyperkalemia (≥5.5mEq/L) especially with renal impairment, elderly, DM; monitor levels frequently. D/C if hyperkalemia occurs. Caution in severely ill in whom respiratory or metabolic acidosis may occur; monitor acid-base balance frequently. Hepatic encephalopathy reported with severe hepatic disease. Increased BUN reported. D/C at least 3 days before glucose tolerance test. Monitor electrolytes and renal function in DM.

ADVERSE REACTIONS: Headache, NV, anorexia, elevated serum potassium, diarrhea, muscle cramps, impotence.

INTERACTIONS: Increased risk of hyperkalemia with ACE inhibitors, angiotensin II receptor antagonists, indomethacin, cyclosporine, and tacrolimus. Risk of lithium toxicity. Decreased effects with NSAIDs. Hyponatremia and hypochloremia with other diuretics.

PREGNANCY: Category B, not for use in nursing.

MECHANISM OF ACTION: Antikaliuretic-diuretic; inhibits Na^+ reabsorption at tubules and collecting duct, decreasing potential of tubular lumen, reducing K^+ and H^+ secretion and excretion.

PHARMACOKINETICS: Absorption: T_{max}=3-4 hrs. **Elimination:** Urine (50%), feces (40%); $T_{1/2}$=6-9 hrs.

NURSING CONSIDERATIONS

Assessment: Assess for hyperkalemia, anuria, renal impairment, DM, possible drug interactions, metabolic or respiratory acidosis. Obtain baseline serum K^+ levels.

Monitoring: Monitor serum electrolytes, renal function, acid-base balance, and serum K^+ levels periodically. Monitor for signs/symptoms of electrolyte imbalance, hyperkalemia, hypersensitivity reactions, and renal dysfunction.

Patient Counseling: Instruct to take with food; avoid use of K^+ supplements or salt substitutes. Advise to seek medical attention if symptoms of hyperkalemia (paresthesias, muscle weakness, fatigue), electrolyte imbalance, or hypersensitivity reactions occur.

Administration: Oral route. **Storage:** 15-30°C (59-86°F).

AMILORIDE/HCTZ
amiloride HCl - hydrochlorothiazide (Various)

RX

THERAPEUTIC CLASS: K^+-sparing diuretic/thiazide diuretic

INDICATIONS: Treatment of hypertension or congestive heart failure if hypokalemia occurs on thiazides or kaliuretic diuretics alone, or if maintenance of normal serum K^+ levels is clinically important.

DOSAGE: *Adults:* Initial: 1 tab qd. Titrate: May increase to 2 tabs qd or in divided doses. Max: 2 tabs/day. May give intermittently once diuresis is achieved. Take with food.

HOW SUPPLIED: Tab: (Amiloride-HCTZ) 5mg-50mg* *scored

CONTRAINDICATIONS: Hyperkalemia, anuria, sulfonamide hypersensitivity, acute or chronic renal insufficiency, diabetic neuropathy. Concomitant K^+-sparing agents (eg, spironolactone, triamterene), K^+ supplements, salt substitutes, K^+-rich diet (except with severe hypokalemia).

WARNINGS/PRECAUTIONS: Risk of hyperkalemia (≥5.5mEq/L), especially with renal impairment or DM; d/c if hyperkalemia occurs. Monitor for fluid/electrolyte imbalance; hyponatremia and hypochloremia may occur. Caution in severely ill (risk of respiratory or metabolic acidosis). Increases BUN, cholesterol, and TG levels. D/C at least 3 days before glucose tolerance test. May precipitate gout or exacerbate SLE. May precipitate azotemia with renal disease.

ADVERSE REACTIONS: Nausea, anorexia, rash, headache, weakness, hyperkalemia, dizziness.

INTERACTIONS: May potentiate other antihypertensives. Risk of lithium toxicity. Increased risk of hyperkalemia with ACE inhibitors, angiotensin II receptor antagonists, indomethacin, cyclosporine, tacrolimus. May increase responsiveness to nondepolarizing muscle relaxants. May decrease response to norepinephrine. Antidiabetic agents may need adjustment. Alcohol, barbiturates, or narcotics may potentiate orthostatic hypotension. NSAIDs may decrease effects. Cholestyramine, colestipol impair absorption. ACTH, corticosteroids intensify electrolyte depletion.

PREGNANCY: Category B, not for use in nursing.

MECHANISM OF ACTION: Amiloride: Antikaliuretic-diuretic; inhibits Na^+ reabsorption at tubules and collecting duct, decreasing potential of tubular lumen, reducing K^+ and H^+ secretion and excretion. HCTZ: Thiazide diuretic; affects distal renal tubular mechanism of electrolyte reabsorption, increasing Na^+ and Cl^- excretion.

PHARMACOKINETICS: Absorption: Amiloride: T_{max}=3-4 hrs. **Distribution:** HCTZ: Crosses placenta; excreted in breast milk. **Elimination:** Amiloride: Urine (50%), feces (40%); $T_{1/2}$=6-9 hrs. HCTZ: Kidney (61%); $T_{1/2}$=5.6-14.8 hrs.

NURSING CONSIDERATIONS

Assessment: Assess for hyperkalemia, anuria, renal impairment, DM, systemic lupus erythematosus (SLE), sulfonamide hypersensitivity, possible drug interactions, metabolic or respiratory acidosis, and history of allergy or bronchial asthma. Obtain baseline serum K^+ levels.

Monitoring: Monitor serum electrolytes, renal function, acid-base balance, and serum K^+ levels periodically. Monitor for signs/symptoms of electrolyte imbalance, hyper/hypokalemia, hypersensitivity reactions, renal dysfunction, hypo/hyperglycemia, hyperuricemia or precipitation of gout, and exacerbation or activation of SLE.

Patient Counseling: Instruct to take with food; avoid use of K^+ supplements or salt substitutes. Seek medical attention if symptoms of hyperkalemia (paresthesias, muscle weakness, fatigue), electrolyte imbalance, or hypersensitivity reactions occur.

Administration: Oral route. **Storage:** 15-30°C (59-86°). Protect from light.

AMITIZA

RX

lubiprostone (Sucampo/Takeda)

THERAPEUTIC CLASS: Chloride channel activator

INDICATIONS: Treatment of chronic idiopathic constipation in adults. Treatment of the irritable bowel syndrome with constipation (IBS-C) in women ≥18 yrs.

DOSAGE: *Adults:* Chronic Idiopathic Constipation: 24mcg bid with food. IBS-C: 8mcg bid with food.

HOW SUPPLIED: Cap: 8mcg, 24mcg

CONTRAINDICATIONS: History of mechanical gastrointestinal obstruction.

WARNINGS/PRECAUTIONS: Potential to cause fetal loss; women who could become pregnant should have a negative pregnancy test prior to initiation of therapy and comply with effective contraceptive measures. May cause nausea. Do not prescribe to patients with severe diarrhea. Dyspnea reported. Confirm absence of mechanical GI obstruction prior to initiating therapy.

ADVERSE REACTIONS: Nausea, diarrhea, abdominal distention/pain/discomfort, flatulence, vomiting, loose stools, sinusitis, urinary/upper respiratory tract infections, headache, dizziness, peripheral edema, arthralgia.

PREGNANCY: Category C, not for use in nursing.

MECHANISM OF ACTION: Chloride channel activator; enhances chloride-rich intestinal fluid secretion, increasing motility in the intestine, thereby facilitating the passage of stool.

PHARMACOKINETICS: Absorption: (M3) C_{max}=41.5pg/mL, T_{max}=1.1 hrs, AUC=57.1pg•hr/mL. **Distribution:** Plasma protein binding (94%). **Metabolism:** Stomach, jejunum (biotransformation via carbonyl reductase). (Metabolite) M3. **Elimination:** (M3) $T_{1/2}$=0.9-1.4hrs.

NURSING CONSIDERATIONS

Assessment: Assess for known mechanical GI obstruction, severe diarrhea, and pregnancy status. Perform pregnancy test and thorough evaluation to confirm absence of obstruction (if symptoms suggestive of mechanical obstruction) prior to therapy.

Monitoring: Monitor for symptoms of hypersensitivity reactions and severe diarrhea.

Patient Counseling: Advise to take with food to reduce symptoms of nausea. Report severe nausea or diarrhea to physician.

Administration: Oral route. **Storage:** 25°C (77°F); excursions permitted to 15-30°C (59-86°F). Protect from extreme temperatures.

AMITRIPTYLINE RX

amitriptyline HCl (Various)

Antidepressants increased the risk of suicidal thinking and behavior (suicidality) in short-term studies in children, adolescents, and young adults with major depressive disorder (MDD) and other psychiatric disorders.

THERAPEUTIC CLASS: Tricyclic antidepressant

INDICATIONS: Treatment of depression, especially endogenous depression.

DOSAGE: *Adults:* PO: Initial: (Outpatient) 75mg/day in divided doses or 50-100mg qhs. (Inpatient) 100mg/day. Titrate: (Outpatient) Increase by 25-50mg qhs. (Inpatient) Increase to 200mg/day. Maint: 50-100mg qhs. Max: (Outpatient) 150mg/day. (Inpatient) 300mg/day. IM: Initial: 20-30mg qid. Elderly: 10mg tid and 20mg qhs.

HOW SUPPLIED: Inj: 10mg/mL; Tab: 10mg, 25mg, 50mg, 75mg, 100mg, 150mg

CONTRAINDICATIONS: MAOI use or within 14 days; acute recovery period following MI; concurrent cisapride.

WARNINGS/PRECAUTIONS: Caution with history of seizures, urinary retention, angle-closure glaucoma, increased IOP, hyperthyroidism, cardiovascular disorders, liver dysfunction. Increases symptoms with schizophrenia and bipolar disorder. D/C several weeks before elective surgery. May alter blood glucose levels.

ADVERSE REACTIONS: MI, stroke, seizure, paralytic ileus, urinary retention, constipation, blurred vision, dry mouth, hyperpyrexia, rash, bone marrow depression, testicular swelling, gynecomastia (male), breast enlargement (female), alopecia, edema.

INTERACTIONS: See Contraindications. May block antihypertensive effects of guanethidine. Potentiates other CNS depressants, alcohol, barbiturates. Increased levels with CYP2D6 inhibitors (eg, quinidine, cimetidine, SSRIs) and enzyme substrates (eg, phenothiazines, propafenone, flecainide). Avoid within 5 weeks of fluoxetine use. Caution with thyroid drugs. Delirium reported with disulfiram and ethchlorvynol. Paralytic ileus and hyperpyrexia with anticholinergics. Monitor with sympathomimetics and neuroleptics. Increased plasma levels with cimetidine.

PREGNANCY: Category C, not for use in nursing.

MECHANISM OF ACTION: Dibenzocycloheptadiene derivative; suspected to inhibit the membrane pump mechanism responsible for uptake of norepinephrine and serotonin in adrenergic and serotonergic neurons.

PHARMACOKINETICS: Absorption: Rapid. **Distribution:** Excreted in breast milk. **Metabolism:** N-demethylation and hydroxylation.

NURSING CONSIDERATIONS

Assessment: Assess if acute recovery period after MI, for bipolar disorder risk, history of mania, paranoia, seizures, unrecognized/history of schizophrenia, possible drug interactions, CVD, hyperthyroidism, IOP, narrow-angle glaucoma, urinary retention, hepatic impairment.

Monitoring: Periodically monitor LFTs, thyroid function tests, blood glucose, and CBC. Monitor for signs/symptoms of clinical worsening (suicidality, unusual changes in behavior), mania, cardiovascular events, increasing psychosis or paranoia, mydriasis, hypo/hyperglycemia, seizures, hepatic dysfunction, cognitive/motor impairment.

Patient Counseling: Advise to avoid alcohol. Seek medical attention for symptoms of mania, clinical worsening (suicidal ideation, unusual changes in behavior), cardiovascular events, increasing psychosis or paranoia, mydriasis, hypo/hyperglycemia, seizures, and discontinuation symptoms (irritability, agitation, dizziness, anxiety, headache, insomnia). Caution that drug may impair physical/mental abilities.

Administration: Oral route. **Storage:** 20-25°C (68-77°F). Dispense in tight, light-resistant container.

AMOXIL

amoxicillin (GlaxoSmithKline) **RX**

THERAPEUTIC CLASS: Semisynthetic ampicillin derivative

INDICATIONS: Treatment of infections of the ear, nose, throat, genitourinary tract, skin and skin structure, lower respiratory tract (LRTI); acute, uncomplicated gonorrhea due to susceptible (β-lactamase negative) strains of microorganisms. Combination therapy for *H.pylori* eradication to reduce the risk of duodenal ulcer recurrence.

DOSAGE: *Adults:* Ear/Nose/Throat/SSSI/GU: (Mild/Moderate) 500mg q12h or 250mg q8h. (Severe) 875mg q12h or 500mg q8h. LRTI: 875mg q12h or 500mg q8h. Gonorrhea: 3g as single dose. *H.pylori:* (Dual Therapy) 1g + 30mg lansoprazole, both tid x 14 days. (Triple Therapy) 1g + 30mg lansoprazole + 500mg clarithromycin, all q12h x 14 days. (Amoxicillin) CrCl 10-30mL/min: 250-500mg q12h. CrCl <10mL/min: 250-500mg q24h. Hemodialysis: 250-500mg or 250mg q24h, additional dose during and at end of dialysis.
Pediatrics: Neonates: ≤12 weeks: Max: 30mg/kg/day divided q12h. >3 months: Ear/Nose/Throat/SSSI/GU: (Mild/Moderate) 25mg/kg/day given q12h or 20mg/kg/day given q8h. (Severe): 45mg/kg/day given q12h or 40mg/kg/day given q8h. LRTI: 45mg/kg/day given q12h or 40mg/kg/day given q8h. Gonorrhea: (Prepubertal) 50mg/kg with 25mg/kg probenecid as single dose. (Not for <2yrs). >40kg: Dose as adult.

HOW SUPPLIED: (Amoxil) Cap: 500mg; Sus: 50mg/mL [30mL], 250mg/5mL [100mL, 150mL], 400mg/5mL [100mL]. (Generic) Cap: 250mg, 500mg; Sus: 125mg/5mL [80mL, 100mL, 150mL], 200mg/5mL [50mL, 75mL, 100mL], 250mg/5mL [80mL, 100mL, 150mL], 400mg/5mL [50mL, 75mL, 100mL]; Tab: 500mg, 875mg; Tab, Chewable: 125mg, 200mg, 250mg, 400mg

WARNINGS/PRECAUTIONS: Serious, sometimes fatal, hypersensitivity reactions reported with PCN therapy. *Clostridium difficile*-associated diarrhea has been reported. Monitor renal, hepatic, and blood with prolonged use. The 200mg and 400mg chewable tabs contain phenylalanine.

ADVERSE REACTIONS: N/V, diarrhea, pseudomembranous colitis, hypersensitivity reactions, blood dyscrasias, superinfection (prolonged use).

INTERACTIONS: Increased levels with probenecid. Chloramphenicol, macrolides, sulfonamides, tetracyclines may interfere with bactericidal effects. False (+) for urine glucose with Clinitest, Benedict's or Fehling's solution.

PREGNANCY: Category B, caution in nursing.

MECHANISM OF ACTION: Ampicillin analog; has broad-spectrum bactericidal activity against susceptible organisms during active multiplication; acts through inhibition of biosynthesis of cell-wall mucopeptide.

PHARMACOKINETICS: Absorption: Rapid. Cap (500mg): T_{max}=1-2 hrs. Tab (875mg): C_{max}=13.8mcg/mL, AUC=35.4mcg•hr/mL. Oral suspension (400mg): C_{max}=5.92mcg/mL, AUC=17.1mcg•hr/mL. Chewable tab (400mg): C_{max}=5.18mcg/mL, AUC=17.9mcg•hr/mL. Oral suspension (125-250mg) T_{max}=1-2 hrs. **Distribution:** Plasma protein binding, (20%). Diffuses to spinal fluid and brain only if meninges inflamed. **Elimination:** Urine (unchanged); $T_{1/2}$=61.3 min.

NURSING CONSIDERATIONS

Assessment: Assess for history of allergic reaction (to PCNs, cephalosporins, or other allergens), infectious mononucleosis, phenylketonurics, pregnancy/nursing status, and possible drug interactions.

Monitoring: Periodically monitor renal, hepatic, and hematopoietic function. Perform serologic test for syphilis at diagnosis of gonorrhea and after 3 months of treatment with amoxicillin. Monitor for serious anaphylactic reactions, erythematous skin rash, development of drug resistance or superinfection with mycotic or bacterial pathogen, signs/symptoms of *Clostridium difficile*-associated diarrhea (may range from mild diarrhea to fatal colitis). Monitor for false (+) reactions for urinary glucose test if Clinitest, Benedict's/Fehling's Solutions are used, and transient decrease in plasma concentration of total conjugated estriol, estriol-glucuronide, conjugated estrone and estradiol if given to pregnant women.

Patient Counseling: Inform drug treats bacterial, not viral, infections. Take exactly as directed; skipping doses or not completing full course may decrease effectiveness and increase resistance. Inform about potential benefits/risks; notify physician if watery/bloody diarrhea (with/without stomach cramps and fever) develop (may occur as late as 2 months after treatment). Notify if pregnant/nursing.

Administration: Oral route. **Storage:** ≤20°C (68°F) for caps and (250mg) unreconstituted powder; ≤25°C (77°F) for unreconstituted powder (200-400mg), chewable tabs, and tabs. Store in tight container.

AMPHOCIN

RX

amphotericin B (Pharmacia & Upjohn)

Treatment primarily for progressive and potentially life-threatening fungal infections. Not for noninvasive fungal infections (eg, oral thrush, vaginal and esophageal candidiasis) in patients with normal neutrophil counts. Exercise caution to prevent inadvertent OD; verify product name and dose if dose >1.5mg/kg.

THERAPEUTIC CLASS: Polyene antifungal

INDICATIONS: Treatment of potentially life-threatening fungal infections including aspergillosis, cryptococcosis, North American blastomycosis, systemic candidiasis, coccidioidomycosis, histoplasmosis, zygomycosis, sporotrichosis, and infections due to susceptible species of *Conidiobolus* and *Basidiobolus*. May be useful for treatment of American mucocutaneous leishmaniasis.

DOSAGE: *Adults:* Administer by slow IV infusion. Test dose: 1mg in 20mL of D5W over 20-30 min. Treatment: Initial: 0.25mg/kg. Severe Infection: Initial: 0.3mg/kg. Give smaller initial dose if impaired cardio-renal function or severe reaction to test dose. Titrate: May increase by 5-10mg/day, depending on cardio-renal status, up to 0.5-0.7mg/kg/day. Max: 1mg/kg/day or 1.5mg/kg/day when given on alternate days. Sporotrichosis: Therapy has ranged up to 9 months with total dose up to 2.5g. Aspergillosis: Has been treated up to 11 months with total dose up to 3.6g. Rhinocerebral Phycomycosis: Cumulative dose of at least 3g is recommended. Whenever therapy is interrupted for >7 days, resume with lowest dose.

HOW SUPPLIED: Inj: 50mg

WARNINGS/PRECAUTIONS: Acute reactions (eg, fever, shaking chills, hypotension, anorexia, NV, tachypnea) 1-3 hrs after starting infusion may occur. Avoid rapid infusion. Caution with renal impairment. Decreased risk of nephrotoxicity with hydration and sodium repletion. Acute pulmonary reactions reported with leukocyte infusions; separate infusions and monitor pulmonary function. Leukoencephalopathy reported. Monitor renal function, LFTs, electrolytes, blood counts, Hgb.

ADVERSE REACTIONS: Fever, malaise, weight loss, hypotension, tachypnea, anorexia, NV, diarrhea, dyspepsia, normochromic normocytic anemia, injection site pain, renal dysfunction.

INTERACTIONS: Antineoplastics may potentiate renal toxicity, bronchospasm, hypotension. Corticosteroids and corticotropin may potentiate hypokalemia. May increase flucytosine toxicity. Caution with imidazoles (eg, ketoconazole, clotrimazole, miconazole, fluconazole). Increased risk of renal toxicity with nephrotoxic drugs (eg, aminoglycosides, cyclosporine, pentamidine). May enhance curariform effect of skeletal muscle relaxants (eg, tubocurarine) or digitalis toxicity with hypokalemia.

PREGNANCY: Category B, not for use in nursing.

MECHANISM OF ACTION: Fungistatic or fungicidal; binds to sterols in cell membranes of susceptible fungi, resulting in change in membrane permeability, allowing leakage of intracellular components.

PHARMACOKINETICS: Absorption: C_{max} = approximately 0.5-2mcg/mL. **Distribution:** Plasma protein binding (>90%). **Elimination:** Renal excretion. Urine (approximately 40%, urinary output over 7-day period); $T_{1/2}$ = approximately 15 days.

NURSING CONSIDERATIONS

Assessment: Assess cultures, renal function, hematological effects (normocytic anemia), hepatic function, and possible drug interactions.

Monitoring: Monitor for signs/symptoms of acute reaction (fever, shaking, chills, hypotension, tachypnea), serum electrolytes (Mg, K+), liver function, frequent renal function tests, Hgb, CBC, pulmonary function. Monitor temperature, pulse, respiration, and BP every 30 min for 2-4 hrs after initial dose.

Patient Counseling: Advise to seek medical attention if symptoms of acute reactions (fever, shaking, chills, respiratory symptoms) occur. Maintain adequate hydration.

Administration: IV: 1) Reconstitute (add 10mL of Sterile Water for Inj, USP into vial). 2) Shake vial until sol is clear. 3) Dilute using 5% Dextrose Inj, USP. **Storage:** Refrigerate 2-8°C (36-46°F); protect against exposure to light. The concentrate may be stored in dark, at room temperature, for 1 week with minimal loss of potency and clarity. Unused material should be discarded. Protect from light during administration.

AMPHOTEC RX

amphotericin B cholesteryl sulfate (Three Rivers)

THERAPEUTIC CLASS: Polyene antifungal

INDICATIONS: Treatment of invasive aspergillosis in patients with renal impairment, unacceptable toxicity, or previous failure to amphotericin deoxycholate.

DOSAGE: *Adults:* Test Dose: Infuse small amount over 15-30 min. Treatment: 3-4mg/kg/day IV at 1mg/kg/hr.
Pediatrics: Test Dose: Infuse small amount over 15-30 min. Treatment: 3-4mg/kg/day IV at 1mg/kg/hr.

HOW SUPPLIED: Inj: 50mg, 100mg

WARNINGS/PRECAUTIONS: Anaphylaxis may occur. D/C if severe respiratory distress occurs. Acute reactions (eg, fever, shaking chills, hypotension, nausea, tachypnea) 1-3 hrs after starting infusion. Monitor renal/hepatic function, electrolytes, CBC, PT during therapy.

ADVERSE REACTIONS: Chills, fever, headache, hypotension, tachycardia, HTN, nausea, vomiting, thrombocytopenia, increased creatinine, hypokalemia, dyspnea, hypoxia.

INTERACTIONS: Antineoplastics may potentiate renal toxicity, bronchospasm, hypotension. Corticosteroids and corticotropin may potentiate hypokalemia. May increase flucytosine toxicity. Caution with imidazoles (eg, ketoconazole, clotrimazole, miconazole, fluconazole). Increased risk of renal toxicity with nephrotoxic drugs (eg, aminoglycosides, cyclosporine, pentamidine). May enhance curariform effect of skeletal muscle relaxants (eg, tubocurarine) or digitalis toxicity with hypokalemia.

PREGNANCY: Category B, not for use in nursing.

MECHANISM OF ACTION: Polyene antibiotic; binds to sterols (primarily ergosterol) in cell membranes of sensitive fungi, with subsequent leakage of intracellular contents and cell death. Also binds to cholesterol in mammalian cell membranes, which may account for human toxicity.

PHARMACOKINETICS: Administration: Variable doses resulted in altered parameters. **Absorption:** 3mg/kg/day: AUC=29µg/mL•hr, C_{max}=2.6µg/mL. 4mg/kg/day: AUC=36µg/mL•hr, C_{max}=2.9µg/mL. **Distribution:** 3mg/kg/day: V_d=3.8L/kg. 4mg/kg/day: V_d=4.1L/kg. **Metabolism:** Unknown. **Elimination:** 3mg/kg/day: $T_{1/2}$=27.5 hrs. 4mg/kg/day: $T_{1/2}$=28.2 hrs.

NURSING CONSIDERATIONS

Assessment: Assess cultures, renal function, and possible drug interactions.

Monitoring: Monitor for acute infusion reactions (fevers, chills, hypoxia, hypotension), hepatic function, serum electrolytes, CBC, PT, and possible drug interactions.

Patient Counseling: Seek medical attention if symptoms of acute reaction occur (fever, chills, respiratory symptoms).

Administration: IV route. Infusion time may be shortened to 2 hrs for patients who show no evidence of intolerance or infusion-related reactions. If reaction occurs or if infusion is not tolerated, infusion time may be extended. Do not reconstitute lyophilized powder with saline or dextrose solutions, or admix the reconstituted liquid with saline or electrolytes. Do not mix infusion admixture with other drugs. If using an existing IV line, flush with 5% Dextrose prior and following infusion, or administer via a separate line. 1) Reconstitute: Add Sterile Water for Inj, USP to vial. If using 50mg/vial, add 10mL of Sterile Water. If using 100mg/vial, add 20mL of Sterile Water. 2) Shake vial until all solids have dissolved. 3) Further dilute using 5% Dextrose Inj, USP. **Storage:** Unopened vial: 15-30°C (59-86°F). Store in unopened carton. Reconstituted: Refrigerate 2-8°C (36-46°F). Use within 24 hrs, do not freeze. Further diluted with 5% Dextrose: Refrigerate 2-8°C. Use within 24 hrs.

AMPICILLIN INJECTION RX

ampicillin sodium (Various)

THERAPEUTIC CLASS: Semisynthetic penicillin derivative

INDICATIONS: Treatment of respiratory tract, urinary tract, and GI infections, bacterial meningitis, septicemia, and endocarditis caused by susceptible strains of microorganisms.

DOSAGE: *Adults:* IM/IV: Respiratory Tract/Soft Tissues: ≥40kg: 250-500mg q6h. <40kg: 25-50mg/kg/day given q6-8h. GI/GU: ≥40kg: 500mg q6h. <40kg: 50mg/kg/day given q6-8h. Urethritis (Caused by *N.gonorrhoeae* in Males): 500mg q8-12h for 2 doses; may retreat if needed. Bacterial Meningitis: 150-200mg/kg/day given q3-4h. Septicemia: 150-200mg/kg/day IV for 3 days, continue with IM q3-4h. Treatment of all infections should be continued for a minimum of 48-72 hrs after becoming asymptomatic. Minimum of 10 days treatment recommended for Group A β-hemolytic streptococci. *Pediatrics:* Bacterial Meningitis: 150-200mg/kg/day given q3-4h. Septicemia: 150-200mg/kg/day IV given q3-4h for 3 days, continue with IM q3-4h. Treatment of all infections should be continued for a minimum of 48-72 hrs after becoming asymptomatic. Minimum of 10 days treatment recommended for Group A β-hemolytic streptococci.

HOW SUPPLIED: Inj: 250mg, 500mg, 1g, 2g

WARNINGS/PRECAUTIONS: Serious, sometimes fatal, hypersensitivity reactions reported with PCN therapy. Caution with renal impairment. Cross-sensitivity with other β-lactams. May cause skin rash, especially in mononucleosis; avoid use. Pseudomembranous colitis reported. May result in overgrowth of nonsusceptible organisms.

ADVERSE REACTIONS: Headache, N/V, oral and vaginal candidiasis, diarrhea, urticaria, allergic reactions, anaphylaxis, serum sickness-like reactions, exfoliative dermatitis.

INTERACTIONS: Potentiated by probenecid. May decrease effects of oral contraceptives. Allopurinol increases incidence of skin rash.

PREGNANCY: Category B, caution in nursing.

MECHANISM OF ACTION: Penicillin derivative; bactericidal against gram-positive and gram-negative organisms.

PHARMACOKINETICS: Distribution: Plasma protein binding (20%), found in breast milk. Penetrates to CSF and brain only if meninges are inflamed. **Elimination:** Urine (unchanged).

NURSING CONSIDERATIONS

Assessment: Assess for hypersensitivity/allergic reactions to PCNs/cephalosporins or other allergens, infectious mononucleosis, pregnancy/nursing status, and possible drug interactions.

Monitoring: Monitor fetal anaphylactoid reactions, development of superinfection, drug resistance, and skin rash. Perform periodic monitoring of renal, hepatic and hematopoietic function. Monitor urinary false-positive glucose reactions if Clinitest, Benedict's, or Fehling's Solutions are used.

Patient Counseling: Inform that drug treats bacterial, not viral, infections. Instruct to take exactly as directed to prevent drug resistance. Notify if pregnant/nursing.

Administration: IM/IV routes. Administer within 1 hr after preparation. Slow direct IV over at least 10-15 min to avoid convulsive seizures. **Storage:** 20-25°C (68-77°F).

AMPICILLIN ORAL RX

ampicillin (Various)

THERAPEUTIC CLASS: Semisynthetic penicillin derivative

INDICATIONS: Genitourinary tract (GU) infections, including gonorrhea, respiratory and GI tract infections, and meningitis.

DOSAGE: *Adults:* GI/GU: 500mg qid. Use larger doses in chronic or severe infections. Gonorrhea: 3.5g single dose with 1g probenecid. Respiratory: 250mg qid. Treat minimum 48-72 hrs after eradication. Treat minimum 10 days for hemolytic strains of strep.
Pediatrics: >20kg: GI/GU: 500mg qid. Respiratory: 250mg qid. ≤20kg: GI/GU: 25mg/kg qid. Respiratory: 50mg/kg/day given tid-qid. Do not exceed adult doses. Use larger doses in chronic or severe infections. Treat minimum 48-72 hrs after eradication. Treat minimum 10 days for hemolytic strains of strep.

HOW SUPPLIED: Cap: 250mg, 500mg; Sus: 125mg/5mL, 250mg/5mL [100mL, 200mL]

CONTRAINDICATIONS: Infections caused by penicillinase-producing organisms.

WARNINGS/PRECAUTIONS: Possible cross-sensitivity with cephalosporins. Pseudomembranous colitis and anaphylatic reactions may occur.

ADVERSE REACTIONS: Stomatitis, NV, diarrhea, rash, SGOT elevation, blood dyscrasias, eosinophilia, thrombocytopenic purpura, hypersensitivity reactions, superinfection (prolonged use).

INTERACTIONS: Increased risk of rash with allopurinol. Bacteriostatic antibiotics (eg, chloramphenicol, erythromycins, sulfonamides or tetracyclines) may interfere with bactericidal activity. May decrease the effectiveness of oral contraceptives. Increased blood levels with probenecid.

PREGNANCY: Category B, not for use in nursing.

MECHANISM OF ACTION: Penicillin derivative; bactericidal against gram-positive and gram-negative organisms.

PHARMACOKINETICS: Absorption: Well-absorbed; (500mg Cap) C_{max}=3mcg/mL; (250mg Sus) C_{max}=2.3mcg/mL. **Distribution:** Plasma protein binding (20%). **Elimination:** Urine (unchanged).

NURSING CONSIDERATIONS

Assessment: Assess for previous hypersensitivity reactions to PCNs and possible drug interactions. Conduct susceptibility testing as guide to therapy.

Monitoring: Monitor for hypersensitivity reactions, pseudomembranous colitis, overgrowth of nonsusceptible organisms with prolonged use, and renal/hepatic/hematopoietic systems periodically with prolonged therapy. Upon completion, obtain cultures to determine organism eradication.

Patient Counseling: Instruct to notify physician of history of hypersensitivity to PCNs/cephalosporins. Inform diabetics to consult with physician prior to changing diet or dosage of diabetic medication. Instruct to take with full glass of water, 1/2 hr before or 2 hrs after meals. Take exactly as directed; skipping doses or not completing full course decreases effectiveness and increases resistance. D/C and notify physician if side effects occur. Inform that therapy only treats bacterial, not viral, infections.

Administration: Oral route. **Storage:** 20-25°C (68-77°F). Dispense in a tight container.

AMRIX

RX

cyclobenzaprine HCl (Cephalon)

THERAPEUTIC CLASS: Skeletal muscle relaxant (central-acting)

INDICATIONS: Adjunct to rest and physical therapy to relieve muscle spasm associated with acute, painful musculoskeletal conditions. Use for only short periods of time (up to 2-3 weeks).

DOSAGE: *Adults:* Usual: 15mg qd. Titrate: May increase to 30mg qd if needed. Use for longer than 2-3 weeks not recommended.

HOW SUPPLIED: Cap, Extended-Release: 15mg, 30mg

CONTRAINDICATIONS: MAOI use during or within 14 days. Hyperpyretic crisis seizures and deaths associated with concomitant use of cyclobenzaprine (or structurally similar to TCAs) and MAOIs reported. Acute recovery phase of MI, arrhythmias, heart block conduction disturbances, CHF, hyperthyroidism.

WARNINGS/PRECAUTIONS: Avoid in hepatic impairment and elderly patients. Caution with history of urinary retention, angle-closure glaucoma, increased IOP, and use of anticholinergic medication. May impair mental and/or physical performance.

ADVERSE REACTIONS: Drowsiness, dry mouth, dizziness, somnolence, headache.

INTERACTIONS: Contraindicated with MAOIs. Enhances effects of alcohol, barbiturates and other CNS depressants. TCAs may block antihypertensive action of guanethidine and similar compounds and may enhance seizure risk with tramadol.

PREGNANCY: Category B, caution in nursing.

MECHANISM OF ACTION: Skeletal muscle relaxant; acts primarily within the CNS at brain stem as opposed to spinal cord level, although overlapping action on the latter may contribute to its overall skeletal muscle relaxant activity; suggested to reduce tonic somatic motor activity influencing both gamma and α motor systems.

PHARMACOKINETICS: Absorption: C_{max}=8.3ng/mL, T_{max}=8.1 hrs, AUC=354.1ng•h/mL; see Full PI for more detailed information. **Metabolism:** Extensive; via CYP3A4, 1A2, and 2D6 through N-demethylation pathway. **Elimination:** Urine (glucuronides); $T_{1/2}$=33.4 hrs.

NURSING CONSIDERATIONS

Assessment: Assess for hepatic impairment, seizures, hyperthyroidism, urinary retention, angle-closure glaucoma, IOP, recent MI, arrhythmias, heart block, CHF, alcohol intake, pregnancy/nursing status, and possible drug interactions (eg, MAOIs if concomitant use or within 14 days after d/c, and anticholinergic medications).

Monitoring: Monitor for cardiac arrhythmias, sinus tachycardia, MI, stroke, IOP, CBC, and LFTs.

Patient Counseling: Caution against performing hazardous tasks (eg, operating machinery/driving); avoid alcohol and other CNS depressants. Notify if pregnant/nursing.

Administration: Oral route; take at same time each day. **Storage:** 25°C (77°F); excursions permitted to 15-30°C (59-86°F); in tight, light-resistant container. Keep out of reach of children.

Anaprox DS — RX

naproxen sodium (Roche Labs)

> **NSAIDs may cause an increased risk of serious cardiovascular thrombotic events, MI, stroke, and serious GI adverse events including bleeding, ulceration, and perforation of the stomach or intestines. Contraindicated for the treatment of perioperative pain in the setting of coronary artery bypass graft (CABG) surgery.**

OTHER BRAND NAMES: Anaprox (Roche Labs)

THERAPEUTIC CLASS: NSAID

INDICATIONS: Relief of signs and symptoms of rheumatoid arthritis (RA), osteoarthritis (OA), ankylosing spondylitis, juvenile arthritis (JA), tendinitis, bursitis, and acute gout. Management of pain and primary dysmenorrhea.

DOSAGE: *Adults:* RA/OA/AS: 275mg bid or 550mg bid. Max: 1650mg/day. Acute Gout: 825mg followed by 275mg q8h. Pain/Dysmenorrhea/Tendinitis/Bursitis: 550mg followed by 550mg q12h or 275mg q6-8h prn. Max: 1375mg on Day 1, then 1100mg/day.

HOW SUPPLIED: (Anaprox) Tab: 275mg; (Anaprox DS) Tab: 550mg* *scored

CONTRAINDICATIONS: History of ASA or NSAID allergy that caused symptoms of asthma, rhinitis, nasal polyps, and hypotension. Treatment of perioperative pain in the setting of CABG surgery.

WARNINGS/PRECAUTIONS: May lead to onset of new HTN or worsening of pre-existing HTN; monitor BP closely. Fluid retention, edema, and peripheral edema reported; caution with fluid retention, HTN, or heart failure. Renal papillary necrosis and other renal injury reported after long-term use. Not recommended for use with advanced renal disease; if therapy must be initiated, monitor renal function. Anaphylactoid reactions may occur. May cause serious skin adverse events (eg, exfoliative dermatitis, Stevens-Johnson syndrome, and toxic epidermal necrolysis). Avoid in late pregnancy; may cause premature closure of ductus arteriosus. Monitor Hgb levels with long-term therapy if initial Hgb ≤10g. Monitor for visual changes or disturbances. May cause elevations of LFTs; d/c if liver disease develops or systemic manifestations occur. Caution with high doses in chronic alcoholic liver disease and elderly. Anemia may occur; with long-term use, monitor Hgb/Hct if signs or symptoms of anemia develop. May inhibit platelet aggregation and prolong bleeding time; monitor with coagulation disorders. Caution with asthma and avoid with ASA-sensitive asthma.

ADVERSE REACTIONS: Edema, drowsiness, dizziness, constipation, heartburn, abdominal pain, nausea, headache, tinnitus, dyspnea, pruritus, skin eruptions, ecchymoses.

INTERACTIONS: Avoid other products containing naproxen. Decreased plasma levels with ASA. May reduce tubular secretion of methotrexate; monitor for toxicity. May diminish antihypertensive effect and potentiate renal disease with ACE inhibitors. May reduce natriuretic effect of furosemide and thiazides. May increase lithium levels; monitor for toxicity. Synergistic effects on GI bleeding with warfarin. Observe for dose adjustment with hydantoins, sulfonamides, or sulfonylureas. May reduce antihypertensive effects of propranolol and other β-blockers. Probenecid may increase half-life.

PREGNANCY: Category C, not for use in nursing.

MECHANISM OF ACTION: NSAIDs; unknown, suspected to inhibit prostaglandin synthetase.

PHARMACOKINETICS: Absorption: Rapid and complete. Bioavailability (95%). T_{max}=1-2 hrs. **Distribution:** V_d=0.16 L/kg; plasma protein binding (>99%); excreted in breast milk. **Metabolism:** Hepatic, metabolite (6-O-desmethyl naproxen). **Elimination:** Kidneys, urine (95%), feces (≤3%), $T_{1/2}$=12-17 hrs.

NURSING CONSIDERATIONS

Assessment: Assess for history of asthma, cardiovascular disease (pre-existing HTN, CHF) or risk factors for disease, fluid retention, edema, cardiovascular thrombotic events, MI, stroke, CABG surgery, pregnancy status, risk factors for GI events (bleeding, ulceration, perforation), possible drug interactions, renal/hepatic dysfunction.

Monitoring: Monitor BP, CBC, LFTs, renal function, and chemistries periodically. Monitor for signs/symptoms of GI events (bleeding, ulceration, perforation), CV thrombotic events, CHF, HTN, salt depletion, renal/liver dysfunction.

Patient Counseling: Seek medical attention if symptoms of hepatotoxicity (nausea, fatigue, pruritus), anaphylactic reaction (difficulty breathing, swelling of face/throat), hypersensitivity reaction (rash), CV events (chest pain, SOB, weakness, slurring of speech), GI ulceration and bleeding (epigastric pain, dyspepsia, melena, hematemesis), weight gain, or edema occur. Inform of pregnancy risks. Caution may impair mental/physical abilities if experience drowsiness, dizziness, vertigo, or depression during therapy.

Administration: Oral route. **Storage:** 15-30°C (59-86°F) in well-closed containers.

ANCOBON
flucytosine (Valeant)

RX

Extreme caution with renal dysfunction. Monitor hematologic, renal, and hepatic status closely.

THERAPEUTIC CLASS: 5-fluorocytosine antifungal

INDICATIONS: Treatment of septicemia, endocarditis, and urinary tract infections caused by *Candida*. Treatment of meningitis and pulmonary infection caused by *Cryptococcus*.

DOSAGE: *Adults:* 50-150mg/kg/day given q6h. Renal Impairment: Reduce initial dose. Take a few caps over 15 min to reduce nausea/vomiting.

HOW SUPPLIED: Cap: 250mg, 500mg

WARNINGS/PRECAUTIONS: Caution with renal dysfunction and bone marrow depression. Bone marrow depression can be irreversible and fatal.

ADVERSE REACTIONS: Myocardial toxicity, chest pain, dyspnea, rash, pruritus, urticaria, photosensitivity, NV, jaundice, renal failure, pyrexia, crystalluria, anemia, leukopenia, eosinophilia, thrombocytopenia, ataxia, hearing loss, neuropathy.

INTERACTIONS: Antagonized by cytosine. Drugs that impair glomerular filtration may prolong half-life. Antifungal synergism with polyene antibiotics (eg, amphotericin B).

PREGNANCY: Category C, not for use in nursing.

MECHANISM OF ACTION: Antifungal agent not established; metabolized to 5-fluorouracil by entering the fungal organism via cytosine permease. The 5-fluorouracil is then incorporated into the fungal RNA where it inhibits synthesis of both RNA and DNA, inhibiting fungal growth, leading to fungal death.

PHARMACOKINETICS: Administration: Absolute bioavailability (78%-89%); C_{max}=30-40μg/mL; T_{max}=2 hrs. **Distribution:** Penetrates blood-brain barrier. Clinically significant amounts found in CSF. **Metabolism:** α-fluro-β-ureido-propionic acid (metabolite). **Elimination:** Renal; Urine (90%), feces (small amount); $T_{1/2}$=2.4-4.8 hrs.

NURSING CONSIDERATIONS

Assessment: Assess use with impaired renal function, history of bone marrow depression, or hematologic disease. Assess serum electrolytes and hematologic and renal function prior to treatment.

Monitoring: Monitor blood concentrations of drug in patients with renal impairment. Monitor hematologic (leukocyte and thrombocyte count) function, renal function (Jaffe reaction), and hepatic (alkaline phosphatase, SGOT, and SGPT) status.

Patient Counseling: Counsel to notify physician of all other medications being taken. Counsel females to avoid nursing. If nausea or vomiting develops, divide dosage and administer over a 15-min period.

Administration: PO. **Storage:** 25°C (77°F); excursions permitted to 15-30°C (59-86°F).

ANDRODERM
testosterone (Watson)

CIII

THERAPEUTIC CLASS: Androgen

INDICATIONS: Testosterone replacement therapy in males due to primary or secondary hypogonadism.

DOSAGE: *Adults:* Initial: 5mg/day. Maint: 2.5mg-7.5mg/day. Apply patch nightly to intact skin of back, abdomen, upper arm or thigh. Rotate sites; avoid same site for 7 days. Do not apply to scrotum or oily, damaged, irritated areas. May apply 2 patches at same time.
Pediatrics: ≥15 yrs: Initial: 5mg/day. Maint: 2.5mg-7.5mg/day. Apply patch

nightly to intact skin of back, abdomen, upper arm or thigh. Rotate sites; avoid same site for 7 days. Do not apply to scrotum or oily, damaged, irritated areas. May apply 2 patches at same time.

HOW SUPPLIED: Patch: 2.5mg/24 hrs [60[s]], 5mg/24 hrs [30[s]]

CONTRAINDICATIONS: Breast or prostate cancer in men. Women.

WARNINGS/PRECAUTIONS: Prolonged use is associated with serious hepatic effects. Increased risk for prostatic hyperplasia/carcinoma in elderly. Risk of edema with pre-existing cardiac, renal, or hepatic disease; d/c if edema occurs. Risk of virilization of female sex partner. Monitor LFTs, Hgb, Hct, PSA, cholesterol, lipids.

ADVERSE REACTIONS: Gynecomastia, pruritus/erythema/vesicles/blister at application site, prostate abnormalities, headache, depression.

INTERACTIONS: May potentiate effects of anticoagulants, oxyphenbutazone. May decrease blood glucose and insulin requirements in diabetics. Pretreatment with ointments may reduce testosterone absorption.

PREGNANCY: Category X, not for use in nursing.

MECHANISM OF ACTION: Endogenous androgen; responsible for normal growth and development of male sex organs and for maintenance of secondary sex characteristics.

PHARMACOKINETICS: Absorption: C_{max}=753ng/dL; T_{max}=7.9 hrs. **Distribution:** SHBG and albumin binding. **Metabolism:** Liver, estradiol, and DHT (major metabolite). **Elimination:** (IM) Urine (90% glucuronide and sulfate conjugates), feces (6% unconjugated); $T_{1/2}$=71 min.

NURSING CONSIDERATIONS

Assessment: Assess for breast or prostate carcinoma, cardiac or renal/hepatic disease, pregnancy/nursing status of female partner, and possible drug interactions.

Monitoring: Periodically monitor Hgb, Hct, LFTs, PSA, cholesterol and HDL, serum testosterone levels after initiation of therapy. Monitor for signs/symptoms of hypersensitivity reactions, edema with/without CHF, gynecomastia, prostatic hyperplasia/carcinoma in geriatrics.

Patient Counseling: Advise not to apply to the scrotum or over a bony prominence or any part of the body that could be subject to prolonged pressure during sleep or sitting. Inform to contact physician if notice changes in body hair distribution, increase in acne, virilization of female partner, too frequent or persistent erections, changes in skin color, ankle swelling, unexplained NV, hypersensitivity reactions.

Administration: Transdermal patch system. The adhesive side of the system should be applied to a clean, dry area of the skin on the back, abdomen, upper arms or thighs. Rotate application site with an interval of 7 days between applications to the same site. **Storage:** 25° (77°F); excursions permitted to 15-30°C (59-86°F). Do not store outside pouch provided.

ANDROGEL

CIII

testosterone (Unimed)

THERAPEUTIC CLASS: Androgen

INDICATIONS: Testosterone replacement in males with primary hypogonadism or hypogonadotrophic hypogonadism.

DOSAGE: *Adults:* Apply 5g qd to clean, dry, intact skin of shoulders and upper arms and/or abdomen. Allow to dry prior to dressing. Titrate: May increase to 7.5g qd, then 10g qd if response not achieved. Do not apply to scrotum/genitals. Pump: 4 actuations (5g), 6 actuations (7.5g), 8 actuations (10g).

HOW SUPPLIED: Gel: 1% [2.5g, 5g pkts; 75g pump]

CONTRAINDICATIONS: Breast or prostate carcinoma in men. Women. Pregnant women should avoid skin contact with application sites in men.

WARNINGS/PRECAUTIONS: Prolonged use is associated with serious hepatic effects. Increased risk for prostatic hyperplasia/carcinoma in elderly. Risk of edema with pre-existing cardiac, renal, or hepatic disease; d/c if edema occurs. Risk of virilization of female sex partner. Monitor LFTs, Hgb, Hct, PSA, cholesterol, lipids. May potentiate sleep apnea. Transfer of testosterone can occur with skin to skin contact. Gels are flammable; avoid fire, flame, or smoking during use.

ADVERSE REACTIONS: Acne, application site reaction, abnormal lab tests, prostatic disorders.

INTERACTIONS: May decrease blood glucose and insulin requirements. Concurrent use with ACTH or corticosteroids may enhance edema. Changes in anticoagulant activity may be seen with androgens, increase frequency of monitoring INR and PT with concomitant anticoagulants.

PREGNANCY: Category X, not for use in nursing.

MECHANISM OF ACTION: Endogenous androgen; responsible for normal growth and development of male sex organs and for maintenance of secondary sex characteristics.

PHARMACOKINETICS: Absorption: 10% absorbed systemically. **Distribution:** SHBG binding (40%), albumin binding (2%). **Metabolism:** Estradiol and DHT (active metabolites). **Elimination:** Urine (90% glucuronic and sulfuric acid conjugates), feces (6% unconjugated); $T_{1/2}$=10-100 min.

NURSING CONSIDERATIONS

Assessment: Assess for breast or prostate carcinoma, cardiac or renal/hepatic disease, obesity, chronic lung disease, pregnancy/nursing status of female partner, and possible drug interactions.

Monitoring: Periodically monitor Hgb, Hct, LFTs, PSA, cholesterol and HDL, serum calcium, serum testosterone levels after initiation of therapy. Monitor for signs/symptoms of hypersensitivity reactions, edema with/without CHF, gynecomastia, prostatic hyperplasia/carcinoma in geriatrics, and potentiation of sleep apnea.

Patient Counseling: Inform of pregnancy risks; avoid contact with application sites if pregnant/nursing. Wash area immediately with soap and water if contact occurs. Cover application site after gel dries with clothing; wash application site with soap and water prior to direct skin-to-skin contact. Advise to wash or swim ≥5 hrs after application. Drug is flammable until dry. Instruct not to apply on the scrotum, penis, or abdomen. Inform to contact physician if changes in body hair distribution, increase in acne, virilization of female partner, too frequent or persistent erections, changes in skin color, ankle swelling, unexplained NV, breathing disturbances, or hypersensitivity reactions occur.

Administration: Topical application. If multi-dose pump is used, prime the pump before using it for the first time by depressing pump 3 times and discarding the portion to assure precise dose delivery. Refer to Full Prescribing Information for administration details. **Storage:** 25°C (77°F); excursions permitted to 15-30°C (59-86°F). Keep out of reach of children.

ANGELIQ — RX

drospirenone - estradiol (Bayer Healthcare)

Estrogens and progestins should not be used for prevention of cardiovascular disease or dementia. Increased risk of MI, stroke, invasive breast cancer, PE, and DVT in postmenopausal women (50-79 yrs of age) reported. Increased risk of developing probable dementia in postmenopausal women ≥65 yrs of age reported.

THERAPEUTIC CLASS: Estrogen/progestogen combination

INDICATIONS: Treatment of moderate to severe vasomotor symptoms and/or vulvar/vaginal atrophy associated with menopause.

DOSAGE: *Adults:* 1 tab qd. Re-evaluate after 3-6 months.

HOW SUPPLIED: Tab: (Drospirenone-Estradiol) 0.5mg-1mg

CONTRAINDICATIONS: Pregnancy, undiagnosed abnormal genital bleeding, breast cancer, estrogen-dependent neoplasia, DVT/PE, active or recent (eg, within past year) arterial thromboembolic disease (eg, stroke, MI), liver dysfunction or disease, renal insufficiency, adrenal insufficiency.

WARNINGS/PRECAUTIONS: Not for use in renal insufficiency, hepatic dysfunction, and adrenal insufficiency due to increased risk of hyperkalemia. May increase risk of cardiovascular events (eg, MI, stroke), venous thrombosis, and PE; d/c immediately if any of these events occur or are suspected. May increase risk of breast/endometrial cancer, and gallbladder disease. May lead to severe hypercalcemia with breast cancer and bone metastases; monitor and d/c if hypercalcemia occurs. Retinal vascular thrombosis reported; monitor and d/c if papilledema or retinal vascular lesions occur. May elevate BP; monitor at regular intervals. May cause elevations of plasma triglycerides with pre-existing hypertriglyceridemia. Caution with history of cholestatic jaundice associated with past estrogen use or with pregnancy; d/c with recurrence. May lead to increased thyroid-binding globulin levels; monitor thyroid function. May cause fluid retention; caution with cardiac/renal dysfunction. Caution with severe hypocalcemia. May increase risk of ovarian cancer. May exacerbate endometriosis, asthma, DM, epilepsy, migraine, porphyria, SLE, and hepatic hemangiomas; use with caution.

ADVERSE REACTIONS: Abdominal pain, pain in extremity, back pain, flu syndrome, enlarged abdomen, headache, upper respiratory infection, sinusitis, breast pain, vaginal hemorrhage.

INTERACTIONS: CYP3A4 inducers (eg, St. John's wort, phenobarbital, carbamazepine, rifampin) may decrease levels which may decrease therapeutic effects and/or change uterine bleeding profile. CYP3A4 inhibitors (eg, erythromycin, clarithromycin, ketoconazole, itraconazole, ritonavir, grapefruit juice) may increase levels which may result in side effects. Increased risk of hyperkalemia with ACE inhibitors, angiotensin receptor blockers, NSAIDs, potassium-sparing diuretics, potassium supplements, and heparin.

PREGNANCY: Contraindicated in pregnancy, caution in nursing.

MECHANISM OF ACTION: Estrogen/progestogen combination. Estradiol: Binds to nuclear receptors in estrogen-responsive tissues. Modulates pituitary secretion of gonadotropins, leuteinizing hormone (LH) and follicle stimulating hormone (FSH), through negative feedback mechanism. Drospirenone (DRSP): Synthetic progestin and spironolactone analog with antimineralocorticoid activity. Possesses anti-androgenic activity. Counters estrogenic effects by decreasing number of nuclear estradiol receptors and suppressing epithelial DNA synthesis in endometrial tissue.

PHARMACOKINETICS: Absorption: DRSP: C_{max}=18.3ng/mL; T_{max}=1.0 hr; AUC_{0-24hr}=208ng•hr/mL. Absolute bioavailability (76-85%) Estradiol; C_{max}=43.8pg/mL; T_{max}=2.5 hrs; $AUC_{0-24 hr}$=665pg•hr/mL. Estrone (metabolite): C_{max}=245pg/mL; T_{max}=4 hrs; $AUC_{(0-24 hr}$=3814pg•hr/mL **Distribution:** Estrogens and DRSP found in breast milk. DRSP: V_d=4.2L/kg, serum protein binding (97%). Estradiol: Sex hormone binding globulin (SHBG) (37%); albumin binding (61%). **Metabolism:** DRSP: Extensive; CYP3A4 (minor). Estradiol: Liver to estrone (metabolite); estriol (major urinary metabolite); enterohepatic recirculation via sulfate and glucuronide conjugation in the liver; biliary secretion of conjugates in the intestine; hydrolysis in the gut; reabsorption. **Elimination:** DRSP: Urine (38-47%, glucuronide and sulfate conjugates), feces (17-20%, glucuronide and sulfate conjugates); $T_{1/2}$=36-42 hrs. Estradiol: Urine. Estrone: Urine; $T_{1/2}$=23 hrs.

NURSING CONSIDERATIONS

Assessment: Assess for abnormal genital bleeding, known or history of breast cancer, estrogen-dependent neoplasias, DVT or PE, present or recent (within past yr) arterial thromboembolic disease (eg, stroke, MI), renal insufficiencies, liver dysfunction/disease, adrenal insufficiencies, and known/suspected pregnancy. Assess use in patients undergoing surgeries associated with risk of thromboembolism, with prolonged immobilization, ≥65 yrs old, presence of hypothyroidism or hypocalcemia, and in nursing females. Assess for drug or lab interactions.

Monitoring: Monitor for signs/symptoms of cardiovascular disorders (eg, MI, stroke, venous thrombosis, PE), malignant neoplasms (eg, endometrial, breast, or ovarian cancer), dementia, gallbladder disease, cholestatic jaundice, hypercalcemia, visual abnormalities (eg, retinal vascular thrombosis), increased BP levels, fluid retention, hyponatremia, hypertriglyceridemia, hypothyroidism, exacerbation of endometriosis, and exacerbation of other conditions (eg, asthma, DM, epilepsy, migraines, porphyria, SLE, and hepatic hemangiomas). Periodically monitor BP levels, thyroid function in patients on thyroid hormone replacement therapy, serum potassium levels during first cycle of therapy in patients at risk for hyperkalemia. Perform proper diagnostic testing (eg, endometrial sampling) in patients with undiagnosed, persistent, or recurring vaginal bleeding. Perform annual breast exam (eg, mammography). Monitor use of therapy every 3-6 months.

Patient Counseling: Inform drug may increase risk for heart attack, stroke, breast cancer, blood clots, and dementia. Report any breast lumps, unusual vaginal bleeding, dizziness and faintness, changes in speech, severe headaches, chest pain, SOB, leg pains, changes in vision, or vomiting. Instruct to perform monthly breast exam.

Administration: Oral route. **Storage:** 25°C (77°F); excursions permitted to 15-30°C (59-86°F). Do not store above 30°C (86°F).

ANGIOMAX — RX

bivalirudin (The Medicines Company)

THERAPEUTIC CLASS: Thrombin inhibitor

INDICATIONS: Adjunct to aspirin for anticoagulation in patients with unstable angina undergoing percutaneous transluminal coronary angioplasty (PTCA) or percutaneous coronary intervention (PCI). Patients with, or at risk of, HIT/HITTS undergoing PCI.

DOSAGE: *Adults:* Initial: 0.75mg/kg IV bolus, then 1.75mg/kg/hr for duration of PCI procedure. Additional bolus of 0.3mg/kg can be given if needed based on ACT. Continuation of infusion for up to 4 hrs post-procedure is optional. After 4 hrs, if needed, an additional 0.2mg/kg/hr IV for up to 20 hrs may be initiated. Renal Impairment: CrCl <30mL/min: 1mg/kg/hr infusion. Hemodialysis: 0.25mg/kg/hr infusion. Reduction in bolus dose not necessary; monitor anticoagulation.

HOW SUPPLIED: Inj: 250mg

CONTRAINDICATIONS: Active major bleeding.

WARNINGS/PRECAUTIONS: Not for IM administration. Hemorrhage can occur at any site. D/C with unexplained symptom, fall in BP or Hct. There is no known antidote to treatment, but can be hemodialyzable. Caution when used during brachytherapy procedures.

ADVERSE REACTIONS: Bleeding, back pain, pain, NV, headache, hypotension, HTN, bradycardia, dyspepsia, urinary retention, insomnia, anxiety, abdominal pain, fever, nervousness.

INTERACTIONS: Increased risk of major bleed with heparin, warfarin, thrombolytics, glycoprotein IIb/IIIa inhibitors.

PREGNANCY: Category B, caution in nursing.

MECHANISM OF ACTION: Reversible direct thrombin inhibitor; inhibits thrombin by specifically binding to catalytic site and to anion-binding exosite of circulating and clot-bound thrombin.

PHARMACOKINETICS: Metabolism: Renal mechanisms and proteolytic cleavage. **Elimination:** Urine; $T_{1/2}$=25 min.

NURSING CONSIDERATIONS

Assessment: Assess for active major bleeding, renal impairment, and drug interactions. Assess use in patients with disease states associated with increased risk of bleeding.

Monitoring: Monitor for signs/symptoms of hemorrhage (eg, decreases in BP or Hct), and thrombus formation. For patients with renal impairment, monitor anticoagulant status.

Patient Counseling: Advise about increased risk of bleeding events and instruct to contact physician if any occur.

Administration: IV route. Not for IM administration. Reconstitute: 1) To each 250mg vial, add 5mL of sterile water for injection. 2) Gently swirl until all material is dissolved. Further dilute: 3) Use 500mL D5W or 0.9% NaCl for injection to yield a final concentration of 0.5mg/mL. 4) Infusion rate to be administered is adjusted according to patient's weight. During brachytherapy, maintain meticulous catheter technique (eg, frequent aspiration and flushing).
Storage: 20-25°C (68-77°F); excursion permitted to 15-30°C. Do not freeze. Reconstituted: May be stored at 2-8°C for up to 24 hrs. Diluted preparation is stable at room temperature for up to 24 hrs.

ANSAID — RX

flurbiprofen (Pharmacia & Upjohn)

NSAIDs may cause an increased risk of serious cardiovascular thrombotic events, MI, stroke, and serious GI adverse events including bleeding, ulceration, and perforation of the stomach or intestines. Contraindicated for the treatment of perioperative pain in the setting of coronary artery bypass graft (CABG) surgery.

THERAPEUTIC CLASS: NSAID

INDICATIONS: Relief of the signs and symptoms of rheumatoid arthritis or osteoarthritis.

DOSAGE: *Adults:* Initial: 200-300mg/day given bid, tid or qid. Max: 300mg/day or 100mg/dose.

HOW SUPPLIED: Tab: 50mg, 100mg

CONTRAINDICATIONS: ASA, with ASA triad, or other NSAID allergy that precipitates acute asthmatic attack, urticaria, or rhinitis. Treatment of perioperative pain in the setting of CABG surgery.

WARNINGS/PRECAUTIONS: May lead to onset of new HTN or worsening of pre-existing HTN; monitor BP closely. Fluid retention and edema reported; caution with fluid retention or heart failure. Renal papillary necrosis and other renal injury reported after long-term use. Not recommended for use with advanced renal disease; if therapy must be initiated, monitor renal function. Anaphylactoid reactions may occur. Avoid in late pregnancy; may cause premature closure of ductus arteriosus. May cause elevations of LFTs; d/c if liver disease develops or systemic manifestations occur. Caution in elderly. Anemia may occur; monitor Hgb/Hct with long-term use. May inhibit platelet aggregation and prolong bleeding time; monitor with coagulation disorders. Caution with asthma and avoid with ASA-sensitive asthma. Monitor for visual changes or disturbances. Risk of GI ulceration, bleeding, and perforation. May cause serious skin adverse events (eg, exfoliative dermatitis, Stevens-Johnson syndrome, toxic epidermal necrolysis).

ADVERSE REACTIONS: Dyspepsia, diarrhea, abdominal pain, constipation, headache, nausea, edema.

INTERACTIONS: Caution with anticoagulants; serious bleeding reported. Concomitant ASA is not recommended. May decrease hypotensive effects of β-blockers, decrease diuretic effects and diminish the antihypertensive effects of ACE inhibitors. May elevate plasma lithium levels and could enhance the toxicity of methotrexate.

PREGNANCY: Category C, not for use in nursing.

MECHANISM OF ACTION: NSAID; suspected to inhibit prostaglandin synthetase and exerts anti-inflammatory, analgesic, and antipyretic actions.

PHARMACOKINETICS: Absorption: Rapid; bioavailability 96%; T_{max}=2 hrs. **Distribution:** V_d=0.12L/kg; plasma protein binding (99%); found in breast milk. **Metabolism:** CYP2C9. 4'-hydroxy-flurbiprofen (major metabolite).

Elimination: Urine (≤3% unchanged) (70% parent drug and metabolites); $T_{1/2}$=4.7 hrs (R-flurbiprofen), 5.7 hrs (S-flurbiprofen).

NURSING CONSIDERATIONS

Assessment: Assess LFTs, renal function, CBC, and coagulation profile. Assess for history of CABG surgery, asthma and allergic reactions to aspirin or other NSAIDs, active ulceration or chronic inflammation of GI tract, CVD, asthma, pregnancy status. Note other diseases/conditions and drug therapies.

Monitoring: Monitor for hypersensitivity reactions, cardiac complications, stroke, GI bleeding, asthma, skin side effects, BP, LFTs, renal function, CBC with differential and platelet count, coagulation profile, ophthalmic exams.

Patient Counseling: Counsel about side effects; seek medical attention if any develop. Avoid alcohol and smoking during treatment. Instruct to take exactly as prescribed. Caution women against using medication late in pregnancy.

Administration: Oral route. **Storage:** 20-25°C (68-77°F).

ANTABUSE RX

disulfiram (Odyssey)

Do not give if in a state of alcohol intoxication, or without full knowledge. Instruct relatives accordingly.

THERAPEUTIC CLASS: Alcohol oxidation inhibitor

INDICATIONS: Aid in the management of selected chronic alcoholics who want to remain sober for supportive and psychotherapeutic treatment.

DOSAGE: *Adults:* Initial: Up to 500mg/day as a single dose for 1-2 weeks. Maint: 125-500mg/day. Max: 500mg/day. Abstain from alcohol at least 12 hours prior to therapy.

HOW SUPPLIED: Tab: 250mg

CONTRAINDICATIONS: Severe myocardial disease, coronary occlusion, psychoses, hypersensitivity to thiuram derivatives in pesticides and rubber vulcanization, and if receiving or recently received metronidazole, paraldehyde, alcohol, or alcohol-containing preparations (eg, cough syrups).

WARNINGS/PRECAUTIONS: Avoid in alcohol intoxication or without patients full knowledge. Antabuse-alcohol reaction; can cause respiratory and cardiovascular problems. Avoid alcohol-containing products (eg, sauces, vinegars, cough mixtures, after shave lotions, back rubs) and ethylene dibromide or its vapors. Reactions with alcohol up to 14 days after ingestion. Evaluate for hypersensitivity if history of rubber contact dermatitis. Hepatic toxicity/failure has been reported. Perform baseline and follow-up LFTs (10-14 days) and monitor CBC and SMA-12. Caution with diabetes mellitus, hypothyroidism, epilepsy, cerebral damage, chronic and acute nephritis, hepatic cirrhosis or insufficiency.

ADVERSE REACTIONS: Optic neuritis, peripheral neuritis, polyneuritis, peripheral neuropathy, hepatitis, skin eruptions, drowsiness, fatigability, impotence, headache, acneiform eruptions, allergic dermatitis, metallic or garlic-like aftertaste.

INTERACTIONS: Increases phenytoin level; monitor for toxicity. May prolong PT; adjust oral anticoagulants. Stop therapy if unsteady gait or marked changes in mental status with isoniazid.

PREGNANCY: Safety not known in pregnancy, not for use in nursing.

MECHANISM OF ACTION: Alcohol antagonist; blocks alcohol oxidation at the acetaldehyde stage.

PHARMACOKINETICS: Absorption/Elimination: Slow.

NURSING CONSIDERATIONS

Assessment: Assess for alcohol intoxication, possible drug interactions, cardiac diseases, prior history of drug abuse, psychoses, hypersensitivity to drug or other thiuram derivatives, history of rubber contact dermatitis. Obtain baseline LFTs.

Monitoring: Monitor for hepatic toxicity, manifestations of hepatitis (eg, fatigue, weakness, malaise, anorexia, NV, jaundice, dark urine), LFTs after 10-14 days of initiation then periodically, CBC and serum chemistries, PT with anticoagulants, and serum phenytoin with concurrent phenytoin.

Patient Counseling: Counsel to avoid alcohol in disguised forms (eg, sauces, vinegar, cough mixtures, aftershave lotions, back rubs). Advise that reactions with alcohol may occur up to 14 days after ingesting drug. Instruct not to be exposed to ethylene dibromide or its vapors while on medication.

Administration: Oral route. **Storage:** 20-25°C (68-77°F). Dispense in tight, light-resistant container.

ANTARA — RX

fenofibrate (Oscient)

THERAPEUTIC CLASS: Fibric acid derivative

INDICATIONS: Adjunct to diet, for treatment of hypertriglyceridemia (Types IV and V) and to reduce elevated LDL-C, Total-C, TG, Apo B, and to increase HDL-C in primary hypercholesterolemia or mixed dyslipidemia (Types IIa and IIb).

DOSAGE: *Adults:* Hypercholesterolemia/Mixed Dyslipidemia: Initial: 130mg qd. Hypertriglyceridemia: Initial: 43-130mg/day. Titrate: Adjust if needed after repeat lipid levels at 4-8 week intervals. Max: 130mg/day. Renal Dysfunction/ Elderly: Initial: 43mg/day. Take with meals.

HOW SUPPLIED: Cap: 43mg, 130mg

CONTRAINDICATIONS: Hepatic or severe renal dysfunction (including primary cirrhosis), unexplained persistent hepatic function abnormality, pre-existing gallbladder disease.

WARNINGS/PRECAUTIONS: Monitor LFTs regularly; d/c if >3x ULN. May cause cholelithiasis; d/c if gallstones found. D/C if myopathy or marked CPK elevation occurs. Decreased Hgb, Hct, WBCs, thrombocytopenia, and agranulocytosis reported; monitor CBCs during first 12 months of therapy. Acute hypersensitivity reactions (rare) and pancreatitis reported. Rare cases of rhabdomyolysis. Evaluate for myopathy. Monitor lipids periodically initially, d/c if inadequate response after 2 months on 130mg/day. Minimize dose in severe renal impairment. Caution in elderly.

ADVERSE REACTIONS: Abdominal pain, back pain, headache, abnormal LFTs, respiratory disorder, increased creatinine phosphokinase, increased SGPT/ SGOT.

INTERACTIONS: May potentiate coumarin anticoagulants; reduce anticoagulant dose and monitor PT/INR. Avoid HMG-CoA reductase inhibitors unless benefits outweigh risks. Bile acid sequestrants may impede absorption; take at least 1 hr before or 4-6 hrs after the resin. Evaluate benefits/risks with immunosuppressants (eg, cyclosporine) and other nephrotoxic agents.

PREGNANCY: Category C, not for use in nursing.

MECHANISM OF ACTION: Fenofibric acid; increases lipolysis and elimination of triglyceride-rich particles from plasma by activating lipoprotein lipase and reducing production of apoprotein C-III. Reduces serum uric acid levels in hyperuricemic and normal individuals by increasing urinary excretion of uric acid.

PHARMACOKINETICS: Absorption: Well; T_{max}=4.8 hrs. **Distribution:** Plasma protein binding (99%). **Metabolism:** Rapid, via esterase. Fenofibric acid (active metabolite). **Elimination:** Urine (60%), feces (25%); $T_{1/2}$=23 hrs.

NURSING CONSIDERATIONS

Assessment: Assess for severe renal/hepatic impairment, primary biliary cirrhosis, pre-existing gallbladder disease, persistent unexplained LFTs, lipid level abnormalities, pregnancy/nursing status, and possible drug interactions.

Control serum lipids (eg, with appropriate diet, exercise, weight loss in obese patients) and medical problems (eg, DM and hypothyroidism) before therapy.

Monitoring: Periodically monitor LFTs, lipid levels, CPK, CBC, INR, and PT. Monitor for signs/symptoms of myopathy/rhabdomyolysis, pancreatitis, cholelithiasis, hepatocellular/chronic active or cholestatic jaundice, hypersensitivity reactions (eg, severe skin rashes).

Patient Counseling: Inform about risks/benefits; promptly report signs of myopathy (eg, unexplained muscle pain, weakness, or tenderness). Notify if pregnant/nursing.

Administration: Oral route. **Storage:** 25°C (77°F); excursions permitted to 15-30°C (59-86°F).

ANTIVERT RX

meclizine HCl (Pfizer)

THERAPEUTIC CLASS: Antihistamine

INDICATIONS: Management of nausea, vomiting and dizziness associated with motion sickness. Management of vertigo associated with diseases affecting the vestibular system.

DOSAGE: *Adults:* Motion Sickness: 25-50mg 1 hr prior to trip/departure, repeat q24h prn. Vertigo: 25-100mg/day in divided doses.
Pediatrics: ≥12 yrs: Motion Sickness: 25-50mg 1 hr prior to trip/departure, repeat q24h prn. Vertigo: 25-100mg/day in divided doses.

HOW SUPPLIED: Tab: 12.5mg, 25mg, 50mg* *scored

WARNINGS/PRECAUTIONS: Caution with asthma, glaucoma, prostatic hypertrophy.

ADVERSE REACTIONS: Drowsiness, dry mouth, blurred vision (rare).

INTERACTIONS: Avoid alcoholic beverages.

PREGNANCY: Category B, safety in nursing is not known.

MECHANISM OF ACTION: Antihistaminic agent; blocks vasodepressor response to histamine; slight blocking against acetylcholine.

NURSING CONSIDERATIONS

Assessment: Assess for asthma, glaucoma, prostate enlargement, alcohol intake, and possible drug interactions.

Monitoring: Monitor for drowsiness.

Patient Counseling: Caution against performing hazardous tasks (eg, operating machinery/driving).

Administration: Oral route.

ANZEMET RX

dolasetron mesylate (Sanofi-Aventis)

THERAPEUTIC CLASS: 5-HT_3 receptor antagonist

INDICATIONS: (Inj) Prevention of nausea/vomiting associated with emetogenic cancer chemotherapy including high-dose cisplatin. Prevention and treatment of post-op nausea/vomiting. (Tab) Prevention of nausea/vomiting associated with moderately emetogenic cancer chemotherapy and prevention of post-op nausea/vomiting.

DOSAGE: *Adults:* (Inj) Prevention of Chemotherapy Nausea/Vomiting: 1.8mg/kg IV single dose or 100mg IV 30 min before chemotherapy. Prevention/Treatment of Post-op Nausea/Vomiting: 12.5mg IV single dose 15 min before cessation of anesthesia or as soon as nausea/vomiting presents. (Tab) Prevention of Chemotherapy-Induced Nausea/Vomiting: 100mg PO within 1 hr before chemotherapy. Prevention of Postoperative Nausea/Vomiting: 100mg PO within 2 hrs before surgery.
Pediatrics: 2-16 yrs: (Inj) Prevention of Chemotherapy Nausea/Vomiting:

1.8mg/kg IV single dose 30 min before chemotherapy. Max: 100mg. May mix inj in apple or grape juice and take orally within 1 hr before chemotherapy. Prevention/Treatment of Post-op Nausea/Vomiting: 0.35mg/kg IV single dose 15 min before cessation of anesthesia or as soon as nausea/vomiting presents. Max: 12.5mg single dose. May mix 1.2mg/kg inj in apple or grape juice and take orally within 2 hrs before surgery. Max: 100mg/dose. (Tab) Prevention of Chemotherapy-Induced Nausea/Vomiting: 1.8mg/kg PO within 1 hr before chemotherapy. Max: 100mg. Prevention of Postoperative Nausea/Vomiting: 1.2mg/kg PO within 2 hrs before surgery. Max: 100mg.

HOW SUPPLIED: Inj: 20mg/mL; Tab: 50mg, 100mg

WARNINGS/PRECAUTIONS: Caution in patients with or who may develop cardiac conduction interval prolongation, especially those with congenital QT syndrome, hypokalemia and hypomagnesemia. Cross sensitivity may occur with other 5-HT_3 antagonists. Can cause ECG interval changes.

ADVERSE REACTIONS: Headache, diarrhea, fever, fatigue, dizziness, abnormal hepatic function, chills/shivering, urinary retention, abdominal pain, HTN, wide complex tachycardia or ventricular tachycardia, ventricular fibrillation.

INTERACTIONS: Increased risk of prolongation of cardiac conduction intervals with diuretics, antiarrhythmics, drugs that prolong QTc interval and cumulative high dose anthracycline therapy. Increased levels with cimetidine. Decreased levels with rifampin. Decreased clearance with IV atenolol.

PREGNANCY: Category B, caution in nursing.

MECHANISM OF ACTION: 5-HT_3 receptor antagonist.

PHARMACOKINETICS: Absorption: T_{max}=0.6 hr. **Distribution:** V_d=5.8L/Kg; plasma protein binding (77%). **Metabolism:** Complete. Via carbonyl reductase CYP2D6 and flavin monooxygenase through reduction, hydroxylation, and N-oxidation. **Elimination:** Urine 53% (unchanged), feces; $T_{1/2}$=7.3 hrs.

NURSING CONSIDERATIONS

Assessment: Assess for possibility of cardiac prolongation of conduction interval (particularly QT), hypokalemia/hypomagnesemia, if taking diuretics/antiarrhythmics, congenital QT syndrome, and possible drug interactions.

Monitoring: Monitor for ECG interval changes (PR, QT, JT prolongation, and QRS widening), heart block or cardiac arrhythmia, cross-hypersensitivity reactions.

Patient Counseling: Inform about potential risks/benefits and to report adverse reactions. Notify if pregnant/nursing. Do not exceed recommended dose.

Administration: IV. **Storage:** 20-25°C (68-77°F); protect from light.

APIDRA — RX

insulin glulisine, rdna (Sanofi-Aventis)

THERAPEUTIC CLASS: Insulin

INDICATIONS: Treatment of adults and children ≥4 yrs with DM for the control of hyperglycemia.

DOSAGE: *Adults:* Individualize dose. Inject SQ within 15 min before a meal or within 20 min after starting a meal. Rotate inj site (abdomen, thigh, or deltoid).
Pediatrics: ≥4 yrs: Individualize dose. Inject SQ within 15 min before a meal or within 20 min after starting a meal. Rotate inj site (abdomen, thigh, or deltoid).

HOW SUPPLIED: Inj: 100 U/mL

CONTRAINDICATIONS: Episodes of hypoglycemia.

WARNINGS/PRECAUTIONS: Hypoglycemia and hypokalemia may occur; monitor glucose and potassium levels. Rapid onset and short duration of action; follow dosage directions. Adjust dose if change in physical activity or usual meal plan. Longer-acting insulin or insulin infusion pump may be required to maintain glucose control. When used in an external pump for SQ infusion, do not dilute or mix with any other insulin. Caution when changing insulin strength, manufacturer, type, or species. Concomitant antidiabetic therapy may need adjustment. As with other insulin therapy, hypoglycemic reactions and local/systemic allergic reactions may occur. May be given IV under proper medical supervision. Caution in renal/hepatic impairment.

ADVERSE REACTIONS: Allergic reactions, injection-site reactions, lipodystrophy, pruritus, rash, hypoglycemia.

INTERACTIONS: Decreased effect with corticosteroids, danazol, diazoxide, diuretics, sympathomimetic agents (eg, epinephrine, albuterol, terbutaline), glucagon, isoniazid, phenothiazine derivatives, somatropin, thyroid hormones, estrogens, progestogens (eg, in oral contraceptives), protease inhibitors, and atypical antipsychotic medications (eg, olanzapine and clozapine). Increased effect with ACEIs, MAOIs, oral antidiabetics, disopyramide, fibrates, fluoxetine, pentoxifylline, propoxyphene, salicylates, sulfonamide antibiotics. Decreased or increased effect with β-blockers, clonidine, lithium salts, and alcohol. Pentamidine may cause hypoglycemia followed by hyperglycemia. β-blockers, clonidine, guanethidine, and reserpine may reduce or mask signs of hypoglycemia.

PREGNANCY: Category C, caution in nursing.

MECHANISM OF ACTION: Insulin glulisine (rDNA origin); lowers blood glucose by stimulating peripheral glucose uptake by skeletal muscle and fat and by inhibiting hepatic glucose production.

PHARMACOKINETICS: Absorption: C_{max}=82, 81, 199μU/mL (0.15, 0.2, 0.3 IU/kg); T_{max}=55, 89, 76 min (0.15, 0.2, 0.3 IU/kg). **Distribution:** V_d=13L. **Elimination:** Rapidly eliminated; $T_{1/2}$=42 min.

NURSING CONSIDERATIONS

Assessment: Assess FPG, HbA_{1c}, renal function, LFTs, pregnancy status, infections, alcohol consumption, exercise routines, and possible drug interactions.

Monitoring: Monitor FPG, HbA_{1c}, hypokalemia, renal function, diabetic ketoacidosis, vision changes, lipodystrophy, allergic reactions. Monitor for signs of hypoglycemia (sweating, palpitations, seizures, disorientation, tremors).

Patient Counseling: Use only if the solution is clear and colorless with no visible particles. Do not dilute or mix with other insulins or solutions. Counsel about signs/symptoms of hypoglycemia, hyperglycemia, diabetic ketoacidosis, the importance of frequent monitoring of blood glucose levels, and the need for eating a balanced diet and exercising regularly. Advise to avoid excessive alcohol use. During periods of stress (eg, trauma, infection, surgery), insulin requirements may be changed; advise patients to seek prompt medical advice. Counsel on proper administration techniques.

Administration: SQ route, administered within 15 min before a meal or within 20 min after starting a meal. Refer to Full Prescribing Information for administration techniques. **Storage:** Unopened vial: 2-8°C (36-46°F). Open (in-use) vial: 25°C (77°F). Opened vials must be used within 28 days. Discard vials after 28 days. Protect from light. Insulin exposed to temperatures >37°C (98°F) should be discarded.

APLENZIN — RX

bupropion hydrobromide (Biovail)

Antidepressants increased the risk of suicidal thinking and behavior (suicidality) in short-term studies in children, adolescents, and young adults with major depressive disorder (MDD) and other psychiatric disorders. Bupropion is not approved for use in pediatric patients.

THERAPEUTIC CLASS: Aminoketone

INDICATIONS: Treatment of major depressive disorder (MDD).

DOSAGE: *Adults:* ≥18 yrs: Give in morning. Swallow whole. Initial: 174mg qd. Titrate: May increase to 348mg qd on Day 4 if tolerated. Max: 522mg/day given as single dose if no clinical improvement after several weeks. Switching from Wellbutrin, Wellbutrin SR, or Wellbutrin XL: Give equivalent dose. 522mg bupropion HBr = 450mg bupropion HCl, 348mg bupropion HBr = 300mg bupropion HCl, 174mg bupropion HBr = 150mg bupropion HCl. Mild-Moderate Hepatic Cirrhosis/Renal Impairment: Reduce frequency and/or dose. Severe Hepatic Cirrhosis: Max: 174mg every other day.

HOW SUPPLIED: Tab, Extended-Release: 174mg, 348mg, 522mg

CONTRAINDICATIONS: Seizure disorder, bulimia or anorexia nervosa, within 14 days of MAOIs, other forms of bupropion, abrupt discontinuation of alcohol or sedatives (including benzodiazepines).

WARNINGS/PRECAUTIONS: May worsen depression and/or emergence of suicidal ideation and behavior; monitor closely. May precipitate manic episodes in bipolar disorder. Dose-related risk of seizures; d/c and do not restart if seizure occurs. Extreme caution with history of seizure, cranial trauma, severe hepatic cirrhosis, concomitant medications that lower seizure threshold. Agitation, insomnia, psychosis, confusion and other neuropsychiatric signs reported. Caution with hepatic impairment (including mild to moderate hepatic cirrhosis). Anorexia/weight loss may occur. HTN reported; caution with recent history of MI or unstable heart disease. Anaphylactoid/anaphylactic reactions reported; d/c if any occur.

ADVERSE REACTIONS: Dry mouth, nausea, insomnia, dizziness, pharyngitis, abdominal pain, agitation, anxiety, tremor, palpitation, tremor, sweating, tinnitus, myalgia, anorexia, urinary frequency, rash.

INTERACTIONS: See Contraindications. Extreme caution with drugs that lower seizure threshold (eg, antidepressants, antipsychotics, theophylline, systemic steroids). Increased seizure risk with opioids, cocaine, or stimulant addiction, OTC stimulants or anorectics, oral hypoglycemics, insulin, excessive use or abrupt discontinuation of alcohol or sedatives. Caution with levodopa, amantadine, and drugs that are metabolized by CYP2D6 (eg, SSRIs, TCAs, antipsychotics, β-blockers, type 1C antiarrhythmics); use low initial dose and gradually titrate. Monitor HTN with transdermal nicotine. Caution with CYP2B6 substrates or inhibitors (eg, orphenadrine, cyclophosphamide, thiotepa). Carbamazepine, phenytoin, cimetidine, and phenobarbital may induce metabolism of bupropion. Minimize or avoid alcohol.

PREGNANCY: Category C, not for use in nursing.

MECHANISM OF ACTION: Aminoketone antidepressant; MOA not established, presumed that action is mediated by noradrenergic and/or dopaminergic mechanisms.

PHARMACOKINETICS: Absorption: T_{max}=5 hrs. **Distribution**: Plasma protein binding (84%). **Metabolism**: Extensive to hydroxybupropion (CYP2B6) via hydroxylation; threohydrobupropion, erythrohydrobupropion via reduction of carbonyl group. **Elimination**: Urine (87%), feces (10%), (0.5% unchanged). $T_{1/2}$= 21 hrs, 24 hrs, 31 hrs, 50 hrs (bupropion, hydroxybupropion, erythrohydrobupropion, threohydrobupropion respectively).

NURSING CONSIDERATIONS

Assessment: Assess for history of seizures, bulimia/anorexia nervosa, LFTs, renal function tests, DM, head trauma, use of alcohol, opiate sedatives, history of MI or unstable heart disease, psychosis, mixed/manic eposodes. Note other diseases/conditions and drug therapies especially other bupropion products.

Monitoring: Monitor for clinical worsening, suicidality, or unusual changes in behavior, seizures, increased restlessness, agitation, anxiety, insomnia, neuropsychiatric signs/symptoms (eg, delusions, hallucinations, psychosis, concentration disturbances, paranoia, and confusion), weight loss, loss of appetite, arthralgia, myalgia, HTN, and fever with rash.

Patient Counseling: Advise families and caregivers of need for close observation of clinical worsening and suicidal risks. Avoid alcohol, sedatives, and OTC drugs. Exercise caution while driving or operating machinery. Report adverse reactions and inform physician before taking any other medications or plan to become pregnant. Advise to swallow tablets whole; do not chew, divide or crush tablets. May notice in stool something that looks like a tablet. D/C and do not restart if experience seizure while on treatment.

Administration: Oral route. **Storage**: 25°C (77°F); excursions permitted to 15-30°C (59-86°F).

APRISO
mesalamine (Salix)

RX

THERAPEUTIC CLASS: Anti-inflammatory Agent

INDICATIONS: Maintenance of remission of ulcerative colitis in patients ≥18 yrs.

DOSAGE: *Adults:* 1.5g (4 caps) qam. Take with or without food.

HOW SUPPLIED: Cap, Extended Release: 0.375g

WARNINGS/PRECAUTIONS: Renal impairment, including minimal change nephropathy, acute and chronic interstitial nephritis, renal failure (rare), reported. Evaluate renal function prior to initiation of therapy and periodically while on therapy. Caution in patients with known renal dysfunction or a history of renal disease. D/C if acute intolerance syndrome occurs (eg, acute abdominal pain, cramping, bloody diarrhea). Re-evaluate periodically. Caution with sulfasalazine hypersensitivity. Caution in patients with liver disease and elderly.

ADVERSE REACTIONS: Headache, diarrhea, upper abdominal pain, nausea, nasopharyngitis, influenza or influenza-like illness, and sinusitis.

INTERACTIONS: Avoid co-administration with antacids.

PREGNANCY: Category B, caution in nursing.

MECHANISM OF ACTION: Anti-inflammatory agent; not established; possible that 5-ASA diminishes inflammation by blocking production of arachidonic acid metabolites.

PHARMACOKINETICS: Absorption: T_{max}=4 hrs, C_{max}=2.1µg/mL, AUC_{0-24}=11µg*h/mL. AUC_{0-inf}= 14 µg*h/mL. **Distribution:** Plasma protein binding (43%). **Metabolism:** Liver and intestinal mucosa via N-acetyltransferase activity; N-acetyl-5-aminosalicylic acid (major metabolite). **Elimination:** $T_{1/2}$=9 hrs. Urine (2%, unchanged).

NURSING CONSIDERATIONS

Assessment: Assess for pre-existing renal/liver disease, hepatic/renal impairment, obtain baseline LFTs, BUN, creatinine, and urinalysis (protein).

Monitoring: Monitor LFTs, BUN, creatinine, and urinalysis (protein) periodically. Monitor acute intolerance syndrome, hypersensitivity, and allergic reactions.

Patient Counseling: Instruct not to take with antacids. Seek medical consultation if ulcerative colitis symptoms worsen.

Administration: Oral route. **Storage:** Store at 20-25°C (68-77°F); excursions permitted between 15-30°C (59-86°F).

APTIVUS
tipranavir (Boehringer Ingelheim)

RX

Both fatal and non-fatal intracranial hemorrhage, clinical hepatitis, and hepatic decompensation, including some fatalities, have been reported. Extra vigilance is warranted in patients with chronic hepatitis B or hepatitis C co-infection, as these patients have an increased risk of hepatotoxicity.

THERAPEUTIC CLASS: Protease inhibitor

INDICATIONS: Co-administered with 200mg of ritonavir for treatment of HIV-1 infected patients with evidence of viral replication, who are highly treatment-experienced or have HIV-1 strains resistant to multiple protease inhibitors.

DOSAGE: *Adults:* 500mg with 200mg ritonavir bid with food.
Pediatrics: 2-18 yrs: 14mg/kg with 6mg/kg ritonavir (or 375mg/m² with ritonavir 150mg/m²) bid. Max: 500mg with ritonavir 200mg bid. If Intolerance

or Toxicity Develops: Decrease dose to 12mg/kg with 5mg/kg ritonavir or 290mg/m² with ritonavir 115mg/m² bid. If unable to swallow caps; may switch to oral sol.

HOW SUPPLIED: Cap: 250mg; Sol: 100mg/mL

CONTRAINDICATIONS: Moderate to severe (Child-Pugh Class B and C) hepatic insufficiency. Concomitant administration with amiodarone, bepridil, flecainide, propafenone, quinidine, rifampin, dihydroergotamine, ergonovine, ergotamine, methylergonovine, cisapride, St. John's wort, lovastatin, simvastatin, pimozide, midazolam, and triazolam.

WARNINGS/PRECAUTIONS: Must be co-administered with ritonavir. Not recommended for use in treatment-naive patients. Caution with mild hepatic impairment (Child-Pugh Class A); monitor LFTs prior to therapy and during therapy. D/C for signs and symptoms of clinical hepatitis. D/C if asymptomatic elevations in AST or ALT >10 times the upper limit of normal or if asymptomatic elevations in AST or ALT between 5-10 times the upper limit of normal and increases in total bilirubin >2.5 times the upper limit of normal occur. Caution in patients at risk of increased bleeding from trauma, surgery, or other medical conditions, or who are receiving medications known to increase risk of bleeding (eg, antiplatelet agents, anticoagulants, high doses of vitamin E). Reports of new-onset DM, exacerbation of pre-existing DM, hyperglycemia; rash (urticarial rash, maculopapular rash, and possible photosensitivity) and rash accompanied with joint pain/stiffness, throat tightness, generalized pruritus; increased bleeding with hemophilia Types A and B; and increased total cholesterol and triglycerides. Caution with known sulfonamide allergy. D/C with severe rash. Possible redistribution/accumulation of body fat. Immune reconstitution syndrome reported with combination therapy.

ADVERSE REACTIONS: Diarrhea, N/V, abdominal pain, pyrexia, fatigue, asthenia, bronchitis, headache, depression, insomnia, cough, rash.

INTERACTIONS: See Contraindications. Do not use with rifampin, St. John's wort, lovastatin, simvastatin, amiodarone, bepridil, flecainide, propafenone, quinidine, ergot derivatives, cisapride, pimozide, midazolam, and triazolam. Decreased levels of abacavir, atazanavir, didanosine, zidovudine, amprenavir, lopinavir, saquinavir, valproic acid, methadone, meperidine, and omeprazole. Increased levels of fluoxetine, paroxetine, sertraline, tipranavir, rosuvastatin, tadalafil. Caution with carbamazepine, phenobarbital, phenytoin, valproic acid, trazodone, itraconazole, ketoconazole, voriconazole, diltiazem, felodipine, nicardipine, nisoldipine, verapamil, disulfiram/metronidazole, atorvastatin, rosuvastatin, fluticasone, omeprazole, cyclosporine, sirolimus, and tacrolimus. Starting dose of sildenafil should not exceed 25mg within 48 hours, tadalfil 10mg every 72 hours, and vardenafil 2.5mg every 72 hours. Decreased levels of ethinyl estradiol; use alternative forms of birth control. Dosage reduction needed for clarithromycin by 50% if CrCl 30-60mL/min and 75% if <30mL/min; rifabutin by 75%; desipramine. Increased levels with fluconazole. Monitor glucose with glimepiride, glipizide, glyburide, pioglitazone, repaglinide, or tolbutamine. Monitor INR with warfarin.

PREGNANCY: Category C, not for use in nursing.

MECHANISM OF ACTION: HIV-1 protease inhibitor; inhibits processing of Gag and Gag-Pol polyproteins, preventing formation of mature virions.

PHARMACOKINETICS: Absorption: Tipranavir/Ritonavir: C_{max}=94.8μM (female), 77.6μM (male). T_{max}=2.9 hrs (female), 3.0 hrs (male). **Distribution:** Plasma protein binding (≥99.9%). **Metabolism:** Hepatic via CYP3A4. **Elimination:** Urine (0.5%), feces (79.9%). Tipranavir/Ritonavir: $T_{1/2}$=4.8 hrs (healthy), 6.0 hrs (HIV-infected).

NURSING CONSIDERATIONS

Assessment: Assess for HBV or HCV co-infection, hepatic impairment, hemophilia, sulfonamide allergy, contraceptive use, baseline LFTs, and possible drug interaction.

Monitoring: Monitor for possible hepatotoxicity, intracranial hemorrhage, risk of increased bleeding, rash, elevation of total cholesterol and triglycerides, immune reconstitution syndrome, exacerbation of DM, hyperglycemia, fat redistribution/accumulation. LFTs should be monitored prior to and throughout treatment.

Patient Counseling: Inform to seek medical attention for symptoms of hepatitis (fatigue, malaise, anorexia, nausea), intracranial hemorrhage (unusual or unexplained bleeding), rash, fat redistribution/accumulation, infections, and hyperglycemia. Instruct that additional or alternative contraceptive measures should be used for patients receiving estrogen-based hormonal contraceptives. Do not alter or d/c therapy without consulting physician. If a dose is missed, take as soon as possible and then return to normal schedule. Take with food.

Administration: Oral route. **Storage:** Store at 2-8°C (36-46°F); excursions permitted to 15-30°C (59-86°F). Must be used within 60 days after opening.

ARANESP **RX**
darbepoetin alfa (Amgen)

Increased mortality, serious cardiovascular/thromboembolic events, and increased risk of tumor progression or recurrence. (Renal Failure) Patients experienced greater risks for death and serious cardiovascular events when administered erythropoiesis-stimulating agents (ESAs) to target higher vs lower Hgb levels (13.5 vs 11.3 g/dL; 14 vs 10 g/dL) in 2 clinical studies. Individualize dosing to achieve and maintain Hgb levels within range of 10-12g/dL. (Cancer) ESAs shortened overall survival and/or increased risk of tumor progression or recurrence in clinical studies in patients with breast, non-small cell lung, head and neck, lymphoid, and cervical cancers. To decrease these risks, as well as risk of serious cardio- and thrombovascular events, use lowest dose needed to avoid RBC transfusions. Use ESAs only for treatment of anemia due to concomitant myelosuppressive chemotherapy. ESAs are not indicated for patients receiving myelosuppressive therapy when anticipated outcome is cure. D/C following completion of chemotherapy course.

THERAPEUTIC CLASS: Erythropoiesis stimulator

INDICATIONS: Treatment of anemia associated with chronic renal failure (CRF), and anemia in patients with non-myeloid malignancies due to chemotherapy.

DOSAGE: *Adults:* CRF: Initial: 0.45mcg/kg IV/SQ weekly. Titrate: Adjust to target Hgb <12g/dL. If Hgb increases >1g/dL in a 2-week period or is approaching 12g/dL, decrease dose by 25%. If Hgb continues to increase, hold dose until Hgb begins to decrease, and reinitiate at 25% below previous dose. Do not increase more than once monthly. Conversion from Epoetin Alfa: Base dose on weekly epoetin dose. Give once weekly if receiving epoetin 2-3x/week. Give every 2 weeks if receiving epoetin once weekly. (See PI for details). Malignancy: Initial: 2.25mcg/kg SQ weekly or 500mcg once every 3 weeks. Titrate: Increase to 4.5mcg/kg if Hgb increases <1g/dL after 6 weeks of therapy. If Hgb increases by >1g/dL in a 2-week period or if Hgb >12g/dL, decrease dose by 40%. If Hgb >12g/dL, hold dose until Hgb approaches a level where transfusions may be required. Reinitiate at 40% below previous dose. *Pediatrics:* ≥1 year: CRF: Conversion from Epoetin Alfa: Base dose on weekly epoetin dose. Give once weekly if receiving epoetin 2-3x/week. Give every 2 weeks if receiving epoetin once weekly. (See Full Prescribing Information for details).

HOW SUPPLIED: Inj: Syringe: 0.025mg/0.42mL, 0.04mg/0.4mL, 0.06mg/0.3mL, 0.1mg/0.5mL, 0.15mg/0.3mL, 0.2mg/0.4mL, 0.3mg/0.6mL, 0.5mg/mL; SDV: 0.025mg/mL, 0.04mg/mL, 0.06mg/mL, 0.1mg/mL, 0.15mg/0.75mL, 0.2mg/mL, 0.3mg/mL

CONTRAINDICATIONS: Uncontrolled HTN.

WARNINGS/PRECAUTIONS: Pure red cell aplasia and severe anemia (with or without other cytopenias) may occur. Due to increased Hgb, increased risk of cardiovascular events including death may occur. This includes MI, stroke, CHF, and hemodialysis vascular access thrombosis. Control BP before therapy. Seizures reported. Increased risk of thrombotic events. Evaluate etiology if lack/loss of response occurs. Permanently d/c if serious allergic reaction occurs. Monitor renal function, fluid, and electrolytes. Albumin solution carries risk of transmission of viral diseases. May need interval of 2-6 weeks between dose adjustment and response. Monitor Hgb weekly until stabilized and maintenance dose is established, and for at least 4 weeks after dosage change. Monitor iron status before and during therapy. Increases RBCs and decreases plasma volume. ESAs shortened time to tumor progression in patients with advanced head and neck cancer receiving radiation therapy.

ADVERSE REACTIONS: Thrombic events, infection, myalgia, HTN, hypotension, headache, diarrhea, fatigue, edema, NV, fever, dyspnea.

PREGNANCY: Category C, caution in nursing.

MECHANISM OF ACTION: Erythropoiesis stimulating protein; stimulates erythropoiesis (same mechanism as endogenous erythropoietin) in response to hypoxia by interacting with progenitor stem cells to increase RBC production.

PHARMACOKINETICS: Absorption: Adults: (SQ) Bioavailability (37%). (2.25mcg/kg; 6.75mcg/kg) T_{max}=90 hrs; 71 hrs. **Pediatrics:** Bioavailability (54%). **Elimination:** (IV, SQ): $T_{1/2}$=21 hrs; 74 hrs.

NURSING CONSIDERATIONS

Assessment: Assess for uncontrolled HTN, latex allergy, underlying hematologic disease (hemolytic anemia, sickle cell anemia, thalassemia, porphyria), history of seizures, and possible drug interactions. Obtain baseline iron status, Hgb, BP, renal function, and electrolytes.

Monitoring: Monitor Hgb weekly and iron status, BP, renal function, and electrolytes periodically. Monitor for signs/symptoms of anaphylactic reactions, lack/loss of response, pure red cell aplasia, viral diseases, HTN, CV events, thrombosis, and seizures.

Patient Counseling: Counsel on importance of compliance with treatment, dietary and dialysis prescription; stress importance of judicious monitoring of BP and Hgb concentrations. Advise to seek medical attention if symptoms of anaphylactic reactions, lack/loss of response, pure red cell aplasia, viral diseases, HTN, CV events, thrombosis, or seizures occur.

Administration: IV route. **Storage:** 2-8°C (36-46°F). Do not freeze or shake. Protect from light.

ARAVA — RX

leflunomide (Sanofi-Aventis)

Avoid pregnancy during treatment or before completion of drug elimination procedure after treatment.

THERAPEUTIC CLASS: Pyrimidine synthesis inhibitor

INDICATIONS: Treatment of active rheumatoid arthritis to reduce signs/symptoms, inhibit structural damage, or improve physical function.

DOSAGE: *Adults:* LD: 100mg qd for 3 days. Maint: 20mg qd. If not tolerated and/or ALT elevations >2 but ≤3x ULN: Reduce to 10mg qd. If elevations persist or >3x ULN, d/c and give cholestyramine or charcoal. Max: 20mg/day.

HOW SUPPLIED: Tab: 10mg, 20mg, 100mg

CONTRAINDICATIONS: Pregnancy.

WARNINGS/PRECAUTIONS: May cause immunosuppression. Avoid with severe immunodeficiency, bone marrow dysplasia, severe, uncontrolled infections, significant hepatic impairment, or evidence of hepatitis B or C. *Pneumocystis jiroveci* pneumonia, tuberculosis, aspergillosis, and sepsis reported. Rare reports of pancytopenia, agranulocytosis, thrombocytopenia, Stevens-Johnson syndrome, toxic epidermal necrolysis, and potentially fatal severe liver injury. Monitor WBCs, platelets, Hgb, Hct, LFTs (esp ALT) at baseline then monthly for 6 months, and every 6-8 weeks thereafter; monitor monthly with concomitant MTX and/or other immunosuppressive agents. D/C with evidence of bone marrow suppression. Women of childbearing potential must have negative pregnancy test. Interstitial lung disease reported. Caution with renal impairment.

ADVERSE REACTIONS: Diarrhea, respiratory infections, HTN, alopecia, rash, nausea, bronchitis, abdominal/back pain, abnormal liver enzymes, urinary tract infections, dyspepsia.

INTERACTIONS: Decreased levels with cholestyramine or activated charcoal. Increased side effects with hepatotoxic substances. Increased levels with rifampin; caution with concomitant use. May increase levels of diclofenac, ibuprofen, or tolbutamide. Avoid vaccination with live vaccines.

PREGNANCY: Category X, not for use in nursing.

MECHANISM OF ACTION: Pyrimidine synthesis inhibitor; immunomodulatory agent. Inhibits dihydroorotate dehydrogenase. Produces antiproliferative activity.

PHARMACOKINETICS: Absorption: A77 1726 (M1) (major active metabolite): T_{max}=6-12 hrs. Oral administration of various doses led to different parameters. **Distribution**: (M1) V_d=0.13L/kg; plasma protein binding (>99.3%). **Metabolism**: M1 and many minor metabolites. **Elimination**: Urine (43%), feces (48%).

NURSING CONSIDERATIONS

Assessment: Assess pregnancy status and that women of childbearing potential are able to maintain reliable contraception while on therapy. Assess for severe immunodeficiency, bone marrow dysplasia, severe infections, hepatic dysfunction or evidence of hepatitis B or C, renal insufficiencies, nursing status, and possible drug interactions. Obtain baseline platelet, WBC count, Hgb, Hct, and ALT levels.

Monitoring: Monitor for signs/symptoms of immunosuppression and opportunistic infections (eg, *Pneumocystis jiroveci* pneumonia, TB, aspergillosis), sepsis, bone marrow suppression, pancytopenia, agranulocytosis, thrombocytopenia, severe liver injury, skin reactions (eg, Stevens-Johnson syndrome, toxic epidermal necrolysis), interstitial lung disease. Monitor platelet, WBC count, Hgb/Hct, and ALT levels monthly for 6 months and every 6-8 weeks thereafter.

Patient Counseling: Advise women of increased risks of having a child with birth defects if taking medication while pregnant or if become pregnant when medication has not been completely eliminated from body. Instruct patient must use reliable form of contraception while on therapy. Advise to promptly inform physician if there is any possibility of pregnancy. Advise to contact physician if develop any type of skin rash or mucous membrane lesions, hepatotoxicity (eg, tiredness, abdominal pain or jaundice), pancytopenia (eg, easy bruising, bleeding, recurrent infections), and interstitial lung disease. Inform that will need periodic lab monitoring of liver enzymes and hematological parameters while on therapy.

Administration: Oral route. **Storage**: 25°C (77°F); excursions permitted to 15-30°C (59-86°F). Protect from light.

AREDIA — RX

pamidronate disodium (Novartis)

THERAPEUTIC CLASS: Bisphosphonate

INDICATIONS: Treatment of moderate to severe hypercalcemia of malignancy, Paget's disease. Adjunct to standard antineoplastic therapy for treatment of osteolytic bone metastases of breast cancer and osteolytic lesions of multiple myeloma.

DOSAGE: *Adults:* Moderate Hypercalcemia: 60-90mg IV single dose over 2-24 hrs. Severe Hypercalcemia: 90mg IV single dose over 2-24 hrs. Retreatment: May repeat after 7 days. Paget's Disease: 30mg IV over 4 hrs for 3 consecutive days. Osteolytic Bone Lesions of Multiple Myeloma: 90mg IV over 4 hrs once a month. Osteolytic Bone Metastases of Breast Cancer: 90mg IV over 2 hrs every 3-4 weeks. Max: 90mg/single dose for all indications. Renal Dysfunction With Bone Metastases: Withhold dose if SrCr increases by 0.5mg/dL (normal baseline) or by 1mg/dL (abnormal baseline). Resume when SrCr returns to within 10% of baseline.

HOW SUPPLIED: Inj: 30mg, 90mg

WARNINGS/PRECAUTIONS: Associated with renal toxicity; monitor SrCr prior to each treatment. Do not use during pregnancy. Monitor serum calcium, electrolytes, phosphate, magnesium, CBC with differential, Hct/Hgb closely. Monitor for 2 weeks post-treatment if pre-existing anemia, leukopenia, thrombocytopenia. Increased risk of renal adverse reactions with renal impairment; monitor renal function. Avoid treatment of bone metastases in severe renal impairment. Reports of osteonecrosis of jaw in cancer patients treated with bisphosphonates; avoid invasive dental procedures.

ADVERSE REACTIONS: Malaise, fever, convulsions, hypomagnesemia, hypocalcemia, hypokalemia, fluid overload, hypophosphatemia, nausea, diarrhea, constipation, anorexia, abnormal hepatic function, bone pain, dyspnea.

INTERACTIONS: Concurrent use with thalidomide increase risk of renal dysfunction in multiple myeloma. Caution with other potential nephrotoxic drugs.

PREGNANCY: Category D, caution in nursing.

MECHANISM OF ACTION: Bone resorption inhibitor; mechanism of antiresorptive action not established. Absorbs to calcium phosphate crystals in bone and may directly block dissolution of this mineral component of bone. Inhibition of osteoclast activity contributes to inhibition of bone resorption.

PHARMACOKINETICS: Elimination: Urine (46% unchanged); $T_{1/2}$=28 hrs.

NURSING CONSIDERATIONS

Assessment: Assess for hypersensitivity to other bisphosphonates, renal impairment (eg, CrCl<30mL/min), history of thyroid surgery, pregnancy/nursing status, and possible drug interactions. Assess SrCr prior to each treatment. Obtain dental exam for patients at risk for osteonecrosis of the jaw (eg, cancer chemotherapy, corticosteroids, poor dental hygiene).

Monitoring: Monitor for signs/symptoms of hypercalcemia, hypocalcemia, hypophosphatemia, hypokalemia, hypomagnesemia, renal toxicity, osteonecrosis of the jaw, and musculoskeletal pain. Monitor serum levels of calcium, phosphate, magnesium, and potassium. Monitor CBC, differential, and Hct/Hgb.

Patient Counseling: Instruct avoid pregnancy/nursing and invasive dental procedures while on medication. Inform periodic laboratory monitoring required.

Administration: IV route. Reconstitute. 1) Add 10mL of SWFI to each vial resulting in a solution of 30mg/10mL or 90mg/10mL. Do not mix with calcium-containing infusion solutions (eg, Ringer's solution); administer in single IV sol and line separate from all other drugs. **Storage**: Vial: Do not store above 30°C (86°F). Reconstituted: Refrigerate at 2-8°C (36-46°F) for up to 24 hrs.

ARGATROBAN — RX

argatroban (GlaxoSmithKline)

THERAPEUTIC CLASS: Direct thrombin inhibitor

INDICATIONS: Prophylaxis or treatment of thrombosis in heparin-induced thrombocytopenia (HIT). As an anticoagulant in patients with or at risk for HIT undergoing percutaneous coronary intervention (PCI).

DOSAGE: *Adults:* Thrombosis: D/C heparin and obtain baseline aPTT. Initial: 2mcg/kg/min IV. Check aPTT after 2 hrs. Titrate: Increase dose until aPTT is 1.5-3x initial baseline. Max: 10mcg/kg/min. Moderate Hepatic Impairment: Initial: 0.5mcg/kg/min. PCI: Initial: 350mcg/kg bolus with 25mcg/kg/min IV. Check activated clotting time (ACT) 5-10 min after bolus. Proceed with PCI if ACT >300 sec. If ACT <300 sec, give additional 150mcg/kg bolus and increase infusion to 30mcg/kg/min. Check ACT 5-10 min later. If ACT >450 sec, decrease to 15mcg/kg/min and check ACT 5-10 min later. Continue infusion dose at therapeutic ACT (300-450 sec) during procedure. May give additional 150mcg/kg bolus and increase infusion to 40mcg/kg/min if dissection, impending abrupt closure, thrombus formation, or inability to achieve/maintain

ACT >300 sec. After PCI, may use lower infusion rate if anticoagulation is needed.

HOW SUPPLIED: Inj: 100mg/mL

CONTRAINDICATIONS: Overt major bleeding.

WARNINGS/PRECAUTIONS: D/C all parenteral anticoagulants before administering. Extreme caution in conditions associated with an increased danger of hemorrhage (eg, severe HTN, immediately following lumbar puncture, bleeding disorder, GI lesions, spinal anesthesia, major surgery, etc). Caution in hepatic impairment. Avoid high doses in PCI patients with significant hepatic disease or AST/ALT ≥3x ULN. Monitor aPTT. For PCI, obtain ACT before dose, 5-10 min after bolus and infusion rate change, at the end of PCI, and every 20-30 min during prolonged procedures.

ADVERSE REACTIONS: GI bleed, GU bleed, Hct/Hgb decrease, hypotension, fever, diarrhea, sepsis, cardiac arrest, NV, ventricular tachycardia, allergic reactions, chest pain (in PCI).

INTERACTIONS: Initiate after cessation of heparin therapy; allow time for heparin's effect on the aPTT to decrease. Prolongation of PT/INR with warfarin. Antiplatelets, thrombolytics, and other anticoagulants may increase risk of bleeding. Discontinue all anticoagulants before argatroban administration.

PREGNANCY: Category B, not for use in nursing.

MECHANISM OF ACTION: Direct thrombin inhibitor; reversibly binds to thrombin active site. Exerts anticoagulant effects by inhibiting thrombin-catalyzed or thrombin-induced reactions, including fibrin formation; activation of coagulation factors V, VIII, XIII; activation of protein C; and platelet aggregation. Capable of inhibiting both free and clot-associated thrombin.

PHARMACOKINETICS: Distribution: V_d=174mL/Kg; plasma protein binding (54%). **Metabolism:** Liver, via hydroxylation and aromatization; CYP3A4/5; M1 (primary metabolite). **Elimination:** Feces (primary), urine; $T_{1/2}$=39-51 min.

NURSING CONSIDERATIONS

Assessment: Assess for hepatic impairment, overt major bleeding, and for drug interactions. Assess use in patients with disease states at risk for a hemorrhagic event (eg, severe HTN). Obtain baseline aPTT and activated clotting time (ACT).

Monitoring: Monitor for signs/symptoms of hemorrhagic events (eg, unexplained fall in Hct, decrease in BP) and for allergic reactions. Monitor aPTT 2 hrs after initiation of therapy to confirm desired therapeutic range. Monitor ACT 5-10 min after bolus dosing, after changes in infusion rate, and at end of PCI procedure.

Patient Counseling: Inform about risk of hemorrhagic events. Instruct to contact physician if unusual bleeding or allergic reactions occur.

Administration: IV route. Do not mix with other drugs prior to dilution. 2.5 mL vial: 1) Dilute (0.9% NS, D5W, or LR) to a final concentration of 1 mg/mL. Each 2.5mL vial should be diluted 100-fold by mixing with 250mL of diluent. 2) Mix repeatedly by inversion for 1 min. **Storage:** Vial: 25°C (77°F); excursions permitted to 15-30°C. Retain in original carton to protect from light. Prepared Solution: 25°C (77°F); excursions permitted to 15-30° (59-86°F) in ambient indoor light for 24 hrs. Stable for 96 hrs when protected from light and stored at controlled room temperature, 20-25°C (68-77°F) or refrigerated, 5°C ± 3°C (41°F ± 5°F).

ARICEPT — RX

donepezil HCl (Eisai/Pfizer)

OTHER BRAND NAMES: Aricept ODT (Eisai/Pfizer)

THERAPEUTIC CLASS: Acetylcholinesterase inhibitor

INDICATIONS: Treatment of dementia of the Alzheimer's type.

DOSAGE: *Adults:* Mild to Moderate Alzheimer's Disease: Initial: 5mg qd. Titrate: May increase to 10mg after 4-6 weeks. Severe Alzheimer's Disease: 10mg qd. Start with 5mg qd and increase to 10mg after 4-6 weeks.

HOW SUPPLIED: Tab: 5mg, 10mg; Tab, Disintegrating: 5mg, 10mg

CONTRAINDICATIONS: Hypersensitivity to piperidine derivatives.

WARNINGS/PRECAUTIONS: May exaggerate succinylcholine-type muscle relaxation during anesthesia. May have vagotonic effects on sinoatrial and atrioventricular node; may cause bradycardia or heart block. May increase gastric acid secretion; monitor for GI bleeding. May cause bladder outflow obstruction or seizures. Caution with asthma or COPD.

ADVERSE REACTIONS: Nausea, diarrhea, insomnia, vomiting, muscle cramps, fatigue, anorexia, dizziness, depression, weight decrease, infection, HTN, back pain, abnormal dreams, ecchymosis.

INTERACTIONS: Synergistic effect with neuromuscular blocking agents (eg, succinylcholine) and cholinergic agonists (eg, bethanechol). May interfere with anticholinergic medications. CYP2D6 and CYP3A4 inducers (eg, phenytoin, carbamazepine, dexamethasone, rifampin, phenobarbital) may increase elimination rate. Ketoconazole and quinidine inhibitors of CYP450, 3A4, and 2D6, respectively, inhibit donepezil metabolism.

PREGNANCY: Category C, not for use in nursing.

MECHANISM OF ACTION: Acetylcholinesterase inhibitor; postulated to exert effect by increasing acetylcholine concentrations through inhibition of its hydrolysis by AChE.

PHARMACOKINETICS: Absorption: Absolute bioavailability (complete); T_{max}=3-4 hrs. **Distribution:** Plasma protein binding (96%). **Metabolism:** Hepatic (glucoronidation) via CYP2D6 and CYP3A4. **Elimination:** Urine (57%), feces (15%); $T_{1/2}$=70 hrs.

NURSING CONSIDERATIONS

Assessment: Assess for history of cardiovascular conditions, ulcer disease, NSAID usage, GI bleed, asthma, obstructive pulmonary disease, possible drug interactions, renal/hepatic function.

Monitoring: Monitor renal/hepatic function, signs/symptoms of GI bleeding.

Patient Counseling: Can be taken without regard to meals. Seek medical attention if symptoms of GI bleeding occur. Caution with use of NSAIDs.

Administration: Oral route. **Storage:** 15-30°C (59-86°F).

ARIMIDEX RX

anastrozole (AstraZeneca)

THERAPEUTIC CLASS: Aromatase inhibitor (non-steroidal)

INDICATIONS: Adjuvant treatment of postmenopausal women with hormone receptor-positive early breast cancer. First-line treatment of postmenopausal women with hormone receptor positive or hormone receptor-unknown locally advanced or metastatic breast cancer. Treatment of advanced breast cancer in postmenopausal women with disease progression following tamoxifen therapy. Patients with ER-negative disease and patients who did not respond to previous tamoxifen therapy rarely respond.

DOSAGE: *Adults:* 1mg qd. Continue until tumor progression with advanced breast cancer.

HOW SUPPLIED: Tab: 1mg

CONTRAINDICATIONS: Pregnancy and premenopausal women.

WARNINGS/PRECAUTIONS: Increase incidence of ischemic cardiovascular events in patients with pre-existing ischemic heart disease reported. May cause reduction in bone mineral density. May elevate serum cholesterol.

ADVERSE REACTIONS: Hot flashes, asthenia, arthritis, pain, arthralgia, pharyngitis, HTN, depression, NV, rash, osteoporosis, fractures, back pain, insomnia, headache, bone pain, peripheral edema, increased cough, dyspnea, pharyngitis, and lymphedema.

INTERACTIONS: Concurrent use with tamoxifen decrease plasma levels. Avoid with estrogen-containing therapies.

PREGNANCY: Category X, not for use in nursing.

MECHANISM OF ACTION: Nonsteroidal aromatase inhibitor; lowers estradiol concentrations and has no detectable effect on formation of adrenal corticosteroids or aldosterone.

PHARMACOKINETICS: Distribution: Plasma protein binding (40%). **Metabolism:** Liver via N-dealkylation, hydroxylation, and glucuronidation. **Elimination**: Hepatic (major), renal (minor); urine (10%); $T_{1/2}$=50 hrs.

NURSING CONSIDERATIONS

Assessment: Assess for pre-existing ischemic cardiac disease, pregnancy/nursing status, menopausal status, and hepatic/renal impairment.

Monitoring: Monitor bone mineral density and LFTs.

Patient Counseling: Instruct to notify physician if pregnant/nursing or intend to become pregnant.

Administration: Oral route. **Storage:** 20-25°C (68-77°F).

ARIXTRA

fondaparinux sodium (GlaxoSmithKline) **RX**

Risk of paralysis by spinal/epidural hematoma with neuraxial anesthesia or spinal puncture. Increased risk with indwelling epidural catheters for analgesia, drugs affecting hemostasis (eg, NSAIDs, platelet inhibitors, anticoagulants), and traumatic or repeated epidural or spinal puncture.

THERAPEUTIC CLASS: Specific factor Xa inhibitor

INDICATIONS: Prophylaxis of DVT in patients undergoing hip fracture surgery, including extended prophylaxis; hip replacement surgery; knee replacement surgery; abdominal surgery who are at risk of thromboembolic complications. With concomitant warfarin, treatment of acute PE when initial therapy is administered in hospital and acute DVT.

DOSAGE: *Adults:* DVT Prophylaxis: 2.5mg SQ qd, starting 6-8 hrs post-op for 5-9 days (up to 11 days). Hip Fracture Surgery: Extended prophylaxis up to 24 additional days is recommended. DVT/PE Treatment: <50kg: 5mg SQ qd. 50-100kg: 7.5mg SQ qd. >100kg: 10mg SQ qd. Add concomitant warfarin ASAP (usually within 72 hrs) and continue for 5-9 days (up to 26 days) until INR=2-3.

HOW SUPPLIED: Inj: (Syringe) 2.5mg/0.5mL, 5mg/0.4mL, 7.5mg/0.6mL, 10mg/0.8mL

CONTRAINDICATIONS: Severe renal impairment (CrCl <30mL/min), body weight <50kg undergoing hip fracture, hip/knee replacement or abdominal surgery, bacterial endocarditis, active major bleeding, thrombocytopenia with a positive *in vitro* test for anti-platelet antibody.

WARNINGS/PRECAUTIONS: Not for IM injection. Cannot use interchangeably unit for unit with heparin or other low molecular weight heparins. Risk of hemorrhage increases with renal impairment. Caution with moderate renal dysfunction, elderly, history of HIT, bleeding diathesis, uncontrolled arterial HTN, recent GI ulceration, diabetic retinopathy, hemorrhage. Monitor renal function periodically. Extreme caution in conditions with an increased risk of hemorrhage (eg, bleeding disorders, hemorrhagic stroke, etc). Perform routine CBC, SCr, stool occult blood tests. D/C if platelets <100,000/mm^3. Thrombocytopenia reported. Major bleeding with abdominal surgery reported.

ADVERSE REACTIONS: Bleeding complications, thrombocytopenia, local reactions (eg, rash, pruritus), anemia, fever, NV, edema, constipation, insomnia, hypokalemia, UTI, dizziness, purpura, hypotension.

INTERACTIONS: Discontinue agents that may enhance risk of hemorrhage (eg, platelet inhibitors); monitor closely if co-administered.

PREGNANCY: Category B, caution in nursing.

MECHANISM OF ACTION: Specific factor Xa inhibitor; selectively binds to antithrombin III (ATIII). Potentiates the innate neutralization of Factor Xa by ATIII. Neutralization of Factor Xa interrupts the blood coagulation cascade and thus inhibits thrombin formation and thrombus development.

PHARMACOKINETICS: Absorption: Rapid, complete; absolute bioavailability (100%); C_{max}=0.39-0.5 mg/L (2.5 mg QD); 1.2-1.26mg/L (5mg, 7.5mg, 10mg QD); T_{max}=3 hrs (2.5 mg QD). **Distribution:** V_d=7-11L; bound to ATIII (94%). **Metabolism:** Not investigated. **Elimination:** Urine (77%); $T_{1/2}$=17-21 hrs.

NURSING CONSIDERATIONS

Assessment: Assess for severe renal impairment (CrCl<30mL/min), presence of active major bleeding, bacterial endocarditis, and thrombocytopenia. Assess use for prophylactic therapy in patients who weigh <50kg and are undergoing hip fracture, hip/knee replacement, or abdominal surgery. Assess use with bleeding diathesis, uncontrolled arterial HTN, history or recent GI ulceration, diabetic retinopathy, recent hemorrhage, nursing/pregnancy status, and in elderly (≥65 yrs) patients. Assess for drug interactions.

Monitoring: Monitor for signs/symptoms of bleeding and thrombocytopenia. In patients undergoing neuraxial anesthesia, monitor for epidural or spinal hematomas and neurologic impairment. Perform periodic monitoring of renal function (SrCr), CBC with platelet count, and stool occult blood tests.

Patient Counseling: Counsel that medication is to be injected subcutaneously once daily. Instruct to report any abnormal bleeding. Advise that periodic laboratory monitoring is required during therapy.

Administration: SQ route. Do not inject IM. Do not inject with other injections or infusions. Do not expel air bubble in pre-filled syringe. Administer in fatty tissue, alternating injection sites. 1) Wipe injection site with alcohol swab. 2) Pinch fold of skin at injection site between thumb and forefinger; hold throughout injection. 3) Insert full length of syringe needle perpendicularly into skin fold. 4) Inject full contents, pushing plunger as far as it will go; plunger should then rise automatically while needle withdraws from skin. **Storage:** 25°C (77°F); excursions permitted to 15-30°C (59-86°F). Keep out of reach of children.

ARMOUR THYROID — RX

thyroid (Forest)

THERAPEUTIC CLASS: Thyroid replacement hormone

INDICATIONS: Treatment of hypothyroidism. As a pituitary TSH suppressant in the treatment or prevention of various types of euthyroid goiters. Diagnostic agent in suppression tests to differentiate suspected mild hyperthyroidism or thyroid gland autonomy. Management of thyroid cancer.

DOSAGE: *Adults:* Hypothyroidism: Initial: 30mg qd. Titrate: Increase by 15mg q2-3 weeks. Myxedema with Cardiovascular Disorder: 15mg qd. Maint: 60-120mg/day. Thyroid Cancer: Higher doses than replacement therapy are required. Myxedema Coma: Levothyroxine Sodium: Initial: 400mcg IV then 100-200mcg/day IV. Continue with oral therapy when stabilized. Thyroid Suppression: 1.56mg/kg/day for 7-10 days. Elderly: Initial: Use lower dose (eg, 15-30mg qd).

Pediatrics: Hypothyroidism: 0-6 months: 4.8-6mg/kg/day; 6-12 months: 3.6-4.8mg/kg/day; 1-5 yrs: 3-3.6mg/kg/day; 6-12 yrs: 2.4-3mg/kg/day; >12 yrs: 1.2-1.8mg/kg/day.

HOW SUPPLIED: Tab: 15mg, 30mg, 60mg, 90mg, 120mg, 180mg, 240mg, 300mg

CONTRAINDICATIONS: Untreated thyrotoxicosis; uncorrected adrenal cortical insufficiency.

WARNINGS/PRECAUTIONS: Do not use in the treatment of obesity; larger doses in euthyroid patients can cause serious or even life-threatening toxicity. Caution with cardiovascular disease, DM, diabetes insipidus, elderly, and adrenal cortical insufficiency.

INTERACTIONS: May increase insulin or oral hypoglycemic requirements. Reduced absorption with cholestyramine and colestipol; space dosing by 4-5 hrs. Altered effect of oral anticoagulants; monitor PT/INR. Estrogens increase thyroxine-binding globulin; increase in thyroid dose may be needed. Serious or life-threatening side effects can occur with sympathomimetic amines. Androgens, corticosteroids, estrogens, iodine-containing preparations, and salicylates may interfere with thyroid lab tests.

PREGNANCY: Category A, caution in nursing.

MECHANISM OF ACTION: Thyroid hormone; not established, suspected to enhance oxygen consumption by most body tissues, increase the basal metabolic rate and metabolism of carbohydrates, lipids, and proteins.

PHARMACOKINETICS: Abosrption: (T_3) Completely absorbed; T_{max}=4 hrs; (T_4) partially absorbed. **Distribution:** Plasma protein binding (>99%), found in breast milk. **Metabolism:** Deiodination in liver, kidneys, other tissues.

NURSING CONSIDERATIONS

Assessment: Assess for diagnosed but uncorrected adrenal cortical insufficiency, untreated thyrotoxicosis, hypersensitivity to any of its active or extraneous constituents, cardiovascular system, angina, DM, myxedema coma, and possible drug and test interactions.

Monitoring: Monitor urinary glucose levels in patients with DM, PT in patients receiving anticoagulants, and periodic assessment of thyroid status (TSH suppression test, serum T_4 levels, free T_4; if TSH is normal, total T_4 is low), free T_3, T_4, signs/symptoms of thyroid hormone toxicity (chest pain, increased pulse rate, palpitations, excessive sweating, heat intolerance, and nervousness), partial hair loss in children.

Patient Counseling: Inform that replacement therapy is to be taken essentially for life, with the exception of cases of transient hypothyroidism, which associated with thyroiditis, and those patients receiving a therapeutical trial of the drug. Report immediately any signs/symptoms of thyroid toxicity.

Administration: Oral route. **Storage**: Store at 15-30°C (59-86°F).

AROMASIN RX

exemestane (Pharmacia & Upjohn)

THERAPEUTIC CLASS: Aromatase inactivator

INDICATIONS: In postmenopausal women, treatment of advanced breast cancer that has progressed after tamoxifen therapy. Adjuvant treatment of postmenopausal women with estrogen-receptor positive early breast cancer who have received 2-3 yrs of tamoxifen and are switched to exemestane for a total completion of 5 consecutive yrs to adjuvant hormonal therapy.

DOSAGE: *Adults:* Early/Advanced: 25mg qd after a meal. Continue in the absence of recurrence of contralateral breast cancer until completion of 5 yrs of adjuvant endocrine therapy in postmenopausal women with early breast cancer treated with 2-3 yrs of tamoxifen. Continue until tumor progression is evident. Concomitant Potent CYP3A4 Inducers (eg, rifampicin, phenytoin): 50mg qd after a meal.

HOW SUPPLIED: Tab: 25mg

WARNINGS/PRECAUTIONS: Fetal harm in pregnancy. Avoid in premenopausal women.

ADVERSE REACTIONS: Fatigue, NV, hot flashes, pain, depression, insomnia, anxiety, dyspnea, dizziness, headache, increased sweating, edema, HTN, anorexia.

INTERACTIONS: Avoid coadministration with estrogen-containing agents. Potent CYP3A4 inducers (eg, rifampin, phenytoin, carbamazepine, phenobarbital, St. John's wort) may decrease plasma levels.

PREGNANCY: Category D, caution in nursing.

MECHANISM OF ACTION: Irreversible steroidal aromatase inactivator; acts as false substrate for aromatase enzyme; processed to intermediate that binds irreversibly to active site of enzyme, causing inactivation.

PHARMACOKINETICS: Absorption: Rapid. (Healthy) T_{max}=2.9 hrs; AUC=41.4ng•h/mL. (Breast cancer) T_{max}=1.2 hrs; AUC=75.4ng•h/mL. **Distribution:** Plasma protein binding (90%). **Metabolism:** Oxidation via CYP3A4; reduction. **Elimination:** Urine (<1%), $T_{1/2}$=24 hrs.

NURSING CONSIDERATIONS

Assessment: Assess for possible drug interactions, renal/hepatic functions.

Monitoring: Monitor for hematological abnormalities, LFTs, creatinine, and bone mineral density.

Patient Counseling: Inform of pregnancy risks. Advise to take after meal.

Administration: Oral route. **Storage:** 25°C (77°F); excursions permitted to 15-30°C (59-86°F).

ARTHROTEC RX

diclofenac sodium - misoprostol (Pfizer)

Contraindicated in pregnancy. Must have negative pregnancy test 2 weeks before therapy. Provide oral and written hazards of misoprostol. Begin on 2nd or 3rd day of the next normal menstrual period. Use reliable contraception. NSAIDs may cause an increased risk of serious cardiovascular thrombotic events, MI, stroke, and serious GI adverse events including bleeding, ulceration, and perforation of the stomach or intestines. Contraindicated for the treatment of perioperative pain in the setting of coronary artery bypass graft (CABG) surgery.

THERAPEUTIC CLASS: NSAID/prostaglandin E_1 analogue

INDICATIONS: Treatment of the signs and symptoms of osteoarthritis (OA) or rheumatoid arthritis (RA) in patients at high risk of developing NSAID-induced gastric and duodenal ulcers.

DOSAGE: *Adults:* OA: 50mg tid. RA: 50mg tid-qid. OA/RA: If not tolerable, give 50-75mg bid (less effective in preventing ulcers). Do not crush, chew, or divide.

HOW SUPPLIED: Tab: (Diclofenac-Misoprostol) 50mg-0.2mg, 75mg-0.2mg

CONTRAINDICATIONS: Pregnancy. ASA or other NSAID allergy that precipitates asthma, urticaria, or other allergic reactions. Treatment of perioperative pain in the setting of CABG surgery.

WARNINGS/PRECAUTIONS: May lead to onset of new HTN or worsening of pre-existing HTN; monitor BP closely. Fluid retention and edema reported; caution with fluid retention or heart failure. Renal papillary necrosis and other renal injury reported after long-term use. Not recommended for use with advanced renal disease; if therapy must be initiated, monitor renal function. May cause elevations of LFTs; d/c if abnormal LFTs persist/worsen, liver disease develops or systemic manifestations occur. Anaphylactoid reactions may occur. May cause serious skin adverse events (eg, exfoliative dermatitis, Stevens-Johnson syndrome, and toxic epidermal necrolysis). Avoid in late pregnancy; may cause premature closure of ductus arteriosis. Caution in elderly. Anemia may occur; with long-term use, monitor Hgb/Hct if signs or symptoms of anemia. May inhibit platelet aggregation and prolong bleeding time; monitor with coagulation disorders. Caution with asthma and avoid with ASA-sensitive asthma. Aseptic meningitis with fever and coma reported. Avoid with hepatic porphyria.

ADVERSE REACTIONS: Abdominal pain, diarrhea, dyspepsia, nausea, flatulence, GI disorders.

INTERACTIONS: Avoid magnesium-containing antacids, salicylates, ASA, other NSAIDs. Caution with anticoagulants; may have synergistic GI bleeding effects with warfarin. May decrease effects of antihypertensives, diuretics. Increased serum potassium with K^+-sparing diuretics. May alter response to insulin or oral hypoglycemics. Monitor for digoxin, methotrexate, cyclosporine, phenobarbital, and lithium toxicities.

PREGNANCY: Category X, not for use in nursing.

MECHANISM OF ACTION: Diclofenac: NSAID; not established. May be related to prostaglandin synthetase inhibition. Possesses anti-inflammatory, analgesic, and antipyretic properties. Misoprostol: Prostaglandin E_1 analog with gastric antisecretory and mucosal protective properties.

PHARMACOKINETICS: Absorption: Oral administration of a single dose or multiple doses of medication are similar to pharmacokinetics of two individual components. Refer to PI for further information. **Distribution:** Diclofenac: V_d=550mL/kg; albumin binding (99%); found in breast milk. Misoprostol: Plasma protein binding (<90%). **Metabolism:** Diclofenac: Glucuronide and sulfate conjugation. Misoprostol: Rapidly, to misoprostol acid (active metabolite). **Elimination:** Diclofenac: Urine (65%), bile (35%); $T_{1/2}$=2 hrs. Misoprostol: Urine (70%); $T_{1/2}$=30 min.

NURSING CONSIDERATIONS

Assessment: Assess for pain, hypersensitivity to aspirin or other NSAIDs, CV disease, risk of HTN, fluid retention, HF, previous history of peptic ulcer disease or GI bleeding, impaired renal/hepatic function, coagulation disorders, asthma, hepatic porphyria, and possible drug interactions. Assess that women have had negative pregnancy test within 2 weeks prior to therapy and are capable to comply with effective contraceptive measures.

Monitoring: Monitor for signs/symptoms of cardiovascular thrombotic events, HTN, fluid retention and edema, GI effects (eg, bleeding, ulceration, perforation of stomach, small intestine, or large intestine), renal papillary necrosis, elevations in liver enzymes or severe hepatic reactions (eg, liver necrosis, jaundice), anaphylactoid reactions, skin reactions, hematological effects (eg, anemia), bronchospasm, aseptic meningitis, and porphyria. Monitor BP at initiation of and during therapy. Monitor renal function if renal disease present. If on long term therapy, monitor transaminases 4-8 weeks after initiating therapy. If anemia is suspected, monitor Hgb/Hct.

Patient Counseling: Instruct females they must not be pregnant when therapy is initiated and must remain on an effective form of contraception during treatment. This drug may cause abortion, premature labor, or birth defects if given while pregnant. Do not give medication to other individuals. Contact physician if signs/symptoms of CV effects (eg, chest pain, SOB, slurring of speech), GI effects (eg, epigastric pain, dyspepsia, melena, hematemesis), or unexplained weight gain and edema occur. Contact physician and d/c treatment if signs of skin reactions or hepatotoxicity (eg, nausea, fatigue, jaundice, right upper quadrant tenderness) occur. Seek emergency attention if breathing difficulty, facial or throat swelling develops. Inform that medication cannot be substituted for corticosteroids or treat corticosteroid insufficiency.

Administration: Oral route. **Storage:** At or below 25°C (77°F), in a dry area.

ASACOL — RX

mesalamine (Procter & Gamble)

THERAPEUTIC CLASS: Anti-inflammatory Agent

INDICATIONS: Treatment of mild to moderately active ulcerative colitis and maintenance of remission of ulcerative colitis.

DOSAGE: *Adults:* Mild-Moderate Active Ulcerative Colitis: Usual: 800mg tid for 6 weeks. Maintenance of Remission: 1.6g/day in divided doses.

HOW SUPPLIED: Tab, Delayed-Release: 400mg

CONTRAINDICATIONS: Hypersensitivity to salicylates.

WARNINGS/PRECAUTIONS: Exacerbation of colitis reported upon initiation of therapy; symptoms abate with discontinuation. Caution with sulfasalazine hypersensitivity. Caution with renal dysfunction or history of renal disease.

Monitor renal function prior to therapy and periodically after. Pyloric stenosis could delay mesalamine release in the colon.

ADVERSE REACTIONS: Diarrhea, headache, NV, pharyngitis, abdominal pain, pain, eructation, dizziness, asthenia, fever, dysmenorrhea, arthralgia, dyspepsia.

PREGNANCY: Category B, caution in nursing.

MECHANISM OF ACTION: Unknown; possibly diminishes inflammation by blocking cyclooxygenase and inhibiting prostaglandin production in the colon.

PHARMACOKINETICS: Absorption: T_{max}=4-12 hrs. **Metabolism:** Gut mucosal wall and liver via rapid acetylation. Metabolite (N-acetyl-5-aminosalicylic acid). **Elimination:** $T_{1/2}$=2-15 hrs. Renally excreted as metabolite.

NURSING CONSIDERATIONS

Assessment: Assess for history of renal dysfunction/disease and pyloric stenosis. Obtain baseline renal function, LFTs, CBC, and cardiac function.

Monitoring: Monitor renal function, LFTs, and CBC periodically. Monitor for signs/symptoms of prolonged gastric retention (pyloric stenosis), exacerbation of colitis (cramping, abdominal pain, bloody diarrhea), renal impairment, hypersensitivity and allergic reactions.

Patient Counseling: Instruct to swallow whole, do not break outer coating. Advise to report if intact or partially intact tablet is seen in stool. Inform that ulcerative colitis rarely remits completely, and the risk of relapse can be subtantially reduced by continued administration of medication. Seek medical attention if symptoms of prolonged gastric retention, exacerbation of colitis (cramping, abdominal pain, bloody diarrhea), hypersensitivity and allergic reactions occur.

Administration: Oral route. **Storage:** 20-25°C (68-77°F).

ASMANEX — RX

mometasone furoate (Schering)

THERAPEUTIC CLASS: Corticosteroid

INDICATIONS: Maintenance treatment of asthma as prophylactic therapy in patients ≥4 yrs.

DOSAGE: *Adults:* Previous Therapy with Bronchodilators Alone or Inhaled Corticosteroids: Initial: 220mcg qpm. Max: 440mcg qpm or 220mcg bid. Previous Therapy with Oral Corticosteroids: Initial: 440mcg bid. Max: 880mcg/day. Titrate to lowest effective dose once asthma stability achieved. *Pediatrics:* ≥12 yrs: Previous Therapy with Bronchodilators Alone or Inhaled Corticosteroids (CS): Initial: 220mcg qpm. Max: 440mcg qpm or 220mcg bid. Previous Therapy with Oral CS: Initial: 440mcg bid. Max: 880mcg/day. 4-11 yrs: 110mcg qpm regardless of prior therapy. Titrate to lowest effective dose once asthma stability achieved.

HOW SUPPLIED: Twisthaler: 110mcg/inh, 220mcg/inh

CONTRAINDICATIONS: Primary treatment of status asthmaticus or other acute episodes of asthma where intensive measures are required.

WARNINGS/PRECAUTIONS: Deaths due to adrenal insufficiency have occurred with transfer from systemic corticosteroids to inhaled corticosteroids. Wean slowly from systemic corticosteroid therapy. Resume oral corticosteroids during stress or severe asthma attack. May unmask allergic conditions previously suppressed by systemic corticosteroid therapy. May increase susceptibility to infections. Not for rapid relief of bronchospasm or other acute episodes of asthma. D/C if bronchospasm occurs after dosing. Observe for systemic corticosteroid withdrawal effects, hypercorticism, reduced bone mineral density, and adrenal suppression; reduce dose slowly if needed. Decreased growth velocity may occur in pediatrics. *Candida* infections in the mouth and pharynx reported. Caution with active or quiescent TB infection of respiratory tract; untreated systemic fungal, bacterial, viral, or parasitic infections; or ocular herpes simplex. Glaucoma, increased IOP, and cataracts reported.

ADVERSE REACTIONS: Headache, allergic rhinitis, pharyngitis, upper respiratory tract infection, sinusitis, oral candidiasis, dysmenorrhea, musculoskeletal pain, back pain, dyspepsia, myalgia, abdominal pain, nausea.

INTERACTIONS: Ketoconazole may increase plasma levels.

PREGNANCY: Category C, caution in nursing.

MECHANISM OF ACTION: Corticosteroid; shown to have inhibitory effects on multiple cell types (mast cells, eosinophils, neutrophils, macrophages, and lymphocytes) and mediators (histamine, eicosanoids, leukotrienes and cytokines), involved in inflammatory and asthmatic response.

PHARMACOKINETICS: Absorption: Absolute bioavailability (≤1%); C_{max}=94-114pcg/mL; T_{max}=1.0-2.5 hrs. **Distribution:** V_d=152L; plasma protein binding (98-99%). **Metabolism:** Liver, via CYP3A4. **Elimination:** $T_{1/2}$=5 hrs.

NURSING CONSIDERATIONS

Assessment: Assess for risk factors for decreased bone mineral content (eg, prolonged immobilization, family history of osteoporosis, drugs that decrease bone mass), history of increased IOP, glaucoma, cataracts, concomitant diseases such as status asthmaticus, active or quiescent pulmonary TB, ocular herpes simplex, untreated systemic fungal, bacterial, parasitic or viral infections, and possible drug interactions.

Monitoring: Monitor for localized oral infections with *Candida albicans*, decreased bone mass, asthma instability (serial objective measures of airflow), body height in children, development of glaucoma, increased IOP, posterior subcapsular cataracts, adrenal insufficiency (eg, fatigue, weakness, NV, hypotension), paradoxical bronchospasm, and hypersensitivity reactions.

Patient Counseling: Instruct to discard inhaler 45 days after opening foil pouch or when dose counter reads "00" and final dose inhaled, whichever comes first. If dose counter not working correctly, do not use and bring to physician or pharmacist. Inform that medication is not a bronchodilator and should not be used for sudden symptoms of SOB or acute bronchospasm. Advise to rinse mouth after inhalation. Inform drug may cause reduction in growth rate (pediatrics) and may also unmask allergies (eg, rhinitis, conjunctivitis, eczema). Avoid exposure to chickenpox or measles; seek medical attention if exposed to chickenpox or measles, worsening of existing TB, infections, or ocular herpes simplex, symptoms do not improve or worsen, during periods of stress or severe asthmatic attack, adrenal insufficiency (eg, fatigue, weakness, NV and hypotension), paradoxical bronchospasm or hypersensitivity reactions occur.

Administration: Oral inhalation. Inhale rapidly and deeply. **Storage:** Dry place at 25°C (77°F); excursions permitted to 15-30°C (59-86°F). Discard inhaler 45 days after opening foil pouch or when dose counter reads "00" and final dose has been inhaled, whichever comes first.

ASTELIN

azelastine HCl (Meda) **RX**

THERAPEUTIC CLASS: Antihistamine

INDICATIONS: Treatment of the symptoms of seasonal allergic rhinitis and vasomotor rhinitis.

DOSAGE: *Adults:* 2 sprays per nostril bid.
Pediatrics: Seasonal Allergic/Vasomotor Rhinitis: ≥12 yrs: 2 sprays per nostril bid. Seasonal Allergic Rhinitis: 5-11 yrs: 1 spray per nostril bid.

HOW SUPPLIED: Spray: 137mcg/spray [30mL]

ADVERSE REACTIONS: Bitter taste, somnolence, weight increase, headache, nasal burning, pharyngitis, paroxysmal sneezing, dry mouth, nausea, atrial fibrillation, palpitations.

INTERACTIONS: Avoid alcohol or other CNS depressants; additive CNS impairment may occur. Increased azelastine levels with cimetidine.

PREGNANCY: Category C, caution in nursing.

MECHANISM OF ACTION: Phthalazinone derivative; inhibits histamine H_1 receptor activity.

PHARMACOKINETICS: Absorption: T_{max}=2-3 hrs. **Distribution:** Azelastine: plasma protein binding (88%). Desmethylazelastine: V_d=14.5L/kg; plasma protein binding (97%).

NURSING CONSIDERATIONS

Assessment: Assess for liver/renal functions, alcohol intake, and possible drug interactions.

Monitoring: Monitor for somnolence.

Patient Counseling: Caution against hazardous activities (eg, operating machinery/driving). Avoid concomitant use of drugs (eg, other antihistamines, CNS depressants) or alcohol. Avoid spraying in eyes. Consult physician if pregnant/nursing or planning to become pregnant.

Administration: Intranasal route. **Storage:** 20-25°C (68-77F°). Protect from freezing. Store bottle upright with pump tightly closed.

ASTEPRO RX

azelastine HCl (Meda)

THERAPEUTIC CLASS: H_1-antagonist

INDICATIONS: Relief of seasonal allergic rhinitis symptoms in patients >12 yrs.

DOSAGE: *Adults:* 1 or 2 sprays per nostril bid.
Pediatrics: >12 yrs: 1 or 2 sprays per nostril bid.

HOW SUPPLIED: Spray: 137mcg [30mL]

WARNINGS/PRECAUTIONS: Somnolence reported. May impair physical/mental abilities.

ADVERSE REACTIONS: Bitter taste, somnolence, epistaxis, headache, nasal discomfort, and fatigue.

INTERACTIONS: Avoid concurrent use with alcohol or other CNS depressants. Increased levels with cimetidine.

PREGNANCY: Category C, caution in nursing.

MECHANISM OF ACTION: H_1 receptor antagonist; inhibits histamine H_1 receptor activity in isolated tissues, animal models, and humans.

PHARMACOKINETICS: Absorption: Bioavailability (40%); C_{max}=200pg/mL; T_{max}=3 hrs; AUC =5122 pg.hr/mL. **Distribution:** Plasma protein binding [azelastine, desmethylazelastine (major metabolite)]: (88%, 97% respectively). V_d=14.5L/kg. **Metabolism:** Oxidation via CYP450 enzyme system. Desmethylazelastine (major). **Elimination:** Azelastine: Feces (75%, 10% unchanged); $T_{1/2}$=22 hrs. Desmethylazelastine: $T_{1/2}$=52 hrs.

NURSING CONSIDERATIONS

Assessment: Assess for liver/renal functions, alcohol intake, and possible drug interactions.

Monitoring: Monitor for somnolence, bitter taste, epistaxis, headache, nasal discomfort, and fatigue.

Patient Counseling: Use exactly as prescribed. Use caution while engaging in hazardous activities (eg, operating machinery/driving) requiring complete mental alertness and motor coordination. Avoid alcohol or other CNS depressants. Avoid spraying in eyes. Notify physician if pregnant/nursing or planning to become pregnant. Advise to prime medication before intial spray by releasing 6 sprays or until a fine mist appears. When medication has not been used for >3 days, reprime with 2 sprays or until a fine mist appears.

Administration: Intranasal route. **Storage:** 20°-25°C (68°-77°F). Protect from freezing. Store bottle upright with pump tightly closed.

ASTRAMORPH PF

CII

morphine sulfate (Abraxis)

THERAPEUTIC CLASS: Opioid analgesic

INDICATIONS: Management of pain unresponsive to non-narcotic analgesics.

DOSAGE: *Adults:* IV: Initial: 2-10mg/70kg. Epidural Injection: Initial: 5mg in lumbar region. Titrate: If inadequate pain relief within 1 hr, increase by 1-2mg. Max: 10mg/24hrs. Continuous Epidural: Initial: 2-4mg/24hrs. Give additional 1-2mg if needed. Intrathecal: 0.2-1mg single dose, do not repeat; may follow with 0.6mg/hr naloxone infusion to reduce incidence of side effects. Elderly/Debilitated: Epidural: <5mg/24hrs. Intrathecal: Lower dose.

HOW SUPPLIED: Inj: 0.5mg/mL, 1mg/mL

CONTRAINDICATIONS: Allergy to opiates, acute bronchial asthma, upper airway obstruction. Epidural/intrathecal routes with injection site infection, anticoagulants, bleeding diathesis, within 2 weeks of IV corticosteroids.

WARNINGS/PRECAUTIONS: Have resuscitation equipment, trained personnel and narcotic antagonists available; severe respiratory depression may occur. Avoid rapid administration. May be habit-forming. Caution with head injury, increased intracranial/intraocular pressure, decreased respiratory reserve, hepatic/renal dysfunction, elderly, debilitated. High doses may cause seizures. Smooth muscle hypertonicity may cause biliary colic, urinary difficulty or retention. Orthostatic hypotension may occur with hypovolemia or myocardial dysfunction. Acute respiratory failure reported with COPD or acute asthmatic attack. Limit epidural/intrathecal route to lumbar area.

ADVERSE REACTIONS: Respiratory depression, hypotension, pruritus, urinary retention, NV, constipation, anxiety, cough reflex depression, oliguria.

INTERACTIONS: CNS depressants (eg, alcohol, sedatives, antihistamines) and psychotropics (eg, MAOIs, phenothiazines, TCAs) potentiate CNS depression. Neuroleptics may increase respiratory depression.

PREGNANCY: Category C, safety in nursing not known.

MECHANISM OF ACTION: Opioid analgesic. Analgesic effect involves 3 areas of CNS; periaqueductal periventricular gray matter, ventromedial medulla, and spinal cord. Interacts predominantly with the µ-receptor to produce analgesic effects; µ-binding sites are found in the brain, spinal cord, and in the trigeminal nerve.

PHARMACOKINETICS: Absorption: (Epidural) C_{max}=33-40ng/mL; (intrathecal) $C_{max} \leq$1-7.8ng/mL; (epidural, intrathecal) T_{max}=5-10 min. **Distribution:** (IV) V_d= 1-4.7L/kg; (intrathecal) V_d=22 mL. Plasma protein binding (36%), muscle tissue binding (54%). **Metabolism:** Hepatic glucuronidation. Found in breast milk. **Elimination:** Urine (major), feces (10%). (IV) $T_{1/2}$=1.5-2 hrs; (Epidural) $T_{1/2}$=39-249 min.

NURSING CONSIDERATIONS

Assessment: Assess for hypersensitivity to other opioids, acute bronchial asthma or COPD, infection at the injection site, bleeding diathesis, hypotension, seizure disorder, head injury or increased intracranial pressure, age of patient, renal/hepatic function, biliary tract disorders, nursing/pregnancy status, and drug interactions.

Monitoring: Monitor for signs/symptoms of respiratory depression, hypotension, myoclonic-like spasms, seizures, urinary retention, and drug dependence. If administered via epidural intrathecally, monitor patients for 24 hrs for signs of respiratory depression.

Patient Counseling: Instruct to report if any signs/symptoms of respiratory depression (eg, difficulty breathing) occur. Inform physician of all medications currently taking. Advise to avoid consumption of alcohol or other CNS depressants. Inform drug may be habit forming. Avoid abrupt withdrawal.

Administration: IV, epidural, or intrathecal route. Administer in a setting where proper monitoring and resuscitative equipment are available. For epidural administration, proper placement of the needle or catheter in the epidural space should be verified before medication is injected. **Storage:** Store in a carton 20-25°C (68-77°F); excursions permitted to 15-30°C (59-86°F). Do not freeze. Discard any unused portion. Do not heat-sterilize.

ATACAND RX

candesartan cilexetil (AstraZeneca)

Can cause injury/death to developing fetus during 2nd and 3rd trimesters. D/C therapy if pregnancy is detected.

THERAPEUTIC CLASS: Angiotensin II receptor antagonist

INDICATIONS: Treatment of hypertension, alone or with other antihypertensives. Treatment of heart failure (NYHA class II-IV, ejection fraction ≤40%) to reduce risk of death and hospitalizations.

DOSAGE: *Adults:* HTN: Monotherapy Without Volume Depletion: Initial: 16mg qd. Usual: 8-32mg/day given qd-bid. May add diuretic if BP not controlled. Intravascular Volume Depletion/Moderate Hepatic Impairment: Lower initial dose. Heart Failure: Initial: 4mg qd. Usual: 32mg qd. Titrate: Double dose every 2 weeks, as tolerated.

HOW SUPPLIED: Tab: 4mg, 8mg, 16mg, 32mg

WARNINGS/PRECAUTIONS: Can cause fetal injury/death. Correct volume or salt depletion before therapy or monitor closely. Changes in renal function may occur; caution with renal artery stenosis, CHF. Risk of hypotension; caution in major surgery and anesthesia, or when initiating therapy in heart failure. May cause hyperkalemia in heart failure patients; monitor serum potassium.

ADVERSE REACTIONS: Back pain, dizziness, upper respiratory infection, pharyngitis, rhinitis, headache.

INTERACTIONS: Increases lithium levels.

PREGNANCY: Category C (1st trimester) and D (2nd and 3rd trimesters), not for use in nursing.

MECHANISM OF ACTION: Angiotensin II receptor antagonist; selective for AT_1 receptors, with tight binding to and slow dissociation from receptor.

PHARMACOKINETICS: Absorption: Absolute bioavailability (14%); T_{max}=3-4 hrs. **Distribution:** V_d=0.1L/kg; plasma protein binding (>99%). **Metabolism:** Ester hydrolysis (metabolite: candesartan); CYP2C9 (minor). **Elimination:** Feces (56%), urine (26%); $T_{1/2}$=9 hrs.

NURSING CONSIDERATIONS

Assessment: Assess for renal impairment, CHF, CVD, aortic or mitral valve stenosis, obstructive hypertrophic cardiomyopathy, primary hyperaldosteronism, galactose intolerance, Lapp lactase deficiency, glucose-galactose malabsorption, pregnancy/nursing status, hepatic impairment (cholestasis), and possible drug interactions.

Monitoring: In renal impairment, monitor serum K^+, creatinine, and BP periodically. Monitor for signs/symptoms of hypotension, CV events, hypersensitivity reactions, liver/renal dysfunction.

Patient Counseling: Inform of pregnancy/nursing risks. Caution may impair physical/mental abilities. Advise to seek medical attention if symptoms of hypotension, CV events, or hypersensitivity reactions occur.

Administration: Oral route. **Storage:** Below 30°C.

ATACAND HCT RX

candesartan cilexetil - hydrochlorothiazide (AstraZeneca)

Can cause injury/death to developing fetus during 2nd and 3rd trimesters. D/C therapy if pregnancy detected.

ATACAND HCT

THERAPEUTIC CLASS: Angiotensin II receptor antagonist/thiazide diuretic

INDICATIONS: Treatment of hypertension. Not for initial therapy.

DOSAGE: *Adults:* Initial: If BP not controlled on HCTZ 25mg/day or controlled but serum K^+ decreased: 16mg-12.5mg tab qd. If BP not controlled on 32mg candesartan/day, give 32mg-12.5mg qd; may increase to 32mg-25mg qd.

HOW SUPPLIED: Tab: (Candesartan-HCTZ) 16mg-12.5mg, 32mg-12.5mg, 32mg-25mg

CONTRAINDICATIONS: Anuria, sulfonamide hypersensitivity.

WARNINGS/PRECAUTIONS: Can cause fetal injury/death. Correct volume or salt depletion before therapy. Caution with hepatic or renal dysfunction, renal artery stenosis, severe CHF, history of allergies, and asthma. May exacerbate or activate SLE. Monitor serum electrolytes. Avoid if CrCl ≤30mL/min. Hyperuricemia, hyperglycemia, hypokalemia, hypomagnesemia, hyponatremia, hypercalcemia may occur. Enhanced effects in post-sympathectomy patient. May increase cholesterol and triglyceride levels. Risk of hypotension; caution in major surgery or anesthesia.

ADVERSE REACTIONS: Upper respiratory infection, back pain, influenza-like symptoms, dizziness, headache.

INTERACTIONS: Potentiates orthostatic hypotension with alcohol, barbiturates, and narcotics. Adjust insulin and antidiabetic drugs. Impaired absorption with cholestyramine, colestipol. Corticosteroids and ACTH deplete electrolytes. May decrease response to pressor amines. Potentiates other antihypertensives. May increase responsiveness to skeletal muscle relaxants. Risk of lithium toxicity; monitor lithium levels during concomitant use. NSAIDs decrease diuretic effects.

PREGNANCY: Category C (1st trimester) and D (2nd and 3rd trimesters), not for use in nursing.

MECHANISM OF ACTION: Candesartan: Angiotensin II receptor antagonist; blocks vasoconstrictor and aldosterone-secreting effects of angiotensin II by blocking binding of angiotensin II to AT_1 receptor. HCTZ: Thiazide diuretic; affects renal tubular mechanism of electrolyte reabsorption, directly increasing excretion of Na^+ and Cl^-, and indirectly reducing plasma volume.

PHARMACOKINETICS: Absorption: Candesartan: Rapid and complete; absolute bioavailability (15%); T_{max}=3-4 hrs. **Distribution:** Candesartan: Plasma protein binding (>99%); V_d=0.13L/kg; crosses placenta. HCTZ: Crosses placenta; excreted in breast milk. **Metabolism:** Candesartan: Ester hydrolysis (GIT); O-deethylation (liver). **Elimination:** Candesartan: Urine (26%), feces; $T_{1/2}$=9 hrs. HCTZ: Kidney; urine (61%); $T_{1/2}$=5.6-14.8 hrs.

NURSING CONSIDERATIONS

Assessment: Assess for pregnancy status, possible drug interactions, volume/salt depletion, systemic lupus erythematosus (SLE), DM, anuria, sulfonamide hypersensitivity, history of allergy or bronchial asthma, hepatic/renal impairment.

Monitoring: Monitor serum electrolytes periodically. Monitor for signs/symptoms of electrolyte imbalance, exacerbation or activation of SLE, hypotension, hyperglycemia, hyperuricemia or precipitation of gout, hypersensitivity reactions, renal/hepatic dysfunction.

Patient Counseling: Instruct not to use K^+ supplements or salt substitutes. Inform of pregnancy risks. Advise that inadequate fluid intake or loss of fluids may result in drop of BP leading to lightheadedness or syncope. Advise to seek medical attention if syncope, symptoms of electrolyte imbalance (dry mouth, thirst, weakness, lethargy), or hypersensitivity reactions occur.

Administration: Oral route. **Storage:** 25°C (77°F), excursions permitted to 15-30°C (59-86°F).

Ativan CIV

lorazepam (Biovail)

THERAPEUTIC CLASS: Benzodiazepine

INDICATIONS: Management of anxiety disorders or for short-term relief of the symptoms of anxiety or anxiety associated with depressive symptoms.

DOSAGE: *Adults:* Initial: 2-3mg/day given bid-tid. Usual: 2-6mg/day in divided doses. Insomnia: 2-4mg qhs. Elderly/Debilitated: 1-2mg/day in divided doses. *Pediatrics:* >12 yrs: Initial: 2-3mg/day given bid-tid. Usual: 2-6mg/day in divided doses. Insomnia: 2-4mg qhs.

HOW SUPPLIED: Tab: 0.5mg, 1mg*, 2mg* *scored

CONTRAINDICATIONS: Acute narrow-angle glaucoma.

WARNINGS/PRECAUTIONS: Avoid with primary depression or psychosis. Withdrawal symptoms with abrupt discontinuation. Careful supervision if addiction-prone. Caution in patients with compromised respiratory function. Caution with elderly, and renal or hepatic dysfunction. Monitor for GI disease with prolonged therapy. Periodic blood counts and LFTs with long-term therapy.

ADVERSE REACTIONS: Sedation, dizziness, weakness, unsteadiness, transient amnesia, memory impairment, visual disturbance, depression, respiratory depression, constipation, vertigo, change in appetite, headache.

INTERACTIONS: CNS-depressant effects with barbiturates, alcohol. Diminished tolerance to alcohol and other CNS depressants. Increased plasma levels with valproate and probenecid, decrease dose by 50%.

PREGNANCY: Not for use in pregnancy or nursing.

MECHANISM OF ACTION: Benzodiazepine; antianxiety agent, interacts with GABA-benzodiazepine receptor complex.

PHARMACOKINETICS: Absorption: Absolute bioavailability (90%); C_{max}=20ng/mL (2mg PO); T_{max}=2 hrs. **Distribution:** Plasma protein binding (85%). **Metabolism:** Glucuronidation. **Elimination:** Urine; $T_{1/2}$=12 hrs.

NURSING CONSIDERATIONS

Assessment: Assess for acute narrow-angle glaucoma, pre-existing depression and/or psychosis, compromised respiratory function (eg, COPD, sleep apnea syndrome), impaired renal/hepatic function, and possible drug interactions. Assess addiction-prone individuals (eg, drug addicts, alcoholics).

Monitoring: Monitor worsening of depression and/or suicidal thinking, physical/psychological dependence, paradoxical reactions, CNS depression, lab tests (CBC, LFTs, LDH).

Patient Counseling: Inform that psychological/physical dependence may result; consult physician before increasing dose or abruptly d/c drug. Caution with hazardous tasks (eg, operating machinery/driving); do not drink alcohol or take other CNS depressants concomitantly.

Administration: Oral route. **Storage:** 20-25°C (68-77°F). Keep tightly closed.

Ativan Injection CIV

lorazepam (Baxter)

THERAPEUTIC CLASS: Benzodiazepine

INDICATIONS: Treatment of status epilepticus and preanesthetic medication in adults.

DOSAGE: *Adults:* ≥18 yrs: Status Epilepticus: 4mg IV (given slowly at 2mg/min); may repeat 1 dose after 10-15 min if seizures recur or fail to cease. Preanesthetic Sedation: Usual: 0.05mg/kg IM; 2mg or 0.044mg/kg IV (whichever is smaller). Max: 4mg IM/IV.

HOW SUPPLIED: Inj: 2mg/mL, 4mg/mL

CONTRAINDICATIONS: Acute narrow-angle glaucoma, sleep apnea syndrome, severe respiratory insufficiency. Not for intra-arterial injection.

WARNINGS/PRECAUTIONS: Monitor all parameters to maintain vital function. Risk of respiratory depression or airway obstruction in heavily sedated patients. May cause fetal damage during pregnancy. Increased risk of CNS and respiratory depression in elderly. Avoid with hepatic/renal failure. Caution with mild to moderate hepatic/renal disease. Avoid outpatient endoscopic procedures. Possible propylene glycol toxicity in renal impairment. Extreme caution when administering injections to elderly, very ill, or to patients with limited pulmonary reserve as hypoventilation and/or hypoxic cardiac arrest may occur. Gasping syndrome, characterized by CNS depression, metabolic acidosis, gasping respirations, and high levels of benzyl alcohol may occur.

ADVERSE REACTIONS: Respiratory depression/failure, hypotension, somnolence, headache, hypoventilation.

INTERACTIONS: Additive CNS depression with other CNS depressants (eg, ethyl alcohol, phenothiazines, barbiturates, MAOIs). Increased sedation, hallucinations and irrational behavior with scopolamine. Decreased clearance with valproate, probenecid. Increased clearance with oral contraceptives. Severe adverse effects with clozapine and haloperidol reported.

PREGNANCY: Category D, not for use in nursing.

MECHANISM OF ACTION: Benzodiazepine; antianxiety, sedative and anticonvulsant effects. Interacts with GABA-benzodiazepine receptor complex in human brain. Exhibits relatively high and specific affinity for its recognition site but does not displace GABA. Attachment to the specific binding site enhances the affinity of GABA for its receptor site on the same receptor complex.

PHARMACOKINETICS: Absorption: Completely, rapidly absorbed, C_{max}=48ng/mL, T_{max}=within 3 hrs. **Distribution:** V_d=approximately 1.3L/kg, plasma protein binding (91%), crosses blood brain barrier. **Elimination:** Urine (88%), feces (7%), (0.3% unchanged); $T_{1/2}$=14 hrs.

NURSING CONSIDERATIONS

Assessment: Comprehensive review of benefits/risks in status epilepticus. Assess for hypersensitivity to benzodiazepine or its vehicle, acute-angle glaucoma, pre-existing respiratory impairment, hepatic/renal impairment, and possible drug interactions.

Monitoring: Gasping syndrome in very low body weight neonates, which manifests by CNS depression, metabolic acidosis, gasping respiration. Monitor for respiratory depression, airway obstruction, heavy sedation, drowsiness, excessive sleepiness, hypogylcemia and hyponatremia in status epilepticus, seizures, myoclonus, somnolence, injection site reactions (pain, burning sensation, and redness), and paradoxical reactions (mania, agitation, psychosis). Signs of toxicity to the vehicle's components (eg, lactic acidosis, hyperosmolarity, hypotension, and acute tubular necrosis).

Patient Counseling: Inform of risks/benefits. Caution with hazardous tasks (eg, operating machinery/driving). Do not get out of bed unassisted. Avoid alcoholic beverages for at least 24-48 hrs after receiving drug. Advise about potential for physical/psychological dependence and withdrawal symptoms.

Administration: IM/IV route. **Storage:** Refrigerate; protect from light.

ATRIPLA RX

tenofovir disoproxil fumarate - emtricitabine - efavirenz (Bristol-Myers Squibb/ Gilead Sciences)

Lactic acidosis and severe hepatomegaly with steatosis, including fatal cases, have been reported with the use of nucleoside analogs alone or in combination with other antiretrovirals. Not indicated for the treatment of chronic hepatitis B virus (HBV) infection and the safety and efficacy have not been established in patients co-infected with HBV and HIV. Severe acute exacerbations of hepatitis B have been reported in patients who have discontinued Emtriva or Viread. Hepatic function should be monitored closely with both clinical and laboratory follow-up for at least several months in patients who discontinue Atripla and are co-infected with HIV and HBV. If appropriate, initiation of anti-hepatitis B therapy may be warranted.

THERAPEUTIC CLASS: Non-nucleoside reverse transcriptase inhibitor/nucleoside analog combination

INDICATIONS: For use alone as a complete regimen or in combination with other antiretroviral agents for the treatment of HIV-1 infection in adults.

DOSAGE: *Adults:* ≥18 yrs: 1 tab qd on empty stomach. Bedtime dosing may improve tolerability of nervous system effects. Moderate or Severe Renal Impairment: Should not be administered with CrCl <50mL/min.

HOW SUPPLIED: Tab: (Efavirenz-Emtricitabine-Tenofovir DF) 600mg-200mg-300mg

CONTRAINDICATIONS: Concomitant astemizole, cisapride, midazolam, triazolam, ergot derivatives, voriconazole, bepridil, pimozide.

WARNINGS/PRECAUTIONS: Obesity and prolonged nucleoside exposure may be risk factors for lactic acidosis and severe hepatomegaly with steatosis. Suspend treatment if clinical or laboratory findings suggestive of lactic acidosis or pronounced hepatotoxicity. Test for presence of HBV prior to initiation; post-treatment exacerbations reported. Monitor hepatic function for several months with discontinuation and with co-infection with HIV and HBV. Serious psychiatric adverse experiences reported. CNS symptoms reported. May impair mental/physical abilities. May cause renal impairment. Avoid with moderate or severe renal impairment (CrCl <50mL/min). Monitor SrCr and phosphorous with risk or with a history of renal dysfunction and with concomitant nephrotoxic agents. Avoid in pregnancy; use barrier contraception with other contraception methods and obtain negative pregnancy test before therapy. Severe skin rash reported. Monitoring of liver enzymes recommended with known or suspected history of hepatitis B or C infection and with other medications associated with liver toxicity. Bone density monitoring should be considered for HIV infected patients with a history of pathologic bone fracture or are at risk for osteopenia. Caution with history of seizures. Possible redistribution/accumulation of body fat. Immune reconstitution syndrome reported.

ADVERSE REACTIONS: Diarrhea, nausea, fatigue, sinusitis, upper respiratory tract infections, drowsiness, headache, dizziness, depression, insomnia, abnormal dreams, rash, laboratory abnormalities.

INTERACTIONS: Efavirenz is a CYP3A4 inducer *in vivo*, increasing the biotransformation of some drugs metabolized by CYP3A4. Co-administration of efavirenz with drugs primarily metabolized by 2C9, 2C19, and 3A4 isozymes may result in altered plasma concentrations of the co-administered drug. Drugs which induce CYP3A4 activity (eg, phenobarbital, rifampin, rifabutin) may increase clearance of efavirenz resulting in lowered plasma concentrations. Levels of efavirenz may be decreased by lopinavir/ritonavir, nelfinavir, SGC, rifabutin, rifampin, carbamazepine. St. John's wort to suboptimal levels, leading to loss of virologic response and possible resistance. Levels of efavirenz are increased by ritonavir, clarithromycin, sertraline, voriconazole, diltiazem. Efavirenz decreased levels of atazanavir, indinavir, lopinavir/ritonavir, saquinavir, clarithromycin, rifabutin, carbamazepine, methadone, sertraline and significantly reduced levels of voriconazole, itraconazole, atorvastatin, pravastatin, simvastatin, diltiazem. Efavirenz increased levels of nelfinavir, ritonavir, ethinyl estradiol. Co-administration of emtricitabine and tenofovir

DF with drugs that are eliminated by active tubular secretion may increase concentrations of emtricitabine, tenofovir, and/or the co-administered drug. Drugs that decrease renal function may increase concentrations of emtricitabine and/or tenofovir. Levels of tenofovir increased by atazanavir, lopinavir/ritonavir may potentiate tenofovir-associated adverse events, including renal disorders. Tenofovir decreased levels of atazanavir, atazanavir/ritonavir. Co-administration of tenofovir DF with didanosine buffered tablets or EC capsules significantly increases the C_{max} and AUC of didanosine; patients receiving this combination should be monitored closely for didanosine-associated adverse events. Related drugs not for co-administration include Emtriva, Viread, Truvada, and Sustiva. Should not be co-administered with drugs containing lamivudine, including Combivir, Epivir, Epivir-HBV, Epzicom, and Trizivir.

PREGNANCY: Category D, not for use in nursing.

MECHANISM OF ACTION: Efavirenz: Non-nucleoside reverse transcriptase inhibitor; noncompetitive inhibition of HIV-1 reverse transcriptase (RT). Emtricitabine: Nucleoside analog of cytidine; inhibits activity of HIV-1 RT by competing with natural substrate deoxycytidine 5'-triphosphate and incorporating into nascent viral DNA, resulting in chain termination. Tenofovir disoproxil: Acyclic nucleoside phosphonate diester analog of adenosine monophosphate; inhibits activity of HIV-1 RT by competing with natural substrate deoxyadenosine 5'-triphosphate and incorporating into DNA by DNA chain termination.

PHARMACOKINETICS: Absorption: Efavirenz: C_{max}=12.9μM, T_{max}=3-5 hrs, AUC=184μM•hr. Emtricitabine: Rapid; absolute bioavailability (93%), C_{max}=1.8μg/mL, T_{max}=1-2 hrs, AUC=10μg•hr/mL. Tenofovir disoproxil: Absolute bioavailability (25%); C_{max}=296ng/mL, T_{max}=1hr, AUC=2287ng•hr/mL. **Distribution:** Efavirenz: Plasma protein binding (99.5%-99.75%). Emtricitabine: Plasma protein binding (<4%). Tenofovir disoproxil: Plasma protein binding (<0.7%). **Metabolism:** Efavirenz: Hepatic via CYP3A4 and CYP2B6. **Elimination:** Efavirenz: $T_{1/2}$=52-76 hrs. Emtricitabine: Urine (86%); $T_{1/2}$=10 hrs. Tenofovir disoproxil: Urine (70-80%); $T_{1/2}$=17 hrs.

NURSING CONSIDERATIONS

Assessment: Assess for liver dysfunction, history of injection drug use, psychiatric history (including receipt of psychiatric medication), risk or history of renal dysfunction, history of HBV or HCV, history of pathologic bone fracture, seizures, risk factors for lactic acidosis, pregnancy status, and possible drug interactions.

Monitoring: Monitor for lactic acidosis, severe hepatomegaly with steatosis, hepatic function, cardiac adverse events, immune reconstitution syndrome, renal dysfunction, and fat redistribution. Monitor CD4 cell count, HIV-1 RNA, LFTs, SrCr, serum phosphorus, bone density monitoring, drug plasma level monitoring.

Patient Counseling: Inform not to change or stop medicine without consulting physician; take exact amount prescribed. Seek medical attention if symptoms of lactic acidosis (weakness, muscle pain, breathing trouble, cold extremities, dizziness), liver toxicity (jaundice, no appetite, nausea, stomach pain), infections, pregnancy risks, psychiatric symptoms (aggressive behavior, depression, suicide attempts, delusions, paranoia), CNS symptoms (dizziness, insomnia, somnolence, abnormal dreams), flare-ups of HBV infection, kidney problems, and fat redistribution or accumulation occur. Take on empty stomach. Caution against potentially hazardous tasks (eg, driving or operating machinery).

Administration: Oral route. **Storage:** 25°C (77°F); excursions permitted to 15-30°C (59-86°F). Keep in original container, tightly closed.

Atrovent HFA — RX

ipratropium bromide (Boehringer Ingelheim)

THERAPEUTIC CLASS: Anticholinergic bronchodilator

INDICATIONS: Maintenance treatment of bronchospasm associated with COPD, including chronic bronchitis and emphysema.

DOSAGE: *Adults:* Initial: 2 inh qid. Max: 12 inh/24hrs.

HOW SUPPLIED: MDI: 0.017mg/inh [12.9g]

CONTRAINDICATIONS: Hypersensitivity to atropine or its derivatives.

WARNINGS/PRECAUTIONS: Not for acute episodes. Immediate hypersensitivity reaction reported. Caution with narrow-angle glaucoma, prostatic hypertrophy or bladder-neck obstruction.

ADVERSE REACTIONS: Back pain, bronchitis, dyspnea, dizziness, headache, nausea, blurred vision, dry mouth, exacerbation of symptoms.

INTERACTIONS: Caution with anticholinergic-containing drugs.

PREGNANCY: Category B, caution in nursing.

MECHANISM OF ACTION: Anticholinergic; inhibits vagally-mediated refluxes by antagonizing the action of acetylcholine; prevents increase in intracellular concentration of cGMP caused by interaction of acetylcholine with muscarinic receptors on bronchial smooth muscle (animal studies).

PHARMACOKINETICS: Absorption: C_{max}=59pg/mL. **Distribution:** Plasma protein binding (0-9%). **Metabolism:** Partial. **Elimination:** $T_{1/2}$=2 hrs.

NURSING CONSIDERATIONS

Assessment: Assess for hypersensitivity to atropine or derivative, narrow-angle glaucoma, prostatic hyperplasia, bladder-neck obstruction, and possible drug interactions.

Monitoring: Monitor for urinary retention, mydriasis, GI distress (diarrhea, NV), paradoxical bronchospasm and allergic type-reaction (pruritus, angioedema of tongue, lips and face, urticaria, laryngospasm, anaphylaxis).

Patient Counseling: Advise not to increase dose or frequency. Not for acute periods of bronchospasm. Avoid spraying in the eyes. Seek medical attention if symptoms of precipitation or worsening of narrow-angle glaucoma, mydriasis, increased IOP, acute eye pain/discomfort, blurring of vision, visual halos or colored images with red eyes from conjunctival and corneal congestion, or allergic/hypersensitivity reactions occur.

Administration: Oral inhalation. Prime pump: Before first use, prime with 2 sprays. If not used for >3 days, reprime with 2 sprays. **Storage:** 25°C (77°F); excursions permitted to 15-30°C (59-86°F). Do not puncture, use or store near heat or open flame.

ATROVENT NASAL — RX

ipratropium bromide (Boehringer Ingelheim)

THERAPEUTIC CLASS: Anticholinergic

INDICATIONS: (0.03%) Relief of rhinorrhea associated with allergic and nonallergic perennial rhinitis in adults and children ≥6 yrs. (0.06%) Relief of rhinorrhea associated with the common cold or seasonal allergic rhinitis in adults and children ≥5 yrs.

DOSAGE: *Adults:* Rhinorrhea w/Allergic/Nonallergic Perennial Rhinitis: (0.03%) 2 sprays per nostril bid-tid. Rhinorrhea w/Common Cold: (0.06%) 2 sprays per nostril tid-qid. Rhinorrhea w/Seasonal Allergic Rhinitis: (0.06%) 2 sprays per nostril qid.
Pediatrics: Rhinorrhea w/Allergic/Nonallergic Perennial Rhinitis: ≥6 yrs: (0.03%) 2 sprays per nostril bid-tid. Rhinorrhea w/Common Cold: ≥12 yrs: (0.06%) 2 sprays per nostril tid-qid. 5-11 yrs: (0.06%) 2 sprays per nostril tid. Rhinorrhea w/Seasonal Allergic Rhinitis: ≥5 yrs: (0.06%) 2 sprays per nostril qid.

HOW SUPPLIED: Spray: (0.03%) 21mcg/spray [31g], (0.06%) 42mcg/spray [16.6g]

CONTRAINDICATIONS: Hypersensitivity to atropine or its derivatives.

WARNINGS/PRECAUTIONS: Immediate hypersensitivity reaction reported. Caution with narrow-angle glaucoma, prostatic hyperplasia or bladder-neck obstruction.

ADVERSE REACTIONS: Epistaxis, nasal dryness, dry mouth, dry throat, headache, upper respiratory infection, pharyngitis.

INTERACTIONS: May produce additive effects with other anticholinergic agents.

PREGNANCY: Category B, caution in nursing.

MECHANISM OF ACTION: Anticholinergic; inhibits secretions from serous and seromucous glands lining the nasal mucosa.

PHARMACOKINETICS: Absorption: 6-18 yrs old: C_{max}=undetectable up to 0.49 ng/mL. **Distribution:** Plasma protein binding (0-9%). **Elimination:** 6-18 yrs old: Urine (8.6-11.1% unchanged). **Adults:** Urine (3.7-5.6% unchanged).

NURSING CONSIDERATIONS

Assessment: Assess for hypersensitivity to atropine or its derivatives, prostatic hyperplasia, narrow-angle glaucoma, bladder-neck obstruction, hepatic/renal insufficiency, pregnancy/nursing status, and possible drug interactions.

Monitoring: Monitor for blurring of vision, precipitation or worsening of narrow-angle glaucoma, increased IOP, mydriasis, acute eye pain/discomfort, visual halos or colored images in association with red eyes from conjunctival and corneal congestion, epistaxis, excessive nasal dryness, and hypersensitivity reactions.

Patient Counseling: Advise not to alter size of nasal spray opening. Notify physician if symptoms such as eye pain, blurred vision, excessive nasal dryness, or epistaxis occur. Avoid spraying into eyes.

Administration: Intranasal. Prime the nasal spray pump and blow nose to clear nostrils before first use. **Storage:** 25°C (77°F); excursions permitted to 15-30°C (59-86°F). Avoid freezing.

AUGMENTIN — RX

clavulanate potassium - amoxicillin (GlaxoSmithKline)

THERAPEUTIC CLASS: Aminopenicillin/beta lactamase inhibitor

INDICATIONS: Treatment of lower respiratory tract (LRTI), skin and skin structure (SSSI), and urinary tract infections (UTI), otitis media (OM), sinusitis caused by susceptible strains of microorganisms.

DOSAGE: *Adults:* (Dose based on amoxicillin) 500mg q12h or 250mg q8h. Severe Infections/RTI: 875mg q12h or 500mg q8h. May use 125mg/5mL or 250mg/5mL sus in place of 500mg tab and 200mg/5mL sus or 400mg/5mL sus in place of 875mg tab. CrCl <30mL/min: Do not give 875mg tab. CrCl 10-30mL/min: 250-500mg q12h. CrCl <10mL/min: 250-500mg q24h. Hemodialysis: 250-500mg q24h, give additional dose during and at end of dialysis.

Pediatrics: (Dose based on amoxicillin) ≥40kg: Use adult dose. ≥12 weeks: Sinusitis/Otitis Media/LRTI/Severe Infections: (Sus/Tab, Chewable) 45mg/kg/day given q12h or 40mg/kg/day given q8h. Treat otitis media for 10 days. Less Severe Infections: 25mg/kg/day given q12h or 20mg/kg/day given q8h. <12 weeks: 15mg/kg q12h (use 125mg/5mL sus).

HOW SUPPLIED: (Amoxicillin-Clavulanate) Sus: 125-31.25mg/5mL [75mL, 100mL, 150mL], 200-28.5mg/5mL [50mL, 75mL, 100mL], 250-62.5mg/5mL [75mL, 100mL, 150mL], 400-57mg/5mL [50mL, 75mL, 100mL]; Tab: 250-125mg, 500-125mg, 875-125mg*; Tab, Chewable: 125-31.25mg, 200-28.5mg, 250-62.5mg, 400-57mg *scored

CONTRAINDICATIONS: History of PCN allergy or amoxicillin-clavulanate associated cholestatic jaundice/hepatic dysfunction.

WARNINGS/PRECAUTIONS: Serious, sometimes fatal, hypersensitivity reactions reported with PCN therapy. *Clostridium difficile*-associated diarrhea reported. Possibility of superinfection. Caution with hepatic dysfunction.

Monitor renal, hepatic, and hematopoietic functions with prolonged use. Avoid with mononucleosis. Take with food to reduce GI upset. The 200mg and 400mg chewable tabs and 200mg/5mL and 400mg/5mL sus contain phenylalanine. The 250mg tab and chewable tab are not interchangeable due to unequal clavulanic acid amounts. Only use 250mg tab in pediatrics ≥40kg. False (+) for urine glucose with Clinitest and Benedict's or Fehling's solution.

ADVERSE REACTIONS: Diarrhea/loose stools, nausea, skin rashes, urticaria, pruritus, angioedema, serum sickness-like reactions, erythema multiforme, acute generalized exanthematous pustulosis, hypersensitivity vasculitis, and exfoliative dermatitis.

INTERACTIONS: Increased and prolonged plasma levels with probenecid. May reduce effects of oral contraceptives. Allopurinol may increase incidence of rash. May increase PT with anticoagulant therapy.

PREGNANCY: Category B, caution in nursing.

MECHANISM OF ACTION: Amoxicillin: Semisynthetic antibiotic with broad-spectrum of bactericidal activity against gram-positive and gram-negative organisms. Clavulanate: β-lactamase inhibitor; possesses ability to inactivate a wide range of β-lactamase enzymes commonly found in microorganisms resistant to PCN and cephalosporins.

PHARMACOKINETICS: Absorption: Well absorbed from GI tract. C_{max} and AUC varied according to dose and regimen; see Full PI for more information. (Tab, Sol) T_{max}=1.5 hrs, 1 hr. **Distribution:** Found in breast milk. Amoxicillin: Diffuses readily in body tissues and fluids. Clavulanic: Well distributed in body tissues. Plasma protein binding: Amoxicillin (18%), clavulanic (25%). **Elimination:** Urine, (amoxicillin) (50-70% unchanged), (clavulanic) (25-40% unchanged); $T_{1/2}$=1.3 hrs (amoxicillin), 1 hr (clavulanic).

NURSING CONSIDERATIONS

Assessment: Assess for history of allergic reactions to penicillins or cephalosporins or other allergens, hepatic or renal or hematopoietic function, pregnancy/nursing status, and possible drug interactions.

Monitoring: Periodically monitor renal, hepatic, and hematopoietic functions. Monitor for anaphylactic reactions, hepatic toxicity, cholestatic jaundice, superinfection with mycotic or bacterial pathogen, drug resistance, and pseudomembranous colitis/CDAD.

Patient Counseling: Inform drug only treats bacterial, not viral, infections. Instruct to take as directed; skipping doses or not completing full course may decrease effectiveness and increase resistance. Inform about potential benefits/risks of therapy. Advise to d/c therapy and consult physician if allergic reactions or watery/bloody diarrhea (with/without stomach cramps) occur (may occur up to 2 months after therapy). Advise to notify physician if pregnant/nursing.

Administration: Oral route. Take at start of meals or snacks. **Storage:** Tabs/Dry Powder at or below 25°C (77°F); store in original containers. Refrigerate reconstituted sus; shake well before using; discard after 10 days.

AUGMENTIN ES-600 RX

clavulanate potassium - amoxicillin (GlaxoSmithKline)

THERAPEUTIC CLASS: Aminopenicillin/beta lactamase inhibitor

INDICATIONS: Treatment of pediatric patients with recurrent or persistent acute otitis media due to susceptible strains of microorganisms.

DOSAGE: *Pediatrics:* 3 months-12 yrs: <40kg: (Dose based on amoxicillin content) 45mg/kg q12h for 10 days.

HOW SUPPLIED: Sus: (Amoxicillin-Clavulanate) 600mg-42.9mg/5mL [75mL, 125mL, 200mL]

CONTRAINDICATIONS: History of PCN allergy or amoxicillin-clavulanate associated cholestatic jaundice/hepatic dysfunction.

WARNINGS/PRECAUTIONS: Serious, sometimes fatal, hypersensitivity reactions reported with PCN therapy. *Clostridium difficile*-associated diarrhea reported. Possibility of superinfection. Caution with hepatic dysfunction. Monitor renal, hepatic, and hematopoietic functions with prolonged use. Avoid with mononucleosis. Contains phenylalanine. False (+) for urine glucose with Clinitest and Benedict's or Fehling's solution.

ADVERSE REACTIONS: Diaper rash, diarrhea, vomiting, moniliasis, rash.

INTERACTIONS: Increased and prolonged plasma levels with probenecid. May reduce effects of oral contraceptives. Allopurinol may increase incidence of rash. May increase PT with anticoagulant therapy.

PREGNANCY: Category B, caution in nursing.

MECHANISM OF ACTION: Amoxicillin: Semisynthetic antibiotic with broad spectrum of bactericidal activity against gram-positive and gram-negative organisms. Clavulanate: β-lactamase inhibitor. Possesses ability to inactivate a wide range of β-lactamase enzymes commonly found in microorganisms resistant to PCN and cephalosporins.

PHARMACOKINETICS: Absorption: Amoxicillin: C_{max}=15.7mcg/mL; T_{max}=2.0 hr; AUC=59.8mcg•hr/mL. Clavulanic acid: C_{max}=1.7mcg/mL; T_{max}=1.1 hr; AUC=4.0mcg•hr/mL. **Distribution:** Plasma protein binding 18% (amoxicillin), 25% (clavulanic acid). Well distributed in bodily tissues except brain and spinal fluid. **Elimination:** Urine (unchanged) amoxicillin (50-70%); clavulanic acid (25-40%).

NURSING CONSIDERATIONS

Assessment: Assess for history of allergic reactions to PCNs, cephalosporins or other allergens, cholestatic jaundice, hepatic dysfunction, infectious mononucleosis, phenylketonuria, pregnancy/nursing status, and possible drug interactions.

Monitoring: Periodically monitor renal, hepatic and hematopoietic organ functions. Monitor for anaphylactic reactions, hepatic toxicity, cholestatic jaundice, development of superinfection with mycotic or bacterial pathogen, development of drug resistance, skin rash, diarrhea, pseudomembranous colitis/*C.difficile* colitis, false-positive reaction of urinary glucose if Benedict's or Fehling's solution or Clinitest are used, and for transient decrease in plasma concentration of total conjugated estriol, estriol-glucuronide, conjugated estrone and estradiol if given to pregnant women.

Patient Counseling: Inform drug only treats bacterial, not viral, infections. Instruct to take as directed; skipping doses or not completing full course may decrease effectiveness and increase resistance. Inform about potential benefits/risks of therapy. Advise to d/c therapy and consult physician if allergic reactions or watery/bloody diarrhea (with or without stomach cramps) occur (may occur up to 2 months or more after treatment). Advise to notify physician if pregnant/nursing.

Administration: Oral route. Take at start of meals or snacks to prevent gastric upset. Shake well before using. **Storage:** Dry powder at or below 25°C (77°F); original container. Refrigerate reconstituted sus; discard after 10 days.

AUGMENTIN XR — RX

clavulanate potassium - amoxicillin (GlaxoSmithKline)

THERAPEUTIC CLASS: Aminopenicillin/beta lactamase inhibitor

INDICATIONS: Treatment of community-acquired pneumonia (CAP) or acute bacterial sinusitis due to confirmed or suspected β-lactamase producing pathogens and *S.pneumoniae* with reduced susceptibility to PCN.

DOSAGE: *Adults:* Sinusitis: 2 tabs q12h for 10 days. CAP: 2 tabs q12h for 7-10 days. Take at start of a meal.
Pediatrics: ≥16 yrs: Sinusitis: 2 tabs q12h for 10 days. CAP: 2 tabs q12h for 7-10 days. Take at the start of a meal.

HOW SUPPLIED: Tab, Extended-Release: (Amoxicillin-Clavulanate) 1000mg-62.5mg

CONTRAINDICATIONS: History of PCN allergy or amoxicillin-clavulanate associated cholestatic jaundice/hepatic dysfunction, severe renal impairment (CrCl <30mL/min), hemodialysis.

WARNINGS/PRECAUTIONS: Serious, sometimes fatal, hypersensitivity reactions reported with PCN therapy. *Clostridium difficile*-associated diarrhea reported. Possibility of superinfection. Caution with hepatic dysfunction. Monitor renal, hepatic, and hematopoietic functions with prolonged use. Avoid with mononucleosis. False (+) for urine glucose with Clinitest and Benedict's or Fehling's solution.

ADVERSE REACTIONS: Diarrhea, nausea, genital moniliasis, abdominal pain, vaginal mycosis, skin rashes, pruritus, urticaria, angioedema, serum sickness-like reactions, erythema multiforme, acute generalized exanthematous pustulosis, hypersensitivity vasculitis, and exfoliative dermatitis.

INTERACTIONS: Increased and prolonged plasma levels with probenecid. May reduce effects of oral contraceptives. Allopurinol may increase incidence of rash. May increase PT with anticoagulant therapy.

PREGNANCY: Category B, caution in nursing.

MECHANISM OF ACTION: Amoxicillin: Semisynthetic antibiotic with broad spectrum of bactericidal activity against gram-positive and gram-negative organisms. Clavulanate: β-lactamase inhibitor; possesses ability to inactivate a wide range of β-lactamase enzymes commonly found in microorganisms resistant to PCN and cephalosporins.

PHARMACOKINETICS: Absorption: Well-absorbed. Amoxicillin: C_{max}=17 mcg/mL, T_{max}=1.5 hrs, AUC=71.6mcg•hr/mL. Clavulanate potassium: C_{max}=2.05mcg/mL, T_{max}=1.03 hrs, AUC=5.29mcg•hr/mL. **Distribution:** Plasma protein binding: Amoxicillin (18%); Clavulanate potassium (25%). Found in breast milk. Well distributed to body tissues except brain and spinal fluid. **Elimination:** Urine: Amoxicillin (60-80% unchanged); $T_{1/2}$=1.27 hrs. Clavulanate potassium: (30-50% unchanged); $T_{1/2}$=1.03 hrs.

NURSING CONSIDERATIONS

Assessment: Assess for history of allergic reactions to PCNs, cephalosporins or other allergens, cholestatic jaundice, hepatic/renal impairment or hemodialysis patients, infectious mononucleosis, pregnancy/nursing status, and possible drug interactions.

Monitoring: Periodically monitor renal, hepatic and hematopoietic organ functions. Monitor for anaphylactic reactions, hepatic toxicity, cholestatic jaundice, development of superinfection with mycotic or bacterial pathogen, development of drug resistance, skin rash, diarrhea, pseudomembranous colitis/*C.difficile* colitis, false-postive reaction of urinary glucose if Benedict's, Fehling's solution or Clinitest are used. Monitor for transient decrease in plasma concentration of total conjugated estriol, estriol-glucuronide, conjugated estrone and estradiol if given to pregnant women.

Patient Counseling: Inform drug only treats bacterial, not viral, infections. Instruct to take as directed; skipping doses or not completing full course may decrease effectiveness and increase resistance. Inform about potential benefits/risks of therapy. Advise to d/c and consult physician if allergic reactions or watery/bloody diarrhea (with/without stomach cramps) occur (may occur up to 2 months or more after treatment). Advise to notify physician if pregnant/nursing.

Administration: Oral route. Take at start of meals or snacks to reduce possible GI upset. **Storage:** At or below 25°C (77°F); store in original container; discard unused medicine.

AVAGE — RX

tazarotene (Allergan)

THERAPEUTIC CLASS: Retinoid

INDICATIONS: Adjunct to a comprehensive skin care and sunlight avoidance program, in the mitigation (palliation) of facial fine wrinkling, facial mottled hyper- and hypopigmentation, and benign facial lentigines.

DOSAGE: *Adults:* ≥17 yrs: Cleanse and dry skin. Apply a pea-sized (1/4 inch or 5mm diameter) amount to face (including eyelids, if desired) qhs.

HOW SUPPLIED: Cre: 0.1% [30g]

CONTRAINDICATIONS: Women who are or may become pregnant.

WARNINGS/PRECAUTIONS: Use adequate birth control measures. Obtain negative pregnancy test within 2 weeks before therapy. Begin therapy during normal menstrual period. Avoid mouth, eyes, sunlight exposure (including sunlamps), or sunburned or eczematous skin. Stop therapy or reduce dosing interval with pruritus, burning, skin redness, or peeling. Weather extremes (eg, wind, cold) may be irritating. Sunscreen (minimum SPF 15) and protective clothing should be used.

ADVERSE REACTIONS: Desquamation, erythema, burning sensation, dry skin, skin irritation, pruritus, irritant contact dermatitis.

INTERACTIONS: Avoid topical agents that have a strong drying effect. Caution with photosensitizers (eg, thiazides, tetracyclines, fluoroquinolones, phenothiazines, sulfonamides).

PREGNANCY: Category X; caution in nursing.

MECHANISM OF ACTION: Retinoic acid derivative; binds to all 3 members of the retinoic acid receptor (RAR family): RARα, RARβ, and RAR-gamma, but shows relative selectivity for RARβ and RAR-gamma and may modify gene expression. Amelioration of fine wrinkling, facial mottled hypo- and hyperpigmentation, and benign facial lentigines not established.

PHARMACOKINETICS: Distribution: Plasma protein binding (>99%). **Metabolism:** Undergoes esterase hydrolysis. Tazarotenic acid (active metabolite). Tazarotene and tazarotenic acid are metabolized to sulfoxides, sulfones, and other polar metabolites. **Elimination:** Urine, feces; $T_{1/2}$=approximately 18 hrs.

NURSING CONSIDERATIONS

Assessment: Obtain a negative pregnancy test within 2 weeks prior to therapy. Assess for eczematous skin, lentigo maligna, nursing status, and for possible drug interactions as photosensitizers (eg, thiazides, tetracyclines, fluoroquinolones, phenothiazines, and sulfonamides).

Monitoring: Monitor for irritation, excessive pruritus, burning, redness, or peeling.

Patient Counseling: Caution women of childbearing potential of the potential risks and to use adequate birth control measures during therapy. Apply only to the affected areas. Advise to avoid excessive exposure to sunlight and to use sunscreens/protective clothing. Not for ophthalmic, oral, or intravaginal use. Not be used by nursing women.

Administration: Topical route. **Storage:** 25°C (77°F); excursions permitted from -5-30°C (23-86°F).

AVALIDE — RX

irbesartan - hydrochlorothiazide (Bristol-Myers Squibb/Sanofi-Aventis)

Can cause death/injury to developing fetus during 2nd and 3rd trimesters. Stop therapy if pregnancy detected.

THERAPEUTIC CLASS: Angiotensin II receptor antagonist/thiazide diuretic

INDICATIONS: Treatment of hypertension in patients not adequately controlled with monotherapy. As initial therapy in patients likely to need multiple drugs.

DOSAGE: *Adults:* Not controlled on Monotherapy: 150mg/12.5mg qd. Titrate: May increase to 300mg/12.5mg, then 300mg/25mg qd if needed. Initial Therapy: Initiate with 150mg/12.5mg qd for 1 to 2 weeks. Titrate: As needed to maximum 300mg/25mg qd. Replacement Therapy: May substitute for titrated components. Elderly: Start at low end of dosing range. Avoid with CrCl ≤30mL/min.

HOW SUPPLIED: Tab: (Irbesartan-HCTZ) 150mg-12.5mg, 300mg-12.5mg, 300mg-25mg

CONTRAINDICATIONS: Anuria, sulfonamide hypersensitivity.

WARNINGS/PRECAUTIONS: Can cause fetal injury/death when administered to pregnant women. Correct volume or salt depletion before therapy. Caution in elderly or with hepatic or renal dysfunction, renal artery stenosis, severe CHF, history of allergies, elderly, and asthma. May exacerbate or activate SLE. Monitor serum electrolytes. Avoid if CrCl ≤30mL/min. Hyperuricemia, hyperglycemia, hypokalemia, hypomagnesemia, and hypercalcemia may occur. Enhanced effects in post-sympathectomy patient. May increase cholesterol and triglyceride levels. Caution in elderly.

ADVERSE REACTIONS: Dizziness, fatigue, musculoskeletal pain, influenza, edema, nausea, vomiting, fever, chills, flushing, HTN, pruritus, sexual dysfunction, diarrhea, anxiety, vision disturbance, pancreatitis, aplastic anemia.

INTERACTIONS: Potentiation of orthostatic hypotension may occur with alcohol, barbiturates, and narcotics. Dosage adjustment of insulin or oral hypoglycemic agents may be required. Impaired absorption with cholestyramine, colestipol. Corticosteroids and ACTH deplete electrolytes. May decrease response to pressor amines. Potentiates other antihypertensives. May increase responsiveness to skeletal muscle relaxants. Increased risk of lithium toxicity. NSAIDs may reduce diuretic effects.

PREGNANCY: Category D, not for use in nursing.

MECHANISM OF ACTION: Irbesartan: Angiotensin II receptor antagonist; blocks vasoconstrictor and aldosterone-secreting effects of angiotensin II by blocking binding of angiotensin II to AT_1 receptor. HCTZ: Thiazide diuretic; affects renal tubular mechanism of electrolyte reabsorption, directly increasing Na^+ and Cl^- and indirectly reducing plasma volume.

PHARMACOKINETICS: Absorption: Irbesartan: Rapid, complete; absolute bioavailability (60-80%); T_{max}=1.5-2 hrs. **Distribution:** Irbesartan: V_d=53-93L; plasma protein binding (90%); crosses placenta; excreted in breast milk. HCTZ: Crosses placenta, excreted in breast milk. **Metabolism:** Irbesartan: CYP2C9 (oxidation), glucuronide conjugation. **Elimination:** Irbesartan: $T_{1/2}$=11-15 hrs. HCTZ: Kidney (61%); $T_{1/2}$=5.6-14.8 hrs.

NURSING CONSIDERATIONS

Assessment: Assess for pregnancy status, possible drug interactions, volume/salt depletion, systemic lupus erythematosus (SLE), DM, anuria, sulfonamide hypersensitivity, history of allergy or bronchial asthma, hepatic/renal impairment.

Monitoring: Monitor serum electrolytes periodically. Monitor for signs/symptoms of electrolyte imbalance, exacerbation or activation of SLE, hypotension, hyperglycemia, hyperuricemia or precipitation of gout, hypersensitivity reactions, hepatic/renal dysfunction.

Patient Counseling: Inform of pregnancy risks. Advise that inadequate fluid intake or loss of fluids may result in drop of BP leading to lightheadedness or syncope. Advise to seek medical attention if symptoms of hypersensitivity reactions, electrolyte imbalance (dry mouth, thirst, weakness, lethargy), lightheadedness, or syncope occur.

Administration: Oral route. **Storage:** 25°C (77°F); excursions permitted 15-30°C (59-86°F).

AVANDAMET RX

metformin HCl - rosiglitazone maleate (GlaxoSmithKline)

Thiazolidinediones may cause or exacerbate CHF in some patients. Avandamet is not recommended in patients with symptomatic heart failure. Meta-analysis of studies has shown rosiglitazone to be associated with an increased risk of myocardial ischemic events. Lactic acidosis may occur due to metformin accumulation.

THERAPEUTIC CLASS: Thiazolidinedione/biguanide

INDICATIONS: Adjunct to diet and exercise, to improve glycemic control in type 2 diabetes mellitus when treatment with dual rosiglitazone and metformin therapy is appropriate.

DOSAGE: *Adults:* Prior Metformin Therapy of 1000mg/day: Initial: 2mg-500mg tab bid. Prior Metformin Therapy of 2000mg/day: Initial: 2mg-1000mg tab bid. Prior Rosiglitazone Therapy of 4mg/day: Initial: 2mg-500mg tab bid. Prior Rosiglitazone Therapy of 8mg/day: 4mg-500mg tab bid. Titrate: May increase by increments of 4mg rosiglitazone and/or 500mg metformin. Max: 8mg-2000mg/day. Drug-Naive Patients: Initial: 2mg-500mg qd-bid. If HbA_{1c} >11% and FPG >270mg/dL: Initial: 2mg-500mg bid. Titrate: After 4 weeks, may increase by increments of 2mg-500mg per day. Max: 8mg-2000mg per day. Elderly/Debilitated/Malnourished: Conservative dosing; do not titrate to max dose. Take with meals.

HOW SUPPLIED: Tab: (Rosiglitazone-Metformin) 2mg-500mg, 4mg-500mg, 2mg-1000mg, 4mg-1000mg

CONTRAINDICATIONS: Established NYHA Class III or IV heart failure, renal disease/dysfunction (SrCr ≥1.5mg/dL [males], ≥1.4mg/dL [females], or abnormal CrCl), metabolic acidosis, including diabetic ketoacidosis. D/C temporarily (48 hrs) for radiologic studies with intravascular iodinated contrast materials.

WARNINGS/PRECAUTIONS: Lactic acidosis reported; increased risk with renal dysfunction, increased age, DM, CHF, and other conditions with risk of hypoperfusion and hypoxemia. Avoid use in patients ≥80 yrs unless renal function is normal. Monitor renal function and for ketoacidosis and metabolic acidosis. D/C in hypoxic states (eg, CHF, shock, acute MI), loss of blood glucose control due to stress, acidosis and prior to surgical procedures (due to restricted food intake). May decrease serum vitamin B_{12} levels. Increased risk of hypoglycemia with concomitant use with other hypoglycemic agents, elderly, debilitated/malnourished, adrenal or pituitary insufficiency, or alcohol intoxication. May cause fluid retention and exacerbation/initiation of heart failure; d/c if cardiac status deteriorates. Initiation not recommended in patients experiencing an acute coronary event. Avoid with NYHA Class III or IV cardiac status. Not for use in type 1 diabetes or for diabetic ketoacidosis treatment. Caution with edema. Dose-related wt gain reported. Ovulation in premenopausal anovulatory patients may occur; risk of pregnancy with inadequate contraception. May decrease Hgb and Hct. Avoid with active liver disease, if ALT levels >2.5x ULN, or if jaundice occurred with troglitazone. Check LFTs before therapy, every 2 months for 1 year, and periodically thereafter, or if hepatic dysfunction symptoms occur. D/C if ALT >3x ULN on therapy. Not for use with insulin. Increased incidence of bone fracture was noted in female patients.

ADVERSE REACTIONS: Upper respiratory tract infection, headache, back pain, hyperglycemia, fatigue, sinusitis, diarrhea, viral infection, arthralgia, anemia, dyspepsia, dizziness, abdominal pain, NV.

INTERACTIONS: Furosemide, nifedipine, cimetidine, and cationic drugs (eg, digoxin, amiloride, procainamide, quinidine, quinine, ranitidine, trimethoprim, vancomycin, triamterene, morphine) may increase metformin levels. Thiazides and other diuretics, corticosteroids, phenothiazines, thyroid products, estrogens, oral contraceptives, phenytoin, nicotinic acid, sympathomimetics, CCBs, and isoniazid may cause hyperglycemia. Risk of hypoglycemia with alcohol. Excess alcohol may increase potential for lactic acidosis. May decrease furosemide levels. Inhibitors of CYP2C8 (eg, gemfibrozil) may increase rosiglitazone AUC. Inducers of CYP2C8 (eg, rifampin) may decrease rosiglitazone AUC. Co-administration with insulin or nitrates is not recommended.

PREGNANCY: Category C, not for use in nursing.

MECHANISM OF ACTION: Rosiglitazone: Thiazolidinedione; insulin sensitizing agent that acts by enhancing peripheral glucose utilization. Metformin: Biguanide; decreases hepatic glucose production, decreases intestinal absorption of glucose, and increases peripheral glucose uptake and utilization.

PHARMACOKINETICS: Absorption: Rosiglitazone: Absolute bioavailability (99%). (4mg) C_{max}=242ng/mL. T_{max}=1 hr. Metformin: Absolute bioavailability (50-60%). (500mg) C_{max}=1106ng/mL; T_{max}=3 hrs. **Distribution:** Rosiglitazone: V_d=17.6L; plasma protein binding (99.8%). Metformin: V_d=654L. **Metabolism:** Rosiglitazone: Liver (extensive); CYP2C8 (major), 2C9 (minor). Metformin: No hepatic metabolism. **Elimination:** Rosiglitazone: Urine (64%), feces (23%); $T_{1/2}$=3-4 hrs. Metformin: Urine (unchanged); $T_{1/2}$=6.2 hrs (plasma).

NURSING CONSIDERATIONS

Assessment: After initiation or dose increases, observe carefully for signs/symptoms of heart failure (including excessive and rapid weight gain, dyspnea, edema). Prior to initiation or escalation, investigate and treat secondary causes of poor glycemic control (eg, infection). Before initiation and at least annually thereafter, assess renal function and liver enzymes and verify as normal.

Monitoring: Measure fasting blood glucose and glycosylated hemoglobin to monitor therapeutic response. Monitor liver enzymes, hematologic parameters (Hct/Hgb), and renal function periodically. Monitor for signs/symptoms of lactic acidosis.

Patient Counseling: Inform of importance of diet and regular exercise, regular testing of blood glucose, HbA_{1c}, renal function, and hematologic parameters. Advise to d/c and notify physician if unexplained hyperventilation, myalgia, malaise, unusual somnolence, or nonspecific symptoms occur. Warn against excessive alcohol intake.

Administration: Oral route. **Storage:** Store at 25°C (77°F); excursions permitted to 15-30°C (59-86°F). Keep out of reach of children.

AVANDARYL RX

rosiglitazone maleate - glimepiride (GlaxoSmithKline)

Thiazolidinediones may cause or exacerbate CHF in some patients. Avandaryl is not recommended in patients with symptomatic heart failure. Meta-analysis of studies has shown rosiglitazone to be associated with an increased risk of myocardial ischemic events.

THERAPEUTIC CLASS: Thiazolidinedione/sulfonylurea

INDICATIONS: Adjunct to diet and exercise to improve glycemic control in type 2 DM when treatment with dual rosiglitazone and glimepiride therapy is appropriate.

DOSAGE: *Adults:* Initial: 4mg-1mg qd with 1st meal of day. With Sulfonylurea or Thiazolidinedione: Initial: 4mg-2mg qd. Switching From Prior Combination Therapy: Same dose of each component already being taken. Prior Thiazolidinedione Monotherapy: Titrate dose. After 1-2 weeks with inadequate control, increase glimepiride component in no more than 2mg increments at 1-2 week intervals. Max: 8mg-4mg qd. Prior Sulfonylurea Monotherapy: May take 2-3 months for full effect of rosiglitazone; do not exceed 8mg of rosiglitazone daily. Titrate: May increase glimepiride component. Elderly/Debilitated/Malnourished/Renal, Hepatic, or Adrenal Insufficiency: Initial: 4mg-1mg qd. Titrate carefully.

HOW SUPPLIED: Tab: (Rosiglitazone-Glimepiride) 4mg-1mg, 4mg-2mg, 4mg-4mg, 8mg-2mg, 8mg-4mg

CONTRAINDICATIONS: Established NYHA Class III or IV heart failure.

WARNINGS/PRECAUTIONS: Should not be used in patients with type 1 diabetes or for the treatment of diabetic ketoacidois. (Glimepiride) Increased cardiovascular mortality. Hypoglycemia risk if debilitated, malnourished, or with adrenal, pituitary, renal or hepatic insufficiency. Hypoglycemia may be masked in elderly. May lose blood glucose control with stress. Secondary failure may occur. D/C if skin reactions persist or worsen. (Rosiglitazone) May cause fluid retention and exacerbation/initiation of heart failure; d/c if cardiac status deteriorates. Increased risk of CV events with NYHA Class I and II heart failure. Initiation not recommended for patients experiencing an acute coronary event and d/c during this acute phase. Caution with edema. May cause macular edema. Dose-related wt gain reported. Ovulation in premenopausal anovulatory patient may occur; risk of pregnancy with inadequate contraception. May decrease Hgb and Hct. Avoid with active liver disease, if ALT levels >2.5x ULN, or if jaundice occurred with rosiglitazone. Check LFTs before therapy, every 2 months for 1 yr, and periodically thereafter, or if hepatic dysfunction symptoms occur. D/C if ALT >3x ULN on therapy. Increased incidence of bone fracture was noted in female patients. Combination use with insulin not recommended.

ADVERSE REACTIONS: Upper respiratory tract infection, injury, headache, hypoglycemia, anemia, edema.

INTERACTIONS: Rosiglitazone: CYP2C8 inhibitors (eg, gemfibrozil) may increase the AUC. CYP2C8 inducers (eg, rifampin) may decrease the AUC. Glimepiride: Risk of hyperglycemia with thiazides, corticosteroids, phenothiazines, thyroid products, estrogens, oral contraceptives, phenytoin, nicotinic acid, sympathomimetics, and isoniazid. Risk of severe hypoglycemia with oral miconazole. β-blockers may mask symptoms of hypoglycemia. Use with insulin or nitrates is not recommended.

PREGNANCY: Category C, not for use in nursing.

MECHANISM OF ACTION: Rosiglitazone: Thiazolidinedione; insulin sensitizing agent that acts by enhancing peripheral glucose utilization. Glimepiride: Sulfonylurea; stimulates insulin release from functional pancreatic β cells.

PHARMACOKINETICS: Absorption: Rosiglitazone: Absolute bioavailability (99%); T_{max}=1 hr; (4mg) C_{max}=257ng/mL. Glimepiride: Complete; T_{max}=2-3 hrs; (4mg) C_{max}=151ng/mL. **Distribution:** Rosiglitazone: V_d=17.6L; plasma protein binding (99.8%). Glimepiride: (IV) V_d=8.8L; protein binding (>99.5%). **Metabolism:** Rosiglitazone: N-demethylation & hydroxylation followed by conjugation; CYP2C8 (major), 2C9 (minor). Glimepiride: Liver (complete); major metabolites M1 & M2; CYP2C9. **Elimination:** Rosiglitazone: Urine (64%), feces (23%); $T_{1/2}$=3-4 hrs. Glimepiride: Urine (60%), feces (40%); $T_{1/2}$=5-7 hrs.

NURSING CONSIDERATIONS

Assessment: Assess for signs/symptoms of heart failure (excessive and rapid weight gain, dyspnea, and edema), liver failure (NV, loss of appetite, dark urine, unusual fatigue, and jaundice). Check liver enzymes prior to therapy.

Monitoring: Monitor fasting blood glucose, glycosylated hemoglobin to check therapeutic response, and liver enzymes periodically.

Patient Counseling: Inform of importance of adherence to dietary instructions, weight loss, and exercise program. Instruct regarding regular blood glucose testing and HbA_{1c}. Inform to report unexplained NV, anorexia, abdominal pain, or dark urine. Instruct to also report any edema, SOB, or other symptoms of heart failure.

Administration: Oral route. **Storage:** Store at 25°C (77°F); excursions permitted to 15-30°C (59-86°F).

AVANDIA RX

rosiglitazone maleate (GlaxoSmithKline)

Thiazolidinediones may cause or exacerbate CHF in some patients. Rosiglitazone is not recommended in patients with symptomatic heart failure. Studies have shown rosiglitazone to be associated with an increased risk of myocardial ischemic events, such as angina or MI.

THERAPEUTIC CLASS: Thiazolidinedione

INDICATIONS: Adjunct to diet and exercise to improve glycemic control in type 2 diabetes mellitus. Coadministration with insulin or nitrates is not recommended.

DOSAGE: *Adults:* ≥18 yrs: Initial: 2mg bid or 4mg qd. Titrate: May increase after 8-12 weeks to 8mg daily as monotherapy or in combination with metformin, sulfonylurea, or sulfonylurea plus metformin. Max: 8mg/day.

HOW SUPPLIED: Tab: 2mg, 4mg, 8mg

CONTRAINDICATIONS: Established NYHA Class III or IV heart failure.

WARNINGS/PRECAUTIONS: May cause fluid retention and exacerbation/initiation of heart failure; d/c if cardiac status deteriorates. Increased risk of CV events with NYHA Class I or II cardiac status; avoid with NYHA Class III or IV cardiac status. An increased risk of myocardial ischemic events has been observed. CHF and MI during coadministration with insulin. Coadministration with insulin or nitrates is not recommended. Not for use in type 1 diabetes or diabetic ketoacidosis treatment. Caution with edema. Macular edema reported. Dose-related wt gain and anemia reported. Avoid with active liver disease, if ALT levels >2.5x ULN, or if jaundice occurred with troglitazone. Check LFTs before therapy, every 2 months for 1 year, and periodically thereafter, or if hepatic dysfunction symptoms occur. D/C if ALT >3x ULN on therapy. Increased incidence of bone fracture in female patients. May decrease Hgb and Hct. Risk for hypoglycemia. Monitor blood glucose and HbA_{1c} measurements. Ovulation in premenopausal anovulatory patients may occur; risk of pregnancy with inadequate contraception.

ADVERSE REACTIONS: Upper respiratory tract infection, injury, headache, back pain, hyperglycemia, fatigue, sinusitis, anemia, edema.

INTERACTIONS: Risk of hypoglycemia when used in combination with other hypoglycemic agents. CYP2C8 inhibitors (eg, gemfibrozil) may increase AUC of rosiglitazone. CYP2C8 inducers (eg, rifampin) may decrease AUC of rosiglitazone.

PREGNANCY: Category C, not for use in pregnancy or nursing.

MECHANISM OF ACTION: Thiazolidinedione; acts by improving insulin sensitivity.

PHARMACOKINETICS: Absorption: Absolute bioavailability (99%); T_{max}=1 hr. **Distribution:** V_d=17.6L; plasma protein binding (99.8%). **Metabolism:** CYP450, 2C8 (major) & 2C9 (minor); N-demethylation & hydroxylation then conjugation. **Elimination**: Urine (64%), feces (23%); $T_{1/2}$=3-4 hrs.

NURSING CONSIDERATIONS

Assessment: Check liver enzymes prior to initiation and periodically after initiation; assess for elevated liver enzymes prior to therapy. Assess for risk of hypoglycemia, its symptoms, and its predisposing conditions.

Monitoring: Regularly monitor fasting blood glucose and glycosylated hemoglobin levels to measure therapeutic response. Monitor liver function tests periodically. Monitor for signs/symptoms of heart failure (eg, excessive rapid weight gain, dyspnea, edema).

Patient Counseling: Instruct to report any rapid increase in weight or edema, SOB, or other symptoms of heart failure. Instruct to report anorexia, NV, dark urine, abdominal pain. Inform of importance of caloric restriction, weight loss, and exercise for glycemic control. Educate on importance of testing blood glucose and glycosylated hemoglobin regularly.

Administration: Oral route. **Storage**: 25°C (77°F). Dispense in tight, light-resistant container.

AVAPRO RX

irbesartan (Bristol-Myers Squibb/Sanofi-Aventis)

Can cause death/injury to developing fetus during 2nd and 3rd trimesters. Stop therapy if pregnancy detected.

THERAPEUTIC CLASS: Angiotensin II receptor antagonist

INDICATIONS: Hypertension, alone or with other antihypertensives. Diabetic nephropathy with an elevated serum creatinine and proteinuria (>300mg/day) in patients with type 2 diabetes and hypertension.

DOSAGE: *Adults:* HTN: Initial: 150mg qd. Titrate: May increase to 300mg qd. Intravascular Volume/Salt Depletion: Initial: 75mg qd. Nephropathy: Maint: 300mg qd.
Pediatrics: HTN: ≥17 yrs: Initial: 150mg qd. Titrate: May increase to 300mg qd. Intravascular Volume/Salt Depletion: Initial: 75mg qd.

HOW SUPPLIED: Tab: 75mg, 150mg, 300mg

WARNINGS/PRECAUTIONS: Can cause fetal injury/death. Correct volume or salt depletion before therapy. Changes in renal function may occur; caution with renal artery stenosis, severe CHF. Angioedema reported.

ADVERSE REACTIONS: Diarrhea, dyspepsia/heartburn, musculoskeletal trauma, fatigue, upper respiratory infection.

PREGNANCY: Category C (1st trimester) and D (2nd and 3rd trimesters), not for use in nursing.

MECHANISM OF ACTION: Angiotensin II receptor antagonist; blocks vasoconstrictor and aldosterone-secreting effects of angiotensin II by selectively binding to AT_1 angiotensin II receptor.

PHARMACOKINETICS: Absorption: Rapid and complete, absolute bioavailability (60-80%); T_{max}=1.5-2 hrs. **Distribution:** V_d=53-93L; plasma protein binding (90%); crosses placenta; excreted in breast milk. **Metabolism:** CYP29C (oxidation), glucuronide conjugation. **Elimination:** Urine, feces; $T_{1/2}$=11-15 hrs.

NURSING CONSIDERATIONS

Assessment: Assess for pregnancy status, renal impairment, possible drug interactions, and volume/salt depletion.

Monitoring: Monitor renal function periodically. Monitor for signs/symptoms of hypotension, hypersensitivity reactions, and renal dysfunction.

Patient Counseling: Inform of pregnancy risks. Advise to seek medical attention if symptoms of hypotension or hypersensitivity reactions occur.

Administration: Oral route. **Storage:** 25°C (77°F); excursions permitted to 15-30°C (59-86°F).

AVASTIN — RX

bevacizumab (Genentech)

Severe or fatal hemorrhage including hemoptysis, gastrointestinal (GI) bleeding, central nervous systems (CNS) hemorrhage, epistaxis, and vaginal bleeding occurred; avoid with serious hemorrhage or recent hemoptysis. Avoid if GI perforation or wound dehiscence develops; may be fatal.

THERAPEUTIC CLASS: Vascular endothelial growth factor (VEGF) inhibitor

INDICATIONS: 1st- or 2nd-line treatment of metastatic colorectal cancer (CRC), in combination with 5-fluorouracil-based chemotherapy. 1st-line treatment of unresectable, locally advanced, recurrent or metastatic non-squamous non-small cell lung cancer (NSCLC), in combination with carboplatin and paclitaxel. Treatment of patients who have not received chemotherapy for metastatic HER2-negative breast cancer, in combination with paclitaxel. Treatment of glioblastoma with progressive disease following prior therapy as a single agent.

DOSAGE: *Adults:* CRC: 5mg/kg (in combination with bolus IFL) or 10mg/kg (in combination with FOLFOX4) every 2 weeks. Non-squamous NSCLC: 15mg/kg (in combination with carboplatin/paclitaxel) every 3 weeks.
Breast Cancer: 10mg/kg (in combination with paclitaxel) every 2 weeks.
Glioblastoma: 10mg/kg every 2 weeks. Give as IV infusion over 90 min; if 1st infusion is well tolerated, give 2nd infusion over 60 min and subsequent doses over 30 min.

HOW SUPPLIED: Inj: 25mg/mL [4mL, 16mL]

WARNINGS/PRECAUTIONS: D/C with nephrotic syndrome, serious hemorrhage, and arterial thromboembolic events. Increased risk of HTN; permanently d/c if hypertensive crisis or hypertensive encephalopathy occurs. Monitor BP every 2-3 weeks during treatment. Increased incidence/severity of proteinuria. Potential for immunogenicity. CHF and neutropenia reported. Avoid initiation of therapy for at least 28 days following major surgery; surgical incision must be fully healed prior to start of therapy. Suspend treatment prior to elective surgery. Intracranial hemorrhage (Grade 3-4) reported in patients with previously treated glioblastoma. Reversible posterior leukoencephalopathy syndrome reported; d/c if symptoms occur. Non-GI fistula formation reported.

ADVERSE REACTIONS: Epistaxis, headache, hypertension, rhinitis, proteinuria, taste alteration, dry skin, rectal hemorrhage, lacrimation disorder, exfoliative dermatitis, GI perforations, wound healing complications (eg, wound dehiscence), hemoptysis, CNS hemorrhage, and vaginal bleeding.

INTERACTIONS: Increased risk of thromboembolic events when co-administered with chemotherapy; d/c if severe arterial thromboembolic event occurs. Serious fatal pulmonary hemorrhage may occur with chemotherapy in patients with NSCLC.

PREGNANCY: Category C, not for use in nursing.

MECHANISM OF ACTION: VEGF inhibitor; monoclonal IgG_1 antibody that binds to VEGF and prevents interaction with receptors (Flt-1, KDR) on surface of endothelial cells, inhibiting endothelial cell proliferation and new blood vessel formation.

PHARMACOKINETICS: Absorption: T_{max}=100 days. **Distribution:** V_d=3.25L (male) and 2.66L (female). **Elimination:** $T_{1/2}$=20 days.

NURSING CONSIDERATIONS

Assessment: Assess for history of hemoptysis (≥1/2 tsp of red blood), CVD, HTN, hepatic/renal dysfunction (proteinuria, nephrotic syndrome), and possible drug interactions. Therapy should not be initiated for at least 28 days following major surgery. Obtain baseline urinalysis, BP, and CBC.

Monitoring: Monitor BP every 2-3 weeks and perform serial urinalysis and CBC. Monitor signs/symptoms of GI perforation, fistula formation, wound-healing complications, serious hemorrhage, arterial thromboembolic events, hypertensive events (eg, crisis, encephalopathy), reversible posterior leukoencephalopathy syndrome, neutropenia, proteinuria, nephrotic syndrome, severe infusion reactions, CHF, and hypersensitivity reactions.

Patient Counseling: Inform of pregnancy risks and to d/c nursing. Counsel to seek medical attention if symptoms of the following occur: GI perforation (abdominal pain, constipation, vomiting), fistula formation, wound healing complications, serious hemorrhage, arterial thromboembolic events, hypertensive events, reversible posterior leukoencephalopathy syndrome (headache, seizures, lethargy, confusion, blindness), neutropenia (fever, infection), proteinuria, nephrotic syndrome, severe infusion reactions, CHF, and hypersensitivity reactions.

Administration: IV route. Do not administer as an IV push or bolus. **Storage**: Refrigerate at 2-8°C (36-46°F). (Diluted): 2-8°C (36-46°F) for up to 8 hrs. Protect from light. Do not freeze or shake.

AVELOX RX

moxifloxacin HCl (Schering)

Fluoroquinolones are associated with an increased risk of tendinitis and tendon rupture in all ages. Risk further increased in patients >60 yrs, patients taking corticosteroid drugs, and patients with kidney, heart or lung transplants.

THERAPEUTIC CLASS: Fluoroquinolone

INDICATIONS: Treatment of acute bacterial sinusitis, acute bacterial exacerbation of chronic bronchitis (ABECB), uncomplicated skin and skin structure infections (SSSI), community-acquired pneumonia (CAP), complicated intra-abdominal infections, and complicated SSSI caused by susceptible strains of microorganisms.

DOSAGE: *Adults:* ≥18 yrs: Sinusitis: 400mg PO/IV q24h for 10 days. ABECB: 400mg PO/IV q24h for 5 days. Uncomplicated SSSI: 400mg PO/IV q24h for 7 days. Complicated SSSI: 400mg PO/IV q24h for 7-21 days. CAP: 400mg PO/IV q24h for 7-14 days. Complicated Intra-Abdominal Infections: 400mg PO/IV q24h for 5-14 days.

HOW SUPPLIED: Inj: 400mg/250mL; Tab: 400mg

WARNINGS/PRECAUTIONS: Not for intra-arterial, IM, intrathecal, intraperitoneal, or SQ use. Avoid with known QT interval prolongation, and uncorrected hypokalemia. Caution with ongoing proarrhythmic conditions (eg, significant bradycardia, acute MI). QT-prolongation may be dose or infusion-rate dependent; do not exceed recommended dose. QT prolongation may increase risk of ventricular arrhythmias (eg, torsade de pointes). Caution in patients with mild, moderate, or severe liver cirrhosis. *Clostridium difficile*-associated diarrhea reported. Caution with CNS disorders (eg, severe cerebral arteriosclerosis, epilepsy). Tendon ruptures reported. D/C if convulsions, CNS effects, hypersensitivity reaction, or tendon rupture occurs. Rare cases of peripheral neuropathy reported.

ADVERSE REACTIONS: Nausea, diarrhea, dizziness.

INTERACTIONS: Take oral formulation at least 4 hrs before or 8 hrs after aluminum-, magnesium-, or calcium-containing antacids, sucralfate, multivitamins with iron or zinc, and didanosine chewable/buffered tablets or oral solution. Avoid Class IA (eg, quinidine, procainamide) or Class III (eg, amiodarone, sotalol) antiarrhythmics. Caution with drugs that prolong the QT interval (eg, cisapride, erythromycin, antipsychotics, TCAs). NSAIDs may increase risk of CNS stimulation and convulsions. Monitor PT with warfarin. Corticosteroids in elderly may increase risk of tendon rupture. Do not add other substances, additives, or medications to injection or infuse simultaneously through same IV line.

PREGNANCY: Category C, not for use in nursing.

MECHANISM OF ACTION: Fluoroquinolone; synthetic broad-spectrum antibiotic with activity against gram-positive and gram-negative microorganisms. Inhibits topoisomerase II (DNA gyrase) and topoisomerase IV, which are required for bacterial DNA replication, transcription, repair, and recombination.

PHARMACOKINETICS: Absorption: Well-absorbed; absolute bioavailability (90%). Single dose: (Oral) C_{max}=3.1mg/L, AUC=36.1mg•hr/L; (IV) C_{max}= 3.9mg/L, AUC=39.3mg•hr/L. Multiple dose: (Oral) C_{max}=4.5mg/L, AUC=48.0mg•hr/L; (IV) C_{max}= 4.2mg/L, AUC=38.0mg•hr/L. Refer to PI for further info. **Distribution:** V_d=1.7-2.7L/kg; plasma protein binding (50%); widely distributed. **Metabolism:** Glucuronide and sulfate conjugation. **Elimination:** 45% unchanged; urine (20%), feces (25%); $T_{1/2}$=11.5-15.6 hrs (oral), 8.2-15.4 hrs (IV).

NURSING CONSIDERATIONS

Assessment: Assess for QT interval prolongation, uncorrected hypokalemia, patients receiving Class IA (eg, quinidine, procainamide) or Class III (eg, amiodarone, sotalol) antiarrhythmic agents, ongoing proarrhythmic conditions (eg, bradycardia, acute MI), CNS disorders (eg, severe cerebral arteriosclerosis, epilepsy), or risk factors that may predispose to seizures or lower seizure threshold. Assess pregnancy/nursing status and possible drug interactions.

Monitoring: Monitor ECG and lab changes (eg, CBC, PT, Ca, glucose, bilirubin, and amylase). Monitor for signs/symptoms of anaphylactic reactions (eg, fever, rash, toxic epidermal necrolysis, Stevens-Johnson syndrome, allergic pneumonitis, interstitial nephritis, hepatitis, anemia, and vasculitis), prolongation of QT interval, ventricular arrhythmia/torsade de pointes, CNS events (eg, dizziness, confusion, tremors, hallucinations, depression, suicidal thoughts or acts, and seizures), drug resistance, *C.difficile*-associated diarrhea that ranges from mild diarrhea to fatal colitis, peripheral neuropathy (eg, paresthesia, hypoesthesia, dysesthesia, weakness), tendon rupture (eg, shoulder, hand, Achilles, or other tendons), and photosensitivity.

Patient Counseling: Notify healthcare provider if experience symptoms of pain, swelling, or inflammation of a tendon, or weakness or inability to move joints; rest and refrain from exercise and d/c therapy. Inform that drug treats bacterial, not viral, infections. Take exactly as directed; skipping doses or not completing full course may decrease effectiveness and increase resistance. Inform about potential benefits/risks. D/C and notify physician if allergic reaction, skin rash, and watery and bloody stools (with or without stomach cramps and fever) occur. Notify if pregnant/nursing or taking antiarrhythmics, OTC drugs, multivitamins, antacids, or sucralfate. Use caution while performing hazardous tasks (eg, operating machinery/driving). Avoid excessive exposure to sunlight and wear protective clothes. Contact physician if sunburn-like reaction occurs.

Administration: Oral, IV routes. Avoid rapid or bolus IV infusion. Inspect visually for particulate matter in vial prior to administration. **Storage:** 25°C (77°F); excursions permitted to 15-30°C (59-86°F). Avoid high humidity. Do not refrigerate.

AVINZA

morphine sulfate (King)

CII

Swallow capsules whole or sprinkle contents on applesauce. Do not crush, chew, or dissolve capsule beads. Avoid alcohol and alcohol-containing medications; consumption of alcohol may result in the rapid release and absorption of potentially fatal dose of morphine.

THERAPEUTIC CLASS: Opioid analgesic

INDICATIONS: Relief of moderate to severe pain requiring continuous opioid therapy for an extended period of time.

DOSAGE: *Adults:* ≥18 yrs: Conversion from Other Oral Morphine Products: Give total daily morphine dose as a single dose q24h. Conversion from Parenteral Morphine: Initial: Give about 3x the previous daily parenteral morphine requirement. Conversion from Other Parenteral or Oral Non-Morphine Opioids: Initial: Give 1/2 of estimated daily morphine requirement q24h. Supplement with immediate-release morphine or short-acting analgesics if needed. Titrate: Adjust dose as frequently as every other day. Non-Opioid Tolerant: 30mg q24h. Titrate: Increase by increments ≤30mg every 4 days. The 60, 90, and 120mg caps are for opioid-tolerant patients. Max: 1600mg/day. Doses >1600mg/day contain a quantity of fumaric acid, which may cause renal toxicity.

HOW SUPPLIED: Cap, Extended-Release: 30mg, 60mg, 90mg, 120mg

CONTRAINDICATIONS: Respiratory depression in the absence of resuscitative equipment, acute or severe bronchial asthma, paralytic ileus.

WARNINGS/PRECAUTIONS: Abuse potential. Extreme caution with COPD, cor pulmonale, decreased respiratory reserve (eg, severe kyphoscoliosis), hypoxia, hypercapnia, pre-existing respiratory depression, increased ICP, head injury. May cause orthostatic hypotension, syncope, severe hypotension with depleted blood volume. Caution with circulatory shock, biliary tract disease, severe renal/hepatic insufficiency, Addison's disease, hypothyroidism, prostatic hypertrophy, urethral stricture, elderly or debilitated, CNS depression, toxic psychosis, acute alcoholism, delirium tremens, seizure disorders. Avoid with GI obstruction. Withdrawal symptoms with abrupt discontinuation. Tolerance and physical dependence may develop. Potential for severe constipation; use laxatives, stool softeners at onset of therapy.

ADVERSE REACTIONS: Constipation, NV, somnolence, dehydration, headache, peripheral edema, diarrhea, abdominal pain, infection, UTI, flu syndrome, back pain, rash, sweating, fever, insomnia, depression, paresthesia, anorexia, dry mouth, asthenia, dyspnea.

INTERACTIONS: See Black Box Warning. Additive effects with alcohol, other opioids, illicit drugs that cause CNS depression. Reduce dose with other CNS depressants (eg, sedatives, hypnotics, general anesthetics, antiemetics, phenothiazines, tranquilizers, alcohol). May enhance neuromuscular blocking action of skeletal muscle relaxants. Avoid with mixed agonist/antagonists (eg, pentazocine, nalbuphine, butorphanol) and within 14 days of MAOI use. Monitor for increased respiratory and CNS depression with cimetidine.

PREGNANCY: Category C, not for use in nursing.

MECHANISM OF ACTION: Opioid analgesic; pure opioid agonist that is relatively selective for μ-receptor but may interact with other opioid receptors at higher doses. Analgesic effects not established. Specific CNS opiate receptors (eg, μ-receptors) and endogenous compounds with morphine-like activity are found throughout brain and spinal cord and are likely to play a role in analgesic effects.

PHARMACOKINETICS: Absorption: C_{max}=18.65ng/mL; AUC=273.25ng/mL•h. **Distribution:** Plasma protein binding (20-35%), V_d=1-6L/kg, distributed to skeletal muscle, kidneys, liver, GI tract, lung, spleen and brain. Small quantities cross the blood-brain barrier. Found in placental membranes and human breast milk. **Metabolism:** Hepatic conjugation; 3-glucuronide (M3G) (metabolite); 6-glucuronide (M6G) (active metabolite). **Elimination:** Urine (major), feces (7-10%), bile (small); (IV) $T_{1/2}$=2 hrs.

NURSING CONSIDERATIONS

Assessment: Assess for respiratory depression, GI obstruction (eg, paralytic ileus), acute or severe bronchial asthma, COPD, presence of head injury or increased ICP, biliary tract disease, acute pancreatitis, Addison's disease, hypothyroidism, prostatic hypertrophy, urethral stricture, CNS depression, toxic psychosis, seizure disorders, acute alcoholism, hepatic/renal function, age, nursing/pregnancy status, and possible drug interactions.

Monitoring: Monitor for signs/symptoms of respiratory depression, orthostatic hypotension, syncope, drug dependence and tolerance, and withdrawal syndrome (eg, restlessness, lacrimation, rhinorrhea, myalgia, mydriasis). Monitor for signs of increased ICP with head injuries.

Patient Counseling: Counsel drug may be taken with/without food. Instruct to swallow whole (not to chew, crush, or dissolve) or open and sprinkle onto small amount of applesauce. Instruct not to consume alcohol during therapy, including Rx/OTC drugs containing alcohol. Notify physician of all concurrently taken medications and avoid use of other CNS depressants. Inform drug may impair mental/physical abilities and to exercise caution when performing hazardous tasks (eg, operating machinery/driving). Do not adjust dose or abruptly d/c medication without consulting physician. Advise that medication has potential for abuse. Instruct to keep out of reach of children. Advise to dispose of any unused medication via toilet. Advise drug may cause severe constipation; take appropriate laxatives or stool softeners at start of therapy.

Administration: Oral route. **Storage:** 25°C (77°F); excursions permitted to 15-30°C (59-86°F). Protect from moisture; dispense in a tight, light-resistant container.

AVODART RX

dutasteride (GlaxoSmithKline)

THERAPEUTIC CLASS: Type I and II 5 alpha-reductase inhibitor (2nd generation)

INDICATIONS: Treatment of symptomatic benign prostatic hyperplasia (BPH) either as monotherapy or in combination with the α-blocker tamsulosin.

DOSAGE: *Adults:* Monotherapy: 0.5mg qd. Combination Therapy with Tamsulosin: 0.5mg qd and tamsulosin 0.4mg qd. Swallow whole.

HOW SUPPLIED: Cap: 0.5mg

CONTRAINDICATIONS: Women and children.

WARNINGS/PRECAUTIONS: Risk to male fetus; should not be handled by pregnant women. Monitor for obstructive uropathy with large residual urinary volume and/or severely diminished urinary flow. Avoid donating blood until 6 months after last dose. Caution with liver disease. Decreases serum PSA levels by about 40%-50%; adjust (double) PSA results after 6 months or more of therapy to compare with normal values.

ADVERSE REACTIONS: Impotence, decreased libido.

INTERACTIONS: CYP3A4 inhibitors (eg, ritonavir, ketoconazole, verapamil, diltiazem, cimetidine, ciprofloxacin) may increase blood levels.

PREGNANCY: Category X, not for use in nursing.

MECHANISM OF ACTION: Type I, II 5α-reductase inhibitor; inhibits conversion of testosterone to 5α-dihydrotestosterone, androgen responsible for development and enlargement of prostate gland.

PHARMACOKINETICS: Absorption: Absolute bioavailability (60%); T_{max}=2-3 hrs. **Distribution:** V_d=300-500L; plasma protein binding (99%). **Metabolism:** CYP3A4, 3A5. **Elimination:** Feces (5%), urine (<1%); $T_{1/2}$=5 weeks.

NURSING CONSIDERATIONS

Assessment: Assess for liver disease, possible drug interactions, large residual urinary volume or severely diminished urinary flow. Rule out prostate cancer. Perform digital rectal exam (DRE) prior to therapy.

Monitoring: Perform DRE periodically. Obtain new baseline PSA after 3-6 months of treatment. Monitor for obstructive uropathy, hepatic dysfunction, and hypersensitivity reactions.

Patient Counseling: Advise not to donate blood for at least 6 months after d/c therapy. Inform females who are pregnant, or intend to become pregnant, not to handle drug due to potential risk to fetus. If contact made, wash area immediately with soap and water. Inform males that volume of ejaculate may decrease.

Administration: Oral route. **Storage:** 25°C (77°F); excursions permitted to 15-30°C (59-86°F).

AXERT — RX

almotriptan malate (Ortho-McNeil)

THERAPEUTIC CLASS: 5-$HT_{1B/1D}$ agonist

INDICATIONS: Acute treatment of migraine with or without aura.

DOSAGE: *Adults:* ≥18 yrs: Initial: 6.25-12.5mg at onset of headache. May repeat after 2 hrs. Max: 2 doses/24 hrs. Hepatic/Renal Impairment: 6.25mg at onset of headache. Max: 12.5mg/24 hrs. Safety of treating >4 headaches/30 days not known.

HOW SUPPLIED: Tab: 6.25mg, 12.5mg

CONTRAINDICATIONS: Ischemic heart disease, coronary artery vasospasm, other significant CVD, uncontrolled HTN, within 24 hrs of another 5-HT_1 agonist or ergot-type agent, hemiplegic or basilar migraine.

WARNINGS/PRECAUTIONS: Confirm diagnosis. Supervise first dose and monitor cardiac function in those at risk of CAD (eg, HTN, hypercholesterolemia, smoker, obesity, diabetes, CAD family history, postmenopausal women, males >40 yrs). Monitor cardiovascular function with long-term intermittent use. May cause vasospastic reactions or cerebrovascular events. Serotonin syndrome symptoms (eg, mental status changes, autonomic instability, neuromuscular aberrations, and GI symptoms) reported. Caution with renal or hepatic dysfunction. Avoid in elderly.

ADVERSE REACTIONS: Nausea, somnolence, headache, paresthesia, dry mouth, coronary artery vasospasm, MI, ventricular tachycardia, fibrillation.

INTERACTIONS: Additive vasospastic reactions with ergotamines. SSRIs may cause weakness, hyperreflexia, and incoordination. Serotonin syndrome reported with combined use of an SSRI or SNRI. Avoid other 5-HT_1 agonist drugs within 24-hr period. Clearance may be decreased by MAOIs. Increased levels possible with CYP3A4 inhibitors (eg, ketoconazole).

PREGNANCY: Category C, caution in nursing.

MECHANISM OF ACTION: Selective 5-$HT_{1B/1D}$ receptor agonist; binds with high affinity to 5-$HT_{1B/1D/1F}$ receptors and weak affinity to 5-$HT_{1A/7}$ receptors. Attributed to agonist effects at 5-$HT_{1B/1D}$ receptors on extracerebral, intracranial blood vessels that become dilated during migraine attack and on nerve terminal in trigeminal system. Activation of these receptors results in cranial nerve constriction, inhibition of neuropeptide release, and reduced transmission in trigeminal pain pathways.

PHARMACOKINETICS: Absorption: Well-absorbed; absolute bioavailability (70%); T_{max}=1-3 hrs. **Distribution:** V_d=180-200L; plasma protein binding (35%). **Metabolism:** Monoamine oxidase (MAO)-mediated oxidative deamination and CYP450-mediated oxidation (major pathways); indoleacetic acid, gamma-aminobutyric acid (inactive metabolites). **Elimination:** Urine (40% unchanged), feces (13%, unchanged and metabolite); $T_{1/2}$=3-4 hrs.

NURSING CONSIDERATIONS

Assessment: Confirm diagnosis of migraine before therapy. Assess for cluster headache, ischemic heart disease (eg, angina pectoris, Prinzmetal's variant angina, MI or documented silent MI), HTN, hemiplegic or basilar migraine, presence of risk factors (eg, hypercholesterolemia, smoking, obesity, DM, strong family history of CAD, female with surgical or physiological menopause, or male >49 yrs), ECG changes, hepatic/renal impairment, pregnancy/nursing status, and possible drug interactions.

Monitoring: Administration of 1st dose should be in physician's office or medically staffed and equipped facility as cardiac ischemia may occur in absence of clinical symptoms; ECG should be obtained immediately during interval in those with risk factors. Monitor for signs/symptoms of cardiac events (eg, coronary vasospasm, acute MI, arrhythmia, ECG changes, follow-up coronary angiography), cerebrovascular events (eg, hemorrhage, stroke, TIAs), peripheral vascular ischemia, colonic ischemia with bloody diarrhea and abdominal pain, serotonin syndrome (eg, mental status changes, autonomic instability, neuromuscular aberrations and/or GI symptoms), ophthalmic effects, and increased BP.

Patient Counseling: Inform about potential benefits/risks (eg, serotonin syndrome manifestations such as confusion, hallucinations, fast heartbeat, fever, sweating, muscle spasm, and diarrhea), especially if taken with SSRIs or SNRIs. Instruct to report adverse reactions to physician. Advise to take exactly as directed. Counsel to use caution during hazardous tasks (eg, driving/operating machinery). Instruct to notify if pregnant/nursing or planning to become pregnant.

Administration: Oral route. **Storage:** 25°C (77°F); excursions permitted to 15-30°C (59-86°F).

AXID

nizatidine (GlaxoSmithKline) **RX**

OTHER BRAND NAMES: Axid Oral Solution (Braintree)

THERAPEUTIC CLASS: H_2-blocker

INDICATIONS: Short term treatment of active duodenal ulcer (DU) and benign gastric ulcer (GU). Maintenance therapy for duodenal ulcers. Treatment of endoscopically diagnosed esophagitis, including erosive and ulcerative esophagitis, and heartburn due to GERD.

DOSAGE: *Adults:* Active DU/Active Benign GU: Usual: 300mg qhs or 150mg bid up to 8 weeks. Healed DU: Maint: 150mg qhs, up to 1 year. GERD: 150mg bid up to 12 weeks. Renal Impairment: Treatment: CrCl 20-50mL/min: 150mg/day. CrCl <20mL/min: 150mg every other day. Maint: CrCl 20-50mL/min: 150mg every other day. CrCl <20mL/min: 150mg every 3 days. *Pediatrics:* ≥12 yrs: (Sol) Erosive Esophagitis/GERD: 150mg bid up to 8 weeks. Max: 300mg/day. Renal Impairment: Treatment: CrCl 20-50mL/min: 150mg/day. CrCl <20mL/min: 150mg every other day. Maint: CrCl 20-50mL/min: 150mg every other day. CrCl <20mL/min: 150mg every 3 days.

HOW SUPPLIED: Cap: 150mg, 300mg; Sol: 15mg/mL

WARNINGS/PRECAUTIONS: Caution with renal dysfunction; reduce dose. Symptomatic response does not preclude the presence of gastric malignancy. False positive tests for urobilinogen with Multistix.

ADVERSE REACTIONS: Headache, abdominal pain, pain, asthenia, diarrhea, NV, flatulence, dyspepsia, rhinitis, pharyngitis, dizziness.

INTERACTIONS: May elevate serum salicylate levels with high dose ASA.

PREGNANCY: Category B, not for use in nursing.

MECHANISM OF ACTION: H_2 receptor antagonist; competitive, reversible inhibitor of histamine at the histamine H_2 receptors, particularly those in gastroparietal cells.

PHARMACOKINETICS: Absorption: Absolute bioavailability (>70%); (150mg, 300mg) C_{max}=700-1800mcg/L, 1400-3600mcg/L; T_{max}=0.5-3 hrs. (12-18 yrs, 150mg) C_{max}=1422.9ng/mL; T_{max}=1.3 hrs; AUC=3764ng•hr/mL. **Distribution:** (Adult) V_d=0.8-1.5L/kg; (12-18 yrs) V_d=71.4L. Plasma protein binding (35%); found in breast milk. **Metabolism:** N_2-monodesmethylnizatidine (major). **Excretion:** Urine (90%, 60% unchanged); feces (6%). (Adult) $T_{1/2}$=1-2 hrs; (12-18 yrs) $T_{1/2}$=1.2 hrs.

NURSING CONSIDERATIONS

Assessment: Assess for hypersensitivity to other H_2 receptor antagonists, renal dysfunction, presence of gastric malignancy, pregnancy/nursing status, and possible drug interactions.

Monitoring: Monitor for signs/symptoms of hepatocellular injury (eg, elevation in liver enzymes), hematological effects (eg, anemia), hypersensitivity reactions (eg, anaphylaxis), and for signs of clinical improvement. If treatment is for active duodenal ulcer, monitor for signs of healing after 4 weeks and for complete healing by 8 weeks.

Patient Counseling: Advise if taking single dosing, take at bedtime. Contact physician if hypersensitivity reaction develops. Notify pregnant/nursing females about risks of use.

Administration: Oral route. **Storage:** Dispense in tightly closed container. Cap: 20-25° (68-77°F). Sol: 25° (77°F); excursions permitted to 15-30°C (59-86°F).

AYGESTIN — RX

norethindrone acetate (Duramed)

THERAPEUTIC CLASS: Progestogen

INDICATIONS: Treatment of secondary amenorrhea, endometriosis, and abnormal uterine bleeding due to hormonal imbalance in the absence of organic pathology.

DOSAGE: *Adults:* Assume interval between menses is 28 days. Secondary Amenorrhea/Abnormal Uterine Bleeding: 2.5-10mg qd for 5-10 days during second half of menstrual cycle. Endometriosis: Initial: 5mg qd for 2 weeks. Titrate: Increase by 2.5mg qd every 2 weeks until 15mg/day. Continue for 6-9 months or until breakthrough bleeding demands temporary termination.

HOW SUPPLIED: Tab: 5mg* *scored

CONTRAINDICATIONS: Pregnancy, thrombophlebitis, thromboembolic disorders, cerebral apoplexy, liver impairment, breast carcinoma, undiagnosed vaginal bleeding, missed abortion, use as a pregnancy diagnostic test.

WARNINGS/PRECAUTIONS: D/C with migraine, vision loss, proptosis, diplopia, papilledema, or retinal vascular lesions. May cause thrombophlebitis, pulmonary embolism, and fluid retention. Caution with epilepsy, migraine, psychic depression, asthma, cardiac or renal dysfunction, depression, DM, and hyperlipidemia. May mask onset of climacteric. Not for use during the first trimester of pregnancy; risk to the fetus.

ADVERSE REACTIONS: Breakthrough bleeding, spotting, change in menstrual flow, amenorrhea, edema, weight changes, cervical changes, cholestatic jaundice, rash, melasma, chloasma, depression.

PREGNANCY: Category X, safety in nursing is not known.

MECHANISM OF ACTION: Progestogen; induces secretory changes in estrogen-primed endometrium.

PHARMACOKINETICS: Absorption: Rapid; C_{max}=26.19ng/mL; T_{max}=1.83 hrs; AUC=166.9ng/mL•hr. **Distribution:** V_d=4L/kg; sex hormone binding globulin (SHBG) (36%); albumin binding (61%); found in breast milk. **Metabolism:**

Extensive, via reduction; sulfate and glucuronide conjugation. **Elimination:** Urine, feces (metabolites); $T_{1/2}$=9 hrs.

NURSING CONSIDERATIONS

Assessment: Assess for known/suspected pregnancy, vaginal bleeding, presence or history of breast cancer, DVT, PE, active or recent (within past yr) arterial thromboembolic disease (eg, stroke, MI), and impaired renal/hepatic function. Assess use in nursing females, history of depression, and those at risk for arterial vascular disease (eg, presence of HTN, hypercholesterolemia, DM, obesity, tobacco use) and for VTE (eg, family history, obesity, SLE). Assess for possible lab interactions.

Monitoring: Monitor for signs/symptoms of cardiovascular disorders (eg, thromboembolic events), visual abnormalities (eg, loss of vision, proptosis, diplopia), fluid retention, and breakthrough bleeding. Monitor for signs of worsening depression in patients with previous history. Monitor with hyperlipidemias and DM for changes in lipid and carbohydrate metabolism.

Patient Counseling: Counsel to contact physician if breast lumps, dizziness or faintness, changes in speech, severe headaches, chest pain, SOB, leg pain, or changes in vision occur. Advise to have annual breast exam and mammography unless otherwise directed by physician. Counsel to avoid using tobacco.

Administration: Oral route. **Storage:** 20-25°C (68-77°F).

AZACTAM — RX

aztreonam (Elan)

THERAPEUTIC CLASS: Monobactam

INDICATIONS: Treatment of septicemia and lower respiratory tract (eg, pneumonia, bronchitis), skin and skin-structure, urinary tract (UTI), gynecologic (eg, endometritis), and intra-abdominal (eg, peritonitis) infections caused by susceptible microorganisms. Adjunct therapy to surgery for management of infections caused by susceptible microorganisms.

DOSAGE: *Adults:* UTI: 500mg-1g IM/IV q8-12h. Moderately Severe Systemic Infections: 1-2g IM/IV q8-12h. Severe Systemic/Life-Threatening Infections/ *Pseudomonas aeruginosa*: 2g IV q6-8h. Max: 8g/day. CrCl 10-30mL/min/1.73m²: Initial: LD: 1 or 2g. Maint: 50% of usual dose. CrCl <10mL/min/1.73m²: Initial: LD: 500mg, 1g or 2g. Maint: 25% of usual initial dose at usual intervals. Serious/Life-Threatening Infections: In addition to maint dose, give 1/8 initial dose after each hemodialysis session. IV route recommended for single doses >1g or for bacterial septicemia, localized parenchymal abscess (eg, intra-abdominal abscess), peritonitis, or other severe systemic or life-threatening infections. Continue for at least 48 hrs after patient is asymptomatic or evidence of bacterial eradication.

Pediatrics: 9 months-16 yrs: Mild-Moderate Infections: 30mg/kg IV q8h. Moderate-Severe Infections: 30mg/kg IV q6-8h. Max: 120mg/kg/day. IV route is recommended for single doses >1g or for bacterial septicemia, localized parenchymal abscess (eg, intra-abdominal abscess), peritonitis, or other severe systemic or life-threatening infections. Continue for at least 48 hrs after patient is asymptomatic or evidence of bacterial eradication.

HOW SUPPLIED: Inj: 1g, 2g, 1g/50mL, 2g/50mL

WARNINGS/PRECAUTIONS: Caution with hypersensitivity to other β-lactams or allergens. *Clostridium difficile*-associated diarrhea reported. May promote overgrowth of nonsusceptible organisms. Monitor with renal or hepatic impairment. Toxic epidermal necrolysis reported (rarely) in bone marrow transplant with multiple risk factors including sepsis.

ADVERSE REACTIONS: Diarrhea, NV, rash, abdominal cramps, vaginal candidiasis, discomfort/swelling at injection site, hypersensitivity reaction.

INTERACTIONS: Monitor renal function with aminoglycosides; increased risk of nephrotoxicity, ototoxicity. Toxic epidermal necrolysis reported (rarely) in bone marrow transplant with radiation therapy and other drugs associated with toxic epidermal necrolysis.

PREGNANCY: Category B, not for use in nursing.

MECHANISM OF ACTION: Monobactam; synthetic bactericidal antibiotic. Inhibits bacterial cell-wall synthesis due to high affinity of aztreonam for penicillin-binding protein 3 (PBP3).

PHARMACOKINETICS: Absorption: C_{max}=90μ/ml (1g dose), 204μ/ml (2g dose); T_{max}=1 hr. **Distribution:** V_d=12.6L; found in breast milk. **Elimination:** Urine; $T_{1/2}$=1.7 hr.

NURSING CONSIDERATIONS

Assessment: Assess for hypersensitivity reaction to PCNs, cephalosporins, and/or carbapenems, hepatic/renal impairment, pregnancy/nursing status, patients undergoing bone marrow transplant with multiple risk factors (sepsis or radiation therapy) and possible drug interactions.

Monitoring: Monitor for anaphylactic reactions, overgrowth of non-susceptible organisms, development of drug resistance, *C.difficile*-associated diarrhea, toxic epidermal necrolysis, and hepatic/renal functions.

Patient Counseling: Inform that drug treats bacterial, not viral, infections. Take exactly as directed; skipping doses or not completing full course may decrease effectiveness and increase resistance. Inform about potential benefits/risks. D/C and notify physician if allergic reactions, watery/bloody diarrhea (with/without stomach cramps) occur (may occur as late as 2 or more months after therapy). Notify if pregnant/nursing.

Administration: IM/IV routes. **Storage:** Room temperature; avoid excessive heat.

AZASITE RX

azithromycin (Inspire)

THERAPEUTIC CLASS: Macrolide

INDICATIONS: Treatment of bacterial conjunctivitis caused by susceptible strains of microorganisms.

DOSAGE: *Adults:* Initial: 1 drop bid, 8 to 12 hrs apart, for first 2 days. Maint: 1 drop qd for next 5 days.
Pediatrics: ≥1 yr: Initial: 1 drop bid, 8 to 12 hrs apart, for first 2 days. Maint: 1 drop qd for next 5 days.

HOW SUPPLIED: Sol: 1% [2.5mL]

WARNINGS/PRECAUTIONS: Not for injection; do not give systemically, inject subconjunctivally or into chamber of eye. Caution may cause hypersensitivity reactions. Growth of resistant organisms including fungi may occur with prolonged use. Avoid contact lens use.

ADVERSE REACTIONS: Eye irritation, burning, stinging and irritation upon instillation, contact dermatitis, corneal erosion, dry eye, dysgeusia, nasal congestion, ocular discharge, punctate keratitis, sinusitis.

PREGNANCY: Category B, caution in nursing.

MECHANISM OF ACTION: Macrolide; binds to the 50S ribosomal subunit of susceptible microorganisms and interferes with microbial protein synthesis.

PHARMACOKINETICS: Absorption: C_{max}≤10ng/mL.

NURSING CONSIDERATIONS

Assessment: Assess proper diagnosis of causative bacteria.

Monitoring: Monitor for signs/symptoms of anaphylaxis (angioedema, Stevens-Johnson syndrome), development of growth of resistant organisms, and eye irritation.

Patient Counseling: Advise patients with signs/symptoms of bacterial conjuctivitis to avoid wearing contact lenses. Instruct not to allow applicator tip to touch the eye, fingers, or other sources. Take exactly as directed. Advise if doses are skipped or medication is stopped early, treatment effectiveness will be decreased and bacteria may develop resistance. Direct to d/c and contact physician if signs of allergic reaction occur.

Administration: Ocular route. **Storage:** Store unopened bottle under refrigeration at 2-8°C (36-46°F). Once bottle is opened, store at 2-25°C (36-77°F) for up to 14 days. Discard after 14 days.

AZELEX

azelaic acid (Allergan)

RX

THERAPEUTIC CLASS: Dicarboxylic acid antimicrobial

INDICATIONS: Mild to moderate inflammatory acne vulgaris.

DOSAGE: *Adults:* Wash and dry skin. Massage gently into affected area bid (am and pm).
Pediatrics: ≥12 yrs: Wash and dry skin. Massage gently into affected area bid (am and pm).

HOW SUPPLIED: Cre: 20% [30g, 50g]

WARNINGS/PRECAUTIONS: Avoid mouth, eyes, mucous membranes, and occlusive dressings.

ADVERSE REACTIONS: Pruritus, burning, stinging, tingling, hypopigmentation.

PREGNANCY: Category B, caution in nursing.

MECHANISM OF ACTION: Dicarboxylic acid antimicrobial; not established. Possesses antimicrobial activity that may be attributable to inhibition of microbial cellular protein synthesis. A normalization of keratinization leading to an anticomedonal effect of azelaic acid may also contribute to clinical activity.

PHARMACOKINETICS: Absorption: Penetrates stratum corneum (3-5%), up to 10% of dose found in dermis and epidermis; systemic absorption (4%); C_{max}=20-80ng/mL. **Metabolism:** Cutaneous (negligible), beta-oxidation. **Elimination:** Urine (mainly unchanged); $T_{1/2}$=12 hrs (after topical dosing).

NURSING CONSIDERATIONS

Assessment: Assess proper diagnosis of acne vulgaris. Assess use in nursing females.

Monitoring: Monitor for signs/symptoms of hypopigmentation (especially in patients with dark complexions), sensitivity reactions, and severe skin irritation.

Patient Counseling: Counsel to use medication for the full prescribed treatment period. Instruct to avoid using occlusive dressings with medication. Advise to keep medication away from mouth, eyes, and mucous membranes. If contact occurs with eyes, instruct to wash eyes with large amounts of water and consult physician if problem persists. Instruct that temporary skin irritation may occur when applied to broken or inflamed skin; if irritation persists, consult physician immediately. Counsel patients with dark complexions to notify physician if they notice pigment changes.

Administration: Topical. **Storage:** 15-30°C (59-86°F). Protect from freezing.

AZILECT

rasagiline mesylate (Teva)

RX

THERAPEUTIC CLASS: Monoamine oxidase inhibitor (Type B)

INDICATIONS: Treatment of signs and symptoms of idiopathic Parkinson's disease as initial monotherapy and adjunct therapy to levodopa.

DOSAGE: *Adults:* Monotherapy: 1mg qd. Adjunctive Therapy: Initial: 0.5mg qd. Titrate: May increase to 1mg qd. Adjust dose of levodopa with concomitant use. Concomitant Ciprofloxacin or Other CYP1A2 Inhibitors/Hepatic Impairment: 0.5mg qd.

HOW SUPPLIED: Tab: 0.5mg, 1mg

CONTRAINDICATIONS: Pheochromocytoma. Concomitant use with meperidine, tramadol, methadone, propoxyphene, dextromethorphan, St. John's wort, mirtazapine, cyclobenzaprine, sympathomimetic amines (eg, amphetamines, cold products containing pseudoephedrine, phenylephrine, phenylpropanolamine, and ephedrine), other MAOIs, cocaine, general anesthesia, local anesthesia containing vasoconstrictors.

WARNINGS/PRECAUTIONS: May increase incidence of melanoma. Concomitant use with levodopa may potentiate dopaminergic side effects and exacerbate pre-existing dyskinesia. Postural hypotension reported. Patients should be warned to restrict dietary tyramines and avoid amine-containing medications for 2 weeks after discontinuation.

ADVERSE REACTIONS: Headache, arthralgia, depression, fall, flu syndrome, dyskinesia, accidental injury, nausea, weight loss, constipation, postural hypotension, vomiting, dry mouth, rash, somnolence.

INTERACTIONS: See Contraindications. Concomitant use with SSRIs, SNRIs, tricyclic and tetracyclic antidepressants is not recommended due to severe CNS toxicity. Increased plasma concentrations up to 2-fold with concomitant ciprofloxacin and other CYP1A2. Severe hypertensive reactions reported with concomitant use of sympathomimetics.

PREGNANCY: Category C, caution in nursing.

MECHANISM OF ACTION: MAO-B inhibitor; suspected to inhibit MAO type B, which causes an increase in extracellular dopamine levels in the striatum and increases dopaminergic activity.

PHARMACOKINETICS: Absorption: Rapid. Absolute bioavailability (36%); T_{max}=approximately 1 hr. **Distribution**: V_d=87L; plasma protein binding (88-94%). **Metabolism**: N-dealkylation, hydroxylation; CYP1A2: 1-aminoindan (AI), 3-hydroxy-N-propargyl-1 aminoindan (1-OH-PAI) and 3-hydroxy-1-aminoindan (3-OH-AI). **Elimination**: Urine (62% over 7 days), (84% over 38 days), (<1% unchanged), feces (7%); $T_{1/2}$=3 hrs.

NURSING CONSIDERATIONS

Assessment: Assess LFTs, renal function tests, pheochromocytoma, and dyskinesia. Note other diseases/conditions and drug therapies.

Monitoring: Monitor LFTs, renal function test, BP, melanomas, hallucinations, postural hypotension, diarrhea, weight loss, rash, dyskinesia.

Patient Counseling: Instruct to take with/without food. Restrict tyramine-rich foods (aged cheeses, pickled herring, yeast extract, air-dried meats) and beverages (certain red wines and beers). Avoid amine-containing medications (pseudoephedrine, phenylephrine, phenylpropanolamine, and ephedrine) during and 2 weeks following d/c of treatment. Report adverse side effects.

Administration: Oral route, with/without food. **Storage**: 25°C (77°F); excursions permitted to 15-30°C (59-86°F).

AZMACORT RX

triamcinolone acetonide (Abbott)

THERAPEUTIC CLASS: Corticosteroid

INDICATIONS: Maintenance treatment of asthma as prophylactic therapy in patients ≥6 yrs; to reduce or eliminate the need for oral corticosteroidal therapy.

DOSAGE: *Adults:* 2 inh (150mcg) tid-qid or 4 inh (300mcg) bid. Severe Asthma: Initial: 12-16 inh/day. Max: 16 inh/day (1200mcg). Rinse mouth after use.

Pediatrics: >12 yrs: 2 inh (150mcg) tid-qid or 4 inh (300mcg) bid. Severe Asthma: Initial: 12-16 inh/day. Max: 16 inh/day (1200mcg). 6-12 yrs: 1-2 inh (75-150mcg) tid-qid or 2-4 (150-300mcg) inh bid. Max: 12 inh/day (900mcg). Rinse mouth after use.

HOW SUPPLIED: MDI: 75mcg/inh [20g]

CONTRAINDICATIONS: Primary treatment of status asthmaticus or other acute asthma attacks.

WARNINGS/PRECAUTIONS: Deaths due to adrenal insufficiency have occurred with transfer from systemic corticosteroids to inhaled corticosteroids. Resume oral corticosteroids during stress or severe asthma attack. Observe for adrenal insufficiency, systemic corticosteroid withdrawal effects, hypercorticoidism and growth suppression (children). More susceptible to infections. Not for acute bronchospasm. D/C if bronchospasm occurs after dosing. Caution with TB of respiratory tract; untreated systemic fungal, bacterial, viral or parasitic infections; or ocular herpes simplex. *Candida* infection of mouth and pharynx reported.

ADVERSE REACTIONS: Pharyngitis, sinusitis, headache, flu syndrome.

INTERACTIONS: Caution with prednisone.

PREGNANCY: Category C, caution in nursing.

MECHANISM OF ACTION: Corticosteroid; not established. Inhaled route makes possible to provide local anti-inflammatory activity.

PHARMACOKINETICS: Absorption: T_{max}=1.5-2 hrs. **Distribution:** V_d=99.5L; plasma protein binding (68%). **Elimination:** Urine (40%), feces (60%); $T_{1/2}$=88 min.

NURSING CONSIDERATIONS

Assessment: Assess for concomitant diseases such as status asthmaticus, active or quiescent pulmonary TB, untreated systemic fungal, bacterial, parasitic or viral infections, and possible drug interactions (prednisone).

Monitoring: Monitor for localized oral infections with *Candida albicans*, body height in children, adrenal insufficiency, paradoxical bronchospasm, and hypersensitivity reactions.

Patient Counseling: Inform not for relief of acute bronchospasm. Advise that drug may unmask allergies (rhinitis, conjunctivitis, eczema). Instruct to track use of drug and dispose canister after 240 actuations since reliable dose delivery not assured after 240 doses. Warn to avoid exposure to chickenpox or measles. Advise to seek medical attention if exposed to chickenpox or measles, symptoms do not improve or worsen, during periods of stress or severe asthmatic attack, paradoxical bronchospasm or hypersensitivity reaction occurs. Counsel to avoid spraying in eyes and shake well before each use.

Administration: Oral inhalation. **Storage:** 20-25°C (68-77°F). Do not puncture, use, or store near heat or open flame; do not freeze.

AZOPT RX

brinzolamide (Alcon)

THERAPEUTIC CLASS: Carbonic anhydrase inhibitor

INDICATIONS: Open-angle glaucoma. Ocular hypertension.

DOSAGE: *Adults:* 1 drop tid. Space dosing with other ophthalmic drugs by 10 min.

HOW SUPPLIED: Sus: 1% [5mL, 10mL, 15mL]

WARNINGS/PRECAUTIONS: Systemically absorbed. Avoid with sulfonamide allergy or severe renal impairment. Caution with hepatic impairment. Not studied in acute angle-closure glaucoma.

ADVERSE REACTIONS: Blurred vision, taste disturbances, blepharitis, dermatitis, dry eye, foreign body sensation, headache, hyperemia, ocular discharge, ocular discomfort, ocular keratitis, ocular pain, ocular pruritus, rhinitis.

INTERACTIONS: Caution with high-dose salicylates. Acid-base disturbances with oral carbonic anhydrase inhibitors. Avoid oral carbonic anhydrase inhibitors due to additive effects. Wait 10 min before using another ophthalmic drug.

PREGNANCY: Category C, not for use in nursing.

MECHANISM OF ACTION: Carbonic anhydrase II inhibitor; inhibits aqueous humor formation and reduces elevated IOP.

PHARMACOKINETICS: Distribution: Plasma protein binding (60%). **Elimination:** Urine (unchanged).

NURSING CONSIDERATIONS

Assessment: Assess for allergy to sulfonamides, hepatic/renal function prior to therapy, and possible drug interactions.

Monitoring: Monitor for signs/symptoms of Stevens-Johnson syndrome, toxic epidermal necrolysis, fulminant hepatic necrolysis, agranulocytosis, aplastic anemia, and other blood dyscrasias.

Patient Counseling: Advise to contact physician if any serious or unusual ocular or systemic reactions occur while on medication. Instruct to avoid touching container tip to the eye or any other surfaces. Instruct if having ocular surgery or if an intercurrent ocular condition (eg, trauma, infection) develops, to contact physician prior to using present multidose container. Instruct to remove contact lenses prior to administration; wait 15 min after administration to wear contact lenses. Advise that if using more than 1 topical ophthalmic medication, separate medication by at least 10 min.

Administration: Ocular route. **Storage:** 4-30°C (39-86°F).

AZOR — RX

amlodipine besylate - olmesartan medoxomil (Daiichi Sankyo)

> **When used in pregnancy during 2nd and 3rd trimesters, drugs that act directly on the renin-angiotensin system can cause injury and even death to developing fetus. When pregnancy is detected, d/c therapy asap.**

THERAPEUTIC CLASS: ARB/Calcium channel blocker (dihydropyridine)

INDICATIONS: Treatment of hypertension, alone or with other antihypertensive agents.

DOSAGE: *Adults:* Replacement Therapy: May substitute for individually titrated components for patients on amlodipine and olmesartan. When substituting for individual components, the dose of 1 or both components may be increased if needed. Add-On Therapy: May use as add-on therapy when not adequately controlled on amlodipine or olmesartan. May increase dose after 2 weeks to maximum dose of 10mg-40mg qd.

HOW SUPPLIED: Tab: (Amlodipine-Olmesartan) 5mg-20mg, 10mg-20mg, 5mg-40mg, 10mg-40mg

WARNINGS/PRECAUTIONS: Hypotension, especially in volume- or salt-depleted patients, may occur with treatment initiation; monitor closely. Caution with severe aortic stenosis, heart failure, or severe hepatic impairment. Increased angina or MI with CCBs may occur with dosage initiation or increase. Changes in renal function, oliguria, progressive azotemia, or acute renal failure may occur.

ADVERSE REACTIONS: Edema.

PREGNANCY: Category C (1st trimester) and D (2nd and 3rd trimester), not for use in nursing.

MECHANISM OF ACTION: Amlodipine: Calcium channel receptor blocker (dihydropyridine); inhibits transmembrane influx of calcium ions. Olmesartan: Angiotensin II receptor blocker; blocks vasoconstrictor effect of angiotensin II.

PHARMACOKINETICS: Absorption: Amlodipine: T_{max}=6-12 hrs, absolute bioavailability (64-90%). Olmesartan: Rapid and complete, absolute bioavailability (26%), T_{max}=1-2 hrs. **Distribution:** Amlodipine: Plasma protein binding (93%). Olmesartan: V_d=17L, plasma protein binding (99%), crosses placental barrier; excreted in breast milk. **Metabolism:** Amlodipine: Liver. Olmesartan: Ester hydrolysis. **Elimination:** Amlodipine: Urine (10%); $T_{1/2}$=30-50 hrs. Olmesartan: Urine (35-50%), feces; $T_{1/2}$=13 hrs.

NURSING CONSIDERATIONS

Assessment: Assess for severe obstructive CAD, CHF, severe aortic stenosis, pregnancy status, volume/salt depletion, renal/hepatic impairment.

Monitoring: Monitor for signs/symptoms of hypotension, hypersensitivity reactions, renal/hepatic dysfunction. Monitor for symptoms of angina or MI after dosage initiation or increase.

Patient Counseling: Inform of pregnancy risks. Advise to seek medical attention if symptoms of hypotension or hypersensitivity reactions occur.

Administration: Oral route. **Storage:** 25°C (77°F); excursions permitted to 15-30°C (59-86°F).

AZULFIDINE — RX

sulfasalazine (Pharmacia & Upjohn)

THERAPEUTIC CLASS: 5-Aminosalicylic acid derivative/sulfapyridine

INDICATIONS: Treatment of mild to moderate ulcerative colitis. Adjunct therapy in severe ulcerative colitis. To prolong remission period between acute attacks of ulcerative colitis.

DOSAGE: *Adults:* Initial: 3-4g/day in divided doses. May initiate at 1-2g/day to reduce GI intolerance. Maint: 2g/day.
Pediatrics: ≥2 yrs: 40-60mg/kg/day divided into 3-6 doses. Maint: 7.5mg/kg qid.

HOW SUPPLIED: Tab: 500mg* *scored

CONTRAINDICATIONS: <2 yrs, intestinal or urinary obstruction, porphyria, hypersensitivity to sulfonamides, salicylates.

WARNINGS/PRECAUTIONS: Caution with hepatic/renal impairment, blood dyscrasias, severe allergy, bronchial asthma, G6PD deficiency. Monitor CBC, WBC, LFTs, at baseline, every 2nd week for 1st 3 months, monthly for next 3 months, and every 3 months thereafter. Monitor renal function periodically. Maintain adequate fluid intake to prevent crystalluria and stone formation. D/C if hypersensitivity or toxic reaction occurs.

ADVERSE REACTIONS: Anorexia, headache, NV, gastric distress, reversible oligospermia.

INTERACTIONS: Reduces absorption of folic acid, digoxin.

PREGNANCY: Category B, caution in nursing.

MECHANISM OF ACTION: 5-aminosalicylic acid (5-ASA) derivative/sulfapyridine (SP); not established, may be related to anti-inflammatory and/or immunomodulatory properties of sulfasalazine (SSZ) or its metabolites (5-ASA and SP), its affinity for connective tissue, and/or to relatively high concentration reached in serous fluids, liver, and intestinal wall.

PHARMACOKINETICS: Absorption: SSZ: C_{max}=6mcg/mL, T_{max}=6 hrs; 5-ASA; SP: T_{max}=10 hrs. SSZ: Absolute bioavailability <15%; SP: Well absorbed from colon, estimated bioavailability 60%. 5-ASA: Much less well absorbed from GI tract, estimated bioavailability 10-30%. **Distribution:** SSZ: V_d=7.5L; plasma protein binding >99.3%. SP: Plasma protein binding 70%. **Metabolism:** Intestinal bacteria to 5-ASA and SP; liver (acetylation). **Elimination:** Urine (37%), feces. SSZ: $T_{1/2}$=7.6 hrs; SP: $T_{1/2}$=10.4 hrs (slow acetylators), 14.8 hrs (fast acetylators).

NURSING CONSIDERATIONS

Assessment: Assess for intestinal or urinary obstruction, porphyria, blood dyscrasias, renal/liver damage, severe allergy or bronchial asthma, glucose 6-phosphate dehydrogenase deficiency and drug interactions. Obtain baseline CBC, including WBC, LFTs.

Monitoring: Perform CBC, including differential WBC and LFTs before start, every 2 weeks during the first 3 months, every month for second 3 months, then every 3 months. Monitor serum SP levels, urinalysis and renal function test periodically. Monitor for signs/symptoms of serious blood disorder (sore throat, fever, pallor, purpura, jaundice), hypersensitivity/allergic reactions, renal/hepatic dysfunction.

Patient Counseling: Inform that ulcerative colitis rarely remits completely and that risk of relapse can be substantially reduced by continued administration at maintenance dosage. Instruct to take in evenly divided doses after meals and to swallow tablet whole. Orange-yellow discoloration of urine or skin may occur. Inform to seek medical attention if sore throat, fever, pallor, purpura, or jaundice, allergic reactions or hypersensitivity occur.

Administration: Oral route. **Storage:** 25°C (77°F); excursions permitted to 15-30°C (59-86°F).

AZULFIDINE EN — RX

sulfasalazine (Pharmacia & Upjohn)

THERAPEUTIC CLASS: 5-Aminosalicylic acid derivative/sulfapyridine

INDICATIONS: Mild to moderate ulcerative colitis, as an adjunct treatment of severe ulcerative colitis, and for the prolongation of the remission period between acute attacks of ulcerative colitis. Rheumatoid arthritis and polyarticular-course juvenile rheumatoid arthritis that has responded inadequately to salicylates or other NSAIDs.

DOSAGE: *Adults:* Ulcerative Colitis: Initial: 1-4g/day in divided doses at intervals not exceeding 8 hrs. Maint: 2g/day. Rheumatoid Arthritis: Initial: 0.5-1g/day. Maint: 2g/day given bid. Swallow tabs whole after meals.
Pediatrics: ≥6 yrs: Ulcerative Colitis: Initial: 40-60mg/kg/24 hrs in 3-6 divided doses. Maint: 7.5mg/kg qid. Juvenile Rheumatoid Arthritis: 30-50mg/kg/day given bid. To reduce GI effects give 1/4 to 1/3 initial dose; increase weekly for 1 month. Max: 2g/day. Swallow tabs whole after meals.

HOW SUPPLIED: Tab, Delayed-Release: 500mg

CONTRAINDICATIONS: Intestinal or urinary obstruction, porphyria, hypersensitivity to sulfonamides or salicylates.

WARNINGS/PRECAUTIONS: Caution with hepatic or renal impairment, blood dyscrasias, severe allergy, bronchial asthma or G6PD deficiency. Monitor CBC, WBC, and LFTs prior to therapy and every other week for the 1st 3 months, once monthly for next 3 months, then every 3 months. Monitor renal function periodically. Maintain adequate fluid intake. Fatal hypersensitivity reactions reported. D/C if tabs pass undisintegrated or if hypersensitivity reactions occur.

ADVERSE REACTIONS: Anorexia, headache, nausea, vomiting, gastric distress, oligospermia, rash, pruritus, urticaria, fever, orange-yellow urine or skin.

INTERACTIONS: Reduces absorption of folic acid and digoxin. Increased incidence of GI adverse events with combination of sulfasalazine (2g/day) and MTX (7.5mg/week).

PREGNANCY: Category B, caution in nursing.

MECHANISM OF ACTION: 5-aminosalicylic acid (5-ASA) derivative/sulfapyridine (SP); not established, may be related to the anti-inflammatory and/or immunomodulatory properties of sulfasalazine (SSZ) or its metabolites (5-ASA and SP), its affinity for connective tissue, and/or to relatively high concentration reached in serous fluids, liver and intestinal wall.

PHARMACOKINETICS: Absorption: SSZ: C_{max}=6mcg/mL, T_{max}=6 hrs; 5-ASA. SP: T_{max}=10 hrs. SSZ: Absolute bioavailability <15%; SP: Well absorbed from colon, estimated bioavailability 60%. 5-ASA: Much less well absorbed from GI tract, estimated bioavailability 10-30%. **Distribution:** SSZ: V_d=7.5L; plasma protein binding >99.3%. SP: Plasma protein binding 70%. **Metabolism:** Intestinal bacteria to 5-ASA and SP; liver (acetylation). **Elimination:** Urine (37%), feces. SSZ: $T_{1/2}$=7.6 hrs, SP: $T_{1/2}$=10.4 hrs (slow acetylators), 14.8 hrs (fast acetylators).

NURSING CONSIDERATIONS

Assessment: Assess for intestinal or urinary obstruction, porphyria, blood dyscrasias, renal/liver damage, severe allergy or bronchial asthma, glucose 6-phosphate dehydrogenase deficiency and drug interactions. Obtain baseline CBC, including WBC, LFTs.

Monitoring: Perform CBC, including differential WBC and LFTs before start, every 2 weeks during the first 3 months, every month for second 3 months, then every 3 months. Monitor serum SP levels, urinalysis and renal function test periodically. Monitor for signs/symptoms of serious blood disorder (sore throat, fever, pallor, purpura, jaundice), hypersensitivity/allergic reactions, renal/hepatic dysfunction.

Patient Counseling: Inform that ulcerative colitis rarely remits completely and that risk of relapse can be substantially reduced by continued administration at maintenance dosage. Instruct take in evenly divided doses after meals and to swallow tablet whole. Orange-yellow discoloration of urine or skin may occur. Inform to seek medical attention if sore throat, fever, pallor, purpura, or jaundice, allergic reactions or hypersensitivity occur.

Administration: Oral route. **Storage:** 25°C (77°F); excursions permitted to 15-30°C (59-86°F).

BACLOFEN **RX**

baclofen (Various)

OTHER BRAND NAMES: Kemstro (Schwarz)

THERAPEUTIC CLASS: GABA analog

INDICATIONS: Treatment of spasticity associated with multiple sclerosis. May be effective in spinal cord injuries and other spinal cord diseases.

DOSAGE: *Adults:* Initial: 5mg tid for 3 days. Titrate: May increase dose by 5mg tid every 3 days. Usual: 40-80mg/day. Max: 80 mg/day (20mg qid). Renal Impairment: Reduce dose.
Pediatrics: ≥12 yrs: Initial: 5mg tid for 3 days. Titrate: May increase dose by 5mg tid every 3 days. Usual: 40-80mg/day. Max: 80 mg/day (20mg qid). Renal Impairment: Reduce dose.

HOW SUPPLIED: Tab: (Generic) 10mg, 20mg; Tab, Disintegrating (ODT): (Kemstro) 10mg, 20mg

WARNINGS/PRECAUTIONS: Caution with psychosis, schizophrenia, confused states; may exacerbate conditions. Caution with bladder sphincter hypertonia, peptic ulceration, seizures, elderly, cerebrovascular disorder, respiratory failure, hepatic or renal failure. Abnormal AST, alkaline phosphatase and blood glucose reported. Caution when used to maintain locomotion or to obtain increased function. Decreased alertness with operating machinery. Has not significantly benefited stroke patients. Avoid abrupt discontinuation; reduce dose slowly over 1-2 weeks.

ADVERSE REACTIONS: Drowsiness, dizziness, weakness, fatigue, confusion, daytime sedation, headache, insomnia, hypotension, nausea, constipation, urinary frequency.

INTERACTIONS: May potentiate antihypertensives. May increase CNS depressant effects with MAO inhibitors. Potentiated by TCAs. Mental confusion, hallucinations and agitation with levodopa plus carbidopa therapy. May increase blood glucose and require dosage adjustment of antidiabetic agents. Synergistic effects with magnesium sulfate and other neuromuscular blockers. Additive CNS effects with alcohol and other CNS depressants.

PREGNANCY: Category C, caution in nursing.

MECHANISM OF ACTION: A GABA analog; muscle relaxant/antispastic agent; not fully known; capable of inhibiting both monosynaptic and polysynaptic reflexes at the spinal level, possibly by hyperpolarization of afferent terminals, although actions at supraspinal sites may also occur and contribute to its clinical effect.

NURSING CONSIDERATIONS

Assessment: Assess for renal dysfunction, pregnancy/nursing status, epilepsy, and possible drug interactions.

Monitoring: Monitor for CNS depression, deterioration of seizure control, EEG changes, and ovarian cysts.

Patient Counseling: Caution against performing hazardous tasks (eg, operating machinery/driving). Notify if pregnant/nursing; not for use by children.

Administration: Oral route. **Storage:** 20-25°C (68-77°F); excursions permitted to 15-30°C (59-86°F); avoid moisture.

BACTRIM — RX

sulfamethoxazole - trimethoprim (AR Scientific)

OTHER BRAND NAMES: Bactrim DS (AR Scientific)

THERAPEUTIC CLASS: Sulfonamide/tetrahydrofolic acid inhibitor

INDICATIONS: Treatment of urinary tract infection (UTI), acute otitis media, acute exacerbation of chronic bronchitis (AECB), traveler's diarrhea, shigellosis, and *Pneumocystis carinii* pneumonia (PCP).

DOSAGE: *Adults:* UTI: 800mg SMX-160mg TMP or 2 tabs of 400mg SMX-80mg TMP q12h for 10-14 days. Shigellosis: 800mg SMX-160mg TMP or 2 tabs of 400mg SMX-80mg TMP q12h for 5 days. AECB: 800mg SMX-160mg TMP or 2 tabs of 400mg SMX-80mg TMP q12h for 14 days. PCP Treatment: 15-20mg/kg TMP and 75-100mg/kg SMX per 24 hrs given q6h for 14-21 days. PCP Prophylaxis: 800mg SMX-160mg TMP qd. Traveler's Diarrhea: 800mg SMX-160mg TMP q12h for 5 days. CrCl: 15-30mL/min: 50% usual dose. CrCl: <15mL/min: Not recommended.
Pediatrics: ≥2 months: UTI/Otitis Media: 4mg/kg TMP and 20mg/kg SMX q12h for 10 days. Shigellosis: 8mg/kg TMP and 40mg/kg SMX per 24 hrs given q12h for 5 days. PCP Treatment: 15-20mg/kg TMP and 75-100mg/kg SMX per 24 hrs given q6h for 14-21 days. PCP Prophylaxis: 150mg/m^2/day TMP with 750mg/m^2/day SMX given bid, on 3 consecutive days/week. Max: 320mg TMP/1600mg SMX/day. CrCl: 15-30mL/min: 50% usual dose. CrCl: <15mL/min: Not recommended.

HOW SUPPLIED: (Sulfamethoxazole [SMX]-Trimethoprim [TMP]) Tab: 400mg-80mg*; Tab, DS: 800mg-160mg* *scored

CONTRAINDICATIONS: Megaloblastic anemia due to folate deficiency, pregnancy, nursing, infants <2 months, marked hepatic damage, severe renal insufficiency if cannot monitor renal status.

WARNINGS/PRECAUTIONS: Fatal hypersensitivity reactions (eg, Stevens-Johnson syndrome, toxic epidermal necrolysis, fulminant hepatic necrosis, agranulocytosis, aplastic anemia) may occur. Pseudomembranous colitis, cough, SOB, and pulmonary infiltrates reported. Avoid with group A β-hemolytic streptococcal infections. Caution with hepatic/renal impairment, elderly, folate deficiency (eg, chronic alcoholics, anticonvulsants, malabsorption, malnutrition), bronchial asthma, and other allergies. In G6PD deficiency, hemolysis may occur. Increased incidence of adverse events with AIDS. Ensure adequate fluid intake and urinary output. Caution with porphyria, thyroid dysfunction.

ADVERSE REACTIONS: NV, anorexia, rash, urticaria.

INTERACTIONS: Diuretics (especially thiazides) may increase risk of thrombocytopenia with purpura in elderly patients. Caution with warfarin, may prolong PT. Increased effects of phenytoin, oral hypoglycemics. Increased plasma levels of methotrexate, digoxin (especially in elderly). Marked but reversible nephrotoxicity reported with cyclosporine. May develop megaloblastic anemia with pyrimethamine >25mg/week. Increased levels with indomethacin. May decrease effects of TCAs. Single case of toxic delirium with amantadine.

PREGNANCY: Category C, contraindicated in nursing.

MECHANISM OF ACTION: Sulfamethoxazole: Inhibits bacterial synthesis of dyhydrofolic acid by competing with PABA. Trimethoprim: Blocks the production of tetrahydrofolic acid from dihydrofolic acid by binding to and reversibly inhibiting the required enzyme, dihydrofolate reductase.

PHARMACOKINETICS: Absorption: Rapid; T_{max}=1-4 hrs; Sulfamethoxazole: C_{max}=57.4mcg/mL (free), 68.0mcg/mL (total); Trimethoprim: C_{max}=1.72mcg/mL. **Distribution:** Sulfamethoxazole: Plasma protein binding (70%); Trimethoprim: Plasma protein binding (44%). Both pass placental barrier and excreted in breast milk. **Metabolism:** Sulfamethoxazole: N_4-acetylation; Trimethoprim: 1- and 3-oxides, 3'-4'-hydroxy derivatives (principal metabolites). **Elimination:** Sulfamethoxazole: $T_{1/2}$=0.72 hrs. Urine: Total sulfonamide (84.5%), 30% (free), and the remaining (N_4-acetylated metabolite); 66.8% (trimethoprim); $T_{1/2}$=10 hrs (sulfamethoxazole), 8-10 hrs (trimethoprim).

NURSING CONSIDERATIONS

Assessment: Assess for hypersensitivity reaction to drug components, documented megaloblastic anemia due to folate deficiency (eg, malabsorption syndrome, chronic alcoholic, malnutrition status, elderly, receiving anticonvulsant therapy), marked hepatic/renal insufficiency, pregnancy/nursing status, severe allergies or bronchial asthma, glucose-6-phosphate dehydrogenase deficiency, phenylketonuria patients, porphyria or thyroid dysfunction, and possible drug interactions.

Monitoring: Monitor for severe allergic reactions (eg, Stevens-Johnson syndrome, toxic epidermal necrolysis, fulminant hepatic necrosis, agranulocytosis, aplastic anemia and other blood dyscrasias) and their clinical signs (eg, rash, sore throat, fever, arthralgia, pallor, purpura or jaundice), *C.difficile*-associated diarrhea (may range from mild diarrhea to fatal colitis), development of drug resistance, overgrowth of nonsusceptible microorganisms, hypersensitivity reactions of respiratory tract (eg, cough, SOB, pulmonary infiltrates), kernicterus if given to infants, hypogylcemia, signs of bone marrow depression after chronic use, and interference with serum methotrexate assay and with the Jaffe alkaline picrate reaction assay for creatinine. Periodically monitor CBC, renal function, LFTs and K^+ levels, and perform urinalysis with careful microscopic exam.

Patient Counseling: Inform that drug only treats bacterial, not viral, infections. Instruct to take exactly as directed; skipping doses or not completing full course may decrease effectiveness and increase resistance. Inform about potential benefits/risks of therapy. D/C and notify physician if allergic reaction, watery/bloody diarrhea (with/without stomach cramps) occur (may occur up to 2 or more months after treatment). Counsel to drink adequate fluids to prevent crystalluria and stone formation. Notify physician if pregnant/nursing or planning to become pregnant. Instruct medication is not recommended for use in pediatrics <2 months of age.

Administration: Oral route. **Storage:** 20-25°C (68-77°F); tight, light-resistant container.

BACTROBAN — RX

mupirocin (GlaxoSmithKline)

THERAPEUTIC CLASS: Bacterial protein synthesis inhibitor

INDICATIONS: (Oint) Topical treatment of impetigo due to *S.aureus* and *S.pyogenes*. (Cre) Treatment of secondarily infected traumatic skin lesions (up to 10cm in length or 100cm²) due to *S.aureus* and *S.pyogenes*.

DOSAGE: *Adults:* (Oint) Apply tid. (Cre) Apply tid for 10 days. May cover with gauze. Re-evaluate if no response within 3-5 days.
Pediatrics: (Oint) 2 months -16 yrs: Apply tid. (Cre) 3 months-16 yrs: Apply tid for 10 days. May cover with gauze. Re-evaluate if no response within 3-5 days.

HOW SUPPLIED: Cre: 2% [15g, 30g]; Oint: 2% [22g]

WARNINGS/PRECAUTIONS: Avoid eyes. D/C if sensitization or irritation occurs. May cause superinfection with prolonged use. Caution with oint in renal dysfunction. Avoid mucosal surfaces. Avoid open wounds or damaged skin with oint.

ADVERSE REACTIONS: Burning, pain, pruritus, headache, rash, nausea.

PREGNANCY: Category B, caution in nursing.

MECHANISM OF ACTION: Bacterial protein synthesis inhibitor; inhibits bacterial protein synthesis by reversibly and specifically binding to bacterial isoleucyl transfer-RNA synthetase. Active against a wide range of gram-positive bacteria including methicillin-resistant *Staphylococcus aureus* (MRSA). Also active against certain gram-negative bacteria.

PHARMACOKINETICS: Absorption: Minimal percutaneous absorption. **Metabolism:** Rapid. Monic acid (inactive metabolite). **Elimination:** Renal (metabolite).

NURSING CONSIDERATIONS

Assessment: Perform proper diagnosis of skin infection. Assess use in pregnant/nursing females.

Monitoring: Monitor for sensitization or severe local irritation of the skin. In patients on prolonged therapy, monitor for possible overgrowth of nonsusceptible microorganisms, including fungi.

Patient Counseling: Inform that medication is for external use only and to avoid contact of medication with the eyes. Counsel that treated area can be covered with a gauze dressing. Advise to contact physician and d/c medication if any signs of local adverse reactions (eg, irritation, severe itching, rash) develop. Notify if no clinical improvement is seen within 3-5 days.

Administration: Topical. **Storage:** Store at or below 25°C (77°F). Do not freeze.

BACTROBAN NASAL — RX

mupirocin calcium (GlaxoSmithKline)

THERAPEUTIC CLASS: Antibacterial agent

INDICATIONS: Eradication of nasal colonization of MRSA in adults and health-care workers in certain institutional settings during outbreaks of MRSA.

DOSAGE: *Adults:* Apply 1/2 of the single-use tube into each nostril bid for 5 days. Spread oint by pressing together and releasing the sides of the nose repetitively for 1 min. Do not re-use tube.
Pediatrics: ≥12 yrs: Apply 1/2 of the single-use tube into each nostril bid for 5 days. Spread oint by pressing together and releasing the sides of the nose repetitively for 1 min. Do not re-use tube.

HOW SUPPLIED: Oint: 2% [1g pkt]

WARNINGS/PRECAUTIONS: Avoid eyes. D/C if sensitization or irritation occur. May cause superinfection with prolonged use.

ADVERSE REACTIONS: Headache, rhinitis, respiratory disorder, pharyngitis, taste perversion.

INTERACTIONS: Avoid use with other intranasal products.

PREGNANCY: Category B, caution in nursing.

MECHANISM OF ACTION: Antibacterial agent; inhibits protein synthesis by reversibly and specifically binding to bacterial isoleucyl transfer-RNA synthetase.

PHARMACOKINETICS: Absorption: Significant in neonates and premature infants. **Elimination:** Urine.

NURSING CONSIDERATIONS

Assessment: Assess for drug hypersensitivity, high-risk health care workers during institutional outbreaks of methicillin-resistant *S.aureus,* possible drug interactions.

Monitoring: Monitor for sensitization, severe local irritation, tearing, and for overgrowth of nonsusceptible microorganisms (eg, fungi).

Patient Counseling: Avoid contact with eyes. Consult physician if sensitization or severe irritation occurs.

Administration: Intranasal route. Apply approximately half of ointment from single-use tube directly into 1 nostril and other half into other nostril; discard tube after using. Press sides of nose together and gently massage after application to spread ointment throughout inside of nostril. **Storage:** 20-25°C (68-77°F); excursions permitted to 15-30°C (59-86°F). Do not refrigerate.

BANZEL — RX

rufinamide (Eisai)

THERAPEUTIC CLASS: Triazole derivative

INDICATIONS: Adjunctive treatment of seizures associated with Lennox-Gastaut syndrome in adults and children ≥4 yrs.

DOSAGE: *Adults:* Initial: 400-800mg/day in two equally divided doses. Titrate: May increase by 400-800mg/day every two days until max of 3200mg/day, given in two equally divided doses, is reached. Max: 3200mg/day. Take with food. May give as whole tabs, half-tabs, or crushed. *Pediatrics:* ≥4 yrs: Initial: 10mg/kg/day in two equally divided doses. Titrate: May increase by 10mg/kg increments every other day to target dose of 45mg/kg/day or 3200mg/day, whichever is less, given in two equally divided doses. Max: 45mg/kg/day or 3200mg/day. Take with food. May give as whole tabs, half-tabs, or crushed.

HOW SUPPLIED: Tab: 200mg*, 400mg* *scored

CONTRAINDICATIONS: Familial short QT syndrome.

WARNINGS/PRECAUTIONS: May increase risk of suicidal thoughts or behavior; monitor for emergence or worsening of depression, or any unusual changes in mood or behavior. Caution with other drugs that shorten QT interval. Multi-organ hypersensitivity syndrome reported; d/c therapy and start alternative treatment. Monitor closely if rash develops. Withdraw gradually to minimize risk of precipitating seizures, seizure exacerbation, or status epilepticus.

ADVERSE REACTIONS: Somnolence, N/V, headache, fatigue, dizziness, tremor, nystagmus, nasopharyngitis, rash, ataxia, diplopia, bronchitis, blurred vision.

INTERACTIONS: Potent cytochrome P450 inducers (eg, carbamazepine, phenytoin, primodone, phenobarbital) may increase clearance of rufinamide. Valproate may reduce clearance and increase levels; initiate valproate at low dose and titrate to clinically effective dose. May decrease levels of hormonal contraceptives; additional forms of contraception are recommended during co-administration. May decrease levels of drugs that are substrates of CYP3A4 (eg, triazolam).

PREGNANCY: Category C, not for use in nursing.

MECHANISM OF ACTION: Precise MoA not established; may modulate activity of sodium channels and, in particular, prolongation of the inactive state of the channel. Slows channel recovery from inactivation after prolonged prepulse in cultured cortical neurons, and limited sustained repetitive firing of sodium-dependent action potentials (in-vitro studies).

PHARMACOKINETICS: Absorption: Well-absorbed, T_{max}=4-6 hrs. **Distribution:** Plasma protein binding (34%); V_d=50L (3200mg/day). **Metabolism:** Via hydrolysis; CGP 47292, CYP 2E1 (weak inhibitor), CYP3A4 (weak inducer). **Elimination:** $T_{1/2}$=6-10 hrs; urine (2%, unchanged).

NURSING CONSIDERATIONS

Assessment: Assess for suicidal behavior or ideation, QT interval, familial short QT syndrome, ventricular arrhythmias, multi-organ hypersensitivity syndrome, rash, urticaria, facial edema, fever, elevated eosinophils, stuporous state, severe hepatitis, history of seizures, status epilepticus, possible drug interactions, and pregnancy/nursing status.

Monitoring: Monitor for somnolence, N/V, headache, fatigue, dizziness, convulsion, tremor, nystagmus, nasopharyngitis, rash, ataxia, diplopia, bronchitis, blurred vision, leukopenia.

Patient Counseling: Inform patients, caregivers, and families of the high risk of suicidal thoughts and behavior and to be alert for emergence or worsening of signs/symptoms of depression, unusual changes in mood or behavior, suicidal thoughts and behavior, and thoughts of self-harm. Instruct to take only as prescribed and to avoid alcohol. Counsel about potential somnolence or dizziness. Advise not to drive or operate machinery until gaining sufficient experience to gauge whether therapy adversely affects mental and/or motor performance. Notify physician if pregnant or intend to become pregnant, and if breastfeeding or intend to breastfeed. Instruct to seek consultation if rash with fever occurs. Tabs are scored on both sides and may be cut in half for dosing flexibility; swallow as whole, as half tabs or crushed.

Administration: Oral route. **Storage:** Store at 25°C (77°F); excursions permitted to 15°-30°C (59°F-86°F). Protect from moisture.

BARACLUDE RX

entecavir (Bristol-Myers Squibb)

Lactic acidosis and severe, possibly fatal, hepatomegaly with steatosis reported. Reports of severe acute exacerbations of hepatitis B upon discontinuation of therapy. Follow-up liver function monitoring required. Limited clinical experience suggests there is a potential for the development of resistance to HIV nucleoside reverse transcriptase inhibitors if Entecavir is used to treat chronic hepatitis B virus infection in patients with HIV infection that is not being treated. Not recommended for HIV/HBV coinfected who are not receiving highly active antiretroviral therapy (HAART).

THERAPEUTIC CLASS: Guanosine nucleoside analogue

INDICATIONS: Treatment of chronic hepatitis B virus (HBV) infection with active viral replication and persistent elevations in serum aminotransferases (ALT or AST) or histologically active disease.

DOSAGE: *Adults:* Nucleoside-Treatment-Naive: 0.5mg qd. CrCl 30 to <50mL/min: 0.25mg qd or 0.5mg q48h. CrCl 10 to <30mL/min: 0.15mg qd or 0.5mg q72h. CrCl <10mL/min: 0.05mg qd or 0.5mg q7 days. Receiving Lamivudine or Known Lamivudine Resistance Mutation: 1mg qd. CrCl 30 to <50mL/min: 0.5mg qd or 1mg q48h. CrCl 10 to <30mL/min: 0.3mg qd or 1mg q72h. CrCl <10mL/min: 0.1mg qd or 1mg q7 days. Take on empty stomach. *Pediatrics:* ≥16 yrs: Nucleoside-Treatment-Naive:0.5mg qd. CrCl 30 to <50mL/min: 0.25mg qd or 0.5mg q48h. CrCl 10 to <30mL/min: 0.15mg qd or 0.5mg q72h. CrCl <10mL/min: 0.05mg qd or 0.5mg q7 days. Receiving Lamivudine or Known Lamivudine Resistance Mutation: 1mg qd. CrCl 30 to <50mL/min: 0.5mg qd or 1mg q48h. CrCl 10 to <30mL/min: 0.3mg qd or 1mg q72h. CrCl <10mL/min: 0.1mg qd or 1mg q7 days. Take on empty stomach.

HOW SUPPLIED: Sol: 0.05mg/mL; Tab: 0.5mg, 1mg

WARNINGS/PRECAUTIONS: Reduce dose in renal dysfunction (CrCl <50mL/min) including patients on hemodialysis or CAPD (continuous ambulatory peritoneal dialysis). Exacerbations of hepatitis after discontinuation of treatment. Caution with known risk factors of liver disease. D/C with lactic acidosis and hepatotoxicity.

ADVERSE REACTIONS: Headache, fatigue, dizziness, nausea, hyperglycemia, ALT >5.0 X ULN, lipase ≥2.1 X ULN, glycosuria, hematuria, anaphylactoid reactions, alopecia, rash, acute hepatitis exacerbation, lactic acidosis, and severe hepatomegaly with steatosis.

INTERACTIONS: May increase serum concentrations of entecavir or coadministered drug with drugs that reduce renal function or compete for active tubular secretion.

PREGNANCY: Category C, not for use in nursing.

MECHANISM OF ACTION: Guanosine nucleoside analogue; inhibits base priming, reverse transcription of negative strand from pregenomic mRNA, and synthesis of positive strand of HBV DNA.

PHARMACOKINETICS: Absorption: (0.5mg) C_{max}=4.2ng/mL; T_{max}=0.5-1.5 hrs. (1.0mg) C_{max}=8.2ng/mL. Bioavailability (100%). **Distribution:** Plasma protein binding (13%). **Metabolism:** Hepatic. **Elimination:** Kidneys; urine (62-73%); $T_{1/2}$=128-149 hrs.

NURSING CONSIDERATIONS

Assessment: Assess for hepatic/renal impairment, HIV antibody testing, pregnancy/nursing status and possible drug interactions.

Monitoring: Periodic monitoring of hepatic/renal function is recommended during treatment and for those who d/c anti-hepatitis B therapy for at least several months.

Patient Counseling: Advise to take on an empty stomach (≥2 hrs pc and 2 hrs before next meal). Inform that deterioration of liver disease may occur in some cases if treatment is discontinued, and should discuss any change in regimen. Inform that treatment has not shown to reduce risk of transmission of HBV. Advise to remain under care of physician; discuss new symptoms or concurrent medications. Offer HIV antibody testing before starting therapy.

Administration: Oral route. **Storage:** 25°C (77°F); excursion permitted between 15-30°C (59-86°F). Protect from light.

BAYER ASPIRIN — OTC

aspirin (Bayer Healthcare)

OTHER BRAND NAMES: Bayer Aspirin Children's (Bayer Healthcare) - Bayer Aspirin Regimen with Calcium (Bayer Healthcare) - Bayer Aspirin Regimen (Bayer Healthcare) - Genuine Bayer Aspirin (Bayer Healthcare)

THERAPEUTIC CLASS: Salicylate

INDICATIONS: To reduce the risk of death and nonfatal stroke with previous ischemic stroke or transient ischemia of the brain. To reduce risk of vascular mortality with suspected acute MI. To reduce risk of death and nonfatal MI with previous MI or unstable angina. To reduce risk of MI and sudden death in chronic stable angina pectoris. For patients who have undergone revascularization procedures with a pre-existing condition for which ASA is indicated. Relief of signs of rheumatoid arthritis (RA), juvenile rheumatoid arthritis (JRA), osteoarthritis (OA), spondyloarthropathies, arthritis, and pleurisy associated with systemic lupus erythematosus (SLE). For minor aches and pains.

DOSAGE: *Adults:* Ischemic Stroke/TIA: 50-325mg qd. Suspected Acute MI: Initial: 160-162.5mg qd as soon as suspect MI. Maint: 160-162.5mg qd for 30 days post-infarction, consider further therapy for prevention/recurrent MI. Prevention or Recurrent MI/Unstable Angina/Chronic Stable Angina: 75-325mg qd. CABG: 325mg qd, start 6 hrs post-surgery. Continue for 1 yr. PTCA: Initial: 325mg, 2 hrs pre-surgery. Maint: 160-325mg qd. Carotid Endarterectomy: 80mg qd to 650mg bid, start pre-surgery. RA: Initial: 3g qd in divided doses. Increase for anti-inflammatory efficacy to 150-300mcg/mL plasma salicylate level. Spondyloarthropathies: Up to 4g/day in divided doses. OA: Up to 3g/day in divided doses. Arthritis/SLE Pleurisy: Initial: 3g/day in divided doses. Increase for anti-inflammatory efficacy to 150-300mcg/mL plasma salicylate level. Pain: 325-650mg q4-6h. Max: 4g/day.
Pediatrics: JRA: Initial: 90-130mg/kg/day in divided doses. Increase for anti-inflammatory efficacy to 150-300mcg/mL plasma salicylate level. Pain: ≥12 yrs: 325-650mg q4-6h. Max: 4g/day.

HOW SUPPLIED: Tab: (Genuine Bayer Aspirin) 325mg; Tab: (Bayer Aspirin Regimen with Calcium) 81mg; Tab, Chewable: (Bayer Aspirin Children's) 81mg; Tab, Delayed-Release: (Bayer Aspirin Regimen) 81mg, 325mg

CONTRAINDICATIONS: NSAID allergy, viral infections in children or teenagers, syndrome of asthma, rhinitis, and nasal polyps.

WARNINGS/PRECAUTIONS: Increased risk of bleeding with heavy alcohol use (≥3 drinks/day). May inhibit platelet function; can adversely affect inherited (hemophilia) or acquired (hepatic disease, vitamin K deficiency) bleeding disorders. Monitor for bleeding and ulceration. Avoid in history of active peptic ulcer, severe renal failure, severe hepatic insufficiency, and sodium restricted diets. Associated with elevated LFTs, BUN, and SrCr; hyperkalemia;

proteinuria; and prolonged bleeding time. Avoid 1 week before and during labor.

ADVERSE REACTIONS: Fever, hypothermia, dysrhythmias, hypotension, agitation, cerebral edema, dehydration, hyperkalemia, dyspepsia, GI bleed, hearing loss, tinnitus, problems in pregnancy.

INTERACTIONS: Diminished hypotensive and hyponatremic effects of ACE inhibitors. May increase levels of acetazolamide, valproic acid. Increased bleeding risk with heparin, warfarin. Decreased levels of phenytoin. Decreased hypotensive effects of β-blockers. Decreased diuretic effects with renal or cardiovascular disease. Decreased methotrexate clearance; increased risk of bone marrow toxicity. Avoid NSAIDs. Increased effects of hypoglycemic agents. Antagonizes uricosuric agents.

PREGNANCY: Avoid in 3rd trimester of pregnancy and nursing.

MECHANISM OF ACTION: Provides temporary relief from arthritis pain and arthritis inflammation.

NURSING CONSIDERATIONS

Assessment: Assess for hypersensitivity, stomach problems, bleeding problems, ulcers, history of chickenpox or flu symptoms, and possible drug interactions.

Monitoring: Monitor for Reye's syndrome, allergic reactions include hives, facial swelling, asthma (wheezing) and shock.

Patient Counseling: Instruct to immediately report worsening of any adverse effects.

Administration: Oral route. **Storage:** Room temperature.

BECONASE AQ RX

beclomethasone dipropionate (GlaxoSmithKline)

THERAPEUTIC CLASS: Corticosteroid

INDICATIONS: Relief of symptoms of seasonal or perennial allergic and nonallergic rhinitis. Prevention of nasal polyp recurrence following surgical removal.

DOSAGE: *Adults:* 1-2 sprays per nostril bid. Max: 2 sprays per nostril bid. *Pediatrics:* ≥6 yrs: 1-2 sprays per nostril bid. Max: 2 sprays per nostril bid.

HOW SUPPLIED: Spray: 42mcg/spray [25g]

WARNINGS/PRECAUTIONS: Risk of adrenal insufficiency and withdrawal symptoms when replacing systemic corticosteroids with topical corticosteroids. Caution with active or quiescent TB, ocular herpes simplex, or untreated bacterial, fungal and systemic viral infections. Avoid with recent nasal trauma/surgery or septum ulcers. Risk for more severe/fatal course of infections (eg, chickenpox, measles) and for *Candida* infections of nose and pharynx. Potential for reduced growth velocity in pediatrics.

ADVERSE REACTIONS: Nasopharyngeal irritation, sneezing, headache, nausea, lightheadedness, irritated/dry nose and throat, unpleasant taste/smell.

INTERACTIONS: Concomitant systemic corticosteroids increase risk of hypercorticism and/or HPA axis suppression.

PREGNANCY: Category C, caution in nursing.

MECHANISM OF ACTION: Corticosteroid; mechanism not established; anti-inflammatory and vasoconstrictor effects.

PHARMACOKINETICS: Absorption: Absolute bioavailability (44%) (for the active metabolite B-17-MP). C_{max}≤50pg/mL. **Distribution:** V_d=20L (parent drug); V_d=424L (B-17-MP). Plasma protein binding (87%). **Metabolism:** B-17-MP (active metabolite) via esterase enzymes.

NURSING CONSIDERATIONS

Assessment: Assess for associated asthma with history of long-term therapy with systemic steroids, active or quiescent TB of upper respiratory tract, untreated local or systemic fungal or bacterial infections, systemic viral or parasitic infections, ocular herpes simplex, nasal polyps or recent nasal septal ulcers, nasal surgery/trauma, and possible drug interactions.

Monitoring: Monitor for reduced growth velocity (in pediatrics), nasal septum perforation, localized infection, *Candida* infection, exacerbation of infections, nasopharyngeal irritation, signs of adrenal insufficiency, and symptoms of hypercorticism.

Patient Counseling: Instruct to take as directed at regular intervals and to avoid exposure to chickenpox or measles. Consult physician immediately if exposed to infection or symptoms do not improve, if the condition worsens, or if sneezing or nasal irritation occurs.

Administration: Intranasal route. **Storage:** 15-30°C (59-86°F).

BENICAR — RX

olmesartan medoxomil (Daiichi Sankyo)

Can cause death/injury to developing fetus during 2nd and 3rd trimesters. Stop therapy if pregnancy detected.

THERAPEUTIC CLASS: Angiotensin II receptor antagonist

INDICATIONS: Hypertension, alone or with other antihypertensives.

DOSAGE: *Adults:* Monotherapy Without Volume Depletion: Initial: 20mg qd. Titrate: May increase to 40mg qd after 2 weeks if needed. May add diuretic if BP not controlled. Intravascular Volume Depletion (eg, with diuretics, impaired renal function): Lower initial dose; monitor closely.

HOW SUPPLIED: Tab: 5mg, 20mg, 40mg

WARNINGS/PRECAUTIONS: Can cause fetal injury/death. Symptomatic hypotension may occur in volume- and/or salt-depleted patients; monitor closely. Changes in renal function may occur; caution with severe CHF. Increases in SrCr or BUN reported with renal artery stenosis.

ADVERSE REACTIONS: Dizziness, transient hypotension, hyperkalemia.

INTERACTIONS: Risk of hypotension with high-dose diuretics.

PREGNANCY: Category C (1st trimester) and D (2nd and 3rd trimesters), not for use in nursing.

MECHANISM OF ACTION: Angiotensin II receptor antagonist; blocks vasoconstrictor effects of angiotensin II by selectively blocking binding of angiotensin II to AT_1 receptor in vascular smooth muscle.

PHARMACOKINETICS: Absorption: Rapid, complete. Absolute bioavailability (26%); T_{max}=1-2 hrs. **Distribution:** V_d=17L; plasma protein binding (99%). Crosses placenta, excreted in breast milk. **Metabolism:** Ester hydrolysis. **Elimination:** Urine (35-50%), feces; $T_{1/2}$=13 hrs.

NURSING CONSIDERATIONS

Assessment: Assess for pregnancy status, possible drug interactions, volume/salt depletion, renal/hepatic impairment.

Monitoring: Monitor LFTs and renal function periodically. Monitor for signs/symptoms of hypotension, hypersensitivity reactions, renal/hepatic dysfunction.

Patient Counseling: Inform of pregnancy risks. Advise to seek medical attention if symptoms of hypotension or hypersensitivity reactions occur.

Administration: Oral route. **Storage:** 20-25°C (68-77°F).

BENICAR HCT — RX

olmesartan medoxomil - hydrochlorothiazide (Daiichi Sankyo)

Can cause death/injury to developing fetus during 2nd and 3rd trimesters. Stop therapy if pregnancy detected.

THERAPEUTIC CLASS: Angiotensin II receptor antagonist/thiazide diuretic

B

INDICATIONS: Hypertension. Not for initial therapy.

DOSAGE: *Adults:* If BP not controlled with olmesartan alone: Add HCTZ 12.5mg qd. May titrate to 25mg qd if BP uncontrolled after 2-4 weeks. If BP not controlled with HCTZ alone: Add olmesartan 20mg qd. May titrate to 40mg qd if BP uncontrolled after 2-4 weeks. Intravascular Volume Depletion (eg, with diuretics, impaired renal function): Lower initial dose; monitor closely. Elderly: Start at lower end of dosing range.

HOW SUPPLIED: Tab: (Olmesartan-HCTZ) 20mg-12.5mg, 40mg-12.5mg, 40mg-25mg

CONTRAINDICATIONS: Sulfonamide hypersensitivity.

WARNINGS/PRECAUTIONS: Can cause fetal injury/death. Correct volume or salt depletion before therapy or monitor closely. Caution with hepatic or severe renal dysfunction, progressive liver disease, history of allergies or asthma, renal artery stenosis, severe CHF. Avoid if CrCl ≤30mL/min. May exacerbate or activate SLE. Monitor serum electrolytes. Hyperuricemia, hyperglycemia, hypercalcemia, hypomagnesemia may occur. May increase cholesterol and triglyceride levels.

ADVERSE REACTIONS: Dizziness, upper respiratory tract infection, hyperuricemia, NV, asthenia, angioedema, hyperkalemia, rhabdomyolysis, ARF, alopecia, urticaria.

INTERACTIONS: Potentiates orthostatic hypotension with alcohol, barbiturates, or narcotics. May need to adjust antidiabetics. Potentiates other antihypertensives. Impaired absorption with cholestyramine, colestipol. Corticosteroids, ACTH deplete electrolytes. May decrease response to pressor amines. May potentiate non-depolarizing skeletal muscle relaxants. Risk of lithium toxicity. NSAIDs decrease diuretic effects.

PREGNANCY: Category C (1st trimester) and D (2nd and 3rd trimesters), not for use in nursing.

MECHANISM OF ACTION: Olmesartan: Angiotensin II receptor antagonist; blocks vasoconstrictor effects of angiotensin II by selectively blocking binding of angiotensin II to AT_1 receptor in vascular smooth muscle. HCTZ: Thiazide diuretic; affects renal tubular mechanism of electrolyte reabsorption, directly increasing excretion of Na^+ and Cl^- and indirectly reducing plasma volume.

PHARMACOKINETICS: Absorption: Olmesartan: Rapid, complete; absolute bioavailability (26%); T_{max}=1-2 hrs. **Distribution:** Olmesartan: V_d=17 L; plasma protein binding (99%). Crosses placenta; excreted in breast milk. HCTZ: Crosses placenta; excreted in breast milk. **Metabolism:** Olmesartan: Ester hydrolysis. **Elimination:** Olmesartan: Urine (35-50%), feces; $T_{1/2}$=13 hrs. HCTZ: Kidney (61%); $T_{1/2}$=5.6-14.8 hrs.

NURSING CONSIDERATIONS

Assessment: Assess for pregnancy status, possible drug interactions, volume/salt depletion, SLE, DM, anuria, sulfonamide hypersensitivity, history of allergy or bronchial asthma, hepatic/renal impairment.

Monitoring: Monitor serum electrolytes periodically. Monitor for signs/symptoms of electrolyte imbalance, exacerbation or activation of systemic lupus erythematosus (SLE), hypotension, hyperglycemia, hyperuricemia or precipitation of gout, hypersensitivity reactions, renal/hepatic dysfunction.

Patient Counseling: Inform of pregnancy risks. Advise that inadequate fluid intake or loss of fluids may result in drop of BP, leading to lightheadedness or syncope. Advise to seek medical attention if syncope, symptoms of electrolyte imbalance (dry mouth, thirst, weakness, lethargy), or hypersensitivity reactions occur.

Administration: Oral route. **Storage:** 20-25°C (68-77°F).

BENTYL RX

dicyclomine HCl (Axcan Scandipharm)

THERAPEUTIC CLASS: Anticholinergic

INDICATIONS: Treatment of functional bowel/irritable bowel syndrome.

DOSAGE: *Adults:* (Tab/Syrup) Initial: 20mg qid. Usual: 40mg qid if tolerated. Discontinue if no improvement after 2 weeks or if doses ≥80mg/day are not tolerated. (Inj) 20mg IM qid for 1-2 days, followed by oral dicyclomine. Not for IV use.

HOW SUPPLIED: Cap: 10mg; Inj: 10mg/mL; Syrup: 10mg/5mL; Tab: 20mg

CONTRAINDICATIONS: GI tract obstruction, obstructive uropathy, severe ulcerative colitis, reflux esophagitis, glaucoma, myasthenia gravis, unstable cardiovascular status and in acute hemorrhage, nursing mothers, infants <6 months of age.

WARNINGS/PRECAUTIONS: Caution in autonomic neuropathy, hepatic/renal impairment, ulcerative colitis, hyperthyroidism, HTN, CHF, cardiac tachyarrhythmia, coronary heart disease, hiatal hernia, and prostatic hypertrophy. Heat prostration may occur in high environmental temperature. Monitor for diarrhea, may be the early symptom of intestinal obstruction. Psychosis reported. Serious respiratory symptoms, seizures, syncope and death reported in infants.

ADVERSE REACTIONS: Dry mouth, NV, blurred vision, dizziness, drowsiness, nervousness, mental confusion/excitement (especially in the elderly), mydriasis, increased ocular tension, urinary retention, dyspnea, apnea, tachycardia, decreased sweating, lactation suppression, impotence.

INTERACTIONS: Potentiated by amantadine, Class I antiarrhythmics (eg, quinidine), antihistamines, antipsychotics (eg, phenothiazines), benzodiazepines, MAOIs, narcotic analgesics (eg, meperidine), nitrates/nitrites, sympathomimetics, TCAs. Antagonizes the effects of antiglaucoma agents; do not give with corticosteroid eye drops. Antagonizes the effect of metoclopramide. May effect the GI absorption of delayed release digoxin. Decreased absorption with antacids. Antagonized by drugs treating achlorhydria and those used to test gastric secretion.

PREGNANCY: Category B, contraindicated in nursing.

MECHANISM OF ACTION: Dicyclomine anticholinergic and antispasmodic agent; relieves smooth muscle spasm of the GI tract, and antagonizes bradykinin- and histamine-induced spasms.

PHARMACOKINETICS: Absorption: Rapidly absorbed; T_{max}=60-90 mins. **Distribution:** V_d=approximately 3.65L/Kg (extensive); excreted in breast milk **Elimination:** Urine (79.5%), feces (8.4%); $T_{1/2}$=1.8 hrs.

NURSING CONSIDERATIONS

Assessment: Assess for glaucoma, obstructive uropathy, obstructive disease of GI tract, paralytic ileus, ulcerative colitis, myasthenia gravis, hiatal hernia associated with reflux esophagitis, renal/hepatic dysfunction, hyperthyroidism, cardiac disorders.

Monitoring: Monitor for heat prostration, drowsiness, blurred vision, increased HR, constipation, diarrhea, urinary hesitancy/retention, hypersensitivity reactions.

Patient Counseling: Review side effects and report if any develop. Exercise caution while operating machinery/driving. Avoid high environmental temperatures.

Administration: PO, IM. IM form should not be used for more than 2 days. **Storage:** Cap/Tab/Syrup/Inj: Room temperature below 30°C (86°F). Syrup: Protect from excessive heat. Inj: Protect from freezing.

BenzaClin — RX

clindamycin - benzoyl peroxide (Dermik)

THERAPEUTIC CLASS: Antibacterial/keratolytic

INDICATIONS: Topical treatment of acne vulgaris.

DOSAGE: *Adults:* Wash face and pat dry. Apply bid (am and pm). *Pediatrics:* ≥12 yrs: Wash face and pat dry. Apply bid (am and pm).

HOW SUPPLIED: Gel: (Clindamycin-Benzoyl Peroxide) 1%-5% [25g, 50g]

CONTRAINDICATIONS: Hypersensitivity to lincomycin. History of regional enteritis, ulcerative colitis, and antibiotic-associated colitis.

WARNINGS/PRECAUTIONS: Severe colitis reported with oral and parenteral clindamycin. D/C if severe diarrhea occurs. Avoid contact with eyes and mucous membranes.

ADVERSE REACTIONS: Dry skin, pruritus, peeling, erythema, sunburn.

INTERACTIONS: Cumulative irritancy possible with other topical acne agents. Avoid erythromycin agents.

PREGNANCY: Category C, not for use in nursing.

MECHANISM OF ACTION: Antibacterial/keratolytic; acts against *Propionibacterium acnes*.

PHARMACOKINETICS: Absorption: Benzoyl peroxide: Systemic bioavailability (<2%). Clindamycin: Systemic bioavailability (≤1%).

NURSING CONSIDERATIONS

Assessment: Assess for drug hypersensitivity, history of regional enteritis, ulcerative or antibiotic-associated colitis, and possible drug interactions.

Monitoring: Monitor for diarrhea, bloody diarrhea, pseudomembranous colitis, application-site reaction, dry skin, pruritus, peeling, erythema, sunburn, and overgrowth of nonsusceptible organisms.

Patient Counseling: Advise to use as directed, for external use only, to avoid contact with eyes and mucous membranes. May bleach hair or colored fabric. Inform to minimize or avoid exposure to natural/artificial sunlight, and to immediately report side effects to physician. Wash skin gently prior to use, then rinse with warm water and pat dry.

Administration: Topical. **Storage:** 25°C (77°F). Do not freeze. Keep tightly closed. Keep out of reach of children. Discard unused product after 3 months.

BENZAMYCIN RX

erythromycin - benzoyl peroxide (Dermik)

THERAPEUTIC CLASS: Antibacterial/keratolytic

INDICATIONS: Topical treatment of acne vulgaris.

DOSAGE: *Adults:* Wash skin and dry. Apply bid (am and pm).
Pediatrics: ≥12 yrs: Wash skin and dry. Apply bid (am and pm).

HOW SUPPLIED: Gel: (Benzoyl Peroxide-Erythromycin) 5%-3% [0.8g/pkt, 60^s]

WARNINGS/PRECAUTIONS: D/C if severe irritation occurs. Avoid eyes, mouth, and mucous membranes. Keep refrigerated after reconstitution and discard after 3 months.

ADVERSE REACTIONS: Dryness, urticaria, skin irritation, skin discoloration, oiliness, tenderness.

INTERACTIONS: Additive irritation with peeling, desquamating, or abrasive agents.

PREGNANCY: Category C, caution in nursing.

MECHANISM OF ACTION: Antibacterial/keratolytic agent; not known. Erythromycin: Antibacterial agent; inhibits protein synthesis by reversibly binding to 50S ribosomal subunits, thereby inhibiting translocation of aminoacyl transfer-RNA and inhibiting polypeptide synthesis. Benzoyl peroxide: Believed to act by releasing active oxygen.

PHARMACOKINETICS: Absorption: Benzoyl peroxide shown to be absorbed by skin, where it is converted to benzoic acid. **Distribution:** Orally and parenterally administered erythromycin found in breast milk.

B

NURSING CONSIDERATIONS

Assessment: Assess proper diagnosis of acne vulgaris. Assess use in patients who are using other concomitant topical acne therapies. Assess use in pregnant/nursing patients.

Monitoring: Monitor for occurrence of cumulative irritancy effect when using other concomitant topical acne agents. Monitor for development of severe skin irritation and for overgrowth of nonsusceptible organisms that is associated with antibiotic usage.

Patient Counseling: Instruct to avoid excessive exposure to sunlight and to use protective clothing when exposed to the sun. Counsel to report to physician signs of local adverse reactions (eg, skin irritation, photosensitivity reaction). Advise not to use any other topical acne preparation unless directed by physician. Advise that contact with hair or fabrics may bleach them.

Administration: Mix thoroughly in palm of hand prior to application. Apply product immediately after mixing, then wash hands after application. Do not mix or apply near open flame. Avoid contact with eyes and all mucous membranes. **Storage**: Store at room temperature, 20-25°C (68-77°F). Keep away from heat and open flame. Keep out of reach of children.

BENZTROPINE — RX

benztropine mesylate (Various)

OTHER BRAND NAMES: Cogentin (Merck)

THERAPEUTIC CLASS: Anticholinergic

INDICATIONS: Adjunct in all forms of parkinsonism. Control of drug-induced extrapyramidal disorders.

DOSAGE: *Adults:* Parkinsonism: Initial: 0.5-1mg PO/IV/IM qhs. Titrate: May increase every 5-6 days by 0.5mg. Usual: 1-2mg PO/IV/IM qhs. Max: 6mg/day. Extrapyramidal Disorders: 1-4mg PO/IV/IM qd-bid. Acute Dystonic Reactions: 1-2mg IM/IV, then 1-2mg PO bid.

HOW SUPPLIED: Inj: 1mg/mL; Tab: 0.5mg, 1mg, 2mg

CONTRAINDICATIONS: Patients <3 yrs.

WARNINGS/PRECAUTIONS: May produce anhidrosis, caution in hot weather. Muscle weakness and dysuria may occur. Caution in pediatrics >3 years of age. Not recommended for tardive dyskinesia. Avoid with angle-closure glaucoma. Caution with CNS disease, mental disorders, tachycardia, prostatic hypertrophy, alcoholics, chronically ill, those exposed to hot environments.

ADVERSE REACTIONS: Tachycardia, paralytic ileus, constipation, vomiting, nausea, dry mouth, confusion, blurred vision, urinary retention, heat stroke, hyperthermia, fever.

INTERACTIONS: Paralytic ileus, hyperthermia and heat stroke reported with phenothiazines and TCAs. Caution with other atropine-like agents.

PREGNANCY: Safety in pregnancy and nursing not known.

MECHANISM OF ACTION: Anticholinergic agent; controls extrapyramidal symptoms in parkinsonism.

NURSING CONSIDERATIONS

Assessment: Assess for tachycardia, prostatic hypertrophy, anhidrosis, TD. Note other diseases/conditions and drug therapy.

Monitoring: Monitor for tachycardia, prostatic hypertrophy, anhidrosis, hyperthermia, constipation, urinary retention, paralytic ileus, toxic psychosis.

Patient Counseling: Caution during hot weather, especially when given concomitantly with other atropine-like drugs to the chronically ill, alcoholics, those who have CNS disease, and those who do manual labor in a hot environment. Caution while operating machinery/driving.

Administration: Oral route, IV, IM. **Storage:** 15-30°C. Dispense in well-closed container.

BETAGAN — RX
levobunolol HCl (Allergan)

THERAPEUTIC CLASS: Nonselective beta-blocker

INDICATIONS: Treatment of elevated IOP in chronic open-angle glaucoma and ocular hypertension.

DOSAGE: *Adults:* (0.5%) 1-2 drops qd; bid for more severe or uncontrolled glaucoma. (0.25%): 1-2 drops bid.

HOW SUPPLIED: Sol: 0.25% [5mL, 10mL], 0.5% [2mL, 5mL, 10mL, 15mL]

CONTRAINDICATIONS: Bronchial asthma, COPD, overt cardiac failure, sinus bradycardia, 2nd- and 3rd-degree AV block, cardiogenic shock.

WARNINGS/PRECAUTIONS: Caution with cardiac failure, DM, COPD, cerebral insufficiency, pulmonary disease, bronchospastic disease, surgery and hepatic impairment. May mask symptoms of hypoglycemia and thyrotoxicosis. Contains sodium metabisulfite. Follow with a miotic in angle-closure glaucoma. Potentiates muscle weakness (eg, diplopia, ptosis).

ADVERSE REACTIONS: Ocular burning, ocular stinging, decreased heart rate, decreased blood pressure.

INTERACTIONS: Mydriasis with epinephrine. Additive effects with catecholamine-depleting drugs (eg, reserpine) and systemic β-blockers. AV conduction disturbance with calcium antagonists and digitalis. Left ventricular failure and hypotension with calcium antagonists also. Additive hypotensive effects with phenothiazine-related drugs. Risk of hypoglycemia with insulin and oral hypoglycemic agents.

PREGNANCY: Category C, caution in nursing.

MECHANISM OF ACTION: Noncardioselective β-adrenoceptor blocking agent; equipotent at both β_1 and β_2 receptors. Responsible for reducing cardiac output, increasing airway resistance, and lowering elevated as well as normal IOP. Presumed to lower IOP through decreasing production of aqueous humor.

PHARMACOKINETICS: Absorption: T_{max}=2 and 6 hrs.

NURSING CONSIDERATIONS

Assessment: Assess for active or history of bronchial asthma, severe COPD, sinus bradycardia, 2nd- and 3rd- degree AV block, overt cardiac failure, and cardiogenic shock. Assess for possible sulfite allergy prior to therapy. Assess use in patients who have DM, hyperthyroidism, diminished pulmonary function, cerebrovascular insufficiencies, patients undergoing major elective surgery, and in pregnant/nursing females. Assess that patients with angle-closure glaucoma are not using this drug as monotherapy. Assess for possible drug interactions.

Monitoring: Monitor for signs/symptoms of muscle weakness (eg, diplopia, ptosis), severe respiratory and cardiac reactions, and anaphylactic reactions. Monitor for occurrence of a thyroid storm in patients who have thyrotoxicosis and withdraw abruptly from medication. Monitor for signs/symptoms of acute hypoglycemia with DM.

Patient Counseling: Counsel to notify physician immediately if any signs of anaphylactic reaction, cardiac or respiratory symptoms develop while on medication. Counsel patients with DM medication may mask symptoms of hypoglycemia.

Administration: Ocular route. **Storage:** 15-25°C (59-77°F), protect from light.

BETAMETHASONE DIPROPIONATE — RX
betamethasone dipropionate (Various)

THERAPEUTIC CLASS: Corticosteroid

INDICATIONS: Corticosteroid-responsive dermatoses.

B

DOSAGE: *Adults:* (Cre, Oint) Apply qd-bid. (Lot) Apply a few drops bid, am and pm.
Pediatrics: (Cre, Oint) Apply qd-bid. (Lot) Apply a few drops bid, am and pm.

HOW SUPPLIED: Cre, Oint: 0.05% [15g, 45g]; Lot: 0.05% [60mL]

WARNINGS/PRECAUTIONS: May produce reversible HPA axis suppression, manifestations of Cushing's syndrome, hyperglycemia, and glucosuria. Avoid occlusive dressings. Pediatrics are more prone to systemic toxicity. D/C if irritation occurs. Avoid eyes.

ADVERSE REACTIONS: Burning, itching, irritation, dryness, folliculitis, hypertrichosis, acneiform eruptions, hypopigmentation, perioral dermatitis, allergic contact dermatitis, skin maceration, secondary infection, skin atrophy, striae, miliaria.

PREGNANCY: Category C, caution in nursing.

MECHANISM OF ACTION: Corticosteroid; not established. Possesses anti-inflammatory, anti-pruritic, and vasoconstrictive actions. Effective in treating corticosteroid-responsive dermatoses.

PHARMACOKINETICS: Absorption: Percutaneous; inflammation, other disease states, and occlusive dressings increase absorption. **Metabolism**: Liver. **Elimination**: Kidney, bile.

NURSING CONSIDERATIONS

Assessment: Assess for hypersensitivity to other corticosteroids. Assess use in pregnant/nursing females, pediatric patients younger than 12 yrs, patients who have conditions which augment the systemic absorption of the medication and those on additional corticosteroid-containing therapies.

Monitoring: Monitor for evidence of HPA-axis suppression, Cushing's syndrome, hyperglycemia, and glycosuria. When applying large doses to large surface areas of the body, perform periodic monitoring using the urinary free cortisol and ACTH stimulation tests to detect evidence of HPA-axis suppression. Monitor for signs of skin irritation; d/c treatment if evident. Monitor for development of infection (eg, bacterial or fungal) and treat appropriately; d/c therapy if infections are not adequately controlled.

Patient Counseling: Instruct to use exactly as directed and for no longer than prescribed time period. Counsel to avoid contact of medication with eyes. Instruct not to use occlusive bandages, coverings, or wrappings on treated skin. Advise to report any signs of local skin reactions. Inform not to use other corticosteroid-containing products during therapy unless directed.

Administration: Apply topically. Treatment should be limited to 45g per week. Not to be used with occlusive dressings. **Storage**: 2-30°C (36-86°F).

BETAPACE RX

sotalol HCl (Bayer Healthcare)

To minimize risk of arrhythmia, place patients initiated or reinitiated on therapy for minimum of 3 days in a facility that can provide ECG monitoring and cardiac resuscitation. Perform CrCl before therapy. Do not substitute Betapace for Betapace AF.

THERAPEUTIC CLASS: Beta-blocker (group II/III antiarrhythmic)

INDICATIONS: Treatment of documented life-threatening ventricular arrhythmias.

DOSAGE: *Adults:* Initial: 80mg bid. Titrate: Increase to 120-160mg bid if needed. Allow 3 days between dose increments. Usual: 160-320mg/day given bid-tid. Refractory Patients: 480-640mg/day. CrCl 30-59mL/min: Dose q24h. CrCl 10-29mL/min: Dose q36-48h. CrCl <10mL/min: Individualize dose. May increase dose with renal impairment after at least 5-6 doses.
Pediatrics: ≥2 yrs: Initial: $30mg/m^2$ tid. Titrate: Wait at least 36 hrs between dose increases. Guide dose by response, HR, and QTc. Max: $60mg/m^2$.
<2 yrs: See dosing chart in PI. Reduce dose or d/c if QTc >550msec. Renal Impairment: Reduce dose or increase interval. Preparation of 5mg/mL Oral Solution: Add five 120mg tabs to 120mL simple syrup in a 6oz plastic, amber

bottle. Shake bottle to wet all tabs. Allow tabs to hydrate for 2 hrs then shake bottle intermittently over 2 hrs until tabs are completely disintegrated. Shake before administration. Store at room temp for 3 months.

HOW SUPPLIED: Tab: 80mg*, 120mg*, 160mg* *scored

CONTRAINDICATIONS: Bronchial asthma, sinus bradycardia, 2nd- and 3rd-degree AV block (unless a functioning pacemaker is present), long QT syndromes, cardiogenic shock, uncontrolled CHF.

WARNINGS/PRECAUTIONS: Caution with heart failure controlled by digitalis and/or diuretics, DM, left ventricular dysfunction, non-allergic bronchospasm, sick sinus syndrome, renal impairment, 2-weeks post-MI. Avoid with hypokalemia, hypomagnesemia, excessive QT interval prolongation (>550msec). Correct electrolyte imbalances before therapy. May provoke new or worsen ventricular arrhythmias. Avoid abrupt withdrawal. Use in surgery is controversial. May mask hypoglycemia, hyperthyroidism symptoms. Proarrhythmic events reported.

ADVERSE REACTIONS: Dyspnea, fatigue, dizziness, bradycardia, chest pain, palpitation, asthenia, abnormal ECG, hypotension, headache, lightheadedness, edema.

INTERACTIONS: May block epinephrine effects. Caution with drugs that prolong the QT interval (eg, Class I and III antiarrhythmics, phenothiazines, TCAs, bepridil, certain quinolones and oral macrolides, astemizole). Avoid within 2 hrs of aluminum- or magnesium-containing antacids. Potentiates rebound HTN with clonidine withdrawal. May potentiate bradycardia or hypotension with catecholamine-depleting drugs (eg, reserpine). Antidiabetic agents may need adjustment. Avoid Class 1A and Class III antiarrhythmics; potential to prolong refractoriness. β_2-agonists (eg, terbutaline) may need dose increase. Additive Class II effects with β-blockers. Additive conduction abnormalities with digoxin and CCBs. Caution with diuretics.

PREGNANCY: Category B, not for use in nursing.

MECHANISM OF ACTION: Has both β-adrenoreceptor blocking and cardiac action potential duration prolongation antiarrhythmic property. It prolongs the plateau phase of the cardiac action potential.

PHARMACOKINETICS: Absorption: T_{max}=2.5-4 hrs. **Distribution:** Crosses blood-brain barrier (poor); found in breast milk. **Elimination:** Urine (unchanged); $T_{1/2}$=12 hrs.

NURSING CONSIDERATIONS

Assessment: Establish creatinine clearance prior to dosing. Assess for bronchial asthma, sinus bradycardia/tachycardia, sick sinus syndrome, second- and third-degree HB, patients with functioning pacemaker, congenital/acquired long QT syndromes, cardiogenic shock, left ventricular dysfunction or uncontrolled CHF, recent MI, IHD, hypokalemia or hypomagnesemia, history of chronic bronchitis and emphysema, DM, episodes of hypoglycemia, upcoming major surgery, hyperthyroidism, renal impairment, nursing status, and for possible drug interactions.

Monitoring: After initiation, stay at least 3 days where continuous ECG monitoring and resuscitation are available if needed. Monitor ECG changes, proarrhythmia (eg, ventricular tachycardia/or fibrillation and torsade de pointes), HR, and creatinine clearance, asystole, new arrhythmias, signs/symptoms of depressed myocardial contractility and more severe HF, anaphylaxis, bronchospasm, MI, hypotension, masking of hypoglycemic signs, exacerbation of hyperthyroidism symptoms and thyroid storm.

Patient Counseling: Do not d/c without consulting physician. Inform of benefits/risks of drug. Report any adverse reactions to physician. Not for use by nursing women.

Administration: Oral route. **Storage:** 15-30°C (59-86°F).

B

BETAPACE AF

RX

sotalol HCl (Bayer Healthcare)

To minimize risk of arrhythmia, place patients initiated or reinitiated on therapy for minimum of 3 days in a facility that can provide CrCl, ECG monitoring, and cardiac resuscitation. Do not substitute Betapace for Betapace AF.

THERAPEUTIC CLASS: Beta-blocker (group II/III antiarrhythmic)

INDICATIONS: Maintenance of normal sinus rhythm with symptomatic atrial fibrillation/atrial flutter (AFIB/AFL) in patients who are currently in sinus rhythm.

DOSAGE: *Adults:* Initiate with continuous ECG monitoring. Give dose qd for CrCl 40-60mL/min and bid for CrCl >60mL/min. Initial: 80mg. Monitor QT 2-4hrs after each dose. Reduce dose or d/c if QT ≥500msec. If QT <500msec after 3 days (after 5th or 6th dose if receiving qd dosing), discharge on current treatment. Alternatively, may increase dose to 120mg during hospitalization, and follow for 3 days with bid dose and for 5 or 6 doses if receiving qd dose. Max: 160mg qd or bid depending on CrCl.
Pediatrics: ≥2 yrs: Initial: $30mg/m^2$ tid. Titrate: Wait at least 36 hrs between dose increases. Guide dose by response, heart rate and QTc. Max: $60mg/m^2$. <2 yrs: See dosing chart in PI. Reduce dose or d/c if QTc >550msec. Renal Impairment: Reduce dose or increase interval. Preparation of 5mg/mL Oral Solution: Add five 120mg tabs to 120mL simple syrup in a 6oz plastic, amber bottle. Shake bottle to wet all tabs. Allow tabs to hydrate for 2 hrs then shake bottle intermittently over 2 hrs until tabs are completely disintegrated. Shake before administration. Store at room temp for 3 months.

HOW SUPPLIED: Tab: 80mg*, 120mg*, 160mg* *scored

CONTRAINDICATIONS: Sinus bradycardia (<50bpm during waking hrs), sick sinus syndrome or 2nd- or 3rd-degree AV block (unless a functioning pacemaker is present), long QT syndromes, baseline QT interval >450msec, cardiogenic shock, uncontrolled heart failure, hypokalemia (<4meq/L), CrCl <40mL/min, bronchial asthma.

WARNINGS/PRECAUTIONS: Can cause serious ventricular arrhythmias. Avoid with hypokalemia, hypomagnesemia. Correct electrolyte imbalances before therapy. Bradycardia reported. Caution with heart failure controlled by digitalis and/or diuretics, non-allergic bronchospasm, sick sinus syndrome, left ventricular dysfunction, DM, renal dysfunction, post-MI. Avoid abrupt withdrawal. Use in surgery is controversial. May mask hypoglycemia, hyperthyroidism symptoms.

ADVERSE REACTIONS: Bradycardia, dyspnea, fatigue, dose-related QT interval prolongation, abnormal ECG, chest pain, diarrhea, NV, hyperhidrosis, dizziness.

INTERACTIONS: May block epinephrine effects. Avoid drugs that prolong the QT interval (eg, antiarrhythmics, phenothiazines, TCAs, bepridil, certain oral macrolides). Avoid within 2 hrs of aluminum- or magnesium-containing antacids. Potentiates rebound HTN with clonidine withdrawal. May potentiate bradycardia or hypotension with catecholamine-depleting drugs (eg, reserpine). Antidiabetic agents may need adjustment. β_2-agonists (eg, terbutaline) may need dose increase. Additive conduction abnormalities with digoxin and CCBs. Caution with diuretics.

PREGNANCY: Category B, not for use in nursing.

MECHANISM OF ACTION: Antiarrhythmic drug (Class II and III properties); has both β-adrenoreceptor blocking and cardiac action potential duration prolongation property.

PHARMACOKINETICS: Absorption: T_{max}=2.5-4 hrs. **Distribution:** Crosses blood brain barrier (poor); found in breast milk. **Elimination**: Urine (unchanged); $T_{1/2}$=12 hrs.

NURSING CONSIDERATIONS

Assessment: Calculate CrCl prior to dosing. Assess for structural heart disease, pre-existing long-QT syndrome, implanted pacemaker, other conduction defects, CHF, renal/hepatic dysfunction, recent MI, IHD, history of chronic bronchitis and emphysema, DM, episodes of hypoglycemia, undergoing major surgery, hyperthyroidism, nursing status, medication history and possible drug/diet interactions. Correct hypokalemia and hypomagnesemia before initiation of therapy.

Monitoring: After initiation monitor patient for at least 3 days. Continuous ECG monitoring and resuscitation should be done if necessary. Monitor ECG changes, HR, and CrCl, asystole, new arrhythmias, signs/symptoms of depressed myocardial contractility and more severe HF, anaphylaxis, bronchospasm, MI, hypotension, masking of hypoglycemic signs, exacerbation of hyperthyroidism symptoms, and signs of electrolyte imbalance.

Patient Counseling: Do not abruptly d/c without consulting physician. Inform of benefits/risks and report any signs of electrolyte imbalance (eg, diarrhea and vomiting). After initiation, patient should stay for 3 days where continuous ECG monitoring and resuscitation are availabe. May experience abnormal heartbeat. Inform physician if taking any other medications or OTC drugs.

Administration: PO. **Storage:** 25°C (77°F); excursions permitted to 15-30°C (59-86°F).

BETIMOL — RX

timolol (Vistakon)

THERAPEUTIC CLASS: Nonselective beta-blocker

INDICATIONS: Treatment of elevated IOP in patients with open-angle glaucoma or ocular hypertension.

DOSAGE: *Adults:* Initial: 1 drop 0.25% bid. May increase to max of 1 drop 0.5% bid. Maint: If adequate control, may try 1 drop 0.25-0.5% qd.

HOW SUPPLIED: Sol: 0.25%, 0.5% [2.5mL, 5mL, 10mL, 15mL]

CONTRAINDICATIONS: Bronchial asthma, history of bronchial asthma, severe COPD, sinus bradycardia, 2nd- or 3rd-degree AV block, overt cardiac failure, cardiogenic shock.

WARNINGS/PRECAUTIONS: Caution with cardiac failure, DM, cerebrovascular insufficiency. Severe cardiac and respiratory reactions reported. May mask symptoms of hypoglycemia and hyperthyroidism. Bacterial keratitis reported with contaminated containers. May reinsert contacts 5 min after applying drops. Avoid with COPD, bronchospastic disease. Not for use alone in angle-closure glaucoma. May potentiate muscle weakness. D/C if cardiac failure develops. Withdrawal before surgery is controversial.

ADVERSE REACTIONS: Burning/stinging on instillation, dry eyes, itching, foreign body sensation, eye discomfort, eyelid erythema, conjunctival injection, headache.

INTERACTIONS: May potentiate systemic β-blockers and catecholamine-depleting drugs (eg, reserpine). Oral/IV calcium antagonists can cause AV conduction disturbances, left ventricular failure, or hypotension. Digitalis can cause additive effects in prolonging AV conduction time. May antagonize epinephrine.

PREGNANCY: Category C, not for use in nursing.

MECHANISM OF ACTION: Nonselective β-adrenergic antagonist; blocks both β_1- and β_2-adrenergic receptors. Thought to reduce IOP through reducing production of aqueous humor.

PHARMACOKINETICS: Elimination: Urine (metabolites); $T_{1/2}$=4 hrs

NURSING CONSIDERATIONS

Assessment: Assess for overt heart failure, cardiogenic shock, sinus bradycardia, 2nd-or 3rd-degree AV block, active or history of bronchial asthma, and severe COPD. Assess use in patients with cerebrovascular insufficiencies, undergoing elective surgery, with DM, with hyperthyroidism, and in pregnant/nursing females. Assess patients with angle-closure glaucoma are not on monotherapy with this drug. Assess for possible drug interactions.

Monitoring: Monitor for signs/symptoms of reduced cerebral blood flow, cardiac failure, muscle weakness, bacterial keratitis when using multi-dose container, severe anaphylactic reactions, and hypoglycemia in patients with DM. Monitor for occurrence of thyroid storm in patients who abruptly withdraw from medication and have thyrotoxicosis.

Patient Counseling: Counsel to immediately notify physician if signs of cardiac, respiratory, or anaphylactic symptoms develop while on medication. Instruct patients with DM medication may mask signs of hypoglycemia. To avoid contaminating solution, avoid touching container tip to the eye or surrounding structures. Counsel that if taking concomitant topical ophthalmic medications, to separate dosing by at least 5 min. Instruct patients who wear soft contact lenses to wait at least 5 min after administration before reinserting.

Administration: Ocular route. **Storage:** 15-25°C (59-77°F). Do not freeze. Protect from light.

Betoptic S

betaxolol HCl (Alcon)

RX

THERAPEUTIC CLASS: Selective $beta_1$-blocker

INDICATIONS: Chronic open-angle glaucoma. Ocular hypertension.

DOSAGE: *Adults:* 1-2 drops bid.

HOW SUPPLIED: Sus: 0.25% [5mL, 10mL, 15mL]

CONTRAINDICATIONS: Sinus bradycardia, greater than 1st-degree AV block, cardiogenic shock or overt cardiac failure.

WARNINGS/PRECAUTIONS: May be absorbed systemically. Caution with cardiac failure, heart block, DM, asthma. May mask hypoglycemic symptoms and signs of hyperthyroidism. May potentiate muscle weakness. D/C before general anesthesia. Avoid abrupt withdrawal. Caution in patients with cerebrovascular insufficiency.

ADVERSE REACTIONS: Transient ocular discomfort, blurred vision, corneal punctate keratitis, foreign body sensation, tearing, photophobia, tearing, itching, dryness of eye, erythema, inflammation, discharge, ocular pain, decreased visual acuity, crusty lashes.

INTERACTIONS: May potentiate systemic β-blockers and catecholamine-depleting drugs (eg, reserpine). May be potentiated by systemic β-blockers. May antagonize adrenergic psychotropics. May increase risk of hypoglycemia with insulin or oral hypoglycemic drugs.

PREGNANCY: Category C, caution with nursing.

MECHANISM OF ACTION: It is a cardioselective (β-1-adrenergic) receptor inhibitor. Responsible for reducing intraocular pressure through a reduction of aqueous production.

PHARMACOKINETICS: Absorption: T_{max}=2 hrs.

NURSING CONSIDERATIONS

Assessment: Assess for sinus bradycardia, >1st-degree atrioventricular block, cardiogenic shock, and overt cardiac failure. Assess use with history of cardiac failure or heart block, cerebrovascular insufficiencies, a history of hypoglycemia or DM, hyperthyroidism, patients undergoing elective surgery, patients with excessive restriction of pulmonary function, and in pregnant/nursing females. Assess that patients with angle-closure glaucoma are not on monotherapy with this drug. Assess for possible drug interactions.

Monitoring: Monitor for signs/symptoms of respiratory reactions, cardiac failure, muscle weakness, reduced cerebral blood flow, and anaphylaxis. Monitor for occurrence of a thyroid storm in patients who have thyrotoxicosis and withdraw abruptly from medication. Monitor for signs/symptoms of acute hypoglycemia with DM. Monitor for development of bacterial keratitis in patients who are using multidose containers. Monitor for occurrence of choroidal detachment.

Patient Counseling: Counsel that if any type of cardiac, respiratory, or anaphylactic reactions develop, to contact physician immediately. Advise patients with DM that medication may mask symptoms of hypoglycemia. Instruct to avoid allowing tip of dispensing container to contact the eye or surrounding structures. Advise if solution handled improperly, may become contaminated and cause bacterial infections. Advise if having ocular surgery or if an intercurrent ocular condition develops, to contact physician before continuing to use the multidose container they were previously using. Patients on concomitant topical ophthalmic medication should be instructed to administer medications at least 10 min apart.

Administration: Ocular route. 1) Wash hands prior to use. 2) Invert container and shake once before use. 3) Tilt head back and position bottle above affected eye. 4) With opposite hand, place finger under eye and gently pull down, creating a "V" pocket between eye and lower lid. 5) With hand holding the bottle, place index finger on bottom of bottle. Push bottom of bottle to dispense 1 drop. Do not squeeze sides of bottle. **Storage**: Store upright at room temperature.

BEXXAR — RX

iodine I 131 tositumomab - tositumomab (GlaxoSmithKline)

Hypersensitivity reactions, including anaphylaxis, and prolonged and severe cytopenias reported. Can cause fetal harm if given during pregnancy. Contains radioactive component.

THERAPEUTIC CLASS: Monoclonal antibody/CD20-blocker

INDICATIONS: Treatment of CD20-positive, follicular, non-Hodgkin's lymphoma (NHL), with and without transformation, in patients refractory to rituximab and who have relapsed following chemotherapy.

DOSAGE: *Adults:* Premedication: Day 1: Begin thyro-protective regimen of either SSKI (4 drops po tid), Lugol's sol (20 drops po tid), or potassium iodide (130mg po qd). Continue until 14 days post-therapeutic dose. Day 0: APAP 650mg and diphenhydramine 50mg. Dosimetric Step: IV: 450mg tositumomab over 60 min followed by 5mCi Iodine I 131 tositumomab (35mg) over 20 min. Day 0 + Day 2, 3, or 4 + Day 6 or 7: Whole body dosimetry and biodistribution. Day 6 or 7: Calculation of patient-specific activity of iodine I 131 tositumomab to deliver 75cGy total body irradiation or 65cGy if platelets ≥100,000 but <150,000 platelets/mm^3. Day 7 (up to Day 14): Premedicate with APAP and diphenhydramine. Therapeutic Step: IV: Do not administer if biodistribution is altered. 450mg tositumomab over 60 min followed by prescribed therapeutic dose of iodine I 131 tositumomab (35mg) over 20 min.

HOW SUPPLIED: Inj: For Dosimetric Dosing: Tositumomab: 225mg [2 single-use vials], 35mg [1 single-use vial]; Iodine I 131 Tositumomab: 1 single-use vial. For Therapeutic Dosing: Tositumomab: 225mg [2 single-use vials], 35mg [1 single-use vial]; Iodine I 131 Tositumomab: 1 or 2 single-use vials.

CONTRAINDICATIONS: Pregnant women.

WARNINGS/PRECAUTIONS: Obtain CBCs weekly for 10-12 weeks. Safety not established with >25% lymphoma marrow involvement, platelet <100,000 cells/mm^3, or neutrophil count <1500 cells/mm^3. Secondary malignancies reported. May cause hypothyroidism; monitor TSH prior to initiation and then annually. Thyroid blocking agents must be used; initiate at least 24 hrs before dosimetric dose and continue until 14 days after therapeutic dose. Caution with impaired renal function. Effective contraceptive methods should be used during, and for 12 months following treatment. Increased risk of serious allergic reactions if positive for human anti-murine antibodies (HAMA).

ADVERSE REACTIONS: Neutropenia, thrombocytopenia, anemia, asthenia, fever, infection, cough, pain, chills, headache, GI effects, myalgia, arthralgia, pharyngitis, dyspnea, rash.

INTERACTIONS: Weigh risks vs benefits of concomitant agents that interfere with platelet function and/or anticoagulation.

PREGNANCY: Category X, not for use in nursing.

MECHANISM OF ACTION: Monoclonal antibody; possibly induces apoptosis, complement-dependent cytotoxicity, antibody-dependent cellular cytotoxicity mediated by the antibody; cell death associated with ionizing radiation from radioisotope. Tositumomab; murine IgG2a lambda monoclonal antibody directed against CD20 antigen found on surface of B lymphocytes. Iodine I 131 Tositumomab; radio-iodinated derivative of Tositumomab, covalently linked to Iodine-131.

PHARMACOKINETICS: Elimination: (Iodine-131): Decay (β and gamma emissions). Physical $T_{1/2}$=8.04 days. Excreted in urine; (Iodine I 131 Tositumomab): Urine; $T_{1/2}$=67 hrs.

NURSING CONSIDERATIONS

Assessment: Assess for known hypersensitivity to murine proteins, lymphoma marrow involvement, impaired bone marrow reserve, renal function, pregnancy status, use of thyroid-blocking agent. Screen for human anti-mouse antibody (prior murine protein use) and possible drug interactions. Obtain baseline CBC, serum creatinine, TSH, and platelet count

Monitoring: Monitor CBC weekly for 10-12 weeks. Monitor renal function (periodically) and TSH (annually). Monitor for signs/symptoms of thrombocytopenia, neutropenia, anemia, secondary malignancies, hypersensitivity reaction (bronchospasm and angioedema), and hypothyroidism.

Patient Counseling: Inform of pregnancy risks and to d/c nursing. Instruct to use effective contraceptive methods during treatment and for 12 months after completion. Advise on importance of compliance with thyroid-blocking agents and need for lifelong monitoring. Seek medical attention if symptoms of thrombocytopenia, neutropenia, anemia, secondary malignancies, hypersensitivity reaction (bronchospasm and angioedema), and hypothyroidism occur.

Administration: IV infusion. Do not administer therapeutic dose if biodistribution is altered. Same IV tubing set and filter must be used throughout all steps. Changes in filter can result in loss of drug. Refer to Full PI for detailed administration. **Storage:** Tositumomab: 2-8°C (36-46°). Do not freeze or shake. Protect from strong light. (Diluted): Stable for 24 hrs if refrigerated 2-8°C (36-46°F); stable for 8 hrs at room temperature. Do not freeze. Iodine I 131 Tositumomab: Frozen in original lead pots at -20°C or below. (Thawed): Stable for 8 hrs at 2-8°C (36-46°), or room temperature. (Diluted): Refrigerate 2-8°C (36-46°).

BIAXIN RX

clarithromycin (Abbott)

THERAPEUTIC CLASS: Macrolide

INDICATIONS: Treatment of the following infections caused by susceptible strains of microorganisms: (Adults): Pharyngitis/tonsillitis, acute maxillary sinusitis, acute bacterial exacerbation of chronic bronchitis (ABECB), community-acquired pneumonia (CAP), uncomplicated skin and skin structure infections (SSSI), and disseminated mycobacterial infections. Combination therapy for *H.pylori* infection with duodenal ulcers. MAC prophylaxis in advanced HIV. (Pediatrics): Pharyngitis/tonsillitis, CAP, acute maxillary sinusitis, acute otitis media, uncomplicated SSSI, disseminated mycobacterial infections. MAC prophylaxis in advanced HIV.

DOSAGE: *Adults:* Pharyngitis/Tonsillitis: 250mg q12h for 10 days. Sinusitis: 500mg q12h for 14 days. ABECB: 250-500mg q12h for 7-14 days. SSSI/CAP: 250mg q12h for 7-14 days. MAC Prophylaxis/Treatment: 500mg bid. CrCl <30mL/min: Give 50% dose or double interval. *H.pylori:* Triple Therapy: 500mg + amoxicillin 1g + omeprazole 20mg, all q12h for 10 days; or 500mg + amoxicillin 1g + lansoprazole 30mg, all q12h for 10-14 days. Give additional

omeprazole 20mg qd for 18 days with active ulcer. Dual Therapy: 500mg q8h + omeprazole 40mg qd for 14 days (give additional omeprazole 20mg qd for 14 days with active ulcer); or 500mg q8h or q12h + ranitidine bismuth citrate 400mg q12h for 14 days (give additional ranitidine bismuth citrate 400mg bid for 14 days with active ulcer). Avoid combination with ranitidine bismuth citrate if CrCl<25mL/min.
Pediatrics: ≥6 months: Usual: 7.5mg/kg q12h for 10 days. MAC Prophylaxis/Treatment: ≥20 months: 7.5mg/kg bid, up to 500mg bid. CrCl <30mL/min: Give 50% dose or double interval.

HOW SUPPLIED: Sus: 125mg/5mL, 250mg/5mL [50mL, 100mL]; Tab: 250mg, 500mg

CONTRAINDICATIONS: Concomitant cisapride, pimozide, astemizole, terfenadine, ergotamine or dihydroergotamine, or other macrolide antibiotics.

WARNINGS/PRECAUTIONS: Avoid in pregnancy. *Clostridium difficile*-associated diarrhea reported. Adjust dose with severe renal impairment. Colchicine toxicity reported; avoid concomitant use especially in elderly.

ADVERSE REACTIONS: Diarrhea, N/V, abnormal taste, dyspepsia, abdominal pain, headache, rash.

INTERACTIONS: See Contraindications. Increases serum levels of theophylline, digoxin, HMG-CoA reductase inhibitors, omeprazole, carbamazepine, drugs metabolized by CYP450. Decreases zidovudine plasma levels. Potentiates oral anticoagulant effects. Decreased clearance of triazolam. Avoid ranitidine, bismuth citrate if CrCl <25mL/min or history of porphyria. Reduce dose with ritonavir if CrCl <60mL/min. Increased levels with fluconazole. Caution with concomitant colchicine use.

PREGNANCY: Category C, caution in nursing.

MECHANISM OF ACTION: Macrolide antibiotic; exerts antibacterial action by binding to the 50S ribosomal subunit of susceptible microorganisms, resulting in inhibition of protein synthesis. Active against aerobic and anaerobic gram-positive and gram-negative microorganisms.

PHARMACOKINETICS: Absorption: Rapid; absolute bioavailability (50%); C_{max}=1-2mcg/mL (250mg tab), 3-4mcg/mL (500mg tab), 2mcg/mL (sus); T_{max}=2-3 hrs. **Metabolism:** 14-OH clarithromycin (principal metabolite). **Elimination:** Urine: 20% (250mg tab), 40% (500mg tab), 10-15% (14-OH). Parent drug; $T_{1/2}$=3-4 hrs (250mg tab, sus), 5-7 hrs (500mg tab). 14-OH: $T_{1/2}$=5-6 hrs (250mg tab, sus), 7-9 hrs (500mg tab).

NURSING CONSIDERATIONS

Assessment: Assess for hepatic/renal impairment, pregnancy/nursing status, acute porphyria, and possible drug interactions.

Monitoring: Monitor for anaphylactic reactions (eg, Stevens-Johnson syndrome, toxic epidermal necrolysis), development of drug-resistant bacteria, *C.difficile*-associated diarrhea ranging from mild diarrhea to fatal colitis, overgrowth of nonsusceptible microorganisms, cardiac arrhythmia if taken concurrently with cisapride, pimozine, astemizole, or terfenadine. Monitor for colchicine toxicity if taken concurrently with colchicine, especially in elderly, and lab changes of LFTs, CBC, PT, and renal function.

Patient Counseling: Inform that drug only treats bacterial, not viral, infection. Take exactly as directed; skipping doses or not completing full course may decrease effectiveness and increase resistance. Inform about potential benefits/risks. D/C and notify physician if allergic reactions or watery/bloody diarrhea (with/without stomach cramps) develop (may occur up to 2 or more months after treatment). Notify if pregnant/nursing.

Administration: Oral route. **Storage:** 15-30°C (59-86°F); well-closed container. Protect from light.

BIAXIN XL

RX

clarithromycin (Abbott)

THERAPEUTIC CLASS: Macrolide

B

INDICATIONS: Treatment of acute maxillary sinusitis, community-acquired pneumonia (CAP), and acute bacterial exacerbation of chronic bronchitis (ABECB).

DOSAGE: *Adults:* Sinusitis: 1000mg qd for 14 days. ABECB/CAP: 1000mg qd for 7 days. CrCl <30mL/min: Give 50% dose or double interval. Take with food.

HOW SUPPLIED: Tab, Extended-Release: 500mg [PAC 14[s]]

CONTRAINDICATIONS: Concomitant cisapride, pimozide, astemizole, terfenadine, ergotamine or dihydroergotamine, or other macrolide antibiotics.

WARNINGS/PRECAUTIONS: Avoid in pregnancy. *Clostridium difficile*-associated diarrhea reported. Adjust dose with severe renal impairment. Colchicine toxicity reported, avoid concomitant use especially in the elderly.

ADVERSE REACTIONS: Diarrhea, NV, abnormal taste, dyspepsia, abdominal pain, headache, rash.

INTERACTIONS: See Contraindications. May increase serum levels of theophylline, digoxin, HMG-CoA reductase inhibitors, omeprazole, carbamazepine and drugs metabolized by CYP450. May decrease zidovudine plasma levels. May potentiate oral anticoagulant effects. May decrease clearance of triazolam. Avoid ranitidine bismuth citrate if CrCl <25mL/min or history of porphyria. Reduce dose with ritonavir if CrCl <60mL/min. Increased levels with fluconazole. Caution with concomitant colchicine use.

PREGNANCY: Category C, caution in nursing.

MECHANISM OF ACTION: Macrolide antibiotic; exerts antibacterial action by binding to 50S ribosomal subunit of susceptible microorganisms resulting in inhibition of protein synthesis. Active against aerobic and anaerobic gram-positive and gram-negativie microorganisms.

PHARMACOKINETICS: Absorption: Rapid. (2 x 500mg dose): (parent drug) C_{max}=2-3µg/mL, T_{max}=5-8 hrs.(14-OH) C_{max}=0.8µg/mL, T_{max}=6-9 hrs. (1 x 500mg dose): (parent drug) C_{max}=1-2µg/mL, T_{max}=5-6 hr; (14-OH) C_{max}=0.6µ/mL, T_{max}=6 hrs. **Distribution:** Body tissues, fluids. **Metabolism:** 14-OH clarithromycin (principal metabolite). **Elimination:** Urine; (40%).

NURSING CONSIDERATIONS

Assessment: Assess for hepatic/renal impairment, pregnancy/nursing status, acute porphyria and possible drug interactions.

Monitoring: Monitor for anaphylactic reactions (eg, Stevens-Johnson syndrome, toxic epidermal necrolysis), development of drug resistant bacteria, *Clostridium difficile*-associated diarrhea ranging from mild diarrhea to fetal colitis, overgrowth of nonsusceptible microorganisms, cardiac arrhythmia if taken concurrently with cisapride, colchicine toxicity if taken concurrently with colchicine especially in elderly, and lab changes of LFTs, CBC, PT, and renal function.

Patient Counseling: Counsel that drug treats bacterial, not viral, infections. Take exactly as directed; skipping doses or not completing full course may decrease effectiveness and increase resistance. Inform about potential benefits/risks. D/C and notify physician if allergic reaction or watery/bloody diarrhea (with/without stomach cramps) occur (may occur as late as 2 or more months after treatment). Notify if pregnant/nursing.

Administration: Oral route. Swallow whole with food; do not chew, crush, or break. **Storage:** 20-25°C (68-77°F); excursions permitted 15-30°C (59-86°F).

BONIVA

RX

ibandronate sodium (Roche)

THERAPEUTIC CLASS: Bisphosphonate

INDICATIONS: (Inj) Treatment of osteoporosis in postmenopausal women. (PO) Treatment and prevention of postmenopausal osteoporosis.

DOSAGE: *Adults:* Inj: 3mg IV over 15-30 sec every 3 months. PO: 2.5mg qd or 150mg once monthly. Swallow whole with 6-8 oz water. Do not lie down for 60

B

min after dose. Take at least 60 min before 1st food, drink (other than water), medication, or supplementation.

HOW SUPPLIED: Inj: 3mg/3mL; Tab: 2.5mg, 150mg

CONTRAINDICATIONS: (Inj, PO) Hypocalcemia. (PO) Inability to stand or sit upright for at least 60 min.

WARNINGS/PRECAUTIONS: (Inj, PO) Not recommended in severe renal impairment (CrCl <30mL/min). Reports of osteonecrosis, primarily in the jaw, and severe, incapacitating bone, joint, and/or muscle pain. (PO) May cause upper GI disorders (eg, dysphagia, esophagitis, esophageal or gastric ulcer).

ADVERSE REACTIONS: (Inj) Influenza, nasopharyngitis, cystitis, gastroenteritis, UTI, abdominal pain, dyspepsia, nausea, constipation, arthralgia, back pain, HTN. (PO) Back pain, extremity pain, infection, dyspepsia, diarrhea, hypercholesterolemia, myalgia, headache, dizziness, upper respiratory infection, bronchitis, pneumonia, UTI.

INTERACTIONS: (PO) Calcium and other multivalent cations may interfere with absorption.

PREGNANCY: Category C, caution in nursing.

MECHANISM OF ACTION: Bisphosphonate; has affinity for hydroxyapatite, a component of the mineral matrix of the bone. Inhibits osteoclast activity and reduces bone resorption and turnover.

PHARMACOKINETICS: Absorption: (PO): T_{max}=0.5-2 hrs. **Distribution:** V_d=90L; serum protein binding (85.7-99.5%). **Elimination:** (IV, PO) Kidney (50-60%); (PO) Feces (unabsorbed dose); (PO)(150mg): $T_{1/2}$=37-157 hrs; (IV, 2mg): $T_{1/2}$=6.6-15.3 hrs; (IV, 4mg): $T_{1/2}$=5-25.5 hrs.

NURSING CONSIDERATIONS

Assessment: For both oral and IV formulations, assess for hypocalcemia and other disturbances of bone and mineral metabolism, severe renal impairment (eg, CrCl<30mL/min), risk of osteonecrosis, pregnancy/nursing status, and possible drug interactions. Oral formulation: Assess for ability to stand or sit upright for at least 60 min. IV formulation: Assess potential for renal impairment and obtain SrCr levels prior to each administration of dose.

Monitoring: For IV and oral formulations, monitor for signs/symptoms of jaw osteonecrosis and musculoskeletal pain. IV formula: Monitor for renal toxicity (eg, increased SrCr) and transient decrease in serum calcium levels. Oral formulation: Monitor for signs/symptoms of upper GI disorders (eg, dysphagia, esophagitis, esophageal or gastric ulcer).

Patient Counseling: Oral formulation: Counsel to take at least 60 min before first food or drink (other than water) and before taking other oral medication or supplementation. Instruct to swallow whole with full glass of plain water while standing or sitting in upright position; avoid lying down for 60 min following administration of drug. Inform not to chew or suck medication. Take supplemental calcium and vitamin D if dietary intake is inadequate; should be delayed by at least 60 min following administration of ibandronate. If taking 150mg tablet, take on the same date each month. Instruct to d/c treatment and seek medical attention if signs of esophageal reaction develop during therapy. IV formulation: Must receive intravenously, only by healthcare professional, once every 3 months.

Administration: Oral or IV route. **Storage:** 25°C (77°F); excursions permitted to 15-30°C (59-86°F).

BOOSTRIX RX

pertussis vaccine, acellular - diphtheria toxoid - tetanus toxoid

(GlaxoSmithKline)

THERAPEUTIC CLASS: Vaccine/toxoid combination

INDICATIONS: Active booster immunization against tetanus, diphtheria, and pertussis as a single dose in individuals 10-64 yrs of age.

DOSAGE: *Adults:* >18-64 yrs: 0.5mL IM into the deltoid muscle. *Pediatrics:* 10-18 yrs: 0.5mL IM into the deltoid muscle.

HOW SUPPLIED: Inj: (Tetanus-Diphtheria-Pertussis) 5LF-2.5LF-18.5mcg/0.5mL.

CONTRAINDICATIONS: Hypersensitivity to any component; serious allergic reaction (eg, anaphylaxis) associated with previous dose. Encephalopathy (eg, coma, decreased level of consciousness, prolonged seizures) within 7 days of administration of a previous pertussis antigen-containing vaccine.

WARNINGS/PRECAUTIONS: Caution if Guillain-Barre syndrome and brachial neuritis within 6 weeks of tetanus toxoid vaccine. Defer Tdap vaccination if progressive neurologic disorder, uncontrolled epilepsy, progressive encephalopathy or unstable neurological conditions (eg, cerebrovascular events, acute encephalopathy) occur; caution in giving pertussis antigen-containing vaccine. Do not give Td, Tdap, or emergency dose of Td more frequently than every 10 yrs if patient has experienced Arthus-type reaction. May cause allergic reactions in latex-sensitive patients. May not obtain expected immune response in immunosuppressed individuals. Hypersensitivity reaction possible; epinephrine injection (1:1000) should be readily available.

ADVERSE REACTIONS: Local: pain, redness, swelling. Systemic: headache, fatigue, fever, nausea, vomiting, diarrhea, abdominal pain.

INTERACTIONS: Concomitant with influenza virus vaccine lowers geometric mean antibody concentrations for antibodies to the pertussis antigens filamentous hemagglutinin and pertactin. Avoid mixing with other vaccines in the same syringe or vial. May give tetanus immune globulin on separate site, syringe, and needle. Immunosuppressive therapies, including irradiation, antimetabolites, alkylating agents, cytotoxic drugs, and corticosteroids may reduce the immune response to vaccines.

PREGNANCY: Category C, caution in nursing.

MECHANISM OF ACTION: Stimulates immune system to elicit immune response, which produces antibodies that may protect against tetanus, diphtheria, and pertussis.

NURSING CONSIDERATIONS

Assessment: Assess immunization history and current health/medical status, previous hypersensitivity, immunization-related complications such as Guillain-Barre syndrome and brachial neuritis, and possible drug interactions. Assess for uncontrolled epilepsy, progressive encephalopathy and neurological disorders, and pregnancy/nursing status.

Monitoring: Monitor for local adverse events (pain, redness, swelling at injection site), increase in arm circumference, and GI symptoms.

Patient Counseling: Inform about benefits/risks; report any adverse reactions to physician. Advise patient, parent or guardian should acquire vaccine information statements given by the national childhood vaccine injury act of 1986 prior to immunization.

Administration: IM (deltoid muscle). **Storage:** Refrigerate at 2-8°C (36-46°F). Do not freeze. Discard if vaccine has been frozen.

BREVIBLOC — RX

esmolol HCl (Baxter)

THERAPEUTIC CLASS: Selective $beta_1$-blocker

INDICATIONS: For rapid control of ventricular rate in atrial fibrillation or atrial flutter in perioperative, postoperative, or other emergent circumstances. For noncompensatory sinus tachycardia. Treatment of tachycardia and hypertension that occur during induction and tracheal intubation, during surgery, on emergence from anesthesia, and in the postoperative period.

DOSAGE: *Adults:* Supraventricular Tachycardia: Titrate dose based on ventricular rate. Load: 0.5mg/kg over 1 min. Maint: 0.05mg/kg/min for next 4 min. May increase by 0.05mg/kg/min at intervals of 4 min or more up to

0.2mg/kg/min. Rapid slowing of ventricular response: Repeat 0.5mg/kg load over 1 min, then 0.1mg/kg/min for 4 min. If needed, another (final) load of 0.5mg/kg over 1 min, then 0.15mg/kg/min for 4 min up to 0.2mg/kg/min. May continue infusions for 24-48hrs. Intraoperative/Postoperative Tachycardia and/or HTN: Immediate Control: Initial: 80mg bolus over 30 sec. Maint: 0.15mg/kg/min. May titrate up to 0.3mg/kg/min. Gradual Control: Initial: 0.5mg/kg over 1 min. Maint: 0.05mg/kg/min for 4 min. Then, if needed, may repeat load and increase to 0.1mg/kg/min.

HOW SUPPLIED: Inj: 10mg/mL [10mL, 250mL], 20mg/mL [5mL, 100mL]

CONTRAINDICATIONS: Sinus bradycardia, heart block greater than first degree, cardiogenic shock or overt heart failure.

WARNINGS/PRECAUTIONS: Hypotension may occur; monitor BP and reduce dose or d/c if needed. May cause cardiac failure; withdraw at 1st sign of impending cardiac failure. Caution with supraventricular arrhythmias when patient is compromised hemodynamically or is taking other drugs that decrease peripheral resistance, myocardial filling/contractility, and/or electrical impulse propagation in the myocardium. Not for HTN associated with hypothermia. Caution in bronchospastic diseases; titrate to lowest possible effective dose and terminate immediately in the event of bronchospasm. Caution in diabetics; may mask tachycardia occurring with hypoglycemia. Caution in impaired renal function. Avoid concentrations >10mg/mL and infusions into small veins or through butterfly catheters. Sloughing of skin and necrosis reported with infiltration and extravasation. Use caution when discontinuing infusion in CAD patients.

ADVERSE REACTIONS: Hypotension, dizziness, diaphoresis, somnolence, confusion, headache, agitation, bronchospasm, nausea, infusion site reactions.

INTERACTIONS: Additive effects with catecholamine-depleting agents (eg, reserpine); monitor for hypotension or bradycardia. Levels increased by warfarin or morphine; titrate with caution. May increase digoxin levels; titrate with caution. May prolong effects of succinylcholine; titrate with caution. Caution when using with verapamil in depressed myocardial function; fatal cardiac arrest may occur. Do not use to control supraventricular tachycardia with vasoconstrictive and inotropic agents (eg, dopamine, epinephrine, norepinephrine) because of the danger of blocking cardiac contractility when systemic vascular resistance is high. Patients with a history of severe anaphylactic reaction may be more reactive to repeated challenge and unresponsive to the usual doses of epinephrine used to treat allergic reaction.

PREGNANCY: Category C, caution in nursing.

MECHANISM OF ACTION: Selective β_1 blocker; inhibits β_1 receptors located chiefly in cardiac muscle, and at higher doses begins to inhibit β_2 receptors located chiefly in the bronchial and vascular musculature.

PHARMACOKINETICS: Distribution: Plasma protein binding (55%). **Metabolism:** Rapid. Through hydrolysis of the ester linkage in red blood cells to methanol and free acid. **Elimination:** Urine (73-88% unchanged); $T_{1/2}$=9 min (Brevibloc), and 3.7 hrs (acid metabolites).

NURSING CONSIDERATIONS

Assessment: Assess for sinus bradycardia, heart block greater than first degree, cardiogenic shock or overt heart failure, hypotension, HTN associated with hypothermia, bronchospastic disease, DM, renal impairment, and possible drug interactions (verapamil).

Monitoring: Monitor BP, HR. Monitor for signs/symptoms of impending cardiac failure, hypotension (eg, diaphoresis or dizziness), postoperative tachycardia/HTN, bronchospasm, and masking signs of hypoglycemia.

Patient Counseling: Inform about benefits/risks. Report any adverse reactions to physician.

Administration: IV route. Prediluted to provide ready-to-use vials. Do not introduce additives to vials. **Storage:** Store at 25°C (77°F); excursions permitted to 15-30°C (59-86°F). Protect from freezing.

B

BREVOXYL — RX
benzoyl peroxide (Stiefel)

THERAPEUTIC CLASS: Antibacterial/keratolytic

INDICATIONS: Topical treatment of mild to moderate acne vulgaris.

DOSAGE: *Adults:* (Gel) Apply qd-bid to clean affected area. (Lot) Shake well. Wet affected area and wash qd for 1st week, then bid thereafter if tolerated. *Pediatrics:* ≥12 yrs: (Gel) Apply qd-bid to clean affected area. (Lot) Shake well. Wet affected area and wash qd for 1st week, then bid thereafter if tolerated.

HOW SUPPLIED: Gel: 4%, 8% [42.5g, 90g]; Lot: (Cleanser) 4%, 8% [297g]; Lot: (Creamy Wash) 4%, 8% [170g]

WARNINGS/PRECAUTIONS: Avoid contact with hair, eyes, mucous membranes, carpeting, and fabrics.

ADVERSE REACTIONS: Erythema, peeling.

PREGNANCY: Category C, caution in nursing.

MECHANISM OF ACTION: Antibacterial/keratolytic agent; not established; demonstrated activity against *Propionibacterium acnes.* Has also shown to have a mild keratolytic effect.

PHARMACOKINETICS: Absorption: Absorbed by skin. **Metabolism:** Metabolized in skin to benzoic acid. **Elimination:** Urine (benzoate; metabolite).

NURSING CONSIDERATIONS

Assessment: Assess proper diagnosis of acne vulgaris. Assess use in pregnant/nursing patients.

Monitoring: Monitor for adequate clinical response and development of contact sensitization reactions, erythema, and peeling.

Patient Counseling: Cleanse affected areas prior to application of medication. Inform that clinically visible improvement will normally occur by third week of therapy and maximum lesion reduction may be expected after approximately 8-12 weeks of use. Avoid medication coming in contact with hair, fabrics, or carpeting to prevent bleaching.

Administration: Topical. For external use only. Avoid contact with eyes and mucous membranes. **Storage:** Store at controlled room temperature; 15-30°C (59-86°F).

BROVANA — RX
arformoterol tartrate (Sepracor)

Long-acting β_2-adrenergic agonists may increase the risk of asthma-related death.

THERAPEUTIC CLASS: $Beta_2$-agonist

INDICATIONS: Long-term maintenance treatment of bronchoconstriction in patients with COPD, including chronic bronchitis and emphysema.

DOSAGE: *Adults:* Usual: 15mcg bid (am and pm). Max: 30mcg/day. Administer via nebulizer.

HOW SUPPLIED: Sol, Inhalation: 15mcg/2mL [30^s, 60^s]

CONTRAINDICATIONS: Hypersensitivity to racemic formoterol

WARNINGS/PRECAUTIONS: Not indicated for treatment of acute episodes of bronchospasm. Should not be initiated or used in children or patients with acutely deteriorating COPD. Fatalities reported with excessive use of inhaled sympathomimetics, avoid use with other long-acting β_2-agonists. D/C regular use of short acting β_2-agonists (eg, qid) before initiating therapy. May produce life-threatening paradoxical bronchospasm. Caution in patients with convulsive disorders, thyrotoxicosis, cardiovascular disorders especially coronary insufficiency, cardiac arrhythmias, and HTN. Immediate hypersensitivity reactions may occur.

ADVERSE REACTIONS: Pain, chest pain, back pain , diarrhea, sinusitis, leg cramps, dyspnea, rash, flu syndrome, peripheral edema.

INTERACTIONS: Sympathetic effects may be potentiated with concomitant use of additional adrenergic agonists. Concomitant use with methylxanthines, steroids, or diuretics may potentiate hypokalemia. Caution with co-administration with non-potassium sparing diuretics may cause ECG changes. Use extreme caution in patients being treated with MAOIs, TCAs, or any drugs known to prolong the QTc interval. Caution with β-blockers.

PREGNANCY: Category C, caution in nursing.

MECHANISM OF ACTION: β_2-adrenergic agonist; stimulates intracellular adenyl cyclase, which catalyzes conversion of ATP to cAMP to produce relaxation of bronchial smooth muscle and inhibition of release of mediators of immediate hypersensitivity from cells (mast cells).

PHARMACOKINETICS: Absorption: C_{max}=4.3pg/mL, T_{max}=30 min, AUC=34.5pg•hr/mL. **Distribution:** Plasma protein binding (52-65%). **Metabolism:** Glucuronidation (major) via uridine diphosphoglucuronosyltransferase (UGT) isoenzymes, O-demethylation (minor) via CYP2D6, CYP2C19. **Elimination:** Urine (1%); $T_{1/2}$=26 hrs.

NURSING CONSIDERATIONS

Assessment: Assess for hepatic impairment, acute deteriorating COPD, CVD (coronary insufficiency, cardiac arrythmias, HTN), convulsive disorders, thyrotoxicosis, and possible drug interactions. D/C inhaled, short-acting β_2-agonists (if using on regular basis) before therapy.

Monitoring: Monitor for signs/symptoms of acute deteriorating COPD, cardiovascular effects (increased BP, palpitations), worsening of symptoms, paradoxical bronchospasm, and hypersensitivity reactions (anaphylactic, urticaria, angioedema, rash, bronchospasm).

Patient Counseling: To be used by nebulizer only, instruct not to inject or swallow. If taking inhaled, short-acting β_2-agonists on regular basis, instruct to d/c before therapy. Inform not for relief of acute respiratory symptoms. Caution drug may increase risk of asthma-related death. Seek medical attention if symptoms of deterioration of COPD, worsening of symptoms, therapy becomes less effective, need more inhalation from short-acting β_2-agonist than usual, paradoxical bronchospasms, and hypersensitivity (anaphylactic, urticaria, angioedema, rash, bronchospasm) occur.

Administration: Oral inhalation. **Storage:** Refrigerate; 2-8°C (36-46°F) or store at 20-25°C (68-77°F) for up to 6 weeks. Use immediately once opened; discard if colored. Protect from light and excessive heat.

BUMETANIDE — RX

bumetanide (Various)

Can lead to profound water and electrolyte depletion with excessive use.

OTHER BRAND NAMES: Bumex (Roche Labs)

THERAPEUTIC CLASS: Loop diuretic

INDICATIONS: Treatment of edema associated with CHF, hepatic disease, and renal disease including nephrotic syndrome.

DOSAGE: *Adults:* ≥18 yrs: PO: Usual: 0.5-2mg qd. Maint: May give every other day or every 3-4 days. Max: 10mg/day. IV/IM: Initial: 0.5-1mg over 1-2 min, may repeat every 2-3 hrs for 2-3 doses. Max: 10mg/day. Elderly: Start at low end of dosing range.

HOW SUPPLIED: Inj: 0.25mg/mL; Tab: 0.5mg*, 1mg*, 2mg* *scored

CONTRAINDICATIONS: Anuria, hepatic coma, severe electrolyte depletion.

WARNINGS/PRECAUTIONS: Monitor for volume/electrolyte depletion, hypokalemia, blood dyscrasias, hepatic damage. Elderly are prone to volume/electrolyte depletion. Caution in elderly, hepatic cirrhosis and ascites. Associated with ototoxicity, hypocalcemia, thrombocytopenia, hypomagnesemia, hypokalemia, and hyperuricemia. Hypersensitivity with sulfonamide allergy. D/C if marked increase in BUN or creatinine or if develop oliguria with progressive renal disease.

ADVERSE REACTIONS: Muscle cramps, dizziness, hypotension, headache, nausea, hyperuricemia, hypokalemia, hyponatremia, hyperglycemia, azotemia, increase serum creatinine.

INTERACTIONS: Avoid aminoglycosides, ototoxic and nephrotoxic drugs, indomethacin. Lithium toxicity. Probenecid reduces effects. Potentiates antihypertensives.

PREGNANCY: Category C, not for use in nursing.

MECHANISM OF ACTION: Loop diuretic; inhibits sodium reabsorption in ascending loop of Henle.

PHARMACOKINETICS: Absorption: (IV) T_{max}=15-30 min. (Tab) T_{max}=1-2 hrs. **Distribution:** Plasma protein binding (94-96%). **Metabolism:** Oxidation. **Elimination:** Urine, bile (2%); $T_{1/2}$=1-1.5 hrs.

NURSING CONSIDERATIONS

Assessment: Assess for progressive renal disease, severe electrolyte depletion, anuria, oliguria, risk for vetricular arrhythmia, possible drug interactions, DM, impaired GI absorption, CHF, sulfonamide allergy, and liver disease (hepatic coma).

Monitoring: Periodically monitor serum potassium, serum electrolytes, CBC, blood glucose, and renal function. Monitor for signs/symptoms of ototoxicity, hypersensitivity reactions, hyperuricemia, oliguria, and thrombocytopenia.

Patient Counseling: Advise to seek medical attention if symptoms of ototoxicity, oliguria, hypersensitivity reactions, or thrombocytopenia occur.

Administration: Oral route. **Storage:** IV: 20-25°C (68-77°F). Protect from light. Tab: 15-30°C (59-86°F).

BUPRENEX

CIII

buprenorphine HCl (Reckitt Benckiser)

THERAPEUTIC CLASS: Opioid analgesic

INDICATIONS: Relief of moderate to severe pain.

DOSAGE: *Adults:* 0.3mg IM/IV q6h prn. Repeat if needed, 30-60 min after initial dose and then prn. High Risk Patients/Concomitant CNS depressants: Reduce dose by approximately 50%. May use single doses ≤0.6mg IM if not at high-risk.
Pediatrics: ≥13 yrs: 0.3mg IM/IV q6h prn. Repeat if needed, 30-60 min after initial dose and then prn. High Risk Patients/Concomitant CNS depressants: Reduce dose by approximately 50%. May use single doses ≤0.6mg IM if not at high-risk. 2-12 yrs: 2-6mcg/kg IM/IV q4-6h.

HOW SUPPLIED: Inj: 0.3mg/mL

WARNINGS/PRECAUTIONS: Significant respiratory depression reported; caution with compromised respiratory function. May increase CSF pressure; caution with head injury, intracranial lesions. Caution with debilitated, BPH, biliary tract dysfunction, myxedema, hypothyroidism, urethral stricture, acute alcoholism, Addison's disease, CNS disease, coma, toxic psychoses, delirium tremens, elderly, pediatrics, kyphoscoliosis or hepatic/renal/pulmonary impairment. May impair mental or physical abilities. May precipitate withdrawal in narcotic-dependence. May lead to psychological dependence.

ADVERSE REACTIONS: Sedation, NV, dizziness, sweating, hypotension, headache, miosis, hypoventilation.

INTERACTIONS: Caution with MAOIs, CNS and respiratory depressants. Respiratory and cardiovascular collapse reported with diazepam. Increased CNS depression with other narcotic analgesics, general anesthetics, antihistamines, benzodiazepines, phenothiazines, other tranquilizers, sedative-hypnotics. Decreased clearance with CYP3A4 inhibitors (eg, macrolides, azole antifungals, protease inhibitors). Increased clearance with CYP3A4 inducers (eg, rifampin, carbamazepine, phenytoin).

PREGNANCY: Category C, not for use in nursing.

MECHANISM OF ACTION: Opioid analgesic; high affinity binding to μ-opiate receptors in CNS. Possesses slow rate of dissociation from its receptor. Also possesses narcotic antagonist activity.

PHARMACOKINETICS: Absorption: T_{max}=1 hr. **Distribution:** Found in breast milk. **Metabolism:** Liver. **Elimination:** $T_{1/2}$=1.2-7.2 hrs.

NURSING CONSIDERATIONS

Assessment: Assess for compromised respiratory function (eg, COPD, hypoxia), head injury, intracranial lesions, age of patient, hepatic/renal function, myxedema or hypothyroidism, adrenal cortical insufficiencies (eg, Addison's disease), CNS depression or coma, toxic psychosis, prostatic hypertrophy or urethral stricture, acute alcoholism, delirium tremens, kyphoscoliosis, biliary tract dysfunction, pregnancy/nursing, and possible drug interactions.

Monitoring: Monitor for signs/symptoms of respiratory depression, CNS depression, elevation of CSF pressure, increased intracholedochal pressure, drug dependence, and withdrawal effects.

Patient Counseling: Inform that medication may impair mental/physicial abilities; use caution when performing dangerous tasks (eg, operating machinery/driving). Advise to notify physician of all medications currently taken. Instruct to avoid use of other CNS depressants and alcohol during therapy. Advise that medication may lead to dependence. Counsel to not exceed prescribed dosage. Advise to avoid abruptly discontinuing medication. Counsel to contact physician if signs/symptoms of respiratory depression develop.

Administration: Deep IM or slow IV route. **Storage:** Avoid excessive heat (over 40°C or 104°F). Protect from prolonged exposure to light.

BuSpar RX

buspirone HCl (Bristol-Myers Squibb)

THERAPEUTIC CLASS: Atypical anxiolytic

INDICATIONS: Management of anxiety disorders, short-term relief of anxiety symptoms.

DOSAGE: *Adults:* Usual: 7.5mg bid. Titrate: May increase by 5mg/day every 2-3 days. Usual: 20-30mg/day. Max: 60mg/day. Use low dose with potent CYP450 3A4 inhibitors (eg, 2.5mg qd with nefazodone). Take consistently with or without food; bioavailability increased with food.

HOW SUPPLIED: Tab: 5mg*, 10mg*, 15mg*, 30mg* *scored

WARNINGS/PRECAUTIONS: Avoid with hepatic or renal impairment.

ADVERSE REACTIONS: Dizziness, nausea, headache, nervousness, lightheadedness, excitement, dystonia, fatigue, parkinsonism, akathisia, restless legs syndrome, restlessness.

INTERACTIONS: Avoid MAOIs and alcohol. Withdraw other CNS depressants gradually before therapy. Caution with psychotropics. Elevated liver transaminases reported with trazodone. Increases haloperidol levels. Verapamil, diltiazem, grapefruit juice, nefazodone, itraconazole, cimetidine, erythromycin increase plasma levels. May increase levels of both drugs with nefazodone; decrease dose of buspirone. Decreased plasma levels and effects with rifampin; may need to adjust buspirone dose. CYP3A4 inhibitors may increase plasma levels and CYP3A4 inducers may increase metabolism of buspirone; may need dose adjustment. Presystemic clearance may be decreased with food. May displace digoxin.

PREGNANCY: Category B, not for use in nursing.

MECHANISM OF ACTION: Atypical antianxiety agent; not fully established. Binds with high affinity to serotonin receptors (5-HT_{1A}) and moderate affinity to dopamine receptors (D_2); may have indirect effects on other neurotransmitter systems.

PHARMACOKINETICS: Absorption: Rapid; C_{max}=1-6ng/mL; T_{max}=40-90 min. **Distribution:** Plasma protein binding (86%). **Metabolism:** CYP3A4; oxidation and hyroxylation; 1-pyrimidinylpiperazine (active metabolite). **Elimination:** Urine (29-63%), feces (18-38%); $T_{1/2}$=2-3 hrs.

NURSING CONSIDERATIONS

Assessment: Assess for hypersensitivity, hepatic/renal functions, and possible drug interactions (eg, MAOIs).

Monitoring: Monitor BP, CNS disturbances, withdrawal symptoms (eg, irritability, anxiety, agitation, insomnia, tremor, abdominal cramps/muscle cramps, vomiting, sweating, flu-like symptoms w/o fever, and seizures), pseudo-parkinsonism, akathisia, TD, dystonia.

Patient Counseling: Counsel to avoid hazardous tasks (eg, operating machinery/driving), ingesting large amounts of grapefruit juice. Advise to notify physician of current medications, alcohol use, and pregnancy status.

Administration: Oral route. **Storage:** 25°C (77°F); excursions permitted to 15-30°C (59-86°F). Dispense in tight, light-resistant container.

BYETTA — RX

exenatide (Amylin/Lilly)

THERAPEUTIC CLASS: Incretin mimetic

INDICATIONS: Adjunctive therapy to improve glycemic control in patients with type 2 DM who are taking metformin, a sulfonylurea, a thiazolidinedione, a combination of metformin/sulfonylurea or metformin/thiazolidinedione, but have not achieved adequate glycemic control.

DOSAGE: *Adults:* 5mcg SQ bid, 60 min before am & pm meals. Titrate: May increase to 10mcg bid after 1 month. Reduction of sulfonylurea dose may be considered to reduce risk of hypoglycemia.

HOW SUPPLIED: Inj: 5mcg/dose, 10mcg/dose [60-dose prefilled pen]

WARNINGS/PRECAUTIONS: Not a substitute for insulin. Avoid with type 1 DM, treatment of diabetic ketoacidosis, ESRD, severe renal impairment (CrCl <30mL/min), or severe GI disease. Acute pancreatitis reported. Increased incidence of hypoglycemia with sulfonylureas. Observe for signs and symptoms of hypersensitivity reactions; patients with abdominal pain should be investigated. When used with thiazolidinediones possible CP and/or chronic hypersensitivity pneumonitis.

ADVERSE REACTIONS: NV, diarrhea, feeling jittery, dizziness, headache, dyspepsia, injection-site reactions; dysgeusia, somnolence, generalized pruritus and/or urticaria, macular or papular rash, angioedema, rare reports of anaphylactic reaction, abdominal pain, hypoglycemia.

INTERACTIONS: Caution with drugs that require rapid GI absorption. Drugs dependent on threshold concentrations for efficacy (eg, contraceptives, antibiotics) should be taken 1 hr before. Caution with concomitant use of warfarin; may lead to increased INR and possible bleeding.

PREGNANCY: Category C, caution in nursing.

MECHANISM OF ACTION: Antihyperglycemic, incretin-mimetic agent; enhances glucose-dependent insulin secretion by the pancreatic β-cell, suppresses inappropriately elevated glucagon secretion and slows gastric emptying.

PHARMACOKINETICS: Absorption: (SQ) C_{max}=211pg/mL, T_{max}=2.1 hrs. **Distribution:** V_d=28.3L. **Elimination:** $T_{1/2}$=2.4 hrs.

NURSING CONSIDERATIONS

Assessment: Assess for type 1 DM, pancreatitis, renal function test, gastroparesis, HbA_{1c}.

Monitoring: Monitor for symptoms of acute pancreatitis (severe abdominal pain, vomiting), renal function, and fasting blood glucose, HbA_{1c}, hypoglycemia, and body weight.

Patient Counseling: Take drug within 60-min period before morning and evening meals. Do not administer after a meal. If a dose is missed, resume treatment regimen as prescribed with the next scheduled dose. Report side effects.

Administration: SQ injection (thigh, abdomen, or upper arm). **Storage:** Prior to first use, keep at 2-8°C (36-46°F). After first use, keep at ≤25°C (77°F). Do not freeze. Protect from light. Discard pen 30 days after the first use, even if some drug remains.

BYSTOLIC RX

nebivolol (Forest)

THERAPEUTIC CLASS: Selective $beta_1$-blocker

INDICATIONS: Treatment of hypertension. May be used alone or in combination with other antihypertensive agents.

DOSAGE: *Adults:* Monotherapy/Combination Therapy: Initial: 5mg qd. Titrate: May increase dose if needed at 2-week intervals. Max: 40mg. Hepatic Impairment/CrCl <30mL/min: 2.5mg qd; upward titration may be performed cautiously.

HOW SUPPLIED: Tab: 2.5mg, 5mg, 10mg, 20mg

CONTRAINDICATIONS: Severe bradycardia, heart block >1st degree, cardiogenic shock, decompensated cardiac failure, sick sinus syndrome (unless permanent pacemaker in place), severe hepatic impairment (Child-Pugh >B).

WARNINGS/PRECAUTIONS: Exacerbation of angina, and occurrence of MI and ventricular arrhythmias reported in patients with CAD following abrupt withdrawal; taper over 1-2 weeks when possible. Avoid with bronchospastic disease. Caution with compensated CHF; consider d/c if heart failure worsens. Caution with PVD, severe renal/moderate hepatic impairment. May mask signs/symptoms of hypoglycemia or hyperthyroidism. Abrupt withdrawal may also exacerbate symptoms of hyperthyroidism or precipitate a thyroid storm. Caution with history of severe anaphylactic reactions. Patients with known/suspected pheochromocytoma should initially receive an α-blocker prior to use of any β-blocker. No studies done in patients with angina pectoris, recent MI, or severe hepatic impairment.

ADVERSE REACTIONS: Headache, fatigue, dizziness, diarrhea, nausea.

INTERACTIONS: CYP2D6 inhibitors (eg, fluoxetine, quinidine, propafenone, paroxetine) may increase nebivolol levels; monitor and consider dosage adjustment. Sildenafil may decrease nebivolol levels. May depress myocardial function with anesthetic agents (eg, ether, cyclopropane, trichloroethylene); monitor closely. May potentiate hypoglycemic effect of glucose-lowering agents (eg, insulin, oral hypoglycemic agents); use with caution. Caution with calcium antagonists (particularly verapamil and diltiazem type) or antiarrhythmic agents (eg, disopyramide). Excessive reduction of sympathetic activity may occur with catecholamine-depleting drugs (eg, reserpine, guanethidine); monitor closely. D/C for several days before gradually tapering clonidine.

PREGNANCY: Category C, not for use in nursing.

MECHANISM OF ACTION: A β-adrenergic receptor blocking agent.

PHARMACOKINETICS: Administration: Bioavailability not yet determined; C_{max}=2mg; T_{max}=1-4 hrs. **Distribution:** Plasma protein binding 98%. **Metabolism**: N-dealkylation and oxidation via P450 2D6. **Elimination**: Urine (38%), feces (44%).

NURSING CONSIDERATIONS

Assessment: Assess for severe bradycardia, heart block, cardiogenic shock, cardiac failure, sick sinus syndrome, angina, MI, severe hypotension, severe hepatic impairment, hypersensitivity, and any drug interactions.

Monitoring: Monitor diastolic BP, HR, renal clearance, serum glucose level, breathing, and weight gain.

Patient Counseling: Advise patient with CAD not to abruptly d/c therapy. Use with caution with severe renal impairment. Inform that drug can be taken with/without food. Instruct not to interrupt or d/c therapy without consulting physician.

Administration: Oral route. **Storage:** 20-25°C (68-77°F).

CADUET — RX

atorvastatin calcium - amlodipine besylate (Pfizer)

THERAPEUTIC CLASS: Calcium channel blocker/HMG-CoA reductase inhibitor

INDICATIONS: When treatment with both amlodipine and atorvastatin is appropriate. (Amlodipine) Treatment of hypertension, chronic stable or vasospastic angina (Prinzmetal's or Variant Angina). (Atorvastatin) Adjunct to diet to reduce total cholesterol (total-C), LDL-C, TG, and Apo B levels, and to increase HDL-C in primary hypercholesterolemia (heterozygous familial and nonfamilial) and mixed dyslipidemia (Types IIa and IIb). Adjunct to diet for elevated serum TG levels (Type IV). Treatment of primary dysbetalipoproteinemia (Type III) inadequately responding to diet. Adjunct to other lipid-lowering treatments or if treatments are unavailable, to reduce total-C and LDL-C in homozygous familial hypercholesterolemia. Adjunct to diet to lower total-C, LDL-C, and Apo B in boys and postmenarchal girls with heterozygous familial hypercholesterolemia.

DOSAGE: *Adults:* Dosing should be individualized and based on the appropriate combination of recommendations for the monotherapies. (Amlodipine): HTN: Initial: 5mg qd. Titrate over 7-14 days. Max: 10mg qd. Small, Fragile, or Elderly/Hepatic Dysfunction/Concomitant Antihypertensive: Initial: 2.5mg qd. Angina: 5-10mg qd. Elderly/Hepatic Dysfunction: 5mg qd. (Atorvastatin): Hypercholesterolemia/Mixed Dyslipidemia: Initial: 10-20mg qd (or 40mg qd for LDL-C reduction >45%). Titrate: Adjust dose if needed at 2-4 week intervals. Usual: 10-80mg qd. Homozygous Familial Hypercholesterolemia: 10-80mg qd.

Pediatrics: ≥10 yrs (postmenarchal): (Amlodipine): HTN: 2.5-5mg qd. 10-17 yrs (postmenarchal): (Atorvastatin): Heterozygous Familial Hypercholesterolemia: Initial: 10mg/day. Titrate: Adjust dose if needed at intervals of ≥4 weeks. Max: 20mg/day.

HOW SUPPLIED: Tab: (Amlodipine-Atorvastatin) 2.5mg-10mg, 2.5mg-20mg, 2.5mg-40mg, 5mg-10mg, 5mg-20mg, 5mg-40mg, 5mg-80mg, 10mg-10mg, 10mg-20mg, 10mg-40mg, 10mg-80mg

CONTRAINDICATIONS: Active liver disease, unexplained persistent elevations of serum transaminases, pregnancy, nursing mothers.

WARNINGS/PRECAUTIONS: May rarely increase angina or MI with severe obstructive CAD. Monitor LFTs prior to therapy, at 12 weeks after initiation, with dose elevation, and periodically thereafter. Reduce dose or withdraw if AST or ALT >3x ULN persists. Caution with heavy alcohol use and/or history of hepatic disease, severe aortic stenosis, CHF. D/C if markedly elevated CPK levels occur, if myopathy is diagnosed or suspected, or if predisposition to renal failure secondary to rhabdomyolysis. Increased risk of hemorrhagic stroke in patients with recent stroke or TIA.

ADVERSE REACTIONS: Headache, edema, palpitation, dizziness, fatigue, constipation, flatulence, dyspepsia, abdominal pain.

INTERACTIONS: Increases levels with erythromycin. Increases levels of oral contraceptives (norethindrone, ethinyl estradiol), digoxin. Cyclosporine, fibric acid derivatives, niacin, erythromycin, azole antifungals may increase risk of myopathy. Caution with drugs that decrease levels or activity of endogenous steroid hormones (eg, ketoconazole, spironolactone, cimetidine). Decreased levels with Maalox TC, but LDL-C reduction not altered. Colestipol decreases levels when coadministered, but greater LDL-C reduction with coadministration than when each given alone. Avoid fibrates.

PREGNANCY: Category X, not for use in nursing

NURSING CONSIDERATIONS

Assessment: Assess for severe aortic stenosis, CHF, pregnancy/nursing status, liver disease, obstructive CAD, alcoholism, and possible drug interactions. Obtain baseline LFTs.

Monitoring: Monitor LFTs at 12 weeks following initiation of therapy and any drug dose elevation, then periodically thereafter. Monitor for signs/symptoms of hypotension, hypersensitivity reaction, angina, and myopathy.

Patient Counseling: Advise to seek medical attention if symptoms of hypotension, hypersensitivity reaction, angina, or myopathy (unexplained muscle pain, tenderness, fever, malaise) occur. Instruct to avoid alcohol consumption.

Administration: Oral route. **Storage:** 25°C (77°F); excursions permitted to 15-30°C (59-86°F).

CALAN

RX

verapamil HCl (Pharmacia & Upjohn)

THERAPEUTIC CLASS: Calcium channel blocker (nondihydropyridine)

INDICATIONS: Treatment of hypertension and vasospastic, unstable and chronic stable angina. With digitalis, for control of ventricular rate at rest and during stress in patients with chronic atrial flutter and/or atrial fibrillation. Prophylaxis of repetitive paroxysmal supraventricular tachycardia.

DOSAGE: *Adults:* HTN: Initial: 80mg tid. Usual: 360-480mg/day. Elderly/Small Stature: Initial: 40mg tid. Angina: Usual: 80-120mg tid. Elderly/Small Stature: Initial: 40mg tid. Titrate: Increase daily or weekly. A-Fib (Digitalized): Usual: 240-320mg/day given tid-qid. PSVT Prophylaxis (Non-Digitalized): 240-480mg/day given tid-qid. Max: 480mg/day. Severe Hepatic Dysfunction: Give 30% of normal dose.

HOW SUPPLIED: Tab: 40mg, 80mg*, 120mg* *scored

CONTRAINDICATIONS: Severe ventricular dysfunction, hypotension, cardiogenic shock, sick sinus syndrome or 2nd- or 3rd-degree AV block (except with functioning ventricular pacemaker), A-Fib/Flutter with an accessory bypass tract.

WARNINGS/PRECAUTIONS: Avoid with moderate to severe cardiac failure, and ventricular dysfunction if taking a β-blocker. May cause hypotension, AV block, transient bradycardia, PR interval prolongation. Monitor LFTs periodically; hepatocellular injury reported. Caution with hypertrophic cardiomyopathy, renal or hepatic dysfunction. Decrease dose with decreased neuromuscular transmission.

ADVERSE REACTIONS: Constipation, dizziness, nausea, hypotension, headache, edema, CHF, fatigue, elevated liver enzymes, dyspnea, bradycardia, AV block, rash, flushing.

INTERACTIONS: Additive effects on HR, AV conduction, and contractility with β-blockers. Potentiates other antihypertensives. May increase digoxin, carbamazepine, theophylline, cyclosporine, and alcohol levels. Avoid disopyramide within 48 hrs before or 24 hrs after verapamil. Additive negative inotropic effects and AV conduction prolongation with flecainide. Avoid quinidine with hypertrophic cardiomyopathy. Monitor lithium. Increased clearance with phenobarbital. Rifampin may reduce oral bioavailability. May potentiate neuromuscular blockers; both agents may need dose reduction.

PREGNANCY: Category C, not for use in nursing.

MECHANISM OF ACTION: Calcium channel blocker; modulates influx of ionic calcium across cell membrane of arterial smooth muscle, conductile and contractile myocardial cells.

PHARMACOKINETICS: Absorption: Bioavailability (20-35%), T_{max}=1-2 hrs. **Distribution:** Plasma protein binding (90%). **Metabolism:** Biotransformation. Norverapamil (metabolite). **Elimination:** Urine (3-4%), feces; $T_{1/2}$=4.5-12 hrs.

C

NURSING CONSIDERATIONS

Assessment: Assess for severe left ventricular dysfunction, Duchenne's muscular dystrophy, hypotension, sick sinus syndrome, AV block, atrial flutter/fibrillation with accessory bypass tract (WPW), possible drug interactions, hepatic/renal impairment.

Monitoring: Monitor LFTs and renal function periodically. Monitor for abnormal PR interval prolongation for toxicity; signs/symptoms of hepatotoxicity, renal dysfunction, CV events (hypotension), and hypersensitivity reactions.

Patient Counseling: Advise to seek medical attention if symptoms of hepatotoxicity (malaise, fever, RUQ pain), CV events (hypotension), or hypersensitivity reactions occur.

Administration: Oral route. **Storage:** 15-25°C (59-77°F). Protect from light.

CALAN SR — RX

verapamil HCl (Pharmacia & Upjohn)

THERAPEUTIC CLASS: Calcium channel blocker (nondihydropyridine)

INDICATIONS: Treatment of hypertension.

DOSAGE: *Adults:* ≥18 yrs: Initial: 180mg qam. Titrate: If inadequate response, increase to 240mg qam, then 180mg bid; or 240mg qam plus 120mg qpm, then 240mg q12h. Elderly/Small Stature: Initial: 120mg qam. Take with food.

HOW SUPPLIED: Tab, Extended-Release: 120mg, 180mg*, 240mg* *scored

CONTRAINDICATIONS: Severe ventricular dysfunction, hypotension, cardiogenic shock, sick sinus syndrome or 2nd- or 3rd-degree AV block (except with functioning ventricular pacemaker), A-Fib/Flutter with an accessory bypass tract.

WARNINGS/PRECAUTIONS: Avoid with moderate to severe cardiac failure, and ventricular dysfunction if taking a β-blocker. May cause hypotension, AV block, transient bradycardia, PR interval prolongation. Monitor LFTs periodically; hepatocellular injury reported. Caution with hypertrophic cardiomyopathy, renal or hepatic dysfunction. Decrease dose with decreased neuromuscular transmission.

ADVERSE REACTIONS: Constipation, dizziness, nausea, hypotension, headache, edema, CHF, fatigue, elevated liver enzymes, dyspnea, bradycardia, AV block, rash, flushing.

INTERACTIONS: Additive effects on HR, AV conduction, and contractility with β-blockers. Potentiates other antihypertensives. May increase digoxin, carbamazepine, theophylline, cyclosporine, and alcohol levels. Avoid disopyramide within 48 hrs before or 24 hrs after verapamil. Additive negative inotropic effects and AV conduction prolongation with flecainide. Avoid quinidine with hypertrophic cardiomyopathy. Monitor lithium. Increased clearance with phenobarbital. Rifampin may reduce oral bioavailability. May potentiate neuromuscular blockers; both agents may need dose reduction.

PREGNANCY: Category C, not for use in nursing.

MECHANISM OF ACTION: Calcium channel blocker; modulates influx of ionic calcium across cell membrane of arterial smooth muscle and in conductile and contractile myocardial cells.

PHARMACOKINETICS: Absorption: Absolute bioavailability (20-35%); T_{max}=7.7 hrs; C_{max}=79ng/mL; AUC=841ng•h/mL. **Distribution:** Plasma protein binding (90%). **Metabolism:** Biotransformation; norverapamil (metabolite). **Elimination:** $T_{1/2}$=4.5-12 hrs; urine (3-4%), feces.

NURSING CONSIDERATIONS

Assessment: Assess for severe left ventricular dysfunction, Duchenne's muscular dystrophy, severe heart failure, hypotension, sick sinus syndrome, AV block, atrial flutter/fibrillation with accessory bypass tract (eg, Wolff-Parkinson-White), possible drug interactions, hypertrophic cardiomyopathy, hepatic/renal impairment.

Monitoring: Monitor LFTs and renal function periodically; abnormal PR-interval prolongation for toxicity. Monitor for signs/symptoms of hepatotoxicity, renal dysfunction, CV events (hypotension), and hypersensitivity reactions.

Patient Counseling: Advise to seek medical attention if symptoms of hepatotoxicity (malaise, fever, right upper quadrant pain), CV events (hypotension), or hypersensitivity reactions occur.

Administration: Oral route. **Storage:** 15-25°C (59-77°F). Protect from light and moisture.

CAMPATH RX

alemtuzumab (Bayer Healthcare)

Cytopenias such as serious, including fatal, pancytopenia/marrow hypoplasia, autoimmune idiopathic thrombocytopenia, and autoimmune hemolytic anemia may occur; avoid single doses >30mg or cumulative doses >90mg/week. Serious, including fatal, infusion reactions can result; gradually escalate dose to prevent. Serious, including fatal, bacterial, viral, fungal, and protozoan infections can occur; administer prophylaxis against PCP and herpes virus infections.

THERAPEUTIC CLASS: Monoclonal antibody/CD52-blocker

INDICATIONS: As a single agent for the treatment of B-cell chronic lymphocytic leukemia (B-CLL).

DOSAGE: *Adults:* Administer as IV infusion over 2 hours. Initial: 3mg IV qd until tolerated, then increase to 10mg IV qd. Continue until tolerated, then increase to maint dose of 30mg (escalation to 30mg usually takes 3-7 days). Maint: 30mg/day IV 3x/week on alternate days up to 12 weeks. Max: 30mg single dose or 90mg/week. Refer to prescribing information for dose modifications for neutropenia or thrombocytopenia.

HOW SUPPLIED: Inj: 30mg/mL

WARNINGS/PRECAUTIONS: Premedicate with oral antihistamine, APAP to avoid infusion reactions. Monitor BP, hypotensive symptoms in ischemic heart disease, with antihypertensives. If serious infection occurs, withhold treatment until infection resolves. Monitor CBC, platelets weekly during therapy and CD4 counts after therapy. D/C for autoimmune or severe hematologic adverse reactions. Severe, including fatal, autoimmune anemia and thrombocytopenia, and prolonged myelosuppression reported. Hemolytic anemia, pure red cell aplasia, bone marrow aplasia, and hypoplasia reported. D/C for autoimmune cytopenias. Severe and prolonged lymphopenias with increased incidence of opportunistic infections reported. Administer PCP and herpes viral prophylaxis for a minimum of 2 months after completion or until CD4+ count is ≥200 cells/µL and monitor for CMV infection during and for at least 2 months after completion of treatment.

ADVERSE REACTIONS: Cytopenias, infusion reactions, cytomegalovirus (CMV) and other infections, nausea, emesis, diarrhea, insomnia.

INTERACTIONS: Avoid live viral vaccines.

PREGNANCY: Category C, not for use in nursing.

MECHANISM OF ACTION: Monoclonal antibody/CD52-blocker; binds to CD52 on surfaces of B and T lymphocytes, monocytes, macrophages, NK cells, granulocytes and bone marrow cells, causing antibody-dependent cellular-mediated cell death.

PHARMACOKINETICS: Distribution: V_d=0.18L/kg. **Elimination:** (1st dose) $T_{1/2}$=11 hrs. (Last dose) $T_{1/2}$=6 days.

NURSING CONSIDERATIONS

Assessment: Assess pregnancy status. Obtain baseline CBC, CD4, and platelet count.

Monitoring: Monitor CBC and platelet counts weekly; CD4 count after therapy until recovery to >200cells/mL; for CMV infections during therapy and 2 months following completion. Monitor for signs/symptoms of autoimmune anemia, thrombocytopenia, myelosuppression, hemolytic anemia, pure red cell aplasia, bone marrow aplasia, hypoplasia, infusion reactions (pyrexia, chills/rigors, nausea, hypotension, urticaria, dyspnea, rash, emesis, bronchospasm), immunosuppression, and exacerbation of infection.

C

Patient Counseling: Instruct irradiation of blood products required until adequate lymphocyte recovery; use effective contraceptive methods during treatment and at least 6 months following therapy. Inform should not be immunized with live vaccines if recently treated. Counsel on importance of need to take premedications and prophylactic anti-infectives as prescribed. Advise to seek medical attention if symptoms of bleeding, easy bruising, petechiae/purpura, pallor, weakness, fatigue, infusion reactions, or infection (pyrexia) occur.

Administration: IV infusion. **Storage:** 2-8°C (36-46°F). Do not freeze. If frozen, thaw at 2-8°C before administration. Protect from direct sunlight.

CAMPRAL RX
acamprosate calcium (Forest)

THERAPEUTIC CLASS: GABA analog

INDICATIONS: Maintenance of abstinence from alcohol in patients with alcohol dependence who are abstinent at treatment initiation.

DOSAGE: *Adults:* 2 tabs tid. CrCl 30-50mL/min: 1 tab tid.

HOW SUPPLIED: Tab: 333mg

CONTRAINDICATIONS: Severe renal impairment (CrCl ≤30mL/min).

WARNINGS/PRECAUTIONS: Use does not eliminate or diminish withdrawal symptoms. Dose reduction required with renal impairment (CrCl ≤30-50mL/min). Suicidal events reported.

ADVERSE REACTIONS: Accidental injury, asthenia, pain, anorexia, diarrhea, flatulence, nausea, anxiety, depression, dizziness, dry mouth, insomnia, paresthesia, pruritus, sweating.

INTERACTIONS: Naltrexone may increase levels. Weight gain/weight loss may occur with antidepressants.

PREGNANCY: Category C, caution in nursing.

MECHANISM OF ACTION: GABA analogue; not completely understood; suspected to interact with glutamate and GABA neurotransmitter systems centrally, hypothesized that the drug restores this balance.

PHARMACOKINETICS: Absorption: Absolute bioavailability (11%); C_{max}=350ng/mL; T_{max}=3-8 hrs. **Distribution:** V_d=72-109L. **Elimination:** Urine; $T_{1/2}$=20-33 hrs.

NURSING CONSIDERATIONS

Assessment: Assess for renal impairment.

Monitoring: Monitor for emergence of symptoms of depression and suicidality.

Patient Counseling: Caution while performing hazardous tasks (operating machinery/driving). Notify if pregnant/nursing or planning to become pregnant. Alert families/caregivers to look for symptoms of suicidality or depression.

Administration: Oral route. **Storage:** 25°C (77°F); excursions permitted to 15-30°C (59-86°F).

CAMPTOSAR RX
irinotecan HCl (Pharmacia & Upjohn)

Early and/or late forms of diarrhea, severe myelosuppression may occur. Interrupt and reduce subsequent doses if severe diarrhea occurs. Carefully monitor with diarrhea; give fluid/electrolyte replacement if dehydrated or give antibiotics if ileus, fever, or severe neutropenia develop.

THERAPEUTIC CLASS: Topoisomerase I inhibitor

INDICATIONS: First-line therapy in combination with 5-fluorouracil (5-FU) and leucovorin (LV) for metastatic colon or rectal carcinomas, and for disease that has progressed or recurred following initial 5-FU therapy.

DOSAGE: *Adults:* Combination Therapy (5-FU/LV, see PI for dosage): 125mg/m² IV over 90 min on days 1, 8, 15, 22 for 6 weeks; or 180mg/m² IV over 90 min on days 1, 15, and 29 for 6 weeks. Both regimens: Begin next cycle on Day 43. Single Therapy: 125mg/m² IV over 90 min on days 1, 8, 15, 22 followed by a 2 week rest; or 350mg/m² IV over 90 min once every 3 weeks. Premedicate with antiemetics at least 30 min prior to therapy. Dose modifications for reduced UGT1A1 activity, neutropenia, diarrhea, and other toxicities: See PI. All dose modifications should be based on worst preceding toxicity.

HOW SUPPLIED: Inj: 20mg/mL

WARNINGS/PRECAUTIONS: Due to increased toxicity, avoid use of irinotecan with the "Mayo Clinic" regimen of 5-FU/LV (given 4-5 days every 4 weeks). Treat/prevent early diarrhea with atropine IV/SQ and late diarrhea (occurring >24 hrs after dose) with loperamide PO. If late diarrhea occurs, delay therapy until return of pretreatment bowel function for at least 24 hrs without antidiarrheals; decrease subsequent doses if late diarrhea is Grade 2, 3, or 4. Deaths due to sepsis reported following severe neutropenia. Temporarily hold therapy if neutropenic fever occurs or if neutrophils <1000/mm³. Increased risk for neutropenia in patients homozygous for the UGT1A1 28 allele. Consider reduced initial dose. Heterozygous patients may also have increased risk. Hypersensitivity reactions, colitis, ileus, and renal impairment/failure, thromboembolic events reported. May cause fetal harm during pregnancy. Monitor for extravasation at infusion site. Consider atropine for cholinergic symptoms. Caution with modestly elevated baseline bilirubin levels (eg, 1-2mg/dL), abnormal glucuronidation of bilirubin, hepatic insufficiency, elderly with comorbidities, previous pelvic/abdominal irradiation. Careful monitoring of WBC with differential, Hgb, and platelets is recommended before each dose. Avoid in severe bone marrow failure, and fructose intolerant patients.

ADVERSE REACTIONS: NV, diarrhea, abdominal pain, blood dyscrasias, asthenia, mucositis, anorexia, alopecia, fever, pain, constipation, infection, dyspnea, increased bilirubin.

INTERACTIONS: Exacerbated myelosuppression and diarrhea with antineoplastic agents having similar adverse effects. Avoid concurrent irradiation therapy. Possible hyperglycemia and lymphocytopenia with dexamethasone. Akathisia reported with prochlorperazine. Laxatives may worsen diarrhea. Consider withholding diuretics with irinotecan therapy. Decreased levels with CYP3A4 inducing anticonvulsants and St. John's wort. Consider substituting non-enzyme inducing anticonvulsants 2 weeks prior to and during treatment. Increased levels with ketoconazole. Discontinue ketoconazole at least 1 week prior to and during therapy.

PREGNANCY: Category D, not for use in nursing.

MECHANISM OF ACTION: Topoisomerase I inhibitor; binds to topoisomerase I-DNA complex and prevents religation of single-strand breaks induced by the enzyme to relieve torsional strain in DNA.

PHARMACOKINETICS: Absorption: Irinotecan: (125mg/m²); C_{max}=1660ng/mL; AUC_{0-24}=10200ng•h/mL. (340mg/m²); C_{max}=3392ng/mL; AUC_{0-24}=20604ng•h/mL. SN-38: (125mg/m²) C_{max}=26.3ng/mL; AUC_{0-24}=229ng•h/mL. (340mg/m²) C_{max}=56ng/mL; AUC_{0-24}=474ng•h/mL. **Distribution:** Irinotecan: (125mg/m²) V_d=110L/m². (340mg/m²) V_d=234L/m². Plasma protein binding (30-68%). SN-38: Plasma protein binding (95%). **Metabolism:** Liver via carboxyl esterase. Metabolite (SN-38). **Elimination:** Irinotecan: Urine (11-20%). (125mg/m²) $T_{1/2}$=5.8 hrs. (340mg/m²) $T_{1/2}$=11.7 hrs. SN-38: Urine (<1%). (125mg/m²) $T_{1/2}$=10.4 hrs. (340mg/m²) $T_{1/2}$=21 hrs

NURSING CONSIDERATIONS

Assessment: Assess for severe bone marrow failure, bowel obstruction, hereditary fructose intolerance, reduced UDP-glucuronosyl transferase 1A1 activity, pregnancy status, DM, glucose intolerance, pelvic/abdominal radiation. Assess in elderly patients with comorbid conditions. Assess for deficient glucuronidation of bilirubin (Gilbert's syndrome), possible drug interactions, renal/hepatic function. Assess WBC with differential, Hgb, platelet count.

Monitoring: Monitor WBC with differential, Hgb, platelet count before each dose. Monitor for toxicity before each dose. Assess need to premedicate with antiemetics. Monitor for signs/symptoms of renal impairment, colitis/ileus, severe neutropenia (complications, fever), severe myelosuppression, inflammation of infusion site, thromboembolism, early and late form diarrhea (may lead to dehydration, electrolyte imbalance, sepsis), rhinitis, increased salivation, miosis, lacrimation, diaphoresis, flushing, intestinal hyperperistalsis, and anaphylactic reactions.

Patient Counseling: Instruct to avoid vaccinations with live vaccines. Inform of pregancy risks. Inform of toxic effects (GI complications). Instruct not to use with laxative properties and to have loperamide ready to use for treatment of late diarrhea occurring >24 hrs after infusion at 1st episode of poorly formed or loose stool. Inform loperamide not recommended for >48 hrs (risk of paralytic ileus). Premedication of loperamide not recommended. Seek medical attention for symptoms of diarrhea (first time during treatment), black or bloody stools, dehydration (lightheadedness, dizziness, faintness), inability to take fluids by mouth due to NV, inability to get diarrhea under control within 24 hrs, fever, evidence of infection, toxicity, or anaphylactic reactions. Caution dizziness or visual disturbances may occur within 24 hrs; may impair physical/mental abilities.

Administration: IV route. Dilute in 5% Dextrose or 0.9% NaCl to final concentration range of 0.12-2.8mg/mL. **Storage:** 25°C (stable for 24 hrs); 2-8°C (stable for 48 hrs). (Diluted): 15-30°C (59-86°F); (stable for 6 hrs). Protect from light.

CANASA RX

mesalamine (Axcan Scandipharm)

THERAPEUTIC CLASS: Anti-inflammatory Agent

INDICATIONS: Treatment of active ulcerative proctitis.

DOSAGE: *Adults:* 1000mg rectally qhs. Retain suppository for at least 1-3 hrs.

HOW SUPPLIED: Sup: 1000mg

CONTRAINDICATIONS: Hypersensitivity to suppository vehicle (eg, saturated vegetable fatty acid esters) or salicylates.

WARNINGS/PRECAUTIONS: D/C if acute intolerance syndrome develops (eg, cramping, bloody diarrhea, abdominal pain, headache); consider sulfasalazine hypersensitivity. If rechallenge is considered, perform under careful observation. Caution with sulfasalazine hypersensitivity. Carefully monitor with renal dysfunction. Pancolitis, pericarditis (rare) reported.

ADVERSE REACTIONS: Dizziness, rectal pain, fever, acne, colitis, rash, hair loss.

PREGNANCY: Category B, caution in nursing.

MECHANISM OF ACTION: Not fully established; anti-inflammatory drug appears to act topically rather than systemically. Postulated to have a role as free radical scavenger or inhibitor of tumor necrosis factor.

PHARMACOKINETICS: Absorption: Variable; C_{max}=361ng/mL. **Metabolism:** Extensively metabolized to N-acetyl-5-ASA. **Elimination:** Urine; $T_{1/2}$=7 hrs.

NURSING CONSIDERATIONS

Assessment: Assess for hypersensitivity to the suppository vehicle, sulfa allergy, pre-existing renal disease, history of pancreatitis, and pericarditis. Obtain baseline renal function (BUN, creatinine, urinalysis).

Monitoring: Monitor renal function (BUN, creatinine, urinalysis) periodically, signs/symptoms of pericarditis, pancreatitis, acute intolerance syndrome (cramping, abdominal pain, bloody diarrhea), renal dysfunction, hypersensitivity, and allergic reactions.

Patient Counseling: Inform may cause stains. Advise to empty rectum before use and not to handle too much. If miss dose, use as soon as possible, unless almost time for next dose. Do not use 2 doses at once. Seek medical attention if chest pain, SOB, cramping, abdominal pain, bloody diarrhea, hypersensitivity, and allergic reactions occur. Inform to d/c if rash or fever occur.

Administration: Rectal route. 1) Remove plastic wrapper. 2) Avoid excessive handling. 3) Insert completely into rectum. 4) Lubricant may be used to assist insertion. **Storage:** 25°C (77°F), do not freeze. Keep away from direct heat, light or humidity, and out of reach of children.

CANCIDAS — RX

caspofungin acetate (Merck)

THERAPEUTIC CLASS: Glucan synthesis inhibitor

INDICATIONS: For adults and pediatric patients (≥3 months): Empirical therapy for presumed fungal infections in febrile, neutropenic patients. Treatment of candidemia and the following *Candida* infections: intra-abdominal abscesses, peritonitis, and pleural space infections. Treatment of esophageal candidiasis. Treatment of invasive aspergillosis in patients refractory to or intolerant of other therapies (eg, amphotericin B, itraconazole).

DOSAGE: *Adults:* Empirical Therapy: LD: 70mg IV on Day 1. Maint: 50mg IV qd. If 50mg is well tolerated but does not provide adequate clinical response, daily dose can be increased to 70mg. Fungal infections should be treated for a minimum of 14 days. Continue treatment 7 days after neutropenia and clinical symptoms are resolved. Candidemia/*Candida* Infections: LD: 70mg IV on Day 1. Maint: 50mg IV qd. Esophageal Candidiasis: 50mg IV qd. Consider PO suppressive therapy with HIV. Invasive Aspergillosis: LD: 70mg IV on Day 1. Maint: 50mg IV qd. Moderate Hepatic Insufficiency (Child-Pugh Score 7-9): LD: 70mg IV on Day 1. Maint: 35mg IV qd. Concomitant Rifampin: 70mg IV qd. Concomitant Nevirapine/Efavirenz/Carbamazepine/Dexamethasone/Phenytoin: May need to increase dose to 70mg IV qd. Base duration of treatment on severity of disease, clinical response, microbiological response, and recovery from immunosuppression.
Pediatrics: 3 months-17 yrs: LD: 70mg/m^2 IV on Day 1. Maint: 50mg/m^2 IV qd. If 50mg/m^2 is well tolerated but does not provide adequate clinical response, daily dose can be increased to 70mg/m^2. Max: 70mg/day. Concomitant Rifampin/Nevirapine/Efavirenz/Carbamazepine/Dexamethasone/Phenytoin: 70mg/m^2 IV qd. Max: 70mg/day.

HOW SUPPLIED: Inj: 50mg, 70mg

WARNINGS/PRECAUTIONS: LFT abnormalities may be seen; if abnormal LFTs develop, monitor for evidence of worsening hepatic function and re-evaluate.

ADVERSE REACTIONS: Fever, chills, hypotension, diarrhea, NV, abdominal pain, edema, headache, rash, pneumonia, cough, erythema, anaphylaxis.

INTERACTIONS: Reduces blood levels of tacrolimus. Efavirenz, nevirapine, phenytoin, rifampin, dexamethasone, carbamazepine may decrease levels. Increased levels with cyclosporine; use only when benefits outweigh risks. Do not mix or co-infuse with other medications. Do not use with dextrose-containing diluents.

PREGNANCY: Category C, caution in nursing.

MECHANISM OF ACTION: Antifungal; inhibits the synthesis of β (1,3)-D-glucan, a primary component responsible for cell-wall synthesis in susceptible fungi.

PHARMACOKINETICS: Distribution: Plasma protein binding (97%); found in breast milk. **Metabolism:** Hydrolysis and N-acetylation (slowly). **Elimination:** Urine (41%), feces (35%).

NURSING CONSIDERATIONS

Assessment: Assess use in patients who are on concomitant therapy with cyclosporine. Assess hepatic function prior to therapy.

C

Monitoring: Monitor for histamine-related and anaphylaxis reactions (eg, rash, facial swelling, bronchospasm) when administering. Monitor LFTs and CBC while on therapy.

Patient Counseling: Counsel to notify physician if rash or swelling develops. Continue empiric therapy until neutropenia is resolved. Treat patients with a fungal infection for at least 14 days; treatment should continue for at least 7 days after both neutropenia and clinical symptoms are resolved.

Administration: IV infusion. Do not mix or co-infuse with other intravenous substances, additives, or other medications. Do not use diluents containing dextrose. 1) Equilibrate refrigerated vial to room temperature. 2) Reconstitute. Add 10.8mL to compatible solution 0.9% sodium chloride injection, sterile water for injection, bacteriostatic water for injection with methylparaben and propylparaben, or bacteriostatic water for injection with 0.9% benzyl alcohol to the vial. 3) Transfer 10mL of reconstituted solution to a 250mL IV bag containing 0.9%, 0.45%, or 0.225% sodium chloride injection or lactated ringer's injection. Refer to full prescribing information for alternate preparations.
Storage: Vial: Refrigerate at 2-8°C (36-46°F). Reconstituted: May be stored at ≤25°C (≤77°F) for 1 hr prior to preparation of patient infusion solution. Final infusion: ≤25°C (≤77°F) for 24 hrs or at 2-8°C (36-46°F) for 48 hours.

CAPOZIDE **RX**
hydrochlorothiazide - captopril (Par)

ACE inhibitors can cause death/injury to developing fetus during 2nd and 3rd trimesters. Stop therapy if pregnancy detected.

THERAPEUTIC CLASS: ACE inhibitor/thiazide diuretic

INDICATIONS: Treatment of hypertension.

DOSAGE: *Adults:* Initial: 25mg-15mg tab qd. Titrate: Adjust dose at 6-week intervals. Max: 150mg captopril/50mg HCTZ per day. Replacement Therapy: Substitute combination for titrated components. Renal Impairment: Decrease dose or increase interval. Take 1 hr before meals.

HOW SUPPLIED: Tab: (Captopril-HCTZ) 25mg-15mg*, 25mg-25mg*, 50mg-15mg*, 50mg-25mg* *scored

CONTRAINDICATIONS: History of ACE inhibitor-associated angioedema, anuria, sulfonamide hypersensitivity.

WARNINGS/PRECAUTIONS: D/C if angioedema, jaundice, or if marked LFT elevation occurs. Risk of hyperkalemia with DM, renal dysfunction. Monitor WBCs in renal and collagen vascular disease. Fetal/neonatal morbidity and death reported. Monitor for hypotension in high-risk patients (eg, surgery/anesthesia, volume/salt depletion). Caution with renal or hepatic dysfunction. More reports of angioedema in blacks than nonblacks. May exacerbate or activate systemic lupus erythematosus. Monitor electrolytes. Hypercalcemia, hypomagnesemia, hyperuricemia may occur. With renal impairment, monitor WBCs and differential before therapy, every 2 weeks for 3 months, then periodically. Neutropenia with myeloid hypoplasia, persistent nonproductive cough, anaphylactoid reactions, proteinuria reported.

ADVERSE REACTIONS: Cough, hypotension, rash, pruritus, fever, arthralgia, eosinophilia, dysgeusia, neutropenia/thrombocytopenia.

INTERACTIONS: Increased risk of hyperkalemia with K^+-sparing diuretics, K^+ supplements, or K^+-containing salt substitutes. Potentiates orthostatic hypotension with alcohol, barbiturates, and narcotics. Adjust other antihypertensives, anticoagulants, antidiabetic, or antigout drugs. Reduced absorption with cholestyramine, colestipol. Amphotericin B, corticosteroids, ACTH deplete electrolytes. May decrease methenamine effects. May decrease response to pressor amines. May potentiate non-depolarizing skeletal muscle relaxants, anesthetics. Risk of lithium toxicity. NSAIDs (eg, indomethacin) reduce effects. Enhanced hypotensive effects with MAOIs. Probenecid, sulfinpyrazone may need dose increase. Diazoxide enhances hyperglycemic, hyperuricemic, and antihypertensive effects. Monitor serum calcium levels with calcium salts. Monitor potassium levels with cardiac glycosides. Caution with agents affecting sympathetic activity. D/C vasodilators before therapy. Caution and decrease vasodilator dose if resumed during therapy.

PREGNANCY: Category C (1st trimester) and D (2nd and 3rd trimesters), not for use in nursing.

MECHANISM OF ACTION: Captopril: ACE inhibitor; not established. Effects appear to result from suppression of renin-angiotensin-aldosterone system. HCTZ: Thiazide diuretic. Affects renal tubular mechanism of electrolyte reabsorption.

PHARMACOKINETICS: Absorption: Captopril: Rapid; T_{max}=1 hr. **Distribution:** Captopril: Plasma protein binding (25-30%). **Elimination:** Captopril: Urine (40-50%); $T_{1/2}$≤2 hrs. HCTZ: Kidney; $T_{1/2}$=2.5 hrs.

NURSING CONSIDERATIONS

Assessment: Assess for pregnancy status, possible drug interactions, volume/salt depletion, SLE, DM, anuria, sulfonamide hypersensitivity, history of allergy or bronchial asthma, collagen vascular disease, CHF, hepatic/renal impairment. Obtain baseline serum electrolytes, renal function, and WBC with differential (impaired renal function).

Monitoring: Monitor serum electrolytes and renal function periodically. If impaired renal function, monitor WBC with differential before therapy, at 2-week intervals for 3 months, and then periodically during therapy. Monitor for signs/symptoms of electrolyte imbalance, exacerbation or activation of systemic lupus erythematosus (SLE), hypotension, hyperuricemia or precipitation of gout, anaphylactoid or hypersensitivity reactions, head/neck and intestinal angioedema, infection, and neutropenia/agranulocytosis.

Patient Counseling: Instruct to take 1 hr before meal. Inform of pregnancy risks. Advise that inadequate fluid intake or loss of fluids may lead to drop in BP, resulting in lightheadedness or syncope. Instruct not to interrupt or d/c therapy without consulting physician; may cause withdrawal symptoms (eg, angina). Advise to seek medical attention if symptoms of angioedema (head/neck; intestinal; abdominal pain with/without NV), infection (eg, sore throat, fever), syncope, edema, hypersensitivity reactions, or electrolyte imbalance (eg, dry mouth, thirst, lethargy) occur.

Administration: Oral route. **Storage:** Below 30°C (86°F).

CAPTOPRIL — RX

captopril (Various)

ACE inhibitors can cause death/injury to developing fetus during 2nd and 3rd trimesters. Stop therapy if pregnancy detected.

OTHER BRAND NAMES: Capoten (Par)

THERAPEUTIC CLASS: ACE inhibitor

INDICATIONS: Treatment of hypertension alone or in combination with other antihypertensive agents (eg, thiazide-type diuretics) and CHF in combination with diuretics and digitalis. To improve survival in stable post-MI patients with left ventricular dysfunction and to reduce the incidence of overt heart failure or hospitalizations for CHF in these patients. Diabetic nephropathy (proteinuria >500mg/day) and slows progression of renal insufficiency in type 1 diabetes.

DOSAGE: *Adults:* Take 1 hour before meals. HTN: If possible, d/c recent antihypertensive drug for 1 week prior to therapy. Initial: 25mg bid-tid. Titrate: May increase to 50mg bid-tid after 1-2 weeks. With Concomitant Diuretic Therapy: Range: 25-150mg bid-tid. Max: 450mg/day. CHF: Initial: 25mg tid. Titrate: May increase to 50-100mg tid. With Risk of Hypotension or Salt/Volume Depletion: Initial: 6.25mg or 12.5mg tid. Max: 450mg/day. Left Ventricular Dysfunction Post-MI: Initial: 6.25mg single dose, then 12.5mg tid. Titrate: Increase to 25mg tid over next several days, then to 50mg tid over next several weeks. Usual: 50mg tid. Diabetic Nephropathy: 25mg tid. Significant Renal Dysfunction: Decrease initial dose and titrate slowly.

HOW SUPPLIED: Tab: 12.5mg*, 25mg*, 50mg*, 100mg* *scored

CONTRAINDICATIONS: History of ACE inhibitor-associated angioedema.

C

WARNINGS/PRECAUTIONS: Persistent nonproductive cough, anaphylactoid reactions, angioedema, and neutropenia/agranulocytosis with myeloid hypoplasia reported. D/C if jaundice or marked LFT elevation occurs. Risk of hyperkalemia with DM, renal dysfunction. Fetal/neonatal morbidity and death reported. Monitor for hypotension in high-risk patients (surgery/anesthesia, dialysis, heart failure, volume/salt depletion, etc). Caution with CHF, renal dysfunction, renal artery stenosis, collagen vascular disease (especially with renal dysfunction). Monitor WBC before therapy, then every 2 weeks for 3 months, then periodically. Less effective on BP in blacks and more reports of angioedema than nonblacks.

ADVERSE REACTIONS: Proteinuria, neutropenia/agranulocytosis, rash, hypotension, angioedema, dysgeusia, cough, MI, jaundice, pancreatitis, hyponatremia, myalgia, blurred vision.

INTERACTIONS: May increase lithium levels. NSAIDs may decrease antihypertensive effects. Hypotension risk with diuretics. Increased risk of hyperkalemia with K^+-sparing diuretics, K^+-containing salt substitutes, or K^+ supplements. Caution with vasodilators or agents affecting sympathetic activity. Augmented effect by antihypertensives that cause renin release (eg, thiazides). Nitritoid reactions (eg, facial flushing, NV, hypotension) reported rarely with injectable gold.

PREGNANCY: Category C (1st trimester) and D (2nd and 3rd trimesters), not for use in nursing.

MECHANISM OF ACTION: ACE inhibitor; not established. Effects appear to result from suppression of renin-angiotensin-aldosterone system.

PHARMACOKINETICS: Absorption: Rapid; T_{max}=1 hr. **Distribution:** Plasma protein binding (25-30%). **Elimination:** Urine (40-50%); $T_{1/2}$=≤2 hrs.

NURSING CONSIDERATIONS

Assessment: Assess for pregnancy status, possible drug interactions, volume/salt depletion, DM, collagen vascular disease, CHF, aortic stenosis, hepatic/renal impairment. Obtain baseline BP, renal function, and WBC with differential (impaired renal function).

Monitoring: Monitor renal function periodically; BP in first 2 weeks and whenever dosage changes. If impaired renal function, monitor WBC with differential before therapy, at 2-week intervals for 3 months, and then periodically during therapy. Monitor for signs/symptoms of hypotension, anaphylactoid or hypersensitivity reactions, head/neck and intestinal angioedema, infection, and neutropenia/agranulocytosis.

Patient Counseling: Inform of pregnancy risks; inadequate fluid intake or loss of fluids may lead to drop in BP resulting in lightheadedness or syncope. Instruct to take 1 hr before meal. Instruct not to interrupt or d/c therapy without consulting physician; may cause withdrawal symptoms (eg, angina). Advise to seek medical attention if symptoms of angioedema (head/neck; intestinal/abdominal pain with/without N/V), infection (eg, sore throat, fever), syncope, edema, or hypersensitivity reactions occur. Caution patients against excessive perspiration and dehydration to avoid excessive fall in BP.

Administration: Oral route. **Storage:** 20-25°C (68-77°F). Protect from moisture.

CARBATROL — RX

carbamazepine (Shire)

Serious and fatal dermatologic reactions, including toxic epidermal necrolysis (TEN), Stevens-Johnson syndrome (SJS) and presence of HLA-B*1502 allele reported. Aplastic anemia and agranulocytosis reported. Obtain complete pretreatment hematological testing as a baseline. D/C if evidence of bone marrow depression develops.

THERAPEUTIC CLASS: Carboxamide

C

INDICATIONS: Treatment of partial seizures with complex symptomatology, generalized tonic-clonic seizures, and mixed seizure patterns of these or other partial or generalized seizures. Treatment of trigeminal neuralgia pain.

DOSAGE: *Adults:* Epilepsy: Initial: 200mg bid. Titrate: May increase weekly by 200mg/day. Maint: 800-1200mg/day. Max: 1200mg/day. Trigeminal Neuralgia: Initial (Day 1): 200mg qd. Titrate: May increase by 200mg/day q12h. Maint: 400-800mg/day. Max: 1200mg/day. Re-evaluate every 3 months. *Pediatrics:* Epilepsy: >12 yrs: Initial: 200mg bid. Titrate: May increase weekly by 200mg/day. Max: 12-15 yrs: 1000mg/day. >15 yrs: 1200mg/day. 6 months-12 yrs: May convert immediate-release dose ≥400mg/day to equal daily dose using bid regimen. Usual/Max: ≤35mg/kg/day.

HOW SUPPLIED: Cap, Extended-Release: 100mg, 200mg, 300mg

CONTRAINDICATIONS: History of bone marrow depression, MAOI use within 14 days, sensitivity to TCAs.

WARNINGS/PRECAUTIONS: Toxic epidermal necrolysis (Lyell's syndrome), Stevens-Johnson syndrome (SJS), multi-organ hypersensitivity reactions, and presence of HLA-B*1502 reported. Caution with history of adverse hematologic reaction to any drug, increased IOP, the elderly, mixed seizure with atypical absence seizure. Fetal harm with pregnancy. May activate latent psychosis. Caution with cardiac, hepatic, or renal damage. Perform eye exam and monitor LFTs and renal function at baseline and periodically.

ADVERSE REACTIONS: Dizziness, drowsiness, unsteadiness, nausea, vomiting, bone marrow depression, rash, urticaria, hypersensitivity reactions, photosensitivity reactions, CHF, edema, HTN, hypotension.

INTERACTIONS: See Contraindications. Metabolism is inhibited by CYP3A4 inhibitors (eg, cimetidine, macrolides, etc.) and induced by CYP3A4 inducers (eg, rifampin, phenytoin, trazodone, etc.). Decreases oral contraceptive effectiveness. Increases plasma levels of clomipramine, phenytoin, and primidone. Decreases levels of APAP, alprazolam, clonazepam, clozapine, dicumarol, doxycycline, ethosuximide, haloperidol, methsuximide, phensuximide, phenytoin, theophylline, valproate, warfarin. Increased risk of neurotoxic side effects with lithium.

PREGNANCY: Category D, not for use in nursing.

MECHANISM OF ACTION: Carboxamide anticonvulsant; suspected to reduce polysynaptic responses and blocks post-tetanic potentiation.

PHARMACOKINETICS: Absorption: C_{max}=1.9mcg/mL (200mg); T_{max}=19 hrs (200mg). **Distribution:** Plasma protein binding (76%). **Metabolism:** Liver, via CYP3A4 to carbamazepine-10,11-epoxide (metabolite). **Elimination:** Urine (72%), feces (28%); $T_{1/2}$=35-40 hrs.

NURSING CONSIDERATIONS

Assessment: Assess for history of mixed seizure disorders, bone marrow depression, renal function, LFTs, HLA-B 1502 typing, CBC with platelets and differential, serum iron, lipid profile, baseline eye exam, pregnancy status.

Monitoring: Monitor dermatologic reactions (toxic epidermal necrolysis, Stevens-Johnson syndrome), CBC with differential and platelet count, BUN, total cholesterol, LDL, HDL, signs/symptoms of anticholinergic effects, periodic eye exams, cardiovasular complications, LFTs, renal function.

Patient Counseling: Instruct to report toxic signs/symptoms of potential hematologic problems (fever, sore throat, rash, ulcers in mouth, easy bruising, petechial or purpuric hemorrhage). Caution while operating machinery/driving. Instruct to take exactly as directed; do not crush or chew cap.

Administration: Oral route. **Storage:** 25°C (77°F); excursions permitted to 15-30°C (59-86°F). Protect from light and moisture.

CARDENE IV — RX

nicardipine HCl (EKR)

THERAPEUTIC CLASS: Calcium channel blocker (dihydropyridine)

C

INDICATIONS: Short-term treatment of hypertension when oral therapy is not feasible or desirable.

DOSAGE: *Adults:* IV: Individualized dose; Administer by slow continuous infusion at a concentration of 0.1mg/mL. Gradual Reduction: Initial: 50mL/hr (5mg/hr). Titrate: May increase by 25mL/hr (2.5mg/hr) q15 min. Max: 150mL/hr (15mg/hr). Rapid BP Reduction: Initial 50mL/hr (5mg/hr). Titrate: 25mL/hr (2.5mg/hr) q5 min. Max 150mL/hr (15mg/hr). Decrease rate to 30mL/hr (3mg/hr) after BP reduction is achieved. Equiv. PO/IV Dose: 20mg q8h=0.5mg/hr, 30mg q8h=1.2mg/hr, 40mg q8h=2.2mg/hr.

HOW SUPPLIED: Inj: 2.5mg/mL

CONTRAINDICATIONS: Advanced aortic stenosis.

WARNINGS/PRECAUTIONS: May induce or exacerbate angina. Caution with CHF, significant left ventricular dysfunction, or pheochromocytoma. Change IV site every 12 hrs to minimize risk of peripheral venous irritation. Monitor BP during administration. Caution in hepatic/renal impairment or reduced hepatic blood flow.

ADVERSE REACTIONS: Headache, hypotension, tachycardia, NV.

INTERACTIONS: Monitor with other antihypertensive agents. Caution with β-blockers in CHF. Increased levels with cimetidine. Monitor digoxin levels. Caution with fentanyl anesthesia. May increase cyclosporine levels.

PREGNANCY: Category C, not for use in nursing.

MECHANISM OF ACTION: Ca^{2+} channel blocker; inhibits transmembrane influx of Ca^{2+} ions into cardiac muscle and smooth muscles without changing serum Ca^{2+} concentration.

PHARMACOKINETICS: Distribution: V_d=8.3L/kg; plasma protein binding (>95%). **Metabolism:** Liver. **Elimination:** Urine, feces; $T_{1/2}$=14.4 hrs.

NURSING CONSIDERATIONS

Assessment: Assess for advanced aortic stenosis, CHF, left ventricular dysfunction, possible drug interactions, pheochromocytoma, acute cerebral infarction or hemorrhage, portal HTN, liver/renal impairment.

Monitoring: Monitor BP during administration. Monitor for signs/symptoms of hypotension, angina, infusion-site reaction, hypersensitivity reactions, liver/renal dysfunction.

Patient Counseling: Advise to seek medical attention if symptoms of hypotension, angina, infusion-site reaction, or hypersensitivity reactions occur.

Administration: IV infusion. **Storage:** 20-25°C (68-77°F). Avoid elevated temperatures. Protect from light. Diluted: At room temperature, stable for 24 hrs.

CARDENE SR — RX

nicardipine HCl (EKR)

THERAPEUTIC CLASS: Calcium channel blocker (dihydropyridine)

INDICATIONS: Treatment of hypertension.

DOSAGE: *Adults:* Initial: 30mg bid. Usual: 30-60mg bid.

HOW SUPPLIED: Cap, Extended-Release: 30mg, 45mg, 60mg

CONTRAINDICATIONS: Advanced aortic stenosis.

WARNINGS/PRECAUTIONS: Increased angina reported in patients with angina. Caution with CHF when titrating dose. Caution in hepatic/renal impairment, or reduced hepatic blood flow. May cause symptomatic hypotension. Measure BP 2-4 hrs after 1st dose or dose increase.

ADVERSE REACTIONS: Headache, pedal edema, vasodilation, palpitations, nausea, dizziness, asthenia, flushing, increased angina.

INTERACTIONS: Increased levels with cimetidine. Elevates cyclosporine levels. With β-blocker withdrawal, gradually reduce over 8-10 days. Monitor digoxin levels. Caution with fentanyl anesthesia.

PREGNANCY: Category C, not for use in nursing.

MECHANISM OF ACTION: Ca^{2+} channel blocker; inhibits transmembrane influx of Ca^{2+} ions into cardiac muscle and smooth muscle without changing serum Ca^{2+} concentration.

PHARMACOKINETICS: Absorption: Complete; bioavailability (35%); C_{max}=13.4ng/mL (30mg), 34.0ng/mL (45mg), 58.4ng/mL (60mg); T_{max}=1-4 hrs. **Distribution:** Plasma protein binding (>95%). **Metabolism:** Liver. **Elimination:** Urine (<1%), feces; $T_{1/2}$=8.6 hrs.

NURSING CONSIDERATIONS

Assessment: Assess for advanced aortic stenosis, CHF, acute cerebral infarction or hemorrhage, possible drug interactions, liver/renal impairment. Obtain baseline BP.

Monitoring: Monitor BP initally and during titration. Monitor for signs/symptoms of angina, hypersensitivity reactions, hypotension, liver/renal dysfunction.

Patient Counseling: Advise to seek medical attention if symptoms of hypotension, angina, or hypersensitivity reactions occur.

Administration: Oral route. **Storage:** 15-30°C (59-86°F); in light-resistant container.

CARDIZEM RX

diltiazem HCl (Biovail)

THERAPEUTIC CLASS: Calcium channel blocker (nondihydropyridine)

INDICATIONS: Management of chronic stable angina or angina due to coronary artery spasm.

DOSAGE: *Adults:* Initial: 30mg qid (before meals and qhs). Adjust at 1-2 day intervals. Usual: 180-360mg/day.

HOW SUPPLIED: Tab: 30mg, 60mg*, 90mg*, 120mg* *scored

CONTRAINDICATIONS: Sick sinus syndrome and 2nd- or 3rd-degree AV block (except with functioning pacemaker), hypotension (<90mmHg systolic), acute MI, pulmonary congestion.

WARNINGS/PRECAUTIONS: Caution in renal, hepatic, or ventricular dysfunction. Monitor LFTs and renal function with prolonged use. D/C if persistent rash occurs. Symptomatic hypotension may occur. Acute hepatic injury reported.

ADVERSE REACTIONS: Headache, dizziness, asthenia, flushing, 1st-degree AV block, edema, nausea, bradycardia, rash.

INTERACTIONS: Increased levels of propranolol, digoxin, carbamazepine, cyclosporine, lovastatin, quinidine; monitor closely. Increased levels of diltiazem with cimetidine. Potentiates depression of cardiac contractility, conductivity, automaticity and vascular dilation with anesthetics. Additive cardiac conduction effects with digitalis or β-blockers. Potential additive effects with agents known to affect cardiac contractility and/or conduction. May increase levels of midazolam/triazolam. Avoid with CYP3A4 inducers (eg, rifampin). Enhanced effects and increased toxicity of buspirone.

PREGNANCY: Category C, not for use in nursing.

MECHANISM OF ACTION: Calcium channel blocker; still being delineated; believed to be potent dilator of coronary arteries both epicardial and subendocardial. Inhibits spontaneous and ergonovine-induced coronary artery spasm. Increases exercise tolerance by its ability to reduce myocardial oxygen demand; accomplished via reduction in heart rate and systemic BP.

PHARMACOKINETICS: Absorption: Well absorbed, absolute bioavailability (40%). T_{max}=2-4 hrs. **Distribution:** Plasma protein bound (70-80%); found in breast milk. **Metabolism:** Liver (extensive). **Elimination:** Urine (2-4% unchanged), bile.

NURSING CONSIDERATIONS

Assessment: Assess for cardiac conduction disorders (eg, sick sinus syndrome, second- or third-degree AV block and presence of a functioning ventricular pacemaker), presence of Prinzmetal's angina, hypotension, acute MI, pulmonary congestion documented by x-ray, CHF, hepatic/renal impairment, pregnancy/nursing status, and for possible drug interactions as additive effects on cardiac conduction if taken with digoxin or β-blockers.

Monitoring: Monitor LFTs and renal function regularly. Monitor heart rhythm, BP, dermatological events (eg, skin eruptions which may progress to erythema multiform and/or exfoliative dermatitis).

Patient Counseling: Inform about benefits/risks of drug and to report any adverse reactions to physician. Caution about the additive effects on cardiac conduction. Careful titration is needed in those receiving the drug concomitantly with agents known to affect cardiac contractility and/or conduction. Not for use by nursing women. Only use in pregnant women if benefit outweighs risk.

Administration: Oral route. **Storage:** 25°C (77°F), excursions permitted to 15-30°C (59-86°F).

CARDIZEM CD

diltiazem HCl (Biovail)

RX

OTHER BRAND NAMES: Cardizem LA (Abbott) - Cartia XT (Watson)

THERAPEUTIC CLASS: Calcium channel blocker (nondihydropyridine)

INDICATIONS: Treatment of hypertension. Management of chronic stable angina (LA) or angina due to coronary artery spasm.

DOSAGE: *Adults:* HTN: (CD, Cartia XT) Initial (monotherapy): 180-240mg qd. Titrate: Adjust at 2-week intervals. Usual: 240-360mg qd. Max: 480mg qd. (LA) Initial: 180-240mg qd. Adjust at 2-week intervals. Max: 540mg qd. Angina: (CD, Cartia XT) Initial: 120-180mg qd. Adjust at 1-2 week intervals. Max: 480mg/day. (LA) Initial: 180mg qd. Adjust at 1-2 week intervals.

HOW SUPPLIED: Cap, Extended-Release: (Cardizem CD, Cartia XT) 120mg, 180mg, 240mg, 300mg, (Cardizem CD) 360mg; Tab, Extended-Release: (Cardizem LA) 120mg, 180mg, 240mg, 300mg, 360mg, 420mg

CONTRAINDICATIONS: Sick sinus syndrome and 2nd- or 3rd-degree AV block (except with functioning pacemaker), hypotension (<90mmHg systolic), acute MI, pulmonary congestion.

WARNINGS/PRECAUTIONS: Caution in renal, hepatic, or ventricular dysfunction. Monitor LFTs and renal function with prolonged use. D/C if persistent rash occurs. Symptomatic hypotension may occur. Acute hepatic injury reported.

ADVERSE REACTIONS: Headache, dizziness, asthenia, flushing, 1st-degree AV block, edema, nausea, bradycardia, rash.

INTERACTIONS: May require dosage adjustment with concomitant CYP3A4 substrates. Increased levels of propranolol, digoxin, carbamazepine, lovastatin. Increased levels of diltiazem with cimetidine. May increase effects of benzodiazepines. Monitor digoxin, cyclosporine. Potentiates the depression of cardiac contractility, conductivity, automaticity, and vascular dilation with anesthetics. Avoid concurrent use with CYP3A4 inducers (eg, rifampin). Additive cardiac conduction effects with digitalis or β-blockers. Potential additive effects with agents known to affect cardiac contractility and/or conduction.

PREGNANCY: Category C, not for use in nursing.

MECHANISM OF ACTION: Calcium channel blocker; inhibits influx of Ca^{2+} ions during membrane depolarization of cardiac and vascular smooth muscle.

PHARMACOKINETICS: Absorption: CD: Absolute bioavailability (40%); T_{max}=10-14 hrs. LA: T_{max}=11-18 hrs. **Distribution:** Plasma protein binding (70-80%). **Elimination:** CD: Urine (2-4%); $T_{1/2}$=5-8 hrs; LA: $T_{1/2}$=6-9 hrs.

C

NURSING CONSIDERATIONS

Assessment: Assess for sick sinus syndrome, hypotension, AV block, acute MI, pulmonary congestion, pre-existing impairment of ventricular function, possible drug interactions, renal/hepatic impairment.

Monitoring: Monitor renal function and LFTs periodically. Monitor for signs/symptoms of worsening CHF, hypotension, hypersensitivity reactions, renal/hepatic dysfunction.

Patient Counseling: Advise to seek medical attention if symptoms of worsening CHF, hypotension, or hypersensitivity reactions occur.

Administration: Oral route. **Storage:** 25°C (77°F); excursions permitted to 15-30°C (59-86°F). Avoid excessive humidity and temperature.

CARDURA — RX

doxazosin mesylate (Pfizer)

THERAPEUTIC CLASS: Alpha$_1$-blocker (quinazoline)

INDICATIONS: Treatment of hypertension and/or benign prostatic hyperplasia (BPH).

DOSAGE: *Adults:* HTN: Initial: 1mg qd (am or pm). Monitor BP 2-6 hrs and 24 hrs after 1st dose. Titrate: Increase to 2mg qd then upwards as needed. Max: 16mg/day. BPH: Initial: 1mg qd (am or pm). Titrate: May double the dose every 1-2 weeks. Max: 8mg/day.

HOW SUPPLIED: Tab: 1mg*, 2mg*, 4mg*, 8mg* *scored

WARNINGS/PRECAUTIONS: Monitor for orthostatic hypotension and syncope with 1st dose and dose increase. Caution with hepatic dysfunction. Rule out prostate cancer. Priapism (rare), leukopenia/neutropenia reported.

ADVERSE REACTIONS: Fatigue/malaise, hypotension, edema, dizziness, dyspnea, wt gain.

PREGNANCY: Category C, caution with nursing.

MECHANISM OF ACTION: α-adrenergic receptor inhibitor; (BPH) antagonizes phenylephrine-induced contractions in prostate; (HTN) competitively antagonizes pressor effects of phenylephrine and systolic pressor effect of norepinephrine.

PHARMACOKINETICS: Absorption: Absolute bioavailability (65%); T_{max}=2-3 hrs. **Distribution:** Plasma protein binding (98%). **Metabolism:** O-demethylation or hydroxylation. **Elimination:** Feces (4.8%), urine (trace); $T_{1/2}$=22 hrs.

NURSING CONSIDERATIONS

Assessment: Assess for liver impairment and possible drug interactions. Rule out prostate cancer.

Monitoring: Monitor BP periodically. Monitor for signs/symptoms of hypotension, priapism, liver dysfunction, and hypersensitivity reactions.

Patient Counseling: Inform of possibility of syncopal and orthostatic symptoms, especially at initiation of therapy; urge to avoid driving or hazardous tasks for 24 hrs after first dose, dosage increase, and interruption of therapy when treatment is resumed. Caution to avoid situations where injury could result should syncope occur. Advise to sit or lie down when symptoms of low BP occur. Inform of possibility of priapism; advise to seek medical attention if priapism occurs.

Administration: Oral route. **Storage:** Below 30°C (86°F).

CARDURA XL — RX

doxazosin mesylate (Pfizer)

THERAPEUTIC CLASS: Alpha$_1$-blocker (quinazoline)

C

INDICATIONS: Treatment of the signs and symptoms of benign prostatic hyperplasia.

DOSAGE: *Adults:* Initial: 4mg qd with breakfast. Titrate: May increase to 8mg after 3-4 weeks. Max: 8mg. Swallow whole; do not chew, divide, cut, or crush.

HOW SUPPLIED: Tab, Extended-Release: 4mg, 8mg

WARNINGS/PRECAUTIONS: Postural hypotension with or without symptoms (eg, dizziness) may develop; caution with symptomatic hypotension or hypotensive response to other medications. Rule out prostate cancer. Intraoperative Floppy Iris Syndrome has been observed during cataract surgery in some patients on or previously treated with alpha$_1$ blockers. Caution with preexisting severe GI narrowing (pathologic or iatrogenic). Caution with mild or moderate hepatic dysfunction; avoid with severe hepatic dysfunction. D/C with worsening of or new-onset angina pectoris symptoms.

ADVERSE REACTIONS: Dizziness, dyspnea, asthenia, headache, hypotension, postural hypotension, somnolence, respiratory tract infection, backache.

INTERACTIONS: Caution with potent CYP3A4 inhibitors (eg, atanazavir, clarithromycin, indinavir, itraconazole, ketoconazole, nefazodone, nelfinavir, ritonavir, saquinavir, telithromycin, voriconazole).

PREGNANCY: Category C, not for use in nursing.

MECHANISM OF ACTION: Quinazoline; selectively inhibits α_1-subtype of α adrenergic receptors decreasing urethral resistance, which may relieve BPH symptoms and improve urine flow.

PHARMACOKINETICS: Absorption: (4mg) C_{max}=10.1ng/mL, T_{max}=8 hrs, AUC=183ng•hr/mL. (8mg) C_{max}=25.8ng/mL, T_{max}=9 hrs, AUC=472ng-hr/mL. **Distribution:** Plasma protein binding (98%). **Metabolism:** CYP3A4 (major); 2D6, 2C19 (minor). **Elimination:** $T_{1/2}$=15-19 hrs.

NURSING CONSIDERATIONS

Assessment: Assess for hepatic impairment, symptomatic hypotension, severe GI narrowing (chronic constipation), coronary insufficiency, and possible drug interactions. Rule out prostate cancer.

Monitoring: Monitor for signs/symptoms of postural hypotension and coronary insufficiency.

Patient Counseling: Instruct to take with breakfast; swallow whole; do not chew, divide, cut, or crush. Advise symptoms related to postural hypotension may occur; caution may impair physical/mental abilities. Advise to avoid situations where injury could result if syncope occurs. Instruct if considering cataract surgery, to inform ophthalmologist of drug use.

Admininistration: Oral route. **Storage:** 25°C (77°F); excursions permitted to 15-30°C (59-86°F).

CASODEX RX

bicalutamide (AstraZeneca)

THERAPEUTIC CLASS: Nonsteroidal antiandrogen

INDICATIONS: Treatment of stage D_2 metastatic carcinoma of the prostate in combination with a luteinizing hormone-releasing hormone (LHRH) analogue.

DOSAGE: *Adults:* 50mg qd at the same time each day. Initiate with LHRH analogue therapy.

HOW SUPPLIED: Tab: 50mg

CONTRAINDICATIONS: Women, pregnancy.

WARNINGS/PRECAUTIONS: Rare cases of death or hospitalization due to severe liver injury reported. Hepatitis and marked increases in liver enzymes leading to drug discontinuation have occurred. Caution with moderate-severe hepatic impairment; serum transaminase levels should be measured prior to starting treatment, at regular intervals for 1st four months, then periodically. Monitor PSA regularly to assess therapy. For patients who have objective progression of disease together with elevated PSA, a treatment-free period of antiandrogen, while continuing LHRH analogue, may be considered. Gynecomastia, breast pain reported with single agent.

ADVERSE REACTIONS: Hot flushes, pain, back pain, asthenia, constipation, pelvic pain, infection, nausea, dyspnea, peripheral edema, diarrhea, hematuria, nocturia.

INTERACTIONS: Can displace coumarin anticoagulants, such as warfarin, from their protein-binding sites; monitor PT.

PREGNANCY: Category X, caution in nursing.

MECHANISM OF ACTION: Nonsteroidal antiandrogen; inhibits the action of androgens by binding to cytosol androgen receptors in target tissue.

PHARMACOKINETICS: Absorption: Well-absorbed, C_{max}=0.768mcg/mL, T_{max}=31.3 hrs. **Distribution:** Plasma protein binding (96%). **Metabolism:** Liver via oxidation and glucuronidation. **Elimination:** Urine, feces; $T_{1/2}$=5.8 days.

NURSING CONSIDERATIONS

Assessment: Assess for hepatic impairment, pregnancy status, and CBC. Note other diseases/conditions and drug therapies.

Monitoring: Monitor LFTs, CBC, PSA, hot flushes, hypersensitivity reactions, hyperuricemia, BP, and dyspnea.

Patient Counseling: Do not interrupt or d/c without consulting physician. Start treatment at the same time as treatment with an LHRH analogue. Take with/without food.

Administration: Oral route. **Storage:** 20-25°C (68-77°F).

CATAFLAM RX

diclofenac potassium (Novartis)

NSAIDs may cause an increased risk of serious cardiovascular thrombotic events, MI, stroke, and serious GI adverse events including bleeding, ulceration, and perforation of the stomach or intestines. Contraindicated for the treatment of perioperative pain in the setting of coronary artery bypass graft (CABG) surgery.

THERAPEUTIC CLASS: NSAID

INDICATIONS: Relief of signs and symptoms of osteoarthritis (OA) and rheumatoid arthritis (RA). Treatment of primary dysmenorrhea and relief of mild to moderate pain.

DOSAGE: *Adults:* OA: 50mg bid-tid. Max: 150mg/day. RA: 50mg tid-qid. Max: 200mg/day. Pain/Primary Dysmenorrhea: Initial: 50mg tid or 100mg on 1st dose, then 50mg on subsequent doses.

HOW SUPPLIED: Tab: 50mg

CONTRAINDICATIONS: ASA or other NSAID allergy that precipitates asthma, urticaria, or allergic reactions. Treatment of perioperative pain in the setting of CABG surgery.

WARNINGS/PRECAUTIONS: May lead to onset of new HTN or worsening of pre-existing HTN; monitor BP closely. Fluid retention and edema reported; caution with fluid retention or heart failure. Renal papillary necrosis and other renal injury reported after long-term use. Not recommended for use with advanced renal disease; if therapy must be initiated, monitor renal function. Anaphylactoid reactions may occur. May cause serious skin adverse events (eg, exfoliative dermatitis, Stevens-Johnson syndrome, and toxic epidermal necrolysis). Avoid in late pregnancy; may cause premature closure of ductus arteriosis. May cause elevations of LFTs; d/c if liver disease develops or systemic manifestations occur. Caution in elderly. Anemia may occur; with long-term use, monitor Hgb/Hct if signs or symptoms of anemia develop. May inhibit platelet aggregation and prolong bleeding time; monitor with coagulation disorders. Caution with asthma and avoid with ASA-sensitive asthma.

ADVERSE REACTIONS: Fluid retention, dizziness, rash, nausea, abdominal cramps, LFT abnormalities, constipation, diarrhea, heartburn, tinnitus, GI ulceration, HTN, insomnia, stomatitis, pruritus.

INTERACTIONS: Avoid with other diclofenac products. Increased adverse effects with ASA; avoid use. May enhance methotrexate toxicity; caution when co-administering. May increase nephrotoxicity of cyclosporine; caution when co-administering. May diminish antihypertensive effect of ACE-inhibitors. May reduce natriuretic effect of furosemide and thiazides; monitor for renal failure. May increase lithium levels; monitor for toxicity. Synergistic effects on GI bleeding with warfarin.

PREGNANCY: Category C, not for use in nursing.

MECHANISM OF ACTION: NSAID (benzeneacetic acid derivative); suspected to inhibit prostaglandin synthetase, exerts anti-inflammatory, analgesic, and antipyretic actions.

PHARMACOKINETICS: Absorption: Mean absolute bioavailabilty (55%), T_{max}=1 hr. **Distribution**: V_d=1.3L/kg; serum protein binding (>99%). **Metabolism**: Metabolites: 4-hydroxy-, 5-hydroxy-, 3-hydroxy-, 4,'5-dihydroxy-, and 3'-hydroxy-4'-methoxy diclofenac. **Elimination:** Urine (65%), bile (35%); $T_{1/2}$= approximately 2 hrs.

NURSING CONSIDERATIONS

Assessment: Assess LFTs, renal function, CBC and coagulation profile. Assess for history of CABG surgery, asthma and allergic reactions to aspirin or other NSAIDs, active ulceration or chronic inflammation of GI tract, CVD, asthma, pregnancy status. Note other diseases/conditions and drug therapies.

Monitoring: Monitor for hypersensitivity reactions, cardiac complications, stroke, GI bleeding, asthma, skin side effects. Monitor BP, LFTs, renal function, CBC with differential and platelet count, coagulation profile, hyperglycemia.

Patient Counseling: Counsel about potential side effects; seek medical attention if any develop. Avoid alcohol and smoking during treatment. Take drug as prescribed. Caution women against using medication late in pregnancy.

Administration: Oral route. **Storage:** Do not store above 30°C (86°F).

CATAPRES RX

clonidine (Boehringer Ingelheim)

OTHER BRAND NAMES: Catapres-TTS (Boehringer Ingelheim)

THERAPEUTIC CLASS: Central alpha-adrenergic agonist

INDICATIONS: Treatment of hypertension.

DOSAGE: *Adults:* (Patch) Apply to hairless, intact area of upper arm or chest weekly. Taper withdrawal of previous antihypertensive. Initial: 0.1mg/24 hr patch weekly. Titrate: May increase after 1-2 weeks. Max: 0.6mg/24 hr. (Tab) Initial: 0.1mg bid. Titrate: May increase by 0.1mg weekly. Usual: 0.2-0.6mg/day in divided doses. Max: 2.4mg/day. (Patch, Tab) Renal Impairment: Adjust according to degree of impairment.

HOW SUPPLIED: Patch, Extended-Release (TTS): 0.1mg/24 hr [4[s]], 0.2mg/24 hr [4[s]], 0.3mg/24 hr [4[s]]; Tab: 0.1mg*, 0.2mg*, 0.3mg* *scored

WARNINGS/PRECAUTIONS: Avoid abrupt discontinuation. Tabs may cause rash if have allergic reaction to patch. Continue tabs within 4 hrs of surgery and resume as soon as possible thereafter. Do not remove patch for surgery. Caution with severe coronary insufficiency, conduction disturbances, recent MI, cerebrovascular disease, or chronic renal failure. Remove patch before defibrillation or cardioversion due to the potential risk of altered electrical conductivity or MRI due to the occurrence of burns.

ADVERSE REACTIONS: Dry mouth, drowsiness, dizziness, constipation, sedation, impotence/sexual dysfunction, NV, alopecia, weakness, orthostatic symptoms, nervousness, localized skin reactions (patch).

INTERACTIONS: May potentiate CNS depression with alcohol, barbiturates, or other sedatives. Additive bradycardia and AV block with agents that affect sinus node function or AV nodal conduction (eg, digitalis, CCBs, and β-blockers). Hypotensive effect reduced by TCAs.

PREGNANCY: Category C, caution in nursing.

MECHANISM OF ACTION: Central acting α-agonist; stimulates α-adrenoreceptor in brain stem, reducing sympathetic outflow from CNS and decreasing HR, BP, peripheral and renal vascular resistance.

PHARMACOKINETICS: Absorption: T_{max}=3-5 hrs. **Metabolism:** Liver. **Elimination:** Urine (40-60%); $T_{1/2}$=12-16 hrs.

C

NURSING CONSIDERATIONS

Assessment: Assess for coronary insufficiency, conduction disturbances, recent MI, cerebrovascular disease, possible drug interactions, and renal impairment.

Monitoring: Monitor renal function periodically. Monitor for signs of withdrawal symptoms and hypersensitivity reactions.

Patient Counseling: Caution that drug may impair physical/mental abilities. Instruct to avoid alcohol. Inform to remove patch before MRI.

Administration: Oral; transdermal route. **Storage:** Oral: 25°C (77°F); excursions permitted to 15-30°C (59-86°F). Patch: Below 30°C (86°F).

CEFACLOR RX

cefaclor (Various)

THERAPEUTIC CLASS: Cephalosporin (2nd generation)

INDICATIONS: Treatment of otitis media, pharyngitis, tonsillitis, lower respiratory tract, urinary tract, and skin and skin structure infections caused by susceptible strains of microorganisms.

DOSAGE: *Adults:* Usual: 250mg q8h. Severe Infections/Pneumonia: 500mg q8h. Treat β-hemolytic strep for 10 days.
Pediatrics: ≥1 month: Usual: 20mg/kg/day given q8h. Otitis Media/Serious Infections/Infections Caused by Less Susceptible Organisms: 40mg/kg/day. Max: 1g/day. May administer q12h for otitis media and pharyngitis. Treat β-hemolytic strep for 10 days.

HOW SUPPLIED: Cap: 250mg, 500mg; Sus: 125mg/5mL [75mL, 150mL], 250mg/5mL [75mL, 150mL], 375mg/5mL [50mL, 100mL]

WARNINGS/PRECAUTIONS: Cross-sensitivity to PCNs and other cephalosporins may occur. *Clostridium difficile*-associated diarrhea reported. Positive direct Coombs' test reported. Caution with markedly impaired renal function, history of GI disease. False (+) for urine glucose with Benedict's, Fehling's solution, and Clinitest tabs.

ADVERSE REACTIONS: Hypersensitivity reactions, diarrhea, eosinophilia, genital pruritus and vaginitis, serum-sickness-like reactions, superinfection.

INTERACTIONS: Renal excretion inhibited by probenecid. May potentiate warfarin and other anticoagulants; monitor PT/INR.

PREGNANCY: Category B, caution in nursing.

MECHANISM OF ACTION: Cephalosporin; bactericidal agent, inhibits cell-wall synthesis.

PHARMACOKINETICS: Absorption: Well-absorbed; (Fasting): C_{max}=7mcg/mL (250mg), 13mcg (500mg), 23mcg (1g); T_{max}=30-60 min. **Elimination:** Urine (60-85% unchanged); $T_{1/2}$= 0.6-0.9 hrs.

NURSING CONSIDERATIONS

Assessment: Assess for hypersensitivity reactions to cephalosporins, PCNs and other drugs, pregnancy/nursing status, renal impairment, and possible drug interactions.

Monitoring: Monitor for anaphylactic reactions, *C.difficile*-associated diarrhea, superinfection, drug resistance, positive Coombs' test, increased anticoagulant effect when used concomitantly with anticoagulants, false positive reaction for urinary glucose when using Benedict's and Fehling's solutions, and Clinitest tablets.

Patient Counseling: Inform drug only treats bacterial, not viral, infections. Take exactly as directed; skipping doses or not completing full course may decrease effectiveness and increase resistance. Inform about potential benefits/risks. D/C and notify physician if allergic reaction or watery/bloody diarrhea (with/without muscle cramps and fever) occur (as late as 2 months after treatment end). Notify if pregnant/nursing.

Administration: Oral route. **Storage:** 20-25°C (68-77°F).

CEFACLOR ER — RX

cefaclor (Various)

THERAPEUTIC CLASS: Cephalosporin (2nd generation)

INDICATIONS: Treatment of acute bacterial exacerbation of chronic bronchitis (ABECB), secondary bacterial infections of acute bronchitis, pharyngitis, tonsillitis, and uncomplicated skin and skin structure infections (SSSI) caused by susceptible strains of microorganisms.

DOSAGE: *Adults:* ABECB/Acute Bronchitis: 500mg q12h for 7 days. Pharyngitis/Tonsillitis: 375mg q12h for 10 days. SSSI: 375mg q12h for 7-10 days. Take with meals. Do not crush, cut, or chew tab.
Pediatrics: ≥16 yrs: ABECB/Acute Bronchitis: 500mg q12h for 7 days. Pharyngitis/Tonsillitis: 375mg q12h for 10 days. SSSI: 375mg q12h for 7-10 days. Take with meals. Do not crush, cut, or chew tab.

HOW SUPPLIED: Tab, Extended-Release: 500mg

WARNINGS/PRECAUTIONS: Cross-sensitivity to PCNs and other cephalosporins may occur. *Clostridium difficile*-associated diarrhea reported. Positive direct Coombs' test reported. Caution with markedly impaired renal function, history of GI disease. False (+) for urine glucose with Benedict's, Fehling's solution, and Clinitest tabs.

ADVERSE REACTIONS: Headache, rhinitis, diarrhea, nausea, vaginitis, abdominal pain, pharyngitis, increased cough, pruritus, back pain, serum-sickness-like reactions, superinfection (prolonged use).

INTERACTIONS: Decreased absorption with aluminum or magnesium hydroxide-containing antacids; space dose by 1 hr. Potentiated by probenecid. May potentiate warfarin, and other anticoagulants; monitor PT/INR.

PREGNANCY: Category B, caution in nursing.

MECHANISM OF ACTION: Cephalosporin; bactericidal, inhibits cell-wall synthesis.

PHARMACOKINETICS: Absorption: Fed: (375mg) C_{max}=3.7mcg/mL, T_{max}=2.7 hr, AUC=9.9mcg•hr/mL. (500mg) C_{max}=4.2mcg/mL, T_{max}=2.5 hr, AUC=18.1mcg•hr/mL. Fasting: C_{max}=5.4, T_{max}=1.5 hrs, AUC=14.8mcg•hr/mL.

NURSING CONSIDERATIONS

Assessment: Assess for hypersensitivity reactions to cephalosporins, PCNs, and other drugs, pregnancy/nursing status, renal impairment, and possible drug interactions.

Monitoring: Monitor for anaphylactic reactions, pseudomembranous colitis, *C.difficile*-associated diarrhea, superinfection, drug resistance, and false (+) reaction for urinary glucose when using Benedict's/Fehling's solution or Clinitest tab. Monitor for lab events for CBC, LFTs, renal function tests, and blood chemistry.

Patient Counseling: Inform drug only treats bacterial, not viral, infections. Take exactly as directed; skipping doses or not completing full course may decrease effectiveness and increase resistance. Inform about benefits/risks; d/c and notify physician if allergic reaction or diarrhea occurs. Notify if pregnant/nursing.

Administration: Oral route. Take with food. **Storage:** 20-25°C (68-77°F); store in tightly-closed, light-resistant container.

CEFADROXIL RX

cefadroxil monohydrate (Various)

C

THERAPEUTIC CLASS: Cephalosporin (1st generation)

INDICATIONS: Treatment of skin and skin structure (SSSI) and urinary tract infections (UTI), pharyngitis, and tonsillitis caused by susceptible strains of microorganisms.

DOSAGE: *Adults:* Uncomplicated Lower UTI: 1-2g/day given qd or bid. Other UTI: 1g bid. SSSI: 1g qd or 500mg bid. Group A β-hemolytic Strep Pharyngitis/Tonsillitis: 1g qd or 500mg bid for 10 days. CrCl ≤50mL/min: Initial: 1g. Maint: CrCl 25-50mL/min: 500mg q12h; CrCl 10-25mL/min: 500mg q24h; CrCl 0-10mL/min: 500mg q36h.
Pediatrics: UTI/SSSI: 15mg/kg q12h. Pharyngitis/Tonsillitis/Impetigo: 30mg/kg qd or 15mg/kg q12h. Treat β-hemolytic strep infections for at least 10 days.

HOW SUPPLIED: Cap: 500mg; Sus: 250mg/5mL [100mL], 500mg/5mL [75mL, 100mL]; Tab: 1g* *scored

WARNINGS/PRECAUTIONS: Caution with markedly impaired renal function, history of GI disease. Cross-sensitivity with cephalosporins and PCNs. False (+) direct Coombs' tests, colitis, and *Clostridium difficile*-associated diarrhea (CDAD) reported.

ADVERSE REACTIONS: Diarrhea, rash, hypersensitivity reactions, pruritus, hepatic dysfunction, genital moniliasis, vaginitis, fever, superinfection (prolonged use).

PREGNANCY: Category B, caution in nursing.

MECHANISM OF ACTION: Cephalosporin; bactericidal due to inhibition of cell-wall synthesis.

PHARMACOKINETICS: Absorption: Rapid; C_{max} (500, 1000mg)=16mcg/mL, 28mcg/mL. **Elimination:** Urine (90% unchanged).

NURSING CONSIDERATIONS

Assessment: Assess for history of hypersensitivity to cephalosporins/PCNs, pregnancy status, possible drug interactions, renal impairment, colitis. Document indications for therapy, culture, and susceptibility testing.

Monitoring: Monitor for hypersensitivity reactions (toxic epidermal necrolysis), superinfection with other pathogens, renal function tests (creatinine clearance, creatinine, BUN, alkaline phosphatase), LFTs (ALT, AST, bilirubin, LDH) and hematologic parameters (prothrombin time, CBC). Culture and sensitivity tests should be done to monitor drug susceptibility.

Patient Counseling: Inform drug only treats bacterial, not viral, infections. Instruct to take exactly as directed; skipping doses or not completing full course may decrease effectiveness and increase resistance. Inform may experience diarrhea; contact physician if watery/bloody stools, superinfection, or hypersensitivity reactions occur.

Administration: Oral route. **Storage:** 15-30°C (59-86°F). Keep reconstituted sus refrigerated, discard any unused sus after 14 days. Shake well before use. Keep container tightly closed.

CEFAZOLIN RX

cefazolin (Various)

THERAPEUTIC CLASS: Cephalosporin (1st generation)

INDICATIONS: Treatment of respiratory tract, urinary tract (UTI), skin and skin structure, biliary tract, bone and joint, and genital infections, septicemia, and endocarditis caused by susceptible strains of microorganisms. Perioperative prophylaxis for surgical procedures classified as contaminated or potentially contaminated.

DOSAGE: *Adults:* Moderate-Severe Infections: 500mg-1g q6-8h. Mild Gram-Positive Cocci Infection: 250-500mg q8h. Acute, Uncomplicated UTI: 1g q12h.

C

Pneumococcal Pneumonia: 500mg q12h. Severe Life-Threatening Infection (eg, Endocarditis, Septicemia): 1-1.5g q6h; Max: 12g/day (rare). Perioperative Prophylaxis: 1g IM/IV 0.5-1 hr before surgery. For Procedures ≥2 hrs: 500mg-1g IM/IV during surgery. Maint: 500mg-1g IM/IV q6-8h for 24 hrs post-op. Continue for 3-5 days post-op for devastating procedures (eg, open-heart surgery and prosthetic arthroplasty). Renal Impairment: CrCl 35-54mL/min: Full dose q8h. CrCl 11-34mL/min: 1/2 usual dose q12h. CrCl <10mL/min: 1/2 usual dose q18-24h. Apply reduced dosage recommendations after initial LD is given.

Pediatrics: Mild-Moderately Severe Infection: 25-50mg/kg/day in 3-4 equal doses. Severe Infection: 100mg/kg/day in divided doses. Renal Impairment: CrCl 40-70mL/min: 60% of normal daily dose in equally divided doses q12h. CrCl 20-40mL/min: 25% of normal daily dose in equally divided doses q12h. CrCl 5-20mL/min: 10% of normal daily dose q24h. Apply reduced dosage recommendations after initial LD is given.

HOW SUPPLIED: Inj: 500mg, 1g, 10g, 20g

WARNINGS/PRECAUTIONS: Prolonged use may result in overgrowth of nonsusceptible organisms. Possible cross-sensitivity between PCNs, cephalosporins, and other β-lactam antibiotics. Pseudomembranous colitis reported. Elevated levels with renal insufficiency can lead to seizures. Caution with colitis and other GI diseases. Safety in premature infants and neonates not established.

ADVERSE REACTIONS: Diarrhea, oral candidiasis, NV, stomach cramps, anorexia, allergic reactions, blood dyscrasias, renal failure, transient rise in SGOT/SGPT/BUN/SCr/alkaline phosphatase, local reactions.

INTERACTIONS: Decreased renal tubular secretion with probenecid.

PREGNANCY: Category B, caution in nursing.

MECHANISM OF ACTION: Cephalosporin; inhibits cell wall synthesis.

PHARMACOKINETICS: Absorption: C_{max}=185mcg/mL. **Distribution:** Crosses placenta; found in breast milk. **Elimination:** Urine (unchanged); $T_{1/2}$=1.8 hrs.

NURSING CONSIDERATIONS

Assessment: Assess for previous hypersensitivity reaction to cephalosporins, PCNs or other allergens, renal/hepatic impairment, pregnancy/nursing status, GI disease (eg, colitis), nutritional status, and possible drug interactions.

Monitoring: Monitor for signs/symptoms of anaphylactic/anaphylactoid reactions, CDAD, drug resistance or superinfection. Seizures and PT time should be checked in patients at risk.

Patient Counseling: Inform drug only treats bacterial, not viral, infections. Take as directed; skipping doses or not completing full course may decrease effectiveness and increase resistance. Educate about potential benefits/risks. D/C and notify physician if allergic reaction or diarrhea occurs. Notify if pregnant/nursing.

Administration: IV route. **Storage**: -20°C (-4°F). Do not force thaw by immersion in water baths or by microwave irradiation. Thawed solution is stable for 30 days under refrigeration 5°C (41°F) and for 48 hrs at 25°C (77°F). Do not refreeze thawed antibiotics.

CEFOXITIN — RX

cefoxitin sodium (Various)

OTHER BRAND NAMES: Mefoxin (Merck)

THERAPEUTIC CLASS: Cephalosporin (2nd generation)

INDICATIONS: Treatment of lower respiratory tract, urinary tract, intra-abdominal, gynecological, skin and skin structure, and bone and joint infections, and septicemia caused by susceptible strains of microorganisms. Prophylaxis of infection in patients undergoing uncontaminated GI surgery, abdominal/vaginal hysterectomy, or cesarean section.

DOSAGE: *Adults:* Usual: 1-2g IV q6-8h. Uncomplicated Infections: 1g IV q6-8h. Moderate-Severe: 1g IV q4h or 2g IV q6-8h. Gas Gangrene/Other Infections Requiring Higher Dose: 2g IV q4h or 3g IV q6h. Renal Insufficiency: LD: 1-2g IV. Maint: CrCl 30-50mL/min: 1-2g IV q8-12h. CrCl 10-29mL/min: 1-2g IV q12-24h. CrCl 5-9mL/min: 0.5-1g IV q12-24h. CrCl <5mL/min: 0.5-1g IV q24-48h. Hemodialysis: LD: 1-2g IV after dialysis. Maint: See renal insufficiency doses above. Prophylaxis: Uncontaminated GI Surgery/Hysterectomy: 2g IV 0.5-1 hr prior to surgery (1/2-1 hr before initial incision), then 2g IV q6h after 1st dose up to 24 hrs. C-Section: 2g IV single dose as soon as umbilical cord is clamped, or 2g IV as soon as umbilical cord is clamped, followed by 2g IV at 4 and 8 hrs after initial dose.
Pediatrics: ≥3 months: 80-160mg/kg/day divided into 4-6 equal doses. Max: 12g/day. Prophylaxis: Uncontaminated GI Surgery/Hysterectomy: 30-40mg/kg IV 0.5-1 hr prior to surgery, then 30-40mg/kg IV q6h after first dose for up to 24 hrs.

HOW SUPPLIED: Inj: 1g, 1g/50mL, 2g, 2g/50mL, 10g

WARNINGS/PRECAUTIONS: Possible cross-sensitivity between PCNs and cephalosporins. *Clostridium difficile*-associated diarrhea reported. Caution with allergies, GI disease, particularly colitis. Prolonged use may result in overgrowth of nonsusceptible organisms. Monitor renal, hepatic, hematopoietic functions, especially with prolonged therapy. False (+) for urine glucose with Clinitest tabs.

ADVERSE REACTIONS: Thrombophlebitis, rash, pseudomembranous colitis, pruritus, fever, dyspnea, hypotension, diarrhea, blood dyscrasias, elevated LFTs, changes in renal function tests, exacerbation of myasthenia gravis.

INTERACTIONS: Increased nephrotoxicity with concomitant aminoglycosides.

PREGNANCY: Category B, caution in nursing.

MECHANISM OF ACTION: 2nd-generation cephalosporin; inhibits bacterial cell-wall synthesis.

PHARMACOKINETICS: Metabolism: Passes pleural and joint fluids; found in bile and breast milk. **Elimination:** Urine (85% unchanged); $T_{1/2}$=41-59 min.

NURSING CONSIDERATIONS

Assessment: Assess for previous hypersensitivity reactions to cephalosporins, PCNs, or other drugs, renal/hepatic impairment, GI tract disease (particularly colitis), DM or carbohydrate intolerance, pregnancy/nursing status, and possible drug interactions.

Monitoring: Periodically monitor renal function, LFTs, and hematopoietic functions. Monitor for *C.difficile*-associated diarrhea (may range from mild diarrhea to fatal colitis), development of superinfections or drug resistance, allergic reactions (eg, toxic epidermal necrolysis or exfoliative dermatitis). May interfere with lab test measurements of serum/urinary creatinine levels by Jaffe reaction (do not analyze creatinine if drawn within 2 hrs of administration). May interfere with measurement of urinary 17-hydroxy-corticosteroid by Porter-Silber reaction, and may cause false (+) reaction for urinary glucose using Clinitest.

Patient Counseling: Inform drug only treats bacterial, not viral, infections. Take exactly as directed; skipping doses or not completing full course may decrease effectiveness and increase resistance. Inform about potential benefits/risks. D/C therapy and notify physician if allergic reactions, watery/bloody diarrhea (with/without muscle cramps), or fever occurs. May occur up to 2 months or more after therapy. Notify if pregnant/nursing.

Administration: IV route; in DUPLEX container, keep container in folded position to avoid inadvertent activation. Do not use plastic containers in series connections to avoid air embolism. **Storage:** Unactivated unit at 20-25°C (68-77°F); excursions permitted to 15-30°C (59-86°F); use reconstituted product within 12 hrs if stored at room temperature or within 7 days if refrigerated. Can darken depending on storage conditions; do not freeze; discard if leak detected.

CEFTAZIDIME

RX

ceftazidime (Various)

C

THERAPEUTIC CLASS: Cephalosporin (3rd generation)

INDICATIONS: Treatment of lower respiratory tract (eg, pneumonia), skin and skin structure (SSSI), bone and joint, gynecologic, CNS (eg, meningitis), intra-abdominal, and urinary tract infections (UTI), and septicemia caused by susceptible strains of microorganisms. For use in sepsis.

DOSAGE: *Adults:* Usual: 1g IM/IV q8-12h. Uncomplicated UTI: 250mg IM/IV q12h. Complicated UTI: 500mg IM/IV q8-12h. Bone and Joint Infection: 2g IV q12h. Uncomplicated Pneumonia/SSSI: 500mg-1g IM/IV q8h. Gynecological/Intra-Abdominal/Meningitis/Severe Life-Threatening Infection: 2g IV q8h. Lung Infection caused by *Pseudomonas* spp. in Cystic Fibrosis (normal renal function): 30-50mg/kg IV q8h. Max: 6g/day. CrCl 31-50mL/min: 1g q12h. CrCl 16-30mL/min: 1g q24h. CrCl 6-15mL/min: 500mg q24h. CrCl <5mL/min: 500mg q48h. For severe infections (6g/day), increase renal impairment dose by 50% or increase dosing interval. Apply reduced dosage recommendations after initial 1g LD is given. Hemodialysis: Give 1g before then 1g after each hemodialysis. Intra-Peritoneal Dialysis/Continuous Ambulatory Peritoneal Dialysis: Give 1g followed by 500mg q24h.
Pediatrics: ≥12 yrs: Usual: 1g IM/IV q8-12h. Uncomplicated UTI: 250mg IM/IV q12h. Complicated UTI: 500mg IM/IV q8-12h. Bone and Joint Infection: 2g IV q12h. Uncomplicated Pneumonia/SSSI: 500mg-1g IM/IV q8h. Gynecological/Intra-Abdominal/Meningitis/Severe Life-Threatening Infection: 2g IV q8h. Lung Infection caused by *Pseudomonas* spp. in Cystic Fibrosis (normal renal function): 30-50mg/kg IV q8h. Max: 6g/day. CrCl 31-50mL/min: 1g q12h. CrCl 16-30mL/min: 1g q24h. CrCl 6-15mL/min: 500mg q24h. CrCl <5mL/min: 500mg q48h. For severe infections (6g/day), increase renal impairment dose by 50% or increase dosing interval. Apply reduced dosage recommendations after initial 1g LD is given. Hemodialysis: Give 1g before then 1g after each hemodialysis. Intra-Peritoneal Dialysis/Continuous Ambulatory Peritoneal Dialysis: Give 1g followed by 500mg q24h.

HOW SUPPLIED: Inj: 1g, 2g, 6g

WARNINGS/PRECAUTIONS: Monitor renal function; potential for nephrotoxicity. Prolonged use may result in overgrowth of nonsusceptible organisms. Possible cross-sensitivity between PCNs, cephalosporins, and other β-lactam antibiotics. Pseudomembranous colitis reported. Elevated levels with renal insufficiency can lead to seizures, encephalopathy, asterixis, coma, and neuromuscular excitability. Possible decrease in PT; caution with renal or hepatic impairment, poor nutritional state; monitor PT and give vitamin K if needed. Caution with colitis and other GI diseases. Distal necrosis can occur after inadvertent intra-arterial administration. Continue therapy for 2 days after the signs and symptoms of infection have disappeared, but in complicated infections longer therapy may be required. False positive for urine glucose with Benedict's, Fehling's solution, and Clinitest tabs.

ADVERSE REACTIONS: Phlebitis and inflammation at injection site, pruritus, rash, fever, diarrhea.

INTERACTIONS: Nephrotoxicity reported with aminoglycosides or potent diuretics (eg, furosemide). Avoid with chloramphenicol; may decrease effect of β-lactam antibiotics.

PREGNANCY: Category B, not for use in nursing.

MECHANISM OF ACTION: Broad spectrum, β-lactam antibiotic; exerts effects by inhibiting enzymes responsible for cell-wall synthesis.

PHARMACOKINETICS: Absorption: (IV) C_{max}=45mcg/mL (500mg), 90mcg/mL (1g). (IM) C_{max}=17mcg/mL (500mg), 39mcg/mL (1g), T_{max}=1 hr. **Distribution:** Plasma protein binding (<10%); found in breast milk. **Elimination:** Urine, (80-90% unchanged). $T_{1/2}$=1.9 hrs (IV), 2 hrs (IM).

C

NURSING CONSIDERATIONS

Assessment: Assess for previous hypersensitivity to cephalosporins/PCNs or other drugs, renal/hepatic insufficiency, nutritional status, history of GI disease, pregnancy/nursing status, and possible drug interactions.

Monitoring: Periodically monitor PT, with vitamin K administration if indicated. Monitor for allergic reactions (eg, Stevens-Johnson syndrome), signs/symptoms of pseudomembranous colitis or *C.difficile*-associated diarrhea, seizures, encephalopathy, coma, asterixis, neuromuscular excitability, and myoclonia, development of superinfection or drug resistance, renal function tests/urine output for daily dosage, LFTs, hematopoietic function, and lab test interactions.

Patient Counseling: Inform that drug only treats bacterial, not viral, infections. Take exactly as directed; skipping doses or not completing full course may decrease effectiveness and increase resistance. Inform about potential benefits/risks. D/C and notify physician if allergic reactions, watery/bloody diarrhea (with/without muscle cramps), or fever occurs. Notify if pregnant/nursing.

Administration: IV/IM routes. Do not use plastic containers for series connections to avoid development of air embolism. **Storage**: Dry state at 15-30°C (59-86°F); protect from light. As premixed solution not >-20°C; do not force thaw by immersion in water baths or by microwave irradiation; store thawed solutions for up to 24 hrs at room temperature or for 7 days in a refrigerator. Do not refreeze thawed solution.

CEFTIN — RX

cefuroxime axetil (GlaxoSmithKline)

THERAPEUTIC CLASS: Cephalosporin (2nd generation)

INDICATIONS: Treatment of the following infections caused by susceptible strains of microorganisms: (Sus/Tab) Pharyngitis/tonsillitis, acute otitis media, and impetigo. (Tab) Uncomplicated skin and skin structure (SSSI), and urinary tract infection (UTI), gonorrhea, early Lyme disease, acute bacterial maxillary sinusitis, acute bacterial exacerbations of chronic bronchitis (ABECB) and secondary bacterial infections of acute bronchitis.

DOSAGE: *Adults:* (Tab) Pharyngitis/Tonsillitis/Sinusitis: 250mg bid for 10 days. ABECB/SSSI: 250-500mg bid for 10 days. Acute Bronchitis: 250-500mg bid for 5-10 days. UTI: 250mg bid for 7-10 days. Gonorrhea: 1000mg single dose. Lyme Disease: 500mg bid for 20 days.
Pediatrics: ≥13 yrs: (Tab) Pharyngitis/Tonsillitis/Sinusitis: 250mg bid for 10 days. ABECB/SSSI: 250-500mg bid for 10 days. Acute Bronchitis: 250-500mg bid for 5-10 days. UTI: 250mg bid for 7-10 days. Gonorrhea: 1000mg single dose. Lyme Disease: 500mg bid for 20 days. 3 months-12 yrs: (Sus) Pharyngitis/Tonsillitis: 10mg/kg bid for 10 days. Max: 500mg/day. Otitis Media/Sinusitis/Impetigo: 15mg/kg bid for 10 days. Max: 1000mg/day. (Tab-if can swallow whole) Otitis Media/Sinusitis: 250mg bid for 10 days.

HOW SUPPLIED: Sus: 125mg/5mL [100mL], 250mg/5mL [50mL, 100mL]; Tab: 250mg, 500mg

WARNINGS/PRECAUTIONS: Tabs are not bioequivalent to sus. Caution with colitis, renal impairment. Cross-sensitivity with cephalosporins and PCNs. False (+) for urine glucose with Benedict's, Fehling's solution, and Clinitest tabs. May cause fall in PT; risk in patients stable on anticoagulants, if receiving protracted course of antibiotics, renal/hepatic impairment, or a poor nutritional state; give vitamin K as needed. Watery, bloody stools (with or without stomach cramps and fever) may develop after starting treatment; notify physician. *Clostridium difficile*-associated diarrhea (CDAD) reported.

ADVERSE REACTIONS: Diarrhea, N/V, vaginitis, (suspension in peds) taste aversion, superinfection (prolonged use).

INTERACTIONS: Probenecid increases plasma levels. Lower bioavailability with drugs that lower gastric acidity. Caution with agents causing adverse effects on renal function (diuretics). Reduced efficacy of combined oral estrogen/progesterone contraceptives.

PREGNANCY: Category B, not for use in nursing.

MECHANISM OF ACTION: 2nd-generation cephalosporin; binds to essential target proteins and inhibits cell-wall synthesis.

PHARMACOKINETICS: Absorption: Absolute bioavailability (52% with food). PO administration of variable doses resulted in different parameters. **Distribution:** Plasma protein binding (50%). **Metabolism:** Rapid hydrolysis, via nonspecific esterases in the intestinal mucosa and blood. **Elimination:** Urine (50% unchanged).

NURSING CONSIDERATIONS

Assessment: Assess for previous hypersensitivity reactions to cephalosporins/PCNs or other drugs, renal/hepatic impairment, nutritional state, history of colitis, malabsorption, pregnancy/nursing status, phenylketonuria, and possible drug interactions.

Monitoring: Periodically monitor PT; with vitamin K administration if indicated. Monitor for allergic reactions, signs/symptoms of pseudomembranous colitis or *C.difficile*-associated diarrhea, development of superinfection or drug resistance, renal function, and lab test interactions.

Patient Counseling: Inform drug only treats bacterial, not viral, infections. Take exactly as directed; skipping doses or not completing full course may decrease effectiveness and increase resistance. Inform about potential benefits/risks. D/C and notify physician if allergic reactions, watery/bloody diarrhea (with/without muscle cramps), or fever occur. Notify if pregnant/nursing. Pediatrics who can not swallow tab whole should receive oral sus; if tab crushed, has strong/persistent bitter taste. Administer tab immediately after a meal, and suspension with milk or milk products.

Administration: Oral route. Tab and sus not bioequivalent and not substitutable on mg-per-mg basis. Shake sus well before use. **Storage:** Tab: Store at 15-30°C (59-86°F). Sus Powder: Store at 2-30°C (36-86°F). Reconstituted Sus: Store at 2-8°C (36-46°F); discard after 10 days.

CEFZIL — RX

cefprozil (Bristol-Myers Squibb)

THERAPEUTIC CLASS: Cephalosporin (2nd generation)

INDICATIONS: Treatment of mild to moderate pharyngitis/tonsillitis, otitis media, acute sinusitis, secondary bacterial infection of acute bronchitis, acute bacterial exacerbation of chronic bronchitis (ABECB), and uncomplicated skin and skin structure infections (SSSI) caused by susceptible strains of microorganisms.

DOSAGE: *Adults:* Pharyngitis/Tonsillitis: 500mg q24h for 10 days. Acute Sinusitis: 250-500mg q12h for 10 days. ABECB/Acute Bronchitis: 500mg q12h for 10 days. SSSI: 250-500mg q12h or 500mg q24h for 10 days. CrCl <30mL/min: 50% of standard dose.

Pediatrics: ≥13 yrs: Use adult dose. 2-12 yrs: Pharyngitis/Tonsillitis: 7.5mg/kg q12h for 10 days. SSSI: 20mg/kg q24h for 10 days. 6 months-12 yrs: Otitis Media: 15mg/kg q12h for 10 days. Acute Sinusitis: 7.5-15mg/kg q12h for 10 days. Do not exceed adult dose. CrCl <30mL/min: 50% of standard dose.

HOW SUPPLIED: Sus: 125mg/5mL [50mL, 75mL, 100mL], 250mg/5mL [50mL, 75mL, 100mL]; Tab: 250mg, 500mg

WARNINGS/PRECAUTIONS: Cross-sensitivity with cephalosporins and PCNs. False (+) direct Coombs' tests reported. *Clostridium difficile*-associated diarrhea reported. Caution with GI disease, renal impairment, elderly. False (+) for urine glucose with Benedict's, Fehling's solution, and Clinitest tabs. Sus contains phenylalanine.

ADVERSE REACTIONS: Diarrhea, nausea, hepatic enzyme elevations, eosinophilia, genital pruritus, vaginitis, superinfection (prolonged use).

INTERACTIONS: Nephrotoxicity with aminoglycosides reported. Probenecid may increase plasma levels. Caution with agents causing adverse effects on renal function (diuretics).

PREGNANCY: Category B, caution in nursing.

MECHANISM OF ACTION: 2nd-generation cephalosporin; inhibits bacterial cell-wall synthesis.

PHARMACOKINETICS: Absorption: C_{max}=6.1mcg/mL (250mg), 10.5mcg/mL (500mg), 18.3mcg/mL(1g); T_{max}=1.5 hrs (adults), 1-2 hrs (peds). Plasma concentration (peds) at 7.5, 15, and 30mg/kg doses similar to those observed within same time frame in normal adults at 250, 500, and 1000mg doses, respectively. **Distribution:** V_d=0.23L/kg; plasma protein binding (36%); found in breast milk. **Elimination:** Urine (60%); $T_{1/2}$=1.3 hrs (adults), 1.5 hrs (peds).

NURSING CONSIDERATIONS

Assessment: Assess for previous hypersensitivity reactions to PCNs/cephalosporins or other drugs, renal/hepatic impairment, pregnancy/nursing status, and possible drug interactions. Perform renal function tests prior to and during therapy.

Monitoring: Periodically monitor renal function tests, LFTs and hematopoietic functions. Monitor for allergic reactions (eg, Stevens-Johnson syndrome), signs/symptoms of *C.difficile*-associated diarrhea (may range between mild diarrhea to fatal colitis), development of drug resistance or superinfection, nephrotoxicity if given concurrently with aminoglycosides and for lab test interactions (eg, positive Coombs' test, false positive for urinary glucose if copper reduction tests used, false negative in ferricyanide test for blood glucose; no interference in plasma/urinary creatinine by alkaline picrate method).

Patient Counseling: Inform drug only treats bacterial, not viral, infections. Take exactly as directed; skipping doses or not completing full course may decrease effectiveness and increase resistance. Inform about potential benefits/risks. D/C and notify physician if allergic reactions, watery/bloody diarrhea (with/without muscle cramps), or fever occur (up to 2 months after therapy). Notify if pregnant/nursing.

Administration: Oral route. Shake sus well before use. **Storage:** Tab: 15-30°C (59-86°F); prior to reconstitution at 15-25°C (59-77°F), refrigerate after mixing; discard after 14 days.

CELEBREX RX

celecoxib (G.D. Searle)

NSAIDs may cause an increased risk of serious cardiovascular thrombotic events, MI, stroke and serious GI adverse events including bleeding, ulceration, and perforation of the stomach or intestines. Contraindicated for the treatment of perioperative pain in the setting of coronary artery bypass graft (CABG) surgery.

THERAPEUTIC CLASS: COX-2 inhibitor

INDICATIONS: Relief of signs and symptoms of rheumatoid arthritis (RA) in adults, osteoarthritis (OA), and ankylosing spondylitis (AS). Management of acute pain in adults. Treatment of primary dysmenorrhea. Adjunct to usual care (eg, surgical endoscopic surveillance) to reduce the number of adenomatous colorectal polyps in familial adenomatous polyposis (FAP). Relief of signs and symptoms of juvenile rheumatoid arthritis (JRA) in patients ≥2 yrs.

DOSAGE: *Adults:* ≥18 yrs: OA: 200mg qd or 100mg bid. RA: 100-200mg bid. AS: 200mg qd or 100mg bid. Titrate: May increase to 400mg/day after 6 weeks. FAP: 400mg bid with food. Acute Pain/Primary Dysmenorrhea: Day 1: 400mg, then 200mg if needed. Maint: 200mg bid prn. Moderate Hepatic Insufficiency: Reduce daily dose by 50%. Poor Metabolizers of CYP2C9 Substrates: Half the lowest recommended dose.
Pediatrics: JRA: ≥2 yrs: 10-25kg: 50mg bid. >25kg: 100mg bid.

HOW SUPPLIED: Cap: 50mg, 100mg, 200mg, 400mg

C

CONTRAINDICATIONS: Sulfonamide hypersensitivity. Asthma, urticaria, or allergic type reactions after ASA or NSAID use. Treatment of perioperative pain in the setting of CABG surgery.

WARNINGS/PRECAUTIONS: Increased risk of serious adverse cardiovascular thrombotic events, MI, and stroke. May lead to onset of new HTN or worsening of pre-existing HTN; monitor BP closely. Fluid retention and edema reported; caution with fluid retention or heart failure. Renal papillary necrosis and other renal injury reported after long-term use. Not recommended for use with advanced renal disease; if therapy must be initiated, monitor renal function. Greatest risk with those taking diuretics and ACE-inhibitors. Anaphylactoid reactions may occur. May cause serious skin adverse events (eg, exfoliative dermatitis, Stevens-Johnson syndrome, and toxic epidermal necrolysis). Avoid in late pregnancy; may cause premature closure of ductus arteriosus. May cause elevations of LFTs; d/c if liver disease develops or systemic manifestations occur. Anemia may occur; with long-term use, monitor Hgb/Hct if signs or symptoms of anemia or blood loss develop. May inhibit platelet aggregation and prolong bleeding time (prolonged APTT); monitor with coagulation disorders. Caution with asthma and avoid with ASA-sensitive asthma. Caution in pediatric patients with systemic onset JRA due to increased possibility of DIC. Caution in patients to be known or suspected poor CYP2C9 metabolizers based on previous history/experience with other CYP2C9 substrates (eg, warfarin, phenytoin). Caution in elderly.

ADVERSE REACTIONS: Dyspepsia, diarrhea, abdominal pain, nausea, dizziness, headache, sinusitis, upper respiratory infection, rash, fever, cough, arthralgia, HTN, insomnia, pharyngitis.

INTERACTIONS: Monitor oral anticoagulants; reports of serious bleeding, some fatal, with warfarin. Decreased effects of ACE-inhibitors, furosemide, and thiazides. Increased levels with fluconazole. Monitor lithium. Caution with CYP2C9 inhibitors and drugs metabolized by CYP2D6. Celecoxib is not a substitute for ASA for cardiovascular prophylaxis; may use with low-dose ASA but may increase GI complications. Avoid with NSAID.

PREGNANCY: Category C, caution in nursing.

MECHANISM OF ACTION: NSAID; inhibits prostaglandin synthesis primarily via inhibition of COX-2.

PHARMACOKINETICS: Absorption: C_{max}=705ng/mL, T_{max}=2.8 hrs. **Distribution:** V_d=429L; plasma protein binding (97%). **Metabolism:** CYP2C9. Primary alcohol, carboxylic acid, glucuronide conjugate (metabolites). **Elimination:** Urine (27%), feces (57%); $T_{1/2}$=11.2 hrs.

NURSING CONSIDERATIONS

Assessment: Assess for risk of cardiovascular thrombotic events (MI, stroke), CABG surgery, renal/hepatic insufficiency, HTN, history of peptic ulcer disease and/or GI bleeding, allergic-type reactions to sulfonamides, pre-existing asthma, and urticaria.

Monitoring: Monitor renal function, LFTs, chemistries, and CBC periodically. Monitor for signs and symptoms of CV thrombotic events, GI events (bleeding, ulceration, perforation), HTN, fluid retention, edema, CHF, hypersensitivity reactions, renal and hepatic dysfunction.

Patient Counseling: Inform may cause MI or stroke, and GI discomfort; d/c and report immediately if rash develops. Seek medical attention if symptoms of unexplained weight gain or edema, anaphylactoid reactions (difficulty in breathing, swelling of the face or throat), or hepatotoxicity (nausea, fatigue, lethargy, pruritus, jaundice, right upper quadrant tenderness and "flu-like" symptoms) occur. Inform of pregnancy risks.

Administration: Oral route. **Storage:** 25°C (77°F); excursions permitted to 15-30°C (59-86°F).

CELEXA
RX

citalopram hydrobromide (Forest)

Antidepressants increased the risk of suicidal thinking and behavior (suicidality) in short-term studies in children, adolescents, and young adults with major depressive disorder (MDD) and other psychiatric disorders. Citalopram is not approved for use in pediatric patients.

THERAPEUTIC CLASS: Selective serotonin reuptake inhibitor

INDICATIONS: Treatment of depression.

DOSAGE: *Adults:* Initial: 20mg qd, in the am or pm. Titrate: Increase by 20mg at intervals of no less than 1 week. Max: 40mg/day (non-responders may require 60mg/day). Elderly/Hepatic Impairment: 20mg/day. Titrate: Increase to 40mg/day in nonresponders.

HOW SUPPLIED: Sol: 10mg/5mL [240mL]; Tab: 10mg, 20mg*, 40mg* *scored

CONTRAINDICATIONS: Concomitant use of MAOI or pimozide.

WARNINGS/PRECAUTIONS: Avoid abrupt withdrawal. May increase risk of bleeding events. Activation of mania/hypomania, SIADH, hyponatremia reported. Caution with history of mania or seizures, hepatic impairment, severe renal impairment, conditions that alter metabolism or hemodynamic responses. May impair judgment, thinking, or motor skills. Serotonin syndrome may occur. Monitor for clinical worsening and/or suicidality, especially at initiation of therapy or dose changes.

ADVERSE REACTIONS: NV, dyspepsia, diarrhea, dry mouth, somnolence, insomnia, increased sweating, ejaculation disorder, rhinitis, anxiety, anorexia, tremor, and agitation.

INTERACTIONS: See Contraindications. Avoid alcohol, tryptophan. Caution with other centrally acting drugs, SSRIs, SNRIs, TCAs, lithium, carbamazepine, cimetidine. Increased risk of bleeding with warfarin, ASA, NSAIDs. Rare reports of weakness, hyperreflexia, incoordination with SSRIs and sumatriptan. Clearance may be decreased with potent CYP3A4 (eg, ketoconazole, itraconazole, fluconazole, erythromycin) and CYP2C19 (eg, omeprazole) inhibitors. May increase metoprolol levels which leads to decreased cardioselectivity. Concomitant use of serotonergic drugs and with drugs that impair metabolism of serotonin may cause serotonin syndrome. Caution with other agents that may affect serotonergic neurotransmitter systems (eg, triptans, linezolid, tramadol, or St. John's Wort).

PREGNANCY: Category C, not for use in nursing.

MECHANISM OF ACTION: SSRI; inhibits CNS neuronal reuptake of serotonin.

PHARMACOKINETICS: Absorption: Absolute bioavailability (80%); T_{max}=4 hrs. **Distribution:** V_d=12L/kg. **Metabolism:** Hepatic (biotransformation: N-demethylation) via CYP3A4 and CYP2C19 . **Elimination:** Urine (10%); $T_{1/2}$=35 hrs.

NURSING CONSIDERATIONS

Assessment: Assess for risk for bipolar disorder, history of mania, history of seizures, disease/condition that alters metabolism or hemodynamic response, hepatic/renal impairment, pregnancy/nursing status, and possible drug interactions.

Monitoring: Monitor for signs/symptoms of clinical worsening (suicidality, unusual changes in behavior), serotonin syndrome/NMS-like reactions, abnormal bleeding, hyponatremia, seizures, cognitive and motor impairment, and hepatic/renal dysfunction. If therapy is abruptly d/c, monitor for symptoms of dysphoric mood, irritability, agitation, dizziness, sensory disturbances, anxiety, confusion, headache, lethargy, emotional lability, insomnia, and hypomania.

Patient Counseling: Advise to avoid alcohol. Seek medical attention for symptoms of serotonin syndrome (mental status changes, tachycardia, hyperthermia, NV, diarrhea, incoordination), abnormal bleeding (particularly if using NSAID or ASA), hyponatremia, activation of mania, seizures, clinical worsening (suicidal ideation, unusual changes in behavior) and discontinuation of symptoms (irritability, agitation, dizziness, anxiety, headache, insomnia). Caution against hazardous tasks (eg, operating machinery and driving). May notice improvement in 1-4 weeks; continue therapy as directed. Notify physician if pregnant/intend to become pregnant, or breastfeeding. Counsel about benefits and risks of therapy. Inform physician if taking, or plan to take any over-the-counter prescriptions.

Administration: Oral route. **Storage:** 25°C (77°F); excursions permitted to 15-30°C (59-86°F).

CellCept — RX

mycophenolate mofetil (Roche Labs)

Immunosuppression may lead to increased susceptibility to infection and possible development of lymphoma. Female users of childbearing potential must use contraception. CellCept use during pregnancy associated with increased risk of pregnancy loss and congenital malformations.

THERAPEUTIC CLASS: Inosine monophosphate dehydrogenase inhibitor

INDICATIONS: Prophylaxis of organ rejection in allogeneic renal, cardiac, or hepatic transplants. Use with cyclosporine and corticosteroids.

DOSAGE: *Adults:* Renal Transplant: 1g IV/PO bid. Cardiac Transplant: 1.5g IV/PO bid. Hepatic Transplant: 1g IV bid or 1.5g PO bid. Start PO as soon as possible after transplant. Start IV within 24 hrs after transplant; can continue for up to 14 days. Switch to oral when tolerated. Give on an empty stomach. *Pediatrics:* Renal Transplant: (Sus) 600mg/m^2 PO bid. Max: 2g/day (10 mL/day). (Cap) BSA 1.25m^2 to 1.5m^2: 750mg PO bid. (Cap/Tab) BSA >1.5m^2: 1g bid.

HOW SUPPLIED: Cap: 250mg; Inj: 500mg; Sus: 200mg/mL [175mL]; Tab: 500mg

CONTRAINDICATIONS: (Inj) Hypersensitivity to Polysorbate 80 (TWEEN).

WARNINGS/PRECAUTIONS: Risk of lymphomas and other malignancies, especially of the skin. Avoid sunlight to decrease risk of skin cancer. May cause fetal harm during pregnancy. Must have negative serum/urine pregnancy test within 1 week before therapy. Two reliable forms of contraception required before and during therapy, and 6 weeks following discontinuation. Monitor for bone marrow suppression. Risk of GI ulceration, hemorrhage, and perforation; caution with active digestive system disease. Caution with delayed renal graft function post-transplant. Oral suspension contains phenylalanine; caution with phenylketonurics. Monitor CBC weekly during the 1st month, twice monthly for the 2nd and 3rd months, and then monthly through 1st year. Avoid with rare hereditary deficiency of hypoxanthine-guanine phosphoribosyltransferase (eg, Lesch-Nyhan and Kelley-Seegmiller syndrome). Increased susceptibility infections/sepsis.

ADVERSE REACTIONS: Infections, diarrhea, leukopenia, sepsis, vomiting, GI bleeding, pain, abdominal pain, fever, headache, asthenia, chest pain, back pain, anemia, thrombocytopenia.

INTERACTIONS: Additive bone marrow suppression with azathioprine; avoid use. Reduced efficacy with drugs that interfere with enterohepatic recirculation (eg, cholestyramine). Efficacy/safety with other immunosuppressive agents not determined. Avoid live attenuated vaccines. Increased levels of both drugs with acyclovir, ganciclovir. Decreased levels with magnesium- and aluminum-containing antacids; space dosing. Decreased effects of oral contraceptives. Increased levels with probenecid. Other drugs that compete for renal tubular secretion may raise levels of both drugs.

PREGNANCY: Category D, not for use in nursing.

MECHANISM OF ACTION: Prolongs the survival of allogeneic transplants (kidney, heart, liver, intestine, limb, small bowel, pancreatic islets, and bone marrow). Inhibits proliferative arteriopathy in experimental models of aortic and cardiac allografts in rats as well as in primate cardiac xenografts. Inhibits immunologically mediated inflammatory responses and tumor development and prolongs survival in tumor transplant models.

PHARMACOKINETICS: Absorption: Oral; rapid and complete, absolute bioavailability (94%). MPA C_{max} decreased by 40% with food. **Distribution:** V_d=3.6L/kg (IV), 4L/kg (oral); plasma protein binding of MPA (97%), MPAG (82%). **Metabolism:** MPA (active metabolite) metabolized by glucuronyl transferase to MPAG, which is converted to MPA via entrohepatic recirculation. **Elimination:** Oral: Urine (93%), feces (6%). Urine: MPA (<1%) and MPAG (87%). MPA: (Oral) $T_{1/2}$=17.9 hrs. (Oral) and (IV) $T_{1/2}$=16.6 hrs. In pediatrics: Oral administration in different age groups ranging between 1-18 years results in different pharmacokinetics.

NURSING CONSIDERATIONS

Assessment: Assess drug hypersensitivity, hepatic/renal impairment, pregnancy status, vaccination history, phenylketonuria, hereditary deficiency of HGPRT such as Lesch-Nyhan and Kelley-Seegmiller syndrome, active digestive disease, and for possible drug interactions.

Monitoring: Monitor for signs of delayed graft rejection (eg, anemia, thrombocytopenia, and hyperkalemia), lymphomas, skin cancer, GI bleeding/perforation, peptic/duodenal ulcers, infections, opportunistic infections (eg, herpes virus, fatal infection, sepsis), unexpected bruising, bleeding, or any signs of bone marrow suppression. Periodically monitor CBC.

Patient Counseling: Counsel on importance of following dosage instructions and having periodic laboratory tests. Inform about increased risk of the malignancies, infection; notify physician for any signs of infection, bruising, and/or bleeding. Avoid prolonged exposure to sunlight. Not for use in pregnant/nursing women or those planning to become pregnant. Take on empty stomach.

Administration: Oral route and slow IV infusion route. **Storage:** (Tablet) 25°C (77°F); excursions permitted to 15-30°C (59-86°F). Store dry powder and reconstituted/infusion solution at 25°C (77°F); excursions permitted to 15-30°C (59-86°F). Do not freeze.

CENESTIN RX

conjugated estrogens (Duramed)

Estrogens increase risk of endometrial cancer. Estrogens, with or without progestins, should not be used for the prevention of cardiovascular disease. Increased risks of MI, stroke, invasive breast cancer, PE, and DVT in postmenopausal women reported.

THERAPEUTIC CLASS: Estrogen

INDICATIONS: (0.45mg, 0.625mg, 0.9mg, 1.25mg) Treatment of moderate to severe vasomotor symptoms associated with menopause. (0.3mg) Treatment of vulvar and vaginal atrophy.

DOSAGE: *Adults:* Vasomotor Symptoms: Initial: 0.45mg/day. Adjust dose based on response. Discontinue or taper at 3-6 month intervals. Vulvar/Vaginal Atrophy: 0.3mg qd.

HOW SUPPLIED: Tab: 0.3mg, 0.45mg, 0.625mg, 0.9mg, 1.25mg

CONTRAINDICATIONS: Pregnancy, undiagnosed abnormal genital bleeding, breast cancer, estrogen-dependent neoplasia, DVT/PE, active or recent (eg, within past year) arterial thromboembolic disease (eg, stroke, MI), liver dysfunction or disease.

WARNINGS/PRECAUTIONS: May increase risk of cardiovascular events (eg, MI, stroke), venous thrombosis, and PE; d/c immediately if any of these events occur or are suspected. May increase risk of breast/endometrial cancer, and gallbladder disease. May lead to severe hypercalcemia with breast cancer and bone metastases; monitor and d/c if hypercalcemia occurs. Retinal vascular thrombosis reported; monitor and d/c if papilledema or retinal vascular lesions occur. Consider addition of a progestin if no hysterectomy. May elevate BP; monitor at regular intervals. May cause elevations of plasma triglycerides with pre-existing hypertriglyceridemia. Caution with history of cholestatic jaundice associated with past estrogen use or with pregnancy; d/c with recurrence. May lead to increased thyroid-binding globulin levels; monitor thyroid function. May cause fluid retention; caution with cardiac/renal dysfunction.

Caution with severe hypocalcemia. May increase risk of ovarian cancer. May exacerbate endometriosis, asthma, DM, epilepsy, migraine, porphyria, SLE, and hepatic hemangiomas; use with caution.

ADVERSE REACTIONS: Abdominal pain, back pain, pain, headache, infection, vomiting, leg cramps, paresthesia, breast pain, metrorrhagia, endometrial thickening, vaginitis.

INTERACTIONS: CYP3A4 inducers (eg, St. John's wort, phenobarbital, carbamazepine, rifampin) may decrease levels which may decrease therapeutic effects and/or change uterine bleeding profile. CYP3A4 inhibitors (eg, erythromycin, clarithromycin, ketoconazole, itraconazole, ritonavir, grapefruit juice) may increase levels which may result in side effects.

PREGNANCY: Contraindicated in pregnancy; caution in nursing.

MECHANISM OF ACTION: Estrogen; binds to nuclear receptor in estrogen-responsive tissues. Modulates pituitary secretion of gonadotropins, luteinizing hormone (LH) and follicle stimulating hormone (FSH), through negative feedback mechanism.

PHARMACOKINETICS: Absorption: Well-absorbed; conjugated and unconjugated estrogens had altered parameters. **Distribution:** Estrogens found in breast milk; largely bound to sex hormone binding globulin (SHBG) and albumin. **Metabolism:** Liver, to estrone (metabolite); estriol (major urinary metabolite); enterohepatic recirculation, via sulfate and glucuronide conjugation; biliary secretion of conjugates into the intestine; hydrolysis in gut; reabsorption; CYP3A4 (partial). **Elimination:** Urine.

NURSING CONSIDERATIONS

Assessment: Assess for genital bleeding, presence or history of breast cancer, estrogen-dependent neoplasia, DVT, PE, active or recent (within past yr) arterial thromboembolic disease (eg, stroke, MI), liver dysfunction/disease, hypocalcemia, and known/suspected pregnancy. Assess use in nursing females and in patients ≥65 yrs. Assess for drug and lab interactions.

Monitoring: Monitor for signs/symptoms of cardiovascular disorders (eg, MI, stroke, venous thrombosis, PE), malignant neoplasms (eg, cancers of endometrium, breast, ovaries), dementia, gallbladder disease, hypercalcemia, visual abnormalities (eg, retinal vascular thrombosis), cholestatic jaundice, elevated BP, hypertriglyceridemia, hypothyroidism, fluid retention, exacerbation of endometriosis, and exacerbation of other conditions (eg, asthma, DM, epilepsy, migraines or porphyria, SLE, and hepatic hemangiomas). Monitor thyroid function in patients on thyroid hormone replacement therapy. If abnormal genital bleeding occurs, perform proper diagnostic measures (eg, endometrial sampling) to rule out malignancy. Re-evaluate every 3-6 months to evaluate need for therapy.

Patient Counseling: Inform that medication increases risk for uterine cancer and may increase risk for heart attack, stroke, breast cancer, blood clots, and dementia. Advise to notify physician if signs/symptoms of unusual vaginal bleeding, dizziness/faintness, changes in speech, severe headaches, CP, SOB, leg pain, visual changes, or vomiting develop.

Administration: Oral route. **Storage:** 20-25°C (68-77°F); excursions permitted 15-30°C (59-86°F).

CEPHALEXIN — RX

cephalexin (Various)

OTHER BRAND NAMES: Keflex (Middlebrook)

THERAPEUTIC CLASS: Cephalosporin (1st generation)

INDICATIONS: Treatment of otitis media and skin and skin structure (SSSI), bone, genitourinary tract, and respiratory tract infections caused by susceptible strains of microorganisms.

DOSAGE: *Adults:* Usual: 250mg q6h. Streptococcal Pharyngitis/SSSI/Uncomplicated Cystitis (>15 yrs): 500mg q12h. Treat cystitis for 7-14 days. Max: 4g/day.

Pediatrics: Usual: 25-50mg/kg/day in divided doses. Streptococcal Pharyngitis (>1 yr)/SSSI: May divide dose and give q12h. Otitis Media: 75-100mg/kg/day in divided doses. Administer for ≥10 days in β-hemolytic streptococcal infections.

HOW SUPPLIED: (Keflex) Cap: 250mg, 500mg, 750mg; (Generic) Cap: 250mg, 500mg; Sus: 125mg/5mL [100mL, 200mL], 250mg/5mL [100mL, 200mL]

WARNINGS/PRECAUTIONS: Caution with markedly impaired renal function, history of GI disease. Cross-sensitivity with cephalosporins and PCNs. *Clostridium difficile*-associated diarrhea reported. Positive direct Coombs' tests reported. False (+) for urine glucose with Benedict's, Fehling's solution, and Clinitest tabs. May result in overgrowth of nonsusceptible bacteria.

ADVERSE REACTIONS: Diarrhea, allergic reactions, dyspepsia, gastritis, abdominal pain, superinfection (prolonged use).

INTERACTIONS: Probenecid inhibits excretion.

PREGNANCY: Category B, caution in nursing.

MECHANISM OF ACTION: Cephalosporin; bactericidal due to inhibition of cell-wall synthesis.

PHARMACOKINETICS: Absorption: Rapid; oral administration of variable doses resulted in different parameters. T_{max}=1 hr. **Elimination:** Urine (90% unchanged).

NURSING CONSIDERATIONS

Assessment: Assess for history of hypersensitivity to cephalosporins/PCNs, pregnancy status, possible drug interactions, renal impairment. Document indications for therapy, culture and susceptibility testing. Perform incision and drainage in conjunction with antibiotic therapy when indicated.

Monitoring: Monitor for signs/symptoms of hypersensitivity reactions (anaphylaxis), *C. difficile*-associated diarrhea, seizures, aplastic anemia, renal functions, PT, LDH, superinfections.

Patient Counseling: Inform drug only treats bacterial, not viral, infections. Instruct to take exactly as directed; skipping doses or not completing full course may decrease effectiveness and increase resistance. Inform patient may experience diarrhea; contact physician if watery/bloody stools, superinfection, or hypersensitivity reactions occur.

Administration: Oral route. **Storage:** 25°C (77°F); excursions permitted to 15-30°C (59-86°F).

CEREBYX — RX

fosphenytoin sodium (Parke-Davis)

THERAPEUTIC CLASS: Hydantoin

INDICATIONS: Short-term (up to 5 days) parenteral administration when other means of phenytoin administration are unavailable, inappropriate, or less advantageous, including to control general convulsive status epilepticus, prevent or treat seizures during neurosurgery, as a short-term substitute for oral phenytoin.

DOSAGE: *Adults:* Doses, concentration in dosing solutions, and infusion rates are expressed as phenytoin sodium equivalents (PE). Status Epilepticus: LD: 15-20 PE/kg IV at 100-150mg PE/min then switch to maintenance dose. Non-Emergent Cases: LD: 10-20mg PE/kg IV (max 150mg PE/min) or IM. Maint: Initial: 4-6mg PE/kg/day. May substitute for oral phenytoin sodium at the same total daily dose.

HOW SUPPLIED: Inj: 50mg PE/mL (2mL, 10mL)

CONTRAINDICATIONS: Sinus bradycardia, sino-atrial block, 2nd- and 3rd-degree AV block, Adams-Stokes syndrome.

WARNINGS/PRECAUTIONS: Avoid abrupt discontinuation. Not for use in absence seizures. Hypotension and severe cardiovascular reactions and fatalities reported; continuously monitor ECG, BP, and respiration during and for at least 20 min after IV infusion and monitor phenytoin levels at least 2 hrs after IV infusion or 4 hrs after IM injection. Caution with severe myocardial insufficiency, porphyria, hepatic/renal dysfunction, hypoalbuminemia, elderly, and diabetes. Acute hepatotoxicity, lymphadenopathy, hemopoietic complications, hyperglycemia reported. D/C if rash or acute hepatotoxicity occurs. Neonatal postpartum bleeding disorder, congenital malformations, and increased seizure frequency reported with use during pregnancy. Avoid use with seizures due to hypoglycemia or other metabolic causes. Caution with phosphate restriction because of phosphate load (0.0037mmol phosphate/mg PE). May lower folate levels.

ADVERSE REACTIONS: Nystagmus, dizziness, pruritus, paresthesia, headache, somnolence, ataxia, tinnitus, stupor, nausea, hypotension, vasodilation, tremor, incoordination, dry mouth.

INTERACTIONS: Increased levels with acute alcohol intake, amiodarone, chloramphenicol, chlordiazepoxide, cimetidine, diazepam, dicumarol, disulfiram, estrogens, ethosuximide, fluoxetine, H_2-antagonists, halothane, isoniazid, methylphenidate, phenothiazines, phenylbutazone, salicylates, succinimides, sulfonamides, tolbutamide, trazodone. Decreased levels with carbamazepine, chronic alcohol abuse, reserpine. Decreases efficacy of anticoagulants, corticosteroids, coumarin, digitoxin, doxycycline, estrogens, furosemide, oral contraceptives, rifampin, quinidine, theophylline, vitamin D. Variable effects (increase or decrease levels) with phenobarbital, valproic acid, and sodium valproate. Caution with drugs highly bound to serum albumin. TCAs may precipitate seizures.

PREGNANCY: Category D, not for use in nursing.

MECHANISM OF ACTION: Anticonvulsant; prodrug of phenytoin. Modulates voltage-dependent sodium and calcium channels of neurons, inhibits calcium flux across neuronal membranes, and enhances sodium-potassium ATPase activity of neurons and glial cells.

PHARMACOKINETICS: Absorption: Fosphenytoin is completely converted to phenytoin. (IM) T_{max}=30 min. **Distribution:** Plasma protein binding (95-99%); V_d=4.3-10.8L. **Metabolism:** Phosphatases (conversion to phenytoin); liver (phenytoin metabolism). **Elimination:** Urine (1-5% phenytoin and metabolites); $T_{1/2}$=15 min (fosphenytoin), 12-28.9 hrs (phenytoin).

NURSING CONSIDERATIONS

Assessment: Assess LFTs, renal function, CBC with platelets and differential, hypoalbuminemia, porphyria, cardiac conduction defects, pregnancy status, and phosphate levels. Note other diseases/conditions and drug therapies.

Monitoring: Careful cardiac monitoring is needed when administering IV loading doses. Monitor LFTs, renal function, CBC with differential and platelets, hypersensitivity reactions, myasthenia, pneumonia, and hypokalemia.

Administration: IM/IV route. Should be prescribed in phenytoin sodium equivalent units (PE). Rate of IV administration should not exceed 150mg PE/min. **Storage:** Refrigerate at 2-8°C (36-46°F).

CESAMET

CII

nabilone (Valeant)

THERAPEUTIC CLASS: Cannabinoid

INDICATIONS: Treatment of the nausea and vomiting associated with chemotherapy when conventional treatment has failed.

DOSAGE: *Adults:* Initial: 1 or 2mg bid; given 1-3 hrs before chemotherapy. A dose of 1 or 2mg the night before may be useful. Max: 6mg/day given in divided doses tid.

HOW SUPPLIED: Cap: 1mg

WARNINGS/PRECAUTIONS: Patients should remain under the supervision of a responsible adult during treatment, especially during initial use and dose adjustments. Caution when initiating therapy with HTN, heart disease, current or previous psychiatric disorders and with history of substance abuse. Avoid driving, operating heavy machinery, or engaging in any hazardous activity during treatment. May cause dizziness, euphoria, ataxia, anxiety, disorientation, depression, hallucinations, and psychosis. Adverse psychiatric reactions can persist for 48-72 hrs following cessation of treatment. Avoid with alcohol, sedatives, hypnotics, or other psychoactive substances. May cause tachycardia and orthostatic hypotension.

ADVERSE REACTIONS: Drowsiness, vertigo, dry mouth, euphoria, ataxia, headache, concentration difficulties, nausea, dysphoria, sleep/visual disturbance, asthenia, anorexia.

INTERACTIONS: Additive HTN, tachycardia, possibly cardiotoxicity may occur with amphetamines, cocaine, other sympathomimetics. Additive or super-additive tachycardia, drowsiness may occur with atropine, scopolamine, antihistamines, other anticholinergics. Additive tachycardia, HTN, drowsiness may occur with TCAs. Additive drowsiness and CNS depression may occur with barbiturates, benzodiazepines, ethanol, lithium, opioids, buspirone, antihistamines, muscle relaxants, other CNS depressants. Hypomanic reaction reported with disulfiram, fluoxetine. May decrease clearance of antipyrine, barbiturates. May increase metabolism of theophylline. Cross-tolerance and mutual potentiation with opioids. Effects may be enhanced by opioid receptor blockade. Alcohol may increase the positive subjective mood effects.

PREGNANCY: Category C, not for use in nursing.

MECHANISM OF ACTION: Cannabinoid; interacts with the cannabinoid receptor system (CB (1) receptor that has been discovered in neural tissues).

PHARMACOKINETICS: Absorption: Complete, C_{max}=2ng/mL, T_{max}=2.0 hrs. **Distribution:** V_d=12.5L/kg. **Metabolism:** Liver (extensive), via stereospecific enzymes and multiple P450 enzyme isoforms. Isomeric carbinol (metabolite). **Elimination:** Feces (60%), urine (24%); $T_{1/2}$=2 hrs (identified metabolite), 35 hrs (unidentified metabolite).

NURSING CONSIDERATIONS

Assessment: Assess for heart disease, HTN, previous/current psychiatric disorders (Bipolar disorder, depression, and schizophrenia), alcohol intake or substance abuse, concomitant therapy with sedatives, hypnotics, or other psychoactive drugs with potential additive or synergistic CNS effects, hepatic/renal impairment, pregnancy/nursing status, and possible drug interactions.

Monitoring: Monitor for adverse psychiatric reactions or unmasking of symptoms of psychiatric disorders, signs/symptoms of CNS effects (dizziness, drowsiness, euphoria, ataxia, anxiety, disorientation, depression, hallucinations and psychosis), postural hypotension. Monitor BP and HR.

Patient Counseling: Caution against performing hazardous tasks such as driving or operating machinery and inform of possibility of psychological or physical dependence. Avoid concomitant use of alcohol and other CNS depressants; remain under supervision of responsible adult during therapy. Notify if pregnant/nursing; not recommended for children.

Administration: Oral route. **Storage:** 25°C (77°F); excursions permitted to 15-30°C (59-86°F).

CHANTIX — RX

varenicline tartrate (Pfizer)

THERAPEUTIC CLASS: Nicotinic Acetylcholine Receptor Agonist

INDICATIONS: Aid to smoking cessation treatment.

DOSAGE: *Adults:* ≥18 yrs: Days 1-3: 0.5mg qd. Days 4-7: 0.5mg bid. Day 8 to End of Treatment: 1mg bid. Duration: 12 weeks with additional 12 weeks after successful completion to ensure long-term abstinence. Severe Renal Impairment: Initial: 0.5mg qd. Titrate: Max: 0.5mg bid. End-Stage Renal Disease: Max: 0.5mg qd.

HOW SUPPLIED: Tab: 0.5mg, 1mg

C

WARNINGS/PRECAUTIONS: Serious neuropsychiatric symptoms (eg, changes in behavior, agitation, depressed mood, suicidal ideation, suicidal behavior) reported. Physiological changes resulting from smoking cessation may alter pharmacokinetics or pharmacodynamics of some drugs (eg, theophylline, warfarin, insulin). Use caution driving or operating machinery until the effects of varenicline are known.

ADVERSE REACTIONS: Nausea, sleep disturbance, constipation, flatulence, vomiting.

INTERACTIONS: Reduced renal clearance with cimetidine. Increased incidence of side effects (eg, vomiting, headache, nausea) with nicotine replacement therapy.

PREGNANCY: Category C, not for use in nursing.

MECHANISM OF ACTION: Nicotinic acetylcholine receptor agonist; binds with high affinity and selectivity at α4β2 neuronal nicotinic acetycholine receptors, blocking ability of nicotine to activate these receptors, thus stimulating central nervous mesolimbic dopamine system.

PHARMACOKINETICS: Absorption: T_{max}=3-4 hrs. **Distribution:** Plasma protein binding (≤20%). **Metabolism:** Minimal. **Elimination:** Urine (92% unchanged); $T_{1/2}$=24 hrs.

NURSING CONSIDERATIONS

Assessment: Assess for pre-existing psychiatric illness and impaired renal function.

Monitoring: Monitor for neuropsychiatric symptoms (eg, changes in behavior, agitation, depressed mood, suicidal ideation/behavior), worsening of pre-existing psychiatric illness, nausea, and insomnia. Monitor for altered pharmacokinetics or pharmacodynamics of some drugs (eg, theophylline, warfarin, insulin); dosage adjustments may be necessary.

Patient Counseling: Inform to take as prescribed, set a date to quit smoking, and start 1 week before this date. Counsel on dosage titration and to take after eating with full glass of water. Inform about withdrawal symptoms and to report any to physician. Notify if pregnant/nursing or planning to become pregnant. Caution while performing hazardous tasks (eg, operating machinery/driving).

Administration: Oral route. **Storage:** 25°C (77°F); excursions permitted to 15-30°C (59-86°F).

CHLORPROMAZINE — RX

chlorpromazine (Various)

THERAPEUTIC CLASS: Phenothiazine

INDICATIONS: Treatment of schizophrenia. Control of nausea and vomiting. Relief of restlessness and apprehension before surgery. Treatment of acute intermittent porphyria. Adjunct treatment of tetanus. To control the manic type of manic-depressive illness. Relief of intractable hiccups. Treatment of severe behavioral problems in children. Short-term treatment of hyperactivity in children.

DOSAGE: *Adults:* Severe Behavioral Problems: Inpatient: Acute Schizophrenic/Manic State: 25mg IM, then 25-50mg IM in 1 hr if needed. Titrate: Increase over several days up to 400mg q4-6h until controlled then switch to PO. Usual: 500mg/day PO. Max: 1000mg/day PO. Less Acutely Disturbed: 25mg PO tid. Titrate: Increase gradually to 400mg/day. Outpatient: 10mg PO tid-qid or 25mg PO bid-tid. More Severe: 25mg PO tid. Titrate: After 1-2 days, increase by 20-50mg twice weekly until calm. Prompt Control of Severe Symptoms: 25mg IM, may repeat in 1 hr then 25-50mg PO tid. N/V: Usual: 10-25mg PO q4-6h prn; 25mg IM then, if no hypotension, 25-50mg q3-4h prn until vomiting stops then switch to PO; 100mg rectally q6-8h prn. N/V in Surgery: 12.5mg IM, may repeat in 1/2 hr; 2mg IV per fractional inj at 2 min intervals. Max: 25mg. Presurgical Apprehension: 25-50mg PO 2-3 hrs pre-op; 12.5-25mg IM 1-2 hrs pre-op. Intractable Hiccups: 25-50mg PO tid-qid;

if symptoms persist after 2-3 days, give 25-50mg IM; if symptoms still persist, give 25-50mg slow IV. Porphyria: 25-50mg PO tid-qid; 25mg IM tid-qid until PO therapy. Tetanus: 25-50mg IM tid-qid; 25-50mg IV. Elderly: Use lower doses, increase dose more gradually, monitor closely.
Pediatrics: 6 months-12 yrs: Severe Behavioral Problems: Outpatient: 0.25mg/lb PO q4-6h prn; 0.5mg/lb sup rectally q6-8h prn; 0.25mg/lb IM q6-8h prn. Inpatient: Start low and increase gradually to 50-100mg/day; ≥200mg/day in older children. Max: 500mg/day. <5 yrs (<50lbs): Max: ≤40mg/day IM; 5-12 yrs (50-100lbs): Max: ≤75mg/day IM. N/V: 0.25mg/lb PO q4-6h; 0.5mg/lb sup rectally q6-8 prn. 0.25mg/lb IM q6-8h prn. Max: 6 months-5 yrs (or 50 lbs): <40mg/day. 5-12 yrs (or 50-100lbs): <75mg/day except in severe cases. During Surgery: 0.125mg/lb IM repeat in 1/2 hr if needed; 1mg IV per fractional inj at 2 min intervals and not exceeding recommended IM dosage. Presurgical Apprehension: 0.25mg/lb PO 2-3 hrs (or IM 1-2 hrs) before operation. Tetanus: 0.25mg/lb IM/IV q6-8h. <50lbs: Max: ≤40mg/day; 50-100lbs: Max: ≤75mg/day.

HOW SUPPLIED: Cap, Extended-Release: 30mg, 75mg, 150mg; Inj: 25mg/mL; Sup: 25mg, 100mg; Syrup: 10mg/5mL [120mL]; Tab: 10mg, 25mg, 50mg, 100mg, 200mg

CONTRAINDICATIONS: Comatose states, or with large amounts of CNS depressants. Hypersensitivity to phenothiazines.

WARNINGS/PRECAUTIONS: Tardive dyskinesia, NMS may occur. Caution with chronic respiratory disorders, acute respiratory infections (especially in children), glaucoma, cardiovascular, hepatic, or renal disease, history of hepatic encephalopathy due to cirrhosis. Suppresses cough reflex; aspiration of vomitus possible. Caution if exposed to extreme heat or organophosphates. Avoid in children/adolescents with signs of Reye's syndrome. Lowers seizure threshold. Reduce dose gradually to prevent side effects. May mask signs of overdoses to other drugs and obscure diagnosis of other conditions (eg, intestinal obstruction, brain tumor, Reye's syndrome). May produce false-positive PKU test. May elevate prolactin levels. Injection contains sulfites.

ADVERSE REACTIONS: Drowsiness, jaundice, agranulocytosis, hypotensive effects, EKG changes, dystonias, motor restlessness, pseudo-parkinsonism, tardive dyskinesia, anticholinergic effects, NMS, ocular changes.

INTERACTIONS: See Contraindications. May decrease effects of oral anticoagulants, guanethidine. Propranolol increases plasma levels of both agents. Thiazide diuretics may potentiate orthostatic hypotension. Potentiates effects of CNS depressants (eg, anesthetic, barbiturates, narcotics); reduce doses of these drugs by 1/4 to 1/2. Anticonvulsants may need adjustment; phenytoin toxicity reported. Do not use with Amipaque®; discontinue at least 48 hrs before myelography and resume at least 24 hrs after. Can cause α-adrenergic blockade. Caution with atropine or related drugs. Encephalopathic syndrome reported with lithium.

PREGNANCY: Safety in pregnancy not known. Not for use in nursing.

MECHANISM OF ACTION: Phenothiazine; not established. Suspected to act at all levels of CNS, primarily at subcortical levels as well as on multiple organ systems. Exerts psychotropic, sedative, and antiemetic activity. Has strong antiadrenergic and weaker peripheral anticholinergic activity and ganglionic blocking action.

NURSING CONSIDERATIONS

Assessment: Assess for Reye's syndrome in children and adolescents prior to initiation. Evaluate mental status, renal/hepatic and cardiovascular function prior to treatment. Assess for glaucoma, respiratory disorders, or bone marrow depression, use of large amounts of CNS depressants.

Monitoring: Monitor LFTs, CBC, and EKG. Perform periodic eye exams for patients on long-term therapy. Monitor for NMS, TD, EKG changes (reversible Q and T wave distortions), and ocular changes. Monitor for anaphylaxis reactions when administering IM formulation.

Patient Counseling: Counsel to immediately report signs of infection and to avoid exposure to extreme heat. Drug may impair mental/physical abilities, especially during first few days of therapy. Advise to avoid alcohol and abrupt withdrawal of therapy.

C

Administration: Oral/IM. Parenteral administration should be reserved for bedridden patients or patients with acute ambulatory problems. Inject slowly, deep into upper outer quadrant of buttock. Instruct patient to lie down for at least 30 min following injection. If irritation occurs, dilute injection with saline or 2% procaine; mixing with other agents in syringe is not recommended.
Storage: Inj: 20-25°C (68-77°F); excursions permitted to 15-30°C (59-86°F). Protect from light and freezing. Tab: 20-25°C (68-77°F). Protect from moisture. Dispense in a tight, light-resistant container.

CIALIS RX

tadalafil (Lilly ICOS)

THERAPEUTIC CLASS: Phosphodiesterase type 5 inhibitor

INDICATIONS: Treatment of erectile dysfunction (ED).

DOSAGE: *Adults:* Prn Use: Take prior to sexual activity. Initial: 10mg. Range: 5-20mg. Renal Impairment: CrCl 31-50mL/min: Initial: 5mg. Max: 10mg/48 hrs. CrCl <30mL/min/Hemodialysis: Max: 5mg/72 hrs. Mild/Moderate Hepatic Impairment: Max: 10mg. Severe Hepatic Impairment: Avoid use. With Potent CYP3A4 Inhibitors (eg, ketoconazole, itraconazole, ritonavir): Max: 10mg/72 hrs. Once-Daily Use: Initial: 2.5mg qd without regard to timing of sexual activity. Titrate: May increase to 5mg qd based on efficacy and tolerability. CrCl <30mL/min/Hemodialysis/Severe Hepatic Impairment: Avoid use. Mild/Moderate Hepatic Impairment: Use with caution. With Potent CYP3A4 Inhibitors (eg, ketoconazole, itraconazole, ritonavir): Max: 2.5mg.

HOW SUPPLIED: Tab: 2.5mg, 5mg, 10mg, 20mg

CONTRAINDICATIONS: Concomitant nitrates.

WARNINGS/PRECAUTIONS: Avoid in men for whom sexual activity is inadvisable due to underlying CV status. Increased sensitivity to vasodilatory effect with left ventricular outflow obstruction. Avoid with MI (within last 90 days); unstable angina or angina occurring during sexual intercourse; NYHA Class 2 or greater heart failure (in the last 6 months); uncontrolled arrhythmias, hypotension (<90/50mmHg); or uncontrolled HTN (>170/100mmHg); stroke within the last 6 months; severe hepatic impairment (Child-Pugh Class C); degenerative retinal disorders, including retinitis pigmentosa. Prolonged erection reported. Substantial consumption of alcohol with tadalafil can increase HR, decrease BP, cause dizziness and headache. Caution with predisposition to priapism (eg, sickle cell anemia, multiple myeloma, leukemia), anatomical deformation of the penis, bleeding disorders, or active peptic ulceration. May cause transient decrease in BP. Caution with coadministration of PDE5 inhibitors and α-blockers. May cause additive hypotensive effect. Initiate at lowest dose once patient is stable on either therapy. Rare reports of nonarteritic anterior ischemic optic neuropathy (NAION) with PDE5 inhibitors. Sudden decrease or loss of hearing, tinnitus, and dizziness reported. D/C if experienced these symptoms.

ADVERSE REACTIONS: Headache, dyspepsia, back pain, myalgia, nasal congestion, flushing, limb pain, urticaria, Stevens-Johnson syndrome, exfoliative dermatitis, migraine, visual field defect, retinal vein occlusion, retinal artery occlusion, sudden decrease or loss of hearing, tinnitus.

INTERACTIONS: See Contraindications. Increased levels with CYP3A4 inhibitors (eg, ketoconazole, HIV-protease inhibitors, erythromycin, itraconazole, grapefruit juice). Decreased levels with CYP3A4 inducers (eg, rifampin, carbamazepine, phenytoin, phenobarbital). Additive hypotensive effects with alcohol, α-blockers (eg, tamsulosin, doxazosin, alfuzosin), antihypertensives (eg, amlodipine, metoprolol, bendrofluazide, enalapril, angiotensin-II receptor blockers).

PREGNANCY: Category B, not for use in nursing.

MECHANISM OF ACTION: Phosphodiesterase type 5 inhibitor; enhances effect of nitric oxide by inhibiting phosphodiesterase type 5, which is responsible for the degradation of cGMP in the corpus cavernosum.

PHARMACOKINETICS: Absorption: C_{max}=2hrs. **Distribution:** V_d=63L; plasma protein binding (94%). **Metabolism:** Via CYP3A4 to a catechol metabolite which undergoes extensive methylation and glucuronidation; methylcatechol glucuronide (major metabolite). **Elimination:** Urine (36%), feces (61%); $T_{1/2}$=17.5 hrs.

NURSING CONSIDERATIONS

Assessment: Assess for CVD, long QT syndrome, retinitis pigmentosa, bleeding disorders, active peptic ulceration, anatomical deformation of the penis, renal/hepatic impairment, contraindications for sexual activity. Assess potential underlying causes of erectile dysfunction and for possible drug interactions.

Monitoring: Monitor potential for cardiac risk due to sexual activity, postural hypotension, color vision changes, hypersensitivity reactions, stomach ulcers. Monitor therapeutic effect when used in combination with other drugs.

Patient Counseling: Instruct to seek medical assistance if erection persists >4 hrs. Advise of potential BP-lowering effect of α-blockers, other antihypertensive medications, alcohol, and cardiac risk of sexual activity. Counsel about the protective measures necessary to guard against STDs, including HIV. D/C and inform doctor if sudden loss of vision, color vision, or hearing occur. Counsel to take as prescribed.

Administration: 1) Administer PO at least 30 min before anticipated sexual activity. 2) For qd use, take one tablet at the same time of day. **Storage:** 25°C (77°F); excursions permitted to 15-30°C (59-86°F).

CILOXAN — RX

ciprofloxacin HCl (Alcon)

THERAPEUTIC CLASS: Fluoroquinolone

INDICATIONS: Bacterial conjunctivitis and corneal ulcers.

DOSAGE: *Adults:* Bacterial Conjunctivitis: Sol: 1-2 drops q2h while awake for 2 days, then 1-2 drops q4h while awake for 5 days. Oint: 1/2 inch tid for 2 days, then bid for 5 days. Corneal Ulcer: Sol: 2 drops every 15 min for 1st 6 hrs, then 2 drops every 30 min for rest of Day 1, then 2 drops every hr on Day 2, then 2 drops q4h on Days 3-14. May continue if re-epithelialization has not occurred. *Pediatrics:* Bacterial Conjunctivitis: ≥1 yr: Sol: 1-2 drops q2h while awake for 2 days, then 1-2 drops q4h while awake for 5 days. ≥2 yrs: Oint: 1/2 inch tid for 2 days, then bid for 5 days. Corneal Ulcer: Sol: ≥1 yr: 2 drops every 15 min for 1st 6 hrs, then 2 drops every 30 min for rest of Day 1, then 2 drops every hr on Day 2, then 2 drops q4h on Days 3-14. May continue if re-epithelialization has not occurred.

HOW SUPPLIED: Oint: 0.3% [3.5g]; Sol: 0.3% [2.5mL, 5mL, 10mL]

WARNINGS/PRECAUTIONS: Not for injection into eye. Superinfection may result with prolonged use. Fatal hypersensitivity reactions reported after 1st dose of systemic quinolone therapy. Avoid allowing tip of container to contact eye or surrounding structures. Avoid contact lenses with conjunctivitis. Risk of crystalline precipitate in cornea. Ointment may slow corneal healing and cause visual blurring.

ADVERSE REACTIONS: Local burning, white crystalline precipitants, lid margin crusting, crystals/scales, foreign body sensation, itching, conjunctival hyperemia, bad taste.

INTERACTIONS: Systemic quinolone therapy may increase theophylline levels, interfere with caffeine metabolism, enhance warfarin effects, and elevate serum creatinine with cyclosporine.

PREGNANCY: Category C, caution in nursing.

MECHANISM OF ACTION: Fluoroquinolone antibacterial agent; bactericidal, interferes with the enzyme DNA gyrase which is needed for synthesis of bacterial DNA.

PHARMACOKINETICS: Absorption: $C_{max} \leq 5ng/mL$.

NURSING CONSIDERATIONS

Assessment: Assess for proper diagnosis of causative organisms and for hypersensitivity to other quinolones. Assess for possible drug interactions.

Monitoring: During prolonged use, monitor for overgrowth (eg, superinfection) of nonsusceptible organisms, including fungi. Monitor for signs of hypersensitivity or anaphylactic reaction (eg, cardiovascular collapse, loss of consciousness, pharyngeal or facial edema, dyspnea, and urticaria). Monitor for development of precipitate in the superficial portion of the corneal defect.

Patient Counseling: Instruct not to touch dropper tip to any surface; may contaminate solution. Advise to contact physician if any hypersensitivity reaction occurs (eg, rash). Instruct to remove contact lenses prior to therapy.

Administration: Ocular route. **Storage:** 2-25°C (36-77°F). Protect from light.

CIMZIA RX

certolizumab pegol (UCB)

Tuberculosis (TB), invasive fungal infections, and other opportunistic infections have occurred. Evaluate for latent TB and treat if necessary prior to therapy. Monitor all patients for active TB during treatment, even if initial tuberculin skin test is negative.

THERAPEUTIC CLASS: TNF-receptor blocker

INDICATIONS: For reducing signs and symptoms of Crohn's disease and maintaining clinical response in adults with moderately to severely active disease who have had an inadequate response to conventional therapy.

DOSAGE: *Adults:* Initial: 400mg SQ, and at Weeks 2 and 4. Maint: 400mg SQ every 4 weeks

HOW SUPPLIED: Inj: 200mg

WARNINGS/PRECAUTIONS: Serious infections, sepsis, and cases of opportunistic infections, including fatalities reported. Caution with history of recurrent infection, concomitant immunosuppressive therapy, or underlying conditions that may predispose to infections. May increase risk of reactivation of hepatitis B virus; monitor HBV carriers during and several months after therapy. Lymphoma and other malignancies have occurred with TNF-blockers. Anaphylaxis or serious allergic reactions may occur. Caution with pre-existing or recent onset CNS demyelinating disorders. Rare cases of pancytopenia, including aplastic anemia, reported; d/c if significant hematologic abnormalities occur. Caution with heart failure; monitor closely. May cause autoimmune antibodies; d/c if lupus-like syndrome develops.

ADVERSE REACTIONS: Upper respiratory tract infection, UTI, arthralgia.

INTERACTIONS: Avoid combination treatment with anakinra. Do not give live vaccines concurrently.

PREGNANCY: Category B, not for use in nursing

MECHANISM OF ACTION: TNF-blocker; binds to TNF-α and selectively neutralizes and inhibits its central role in inflammatory processes.

PHARMACOKINETICS: Absorption: Bioavailability (80%). **Distribution:** V_d=6.4L. **Elimination:** $T_{1/2}$=14 days.

NURSING CONSIDERATIONS

Assessment: Assess previous medication history, localized or chronic infections, history of recurring infections, heart disease, hematologic disorders, HBV infection, pre-existing or recurrent CNS demyelinating disorders, and possible drug interactions. Assess for active TB and perform tuberculin skin test prior to therapy.

Monitoring: Monitor for signs/symptoms suggestive of development of new infection, TB, worsening CHF, HBV infection, neurologic disorders (seizures, optic neuritis, peripheral neuropathy), hematologic reactions (aplastic anemia, pancytopenia), anaphylactic (angioedema, dyspnea, rash) and injection-site reactions.

Patient Counseling: Inform about risks/benefits of therapy. Issue patient medication guide and allow time to read prior to starting therapy; discuss any questions. Advise on importance of informing health care providers about all aspects of health at each treatment visit. Inform that drug may lower ability to fight infections; seek medical attention if any severe allergic reactions occur. Report any signs of new or worsening medical conditions such as heart disease, neurological or autoimmune disorders, symptoms such as bruising, bleeding or persistent fever, persistent cough, wasting, weight loss, and if any symptoms of TB or hepatitis B develops.

Administration: SQ route. **Storage:** Refrigerate at 2-8°C (36-46°F). Do not freeze.

CINRYZE — RX

c1 inhibitor (human) (Lev Pharmaceuticals)

THERAPEUTIC CLASS: C1 inhibitor

INDICATIONS: Prophylaxis for angioedema attacks in adolescent and adult patients with Hereditary Angioedema (HAE).

DOSAGE: *Adults:* 1,000 U IV every 3 or 4 days. Infusion Rate: Initial/ Maintenance: 1mL/min (10 mins).

HOW SUPPLIED: Inj: 500 U

WARNINGS/PRECAUTIONS: Severe hypersensitivity reactions (eg, hives, urticaria, chest tightness, wheezing, hypotension, and/or anaphylaxis) may occur; d/c therapy immediately. Have epinephrine available. Thrombotic events at high doses reported (animal studies). May carry a risk of transmitting infectious agents [eg, viruses, Creutzfeldt-Jakob (CJD) agent].

ADVERSE REACTIONS: Upper respiratory tract infection, sinusitis, rash, and headache.

PREGNANCY: Category C, caution in nursing.

MECHANISM OF ACTION: C1 inhibitor; regulates the activation of the complement and intrinsic coagulation (contact system) pathway and regulates the fibrinolytic system; increases plasma levels of C1 inhibitor activity.

PHARMACOKINETICS: Absorption: C_{max}=0.68 U/mL (single dose), 0.85 U/mL (double dose); T_{max}=3.9 hrs; $AUC_{(0-t)}$=74.5 U*hr/mL (single dose), 95.9 U*hr/mL (double dose). **Elimination:** $T_{1/2}$=56 hrs.

NURSING CONSIDERATIONS

Assessment: Assess signs and symptoms of hypersensitivity reactions, known risk factors for thrombotic events, and pregnancy/nursing status.

Monitoring: Monitor for hypersensitivity reactions and thrombotic events.

Patient Counseling: Counsel about the risks and benefits of C1 inhibitor prior to treatment. Inform that medication is made from human plasma and may contain infectious agents that can cause disease (eg, viruses, CJD agent).

Administration: IV route. Cinryze must be administered at room temperature within 3 hrs after reconstitution. Use aseptic technique. See PI for detailed reconstitution information. **Storage:** Store at 2-25°C (36-77°F). Do not freeze, mix with other materials, and/or use after expiration date. Protect from light prior to reconstitution.

CIPRO HC — RX

ciprofloxacin HCl - hydrocortisone (Alcon)

THERAPEUTIC CLASS: Antibacterial/corticosteroid combination

INDICATIONS: Acute otitis externa in adults and pediatric patients ≥1 year.

DOSAGE: *Adults:* 3 drops into affected ear bid for 7 days. Warm bottle in hand for 1-2 min to avoid dizziness. Shake well before use.
Pediatrics: ≥1 yr: 3 drops into affected ear bid for 7 days. Warm bottle in hand for 1-2 min to avoid dizziness. Shake well before use.

HOW SUPPLIED: Sus: (Ciprofloxacin-Hydrocortisone) 0.2%-1% [10mL]

CONTRAINDICATIONS: Perforated tympanic membrane, viral infections of external ear canal (eg, varicella and herpes simplex infections).

WARNINGS/PRECAUTIONS: D/C if hypersensitivity reaction occurs. Re-evaluate if no improvement after 1 week.

ADVERSE REACTIONS: Headache, pruritus.

PREGNANCY: Category C, not for use in nursing.

MECHANISM OF ACTION: Broad-spectrum anti-inflammatory antibiotic; exerts antimicrobial activity against gram-positive and gram-negative bacteria.

NURSING CONSIDERATIONS

Assessment: Assess for history of hypersensitivity to hydrocortisone or quinolones, perforated tympanic membrane, and viral infection of the external canal.

Monitoring: Monitor for possible occurrence of superinfection, ear pain, fungal dermatitis, headache, hypersensitivity reactions, and pruritus.

Patient Counseling: Inform that if rash or allergic reactions occur, d/c and contact physician immediately. Counsel to use as directed. Advise to avoid contact with eyes to avoid contaminating dropper. Protect from light, shake well before use, and discard unused portion after completion.

Administration: Otic route. **Storage:** Below 25°C (77°F). Avoid freezing. Protect from light.

CIPRO IV — RX

ciprofloxacin (Bayer/Schering)

> **Fluoroquinolones are associated with an increased risk of tendinitis and tendon rupture in all ages. Risk further increased in patients >60 yrs, patients taking corticosteroid drugs, and patients with kidney, heart or lung transplants.**

THERAPEUTIC CLASS: Fluoroquinolone

INDICATIONS: Treatment of skin and skin structure (SSSI), bone and joint, complicated intra-abdominal infections, lower respiratory tract infections (LRTI), urinary tract infections (UTI), nosocomial pneumonia, acute sinusitis, chronic bacterial prostatitis, postexposure inhalational anthrax, empirical therapy for febrile neutropenia, complicated UTI and pyelonephritis in pediatrics.

DOSAGE: *Adults:* ≥18 yrs: IV: UTI: Mild-Moderate: 200mg q12h for 7-14 days. Complicated/Severe: 400mg q12h for 7-14 days. LRTI/SSSI: Mild-Moderate: 400mg q12h for 7-14 days. Complicated/Severe: 400mg q8h for 7-14 days. Bone and Joint: Mild-Moderate: 400mg q12h for ≥4-6 weeks. Complicated/Severe: 400mg q8h for ≥4-6 weeks. Nosocomial Pneumonia: 400mg q8h for 10-14 days. Complicated Intra-Abdominal: 400mg q12h (w/metronidazole) for 7-14 days. Acute Sinusitis: 400mg q12h for 10 days. Chronic Bacterial Prostatitis: 400mg q12h for 28 days. Febrile Neutropenia: 400mg q8h (w/piperacillin 50mg/kg q4h) for 7-14 days. Max: 24g/day. Inhalational Anthrax: 400mg q12h for 60 days. Administer over 60 min. CrCl 5-29mL/min: 200-400mg q18-24h.
Pediatrics: <18 yrs: Inhalational Anthrax: 10mg/kg q12h for 60 days. Max: 400mg/dose. 1-17 yrs: Complicated UTI/Pyelonephritis: 6-10mg/kg q8h for 10-21 days. Max: 400mg/dose.

HOW SUPPLIED: Inj: 10mg/mL, 200mg/100mL, 400mg/200mL

CONTRAINDICATIONS: Concomitant administration with tizanidine.

C

WARNINGS/PRECAUTIONS: Convulsions, increased ICP, and toxic psychosis reported. Caution with CNS disorders or if predisposed to seizures. Severe, fatal hypersensitivity reactions may occur. *Clostridium difficile*-associated diarrhea, Achilles and other tendon ruptures reported. D/C at first sign of rash/hypersensitivity or if pain, inflammation, or ruptured tendon occur. May permit overgrowth of *Clostridia*. Maintain hydration; avoid alkaline urine. Avoid excessive sunlight and UV light. Do not give via feeding tube. Monitor renal, hepatic, and hematopoietic function with prolonged use. Adjust dose with renal dysfunction. Caution with concomitant drugs that may result in prolongation of QT interval or in patients with risk factors for torsade de pointes. Caution in elderly taking corticosteroids.

ADVERSE REACTIONS: Nausea, diarrhea, CNS disturbances, local IV site reactions, hepatic enzyme abnormalities, eosinophilia, headache, restlessness, and rash.

INTERACTIONS: See Contraindications. May increase theophylline and caffeine levels and prolong effects. May alter serum levels of phenytoin. Severe hypoglycemia with glyburide (rare). Potentiated by probenecid. Transient SrCr elevations with cyclosporine. May enhance oral anticoagulant effects. Caution with drugs that lower seizure threshold. Severe tendon disorder risks are increased with concomitant corticosteroid therapy. Caution with concomitant drugs that may result in prolongation of QT interval.

PREGNANCY: Category C, not for use in nursing.

MECHANISM OF ACTION: Synthetic broad-spectrum antimicrobial agent. Inhibits the enzymes topoisomerase II (DNA gyrase) and topoisomerase IV, which are required for bacterial DNA replication, transcription, repair, and recombination.

PHARMACOKINETICS: Absorption: Absolute bioavailability (70-80%); C_{max}=0.1, 0.2mcg/mL (200mg, 400mg, after 12 hrs). **Distribution:** Plasma protein binding (20-40%). **Metabolism:** CYP1A2. **Elimination:** Urine (unchanged), feces (15%). $T_{1/2}$=5-6 hrs.

NURSING CONSIDERATIONS

Assessment: Assess renal function tests, LFTs, history of seizures, pregnancy/nursing status, and possible drug interactions. Note other diseases/conditions and drug therapies.

Monitoring: Monitor for cardiac arrest, seizures, status epilepticus, respiratory failure, *Clostridium difficile*-associated diarrhea, renal function tests, LFTs, CBC, tendinitis and tendon rupture, peripheral neuropathy, and hypersensitivity reactions.

Patient Counseling: Notify healthcare provider if symptoms of pain, swelling, or inflammation of a tendon, or weakness or inability to move joints; rest and refrain from exercise; and d/c therapy. Inform that drug treats bacterial, not viral infections. Take exactly as directed; skipping doses or not completing full course may decrease effectiveness and increase resistance. Inform about potential benefits/risks. D/C and notify physician if skin rash, other allergic reactions, and watery and bloody stools (with or without stomach cramps, and fever) occur. Inform to use caution in any activity requiring mental alertness and coordination. Avoid excessive sun exposure and wear protective clothes.

Administration: IV route. Slow infusion over a period of 1 hr after reconstitution. **Storage:** Vial: 5-30°C (41-86°F). Flexible container: 5-25°C (41-77°F). Protect from light, avoid excessive heat, protect from freezing.

CIPRO ORAL — RX

ciprofloxacin HCl (Bayer/Schering)

Fluoroquinolones are associated with an increased risk of tendinitis and tendon rupture in all ages. Risk further increased in patients >60 yrs, patients taking corticosteroid drugs, and patients with kidney, heart or lung transplants.

THERAPEUTIC CLASS: Fluoroquinolone

C

INDICATIONS: Treatment of lower respiratory tract (LRTI), complicated intra-abdominal, skin and skin structure (SSSI), bone and joint, and urinary tract infections (UTI), acute exacerbations of chronic bronchitis, acute sinusitis, acute uncomplicated cystitis in females, chronic bacterial prostatitis, infectious diarrhea, typhoid fever, postexposure inhalational anthrax, uncomplicated cervical and urethral gonorrhea, complicated UTI and pyelonephritis in pediatrics.

DOSAGE: *Adults:* ≥18 yrs: Acute Sinusitis/Typhoid Fever: 500mg q12h for 10 days. LRTI/SSSI: Mild-Moderate: 500mg q12h for 7-14 days. Severe/Complicated: 750mg q12h for 7-14 days. Cystitis/Acute Uncomplicated UTI: 250mg q12h for 3 days. Mild-Moderate UTI: 250mg q12h for 7-14 days. Severe/Complicated UTI: 500mg q12h for 7-14 days. Chronic Bacterial Prostatitis: 500mg q12h for 28 days. Intra-Abdominal: 500mg q12h (w/ metronidazole) for 7-14 days. Bone and Joint: Mild-Moderate: 500mg q12h for ≥4-6 weeks. Severe/Complicated: 750mg q12h for ≥4-6 weeks. Infectious Diarrhea: 500mg q12h for 5-7 days. Uncomplicated Urethral/Cervical Gonococcal Infections: 250mg single dose. Inhalational Anthrax: 500mg q12h for 60 days. CrCl 30-50mL/min: 250-500mg q12h. CrCl 5-29mL/min: 250-500mg q18h. Hemodialysis/Peritoneal Dialysis: 250-500mg q24h (after dialysis). Administer at least 2 hrs before or 6 hrs after magnesium- or aluminum-containing antacids, sucralfate, Videx (didanosine) chewable/buffered tablets or pediatric powder, or other products containing calcium, iron, or zinc. *Pediatrics:* <18 yrs: Inhalational Anthrax: 15mg/kg q12h for 60 days. Max: 500mg/dose. 1-17 yrs: Complicated UTI/Pyelonephritis: 10-20mg/kg q12h for 10-21 days. Max: 750mg/dose.

HOW SUPPLIED: Sus: 250mg/5mL, 500mg/5mL [100mL]; Tab: 250mg, 500mg, 750mg

CONTRAINDICATIONS: Concomitant administration with tizanidine.

WARNINGS/PRECAUTIONS: Convulsions, increased ICP, and toxic psychosis reported. Caution with CNS disorders or if predisposed to seizures. Severe, fatal hypersensitivity reactions may occur. *Clostridium difficile*-associated diarrhea, colitis, achilles and other tendon ruptures reported. D/C at first sign of rash or if pain, inflammation, or ruptured tendon occurs. Maintain hydration; avoid alkaline urine. Avoid excessive sunlight and UV light. Do not give via feeding tube. Monitor renal, hepatic, and hematopoietic function with prolonged use. Adjust dose with renal dysfunction. Caution with concomitant drugs that may result in prolongation of the QT interval or in patients with risk factors for torsades de pointes. Caution in elderly taking corticosteroids.

ADVERSE REACTIONS: Nausea, dizziness, headache, CNS disturbances, vomiting, diarrhea, rash, abdominal pain/discomfort, pain, swelling, tendon tears.

INTERACTIONS: See Contraindications. Increases theophylline and caffeine levels and prolongs effects. Fatal reactions have occurred with theophylline. Magnesium- or aluminum-containing antacids, sucralfate, Videx (didanosine) chewable/buffered tablets or pediatric powder, and products containing calcium, iron, or zinc decrease serum and urine levels; space doses at least 2 hrs before or 6 hrs after administration. Altered serum levels of phenytoin. Severe hypoglycemia with glyburide (rare). Potentiated by probenecid. Transient serum creatinine elevations with cyclosporine. Enhances oral anticoagulant effects; monitor PT. Caution with drugs that lower seizure threshold. Severe tendon disorder risks increased with concomitant corticosteroid therapy. Caution with concomitant drugs that may result in prolongation of the QT interval.

PREGNANCY: Category C, not for use in nursing.

MECHANISM OF ACTION: Synthetic broad-spectrum antimicrobial agent; inhibits enzymes topoisomerase II (DNA gyrase) and topoisomerase IV, which are required for bacterial DNA replication.

PHARMACOKINETICS: Absorption: Rapid, well absorb (GIT); absolute bioavailability (70%); C_{max}=0.1, 0.2, 0.4mcg/mL (250mg, 500mg, 750mg, after 12 hrs); T_{max}=1-2 hrs. **Distribution:** Plasma protein binding (20-40%). **Metabolism:** CYP1A2. **Elimination:** Urine (40-50%); $T_{1/2}$=4 hrs.

NURSING CONSIDERATIONS

Assessment: Assess renal function tests, LFTs, history of seizures, pregnancy/nursing status, and possible drug interactions. Note other diseases/conditions and drug therapies.

Monitoring: Monitor for cardiac arrest, seizure, status epilepticus, respiratory failure, *Clostridium difficile*-associated diarrhea, renal function tests, LFTs, CBC, tendon rupture, peripheral neuropathy.

Patient Counseling: Notify healthcare provider if symptoms of pain, swelling, or inflammation of a tendon, or weakness or inability to move joints; rest and refrain from exercise; and d/c therapy. Inform that drug treats bacterial, not viral, infections. Take exactly as directed; skipping doses or not completing full course may decrease effectiveness and increase resistance. Inform to take with or without food, and to drink fluids. Inform about potential benefits/risks. D/C and notify physician if skin rash, other allergic reaction, and watery and bloody stools (with or without stomach cramps and fever) occur. Notify if pregnant/nursing or taking antacids or sucralfate. Use caution in activity requiring mental alertness and coordination. Avoid sun exposure. Take full course as prescribed.

Administration: Oral route. **Storage:** Below 30°C (86°F). Microcapsules and diluent should be stored below 25°C (77°F). Protect from freezing.

Cipro XR

RX

ciprofloxacin (Bayer/Schering)

Fluoroquinolones are associated with an increased risk of tendinitis and tendon rupture in all ages. Risk further increased in patients >60 yrs, patients taking corticosteroid drugs, and patients with kidney, heart or lung transplants.

THERAPEUTIC CLASS: Fluoroquinolone

INDICATIONS: Uncomplicated (acute cystitis) and complicated urinary tract infections (UTI), and acute uncomplicated pyelonephritis due to *E.coli*.

DOSAGE: *Adults:* ≥18 yrs: Uncomplicated UTI: 500mg qd for 3 days. Complicated UTI: 1000mg qd for 7-14 days. CrCl <30mL/min: 500 mg qd. Acute Uncomplicated Pyelonephritis: 1000mg qd for 7-14 days. CrCl <30mL/min: 500mg qd. Take with fluids. Administer at least 2 hrs before or 6 hrs after magnesium-or aluminum- containing antacids, sucralfate, Videx (didanosine) chewable/buffered tablets or pediatric powder, metal cations (eg, iron), multivitamins with zinc. Avoid concomitant administration with dairy products alone, or with calcium-fortified products. Space concomitant calcium intake (>800mg) by at least 2 hrs. Do not split, crush, or chew. Swallow tab whole. Dialysis: Give after procedure is completed.

HOW SUPPLIED: Tab, Extended-Release: 500mg, 1000mg

CONTRAINDICATIONS: Concomitant administration with tizanidine.

WARNINGS/PRECAUTIONS: Convulsions, increased ICP and toxic psychosis reported. Caution with CNS disorders or if predisposed to seizures. Severe, sometimes fatal, hypersensitivity reactions may occur. *Clostridium difficile*-associated diarrhea, colitis, achilles, and other tendon ruptures reported. D/C at first sign of rash or if pain, inflammation, or ruptured tendon occurs. Maintain hydration; avoid alkaline urine. Avoid excessive sunlight and UV light. Not interchangeable with immediate-release tablets. To d/c treatment, rest and refrain from exercise. Caution with concomitant drugs that may result in prolongation of the QT interval or in patients with risk factors for torsades de pointes. Caution in elderly taking corticosteroids.

ADVERSE REACTIONS: Nausea, headache, diarrhea, pain, swelling, tendon tears.

INTERACTIONS: See Contraindications. Increases theophylline and caffeine levels and prolongs effects. Serious/fatal reactions have occurred with theophylline. Magnesium- or aluminum- containing antacids, sucralfate, Videx (didanosine) chewable/buffered tablets or pediatric powder, and products containing calcium, iron, or zinc decrease serum and urine levels; space doses at least 2 hrs before or 6 hrs after administration. Altered serum levels of phenytoin. Severe hypoglycemia with glyburide (rare). Potentiated by probenecid. Transient serum creatinine elevations with cyclosporine. Enhances oral anticoagulant effects. Caution with drugs that lower seizure threshold. Severe tendon disorder risks increased with concomitant corticosteroid therapy. Caution with concomitant drugs that may result in prolongation of the QT interval.

PREGNANCY: Category C, not for use in nursing.

MECHANISM OF ACTION: Synthetic broad-spectrum antimicrobial agent. Inhibits topoisomerase II (DNA gyrase) and topoisomerase IV, which are required for bacterial DNA replication, transcription, repair and recombination.

PHARMACOKINETICS: Absorption: Oral administration of variable doses resulted in different parameters. T_{max}=1-4 hrs. **Distribution:** (IV) V_d= approximately 2.1-2.7L/kg, plasma protein binding (20-40%). **Metabolism:** Primary metabolites: oxociprofloxacin and sulfociprofloxacin. **Elimination:** Urine (approximately 35%, unchanged).

NURSING CONSIDERATIONS

Assessment: Assess renal function tests, LFTs, pregnancy status, history of seizures. Note other diseases/conditions and drug therapies.

Monitoring: Monitor for cardiac arrest, seizure, status epilepticus, respiratory failure, *Clostridium difficile*-associated diarrhea, renal function tests, LFTs, CBC, tendon rupture, peripheral neuropathy, hypersensitivity reactions.

Patient Counseling: Notify healthcare provider if symptoms of pain, swelling, or inflammation of a tendon, or weakness or inability to move joints; rest and refrain from exercise; and d/c therapy. Inform that drug treats bacterial, not viral, infections. Take exactly as directed; skipping doses or not completing full course may decrease effectiveness and increase resistance. Inform to take with or without food, and to drink fluids. Inform about potential benefits/risks. D/C and notify if skin rash, other allergic reaction, and watery and bloody stools (with or without stomach cramps and fever) occur. Notify if pregnant/nursing or taking antacids or sucralfate. Use caution in activity requiring mental alertness and coordination. Avoid sun exposure. Take full course as prescribed. Tablet should not be crushed or chewed.

Administration: Oral route. **Storage**: 25°C (77°F), excursions permitted to 15-30°C (59-86°F).

CIPRODEX — RX

dexamethasone - ciprofloxacin (Alcon)

THERAPEUTIC CLASS: Antibacterial/corticosteroid combination

INDICATIONS: Acute otitis media in pediatric patients with tympanostomy tubes. Acute otitis externa.

DOSAGE: *Adults:* Acute Otitis Externa: 4 drops in affected ear(s) bid for 7 days. Warm bottle in hand for 1-2 min to avoid dizziness. Shake well before use.

Pediatrics: ≥6 months: 4 drops in affected ear(s) bid for 7 days. Warm bottle in hand for 1-2 min to avoid dizziness. Shake well before use.

HOW SUPPLIED: Sus: (Ciprofloxacin-Dexamethasone) 0.3%-0.1% [5mL, 7.5mL]

CONTRAINDICATIONS: Viral infections of external ear canal including herpes simplex infections.

WARNINGS/PRECAUTIONS: D/C if hypersensitivity reaction occurs. Reevaluate if no improvement after one week.

ADVERSE REACTIONS: Ear pain/discomfort/pruritus.

PREGNANCY: Category C, not for use in nursing.

MECHANISM OF ACTION: Fluoroquinolone, corticosteroid; antibacterial/anti-inflammatory; bactericidal action results from interference with the enzyme (DNA gyrase), which is needed for the synthesis of bacterial DNA.

PHARMACOKINETICS: Absorption: Ciprofloxacin: C_{max}=1.39ng/mL; T_{max}=15 min-2 hrs. Dexamethasone: C_{max}=1.14ng/mL; T_{max}=15 min-2 hrs.

NURSING CONSIDERATIONS

Assessment: Assess for history of drug hypersensitivity and viral infection of the external canal, including herpes simplex virus infection.

Monitoring: Monitor for anaphylactic reactions, skin rash, overgrowth of non-susceptible organisms (eg, fungi and yeast) in large doses, lesions or erosions of cartilage in weight-bearing joints, and other signs of arthropathy.

Patient Counseling: Inform drug is for otic use only. Avoid touching dropper tip to ear material or any other surface. D/C if rash or allergic reaction occurs. Instruct to keep infected ear dry and clean. Take as prescribed.

Administration: Otic route. Warm suspension by holding bottle in hand for 1-2 min. Lie with affected ear up, then instill drops. Maintain position for 60 sec and repeat, if necessary, with opposite ear. **Storage:** Store at 15-30°C (59-86°F). Protect from light; avoid freezing.

CLARINEX RX

desloratadine (Schering)

OTHER BRAND NAMES: Clarinex Syrup (Schering) - Clarinex RediTabs (Schering)

THERAPEUTIC CLASS: H_1-antagonist

INDICATIONS: Relief of perennial allergic rhinitis and chronic idiopathic urticaria in patients ≥6 months. Relief of seasonal allergic rhinitis in patients ≥2 yrs.

DOSAGE: *Adults:* 5mg qd. Hepatic/Renal Impairment: 5mg every other day. Dissolve RediTabs on tongue with or without water.
Pediatrics: Tabs: ≥12 yrs: 5mg qd. 6-11 yrs: 2.5mg qd. Syrup: ≥12 yrs: 10mL (5mg) qd. 6-11 yrs: 5mL (2.5mg) qd. 12 months-5 yrs: 2.5mL (1.25mg) qd. 6-11 months: 2mL (1mg) qd. Dissolve RediTabs on tongue with or without water.

HOW SUPPLIED: Tab: 5mg; Tab, Disintegrating: (RediTabs) 2.5mg, 5mg; Syrup: 0.5mg/mL

WARNINGS/PRECAUTIONS: Adjust dose with renal or hepatic impairment. Caution in elderly.

ADVERSE REACTIONS: Pharyngitis, dry mouth, headache, fever, diarrhea, cough, upper respiratory tract infection, irritability, somnolence, bronchitis, otitis media, N/V, fatigue.

INTERACTIONS: Erythromycin, ketoconazole increase plasma levels.

PREGNANCY: Category C, not for use in nursing.

MECHANISM OF ACTION: Long-acting tricyclic histamine antagonist with selective H_1-receptor histamine antagonist activity; inhibits histamine release from human mast cells.

PHARMACOKINETICS: Absorption: T_{max}=3 hrs., C_{max}=4ng/mL, AUC=56.9ng•hr/mL. **Distribution:** Found in breast milk; plasma protein binding (82-87% of desloratadine), (85-89% of 3-hydroxydesloratadine). **Metabolism:** Extensive. Desloratadine (major metabolite), 3-hydroxydesloratadine (active metabolite): **Elimination:** Urine and feces (metabolites); $T_{1/2}$=27 hrs.

NURSING CONSIDERATIONS

Assessment: Assess for renal/hepatic impairment and for possible drug interactions.

Monitoring: Monitor for hypersensitivity reactions.

Patient Counseling: Take drug as directed, without regard to meals. Do not increase dose or dosing frequency.

Administration: Oral route. **Storage:** 25°C (77°F); excursions permitted to 15-30°C (59-86°F).

C

CLARINEX-D RX

pseudoephedrine sulfate - desloratadine (Schering)

THERAPEUTIC CLASS: H_1-antagonist/sympathomimetic amine

INDICATIONS: Relief of nasal and non-nasal symptoms of seasonal allergic rhinitis, including nasal congestion.

DOSAGE: *Adults:* 2.5mg-120mg tab bid or 5mg-240mg tab qd w/ or w/o food. Hepatic Impairment: 12-Hour/24-Hour: Avoid use. Renal Impairment: 12-Hour: Avoid use. 24-Hour: 1 tab qod.
Pediatrics: ≥12 yrs: 2.5mg-120mg tab bid or 5mg-240mg tab qd w/ or w/o food. Hepatic Impairment: 12-Hour/24-Hour: Avoid use. Renal Impairment: 12-Hour: Avoid use. 24-Hour: 1 tab qod.

HOW SUPPLIED: Tab, Extended-Release: (Desloratadine-Pseudoephedrine) (12-Hr) 2.5mg-120mg, (24-Hr) 5mg-240mg

CONTRAINDICATIONS: Narrow-angle glaucoma, urinary retention, MAOI therapy or within 14 days of discontinuation, severe HTN, severe CAD, hypersensitivity or idiosyncrasy to adrenergic agents or to other drugs of similar chemical structures.

WARNINGS/PRECAUTIONS: Caution with HTN, DM, ischemic heart disease, increased intraocular pressure, hyperthyroidism, renal impairment, or prostatic hypertrophy. CNS stimulation with convulsions or cardiovascular collapse with accompanying hypotension may be produced by sympathomimetic amines. Avoid with hepatic insufficiency.

ADVERSE REACTIONS: Dry mouth, headache, insomnia, fatigue, pharyngitis, somnolence.

INTERACTIONS: Do not use with MAOIs or within 14 days of discontinuation. Antihypertensive effects of β-adrenergic blocking agents, methyldopa, mecamylamine, reserpine, and veratrum alkaloids may be reduced by sympathomimetics (eg, pseudoephedrine). Increased ectopic pacemaker activity with digitalis.

PREGNANCY: Category C, not for use in nursing.

MECHANISM OF ACTION: Desloratadine: Long-acting tricyclic histamine antagonist with selective H_1-receptor antagonist activity. Inhibits histamine release from human mast cells *in vitro*. Pseudoephedrine: Orally active sympathomimetic amine, which exerts a decongestant action on nasal mucosa.

PHARMACOKINETICS: Absorption: Desloratadine: (24 hr) C_{max}=1.79ng/mL; T_{max}=6-7 hrs, AUC=61.1ng•hr/mL. (12 hr) C_{max}=1.09ng/mL; T_{max}=4-5 hrs, AUC=31.6ng•hr/mL. Pseudoephedrine: (24 hr) C_{max}=328ng/mL, T_{max}=8-9 hrs, AUC=6438ng•hr/mL. (12 hr) C_{max}=263ng/mL, T_{max}=6-7 hrs, AUC=4588ng•hr/mL. **Distribution:** Desloratadine: Found in breast milk, plasma protein binding (82-87%), 3-hydroxydesloratadine (85-89%). **Metabolism:** Desloratadine (major metabolite): extensive, 3-hydroxydesloratadine (active metabolite) and glucuronidation pathway. Pseudoephedrine: Liver (incomplete), through N-demethylation. **Elimination:** Desloratadine: (24 hr) $T_{1/2}$=24 hrs, (12 hr) $T_{1/2}$=27 hrs. Pseudoephedrine: Urine (55-96% unchanged). If urinary pH=5, ($T_{1/2}$=3-6 hrs); if urinary pH=8, ($T_{1/2}$ =9-16 hrs).

NURSING CONSIDERATIONS

Assessment: Assess for drug hypersensitivity, hepatic/renal impairment, increased IOP, narrow-angle glaucoma, prostatic hypertrophy, urinary retention, HTN, CAD, ischemic heart disease, DM, hyperthyroidism, possible drug interaction (eg, MAO inhibitors).

Monitoring: Monitor idiosyncratic effects (eg, insomnia, dizziness, weakness, tremor, arrhythmias), BP, IOP, cardiac function, somnolence, CNS stimulation effects with convulsions, cardiovascular collapse with hypotension, liver enzymes, renal function.

Patient Counseling: Counsel to take drug as directed. Caution those with HTN, glaucoma, urinary retention, hyperthyroidism, severe coronary disease, patients taking MAOIs. Not to be taken during nursing/pregnancy.

Administration: Oral route. Do not break or chew, swallow tab whole.
Storage: 25°C (77°F); excursions permitted to 15-30°C (59-86°F). Heat sensitive.

CLEOCIN — RX

clindamycin HCl (Pharmacia & Upjohn)

Clostridium difficile-**associated diarrhea (CDAD) reported with use of nearly all antibacterial agents, including clindamycin, and may range in severity from mild diarrhea to fatal colitis. If CDAD is suspected or confirmed, ongoing antibiotic use not directed against** *C.difficile* **may need to be discontinued.**

THERAPEUTIC CLASS: Lincomycin derivative

INDICATIONS: Serious infections caused by anaerobes, streptococci, pneumococci, and staphylococci.

DOSAGE: *Adults:* Serious Infection: 150-300mg PO q6h or 600-1200mg/day IM/IV given bid-qid. More Severe Infection: 300-450mg PO q6h or 1200-2700mg/day IM/IV given bid-qid. Life-Threatening Infections: Up to 4800mg/day IV. Max: 600mg per IM injection. Take caps with full glass of water. Treat β-hemolytic strep for at least 10 days.
Pediatrics: Give tid or qid. Cap: Serious Infections: 8-16mg/kg/day. More Severe Infections: 16-20mg/kg/day. Sol: Serious Infections: 8-12mg/kg/day. Severe Infections: 13-16mg/kg/day. More Severe Infections: 17-25mg/kg/day. IM/IV: 1 month-16 yrs: 20-40mg/kg/day; use the higher dose for more severe infections. <1 month: 15-20mg/kg/day. Take caps with full glass of water. Treat β-hemolytic strep for at least 10 days.

HOW SUPPLIED: Cap: (HCl) 75mg, 150mg, 300mg; Inj: (Phosphate) 150mg/mL, 300mg/50mL, 600mg/50mL, 900mg/50mL; Sol: (Palmitate HCl) 75mg/5mL [100mL]

WARNINGS/PRECAUTIONS: May permit overgrowth of clostridia. Not for treatment of meningitis. Caution with atopic patients, GI disease (eg, colitis), hepatic disease, and the elderly. Monitor blood, hepatic and renal function with long-term use. Do not give injection undiluted as bolus. The 75mg and 100mg caps contain tartrazine.

ADVERSE REACTIONS: Abdominal pain, colitis, esophagitis, NV, diarrhea, hypersensitivity reactions, jaundice, blood dyscrasias, pruritus, vaginitis, superinfection (prolonged use).

INTERACTIONS: Antagonism may occur with erythromycin. May potentiate neuromuscular blockers.

PREGNANCY: Category B, not for use in nursing.

MECHANISM OF ACTION: Inhibits bacterial protein synthesis at the level of the bacterial ribosome and binds preferentially to the 50S ribosomal subunit affecting process of peptide chain initiation.

PHARMACOKINETICS: Absorption: Cap: Rapid, complete; C_{max}=2.5mcg/mL, T_{max}=45 min. Inj: C_{max}=10.8mcg/mL (adults, IV 600mg q8h), 9mcg/mL (adults, IM q12h), 10mcg/mL (peds, IV), 8mcg/mL (peds, IM); T_{max}=3 hrs (adults), 1 hr (peds). Oral Sol: C_{max}=1.24mcg/mL (peds, 8mg/kg/day), 2.25mcg/mL (12mg/kg/day). **Distribution:** Wide; body fluids, tissues, and bones; found in breast milk. **Elimination:** Cap: Urine (10% unchanged), feces (3.6% unchanged); $T_{1/2}$=3.2 hr. Inj: $T_{1/2}$=3 hrs (adults), 2.5 hrs (peds). Oral Sol: $T_{1/2}$=2 hrs (peds).

NURSING CONSIDERATIONS

Assessment: Assess for previous drug hypersensitivity reaction, GI disease particularly colitis, atopic patients, renal/hepatic impairment, pregnancy/nursing status, presence of meningitis, elderly patients with severe illness, upcoming surgical procedure, and for possible drug interactions.

C

Monitoring: Monitor for serious anaphylactoid reaction, pseudomembranous colitis or *C.difficile*-associated diarrhea (mild diarrhea to fatal colitis), development of drug resistance, overgrowth of nonsuspectible organisms, changes in bowel frequency, lab tests (eg, LFTs, renal function, CBC) during prolonged therapy.

Patient Counseling: Inform therapy only treats bacterial, not viral, infections. Take exactly as directed; skipping doses or not completing full course may decrease effectiveness and increase resistance. Inform about potential benefits/risks. D/C and notify physician if allergic reactions, watery/bloody stools (with/without stomach cramps) occur (may occur as late as 2 months after therapy). Notify if pregnant/nursing.

Administration: Oral route: Cap, Oral Solution. Inj: IM, IV. ADD-Vantage vial for IV use only; do not use flexible container in series connections. **Storage:** 20-25°C (68-77°F). Do not refrigerate reconsitituted solution.

CLEOCIN T — RX

clindamycin phosphate (Pharmacia & Upjohn)

THERAPEUTIC CLASS: Lincomycin derivative

INDICATIONS: Acne vulgaris.

DOSAGE: *Adults:* Apply thin film bid.
Pediatrics: ≥12 yrs: Apply thin film bid. May use more than 1 pledget.

HOW SUPPLIED: Gel: 1% [30g, 60g]; Lot: 1% [60mL]; Sol: 1% [30mL, 60mL]; Swab (Pledgets): 1% [60^s]

CONTRAINDICATIONS: Hypersensitivity to lincomycin. History of regional enteritis, ulcerative colitis, or antibiotic-associated colitis.

WARNINGS/PRECAUTIONS: Avoid eyes, abraded skin, mucous membranes, and mouth. Caution in atopic patients. D/C if significant diarrhea occurs.

ADVERSE REACTIONS: Dryness, oily skin, erythema, peeling, burning, itching, pseudomembranous colitis (rare).

INTERACTIONS: May potentiate neuromuscular blockers.

PREGNANCY: Category B, not for use in nursing.

MECHANISM OF ACTION: Inhibits growth of *Propionibacterium acnes* and decreases free fatty acids on the skin surface.

PHARMACOKINETICS: Absorption: Following topical administration of multiple doses, serum levels of clindamycin were measured at 0-3ng/mL. **Distribution:** Orally and parenterally administered clindamycin has been found in breast milk. **Metabolism:** Hydrolysis. **Elimination:** Urine (≤0.2% found as clindamycin).

NURSING CONSIDERATIONS

Assessment: Assess proper diagnosis of acne vulgaris. Assess for history of hypersensitivity to lincomycin; regional, ulcerative, or antibiotic-associated colitis. Assess use in pregnant/nursing patients. Assess for possible drug interactions.

Monitoring: Monitor for signs/symptoms of diarrhea, bloody diarrhea, and colitis (eg, pseudomembranous colitis). Monitor for occurrence of severe abdominal cramps, blood, and mucus discharge. If significant diarrhea occurs, consider large bowel endoscopy, stool culture, and stool assay.

Patient Counseling: Inform that medication contains alcohol base that will cause burning and irritation if contact with eye occurs. If accidental contact with sensitive surfaces (eg, eye, abraded skin, mucous membranes) occurs, bathe affected areas with copious amounts of cold water. Medication has unpleasant taste. Use caution when applying around mouth. Notify physician immediately if any signs of abdominal pain or GI disturbances (eg, diarrhea) occur.

Administration: Topical. **Storage:** 20-25°C (68-77°F). Protect from freezing. Keep all liquid dosage forms in containers tightly closed.

CLEOCIN VAGINAL RX
clindamycin phosphate (Pharmacia & Upjohn)

OTHER BRAND NAMES: Clindamax Vaginal (PharmaDerm) - Cleocin Vaginal Ovules (Pharmacia & Upjohn)

THERAPEUTIC CLASS: Lincomycin derivative

INDICATIONS: (Cream) Treatment of bacterial vaginosis in non-pregnant women and pregnant women during the 2nd and 3rd trimester. (Sup) Treatment of bacterial vaginosis in non-pregnant women.

DOSAGE: *Adults:* (Cream) 1 applicatorful intravaginally qhs. Treat non-pregnant females for 3 or 7 days. Treat pregnant females (2nd and 3rd trimester) for 7 days. (Sup) 1 suppository intravaginally qhs for 3 days.
Pediatrics: Post-Menarchal: (Sup) 1 suppository intravaginally qhs for 3 days.

HOW SUPPLIED: Cre: 2% [40g]; Sup, Vaginal: (Ovules) 100mg [3^s]

CONTRAINDICATIONS: Hypersensitivity to lincomycin. History of regional enteritis, ulcerative colitis, or antibiotic-associated colitis.

WARNINGS/PRECAUTIONS: Do not use condoms or contraceptive diaphragms within 72 hrs following treatment. Monitor for pseudomembranous colitis. Avoid eye contact. Do not engage in vaginal intercourse or use other vaginal products (such as tampons or douches) during treatment. Monitor for pseudomembranous colitis. May result in overgrowth of nonsusceptible organisms in vagina.

ADVERSE REACTIONS: Vaginitis, vulvovaginal disorder, candidiasis, moniliasis, pruritus, abnormal labor.

INTERACTIONS: May potentiate neuromuscular blockers.

PREGNANCY: Category B, not for use in nursing.

MECHANISM OF ACTION: Antibiotic; inhibits bacterial protein synthesis at the level of the bacterial ribosome and binds preferentially to the 50S ribosomal subunit affecting peptide chain initiation.

PHARMACOKINETICS: Absorption: (Day 1) C_{max}=13ng/ml; (Day 7) C_{max}=16ng/mL, T_{max}=14 hrs. **Elimination:** $T_{1/2}$=1.5-2.6 hrs.

NURSING CONSIDERATIONS

Assessment: Assess for history of drug hypersensitivity, regional enteritis, ulcerative colitis, antibiotic-associated colitis, and possible drug interactions.

Monitoring: Monitor for serious anaphylactoid reaction, pseudomembranous colitis or *C.difficile*-associated diarrhea (mild diarrhea to fatal colitis), development of drug resistance, overgrowth of nonsusceptible organisms.

Patient Counseling: Instruct not to engage in vaginal intercourse or use other vaginal products. Do not use latex or rubber products (eg, condoms and diaphragms) within 72 hrs following treatment. Rinse eye and consult physician if accidental eye contact occurs.

Administration: Intravaginal. Insert one prefilled applicator into vagina, push plunger to release cream; discard empty applicator. **Storage:** 20-25°C (68-77°F). Protect from freezing.

CLIMARA RX
estradiol (Bayer Healthcare)

Estrogens increase risk of endometrial cancer. Estrogens, with or without progestins, should not be used for the prevention of cardiovascular disease or dementia. Increased risk of MI, stroke, invasive breast cancer, PE, and DVT in postmenopausal women (50-79 yrs of age) reported. Increased risk of developing probable dementia in postmenopausal women ≥65 yrs of age reported.

THERAPEUTIC CLASS: Estrogen

INDICATIONS: Treatment of moderate to severe vasomotor symptoms and/or vulvar/vaginal atrophy associated with menopause. Treatment of hypoestrogenism due to hypogonadism, castration, or primary ovarian failure. Prevention of postmenopausal osteoporosis.

C

DOSAGE: *Adults:* Apply 1 patch weekly to lower abdomen or upper area of buttocks (avoid breasts and waistline). Rotate application sites. Vasomotor Symptoms: Initial: 0.025mg/day patch once weekly. Titrate: Adjust dose as needed. Wait 1 week after withdrawal of oral therapy before initiating patch. D/C or taper at 3-6 month intervals. Osteoporosis Prevention: Minimum Effective Dose: 0.025mg/day once weekly.

HOW SUPPLIED: Patch: 0.025mg/day, 0.0375mg/day, 0.05mg/day, 0.06mg/day, 0.075mg/day, 0.1mg/day [4[s]]

CONTRAINDICATIONS: Pregnancy, undiagnosed abnormal genital bleeding, breast cancer, estrogen-dependent neoplasia, DVT/PE, active or recent (eg, within 1 year) thromboembolic disease (eg, stroke, MI), liver dysfunction or disease.

WARNINGS/PRECAUTIONS: May increase risk of cardiovascular events (eg, MI, stroke), venous thrombosis, and PE; d/c immediately if any of these events occur or are suspected. May increase risk of breast/endometrial cancer, and gallbladder disease. Retinal vascular thrombosis reported; monitor and d/c if papilledema or retinal vascular lesions occur. Consider addition of a progestin if no hysterectomy. May elevate BP; monitor at regular intervals. May cause elevations of plasma triglycerides with pre-existing hypertriglyceridemia. Caution with history of cholestatic jaundice associated with past estrogen use or with pregnancy; d/c with recurrence. May lead to increased thyroid-binding globulin levels; monitor thyroid function. May cause fluid retention; caution with cardiac/renal dysfunction. Caution with severe hypocalcemia. May increase risk of ovarian cancer. May exacerbate endometriosis, asthma, DM, epilepsy, migraine, porphyria, systemic lupus erythematosus, hepatic hemangiomas; use with caution.

ADVERSE REACTIONS: Skin irritation, headache, arthralgia, depression, breast pain, leukorrhea, upper respiratory tract infection, sinusitis.

INTERACTIONS: CYP3A4 inducers (eg, St. John's wort, phenobarbital, carbamazepine, rifampin) may decrease levels, which may decrease therapeutic effects and/or change uterine bleeding profile. CYP3A4 inhibitors (eg, erythromycin, clarithromycin, ketoconazole, itraconazole, ritonavir, grapefruit juice) may increase levels, which may result in side effects.

PREGNANCY: Contraindicated in pregnancy, caution in nursing.

MECHANISM OF ACTION: Estrogen; binds to nuclear receptors in estrogen-responsive tissues. Modulates pituitary secretion of gonadotrophins, luteinizing hormone (LH) and follicle stimulating hormone (FSH), through negative feedback mechanism.

PHARMACOKINETICS: Absorption: Transdermal administration of different doses resulted in different parameters. **Distribution**: Estrogens are found in breast milk. Wide; largely bound to sex hormone binding globulin (SHBG) and albumin. **Metabolism:** Liver to estrone (metabolite); estriol (major urinary metabolite); enterohepatic recirculation via sulfate and glucuronide conjugation; biliary secretion of conjugates into the intestine; hydrolysis in the gut; and reabsorbtion. CYP3A4 (partial). **Elimination:** Urine.

NURSING CONSIDERATIONS

Assessment: Assess for abnormal genital bleeding, presence or history of breast cancer, DVT, PE, presence of estrogen-dependent neoplasia, active or recent (within past yr) arterial thromboembolic disease (eg, stroke, MI), liver dysfunction/disease, known/suspected pregnancy. Assess use in patients ≥65 yrs, nursing females, hypocalcemia, asthma, DM, epilepsy, migraine or porphyria, SLE, and hepatic hemangiomas. Assess for drug and lab interactions.

Monitoring: Monitor for signs/symptoms of cardiovascular disorders (eg, MI, stroke, venous thrombosis, PE), malignant neoplasms (eg, cancers of endometrium, breast, ovaries), dementia, gallbladder disease, hypercalcemia, visual abnormalities (eg, retinal vascular thrombosis), cholestatic jaundice, increased BP, hypertriglyceridemia, hypothyroidism, hypocalcemia, exacerbation of endometriosis and other conditions (eg, asthma, DM, epilepsy, migraine or porphyria, SLE, and hepatic hemangiomas). Monitor thyroid function in patients on thyroid replacement therapy. Perform proper diagnostic testing (eg, endometrial sampling) to rule out malignancy when undiagnosed, persistent or recurring, abnormal vaginal bleeding occurs. Perform periodic evaluation every 3-6 months to determine need for therapy.

Patient Counseling: Inform that medication increases risk for uterine cancer and may increase chances for heart attack, stroke, breast cancer, and blood clots. Advise to contact physician if breast lumps, unusual vaginal bleeding, dizziness or faintness, changes in speech, severe headaches, chest pain, SOB, leg pain, visual changes, or vomiting occur. Inform once in place, transdermal system should not be exposed to sun for prolonged periods of time. Removal of system should be done carefully and slowly to avoid skin irritation. If patch falls off during dosing interval, apply new patch for remainder of the 7-day period.

Administration: Transdermal application. Site of application should not be oily, damaged, or irritated. Apply patch after opening pouch and removing protective liner. Ensure patch sticks completely, especially around edges. **Storage:** Do not store above 30°C (86°F). Do not store unpouched. Keep out of reach of children.

CLIMARA PRO — RX

levonorgestrel - estradiol (Bayer Healthcare)

Estrogens and progestins should not be used for the prevention of cardiovascular disease or dementia. Increased risks of MI, stroke, invasive breast cancer, PE, and DVT in postmenopausal women (50-79 yrs of age) reported. Increased risk of developing probable dementia in postmenopausal women ≥65 yrs of age reported.

THERAPEUTIC CLASS: Estrogen/progestogen combination

INDICATIONS: Treatment of moderate to severe vasomotor symptoms associated with menopause. Prevention of postmenopausal osteoporosis.

DOSAGE: *Adults:* Apply 1 patch weekly to lower abdomen (avoid breasts and waistline). Rotate application site; allow 1 week between same site. Reevaluate periodically (3-6 month intervals).

HOW SUPPLIED: Patch: (Estradiol-Levonorgestrel): 0.045mg-0.015mg/day [4[s]]

CONTRAINDICATIONS: Pregnancy, undiagnosed abnormal genital bleeding, breast cancer, estrogen-dependent neoplasia, DVT/PE, active or recent (eg, within 1 year) thromboembolic disease (eg, stroke, MI), liver dysfunction or disease.

WARNINGS/PRECAUTIONS: May increase risk of cardiovascular events (eg, MI, stroke), venous thrombosis, and PE; d/c immediately if any of these events occur or are suspected. May increase risk of breast/endometrial cancer, and gallbladder disease. Retinal vascular thrombosis reported; monitor and d/c if papilledema or retinal vascular lesions occur. Consider addition of a progestin if no hysterectomy. May elevate BP; monitor at regular intervals. May cause elevations of plasma triglycerides with pre-existing hypertriglyceridemia. Caution with history of cholestatic jaundice associated with past estrogen use or with pregnancy; d/c with recurrence. May lead to increased thyroid-binding globulin levels; monitor thyroid function. May cause fluid retention; caution with cardiac/renal dysfunction. Caution with severe hypocalcemia. May increase risk of ovarian cancer. May exacerbate endometriosis, asthma, DM, epilepsy, migraine, porphyria; use with caution.

ADVERSE REACTIONS: Application-site reaction, vaginal bleeding, breast pain, upper respiratory infection, back pain, headache, depression, arthralgia, flu syndrome, abdominal pain.

INTERACTIONS: CYP3A4 inducers (eg, St. John's wort, phenobarbital, carbamazepine, rifampin) may decrease levels which may decrease therapeutic effects and/or change uterine bleeding profile. CYP3A4 inhibitors (eg, erythromycin, clarithromycin, ketoconazole, itraconazole, ritonavir, grapefruit juice) may increase levels which may result in side effects.

C

PREGNANCY: Contraindicated in pregnancy, caution in nursing.

MECHANISM OF ACTION: Estradiol: Estrogen. Binds to nuclear receptors in estrogen-responsive tissue. Modulates pituitary secretion of gonadotrophins, luteinizing hormone (LH) and follicle stimulating hormone, through negative feedback mechanism. Levonorgestrel: Progestogen. Inhibits gonadotropin production resulting in retardation of follicular growth and inhibition of ovulation. Counteracts proliferative effects of estrogens in endometrium.

PHARMACOKINETICS: Absorption:(Single dose): Estradiol: C_{max}=54.3pg/mL, T_{max}=42 hrs, AUC=6340pg•hr/mL; Estrone (metabolite): C_{max}=43.9pg/mL, T_{max}=84 hrs, AUC=6890pg•hr/ mL; Levonorgestrel: C_{max}=138pg/mL, T_{max}=90 hrs, AUC=22900pg•hr/mL. **Distribution:** Estrogens and progestin found in breast milk. Estradiol: Widely distributed; largely bound to sex hormone binding globulin (SHBG) and albumin. Levonorgestrel: Bound to SHBG and albumin. **Metabolism:** Estradiol: Hepatic, to estrone (metabolite); estriol (major urinary metabolite); enterohepatic recirculation, via sulfate and glucuronide conjugation; biliary secretion of conjugates into intestine; hydrolysis in gut, reabsorption. CYP3A4 (partial). Levonorgestrel: Reduction, hydroxylation, conjugation. **Elimination:** Estradiol, estrone, estriol: Urine. Estradiol: $T_{1/2}$=3 hrs. Levonorgestrel: Urine; $T_{1/2}$=28 hrs.

NURSING CONSIDERATIONS

Assessment: Assess for abnormal genital bleeding, presence or history of breast cancer, estrogen-dependent neoplasia, DVT or PE, active or recent (within past yr) arterial thromboembolic disease (eg, stroke, MI), liver dysfunction/disease, and known/suspected pregnancy. Assess use in patients undergoing surgery associated with thromboembolism, patients with prolonged immobilization, nursing females, patients ≥65 yrs, presence of hypocalcemia, presence of asthma, DM, epilepsy, migraines or porphyria, SLE, or presence of hepatic hemangiomas. Assess for drug/lab test interactions.

Monitoring: Monitor for signs/symptoms of cardiovascular disorders (eg, stroke, MI, venous thrombosis, pulmonary embolism), malignant neoplasms (eg, cancers of endometrium, breast, ovaries), dementia, gallbladder disease, hypercalcemia, visual abnormalities (eg, retinal vascular thrombosis), elevated BP, hypertriglyceridemia, cholestatic jaundice, hypothyroidism, fluid retention, hypocalcemia, exacerbation of endometriosis and other conditions (eg, asthma, DM, epilepsy, migraines or porphyria, SLE, and hepatic hemangiomas). Periodically monitor BP and thyroid function in patients on thyroid replacement therapy. Periodically reassess use of therapy (every 3-6 months). If abnormal genital bleeding occurs, perform proper diagnostic measures (eg, endometrial sampling) to rule out malignancy.

Patient Counseling: Inform that drug may increase risk for heart attack, stroke, breast cancer, blood clots, and dementia. Instruct to report breast lumps, unusual vaginal bleeding, dizziness/faintness, changes in speech, severe headaches, chest pain, or SOB. Inform once transdermal system is in place, it should not be exposed to sun for prolonged periods of time. Counsel that if patch falls off, may reapply same patch or place new patch on different area. Remove patch carefully and slowly to avoid skin irritation.

Administration: Transdermal route. Site of application should not be oily, damaged, or irritated. Apply patch immediately after opening pouch and removing protective liner. Assure patch sticks, especially around edges. **Storage:** 20-25°C (68-77°F); excursions permitted to 15-30°C (59-86°F). Do not store above 30°C (86°F). Keep out of reach of children. Do not store unpouched.

CLINDAGEL — RX

clindamycin phosphate (Galderma)

THERAPEUTIC CLASS: Lincomycin derivative

INDICATIONS: Acne vulgaris.

DOSAGE: *Adults:* Apply thin film once daily.
Pediatrics: ≥12 yrs: Apply thin film once daily.

C

HOW SUPPLIED: Gel: 1% [40mL, 75mL]

CONTRAINDICATIONS: Hypersensitivity to lincomycin. History of regional enteritis, ulcerative colitis, or antibiotic-associated colitis.

WARNINGS/PRECAUTIONS: D/C if significant diarrhea occurs. Caution in atopic individuals.

ADVERSE REACTIONS: Peeling, pruritus, pseudomembranous colitis (rare).

INTERACTIONS: May potentiate neuromuscular blockers.

PREGNANCY: Category B, not for use in nursing.

MECHANISM OF ACTION: Lincomycin derivative; inhibits bacteria protein synthesis at ribosomal level by binding to the 50S ribosomal subunit and affecting the process of peptide chain initiation.

PHARMACOKINETICS: Absorption: C_{max}≤5.5ng/mL. **Distribution:** Orally and parenterally administered clindamycin appears in breast milk. **Excretion:** Urine (<0.4% of total dose).

NURSING CONSIDERATIONS

Assessment: Assess for hypersensitivity to lincomycin, history of regional or ulcerative colitis, antibiotic-associated colitis, nursing status. Assess use in atopic individuals and for possible drug interactions.

Monitoring: Monitor for signs/symptoms of colitis (pseudomembranous colitis), diarrhea, and bloody diarrhea. In patients with diarrhea, consider stool culture for *C.difficile* and stool assay for *C.difficile* toxin. In patients with significant diarrhea, consider large bowel endoscopy.

Patient Counseling: Instruct to notify physician of significant diarrhea during therapy or up to several weeks following therapy end.

Administration: Topical application. **Storage:** Controlled room temperature, 20-25°C (68-77°F); excursions permitted to 15-30°C (59-86°F). Keep container tightly closed, out of direct sunlight.

CLOBEVATE RX

clobetasol propionate (Stiefel)

THERAPEUTIC CLASS: Corticosteroid

INDICATIONS: Inflammatory and pruritic manifestations of corticosteroid-responsive dermatoses.

DOSAGE: *Adults:* Apply thin layer bid. Limit treatment to 2 consecutive weeks. Max: 50g/week. Avoid with occlusive dressings.
Pediatrics: ≥12 yrs: Apply thin layer bid. Limit treatment to 2 consecutive weeks. Max: 50g/week. Avoid with occlusive dressings.

HOW SUPPLIED: Gel: 0.05% [45g]

WARNINGS/PRECAUTIONS: May produce reversible HPA axis suppression, manifestations of Cushing's syndrome, hyperglycemia, and glucosuria. Pediatrics may be more susceptible to systemic toxicity. D/C if irritation occurs. Use appropriate antifungal or antibacterial with concomitant skin infections; d/c if infection does not clear. Should not be used to treat rosacea or perioral dermatitis. Avoid use on face, groin, or axillae.

ADVERSE REACTIONS: Burning, stinging, irritation, pruritus, erythema, folliculitis, cracking and fissuring of the skin, numbness of fingers, skin atrophy, telangiectasia.

PREGNANCY: Category C, caution in nursing.

MECHANISM OF ACTION: Corticosteroid; not established. Has anti-inflammatory, antipruritic, and vasoconstrictive properties. Anti-inflammatory not established; thought to induct phospholipase A_2 inhibitory proteins called lipocortins. Lipocortins control the biosynthesis of potent mediators of inflammation (eg, prostaglandins, leukotrienes) through inhibition of their common precursor, arachidonic acid. Arachidonic acid is released from membrane phospholipids by phospholipase A_2.

PHARMACOKINETICS: Absorption: Absorbed through skin. Occlusive dressings ≤24 hrs, no effect. Occlusive dressings at 96 hrs, markedly enhances penetration. **Distribution:** Systemically administered corticosteroids appear in breast milk.

NURSING CONSIDERATIONS

Assessment: Assess use in patients who are <12 years old, and in pregnant/nursing females. Prior to therapy, assess patient is not using medication for treatment of rosacea or perioral dermatitis. Assess medication is not for use on the face, groin, or axillae areas.

Monitoring: Monitor for signs of HPA axis suppression, Cushing's syndrome, hyperglycemia, and glucosuria. In patients on high doses of corticosteroids, perform periodic monitoring for HPA-axis suppression using the ACTH stimulation, AM plasma cortisol, and urinary free cortisol tests. Monitor for signs of skin irritation and allergic contact dermatitis (eg, failure to heal). Monitor and treat if signs of concomitant skin infection develops (eg, fungal, bacterial).

Patient Counseling: Counsel to use medication exactly as directed. Instruct medication for external use only and to avoid contact with eyes. Inform not to use occlusive dressings with medication. Instruct to notify physician if any type of skin reaction or infection develops or if surgery is being contemplated while on medication.

Administration: Topical. Treatment should be limited to 2 consecutive weeks, and not to exceed ≥50g per week. **Storage:** Store between 15-30°C (59-86°F). Do not refrigerate.

Clobex RX

clobetasol propionate (Galderma)

THERAPEUTIC CLASS: Corticosteroid

INDICATIONS: (Lot) Relief of corticosteroid responsive dermatoses. Treatment of moderate to severe plaque psoriasis (<10% BSA). (Shampoo) Treatment of moderate to severe scalp psoriasis. (Spray) Treatment of moderate to severe plaque psoriasis affecting up to 20% BSA.

DOSAGE: *Adults:* ≥18 yrs: (Lot) Apply bid for up to 2 consecutive weeks. Psoriasis: Reassess after 2 weeks; may repeat for additional 2 weeks. Max: 50g/week or 50mL/week. (Shampoo) Apply thin film daily to dry scalp for up to 4 consecutive weeks. Leave in place for 15 mins before lathering and rinsing. (Spray) Spray on affected area(s) bid. Rub in gently and completely. Reassess after 2 weeks; may repeat for additional 2 weeks. Limit treatment to 4 weeks. Max: 50g/week.

HOW SUPPLIED: Lot: 0.05% [30mL, 59mL]; Shampoo: 0.05% [118mL]; Spray: 0.05% [2oz]

WARNINGS/PRECAUTIONS: Not for use on the face, groin, axillae, eyes, lips, or for the treatment of rosacea or perioral dermatitis. May produce reversible HPA axis suppression, manifestations of Cushing's syndrome, hyperglycemia, and glucosuria. D/C if irritation occurs. Use appropriate antifungal or antibacterial agent with dermatological infections.

ADVERSE REACTIONS: Burning/stinging, pruritus, folliculitis, skin dryness, skin atrophy, telangiectasia.

PREGNANCY: Category C, caution in nursing.

MECHANISM OF ACTION: Corticosteroid; not fully established. Contains anti-inflammatory, antipruritic, and vasoconstrictive properties. Corticosteroids thought to act by induction of phospholipase A_2 inhibitory proteins, called lipocortins. Lipocortins control the biosynthesis of potent mediators of inflammation (eg, prostaglandins, leukotrienes) through inhibiting the release of their precursor, arachidonic acid. Arachidonic acid is released from membrane phospholipids by phospholipase A_2.

PHARMACOKINETICS: Absorption: Use of occlusive dressings ≥24 hrs, no change in drug penetration; use of occlusive dressings for up to 96 hrs, markedly increased drug penetration. **Distribution:** Systemically administered corticosteroids are found in breast milk. **Metabolism:** Liver **Elimination:** Kidneys, bile.

NURSING CONSIDERATIONS

Assessment: Assess that the medication is not being used for the treatment of rosacea or perioral dermatitis or for the treatment on the face, groin, or underarm areas. Assess for hypersensitivity to other corticosteroids and conditions that increase systemic absorption of the medication. Assess use in pregnancy/nursing.

Monitoring: Monitor for signs/symptoms of HPA-axis suppression, Cushing's syndrome, hyperglycemia, and glucosuria. Monitor for signs of skin irritation, allergic contact dermatitis (eg, failure to heal), and skin infections (eg, bacterial, fungal); treat accordingly.

Patient Counseling: Use as directed; do not exceed the use of drug longer than the prescribed time period. Advise to not bandage, cover, or wrap treated area unless directed to do so. Instruct that drug is for external use only; do not use on face, underarms, groin area, or lips. Instruct to wash hands after applying medication. Advise to notify physician if any signs of local or systemic adverse effects develop, if no improvement is seen within 2 weeks, or if contemplating surgery while on medication.

Administration: Topical application. Do not use >50g per week. **Storage:** 20-25°C (68-77°F). Avoid freezing.

CLODERM — RX

clocortolone pivalate (Healthpoint)

THERAPEUTIC CLASS: Topical corticosteroid

INDICATIONS: Corticosteroid-responsive dermatoses.

DOSAGE: *Adults:* Apply tid. Use with occlusive dressing for management of psoriasis or recalcitrant conditions.
Pediatrics: Apply TID. Use with occlusive dressing for management of psoriasis or recalcitrant conditions.

HOW SUPPLIED: Cre: 0.1% [15g, 45g, 90g]

WARNINGS/PRECAUTIONS: May produce reversible HPA axis suppression, manifestations of Cushing's syndrome, hyperglycemia, glucosuria. Caution when applied to large surface areas or under occlusive dressings. Use appropriate antifungal or antibacterial agent with dermatological infections. D/C if infection is not adequately controlled or if irritation develops.

ADVERSE REACTIONS: Burning, itching, irritation, dryness, folliculitis, hypertrichosis, acneiform eruptions, hypopigmentation, perioral/allergic contact dermatitis, secondary infection, skin atrophy.

PREGNANCY: Category C, caution in nursing.

MECHANISM OF ACTION: Topical corticosteroid; mechanism not established. Possesses anti-inflammatory, anti-pruritic, and vasoconstrictive actions.

PHARMACOKINETICS: Absorption: Percutaneous; occlusion, inflammation, and other skin diseases increase absorption. **Distribution:** Bound to plasma protein to varying degrees. Systemically administered corticosteroids found in breast milk. **Metabolism:** Liver. **Elimination:** Kidney and bile.

NURSING CONSIDERATIONS

Assessment: Assess use in pregnant/nursing females and in pediatric patients.

Monitoring: Monitor for signs/symptoms of HPA-axis suppression, Cushing's syndrome, hyperglycemia, and glucosuria. In patients on large doses of medication or using occlusive dressings, perform periodic testing for HPA-axis suppression by using the urinary free cortisol and ACTH stimulation tests. Monitor for systemic toxicity in pediatric patients. Monitor for signs of skin irritation, dermatological infections (eg, bacterial, fungal), and treat appropriately.

Patient Counseling: Counsel to use as directed; avoid contact with eyes. Advise not to bandage or wrap treated skin areas unless directed. Instruct to report any signs of local adverse reactions. Instruct caregivers of pediatric patients to avoid using tight-fitting diapers or plastic pants on treatment area.

Administration: Topical application. **Storage:** Store at 15-30°C (59-86°F). Avoid freezing.

CLOLAR

clofarabine (Genzyme)

RX

THERAPEUTIC CLASS: Antimetabolite

INDICATIONS: Treatment of pediatric patients 1-21 years old with relapsed or refractory acute lymphoblastic leukemia after at least two prior regimens.

DOSAGE: *Pediatrics:* 1-21 yrs: 52mg/m^2 IV over 2 hours daily for 5 consecutive days. Treatment cycles are repeated following recovery or return to baseline organ function, approximately 2-6 weeks. Continuous IV fluids throughout 5 days of clofarabine therapy is recommended. The use of prophylactic steroids (eg, 100mg/m^2 hydrocortisone on Days 1-3) may be of benefit in preventing signs and symptoms of systemic inflammatory response syndrome (SIRS) or capillary leak. If patient develops signs and symptoms of SIRS or capillary leak, clofarabine therapy should be discontinued and appropriate supportive measures should be provided. Close monitoring of renal and hepatic function is required. If substantial increases in creatine or bilirubin occur, clofarabine therapy should be discontinued.

HOW SUPPLIED: Inj: 1mg/mL

WARNINGS/PRECAUTIONS: Suppression of bone marrow function should be anticipated. Increased risk of infection, including severe sepsis is possible. Monitor for signs and symptoms of tumor lysis syndrome, as well as cytokine release that could develop into SIRS/capillary leak syndrome and organ dysfunction. D/C immediately if SIRS or capillary leak syndrome develop. Severe bone marrow suppression, including neutropenia, anemia and thrombocytopenia have been observed. Dehydration may occur due to vomiting and diarrhea. Clofarabine should be discontinued if patient develops hypotension for any reason during the 5 days of administration. Since clofarabine is excreted primarily by the kidneys, drugs with known renal toxicity should be avoided during the 5 days of administration. Since the liver is a known target of clofarabine, concomitant use of medications known to induce hepatic toxicity should also be avoided. Patients taking medications known to affect BP or cardiac function should be closely monitored during administration.

ADVERSE REACTIONS: NV, diarrhea, anemia, leukopenia, thrombocytopenia, neutropenia, febrile neutropenia, and infection.

PREGNANCY: Category D, not for use in nursing.

MECHANISM OF ACTION: Antimetabolite; inhibits DNA synthesis by decreasing cellular deoxynucleotide triphosphate pools through an inhibitory action on ribonucleotide reductase, and by terminating DNA chain elongation and inhibiting repair through incorporation into DNA chain by competitive inhibition of DNA polymerases.

PHARMACOKINETICS: Distribution: V_d=172L/m^2; plasma protein binding (47%). **Elimination:** Urine (unchanged); $T_{1/2}$=5.2 hrs.

NURSING CONSIDERATIONS

Assessment: Assess for hepatic/renal dysfunction, CBC with platelet count and differential, pregnancy status. Note other diseases/conditions and drug therapies

Monitoring: Monitor CBC, platelet count, BP, LFTs, cardiac and respiratory and kidney functions, sepsis, hyperuricemia, hypersensitivity reactions, and transfusion reactions.

Patient Counseling: Counsel about possible side effects; report any adverse effects. Advise to use effective contraceptive measures to prevent pregnancy and drink adequate fluids to avoid dehydration.

Administration: IV route. Filter drug through a 0.2µm syringe filter, then dilute with D5W or 0.9% NS prior to infusion. Admixture must be used within 24 hrs.
Storage: 25°C (77°F); excursions permitted to 15-30°C (59-86°F).

CLORPRES RX

clonidine HCl - chlorthalidone (Mylan Bertek)

THERAPEUTIC CLASS: Central alpha-agonist/monosulfamyl diuretic

INDICATIONS: Treatment of hypertension. Not for initial therapy.

DOSAGE: *Adults:* Determine dose by individual titration. 0.1mg clonidine-15mg chlorthalidone tab qd-bid. Max: 0.6mg clonidine-30mg chlorthalidone/day.

HOW SUPPLIED: Tab: (Clonidine-Chlorthalidone) 0.1mg-15mg*, 0.2mg-15mg*, 0.3mg-15mg* *scored

CONTRAINDICATIONS: Anuria, sulfonamide hypersensitivity.

WARNINGS/PRECAUTIONS: Caution with severe renal disease, hepatic dysfunction, asthma, severe coronary insufficiency, recent MI, cerebrovascular disease. May develop allergic reaction to oral clonidine if sensitive to clonidine patch. Avoid abrupt withdrawal. Continue therapy to within 4 hrs of surgery and resume after. Monitor for fluid/electrolyte imbalance. Hyperuricemia, hypokalemia, hyponatremia, hypochloremic alkalosis, and hyperglycemia may occur.

ADVERSE REACTIONS: Drowsiness, dizziness, constipation, sedation, NV, blood dyscrasias, hypersensitivity reactions, orthostatic symptoms, impotence.

INTERACTIONS: Potentiates other antihypertensives. May increase response to tubocurarine. May decrease arterial response to norepinephrine. Antidiabetic agents may need adjustment. Risk of lithium toxicity. TCAs may reduce effects of clonidine. Amitriptyline may enhance ocular toxicity. Enhanced CNS-depressive effects of alcohol, barbiturates, or other sedatives. Orthostatic hypotension aggravated by alcohol, barbiturates, narcotics.

PREGNANCY: (Clonidine) Category C, caution in nursing. (Chlorthalidone) Category B, not for use in nursing.

MECHANISM OF ACTION: Clonidine: Imidazoline derivative; stimulates α-adrenoceptor in brain stem, resulting in reduced sympathetic outflow from CNS and decrease in peripheral resistance, renal vascular resistance, HR, and BP. Chlorthalidone: Monosulfamyl diuretic; increases excretion of Na^+ and Cl^-; decreases extracellular fluid volume, plasma volume, cardiac output, total exchangeable sodium, glomerular filtration rate, and renal plasma flow.

PHARMACOKINETICS: Absorption: Clonidine: T_{max}=3-5 hrs. **Distribution:** Chlorthalidone: Plasma protein binding (75%). **Metabolism:** Clonidine: Liver. **Elimination:** Clonidine: Urine (40-60%); $T_{1/2}$=12-16 hrs. Chlorthalidone: Urine; $T_{1/2}$=40-60 hrs.

NURSING CONSIDERATIONS

Assessment: Assess for anuria, sulfonamide hypersensitivity, coronary insufficiency, recent MI, cerebrovascular disease, history of allergy or bronchial asthma, systemic lupus erythematosus (SLE), DM, renal/hepatic impairment.

Monitoring: Periodically monitor serum electrolytes, serum K^+ levels, and renal function. Monitor for signs/symptoms of electrolyte imbalance, hypokalemia, possible exacerbation or activation of SLE, hyperglycemia, withdrawal symptoms, hyperuricemia or precipitation of gout, hypersensitivity reactions, renal/hepatic dysfunction.

Patient Counseling: Caution that drug may impair physical/mental abilities. Inform to avoid alcohol. Instruct not to interrupt or d/c therapy without consulting physician. Seek medical attention if symptoms of electrolyte imbalance (dry mouth, thirst, weakness), hypokalemia (thirst, tiredness, restlessness), withdrawal (nervousness, agitation, headaches), or hypersensitivity reactions occur.

Administration: Oral route. **Storage:** 15-30°C (59-86°F). Avoid excessive humidity.

CLOTRIMAZOLE TOPICAL RX

clotrimazole (Various)

THERAPEUTIC CLASS: Azole antifungal

INDICATIONS: Topical treatment of candidiasis caused by *Candida albicans* and tinea versicolor caused by *Malassezia furfur*.

DOSAGE: *Adults:* Apply bid (am and pm). Re-evaluate if no improvement after 4 weeks.
Pediatrics: Apply bid (am and pm). Re-evaluate if no improvement after 4 weeks.

HOW SUPPLIED: Cre: 1% [15g, 30g]; Sol: 1% [10mL]

WARNINGS/PRECAUTIONS: D/C if irritation or sensitivity occurs. Not for ophthalmic use.

ADVERSE REACTIONS: Erythema, stinging, blistering, peeling, edema, pruritus, urticaria, burning, irritation.

PREGNANCY: Category B, caution in nursing.

MECHANISM OF ACTION: Broad spectrum antifungal agent; primary action is against dividing and growing organisms. Causes leakage of intracellular phosphorus compounds into the ambient medium with concomitant breakdown of cellular nucleic acids and accelerated potassium efflux.

PHARMACOKINETICS: Absorption: Minimally absorbed. **Elimination:** Urine (≤0.5%).

NURSING CONSIDERATIONS

Assessment: Assess for appropriate microbiological studies to confirm diagnosis, pregnancy status, and nursing status.

Monitoring: Monitor for signs/symptoms of irritation or sensitivity at treatment site. Monitor for clinical response; if lack of response, repeat appropriate microbiological studies to confirm diagnosis.

Patient Counseling: Advise to use medication for full treatment period even if symptoms improve. Contact physician if no improvement seen after 4 weeks of therapy. Notify physician if treatment area shows signs of increased irritation (eg, redness, itching, burning, blistering, oozing). Avoid use of occlusive wrappings or dressings; avoid sources of infection or reinfection.

Administration: Topical route. **Storage:** Cre: 2-30°C (36-86°F). Sol: 20-25°C (68-77°F).

CLOZAPINE RX

clozapine (Various)

Risk of agranulocytosis, seizures, myocarditis, and other cardiovascular and respiratory effects. Conduct baseline WBC and differential before therapy, then regularly, and 4 weeks after discontinuation. Elderly patients with dementia-related psychosis treated with atypical antipsychotic drugs are at an increased risk of death; most appeared to be cardiovascular (eg, heart failure, sudden death) or infectious (eg, pneumonia) in nature. Clozapine is not approved for the treatment of patients with dementia-related psychosis.

OTHER BRAND NAMES: Clozaril (Novartis)

THERAPEUTIC CLASS: Dibenzapine derivative

INDICATIONS: Management of severe schizophrenia when response to standard schizophrenia treatment fails. To reduce the risk of recurrent suicidal behavior with schizophrenia or schizoaffective disorder.

DOSAGE: *Adults:* Initial: 12.5mg qd-bid. Titrate: Increase by 25-50mg/day, up to 300-450mg/day by end of 2nd week, then increase weekly or bi-weekly by up to 100mg. Usual: 100-900mg/day given tid. Max: 900mg/day. If at risk of suicidal behavior then treat for at least 2 yrs then assess; reassess thereafter at regular intervals. To d/c, gradually reduce dose over 1-2 weeks. Monitor for psychotic symptoms if abrupt discontinuation warranted (eg, leukopenia).

HOW SUPPLIED: Tab: (Clozapine) 12.5mg, 25mg, 100mg; (Clozaril) 25mg*, 100mg* *scored

CONTRAINDICATIONS: Myeloproliferative disorders, uncontrolled epilepsy, paralytic ileus, history of clozapine induced agranulocytosis or severe granulocytopenia, severe CNS depression, coma, with agents with potential to cause agranulocytosis or suppress bone marrow function.

WARNINGS/PRECAUTIONS: Reserve treatment for severely ill patients unresponsive to other schizophrenia therapies. Monitor for hyperglycemia, worsening of glucose control with DM, FBG levels with diabetes risk. Significant risk of orthostatic hypotension, and tachycardia. May impair alertness with initial doses. May cause high fever, hyperglycemia, or pulmonary embolism. Cardiomyopathy reported; d/c unless benefit outweighs risk. Caution with prostatic enlargement, narrow angle glaucoma, and renal, hepatic, or cardiac/pulmonary disease. NMS and tardive dyskinesia reported. Acquire WBC and ANC at baseline, then weekly for 1st 6 months of therapy, then every 2 weeks for 6 months, and then every 4 weeks thereafter if WBCs and ANC are acceptable. Avoid initiation of treatment if WBCs <3500/mm^3, ANC <2000/mm^3, history of myeloproliferative disorder, previous clozapine-induced agranulocytosis or granulocytopenia. D/C treatment if WBCs <3000/mm^3, ANC <1500/mm^3, eosinophils >4000/mm^3, or if myocarditis develops. D/C over 1-2 weeks. Varying degrees of intestinal peristalsis impairment (eg, constipation, intestinal obstruction, paralytic ileus), ECG changes reported.

ADVERSE REACTIONS: Drowsiness, vertigo, headache, tremor, salivation, sweating, dry mouth, visual disturbances, tachycardia, hypotension, syncope, constipation, nausea, blood dyscrasias, fever.

INTERACTIONS: See Contraindications. Avoid with bone-marrow suppressants, epinephrine, and carbamazepine. Caution with CNS-active drugs, anesthesia, alcohol, paroxetine, sertraline, fluvoxamine, benzodiazepines, other psychotropics, inhibitors/inducers of CYP1A2, 2D6, 3A4. Potentiates hypotensive effects of antihypertensives and anticholinergic effects of atropine-type drugs. Decrease dose with drugs metabolized by CYP2D6. Caution with general anesthesia. CYP450 inducers (eg, phenytoin, nicotine, rifampin) decrease plasma levels. CYP450 inhibitors (eg, cimetidine, caffeine, erythromycin, citalopram) increase plasma levels.

PREGNANCY: Category B, not for use in nursing.

MECHANISM OF ACTION: Atypical antipsychotic agent; interferes with binding of dopamine at D_1, D_2, D_3, and D_5 receptors. Has high affinity for D_4 receptor. Also acts as antagonist at adrenergic, cholinergic, histaminergic, and serotonergic receptors.

PHARMACOKINETICS: Absorption: C_{max}=319ng/mL; T_{max}=2.5 hrs. **Distribution:** Plasma protein binding (97%). **Elimination:** Urine (50%), feces (30%); $T_{1/2}$=8 hrs (after single dose), $T_{1/2}$=12 hrs (after multiple doses).

NURSING CONSIDERATIONS

Assessment: Assess if patient has severe schizophrenic disorder and has failed at least 2 other trials with 2 other standard drugs, schizophrenic disorder and is at risk for suicidal behavior, dementia-related psychosis, myeloproliferative disorders, uncontrolled epilepsy, paralytic ileus, history of clozapine-induced agranulocytosis or severe granulocytopenia, or severe CNS depression prior to therapy. Assess for possible drug interactions. Assess baseline WBC counts and ANC prior to treatment. Assess fasting blood glucose levels in patients who have DM or are at risk for hyperglycemia.

Monitoring: Monitor for clinical response to treatment, WBC counts and ANC during therapy and for at least 4 weeks following discontinuation. Refer to PI for specific scheduling parameters. Monitor for agranulocytosis, myocarditis, other cardiovascular complications (eg, orthostatic hypotension, cardiomyopathy, cardiac arrest), respiratory complications, seizures, NMS, TD, fever, pulmonary embolism, and hepatitis.

C

Patient Counseling: Inform of need for regular monitoring of WBC counts and ANC. Advise to report immediately any lethargy, weakness, fever, sore throat, or any signs/symptoms of infection during therapy. Inform that drug may impair mental/physical abilities. Counsel to avoid alcohol. Advise to contact physician if more than 2 days of doses are missed. Counsel females to avoid nursing.

Administration: Oral route. **Storage:** 20-25°C (68-77°F). Dispense in tight, light-resistant container with child-resistant closure.

Cognex
tacrine HCl (Sciele)

RX

THERAPEUTIC CLASS: Reversible cholinesterase inhibitor

INDICATIONS: Treatment of mild to moderate dementia of the Alzheimer's type.

DOSAGE: *Adults:* Initial: 10mg qid. Titrate: Increase to 20mg qid after 4 weeks, then increase at 4-week intervals to 30mg qid then to 40mg qid. ALT/SGPT: >3 to ≤5x ULN: Reduce dose by 40mg/day and resume dose titration when levels are normal. >5x ULN: Stop therapy and monitor; may rechallenge when ALT/SGPT levels are normal. D/C and do not rechallenge if jaundice and/or signs of hypersensitivity. Rechallenge: 10mg qid, may titrate if normal ALT/SGPT after 6 weeks. Monitor weekly for 16 weeks, then monthly for 2 months, and every 3 months thereafter. Take between meals.

HOW SUPPLIED: Cap: 10mg, 20mg, 30mg, 40mg

CONTRAINDICATIONS: Hypersensitivity to acridine derivatives, history of tacrine-associated jaundice (bilirubin >3mg/dL) or signs of hypersensitivity associated with ALT/SGPT elevations.

WARNINGS/PRECAUTIONS: Vagotonic effects; caution with conduction abnormalities, bradyarrhythmia, sick sinus syndrome. May increase risk of developing ulcers. Monitor LFTs every other week from weeks 4-16 from start of therapy, then every 3 months. Modify LFT monitoring based on LFTs (see dosage). Higher incidence of LFT elevation in females. May cause seizures, bladder outflow obstruction, neutrophil abnormalities. May worsen cognitive function with abrupt withdrawal. Caution with liver disease, ulcers, asthma. D/C with clinical jaundice or hypersensitivity with ALT/SGPT elevations.

ADVERSE REACTIONS: Elevated LFTs, NV, diarrhea, dyspepsia, myalgia, anorexia, ataxia, dizziness.

INTERACTIONS: May potentiate succinylcholine, cholinesterase inhibitors, cholinergic agonists, and theophylline. May interact with drugs metabolized by CYP450. Fluvoxamine increases levels. May antagonize anticholinergics. Monitor for GI disease with NSAIDs. Increased levels with cimetidine.

PREGNANCY: Category C, caution in nursing.

MECHANISM OF ACTION: Reversible cholinesterase inhibitor; suspected to increase acetylcholine concentration through inhibition of its hydrolysis by cholinesterase.

PHARMACOKINETICS: Absorption: Rapid, absolute bioavailability (17%); T_{max}=1-2 hrs. **Distribution:** V_d=349L; plasma protein binding (55%). **Metabolism:** Liver (glucuronidation) via CYP450. **Elimination:** $T_{1/2}$=2-4 hrs.

NURSING CONSIDERATIONS

Assessment: Assess for conduction abnormalities, bradyarrhythmia, sick sinus syndrome, history of asthma, ulcer disease, hepatic dysfunction, and possible drug interactions.

Monitoring: Monitor serum transaminase level every other week from at least Week 4 to Week 16 following treatment initiation. Continue weekly monitoring of the ALT/SGPT level for a total of 16 weeks. Monitor for signs/symptoms of hepatic dysfunction, active or occult GI disease.

Patient Counseling: Inform physician about emergence of new events or any increase in the severity of existing adverse events. Advise that abrupt d/c may cause decline in cognitive function and behavioral disturbances. Seek medical attention if symptoms of hepatic dysfunction (jaundice), active or occult GI disease occur.

Administration: Oral route. **Storage:** 20-25°C (68-77°F); excursions permitted to 15-30°C (59-86°F). Protect from moisture.

COLAZAL — RX
balsalazide disodium (Salix)

THERAPEUTIC CLASS: Anti-inflammatory Agent

INDICATIONS: Treatment of mild-to-moderate active ulcerative colitis in patients ≥5 yrs.

DOSAGE: *Adults:* 3 caps tid for up to 8 weeks (or 12 weeks if needed). May open cap and sprinkle on applesauce.
Pediatrics: 5-17 yrs: 1 or 3 caps tid for 8 weeks. May open cap and sprinkle on applesauce.

HOW SUPPLIED: Cap: 750mg

CONTRAINDICATIONS: Hypersensitivity to salicylates.

WARNINGS/PRECAUTIONS: May exacerbate symptoms of colitis. Prolonged gastric retention with pyloric stenosis. Caution with renal dysfunction or history of renal disease.

ADVERSE REACTIONS: Headache, abdominal pain, diarrhea, NV, respiratory problems, arthralgia, rhinitis, insomnia, fatigue, rectal bleeding, flatulence, fever, dyspepsia.

INTERACTIONS: Oral antibiotics may interfere with the release of mesalamine in the colon.

PREGNANCY: Category B, caution in nursing.

MECHANISM OF ACTION: Not established; a prodrug enzymatically cleaved in colon to produce mesalamine (5-ASA), an anti-inflammatory drug that acts locally to block production of arachidonic acid metabolites in the colon.

PHARMACOKINETICS: Absorption: Different dosing conditions (fasted, fed, sprinkled) resulted in variable parameters. **Distribution:** Plasma protein binding (≥99%). **Metabolism:** Key metabolites: 5-ASA and N-acetyl-5-ASA. **Elimination:** Urine, feces.

NURSING CONSIDERATIONS

Assessment: Assess for pyloric stenosis, possible drug interactions, history of renal/hepatic disease.

Monitoring: Monitor renal function, LFTs, and CBC, signs/symptoms of prolonged gastric retention with pyloric stenosis, worsening of colitis symptoms, and hypersensitivity.

Patient Counseling: Inform can take with/without food or sprinkle on applesauce. Teeth and/or tongue may get stained when using sprinkle form with food. Seek medical attention if diagnosed with pyloric stenosis or renal dysfunction, experience worsening of colitis symptoms or hypersensitivity (eg, anaphylaxis, bronchospasm, skin reaction).

Administration: Oral route. **Storage:** 20-25°C (68-77°F); excursions permitted to 15-30°C (59-86°F).

COLCHICINE — RX
colchicine (Various)

THERAPEUTIC CLASS: Miscellaneous gout agent

INDICATIONS: Treatment and prophylaxis of acute gouty arthritis.

DOSAGE: *Adults:* Acute Treatment: Initial: 1-1.2mg, followed by 0.5-0.6mg q1h, or 1-1.2mg q2h or 0.5-0.6mg q2-3h until pain relief, GI discomfort or diarrhea ensues. Usual: 4-8mg/attack. Wait 3 days before retreatment. Prophylaxis:

<1 attack/yr: 0.5-0.6mg/day given 3-4x/week. >1 attack/yr: 0.5-0.6mg qd. Severe Cases: 2-3 tabs of 0.5mg or 0.6mg daily. Surgical Gout Prophylaxis: 0.5-0.6mg tid 3 days before and 3 days after surgery.

HOW SUPPLIED: Tab: 0.5mg, 0.6mg

CONTRAINDICATIONS: Serious GI, renal, hepatic or cardiac disorders, and blood dyscrasias.

WARNINGS/PRECAUTIONS: Caution in elderly, debilitated, or with GI, renal, hepatic, cardiac and hematologic disorders. D/C if nausea, vomiting, or diarrhea occurs. Monitor blood counts periodically with long-term therapy. May adversely affect spermatogenesis. Elevates SGOT and alkaline phosphatase. May cause false (+) for urine RBC and Hgb.

ADVERSE REACTIONS: Bone marrow depression, peripheral neuritis, purpura, myopathy, alopecia, dermatoses, reversible azoospermia, nausea, vomiting, diarrhea.

INTERACTIONS: Inhibited by acidifying agents. Potentiated by alkalinizing agents. Potentiates sympathomimetics and CNS depressants.

PREGNANCY: Category C, caution in nursing.

MECHANISM OF ACTION: Colchicum alkaloid; not established, but involves reduction in lactic acid production by leukocytes, resulting in a decrease in uric acid deposition and reduction in phagocytosis, abating inflammatory response.

PHARMACOKINETICS: Absorption: Rapid. **Elimination:** Biliary and renal excretion.

NURSING CONSIDERATIONS

Assessment: Assess for serious GI tract, renal/hepatic or cardiac disorders, blood dyscrasias, debilitation, and possible drug interactions.

Monitoring: Monitor blood counts periodically.

Patient Counseling: Inform to learn dose needed and to keep at hand for use at first sign of attack. Advise to d/c if symptoms of NV and diarrhea occur.

Administration: Oral route. **Storage:** 15-30°C (59-86°F). Protect from light.

COLCHICINE/PROBENECID RX

probenecid - colchicine (Various)

THERAPEUTIC CLASS: Uricosuric

INDICATIONS: Chronic gouty arthritis complicated by frequent, recurrent acute gout attacks.

DOSAGE: *Adults:* Initial: 1 tab qd for 1 week, then 1 tab bid. Titrate: May increase by 1 tab/day every 4 weeks. Max: 4 tabs/day. May reduce dose by 1 tab every 6 months if acute attacks have been absent ≥6 months. Decrease dose with gastric intolerance. Renal Impairment: May need to increase dose. May not be effective if CrCl ≤30mL/min.

HOW SUPPLIED: Tab: (Colchicine-Probenecid) 0.5mg-500mg

CONTRAINDICATIONS: Blood dyscrasias, uric acid kidney stones, children <2 yrs and pregnancy. Do not use in acute gout attack.

WARNINGS/PRECAUTIONS: Exacerbation of gout may occur. Use APAP if analgesic needed. Severe allergic reaction and anaphylaxis reported (rare). D/C if hypersensitivity occurs. Caution with peptic ulcer. Monitor for glycosuria. Determine benefit/risk ratio with long-term therapy. Maintain liberal fluid intake and alkalization of urine.

ADVERSE REACTIONS: Headache, dizziness, hepatic necrosis, vomiting, nausea, anorexia, sore gums, uric acid stones, renal colic, anaphylaxis, fever, pruritus, blood dyscrasias, peripheral neuritis, muscular weakness, abdominal pain, diarrhea, alopecia, dermatitis.

INTERACTIONS: Probenecid increases plasma levels of penicillin and other β-lactams; psychic disturbances reported. Salicylates and pyrazinamide antagonize uricosuric effects. Increased plasma levels of methotrexate, sulfonamides, sulfonylureas, thiopental or ketamine-induced anesthesia, some NSAIDs (eg, indomethacin, naproxen), lorazepam, APAP, and rifampin. Possible false high plasma levels of theophylline.

PREGNANCY: Contraindicated in pregnancy; safety in nursing not known.

MECHANISM OF ACTION: Probenecid: Uricosuric/renal tubular blocking agent; inhibits tubular reabsorption of urate, increasing urinary excretion of uric acid and decreasing serum urate levels. Colchicine: Colchicum alkaloid; not been established, has prophylactic, suppressive effect helping to reduce incidence of acute attacks and relieve residual pain and mild discomfort.

NURSING CONSIDERATIONS

Assessment: Assess for known blood dyscrasias, uric acid kidney stones, acute vs chronic attack, history of peptic ulcer, and possible drug interactions.

Monitoring: Monitor for signs/symptoms of gout exacerbation, allergic reactions, hematuria, renal colic, costovertebral pain, and uric acid stone formation.

Patient Counseling: Instruct on importance of liberal fluid intake. Advise to seek medical attention if symptoms of allergic reaction, hematuria, renal colic, or costovertebral pain occur.

Administration: Oral route. **Storage:** 20-25°C (68-77°F). Protect from light.

COLESTID RX

colestipol HCl (Pharmacia & Upjohn)

THERAPEUTIC CLASS: Bile acid sequestrant

INDICATIONS: Adjunct to diet, to reduce elevated serum total and LDL-C in primary hypercholesterolemia.

DOSAGE: *Adults:* Initial: 2g, 1 pkt or 1 scoopful qd-bid. Titrate: Increase by 2g qd or bid at 1-2 month intervals. Usual: 2-16g/day (tab) or 1-6 pkts or scoopfuls qd or in divided doses. Always mix granules with liquid. Swallow tabs whole with plenty of liquid.

HOW SUPPLIED: Granules: 5g/pkt [30^s 90^s], 5g/scoopful [300g, 500g]; Tab: 1g

WARNINGS/PRECAUTIONS: Exclude secondary causes of hypercholesterolemia and perform a lipid profile. May produce hyperchloremic acidosis with prolonged use. Monitor cholesterol and TG based on NCEP guidelines. May cause hypothyroidism. May interfere with normal fat absorption. Chronic use may produce or worsen constipation. Avoid constipation with symptomatic CAD. May increase bleeding tendency due to vitamin K deficiency.

ADVERSE REACTIONS: Constipation, musculoskeletal pain, headache, migraine headache, sinus headache.

INTERACTIONS: May interfere with absorption of folic acid, fat-soluble vitamins (eg, A, D, K), oral phosphate supplements, hydrocortisone. May delay or reduce absorption of concomitant oral medication; take other drugs 1 hr before or 4 hrs after colestipol. Reduces absorption of chlorothiazide, tetracycline, furosemide, penicillin G, hydrochlorothiazide, and gemfibrozil. Caution with digitalis agents, propranolol.

PREGNANCY: Safety in pregnancy not known, caution in nursing.

MECHANISM OF ACTION: Binds to bile acids in the intestine, forming a complex that is excreted in the feces, leading to increased fecal loss of bile acids and increased oxidation of cholesterol to bile acids, a decrease in β lipoprotein or LDL, and a decrease in serum cholesterol levels.

PHARMACOKINETICS: Elimination: Feces.

NURSING CONSIDERATIONS

Assessment: Assess for hypothyroidism, DM, nephrotic syndrome, dysproteinemia, obstructive liver disease, pre-existing constipation, and possible drug interactions.

Monitoring: Monitor serum cholesterol, TG level, signs of vitamin K deficiency (eg, tendency for bleeding), hypersensitivity reactions (eg, urticaria and dermatitis).

Patient Counseling: Advise to mix drug with water or other fluids before ingesting. Inform about benefits/risks of therapy. Report any adverse reactions to physician.

Administration: Oral route.

COMBIGAN — RX

timolol maleate - brimonidine tartrate (Allergan)

THERAPEUTIC CLASS: $Alpha_2$-agonist/beta-blocker

INDICATIONS: Reduction of elevated intraocular pressure (IOP) in patients with glaucoma or ocular hypertension who require adjunctive or replacement therapy due to inadequately controlled IOP.

DOSAGE: *Adults:* 1 drop in affected eye(s) bid approximately 12 hrs apart. Instill other topical ophthalmic products at least 5 min apart.
Pediatrics: ≥2 yrs: 1 drop in affected eye(s) bid approximately 12 hrs apart. Instill other topical ophthalmic products at least 5 min apart.

HOW SUPPLIED: Sol: (Brimonidine-Timolol) 2mg-5mg/mL

CONTRAINDICATIONS: Bronchial asthma, history of bronchial asthma, severe COPD, sinus bradycardia, second- or third-degree AV block, overt cardiac failure, cardiogenic shock.

WARNINGS/PRECAUTIONS: Systemic absorption, leading to adverse reactions (including severe respiratory reactions) may occur. Caution with cardiac failure; d/c if cardiac failure develops. Avoid with bronchospastic disease and/or mild-to-moderate COPD. May potentiate syndromes associated with vascular insufficiency; caution with depression, cerebral or coronary insufficiency, Raynaud's phenomenon, orthostatic hypotension, or thromboangiitis obliterans. May increase reactivity to allergens. May potentiate muscle weakness consistent with certain myasthenic symptoms. May mask signs/symptoms of acute hypoglycemia; caution in patients subject to spontaneous hypoglycemia or diabetic patients receiving insulin or hypoglycemic agents. May mask signs of hyperthyroidism. Bacterial keratitis reported with use of multiple-dose containers of topical ophthalmic products. May need to gradually withdraw β-blocking agents in patients undergoing elective surgery.

ADVERSE REACTIONS: Allergic conjunctivitis, conjunctival folliculosis, conjunctival hyperemia, eye pruritus, ocular burning/stinging.

INTERACTIONS: May reduce BP; caution with antihypertensives and/or cardiac glycosides. Monitor with concomitant oral β-blockers; avoid concomitant use of 2 topical β-blocking agents. Caution with concomitant oral or IV calcium antagonists; avoid concomitant use with impaired cardiac function. Monitor closely with concomitant catecholamine-depleting drugs (eg, reserpine). Possibility of additive or potentiating effect with CNS depressants (eg, alcohol, barbiturates, opiates, sedatives, anesthetics). Concomitant use of β-blockers with digitalis and/or calcium antagonists may have additive effects in prolonging AV-conduction time. Potentiated systemic β-blockade reported with CYP2D6 inhibitors and timolol. Caution with TCAs and/or MAOIs.

PREGNANCY: Category C, not for use in nursing.

MECHANISM OF ACTION: Decreases elevated IOP. Brimonidine: Selective α-2 adrenergic receptor. Timolol: Nonselective β-blocker.

PHARMACOKINETICS: Absorption: Brimonidine: C_{max}=30pg/mL; T_{max}= 1-4 hrs. Timolol: C_{max}=400pg/mL; T_{max}=1-3 hrs. **Distribution:** Timolol: Plasma protein binding (60%). **Metabolism:** Brimonidine: Liver (extensive). Timolol: Liver (partial). **Elimination:** Brimonidine: Urine (74%); $T_{1/2}$=3 hrs. Timolol: Excreted mainly by kidney; $T_{1/2}$=7 hrs.

C

NURSING CONSIDERATIONS

Assessment: Assess for ocular infection; signs/symptoms of systemic absorption of β-adrenergic blockers (eg, potentiation of bronchial asthma, COPD, cerebral or coronary insufficiency, cardiac failure).

Monitoring: Monitor IOP, vital signs, renal function, LFTs, and adverse reactions (eg, allergic conjunctivitis, conjunctival folliculosis, conjunctival hyperemia, eye pruritis, ocular burning and stinging).

Patient Counseling: To avoid ocular infection, avoid contact of container tip to affected eye. If more than 1 ophthalmic drug is being used, administer at least 5 min apart. Remove contact lenses prior to administration; may be reinserted after 15 min.

Administration: Ocular route. **Storage:** 15-25°C (59-77°F). Protect from light.

CombiPatch RX

norethindrone acetate - estradiol (Novartis)

Estrogens and progestins should not be used for prevention of cardiovascular disease or dementia. Increased risks of MI, stroke, invasive breast cancer, PE, and DVT in postmenopausal women (50-79 yrs of age) reported. Increased risk of developing probable dementia in postmenopausal women ≥65 yrs of age reported.

THERAPEUTIC CLASS: Estrogen/progestogen combination

INDICATIONS: In women with an intact uterus, for the treatment of moderate to severe vasomotor symptoms associated with menopause, vulvar/vaginal atrophy. Treatment of hypoestrogenism due to hypogonadism, castration, or primary ovarian failure.

DOSAGE: *Adults:* Continuous Combined Regimen: Apply 0.05mg/0.14mg patch on lower abdomen (avoid breasts and waistline). Apply twice weekly during 28-day cycle. Continuous Sequential Regimen: Wear estradiol-only patch for 1st 14 days of 28-day cycle, replace twice weekly. Apply 0.05mg/0.14mg patch for remaining 14 days, replace twice weekly. For both regimens, use 0.05mg/0.25mg patch if additional progestin required. Re-evaluate at 3-6 month intervals. Rotate sites; allow 1 week between same site.

HOW SUPPLIED: Patch: (Estradiol-Norethindrone) 0.05-0.14mg/day, 0.05-0.25mg/day [8ˢ, 24ˢ]

CONTRAINDICATIONS: Undiagnosed abnormal genital bleeding, breast cancer, estrogen-dependent neoplasia, DVT, PE, arterial thromboembolic disorder (eg, stroke, MI), liver dysfunction or disease.

WARNINGS/PRECAUTIONS: May increase risk of cardiovascular events (eg, MI, stroke), venous thrombosis, and PE; d/c immediately if any of these events occur or are suspected. May increase risk of breast/endometrial cancer, and gallbladder disease. May lead to severe hypercalcemia with breast cancer and bone metastases; monitor and d/c if hypercalcemia occurs. Retinal vascular thrombosis reported; monitor and d/c if papilledema or retinal vascular lesions occur. May elevate BP; monitor at regular intervals. May cause elevations of plasma triglycerides with pre-existing hypertriglyceridemia. Caution with history of cholestatic jaundice associated with past estrogen use or with pregnancy; d/c with recurrence. May lead to increased thyroid-binding globulin levels; monitor thyroid function. May cause fluid retention; caution with cardiac/renal dysfunction. Caution with severe hypocalcemia. May increase risk of ovarian cancer. May exacerbate endometriosis, asthma, DM, epilepsy, migraine, porphyria, SLE, and hepatic hemangiomas; use with caution.

ADVERSE REACTIONS: Abdominal pain, back pain, asthenia, flu syndrome, application site reaction, nausea, nervousness, pharyngitis, respiratory disorder, breast pain, dysmenorrhea, menstrual disorder, vaginitis.

INTERACTIONS: CYP3A4 inducers (eg, St. John's wort, phenobarbital, carbamazepine, rifampin) may decrease levels which may decrease therapeutic effects and/or change uterine bleeding profile. CYP3A4 inhibitors (eg, erythromycin, clarithromycin, ketoconazole, itraconazole, ritonavir, grapefruit juice) may increase levels which may result in side effects.

PREGNANCY: Contraindicated in pregnancy, caution in nursing.

MECHANISM OF ACTION: Estrogen/progestogen. Acts by binding to nuclear receptors in estrogen-responsive tissues. Modulates pituitary secretion of gonadotropins, luteinizing hormone and follicle stimulating hormone, through negative feedback mechanism.

PHARMACOKINETICS: Absorption: Estradiol: Well-absorbed. Administration of various doses led to altered parameters. Norethindrone: Well-absorbed. Administration of various doses led to altered parameters. **Distribution:** Estrogens and progestins found in breast milk. Estradiol: Largely bound to sex hormone binding globulin (SHBG) and albumin. Norethindrone: 90% to SHBG and albumin. **Metabolism:** Liver, to estrone (metabolite); estriol (major urinary metabolite); enterohepatic recirculation, via sulfate and glucuronide conjugation; biliary secretion of conjugates in the intestine; hydrolysis in gut; reabsorption; CYP 3A4 (partial). Norethindrone: Liver. **Elimination:** Estradiol, estrone, estriol: Urine; $T_{1/2}$=2-3 hrs. Norethindrone: $T_{1/2}$=6-8 hrs.

NURSING CONSIDERATIONS

Assessment: Assess for abnormal genital bleeding, presence or history of breast cancer, DVT or PE, estrogen-dependent neoplasias, active or recent (within past yr) arterial thromboembolic disease (eg, stroke, MI), liver dysfunction, and known/suspected pregnancy. Assess use in nursing females, patients ≥65 yrs, presence of severe hypocalcemia, asthma, DM, epilepsy, migraines or porphyria, SLE, or presence of hepatic hemangiomas. Assess for drug or lab interactions.

Monitoring: Monitor for signs/symptoms of cardiovascular events (eg, MI, stroke, venous thromboembolism, pulmonary embolism), malignant neoplasms (eg, endometrial, breast, ovarian cancer), dementia, gallbladder disease, hypercalcemia, visual abnormalities (eg, retinal vascular thrombosis), elevated BP, fluid retention, hypertriglyceridemia, cholestatic jaundice, hypothyroidism, exacerbation of endometriosis and other conditions (eg, asthma, DM, epilepsy, migraines or porphyria, SLE, and hepatic hemangiomas). Periodically monitor BP levels and thyroid function in patients on thyroid replacement therapy. Perform periodic assessment (eg, every 3-6 months) to evaluate need for therapy. If abnormal genital bleeding occurs, perform proper diagnostic measures (eg, endometrial sampling) to rule out malignancies.

Patient Counseling: Inform that drug may increase risk for heart attack, stroke, breast cancer, blood clots, and dementia. Report any breast lumps, unusual vaginal bleeding, dizziness or faintness, changes in speech, chest pain, SOB, leg pain, changes in vision, and vomiting. Counsel that if patch falls off, reapply same patch to different area of lower abdomen or use new patch.

Administration: Transdermal route. **Storage:** Prior to dispensing: Store refrigerated at 2-8°C (36-46°F). After dispensed: May be stored at room temperature below 25°C (77°F). Do not store in areas where extreme temperatures may occur.

COMBIVENT — RX

ipratropium bromide - albuterol sulfate (Boehringer Ingelheim)

THERAPEUTIC CLASS: $Beta_2$-agonist/anticholinergic

INDICATIONS: Adjunct therapy for bronchospasm in COPD if currently on a regular aerosol bronchodilator and require a second bronchodilator.

DOSAGE: *Adults:* 2 inh qid. Max: 12 inh/24 hrs.

HOW SUPPLIED: MDI: (Albuterol-Ipratropium) 0.09mg-0.018mg/inh [14.7g]

CONTRAINDICATIONS: History of hypersensitivity to soya lecithin or related food products (eg, soybeans, peanuts).

WARNINGS/PRECAUTIONS: Paradoxical bronchospasm reported. Hypersensitivity reactions reported. Caution with coronary insufficiency, arrhythmias, narrow-angle glaucoma, prostatic hypertrophy, bladder-neck obstruction, HTN, DM, hyperthyroidism, seizures, renal or hepatic dysfunction, and in those unusually responsive to sympathomimetic amines. May produce transient hypokalemia. Fatalities reported with excessive use.

ADVERSE REACTIONS: Headache, cough, respiratory disorders, pain, dyspnea, bronchitis.

C

INTERACTIONS: Potential additive interactions with other anticholinergic drugs. Increased risk of cardiovascular effects with other sympathomimetics. β-blockers and albuterol inhibit effects of each other. ECG changes and/or hypokalemia may occur with non-K^+-sparing diuretics. Avoid MAOIs and TCAs.

PREGNANCY: Category C, not for use in nursing.

MECHANISM OF ACTION: Ipratropium: Anticholinergic bronchodilator; inhibits vagally mediated reflexes by antagonizing the action of acetylcholine. Albuterol: Selective β_2-adrenergic bronchodilator; activates β_2-receptors on airway smooth muscle, leading to activation of adenylyl cyclase and increase of intracellular cyclic AMP concentrations. This leads to activation of protein kinase A, which inhibits phosphorylation of myosin and lowers intracellular ionic calcium concentrations, resulting in relaxation.

PHARMACOKINETICS: Absorption: Ipratropium: Not readily absorbed. Albuterol: Rapid, complete; C_{max}=492pg/mL; T_{max}=3 hrs. **Distribution:** Ipratropium: Plasma protein binding (0-9%). **Metabolism:** Ipratopium: Partial; ester hydrolysis. Albuterol: Conjugation; albuterol 4'-O-sulfate (metabolite). **Elimination:** Ipratropiuim: Urine (50% unchanged); $T_{1/2}$=2 hrs. Albuterol: Urine (unchanged); $T_{1/2}$=3.9 hrs.

NURSING CONSIDERATIONS

Assessment: Assess for known history of hypersensitivity to soya lecithin or related food products (eg, soybeans, peanuts). Assess for concomitant diseases (eg, narrow-angle glaucoma, prostatic hyperplasia, convulsive disorders, hyperthyroidism, DM, hepatic/renal insufficiency, CVD), and possible drug interactions.

Monitoring: Monitor for hypersensitivity reactions, parodoxical brochospasm, CV effects such as flattening of the T wave, prolongation of the QT interval, and ST segment depression, unexpected development of severe acute asthmatic crisis and hypoxia.

Patient Counseling: Advise to avoid spraying into eyes, not to exceed recommended dose, and to shake canister vigorously for at least 10 seconds before use.

Administration: Inhalation route. 1) Insert metal canister into end of mouthpiece. 2) Remove orange dust cap and shake and test spray into air 3 times. 3) Shake canister for 10 seconds. 4) Inhale and exhale through mouth and at the same time spray product into mouth. 5) Hold breath for 10 seconds and remove mouth piece. 6) Wait for 2 min before next spray. 7) Replace cap and keep mouthpiece clean. 8) Discard after 200 sprays. **Storage:** 25°C (77°F); excursions permitted to 15-30°C (59-86°F). Keep out of reach of children.

COMBIVIR — RX

zidovudine - lamivudine (GlaxoSmithKline)

Zidovudine has been associated with hematologic toxicity (eg, granulocytopenia, severe anemia), especially with advanced HIV disease, and symptomatic myopathy reported with prolonged use. Lactic acidosis and severe, fatal hepatomegaly with steatosis reported with nucleoside analogues. Severe acute exacerbations of hepatitis B reported in patients coinfected with hepatitis B virus and HIV who discontinued lamivudine (a component of Combivir); monitor hepatic function closely after discontinuation.

THERAPEUTIC CLASS: Nucleoside analog combination

INDICATIONS: Treatment of HIV infection in combination with other antiretrovirals.

DOSAGE: *Adults:* 1 tab bid. Do not give if CrCl ≤50mL/min or with dose-limiting adverse events.
Pediatrics: ≥12 yrs: 1 tab bid. Do not give if CrCl ≤50mL/min or with dose-limiting adverse events.

HOW SUPPLIED: Tab: (Lamivudine-Zidovudine) 150mg-300mg

WARNINGS/PRECAUTIONS: Caution with granulocyte count <1000cells/mm^3 or Hgb <9.5g/dL; monitor blood counts frequently with advanced HIV and periodically with asymptomatic or early HIV. Hepatic decompensation occurred when used with interferon alfa w/ or w/o ribavirin. Avoid with CrCl ≤50mL/min, and hepatic impairment. Myopathy, myositis may occur. Post-treatment exacerbation of hepatitis reported. Lamivudine-resistant hepatitis B virus reported. Caution in elderly. Possible redistribution or accumulation of body fat. Immune reconstitution syndrome reported.

ADVERSE REACTIONS: Headache, malaise, fatigue, fever, chills, nausea, diarrhea, anorexia, abdominal pain/cramps, neuropathy, insomnia, dizziness, neutropenia, musculoskeletal pain, myalgia, rash, cough, aplastic anemia, gynecomastia, oral mucosal pigmentation.

INTERACTIONS: Ganciclovir, interferon-α, other bone marrow suppressives and cytotoxic agents may increase the hematologic toxicity of zidovudine. Increased lamivudine exposure with trimethoprim 160mg/sulfamethoxazole 800mg. Avoid with zalcitabine, stavudine, doxorubicin, ribavirin, zidovudine, lamivudine, and fixed-dose combinations of abacavir, lamivudine, and zidovudine.

PREGNANCY: Category C, not for use in nursing.

MECHANISM OF ACTION: Nucleoside analogue; inhibits reverse transcriptase via DNA chain termination.

PHARMACOKINETICS: Absorption: Lamivudine: Rapid. Absolute bioavailabilty (86%). Zidovudine: Rapid. Absolute bioavialiabilty (64%). **Distribution:** Lamivudine: V_d=1.3L/kg; plasma protein binding (<36%). Zidovudine: V_d=1.6L/kg; plasma protein binding (<38%). **Metabolism:** Lamivudine: Trans-sulfoxide (metabolite). Zidovudine: Hepatic. 3'azido-3'-deoxy-5'-*O*-β-D-glucopyranurosylthymidine (metabolite). **Elimination:** Lamivudine: Urine (70%, unchanged), $T_{1/2}$=5-7 hrs. Zidovudine: Urine (14-74%); $T_{1/2}$=0.5-3 hrs.

NURSING CONSIDERATIONS

Assessment: Assess for bone marrow supression, lactic acidosis and hepatomegaly with steatosis, myopathy and myositis, impaired renal/hepatic function, other drug interactions, HIV and HBV co-infection.

Monitoring: Monitor CBC, platelet counts, renal/liver function, and amylase level. Monitor signs/symptoms that suggest pancreatitis, lactic acidosis, or hepatotoxicity including hepatomegaly with steatosis, peripheral neuropathy, myopathy and myositis, exacerbations of hepatitis, immune reconstitution syndrome, and redistibution/accumulation of body fat.

Patient Counseling: Inform that deterioration of liver disease can occur when drug is discontinued. Advise may be administered with/without food. Educate that redistribution/accumulation of fat may occur. Counsel to seek medical attention if symptoms of lactic acidosis, anemia, infection, or myopathy occur.

Administration: Oral route. **Storage:** 2-30°C (36-86°F).

COMBUNOX — CII

oxycodone HCl - ibuprofen (Forest)

NSAIDs may cause an increased risk of serious cardiovascular thrombotic events, MI, stroke, and serious GI adverse events including bleeding, ulceration, and perforation of the stomach or intestines. Contraindicated for the treatment of perioperative pain in the setting of coronary artery bypass graft (CABG) surgery.

THERAPEUTIC CLASS: Opioid analgesic

INDICATIONS: Short term (<7 days) management of acute, moderate to severe pain.

DOSAGE: *Adults:* 1 tab/dose. Do not exceed 4 tabs/day and 7 days.

HOW SUPPLIED: Tab: (Oxycodone-Ibuprofen) 5mg-400mg

CONTRAINDICATIONS: Significant respiratory depression, acute or severe bronchial asthma, hypercarbia, paralytic ileus, or in patients who have experienced asthma, urticaria, allergic-type reactions after taking ASA or NSAIDs. Treatment of perioperative pain in the setting of CABG surgery.

WARNINGS/PRECAUTIONS: May cause drug dependence and tolerance; potential for abuse. Risk of dose-related respiratory depression. May cause severe hypotension. Can lead to HTN or worsening of pre-existing HTN. Fluid retention and edema reported. Capacity to elevate CSF pressure may be exaggerated with head injury, other intracranial lesions or pre-existing increase in ICP. May obscure diagnosis or clinical course with head injuries or acute abdominal conditions. Risk of GI ulceration, bleeding, and perforation. Risk of anaphylactoid reactions. NSAIDs can cause exfoliative dermatitis, Stevens-Johnson syndrome, and toxic epidermal necrolysis (TEN). Caution with severe hepatic impairment, pulmonary or renal dysfunction, hypothyroidism, Addison's disease, acute alcoholism, convulsive disorders, CNS depression or coma, delirium tremens, kyphoscoliosis associated with respiratory depression, toxic psychosis, prostatic hypertrophy, urethral stricture, biliary tract disease, anemia, pre-existing asthma, elderly or debilitated, aseptic meningitis.

ADVERSE REACTIONS: NV, somnolence, dizziness, asthenia, fever, headache, vasodilation, constipation.

INTERACTIONS: (Oxycodone) Respiratory depression, hypotension and profound sedation with other CNS depressants (eg, narcotics, tranquilizers, sedatives, anesthetics, phenothiazines, alcohol). Concurrent use with anticholinergics may produce paralytic ileus. Mixed agonist/antagonist analgesics may reduce the analgesic effect and/or cause withdrawal. Do not use with or within 14 days of discontinuing MAOIs. May enhance skeletal muscle relaxant effects and increase respiratory depression. (Ibuprofen) May diminish antihypertensive effect of ACEIs. Use caution with anticoagulants, such as warfarin. May enhance methotrexate toxicity. May decrease natriuretic effect of furosemide and thiazides. Avoid with ASA. May decrease lithium clearance; monitor for toxicity.

PREGNANCY: Category C, caution in nursing.

MECHANISM OF ACTION: Oxycodone: Opioid analgesic; not established. Suspected to be related to binding to opiate receptors in the CNS. Also may produce sedation and respiratory depression. Ibuprofen: Nonsteroidal anti-inflammatory agent; not established. Possesses analgesic and antipyretic activity. Inhibits cyclooxygenase activity and prostaglandin synthesis, and is a peripherally acting analgesic.

PHARMACOKINETICS: Absorption: Oxycodone: Rapid; C_{max}=9.8-11.7ng/mL; T_{max}=1.3-2.1 hrs. Ibuprofen: Rapid; C_{max}=18.5-34.3mcg/mL; T_{max}=1.6-3.1 hrs. **Distribution:** Oxycodone: Plasma protein binding (45%). Ibuprofen: Plasma protein binding (99%). **Metabolism:** Oxycodone: Liver via CYP2D6 (N-demethylation, O-demethylation, 6-ketoreduction, glucuronidation); oxymorphone (active metabolite). Ibuprofen: Undergoes interconversion in plasma from R- to S-isomer: (+)-2-4'-(2-hydroxy-2-methyl-propyl) phenyl propionic acid, (+)-2-4'-(carboxypropyl) phenylpropionic acid (primary metabolites). **Elimination:** Oxycodone: Urine (4% unchanged); $T_{1/2}$=3.1-3.7 hrs. Ibuprofen: Urine (≤0.2% unchanged); $T_{1/2}$=1.8-2.6 hrs.

NURSING CONSIDERATIONS

Assessment: Assess for respiratory depression, acute or severe bronchial asthma, hypercarbia, paralytic ileus, hypersensitivity to ASA (eg, asthma, urticaria), HTN, fluid retention, heart failure, circulatory shock, previous history of ulcer disease or GI bleeding, presence of head injury, intracranial lesions, pre-existing increase in ICP, acute abdominal conditions, renal dysfunction, liver dysfunction, biliary tract disease, acute pancreatitis, hypothyroidism, Addison's disease, acute alcoholism, convulsive disorders, CNS depression or coma, delirium tremens, toxic psychosis, prostatic hypertrophy, urethral stricture, nursing/pregnancy status, and possible drug interactions. Obtain baseline BP.

Monitoring: Monitor for signs/symptoms of cardiovascular thrombotic effects, HTN, GI effects (eg, ulceration, bleeding, perforation), abuse and dependence, respiratory depression, hypotension, anaphylactoid reactions, renal papillary necrosis, skin reactions (eg, exfoliative dermatitis, Stevens-Johnson syndrome), hematological effects (eg, anemia), liver dysfunction, and aseptic meningitis. Monitor Hgb and Hct in patients previously treated with NSAIDs and currently exhibiting signs/symptoms of anemia. Perform periodic monitoring of BP. For patients on long-term therapy, perform periodic monitoring of CBC and chemistry profile.

Patient Counseling: Inform that drug may impair mental/physical abilities; use caution when performing dangerous tasks (eg, operating machinery/driving). Advise to avoid using other CNS depressants and alcohol during therapy. Counsel that medication has abuse potential; only take for prescribed duration and dose. Notify physician if develop any serious cardiovascular effects (eg, chest pain, SOB), GI effects (eg, ulcers, bleeding), serious skin reactions (eg, exfoliative dermatitis, Stevens-Johnson syndrome), weight gain or edema, hepatotoxicity (eg, nausea, fatigue, jaundice), or anaphylactoid reactions (eg, difficulty breathing, facial swelling).

Administration: Oral route. **Storage:** 25°C (77°F); excursions permitted to 15-30°C (59-86°F).

COMTAN — RX

entacapone (Novartis)

THERAPEUTIC CLASS: COMT inhibitor

INDICATIONS: Adjunct to levodopa/carbidopa for treatment of idiopathic Parkinson's disease if experience signs of end-of-dose "wearing-off."

DOSAGE: *Adults:* 200mg with each levodopa/carbidopa dose. Max: 1600mg/day. Withdraw slowly for discontinuation.

HOW SUPPLIED: Tab: 200mg

WARNINGS/PRECAUTIONS: Hypotension/syncope, diarrhea, hallucinations, dyskinesia, rhabdomyolysis, hyperpyrexia, confusion, and fibrotic complications may occur due to increased dopaminergic activity. Caution with hepatic impairment, biliary obstruction. Avoid rapid withdrawal or abrupt dose reduction. May impair mental and/or motor performance.

ADVERSE REACTIONS: Sweating, back pain, dyskinesia, hyperkinesia, hypokinesia, nausea, diarrhea, abdominal pain, urine discoloration.

INTERACTIONS: Avoid non-selective MAOIs (eg, phenelzine, tranylcypromine). Caution with drugs metabolized by COMT (eg, isoproterenol, epinephrine, norepinephrine, dopamine, dobutamine, α-methyldopa, apomorphine, isoetherine, bitolterol); increased HR, arrhythmias, and BP changes may occur. Additive sedative effects with CNS depressants. Probenecid, cholestyramine, and some antibiotics (eg, erythromycin, rifamipicin, ampicillin, chloramphenicol) may interfere with biliary excretion.

PREGNANCY: Category C, caution with nursing.

MECHANISM OF ACTION: COMT inhibitor; selectively and reversibly inhibits catechol-O-methyltransferase, increasing levodopa levels.

PHARMACOKINETICS: Absorption: (PO) Rapid; absolute bioavailability (35%); C_{max}=1.2mcg/mL; T_{max}=1 hr. **Distribution:** V_d=20L; plasma protein binding (98%). **Metabolism:** Isomerization to *cis*-isomer, and direct glucuronidation. **Elimination:** Urine 10% (0.2% unchanged), feces (90%); $T_{1/2}$=2.4 hrs (levodopa).

NURSING CONSIDERATIONS

Assessment: Assess for dyskinesia, LFTs, hypotension, arrhythmias, biliary obstruction. Note other disease/conditions and drug therapies.

Monitoring: Monitor BP, LFTs, renal function tests, signs/symptoms of rhabdomyolysis, neuroleptic malignant syndrome, melanoma, fibrotic complications, hallucinations.

Patient Counseling: Advise to use caution when engaging in tasks requiring alertness. Instruct to report side effects (eg, postural hypotension, discoloration of urine), and to use caution when discontinuing treatment.

Administration: Oral route. **Storage:** 25°C (77°F); excursions permitted to 15-30°C (59-86°F).

CONCERTA
methylphenidate HCl (McNeil Pediatrics)

CII

C

Caution with previous history of drug dependence or alcoholism. Marked tolerance and psychological dependence with varying degrees of abnormal behavior may occur with chronic abusive use. Careful supervision is necessary during withdrawal from abusive use to avoid severe depression.

THERAPEUTIC CLASS: Sympathomimetic amine

INDICATIONS: Treatment of attention deficit hyperactivity disorder (ADHD) in patients ≥6 yrs.

DOSAGE: *Adults:* Methylphenidate-Naive or Receiving Other Stimulant: Initial: 18mg qam with food. Titrate: Adjust dose at weekly intervals. Previous Methylphenidate Use: Initial: 18mg qam if previous dose 10-15mg/day; 36mg qam if previous dose 20-30mg/day; 54mg qam if previous dose 30-45mg/day. Initial conversion should not exceed 54mg/day. Titrate: Adjust dose at weekly intervals. Max: 72mg/day. Reduce dose or discontinue if paradoxical aggravation of symptoms occurs. Discontinue if no improvement after appropriate dosage adjustments over 1 month. Swallow whole with liquids. Do not crush, chew, or divide.
Pediatrics: ≥6 yrs: Methylphenidate-Naive or Receiving Other Stimulant: Initial: 18mg qam with food. Titrate: Adjust dose at weekly intervals. Max: 6-12 yrs: 54mg/day; 13-17 yrs: 72mg/day not to exceed 2mg/kg/day. Previous Methylphenidate Use: Initial: 18mg qam if previous dose 10-15mg/day; 36mg qam if previous dose 20-30mg/day; 54mg qam if previous dose 30-45mg/day. Initial conversion should not exceed 54mg/day. Titrate: Adjust dose at weekly intervals. Max: 72mg/day. Reduce dose or discontinue if paradoxical aggravation of symptoms occurs. Discontinue if no improvement after appropriate dosage adjustments over 1 month. Swallow whole with liquids. Do not crush, chew, or divide.

HOW SUPPLIED: Tab, Extended-Release: 18mg, 27mg, 36mg, 54mg

CONTRAINDICATIONS: Marked anxiety, tension, and agitation; glaucoma; motor tics or family history or diagnosis of Tourette's syndrome, during or within 14 days of MAOI use.

WARNINGS/PRECAUTIONS: Monitor growth during treatment in children. Not for severe depression or fatigue. Difficulties with accommodation and blurring of vision reported. May exacerbate symptoms of behavior disturbance and thought disorder in psychotic patients. Avoid with severe GI narrowing (eg, esophageal motility disorders, small bowel inflammatory disease, short-gut syndrome). May lower seizure threshold, especially in known EEG abnormalities. Caution with HTN, conditions affected by BP or HR elevation, history of drug abuse or alcoholism. Monitor during withdrawal from abusive use. Visual disturbances may occur (rare). Monitor CBC, differential, and platelets with prolonged use. Caution when using stimulants to treat patients with comorbid bipolar disorder because of concern for possible induction of mixed/manic episode in such patients. Stimulants at usual dose can cause treatment emergent psychotic or manic symptoms (eg, hallucinations, delusional thinking, mania) in children and adolescents without prior history of psychotic illness. Aggressive behavior or hostility reported in clinical trials and postmarketing experience of some medications indicated for the treatment of ADHD. Avoid with known structural cardiac abnormalities or other serious cardiac problems.

ADVERSE REACTIONS: Loss of appetite, headache, dry mouth, nausea, insomnia, tics, anxiety, dizziness, weight reduction, irritability, upper abdominal pain, hyperhidrosis, tachycardia, and palpitations.

INTERACTIONS: Avoid MAOIs. Potentiates anticoagulants, anticonvulsants (eg, phenobarbital, phenytoin, primidone), TCAs, and SSRIs. Caution with α_2-agonists (eg, clonidine) and pressor agents.

C

PREGNANCY: Category C, caution in nursing.

MECHANISM OF ACTION: Sympathomimetic amine; blocks reuptake of norepinephrine and dopamine into presynaptic neuron and increases release of these monoamines into extraneuronal space.

PHARMACOKINETICS: Absorption: (PO) Readily absorbed; T_{max}=6-10 hrs. **Metabolism:** De-esterification; α-phenyl-piperidine acetic acid (metabolite). **Elimination:** Urine (90%); $T_{1/2}$=3.5 hrs.

NURSING CONSIDERATIONS

Assessment: Assess for agitation, glaucoma, tics, family history of Tourette's syndrome, cardiovascular conditions (HTN, angina pectoris, cardiac arrhythmias, heart failure, recent MI), hyperthyroidism or thyrotoxicosis, bipolar illness, history of drug dependence or alcoholism, and severe GI narrowing (eg, esophageal motility disorders, small bowel inflammatory disease, and short-gut syndrome).

Monitoring: Monitor for cardiac abnormalities, exacerbations of behavior disturbances and thought disorder, bipolar illness, aggression, seizures, and visual disturbances. Monitor periodic CBC, differential and platelet count, LFTs, and height and weight in children.

Patient Counseling: Inform about risks of therapy, appropriate use, and drug abuse/dependence. Counsel to swallow tablet whole, do not crush or chew; take last dose before 6 pm to avoid insomnia.

Administration: Oral route. **Storage:** 25°C (77°F); excursions permitted to 15-30°C (59-86°F). Protect from humidity.

COPAXONE RX

glatiramer acetate (Teva Neuroscience)

THERAPEUTIC CLASS: Immunomodulatory agent

INDICATIONS: To reduce the frequency of relapses with relapsing-remitting multiple sclerosis.

DOSAGE: *Adults:* Usual: 20mg SQ qd.

HOW SUPPLIED: Inj: 20mg/mL

CONTRAINDICATIONS: Hypersensitivity to mannitol.

WARNINGS/PRECAUTIONS: Do not administer IV. May interfere with normal functioning of immune system. Rotate sites; do not use any site more than once a week. Administer first injection under professional supervision.

ADVERSE REACTIONS: Flushing, chest pain, palpitations, anxiety, dyspnea, constriction of throat, pruritus, rash, asthenia, back pain, infection, flu, nausea, arthralgia, injection site reactions.

PREGNANCY: Category B, caution in nursing.

MECHANISM OF ACTION: Immunomodulatory agent; not fully established. Thought to act by modifying immune processes that are currently responsible for the pathogenesis of MS.

NURSING CONSIDERATIONS

Assessment: Assess for drug hypersensitivity.

Monitoring: Monitor for immediate post-injection reactions (eg, flushing, chest pain, palpitations, anxiety, dyspnea, constriction of throat, urticaria).

Patient Counseling: Educate on self-injection techniques. Advise not to change dosing schedule or stop drug without medical consultation. Inform about adverse reactions. Notify if pregnant/nursing or planning to become pregnant.

Administration: SQ route. **Storage:** 2-8°C (36-46°F); 15-30°C (59-86°F) for up to 1 week. Use immediately after reconstituting.

COPEGUS

RX

ribavirin (Roche Labs)

Not for monotherapy treatment of chronic hepatitis C. Primary toxicity is hemolytic anemia. Avoid with significant or unstable cardiac disease. Contraindicated in pregnancy and male partners of pregnant women. Use 2 forms of contraception during therapy and for 6 months after discontinuation.

THERAPEUTIC CLASS: Nucleoside analogue

INDICATIONS: Treatment of chronic hepatitis C, in combination with Pegasys, in adults with compensated liver disease not previously treated with interferon alpha. Patients in whom efficacy was demonstrated included patients with compensated liver disease and histological evidence of cirrhosis (Child-Pugh class A) and patients with HIV disease that is clinically stable.

DOSAGE: *Adults:* HCV: Give bid in divided doses. Treat for 24-48 weeks with Pegasys 180mcg. Genotypes 1 and 4: <75kg: 1000mg/day for 48 weeks. ≥75kg: 1200mg/day for 48 weeks. Genotypes 2 and 3: 800mg/day for 24 weeks. HCV/HIV: 800mg qd. Treat for 48 weeks with Pegasys 180mcg. Dose Modifications: Reduce to 600mg/day if Hgb <10g/dL with no cardiac history, or if Hgb decreases by ≥2g/dL during a 4-week period with stable cardiac disease. D/C if Hgb <8.5g/dL with no cardiac history or if Hgb <12g/dL after 4 weeks of dose reduction with stable cardiac disease. After dose modification, may restart at 600mg/day, then may increase to 800mg/day. CrCl <50mL/min: Avoid use.

HOW SUPPLIED: Tab: 200mg

CONTRAINDICATIONS: Pregnancy, male partners of pregnant women, hemoglobinopathies (eg, thalassemia major, sickle cell anemia). Autoimmune hepatitis, and hepatic decompensation (Child-Pugh score greater than 6, Class B and C) in cirrhotic CHC patients, and in cirrhotic CHC patients co-infected with HIV before or during treatment when used in combination with Pegasys.

WARNINGS/PRECAUTIONS: D/C with hepatic decompensation, confirmed pancreatitis, and hypersensitivity reaction. Severe depression, suicidal ideation, hemolytic anemia, bone marrow suppression, autoimmune and infectious disorders, pancreatitis, and diabetes reported. Pulmonary symptoms reported; monitor closely with evidence of pulmonary infiltrates or pulmonary function impairment and d/c if appropriate. Assess for underlying cardiac disease (obtain EKG); fatal and nonfatal MI reported with anemia. Caution with cardiac disease, d/c if cardiovascular status deteriorates. Hemolytic anemia reported; monitor Hgb or Hct initially then at week 2 and 4 (or more if needed) of therapy. Suspend therapy if symptoms of pancreatitis arise. Avoid if CrCl <50mL/min. Obtain negative pregnancy test prior to initiation then monthly, and for 6 months post-therapy.

ADVERSE REACTIONS: Injection-site reaction, fatigue/asthenia, pyrexia, rigors, NV, neutropenia, anorexia, myalgia, headache, irritability/anxiety/nervousness, insomnia, alopecia.

INTERACTIONS: Avoid concomitant use with didanosine and zidovudine. Hepatic decompensation can occur with concomitant use of NRTIs and Pegasys/Copegus.

PREGNANCY: Category X, not for use in nursing.

MECHANISM OF ACTION: Nucleotide analogue; unknown.

PHARMACOKINETICS: Absorption: C_{max}=2748ng/mL; T_{max}=2 hrs; AUC=25361ng•hr/mL. **Elimination:** $T_{1/2}$=120-170 hrs.

NURSING CONSIDERATIONS

Assessment: Assess for known hypersensitivity, history of hemoglobinopathies (eg, thalassemia major or sickle cell anemia), cardiac disease, hepatic/renal dysfunction, DM, pulmonary dysfunction/disease, pancreatitis, pregnancy status (including female partners of male patients), and possible drug interactions. Assess baseline LFTs, renal function, CBC, ECG, thyroid function, Hgb, Hct, and CD4 count in HIV/AIDS.

C

Monitoring: Pregnancy testing should occur at initiation, monthly during therapy, and for 6 months after therapy (including female partners of male patients). Monitor for significant events including severe depression, suicidal ideation, hemolytic anemia, suppresion of bone marrow function, autoimmune/infection disorder, pulmonary dysfunction, pancreatitis and DM. Monitor Hct and Hgb (before treatment, Weeks 2 and 4, and more if needed). Appropriately monitor ECG with pre-existing cardiac disease for deterioration of cardiac function. Monitor for signs/symptoms of pancreatitis, hepatic decompensation, hypersensitivity reaction, anemia, hyperglycemia, and pulmonary dysfunction (including exacerbation of sarcoidosis).

Patient Counseling: Inform of pregnancy risks; use 2 forms of effective contraception. Seek medical attention if symptoms of pancreatitis, hypersensitivity reaction, anemia, hepatic decompensation, deterioration of cardiac function, hyperglycemia, and pulmonary dysfunction (dyspnea) occur. Caution against operating machinery/driving if symptoms of dizziness, confusion, somnolence, or fatigue occur. Counsel to take with food and to keep well-hydrated.

Administration: Oral route. **Storage:** 25°C (77°F); excursions permitted between 15-30°C (59-86°F).

CORDARONE — RX

amiodarone HCl (Wyeth)

THERAPEUTIC CLASS: Class III antiarrhythmic

INDICATIONS: Treatment of documented, life-threatening recurrent ventricular fibrillation and recurrent hemodynamically unstable ventricular tachycardia.

DOSAGE: *Adults:* Give LD in hospital. LD: 800-1600mg/day in divided doses for 1-3 weeks. After control is achieved, then 600-800mg/day for 1 month. Maint: 400mg/day; up to 600mg/day if needed. Use lowest effective dose. Take with meals. Elderly: Start at low end of dosing range.

HOW SUPPLIED: Tab: 200mg* *scored

CONTRAINDICATIONS: Severe sinus-node dysfunction causing marked sinus bradycardia; 2nd- and 3rd-degree AV block; when episodes of bradycardia have caused syncope (except when used with a pacemaker); cardiogenic shock. Hypersensitivity to iodine.

WARNINGS/PRECAUTIONS: Only for life-threatening arrhythmias due to its substantial toxicity (eg, pulmonary toxicity including pulmonary alveolar hemorrhage, hepatic injury, arrhythmia exacerbation). Hospitalize when giving LD. May cause a clinical syndrome of cough and progressive dyspnea. D/C if LFTs are 3x ULN or if elevated baseline doubles; monitor LFTs regularly. Optic neuropathy, optic neuritis reported. Fetal harm in pregnancy. May develop reversible corneal micro deposits (eg, visual halos, blurred vision), photosensitivity, peripheral neuropathy (rare). May decrease T_3 levels, increase thyroxine levels, increase inactive reverse T_3 levels and can cause hypo- or hyperthyroidism. Hyperthyroidism may result in thyrotoxicosis and/or the possibility of arrhythmia breakthrough or aggravation. ARDS reported with surgery. Correct K^+ or magnesium deficiency before therapy. Caution in elderly.

ADVERSE REACTIONS: Pulmonary toxicity (eg, inflammation, fibrosis), arrhythmia exacerbation, hepatic injury, malaise, fatigue, tremor, poor coordination, paresthesia, nausea, vomiting, constipation, anorexia, ophthalmic abnormalities, photosensitivity, akinesia, bradykinesia.

INTERACTIONS: Risk of interactions after discontinuation due to its long half-life. May increase sensitivity to myocardial depressant and conduction effects of halogenated inhalation anesthetics. Elevates cyclosporine plasma levels. D/C or reduce digoxin dose by 50%. D/C or decrease warfarin dose by 1/3-1/2. Avoid grapefruit juice. Caution with β-blockers, CCBs, lidocaine, methotrexate. May increase levels of quinidine, procainamide, phenytoin, flecainide. Initiate added antiarrhythmic drug at lower than usual dose. D/C or decrease quinidine dose by 1/3-1/2. D/C or decrease procainamide dose by 1/3. Caution with loratadine, trazadone, disopyramide, fluoroquinolones, macrolides, azoles;

QT prolongation reported. Decreased levels with cholestyramine, rifampin, phenytoin, St. John's wort. Rhabdomyolysis/myopathy reported with HMG-CoA reductase inhibitors (simvastatin and atorvastatin). Ineffective inhibition of platelet aggregation with clopidogrel. Fentanyl may cause hypotension, bradycardia, and decreased cardiac output. Increased levels with protease inhibitors; monitor for toxicity. Increased levels of CYP1A2, CYP2C9, CYP2D6, CYP3A4 substrates reported. Interactions reported with CYP3A4 inducers. CYP2C8 and CYP3A4 inhibitors may increase amiodarone levels.

PREGNANCY: Category D, not for use in nursing.

MECHANISM OF ACTION: Class III antiarrhythmic; prolongs myocardial cell-action potential duration and refractory period, and causes noncompetitive α- and β-adrenergic inhibition.

PHARMACOKINETICS: Absorption: Slow and variable; T_{max}=3-7 hrs. **Distribution:** V_d=60L/kg; plasma protein binding (96%); found in breast milk. **Metabolism:** CYP3A4, 2C8; desethylamiodarone (major metabolite). **Elimination:** Bile, urine; $T_{1/2}$=58 days, 36 days (metabolite).

NURSING CONSIDERATIONS

Assessment: Assess for life threatening arrhythmias, ventricular arrhythmia, optic neuropathy or optic neuritis, hepatic impairment, pregnancy/nursing status, thyroid function, pre-exsisting pulmonary disease, recent MI, and possible drug interactions. Correct hypokalemia and hypomagnesemia prior to initiation.

Monitoring: Monitor for pulmonary toxicities (eg, hypersensitivity pneumonitis, or interstitial/alveolar pneumonitis) manifested by cough, progressive dyspnea, and fatalities, accompanied by functional, radiological, gallium-scan, and pathological data. Perform history, physical exam, and chest X-ray every 3-6 months. Monitor for sinus bradycardia, sinus arrest, and heart block. Monitor induced hyperthyroidism/thyrotoxicosis, hepatic failure, optic neuritis/neuropathy, corneal microdeposits, vision loss, fetal harm, peripheral neuropathy, photosensitivity, LFTs, T_4, T_3 and reverse T_3. Perioperative monitoring for hypotension and ARDS recommended.

Patient Counseling: Advise to notify physician if pregnant/nursing. Inform about benefits/risks, including possibility of vision impairment, thyroid abnormalities, peripheral neuropathy, and photosensitivity. Report any adverse reactions to physician. Counsel to take as directed. Do not take with grapefruit juice. Avoid prolonged sunlight exposure. Advise that corneal refractive laser surgery is contraindicated with concurrent use.

Administration: Oral route. **Storage:** 20-25°C (68-77°F). Protect from light.

CORDARONE IV

RX

amiodarone HCl (Wyeth)

THERAPEUTIC CLASS: Class III antiarrhythmic

INDICATIONS: Initiation of treatment and prophylaxis of frequently recurring ventricular fibrillation and hemodynamically unstable ventricular tachycardia refractory to other therapies.

DOSAGE: *Adults:* LD: 150mg over 1st 10 min (15mg/min), then 360mg over next 6 hrs (1mg/min), then 540mg over remaining 18 hrs (0.5mg/min). Maint: 0.5mg/min for 2-3 weeks. Breakthrough Ventricular Tachycardia/Ventricular Fibrillation: 150mg supplement IV over 10 min. Increase rate to achieve suppression. Elderly: Start at low end of dosing range. Administer infusions >2 hrs in a glass or polyolefin bottle containing D_5W. Amiodarone leaches out plasticizers (eg, DEHP from IV tubing) especially at higher infusion concentrations, and lower flow rates.

HOW SUPPLIED: Inj: 50mg/mL [3mL]

CONTRAINDICATIONS: Cardiogenic shock, marked sinus bradycardia, 2nd- or 3rd-degree AV block (unless a functioning pacemaker is available). Hypersensitivity to iodine.

C

WARNINGS/PRECAUTIONS: Bradycardia and AV block reported. Hypotension reported; do not exceed initial rate of infusion. Correct hypokalemia or hypomagnesemia before therapy to prevent exaggeration of QT_c prolongation. Congenital goiter/hypothyroidism, hyperthyroidism, postoperative ARDS reported with oral therapy. Hyperthyroidism may result in thyrotoxicosis and/or the possibility of arrhythmia breakthrough or aggravation. Elevations of hepatic enzymes reported. May worsen or precipitate a new arrhythmia; monitor for QT_c prolongation. Adult respiratory distress syndrome (ARDS) reported. Pulmonary toxicity with long-term use. Contains benzyl alcohol. Caution in elderly.

ADVERSE REACTIONS: Hypotension, fever, bradycardia, CHF, heart arrest, ventricular tachycardia, abnormal LFTs, nausea.

INTERACTIONS: Risk of interactions may persist after discontinuation due to long half-life. May increase PT with warfarin. May elevate plasma levels of cyclosporine, digoxin, quinidine, procainamide, phenytoin, disopyramide, HMG-CoA reductase inhibitors. May increase QT prolongation with disopyramide. Reduce flecainide dose to maintain therapeutic plasma levels. Cholestyramine may decrease levels and half-life. Decreased levels with phenytoin. Risk of bradycardia, hypotension with β-blockers, fentanyl. Increased risk of AV block with verapamil or diltiazem and hypotension with CCBs. May increase sensitivity to myocardial depressant and conduction defects of halogenated inhalational anesthetics. CYP3A4 inhibitors (eg, protease inhibitors, cimetidine, grapefruite juice) may increase levels. QT prolongation and torsades de pointes with H_1 antagonists (eg, loratadine) and antidepressants (eg, trazodone) reported. Concomitant use with clopidogrel may result in ineffective inhibition of platelet aggregation. CYP3A4 inducers (eg, rifampin, St. John's wort) may decrease levels. Concomitant use with fentanyl may cause hypotension, bradycardia, and decreased cardiac output. QT_c prolongation reported with fluoroquinolones, macrolides, and azoles. Concomitant administration with propranolol, diltiazem, and verapamil may result in hemodynamic and electrophysiologic interactions.

PREGNANCY: Category D, not for use in nursing.

MECHANISM OF ACTION: Class III antiarrhythmic; blocks sodium, calcium, and potassium channels; exerts noncompetitive antisympathetic action, and negative chronotropic and dromotropic effects; lengthens cardiac action potential, decreases cardiac workload and myocardial oxygen consumption.

PHARMACOKINETICS: Absorption: C_{max}=5-41mg/L. **Distribution:** Plasma protein binding (>96%). **Metabolism:** CYP3A4, 2C8; N-desethylamiodarone (major active metabolite). **Elimination:** Urine, bile; $T_{1/2}$=20-47 days.

NURSING CONSIDERATIONS

Assessment: Assess for cardiogenic shock, marked sinus bradycardia, 2nd- or 3rd-degree AV block, functioning pacemaker, thyroid dysfunction, pulmonary disorders, pregnancy/nursing status, and possible drug interaction. Prior to initiation, hypokalemia and hypomagnesemia should be corrected with special attention to electrolyte and acid base balance in patients experiencing severe/prolonged diarrhea or concomitantly receiving diuretics.

Monitoring: Monitor for hypotension, bradycardia, AV block, acute/centrolobular confluent hepatocelluar necrosis, hepatic coma, acute renal failure, worsening of existing or precipitation of new arrhythmia, ARDS, pulmonary fibrosis, optic neuropathy/neuritis, visual impairment, thyrotoxicosis, and congenital goiter/hypothyroidism in infants. Monitor LFTs and thyroid function. Perioperative monitoring for myocardial depression recommended.

Patient Counseling: Advise that corneal refractive laser surgery is contraindicated with concurrent use. Inform about benefits/risks and report any adverse reactions promptly.

Administration: IV route. **Storage:** 15-25°C (59-77°F). Protect from light.

Cordran

RX

flurandrenolide (Watson)

OTHER BRAND NAMES: Cordran SP (Watson)

THERAPEUTIC CLASS: Corticosteroid

INDICATIONS: Treatment of corticosteroid-responsive dermatoses.

DOSAGE: *Adults:* (Cre, Lot) Apply qd-qid depending on severity. For moist lesions, apply cream bid-tid. Apply lotion bid-tid. (Tape) Clean and dry skin. Shave or clip hair. Apply tape q12-24h.
Pediatrics: (Cre, Lot) Apply qd-qid depending on severity. For moist lesions, apply cream bid-tid. Apply lotion bid-tid. (Tape) Clean and dry skin. Shave or clip hair. Apply tape q12-24h.

HOW SUPPLIED: Cre (SP): 0.05% [15g, 30g, 60g]; Lot: 0.05% [15mL, 60mL]; Tape: $4mcg/cm^2$

CONTRAINDICATIONS: (Tape) Not for lesions exuding serum or in intertriginous areas.

WARNINGS/PRECAUTIONS: Systemic absorption may produce reversible HPA axis suppression, manifestations of Cushing's syndrome, hyperglycemia, and glucosuria. Application of more potent steroids, use on large surfaces, prolonged use, or occlusive dressings may augment systemic absorption. Evaluate periodically for HPA suppression if large dose applied to large area or with occlusive dressings. Pediatrics are more susceptible to toxicity. D/C if irritation develops. May use occlusive dressing for psoriasis or recalcitrant conditions.

ADVERSE REACTIONS: Burning, itching, irritation, dryness, folliculitis, hypertrichosis, acneiform eruptions, hypopigmentation, dermatitis. Occlusive dressing may cause skin maceration, secondary infection, skin atrophy, miliaria.

PREGNANCY: Category C, caution in nursing.

MECHANISM OF ACTION: Corticosteroid; possesses anti-inflammatory, antipruritic, and vasoconstrictive properties. Suspected to stabilize cellular and lysosomal membranes, thereby preventing release of proteolytic enzymes, and consequently reducing inflammation.

PHARMACOKINETICS: Absorption: Extent of percutaneous absorption depends on integrity of skin, vehicle, and use of occlusive dressings. **Distribution:** Plasma protein binding (variable). **Metabolism:** Liver. **Elimination:** Kidney (major), bile.

NURSING CONSIDERATIONS

Assessment: Assess pregnancy/nursing status.

Monitoring: Monitor for signs/symptoms of reversible hypothalamic-pituitary-adrenal (HPA) axis suppression, Cushing's syndrome, hyperglycemia, glucosuria, skin irritation, and for development of dermatological infections (eg, bacterial, fungal). In patients on large doses or using occlusive dressings, perform periodic testing for HPA-axis suppression by using urinary free cortisol, and ACTH stimulation tests. Following d/c of therapy, monitor for signs/symptoms of steroid withdrawal. In pediatric patients, monitor for systemic toxicity, HPA-axis suppression, Cushing's syndrome, and intracranial HTN.

Patient Counseling: Inform to use exactly as directed, externally. Avoid contact with eyes. Counsel not to bandage or wrap treated skin unless directed by physician. (Tape) Cleanse treatment area and allow it to dry for 1 hour prior to application. Report adverse reactions. Instruct parents of pediatric patients to avoid using tight-fitting diapers or plastic pants on children receiving treatment in diaper area.

Administration: Topical. Application of Tape: 1) Clean treatment area so that scales, crusts, dried exudates, and previously used ointments or creams are removed. Use germicidal soap or cleanser to prevent odor from developing under tape. Shave or clip hair in treatment area. If shower or tub bath is to be taken, complete before application of tape. Dry skin prior to application.

2) Apply tape, keeping skin smooth; press tape into place. **Storage:** 15-30°C (59-86°F).

C

Coreg CR RX

carvedilol (GlaxoSmithKline)

OTHER BRAND NAMES: Coreg (GlaxoSmithKline)

THERAPEUTIC CLASS: Alpha$_1$/Beta-blocker

INDICATIONS: Treatment of mild to severe heart failure of ischemic or cardiomyopathic origin; left ventricular dysfunction (LVD) following MI; essential hypertension.

DOSAGE: *Adults:* Individualize dose. Take with food. Monitor dose increases. Take extended-release capsules in am and swallow whole. CHF: Tab: Initial: 3.125mg bid for 2 weeks. Titrate: May double dose every 2 weeks as tolerated. Max: 50mg bid if >85kg. Reduce dose if HR <55 beats/min. Cap, Extended-Release: Initial: 10mg qd for 2 weeks. Titrate: May double dose every 2 weeks as tolerated. Max: 80mg/day. Reduce dose if HR <55 beats/min. HTN: Tab: Initial: 6.25mg bid for 7-14 days. Titrate: May double dose at 7-14 day intervals. Max: 50mg/day. Cap, Extended-Release: Initial: 20mg qd for 7-14 days. Titrate: May double dose every 7-14 days as tolerated. Max: 80mg/day. LVD Post-MI: Tab: Initial: 6.25mg bid for 3-10 days. Titrate: May double dose every 3-10 days to target of 25mg bid. May begin with 3.125mg bid and slow up-titration rate if clinically indicated. Cap, Extended-Release: Initial: 20mg qd for 3-10 days. Titrate: May double dose every 3-10 days to target of 80mg qd.

HOW SUPPLIED: Tab: 3.125mg, 6.25mg, 12.5mg, 25mg; Cap, Extended-Release: 10mg, 20mg, 40mg, 80mg

CONTRAINDICATIONS: Bronchial asthma or related bronchospastic conditions, 2nd- or 3rd-degree AV block, sick sinus syndrome, severe bradycardia (without permanent pacemaker), cardiogenic shock, decompensated heart failure requiring IV inotropic therapy, severe hepatic impairment.

WARNINGS/PRECAUTIONS: Avoid abrupt discontinuation; taper over 1-2 weeks. Hepatic injury reported; d/c and do not restart if develops hepatic injury. Bradycardia reported; if pulse rate drops below 55 beats/min; reduce dose. Hypotension and syncope reported, most commonly during up-titration period; avoid driving or hazardous tasks during initiation period. May mask hypoglycemia and hyperthyroidism. May potentiate insulin-induced hypoglycemia and delay recovery of serum glucose levels. Decrease dose if pulse <55 beats/min. Monitor renal function during up-titration with low BP (SBP <100mmHg), ischemic heart disease, diffuse vascular disease, and/or renal insufficiency. Worsening heart failure or fluid retention may occur with up-titration. Caution in pheochromocytoma, peripheral vascular disease, major surgery with anesthesia, Prinzmetal's variant angina, and bronchospastic disease. Effectiveness of carvedilol in patients <18 years of age has not been established.

ADVERSE REACTIONS: Bradycardia, fatigue, edema, hypotension, dizziness, headache, diarrhea, NV, hyperglycemia, weight increase, dyspnea, anemia, increased cough, arthralgia.

INTERACTIONS: CYP2D6 inhibitors (eg, quinidine, fluoxetine, paroxetine, and propafenone) may increase levels. Monitor for hypotension and bradycardia with catecholamine-depleting agents (eg, reserpine, MAOIs). Clonidine may potentiate BP and HR lowering effects. Rifampin may reduce plasma levels. Cimetidine may increase AUC. Monitor ECG and BP with CCBs (eg, verapamil, diltiazem). Monitor with insulin, oral hypoglycemics, cyclosporine, and digoxin. Caution with anesthetic agents that may depress myocardial function (eg, cyclopropane, trichloroethylene). Alcohol may affect release properties of extended-release caps; separate administration by ≥2 hrs. Digitalis glycosides and β-blockers slow atrioventricular conduction and decrease heart rate. Concomitant use can increase the risk of bradycardia. Amiodarone may increase plasma levels resulting in further slowing of the HR or cardiac conduction.

PREGNANCY: Category C, not for use in nursing.

MECHANISM OF ACTION: Nonselective β-adrenergic and α_1 blocker.

PHARMACOKINETICS: Absorption: Rapid; absolute bioavailability (25-35%). Cap: T_{max}=5 hrs. **Distribution:** Plasma protein binding (>98%); V_d=115L. **Metabolism**: Oxidation and glucuronidation; CYP2D6, 2C9 (primary); CYP3A4, 2C19, 1A2, 2E1 (minor). **Elimination**: Urine (<2% unchanged); $T_{1/2}$=7-10 hrs.

NURSING CONSIDERATIONS

Assessment: Assess for bronchial asthma, bronchospastic disease, AV block, sick sinus syndrome, severe bradycardia, cardiogenic shock, CHF, Prinzmetal's angina, CAD, DM, pheochromocytoma, peripheral vascular disease, hyperthyroidism, possible drug interactions, hepatic/renal impairment. Obtain baseline blood glucose levels, LFTs, and renal function.

Monitoring: Monitor blood glucose during initiation/dosage adjustments, and upon d/c of therapy; LFTs and renal function periodically. Monitor for signs/symptoms of cardiac failure, hypo/hyperglycemia, thyrotoxicosis, withdrawal symptoms, precipitation or aggravation of arterial insufficiency, hypotension, and hypersensitivity reactions.

Patient Counseling: Inform not to d/c or interrupt therapy without consulting physician and to avoid situations where injury could result should syncope occur. Contact lens wearers may experience decreased lacrimation; may mask signs of thyrotoxicosis or hypoglycemia. Caution drug may impair physical/mental abilities. Instruct to take with food; do not crush or chew. Advise to seek medical attention if symptoms of heart failure (difficulty breathing), hypotension (syncope), withdrawal symptoms (angina), or hypersensitivity reactions occur.

Administration: Oral route. **Storage:** Tab: 25°C (77°F); excursions to 15-30°C (59-86°F). Cap, Extended-Release: Below 30°C (86°F); protect from moisture.

CORMAX — RX

clobetasol propionate (Watson)

OTHER BRAND NAMES: Cormax Scalp (Watson)

THERAPEUTIC CLASS: Corticosteroid

INDICATIONS: Corticosteroid-responsive dermatoses.

DOSAGE: *Adults:* Apply bid. Limit treatment to 2 consecutive weeks. Max: 50g/week or 50mL/week.
Pediatrics: ≥12 yrs: (Cre, Sol) Apply bid. Limit treatment to 2 consecutive weeks. Max: 50g/week or 50mL/week.

HOW SUPPLIED: Cre: 0.05% [15g, 30g, 45g]; Sol (Scalp): 0.05% [25mL, 50mL]

CONTRAINDICATIONS: Primary infections of the scalp with solution.

WARNINGS/PRECAUTIONS: Not for treatment of rosacea or perioral dermatitis. May produce reversible HPA axis suppression, manifestations of Cushing's syndrome, hyperglycemia, and glucosuria. Reassess diagnosis if no improvement after 2 weeks. D/C if irritation occurs. Pediatrics may be more susceptible to systemic toxicity. Use appropriate antifungal or antibacterial agent with dermatological infections. Avoid occlusive dressings.

ADVERSE REACTIONS: Burning, stinging, pruritus, skin atrophy, cracking/fissuring of skin, irritation, (sol) tingling, (sol) folliculitis.

PREGNANCY: Category C, caution in nursing.

MECHANISM OF ACTION: Corticosteroid; possesses anti-inflammatory, antipruritic, and vasoconstrictive properties. Suspected to stabilize cellular and lysosomal membranes, thereby preventing release of proteolytic enzymes, and consequently reducing inflammation.

PHARMACOKINETICS: Absorption: Extent of percutaneous absorption depends on integrity of skin, vehicle, and use of occlusive dressings. **Distribution:** Plasma protein binding (variable). **Metabolism:** Liver. **Elimination:** Kidney (major), bile.

C

NURSING CONSIDERATIONS

Assessment: Assess for known hypersensitivity to other corticosteroids. Assess that medication is not for treatment of rosacea, or perioral dermatitis. Assess use in treatment of acne, and pregnancy/nursing status.

Monitoring: Monitor for signs/symptoms of HPA-axis suppression, Cushing's syndrome, hyperglycemia, and glucosuria. In patients taking large doses, perform periodic monitoring for HPA-axis suppression by using the urinary free cortisol and ACTH stimulation tests. Monitor for signs of skin irritation and infection (eg, bacterial, fungal), and treat accordingly. In patients using the medication on the face, groin, or underarm areas, monitor for atrophic changes. In pediatric patients, monitor for signs of HPA-axis suppression (eg, linear growth retardation, delayed weight gain, low plasma cortisol levels, and absence of response to ACTH), Cushing's syndrome, and intracranial HTN.

Patient Counseling: Instruct to use as directed and avoid contact with eyes. Counsel not to bandage, cover, or wrap treated skin areas. Inform to report any signs of local adverse reactions.

Administration: Topical. Treatment must be limited to 2 consecutive weeks, and should not exceed >50g per week. Not to be used with occlusive dressings. **Storage**: 15-30°C (59-86°F).

CORTEF — RX

hydrocortisone (Pharmacia & Upjohn)

THERAPEUTIC CLASS: Corticosteroid

INDICATIONS: Steroid-responsive disorders.

DOSAGE: *Adults:* Initial: 20-240mg/day depending on disease. Adjust until a satisfactory response. Maint: Decrease in small amounts to lowest effective dose. Acute Exacerbations of Multiple Sclerosis: (Tab) Initial: 200mg/day of prednisolone for 1 week, then 80mg every other day for 1 month (20mg hydrocortisone=5mg prednisolone).
Pediatrics: Initial: 20-240mg/day depending on disease. Adjust until a satisfactory response. Maint: After favorable response, decrease in small amounts to lowest effective dose. Acute Exacerbations of Multiple Sclerosis: Initial: (Tab) 200mg/day of prednisolone for 1 week, then 80mg every other day for 1 month (20mg hydrocortisone=5mg prednisolone).

HOW SUPPLIED: Sus: (Hydrocortisone Cypionate) 10mg/5mL [120mL]; Tab: (Hydrocortisone) 5mg, 10mg, 20mg

CONTRAINDICATIONS: Systemic fungal infections.

WARNINGS/PRECAUTIONS: May need to increase dose before, during, and after stressful situations. May mask signs of infections. Avoid abrupt withdrawal. Prolonged use may produce glaucoma, optic nerve damage, secondary ocular infections. Increases BP, salt/water retention, potassium excretion. More severe/fatal course of infections reported with chickenpox, measles. Caution with TB, hypothyroidism, cirrhosis, ocular herpes simplex, HTN, diverticulitis, fresh intestinal anastomosis, ulcerative colitis, osteoporosis, myasthenia gravis, renal insufficiency, peptic ulcer disease. Growth and development of children on prolonged therapy should be monitored. Monitor for psychic disturbances. Kaposi's sarcoma reported.

ADVERSE REACTIONS: Fluid and electrolyte disturbances, HTN, osteoporosis, muscle weakness, cushingoid state, menstrual irregularities, nervousness, insomnia, impaired wound healing, DM, ulcerative esophagitis, excessive sweating, increased ICP, carbohydrate intolerance, glaucoma, cataracts.

INTERACTIONS: Reduced efficacy and increased clearance with hepatic enzyme inducers (eg, phenobarbital, phenytoin, and rifampin). Decreased clearance with ketoconazole and troleandomycin. Increases clearance of chronic high-dose ASA; caution with hypoprothrombinemia. Effects on oral anticoagulants are variable; monitor PT. Increased insulin and oral hypoglycemic requirements in DM. Avoid live vaccines with immunosuppressive doses. Possible decreased vaccine response with killed or inactivated vaccines with immunosuppressive doses.

PREGNANCY: Safety in pregnancy and nursing not known.

MECHANISM OF ACTION: Anti-inflammatory glucocorticoid; causes profound and varied metabolic effects and modifies the body's immune responses to diverse stimuli.

NURSING CONSIDERATIONS

Assessment: Assess systemic fungal infections, current infections, active TB, vaccination history, ulcerative colitis, diverticulitis, peptic ulcer, renal/hepatic insufficiency, septic arthritis/unstable joint, HTN, osteoporosis, myasthenia gravis, thyroid status, psychotic tendencies, and possible drug interactions.

Monitoring: Monitor for adrenocortical insufficiency, occurrence of infections, psychic derangement, cataracts, acute myopathy, Kaposi's sarcoma, fluid retention, and measurement of serum electrolytes, TSH, LFTs, IOP, and BP. Monitor urinalysis, blood sugar, weight, chest X-ray, and upper GI X-ray (if ulcer history) regularly during prolonged therapy.

Patient Counseling: Inform that susceptibility to infections may increase. Avoid exposure to chickenpox and measles; report immediately if exposed. Do not d/c abruptly or without medical supervision. Dietary salt restriction and supplementation of potassium is advised.

Administration: Oral route. **Storage:** 20-25°C (68-77°F).

Cortisporin-TC Otic — RX

hydrocortisone acetate - thonzonium bromide - neomycin sulfate - colistin sulfate (King)

THERAPEUTIC CLASS: Antibacterial/corticosteroid combination

INDICATIONS: Treatment of infections of the external auditory canal, mastoidectomy and fenestration cavities.

DOSAGE: *Adults:* Clean and dry ear canal. Dropper: 5 drops (calibrated dropper) or 4 drops (dropper bottle) tid-qid. Alternate Regimen: Insert cotton wick into ear canal, then saturate cotton. Repeat q4h to keep cotton moist. Replace wick q24h.

Pediatrics: Clean and dry ear canal. Dropper: 4 drops (calibrated dropper) or 3 drops (dropper bottle) tid-qid. Alternate Regimen: Insert cotton wick into ear canal, then saturate cotton. Repeat q4h to keep cotton moist. Replace wick q24h.

HOW SUPPLIED: (Colistin-Hydrocortisone-Neomycin-Thonzonium) Sus: 3mg-10mg-3.3mg-0.5mg/mL [10mL]

CONTRAINDICATIONS: Herpes simplex, vaccinia, and varicella infections.

WARNINGS/PRECAUTIONS: Caution with perforated eardrum, chronic otitis media. Prolonged use may result in secondary infection. Re-evaluate if no improvement after 1 week. D/C after 10 days.

ADVERSE REACTIONS: Cutaneous sensitization.

PREGNANCY: Safety in pregnancy and nursing not known.

MECHANISM OF ACTION: Colistin: Polypeptide antibiotic; penetrates into and disrupts bacterial cell membrane. Neomycin: Aminoglycoside antibiotic; inhibits protein synthesis, disrupting normal cycle of ribosomal function. Hydrocortisone: Corticosteroid hormone; thought to act by regulating rate of protein synthesis and controls inflammation. Thonzonium: Surfactant; promotes tissue contact by dispersion and penetration of the cellular debris and exudate.

NURSING CONSIDERATIONS

Assessment: Assess for hypersensitivity, external auditory canal disorder due to cutaneous viral infection, perforated tympanic membrane, chronic otitis media, stasis dermatitis and pregnancy/nursing status.

Monitoring: Monitor for allergic cross-reactions, cutaneous sensitization as in chronic dermatoses manifested by low-grade reddening with swelling, dry scaling and itching, auditory function, ototoxicity, overgrowth of nonsusceptible organisms and fungi, and lab monitoring of eosinophils and urinary 17-hydroxycorticosteroids.

C

Patient Counseling: Avoid contaminating dropper with material from the ear or any other surface. D/C and contact physician if sensitization or irritation occurs. Do not use in eyes.

Administration: Otic route. Shake well before use. **Storage:** 20-25°C (68-77°F).

CORVERT RX

ibutilide fumarate (Pharmacia & Upjohn)

THERAPEUTIC CLASS: Class III antiarrhythmic

INDICATIONS: For rapid conversion of atrial fibrillation or flutter (A-Fib/Flutter) of recent onset to sinus rhythm.

DOSAGE: *Adults:* ≥60kg: 1mg over 10 min. <60kg: 0.01mg/kg over 10 min. If arrhythmia still present within 10 min after the end of the initial infusion, repeat infusion 10 min after completion of 1st infusion.

HOW SUPPLIED: Inj: 0.1mg/mL

WARNINGS/PRECAUTIONS: Proarrhythmic; can cause potentially fatal arrhythmias. Administer in setting with continuous ECG monitoring and person able to treat acute ventricular arrhythmia. Adequately anticoagulate if A-Fib >2-3 days. Correct hypokalemia and hypomagnesemia before therapy. Caution in elderly.

ADVERSE REACTIONS: Sustained and nonsustained polymorphic ventricular tachycardia, sustained and nonsustained monomorphic ventricular tachycardia, bundle branch and AV block, ventricular and supraventricular extrasystoles, hypotension, bradycardia.

INTERACTIONS: Avoid Class IA (eg, disopyramide, quinidine, procainamide) and other Class III (eg, amiodarone, sotalol) antiarrhythmics with or within 4 hrs postinfusion of ibutilide. Increase proarrhythmia potential with drugs that prolong the QT interval (eg, phenothiazines, TCAs). Supraventricular arrhythmias may mask cardiotoxicity associated with excessive digoxin levels.

PREGNANCY: Category C, not for use in nursing.

MECHANISM OF ACTION: Class III antiarrhythmic agent; prolongs atrial and ventricular action potential duration and refractoriness. Delays repolarization by activation of a slow, inward current, rather than blocking outward potassium currents.

PHARMACOKINETICS: Distribution: V_d=11 L/kg; plasma protein binding (40%). **Metabolism:** Omega-oxidation and β-oxidation; omega-hydroxy metabolite (active). **Elimination:** Urine 82% (7% unchanged) feces (19%); $T_{1/2}$=6 hrs.

NURSING CONSIDERATIONS

Assessment: Assess for arrhythmia, bradycardia, hypokalemia, renal/hepatic impairment, and possible drug interactions.

Monitoring: Monitor for worsening of induction of new ventricular arrhythmia, torsade de pointes (a polymorphic ventricular tachycardia), and HR.

Patient Counseling: Inform about benefits/risks. Report any adverse reactions to physician. Patients with chronic A-Fib of ≥2-3 days duration must be adequately anticoagulated for at least 2 weeks. May cause potentially fatal arrhythmia, particularly sustained polymorphic ventricular tachycardia.

Administration: IV route. **Storage:** 20-25°C (68-77°F).

Cosopt RX

dorzolamide HCl - timolol maleate (Merck)

THERAPEUTIC CLASS: Carbonic anhydrase inhibitor/nonselective beta-blocker

INDICATIONS: Treatment of ocular hypertension and open-angle glaucoma insufficiently responsive to β-blockers.

DOSAGE: *Adults:* 1 drop bid. Space dosing of other ophthalmic drugs by 10 min.
Pediatrics: ≥2 yrs: 1 drop bid. Space dosing of other ophthalmic drugs by 10 min.

HOW SUPPLIED: Sol: (Dorzolamide-Timolol) 2%-0.5% [5mL, 10mL]

CONTRAINDICATIONS: Bronchial asthma, history of bronchial asthma, severe COPD, sinus bradycardia, 2nd- or 3rd-degree AV block, overt cardiac failure, cardiogenic shock.

WARNINGS/PRECAUTIONS: Caution with sulfonamide allergy, cardiac failure, DM, COPD, bronchospastic disease, surgery and hepatic impairment. May mask symptoms of hypoglycemia and thyrotoxicosis. Bacterial keratitis reported with contaminated containers. Avoid in severe renal impairment. D/C if hypersensitivity or ocular reaction occur. Reinsert contact lenses 15 minutes after applying drops.

ADVERSE REACTIONS: Taste perversion, ocular burning, conjunctival hyperemia, blurred vision, superficial punctate keratitis, eye itching.

INTERACTIONS: Avoid oral carbonic anhydrase inhibitors, oral β-blockers, or topical β-blockers due to potential additive effects. Oral/IV calcium antagonists can cause AV-conduction disturbances, left ventricular failure or hypotension. Potentiated systemic β-blockade with concomitant CYP2D6 inhibitors. Reserpine can cause additive effects, hypotension and/or bradycardia. AV conduction time prolonged with digitalis. Quinidine may potentiate β-blockade. Increased risk of hypoglycemia with insulin or oral hypoglycemic agents. Wait 10 minutes before using another ophthalmic drug.

PREGNANCY: Category C, not for use in nursing.

MECHANISM OF ACTION: Dorzolamide: Inhibitor of human carbonic anhydrase II; decreases aqueous humor secretion, presumably by slowing formation of bicarbonate ions with subsequent reduction in Na^+ and fluid transport. Timolol: β_1 and β_2 (non-selective) adrenergic receptor blocking agent; decrease elevated IOP by reducing aqueous humor secretion.

PHARMACOKINETICS: Absorption: Timolol: C_{max}=0.46ng/mL. **Distribution:** Dorzolamide: Plasma protein binding (33%). **Elimination:** Dorzolamide: Urine (unchanged).

NURSING CONSIDERATIONS

Assessment: Assess for history of bronchial asthma, severe COPD, sinus bradycardia, 2nd- or 3rd-degree AV block, overt cardiac failure, and cardiogenic shock. Assess sulfonamide allergy, use when undergoing elective surgery, risk for hypoglycemia with DM, with hyperthyroidism, with acute angle-closure glaucoma, with severe renal impairment (CrCl <30mL/min), with hepatic impairment, in pregnancy/nursing, and for possible drug interactions.

Monitoring: Monitor for signs/symptoms of anaphylaxis, severe respiratory reactions, cardiac reactions, Stevens-Johnson syndrome, toxic epidermal necrolysis, fulminant hepatic necrosis, agranulocytosis, aplastic anemia and other blood system dyscrasias, muscle weakness, choroidal detachment, acute hypoglycemia with DM, occurrence of thyroid storm with thyrotoxicosis and abrupt withdrawal, primary conjunctivitis and lid reactions with chronic therapy, and bacterial keratitis with use of multi-dose containers.

Patient Counseling: Contact physician immediately if any type of cardiac, respiratory, or anaphylactic reactions occur. Advise to d/c and report if ocular reactions (eg, conjunctivitis, lid reactions) occur. Handle solution properly. Do not touch container tip to eye or surrounding structures; may become contaminated. Immediately contact physician concerning use of present multidose container if undergoing ocular surgery or develop a concomitant ocular condition (eg, trauma, infection). Remove contact lenses prior to administration; may be reinserted 15 min after. Inform to administer at least 10 min apart if using other ophthalmic medications.

Administration: Ocular route. 1) Tilt head back and pull lower eyelid down to form pocket between eyelid and eye. 2) Invert bottle and press lightly until single drop is released. **Storage:** 15-30°C (59-86°F). Protect from light.

COUMADIN — RX

warfarin sodium (Bristol-Myers Squibb)

May cause major or fatal bleeding; monitor INR regularly.

OTHER BRAND NAMES: Jantoven (Upsher-Smith)

THERAPEUTIC CLASS: Vitamin K-dependent coagulation factor inhibitor

INDICATIONS: Prophylaxis and treatment of venous thrombosis, PE, and thromboembolic disorders associated with atrial fibrillation and/or cardiac valve replacement. To reduce risk of death, recurrent MI, and thromboembolic events after MI.

DOSAGE: *Adults:* ≥18 yrs: Adjust dose based on PT/INR. Give IV as alternate to PO. Initial: 2-5mg qd. Usual: 2-10mg qd. Venous Thromboembolism (including pulmonary embolism): INR 2-3. Atrial Fibrillation: INR 2-3. Post-MI: Initiate 2-4 weeks post-infarct and maintain INR 2.5-3.5. Mechanical/Bioprosthetic Heart Valve: INR 2-3 for 12 weeks after valve insertion, then INR 2.5-3.5 long term.

HOW SUPPLIED: Inj: (Coumadin) 5mg; Tab: (Coumadin, Jantoven) 1mg*, 2mg*, 2.5mg*, 3mg*, 4mg*, 5mg*, 6mg*, 7.5mg*, 10mg* *scored

CONTRAINDICATIONS: Hemorrhagic tendencies, blood dyscrasias, CNS surgery, ophthalmic or traumatic surgery, inadequate lab facility, threatened abortion, eclampsia, preeclampsia, major regional lumbar block anesthesia, malignant HTN, pregnancy and unsupervised senile, alcoholic or psychotic patients. Bleeding of GI, GU or respiratory tract, aneurysms, pericarditis and pericardial effusion, bacterial endocarditis, cerebrovascular hemorrhage, spinal puncture, procedures with potential for uncontrollable bleeding.

WARNINGS/PRECAUTIONS: Monitor PT/INR; many endogenous and exogenous factors may affect PT/INR. Weigh benefits/risks with severe-moderate hepatic or renal insufficiency, infectious disease, intestinal flora disturbance, lactation, surgery, trauma, severe-moderate HTN, protein C deficiency, polycythemia vera, vasculitis, severe DM, indwelling catheters. D/C if tissue necrosis, systemic cholesterol microembolization ("purple toe syndrome") occurs. Caution with HIT, DVT, elderly. Warfarin resistance, allergic reactions reported.

ADVERSE REACTIONS: Tissue or organ hemorrhage/necrosis, paresthesia, vasculitis, fever, rash, abdominal pain, hepatic disorders, fatigue, headache, alopecia.

INTERACTIONS: Interacts with protein bound drugs, hepatic enzyme inducers and inhibitors. Avoid streptokinase and urokinase. Caution with drugs that may cause hemorrhage (eg, NSAIDs, ASA). Potentiates hypoglycemic, anticonvulsant drugs, and antihyperlipidemic drugs like ezetimibe. See PI for extensive list.

PREGNANCY: Category X, weigh benefits/risks with nursing.

MECHANISM OF ACTION: Vitamin K-dependent coagulation factor inhibitor; interferes with clotting factor synthesis by inhibition of the C1 subunit of the vitamin K epoxide enzyme complex, thereby reducing the regeneration of vitamin K_1 epoxide.

PHARMACOKINETICS: Absorption: (PO) Complete; T_{max}=4 hrs. **Distribution:** V_d=0.14 L/kg; plasma protein binding (99%); found in fetal plasma. **Metabolism:** Hepatic via CYP2C9, 2C19, 2C8, 2C18, 1A2, 3A4. **Elimination:** Urine (major), bile; $T_{1/2}$=1 week.

C

NURSING CONSIDERATIONS

Assessment: Assess pregnancy status, presence of hemorrhagic tendencies or blood dyscrasias, bleeding tendencies associated with active ulceration, overt bleeding (eg, genitourinary, cerebrovascular hemorrhage, pericarditis), senility (psychosis), alcoholism, presence of major regional lumbar block anesthesia, and malignant HTN. Assess use in nursing females, severe to moderate hepatic/renal insufficiencies, presence of infectious diseases, disturbances in the intestinal flora, indwelling catheters, severe to moderate HTN, known or suspected deficiency in protein C-mediated anticoagulant response, presence of polycythemia vera, vasculitis, and severe DM. Assess for drug and drug-disease interactions.

Monitoring: Monitor for signs/symptoms of bleeding, necrosis of the skin and other organs, and systemic atheroemboli or cholesterol microemboli (eg, "purple toe syndrome," livedo reticularis, rash). Periodically monitor INR/PT.

Patient Counseling: Counsel to maintain strict adherence to dosing regimen. Instruct to notify physician of all medications (OTC, herbals) currently taken. Advise not to start or stop other medications before contacting physician. Instruct to avoid any activity or sport that may result in traumatic injury. Inform females about risk during pregnancy. Instruct that regular prothrombin time tests are required. Advise patient to carry ID card stating drug is being taken. Inform that vitamin K in diet may affect medication. Instruct to eat normal, balanced diet; avoid drastic changes in diet such as eating large amounts of leafy green vegetables. Instruct to avoid alcohol consumption, cranberry juice, and cranberry products. Inform to contact physician if dose is missed. Take missed dose as soon as possible, however, do not take two doses in one day. Advise to immediately report unusual bleeding.

Administration: Oral or IV route. IV: Reconstitute with 2.7 mL of sterile Water for Inj to yield 2mg/mL. **Storage:** Tab: 15-30°C (59-86°F). Dispense in tight, light-resistant container. Inj: 15-30°C (59-86°F). Use within 4 hrs after reconstitution. Do not refrigerate.

COVERA-HS — RX

verapamil HCl (G.D. Searle)

THERAPEUTIC CLASS: Calcium channel blocker (nondihydropyridine)

INDICATIONS: Management of hypertension and angina.

DOSAGE: *Adults:* Initial: 180mg qhs. Titrate: May increase to 240mg qhs, then 360mg qhs, then 480mg qhs, if needed. Swallow tab whole. Elderly: Start at the low end of the dosing range.

HOW SUPPLIED: Tab, Extended-Release: 180mg, 240mg

CONTRAINDICATIONS: Severe ventricular dysfunction, hypotension, cardiogenic shock, sick sinus syndrome or 2nd- or 3rd-degree AV block (except with functioning ventricular pacemaker), A-Fib/Flutter with an accessory bypass tract.

WARNINGS/PRECAUTIONS: Avoid with moderate to severe cardiac failure, and ventricular dysfunction if taking a β-blocker. May cause hypotension, AV block, transient bradycardia, PR interval prolongation. Monitor LFTs periodically; hepatocellular injury reported. Give 30% of normal dose with severe hepatic dysfunction. Caution with hypertrophic cardiomyopathy, renal or hepatic dysfunction. Decrease dose with decreased neuromuscular transmission.

ADVERSE REACTIONS: Constipation, dizziness, nausea, hypotension, headache, edema, CHF, pulmonary edema, fatigue, dyspnea, bradycardia, AV block, rash, flushing.

INTERACTIONS: Additive effects on HR, AV conduction, and contractility with β-blockers. Potentiates other antihypertensives. May increase digoxin, carbamazepine, theophylline, cyclosporine, and alcohol levels. Avoid disopyramide within 48 hrs before or 24 hrs after verapamil. Additive negative inotropic effects and AV conduction prolongation with flecainide. Avoid quinidine with hypertrophic cardiomyopathy. Monitor lithium. CYP3A4 inhibitors (eg, erythromycin, ritonavir) and grapefruit juice may increase levels. CYP3A4 inducers (eg, rifampin, phenobarbital) may decrease levels. Increased bleeding time with ASA. May potentiate neuromuscular blockers; both agents may need dose reduction. Caution with inhalation anesthetics.

PREGNANCY: Category C, not for use in nursing.

MECHANISM OF ACTION: Calcium channel blocker; inhibits transmembrane influx of calcium ions into arterial smooth muscle and conductile and contractile myocardial cells.

PHARMACOKINETICS: Absorption: T_{max}=11 hrs. R-Enantiomer: Bioavailability (33-65%). S-Enantiomer: Bioavailability (13-34%). Oral administration of variable doses resulted in different parameters. **Distribution:** R: Plasma protein binding (94%). S: Plasma protein binding (88%). **Metabolism:** Liver; norverapamil (active metabolite). **Elimination:** Urine 70% (3-4% unchanged).

NURSING CONSIDERATIONS

Assessment: Assess for left ventricular dysfunction, hypotension, sick sinus syndrome, AV block, atrial flutter/fibrillation with accessory bypass tract (eg, WPW), possible drug interactions, hypertrophic cardiomyopathy, severe GI narrowing, hepatic/renal impairment.

Monitoring: Periodically monitor LFTs and renal function; monitor abnormal PR interval prolongation for toxicity. Monitor for signs/symptoms of hepatotoxicity, renal dysfunction, CV events (hypotension), and hypersensitivity reactions.

Patient Counseling: Instruct to swallow tablet whole; do not chew, break, or crush. Advise to seek medical attention if symptoms of hepatotoxicity (malaise, fever, RUQ pain), CV events (hypotension), or hypersensitivity reactions occur.

Administration: Oral route. **Storage:** 20-25°C (68-77°F); keep in a light-resistant container.

COZAAR — RX

losartan potassium (Merck)

Can cause death/injury to developing fetus during 2nd and 3rd trimesters. Stop therapy if pregnancy detected.

THERAPEUTIC CLASS: Angiotensin II receptor antagonist

INDICATIONS: Treatment of hypertension (HTN), alone or with other antihypertensives. To reduce the risk of stroke in patients with HTN and left ventricular hypertrophy (LVH), but evidence shows this does not apply to black patients. Diabetic nephropathy with an elevated serum creatinine and proteinuria (urinary albumin to creatinine ratio ≥300mg/g) in patients with type 2 diabetes and HTN.

DOSAGE: *Adults:* HTN: Initial: 50mg qd. Usual: 25-100mg/day given qd-bid. Intravascular Volume Depletion/Hepatic Impairment: Initial: 25mg qd. HTN with LVH: Initial: 50mg qd. Add hydrochlorothiazide (HCTZ) 12.5mg qd and/or increase losartan to 100mg qd, followed by an increase in HCTZ to 25mg qd based on BP response. Nephropathy: Initial: 50 mg qd. Titrate: Increase to 100mg qd based on BP response.
Pediatrics: ≥6 yrs: HTN: Initial: 0.7mg/kg qd (up to 50mg/day). Max: 1.4mg/kg/day (100mg/day).

HOW SUPPLIED: Tab: 25mg, 50mg, 100mg

WARNINGS/PRECAUTIONS: Can cause fetal injury/death. Correct volume or salt depletion before therapy. Changes in renal function may occur; caution with renal artery stenosis, severe CHF. Angioedema reported. Consider dose adjustment with hepatic dysfunction.

ADVERSE REACTIONS: Dizziness, cough, upper respiratory infection, diarrhea.

INTERACTIONS: K^+-sparing diuretics (eg, spironolactone, triamterene, amiloride), K^+ supplements, or K^+-containing salt substitutes may increase serum K^+. May reduce excretion of lithium; monitor lithium levels. Combination with NSAIDs, including COX-2 inhibitors, may lead to further deterioration of renal function and diminish antihypertensive effect.

PREGNANCY: Category C (1st trimester) and D (2nd and 3rd trimesters), not for use in nursing.

MECHANISM OF ACTION: Angiotensin II receptor antagonist; blocks vasoconstrictor and aldosterone-secreting effects of angiontensin II by selectively blocking binding of angiotensin II to AT_1 receptor.

PHARMACOKINETICS: Absorption: Bioavailability (33%). **Adults:** C_{max}=224ng/mL, T_{max}=0.9 hrs, AUC=442ng•h/mL. (Metabolite) C_{max}=212ng/mL, T_{max}=3.5 hrs, AUC= 1685 ng•h/mL. **Pediatrics:** C_{max}=141ng/mL, T_{max}=2 hrs, AUC=368ng•h/mL. (Metabolite) C_{max}=222ng/mL, T_{max}=4.1 hrs, AUC=1866ng•h/mL. **Distribution:** V_d=34L, 12L (metabolite). **Metabolism:** Liver via CYP2C9, 3A4; carboxylic acid (active metabolite). **Elimination:** Urine (4% unchanged; 6% metabolite). **Adults:** $T_{1/2}$=2.1 hrs, 7.4 hrs (metabolite). **Pediatrics:** $T_{1/2}$=2.3 hrs, 5.6 hrs (metabolite).

NURSING CONSIDERATIONS

Assessment: Assess pregnancy status, volume depletion, possible drug interactions, DM, hepatic/renal impairment.

Monitoring: Monitor serum electrolytes and renal function periodically. Monitor for signs/symptoms of electrolyte imbalance, hypotension, hypersensitivity reactions, renal/hepatic dysfunction.

Patient Counseling: Inform of pregnancy risks. Advise to seek medical attention if symptoms of electrolyte imbalance, hypotension, or hypersensitivity reactions (angioedema) occur.

Administration: Oral route. Refer to PI for preparation of suspension. **Storage:** 25°C (77°F); excursions permitted to 15-30°C (59-86°F). Keep container tightly closed. Protect from light.

CRESTOR RX

rosuvastatin calcium (AstraZeneca)

THERAPEUTIC CLASS: HMG-CoA reductase inhibitor

INDICATIONS: Adjunct to diet in primary hyperlipidemia and mixed dyslipidemia to reduce elevated total-C, LDL-C, ApoB, non-HDL-C, and triglyceride (TG) levels and to increase HDL-C. Adjunct to diet for the treatment of hypertriglyceridemia and/or primary dysbetalipoproteinemia (Type III hyperlipoproteinemia). Adjunct to other lipid-lowering treatments (eg, LDL apheresis) or alone if such treatments are unavailable, to reduce LDL-C, total-C, and ApoB in homozygous familial hypercholesterolemia. Adjunct to diet to slow the progression of atherosclerosis as part of a treatment strategy to lower total-C and LDL-C to target levels.

DOSAGE: *Adults:* Hypercholesterolemia/Mixed Dyslipidemia/Hypertriglyceridemia/Primary Dysbetalipoproteinemia/Slowing Progression of Atherosclerosis: Initial: 10mg qd. (20mg qd with LDL-C >190mg/dL). Titrate: Adjust dose if needed at 2-4 week intervals. Range: 5-40mg qd. Homozygous Familial Hypercholesterolemia: 20mg qd. Max: 40mg qd. Asian Patients: 5mg qd. Concomitant Cyclosporine: Max: 5mg qd. Concomitant Lopinavir/Ritonavir: Max 10mg qd. Concomitant Gemfibrozil: Max: 10mg qd. Severe Renal Impairment: CrCl <30mL/min/1.73m^2 (not on hemodialysis): Initial: 5mg qd. Max: 10mg qd.

HOW SUPPLIED: Tab: 5mg, 10mg, 20mg, 40mg

CONTRAINDICATIONS: Active liver disease, unexplained persistent elevations of hepatic transaminase levels, pregnancy, nursing mothers.

WARNINGS/PRECAUTIONS: Increased risk of myopathy with other lipid-lowering therapies, cyclosporine, or lopinavir/ritonavir. Rare cases of rhabdomyolysis with acute renal failure secondary to myoglobinuria reported. Monitor LFTs prior to therapy, at 12 weeks or with dose elevation, and periodically thereafter. Reduce dose or d/c if AST/ALT ≥3x ULN persists. Caution with heavy alcohol use, history of hepatic disease, renal impairment, hypothyroidism, elderly. D/C if markedly elevated CPK levels occur, if myopathy is diagnosed or suspected, or if predisposition to renal failure secondary to rhabdomyolysis. Approximately two-fold elevation in median exposure in Asian subjects. Persistent elevations in hepatic transaminase occurred. Monitor liver enzymes.

ADVERSE REACTIONS: Headache, myalgia, abdominal pain, asthenia, constipation, nausea, rhabdomyolysis with myoglobinuria, acute renal failure, myopathy, liver enzyme abnormalities.

INTERACTIONS: Increased levels and risk of myopathy with cyclosporine, fibrates (eg, gemfibrozil), niacin, and lopinavir/ritonavir. Caution with drugs that decrease levels or activity of endogenous steroid hormones (eg, ketoconazole, spironolactone, cimetidine). Increases levels of oral contraceptives (norgestrel, ethinyl estradiol). Increases INR with warfarin. Space antacid dosing by 2 hrs.

PREGNANCY: Category X, not for use in nursing.

MECHANISM OF ACTION: HMG-CoA reductase inhibitor; increases the number of hepatic LDL receptors on the cell surface and inhibits hepatic synthesis of VLDL, which reduces the total number of VLDL and LDL particles.

PHARMACOKINETICS: Absorption: Absolute bioavailability (20%). T_{max}=3-5 hrs. **Distribution:** V_d=134L, plasma protein binding (88%). **Metabolism:** CYP2C9; N-desmethyl rosuvastatin (active metabolite). **Elimination:** Feces (90%); $T_{1/2}$=19 hrs.

NURSING CONSIDERATIONS

Assessment: Assess for active liver disease, unexplained persistent LFTs and lipid-level abnormalities, pregnancy/nursing status, renal impairment, hypothyroidism, alcohol intake, and possible drug interactions. Perform LFTs prior to therapy, at 12 weeks and periodically thereafter.

Monitoring: Periodically monitor LFTs, creatinine kinase, hematuria and proteinuria (via urine analysis), signs of myopathy/rhabdomyolysis (eg, muscle pain, tenderness, or weakness, acute renal failure and endocrine effects).

Patient Counseling: Notify physician if pregnant/nursing or planning to become pregnant. Inform about potential risks/benefits. Report promptly any signs of myopathy (eg, unexplained muscle pain, tenderness or weakness, fever or malaise). Counsel to take at least 2 hrs after antacids. May take without regards to food.

Administration: Oral route. **Storage:** 20-25°C (68-77°F).

CRIXIVAN — RX

indinavir sulfate (Merck)

THERAPEUTIC CLASS: Protease inhibitor

INDICATIONS: Treatment of HIV infection in combination with other antiretrovirals.

DOSAGE: *Adults:* 800mg q8h on empty stomach. Hepatic Insufficiency or Concomitant Delavirdine, Itraconazole, Ketoconazole: 600mg every 8 hrs. Concomitant Efavirenz or Rifabutin: 1g every 8 hrs (reduce rifabutin dose by 1/2). Maintain adequate hydration (1.5L fluid/24 hrs).

HOW SUPPLIED: Cap: 100mg, 200mg, 333mg, 400mg

CONTRAINDICATIONS: Concomitant pimozide, cisapride, amiodarone, triazolam, midazolam, alprazolam, ergot derivatives.

WARNINGS/PRECAUTIONS: D/C or suspend during acute nephrolithiasis/urolithiasis. Tubulointerstitial nephritis seen with asymptomatic severe leukocyturia; monitor frequently with urinalyses. Consider discontinuation with severe leukocyturia. Immune reconstitution syndrome, hemolytic anemia, hyperglycemia, hyperbilirubinemia, hepatitis and liver failure reported. Spontaneous bleeding may occur with hemophilia A and B. Monitor hepatic function. Maintain adequate hydration. Possible redistribution or accumulation of body fat. Caution in elderly.

ADVERSE REACTIONS: Nephrolithiasis, GI discomfort, headache, fatigue, insomnia, hyperbilirubinemia, hepatitis, hyperglycemia, hemolytic anemia, renal failure, hematuria, nausea.

INTERACTIONS: See Contraindications. Increased risk of myopathy with HMG-CoA reductase inhibitors metabolized by CYP3A4. Increased levels with delavirdine, itraconazole, ketoconazole; reduce dose. Decreased levels with efavirenz, rifabutin, St. John's wort, rifampin. Avoid coadministration with atazanavir, lovastatin, simvastatin, or rosuvastatin. May increase rifabutin and CCB levels. Administer didanosine 1 hr apart on empty stomach. Caution with phenobarbital, phenytoin, carbamazepine, dexamethasone, atorvastatin. Substantially increases sildenafil plasma levels; increased risk of sildenafil adverse events (eg, hypotension, visual changes, priapism). Decreases metabolism of alprazolam; increased risk of alprazolam adverse effects (eg, sedation, respiratory depression)

PREGNANCY: Category C, not for use in nursing.

MECHANISM OF ACTION: HIV protease inhibitor; prevents cleavage of viral polyproteins, forming immature, non-infectious viral particles.

PHARMACOKINETICS: Absorption: Rapid; C_{max}=12617nM; T_{max}=0.8 hrs; AUC=30691nM•hr. **Distribution:** Plasma protein binding (60%). **Metabolism:** Hepatic via CYP3A4. **Elimination:** Urine (<20%), feces (83%); $T_{1/2}$=1.8 hrs.

NURSING CONSIDERATIONS

Assessment: Assess for asymptomatic severe leukocyturia, hemophilia, hepatic/renal dysfunction, anemia, DM, pregnancy/nursing status, and possible drug interactions.

Monitoring: Monitor for possible indirect hyperbilirubinemia, increase in serum transaminase, triglycerides, cholesterol, immune reconstitution syndrome, nephrolithiasis/urolithiasis, hemolytic anemia, hepatitis, fat redistribution, exacerbation of DM (hyperglycemia). Monitor urinalysis frequently for patients with severe leukocyturia and for possible tubulointerstitial nephritis with medullary calcification and cortical atrophy.

Patient Counseling: Seek medical attention if symptoms of infection, nephrolithiasis/urolithiasis (flank pain, with or without hematuria), anemia, hepatitis, fat redistribution/accumulation and hyperglycemia occur. Advise not to modify or d/c treatment without consulting physician. If a dose is missed, take the next dose at the regularly scheduled time; do not double dose. Take without food (1 hr before or 2 hrs after a meal) and keep well hydrated.

Administration: Oral route. **Storage:** 15-30°C (59-86°F). Store in a tightly closed container; protect from moisture.

CROMOLYN SODIUM INHALATION RX

cromolyn sodium (Various)

OTHER BRAND NAMES: Intal (King)

THERAPEUTIC CLASS: Mast cell stabilizer

INDICATIONS: Prophylactic treatment of bronchial asthma and of acute bronchoconstriction due to exercise, environmental agents, and known antigens.

DOSAGE: *Adults:* Asthma: (Inhaler) Usual/Max: 2 inh qid. (Sol) 20mg nebulized qid. Acute Bonchospasm Prevention: (Inhaler) Usual: 2 inh 10-60 min before exposure to precipitant. (Sol) 20mg nebulized shortly before exposure to precipitant. Renal/Hepatic Dysfunction: Decrease inhaler dose.
Pediatrics: Asthma: (Inhaler) ≥5 yrs: Usual/Max: 2 inh qid. (Sol) ≥2 yrs: 20mg nebulized qid. Acute Bronchospasm Prevention: (Inhaler) ≥5 yrs: Usual: 2 inh 10-60 min before exposure to precipitant. (Sol) ≥2 yrs: 20mg nebulized shortly before exposure to precipitant. Renal/Hepatic Dysfunction: Decrease inhaler dose.

HOW SUPPLIED: MDI: (Intal) 0.8mg/inh [8.1g, 14.2g]; Sol: (Cromolyn, neb) 10mg/mL [2mL, 10^s 60^s]

WARNINGS/PRECAUTIONS: Not for treatment of acute attack. Severe anaphylaxis may occur. D/C if eosinophilic pneumonia or pulmonary infiltrates with eosinophilia develop. May experience cough and/or bronchospasm. Caution with inhaler in CAD or history of cardiac arrhythmias. Decrease dose or d/c with renal/hepatic dysfunction.

ADVERSE REACTIONS: Throat irritation/dryness, bad taste, cough, nausea, bronchospasm, sneezing, wheezing.

INTERACTIONS: Avoid with isoproterenol during pregnancy.

PREGNANCY: Category B, caution in nursing.

MECHANISM OF ACTION: Mast cell stabilizer; inhibits sensitized mast cell degranulation, release of mediators from mast cells, and both immediate and non-immediate bronchoconstrictive reactions to inhaled antigen.

PHARMACOKINETICS: Absorption: 8% absorbed. **Elimination:** Urine, bile.

NURSING CONSIDERATIONS

Assessment: Assess for drug hypersensitivity to cromolyn sodium, impaired renal/hepatic function, respiratory function, CVD.

Monitoring: Monitor LFTs, renal function, hypersensitivity reactions, eosinophilic pneumonia, CVD. Maintain close supervision of concomitant therapy to avoid exacerbation of asthma.

Patient Counseling: Advise that effect of therapy depends on administration at regular intervals. Take as directed. Take at least 10-15 min before exposure to precipitating factor.

Administration: Oral inhalation. 1) Ensure canister properly inserted into inhaler unit. 2) Take cover off and shake inhaler. 3) Hold inhaler and breathe out while depressing top of metal canister with index finger. 4) Remove inhaler from mouth and hold breath for several seconds before next inhalation. 5) Replace cover when done. **Storage:** Store between 15-30°C (59-86°F). Do not puncture, incinerate, or place near sources of heat. Exposure to temps above 120°F may cause bursting.

CUBICIN — RX

daptomycin (Cubist)

THERAPEUTIC CLASS: Cyclic lipopeptide

INDICATIONS: Susceptible complicated skin and skin structure infections (cSSSI). *Staphylococcus aureus* bloodstream infections (bacteremia).

DOSAGE: *Adults:* ≥18 yrs: Administer as IV infusion over 30 min. cSSSI: 4mg/kg q24h for 7-14 days. *S.aureus* Bacteremia: 6mg/kg q24h for minimum 2-6 weeks. Renal impairment: CrCl <30mL/min, HD, or CAPD: 4mg/kg (cSSSI) or 6mg/kg (*S.aureus* bacteremia) once q48h.

HOW SUPPLIED: Inj: 500mg

WARNINGS/PRECAUTIONS: *Clostridium difficile*-associated diarrhea reported. D/C if CDAD confirmed. Monitor CPK levels weekly; d/c with unexplained signs and symptoms of myopathy and CPK elevation >1000 U/L (~5x ULN), or with CPK levels ≥10x ULN. Persisting or relapsing *S.aureus* infection or poor clinical response should have repeat blood cultures.

ADVERSE REACTIONS: Constipation, NV, injection site reactions, headache, diarrhea, insomnia, rash, abnormal LFTs, superinfection, pharyngolaryngeal pain, pain in extremity and pulmonary eosinophilia.

INTERACTIONS: Caution with tobramycin; may affect levels. Monitor PT/INR for first several days with warfarin. Consider temporarily suspending statins. HMG-CoA reductase inhibitors may cause myopathy; consider suspending these agents with concomitant therapy.

PREGNANCY: Category B, caution in nursing.

MECHANISM OF ACTION: Cyclic lipopeptide; binds to bacterial membranes and causes a rapid depolarization of membrane potential, causing inhibition of protein, DNA, RNA synthesis, which results in bacterial cell death.

PHARMACOKINETICS: Absorption: (6mg/kg) C_{max}=93.9µg/mL, AUC=632µg•h/mL. **Distribution:** Plasma protein binding (90-93%); V_d=0.1L/kg. **Elimination:** Urine (78%), feces (5.7%); $T_{1/2}$=7.7-8.3 hrs.

NURSING CONSIDERATIONS

Assessment: Assess renal fuction, LFTs, CBC and possible drug interactions with HMG-CoA reductase inhibitors.

Monitoring: Monitor renal function tests, CPK, fluid electrolyte balance, CBC, PT/INR evaluation, CDAD, neuropathy, myopathy.

Patient Counseling: Counsel to immediately report development of watery/bloody diarrhea (with/without stomach cramps) and fever, (may occur as late as 2 months after therapy).

Administration: Reconstituted solution should be further diluted with 0.9% NaCl injection to be administered by IV infusion over a period of 30 min. **Storage:** 2-8°C (36-46°F). Avoid excessive heat.

CUTIVATE — RX

fluticasone propionate (PharmaDerm)

THERAPEUTIC CLASS: Corticosteroid

INDICATIONS: (Cre, Oint) Relief of the inflammatory and pruritic manifestations of corticosteroid-responsive dermatoses. Cre may be used with caution in pediatric patients ≥3 months of age. (Lot) Relief of the inflammatory and pruritic manifestations of atopic dermatitis in patients ≥1 yr of age.

DOSAGE: *Adults:* Atopic Dermatitis: (Cre) Apply qd-bid. (Lot) Apply qd. Other Dermatoses: (Cre) Apply bid. (Oint) Apply bid. (Cre, Lot, Oint) Avoid occlusive dressings and re-evaluate if no improvement after 2 weeks.
Pediatrics: ≥3 months: Atopic Dermatitis: (Cre) Apply qd-bid. Other Dermatoses: (Cre) Apply bid. Avoid in diaper area. ≥1 yr: Atopic Dermatitis: (Lot) Apply qd. (Cre, Lot): Avoid occlusive dressings and re-evaluate if no improvement after 2 weeks. Oint not approved in peds.

HOW SUPPLIED: Cre: 0.05% [30g, 60g]; Lot: 0.05% [120mL]; Oint: 0.005% [30g, 60g]

WARNINGS/PRECAUTIONS: Caution with cre in peds. May produce reversible HPA axis suppression, manifestations of Cushing's syndrome, hyperglycemia, and glucosuria. D/C if irritation occurs. Use appropriate antifungal or antibacterial agent with dermatological infections. Peds may be more susceptible to systemic toxicity. Caution when applied to large surface areas. Avoid with pre-existing skin atrophy. Not for use in rosacea or perioral dermatitis.

ADVERSE REACTIONS: (Cre) Pruritus, dryness, numbness of fingers, burning. (Oint) Pruritus, burning, hypertrichosis, increased erythema, hives, irritation, light-headedness. (Lot) Burning, stinging, dryness, common cold, upper respiratory tract infection, cough, fever.

PREGNANCY: Category C, caution in nursing.

MECHANISM OF ACTION: Corticosteroid; not fully established. Possesses anti-inflammatory, antipruritic, and vasoconstrictive properties. Suspected to act by the induction of phospholipase A_2 inhibitory proteins, called lipocortins. Lipocortins control biosynthesis of potent mediators of inflammation (eg, prostaglandins, leukotrienes) by inhibiting release of common precursor, arachidonic acid. Arachidonic acid is released from membrane phospholipids by phospholipase A_2.

PHARMACOKINETICS: Absorption: Extent of percutaneous absorption depends on skin integrity, vehicle, and use of occlusive dressings. **Distribution**: (IV) V_d=4.2L/kg; plasma protein binding (91%). **Metabolism**: Liver via CYP3A4 (hydrolysis). **Elimination**: (IV) $T_{1/2}$=7.2 hrs.

NURSING CONSIDERATIONS

Assessment: Assess for pre-existing skin atrophy, presence of skin infection at treatment site, rosacea, and perioral dermatitis. Assess use in pediatrics and in pregnant/nursing patients.

Monitoring: Monitor for signs/symptoms of HPA-axis suppression, Cushing's syndrome, hyperglycemia, and glucosuria. With large doses or occlusive dressings, monitor for HPA-axis suppression by using the ACTH stimulation, plasma cortisol, and urinary free cortisol tests. Monitor for signs/symptoms of local cutaneous reactions and for allergic contact dermatitis (eg, failure to heal). Monitor for signs of skin infections (eg, bacterial, fungal), and treat accordingly. In pediatrics, monitor for signs/symptoms of HPA-axis suppression, Cushing's syndrome, linear growth retardation, delayed weight gain, and intracranial HTN.

Patient Counseling: Counsel to use as directed, avoid contact with eyes, not to bandage or cover or wrap treated skin, and avoid using on face, underarms, or groin areas unless directed by physician. Advise to contact physician if any signs of adverse reactions or no clinical improvement within 2 weeks of therapy occurs.

Administration: Topical. For external use only. **Storage**: 2-30°C (36-86°F).

CYCLESSA **RX**

desogestrel - ethinyl estradiol (Organon)

OTHER BRAND NAMES: Velivet (Duramed Pharms Barr)

THERAPEUTIC CLASS: Estrogen/progestogen combination

INDICATIONS: Prevention of pregnancy.

DOSAGE: *Adults:* 1 tab qd for 28 days, then repeat. Start 1st Sunday after menses begin or 1st day of menses.

HOW SUPPLIED: Tab: (Ethinyl Estradiol-Desogestrel) 0.025mg-0.1mg, 0.025mg-0.125mg, 0.025mg-0.15mg

CONTRAINDICATIONS: Thrombophlebitis, DVT or thromboembolic disorders, pregnancy, cerebrovascular or coronary artery disease, undiagnosed abnormal genital bleeding, cholestatic jaundice of pregnancy or jaundice with prior pill use, hepatic adenomas or carcinomas, breast cancer or other estrogen-dependent neoplasia, hepatic tumors, active liver disease, and heavy smoking (≥15 cigarettes/day) and over age 35.

WARNINGS/PRECAUTIONS: Cigarette smoking increases risk of serious cardiovascular side effects; risk increases with age (especially >35 yrs) and heavy smoking. Increased risk of MI, vascular disease, thromboembolism, stroke and gallbladder disease. Retinal thrombosis, hepatic neoplasia, carcinoma of breast and reproductive organs reported. May cause glucose intolerance. May increase BP, elevate LDL levels or cause other lipid changes, fluid retention, breakthrough bleeding, and spotting. May cause or exacerbate migraine. May develop visual changes with contact lens. Increased risk of MI with HTN, hyperlipidemia, obesity, and diabetes. Increased risk of stroke with thrombophilias, hyperlipidemias, obesity, and migraine (especially with aura). D/C if jaundice, significant depression or ophthalmic irregularities develop. Perform annual physical exam. Use before menarche is not indicated. May affect certain endocrine, LFT and blood components. Should not be used if pregnant. Does not protect against STDs. Caution in nursing mothers and those with lipid disorders.

ADVERSE REACTIONS: Nausea, vomiting, breakthrough bleeding, spotting, amenorrhea, migraine headache, mood changes (including depression), vaginal candidiasis, edema, weight or appetite changes, and fluid retention.

INTERACTIONS: Reduced effects, increased breakthrough bleeding, and menstrual irregularities with some antibiotics, antifungals, anticonvulsants. Anti-HIV protease inhibitors may affect safety and efficacy. St. John's wort may induce hepatic enzymes and reduce effectiveness as well as resulting in breakthrough bleeding. Increased plasma concentrations of cyclosporine, prednisolone, and theophylline.

C

PREGNANCY: Category X, not for use in nursing.

MECHANISM OF ACTION: Triphasic oral contraceptive; acts by suppression of gonadotropins and inhibition of ovulation. Also causes changes in the cervical mucus and in the endometrium.

PHARMACOKINETICS: Absorption: Desogestrel and ethinyl estradiol: Rapid and complete. **Distribution:** Etonogestrel: Plasma protein binding (98%). **Metabolism:** Desogestrel: Liver; hydroxylation in intestinal mucosa; CYP3A4, 2C9; etonogestrel (active metabolite). Ethinyl estradiol: Hepatic conjugation. **Elimination:** Urine, bile, feces. Etonogestrel: $T_{1/2}$=37.1 hrs. Ethinyl estradiol: $T_{1/2}$=28.2 hrs.

NURSING CONSIDERATIONS

Assessment: Assess for presence or history of thrombophlebitis, thromboembolic disorders, CVD, CAD, valvular heart disease with thrombogenic complications, severe HTN, DM with vascular involvement, headaches with focal neurological symptoms, major surgery with prolonged immobilization, known or suspected carcinoma of the breast/endometrium, undiagnosed genital bleeding, cholestatic jaundice of pregnancy or jaundice with prior pill use, hepatic tumors, active liver disease, and pregnancy prior to therapy. Assess for possible drug interactions and use with concurrent smoking.

Monitoring: Monitor for venous and arterial thrombotic and thromboembolic events (eg, MI, thromboembolism, stroke), hepatic neoplasia, gallbladder disease, HTN, development of ocular lesions, ocular changes in patients who wear contact lenses, signs of hepatotoxicity (eg, jaundice). Monitor serum glucose levels with DM, BP with history of HTN, onset or exacerbations of migraines or headaches, lipid levels with hyperlipidemia, signs of depression (with a previous history), and bleeding irregularities.

Patient Counseling: Counsel about possible side effects, and to avoid smoking while on therapy. Inform that medication does not protect against STDs, and to use other forms of contraception to protect against such diseases. Inform not to skip pills and to take at the same time everyday, and that there is a risk of pregnancy if pills are missed. If a dose is missed, take as soon as possible; take next dose at regular time, or may take two pills in one day. Instruct to continue taking medication, even if irregular vaginal bleeding occurs; notify physician if bleeding occurs in more than one cycle or lasts for more than a few days. Instruct to go for annual physical while on therapy.

Administration: Oral route. **Storage:** 25°C (77°F); excursions permitted to 15-30°C (59-86°F).

CYMBALTA RX

duloxetine HCl (Lilly)

Antidepressants increased the risk of suicidal thinking and behavior (suicidality) in short-term studies in children, adolescents, and young adults with major depressive disorder (MDD) and other psychiatric disorders. Not approved for use in pediatric patients.

THERAPEUTIC CLASS: Serotonin and norepinephrine reuptake inhibitor

INDICATIONS: Acute and maintenance treatment of MDD in adults. Management of neuropathic pain associated with diabetic peripheral neuropathy. Acute treatment of generalized anxiety disorder (GAD). Management of fibromyalgia (FM).

DOSAGE: *Adults:* MDD: Initial: 40mg/day (given as 20mg bid) to 60mg/day (given qd or as 30mg bid) or 30mg qd for 1 week before increasing to 60mg qd. Max:120mg. Re-evaluate periodically. Diabetic Peripheral Neuropathic Pain: 60mg/day given qd. May lower starting dose if tolerability a concern. Renal Impairment: Consider lower starting dose with gradual increase. GAD: Initial: 60mg qd or 30mg qd for 1 week to adjust before increasing to 60mg qd. Titrate: May increase by increments of 30mg qd if needed. Max: 120 mg qd. FM: Initial: 30mg qd for 1 week to adjust before increasing to 60mg qd. Max: 60mg qd. Do not chew or crush.

HOW SUPPLIED: Cap, Delayed-Release: 20mg, 30mg, 60mg

CONTRAINDICATIONS: Concomitant use of MAOIs, uncontrolled narrow-angle glaucoma.

WARNINGS/PRECAUTIONS: Monitor for clinical worsening and/or suicidality. May cause hepatotoxicity. Avoid with chronic liver disease. May increase BP; obtain baseline and monitor periodically. Orthostatic hypotension and syncope reported. Avoid abrupt cessation and with severe renal impairment/ESRD or hepatic insufficiency. Caution with conditions that may slow gastric emptying, history of mania or seizures. May increase risk of mydriasis; caution in patients with controlled narrow-angle glaucoma. Serotonin syndrome may occur; caution with concomitant use of serotonergic drugs. Hyponatremia reported. May affect urethral resistance. May increase risk of abnormal bleeding; caution with aspirin, NSAIDs, warfarin. May increase risk of serum transaminase elevations.

ADVERSE REACTIONS: Nausea, dry mouth, constipation, diarrhea, vomiting, decreased appetite, fatigue, dizziness, somnolence, increased sweating, blurred vision, insomnia, agitation, erectile dysfunction.

INTERACTIONS: See Contraindications. Avoid within 14 days of MAOI therapy. Upon discontinuation, wait at least 5 days before starting MAOI therapy. Avoid thioridazine, CYP1A2 inhibitors (eg, fluvoxamine, some quinolone antibiotics), substantial alcohol use. Increased levels with potent CYP2D6 inhibitors (eg, paroxetine, fluoxetine, quinidine). Caution with drugs metabolized by CYP2D6 having a narrow therapeutic index (eg, TCAs, phenothiazines, type 1C antiarrhythmics), and CNS-active drugs. May increase free concentration levels of highly protein-bound drugs. Potential for interaction with drugs that affect gastric acidity. Caution with serotonergic drugs (including triptans, tramadol, SNRIs).

PREGNANCY: Category C, not for use in nursing.

MECHANISM OF ACTION: Selective serotonin and norepinephrine reuptake inhibitor; actions may be related to potentiation of serotonergic and noradrenergic activity in the CNS.

PHARMACOKINETICS: Absorption: T_{max}=6 hrs. **Distribution:** V_d=1640L; plasma protein binding (>90%). **Metabolism:** Hepatic via CYP1A2, 2D6; oxidation and conjugation. **Elimination:** Urine 70% (<1% unchanged), feces (20%); $T_{1/2}$=12 hrs.

NURSING CONSIDERATIONS

Assessment: Assess for bipolar disorder risk, history of mania, chronic liver disease, chronic alcohol use, history of seizures, disease/condition that slows gastric emptying (eg, DM), uncontrolled narrow-angle glaucoma, risk factors for hyponatremia, history of urinary retention, hepatic/renal impairment, and possible drug interactions. Assess baseline BP, LFTs, renal function tests, and blood glucose.

Monitoring: Perform periodic BP, LFTs, and renal function tests. Monitor for signs/symptoms of clinical worsening (suicidality, unusual changes in behavior), hepatotoxicity, serotonin syndrome, abnormal bleeding, hyponatremia, seizures, orthostatic hypotension, decreased glycemic control, urinary hesitation/retention, mydriasis, cognitive/motor impairment, and hepatic/renal dysfunction. If abruptly d/c, monitor for symptoms of dysphoric mood, irritability, agitation, dizziness, sensory disturbances, anxiety, confusion, headache, lethargy, emotional lability, insomnia, and hypomania.

Patient Counseling: Counsel to swallow whole, not to chew, crush, or open. Advise to avoid alcohol. Seek medical attention for symptoms of serotonin syndrome (mental status changes, tachycardia, hyperthermia, NV, diarrhea, incoordination), abnormal bleeding (particularly if using NSAIDs or ASA), hyponatremia, activation of mania, mydriasis, decreased glycemic control, orthostatic hypotension, hepatotoxicity, urinary hesitation/retention, seizures, clinical worsening (suicidal ideation, unusual changes in behavior), or discontinuation symptoms (irritability, agitation, dizziness, anxiety, headache, insomnia). Caution may impair physical/mental abilities. May notice improvement within 1-4 weeks; continue therapy as directed.

Administration: Oral route. **Storage:** 25°C (77°F); excursions permitted to 15-30°C (59-86°F).

CYTOMEL RX

liothyronine sodium (King)

THERAPEUTIC CLASS: Thyroid replacement hormone

INDICATIONS: Hypothyroidism. As a pituitary TSH suppressant in the treatment and prevention of euthyroid goiters, including thyroid nodules, and Hashimoto's and multinodular goiter. Diagnostic agent in suppression tests to differentiate mild hyperthyroidism or thyroid gland autonomy.

DOSAGE: *Adults:* Mild Hypothyroidism: Initial: 25mcg qd. Titrate: May increase by up to 25mcg qd every 1-2 weeks. Maint: 25-75mcg qd. Myxedema: Initial: 5mcg qd. Titrate: May increase by 5-10mcg qd every 1-2 weeks up to 25mcg qd, then increase by 5-25mcg qd every 1-2 weeks. Maint: 50-100mcg/day. Goiter: Initial: 5mcg/day. Titrate: May increase by 5-10mcg qd every 1-2 weeks up to 25mcg qd, then by 12.5-25mcg qd every 1-2 weeks. Maint: 75mcg qd. Elderly/Coronary Artery Disease: Initial: 5mcg qd. Titrate: Increase by no more than 5mcg qd every 2 weeks. Thyroid Suppression Therapy: 75-100mcg qd for 7 days. Radioactive iodine uptake is determined before and after administration of hormone.
Pediatrics: Congenital Hypothyroidism: Initial: 5mcg qd. Titrate: Increase by 5mcg qd every 3-4 days until desired response. Maint: <1 yr: 20mcg qd. 1-3 yrs: 50mcg qd. >3 yrs: 25-75mcg/day.

HOW SUPPLIED: Tab: 5mcg, 25mcg*, 50mcg* *scored

CONTRAINDICATIONS: Uncorrected adrenal cortical insufficiency and untreated thyrotoxicosis.

WARNINGS/PRECAUTIONS: Do not use in the treatment of obesity; larger doses in euthyroid patients can cause serious or even life threatening toxicity. Caution with angina pectoris and elderly; use lower doses. Rule out hypogonadism and nephrosis prior to therapy. With prolonged and severe hypothyroidism supplement with adrenocortical steroids. May aggravate diabetes mellitus or insipidus and adrenal cortical insufficiency. Add glucocorticoid with myxedema coma. Excessive doses may cause craniosynostosis in infants.

ADVERSE REACTIONS: Allergic skin reactions (rare).

INTERACTIONS: Hypothyroidism decreases and hyperthyroidism increases sensitivity to oral anticoagulants; monitor PT/INR. Monitor insulin and oral hypoglycemic requirements. Decreased absorption with cholestyramine; space dosing by 4-5 hrs. Large dose may cause life-threatening toxicities with sympathomimetic amines. Estrogens increase thyroxine-binding globulin; increase in thyroid dose may be needed. Additive effects of both agents with TCAs. HTN and tachycardia with ketamine. May potentiate digitalis toxicity. Increased adrenergic effects of catecholamines; caution with CAD.

PREGNANCY: Category A, caution in nursing.

MECHANISM OF ACTION: Synthetic thyroid hormone; not established, suspected to enhance oxygen consumption by tissues, increases the basal metabolic rate and metabolism of carbohydrates, lipids, and proteins.

PHARMACOKINETICS: Elimination: $T_{1/2}$=2.5 days.

NURSING CONSIDERATIONS

Assessment: Assess for possible drug interactions, CV disease (eg, CAD, angina pectoris), DM, adrenal cortical insufficiency, thyrotoxicosis, myxedema, hypogonadism, and nephrosis.

Monitoring: Periodically monitor thyroid function and urinary glucose with DM. Monitor for signs/symptoms of precipitation of adrenocortical insufficiency, aggravation of DM and diabetes insipidus, hypoglycemia, toxicity, and hypersensitivity reactions.

Patient Counseling: Inform that replacement therapy is taken for life. Warn that partial hair loss may be seen in pediatrics. Instruct to seek medical attention if symptoms of toxicity (eg, CP, increased HR, palpitations, excessive sweating, heat intolerance, nervousness), hypoglycemia, aggravation of DM and diabetes insipidus, or hypersensitivity reactions occur.

Administration: Oral route. **Storage:** 15-30°C (59-86°F).

C

CYTOVENE

ganciclovir (Roche Labs)

RX

Risk of granulocytopenia, anemia, and thrombocytopenia. More rapid rate of CMV retinitis progression with caps; only use as maintenance treatment when the risk is balanced by the benefit of avoiding daily IV infusions.

THERAPEUTIC CLASS: Synthetic guanine derivative

INDICATIONS: (Caps) Prevention of cytomegalovirus (CMV) in solid organ transplants and in advanced HIV patients at risk for CMV disease. Alternative to IV for maintenance treatment of CMV retinitis in immunocompromised patients, in whom retinitis is stable. (IV) Treatment of CMV retinitis in immunocompromised patients. Prevention of CMV disease in transplant recipients at risk for CMV disease.

DOSAGE: *Adults:* CMV Retinitis Treatment: Initial: 5mg/kg IV q12h for 14-21 days. Maint: 5mg/kg IV qd for 7 days or 6mg/kg IV qd for 5 days/week or 1000mg PO tid or 500mg PO 6 times daily q3h, while awake. CMV Retinitis Prevention in HIV Patients: 1000mg PO tid. CMV Retinitis Prevention in Transplant Patients: Initial: 5mg/kg IV q12h for 7-14 days. Maint: 5mg/kg IV qd for 7 days or 6mg/kg IV for 5 days/week or 1000mg PO tid. Renal Impairment: See PI for details. Take caps with food.

HOW SUPPLIED: Cap: 250mg; Inj: 500mg

CONTRAINDICATIONS: Hypersensitivity to acyclovir.

WARNINGS/PRECAUTIONS: Avoid if ANC <500 cells/mcL, or platelets <25,000 cells/mcL. Caution in pre-existing cytopenias and history of cytopenic reactions to drugs, chemicals, and irradiation. Reduce dose in renal impairment. High frequency of renal dysfunction in transplant recipients. Women of childbearing potential should use effective contraception during treatment due to fetal mutagenic/teratogenic potential. Men should practice barrier contraception during and ≥90 days after therapy.

ADVERSE REACTIONS: Fever, diarrhea, anorexia, vomiting, leukopenia, anemia, sweating.

INTERACTIONS: Decreased effects with zidovudine; combination may potentiate zidovudine and cause severe neutropenia. Potentiated by probenecid. Avoid imipenem-cilastatin; may precipitate seizures. Extreme caution with other nucleoside analogues, dapsone, pentamidine, flucytosine, vincristine, vinblastine, adriamycin, cyclosporine, amphotericin B, Bactrim; potential additive toxicity. Increased didanosine serum levels.

PREGNANCY: Category C, not for use in nursing.

MECHANISM OF ACTION: Guanine derivative; inhibits viral DNA synthesis by inhibiting viral DNA polymerase, incorporating into viral DNA, resulting in eventual termination of viral DNA elongation.

PHARMACOKINETICS: Absorption: C_{max}=8.27-9mcg/mL; AUC=22.1-26.8mcg•hr/mL. **Distribution:** V_d=0.74L/kg; plasma protein binding (1-2%). **Elimination:** Urine (91.3%); $T_{1/2}$=3.5 hrs (IV), 4.8 hrs (PO).

NURSING CONSIDERATIONS

Assessment: Assess for hypersensitivity to acyclovir, pregnancy/nursing status, renal impairment, pre-existing cytopenias, and possible drug interactions. Obtain baseline renal function (creatinine); neutrophil (>500 cells/mcL), and platelet (>25,000 cells/mcL) counts.

Monitoring: Monitor CBC; serum creatinine (renal impairment) periodically. Monitor for signs/symptoms of hypersensitivity reactions, infusion-site reactions, infertility, anemia, granulocytopenia, and thrombocytopenia.

Patient Counseling: Instruct to use effective contraception and practice barrier contraception during and for ≥90 days following therapy due to pregnancy risks. Inform to keep well hydrated. Advise to seek medical attention if symptoms of hypersensitivity reactions, infusion-site reactions, anemia, granulocytopenia, or thrombocytopenia occur.

Administration: IV. **Storage:** Below 40°C (104°F).

CYTOXAN RX

cyclophosphamide (Bristol-Myers Squibb)

THERAPEUTIC CLASS: Nitrogen mustard alkylating agent

INDICATIONS: Treatment of malignant lymphomas, Hodgkin's disease, lymphocytic lymphoma, mixed-cell type or histiocytic lymphoma, Burkitt's lymphoma, multiple myeloma, chronic lymphocytic leukemia, chronic granulocytic leukemia, acute myelogenous and monocytic leukemia, acute lymphoblastic leukemia in children, mycosis fungoides, neuroblastoma, ovary adenocarcinoma, retinoblastoma, breast carcinoma. Treatment of biopsy proven "minimal change" nephrotic syndrome in children, but not as primary therapy.

DOSAGE: *Adults:* Malignant Diseases (Without Hematologic Deficiency): Monotherapy: Initial: 40-50mg/kg IV in divided doses over 2-5 days, or 10-15mg/kg IV given every 7-10 days, or 3-5mg/kg twice weekly. Oral Dosing: Initial/Maint: 1-5mg/kg/day PO. Adjust dose according to antitumor activity and/or leukopenia. May need to reduce dose when combined with other cytotoxic drugs.

Pediatrics: Malignant Diseases (Without Hematologic Deficiency): Monotherapy: Initial: 40-50mg/kg IV in divided doses over 2-5 days, or 10-15mg/kg IV given every 7-10 days, or 3-5mg/kg twice weekly. Oral Dosing: Initial/Maint: 1-5mg/kg/day PO. Adjust dose according to antitumor activity and/or leukopenia. May need to reduce dose when combined with other cytotoxic drugs. Nephrotic Syndrome: 2.5-3mg/kg/day PO for 60-90 days.

HOW SUPPLIED: Inj (Lyophilized): 500mg, 1g, 2g; Tab: 25mg, 50mg

CONTRAINDICATIONS: Severely depressed bone marrow function.

WARNINGS/PRECAUTIONS: Second malignancies, cardiac dysfunction, and hemorrhagic cystitis reported. May cause fetal harm in pregnancy. Serious, fatal infections may develop if severely immunosuppressed. Monitor for toxicity with leukopenia, thrombocytopenia, tumor cell infiltration of bone marrow, previous x-ray therapy or cytotoxic therapy, and impaired hepatic and/or renal function. Monitor hematologic profile for hematopoietic suppression. Examine urine for red blood cells. Anaphylactic reactions reported. Possible cross-sensitivity with other alkylating agents. May cause sterility. May interfere with normal wound healing. Consider dose adjustment with adrenalectomy.

ADVERSE REACTIONS: Impairment of fertility, amenorrhea, NV, anorexia, abdominal discomfort, diarrhea, alopecia, leukopenia, thrombocytopenia, hemorrhagic ureteritis, interstitial pneumonitis, malaise, asthenia, renal tubular necrosis.

INTERACTIONS: Chronic, high doses of phenobarbital increase metabolism and leukopenic activity. Potentiates succinylcholine chloride effects and doxorubicin-induced cardiotoxicity. Alert anesthesiologist if treated within 10 days of general anesthesia.

PREGNANCY: Category D, not for use in nursing.

MECHANISM OF ACTION: Nitrogen mustard alkylating agent; exerts action by cross linking of tumor cell DNA.

PHARMACOKINETICS: Absorption: Well absorbed; bioavailability (≥75%). **Distribution:** Plasma protein binding (≥60% as metabolites). **Metabolism:** Liver; active metabolites. **Elimination:** Urine (5-25% unchanged); $T_{1/2}$=3-12 hrs.

NURSING CONSIDERATIONS

Assessment: Assess for severely depressed bone marrow function, leukopenia, thrombocytopenia, tumor cell infiltration of bone marrow, previous X-ray therapy, previous therapy with other cytotoxic agents, impaired hepatic/renal function.

Monitoring: Monitor for second malignancies, amenorrhea, sterility, ovarian fibrosis, oligospermia or azoospermia, hemorrhagic cystitis, cardiac dysfunction, infection, anaphylactic reactions, CBC with differential and platelets.

Patient Counseling: Counsel about possible side effects and required contraceptive methods while on therapy. Take in the morning and drink adequate fluids. Report adverse side effects.

Administration: Oral, IV, IM, intraperitoneal, intrapleural route. Inspect drug product visually for particulate matter and discoloration prior to parenteral administration. **Storage:** Vial: Below 25°C (77°F). Tab: Below 25°C (77°F); excursions permitted to 30°C (86°F); protect from temperatures above 30°C (86°F).

D.H.E. 45 — RX

dihydroergotamine mesylate (Valeant)

Serious and life-threatening peripheral ischemia reported with potent CYP3A4 inhibitors (eg, protease inhibitors, macrolides). Elevated levels of dihydroergotamine increases risk of vasospasm leading to cerebral ischemia or ischemia of the extremities. Concomitant use with CYP3A4 inhibitors is contraindicated.

THERAPEUTIC CLASS: Ergot alkaloid

INDICATIONS: Acute treatment of migraine with or without aura. Acute treatment of cluster headache episodes.

DOSAGE: *Adults:* 1mL IV/IM/SQ. May repeat at 1 hr intervals. Max: 3mL/24hrs IM/SC or 2mL/24hrs IV and 6mL/week.

HOW SUPPLIED: Inj: 1mg/mL

CONTRAINDICATIONS: Ergot alkaloids hypersensitivity, ischemic heart disease, coronary artery vasospasm (eg, Prinzmetal's variant angina), uncontrolled HTN, hemiplegic or basilar migraine, peripheral artery disease, sepsis, following vascular surgery, severe renal/hepatic dysfunction, pregnancy, nursing, with potent CYP3A4 inhibitors (eg, ritonavir, nelfinavir, indinavir, erythromycin, clarithromycin, troleandomycin, ketoconazole, itraconazole), concomitant peripheral and central vasoconstrictors, and within 24 hrs after taking 5-HT_1 agonists, methysergide, ergotamine-containing, or ergot-type agents.

WARNINGS/PRECAUTIONS: Confirm migraine diagnosis. Inform of risks of adverse cardiac, cerebrovascular, and vasospastic events and fatalities. Avoid with cardiac risk factors (eg, HTN, hypercholesterolemia, smoker, obesity, DM, strong family history of CAD, females who are surgically/physiologically postmenopausal, or males >40 yrs) unless cardiovascular evaluation is done. Perform cardiovascular monitoring with long-term use. Significant BP elevations reported.

ADVERSE REACTIONS: Vasospasm, angina, paresthesia, HTN, dizziness, anxiety, dyspnea, headache, flushing, diarrhea, rash, increased sweating.

INTERACTIONS: Potentiated BP elevation with peripheral and central vasoconstrictors. Additive coronary vasospastic effect with sumatriptan; avoid within 24 hrs of each other. Propranolol and nicotine may potentiate the vasoconstrictive action. Increased plasma levels and peripheral vasoconstriction with macrolides. Contraindicated with CYP3A4 inhibitors (eg, macrolides, protease inhibitors). Caution with less potent CYP3A4 inhibitors (eg, saquinavir, nefazodone, fluconazole, grapefruit juice, fluoxetine, fluvoxamine, zileuton, clotrimazole).

PREGNANCY: Category X, contraindicated in nursing.

MECHANISM OF ACTION: Ergotamine; binds with high affinity to 5-HT_{1D} receptors on intracranial blood vessels, causing vasoconstriction, or activates 5-HT_{1D} receptors on sensory nerve endings of trigeminal system, resulting in inhibition of proinflammatory neuropeptide release.

PHARMACOKINETICS: Distribution: V_d=800L; plasma protein binding (93%). **Metabolism:** Liver; 8'-β-hydroxydihydroergotamine (major metabolite). **Elimination:** Feces (major), urine (6-7%); $T_{1/2}$=9 hrs.

NURSING CONSIDERATIONS

Assessment: Assess for ischemic heart disease (angina pectoris, history of MI, documented silent ischemia), coronary artery vasospasm, Prinzmetal's variant angina, uncontrolled HTN, hemiplegic or basilar migraine, peripheral arterial disease, sepsis, pregnancy/nursing status, possible drug interactions, CAD, renal/hepatic impairment.

Monitoring: Monitor for signs/symptoms of vasospastic reactions, HTN, fibrosis, CV events, and hypersensitivity reactions.

Patient Counseling: Advise to seek medical attention if numbness or tingling in fingers and toes, muscle pain in arms and legs, weakness in legs, pain in chest, temporary speeding or slowing of HR, swelling, or itching occur.

Administration: SQ, IV, IM route. **Storage:** Below 25°C (77°F). Do not refrigerate or freeze. Protect from light and heat.

DACOGEN — RX

decitabine (Eisai)

THERAPEUTIC CLASS: DNA methyltransferase inhibitor

INDICATIONS: Treatment of myelodysplastic syndromes.

DOSAGE: *Adults*: Initial: 15mg/m^2 IV over 3 hrs q8h for 3 days. Repeat cycle every 6 weeks. Treat for ≥4 cycles. Adjust dose based on hematology lab values, renal function, and serum electrolytes.

HOW SUPPLIED: Inj: 50mg

WARNINGS/PRECAUTIONS: May cause fetal harm. Avoid pregnancy in women of childbearing potential. Men should be advised not to father a child while receiving treatment and for 2 months afterwards. Neutropenia and thrombocytopenia may occur; monitor CBC and platelets periodically (at minimum, before each cycle). Caution with renal and hepatic dysfunction. Avoid with SrCr >2mg/dL, transaminase >2x normal, or serum bilirubin >1.5mg/dL.

ADVERSE REACTIONS: Neutropenia, thrombocytopenia, anemia, fatigue, pyrexia, nausea, cough, petechiae, constipation, diarrhea, hyperglycemia, febrile neutropenia, leukopenia, headache, insomnia.

PREGNANCY: Category D, not for use in nursing.

MECHANISM OF ACTION: DNA methyltransferase inhibitor. Inhibition of methyltransferase causes hypomethylation of DNA and cellular differentiation or apoptosis.

PHARMACOKINETICS: Distribution: Plasma protein binding (<1%). **Metabolism:** Deamination in liver, granulocytes, intestinal epithelium, and blood. **Elimination:** $T_{1/2}$=0.51 hrs.

NURSING CONSIDERATIONS

Assessment: Assess CBC with platelets, renal/hepatic functions, pregnancy status. Note other diseases/condition and drug therapies.

Monitoring: Monitor hypersensitivity reactions, CBC with platelets, renal/hepatic impairment, cardiac disorders, infections and infestations, intracranial hemorrhage, mental status change, cholecystitis, and hyperglycemia.

Patient Counseling: Counsel about contraception while on treatment, to avoid crowds and those with active infections, and to report abnormal bleeding or bruising and any adverse effects.

Administration: IV route. Reconstitute aseptically with 10mL of SWFI. Dilute with 0.9% NS, D5W, or LR to final concentration of 0.1-1.0mg/mL. Unless used within 15 min of reconstitution, diluted sol must be prepared using cold (2-8°C) infusion fluids. **Storage**: 2-8°C (36-46°F) for up to a maximum of 7 hrs, until administration. Vials: 25°C (77°F); excursions permitted to 15-30°C (59-86°F). Diluted solution: 2-8°C (36-46°F) for up to maximum of 7 hrs, until administration.

DALMANE

CIV

flurazepam HCl (Valeant)

D

THERAPEUTIC CLASS: Benzodiazepine

INDICATIONS: Treatment of insomnia.

DOSAGE: *Adults:* Usual: 15-30mg at bedtime. Elderly/Debilitated: Initial: 15mg at bedtime.
Pediatrics: ≥15 yrs: Usual: 15-30mg at bedtime.

HOW SUPPLIED: Cap: 15mg, 30mg

CONTRAINDICATIONS: Pregnancy.

WARNINGS/PRECAUTIONS: Caution in elderly, debilitated, severely depressed, those with suicidal tendencies, hepatic/renal impairment, respiratory disease. Ataxia and falls reported in elderly and debilitated.Withdrawal symptoms after discontinuation; avoid abrupt discontinuation. Rare cases of angioedema involving the tongue, glottis, or larynx reported. Complex behaviors such as sleep driving, and other complex behaviors (eg, preparing and eating food, making phone calls, and having sex) reported.

ADVERSE REACTIONS: Confusion, dizziness, drowsiness, lightheadedness, ataxia.

INTERACTIONS: Additive effects with alcohol and other CNS depressants.

PREGNANCY: Not for use in pregnancy or nursing.

MECHANISM OF ACTION: Benzodiazepine; hypnotic.

PHARMACOKINETICS: Absorption: Rapid; C_{max}=4.0ng/mL; T_{max}=1 hr. **Metabolism:** N_1-desalkyl-flurazepam (active metabolite); conjugation. **Elimination:** Urine; $T_{1/2}$=2.3 hrs, 47-100 hrs (active metabolite).

NURSING CONSIDERATIONS

Assessment: Assess for primary psychiatric illness, impaired renal/hepatic function, chronic pulmonary insufficiency, depression, possible drug interactions, and history of drug abuse.

Monitoring: Monitor for anaphylactic and anaphylactoid reactions, worsening of insomnia, complex behaviors (eg, sleep driving), lab abnormalities (eg, LFTs).

Patient Counseling: Caution about hazardous tasks (eg, operating machinery/driving). Advise to consult physician before increasing dose or abruptly d/c, avoid concomitant alcohol consumption or other sedative-hypnotics, and do not take if pregnant.

Administration: Oral route. **Storage:** 25°C (77°F); excursions permitted to 15-30°C (59-86°F).

DANTRIUM

RX

dantrolene sodium (Procter & Gamble Pharmaceuticals)

Associated with hepatotoxicity; monitor hepatic function. Discontinue if no benefit after 45 days.

THERAPEUTIC CLASS: Direct acting skeletal muscle relaxant

INDICATIONS: To control manifestations of clinical spasticity from upper motor neuron disorders (eg, spinal cord injury, stroke, cerebral palsy, multiple sclerosis). Preoperatively to prevent or attenuate development of malignant hyperthermia, and after a malignant hyperthermia crisis.

DOSAGE: *Adults:* Chronic Spasticity: Initial: 25mg qd for 7 days. Titrate: Increase to 25mg tid for 7 days, then 50mg tid for 7 days, then 100mg tid. Max: 100mg qid. If no further benefit at next higher dose, decrease to previous lower dose. Malignant Hyperthermia: Pre-Op: 4-8mg/kg/day given tid-qid for 1-2 days before surgery, with last dose given 3-4 hrs before surgery. Post-Op Following Malignant Hyperthermia Crisis: 4-8mg/kg/day given qid for 1-3 days.

Pediatrics: ≥5 yrs: Chronic Spasticity: Initial: 0.5mg/kg qd for 7 days. Titrate: Increase to 0.5mg/kg tid for 7 days, then 1mg/kg tid for 7 days, then 2mg/kg tid. Max: 100mg qid. If no further benefit at next higher dose, decrease to previous lower dose.

HOW SUPPLIED: Cap: 25mg, 50mg, 100mg

CONTRAINDICATIONS: Active hepatic disease, where spasticity is utilized to sustain upright posture and balance in locomotion, when spasticity is utilized to obtain or maintain increased function.

D

WARNINGS/PRECAUTIONS: Monitor LFTs at baseline, then periodically. Increased risk of hepatocellular disease in females and patients >35 yrs. Caution with pulmonary, cardiac, and liver dysfunction. Photosensitivity reaction may occur; limit sunlight exposure.

ADVERSE REACTIONS: Drowsiness, dizziness, weakness, malaise, fatigue, diarrhea, hepatitis, tachycardia, aplastic anemia, thrombocytopenia, depression, seizure.

INTERACTIONS: Increased drowsiness with CNS depressants. Caution with estrogens; risk of hepatotoxicity. Avoid with CCBs; risk of cardiovascular collapse. May potentiate vecuronium-induced neuromuscular block.

PREGNANCY: Safety in nursing not known. Not for use in nursing.

MECHANISM OF ACTION: Direct-acting skeletal muscle relaxant; interferes with release of calcium ions from the sarcoplasmic reticulum.

PHARMACOKINETICS: Absorption: Incomplete/slow but consistent. **Metabolism:** Hepatic microsomal enzymes; 5-hydroxy and acetamido analog (major metabolites). **Elimination:** Urine; $T_{1/2}$=8.7 hrs.

NURSING CONSIDERATIONS

Assessment: Assess for active hepatic disease (eg, hepatitis and cirrhosis), pregnancy/nursing status, impaired pulmonary/cardiac function due to myocardial disease, and possible drug interactions. Perform baseline LFTs to establish pre-existing liver disease. Assess use in patients >35 yrs due to increased risk of drug-induced hepatocellular disease.

Monitoring: Monitor LFTs regularly, photosensitivity reactions, and signs/symptoms of hepatitis; d/c if abnormalities of LFTs or jaundice appear.

Patient Counseling: Caution against performing hazardous tasks (eg, operating machinery/driving), and avoid prolonged sunlight exposure. Notify if pregnant/nursing.

Administration: Oral route. **Storage:** Avoid excessive heat, over 40°C (104°F).

DANTRIUM IV — RX

dantrolene sodium (Procter & Gamble Pharmaceuticals)

THERAPEUTIC CLASS: Direct acting skeletal muscle relaxant.

INDICATIONS: Adjunct management of fulminant hypermetabolism of skeletal muscle characteristic of malignant hyperthermia crises. For pre- and post-operative use to prevent or attenuate development of malignant hyperthermia.

DOSAGE: *Adults:* Malignant Hyperthermia: Initial: Minimum 1mg/kg IV push. Continue until symptoms subside or max cumulative dose 10mg/kg. Pre-Op Malignant Hyperthermia Prophylaxis: 2.5mg/kg 1.25 hrs before anesthesia and infuse over 1 hr. May need additional therapy during anesthesia/surgery if symptoms arise. Post-Op Prophylaxis: Initial: 1mg/kg or more as clinical situation dictates.

Pediatrics: Malignant Hyperthermia: Initial: Minimum 1mg/kg IV push. Continue until symptoms subside or max cumulative dose 10mg/kg.

HOW SUPPLIED: Inj: 20mg

WARNINGS/PRECAUTIONS: Use with supportive therapies to treat malignant hyperthermia. Take steps to prevent extravasation. Fatal and non-fatal hepatic disorders reported. Do not operate automobile or engage hazardous activity for 48 hrs after therapy. Caution at meals on day of administration because difficulty in swallowing/choking reported. Monitor vital signs if receive pre-operatively.

ADVERSE REACTIONS: Loss of grip strength, weakness in legs, drowsiness, dizziness, pulmonary edema, thrombophlebitis, urticaria, erythema.

INTERACTIONS: Plasma protein-binding reduced by warfarin and clofibrate, and increased by tolbutamide. Avoid with CCBs; possible risk of cardiovascular collapse. Caution with tranquilizers. Possible increased metabolism by drugs known to induce hepatic microsomal enzymes. May potentiate vecuronium-induced neuromuscular block.

PREGNANCY: Category C, safety in nursing not known.

MECHANISM OF ACTION: Direct acting skeletal muscle relaxant; interferes with release of calcium ions from sarcoplasmic reticulum.

PHARMACOKINETICS: Distribution: Found in breast milk. **Metabolism:** Hydrolysis and oxidation; 5-hydroxy dantrolene and acetylamino analog (major metabolites). **Elimination:** Urine; $T_{1/2}$=4-8 hrs.

NURSING CONSIDERATIONS

Assessment: Assess for active hepatic disease (hepatitis and cirrhosis), pregnancy/nursing status, and possible drug interactions.

Monitoring: Monitor for vital signs, tissue necrosis, LFTs. Monitor for cardiovascular collapse if given concomitantly with CCBs.

Patient Counseling: Caution against performing hazardous tasks (eg, operating machinery/driving). Inform that at meals, on administration day, choking and difficulty swallowing have been reported. Inform about postop muscle weakness, reduced grip strength, and lightheadedness. Notify if pregnant/nursing.

Administration: IV route. **Storage:** 15-30°C (59-86°F); avoid prolonged light exposure.

DARVOCET A500 CIV

propoxyphene napsylate - acetaminophen (Xanodyne)

THERAPEUTIC CLASS: Opioid analgesic

INDICATIONS: Relief of mild to moderate pain.

DOSAGE: *Adults:* Usual: 1 tab q4h prn for pain. Max: 6 tabs/24 hrs. Elderly: Increase dosing interval. Hepatic/Renal Impairment: Reduce daily dose.

HOW SUPPLIED: Tab: (Propoxyphene-APAP) 100mg-500mg

WARNINGS/PRECAUTIONS: Drug dependence potential. Not for suicidal or addiction-prone patients. Caution with hepatic or renal impairment, elderly.

ADVERSE REACTIONS: Dizziness, sedation, NV, liver dysfunction.

INTERACTIONS: Additive CNS-depressant effects with alcohol, sedatives, tranquilizers, muscle relaxants, antidepressants. Increases plasma levels of antidepressants, anticonvulsants, coumarins. Severe neurologic signs, including coma reported with carbamazepine.

PREGNANCY: Not for use in pregnancy, safety not known in nursing.

MECHANISM OF ACTION: Propoxyphene: Centrally acting narcotic analgesic. Acetaminophen: Produces antipyretic and analgesic activity.

PHARMACOKINETICS: Absorption: T_{max}=2-2.5 hrs; (100mg) C_{max}=0.05-0.1mcg/mL. **Distribution:** Found in breast milk. **Metabolism:** Liver; norpropoxyphene (active metabolite). **Elimination:** $T_{1/2}$=6-12 hrs, 30-36 hrs (active metabolite).

NURSING CONSIDERATIONS

Assessment: Assess for suicidal tendencies, emotional disturbances, hepatic/renal impairment, history of ulcers, patient's age, proneness to addiction, alcoholism, pregnancy/nursing status, and possible drug interactions.

Monitoring: Monitor for signs/symptoms of CNS depression, drug dependence, liver dysfunction, and renal papillary necrosis. Monitor for subacute painful myopathy if chronic overdosage occurs.

Patient Counseling: Counsel that medication may impair mental/physical abilities; use caution when performing dangerous tasks (eg, operating machinery/driving). Avoid using other CNS depressants and alcohol during therapy, and instruct not to take >6 tablets in 24-hr period. Inform dependence may develop if higher than recommended dose is taken for a longer period of time.

Administraion: Oral route. **Storage**: 20-25°C (68-77°F); dispense in tight, light-resistant container with child-resistant closure.

DARVOCET-N

CIV

propoxyphene napsylate - acetaminophen (Xanodyne)

THERAPEUTIC CLASS: Opioid analgesic

INDICATIONS: Relief of mild to moderate pain.

DOSAGE: *Adults:* Usual: 100mg propoxyphene napsylate and 650mg APAP q4h prn for pain. Max: 600mg propoxyphene napsylate/day. Elderly: Increase dosing interval. Hepatic/Renal Impairment: Reduce daily dose.

HOW SUPPLIED: Tab: (Propoxyphene-APAP) 50mg-325mg, 100mg-650mg

WARNINGS/PRECAUTIONS: Drug dependence potential. Not for suicidal or addiction-prone patients. Caution with hepatic/renal impairment, elderly. May impair mental/physical abilities.

ADVERSE REACTIONS: Dizziness, sedation, NV, liver dysfunction.

INTERACTIONS: Additive CNS-depressant effects with alcohol, sedatives, tranquilizers, muscle relaxants, antidepressants. Increases plasma levels of antidepressants, anticonvulsants, coumarins. Severe neurologic signs, including coma reported with carbamazepine.

PREGNANCY: Not for use in pregnancy, safety not known in nursing.

MECHANISM OF ACTION: Propoxyphene: Centrally acting narcotic analgesic. Acetaminophen: Produces antipyretic-analgesic activity.

PHARMACOKINETICS: Absorption: C_{max}=0.05-0.1mcg/mL; T_{max}=2-2.5 hrs. **Distribution:** Found in breast milk. **Metabolism:** Liver; norpropoxyphene (active metabolite). **Elimination:** $T_{1/2}$=6-12 hrs, 30-36 hrs (norpropoxyphene).

NURSING CONSIDERATIONS

Assessment: Assess for suicidal tendencies, proneness to addiction, history of emotional disturbances, alcoholism, hepatic/renal impairment, ulcers, age of patient, pregnancy/nursing status, and possible drug interactions.

Monitoring: Monitor for signs/symptoms of CNS depression, drug dependence (eg, psychic dependence), liver dysfunction, renal papillary necrosis. Monitor for signs/symptoms of subacute painful myopathy if chronic overdosage occurs.

Patient Counseling: Inform drug may impair mental/physical abilities; use caution when performing hazardous tasks (eg, operating machinery/driving). Instruct to notify physician of all medications currently taken (eg, CNS depressants). Avoid use of alcohol during therapy. Inform dependence may develop if higher than recommended dose is taken for a longer period of time.

Administration: Oral route. **Storage:** 25°C (77°F); excursions permitted to 15-30°C (59-86°F).

DARVON

CIV

propoxyphene HCl (Xanodyne)

THERAPEUTIC CLASS: Opioid analgesic

INDICATIONS: Relief of mild to moderate pain.

DOSAGE: *Adults:* Usual: 65mg q4h as needed for pain. Max: 390mg/day. Elderly: Increase dose interval. Hepatic/Renal Impairment: Reduce daily dose.

HOW SUPPLIED: Cap: 65mg

WARNINGS/PRECAUTIONS: Drug dependence potential. May impair mental/physical ability for operating machinery. Caution with hepatic or renal impairment and the elderly. Not for suicidal or addiction-prone patients. Do not exceed recommended dose.

D

ADVERSE REACTIONS: Dizziness, sedation, NV, liver dysfunction.

INTERACTIONS: Additive CNS-depressant effect with other CNS depressants, including alcohol. Increases plasma levels of antidepressants, anticonvulsants, and coumarins. Severe neurologic signs, including coma reported with carbamazepine. Caution with tranquilizers, antidepressants, and with excessive alcohol use.

PREGNANCY: Not for use in pregnancy, unknown use in nursing.

MECHANISM OF ACTION: Centrally acting narcotic analgesic agent.

PHARMACOKINETICS: Absorption: C_{max}=0.05-0.1mcg/mL; T_{max}=2-2.5 hrs. **Distribution:** Found in breast milk. **Metabolism:** Liver; norpropoxyphene (active metabolite). **Elimination:** $T_{1/2}$=6-12 hrs, 30-36 hrs (norpropoxyphene).

NURSING CONSIDERATIONS

Assessment: Assess for suicidal tendencies, history of emotional disturbances, alcoholism, proneness to addiction, renal/hepatic impairment, age of patient, history of ulcers, pregnancy/nursing status, and possible drug interactions.

Monitoring: Monitor for signs/symptoms of CNS depression, drug dependence, and liver dysfunction. In cases of chronic overdosage, monitor for subacute painful myopathy.

Patient Counseling: Inform that drug may impair mental/physical abilities; use caution when performing hazardous tasks (eg, operating machinery/driving). Counsel to avoid using other CNS depressants and alcohol. Advise to notify physician of all medications currently taken. Inform that dependence may occur if higher than recommended doses taken for a long period of time. Advise to lie down and rest if any signs/symptoms of drowsiness, dizziness, or NV occur.

Administration: Oral route. **Storage:** 20-25°C (86-77° F); keep out of reach of children.

DARVON-N

CIV

propoxyphene napsylate (Xanodyne)

THERAPEUTIC CLASS: Opioid analgesic

INDICATIONS: Relief of mild to moderate pain.

DOSAGE: *Adults:* Usual: 100mg q4h prn pain. Max: 600mg/day. Elderly: Increase dose interval. Hepatic/Renal Impairment: Reduce daily dose.

HOW SUPPLIED: Tab: 100mg

WARNINGS/PRECAUTIONS: Avoid in suicidal or addiction-prone patients. May produce drug dependence in higher than recommended doses. May impair mental/physical ability. Caution with hepatic or renal impairment. Do not exceed recommended dose and limit alcohol intake.

ADVERSE REACTIONS: Dizziness, sedation, NV, constipation, abdominal pain, skin rashes, lightheadedness, headache, weakness, euphoria, dysphoria, hallucinations.

INTERACTIONS: Additive CNS-depressant effect with other CNS depressants, including alcohol. Increases plasma levels of antidepressants, anticonvulsants, and warfarin-like drugs. Severe neurologic signs, including coma, reported with carbamazepine. Caution with tranquilizers, antidepressants, and excessive alcohol use.

PREGNANCY: Safety in pregnancy and nursing not known.

MECHANISM OF ACTION: Centrally acting narcotic analgesic agent.

PHARMACOKINETICS: Absorption: C_{max}=0.05-0.1mcg/mL; T_{max}=2-2.5 hrs. **Distribution:** Found in breast milk. **Metabolism:** Liver; norpropoxyphene (active metabolite). **Elimination:** $T_{1/2}$=6-12 hrs, 30-36 hrs (active metabolite).

NURSING CONSIDERATIONS

Assessment: Assess for abuse potential, suicidal tendencies, previous history of emotional disorders, alcoholism, renal/hepatic function, age of patient, pregnancy/nursing status, and possible drug interactions.

Monitoring: Monitor for signs/symptoms of CNS depression, drug dependence, liver dysfunction. Monitor for subacute painful myopathy if chronic overdosage occurs.

Patient Counseling: Counsel that drug may impair mental/physical abilities; use caution when performing hazardous tasks (eg, operating machinery/driving). Advise to avoid using other CNS depressants and alcohol during therapy. Counsel to notify physician of all medications currently taken. Inform that dependence may occur if higher than recommended dose taken for a longer period of time.

Storage: Oral route. **Storage:** 25°C (77°F); excursions permitted to 15-30°C (59-86°F).

D

DAYTRANA

methylphenidate (Shire)

CII

THERAPEUTIC CLASS: Sympathomimetic amine

INDICATIONS: Treatment of attention deficit hyperactivity disorder (ADHD).

DOSAGE: *Adults:* Individualize dose. Apply to hip area 2 hrs before effect is needed and remove 9 hrs after application. Recommended Titration Schedule: Week 1: 10mg/9 hrs. Week 2: 15mg/9 hrs. Week 3: 20mg/9 hrs. Week 4: 30mg/9 hrs.
Pediatrics: ≥6 yrs: Individualize dose. Apply to hip area 2 hrs before effect is needed and remove 9 hrs after application. Recommended Titration Schedule: Week 1: 10mg/9 hrs. Week 2: 15mg/9 hrs. Week 3: 20mg/9 hrs. Week 4: 30mg/9 hrs.

HOW SUPPLIED: Patch: 10mg/9 hrs, 15mg/9 hrs, 20mg/9 hrs, 30mg/9 hrs [10^s, 30^s]

CONTRAINDICATIONS: Marked anxiety, tension, and agitation; glaucoma; motor tics or family history or diagnosis of Tourette's syndrome; treatment with MAOIs and within minimum of 14 days following discontinuation.

WARNINGS/PRECAUTIONS: Avoid use with known structural cardiac abnormalities; sudden death reported. D/C if contact sensitization is suspected. Monitor growth during treatment. May exacerbate symptoms of behavior disturbance and thought disorder in psychotic patients. Caution when using stimulants to treat patients with comorbid bipolar disorder because of concern for possible induction of mixed/manic episode in such patients. Stimulants at usual doses can cause treatment emergent psychotic or manic symptoms (eg, hallucinations, delusional thinking, mania) in children and adolescents without prior history of psychotic illness. Aggressive behavior or hostility reported in clinical trials and postmarketing experience of some medications indicated for the treatment of ADHD. May lower convulsive threshold; d/c in the presence of seizures. Caution with HTN; monitor BP. Caution when underlying medical conditions might be compromised by increases in BP or HR (eg, pre-existing HTN, heart failure, recent MI, or hyperthyroidism). Visual disturbances reported. Caution with history of drug dependence or alcoholism. Avoid exposing application site to external heat sources (eg, heating pads, electric blankets, heated water beds, etc). Monitor CBC, differential, and platelet counts during prolonged therapy.

ADVERSE REACTIONS: NV, nasopharyngitis, weight decrease, anorexia, decreased appetite, affect lability, insomnia, tics, nasal congestion.

D

INTERACTIONS: See Contraindications. Caution with pressor agents. May decrease effectiveness of antihypertensive agents. May inhibit metabolism of coumarin anticoagulants, anticonvulsants (eg, phenobarbital, phenytoin, primidone), some tricyclic drugs (eg, imipramine, clomipramine, desipramine), and SSRIs. Monitor drug levels (or coagulation times with coumarin) and consider dose adjustments with concomitant use. Serious adverse events reported with concomitant clonidine use.

PREGNANCY: Category C, caution in nursing.

MECHANISM OF ACTION: Sympathomimetic amine; CNS stimulant. Suspected to block reuptake of norepinephrine and dopamine into presynaptic neuron and increase release of these monoamines into neuronal spaces.

PHARMACOKINETICS: Absorption: C_{max}=39ng/mL; T_{max}=7.5-10.5 hrs. **Distribution:** Plasma concentrations decline in biexponential manner due to continued distribution from skin after patch removal. **Metabolism:** De-esterification; ritalinic acid (metabolite). **Elimination:** $T_{1/2}$=3-4 hrs (*d*-methylphenidate); $T_{1/2}$=1.4-2.9 hrs (*l*-methylphenidate).

NURSING CONSIDERATIONS

Assessment: Assess for marked anxiety, tension, agitation, known hypersensitivity to methylphenidate, glaucoma, motor tics, family history or diagnosis of Tourette's syndrome, behavior disturbances, thought disorder, bipolar disorder, depression, family history of suicide, pre-existing structural cardiac abnormalities, cardiomyopathy, heart rhythm abnormalities, CAD, HTN, heart failure, recent MI, psychiatric history, history of seizures, prior EEG abnormalities in absence of seizures, and patients without history of seizures and with no prior EEG evidence of seizures. Assess for history of drug dependence or alcoholism.

Monitoring: Monitor periodically for long-term usefulness, possible drug interactions, BP, HR, contact sensitization evidenced by erythema, edema, papules, vesicles, psychotic or manic symptoms such as hallucinations, delusional thinking, mania, confused state, crying, tics, headaches, irritability, anorexia, insomnia, infectious mononucleosis, and viral infection. Monitor for appearance of or worsening aggressive behavior or hostility. Perform follow-up weight and height in children 7-10 yrs. Periodic CBC, differential, and platelet counts are advised during prolonged therapy.

Patient Counseling: Counsel about drug abuse/dependence potential. Advise to avoid exposing application site to direct external heat sources while wearing the patch. Inform to apply patch to a clean, dry site on hip. Site of application must be alternated daily and patch should not be applied to waistline, where tight clothing may rub the patch. Encourage patient or caregiver to use administration chart to monitor application and removal time, and method of disposal. Patient or caregiver should avoid touching adhesive side of patch during application; if touched, wash hands after application. If any swelling or blistering occurs, remove patch; inform physician. Do not apply hydrocortisone or other solutions, creams, ointments, or emollients immediately prior to patch application. Inform of drug's side effects (heart-related problems, mental problems); notify physician if any occur.

Administration: Transdermal. Once tray is opened, use contents within 2 months. Apply patch immediately upon removal from protective pouch. If patch does not fully adhere to skin, or is partially or fully detached during wear time, discard patch and apply a new one. Inspect release liner to ensure no adhesive-containing medication has transferred to liner; if adhesive transfer has occurred, discard patch. If a patch is replaced, total recommended wear time for the day should remain 9 hrs. Peel patches off slowly. Patches should not be applied or re-applied with dressings, tape, or other common adhesives. **Storage:** Store at 25°C (77°F); excursions permitted to 15-30°C (59-86°F). Do not store patches unpouched. Do not refrigerate or freeze patches.

DDAVP

RX

desmopressin acetate (Sanofi-Aventis)

OTHER BRAND NAMES: DDAVP Nasal Spray (Sanofi-Aventis) - DDAVP Rhinal Tube (Sanofi-Aventis)

THERAPEUTIC CLASS: Synthetic vasopressin analog

INDICATIONS: (Tab) Management of primary nocturnal enuresis. (Inj/Nasal Spray/Rhinal Tube/Tab) As antidiuretic replacement therapy in management of central (cranial) diabetes insipidus. Management of temporary polyuria and polydipsia following head trauma or surgery in pituitary region. (Inj) Hemophilia A with factor VIII coagulant activity levels >5% and mild to moderate classic von Willebrand's disease (Type I) with factor VIII levels >5%.

DOSAGE: *Adults:* Diabetes Insipidus: (Tab) Initial: 0.05mg bid. Titrate: May increase/decrease by 0.1-1.2mg/day given bid-tid. Maint: 0.1-0.8mg/day in divided doses. (Spray/Tube) Usual: 0.1-4mL/day given qd-tid. (Inj) 0.5-1mL/day IV/SQ given bid. Hemophilia A/von Willebrand's Disease: (Inj) 0.3mcg/kg IV over 15-30 min. Add 50mL diluent. If used pre-op, give 30 min before procedure.
Pediatrics: Diabetes Insipidus: (Tab) ≥4 yrs: Initial: 0.05mg bid. Titrate: May increase/decrease by 0.1-1.2mg/day given bid-tid. Maint: 0.1-0.8mg/day in divided doses. (Spray/Tube) 3 months-12 yrs: Usual: 0.05-0.3mL/day given qd-bid. (Inj) ≥12 yrs: 0.5-1mL/day IV/SQ given bid. Hemophilia A/von Willebrand's Disease: (Inj) ≥3 months: 0.3mcg/kg IV over 15-30 min. Add 50mL diluent (>10kg) or 10mL diluent (≤10kg). If used pre-op, give 30 min before procedure.

HOW SUPPLIED: Inj: 4mcg/mL; Nasal Spray: 10mcg/inh [5mL]; Tab: 0.1mg*, 0.2mg*; Rhinal Tube: 0.01% [2.5mL] *scored

CONTRAINDICATIONS: Moderate to severe renal impairment (CrCL<50mL/min), hyponatremia, or history of hyponatremia.

WARNINGS/PRECAUTIONS: Mucosal changes with nasal forms may occur; d/c until resolved. Decrease fluid intake in pediatrics and elderly to decrease risk of water intoxication and hyponatremia; monitor osmolality. Caution with coronary artery insufficiency, hypertensive cardiovascular disease, fluid and electrolyte imbalance (eg, cystic fibrosis). Anaphylaxis reported with IV use. Caution with IV use if history of thrombus formation. For diabetes insipidus, dosage must be adjusted according to diurnal pattern of response; estimate response by adequate duration of sleep and adequate, not excessive, water turnover.

ADVERSE REACTIONS: Inj: Headache, nausea, abdominal cramps, vulval pain, injection site reactions, facial flushing, BP changes. Spray: Headache, dizziness, rhinitis, nausea, nasal congestion, sore throat, cough, respiratory infection, epistaxis. Tab: Nausea, flushing, abdominal cramps, headache, increased SGOT, water intoxication, hyponatremia.

INTERACTIONS: Caution with other pressor agents.

PREGNANCY: Category B, caution in nursing.

MECHANISM OF ACTION: Synthetic vasopressin analog; antidiuretic affecting renal water conservation.

PHARMACOKINETICS: Absorption: (Inj) Rapid, T_{max}=90 min-2 hrs. (Tab, Nasal) Rapid, T_{max}=0.9-1.5 hrs. **Elimination:** Urine; (Inj, Nasal) $T_{1/2}$=3 hrs; (Tab) 1.5-2.5 hrs.

NURSING CONSIDERATIONS

Assessment: Assess for hypersensitivity, factor VIII (antibodies, coagulant activity levels, abnormal molecular form of antigen), hemophilia A or B, von Willebrand's disease, renal impairment, hyponatremia, habitual or psychogenic polydipsia, coronary artery insufficiency, HTN, electrolyte imbalance disorders (eg, CF, CHF, renal disorders), risk factors for thrombus formation, and possible drug interactions. (Nasal, Rhinal Tube) Assess for factors against nasal insufflation (eg, nasal congestion, blockage, discharge, atrophy, severe rhinitis, impaired level of consciousness). Obtain baseline bleeding time, ristocetin cofactor activity, renal function, urine volume, and osmolality.

Monitoring: Monitor bleeding time, factor VIII coagulant activity, ristocetin cofactor activity, von Willebrand's factor, diabetes insipidus, renal function, urine volume and osmolality periodically. (Nasal, Rhinal tube) Changes in nasal mucosa (eg, scarring, edema, blockage, congestion, discharge, impaired level of consciousness), signs/symptoms of renal dysfunction, hyponatremia (eg, headache, NV, weight gain, fatigue), coronary artery insufficiency, HTN, electrolyte imbalance, thrombus formation, water intoxication, hypersensitivity, and allergic reactions.

Patient Counseling: Counsel to seek medical attention if flushing, headache, NV, abdominal pain, weight gain, fatigue, dizziness, cough, chills, HTN, thrombus formation, water intoxication, hypersensitivity, or allergic reactions occur. If using nasal spray or rhinal tube, inform that administration should be under adult supervision to control dose intake, and to contact physician if symptoms of nasal blockage, discharge, or congestion occur.

Administration: Intranasal/IV/SQ/Oral routes. Refer to PI for specific administration techniques. **Storage:** Inj: 2-8°C (36-46°F). Tab: 20-25°C (68-77°F); avoid exposure to excessive light or heat. Nasal Spray: 20-25°C (68-77°F) in upright position. Rhinal Tube: 2-8°C (36-46°F); closed bottles stable for 3 weeks at 20-25°C (68-77°F).

DEMADEX — RX

torsemide (Roche Labs)

THERAPEUTIC CLASS: Loop diuretic

INDICATIONS: Treatment of edema associated with CHF, renal disease, chronic renal failure or hepatic disease. Treatment of hypertension.

DOSAGE: *Adults:* PO/IV (bolus over 2 min or continuous): CHF: Initial: 10-20mg qd. Max: 200mg single dose. Chronic Renal Failure: Initial: 20mg qd. Max: 200mg single dose. Hepatic Cirrhosis: Initial: 5-10mg qd with aldosterone antagonist or K^+-sparing diuretic. Titrate: Double dose. Max: 40mg single dose. HTN: Initial: 5mg qd. Titrate: May increase to 10mg qd in 4-6 weeks, then may add additional antihypertensive agent.

HOW SUPPLIED: Inj: 10mg/mL; Tab: 5mg*, 10mg*, 20mg*, 100mg* *scored

CONTRAINDICATIONS: Anuria, sulfonamide hypersensitivity.

WARNINGS/PRECAUTIONS: Caution with cirrhosis and ascites in hepatic disease. Tinnitus and hearing loss (usually reversible) reported. Avoid excessive diuresis, especially in elderly. Caution with brisk diuresis, inadequate oral intake of electrolytes, and cardiovascular disease, especially with digitalis glycosides. Monitor for electrolyte/volume depletion. Hyperglycemia, hypokalemia, hypermagnesemia, hypercalcemia, gout reported. May increase cholesterol and TG.

ADVERSE REACTIONS: Headache, excessive urination, dizziness, cough, ECG abnormality, asthenia, rhinitis, diarrhea.

INTERACTIONS: Caution with high-dose salicylates, aminoglycosides. Lithium toxicity. Indomethacin partially inhibits natriuretic effect. Avoid simultaneous cholestyramine administration. Probenecid decreases effects. Reduces spironolactone clearance. Risk of hypokalemia with ACTH, corticosteroids. Possible renal dysfunction with NSAIDs.

PREGNANCY: Category B, caution in nursing.

MECHANISM OF ACTION: Pyridine-sulfonylurea diuretic; acts within lumen of thick ascending part of loop of Henle, inhibiting $Na^+/K^+/2Cl^-$ carrier system.

PHARMACOKINETICS: Absorption: Absolute bioavailability (80%); T_{max}=1 hr. **Distribution:** V_d=12-15L; plasma protein binding (>99%). **Metabolism:** Carboxylic acid (major metabolite). **Elimination:** Urine; $T_{1/2}$=3.5 hrs.

NURSING CONSIDERATIONS

Assessment: Assess for sulfonamide hypersensitivity, anuria, CVD, possible drug interactions, renal/hepatic impairment.

Monitoring: Monitor serum electrolytes, serum K^+ levels, and renal function. Monitor for signs/symptoms of hypokalemia, electrolyte imbalance, arrhythmias, ototoxicity, hypersensitivity reactions, renal/hepatic dysfunction.

Patient Counseling: Advise to seek medical attention if symptoms of hypokalemia, electrolyte imbalance, hypersensitivity reactions, hearing loss or tinnitus occur.

Administration: IV, oral route. **Storage:** 15-30°C (59-86°F). Do not freeze.

Demerol Injection

CII

meperidine HCl (Hospira)

THERAPEUTIC CLASS: Opioid analgesic

INDICATIONS: For relief of moderate to severe pain. For preoperative medication, anesthesia support, and obstetrical analgesia.

DOSAGE: *Adults:* Pain: Usual: 50-150mg IM/SQ q3-4h prn. Preoperative: Usual: 50-100mg IM/SQ 30-90 min before anesthesia. Anesthesia Support: Use repeated slow IV inj of fractional doses (eg, 10mg/mL) or continuous IV infusion of a more dilute solution (eg, 1mg/mL). Titrate as needed. Obstetrical Analgesia: Usual: 50-100mg IM/SQ when pain is regular, may repeat at 1- to 3-hr intervals. Elderly: Start at lower end of dosage range and observe. With Phenothiazines/Other Tranquilizers: Reduce dose by 25 to 50%. IM method preferred with repeated use. For IV injection: Reduce dose and administer slowly, preferably using diluted solution.
Pediatrics: Pain: Usual: 0.5-0.8mg/lb IM/SQ, up to 50-150mg, q3-4h prn. Preoperative: Usual: 0.5-1mg/lb IM/SQ, up to 50-100mg, 30-90 min before anesthesia. With Phenothiazines/Other Tranquilizers: Reduce dose by 25 to 50%. IM method preferred with repeated use. For IV injection: Reduce dose and administer slowly, preferably using diluted solution.

HOW SUPPLIED: Inj: 25mg/mL, 50mg/mL, 75mg/mL, 100mg/mL

CONTRAINDICATIONS: MAOIs during or within 14 days of use.

WARNINGS/PRECAUTIONS: May develop tolerance and dependence; abuse potential. Extreme caution with head injury, increased ICP, intracranial lesions, acute asthmatic attack, chronic COPD or cor pulmonale, decreased respiratory reserve, respiratory depression, hypoxia, and hypercapnia. Rapid IV infusion may result in increased adverse reactions. Caution with acute abdominal conditions, atrial flutter, supraventricular tachycardias. May aggravate convulsive disorders. Caution and reduce initial dose with elderly or debilitated, renal/hepatic impairment, hypothyroidism, Addison's disease, prostatic hypertrophy or urethral stricture. Severe hypotension may occur post-op or if depleted blood volume. Orthostatic hypotension may occur. May impair mental/physical abilities. Not for use in pregnancy prior to labor. May produce depression of respiration and psychophysiologic functions in newborn when used as an obstetrical analgesic.

ADVERSE REACTIONS: Lightheadedness, dizziness, sedation, NV, sweating, respiratory/circulatory depression.

INTERACTIONS: See Contraindications. Caution and reduce dose with other CNS depressants (eg, narcotics, anesthetics, phenothiazines, tranquilizers, sedative-hypnotics, TCAs, alcohol).

PREGNANCY: Safety in pregnancy and nursing not known.

MECHANISM OF ACTION: Narcotic analgesic; produces actions similiar to morphine. Principle actions involve the CNS and organs composed of smooth muscle. Produces analgesic and sedative effects.

PHARMACOKINETICS: Distribution: Crosses placental barrier; found in breast milk.

NURSING CONSIDERATIONS

Assessment: Assess for presence of head injury, intracranial lesions, presence of elevated intracranial pressure, nursing/pregnancy status, presence of acute asthmatic attack, COPD or cor pulmonale, respiratory depression, hypotension, atrial flutter and other supraventricular tachycardias, convulsive disorders, acute abdominal conditions, hepatic/renal impairment, hypothyroidism, Addison's disease, prostatic hypertrophy or urethral stricture, and drug interactions (eg, MAO inhibitors).

Monitoring: Monitor for signs/symptoms of drug dependence (eg, psychic dependence, physical dependence), respiratory depression, circulatory depression (eg, hypotension), and convulsions.

Patient Counseling: Inform that medication may impair mental/physical abilities; use caution when performing hazardous tasks (eg, operating machinery/driving). Advise to notify physician of all medications currently taken. Instruct patient cannot take medication if an MAO inhibitor was used within previous 14 days. Avoid using other CNS depressants and alcohol during medication. Advise about potential for dependence upon repeated administration. Inform women in labor that medication crosses placental barrier and can produce depression of respiration and psychophysiologic function in newborn.

Administration: SQ, IM, IV route. SQ route is suitable for occasional use, IM administration is preferred if repeated doses are required. IM injection should be injected well into the body of a large muscle. If IV route is required, dosage should be decreased and injection should be made very slowly, preferably using a diluted solution. Dosage should be adjusted according to severity of pain. **Storage:** 20-25°C (68-77°F).

DEMEROL ORAL

CII

meperidine HCl (Sanofi-Aventis)

THERAPEUTIC CLASS: Opioid analgesic

INDICATIONS: Moderate to severe pain.

DOSAGE: *Adults:* Usual: 50-150mg q3-4h prn. Concomitant Phenothiazines/Other Tranquilizers: Reduce dose by 25-50%. Dilute syrup in 1/2 glass of water. *Pediatrics:* Usual: 1.1-1.8mg/kg up to 50-150mg q3-4h prn. Concomitant Phenothiazines/Other Tranquilizers: Reduce dose by 25-50%. Dilute syrup in 1/2 glass of water.

HOW SUPPLIED: Syrup: 50mg/5mL; Tab: 50mg*, 100mg *scored

CONTRAINDICATIONS: MAOI during or within 14 days of use.

WARNINGS/PRECAUTIONS: May develop tolerance and dependence; abuse potential. Extreme caution with head injury, increased ICP, intracranial lesions, acute asthma attack, chronic COPD, cor pulmonale, decreased respiratory reserve, respiratory depression, hypoxia, and hypercapnia. Caution with sickle cell anemia, pheochromocytoma, acute alcoholism, Addison's disease, CNS depression or coma, delirium tremens, elderly or debilitated, kyphoscoliosis associated with respiratory depression, myxedema, hypothyroidism, acute abdominal conditions, epilepsy, atrial flutter, other supraventricular tachycardias, renal/hepatic impairment, prostatic hypertrophy, urethral stricture, drug dependencies, neonates, and young infants. Severe hypotension may occur post-op or if depleted blood volume. Orthostatic hypotension may occur. Not for use in pregnancy prior to labor.

ADVERSE REACTIONS: Lightheadedness, dizziness, sedation, N/V, sweating, respiratory depression.

INTERACTIONS: See Contraindications. Reduce dose with other CNS depressants (eg, narcotics, anesthetics, phenothiazines, tranquilizers, sedative-hypnotics, TCAs, alcohol). Mixed agonist/antagonist analgesics (eg, pentazocine, nalbuphine, butorphanol, buprenorphine) may reduce analgesic effects and/or precipitate withdrawal symptoms. Caution with acyclovir, cimetidine. Phenytoin may enhance hepatic metabolism. May enhance neuroblocking action of skeletal muscle relaxants. Increased levels with ritonavir; avoid concurrent administration.

PREGNANCY: Category C, not for use in nursing.

MECHANISM OF ACTION: Narcotic analgesic; produces actions similiar to morphine. Principle actions involve the CNS and organs composed of smooth muscle. Produces analgesic and sedative effects.

PHARMACOKINETICS: Distribution: Crosses placental barrier; found in breast milk.

NURSING CONSIDERATIONS

Assessment: Assess for abuse potential, head injury or intracranial lesions, presence of elevated ICP, presence of acute asthmatic attack, COPD, respiratory depression, hypotension, atrial flutter and other supraventricular tachycardias, pregnancy/nursing status, hepatic/renal impairment, sickle cell anemia, pheochromocytoma, acute alcoholism, adrenocortical insufficiency (eg, Addison's disease), CNS depression or coma, delirium tremens, convulsive disorders, presence of debilitation, myxedema or hypothyroidism, acute abdominal conditions, prostatic hypertrophy or urethral stricture, toxic psychosis, and possible drug interactions (eg, MAO inhibitors).

Monitoring: Monitor for signs/symptoms of tolerance or dependence, misuse or abuse, increase in CSF pressure, circulatory depression (eg, hypotension), respiratory depression, and convulsions.

Patient Counseling: Counsel to notify physician of all medications currently taken. Inform patient cannot take medication if MAO inhibitor was used within previous 14 days. Notify physician of any adverse events. Do not adjust dosage without consulting physician. Medication has potential of drug abuse. Avoid abrupt withdrawal if on chronic therapy. Drug may impair mental/physical abilities; use caution when performing hazardous tasks (eg, operating machinery, driving). Avoid using other CNS depressants and alcohol. Inform pregnant women about effects of medication on pregnancy. Instruct that if taking oral sol formulation, to take medication in half glass of water to prevent slight anesthetic effect on mucous membranes.

Administration: Oral route. **Storage:** 25°C (77°F); excursions permitted to 15-30°C (59-86°F).

DENAVIR — RX

penciclovir (Novartis)

THERAPEUTIC CLASS: Nucleoside analogue

INDICATIONS: Treatment of recurrent herpes labialis (cold sores) in adults and children ≥12 yrs.

DOSAGE: *Adults:* Apply q2h while awake for 4 days. Start with earliest sign or symptom.
Pediatrics: ≥12 yrs: Apply q2h while awake for 4 days. Start with earliest sign or symptom.

HOW SUPPLIED: Cre: 1% [1.5g]

WARNINGS/PRECAUTIONS: Only use on herpes labialis on the lips and face. Avoid mucous membranes or near the eyes. Effectiveness not established in immunocompromised patients.

ADVERSE REACTIONS: Headache, application site reaction, local anesthesia, taste perversion, rash.

PREGNANCY: Category B, not for use in nursing.

MECHANISM OF ACTION: Antiviral agent; active against herpes simplex virus types 1 (HSV-1) and 2 (HSV-2). Inhibits HSV polymerase competitively with deoxyguanosine triphosphate. Consequently, herpes viral DNA synthesis and replication are selectively inhibited.

NURSING CONSIDERATIONS

Assessment: Assess use in pregnancy/nursing.

Monitoring: Monitor lesions for clinical response. If lesions worsen or do not improve, monitor for secondary bacterial infection.

Patient Counseling: Counsel to avoid applying medication in or near eyes. Instruct to wash hands with soap and water after applying product. Advise females to notify physician if they become pregnant or are nursing.

Administration: Topical. **Storage**: 20-25°C (68-77°F).

DEPACON
RX

valproate sodium (Abbott)

Fatal hepatic failure (<2 yrs at considerable risk), teratogenic effects (eg, neural tube defects), and life-threatening pancreatitis reported.

D

THERAPEUTIC CLASS: Carboxylic acid derivative

INDICATIONS: Monotherapy and adjunctive therapy for treatment of simple and complex absence seizures, and complex partial seizures. Adjunct therapy for multiple seizure types.

DOSAGE: *Adults:* Simplex/Complex Absence Seizure: Initial: 15mg/kg/day. Titrate: Increase weekly by 5-10mg/kg/day until optimal response. Max: 60mg/kg/day. Complex Partial Seizure: Initial: 10-15mg/kg/day. Titrate: Increase weekly by 5-10mg/kg/day until optimal response. Max: 60mg/kg/day. Elderly: Reduce initial dose and titrate slowly. If dose >250mg/day, give in divided doses. Administer as 60 min IV infusion, not >20mg/min. Not for use >14 days; switch to oral route as soon as clinically feasible. Decrease dose or d/c if decreased food or fluid intake or if excessive somnolence occurs.
Pediatrics: ≥2 yrs: Simplex/Complex Absence Seizure: Initial: 15mg/kg/day. Titrate: Increase weekly by 5-10mg/kg/day until optimal response. Max: 60mg/kg/day. ≥10 yrs: Complex Partial Seizure: Initial: 10-15mg/kg/day. Titrate: Increase weekly by 5-10mg/kg/day until optimal response. Max: 60mg/kg/day. If dose >250mg/day, give in divided doses. Administer as 60 min IV infusion, not >20mg/min. Not for use >14 days; switch to oral route as soon as clinically feasible. Decrease dose or d/c with decreased food or fluid intake and if excessive somnolence.

HOW SUPPLIED: Inj: 100mg/mL

CONTRAINDICATIONS: Hepatic disease, significant hepatic dysfunction, known urea cycle disorders (UCD).

WARNINGS/PRECAUTIONS: Hyperammonemic encephalopathy in UCD patients; d/c if this occurs. Prior to therapy, evaluate for UCD in high risk patients (eg, history of unexplained encephalopathy, coma, etc). Measure ammonia levels if develop unexplained lethargy, vomiting, or mental status changes. Caution in elderly; monitor for fluid/nutritional intake, dehydration, somnolence. Monitor LFTs before therapy and during 1st 6 months. D/C if develop hepatic dysfunction, pancreatitis. Increased risk of hepatotoxicity with multiple anticonvulsants, congenital metabolic disorders, severe seizure disorder with mental retardation, organic brain disease, children <2 yrs. Avoid abrupt withdrawal. Monitor platelets and coagulation tests before therapy and periodically thereafter. Elevated liver enzymes and thrombocytopenia may be dose-related. Not for prophylaxis of post-traumatic seizures in acute head trauma. May interfere with urine ketone and thyroid function tests.

ADVERSE REACTIONS: Dizziness, headache, nausea, local reactions.

INTERACTIONS: Clonazepam may induce absence status in patients with absence seizures. Potentiates amitriptyline, nortriptyline, carbamazepine, diazepam, ethosuximide, lamotrigine, phenobarbital, primidone, phenytoin, tolbutamide, warfarin, zidovudine. Potentiated by ASA and felbamate. Antagonized by rifampin, carbamazepine, phenobarbital, phenytoin. Additive CNS depression with other CNS depressants (eg, alcohol).

PREGNANCY: Category D, not for use in nursing.

MECHANISM OF ACTION: Anticonvulsant; increases GABA concentrations in the brain.

PHARMACOKINETICS: Absorption: T_{max}=1 hr. **Distribution:** Plasma protein binding (10%-18.5%). **Metabolism:** Liver; glucuronidation, mitochondrial β-oxidation. **Elimination:** Urine (<3% unchanged); $T_{1/2}$=16 hrs.

NURSING CONSIDERATIONS

Assessment: Assess LFTs, CBC with platelets, pancreatitis, plasma ammonia levels, and pregnancy status. Note other diseases/conditions and drug therapies.

Monitoring: Monitor LFTs, CBC with platelets, coagulation parameters, pancreatitis, hypersensitivity reactions, hyperammonemia, thyroid function tests.

Patient Counseling: Advise to avoid alcohol, sedatives, and other OTCs; caution while operating machinery/driving. Counsel about signs/symptoms of pancreatitis, hyperammonemia; report any symptoms.

Administration: IV route. Give as a 60-min infusion after diluting with at least 50mL of a compatible diluent. **Storage:** 15-30°C (59-86°F).

DEPAKENE RX

valproic acid (Abbott)

Fatal hepatic failure (<2 yrs at considerable risk), teratogenic effects (eg, neural tube defects), and life-threatening pancreatitis reported.

THERAPEUTIC CLASS: Carboxylic acid derivative

INDICATIONS: Monotherapy and adjunctive therapy for treatment of simple and complex absence seizures, and complex partial seizures. Adjunct therapy for multiple seizure types.

DOSAGE: *Adults:* Simplex/Complex Absence Seizure: Initial: 15mg/kg/day. Titrate: Increase weekly by 5-10mg/kg/day until optimal response. Max: 60mg/kg/day. Complex Partial Seizure: Initial: 10-15mg/kg/day. Titrate: Increase weekly by 5-10mg/kg/day until optimal response. Max: 60mg/kg/day. If dose >250mg/day, give in divided doses. Elderly: Reduce initial dose. Swallow caps whole, do not chew.
Pediatrics: ≥10 yrs: Complex Partial Seizure: Initial: 10-15mg/kg/day. Titrate: Increase weekly by 5-10mg/kg/day until optimal response. Max: 60mg/kg/day. If dose >250mg/day, give in divided doses. Swallow caps whole, do not chew.

HOW SUPPLIED: Cap: 250mg; Syrup: 250mg/5mL

CONTRAINDICATIONS: Hepatic disease, significant hepatic dysfunction, known urea cycle disorders (UCD).

WARNINGS/PRECAUTIONS: Hyperammonemic encephalopathy in UCD patients; d/c if this occurs. Prior to therapy, evaluate for UCD in high risk patients (eg, history of unexplained encephalopathy, coma, etc). Measure ammonia levels if develop unexplained lethargy, vomiting, or mental status changes. Caution in elderly; monitor for fluid/nutritional intake, dehydration, somnolence. Monitor LFTs before therapy and during 1st 6 months. D/C if develop hepatic dysfunction, pancreatitis. Increased risk of hepatotoxicity with multiple anticonvulsants, congenital metabolic disorders, severe seizure disorder with mental retardation, organic brain disease, children <2 yrs. Avoid abrupt withdrawal. Hyperammonemia reported. Monitor platelets and coagulation tests before therapy and periodically thereafter. Elevated liver enzymes and thrombocytopenia may be dose-related. May interfere with urine ketone and thyroid function tests.

ADVERSE REACTIONS: Headache, asthenia, nausea, vomiting, diarrhea, abdominal pain, somnolence, tremor, dizziness, thrombocytopenia, ecchymosis, nystagmus, alopecia.

INTERACTIONS: Clonazepam may induce absence status in patients with absence seizures. Potentiates amitriptyline, nortriptyline, carbamazepine, diazepam, ethosuximide, lamotrigine, phenobarbital, primidone, phenytoin, tolbutamide, warfarin, zidovudine. Potentiated by ASA and felbamate. Antagonized by rifampin, carbamazepine, phenobarbital, phenytoin. Additive CNS depression with other CNS depressants (eg, alcohol).

PREGNANCY: Category D, not for use in nursing.

MECHANISM OF ACTION: Anticonvulsant; increases GABA concentration in the brain.

PHARMACOKINETICS: Absorption: T_{max}=4-8 hrs (tab), T_{max}=3.3-4.8 hrs (caps). **Distribution:** V_d=11L/1.73m²; plasma protein binding (10%-18.5%). **Metabolism:** Liver; glucuronidation, mitochondrial β-oxidation. **Elimination:** Urine (<3% unchanged); $T_{1/2}$=9-16 hrs.

NURSING CONSIDERATIONS

D

Assessment: Assess LFTs, CBC with platelets, pancreatitis, plasma ammonia levels, pregnancy status. Note other diseases/conditions and drug therapies.

Monitoring: Monitor LFTs, CBC with platelets, coagulation parameters, pancreatitis, thyroid disorders, hypersensitivity reactions, hyperammonemia, and thyroid function tests.

Patient Counseling: Counsel to avoid alcohol, sedatives, OTCs. Caution while operating machinery/driving. Counsel about signs/symptoms of pancreatitis, hyperammonemia; notify if symptoms occur, report any adverse effects.

Administration: Oral route. **Storage:** Capsule: 15-25°C (59-77°F). Oral solution: Below 30°C (86°F).

DEPAKOTE — RX

divalproex sodium (Abbott)

Fatal hepatic failure (<2 yrs at considerable risk), teratogenic effects (eg, neural tube defects), and life-threatening pancreatitis reported.

THERAPEUTIC CLASS: Valproate compound

INDICATIONS: (Tab, Cap) Management of simple and complex absence seizures; complex partial seizures; and adjunctively with multiple seizure types including absence seizures. (Tab) Treatment of mania associated with bipolar disorder and migraine prophylaxis.

DOSAGE: *Adults:* (Cap/Tab) Complex Partial Seizures: Initial: 10-15mg/kg/day. Titrate: Increase by 5-10mg/kg/week. Max: 60mg/kg/day. Absence Seizures: Initial: 15mg/kg/day. Titrate: Increase weekly by 5-10mg/kg/day. Max: 60mg/kg/day. Give in divided doses if >250mg/day. (Tab) Migraine: Initial: ≥16 yrs: 250mg bid. Max: 1000mg/day. Mania: 750mg daily in divided doses. Titrate: Increase dose rapidly to clinical effect. Max: 60mg/kg/day. Elderly: Reduce initial dose and titrate slowly. Decrease dose or d/c if decreased food or fluid intake or if excessive somnolence occurs.
Pediatrics: ≥10 yrs: (Cap/Tab) Complex Partial Seizures: Initial: 10-15mg/kg/day. Titrate: Increase by 5-10mg/kg/week. Max: 60mg/kg/day. Absence Seizures: Initial: 15mg/kg/day. Titrate: Increase weekly by 5-10mg/kg/day. Max: 60mg/kg/day. Give in divided doses if >250mg/day.

HOW SUPPLIED: Cap, Delayed-Release: (Sprinkle) 125mg; Tab, Delayed-Release: 125mg, 250mg, 500mg

CONTRAINDICATIONS: Hepatic disease, significant hepatic dysfunction, known urea cycle disorders (UCD).

WARNINGS/PRECAUTIONS: Hyperammonemic encephalopathy in UCD patients; d/c if this occurs. Prior to therapy, evaluate for UCD in high risk patients (eg, history of unexplained encephalopathy, coma, etc). Measure ammonia levels if develop unexplained lethargy, vomiting, or mental status changes. Caution with hepatic disease. Check LFTs prior to therapy, then frequently during 1st six months. Dose-related thrombocytopenia and elevated liver enzymes reported. Monitor platelet and coagulation tests prior to therapy, then periodically. Altered thyroid function tests and urine ketone test. May stimulate replication of HIV and CMV viruses. Avoid abrupt discontinuation.

ADVERSE REACTIONS: Diarrhea, N/V, somnolence, dyspepsia, thrombocytopenia, asthenia, abdominal pain, tremor, headache, anorexia, diplopia, blurred vision, weight gain, ataxia, nystagmus.

INTERACTIONS: Potentiates carbamazepine, amitriptyline, nortriptyline, diazepam, ethosuximide, primidone, lamotrigine, phenobarbital, phenytoin, tolbutamide, zidovudine, lorazepam. Efficacy potentiated by ASA, felbamate. Efficacy reduced by rifampin, carbamazepine, phenobarbital, phenytoin, primidone. Clonazepam may induce absence status in patients with absence type seizures. CNS depression with alcohol and other CNS depressants. Monitor PT/INR with warfarin.

PREGNANCY: Category D, not for use in nursing.

MECHANISM OF ACTION: Anticonvulsant; increases GABA concentrations in the brain.

PHARMACOKINETICS: Absorption: T_{max}=4-8 hrs (tab), T_{max}=3.3-4.8 hrs (cap). **Distribution:** Plasma protein binding (10%-18.5%). **Metabolism:** Liver; glucuronidation, mitochondrial β-oxidation. **Elimination:** Urine (<3% unchanged); $T_{1/2}$=9-16 hrs.

NURSING CONSIDERATIONS

Assessment: Assess LFTs, CBC with platelets, pancreatitis, plasma ammonia levels, pregnancy status. Note other diseases/conditions and drug therapies.

Monitoring: Monitor LFTs, CBC with platelets, coagulation parameters, pancreatitis, hypersensitivity reactions, hyperammonemia, thyroid function tests.

Patient Counseling: Counsel to avoid alcohol, sedatives, OTC agents. Advise to exercise caution while driving/operating machinery. Counsel about signs/symptoms of pancreatitis, hyperammonemia; notify physician if any symptoms or adverse effects occur.

Administration: Oral route. **Storage:** Store below 30°C (86°F).

DEPAKOTE ER — RX

divalproex sodium (Abbott)

Fatal hepatic failure (<2 yrs at considerable risk), teratogenic effects (eg, neural tube defects), and life-threatening pancreatitis reported.

THERAPEUTIC CLASS: Valproate compound

INDICATIONS: Migraine prophylaxis. Monotherapy and adjunct therapy for treatment of complex partial seizures, and simple and complex absence seizures. Adjunct for multiple seizure types that include absence seizures. Acute manic or mixed episodes associated with bipolar disorder.

DOSAGE: *Adults:* For qd dosing. Migraine: Initial: 500mg qd for 1 week. Titrate: Increase to 1000mg qd. Max: 1000mg/day. Complex Partial Seizures: Monotherapy/Adjunct Therapy: Initial: 10-15mg/kg/day. Titrate: Increase by 5-10mg/kg/week to optimal response. Usual: Less than 60mg/kg/day (accepted therapeutic range 50-100mcg/mL). When converting to monotherapy, reduce concomitant antiepilepsy drug by 25% every 2 weeks starting at initiation or delay 1-2 weeks after start of therapy. Simple and Complex Absence Seizures: Initial: 15mg/kg/day. Titrate: Increase weekly by 5-10mg/kg/day to optimal response. Max: 60mg/kg/day. Bipolar Disorder: Initial: 25mg/kg/day given once daily. Titrate: Increase dose rapidly to clinical effect. Max: 60mg/kg/day. Conversion from Depakote: Administer Depakote ER qd using a dose 8-20% higher than the total daily dose of Depakote. If cannot directly convert to Depakote ER, consider increasing to next higher Depakote total daily dose before converting to appropriate total daily Depakote ER dose. Elderly: Give lower initial dose and titrate slowly. Decrease dose or d/c if decreased food or fluid intake or if excessive somnolence occurs. Swallow whole; do not crush or chew.

Pediatrics: ≥10yrs: For qd dosing. Complex Partial Seizures: Monotherapy/Adjunct Therapy: Initial: 10-15mg/kg/day. Titrate: Increase by 5-10mg/kg/week to optimal response. Usual: Less than 60mg/kg/day (accepted therapeutic range 50-100mcg/mL). When converting to monotherapy, reduce concomitant antiepilepsy drug by 25% every 2 weeks starting at initiation or delay 1-2 weeks after start of therapy. Simple and Complex Absence Seizures: Initial: 15mg/kg/day. Titrate: Increase weekly by 5-10mg/kg/day to optimal response. Max: 60mg/kg/day. Conversion from Depakote: Administer Depakote ER qd using a dose 8-20% higher than the total daily dose of Depakote. If cannot directly convert to Depakote ER, consider increasing to next higher Depakote total daily dose before converting to appropriate total daily Depakote ER dose. Swallow whole; do not crush or chew.

HOW SUPPLIED: Tab, Extended-Release: 250mg, 500mg

CONTRAINDICATIONS: Hepatic disease, significant hepatic dysfunction, known urea cycle disorders (UCD).

D

WARNINGS/PRECAUTIONS: Hyperammonemic encephalopathy in UCD patients; d/c if this occurs. Prior to therapy, evaluate for UCD in high risk patients (eg, history of unexplained encephalopathy, coma, etc). If unexplained lethargy, vomiting, or mental status changes occur measure ammonia levels. Caution with hepatic disease and elderly. Check LFTs prior to therapy, then frequently during 1st 6 months. Dose-related thrombocytopenia and elevated liver enzymes reported. Thrombocytopenia significantly increases with plasma trough levels >110mcg/mL in females and >135mcg/mL in males. Monitor platelet and coagulation tests prior to therapy, then periodically. Altered thyroid function tests and urine ketone test. May stimulate replication of HIV and CMV viruses. Avoid abrupt discontinuation.

ADVERSE REACTIONS: NV, dyspepsia, diarrhea, abdominal pain, increased appetite, asthenia, somnolence, infection, dizziness, tremor, weight gain, back pain, alopecia.

INTERACTIONS: Potentiates carbamazepine, amitriptyline, nortriptyline, diazepam, ethosuximide, primidone, lamotrigine, phenobarbital, phenytoin, tolbutamide, zidovudine, lorazepam. Efficacy potentiated by ASA, felbamate. Efficacy reduced by rifampin, carbamazepine, phenobarbital, phenytoin, primidone. Clonazepam may induce absence status in patients with history of absence type seizures. CNS depression with alcohol and other CNS depressants. Monitor PT/INR with warfarin.

PREGNANCY: Category D, not for use in nursing.

MECHANISM OF ACTION: Anti-convulsant; increases GABA concentrations in the brain.

PHARMACOKINETICS: Absorption: Bioavailability (90%); T_{max}=4-17 hrs. **Distribution:** Plasma protein binding (10-18.5%). **Metabolism:** Liver; glucuronidation, mitochondrial β-oxidation. **Elimination:** Urine (<3% unchanged); $T_{1/2}$=9-16 hrs.

NURSING CONSIDERATIONS

Assessment: Assess LFTs, CBC with platelets, pancreatitis, plasma ammonia levels, pregnancy status. Note other diseases/conditions and drug therapies.

Monitoring: Monitor LFTs, CBC with platelets, coagulation parameters, pancreatitis, hypersensitivity reactions, hyperammonemia, thyroid function tests.

Patient Counseling: Counsel to avoid alcohol, sedatives, OTC agents. Advise to exercise caution while driving/operating machinery. Counsel about signs/symptoms of pancreatitis, hyperammonemia; notify physician if any symptoms or adverse effects occur.

Administration: Oral route. **Storage:** 25°C (77°F); excursions permitted to 15-30°C (59-86°F).

DEPO-ESTRADIOL RX

estradiol cypionate (Pharmacia & Upjohn)

Estrogens increase the risk of endometrial cancer. Estrogens, with or without progestins, should not be used for the prevention of cardiovascular disease or dementia. Increased risks of MI, stroke, invasive breast cancer, PE, and DVT in postmenopausal women (50-79 yrs of age) reported. Increased risk of developing probable dementia in postmenopausal women ≥65 yrs of age reported.

THERAPEUTIC CLASS: Estrogen

INDICATIONS: Treatment of moderate to severe vasomotor symptoms associated with menopause and hypoestrogenism due to hypogonadism.

DOSAGE: *Adults:* Vasomotor Symptoms/Vaginal/Vulval Atrophy: 1-5mg IM every 3-4 weeks cyclically. Discontinue or taper at 3-6 month intervals. Hypoestrogenism: 1.5-2mg IM every month.

HOW SUPPLIED: Inj: 5mg/mL

CONTRAINDICATIONS: Pregnancy, undiagnosed abnormal genital bleeding, breast cancer, estrogen-dependent neoplasia, DVT/PE, active or recent (eg, within past year) arterial thromboembolic disease (eg, stroke, MI), liver dysfunction or disease.

WARNINGS/PRECAUTIONS: May increase risk of cardiovascular events (eg, MI, stroke), venous thrombosis, and PE; d/c immediately if any of these events occur or are suspected. May increase risk of breast/endometrial cancer, and gallbladder disease. May lead to severe hypercalcemia with breast cancer and bone metastases; monitor and d/c if hypercalcemia occurs. Retinal vascular thrombosis reported; monitor and d/c if papilledema or retinal vascular lesions occur. Consider addition of a progestin if no hysterectomy. May elevate BP; monitor at regular intervals. May cause elevations of plasma triglycerides with pre-existing hypertriglyceridemia. Caution with history of cholestatic jaundice associated with past estrogen use or with pregnancy; d/c with recurrence. May lead to increased thyroid-binding globulin levels; monitor thyroid function. May cause fluid retention; caution with cardiac/renal dysfunction. Caution with severe hypocalcemia. May increase risk of ovarian cancer. May exacerbate endometriosis, asthma, DM, epilepsy, migraine, porphyria, SLE, and hepatic hemangiomas; use with caution.

ADVERSE REACTIONS: Changes in vaginal bleeding pattern, breakthrough bleeding, vaginal candidiasis, breast tenderness/enlargement, NV, abdominal cramps, headache, migraine, dizziness, increase/decrease in weight.

INTERACTIONS: CYP3A4 inducers (eg, St. John's wort, phenobarbital, carbamazepine, rifampin) may decrease levels which may decrease therapeutic effects and/or change uterine bleeding profile. CYP3A4 inhibitors (eg, erythromycin, clarithromycin, ketoconazole, itraconazole, ritonavir, grapefruit juice) may increase levels which may result in side effects.

PREGNANCY: Contraindicated in pregnancy, caution in nursing.

MECHANISM OF ACTION: Estrogen; binds to nuclear receptors in estrogen-responsive tissues. Modulates pituitary secretion of gonadotrophins, luteinizing hormone (LH) and follicle stimulating hormone (FSH), through negative feedback mechanism.

PHARMACOKINETICS: Absorption: Slow. **Distribution:** Wide; bound to sex hormone-binding globulin and albumin; found in breast milk. **Metabolism:** Liver via CYP3A4 (partial); estrone (active metabolite); estriol (major urinary metabolite); enterohepatic recirculation via sulfate and glucuronide conjugation. **Elimination:** Urine (estradiol, estrone, estriol, conjugates).

NURSING CONSIDERATIONS

Assessment: Assess for abnormal genital bleeding, breast cancer, estrogen-dependent neoplasia, presence or history of DVT or PE, active or recent (within past yr) arterial thromboembolic disease (eg, stroke, MI), liver dysfunction/disease, known/suspected pregnancy. Assess use in patients undergoing surgeries associated with risk of thromboembolism, prolonged immobilization, presence of hypocalcemia, asthma, DM, epilepsy, migraines or porphyria, SLE, presence of hepatic hemangiomas, nursing status, and in patients ≥65 yrs old. Assess for possible drug/lab test interactions.

Monitoring: Monitor for signs/symptoms of cardiovascular disorders (eg, MI, stroke), venous thrombosis, PE, malignant neoplasms (eg, endometrial, breast, ovarian cancer), dementia, gallbladder disease, hypercalcemia, visual abnormalities (eg, retinal vascular thrombosis), cholestatic jaundice, elevated BP, hypertriglyceridemia, hypothyroidism, fluid retention, exacerbation of endometriosis and other conditions (eg, asthma, DM, epilepsy, migraines or porphyria, SLE, and hepatic hemangiomas). Perform periodic BP monitoring. Monitor thyroid function in patients on thyroid replacement therapy. Perform annual breast exams. Perform periodic assessment (every 3-6 months) to determine therapy need. If abnormal genital bleeding occurs, perform proper diagnostic measures (eg, endometrial sampling) to rule out malignancies.

Patient Counseling: Inform that drug increases risk of uterine and breast cancer, heart attack, stroke, and blood clots. Advise to report breast lumps, unusual vaginal bleeding, dizziness or faintness, changes in speech, severe headaches, chest pain, SOB, leg pains, changes in vision, or vomiting. Instruct to perform monthly self breast exams.

Administration: IM route. **Storage:** 20-25°C (68-77°F).

DEPO-MEDROL

methylprednisolone acetate (Pharmacia & Upjohn) **RX**

THERAPEUTIC CLASS: Glucocorticoid

INDICATIONS: Steroid-responsive disorders.

DOSAGE: *Adults:* Local Effect: Rheumatoid/Osteoarthritis: Large Joint: 20-80mg. Medium Joint: 10-40mg. Small Joint: 4-10mg. Administer intra-articularly into synovial space every 1-5 weeks or more depending on relief. Ganglion/Tendinitis/Epicondylitis: 4-30mg into cyst/area of greatest tenderness. May repeat if necessary. Dermatologic Conditions: Inject 20-60mg into lesion. Distribute 20-40mg doses by repeated injections into large lesions. Usual: 1-4 injections. Systemic Effect: Substitute for Oral Therapy: IM dose should equal total daily PO methylprednisolone dose q24h. Prolonged Therapy: Administer weekly PO dose as single IM injection. Androgenital Syndrome: 40mg IM every 2 weeks. Rheumatoid Arthritis: 40-120mg IM weekly. Dermatologic Lesions: 40-120mg IM weekly for 1-4 weeks. Acute Severe Dermatitis (Poison Ivy): 80-120mg IM single dose. Chronic Contact Dermatitis: May repeat injections every 5-10 days. Seborrheic Dermatitis: 80mg IM weekly. Multiple Sclerosis: 200mg/day prednisolone for 1 week, then 80mg every other day for 1 month (4mg methylprednisolone=5mg prednisolone). Asthma/Allergic Rhinitis: 80-120mg IM.
Pediatrics: Use lower adult doses. Determine dose by severity of condition and response.

HOW SUPPLIED: Inj: 20mg/mL, 40mg/mL, 80mg/mL

CONTRAINDICATIONS: Intrathecal administration, systemic fungal infections.

WARNINGS/PRECAUTIONS: Dermal and subdermal atrophy reported; do not exceed recommended doses. May need to increase dose before, during, and after stressful situations. May mask signs of infection or cause new infections. Prolonged use may produce cataracts, glaucoma, secondary ocular infections. Increases BP, salt/water retention, potassium and calcium excretion. More severe/fatal course of infections reported with chickenpox, measles. Caution with *Strongyloides*, latent TB, hypothyroidism, cirrhosis, ocular herpes simplex, HTN, diverticulitis, fresh intestinal anastomoses, ulcerative colitis, osteoporosis, myasthenia gravis, renal insufficiency, peptic ulcer disease. Kaposi's sarcoma reported. Growth and development of children on prolonged therapy should be monitored. Monitor for psychic disturbances. Avoid abrupt withdrawal. Do not use intra-articularly, intrabursally, or for intratendinous administration in acute infection. Avoid injection into unstable and previously infected joints. Monitor urinalysis, blood sugar, BP, weight, chest X-ray, and upper GI X-ray (if ulcer history) regularly during prolonged therapy.

ADVERSE REACTIONS: Fluid and electrolyte disturbances, HTN, osteoporosis, muscle weakness, Cushingoid state, menstrual irregularities, impaired wound healing, DM, ulcerative esophagitis, excessive sweating, increases ICP, carbohydrate intolerance, glaucoma, cataracts, urticaria, subcutaneous/cutaneous atrophy.

INTERACTIONS: Reduced efficacy with hepatic enzyme inducers (eg, phenobarbital, phenytoin, and rifampin). Increases clearance of chronic high-dose ASA. Caution with ASA in hypoprothrombinemia. Effects on oral anticoagulants are variable; monitor PT. Increased insulin and oral hypoglycemic requirements in DM. Avoid live vaccines with immunosuppressive doses. Possible decreased vaccine response with killed or inactivated vaccines with immunosuppressive doses. Mutual inhibition of metabolism with cyclosporine; convulsions reported. Potentiated by ketoconazole and troleandomycin. Do not dilute or mix with other solutions.

PREGNANCY: Safety in pregnancy and nursing not known.

MECHANISM OF ACTION: Anti-inflammatory glucocorticoid; causes profound and varied metabolic effects and modifies the body's immune responses to diverse stimuli.

PHARMACOKINETICS: Absorption: C_{max}=11.8ng/mL; AUC=1286ng•hr/mL. **Elimination:** 139 hrs.

D

NURSING CONSIDERATIONS

Assessment: Assess systemic fungal infections, current infections, active TB, vaccination history, ulcerative colitis, diverticulitis, peptic ulcer with impending perforation, renal/hepatic insufficiency, septic arthritis/unstable joint, HTN, osteoporosis, myasthenia gravis, thyroid status, psychotic tendencies, and possible drug interactions.

Monitoring: Monitor for adrenocortical insufficiency, occurrence of infections, psychic derangement, cataracts, acute myopathy, Kaposi's sarcoma, fluid retention, measurement of serum electrolytes, TSH, LFTs, IOP, and BP. Monitor urinalysis, blood sugar, weight, chest X-ray, and upper GI X-ray (if ulcer history) regularly during prolonged therapy.

Patient Counseling: Inform that susceptibility to infections may increase. Avoid exposure to chickenpox and measles; report immediately if exposed.

Administration: IM, intrasynovial, or intralesional. **Storage:** 20-25°C (68-77°F).

DEPO-PROVERA — RX

medroxyprogesterone acetate (Pharmacia & Upjohn)

THERAPEUTIC CLASS: Progestogen

INDICATIONS: Adjunct and palliative treatment of inoperable, recurrent, and metastatic endometrial or renal carcinoma.

DOSAGE: *Adults:* Initial: 400-1000mg IM weekly. Maint: 400mg/month if disease stabilizes and/or improves within a few weeks or months.

HOW SUPPLIED: Inj: 400mg/mL [2.5mL]

CONTRAINDICATIONS: Pregnancy, undiagnosed vaginal bleeding, breast malignancy, thrombophlebitis, thromboembolic disorders, cerebral vascular disease, liver dysfunction.

WARNINGS/PRECAUTIONS: Avoid during first 4 months of pregnancy. May cause thromboembolic disorders, ocular disorders, fluid retention. Caution with depression, family history of breast cancer or patients with breast nodules. May mask the onset of climacteric.

ADVERSE REACTIONS: Menstrual irregularities, nervousness, dizziness, edema, wt changes, cervical changes, cholestatic jaundice, breast tenderness, galactorrhea, rash, acne, alopecia, hirsutism, depression, pyrexia, fatigue, insomnia, nausea.

INTERACTIONS: Aminoglutethimide may decrease serum levels. Caution with estrogen.

PREGNANCY: Safety in pregnancy and nursing not known.

MECHANISM OF ACTION: Progestogen; inhibits secretion of gonadotropins which prevents follicular maturation and ovulation resulting in endometrial thinning, thus producing its contraceptive effect.

PHARMACOKINETICS: Absorption: C_{max}=1-7ng/mL; T_{max}=3 weeks. **Distribution:** Found in breast milk. **Elimination**: $T_{1/2}$=50 days.

NURSING CONSIDERATIONS

Assessment: Physical exam of BP, breast, abdominal, pelvic exam, including cervical cytology and relevant lab tests should be done, with assessment of pregnancy status, vaginal bleeding, breast cancer, thromboembolic disorders/active thrombophlebitis and/or cerebrovascular disease, drug hypersensitivity, risk of osteoporosis (eg, metabolic bone disease, chronic alcohol or tobacco use, anorexia nervosa, strong family history and chronic use of anticonvulsants and/or corticosteroids), psychic depression, DM, hepatic/renal impairment, cardiovascular disease, and possible drug/lab test interactions.

Monitoring: Monitor for amenorrhea, menstrual irregularity, breast cancer risk, manifestations of thrombotic disorders (eg, thrombophlebitis, PE, cerebrovascular disorders, retinal thrombosis), ocular disorders (eg, partial/complete vision loss, proptosis, diplopia, migraine), ectopic pregnancy, anaphylaxis/anaphylactoid reaction, manifestations of fluid retentions, epilepsy, abdominal pain, weight changes. Lab monitoring of bone mineral densitometry for osteoporosis/osteoporotic fractures, plasma/urinary steroid levels, gonadotropin level, sex hormone-binding globulin level, LFTs, glucose, lipid profile, and coagulation tests.

Patient Counseling: Counsel on risk/benefits. Notify if pregnant/nursing.

Administration: IM route. **Storage:** 20-25°C (68-77°F).

DEPO-PROVERA CONTRACEPTIVE RX

medroxyprogesterone acetate (Pharmacia & Upjohn)

May cause significant loss of bone mineral density (BMD); greater with increasing duration of use and may not be completely reversible. Should be used as long-term birth control (>2yrs) only if other birth control methods are inadequate. Unknown if use during adolescence or early adulthood will reduce peak bone mass and increase risk of osteoporotic fractures in later life.

THERAPEUTIC CLASS: Progestogen

INDICATIONS: Prevention of pregnancy.

DOSAGE: *Adults:* 150mg IM every 3 months (13 weeks) in gluteal or deltoid muscle. Give 1st injection during 1st 5 days of menses; within 1st 5 days postpartum if not nursing; or 6 weeks postpartum if nursing.

HOW SUPPLIED: Inj: 150mg/mL

CONTRAINDICATIONS: Pregnancy, undiagnosed vaginal bleeding, breast malignancy, thrombophlebitis, thromboembolic disorders, cerebral vascular disease, liver dysfunction.

WARNINGS/PRECAUTIONS: Loss of BMD, may cause bleeding irregularities, cancer risk, thromboembolic disorders, ocular disorders, unexpected pregnancies, ectopic pregnancy, anaphylaxis and anaphylactoid reaction, fluid retention, return of fertility, decrease in glucose metabolism. Caution with CNS or convulsive disorders. D/C if jaundice develops.

ADVERSE REACTIONS: Menstrual irregularities, weight changes, abdominal pain, dizziness, headache, asthenia, nervousness, decreased libido, depression, nausea, insomnia, leukorrhea, acne, vaginitis, pelvic pain.

INTERACTIONS: Aminoglutethimide may decrease serum levels.

PREGNANCY: Category X, safety in nursing not known.

MECHANISM OF ACTION: Progestogen; inhibits secretion of gonadotropins, preventing follicular maturation and ovulation, resulting in endometrial thinning and producing a contraceptive effect.

PHARMACOKINETICS: Absorption: C_{max}=1-7ng/mL; T_{max}=3 weeks. **Distribution:** Found in breast milk. **Elimination**: $T_{1/2}$=50 days.

NURSING CONSIDERATIONS

Assessment: Assess BP. Perform physical exam of breast, abdomen, pelvis, cervical cytology and relevant lab tests. Assess pregnancy status, vaginal bleeding, breast cancer, thromboembolic disorders, active thrombophlebitis and/or cerebrovascular disease, drug hypersensitivity, risk of osteoporosis (eg, metabolic bone disease, chronic alcohol or tobacco use, anorexia nervosa, strong family history of osteoporosis, and chronic use of anticonvulsants and/or corticosteroids), depression, DM, hepatic/renal impairment, CV disease, and possible drug/lab test interactions.

Monitoring: Monitor for amenorrhea, menstrual irregularity, breast cancer risk in women, manifestations of thrombotic disorders (eg, thrombophlebitis,

PE, cerebrovascular disorders, and retinal thrombosis), ocular disorders (eg, partial/complete loss of vision, proptosis, diplopia, migraine), ectopic pregnancy, anaphylaxis/anaphylactoid reaction, manifestations of fluid retention, epilepsy, abdominal pain, weight changes, lab monitoring of bone minerals, densitometry for osteoporosis/osteoporotic fractures, plasma/urinary steroid levels, gonadotropin levels, sex hormone-binding globulin level, LFTs, glucose, lipid profile, and coagulation tests.

Patient Counseling: Counsel about risk/benefits of drug; inform drug does not protect against HIV infection and other STDs.

Administration: IM route. Gluteal or deltoid muscle; 1st injection must be given only during first 5 days of normal menstrual period or 5 days postpartum if not breast-feeding. If exclusively breast-feeding, give at 6th postpartum week. **Storage:** 20-25°C (68-77°F).

DEPO-SUBQ PROVERA 104 — RX

medroxyprogesterone acetate (Pharmacia & Upjohn)

May cause significant loss of bone mineral density (BMD); greater with increasing duration of use and may not be completely reversible. Should be used as long-term birth control (>2yrs) only if other birth control methods are inadequate. Unknown if use during adolescence or early adulthood will reduce peak bone mass and increase risk of osteoporotic fractures in later life.

THERAPEUTIC CLASS: Progestogen

INDICATIONS: Prevention of pregnancy. Management of endometriosis-associated pain.

DOSAGE: *Adults:* 104mg SQ once every 3 months in the anterior thigh or abdomen. Give 1st injection during 1st 5 days of menses or 6 weeks postpartum if nursing.

HOW SUPPLIED: Inj: 104mg/0.65mL

CONTRAINDICATIONS: Pregnancy, undiagnosed vaginal bleeding, breast malignancy, thrombophlebitis, thromboembolic disorders, cerebral vascular disease, liver dysfunction.

WARNINGS/PRECAUTIONS: Loss of BMD, may cause bleeding irregularities, cancer risk, thromboembolic disorders, ocular disorders, unexpected pregnancies, ectopic pregnancy, anaphylaxis and anaphylactoid reaction, fluid retention, return of fertility, decrease in glucose metabolism. Caution with CNS or convulsive disorders. D/C if jaundice develops.

ADVERSE REACTIONS: Uterine bleeding irregularities, increased weight, decreased libido, acne, injection site reactions, headache, amenorrhea.

INTERACTIONS: Amioglutethimide may decrease serum levels.

PREGNANCY: Not for use in pregnancy, safety in nursing not known.

MECHANISM OF ACTION: Progestogen; inhibits secretion of gonadotropins, which prevents follicular maturation and ovulation, resulting in endometrial thinning and producing a contraceptive effect.

PHARMACOKINETICS: Absorption: C_{max}=1.56ng/mL; T_{max}=8.8 days; AUC=66.98ng•day/mL. **Distribution:** Plasma protein binding (86%); found in breast milk. **Metabolism:** Liver (extensive); reduction and hydroxylation. **Elimination:** Urine; $T_{1/2}$=43 days.

NURSING CONSIDERATIONS

Assessment: Perform physical exam of breast, abdomen, pelvis, cervical cytology and relevant lab tests, pregnancy status, vaginal bleeding, breast cancer, thromboembolic disorders, active thrombophlebitis and/or cerebrovascular diseases. Monitor for osteoporosis, history of depression, DM, hepatic/renal impairment, CV disease, BP, and for possible drug/lab test interactions.

Monitoring: Monitor for amenorrhea, menstrual irregularity, manifestations of thromboembolic disorders (eg, thrombophlebitis, PE, cerebrovascular disorders, retinal thrombosis), ocular disorders (eg, partial/complete loss of vision, proptosis, diplopia, migraine), manifestations of fluid retention, epilepsy, abdominal pain, weight changes. Lab monitoring of bone mineral density for osteoporosis/osteoporotic fractures, LFTs, glucose, lipid profile, and coagulation tests.

Patient Counseling: Counsel about benefits/risks of drug; inform drug does not protect against HIV infection and other STDs. Advise to avoid smoking while taking drug.

Administration: SQ route; anterior thigh or abdomen. 1st injection should be given only during first 5 days of normal menstrual period, or during/after 6th postpartum week if breast-feeding. **Storage:** 20-25°C (68-77°F).

DEPO-TESTOSTERONE

CIII

testosterone cypionate (Pharmacia & Upjohn)

THERAPEUTIC CLASS: Androgen

INDICATIONS: Testosterone replacement in males with primary hypogonadism and hypogonadotropic hypogonadism.

DOSAGE: *Adults:* Male Hypogonadism: 50-400mg IM every 2-4 weeks. Dose based on age, sex, and diagnosis. Adjust dose according to response and adverse reactions.
Pediatrics: ≥12 yrs: Male Hypogonadism: 50-400mg IM every 2-4 weeks. Dose based on age, sex, and diagnosis. Adjust dose according to response and adverse reactions.

HOW SUPPLIED: Inj: 100mg/mL, 200mg/mL

CONTRAINDICATIONS: Severe renal, hepatic and cardiac disease. Males with carcinoma of the breast or prostate gland. Pregnancy.

WARNINGS/PRECAUTIONS: May accelerate bone maturation without linear growth; monitor bone growth every 6 months. Risk of hepatic damage with long-term use. D/C if hypercalcemia occurs in immobilized patients. D/C with acute urethral obstruction, priapism, excessive sexual stimulation, or oligospermia; restart at lower doses. Risk of edema; caution with pre-existing cardiac, renal or hepatic disease. Caution in the elderly; increased risk of prostatic hypertrophy and prostatic carcinoma. Caution with BPH. Should not be used for enhancement of athletic performance. Do not administer IV. Monitor Hct, Hgb, cholesterol periodically.

ADVERSE REACTIONS: Gynecomastia, excessive frequency/duration of penile erections, male pattern baldness, increased/decreased libido, oligospermia, hirsutism, acne, fluid and electrolyte disturbances, nausea, hypercholesterolemia, clotting factor suppression, polycythemia, altered LFTs, priapism, anxiety, depression.

INTERACTIONS: May potentiate oral anticoagulants (eg, warfarin) and oxyphenbutazone. May decrease blood glucose and insulin requirements in diabetics.

PREGNANCY: Category X, not for use in nursing.

MECHANISM OF ACTION: Endogenous androgen; responsible for normal growth and development of male sex organs and for maintenance of secondary sex characteristics.

PHARMACOKINETICS: Distribution: Plasma protein binding (98%). **Elimination:** Urine (90%), feces (6%); $T_{1/2}$=8 days.

NURSING CONSIDERATIONS

Assessment: Assess for known hypersensitivity to drug, males with carcinoma of the breast, males with known or suspected carcinoma of the prostate gland, hepatic/renal disease, delayed puberty, and benign prostatic hypertrophy.

Monitoring: Periodically monitor Hgb, Hct, LFTs, PSA, cholesterol and HDL, serum testosterone levels, serum calcium after initiation of therapy. Monitor for signs/symptoms of hypersensitivity reactions, edema with/without CHF, gynecomastia, prostatic hyperplasia/carcinoma, hepatocellular carcinoma. Assess bone development every 6 months in male adolescents.

Patient Counseling: Inform to contact physician if notice changes in body hair distribution, increase in acne, virilization, too frequent or persistent erections, changes in skin color, ankle swelling, unexplained NV, hypersensitivity reactions.

Administration: IM route, preferably gluteal muscle. **Storage:** Controlled temperature, 20-25°C (68-77°F). Protect from light.

DESOGEN RX

desogestrel - ethinyl estradiol (Organon)

OTHER BRAND NAMES: Apri (Barr)

THERAPEUTIC CLASS: Estrogen/progestogen combination

INDICATIONS: Prevention of pregnancy.

DOSAGE: *Adults:* Start 1st Sunday after onset of menstruation or 1st day of menstruation. 1 tab qd for 28 days continuously, then repeat.

HOW SUPPLIED: Tab: (Ethinyl Estradiol-Desogestrel) 0.03mg-0.15mg

CONTRAINDICATIONS: Thrombophlebitis, DVT or thromboembolic disorders, pregnancy, cerebrovascular or coronary artery disease (current or history), undiagnosed abnormal genital bleeding, cholestatic jaundice of pregnancy or jaundice with prior hormonal contraceptive use, hepatic adenomas or carcinomas, breast cancer or other estrogen-dependent neoplasia, valvular heart disease with thrombogenic complications, hepatic tumors (benign or malignant) or active liver disease, heavy smoking (≥ 15 cigarettes per day) and over age 35.

WARNINGS/PRECAUTIONS: Cigarette smoking increases risk of serious cardiovascular side effects. This risk increases with age (especially >35 yrs) and heavy smoking. Increased risk of MI, vascular disease, thromboembolism, stroke and gallbladder disease. Retinal thrombosis, hepatic neoplasia, carcinoma of breast and reproductive organs reported. May cause glucose intolerance. May increase BP, elevate LDL levels or cause other lipid changes, fluid retention, breakthrough bleeding, and spotting. May cause or exacerbate migraine. May develop visual changes with contact lenses. Increased risk of MI with HTN, hyperlipidemia, certain inherited or acquired thrombophilias, obesity, and diabetes. D/C if jaundice, significant depression or ophthalmic irregularities develop. Perform annual physical exam. Use before menarche is not indicated. May affect certain endocrine, LFTs and blood components. D/C if pregnancy is confirmed.

ADVERSE REACTIONS: NV, breakthrough bleeding, spotting, amenorrhea, migraine, mood changes including depression, vaginitis including candidiasis, edema, weight changes.

INTERACTIONS: Reduced effects, increased breakthrough bleeding, and menstrual irregularities with rifampin, barbiturates, phenylbutazone, phenytoin, and possibly with griseofulvin, ampicillin, and tetracyclines. Possible interaction with CYP2C9 substrates or inhibitors. St. John's wort may reduce the effectiveness of contraceptive steroids.

PREGNANCY: Category X, not for use in nursing.

MECHANISM OF ACTION: Estrogen/progestogen combination oral contraceptive; acts by suppression of gonadotropins. Also inhibits ovulation and causes changes in cervical mucus (increasing difficulty of sperm entry into uterus) and changes in endometrium (reducing likelihood of implantation) .

PHARMACOKINETICS: Absorption: Desogestrel: Rapid, complete; Etonogestrel: C_{max}=2805pg/mL (single dose), 5840pg/mL (multiple doses), T_{max}=1.4 hrs, AUC=33858pg/mL•hr (single dose), 52299pg/mL•hr (multiple doses). Ethinyl Estradiol: Rapid and complete, C_{max}=95pg/mL (single dose), 141pg/mL (multiple doses), T_{max}=1.5 hrs; AUC=1471pg/mL•hr (single dose), 1117pg/mL•hr (multiple doses). **Distribution:** Etonogestrel: Protein binding (98%). **Metabolism:** Desogestrel: Hepatic, hydroxylation in intestinal mucosa; CYP2C9, 3A4; Etonogestrel (major active metabolite). Ethinyl estradiol: Hepatic conjugation. **Elimination:** Urine, bile, feces. Desogestrel: $T_{1/2}$=38 hrs. Ethinyl Estradiol: $T_{1/2}$=26 hrs.

NURSING CONSIDERATIONS

Assessment: Assess for current or history of thrombophlebitis or thromboembolic disorders, cerebral vascular disease, CAD, valvular heart disease with thrombogenic complications, severe HTN, DM with vascular involvement, headaches with focal neurological problems, recent major surgery with prolonged immobilization, known/suspected carcinoma of breast, endometrium or other known/suspected estrogen-dependent neoplasia, undiagnosed abnormal genital bleeding, cholestatic jaundice of pregnancy or jaundice with prior hormonal contraceptive use, hepatic tumors, active liver disease. Assess pregnancy status, use in patients >35 yrs old who smoke ≥15 cigarettes/day, and for possible drug interactions.

Monitoring: Monitor for venous and arterial thrombotic and thromboembolic events (eg, MI, thromboembolism, stroke), hepatic neoplasia, gallbladder disease, onset of headaches or migraines, HTN, fluid retention, ocular lesions, and bleeding irregularities. Refer patients with contact lenses to ophthalmologist if visual changes develop. Monitor serum glucose levels in DM and prediabetic patients, BP with history of HTN, lipid levels with history of hyperlipidemia. Monitor for signs/symptoms of liver dysfunction and worsening depression in patients with previous history.

Patient Counseling: Inform that drug does not protect against HIV infection and other STDs. Instruct not to smoke while using oral contraceptives. Advise to undergo annual physical exam while on medication. Inform may experience spotting or light bleeding, or may feel sick to stomach during first 1-3 packs of pill; advise this will usually subside and if not, to contact physician. Inform about pregnancy risk if pills are missed. Instruct to take same time every day. Instruct if one "active" pill is missed to take as soon as remembered; take next pill at regular time.

Administration: Oral route. **Storage:** 20-25°C (68-77°F).

DesOwen — RX

desonide (Galderma)

THERAPEUTIC CLASS: Corticosteroid

INDICATIONS: Corticosteroid responsive dermatoses.

DOSAGE: *Adults:* Apply bid-tid, depending on severity. Reassess if no improvement after 2 weeks.

HOW SUPPLIED: Cre, Oint: 0.05% [15g, 60g]; Lot: 0.05% [60mL, 120mL]

WARNINGS/PRECAUTIONS: May produce reversible HPA axis suppression, manifestations of Cushing's syndrome, hyperglycemia, and glucosuria. D/C if irritation occurs. Use appropriate antifungal or antibacterial agent with dermatological infections. Peds may be more susceptible to systemic toxicity. Caution when applied to large surface areas. Avoid occlusive dressings.

ADVERSE REACTIONS: Stinging, burning, irritation, erythema, contact dermatitis, worsening condition, skin peeling, dryness/scaliness.

PREGNANCY: Category C, caution in nursing.

MECHANISM OF ACTION: Corticosteroid; possesses anti-inflammatory, antipruritic, and vasoconstrictive properties. Suspected to act by induction of phospholipase A_2 inhibitory proteins called lipocortins. Lipocortins control biosynthesis of potent mediators of inflammation (eg, prostaglandins, leukotrienes) by inhibiting the release of their common precursor, arachidonic acid.

PHARMACOKINETICS: Absorption: Extent of percutaneous absorption depends on skin integrity, vehicle, and use of occlusive dressings.

NURSING CONSIDERATIONS

Assessment: Assess pregnancy/nursing status.

Monitoring: Monitor for signs/symptoms of reversible hypothalamic-pituitary-adrenal (HPA) axis suppression, Cushing's syndrome, hyperglycemia, and glucosuria. Following withdrawal of treatment, monitor for glucocorticosteroid insufficiency. In patients applying medication to a large surface area or using occlusive dressings, monitor for HPA-axis suppression through ACTH stimulation, AM plasma cortisol, and urinary free cortisol tests.

Patient Counseling: Instruct to use exactly as directed, externally, and to avoid contact with eyes. Instruct not to bandage, cover, or wrap treatment area so as to be occlusive, unless directed by physician. Counsel to report any local adverse reactions.

Administration: Topical. **Storage:** Lotion: 2-30°C (36-86°F). Ointment: Below 30°C (86°F), avoid freezing. Cream: 15-30°C (59-86°F).

DESOXYN

methamphetamine HCl (Ovation)

CII

High potential for abuse. Avoid prolonged therapy in obesity.

THERAPEUTIC CLASS: Sympathomimetic amine

INDICATIONS: Attention deficit disorder with hyperactivity. Short-term adjunct to treat exogenous obesity.

DOSAGE: *Adults:* Obesity: 5mg, 1/2 hr before each meal. Do not exceed a few weeks of treatment.
Pediatrics: ADHD: ≥6 yrs: Initial: 5mg qd-bid. Titrate: Increase weekly by 5mg/day until optimum response. Usual: 20-25mg/day given bid. Obesity: ≥12 yrs: 5mg, 1/2 hr before each meal. Do not exceed a few weeks of treatment.

HOW SUPPLIED: Tab: 5mg

CONTRAINDICATIONS: Advanced arteriosclerosis, symptomatic cardiovascular disease, moderate to severe HTN, hyperthyroidism, glaucoma, agitated states, history of drug abuse, during or within 14 days of MAOI use.

WARNINGS/PRECAUTIONS: Tolerance to anorectic effect develops within a few weeks, do not exceed recommended dose to increase effect. Monitor growth in children. Caution with HTN. Do not use to combat fatigue or replace rest. Exacerbation of motor and phonic tics and Tourette's syndrome. May exacerbate behavior disturbance and thought disorder in psychotic pediatrics. Emergence of new psychotic symptoms may warrant discontinuation of therapy. Monitor for the appearance or worsening of aggressive behavior in children. Therapy may lower the convulsive threshold and cause blurred vision and difficulty with accommodation. Interrupt occasionally to determine if patient requires continued therapy. Misuse may cause sudden death and serious cardiovascular adverse events. Caution in patients with underlying cardiovascular conditions and comorbid bipolar disorder.

ADVERSE REACTIONS: BP elevation, tachycardia, palpitations, dizziness, insomnia, tremor, diarrhea, constipation, dry mouth, urticaria, impotence, changes in libido.

INTERACTIONS: May alter insulin requirements. May decrease hypotensive effect of guanethidine. Avoid MAOIs. Caution with TCAs and indirect acting sympathomimetic amines. Antagonized by phenothiazines.

PREGNANCY: Category C, not for use in nursing.

MECHANISM OF ACTION: Sympathomimetic amine; CNS stimulant. Peripheral actions involve elevation of BP, weak bronchodilation, and respiratory stimulant actions.

PHARMACOKINETICS: Absorption: Rapid. **Metabolism:** Liver; aromatic hydroxylation, N-dealkylation and deamination. **Elimination:** Urine (62%); $T_{1/2}$=4-5 hrs.

NURSING CONSIDERATIONS

Assessment: Assess for agitation, glaucoma, tics, family history of Tourette's syndrome, cardiovascular conditions (eg, severe HTN, angina pectoris, cardiac arrhythmias, heart failure, recent MI), hyperthyroidism or thyrotoxicosis, bipolar illness, history of drug dependence or alcoholism.

Monitoring: Monitor for cardiac abnormalities, exacerbations of behavior disturbances and thought disorder, bipolar disorder, aggression, seizures, and visual disturbances. Height and weight follow-up in children.

Patient Counseling: Inform about risks of treatment, appropriate use, drug abuse/dependence. Caution while operating machinery/driving. Avoid late evening doses; insomnia may result.

Administration: Oral route. **Storage**: Store below 30°C (86°F). Protect from light.

Detrol LA RX

tolterodine tartrate (Pharmacia & Upjohn)

OTHER BRAND NAMES: Detrol (Pharmacia & Upjohn)

THERAPEUTIC CLASS: Muscarinic antagonist

INDICATIONS: Treatment of overactive bladder with symptoms of urinary frequency, urgency, or urge incontinence.

DOSAGE: *Adults:* (LA Cap) Usual: 4mg qd, may lower to 2mg. (Tab) Initial: 2mg bid, may lower to 1mg bid. (LA Cap, Tab) Significant Hepatic/Renal Dysfunction/Concomitant CYP3A4 Inhibitors: 1mg bid or 2mg LA cap qd.

HOW SUPPLIED: Cap, Extended-Release: 2mg, 4mg; Tab: 1mg, 2mg

CONTRAINDICATIONS: Urinary retention, gastric retention, uncontrolled narrow-angle glaucoma.

WARNINGS/PRECAUTIONS: Risk of urinary retention with significant bladder outflow obstruction and risk of gastric retention with GI obstructive disorders. Caution with renal impairment and narrow-angle glaucoma. Reduce dose with significant hepatic or renal dysfunction. May cause blurred vision, drowsiness, or dizziness. Caution with decreased gastrointestinal motility and myasthenia gravis.

ADVERSE REACTIONS: Dry mouth, dizziness, headache, abdominal pain, constipation, diarrhea, dyspepsia, fatigue, somnolence, aggravation of symptoms of dementia reported.

INTERACTIONS: Reduce dose with concomitant CYP3A4 inhibitors (eg, erythromycin, clarithromycin, ketoconazole, itraconazole, and miconazole).

PREGNANCY: Category C, not for use in nursing.

MECHANISM OF ACTION: Muscarinic receptor antagonist; inhibits cholinergic muscarinic receptors mediating urinary bladder contraction and salivation.

PHARMACOKINETICS: Absorption: (Tab) Extensive metabolizers (EM): C_{max}=2.6mcg/L; T_{max}=1.2 hrs. Poor metabolizers (PM) C_{max}=19mcg/L; T_{max}=1.9 hrs. (Cap, Extended-Release) EM: C_{max}=3.4mcg/L; T_{max}=4 hrs. PM: C_{max}=19mcg/L; T_{max}=4 hrs. **Distribution:** V_d=113 L; high plasma protein binding. **Metabolism:** EM: CYP2D6 (oxidation); 5-hydroxymethyl (active metabolite). PM: CYP3A4 (dealkylation). **Elimination:** Urine (<1% unchanged), feces. (Tab) EM: $T_{1/2}$=2.2 hrs. PM: $T_{1/2}$=9.6 hrs. (Cap, Extended-Release) EM: $T_{1/2}$=6.9 hrs. PM: $T_{1/2}$=18 hrs.

NURSING CONSIDERATIONS

Assessment: Assess for bladder outflow obstruction (urinary retention), GI obstructive disorder (gastric retention), narrow-angle glaucoma, history of QT prolongation, possible drug interaction, hepatic/renal impairment.

Monitoring: Monitor for signs/symptoms of urinary retention, gastric retention, hypersensitivity reactions, hepatic/renal impairment.

Patient Counseling: Inform may produce blurred vision, dizziness, or drowsiness. Caution may impair physical/mental abilities. Notify physician if pregnant/nursing or planning to become pregnant.

Administration: Oral route. **Storage:** 25°C (77°F); excursions permitted to 15-30°C (59-86°F). Protect from light.

DEXAMETHASONE RX

dexamethasone (Various)

OTHER BRAND NAMES: Decadron (Merck)

THERAPEUTIC CLASS: Glucocorticoid

INDICATIONS: (PO) Treatment of steroid-responsive disorders. (Inj) Treatment of steroid-responsive disorders when oral therapy not feasible.

DOSAGE: *Adults:* Individualize for disease and patient response. Withdraw gradually. (Tab) Initial: 0.75-9mg/day PO. Maint: Decrease in small amounts to lowest effective dose. Cushing's Syndrome Test: 1mg PO at 11pm; draw blood at 8am next morning. Or, 0.5mg PO q6h for 48 hrs; or 2mg (to distinguish if excess pituitary ACTH or other causes) PO q6h for 48 hrs; obtain 24-hr urine collections. (Inj) Initial: 0.5-9mg/day IV/IM. Cerebral Edema: Initial: 10mg IV, then 4mg IM q6h until edema subsides. Reduce dose after 2-4 days and gradually d/c over 5-7 days. Palliative Management of Recurrent/Inoperable Brain Tumors: Maint: 2mg IV/PO bid-tid. Acute Allergic Disorders: 4-8mg IM on 1st day, then 1.5mg PO bid for 2 days, then 0.75mg PO bid for 1 day, then 0.75mg PO qd for 2 days. (Inj) Usual: 0.2-9mg. Maint: Decrease in small amounts to lowest effective dose. Intra-Articular/Intralesional/Soft Tissue Injection: Usual: 0.2-6mg once every 3-5 days to once every 2-3 weeks. See PI for Shock Treatment. Take with meals and antacids to prevent peptic ulcer.
Pediatrics: Individualize for disease and patient response. Withdraw gradually. (Tab) Initial: 0.75-9mg/day PO. Maint: Decrease in small amounts to lowest effective dose. Cushing's Syndrome Test: 1mg PO at 11pm; draw blood at 8am next morning. Or, 0.5mg PO q6h for 48 hrs; or 2mg (to distinguish if excess pituitary ATCH or other causes) PO q6h for 48 hrs; obtain 24-hr urine collections. (Inj) Initial: 0.5-9mg/day IV/IM. Cerebral Edema: Initial: 10mg IV, then 4mg IM q6h until edema subsides. Reduce dose after 2-4 days and gradually d/c over 5-7 days. Palliative Management of Recurrent/Inoperable Brain Tumors: Maint: 2mg IV/PO bid-tid. Acute Allergic Disorders: 4-8mg IM on 1st day, then 1.5mg PO bid for 2 days, then 0.75mg PO bid for 1 day, then 0.75mg PO qd for 2 days. (Inj) Usual: 0.2-9mg. Maint: Decrease in small amounts to lowest effective dose. Intra-Articular/Intralesional/Soft Tissue Injection: Usual: 0.2-6mg once every 3-5 days to once every 2-3 weeks. See PI for shock treatment. Take with meals and antacids to prevent peptic ulcer.

HOW SUPPLIED: Inj: (Dexamethasone Sodium Phosphate) 4mg/mL, 10mg/mL; Sol: (Dexamethasone) 0.5mg/5mL, 1mg/mL; Tab: (Dexamethasone) 0.5mg*, 0.75mg*, 1mg*, 1.5mg*, 2mg*, 4mg*, 6mg* *scored

CONTRAINDICATIONS: Systemic fungal infections.

WARNINGS/PRECAUTIONS: Increase dose before, during, and after stressful situations. Avoid abrupt withdrawal. May mask signs of infection, activate latent amebiasis, elevate BP, cause salt/water retention, increase excretion of potassium and calcium. Prolonged use may produce cataracts, glaucoma, secondary ocular infections. Caution with recent MI, ocular herpes simplex, emotional instability, nonspecific ulcerative colitis, diverticulitis, peptic ulcer, renal insufficiency, HTN, osteoporosis, myasthenia gravis, threadworm infection, active tuberculosis. Enhanced effect with hypothyroidism, cirrhosis. Consider prophylactic therapy if exposed to measles or chickenpox. Risk of glaucoma, cataracts, and eye infections. False negative dexamethasone suppression test with indomethacin.

ADVERSE REACTIONS: Fluid/electrolyte disturbances, muscle weakness, osteoporosis, peptic ulcer, pancreatitis, ulcerative esophagitis, impaired wound healing, headache, psychic disturbances, growth suppression (pediatrics), glaucoma, hyperglycemia, weight gain, nausea, malaise.

INTERACTIONS: Caution with ASA. Inducers of CYP3A4 (eg, phenytoin, phenobarbital, carbamazepine, rifampin) and ephedrine enhance clearance; increase steroid dose. Inhibitors of CYP3A4 (ketoconazole, macrolides) may increase plasma levels. Drugs that affect metabolism may interfere with dexamethasone suppression tests. Increased clearance of drugs metabolized by CYP3A4 (eg, indinavir, erythromycin). May increase or decrease phenytoin levels. Ketoconazole may inhibit adrenal corticosteroid synthesis and cause adrenal insufficiency during corticosteroid withdrawal. Antagonizes or potentiates coumarins. Hypokalemia with potassium-depleting diuretics. Live virus vaccines are contraindicated with immunosuppressive doses.

PREGNANCY: Category C, not for use in nursing.

MECHANISM OF ACTION: Adrenocortical steroid; produces anti-inflammatory effects.

PHARMACOKINETICS: Distribution: Found in breast milk. **Metabolism**: Liver; CYP3A4.

NURSING CONSIDERATIONS

Assessment: Assess for hypersensitivity to drug, systemic fungal or current infections, active TB, vaccination, unusual stress, hypothyroidism, hepatic/renal impairment, ulcerative colitis, diverticulitis, peptic ulcer with/without impending perforation, fresh intestinal anastomoses, HTN, recent MI, osteoporosis, myasthenia gravis, unstable joints, septic arthritis, existing psychotic tendencies, and for possible drug interactions (eg, indomethacin).

Monitoring: Monitor for anaphylactoid reactions, appearance/exacerbation of infections, cataracts, fluid retention, psychic derangement. Monitor infants for hypoadrenalism and growth development. Monitor for fat embolism, adrenocortical insufficiency, LFTs, TSH, PT, glucose with IOP, BP, and ECG.

Patient Counseling: Inform that susceptibility to infection may increase. Avoid exposure to chickenpox or measles; report immediately if exposed. Advise to restrict dietary sodium and potassium supplements. Counsel not to overuse joint after intra-articular injection, and not to d/c abruptly without medical supervision.

Administration: Oral route. Parenteral: IM, IV, intra-articular, intralesional, and soft-tissue injection. **Storage:** Inj: 20-25°C (68-77°F); excursions permitted to 15-30°C (59-86°F).

DEXEDRINE **CII**

dextroamphetamine sulfate (GlaxoSmithKline)

High potential for abuse. Avoid prolonged use. Misuse may cause sudden death and serious CV adverse events.

OTHER BRAND NAMES: Dexedrine Spansules (GlaxoSmithKline)

THERAPEUTIC CLASS: Sympathomimetic amine

INDICATIONS: Treatment of attention deficit disorder with hyperactivity (ADHD) and narcolepsy.

DOSAGE: *Adults:* Narcolepsy: Initial: 10mg/day. Titrate: May increase by 10mg/day every week. Usual: 5-60mg/day. For tabs, give 1st dose upon awakening and additional every 4-6 hrs. May give caps once daily.
Pediatrics: Narcolepsy: 6-12 yrs: Initial: 5mg qd. Titrate: Increase weekly by 5mg/day. ≥12 yrs: Initial: 10mg qd. Titrate: Increase weekly by 10mg/day. Usual: 5-60mg/day in divided doses. ADHD: Initial: 3-5 yrs: 2.5mg qd. Titrate: Increase weekly by 2.5mg/day. ≥6 yrs: 5mg qd-bid. Titrate: Increase weekly by 5mg/day. Max: 40mg/day. For tabs, give 1st dose upon awakening and additional every 4-6 hrs. May give caps once daily.

HOW SUPPLIED: Cap, Extended-Release: (Spansules) 5mg, 10mg, 15mg; Tab: 5mg* *scored

CONTRAINDICATIONS: Advanced arteriosclerosis, symptomatic cardiovascular disease, moderate to severe HTN, hyperthyroidism, glaucoma, agitated states, history of drug abuse, during or within 14 days of MAOI use.

WARNINGS/PRECAUTIONS: May exacerbate symptoms of behavior disturbance and thought disorder in psychotic patients. Caution when using stimulants to treat patients with comorbid bipolar disorder because of concern for possible induction of mixed/manic episode in such patients. Stimulants at usual doses can cause treatment emergent psychotic or manic symptoms (eg, hallucinations, delusional thinking, mania) in children and adolescents without prior history of psychotic illness. Aggressive behavior or hostility reported in clinical trials and the postmarketing experience of some medications indicated for the treatment of ADHD. Caution with HTN. Tablets contain tartrazine; may cause allergy reactions. Exacerbation of motor and phonic tics and Tourette's syndrome. Monitor growth in children. Avoid with serious structural cardiac abnormalities, cardiomyopathy, serious heart rhythm abnormalities, CAD, or other serious cardiac problems. Avoid use in the presence of seizure. Visual disturbances reported with stimulant treatment.

ADVERSE REACTIONS: Palpitations, tachycardia, BP elevation, CNS overstimulation, restlessness, insomnia, dry mouth, GI disturbances, anorexia, urticaria, impotence.

INTERACTIONS: GI acidifying agents (guanethidine, reserpine, glutamic acid, etc.) and urinary acidifying agents (ammonium chloride, etc) decrease efficacy. MAOIs may cause hypertensive crisis. Potentiated by GI and urinary alkalinizers, propoxyphene overdose. Potentiated effects of both agents with TCAs. May delay absorption of phenytoin, ethosuximide, phenobarbital. Potentiates meperidine, norepinephrine, phenobarbital, phenytoin. Antagonized by haloperidol, chlorpromazine, lithium. Antagonizes adrenergic blockers, antihistamines, antihypertensives, veratrum alkaloids (antihypertensive).

PREGNANCY: Category C, not for use in nursing.

MECHANISM OF ACTION: Amphetamine; noncatecholamine sympathomimetic amine with CNS stimulant activity. Peripheral actions involve elevation of BP, weak bronchodilation, and respiratory stimulant actions.

PHARMACOKINETICS: Absorption: (15mg Tab) C_{max}=36.6ng/mL, T_{max}=3 hrs. (15mg Cap-ER) C_{max}=23.5ng/mL, T_{max}=8 hrs. **Elimination:** $T_{1/2}$=12 hrs.

NURSING CONSIDERATIONS

Assessment: Assess for agitation, glaucoma, tics, family history of Tourette's syndrome, CV conditions (severe HTN, angina pectoris, cardiac structural abnormalities, arrhythmias, heart failure, recent MI), hyperthyroidism or thyrotoxicosis, bipolar illness, history of drug dependence or alcoholism, and possible drug interactions.

Monitoring: Monitor for cardiac abnormalities, exacerbations of behavior disturbances and thought disorder, bipolar illness, aggression, seizures, and visual disturbances. Height and weight follow-up in children.

Patient Counseling: Inform about risks of treatment, appropriate use, drug abuse/dependence. Caution while operating machinery/driving. Avoid late evening dose; may result in insomnia.

Administration: Oral route. **Storage:** Cap: 20-25°C (68-77°F); Tab: 15-30°C (59-86°F).

DEXTROSTAT

CII

dextroamphetamine sulfate (Shire)

High potential for abuse. Avoid prolonged use.

THERAPEUTIC CLASS: Sympathomimetic amine

INDICATIONS: Treatment of narcolepsy and attention deficit disorder with hyperactivity (ADHD).

DOSAGE: *Adults:* Narcolepsy: Initial: 10mg/day. Titrate: May increase by 10mg/day every week. Usual: 5-60mg/day. Give 1st dose upon awakening, and additional doses every 4-6 hrs.
Pediatrics: Narcolepsy: 6-12 yrs: Initial: 5mg/day. Titrate: Increase weekly by 5mg/day. ≥12 yrs: Initial: 10mg/day. Titrate: Increase weekly by 10mg/day. Usual: 5-60mg/day in divided doses. ADHD: 3-5 yrs: Initial: 2.5mg/day. Titrate: Increase weekly by 2.5mg/day until optimum response. 6-16 yrs: Initial 5mg qd-bid. Titrate: Increase weekly by 5mg/day until optimum response. Give 1st dose upon awakening, and additional doses q4-6h.

HOW SUPPLIED: Tab: 5mg*, 10mg* *scored

CONTRAINDICATIONS: Advanced arteriosclerosis, symptomatic cardiovascular disease, moderate to severe HTN, hyperthyroidism, glaucoma, agitated states, history of drug abuse, during or within 14 days of MAOI use.

WARNINGS/PRECAUTIONS: Caution in HTN. Contains tartrazine, may cause allergic reactions. Exacerbation of motor and phonic tics and Tourette's syndrome. May exacerbate behavior disturbance and thought disorder in psychotic pediatrics. Interrupt occasionally to determine if patient requires continued therapy. Monitor growth in children.

ADVERSE REACTIONS: BP elevation, tachycardia, palpitations, dizziness, insomnia, tremor, diarrhea, constipation, dry mouth, urticaria, impotence, changes in libido.

INTERACTIONS: GI acidifying agents (guanethidine, reserpine, glutamic acid, etc.) and urinary acidifying agents (ammonium chloride, etc.) decrease efficacy. MAOIs may cause hypertensive crisis. Potentiated by GI and urinary alkalinizers, propoxyphene overdose. Potentiated effects of both agents with TCAs. May delay absorption of phenytoin, ethosuximide, phenobarbital. Potentiates meperidine, norepinephrine, phenobarbital, phenytoin. Antagonized by haloperidol, chlorpromazine, lithium. Antagonizes adrenergic blockers, antihistamines, antihypertensives, veratrum alkaloids (antihypertensive).

PREGNANCY: Category C, not for use in nursing.

MECHANISM OF ACTION: Sympathomimetic amine; CNS stimulant activity. Peripheral actions involve elevation of BP, weak bronchodilation, and respiratory stimulant actions.

PHARMACOKINETICS: Absorption: C_{max}=29.2ng/mL, T_{max}=2 hrs. **Elimination:** Urine (45%); $T_{1/2}$=10.25 hrs.

NURSING CONSIDERATIONS

Assessment: Assess for agitation, glaucoma, tics, family history of Tourette's syndrome, cardiovascular conditions (eg, severe HTN, angina pectoris, cardiac structural abnormalities, arrhythmias, HF, recent MI), hyperthyroidism or thyrotoxicosis, bipolar disorder, psychosis, history of drug dependence or alcoholism.

Monitoring: Monitor for cardiac abnormalities, exacerbations of behavior disturbances and thought disorder, bipolar disorder, aggression, seizures, and visual disturbances. Monitor growth in children.

Patient Counseling: Inform about risks of treatment, its appropriate use, drug abuse/dependence. Caution while operating machinery/driving. Avoid late evening doses to prevent insomnia.

Administration: Oral route. **Storage:** 25°C (77°F); excursions permitted to 15-30°C (59-86°F).

DIABETA — RX

glyburide (Sanofi-Aventis)

THERAPEUTIC CLASS: Sulfonylurea (2nd generation)

INDICATIONS: Adjunct to diet and exercise, to improve glycemic control in type 2 diabetes mellitus.

DOSAGE: *Adults:* Initial: 2.5-5mg qd with breakfast or first main meal; give 1.25mg if sensitive to hypoglycemia. Titrate: Increase by no more than 2.5mg/day at weekly intervals. Maint: 1.25-20mg given qd or in divided doses. Max: 20mg/day. May give bid with >10mg/day. Renal/Hepatic Disease, Elderly, Debilitated, Malnourished, Adrenal or Pituitary Insufficiency: Initial: 1.25mg qd. Transfer From Other Oral Antidiabetic Agents: Initial: 2.5-5mg/day. Switch From Insulin: If <20 U/day: 2.5-5mg qd. If 20-40 U/day: 5mg qd. If >40 U/day: Decrease insulin dose by 50% and give 5mg qd. Titrate: Progressive withdrawal of insulin and increase by 1.25-2.5mg/day every 2-10 days.

HOW SUPPLIED: Tab: 1.25mg*, 2.5mg*, 5mg* *scored

CONTRAINDICATIONS: Diabetic ketoacidosis.

WARNINGS/PRECAUTIONS: Increased risk of cardiovascular mortality. Risk of hypoglycemia, especially with renal and hepatic disease; elderly, debilitated, or malnourished patients; and those with adrenal or pituitary insufficiency. May need to d/c and give insulin with stress (eg, fever, trauma). Secondary failure may occur. D/C if jaundice, hepatitis, or persistent skin reaction occur. Hematologic reactions and hyponatremia reported.

ADVERSE REACTIONS: Hypoglycemia, nausea, epigastric fullness, heartburn, allergic skin reactions, disulfiram-like reactions (rarely), hyponatremia, liver function abnormalities, photosensitivity reactions.

INTERACTIONS: Potentiated hypoglycemia with alcohol, NSAIDs, miconazole, fluoroquinolones, highly protein-bound drugs, salicylates, sulfonamides, chloramphenicol, probenecid, coumarins, MAOIs, and β-blockers. Risk of hyperglycemia with diuretics, corticosteroids, phenothiazines, thyroid products, estrogens, oral contraceptives, phenytoin, nicotinic acid, sympathomimetics, CCBs, and INH. β-blockers may mask hypoglycemia. Increased or decreased coumarin effects. Disulfiram-like reactions (rarely) with alcohol.

PREGNANCY: Category C, not for use in nursing.

MECHANISM OF ACTION: Sulfonylurea; acts by stimulating the release of insulin from functioning β-cell in pancreas.

PHARMACOKINETICS: Absorption: T_{max}=4 hrs. **Distribution:** Plasma protein binding (extensive). **Metabolism**: Hydroxylation. **Elimination:** Bile (50%), urine (50%); $T_{1/2}$=10 hrs.

NURSING CONSIDERATIONS

Assessment: Assess for cardiovascular complications and hypoglycemia risk factors. Assess for renal/hepatic impairment and DM complications.

Monitoring: Monitor fasting blood glucose levels regularly and glycosylated hemoglobin periodically. Monitor GI, dermatologic, hematologic, metabolic reactions and vision.

Patient Counseling: Stress importance of caloric restriction, weight loss, exercise programs, and regular testing of blood glucose levels. Take with breakfast or first meal.

Administration: Oral route. **Storage:** 25°C (77°F); excursions permitted to 15-30°C (59-86°F).

DIABINESE — RX

chlorpropamide (Pfizer)

THERAPEUTIC CLASS: Sulfonylurea (1st generation)

INDICATIONS: Adjunct to diet and exercise, to improve glycemic control in type 2 diabetes mellitus.

DOSAGE: *Adults:* Initial: 250mg qd. Titrate: After 5-7 days, adjust by 50-125mg/day every 3-5 days for control. Maint: 100-500mg qd. Max: 750mg qd. Elderly/Debilitated/Malnourished/Renal or Hepatic Dysfunction: Initial: 100-125mg qd. Maint: Conservative dosing. Take with breakfast. Divide dose with GI intolerance. If <40U/day insulin, discontinue therapy. If ≥40U/day insulin, decrease dose by 50% and start chlorpropamide therapy. Adjust insulin dose depending on response.

HOW SUPPLIED: Tab: 100mg*, 250mg* *scored

CONTRAINDICATIONS: Diabetic ketoacidosis and Type I diabetes.

WARNINGS/PRECAUTIONS: Increased risk of cardiovascular mortality. Hypoglycemia risk especially with renal/hepatic insufficiency, elderly, debilitated, malnourished, and adrenal/pituitary insufficiency. Loss of blood glucose control when exposed to stress (fever, trauma, infection, or surgery); d/c therapy and start insulin. Secondary failure can occur over a period of time.

ADVERSE REACTIONS: Hypoglycemia, cholestatic jaundice, diarrhea, nausea, vomiting, anorexia, pruritus, photosensitivity reactions, skin eruptions, blood dyscrasias, hepatic porphyria, disulfiram-like reactions.

INTERACTIONS: Potentiated hypoglycemia with NSAIDs, highly protein-bound drugs, salicylates, sulfonamides, chloramphenicol, probenecid, coumarins, MAOIs, and β-blockers. Risk of hyperglycemia with diuretics, corticosteroids, phenothiazines, thyroid products, estrogens, oral contraceptives, phenytoin, nicotinic acid, sympathomimetics, CCBs, and isoniazid. Alcohol may produce disulfiram-like reaction. β-blockers may mask signs of hypoglycemia. Caution with barbiturates and miconazole.

PREGNANCY: Category C, not for use in nursing.

MECHANISM OF ACTION: Sulfonylurea; acts by stimulating release of insulin from functional β-cells in the pancreas.

PHARMACOKINETICS: Absorption: Rapid; T_{max}=2-4 hrs. **Metabolism:** Extensive via hydroxylation. **Elimination:** Urine (80-90%); $T_{1/2}$=36 hrs.

NURSING CONSIDERATIONS

Assessment: Assess cardiovascular risk factors prior to therapy. Assess for signs/symptoms of hyperglycemia, drug hypersensitivity, diabetic ketoacidosis with/without coma, type 1 DM, adrenal or pituitary insufficiency, and possible drug interactions.

Monitoring: Monitor blood glucose and HbA_{1c} levels regularly. Monitor for hypoglycemia.

Patient Counseling: Inform of importance of caloric restriction, weight loss, and regular exercise. Discuss primary and secondary therapy failure with patients. Counsel on signs/symptoms of cardiovascular mortality and hypoglycemia and its management. Instruct to take therapy once daily with breakfast. Promptly notify physician if symptoms of hypoglycemia or other adverse reactions occur.

Administration: Oral route. **Storage:** Below 30°C (86°F).

DIASTAT

diazepam (Valeant)

CIV

THERAPEUTIC CLASS: Benzodiazepine

INDICATIONS: Management of refractory patients with epilepsy, on stable regimens of anti-epileptic drugs, who require intermittent use to control bouts of increased seizure activity.

DOSAGE: *Adults:* 0.2mg/kg rectally. Calculate amount and round upwards to next available dose. May give 2nd dose 4-12 hrs later. Max: 5 episodes/month or 1 episode every 5 days.
Pediatrics: ≥12 yrs: 0.2mg/kg. 6-11yrs: 0.3mg/kg. 2-5 yrs: 0.5mg/kg. Calculate amount and round upwards to next available dose. May give 2nd dose 4-12 hrs later. For rectal administration. Max: 5 episodes/month and 1 episode every 5 days.

HOW SUPPLIED: Kit: 2.5mg, 5mg, 10mg, 15mg, 20mg

CONTRAINDICATIONS: Acute narrow angle glaucoma, untreated open angle glaucoma.

WARNINGS/PRECAUTIONS: Produces CNS depression. Avoid abrupt withdrawal. Caution with elderly, hepatic/renal dysfunction, compromised respiratory function, neurologic damage. Not for daily chronic use. Withdrawal symptoms reported with discontinuation.

ADVERSE REACTIONS: Somnolence, dizziness, headache, pain, abdominal pain, nervousness, vasodilation, diarrhea, ataxia, euphoria, incoordination, asthma, rhinitis, rash.

INTERACTIONS: Potentiated by phenothiazines, narcotics, barbiturates, valproate, MAOIs, and other antidepressants. Potential inhibitors of CYP450 2C19 (eg, cimetidine, quinidine, tranylcypromine) and CYP450 3A4 (eg, ketoconazole, troleandomycin, clotrimazole) may decrease elimination. CYP450 2C19 (eg, rifampin) and CYP450 3A4 (eg, carbamazepine, phenytoin, dexamethasone, phenobarbital) inducers could increase elimination. May interfere with metabolism of substrates for CYP450 2C19 (eg, omeprazole, propranolol, imipramine) and CYP450 3A4 (eg, cyclosporine, paclitaxel, terfenadine, theophylline, warfarin).

PREGNANCY: Category D, not for use in nursing.

MECHANISM OF ACTION: Benzodiazepine; unknown, suspected to suppress seizures through an interaction with GABA receptors (A-type). GABA acts at this receptor to allow entry of chloride ions, which causes an inhibitory potential that reduces the ability of neurons to depolarize to the threshold potential necessary to produce action potentials.

PHARMACOKINETICS: Absorption: Absolute bioavailability (90%); T_{max}=1.5 hrs. **Distribution:** V_d=1L/kg; plasma protein binding (95-98%). **Metabolism:** Hepatic (CYP3A4, CYP2C19) to form desmethyldiazepam (major active metabolite), temazepam and oxazepam (minor active metabolites). **Elimination:** $T_{1/2}$=46 hrs (15mg rectal).

NURSING CONSIDERATIONS

Assessment: Assess for acute narrow-angle glaucoma, renal/hepatic and pulmonary function, and pregnancy status. Note other diseases/conditions and drug therapies.

Monitoring: Monitor for hypersensitivity reactions, rebound or withdrawal symptoms, seizures, HR, insomnia, LFTs, renal and pulmonary function tests.

Patient Counseling: Advise to take as directed. Avoid alcohol and other sedatives; use caution while operating machinery/driving. Counsel about drug abuse/dependence, side effects, and report if any occur.

Administration: Rectal gel. 1) Lubricate tip with jelly. 2) Turn person on side and bend upper leg forward. 3) Gently insert syringe tip into rectum and slowly push plunger in until it stops. 4) Slowly remove syringe from rectum and hold buttocks together to prevent leakage. **Storage:** 25°C (77°F); excursions permitted to 15-30°C (59-86°F).

DIAZEPAM INJECTION

CIV

diazepam (Various)

THERAPEUTIC CLASS: Benzodiazepine

INDICATIONS: Management of anxiety disorders and short-term relief of anxiety symptoms. Symptomatic relief of acute alcohol withdrawal. Adjunct prior to endoscopic procedures, surgical procedures and cardioversion. Adjunct therapy in skeletal muscle spasm (eg, tetanus, etc), status epilepticus and severe recurrent convulsive disorders.

DOSAGE: *Adults:* Anxiety (moderate): 2-5mg IM/IV, may repeat in 3-4 hrs. Anxiety (severe): 5-10mg IM/IV, may repeat in 3-4 hrs. Alcohol Withdrawal (acute): 10mg IM/IV, then 5-10mg in 3-4 hrs if needed. Endoscopic Procedures: Usual: ≤10mg IV (up to 20mg) or 5-10mg IM 30 min prior to procedure. Muscle Spasm: 5-10mg IM/IV, then 5-10mg in 3-4 hrs if needed. Status Epilepticus/Severe Seizures: Initial: 5-10mg IV. Maint: May repeat at 10-15 min intervals. Max: 30mg. Preoperative: 10mg IM. Cardioversion: 5-15mg IV, 5-10 min prior to procedure. Elderly/Debilitated: Usual: 2-5mg.
Pediatrics: Tetanus: 30 days-5 yrs: 1-2mg IM/IV (slowly), may repeat every 3-4 hrs prn. ≥5 yrs: 5-10mg IM/IV, may repeat every 3-4 hrs. Status Epilepticus/Severe Seizures: 30 days-5 yrs: 0.2-0.5mg IV (slowly) every 2-5 min up to 5mg. ≥5 yrs: 1mg IV (slowly) every 2-5 min up to 10mg, may repeat in 2-4 hrs.

HOW SUPPLIED: Inj: 5mg/mL

CONTRAINDICATIONS: Acute narrow angle glaucoma, untreated open angle glaucoma.

WARNINGS/PRECAUTIONS: Inject slowly and avoid small veins with IV. Do not mix or dilute with other products in syringe or infusion flask. Extreme caution in elderly, severely ill and those with limited pulmonary reserve. Avoid if in shock, coma or acute alcohol intoxication with depressed vital signs. May impair mental/physical abilities. Increase in grand mal seizures reported. Caution with kidney or hepatic dysfunction. Not for obstetrical use. Withdrawal symptoms may occur. Hypotension and muscular weakness reported. Monitor blood counts and LFTs. Not for maintenance of seizures once controlled.

ADVERSE REACTIONS: Drowsiness, fatigue, ataxia, venous thrombosis and phlebitis (injection site).

INTERACTIONS: Phenothiazines, narcotics, barbiturates, MAOIs, and other antidepressants may potentiate effects. Delayed clearance with cimetidine. Reduce narcotic dose by at least one-third. Risk of apnea with concomitant barbiturates, alcohol, or other CNS depressants.

PREGNANCY: Not for use during pregnancy, safety in nursing unknown.

MECHANISM OF ACTION: Antianxiety/hypnotic agent; induces calming effect on parts of the limbic system, thalamus, and hypothalamus (animal study).

NURSING CONSIDERATIONS

Assessment: Assess for acute narrow-angle glaucoma, open-angle glaucoma, acute alcoholic intoxication, shock, coma, cardiac arrest, apnea, hypotension, hypersensitivity, and for possible drug interactions.

Monitoring: Monitor injection site for thrombosis and phlebitis, tonic status epilepticus, drowsiness, fatigue, ataxia, CNS depression, and for habituation and dependence.

Patient Counseling: Caution against hazardous tasks (operating machinery/driving).

Administration: IV, IM route. **Storage:** 20-25°C (6°-77°F). Protect from light.

DICLOXACILLIN RX

dicloxacillin sodium (Various)

THERAPEUTIC CLASS: Penicillin (penicillinase-resistant)

INDICATIONS: Infections caused by penicillinase-producing staphylococci.

DOSAGE: *Adults:* Mild-Moderate Infection: 125mg q6h. Severe Infection: 250mg q6h for at least 14 days.
Pediatrics: <40kg: Mild-Moderate Infection: 12.5mg/kg/day in divided doses q6h. Severe Infection: 25mg/kg/day in divided doses q6h for at least 14 days.

HOW SUPPLIED: Cap: 250mg, 500mg

WARNINGS/PRECAUTIONS: Serious, fatal hypersensitivity reactions reported. Pseudomembranous colitis has been reported; toxin produced by *Clostridium difficile* is the primary cause. Caution with history of allergy and/or asthma. Monitor renal, hepatic, and hematopoietic function with prolonged use. Not for use as initial therapy with serious, life-threatening infections, or with nausea, vomiting, gastric dilation, cardiospasm, or intestinal hypermotility.

ADVERSE REACTIONS: Allergic reactions, NV, diarrhea, stomatitis, black or hairy tongue, superinfection (prolonged use), hepatotoxicity.

INTERACTIONS: Tetracycline may antagonize the bactericidal effects. Potentiated by probenecid.

PREGNANCY: Category B, caution in nursing.

MECHANISM OF ACTION: Penicillin (penicillinase-resistant); bactericidal against penicillin-susceptible microorganisms during state of active multiplication. Inhibits biosynthesis of bacterial cell-wall.

PHARMACOKINETICS: Absorption: Rapid, incomplete; C_{max}=1-1.5 hrs; T_{max}=10-17mcg/mL. **Distribution:** Serum protein binding (95%-99%); found in breast milk. **Elimination:** Urine (unchanged); $T_{1/2}$=0.7 hrs.

NURSING CONSIDERATIONS

Assessment: Assess for comprehensive drug/allergy history (hypersensitivity to PCNs/cephalosporins, cephamycins and other 1-oxa-β-lactams, history of allergy or asthma), presence of severe illness or with NV, gastric dilation, cardiospasm and intestinal hypermotility, pregnancy/nursing status, and possible drug interactions. Perform blood cultures, WBC with differential prior to therapy and weekly thereafter.

Monitoring: Monitor for anaphylactic shock with collapse, pseudomembranous colitis or *C.difficile*-associated diarrhea (can range from mild diarrhea to fatal colitis), development of drug resistance, overgrowth of nonsusceptible organisms and lab monitoring for urine analysis, BUN, creatinine, SGOT, SGPT during therapy with dosage alteration if values elevated. Evaluate renal, hepatic, and hematopoietic functions during prolonged therapy.

Patient Counseling: Advise not to take drug if previous allergic reaction occurred. Counsel to take 1 hr before or 2 hrs after meal. Take exactly as prescribed to avoid developing drug resistance and to maintain effectiveness. Advise to notify physician if pregnant/nursing or experience SOB, wheezing, skin rash, mouth irritation, black tongue, sore throat, NV, diarrhea, fever, swollen joints, or any unusual bleeding or bruising. Instruct to notify if taking additional medications. Counsel that drug only treats bacterial, not viral, infections.

Administration: Oral route. **Storage:** 20-25°C (68-77°F).

DIDRONEL — RX

etidronate disodium (Procter & Gamble)

THERAPEUTIC CLASS: Bisphosphonate

INDICATIONS: Treatment of Paget's disease. Treatment and prevention of heterotopic ossification following total hip replacement or due to spinal cord injury.

DOSAGE: *Adults:* Give as single dose (preferred) or in divided doses. Paget's disease: Initial: 5-10mg/kg/day up to 6 months or 11-20mg/kg/day up to 3 months. May retreat after drug free period of 90 days only if evidence of active disease process. Heterotopic Ossification: Hip Replacement: 20mg/kg/day 1 month before and 3 months after surgery. Spinal Cord: 20mg/kg/day for 2 weeks, followed by 10mg/kg/day for 10 weeks.

HOW SUPPLIED: Tab: 200mg, 400mg* *scored

CONTRAINDICATIONS: Overt osteomalacia.

WARNINGS/PRECAUTIONS: Therapy response in Paget's Disease may be of slow onset and continue for months after stopping. Maintain adequate dietary intake of calcium and vitamin D. Diarrhea reported with enterocolitis. Monitor with renal impairment. Reduce dose with decreased GFR. Max dose (20mg/day) or long-term therapy (>6 months) may increase fracture risk. Rachitic syndrome reported in children at doses of 10mg/kg/day for prolonged periods (approaching or exceeding 1 year).

ADVERSE REACTIONS: Diarrhea, nausea, increased bone pain in Paget's, alopecia, arthropathy, esophagitis, hypersensitivity reactions, osteomalacia, amnesia, confusion.

INTERACTIONS: Vitamins with mineral supplements or antacids that contain calcium, iron, aluminum, or magnesium reduce absorption (separate dosing by 2 hours). Monitor PT with warfarin.

PREGNANCY: Category C, caution with nursing.

MECHANISM OF ACTION: Bone metabolism regulator; inhibits the formation, growth, and dissolution of hydroxyapatite crystals and their amorphous precursors by chemisorption to calcium phosphate surfaces.

PHARMACOKINETICS: Metabolism: Not metabolized. **Elimination:** Urine (50% of absorbed drug); feces (unabsorbed drug).

NURSING CONSIDERATIONS

Assessment: Assess for clinically overt osteomalacia, renal impairment, enterocolitis, presence of fractures, upcoming dental procedures, pregnancy/nursing status, and possible drug interactions.

Monitoring: Monitor for signs/symptoms of osteonecrosis (eg, jaw), musculoskeletal pain, osteomalacia and fractures, diarrhea, and hyperphosphatemia.

Monitor renal function in patients with renal impairment. In patients with lytic lesions, monitor radiographically and biochemically to determine if responsive to therapy.

Patient Counseling: Counsel to maintain adequate nutritional status, particularly adequate intake of calcium and vitamin D. Advise food high in calcium, vitamins with mineral supplements, or antacids which are high in metals (eg, calcium, iron, magnesium, aluminum) should be separated from dose administration by 2 hrs. Advise dose may be divided if GI discomfort occurs. Instruct that a 90-day drug-free interval should be provided between therapy courses.

Administration: Oral route. **Storage:** 25°C (77°F); excursions permitted to 15-30°C (59-86°F).

DIFFERIN RX

adapalene (Galderma)

THERAPEUTIC CLASS: Naphthoic acid derivative (retinoid-like)

INDICATIONS: Topical treatment of acne vulgaris.

DOSAGE: *Adults:* Apply qhs after washing.
Pediatrics: ≥12 yrs: Apply qhs after washing.

HOW SUPPLIED: Cre: 0.1% [45g]; Gel: 0.1%, 0.3% [45g, 75g]

WARNINGS/PRECAUTIONS: Avoid contact with eyes, lips, paranasal creases, mucous membranes, cuts, abrasions, eczematous or sunburned skin. Minimize sun exposure. Extreme weather may increase skin irritation.

ADVERSE REACTIONS: Erythema, scaling, dryness, pruritus, burning, sunburn, acne flares.

INTERACTIONS: Caution with other topicals with strong drying effects, high concentration of alcohol, astringents, spices, or lime. Allow effects of sulfur, resorcinol, or salicylic acid to subside before use.

PREGNANCY: Category C, caution in nursing.

MECHANISM OF ACTION: Naphthoic acid derivative; not established. Suspected to normalize differentiation of follicular epithelial cells resulting in decreased microcomedone formation.

PHARMACOKINETICS: Absorption: Low. **Elimination:** Bile.

NURSING CONSIDERATIONS

Assessment: Assess for sunburn. Assess use in pregnant/nursing patients and for possible drug interactions.

Monitoring: Monitor for sensitivity or chemical irritation, cutaneous signs/symptoms (eg, erythema, dryness, scaling, burning, or pruritus).

Patient Counseling: Instruct to avoid exposure to sunlight and sunlamps; use sunscreen and protective clothing over treated areas when exposed. Medication may also cause skin irritation when exposed to wind or cold. Avoid contact with eyes, lips, angles of the nose, and mucous membranes. Do not apply medication to cuts, abrasions, eczematous or sunburned skin.

Administration: Topical application. **Storage:** 20-25°C (68-77°F), excursions permitted to 15-30°C (59-86°F). Protect from freezing.

DIFLUCAN RX

fluconazole (Pfizer)

THERAPEUTIC CLASS: Azole antifungal

INDICATIONS: Treatment of vaginal, oropharyngeal, and esophageal candidiasis. Treatment of systemic *Candida* infections. Treatment of peritonitis and UTI caused by *Candida*. Treatment of cryptococcal meningitis. Prophylaxis in patients undergoing BMT.

DOSAGE: *Adults:* Vaginal Candidiasis: 150mg PO single dose. IV/PO: Oropharyngeal Candidiasis: 200mg on 1st day, then 100mg qd for at least

2 weeks. Esophageal Candidiasis: 200mg on 1st day, then 100mg qd for at least 3 weeks and for at least 2 weeks following resolution of symptoms. Max: 400mg/day. Systemic *Candida* Infections: Up to 400mg/day. UTI/Peritonitis: 50-200mg/day. Cryptococcal Meningitis: 400mg on 1st day, then 200mg qd for 10-12 weeks after negative CSF culture. Suppression of Cryptococcal Meningitis Relapse in AIDS: 200mg qd. Prophylaxis in BMT: 400mg qd. Renal Impairment: CrCl ≤50mL/min (no dialysis): Initial: LD 50-400mg. Maint: Give 50% of recommended dose. Dialysis: Give 100% of dose after each dialysis. *Pediatrics:* IV/PO: Oropharyngeal Candidiasis: 6mg/kg on 1st day, then 3mg/kg/day for at least 2 weeks. Esophageal Candidiasis: 6mg/kg on 1st day, then 3mg/kg/day for at least 3 weeks and for at least 2 weeks following resolution of symptoms. Max: 12mg/kg/day. Systemic *Candida* Infections: 6-12mg/kg/day. Cryptococcal Meningitis: 12mg/kg 1st day, then 6mg/kg/day for 10-12 weeks after negative CSF culture. Suppression of Cryptococcal Meningitis Relapse in AIDS: 6mg/kg qd. Renal Impairment: CrCl <50mL/min (no dialysis): Initial: LD: 50-400mg. Maint: Give 50% of recommended dose. Dialysis: Give 100% of dose after each dialysis.

D

HOW SUPPLIED: Inj: 200mg/100mL, 400mg/200mL; Sus: 50mg/5mL, 200mg/5mL [35mL]; Tab: 50mg, 100mg, 150mg, 200mg

CONTRAINDICATIONS: Coadministration with cisapride or terfenadine (with multiple fluconazole doses of ≥400mg). Caution if hypersensitive to other azoles.

WARNINGS/PRECAUTIONS: Monitor LFTs. D/C if hepatic dysfunction develops or exfoliative skin disorder progresses. Anaphylaxis reported. Rare cases of QT prolongation and torsade de pointes reported.

ADVERSE REACTIONS: Headache, NV, abdominal pain, diarrhea, skin rash.

INTERACTIONS: See Contraindications. Severe hypoglycemia with oral hypoglycemics. May increase PT with coumarin-type drugs. Increases levels of phenytoin, cyclosporine, cisapride, astemizole, zidovudine and theophylline. Rifampin enhances metabolism of fluconazole. Cimetidine may decrease levels. HCTZ may increase levels. Contraindicated with terfenadine and cisapride due to prolongation of QTc interval. Cardiac events (torsades de pointes) reported with cisapride. Uveitis reported with rifabutin. Nephrotoxicity reported with tacrolimus. May increase or decrease levels of ethinyl estradiol- and levonorgestrel-containing oral contraceptives.

PREGNANCY: Category C, not for use in nursing.

MECHANISM OF ACTION: Antifungal; inhibits fungal CYP450 sterol C-14 α-demethylation. Subsequent loss of normal sterol correlates with accumulation of 14 α-methyl sterols in fungi and may be responsible for its fungistatic activity.

PHARMACOKINETICS: Absorption: Oral: Absolute bioavailability (90%); C_{max}=6.72mcg/mL (50-400mg), T_{max}=1-2 hrs (fasted). **Distribution:** Plasma protein binding (11-12%). **Elimination:** Urine (80% unchanged and 11% metabolites); $T_{1/2}$=30 hrs. Refer to PI for pediatric pharmacokinetic parameters.

NURSING CONSIDERATIONS

Assessment: Assess for proper clinical diagnosis of fungal infection. Assess for possible drug interactions prior to therapy (eg, terfenadine, cisapride, other azole antifungal agents). Assess renal function prior to administration. Assess use of medication in patients who are at risk for developing proarrhythmic conditions.

Monitoring: Monitor LFTs for signs of hepatotoxicity. Monitor for anaphylaxis reactions (eg, angioedema, face edema, pruritus) and dermatological reactions (exfoliative skin disorders) while on therapy. Monitor for ECG for QT prolongation and torsade de pointes. Monitor renal function.

Patient Counseling: Counsel about signs/symptoms of hepatoxicity and anaphylaxis reactions. D/C therapy if skin rash occurs or lesions develop.

Administration: IV infusion and oral route. IV infusion max rate is 200mg/hr. **Storage:** Tablet: Below 30°C (86°F). Oral susp: Store dry powder below 30°C (86°F). Store reconstituted suspension between 30°C (86°F) and 5°C (41°F) and discard unused portion after 2 weeks. Protect from freezing. Inj. in glass bottles: Between 30°C (86°F) and 5°C (41°F), protect from freezing. Inj. in Viaflex Plus plastic container: Between 25°C (77°F) and 5°C (41°F). Brief exposure up to 40°C (104°F) does not adversely affect the product. Protect from light.

DIGIBIND RX

digoxin immune fab (ovine) (GlaxoSmithKline)

THERAPEUTIC CLASS: Antidote, digoxin toxicity

INDICATIONS: Treatment of life-threatening digoxin intoxication. Also has been successfully used to treat digitoxin overdose.

DOSAGE: *Adults:* Acute Ingestion of Unknown Amount: Usual: Administer 10 vials, observe response, then additional 10 vials if clinically indicated. Calculation: # vials = total digitalis body load (mg)/0.5mg of digitalis bound per vial. 1 vial will bind approximately 0.5mg of digoxin (or digitoxin). Steady-State Serum Digoxin Concentrations: # of vials = (serum dig conc in ng/mL) x (wt in kg)/100. Steady-State Digitoxin Concentrations: # of vials = (serum digitoxin conc in ng/mL) x (wt in kg)/1000. If toxicity not adequately reversed after several hrs or appears to recur, may need readministration. See PI for details.
Pediatrics: Acute Ingestion of Unknown Amount: Usual: Administer 10 vials, observe response, then additional 10 vials if clinically indicated. Calculation: # vials = total digitalis body load (mg)/0.5mg of digitalis bound per vial. 1 vial will bind approximately 0.5mg of digoxin (or digitoxin). Steady-State Serum Digoxin Concentrations: Dose (mg) = (# vials) (38mg/vial). Steady-State Digitoxin Concentrations: # of vials = (serum digitoxin conc in ng/mL) x (wt in kg)/1000. If toxicity not adequately reversed after several hrs or appears to recur, may need readministration. See PI for details.

HOW SUPPLIED: Inj: 38mg

WARNINGS/PRECAUTIONS: Obtain digoxin level before initiation. Do not overlook possibility of multiple drug overdose. Risk of hypersensitivity is greater with allergies to papain, chymopapain, or other papaya extracts; skin testing may be appropriate for high-risk individuals. K^+ levels may drop rapidly after administration; monitor closely. Digitalis toxicity may recur with renal dysfunction; caution and monitor closely. Caution with cardiac dysfunction, further deterioration may occur from digoxin withdrawal. Consider additional support with inotropes or vasodilators. Monitor for volume overload in children. D/C if anaphylactoid reaction occurs and treat appropriately.

ADVERSE REACTIONS: Allergic reactions, exacerbation of low cardiac output, CHF, hypokalemia.

PREGNANCY: Category C, caution in nursing.

MECHANISM OF ACTION: Antidote; digoxin toxicity. Binds to molecules of digoxin, making them unavailable for binding at their site of action on cells.

PHARMACOKINETICS: Elimination: Urine; $T_{1/2}$=15-20 hrs.

NURSING CONSIDERATIONS

Assessment: Assess for serum digoxin or digitoxin concentration, serum electrolytes, hypoxia, acid base disturbances, CVD, and renal functions. Note other diseases/conditions and drug therapies.

Monitoring: Monitor for serum potassium concentration, arrhythmias, and renal function.

Patient Counseling: Counsel about adverse effects.

Administration: IV route. Refer to PI for further information. **Storage:** 2-8°C (36-46°F). Unreconstituted vials can be stored at up to 30°C (86°F) for 30 days.

D

DILACOR XR
diltiazem HCl (Watson)

RX

OTHER BRAND NAMES: Diltia XT (Andrx)

THERAPEUTIC CLASS: Calcium channel blocker (nondihydropyridine)

INDICATIONS: Treatment of hypertension and management of chronic stable angina.

DOSAGE: *Adults:* HTN: Initial: 180-240mg qd. Usual: 180-480mg qd. Max: 540mg qd. ≥60 yrs: Initial: 120mg qd. Angina: Initial: 120mg qd. Titrate: Adjust at 1-2 week intervals. Max: 480mg/day. Swallow whole on an empty stomach in the am.

HOW SUPPLIED: Cap, Extended-Release: 120mg, 180mg, 240mg

CONTRAINDICATIONS: Sick sinus syndrome, 2nd- or 3rd-degree AV block (except with functioning pacemaker), hypotension (<90mmHg systolic), acute MI, pulmonary congestion.

WARNINGS/PRECAUTIONS: Caution in renal, hepatic, or ventricular dysfunction. Monitor LFTs and renal function with prolonged use. D/C if persistent rash occurs. Symptomatic hypotension may occur. Acute hepatic injury reported.

ADVERSE REACTIONS: Rhinitis, pharyngitis, cough, flu syndrome, peripheral edema, myalgia, NV, sinusitis, asthenia, vasodilation, headache, constipation, diarrhea.

INTERACTIONS: Increased levels of propranolol. Increased levels of diltiazem with cimetidine. Monitor digoxin, cyclosporine. Potentiates cardiac contractility, conductivity, and automaticity; and vascular dilation with anesthetics. Additive cardiac conduction effects with digitalis or β-blockers. Potential additive effects with agents known to affect cardiac contractility and/or conduction.

PREGNANCY: Category C, not for use in nursing.

MECHANISM OF ACTION: Ca^{2+} channel blocker; inhibits influx of calcium ion during membrane depolarization of cardiac and vascular smooth muscle with resultant decrease in peripheral vascular resistance.

PHARMACOKINETICS: Absorption: Absolute bioavailability (41%); T_{max}=4-6 hrs. **Distribution:** Plasma protein binding (70-80%). **Metabolism:** Liver. Desacetyldiltiazem (major metabolite). **Elimination:** Urine (2-4%); $T_{1/2}$=5-10 hrs.

NURSING CONSIDERATIONS

Assessment: Assess for sick sinus syndrome, hypotension, AV block, AMI, pulmonary congestion, pre-existing impairment of ventricular function, possible drug interactions, pre-existing GI narrowing, renal/hepatic impairment.

Monitoring: Monitor renal function and LFTs periodically. Monitor for signs/symptoms of worsening of CHF, hypotension, obstruction from strictures, hypersensitivity reactions, renal/hepatic dysfunction.

Patient Counseling: Instruct to take on empty stomach; not to open capsule; swallow whole, do not chew or crush. Advise to seek medical attention if symptoms of GI obstruction, worsening of CHF, hypotension, or hypersensitivity reactions occur.

Administration: Oral route. **Storage:** 20-25°C (68-77°F).

DILANTIN
phenytoin (Parke-Davis)

RX

THERAPEUTIC CLASS: Hydantoin

INDICATIONS: (CER, CTB) Control of generalized tonic-clonic (grand mal) and complex partial (psychomotor, temporal lobe) seizures. Prevention and

D

treatment of neurosurgically induced seizures. (Sus) Control of tonic-clonic (grand mal) and psychomotor (temporal lobe) seizures.

DOSAGE: *Adults:* (CER) Initial: 100mg tid. Titrate: May increase at 7-10 day intervals. Max: 200mg tid. May give once daily with extended-release if controlled on 300mg daily. LD (clinic/hospital): 1g in 3 divided doses (400mg, 300mg, 300mg) given 2 hrs apart. Start maintenance 24 hrs later. (CTB) Initial: 100mg tid. Titrate: May increase at 7-10 day intervals. Usual: 300-400mg/day. Max: 600mg/day. May chew or swallow tab whole. Not for once daily dosing. (Sus) Initial: 125mg tid. Titrate: May increase at 7-10 day intervals. Max: 625mg/day.
Pediatrics: (CER, CTB, Sus) Initial: 5mg/kg/day given bid-tid. Titrate: May increase at 7-10 day intervals. Maint: 4-8mg/kg/day. Max: 300mg/day. >6 yrs: May require the minimum adult dose (300mg/day).

HOW SUPPLIED: Cap, Extended-Release (CER): 30mg, 100mg; Sus: 125mg/5mL [237mL]; Tab, Chewable (CTB): 50mg* *scored

WARNINGS/PRECAUTIONS: Avoid abrupt discontinuation. Caution with porphyria, hepatic dysfunction, elderly, diabetes, debilitated. D/C if rash occurs. Lymphadenopathy reported. Serum sickness may occur with lymph node involvement. Gingival hyperplasia reported; maintain proper dental hygiene. Hyperglycemia, birth defects and osteomalacia reported. Monitor levels. Confused states reported with increased levels. Increased seizure frequency during pregnancy. Neonatal coagulation defects reported within first 24 hrs of birth. Give vitamin K to mother before delivery and to neonate after birth. Avoid use with seizures due to hypoglycemia or other metabolic causes.

ADVERSE REACTIONS: Nystagmus, ataxia, slurred speech, decreased coordination, confusion, dizziness, insomnia, transient nervousness, motor twitchings, headaches, nausea, vomiting, constipation, rash, hypersensitivity reactions.

INTERACTIONS: Increased levels with acute alcohol intake, amiodarone, chloramphenicol, chlordiazepoxide, diazepam, dicumarol, disulfiram, estrogens, H_2-antagonists, halothane, isoniazid, methylphenidate, phenothiazines, phenylbutazone, salicylates, succinamides, sulfonamides, tolbutamide, trazodone. Decreased levels with chronic alcohol abuse, carbamazepine, reserpine, sucralfate. Decreases effects of corticosteroids, coumarin anticoagulants, digitoxin, doxycycline, estrogens, furosemide, oral contraceptives, quinidine, rifampin, theophylline, vitamin D. Phenobarbital, sodium valproate, valproic acid may increase or decrease levels. May increase or decrease levels of phenobarbital, sodium valproate, valproic acid. Calcium antacids decrease absorption; space dosing. Moban contains calcium ions that interfere with absorption. TCAs may precipitate seizures. Increased risk of phenytoin hypersensitivity with barbiturates, succinamides, oxazolidinediones.

PREGNANCY: Possibly teratogenic, weigh benefits versus risk; not for use in nursing.

MECHANISM OF ACTION: Anticonvulsant; inhibits seizure activity by promoting sodium efflux from neurons, stabilizing threshold against hyperexcitability caused by excessive stimulation of environmental changes capable of reducing membrane sodium gradient.

PHARMACOKINETICS: Absorption: T_{max}=1.5-3 hrs. **Distribution:** Highly protein bound. **Metabolism:** Liver (hydroxylation). **Elimination:** Bile, urine; $T_{1/2}$=22 hrs.

NURSING CONSIDERATIONS

Assessment: Assess that seizure is not due to hypoglycemia or other metabolic causes and that seizure is not an absence seizure. Assess use with impaired hepatic function and status porphyria. Assess pregnancy status prior to therapy and for possible drug interactions.

Monitoring: Monitor for signs/symptoms of skin rash (Stevens-Johnson syndrome, toxic epidermal necrolysis) and lymphadenopathy (benign lymph node hyperplasia, pseudolymphoma, Hodgkin's disease). Monitor for hyperglycemia in diabetic patients, serum phenytoin levels in pregnant women or if confused states occur (delirium, psychosis, encephalopathy), and for osteomalacia.

Patient Counseling: Inform of importance of strictly adhering to prescribed dosage regimen. Caution on use of other drugs or alcoholic beverages without consulting physician. Instruct to immediately contact physician if skin rash develops. Instruct to maintain proper dental hygeine while on medication to minimize risk of gingival hyperplasia. Advise females about dangers of using medication during pregnancy. Inform pregnant women they will need to receive vitamin K prior to delivery.

Administration: Oral route. Dilantin Infatabs can either be chewed throughly before swallowing or swallowed whole. **Storage:** (Tab) 15-30°C (59-86°F); (Cap/Sus) 20-25°C (68-77°F). Protect from moisture.

DILAUDID

CII

hydromorphone HCl (Abbott)

Contains hydromorphone, a potent Schedule II opioid agonist which has the highest potential for abuse and risk of producing respiratory depression. HP formulation is a highly concentrated solution of hydromorphone; do not confuse with standard parenteral formulations of hydromorphone or other opioids as overdose and death could result. Alcohol, other opioids, CNS depressants potentiate respiratory depressant effects, increasing risk of respiratory depression which may result in death.

OTHER BRAND NAMES: Dilaudid-HP (Abbott)

THERAPEUTIC CLASS: Opioid analgesic

INDICATIONS: Management of pain. (HP) Relief of moderate to severe pain in opioid-tolerant patients who require larger than usual doses of opioids to provide adequate pain relief.

DOSAGE: *Adults:* Individualize dose. Initial: 1-2mg SQ/IM/IV q4-6h prn. (HP) Range: 1-14mg IM/SQ; adjust dose based on response. (Sol) 2.5-10mg PO q3-6h prn. (Tab) 2-4mg PO q4-6h prn. (Sup) Insert 1 PR q6-8h prn. Titrate: Increase dose as needed. Elderly: Start at lower end of dosing range.

HOW SUPPLIED: Inj: 1mg/mL, 2mg/mL, 4mg/mL, (HP) 10mg/mL, 250mg; Sol: 1mg/mL; Sup: 3mg; Tab: 2mg, 4mg, 8mg* *scored

CONTRAINDICATIONS: Intracranial lesions associated with increased ICP, COPD, cor pulmonale, emphysema, kyphoscoliosis, and in status asthmaticus. (HP-Inj) Obstetrical analgesia.

WARNINGS/PRECAUTIONS: Increased respiratory depression with head injury and/or increased ICP. May mask acute abdominal conditions. Caution with elderly/debilitated, seizures, biliary tract surgery, renal/hepatic impairment, hypothyroidism, Addison's disease, BPH, and urethral stricture; initial dose should be reduced in these patients. May suppress cough reflex. Potential for physical/psychological tolerance or dependence, especially in patients with alcoholism and drug dependencies; monitor closely. Seizures reported in compromised patients receiving high doses. Dilaudid-HP should only be used in patients already receiving large doses of narcotics. 8mg tab and sol contains sulfites.

ADVERSE REACTIONS: Excessive sedation, lethargy, mental clouding, anxiety, dysphoria, NV, constipation, urinary retention, respiratory depression. Orthostatic hypotension and fainting reported with injection.

INTERACTIONS: Additive CNS depression with other narcotic analgesics, neuromuscular blocking agents, general anesthetics, phenothiazines, tranquilizers, sedative hypnotics, TCAs, alcohol, or other CNS depressants. Mixed agonist/antagonist analgesics (eg, pentazocine, nalbuphine, butorphanol, buprenorphine) may reduce the analgesic effect of hydromorphone and/or may precipitate withdrawal symptoms.

PREGNANCY: Category C, not for use in nursing.

MECHANISM OF ACTION: Opioid analgesic; not established. Suspected to bind to specific opiate receptors in the CNS to produce analgesia.

PHARMACOKINETICS: Absorption: (PO) Rapid; (Tab) C_{max}=5.5ng, T_{max}=0.74 hrs; (Sol) C_{max}=5.7ng, T_{max}=0.73 hrs. Distribution: Plasma protein binding (8-19%); (IV Bolus) V_d=302.9 L; crosses placenta, found in breast milk. Metabolism: Liver; glucuronidation (extensive); hydromorphone-3-glucuronide (metabolite). Elimination: Urine; (IV) $T_{1/2}$=2.3 hrs; (Tab) $T_{1/2}$=2.6 hrs; (Sol) $T_{1/2}$=2.8 hrs.

NURSING CONSIDERATIONS

Assessment: Assess for respiratory depression, presence of status asthmaticus, COPD, potential for opioid abuse (eg, family history, mental illness), nursing/pregnancy status, presence of obstetrical pain, age of patient, head injury, intracranial lesions, elevated intracranial pressure, circulatory shock, sulfite sensitivity, renal/hepatic impairment, myxedema or hypothyroidism, adrenocortical insufficiency (eg, Addison's disease), CNS depression or coma, toxic psychosis, convulsive disorder, prostatic hypertrophy or urethral stricture, gallbladder disease, upcoming surgery on the biliary tract, presence of acute abdominal conditions, acute alcoholism, delirium tremens, kyphoscoliosis, and possible drug interactions.

Monitoring: Monitor for signs/symptoms of respiratory depression, circulatory depression (eg, hypotension), misuse or abuse, tolerance or dependence, seizures, and for alleviation of pain.

Patient Counseling: Inform that medication may cause respiratory depression if not taken as directed. Instruct not to adjust dosage without physician's consent. Medication may impair mental/physical abilities; use caution when performing hazardous tasks (eg, operating machinery/driving). Avoid using other CNS depressants and alcohol. Inform pregnant women about effects of medication on pregnancy. Instruct to avoid abrupt withdrawal; dosage should be tapered. Educate that medication has abuse potential. Advise to keep out of reach of children and to dispose unused tablets via toilet.

Administration: Subcutaneous, IM, IV, oral, and rectal route. IV administration should be given slowly over at least 2-3 min, depending on dose. **Storage:** Parenteral and oral: 25°C (77°F); excursions permitted to 15-30° (59-86°F), protect from light. Suppository: Refrigerate between 2-8°C (36-46°F).

DILTIAZEM INJECTION — RX

diltiazem HCl (Various)

THERAPEUTIC CLASS: Calcium channel blocker (nondihydropyridine)

INDICATIONS: Temporary control of rapid ventricular rate in atrial fibrillation/flutter (A-Fib/Flutter). Rapid conversion of paroxysmal supraventricular tachycardia (PSVT) to sinus rhythm.

DOSAGE: *Adults:* Bolus: 0.25mg/kg IV over 2 min. If no response after 15 min, may give 2nd dose of 0.35mg/kg over 2 min. Continuous Infusion: 0.25-0.35mg/kg IV bolus, then 10mg/hr. Titrate: Increase by 5mg/hr. Max: 15mg/hr and duration up to 24 hrs.

HOW SUPPLIED: Inj: 5mg/mL

CONTRAINDICATIONS: Sick sinus syndrome and 2nd- or 3rd-degree AV block (except with functioning pacemaker), severe hypotension, cardiogenic shock, concomitant IV β-blockers or within a few hrs of use, A-Fib/Flutter associated with accessory bypass tract (eg, Wolff-Parkinson-White syndrome, short PR syndrome), ventricular tachycardia.

WARNINGS/PRECAUTIONS: Initiate in setting with resuscitation capabilities. Caution if hemodynamically compromised, and renal, hepatic, or ventricular dysfunction. Monitor ECG continuously and BP frequently. Symptomatic hypotension, acute hepatic injury reported. D/C if high-degree AV block occurs in sinus rhythm or if persistent rash occurs. Ventricular premature beats may be present on conversion of PSVT to sinus rhythm.

ADVERSE REACTIONS: Hypotension, injection site reactions (eg, itching, burning), vasodilation (flushing), arrhythmias.

INTERACTIONS: Caution with drugs that decrease peripheral resistance, intravascular volume, myocardial contractility or conduction. Increased AUC of midazolam, triazolam, buspirone, quinidine, and lovastatin; which may require a dose adjustment due to increased clinical effects or increased adverse events. Elevates carbamazepine levels, which may result in toxicity.

Cyclosporine may need dose adjustment. Potentiates the depression of cardiac contractility, conductivity, automaticity and vascular dilation with anesthetics. Possible bradycardia, AV block, and contractility depression with oral β-blockers. Possible competitive inhibition of metabolism with drugs metabolized by CYP450. Avoid IV β-blockers and rifampin. Monitor for excessive slowing of HR and/or AV block with digoxin. Cimetidine increases peak diltiazem plasma levels and AUC.

D

PREGNANCY: Category C, not for use in nursing.

MECHANISM OF ACTION: Calcium channel blocker; inhibits influx of Ca^{2+} ions during membrane depolarization of cardiac and vascular smooth muscle. Has ability to slow AV nodal conduction time and prolong AV nodal refractoriness, which has therapeutic benefits on supraventricular tachycardia. Decreases peripheral resistance, resulting in decreased systolic and diastolic BP.

PHARMACOKINETICS: Distribution: V_d=305-391L; plasma protein binding (70-80%); found in breast milk. **Metabolism:** Liver (extensive) via CYP450; deacetylation, N-demethylation, O-demethylation, and conjugation; N-monodesmethyldiltiazem and desacetyldiltiazem (major metabolites). **Elimination:** Urine and bile; $T_{1/2}$=3.4 hrs (single IV inj), 4.1-4.9 hrs (constant IV infusion).

NURSING CONSIDERATIONS

Assessment: Assess for sick sinus syndrome and 2nd- or 3rd-degree AV block, presence of functioning pacemaker, severe hypotension, cardiogenic shock, AF or atrial flutter associated with accessory bypass tract (eg, Wolff-Parkinson-White syndrome, short PR syndrome), ventricular tachycardia, wide complex tachycardia, AMI, CHF, pulmonary congestion documented by X-ray, hypertrophic cardiomyopathy, renal/hepatic impairment, pregnancy/nursing status, and possible drug interactions.

Monitoring: Initiation of therapy should be done in setting where monitoring and resuscitation capabilities, including DC cardioversion/defibrillation, are present. Monitor BP, HR, LFTs, and ECG. Monitor for hemodynamic deterioration, ventricular fibrillation, cardiac conduction abnormalities (eg, 2nd- or 3rd-degree AV block), hypotension, bradycardia, ventricular premature beats, dermatologic events (erythema multiforme/exfoliative dermatitis), and acute hepatic injury.

Patient Counseling: Initiation of therapy should be done in a setting where monitoring and resuscitation capabilities, including DC cardioversion/defibrillation, are present. Inform risks/benefits; report adverse reactions. Notify if pregnant/nursing.

Administration: IV. **Storage:** 2-8°C (36-46°F). Do not freeze. Room temperature for up to 1 month. Destroy after 1 month.

DIOVAN — RX

valsartan (Novartis)

When used in pregnancy, drugs that act directly on the renin-angiotensin system can cause injury and even death to the developing fetus. D/C therapy when pregnancy is detected.

THERAPEUTIC CLASS: Angiotensin II receptor antagonist

INDICATIONS: Treatment of hypertension, alone or with other antihypertensives. Treatment of heart failure (NYHA Class II-IV). Reduction of cardiovascular mortality in clinically stable patients with left ventricular failure or dysfunction following MI.

DOSAGE: *Adults:* HTN: Monotherapy Without Volume Depletion: Initial: 80mg or 160mg qd. Titrate: May increase to 320mg qd or add diuretic (greater effect than increasing dose >80mg). Hepatic/Severe Renal Dysfunction: Use with caution. Heart Failure: Initial: 40mg bid. Titrate: May increase to 80mg or 160mg bid (use highest dose tolerated). Max: 320mg/day in divided doses. Post-MI: Initial: 20mg bid. Titrate: May increase to 40mg bid within 7 days, with subsequent titrations up to 160mg bid.
Pediatrics: 6-16 yrs: HTN: Initial: 1.3mg/kg qd (up to 40mg total). Adjust dose

according to BP response. Max: 2.7mg/kg (up to 160mg) qd. Use of a sus recommended for children who cannot swallow tabs, or children for whom calculated dosage (mg/kg) does not correspond to available tab strengths. Adjust dose accordingly when switching dosage forms. Hepatic/Severe Renal Impairment: Use with caution. Avoid use in pediatrics with GFR <30mL/min/1.73m².

D

HOW SUPPLIED: Tab: 40mg*, 80mg, 160mg, 320mg *scored

WARNINGS/PRECAUTIONS: Changes in renal function may occur; caution with renal artery stenosis, severe CHF. Caution with hepatic dysfunction, renal dysfunction, and obstructive biliary disorder. Risk of hypotension; caution when initiating therapy in heart failure or post-MI. Correct volume or salt depletion before therapy. Avoid use in pediatric patients with GFR <30mL/min/1.73m². May cause fetal harm when administered to pregnant women.

ADVERSE REACTIONS: (HTN) Headache, dizziness, viral infection, fatigue, abdominal pain. (Heart Failure) Dizziness, hypotension, diarrhea, arthralgia, fatigue, back pain, hyperkalemia. (Post-MI) Hypotension, cough, increased blood creatinine.

INTERACTIONS: Concomitant use of K^+-sparing diuretics, K^+ supplements, or salt substitutes containing K^+ may increase serum K^+ levels, and in heart failure patients increase SrCr.

PREGNANCY: Category D, not for use in nursing.

MECHANISM OF ACTION: Angiotensin II receptor antagonist; blocks vasoconstrictor and aldosterone-secreting effects of angiotensin II by selectively blocking binding of angiotensin II to AT_1 receptor.

PHARMACOKINETICS: Absorption: Absolute bioavailability (25%); T_{max}=2-4 hrs. **Distribution:** (IV) V_d=17L; plasma protein binding (95%). **Metabolism:** Valeryl 4-hydroxy valsartan (metabolite). **Elimination:** Feces, urine; $T_{1/2}$=6 hrs.

NURSING CONSIDERATIONS

Assessment: Assess for pregnancy status, possible drug interactions, volume/salt depletion, CHF, renal/hepatic impairment.

Monitoring: Monitor renal function periodically. Monitor for signs/symptoms of hypotension, hypersensitivity reactions, renal/hepatic dysfunction.

Patient Counseling: Inform of pregnancy risks. Advise to seek medical attention if symptoms of hypotension or hypersensitivity reaction occurs.

Administration: Oral route. Refer to PI for preparation of suspension. **Storage:** Tab: 25°C (77°F); excursions permitted to 15-30°C (59-86°F). Protect from moisture. Sus: Below 30°C (86°F) for 30 days; 2-8°C (35-46°F) for 75 days. Shake well for ≥10 seconds.

DIOVAN HCT RX

hydrochlorothiazide - valsartan (Novartis)

When used in pregnancy, drugs that act directly on the renin-angiotensin system can cause injury and even death to the developing fetus. D/C therapy when pregnancy is detected.

THERAPEUTIC CLASS: Angiotensin II receptor antagonist/thiazide diuretic

INDICATIONS: Treatment of hypertension. May be used in patients whose BP is not adequately controlled on monotherapy. May be used as initial therapy in patients who are likely to need multiple drugs to achieve BP goals.

DOSAGE: *Adults:* Add-On/Initial Therapy: 160mg-12.5mg qd. Titrate: May increase after 1-2 weeks of therapy. Max: 320mg-25mg. Replacement Therapy: May be substituted for titrated components. CrCl ≤30mL/min: Use not recommended.

HOW SUPPLIED: Tab: (Valsartan-HCTZ) 80mg-12.5mg, 160mg-12.5mg, 160mg-25mg, 320mg-12.5mg, 320mg-25mg

CONTRAINDICATIONS: Anuria, sulfonamide hypersensitivity.

WARNINGS/PRECAUTIONS: Correct volume or salt depletion before therapy. Caution with hepatic or renal dysfunction, biliary obstructive disorders, renal artery stenosis, severe CHF, history of allergies, and asthma. May exacerbate or activate SLE. Monitor serum electrolytes. Avoid if CrCl ≤30mL/min. Hyperuricemia, hyperglycemia, hypokalemia, hypomagnesemia, hypercalcemia may occur. Enhanced effects in post-sympathectomy patient. May increase cholesterol and triglyceride levels. May cause fetal and neonatal morbidity and death when given to pregnant women.

D

ADVERSE REACTIONS: Cough, headache, dizziness, fatigue, viral infection, pharyngitis, diarrhea.

INTERACTIONS: Alcohol, barbiturates, and narcotics may potentiate orthostatic hypotension. Insulin and oral antidiabetic agents may require dosage adjustment. Impaired absorption with cholestyramine, colestipol. Corticosteroids and ACTH deplete electrolytes. May decrease response to pressor amines. Potentiates other antihypertensives. May increase responsiveness to skeletal muscle relaxants. Risk of lithium toxicity; avoid concurrent use. NSAIDs may decrease diuretic effects; monitor closely.

PREGNANCY: Category D, not for use in nursing.

MECHANISM OF ACTION: Valsartan: Angiotensin II receptor antagonist; blocks vasoconstrictor and aldosterone-secreting effects of angiotensin II by selectively blocking binding of angiotensin II to AT_1 receptor. HCTZ: Thiazide diuretic; affects renal tubular mechanisms of electrolyte reabsorption, directly increasing excretion of sodium and chloride and indirectly reducing plasma volume.

PHARMACOKINETICS: Absorption: Valsartan: Absolute bioavailability (25%); T_{max}=2-4 hrs. **Distribution:** Valsartan: V_d=17L (IV); plasma protein binding (95%). HCTZ: Crosses placenta; found in breast milk. **Metabolism:** Valsartan: Valeryl 4-hydroxy valsartan (metabolite). **Elimination:** Valsartan: Feces, urine; $T_{1/2}$=6 hrs. HCTZ: Urine (61%); $T_{1/2}$=5.8-18.9 hrs.

NURSING CONSIDERATIONS

Assessment: Assess for pregnancy status, possible drug interactions, volume/salt depletion, SLE, DM, anuria, sulfonamide hypersensitivity, history of allergy or bronchial asthma, hepatic/renal impairment.

Monitoring: Monitor serum electrolytes and renal function periodically. Monitor for signs/symptoms of electrolyte imbalance, exacerbation or activation of SLE, hypotension, hyperglycemia, hyperuricemia or precipitation of gout, hypersensitivity reactions, renal/hepatic dysfunction.

Patient Counseling: Inform of pregnancy risks. Advise that inadequate fluid intake or loss of fluids may result in drop of BP, leading to lightheadedness or syncope. Advise to seek medical attention if syncope, symptoms of electrolyte imbalance (dry mouth, thirst, weakness), or hypersensitivity reactions occur.

Administration: Oral route. **Storage:** 25°C (77°F); excursion permitted to 15-30°C (59-86°F). Protect from moisture.

DIPHENHYDRAMINE HCL INJECTION — RX

diphenhydramine HCl (Various)

THERAPEUTIC CLASS: Antihistamine

INDICATIONS: Amelioration of allergic reactions to blood or plasma. Adjunct to epinephrine in anaphylaxis. For other uncomplicated immediate-type allergic conditions when oral therapy is contraindicated. Treatment of motion sickness. For parkinsonism when oral therapy is not possible or contraindicated.

DOSAGE: *Adults:* Usual: 10-50mg IV or up to 100mg IM if needed. Max: 400mg/day.
Pediatrics: Usual: 5mg/kg/24hrs or 150mg/m²/24hrs IV/IM in 4 divided doses. Max: 300mg/day.

HOW SUPPLIED: Inj: 50mg/mL

CONTRAINDICATIONS: Neonates, premature infants, nursing, as a local anesthetic.

WARNINGS/PRECAUTIONS: Caution with narrow-angle glaucoma, stenosing peptic ulcer, pyloroduodenal obstruction, symptomatic prostatic hypertrophy, or bladder-neck obstruction. May cause excitation in pediatrics. Increased risk of dizziness, sedation, and hypotension in elderly. Caution with lower respiratory diseases, bronchial asthma, increased IOP, hyperthyroidism, cardiovascular disease, or HTN. Local necrosis with SQ or intradermal use.

ADVERSE REACTIONS: Sedation, drowsiness, dizziness, disturbed coordination, epigastric distress, thickening of bronchial secretions.

INTERACTIONS: Additive effects with alcohol, CNS depressants. MAOIs prolong and intensify anticholinergic effects.

PREGNANCY: Category B, contraindicated in nursing.

MECHANISM OF ACTION: Antihistamine; competes with histamine for cell receptor sites on effector cells.

PHARMACOKINETICS: Metabolism: Liver. **Elimination:** Urine.

NURSING CONSIDERATIONS

Assessment: Assess for narrow-angle glaucoma, stenosing peptic ulcer, pyloroduodenal obstruction, prostatic hypertrophy, bladder-neck obstruction, history of bronchial asthma, increased IOP, hyperthyroidism, cardiovascular disease (HTN), lower respiratory disease, possible drug interactions, and nursing status.

Monitoring: Monitor for signs/symptoms of hypersensitivity reactions.

Patient Counseling: Caution may impair physical/mental abilities. Advise to seek medical attention if symptoms of hypersensitivity reactions occur.

Administration: IV, IM route **Storage:** 20-25°C (68-77°F). Protect from freezing and light.

DIPROLENE RX

betamethasone (augmented) dipropionate (Schering)

OTHER BRAND NAMES: Diprolene AF (Schering)

THERAPEUTIC CLASS: Corticosteroid

INDICATIONS: Relief of inflammatory and pruritic manifestations of corticosteroid-responsive dermatoses.

DOSAGE: *Adults:* (Lot) Apply qd-bid for no more than 2 weeks. Max: 50mL/week. (Cre, Oint) Apply qd-bid, up to 45g/week.
Pediatrics: ≥13 yrs: (Cre) Apply qd-bid for no more than 2 weeks. Limit to 45g/week. ≥12 yrs: (Lot) Apply qd-bid for no more than 2 weeks. Limit to 50mL/week. (Oint) Apply qd-bid, up to 45g/week.

HOW SUPPLIED: Cre (AF), Oint: 0.05% [15g, 50g]; Lot: 0.05% [30mL, 60mL]

WARNINGS/PRECAUTIONS: May produce reversible HPA axis suppression, manifestations of Cushing's syndrome, hyperglycemia and glucosuria. D/C if irritation occurs. Use appropriate antifungal or antibacterial agent with dermatological infections. Pediatrics may be more susceptible to systemic toxicity. Caution when applied to large surface areas. Not for use with occlusive dressings. Gel is not for use in rosacea or perioral dermatitis or on the face, groin, or in the axillae.

ADVERSE REACTIONS: Stinging, burning, dry skin, pruritus, folliculitis, acneiform papules, irritation, hypopigmentation, skin maceration, secondary infection, skin atrophy, striae, miliaria.

PREGNANCY: Category C, (Cre, Lot) not for use in nursing; (Oint) caution in nursing.

MECHANISM OF ACTION: Corticosteroid; not established. Possesses anti-inflammatory, antipruritic, and vasoconstrictive actions.

PHARMACOKINETICS: Absorption: Percutaneous. Inflammation, use of occlusive dressings, and/or other disease states may increase absorption. **Distribution:** Systemically administered corticosteroids appear in breast milk. **Metabolism:** Liver. **Elimination:** Kidneys, bile.

NURSING CONSIDERATIONS

Assessment: Assess for hypersensitivity to other corticosteroids. Assess use in pregnancy/nursing. Ensure medication is not being used for treatment of rosacea or perioral dermatitis or being used on face, groin, or in axillae.

Monitoring: Monitor signs/symptoms of HPA-axis suppression, Cushing's syndrome, hyperglycemia, and glucosuria. Perform periodic monitoring of HPA-axis suppression when using large doses, through use of urinary free cortisol and ACTH stimulation tests. Monitor for signs/symptoms of steroid withdrawal and treat accordingly. Monitor for signs of skin irritation and skin infection (eg, bacterial, fungal), and treat accordingly. In pediatric patients, monitor for systemic toxicity, HPA-axis suppression, Cushing's syndrome, and intracranial HTN.

Patient Counseling: Instruct to use externally, exactly as directed. Counsel to avoid contact with eyes. Inform not to bandage, cover, or wrap treated skin. Advise caregivers of pediatric patients not to use medication for treatment of diaper dermatitis and not to apply to diaper area. Advise to avoid using medication on face, underarms, or groin areas unless directed by physician. Instruct to contact physician if any signs of local adverse reactions develop or if there are no signs of clinical improvement within 2 weeks of initiating therapy.

Administration: Topical route. **Storage:** 25°C (77°F); excursions permitted to 15-30°C (59-86°F).

DITROPAN XL — RX

oxybutynin chloride (Ortho-McNeil)

OTHER BRAND NAMES: Ditropan (Ortho-McNeil)

THERAPEUTIC CLASS: Anticholinergic

INDICATIONS: (All) Overactive bladder/bladder instability with symptoms of urge urinary incontinence, urgency, and frequency. (Tab, Extended-Release) Detrusor overactivity associated with a neurological condition in pediatrics ≥6 yrs.

DOSAGE: *Adults:* (Tab, Syrup) Usual: 5mg bid-tid. Max: 5mg qid. Frail Elderly: 2.5mg bid-tid.(Tab, Extended-Release) Initial: 5 or 10mg qd. Titrate: May increase by 5mg weekly. Max: 30mg/day. Swallow XL whole with liquid; do not chew, divide, or crush tab.
Pediatrics: >5 yrs: (Tab, Syrup) Usual: 5mg bid. Max: 5mg tid. ≥6 yrs: (Tab, Extended-Release) Initial: 5mg qd. Titrate: May increase by 5mg weekly. Max: 20mg/day. Swallow XL whole with liquid; do not chew, divide, or crush tab.

HOW SUPPLIED: Syrup: 5mg/5mL; Tab: 5mg*; Tab, Extended-Release: 5mg, 10mg, 15mg *scored

CONTRAINDICATIONS: Urinary retention, gastric retention and other severe decreased GI motility conditions, uncontrolled narrow-angle glaucoma, and in patients at risk for these conditions.

WARNINGS/PRECAUTIONS: Caution with hepatic or renal impairment, bladder outflow obstruction, GI obstruction/narrowing, ulcerative colitis, intestinal atony, myasthenia gravis, hyperthyroidism, CHD, CHF, arrhythmias, HTN, tachycardia, prostatic hypertrophy, and GERD. Heat prostration can occur with high environmental temperatures. Tab, Extended-Release shell may be excreted in the stool. Reduce dose or d/c if anticholinergic CNS effects occur. Caution in preexisting dementia.

ADVERSE REACTIONS: Dry mouth, constipation, somnolence, headache, diarrhea, nausea, blurred vision, dyspepsia, asthenia, pain, dizziness, dry eyes, UTI, insomnia, nervousness.

INTERACTIONS: Increased adverse effects with other anticholinergics. Increased drowsiness with alcohol or other sedatives. May alter GI absorption of other drugs due to GI motility effects. Increased levels with ketoconazole; caution with CYP3A4 inhibitors (eg, antimycotics, macrolides). Caution with bisphosphonates or other drugs that may exacerbate esophagitis.

PREGNANCY: Category B, caution in nursing.

MECHANISM OF ACTION: Antispasmodic/anticholinergic agent; inhibits muscarinic action of acetylcholine on smooth muscle exerting direct antispasmodic effect; relaxes smooth muscle of bladder.

PHARMACOKINETICS: Absorption: (Tab, Syrup) Rapid; absolute bioavailability (6%). Refer to PI for pediatric, isomer, and metabolite parameters. **Distribution:** V_d=193L. **Metabolism:** Liver via CYP3A4; desethyloxybutynin (active metabolite). **Elimination:** Urine (<0.1% unchanged); $T_{1/2}$=13.2 hrs.

NURSING CONSIDERATIONS

Assessment: Assess for bladder outflow obstruction (urinary retention), GI obstructive disorders (gastric retention), decreased GI motility conditions (UC, intestinal atony), GERD, GI narrowing, narrow-angle glaucoma, myasthenia gravis, hyperthyroidism, CAD, CHF, arrhythmias, hiatal hernia, HTN, prostatic hypertrophy, possible drug interactions, hepatic/renal impairment.

Monitoring: Monitor for aggravation of myasthenia gravis, hyperthyroidism, CAD, CHF, arrhythmias, hiatal hernia, HTN, prostatic hypertrophy symptoms, signs/symptoms of hypersensitivity reactions, GI narrowing (strictures), and hepatic/renal impairment.

Patient Counseling: Heat prostration (fever, heat stroke due to decreased sweating), drowsiness, and blurred vision may occur. Avoid concomitant use with alcohol. Swallow tab whole with liquid; do not chew, divide, or crush. Take approximately same time each day, with/without food.

Administration: Oral route. **Storage:** (Tab, Syrup): 15-30°C (59-86°F). (Tab, Extended-Release): 25°C (77°F); excursions permitted to 15-30°C (59-86°F). Protect from moisture and humidity.

DIURIL RX

chlorothiazide (Salix)

OTHER BRAND NAMES: Intravenous Sodium Diuril (Ovation)

THERAPEUTIC CLASS: Thiazide diuretic

INDICATIONS: (PO/IV) Adjunct therapy in edema associated with CHF, hepatic cirrhosis, corticosteroid and estrogen therapy, renal dysfunction. (PO) Management of hypertension.

DOSAGE: *Adults:* (PO/IV) Edema: 0.5-1g qd-bid. May give every other day or 3-5 days/week. Substitute IV for oral using same dosage. (PO) HTN: 0.5-1g qd or in divided doses. Max: 2g/day.
Pediatrics: (PO) Diuresis/HTN: Usual: 10-20mg/kg/day given qd-bid. Max: Infants up to 2 yrs: 375mg/day. 2-12 yrs: 1g/day. <6 months: Up to 15mg/kg bid may be required.

HOW SUPPLIED: Inj: 0.5g; Sus: 250mg/5mL [237mL]

CONTRAINDICATIONS: Anuria, sulfonamide hypersensitivity.

WARNINGS/PRECAUTIONS: Caution in severe renal disease, liver dysfunction, electrolyte/fluid imbalance. Monitor electrolytes. Hyperuricemia, hyperglycemia, hypokalemia, hyponatremia, hypomagnesemia, hypercalcemia may occur. Increases in cholesterol and triglyceride levels reported. May exacerbate SLE. Sensitivity reactions reported. D/C prior to parathyroid test. Enhanced effects in post-sympathectomy patient. IV use not recommended in infants or children.

ADVERSE REACTIONS: Weakness, hypotension, pancreatitis, jaundice, diarrhea, vomiting, blood dyscrasias, rash, photosensitivity, electrolyte imbalance, impotence.

INTERACTIONS: May potentiate orthostatic hypotension with alcohol, barbiturates, narcotics. Adjust antidiabetic drugs. Possible decreased response to pressor amines. Corticosteroids, ACTH increase electrolyte depletion. May potentiate nondepolarizing skeletal muscle relaxants, antihypertensives. Lithium toxicity. NSAIDs, including selective cyclooxygenase-2 (COX-2) inhibitors, decrease effects. Decreased PO absorption with cholestyramine, colestipol.

PREGNANCY: Category C, not for use in nursing.

MECHANISM OF ACTION: Thiazide diuretic; not established. Affects distal renal tubular mechanism of electrolyte reabsorption.

PHARMACOKINETICS: Elimination: Kidney; $T_{1/2}$=45-120 min. PO: Urine (10-15%); IV: Urine (96%).

D

NURSING CONSIDERATIONS

Assessment: Assess for anuria, sulfonamide hypersensitivity, DM, SLE, history of allergy or bronchial asthma, possible drug interactions, hepatic/renal impairment.

Monitoring: Monitor renal function periodically and serum electrolytes. Monitor for signs/symptoms of electrolyte imbalance, exacerbation or activation of SLE, hypotension, hyperglycemia, hyperuricemia or precipitation of gout, hypersensitivity reactions, renal/hepatic dysfunction.

Patient Counseling: Advise to seek medical attention if hypotension, electrolyte imbalance (dry mouth, thirst, weakness), or hypersensitivity reactions occur.

Administration: Oral, IV route. **Storage:** Sus: 15-30°C (59-86°F), protect from freezing. IV: 2-25°C (36-77°F).

DOBUTAMINE RX

dobutamine (Various)

THERAPEUTIC CLASS: Inotropic agent

INDICATIONS: Short-term treatment of cardiac decompensation due to depressed contractility resulting from organic heart disease or from cardiac surgical procedures.

DOSAGE: *Adults:* Initial: 0.5-1mcg/kg/min. Usual: 2-20mcg/kg/min. Max: 40mcg/kg/min (rare). Adjust rate and duration based on BP, urine flow, ectopic activity, HR, and when possible on cardiac output, central venous or pulmonary wedge pressure.

HOW SUPPLIED: Inj: 12.5mg/mL [20mL, 40mL]

CONTRAINDICATIONS: Idiopathic hypertrophic subaortic stenosis.

WARNINGS/PRECAUTIONS: May increase HR or BP, especially systolic pressure; caution with atrial fibrillation and HTN. May precipitate or exacerbate ventricular ectopic activity. Hypersensitivity reactions (eg, skin rash, fever, eosinophilia, bronchospasm) reported. Contains sulfites. Monitor EKG, BP, pulmonary wedge pressure, and cardiac output. Correct hypovolemia prior to infusion. Caution in elderly. May decrease serum K^+ levels. Improvement may not be observed with marked mechanical obstruction (eg, severe valvular aortic stenosis). Safety following acute MI has not been established.

ADVERSE REACTIONS: Increased HR, BP and ventricular ectopic activity, hypotension, infusion site reactions, nausea, headache, anginal pain, palpitations, shortness of breath, decreased K^+ levels.

INTERACTIONS: Recent administration of β-blockers may reduce effectiveness and increase peripheral vascular resistance. Increased cardiac output and lower pulmonary wedge pressure with nitroprusside.

PREGNANCY: Category B, not for use in nursing.

MECHANISM OF ACTION: Direct-acting inotropic agent; stimulates β-receptors of the heart while producing comparatively mild chronotropic, hypertensive, arrhythmogenic, and vasodilative effects.

PHARMACOKINETICS: Metabolism: Methylation of the catechol and conjugation. **Elimination**: Urine (the conjugates of dobutamine and 3-O-methyl dobutamine; inactive metabolite).

NURSING CONSIDERATIONS

Assessment: Assess for idiopathic hypertrophic subaortic stenosis (IHSS), mechanical obstruction (eg, valvular aortic stenosis), HTN, atrial fibrillation, drug or sulfite hypersensitivity and pregnancy status. Prior to treatment, correct hypovolemia if present.

Monitoring: Continuous monitoring of ECG, BP, pulmonary wedge pressure, cardiac output. Monitor for HR and BP, hypersensitivity reactions (eg, skin rash, fever, eosinophilia, and bronchospasm), allergic-type reactions, including anaphylactic symptoms and life-threatening or less severe asthmatic episodes, ectopic activity or ventricular tachycardia, and serum potassium.

Patient Counseling: Inform that drug may increase HR and BP. Report if experience any reactions at infusion site, palpitations, or SOB.

Administration: IV route. **Storage**: Store vial at 15-30°C (59-86°F).

DOLOPHINE

methadone HCl (Roxane)

CII

Only approved hospitals and pharmacies can dispense oral methadone for the treatment of narcotic addiction. Methadone can be dispensed in any licensed pharmacy when used as an analgesic. Deaths, cardiac and respiratory, have been reported during initiation and conversion of pain patients to methadone treatment from treatment with other opioid agonists. Respiratory depression is the main hazard associated with methadone administration. QT interval prolongation and serious arrhythmias have been observed during treatment with methadone.

OTHER BRAND NAMES: Methadone (Various)

THERAPEUTIC CLASS: Opioid analgesic

INDICATIONS: Detoxification and temporary maintenance treatment of narcotic addiction (heroin or other morphine-like drugs). Relief of severe pain.

DOSAGE: *Adults:* Detoxification: Initial: 15-20mg/day (up to 40mg/day may be required). Stabilize for 2-3 days, then may decrease every 1-2 days depending on patient symptoms. Max: 21 days. May not repeat earlier than 4 weeks after completing previous course. Pain: Usual: 2.5-10mg q3-4h PO/IM/SQ prn.

HOW SUPPLIED: Tab: 5mg, 10mg

CONTRAINDICATIONS: Methadone is contraindicated in any patient suspected of having a paralytic ileus, acute bronchial asthma or hypercarbia and respiratory depression.

WARNINGS/PRECAUTIONS: Do not inject agent. Extreme caution if use narcotic antagonists in patients physically dependent on narcotics. Can cause respiratory depression and elevate CSF pressure. Caution with head injuries, acute asthma attacks, COPD, cor pulmonale, decreased respiratory reserve, pre-existing respiratory depression, hypoxia, or hypercapnia. Reduce initial dose in elderly, debilitated, severe hepatic or renal impairment, hypothyroidism, Addison's disease, prostatic hypertrophy, or urethral stricture. Risk of tolerance, dependence, and abuse may occur. Impairs physical and mental abilities. Ineffective in relieving anxiety. May mask symptoms of acute abdominal conditions. May produce hypotension. May cause incomplete cross-tolerance and iatrogenic overdose, interactions with other CNS depressants, alcohol and other drugs of abuse. May cause cardiac conduction effects like prolonged QT interval and serious arrhythmias.

ADVERSE REACTIONS: Lightheadedness, dizziness, sedation, sweating, NV, asthenia, cardiomyopathy, ECG abnormalities, abdominal pain, agitation, seizures, confusion, hallucinations, respiratory depression.

INTERACTIONS: May increase desipramine levels. Pentazocine may precipitate withdrawal. Decreased serum levels with rifampin. Caution and reduce dose with CNS depressants (eg, tranquilizers, sedative-hypnotics, phenothiazines, TCAs, alcohol). MAOIs may cause severe reactions. Use caution with concomitant administration of inducers/inhibitors of CYP450 (eg, azole antifungals, phenytoin).

PREGNANCY: Safety in pregnancy and nursing not known.

MECHANISM OF ACTION: Opioid analgesic; μ-agonist. Produces many actions similiar to morphine. Acts prominently in the CNS and in organs composed of smooth muscle. Also acts as an antagonist at the N-methyl-D-aspartate (NMDA) receptor.

PHARMACOKINETICS: Absorption: C_{max}=124-1255ng/mL; T_{max}=1-7.5 hrs. **Distribution:** V_d=1.0-8.0L/kg; plasma protein binding (85-90%); found in saliva, breast milk, amniotic fluid, and umbilical cord plasma. **Metabolism:** Liver (N-demethylation) via CYP450 enzymes: 3A4 (primary), 2B6 (primary), 2C19 (primary); 2C9; 2D6. **Elimination:** Urine, feces; $T_{1/2}$=8-59 hrs.

NURSING CONSIDERATIONS

Assessment: Assess for respiratory depression, acute bronchial asthma, hypercarbia, COPD, paralytic ileus, CNS depression or coma, age of patient, risk of QT prolongation (eg, cardiac hypertrophy, concomitant diuretic use, hypokalemia), potential for drug abuse, presence of head injury or other intracranial lesions, pre-existing elevation in ICP, hypotension, acute abdominal conditions, renal/hepatic impairment, hypothyroidism, Addison's disease, prostatic hypertrophy or urethral stricture, pregnancy/nursing status, and possible drug interactions.

Monitoring: Monitor for signs/symptoms of respiratory depression, QT prolongation and arrhythmia (eg, torsade de pointes), elevations in CSF pressure, hypotension, misuse or abuse, and tolerance or dependence.

Patient Counseling: Inform that drug may impair mental/physical abilities; use caution when performing hazardous tasks (eg, operating machinery/driving). Avoid use of other CNS depressants and alcohol during therapy. Instruct to notify physician if develop symptoms suggestive of arrhythmia (eg, palpitations, dizziness, lightheadedness, syncope). Medication may produce orthostatic hypotension. Avoid abrupt withdrawal from medication. Instruct that if using for treatment of opioid dependence, discontinuation may lead to relapse of illicit drug use.

Administration: Oral route. **Storage**: 25°C (77°F); excursions permitted to 15-30°C (59-86°F). Dispense in tight, light-resistant container.

DONNATAL — RX

hyoscyamine sulfate - atropine sulfate - scopolamine hydrobromide - phenobarbital (PBM Pharmaceuticals)

OTHER BRAND NAMES: Donnatal Extentabs (PBM Pharmaceuticals)

THERAPEUTIC CLASS: Anticholinergic/barbiturate

INDICATIONS: Adjunct therapy for irritable bowel syndrome, acute enterocolitis, duodenal ulcers.

DOSAGE: *Adults:* (Elixir/Tab) 1-2 tabs or 5-10mL tid-qid. (Extentabs) 1 tab q8-12h. Hepatic Disease: Use lower doses.
Pediatrics: (Elixir) 4.5kg: 0.5mL q4h or 0.75mL q6h. 9.1kg: 1mL q4h or 1.5mL q6h. 13.6kg: 1.5mL q4h or 2mL q6h. 22.7kg: 2.5mL q4h or 3.75mL q6h. 34kg: 3.75mL q4h or 5mL q6h. 45.4kg: 5mL q4h or 7.5mL q6h. Hepatic Disease: Use lower doses.

HOW SUPPLIED: (Atropine-Hyoscyamine-Phenobarbital-Scopolamine) Elixir: 0.0194mg-0.1037mg-16.2mg-0.0065mg/5mL; Tab: 0.0194mg-0.1037mg-16.2mg-0.0065mg; Tab, Extended-Release: (Extentabs) 0.0582mg-0.3111mg-48.6mg-0.0195mg

CONTRAINDICATIONS: Glaucoma, obstructive uropathy, obstructive GI disease, paralytic ileus, intestinal atony in elderly or debilitated, unstable cardiovascular status in acute hemorrhage, severe ulcerative colitis, myasthenia gravis, hiatal hernia with reflux esophagitis, intermittent porphyria, and for patients in whom phenobarbital produces restlessness and/or excitement.

WARNINGS/PRECAUTIONS: Inconclusive whether anticholinergic/antispasmodic drugs aid in duodenal ulcer healing, decrease recurrence rate, or prevent complications. Heat prostration can occur with high environmental temperatures. Avoid with intestinal obstruction. May be habit forming; caution with history of physical and/or psychological drug dependence. Caution with hepatic disease, renal disease, autonomic neuropathy, hyperthyroidism, coronary heart disease, CHF, arrhythmias, tachycardia, HTN. May delay gastric emptying. Diarrhea may be an early symptom of incomplete intestinal obstruction, especially with ileostomy or colostomy; treatment would be inappropriate.

ADVERSE REACTIONS: Xerostomia, urinary hesitancy/retention, blurred vision, tachycardia/palpitation, mydriasis, cycloplegia, increased ocular tension, loss of taste, headache, nervousness, drowsiness, weakness, dizziness, insomnia, nausea, vomiting, impotence, suppression of lactation, constipation, bloated feeling, musculoskeletal pain, allergic reaction/drug idiosyncrasies, decreased sweating.

INTERACTIONS: Phenobarbital may decrease anticoagulant effects; adjust dose.

PREGNANCY: Category C, caution in nursing.

MECHANISM OF ACTION: Anticholinergic/Barbiturate; drug combination provides peripheral anticholinergic, antispasmodic action and mild sedation.

NURSING CONSIDERATIONS

Assessment: Assess for glaucoma, obstructive uropathy, obstructive disease of the GIT, paralytic ileus, ulcerative colitis, myasthenia gravis, hiatal hernia associated with reflux esophagitis, acute intermittent porphyria, renal/hepatic dysfunction, hyperthyroidism, cardiac disorders.

Monitoring: Monitor occurrence of heat prostration, drowsiness, blurred vision, HR, constipation, diarrhea, urinary hesitancy/retention, hypersensitivity reactions.

Patient Counseling: Counsel about side effects; report adverse effects. Counsel about drug abuse/dependence. Exercise caution while operating machinery/driving. Avoid high environmental temperatures.

Administration: Oral route. **Storage**: 20-25°C (68-77°F). Protect from light and moisture. Dispense in well-closed, light-resistant container using child-resistant closure.

DOPAMINE — RX

dopamine HCl (Various)

THERAPEUTIC CLASS: Inotropic agent

INDICATIONS: For correction of hemodynamic imbalances present in shock due to MI, trauma, endotoxic septicemia, open-heart surgery, renal failure, and chronic cardiac decompensation.

DOSAGE: *Adults:* Initial: 2-5mcg/kg/min. Use 5mcg/kg/min in seriously ill. Increase in 5-10mcg/kg/min increments, up to 20-50mcg/kg/min.

HOW SUPPLIED: Inj: 40mg/mL, 80mg/mL, 160mg/mL

CONTRAINDICATIONS: Pheochromocytoma, uncorrected tachyarrhythmias or ventricular fibrillation.

WARNINGS/PRECAUTIONS: Contains sulfites. Monitor BP, urine flow, cardiac output and pulmonary wedge pressure. Correct hypovolemia, hypoxia, hypercapnia, and acidosis prior to use. Reduce infusion rate with increase in diastolic BP/marked decrease in pulse pressure; increase rate if hypotension occurs. D/C if hypotension persists. Reduce dose if increased ectopic beats occurs. Caution with history of occlusive vascular disease (eg, atherosclerosis, arterial embolism, Raynaud's disease, cold injury, diabetic endarteritis, and Buerger's disease); monitor for changes in skin color or temperature. Administer phentolamine if extravasation noted. Avoid abrupt withdrawal.

ADVERSE REACTIONS: Tachycardia, palpitation, ventricular arrhythmia (high doses), dyspnea, nausea, vomiting, headache, anxiety, bradycardia, hypotension, HTN, vasoconstriction.

INTERACTIONS: If treated with MAOIs within 2-3 weeks prior to administration of dopamine, reduce initial dose of dopamine to not greater than 1/10th of usual dose. Potential additive or potentiating effects on urine flow with diuretics. TCAs may potentiate cardiovascular effects of adrenergic agents. Cardiac effects antagonized by β-blockers. Peripheral vasoconstriction antagonized by α-blockers. Butyrophenones (eg, haloperidol) and phenothiazines may suppress renal and mesenteric vasodilation. Extreme caution with cyclopropane or halogenated hydrocarbon anesthetics. Concomitant use with vasopressors, vasoconstricting agents (eg, ergonovine), and some oxytocic drugs may result in severe HTN. Hypotension and bradycardia reported with phenytoin; consider alternatives.

PREGNANCY: Category C, caution in nursing.

MECHANISM OF ACTION: Catecholamine; produces positive chronotropic and inotropic effects on the myocardium, resulting in increased heart rate and cardiac contractility. Acts directly by exerting an agonist action on β-adrenoreceptor and indirectly by causing release of norepinephrine from storage sites in sympathetic nerve endings.

PHARMACOKINETICS: Metabolism: Liver, kidneys, and plasma via MAO and catechol-O-methyltransferase. **Elimination:** Urine (80%).

NURSING CONSIDERATIONS

Assessment: Assess for sulfite hypersensitivity, pheochromocytoma, uncorrected tachyarrhythmias/ventricular fibrillation, history of occlusive vascular disease (eg, atherosclerosis, arterial embolism, Raynaud's disease, cold injury, diabetic endarteritis, and Buerger's disease), pregnancy status, and possible drug interactions. Assess and correct prior to, or concurrently with, administration of therapy for hypovolemia, hypoxia, acidosis, and hypercapnia.

Monitoring: Close monitoring of urine flow, cardiac output, BP, and CVP. Monitor for ventricular arrhythmias, decreased pulse pressure, hypotension, extravasation/peripheral ischemia; sloughing and necrosis of the surrounding tissue and allergic-type reactions, including anaphylactic symptoms and life-threatening or less severe asthmatic episodes. In occlusive vascular disease, monitor for changes in color or temperature of skin in extremities.

Patient Counseling: Inform about benefits/risks of therapy.

Administration: IV infusion route. Not for direct IV injection; drug must be diluted before administration to patient. Avoid injection to sodium bicarbonate or other alkaline and/or amphotericin B solutions. **Storage:** 15-30°C (59-86°F).

DORIBAX — RX

doripenem (Ortho-McNeil)

THERAPEUTIC CLASS: Carbapenem

INDICATIONS: Treatment of complicated intra-abdominal and urinary tract infections, including pyelonephritis, caused by susceptible microorganisms.

DOSAGE: Adults: ≥18 yrs: 500mg IV q8h for 5-14 days (intra-abdominal) or 10 days (UTI). Infuse over 1 hour. Renal Impairment: CrCl: >50mL/min: No dose adjustment. CrCl 30-50mL/min: 250mg IV q8h. CrCl >10 to <30mL/min: 250mg IV q12h.

HOW SUPPLIED: Inj: 500mg

CONTRAINDICATIONS: Anaphylactic reactions to β-lactams.

WARNINGS/PRECAUTIONS: Serious hypersensitivity (anaphylactic) reactions reported. *Clostridium difficile*-associated diarrhea reported (ranging from mild diarrhea to fatal colitis); evaluate if diarrhea occurs.

ADVERSE REACTIONS: Headache, nausea, diarrhea, rash, phlebitis, anemia, pruritus.

INTERACTIONS: May reduce serum valproic acid levels, which may result in loss of seizure control; monitor serum valproic acid levels frequently after initiation of therapy. Probenicid may increase levels; avoid co-administration.

PREGNANCY: Category B, caution in nursing.

MECHANISM OF ACTION: Broad-spectrum carbapenem; exerts bactericidal activity by inhibiting cell wall biosynthesis, resulting in cell death.

PHARMACOKINETICS: Absorption: C_{max}=23mcg/mL, AUC=36.3mcg•hr/mL. **Distribution:** V_d=16.8L; plasma protein binding (8.1%). **Metabolism:** Via dehydropeptidase-1. **Elimination:** Urine (70% unchanged and 15% metabolites), feces (<1%); $T_{1/2}$=1 hr.

NURSING CONSIDERATIONS

Assessment: Assess for previous hypersensitivity reactions to other carbapenems, cephalosporins, PCNs, or other allergens. Assess for renal impairment and possible drug interactions. Document indications for therapy and culture and susceptibility testing.

Monitoring: Monitor for signs/symptoms of anaphylactoid/hypersensitivity reactions, CDAD, superinfection, seizures, anemia, phlebitis, rash.

Patient Counseling: Inform drug only treats bacterial, not viral, infections. Take exactly as directed; skipping doses or not completing full course may decrease effectiveness and increase resistance. May experience diarrhea; notify physician if taking valproic acid or if watery/bloody stools, hypersensitivity reactions, infection, or seizures occur.

Administration: IV route. **Storage:** Store at 25°C (77°F); excursions permitted to 15-30°C (59-86°F).

DORYX — RX

doxycycline hyclate (Warner Chilcott)

THERAPEUTIC CLASS: Tetracycline derivative

INDICATIONS: Treatment of the following infections: respiratory, urinary, lymphogranuloma, psittacosis, trachoma, uncomplicated urethral/endocervical/rectal, nongonococcal urethritis, Rocky Mountain spotted fever, typhus fever and the typhus group, Q fever, rickettsialpox, tick fevers, inclusion conjunctivitis, tularemia, *Campylobacter* fetus infections, bartonellosis, granuloma chancroid, plague, cholera, brucellosis, anthrax (including inhalational anthrax, post-exposure). When penicillin is contraindicated, treatment of uncomplicated gonorrhea, syphilis, yaws, listeriosis, Vincent's infection, actinomycosis, and infections caused by *Clostridium* species. Adjunct therapy for intestinal amebiasis and severe acne. Prophylaxis of malaria in short-term travelers (<4 months) to areas with chloroquine and/or pyrimethamine-sulfadoxine resistant strains.

DOSAGE: *Adults:* Usual: 100mg q12h on 1st day, followed by 100mg/day (single dose or as 50mg q12h). Severe Infections/Chronic UTI: 100mg q12h. Uncomplicated Gonococcal Infections (Men, except anorectal infections): 100mg bid for 7 days, or 300mg followed 300mg 1 hr later. Acute Epididymo-Orchitis: 100mg bid for at least 10 days. Early Syphilis: 100mg bid for 14 days. Syphilis >1 yr: 100mg bid for 28 days. Nongonococcal Urethritis, Uncomplicated Urethral/Endocervical/Rectal Infection: 100mg bid for at least 7 days. Inhalational Anthrax (post-exposure): 100mg bid for 60 days. Treat Strep infections for 10 days. Malaria Prophylaxis: 100mg qd, begin 1-2 days before travel and continue daily during travel and for 28 days after travel to malarious area.

Pediatrics: >8 yrs: >100 lbs: 100mg q12h on 1st day, followed by 100mg/day (single dose or as 50mg q12h). Severe Infections/Chronic UTI: 100mg q12h. ≤100lbs: 2mg/lb in divided doses bid on Day 1, followed by 1mg/lb/day (single dose or divided bid) thereafter. Severe Infections: Up to 2mg/lb. Inhalational Anthrax (post-exposure): <100 lbs: 1mg/lb bid for 60 days. ≥100 lbs: 100mg bid for 60 days. Malaria Prophylaxis: 2mg/kg (up to adult dose) qd, begin 1-2 days before travel and continue daily during travel and for 28 days after travel to malarious area.

HOW SUPPLIED: Tab, Delayed-Release: 75mg, 100mg

WARNINGS/PRECAUTIONS: *Clostridium difficile*-associated diarrhea reported. May decrease bone growth in premature infants, and cause fetal harm during pregnancy. May cause permanent discoloration of the teeth or enamel hypoplasia if used in last half of pregnancy, infancy, or <8 yrs. Photosensitivity, increased BUN, superinfection may occur. Monitor hematopoietic, renal and hepatic values periodically with long-term therapy. Bulging fontanels in infants and benign intracranial HTN in adults reported. May increase incidence of vaginal candidiasis.

ADVERSE REACTIONS: Anorexia, N/V, diarrhea, dysphagia, enterocolitis, rash, inflammatory lesions, exfoliative dermatitis, renal toxicity, hypersensitivity reactions, blood dyscrasias, tooth discoloration (<8 yrs).

INTERACTIONS: May depress plasma PT, adjust anticoagulant dosage. May interfere with bactericidal action of penicillin; avoid concurrent use when possible. Avoid antacids containing aluminum, calcium, or magnesium, sodium bicarbonate, and iron-containing preparations. Reduced absorption with bismuth subsalicylate. Barbiturates, carbamazepine, and phenytoin decrease half-life. Fatal renal toxicity with Penthrane (methoxyflurane). May render oral contraceptives less effective.

PREGNANCY: Category D, not for use in nursing.

MECHANISM OF ACTION: Tetracycline derivative; thought to inhibit protein synthesis.

PHARMACOKINETICS: Absorption: Complete; C_{max}=2.6 mcg/mL; T_{max}=2 hrs. **Distribution:** Crosses placenta. **Metabolism:** Liver. **Elimination:** Urine, feces.

NURSING CONSIDERATIONS

Assessment: Assess for pregnancy, possible drug interactions, hepatic/renal impairment, history of candidiasis prediposition, and severe diarrhea. Document indications for therapy, culture, and susceptibility testing. Perform incision and drainage in conjunction with antibiotic therapy when indicated.

Monitoring: Monitor for hypersensitivity reactions, photosensitivity, superinfection, *C. difficile*-associated diarrhea, vaginal candidiasis, benign intracranial HTN, LFTs, and renal function. In venereal disease with coexistent syphilis, conduct dark field exam before treatment and monthly thereafter for 4 months.

Patient Counseling: Inform of pregnancy risks and to avoid pregnancy. Counsel about photosensitivity reactions and to d/c at first sign of skin erythema. Advise to avoid excessive sunlight/UV light and wear sunscreen or sunblock. Take exactly as directed, skipping doses or not completing full course may decrease effectiveness and increase resistance. Avoid foods with calcium and drink fluids liberally to reduce risk of esophageal irritation or ulceration. Inform that drug only treats bacterial, not viral, infections. Diarrhea may occur; contact physician if watery/bloody stools, hypersensitivity reactions, superinfections, photosensitivity, or benign intracranial HTN occurs. Counsel on malaria prophylaxis to begin therapy 2 days before travel; continue while in the malarious area and for 4 weeks after return. Therapy should not exceed 4 months.

Administration: Oral route. **Storage:** 25°C (77°F); excursions permitted to 15-30°C (59-86°F). Dispense in tight, light-resistant container.

DOVONEX RX

calcipotriene (Warner Chilcott/Bristol-Myers Squibb)

THERAPEUTIC CLASS: Vitamin D_3 derivative

INDICATIONS: Treatment of plaque psoriasis.

DOSAGE: *Adults:* (Cream) Apply bid up to 8 weeks. (Oint) Apply qd-bid. Rub in gently. Wash hands after application.

HOW SUPPLIED: Cre, Oint: 0.005% [60g, 120g]

CONTRAINDICATIONS: Hypercalcemia or vitamin D toxicity. Do not use on the face.

WARNINGS/PRECAUTIONS: Avoid face and eyes. D/C if irritation or hypercalcemia occur; may continue once calcium levels are normal. Avoid excessive exposure to either natural or artificial sunlight.

ADVERSE REACTIONS: Local irritation, rash, pruritus, dermatitis, erythema, itching, worsening of psoriasis.

PREGNANCY: Category C, caution in nursing.

MECHANISM OF ACTION: Calcipotriene monohydrate; synthetic vitamin D_3 derivative.

PHARMACOKINETICS: Metabolism: Liver. **Elimination:** Bile.

NURSING CONSIDERATIONS

Assessment: Assess for drug hypersensitivity reactions, hypercalcemia, evidence of vitamin D toxicity, pregnancy/nursing status.

Monitoring: Monitor for serum calcium concentration, irritation of lesions and surrounding uninvolved skin.

Patient Counseling: Advise to take drug as prescribed; report signs of adverse reactions. Counsel to avoid excessive exposure to natural or artificial sunlight after application. For external use only; avoid contact with eyes or face.

Administration: Topical application. **Storage:** 15-25°C (59-77°F); do not freeze.

DOVONEX SCALP RX

calcipotriene (Warner Chilcott/Bristol-Myers Squibb)

THERAPEUTIC CLASS: Vitamin D_3 derivative

INDICATIONS: Topical treatment of chronic, moderately severe psoriasis of the scalp.

DOSAGE: *Adults:* Comb hair to remove debris. Part hair and apply bid up to 8 weeks. Rub in gently. Avoid uninvolved skin. Wash hands after application.

HOW SUPPLIED: Sol: 0.005% [60mL]

CONTRAINDICATIONS: Acute psoriatic eruptions, hypercalcemia, vitamin D toxicity.

WARNINGS/PRECAUTIONS: Avoid mucous membranes and eyes. D/C if irritation, sensitivity reaction, or hypercalcemia occur; may continue once calcium levels are normal. Avoid excessive exposure to either natural or artificial sunlight.

ADVERSE REACTIONS: Transient burning, stinging, tingling, rash, dry skin, irritation and worsening of psoriasis.

PREGNANCY: Category C, caution in nursing.

MECHANISM OF ACTION: Calcipotriene; not understood. It is roughly equipotent to the natural vitamin in its effects on proliferation and differentiation of a variety of cell types.

PHARMACOKINETICS: Metabolism: Liver. **Elimination:** Bile.

NURSING CONSIDERATIONS

Assessment: Assess for drug hypersensitivity, acute psoriatic eruptions, hypercalcemia, evidence of vitamin D toxicity, pregnancy/nursing status.

Monitoring: Monitor for irritation of both lesions of surrounding uninvolved skin and serum calcium concentration.

Patient Counseling: Advise to use as directed and to d/c and contact physician if any adverse reactions occur. Avoid excessive exposure to natural or artificial sunlight after application. Counsel drug for external use only; avoid contact with face or eyes. Keep away from open flame.

Administration: Topical application. **Storage:** 15-25°C (59-77°F). Do not freeze.

DOXEPIN

RX

doxepin HCl (Various)

Antidepressants increased the risk of suicidal thinking and behavior (suicidality) in short-term studies in children, adolescents, and young adults with major depressive disorder (MDD) and other psychiatric disorders. Doxepin is not approved for use in pediatric patients.

D

OTHER BRAND NAMES: Sinequan (Pfizer)

THERAPEUTIC CLASS: Tricyclic antidepressant

INDICATIONS: Depression and/or anxiety.

DOSAGE: *Adults:* Very Mild Illness: Usual: 25-50mg/day. Mild to Moderate Severity: Initial: 75mg/day. Usual: 75-150mg/day. Severely Ill: May increase up to 300mg/day. Dilute solution with 120mL of water, milk or juice. Give once daily or in divided doses. Divide dose if >150mg. Elderly: Use lower doses and monitor closely.

HOW SUPPLIED: Cap: 10mg, 25mg, 50mg, 75mg, 100mg, 150mg; Sol, Concentrate: 10mg/mL [120mL]

CONTRAINDICATIONS: Glaucoma, urinary retention.

WARNINGS/PRECAUTIONS: Monitor for suicidal tendencies and increased symptoms of psychosis. Avoid abrupt discontinuation.

ADVERSE REACTIONS: Drowsiness, dry mouth, blurred vision, constipation, urinary retention, hypotension, tachycardia, rash, edema, photosensitization, pruritus, eosinophilia, nausea, dizziness.

INTERACTIONS: Caution with drugs metabolized by CYP2D6. Potentiated by inhibitors (eg, cimetidine, quinidine, SSRIs) and substrates (other antidepressants, phenothiazines, propafenone, flecainide) of CYP2D6. Increased danger of overdose with alcohol. Hypoglycemia reported with tolazamide. Avoid within 2 weeks of MAOI therapy. Increased side effects with anticholinergics. Caution when switching from TCAs to SSRIs (≥5 weeks may be needed before initiating TCA treatment after withdrawal from fluoxetine).

PREGNANCY: Safety in pregnancy and nursing not known.

MECHANISM OF ACTION: Dibenzoxepin tricyclic; not established, suspected to influence adrenergic activity at synapse, preventing deactivation of norepinephrine by reuptake into nerve terminals.

PHARMACOKINETICS: Metabolism: CYP2D6 (major); CYP1A2, 3A4 (minor).

NURSING CONSIDERATIONS

Assessment: Assess for bipolar disorder risk, glaucoma, tendency to urinary retention, and possible drug interactions.

Monitoring: Monitor for signs/symptoms of clinical worsening (suicidality, unusual changes in behavior), increasing symptoms of psychosis, mania, withdrawal symptoms (if abruptly d/c), cognitive/motor impairment.

Patient Counseling: Advise to avoid alcohol. Seek medical attention for symptoms of activation of mania, increasing symptoms of psychosis, and clinical worsening (suicidal ideation, unusual changes in behavior). Caution may impair physical/mental abilities. When used with methadone syrup; may dilute with Gatorade, lemonade, orange juice, sugar water, Tang, or water; not grape juice.

Administration: Oral route. **Storage:** 20-25°C (68-77°F). Cap: Protect from light.

D

DOXIL

RX

doxorubicin HCl liposome (Ortho Biotech)

Myocardial damage may lead to CHF when cumulative dose approaches 550mg/m². May lead to cardiac toxicity, consider prior use of anthracyclines or anthracenediones in cumulative dose calculations. Cardiac toxicity may occur at lower cumulative doses with prior mediastinal irradiation or concurrent cardiotoxic agents, such as cyclophosphamide. Acute infusion-associated reactions reported. Severe myelosuppression, myocardial toxicity may occur. Reduce dose with impaired hepatic function. Severe side effects reported with accidental substitution for doxorubicin HCl, do not substitute on mg per mg basis.

THERAPEUTIC CLASS: Anthracycline

INDICATIONS: Treatment of ovarian cancer which has progressed or recurred after platinum-based chemotherapy. Treatment of AIDS-related Kaposi's sarcoma (KS) in patients with disease that has progressed on prior combination chemotherapy or in patients intolerant to such therapy. In combination with bortezomib for the treatment of multiple myeloma (MM) in patients who have not previously received bortezomib and have received at least one prior therapy.

DOSAGE: *Adults:* Administer as IV infusion at initial rate of 1mg/min to minimize risk of infusion-related reactions; if no reactions, may increase rate to complete infusion over 1 hr. Ovarian Cancer: 50mg/m² IV every 4 weeks for minimum of 4 courses. KS: 20mg/m² IV once every 3 weeks. MM: Give bortezomib 1.3mg/m² IV bolus on Days 1, 4, 8 and 11, every 3 weeks. Give doxorubicin 30mg/m² IV on Day 4 following bortezomib. May treat for up to 8 cycles depending on disease progression or unaccepable toxicity. Hepatic Dysfunction: If serum bilirubin 1.2-3mg/dL, give 50% of normal dose. If serum bilirubin >3mg/dL, give 25% of normal dose. Adjust dose based on toxicities (see PI).

HOW SUPPLIED: Inj: 2mg/mL

CONTRAINDICATIONS: Nursing mothers.

WARNINGS/PRECAUTIONS: Monitor cardiac function. Cardiac toxicity may occur after discontinuation. Recall of skin reaction due to radiotherapy reported. Myelosuppression may occur; obtain CBCs, including platelets frequently and at a minimum before each dose. Secondary AML reported with anthracyclines. Evaluate hepatic function before therapy. Avoid extravasation. Can cause fetal harm. Hand-foot syndrome and acute infusion-related reactions reported.

ADVERSE REACTIONS: Neutropenia, leukopenia, anemia, thrombocytopenia, stomatitis, fever, anorexia, fatigue, nausea, asthenia, vomiting, rash, alopecia, diarrhea, constipation, hand-foot syndrome.

INTERACTIONS: See Black Box Warning. May potentiate toxicity of other anticancer therapies. May exacerbate cyclophosphamide-induced hemorrhagic cystitis. May enhance hepatotoxicity of 6-mercaptopurine. May increase radiation-induced toxicity of the myocardium, mucosae, skin, and liver. Hematological toxicity may be more severe with agents that cause bone marrow suppression.

PREGNANCY: Category D, not for use in nursing.

MECHANISM OF ACTION: Anthracycline topoisomerase inhibitor; suspected to bind DNA and inhibit nucleic acid synthesis.

PHARMACOKINETICS: Absorption: (10mg/m²) C_{max}=4.12µg/mL, AUC=277µg/mL•h. (20mg/m²) C_{max}=8.34µg/mL, AUC=590µg/mL•h. **Distribution**: (10mg/m²) V_d=2.83L/m²; (20mg/m²) V_d=2.72L/m². **Metabolism:** Doxorubicinol (metabolite).

NURSING CONSIDERATIONS

Assessment: Assess for history of CVD, radiotherapy, hepatic dysfunction, pregnancy/nursing status, and possible drug interactions. Obtain baseline WBC, neutrophil, platelet count, Hgb/Hct, LFTs, and cardiac function.

Monitoring: Monitor CBCs including platelet counts, Hgb/Hct, LFTs, and cardiac function (EKG, multigated radionuclide scan) periodically. Signs and symptoms of hypersensitivity reaction, infusion reaction (flushing, SOB, facial swelling, headache, chills, back pain, tightness in chest or throat), severe myelosuppression (superinfection, neutropenic fever, hemorrhage), extravasation (stinging or burning sensation), recall reaction (radiotherapy), cardiotoxicity (CHF), impaired hepatic function, hand and foot syndrome (swelling, pain, erythema, and desquamation of skin of hands and feet), and stomatitis.

Patient Counseling: Inform that reddish-orange urine and other body fluids may occur. Inform of pregnancy risks. Advise to seek medical attention if symptoms of hypersensitivity reaction (rash), infusion reaction (flushing, SOB, facial swelling, headache, chills, back pain, tightness in chest or throat), infection, neutropenia, fever, hemorrhage, stinging or burning sensation, N/V, tiredness, weakness, mild hair loss, hand-foot syndrome (swelling, pain, erythema, and desquamation of skin of hands and feet), and stomatitis occur.

Administration: IV route. Do not administer as bolus injection or undiluted solution. Do not use with in-line filters. **Storage:** Refrigerate at 2-8°C (36-46°F). Avoid freezing.

DOXORUBICIN HCL — RX

doxorubicin HCl (Various)

Severe local tissue necrosis will occur if extravasation occurs. Do not give IM/SC route. Myocardial toxicity may occur during or after therapy. Increased risk of CHF with high cumulative doses, previous anthracycline/anthracenedione therapy, pre-existing heart disease, radiotherapy to mediastinal/pericardial area, concomitant cardiotoxic drugs. Increased risk of delayed cardiotoxicity in pediatrics. Secondary acute myelogenous leukemia reported. Reduce dose in hepatic impairment. Severe myelosuppression may occur.

THERAPEUTIC CLASS: Anthracycline

INDICATIONS: To produce regression in disseminated neoplastic conditions such as acute lymphoblastic and myeloblastic leukemias, Wilms' tumor, neuroblastoma, soft tissue/bone sarcomas, breast carcinoma, ovary, bladder and thyroid, gastric and bronchogenic carcinomas, Hodgkin's disease, malignant lymphoma in which the small-cell histologic type is the most responsive compared with other cell types. Adjuvant therapy in women with evidence of axillary lymph node involvement following resection of primary breast cancer.

DOSAGE: *Adults:* Monotherapy: 60-75mg/m^2 IV every 21 days. Use the lower dose with inadequate bone marrow reserves due to old age, prior therapy, or neoplastic marrow infiltration. Concomitant Chemotherapy: 40-60mg/m^2 IV every 21-28 days. Hyperbilirubinemia: Reduce dose by 50% if 1.2-3mg/dL; reduce dose by 75% if 3.1-5mg/dL.

Pediatrics: Monotherapy: 60-75mg/m^2 IV every 21 days. Use the lower dose with inadequate bone marrow reserves due to old age, prior therapy, or neoplastic marrow infiltration. Concomitant Chemotherapy: 40-60mg/m^2 IV every 21-28 days. Hyperbilirubinemia: Reduce dose by 50% if 1.2-3mg/dL; reduce dose by 75% if 3.1-5mg/dL.

HOW SUPPLIED: Inj: (2mg/mL) 10mg, 20mg, 50mg

CONTRAINDICATIONS: Marked myelosuppression induced by previous treatment with other antitumor agents or radiotherapy. Previous therapy with complete cumulative doses of doxorubicin, daunorubicin, idarubicin, or other anthracyclines and anthracenes.

WARNINGS/PRECAUTIONS: Irreversible myocardial toxicity may occur. Bone marrow depression and arrhythmias reported. Enhanced toxicity with hepatic impairment; evaluate hepatic function before dosing. Imparts a red coloration to urine for 1-2 days after administration. May induce tumor lysis syndrome and hyperuricemia with rapidly growing tumors. Periodically monitor CBC, hepatic function, and radionuclide left ventricular ejection fraction. May cause prepubertal growth failure and gonadal impairment.

D

ADVERSE REACTIONS: Myelosuppression, cardiotoxicity, alopecia, nausea, vomiting, mucositis, ulceration and necrosis of colon, fever, chills, urticaria, phlebosclerosis, facial flushing.

INTERACTIONS: May potentiate toxicity of other anticancer therapies. May exacerbate cyclophosphamide-induced hemorrhagic cystitis. May enhance hepatotoxicity of 6-mercaptopurine. May increase radiation induced toxicity of the myocardium, mucosae, skin, and liver. Acute "recall" pneumonitis in pediatrics with actinomycin-D. Paclitaxel infused before doxorubicin may decrease clearance of doxorubicin and increase neutropenia and stomatitis episodes, than the reverse sequence of administration. Enhanced neutropenia and thrombocytopenia reported with concomitant IV progesterone. Cyclosporine may prolong and exacerbate hematologic toxicity. Phenobarbital increases elimination. May decrease phenytoin levels. Streptozocin may inhibit hepatic metabolism. Live vaccines may be hazardous in those undergoing cytotoxic chemotherapy. Necrotizing colitis reported with cytarabine. Seizures and coma reported with cyclosporine, cisplatin or vincristine. Possible increased risk of cardiotoxicity with CCBs. Increased risk of CHF with radiotherapy to mediastinal/pericardial area or cardiotoxic drugs.

PREGNANCY: Category D, not for use in nursing.

MECHANISM OF ACTION: Anthracycline antineoplastic agent; inhibits nucleotide replication and action of DNA and RNA polymerases.

PHARMACOKINETICS: Distribution: V_d=809-1214L/m^2. Plasma protein binding (74-76%), excreted in breast milk. **Metabolism:** Enzymatic reduction; doxorubicinol (major metabolite). **Elimination:** Bile (40%), urine (5-12%); $T_{1/2}$=20-48 hrs.

NURSING CONSIDERATIONS

Assessment: Perform careful baseline assessment of blood counts (WBC, RBC, and platelets); serum levels of total bilirubin, AST, and creatinine; and cardiac function as measured by LVEF should be assessed before therapy. Note other diseases/conditions and drug therapies.

Monitoring: CBC with differential and platelet count, LFTs, cardiac function, hyperuricemia, hypersensitivity reactions, creatinine level, secondary leukemias, injection-site reactions.

Patient Counseling: Inform about adverse effects, including GI symptoms and neutropenic complications. Consult physician if vomiting, dehydration, fever, evidence of infection, symptoms of CHF, or injection-site pain occur. Advise that alopecia will develop, and urine may appear red for 1-2 days after administration. Educate on risk of irreversible myocardial damage and treatment-related leukemia. Counsel men to use effective contraceptive methods while on treatment, and women that irreversible amenorrhea or premature menopause may occur.

Administration: IV route. **Storage:** Unreconstituted vial at 15-30°C (59-86°F). Protect from light. Refrigerate reconstituted solution at 2-8°C (36-46°F); stable for 7 days. Protect from light. Use appropriate handling and disposal techniques.

DUAC — RX

clindamycin - benzoyl peroxide (Stiefel)

THERAPEUTIC CLASS: Antibacterial/keratolytic

INDICATIONS: Topical treatment of inflammatory acne vulgaris.

DOSAGE: *Adults:* Wash face and pat dry. Apply qd in evening.
Pediatrics: ≥12 yrs: Wash face and pat dry. Apply qd in evening.

HOW SUPPLIED: Gel: (Clindamycin-Benzoyl Peroxide) 1%-5% [45g]

CONTRAINDICATIONS: Hypersensitivity to lincomycin. History of regional enteritis, ulcerative colitis, pseudomembranous colitis, or antibiotic-associated colitis.

D

WARNINGS/PRECAUTIONS: Severe colitis reported with oral and parenteral clindamycin. Topical and systemic use of clindamycin may result in absorption of the antibiotic from the skin surface. Diarrhea, bloody diarrhea, and colitis (eg, pseudomembranous) reported; d/c if significant diarrhea occurs. Antiperistaltic agents (eg, opiates, diphenoxylate with atropine) may prolong and/or worsen condition. Avoid contact with eyes and mucous membranes. Minimize sun exposure after application.

ADVERSE REACTIONS: Erythema, peeling, dryness, and burning.

INTERACTIONS: Cumulative irritancy possible with other topical acne agents. Avoid erythromycin agents.

PREGNANCY: Category C, not for use in nursing.

MECHANISM OF ACTION: Clindamycin: Antibacterial; binds to 50S ribosomal subunits of susceptible bacteria and prevents elongation of peptide chains by interfering with peptidyl transfer, thereby suppressing protein synthesis. Benzoyl peroxide: Keratolytic; potent oxidizing agent.

PHARMACOKINETICS: Distribution: Orally and parenterally administered clindamycin found in breast milk.

NURSING CONSIDERATIONS

Assessment: Assess for hypersensitivity to lincomycin, history of regional enteritis, ulcerative colitis, pseudomembranous colitis, antibiotic-associated colitis. Assess use in pregnancy and that females are not nursing. Assess for possible drug interactions.

Monitoring: Monitor for signs/symptoms of diarrhea, bloody diarrhea, and colitis (pseudomembranous colitis). Perform endoscopic exam to ID pseudomembranous colitis. If diarrhea occurs, perform stool culture for *Clostridium difficile* and stool assay for *Clostridium difficile* toxin. If severe diarrhea occurs, perform large bowel endoscopy. Monitor for overgrowth of nonsusceptible organisms (eg, fungi).

Patient Counseling: Inform to notify physician if diarrhea develops during therapy and up to several weeks after. Instruct to take medication exactly as directed, externally. Advise to avoid contact with eyes, inside nose, mouth, and all mucous membranes. Advise to avoid contact with hair or fabrics; drug causes bleaching. Advise to limit exposure to sunlight and to use protection (eg, hats, sunscreen) when exposed to sun.

Administration: Topical route. **Storage:** Prior to dispensing, 2-8°C (36-46°F). Do not freeze. After dispensing: Store up to 25°C (77°F). Do not freeze. Keep tube tightly closed.

DUETACT RX

pioglitazone HCl - glimepiride (Takeda)

Thiazolidinediones may cause or exacerbate CHF in some patients. Duetact is not recommended in patients with symptomatic heart failure.

THERAPEUTIC CLASS: Thiazolidinedione/sulfonylurea

INDICATIONS: Adjunct to diet and exercise to improve glycemic control in type 2 diabetes already being treated with combination of pioglitazone and sulfonylurea, with inadequate control on sulfonylurea alone, or with initial response to pioglitazone alone requiring additional glycemic control.

DOSAGE: *Adults:* Base recommended starting dose on current regimen of pioglitazone and/or sulfonylurea. Give with 1st meal of day. Current Glimepiride Monotherapy or Prior Therapy of Pioglitazone plus Glimepiride Separately: Initial: 30mg-2mg or 30mg-4mg qd. Current Pioglitazone or Different Sulfonylurea Monotherapy or Combination of Both: Initial: 30mg-2mg qd. Adjust dose based on response. Max: Once daily at any strength. Elderly/Debilitated/Malnourished/Renal or Hepatic Insufficiency (ALT ≤2.5x ULN): Initial: 1mg glimepiride prior to prescribing Duetact. Systolic Dysfunction: Initial: 15-30mg of pioglitazone; titrate carefully to lowest Duetact dose.

HOW SUPPLIED: Tab: (Pioglitazone-Glimepiride) 30mg-2mg, 30mg-4mg

CONTRAINDICATIONS: Established NYHA Class III or IV heart failure, diabetic ketoacidosis.

WARNINGS/PRECAUTIONS: Glimepiride: Increased CV mortality. Hypoglycemia risk if debilitated, malnourished, or with adrenal, pituitary, renal, or hepatic insufficiency. Hypoglycemia may be masked in elderly. May lose blood glucose control with stress. Secondary failure may occur. D/C if skin reactions persist or worsen. Pioglitazone: May cause fluid retention and exacerbation/initiation of heart failure; d/c if cardiac status deteriorates. Avoid if NYHA Class III or IV cardiac status. Not for use in type 1 DM or diabetic ketoacidosis treatment. Caution with edema. Dose-related wt gain reported. Ovulation in premenopausal anovulatory patient may occur; risk of pregnancy with inadequate contraception. May decrease Hgb and Hct. Avoid with active liver disease, if ALT levels >2.5x ULN, or if jaundice occurred. Check LFTs before therapy, every 2 months for 1 yr, and periodically thereafter, or if hepatic dysfunction symptoms occur. D/C if ALT >3x ULN on therapy. Macular edema and fractures reported.

ADVERSE REACTIONS: Hypoglycemia, upper respiratory tract infection, increased weight, lower limb edema/pain, headache, UTI, diarrhea, nausea, new onset or worsening diabetic macular edema with decreased visual acuity.

INTERACTIONS: Pioglitazone: CYP3A4 inducer. May decrease levels of ethinyl estradiol and midazolam. CYP2C8 inhibitor. May significantly increase the AUC levels of pioglitiazone. CYP2C8 inducer. May significantly decrease the AUC levels of pioglitiazone. Glimepiride: Risk of hyperglycemia with thiazides, corticosteroids, phenothiazines, thyroid products, estrogens, oral contraceptives, phenytoin, nicotinic acid, sympathomimetics, or isoniazid. Hypoglycemia may be potentiated with β-blockers, MAOIs, salicylates, sulfonamides, and coumarins. Risk of severe hypoglycemia with oral miconazole.

PREGNANCY: Category C, not for use in nursing.

MECHANISM OF ACTION: Pioglitazone: Thiazolidinedione; insulin-sensitizing agent acts by enhancing peripheral glucose utilization. Glimepiride: Sulfonylurea; stimulates release of insulin from functional pancreatic β-cells.

PHARMACOKINETICS: Absorption: Administration of variable doses resulted in different parameters. Glimepiride: T_{max}=2-3 hrs. **Distribution:** Pioglitazone: V_d=0.63 L/kg, plasma protein binding (>99%). Glimepiride: (IV) V_d=8.8L, plasma protein binding (>99.5%). **Metabolism:** Pioglitazone: Extensive (hydroxylation & oxidation), CYP2C8, 3A4. Glimepiride: CYP2C9. **Elimination:** Pioglitazone: Urine (15-30%), feces; $T_{1/2}$=3-7 or 16-24 hrs. Glimepiride: Urine (60%).

NURSING CONSIDERATIONS

Assessment: Obtain baseline LFTs, renal function, CBC. Assess for lactic acidosis, CHF, macular edema, type 1 DM, diabetic ketoacidosis, pregnancy status, and possible drug interactions.

Monitoring: Monitor FPG and HbA_{1c} periodically for glycemic control and therapeutic response. Periodically perform LFTs, hematologic parameters, renal function, and eye exams. Monitor for signs/symptoms of heart failure, edema, diabetic ketoacidosis, fractures.

Patient Counseling: Instruct to d/c with unexplained hyperventilation, myalgia, malaise, unusual somnolence symptoms. Counsel to report unexplained GI symptoms, rapid increase in weight or edema, SOB, NV, abdominal pain, fatigue, anorexia, or dark urine. Advise to avoid excessive alcohol intake. Counsel females about use of reliable contraception. Inform about importance of adherence to meal planning, regular physical activity, regular blood glucose monitoring, periodic HbA_{1c} testing, recognition and management of hypo- and hyperglycemia, and periodic assessment for diabetes complications. Inform that during periods of stress (eg, trauma, infection, surgery), medication requirements may change; seek prompt medical advice.

Administration: Oral route. **Storage:** Store at 25°C (77°F); excursions permitted to 15-30°C (59-86°F). Keep container tightly closed. Protect from moisture and humidity.

DUONEB

RX

ipratropium bromide - albuterol sulfate (Dey)

D

THERAPEUTIC CLASS: Beta$_2$-agonist/anticholinergic

INDICATIONS: Treatment of bronchospasm in COPD in patients requiring more than one bronchodilator.

DOSAGE: *Adults:* 3mL qid via nebulizer. May give 2 additional doses/day.

HOW SUPPLIED: Sol, Inhalation: (Albuterol-Ipratropium) 3mg-0.5mg/3mL [3mL, 30^s 60^s]

CONTRAINDICATIONS: Hypersensitivity to atropine and its derivatives.

WARNINGS/PRECAUTIONS: Paradoxical bronchospasm and hypersensitivity reactions reported. Caution with cardiovascular disorders, convulsive disorders, hyperthyroidism, DM, narrow-angle glaucoma, prostatic hypertrophy, and bladder-neck obstruction.

ADVERSE REACTIONS: Pain, chest pain, diarrhea, dyspepsia, nausea, leg cramps, bronchitis, lung disease, pharyngitis, pneumonia, UTI.

INTERACTIONS: Additive interactions with anticholinergic agents. Increased risk of cardiovascular side effects with sympathomimetics. Use β_1-selective blockers with hyper-reactive airways. Caution within 2 weeks of discontinuation of MAOIs or TCAs.

PREGNANCY: Category C (albuterol) and B (ipratropium), not for use in nursing.

MECHANISM OF ACTION: Albuterol: β_2-adrenergic bronchodilator; stimulates adenyl cylase, enzyme that catalyzes formation of cAMP from ATP. Increased cAMP levels are associated with relaxation of bronchial smooth muscle and inhibition of release of mediators of immediate hypersensitivity. Ipratropium: Anticholinergic bronchodilator; blocks muscarinic receptors of acetylcholine. Prevents the increase in intracellular concentration of cGMP, resulting from interaction of acetylcholine with the muscarinic receptors of bronchial smooth muscle.

PHARMACOKINETICS: Absorption: Albuterol: C_{max}=4.65mg/mL; T_{max}=0.8 hrs; AUC=24.2ng•h/mL. **Distribution:** Ipratropium: Plasma protein binding (0-9%). **Metabolism:** Albuterol: Conjugation. Ipratropium: Ester hydrolysis. **Elimination:** Albuterol: Urine (8.4% unchanged). Ipratropium: Urine (3.9% unchanged); $T_{1/2}$=6.7 hrs.

NURSING CONSIDERATIONS

Assessment: Assess for history of hypersensitivity to atropine or its derivatives. Assess for concomitant diseases such as narrow-angle glaucoma, prostatic hyperplasia, convulsive disorders, hyperthyroidism, DM, hepatic/renal insufficiency, CVD, and possible drug interactions.

Monitoring: Monitor serum potassium, pulse rate and BP, hypersensitivity reactions, parodoxical brochospasm, cardiovascular effects such as flattening of the T wave, prolongation of QT interval, and ST segment depression, severe acute asthmatic crisis, hypoxia, and adverse effects (eg, headache, cough, respiratory disorders, pain, dyspnea, and bronchitis). Monitor for anticholinergic effects.

Patient Counseling: Caution to avoid spraying aerosol into eyes; may cause precipitation or worsening of narrow-angle glaucoma, mydriasis, increased IOP, acute eye pain or discomfort, temporary blurring vision, visual halos or colored images. Advise not to exceed recommended dose. Report lack of response and adverse side effects.

Administration: Oral inhalation. 1) Remove vial and squeeze contents into nebulizer reservoir. 2) Connect nebulizer to mouthpiece and compressor. 3) Place mouthpiece in mouth or put on face mask and turn on compressor. 4) Breathe as calmly as possible through mouth until no more mist is formed (5-15 min). 5) Clean nebulizer. **Storage:** 2-30°C (36-86°F). Protect from light.

DURAGESIC

CII

fentanyl (Ortho-McNeil)

Life-threatening hypoventilation can occur. Contraindicated for acute or post-op pain and mild/intermittent pain. Avoid in patients <2 yrs. Only for use in opioid tolerant patients. Concomitant use with potent CYP450 3A4 inhibitors may result in an increase in fentanyl plasma concentrations which may cause potentially fatal respiratory depression. Monitor patients receiving potent CYP450 3A4 inhibitors.

THERAPEUTIC CLASS: Opioid analgesic

INDICATIONS: Management of persistent, moderate to severe chronic pain when continuous, around-the-clock opioid administration for an extended period of time is required and cannot be managed by other means such as nonsteroidal analgesics, opioid combination products, or immediate-release opioids.

DOSAGE: *Adults:* Individualize dose. Determine dose based on opioid tolerance. Initial: 25mcg/hr for 72 hr.
Pediatrics: ≥2 yrs: Individualize dose. Determine dose based on opioid tolerance. Initial: 25mcg/hr for 72 hr.

HOW SUPPLIED: Patch: 12.5mcg/hr, 25mcg/hr, 50mcg/hr, 75mcg/hr, 100mcg/hr [5[s]]

CONTRAINDICATIONS: Non opioid-tolerant patients, management of acute/post-op pain, mild/intermittent pain. Diagnosis or suspicion of paralytic ileus. Patients who have acute or severe broncial asthma, significant respiratory depression especially in settings where there is lack of resuscitative equipment.

WARNINGS/PRECAUTIONS: Monitor patients with serious adverse events for at least 24 hrs after removal. Avoid exposing application site to direct external heat. Hypoventilation may occur; caution with chronic pulmonary diseases. Caution with brain tumors, bradyarrhythmias, renal/hepatic impairment, pancreatic/biliary tract disease. Avoid with increased ICP, impaired consciousness, or coma. May obscure clinical course of head injury. Tolerance and physical dependence can occur. May impair mental/physical abilities.

ADVERSE REACTIONS: Hypoventilation, HTN, fever, NV, constipation, dry mouth, somnolence, confusion, asthenia, sweating, nervousness, application site reaction, apnea, dyspnea.

INTERACTIONS: See Black Box Warning. Concomitant use with CNS depressants (opioids, sedatives, hypnotics, tranquilizers, general anesthetics, phenothiazines, skeletal muscle relaxants, alcohol) may cause respiratory depression, hypotension, profound sedation, or potentially coma or death. May increase clearance with CYP3A4 inducers (eg, rifampin, carbamazepine, phenytoin). Avoid use within 14 days of MAOI.

PREGNANCY: Category C, not for use in nursing.

MECHANISM OF ACTION: Opioid analgesic; interacts predominantly with the opioid μ-receptor. Exerts principle pharmacological actions on CNS.

PHARMACOKINETICS: Absorption: T_{max}=24-72 hrs. Transdermal administration of variable doses resulted in different parameters. **Distribution**: V_d=6 L/kg; found in breast milk. Accumulates in skeletal muscle and fat; released slowly into the blood; readily crosses placenta. **Metabolism**: Liver via CYP3A4; oxidative N-dealkylation to norfentanyl and other metabolites. **Elimination**: Urine (75%), feces (9%); $T_{1/2}$=3-12 hrs.

NURSING CONSIDERATIONS

Assessment: Assess for opioid tolerance, level of pain intensity, type of pain (eg, postoperative pain, intermittent pain), respiratory depression, acute or severe bronchial asthma, COPD, age of patient, abuse potential, evidence of increased intracranial pressure, impaired consciousness or coma, bradyarrhythmia, hepatic/renal disease, fever, biliary tract disease (eg, acute pancreatitis), presence of paralytic ileus, pregnancy/nursing status, and possible drug interactions.

Monitoring: Monitor for signs/symptoms of respiratory depression, bradycardia, sphincter of Oddi spasms, increases in serum amylase levels, abuse or misuse, and tolerance or physical dependence.

Patient Counseling: Counsel to wear patch continuously for 72 hrs, and apply patch to different intact, nonirritated skin site following removal of previous patch. Following use, advise to fold patch and flush down the toilet. Instruct to apply patch to flat surface of body (eg, chest, back, flank, upper arm). If cognitively impaired, advise to place on upper back, to decrease chance of removal. Advise to clean with water and dry skin prior to application; avoid soaps, oils, lotions, or any skin irritants. Avoid exposing patch to direct external heat sources. Contact physician if fever develops. May impair mental/physical abilities; use caution if performing hazardous tasks (eg, operating machinery/driving). Notify physician of all medications currently taken. Counsel to avoid using other CNS depressants and alcohol. Inform that constipation may develop during therapy. Avoid abrupt withdrawal of medication; taper dose. Medication has high potential for abuse. Instruct to place medication in secure place, away from children. Instruct that if patch sticks to a different person, remove patch and wash exposed area with water, and contact physician.

Administration: Transdermal patch. Apply immediately after removal from individually sealed package. **Storage:** Do not store above 77°F (25°C).

DURAMORPH CII

morphine sulfate (Baxter)

THERAPEUTIC CLASS: Opioid analgesic

INDICATIONS: Management of pain unresponsive to non-narcotic analgesics.

DOSAGE: *Adults:* IV: Initial: 2-10mg/70kg. Epidural Injection: Initial: 5mg in lumbar region. Titrate: If inadequate pain relief within 1 hr, increase by 1-2mg. Max: 10mg/24hrs. Continuous Epidural: Initial: 2-4mg/24hrs. Give additional 1-2mg if needed. Intrathecal: 0.2-1mg single dose, do not repeat; may follow with 0.6mg/hr naloxone infusion to reduce incidence of side effects.

HOW SUPPLIED: Inj: 0.5mg/mL, 1mg/mL, 5mg/mL

CONTRAINDICATIONS: Allergy to opiates, acute bronchial asthma, upper airway obstruction. Severe hypotension may occur in volume depleted patients or with concurrent administration of phenothiazines or general anesthetics.

WARNINGS/PRECAUTIONS: Have resuscitation equipment, oxygen, and antidote (eg, naloxone) available; severe respiratory depression may occur. Avoid rapid administration. May be habit-forming. Caution with head injury, increased intracranial/intraocular pressure, decreased respiratory reserve, hepatic/renal dysfunction, elderly, debilitated. High doses may cause seizures. Smooth muscle hypertonicity may cause biliary colic, urinary difficulty or retention. Orthostatic hypotension may occur with hypovolemia or myocardial dysfunction. Acute respiratory failure reported with COPD or acute asthmatic attack. Limit epidural/intrathecal route to lumbar area.

ADVERSE REACTIONS: Respiratory depression, convulsions, dysphoric reactions, pruritis, urinary retention, constipation, lumbar puncture-type headache, toxic psychoses.

INTERACTIONS: CNS depressants (eg, alcohol, sedatives, antihistamines) and psychotropics potentiate CNS depression. Neuroleptics may increase respiratory depression.

PREGNANCY: Category C, safety in nursing not known.

MECHANISM OF ACTION: Opioid analgesic; analgesic effects are produced via at least 3 areas of the CNS: the periaqueductal-periventricular gray matter, the ventromedial medulla, and the spinal cord. Interacts predominantly with μ-receptors which are found distributed in the brain, spinal cord, and in the trigeminal nerve.

PHARMACOKINETICS: Absorption: (Epidural): Rapid absorption; C_{max}=33-40ng/mL; T_{max}=10-15 min; (Intrathecal): C_{max}<1-7.8ng/mL; T_{max}=5-10 min. **Distribution:** Plasma protein binding (36%); Muscle tissue binding (54%).

Readily passes into fetal circulation, found in breast milk. (IV): V_d=1.0-4.7L/kg. **Metabolism:** Hepatic glucuronidation. **Elimination:** Kidneys (major), urine (2-12% unchanged), feces (10%); (IV, IM) $T_{1/2}$=1.5-4.5 hrs; (epidural) $T_{1/2}$=39-249 min.

NURSING CONSIDERATIONS

D

Assessment: Assess for acute bronchial asthma, upper airway obstruction, hypotension, infection at injection site, bleeding diathesis, seizure disorder, presence of head injury or increased intracranial pressure, age of patient, hepatic/renal dysfunction, biliary tract disorders or recent biliary surgery, urinary system disorders, impaired myocardial function, hypotension, nursing/pregnancy status, and possible drug interactions.

Monitoring: Monitor for signs/symptoms of respiratory depression and/or respiratory arrest, myoclonic events, seizures, dysphoric reactions, toxic psychoses, biliary colic, urinary retention, drug abuse, and drug dependence. If administered intrathecally or via epidural, monitor closely for 24 hrs for signs/symptoms of respiratory depression.

Patient Counseling: Counsel to notify physician immediately if develop signs/symptoms of respiratory depression. Instruct to avoid using other CNS depressants and alcohol during therapy. Inform that medication has potential for abuse and dependence. Counsel to avoid abrupt withdrawal of medication; withdrawal symptoms may occur. Instruct that if accidental skin contact occurs, wash affected area with water.

Administration: Intravenous, epidural, or intrathecal route. Proper placement of needle or catheter should be verified before epidural injection. **Storage:** 20-25°C (68-77°F); excursions permitted to 15-30°C (59-86°F). Protect from light. Do not freeze.

DYAZIDE RX

triamterene - hydrochlorothiazide (GlaxoSmithKline)

THERAPEUTIC CLASS: K^+-sparing diuretic/thiazide diuretic

INDICATIONS: For hypertension or edema if hypokalemia occurs on HCTZ alone, or when a thiazide diuretic is required and cannot risk hypokalemia.

DOSAGE: *Adults:* 1-2 caps qd.

HOW SUPPLIED: Cap: (Triamterene-HCTZ) 37.5mg-25mg

CONTRAINDICATIONS: Hyperkalemia, anuria, acute or chronic renal insufficiency, sulfonamide hypersensitivity, diabetic neuropathy, K^+-sparing agents (eg, diuretics), K^+ supplements (except with severe hypokalemia), K^+ salt substitutes, K^+-rich diet.

WARNINGS/PRECAUTIONS: Risk of hyperkalemia (≥5.5mEq/L), especially with renal impairment, elderly, DM, or severely ill; monitor levels frequently. Caution in severely ill in whom respiratory or metabolic acidosis may occur; monitor acid-base balance frequently. May manifest DM. Caution with hepatic dysfunction, history of renal stones. Increases uric acid levels, BUN, creatinine. May decrease PBI levels. D/C before parathyroid function tests. May potentiate electrolyte imbalance with heart failure, renal disease, cirrhosis.

ADVERSE REACTIONS: Muscle cramps, GI effects, weakness, blood dyscrasias, arrhythmia, impotence, dry mouth, jaundice, paresthesia, renal stones, hypersensitivity reactions.

INTERACTIONS: Hyperkalemia risk with ACE inhibitors, blood from blood bank, low-salt milk, K^+-containing agents (eg, parenteral penicillin G potassium), salt substitutes. Increased risk of hyponatremia with chlorpropamide. Possible renal dysfunction with NSAIDs. Risk of lithium toxicity. Decreases arterial responsiveness to norepinephrine. ACTH, amphotericin B, and corticosteroids intensify electrolyte depletion. Adjust oral anticoagulants, antigout, and antidiabetic drugs. Increases effects of nondepolarizing muscle relaxants, antihypertensives. Overuse of laxatives or sodium polystyrene sulfonate reduces K^+ levels. Reduces methenamine effects.

PREGNANCY: Category C, not for use in nursing.

MECHANISM OF ACTION: Triamterene: Antikaliuretic agent; exerts effect on distal renal tubules to inhibit reabsorption of Na^+ in exchange for K^+ and H^+ ions. HCTZ: Diuretic; blocks reabsorption of Na^+ and Cl^- ions.

PHARMACOKINETICS: Absorption: Triamterene: C_{max}=46.4ng/mL; T_{max}=1.1 hrs; AUC=148.7ng•hrs/mL. HCTZ: C_{max}=135.1ng/mL; T_{max}=2 hrs; AUC=834ng•hrs/mL.

D

NURSING CONSIDERATIONS

Assessment: Assess for anuria, DM, history of renal stones, possible drug interactions, sulfonamide hypersensitivity, renal/hepatic impairment. Obtain baseline serum K^+ levels, renal function and serum electrolytes.

Monitoring: Monitor renal function, serum K^+ levels, and serum electrolytes. Monitor for signs/symptoms of hyperkalemia, hypokalemia, hyperglycemia, renal stones, electrolyte imbalance, hypersensitivity reactions, renal/hepatic dysfunction.

Patient Counseling: Advise to seek medical attention if symptoms of hyperkalemia (paresthesias, muscular weakness, fatigue), hypokalemia, hyperglycemia, renal stones, electrolyte imbalance (dry mouth, thirst, weakness), or hypersensitivity reactions occur.

Administration: Oral route. **Storage:** 20-25°C (68-77°F); excursions permitted to 15-30°C (59-86°F). Protect from light.

DYNACIN — RX

minocycline HCl (Medicis)

THERAPEUTIC CLASS: Tetracycline derivative

INDICATIONS: Treatment of inclusion conjunctivitis, nongonococcal urethritis, and other infections (eg, respiratory tract, endocervical, rectal, urinary tract, skin and skin structure) caused by susceptible strains of microorganisms. Alternative treatment in certain other infections (eg, urethritis, gonococcal, syphilis, anthrax). Adjunctive therapy in acute intestinal amebiasis and severe acne. Treatment of *Mycobacterium marinum* and asymptomatic carriers of *Neisseria meningitidis*.

DOSAGE: *Adults:* Usual: 200mg initially, then 100mg q12h; alternative is 100-200mg initially, then 50mg qid. Uncomplicated Gonococcal Infection (Men, other than urethritis and anorectal infections): 200mg initially, then 100mg q12h for minimum 4 days. Uncomplicated Gonococcal Urethritis (Men): 100mg q12h for 5 days. Syphilis: Administer usual dose for 10-15 days. Meningococcal Carrier State: 100mg q12h for 5 days. *Mycobacterium marinum:* 100mg q12h for 6-8 weeks. Uncomplicated urethral, endocervical, or rectal infection: 100mg q12h for at least 7 days. Renal Dysfunction: Reduce dose and/or extend dose intervals.
Pediatrics: >8 yrs: 4mg/kg initially followed by 2mg/kg q12h. Take with plenty of fluids.

HOW SUPPLIED: Tab: 50mg, 75mg, 100mg

WARNINGS/PRECAUTIONS: May cause fetal harm during pregnancy. Use during tooth development (last half of pregnancy, infancy, <8 yrs) may cause permanent discoloration of the teeth or enamel hypoplasia; avoid use during this period. Renal toxicity, hepatotoxicity, photosensitivity, increased BUN, superinfection, pseudotumor cerebri may occur; perform hematopoietic, renal, and hepatic monitoring. May impair mental/physical abilities. Use alternate form of contraception other than oral contraceptives. May decrease bone growth in premature infants.

ADVERSE REACTIONS: Anorexia, NV, diarrhea, dysphagia, enterocolitis, pancreatitis, increased LFTs, hepatitis, liver failure, renal toxicity, rash, exfoliative dermatitis, Stevens-Johnson syndrome, skin and mucous membrane pigmentation, blood dyscrasias, headache, tooth discoloration.

INTERACTIONS: May require downward adjustments of anticoagulant dosage. May interfere with bactericidal action of penicillin; avoid concurrent use when possible. May decrease efficacy of oral contraceptives. Impaired absorption with antacids containing aluminum, calcium, or magnesium and iron-containing products. Fatal renal toxicity with methoxyflurane has been reported.

PREGNANCY: Category D, not for use in nursing.

MECHANISM OF ACTION: Tetracycline derivative; thought to inhibit protein synthesis.

PHARMACOKINETICS: Absorption: Rapid. **Distribution:** Crosses placenta, excreted in breast milk. **Elimination:** Urine, feces.

NURSING CONSIDERATIONS

Assessment: Assess for pregnancy status, possible drug interactions, and renal impairment. Document indications for therapy, culture, and susceptibility testing. Perform incision and drainage in conjunction with antibiotic therapy when indicated.

Monitoring: Monitor for signs/symptoms of hypersensitivity reactions, photosensitivity, superinfection, benign intracranial HTN, LFTs, renal function, CBC with platelet and differential count. In venereal disease with coexistent syphilis, conduct serologic test before treatment and after 3 months.

Patient Counseling: Inform of pregnancy risks and photosensitivity reactions (d/c at 1st sign of skin erythema). Avoid excessive sunlight/UV light and wear sunscreen/sunblock. Inform therapy treats bacterial, not viral, infections. Take as directed; skipping doses or not completing full course may decrease effectiveness and increase resistance. Notify physician if hypersensitivity reactions, superinfections, photosensitivity, or benign intracranial HTN occur. Advise to avoid foods with calcium. Concomitant use of tetracyclines may render oral contraceptives less effective.

Administration: Oral route. **Storage:** Store at 20-25°C (68-77°F). Protect from light, moisture, and excessive heat.

DynaCirc CR — RX

isradipine (GlaxoSmithKline)

THERAPEUTIC CLASS: Calcium channel blocker (dihydropyridine)

INDICATIONS: Management of hypertension.

DOSAGE: *Adults:* Initial: 5mg qd alone or with a thiazide diuretic. Titrate: May adjust by 5mg/day at 2-4 week intervals. Max: 20mg/day. Swallow whole.

HOW SUPPLIED: Tab, Controlled-Release: 5mg, 10mg.

WARNINGS/PRECAUTIONS: May produce symptomatic hypotension. Caution in CHF, especially with concomitant β-blockers. Caution with pre-existing severe GI narrowing. Peripheral edema reported. Increased bioavailability in elderly.

ADVERSE REACTIONS: Headache, edema, dizziness, constipation, fatigue, flushing, abdominal discomfort.

INTERACTIONS: Additive effects with HCTZ. Severe hypotension possible with fentanyl and β-blockers. Increases AUC and C_{max} of propranolol. Decreased levels with rifampicin.

PREGNANCY: Category C, not for use in nursing.

MECHANISM OF ACTION: Dihydropyridine calcium channel blocker; binds to calcium channels and inhibits calcium flux into cardiac and smooth muscle.

PHARMACOKINETICS: Absorption: Bioavailability (15-24%); C_{max}=3-4ng/mL; AUC=62-73ng•h/mL. **Distribution:** Plasma protein binding (95%). **Metabolism:** Oxidation, ester cleavage; CYP3A4. **Elimination:** Urine, feces.

NURSING CONSIDERATIONS

Assessment: Assess for hypotension, CHF, pre-existing GI narrowing, and possible drug interactions.

Monitoring: Monitor for signs/symptoms of hypotension, peripheral edema, obstruction from strictures, and hypersensitivity reactions.

Patient Counseling: Instruct to swallow whole; do not chew. Inform may see tablet shell in stool.

Administration: Oral route. **Storage:** Below 30°C (86°F); tight container. Protect from moisture and humidity.

DYRENIUM RX

triamterene (WellSpring)

D

Abnormal elevation of serum K^+ levels (≥5.5mEq/L) can occur with all K^+-sparing agents, including triamterene. Hyperkalemia is more likely to occur with renal impairment and diabetes (even without evidence of renal impairment), and in the elderly, or severely ill. Monitor serum K^+ at frequent intervals.

THERAPEUTIC CLASS: K^+-sparing diuretic

INDICATIONS: Treatment of edema associated with congestive heart failure, liver cirrhosis, and nephrotic syndrome. Treatment of steroid induced edema, idiopathic edema and edema due to secondary hyperaldosteronism.

DOSAGE: *Adults:* Initial: 100mg bid pc. Max: 300mg/day.

HOW SUPPLIED: Cap: 50mg, 100mg

CONTRAINDICATIONS: Anuria, severe or progressive kidney disease or dysfunction (except with nephrosis), severe hepatic disease, hyperkalemia, K^+ supplements, K^+ salt substitutes, K^+-sparing agents (eg, diuretics).

WARNINGS/PRECAUTIONS: Check ECG if hyperkalemia occurs. May cause decreased alkali reserve with possibility of metabolic acidosis, mild nitrogen retention. Monitor BUN periodically. May contribute to megaloblastosis in folic acid deficiency. Caution with gouty arthritis; may elevate uric acid levels. May aggravate or cause electrolyte imbalances in CHF, renal disease, or cirrhosis. Caution with history of renal stones.

ADVERSE REACTIONS: Hypersensitivity reactions, hyper- or hypokalemia, azotemia, renal stones, jaundice, NV, diarrhea, weakness, dizziness.

INTERACTIONS: Increased risk of hyperkalemia with ACE inhibitors. Indomethacin may cause renal failure; caution with NSAIDs. Risk of lithium toxicity. Avoid K^+-sparing diuretics, K^+ supplements, K^+-containing agents or salt substitutes, low-salt milk, and blood from blood bank; may potentiate serum K^+ levels. May cause hyperglycemia; adjust antidiabetic agents. Chlorpropamide may increase risk of severe hyponatremia. May potentiate nondepolarizing muscle relaxants, antihypertensives, other diuretics, preanesthetics, and anesthetics.

PREGNANCY: Category C, not for use in nursing.

MECHANISM OF ACTION: K^+ sparing diuretic; inhibits reabsorption of Na^+ ions in exchange for K^+ and H^+ ions at segment of distal tubule under control of adrenal mineralocorticoids.

PHARMACOKINETICS: Absorption: Rapid; C_{max}=30ng/mL, T_{max}=3 hrs. **Distribution:** Crosses placental barrier. **Metabolism:** Hydroxytriamterene (metabolite). **Elimination:** Urine (21%).

NURSING CONSIDERATIONS

Assessment: Assess for anuria, CHF, DM, gout, hyperkalemia, history of kidney stones, possible drug interactions, liver/renal impairment.

Monitoring: Monitor BUN, serum K^+ levels and CBC periodically. Monitor for signs/symptoms of blood dyscrasias, electrolyte imbalance, hyperkalemia, exacerbation of gout, hypersensitivity reactions, liver/renal dysfunction.

Patient Counseling: Advise to take with meals to avoid stomach upset. If single dose prescribed, take in a.m. to minimize frequency of urination during nighttime sleep. Instruct not to take more than prescribed dose at next dosing interval if dose missed. Seek medical attention if symptoms of hyperkalemia, electrolyte imbalance, or hypersensitivity reactions occur.

Administration: Oral route. **Storage:** 25°C (77°F); excursions permitted to 15-30°C (59-86°F); light-resistant container.

E.E.S.

RX

erythromycin ethylsuccinate (Abbott)

E

THERAPEUTIC CLASS: Macrolide

INDICATIONS: Treatment of mild to moderate upper/lower respiratory tract and skin and skin structure infections, listeriosis, pertussis, diphtheria, erythrasma, intestinal amebiasis, acute pelvic inflammatory disease (PID) (*N.gonorrhoeae*), primary syphilis (if PCN allergy), Legionnaires' disease, chlamydial infections (eg, newborn conjunctivitis, pneumonia of infancy, urogenital infections during pregnancy, or urethral, endocervical, or rectal infections when tetracyclines are contraindicated or not tolerated), and nongonococcal urethritis caused by susceptible strains of microorganisms. Prophylaxis of initial and recurrent attacks of rheumatic fever if PCN allergy.

DOSAGE: *Adults:* Usual: 1600mg/day in divided doses given q6h, q8h, or q12h. Max: 4g/day. Treat strep infections for at least 10 days. Streptococcal Infection Prophylaxis with Rheumatic Heart Disease: 400mg bid. Urethritis (*C.trachomatis* or *U.urealyticum*): 800mg tid for 7 days. Primary Syphilis: 48-64g in divided doses over 10-15 days. Intestinal Amebiasis: 400mg qid for 10-14 days. Pertussis: 40-50mg/kg/day in divided doses for 5-14 days. Legionnaires' Disease: 1.6-4g/day in divided doses.
Pediatrics: Usual: 30-50mg/kg/day in divided doses q6h, q8h, or q12h. Severe Infections: May double dose. Treat strep infections for at least 10 days. Streptococcal Infection Prophylaxis with Rheumatic Heart Disease: 400mg bid. Intestinal Amebiasis: 30-50mg/kg/day in divided doses for 10-14 days.

HOW SUPPLIED: Sus: 200mg/5mL, 400mg/5mL; Tab: 400mg

CONTRAINDICATIONS: Concomitant terfenadine, astemizole, cisapride, or pimozide.

WARNINGS/PRECAUTIONS: *Clostridium difficile*-associated diarrhea, hepatic dysfunction reported. Caution with impaired hepatic function. May aggravate weakness of patients with myasthenia gravis.

ADVERSE REACTIONS: N/V, abdominal pain, diarrhea, anorexia, hepatic dysfunction, abnormal LFTs, allergic reactions, superinfection (prolonged use).

INTERACTIONS: See Contraindications. Rhabdomyolysis reported with lovastatin. May increase levels of theophylline, digoxin, drugs metabolized by CYP450 (eg, carbamazepine, cyclosporine, tacrolimus, phenytoin, alfentanil, disopyramide, lovastatin, bromocriptine, valproate, etc). Increases effects of oral anticoagulants, triazolam, midazolam. Risk of acute ergot toxicity with ergotamine or dihydroergotamine. May increase AUC of sildenafil; consider dose reduction of sildenafil.

PREGNANCY: Category B, caution in nursing.

MECHANISM OF ACTION: Macrolide antibiotic; inhibits protein synthesis by binding 50S ribosomal subunits of susceptible organisms.

PHARMACOKINETICS: Absorption: Readily absorbed. **Distribution:** Diffuses into most body fluids, crosses placental barrier. **Metabolism:** Liver. **Elimination:** Biliary excretion, urine (≤5%).

NURSING CONSIDERATIONS

Assessment: Assess for history of impaired hepatic function, myasthenia gravis, hearing loss, arrhythmias. Note other diseases/conditions and drug therapies.

Monitoring: Monitor LFTs, renal function, CK, CDAD, hearing loss, pancreatitis, arrhythmias, infantile hypertrophic pyloric stenosis, hypersensitivity reactions.

Patient Counseling: Inform that therapy treat bacterial, not viral infections. Take as directed; complete entire prescription. Take on empty stomach. Report adverse effects, lack of response, prolonged/persistent diarrhea.

Administration: Oral route. **Storage:** 30°C (86°F).

EFFEXOR

venlafaxine HCl (Wyeth)

RX

Antidepressants increased the risk of suicidal thinking and behavior (suicidality) in short-term studies in children, adolescents, and young adults with major depressive disorder (MDD) and other psychiatric disorders. Venlafaxine is not approved for use in pediatric patients.

E

THERAPEUTIC CLASS: Serotonin and norepinephrine reuptake inhibitor

INDICATIONS: Treatment of MDD.

DOSAGE: *Adults:* ≥18 yrs: Initial: 75mg/day given bid-tid with food. Titrate: Increase by 75mg/day at no less than 4 day intervals. Max: 375mg/day. Hepatic Impairment (moderate): Reduce dose by 50%. Renal Impairment (mild to moderate): Reduce dose by 25%. Hemodialysis: Reduce dose by 50%.

HOW SUPPLIED: Tab: 25mg*, 37.5mg*, 50mg*, 75mg*, 100mg* *scored

CONTRAINDICATIONS: Concomitant use of MAOIs.

WARNINGS/PRECAUTIONS: Avoid abrupt withdrawal. Re-evaluate periodically. Monitor for clinical worsening, suicidality, and/or unusual behavioral changes, especially at initiation of therapy or dose changes. Serotonin syndrome or neuroleptic malignant syndrome (NMS)-like reactions reported. Manage with immediate discontinuation and monitor. May cause sustained increases in BP. Activation of mania/hypomania, mydriasis, hyponatremia, SIADH, altered platelet function, treatment-emergent anxiety, nervousness, insomnia, and anorexia reported. Caution with history of mania or seizures, conditions affecting hemodynamic responses or metabolism. D/C if seizures occur. Monitor increase of IOP or risk of acute narrow angle glaucoma. May increase risk of bleeding events. Elevation of cholesterol levels reported; monitor periodically. Caution with hyperthyroidism, heart failure, recent MI, renal or hepatic impairment. Interstitial lung disease and eosinophilic pneumonia (rare) reported. Caution in elderly.

ADVERSE REACTIONS: Asthenia, sweating, NV, constipation, anorexia, insomnia, somnolence, dry mouth, dizziness, nervousness, anxiety, tremor, blurred vision, abnormal ejaculation/orgasm, impotence in men.

INTERACTIONS: See Contraindications. Avoid alcohol, tryptophan. Increase risk of bleeding with ASA, NSAIDs, warfarin, and other anticoagulants. Caution with cimetidine in elderly, HTN, hepatic dysfunction. Altered coagulation effects with warfarin. Decreases clearance of haloperidol. Increases risperidone and desipramine plasma levels. Caution with potent inhibitors of CYP3A4 and CYP2D6, CNS-active drugs, and serotonergic drugs (eg, triptans, SSRIs, other SNRIs, linezolid, lithium, tramadol, or St. John's Wort).

PREGNANCY: Category C, not for use in nursing.

MECHANISM OF ACTION: 5-HT and NE reuptake inhibitor; potentiates neurotransmitter activity of CNS activity by inhibiting neuronal serotonin and norephinephrine reuptake.

PHARMACOKINETICS: Absorption: Relative bioavailability (100%). **Distribution:** Venlafaxine: V_d=7.5L/kg; plasma protein binding (27%). ODV: V_d=5.7L/kg; plasma protein binding (30%). **Metabolism:** Hepatic; metabolite: O-desmethylvenlafaxine (ODV). **Elimination:** Venlafaxine: Urine (5%); $T_{1/2}$=5 hrs. ODV: Urine; $T_{1/2}$=11 hrs.

NURSING CONSIDERATIONS

Assessment: Assess for bipolar disorder risk, history of mania, hyperthyroidism, heart failure, recent MI, history of glaucoma, increased IOP, risk factors for acute-narrow angle glaucoma, pre-existing HTN, history of seizures, disease/condition that alters metabolism or hemodynamic response, cholesterol levels, hepatic/renal impairment, pregnancy/nursing status, and possible drug interactions.

Monitoring: Monitor HR, BP, LFTs, renal function, serum cholesterol, serum TG and ECG changes. Monitor for signs/symptoms of clinical worsening (suicidality, unusual changes in behavior), serotonin syndrome or NMS-like reactions, mydriasis, severe HTN, lung disease (progressive dyspnea, cough, chest discomfort), abnormal bleeding, allergic reactions (rash, hives), hyponatremia (headache, weakness, unsteadiness), seizures, cognitive/motor impairment, and hepatic/renal dysfunction. If abruptly d/c, monitor for symptoms of dysphoric mood, irritability, agitation, dizziness, sensory disturbances, anxiety, confusion, headache, lethargy, emotional lability, insomnia, and hypomania.

Patient Counseling: Instruct to take with food; swallow whole, or open cap and sprinkle contents on spoonful of applesauce. Advise to avoid alcohol. Seek medical attention for symptoms of serotonin syndrome (mental status changes, tachycardia, hyperthermia, NV, diarrhea, incoordination), abnormal bleeding (particularly if using NSAIDs or ASA), hyponatremia (headache, weakness, unsteadiness), mydriasis, severe HTN, lung disease (progressive dyspnea, cough, chest discomfort), activation of mania, allergic reaction (rash, hives), seizures, clinical worsening (suicidal ideation, unusual changes in behavior) and discontinuation symptoms (irritability, agitation, dizziness, anxiety, headache, insomnia). Caution may impair physical/mental abilities. Notify physician if pregnant or intend to become pregnant, breastfeeding an infant, develop a rash, hives, or related allergic phenomenon. Inform physician if taking, or plan to take, any prescriptions over-the-counter drugs, including herbal preparations and nutritionals supplements.

Administration: Oral route. **Storage:** 20-25°C (68-77°F) in dry place and well-closed container.

EFFEXOR XR — RX

venlafaxine HCl (Wyeth)

Antidepressants increased the risk of suicidal thinking and behavior (suicidality) in short-term studies in children, adolescents, and young adults with major depressive disorder (MDD) and other psychiatric disorders. Venlafaxine is not approved for use in pediatric patients.

THERAPEUTIC CLASS: Serotonin and norepinephrine reuptake inhibitor

INDICATIONS: Treatment of major depressive disorder (MDD), generalized anxiety disorder (GAD), social anxiety disorder (SAD), panic disorder (PD).

DOSAGE: *Adults:* MDD/GAD/SAD: Initial: 75mg qd, or 37.5mg qd increase to 75mg qd after 4-7 days. Titrate: May increase by 75mg/day at no less than 4 day intervals. Max: 225mg/day. PD: Initial: 37.5mg qd for 7 days. Titrate: May increase 75mg/day, as needed at no less than 7 day intervals. Max: 225mg/day. Moderate Hepatic Impairment: Reduce initial dose by 50%. Renal Impairment: Reduce total daily dose by 25-50%. Hemodialysis: Reduce total daily dose by 50%. Withhold dose until after hemodialysis treatment completed. If drug used 6 weeks or longer, taper gradually (over 2 weeks or more) when discontinuing treatment. Periodically reassess need for maintenance therapy. Take with food in the am or pm, the same time each day. May sprinkle on spoonful of applesauce. Do not divide, crush, chew or place in water.

HOW SUPPLIED: Cap, Extended-Release: 37.5mg, 75mg, 150mg

CONTRAINDICATIONS: Concomitant MAOI therapy.

WARNINGS/PRECAUTIONS: May cause sustained increases in BP; monitor BP regularly. Treatment-emergent nervousness, insomnia and anorexia reported. Caution with seizures, conditions affecting hemodynamic responses or metabolism, volume-depletion, the elderly. Risk of mydriasis; monitor those with raised IOP or risk of acute narrow angle glaucoma. Abnormal bleeding (eg, ecchymosis) and activation of mania/hypomania reported. Risk of hyponatremia, SIADH. Caution with recent MI, hyperthyroidism, heart failure, renal or hepatic impairment. Serotonin syndrome may occur; caution with concomitant use of serotonergic drugs. Patients who present with progressive dyspnea, cough or chest discomfort should consider the possibility of interstitial lung disease and eosinophilic pneumonia. D/C if impaired balance occurs. Cases of clinically significant hyponatremia in elderly.

ADVERSE REACTIONS: Asthenia, sweating, headache, nausea, constipation, anorexia, dry mouth, dizziness, insomnia, nervousness, somnolence, abnormal ejaculation, abnormal dreams.

INTERACTIONS: See Contraindications. Avoid within 14 days of MAOI therapy. Upon discontinuation, wait at least 7 days before starting MAOI therapy. Caution with cimetidine in elderly, hepatic dysfunction or pre-existing HTN. Caution with diuretics. Decreases clearance of haloperidol. Increases risperidone and desipramine plasma levels. Decreases indinavir plasma levels. Caution with potent inhibitors of CYP3A4 and CYP2D6, CNS-active drugs (eg, triptans, SSRIs, lithium), and with serotonergic drugs. Avoid alcohol.

PREGNANCY: Category C, not for use in nursing.

MECHANISM OF ACTION: 5-HT and NE reuptake inhibitor; potentiates neurotransmitter activity of CNS by inhibiting neuronal serotonin and norepinephrine reuptake.

PHARMACOKINETICS: Absorption: Venlafaxine: Absolute bioavailability (45%), C_{max}=150ng/mL, T_{max}=5.5 hrs. ODV (metabolite): C_{max}=260ng/mL, T_{max}=9 hrs. **Distribution:** Venlafaxine: V_d=7.5L/kg; plasma protein binding (27%). ODV: V_d=5.7L/kg; plasma protein binding (30%). **Metabolism:** Hepatic via CYP2D6; Active metabolite: O-desmethylvenlafaxine (ODV). **Elimination:** Urine (5% unchanged). Venlafaxine: $T_{1/2}$=5 hrs. ODV: $T_{1/2}$=11 hrs.

NURSING CONSIDERATIONS

Assessment: Assess for bipolar disorder risk, history of mania, possible drug interactions, hyperthyroidism, heart failure, recent MI, acute narrow-angle glaucoma, elevated IOP, HTN, seizures, hypersensitivity, concomitant use of MAOIs, serotonin syndrome, disease/condition that alters metabolism or hemodynamic response, cholesterol levels, hepatic/renal impairment.

Monitoring: Monitor HR, BP, LFTs, renal function, serum cholesterol, serum TG and ECG changes, signs/symptoms of clinical worsening (suicidality, unusual behavior), serotonin syndrome (agitation, hallucinations, coma, incoordination, tachycardia, hyperthermia, labile BP, NV, diarrhea), mydriasis, severe HTN, lung disease (progressive dyspnea, cough, chest discomfort), abnormal bleeding, allergic reactions (rash, hives), hyponatremia (headache, weakness, unsteadiness), seizures, cognitive/motor impairment, and hepatic/renal dysfunction. If abruptly d/c, monitor for dizziness, sensory disturbances, anxiety, confusion, headache, lethargy, emotional lability, insomnia, and hypomania.

Patient Counseling: Counsel to take with food, swallow whole without chewing, or open cap and sprinkle on spoonful of applesauce followed with water. Advise to avoid alcohol; may impair physical/mental abilities. Seek medical attention for symptoms of serotonin syndrome (mental status changes, tachycardia, hyperthermia, NV, diarrhea, incoordination), abnormal bleeding (particularly if using NSAIDs or ASA), hyponatremia (headache, weakness, unsteadiness), mydriasis, severe HTN, lung disease (progressive dyspnea, cough, chest discomfort), activation of mania, allergic reaction (rash, hives), seizures, clinical worsening (suicidal ideation, unusual changes in behavior), or discontinuation symptoms (irritability, agitation, dizziness, anxiety, headache, insomnia).

Administration: Oral route. **Storage:** 20-25°C (68-77°F).

ELDEPRYL — RX

selegiline HCl (Somerset)

THERAPEUTIC CLASS: Monoamine oxidase inhibitor (Type B)

INDICATIONS: Adjunct to levodopa/carbidopa for management of Parkinson's disease.

DOSAGE: *Adults:* 5mg bid, at breakfast and lunch. Max: 10mg/day. May reduce levodopa/carbidopa by 10-30% after 2-3 days of therapy. May reduce further with continued therapy.

HOW SUPPLIED: Cap: 5mg

CONTRAINDICATIONS: Concomitant meperidine, other opioids.

WARNINGS/PRECAUTIONS: Do not exceed 10mg/day due to non-selective MAO inhibition. Decrease levodopa/carbidopa by 10-30% to prevent exacerbation of levodopa side effects.

ADVERSE REACTIONS: Nausea, dizziness, lightheadedness, fainting, abdominal pain, confusion, hallucinations, dry mouth.

INTERACTIONS: See Contraindications. Stupor, muscular rigidity, severe agitation, and elevated temperature reported with meperidine; avoid concomitant use. Avoid SSRIs and TCAs; severe toxicity reported. Allow 2 weeks between discontinuation of selegiline and initiation of TCAs or SSRIs. Allow 5 weeks for fluoxetine due to a longer half-life. Caution with sympathomimetics, tyramine-containing food.

PREGNANCY: Category C, not for use in nursing.

MECHANISM OF ACTION: MAO type inhibitor; increases dopaminergic activity by blocking the catabolism of dopamine.

PHARMACOKINETICS: Absorption: C_{max}=1ng/mL. **Metabolism:** Gut and liver (extensive). Metabolites: N-desmethylselegiline, L-amphetamine, L-methamphetamine. **Elimination:** $T_{1/2}$=2 hrs.

NURSING CONSIDERATIONS

Assessment: Assess BP, HR, dyskinesia. Note other conditions/diseases and drug therapies.

Monitoring: Monitor for hypersensitivity reactions, syncope, angina pectoris, hyperpyrexia, hypertensive crisis, hallucinations, myoclonic jerks.

Patient Counseling: Report adverse side effects. Avoid tyramine-containing foods (aged cheeses, pickled herring, yeast extract, air-dried meats) and beverages (certain red wines and beers).

Administration: Oral route. **Storage:** 15-30°C (59-86°F).

ELESTAT — RX

epinastine HCl (Inspire)

THERAPEUTIC CLASS: H_1-antagonist

INDICATIONS: For the prevention of itching associated with allergic conjunctivitis.

DOSAGE: *Adults:* 1 drop in each eye bid.
Pediatrics: ≥3 yrs: 1 drop in each eye bid.

HOW SUPPLIED: Sol: 0.05% [5mL]

WARNINGS/PRECAUTIONS: Not for contact lens-related irritation. May reinsert contact lens 10 minutes after dosing if eye is not red.

ADVERSE REACTIONS: Burning sensation in the eye, folliculosis, hyperemia, pruritus.

PREGNANCY: Category C, caution in nursing.

MECHANISM OF ACTION: Antihistaminic; topically active; direct H_1-receptor antagonist and an inhibitor of histamine release from the mast cell; selective for the histamine H_1-receptor and has affinity for the histamine H_2-receptor and possesses affinity for the α_1-α_2-and 5-HT_2-receptors.

PHARMACOKINETICS: Absorption: C_{max}=0.04ng/ml; T_{max}=2 hrs. **Distribution:** Plasma protein binding (64%). **Elimination:** Urine, feces; $T_{1/2}$=12 hrs.

NURSING CONSIDERATIONS

Assessment: Assess for drug hypersensitivity.

Monitoring: Monitor adverse events such as burning sensation in the eye, folliculosis, hyperemia, pruritus, and infection (cold symptoms and upper respiratory infections).

Patient Counseling: Counsel not to wear contact lenses if eye is red; remove prior to instillation. Inform that medication is not for treatment of contact lens-related irritation. Instruct to avoid touching tip of container to eye or any other surface to avoid contamination.

Administration: Ocular route. **Storage:** 15-25°C (59-77°F). Keep tightly closed.

ELIDEL

RX

pimecrolimus (Novartis)

THERAPEUTIC CLASS: Macrolactam ascomycin derivative

INDICATIONS: Short-term and intermittent long-term therapy of moderate to severe atopic dermatitis in nonimmunocompromised patients intolerant to or unresponsive to conventional therapy.

DOSAGE: *Adults:* Apply bid. Re-evaluate if symptoms persist after 6 weeks. *Pediatrics:* ≥2 yrs: Apply bid. Re-evaluate if symptoms persist after 6 weeks.

HOW SUPPLIED: Cre: 1% [30g, 60g, 100g]

WARNINGS/PRECAUTIONS: Increased risk of varicella zoster infection, herpes simplex virus infection or eczema herpeticum. Lymphadenopathy reported; d/c if unknown etiology of lymphadenopathy or acute mononucleosis presents. Skin papilloma or warts reported; consider discontinuation if worsening or unresponsive skin papilloma. Minimize or avoid natural or artificial sunlight exposure. Avoid with Netherton's syndrome, areas of active cutaneous viral infections, or occlusive dressings. Long-term safety has not been established. Rare cases of malignancy (eg, skin and lymphoma) reported with topical calcineurin inhibitors; therefore, continuous long-term use should be avoided and application limited to areas of involvement. Not indicated for use in children <2 yrs.

ADVERSE REACTIONS: Application site burning, headache, nasopharyngitis, influenza, pharyngitis, viral infection, pyrexia, cough, skin discoloration.

INTERACTIONS: Caution with CYP3A4 inhibitors (eg, erythromycin, itraconazole, ketoconazole, fluconazole, CCBs, cimetidine) in widespread and/or erythrodermic disease.

PREGNANCY: Category C, not for use in nursing.

MECHANISM OF ACTION: Macrolactam ascomycin derivative; not fully established. Suspected to bind with high affinity to macrophilin-12 (FKBP-12) and inhibit the calcium-dependent phosphatase, calcineurin. Consequently, this inhibits T cell activation by blocking the transcription of early cytokines.

PHARMACOKINETICS: Absorption: C_{max}=1.4ng/mL. **Distribution:** Plasma protein binding (99.5%). **Metabolism:** Liver by CYP3A. **Elimination:** Feces (78.4% metabolites) and (≤1% unchanged).

NURSING CONSIDERATIONS

Assessment: Assess patient is not <2 years of age, immunocompromised, does not have malignant or premalignant skin conditions (eg, cutaneous-cell lymphoma), does not have Netherton's syndrome or other skin diseases that would increase absorption of drug. Assess for absence of viral or bacterial skin infections. Assess use in pregnant/nursing females and in patients with generalized erythroderma. Assess for possible drug interactions.

Monitoring: Monitor for infections (eg, varicella virus infection, herpes simplex virus infection, eczema herpeticum), lymphomas, skin malignancy, and local symptoms (eg, skin burning, pruritus).

Patient Counseling: Inform not to use drug for long continuous periods of time. Advise to d/c medication when signs/symptoms of eczema subside (eg, itching, rash, and redness). Contact physician if symptoms get worse, a skin infection develops, or if symptoms do not improve after 6 weeks of treatment. Instruct to wash hands and dry skin before applying cream. Do not bathe, shower, or swim after applying cream. Instruct not to cover treated skin area with bandages, dressings, or wraps. Advise for external use only; avoid contact with eyes. Avoid natural or artificial sunlight exposure while on therapy.

Administration: Topical. **Storage:** 25°C (77°F); excursions permitted to 15-30°C (59-86°F). Do not freeze.

ELIGARD

RX

leuprolide acetate (Sanofi-Aventis)

THERAPEUTIC CLASS: Synthetic gonadotropin releasing hormone analog

INDICATIONS: Palliative treatment of advanced prostate cancer.

DOSAGE: *Adults:* 7.5mg SQ monthly, 22.5mg SQ every 3 months, 30mg SQ every 4 months, or 45mg SQ every 6 months. Rotate injection sites.

HOW SUPPLIED: Inj: 7.5mg, 22.5mg, 30mg, 45mg

CONTRAINDICATIONS: Women, pregnancy, pediatric patients.

WARNINGS/PRECAUTIONS: Transient worsening of symptoms or onset of new signs/symptoms may occur during 1st few weeks of therapy. Closely monitor patients with metastatic vertebral lesions and/or urinary tract obstruction during first few weeks of therapy. Urethral obstruction and spinal cord compression reported. Monitor serum testosterone, PSA.

ADVERSE REACTIONS: Hot flashes, pain/burning/stinging/erythema/bruising at injection site, malaise/fatigue, atrophy of testes, weakness, gynecomastia, myalgia, dizziness, decreased libido, rigors, lethargy, dyspepsia, scanty urination, limb pain, insomnia, breast soreness, hypertension, clamminess, pituitary aplopexy.

PREGNANCY: Category X, safety in nursing not known.

MECHANISM OF ACTION: LH-RH agonist; acts as a potent inhibitor of gonadotropin secretion and suppresses testicular and ovarian steroidogenesis.

PHARMACOKINETICS: Absorption: (7.5mg, 1st inj) C_{max}=25.3ng/mL, T_{max}=5 hrs. (22.5mg; 1st inj, 2nd inj) C_{max}=127ng/mL, 107ng/mL, T_{max}=5 hrs. (30mg; 1st inj) C_{max}=150ng/mL, T_{max}=3.3 hrs. (45mg; 1st inj, 2nd inj): C_{max}=82ng/mL, 102ng/mL, T_{max}=4.5 hrs. **Distribution**: V_d=27L; plasma protein binding (43%-49%). **Metabolism**: Pentapeptide (major metabolite).

NURSING CONSIDERATIONS

Assessment: Assess for metastatic vertebral lesions and urinary tract obstructions.

Monitoring: Monitor serum testosterone and PSA periodically and for signs/symptoms of worsening, spinal cord compression, renal impairment, and hypersensitivity reactions.

Patient Counseling: Inform may experience worsening of symptoms or onset of new symptoms during first weeks of treatment (bone pain, neuropathy, hematuria, or bladder outlet obstruction). Advise to seek medical attention if symptoms of worsening, spinal cord compression, or hypersensitivity reactions occur.

Administration: SQ. **Storage**: 2-8°C (36-46°F).

ELLENCE

RX

epirubicin HCl (Pharmacia & Upjohn)

Severe local tissue necrosis with extravasation. Not for IM/SQ administration. Risk of myocardial toxicity, severe myelosuppression. Secondary acute myelogenous leukemia reported. Reduce dose with hepatic dysfunction.

THERAPEUTIC CLASS: Anthracycline

INDICATIONS: Adjuvant treatment of primary breast cancer with axillary node tumor involvement following resection of primary breast cancer.

DOSAGE: *Adults:* Initial: 100-120mg/m² IV infusion, repeat at 3-4 week cycles. May give total dose on Day 1 of each cycle or divide equally on Days 1 and 8. Bone Marrow Dysfunction: Initial: 75-90mg/m². Hepatic Dysfunction: Bilirubin 1.2-3mg/dL or AST 2-4X ULN: Give 1/2 of initial dose. Bilirubin >3mg/dL or AST 4X ULN: Give 1/4 of initial dose. Severe Renal Dysfunction: Serum Creatinine >5mg/dL: Lower dose. Give prophylactic therapy with SMZ-TMP or fluoroquinolone with 120mg/m² regimen. Consider pretreatment with antiemetics. Adjust dose after 1st treatment cycle based on hematologic and nonhematologic toxicities (see PI).

HOW SUPPLIED: Inj: 2mg/mL [25mL, 100mL]

CONTRAINDICATIONS: Baseline neutrophils <1500cells/mm^3, severe myocardial insufficiency, recent MI, severe arrhythmias, previous anthracycline therapy with maximum cumulative dose, anthracenedione hypersensitivity, severe hepatic dysfunction.

WARNINGS/PRECAUTIONS: Increased risk of cardiotoxicity with active or dormant cardiovascular disease. Use extreme caution if exceeding cumulative dose of 900mg/m^2. Resolve acute toxicities from other cytotoxic agents prior to initiation. Monitor CBC, total bilirubin, AST, SrCr, and cardiac function before and during each cycle. May induce hyperuricemia. Potential for tumor lysis syndrome. Thrombophlebitis, thromboembolic phenomena reported.

ADVERSE REACTIONS: Hematologic abnormalities, amenorrhea, hot flashes, lethargy, fever, GI disturbances, infection, conjunctivitis/keratitis, alopecia, local toxicity, rash/itch, skin changes.

INTERACTIONS: Increased risk of cardiotoxicity with previous anthracycline or anthracenedione therapy, prior or concomitant radiotherapy to mediastinal/pericardial area, or with concomitant cardiotoxic drugs. Increased risk of refractory secondary leukemia with concurrent DNA-damaging antineoplastics, heavy pretreatment with cytotoxic drugs, or escalated doses of anthracyclines. Additive toxicity with other cytotoxic drugs. Cyclophosphamide and fluorouracil may cause severe leukopenia, neutropenia, thrombocytopenia, and anemia. Monitor closely with cardioactive compounds that could cause heart failure (eg, CCBs). Caution with agents that cause changes in hepatic function. AUC increased with cimetidine; stop cimetidine during therapy. Previous radiation therapy may induce inflammatory recall reaction at irradiation site.

PREGNANCY: Category D, not for use in nursing.

MECHANISM OF ACTION: Anthracycline; complexes with DNA by intercalating its planar rings between nucleotide base pairs, inhibiting nucleic acid (DNA and RNA) and protein synthesis, triggering DNA cleavage by topoisomerase II, inhibits DNA helicase activity, and generates free radicals.

PHARMACOKINETICS: Absorption: IV administration of variable doses resulted in different parameters. **Distribution:** Plasma protein binding (77%). **Metabolism:** Liver (extensive and rapid); reduction, conjugation. Epirubicinol (metabolite). **Elimination:** Biliary (major), urine (minor).

NURSING CONSIDERATIONS

Assessment: Assess for baseline neutrophil count >1500cells/mm^3, CVD (insufficiency, MI, arrhythmias), acute toxicities (prior therapy), hepatic/renal dysfunction, risk factors for cardiac toxicities, pregnancy status, and possible drug interactions. Obtain baseline CBC, total bilirubin, AST, creatinine, and cardiac function (LVEF).

Monitoring: Monitor total and differential WBC, RBC, platelet count, AST, total bilirubin, and cardiac function (MUGA, ECHO) before and during each cycle. Assess need for antiemetics. Monitor for hypersensitivity reaction, CHF, liver dysfunction, myelosuppression, hyperuricemia (tumor lysis syndrome), extravasation, facial flushing or local erythematous streaking, and recall reaction (prior radiation).

Patient Counseling: Inform of red urine 1-2 days after administration. Inform alopecia will develop. Instruct men to use effective contraceptive methods. Inform females may develop premature menopause. Inform of risk of irreversible myocardial damage. Advise to seek medical attention if vomiting, dehydration, fever, evidence of infection, symptoms of CHF, or injection-site pain occur.

Administration: IV route. **Storage:** Refrigerate; 2-8°C (36-46°F). Do not freeze.

E

ELMIRON
pentosan sodium (Ortho-McNeil)

RX

THERAPEUTIC CLASS: Analgesic, urinary

INDICATIONS: Relief of bladder pain/discomfort associated with interstitial cystitis.

DOSAGE: *Adults:* Take 1 hr before or 2 hrs after meals with water. 100mg tid for 3 months. Re-evaluate after 3 months; may continue for another 3 months.
Pediatrics: ≥16 yrs: Take 1 hr before or 2 hrs after meals with water. 100mg tid for 3 months. Re-evaluate after 3 months; may continue for another 3 months.

HOW SUPPLIED: Cap: 100mg

WARNINGS/PRECAUTIONS: Bleeding complications (eg, ecchymosis, epistaxis, gum hemorrhage), alopecia, increased PT/PTT reported. Caution with invasive procedures, coagulopathy, aneurysms, thrombocytopenia, hemophilia, GI ulcers, polyps, diverticula, history of heparin-induced thrombocytopenia, and hepatic impairment. Transient liver enzyme elevation reported.

ADVERSE REACTIONS: Nausea, diarrhea, alopecia, headache, rash, dyspepsia, abdominal pain.

INTERACTIONS: Increased risk of bleeding with anticoagulants, heparin, t-PA, streptokinase, high-dose ASA, and NSAIDs.

PREGNANCY: Category B, caution in nursing.

MECHANISM OF ACTION: Low molecular weight heparin-type compound; not fully established. Possesses anticoagulant and fibrinolytic effects.

PHARMACOKINETICS: Absorption: 3% of administered dose. **Distribution:** Mainly into uroepithelium. **Metabolism:** Liver and spleen, partial desulfation; depolymerization in kidney. **Elimination:** Urine (3% unchanged); $T_{1/2}$=4.8 hrs.

NURSING CONSIDERATIONS

Assessment: Assess for upcoming surgery, pregnancy, liver function, and possible drug interactions (anticoagulants, aspirin, or anti-inflammatory drugs).

Monitoring: Monitor for tendency for bleeding, hair loss, diarrhea, nausea, blood in stool, and abnormal LFTs.

Patient Counseling: Take as prescribed and report any persisting side efffects or presence of blood in stool.

Administration: Oral route.

ELOCON
mometasone furoate (Schering)

RX

THERAPEUTIC CLASS: Corticosteroid

INDICATIONS: Corticosteroid-responsive dermatoses.

DOSAGE: *Adults:* (Cre, Oint) Apply qd. (Lot) Apply a few drops qd. Re-assess if no improvement within 2 weeks.
Pediatrics: (Cre, Oint) ≥2 yrs: Apply qd for up to 3 weeks if needed. Avoid in diaper area. Re-assess if no improvement within 2 weeks.

HOW SUPPLIED: Cre, Oint: 0.1% [15g, 45g]; Lot: 0.1% [30mL, 60mL]

WARNINGS/PRECAUTIONS: May produce reversible HPA axis suppression, manifestations of Cushing's syndrome, hyperglycemia and glucosuria. D/C if irritation occurs. Use appropriate antifungal or antibacterial agent with dermatological infections. Pediatrics may be more susceptible to systemic toxicity. Caution when applied to large surface areas or with occlusive dressings.

ADVERSE REACTIONS: Burning, pruritus, skin atrophy, rosacea, acneiform reaction, tingling, stinging, furunculosis, folliculitis.

PREGNANCY: Category C, caution in nursing.

MECHANISM OF ACTION: Corticosteroid; possesses anti-inflammatory, antipruritic, and vasconstrictive properties. Anti-inflammatory effects not established. Suspected to induce phospholipase A_2 inhibitory proteins, lipocortins. Lipocortins control biosynthesis of potent mediators of inflammation (eg, prostaglandins and leukotrienes) by inhibiting release of their precursor, arachidonic acid.

PHARMACOKINETICS: Absorption: Extent of absorption depends on skin integrity, vehicle, and use of occlusive dressing.

NURSING CONSIDERATIONS

Assessment: Assess use in pregnant/nursing patients.

Monitoring: Monitor for signs/symptoms of hypothalamic-pituitary-adrenal (HPA) axis suppression, glucocorticoid insufficiency, Cushing's syndrome, hyperglycemia, glucosuria, skin irritation, allergic contact dermatitis (eg, failure to heal), and skin infections (eg, fungal, bacterial). In patients applying medication to large surface areas or using occlusive dressings, perform periodic monitoring for HPA-axis suppression by using ACTH stimulation, AM plasma cortisol, and urinary free cortisol tests. In pediatric patients, monitor for systemic toxicity, HPA-axis suppression, Cushing's syndrome, linear growth retardation, delayed weight gain, and intracranial HTN.

Patient Counseling: Counsel to use medication exactly as directed; avoid contact with eyes, face, underarms, and groin. Do not wrap, cover, or bandage treated skin unless directed by physician. Instruct patients to report adverse reactions. Do not apply medication in diaper area. Contact physician if no improvement within 2 weeks. Notify physician before using other corticosteroid therapies.

Administration: Topical route. **Storage:** 25°C (77°F); excursions permitted to 15-30°C (59-86°F).

ELOXATIN — RX

oxaliplatin (Sanofi-Aventis)

Anaphylactic-like reactions may occur within minutes of administration.

THERAPEUTIC CLASS: Organoplatinum complex

INDICATIONS: In combination with infusional 5-fluorouracil (5-FU) and leucovorin (LV) for treatment of advanced metastatic carcinoma of colon or rectum and adjuvant treatment of Stage III colon cancer patients who have undergone complete resection of the primary tumor.

DOSAGE: *Adults:* Advanced Colorectal Cancer: Day 1: 85mg/m² IV with LV 200mg/m²; give over 120 min in separate bags using a Y-line; followed by 5-FU 400mg/m² bolus over 2-4 min, then 5-FU 600mg/m² as a 22 hr infusion. Day 2: LV 200mg/m² over 120 min; followed by 5-FU 400mg/m² bolus over 2-4 min, then 5-FU 600mg/m² as a 22 hr infusion. Repeat cycle every 2 weeks. Persistent Grade 2 Neurosensory Events: Reduce oxaliplatin to 65mg/m². Grade 3 Neurosensory Events: Consider d/c. After Recovery From Grade 3/4 GI or Grade 4 Hematologic Toxicity: Reduce oxaliplatin to 65mg/m² and 5-FU by 20%. Adjuvant Therapy Stage III Colon Cancer: Recommended cycle every 2 weeks for 6 months. Persistent Grade 2 Neurosensory Events: Reduce oxaliplatin to 75mg/m². Persistent Grade 3 Neurosensory Events: Consider d/c. After Recovery From Grade 3/4 GI or Grade 3/4 Hematologic Toxicity: Reduce oxaliplatin to 75mg/m² and 5-FU to 300mg/m² bolus and 500mg/m² 22 hr infusion.

HOW SUPPLIED: Inj: 50mg, 100mg, 200mg

CONTRAINDICATIONS: Hypersensitivity to platinum compounds.

WARNINGS/PRECAUTIONS: Acute and persistent neuropathy reported. Cold may exacerbate acute neurological symptoms; avoid ice for mucositis prophylaxis. Potentially fatal pulmonary fibrosis reported. If unexplained respiratory symptoms develop, d/c until interstitial lung disease or pulmonary fibrosis is ruled out. Monitor WBC with differential, Hgb, platelets, and blood chemistries (including ALT, AST, bilirubin, creatinine) before each cycle. Caution with renal impairment.

ADVERSE REACTIONS: Neuropathy, fatigue, nausea, neutropenia, emesis, diarrhea.

INTERACTIONS: Increased 5-FU plasma levels with doses of 130mg/m² oxaliplatin dosed every 3 weeks; clearance may be decreased with nephrotoxic agents.

PREGNANCY: Category D, not for use in nursing.

MECHANISM OF ACTION: Organoplatinum complex; inhibits DNA replication and transcription.

PHARMACOKINETICS: Absorption: C_{max}=0.814ug/mL. **Distribution**: V_d=440L; plasma protein binding (>90%). **Metabolism:** Rapid, nonenzymatic biotransformation. **Elimination**: Urine (54%), feces (2%).

NURSING CONSIDERATIONS

Assessment: Assess for pre-existing hepatic/renal impairment, pregnancy status, and possible drug interactions.

Monitoring: Monitor LFTs, WBC with differential, Hgb, platelet count, bilirubin, and creatinine periodically and before each dose. Monitor for signs/symptoms of anaphylactic reactions, neuropathy, neurosensory toxicity, portal HTN, liver/renal dysfunction, and pulmonary toxicity.

Patient Counseling: Inform of pregnancy risks; avoid pregnancy. Inform of neurologic effects and persistent neurosensory toxicity that may be precipitated by exposure to cold or cold objects. Avoid cold drinks and ice. Cover exposed skin prior to exposure to cold temperature or cold objects. Advise to seek medical attention if persistent vomiting, diarrhea, fever, signs of dehydration or infection, cough, breathing difficulties, and allergic reactions (rash, urticaria, erythema, pruritus, bronchospasm, and hypotension) occur.

Administration: IV route. Infusion line should be flushed with D5W prior to administration of any concomitant medication. **Storage**: 25°C (77°F); excursions permitted to 15-30°C (59-86°F). Protect from light and do not freeze.

EMCYT RX

estramustine phosphate sodium (Pharmacia & Upjohn)

THERAPEUTIC CLASS: Estradiol/nornitrogen mustard

INDICATIONS: Palliative treatment of metastatic and/or progressive prostate carcinoma.

DOSAGE: *Adults:* Usual: 14mg/kg/day given tid-qid. Take with water at least 1 hr before or 2 hrs after meals.

HOW SUPPLIED: Cap: 140mg

CONTRAINDICATIONS: Active thrombophlebitis, thromboembolic disorders; except when the tumor mass is causing the thromboembolic phenomenon and therapy benefits outweigh risks.

WARNINGS/PRECAUTIONS: Increased risk of thrombosis and MI. Caution with CVD, CAD, metabolic bone disease associated with hypercalcemia, hepatic or renal dysfunction, or with history of thrombophlebitis, thrombosis, or thromboembolic disorders. May decrease glucose tolerance. HTN may occur; monitor BP periodically. May exacerbate pre-existing peripheral edema or CHF. Allergic reactions, angioedema reported. Gynecomastia, impotence may occur.

ADVERSE REACTIONS: Edema, dyspnea, leg cramps, nausea, diarrhea, GI upset, breast tenderness/enlargement, increased hepatic enzymes.

INTERACTIONS: Milk, milk products, and calcium-rich foods or drugs may impair absorption.

PREGNANCY: Safety in pregnancy and nursing not known.

MECHANISM OF ACTION: Estradiol/nornitrogen mustard.

PHARMACOKINETICS: Absorption: Dephosphorylated during absorption. **Metabolism:** Estramustine, estradiol, estrone (major metabolites).

NURSING CONSIDERATIONS

Assessment: Assess for history of thrombophlebitis, thrombosis, thromboembolic disorders, cerebrovascular disease, CAD, metabolic bone diseases, preexisting edema, CHF, DM, epilepsy, migraine, possible drug interactions, pregnancy status, liver/renal dysfunction.

Monitoring: Monitor blood glucose with DM, calcium levels (with metabolic bone disease, renal insufficiency, prostate cancer, osteoblastic metastases), BP, testosterone levels, and LFTs periodically and 2 months after completion. Monitor for signs/symptoms of fluid retention, hypo/hypercalcemia, HTN, allergic reactions (eg, angioedema), thrombosis, liver/renal dysfunction.

Patient Counseling: Advise to use contraceptive measures. Instruct to take at least 1 hr before or 2 hrs after meals, swallowed with water. Avoid simultaneous use with milk, milk products, calcium-rich foods or drugs. Advise to seek medical attention if symptoms of fluid retention, hypo/hypercalcemia, HTN, allergic reactions (eg, angioedema), thrombosis, liver/renal dysfunction occur.

Administration: Oral route. **Storage:** Refrigerate 2-8°C (36-46°F).

EMEND RX

aprepitant (Merck)

THERAPEUTIC CLASS: Substance P/neurokinin 1 receptor antagonist

INDICATIONS: In combination with other antiemetics for prevention of acute and delayed nausea and vomiting associated with initial and repeat courses of highly emetogenic cancer chemotherapy (eg, high-dose cisplatin) and for moderately emetogenic cancer chemotherapy. For the prevention of postoperative nausea and vomiting (PONV).

DOSAGE: *Adults:* Prevention of Chemo-Induced N/V: Day 1: 125mg 1 hr prior to chemotherapy. Days 2 and 3: 80mg qam. Regimen should include a corticosteroid and a 5-HT_3 antagonist. Concomitant Corticosteroid: Reduce dexamethasone PO or methylprednisolone PO by 50% and methylprednisolone IV by 25%. Prevention of Post-Op N/V: 40mg within 3 hrs prior to induction of anesthesia.

HOW SUPPLIED: Cap: 40mg, 80mg, 125mg; Tri-Pak: (one 125mg & two 80mg caps)

CONTRAINDICATIONS: Concurrent treatment with pimozide, terfenadine, astemizole, or cisapride.

WARNINGS/PRECAUTIONS: Chronic continuous use is not recommended. Caution with severe hepatic insufficiency.

ADVERSE REACTIONS: Asthenia/fatigue, NV, constipation, diarrhea, hiccups, anorexia, headache, dizziness, dehydration, heartburn, abdominal pain, epigastric discomfort, gastritis, tinnitis, neutropenia.

INTERACTIONS: See Contraindications. May increase levels of drugs metabolized by CYP3A4 including chemotherapy agents (eg, docetaxel, paclitaxel, etoposide, irinotecan, ifosfamide, imatinib, vinblastine, and vincristine), dexamethasone and methylprednisolone, certain benzodiazepines (eg, midazolam, alprazolam, triazolam). May reduce efficacy of oral contraceptives; use alternative contraception during treatment and for 1 month after last dose. May decrease levels of warfarin, tolbutamide, phenytoin or other drugs metabolized by CYP2C9. Caution with strong CYP3A4 inhibitors (eg, ketoconazole, itraconazole, nefazodone, troleandomycin, clarithromycin, ritonavir, nelfinavir and moderate CYP3A4 inhibitors (eg, diltiazem). Decreased efficacy with CYP3A4 inducers (eg, rifampin, carbamazepine, phenytoin). Concomitant paroxetine may decrease levels of both drugs.

PREGNANCY: Category B, not for use in nursing.

MECHANISM OF ACTION: Substance P/neurokinin 1 receptor antagonist; inhibits emesis induced by cytotoxic chemotherapeutic agents, such as cisplatin, via central actions.

PHARMACOKINETICS: Absorption: (40mg) AUC=7.8mcg•hr/mL, C_{max}=0.7mcg/mL, T_{max}=3 hrs. Refer to PI for detailed information. **Distribution:**

V_d=70L; plasma protein binding (>95%); crosses blood-brain barrier. **Metabolism:** Liver (extensive) via CYP3A4, 1A2, 2C19. **Elimination:** Urine (57%), feces (45%); $T_{1/2}$=9-13 hrs.

NURSING CONSIDERATIONS

Assessment: Assess if receiving concomitant medications primarily metabolized through CYP3A4. Assess other drug interactions, hepatic/renal impairment, and pregnancy/nursing status.

Monitoring: Monitor INR in 2-week period (at 7-10 days if on chronic warfarin therapy).

Patient Counseling: Instruct to take drug as prescribed; first dose (125mg) 1 hr prior to chemotherapy treatment for prevention of chemo-induced nausea and 40mg cap within 3 hrs prior to induction of anesthesia for prevention of PONV. Read patient package insert before starting therapy; reread it each time it is renewed. Patients on chronic warfarin therapy should have clotting status closely monitored. Notify physician if using other Rx/OTC or herbal products.

Administration: Oral route. **Storage:** 20-25°C (68-77°F); original bottle.

EMLA RX

prilocaine - lidocaine (AstraZeneca)

THERAPEUTIC CLASS: Acetamide local anesthetic

INDICATIONS: Topical anesthetic for use on normal intact skin or on genital mucous membranes for minor surgery. Pretreatment for infiltration anesthesia.

DOSAGE: *Adults:* Apply thick layer of cream to intact skin and cover with occlusive dressing. Minor Dermal Procedure: Apply 2.5g (1/2 tube) over 20-25cm² of skin surface for at least 1 hr. Major Dermal Procedure: Apply 2g/10cm² of skin for 2 hrs. Adult Male Genital Skin: Apply 1g/10cm² of skin surface for 15 min. Female External Genitalia: Apply 5-10g for 5-10 min. *Pediatrics:* 7-12 yrs and >20kg: Max: 20g/200cm² for up to 4 hrs. 1-6 yrs and >10 kg: Max:10g/100cm² for up to 4 hrs. 3-12 months and ≥5 kg: Max: 2g/20cm² for up to 4 hrs. 3-12 months and ≥5 kg: Max: 2g/20cm² for up to 4 hrs. 0-3 months or <5kg: Max: 1g/10cm² for up to 1 hr.

HOW SUPPLIED: Cre: (Lidocaine-Prilocaine) 2.5%-2.5%

WARNINGS/PRECAUTIONS: Avoid application for longer than recommended times or on large areas. Avoid with methemoglobinemia. Risk of methemoglobinemia in very young or with G6P deficiency. Avoid eye contact, use in ear. Caution with severe hepatic disease, acutely ill, debilitated, elderly, history of drug sensitivities. Avoid in neonates with a gestational age <37 weeks and infants <12 months receiving treatment with methemoglobin-inducing agents.

ADVERSE REACTIONS: Local reactions such as erythema, edema, abnormal sensations, paleness (pallor or blanching), altered temperature sensations, itching, rash.

INTERACTIONS: Caution with Class I antiarrhythmic drugs (eg, tocainide, mexiletine). Avoid drugs associated with drug-induced methemoglobinemia (eg, sulfonamides, APAP, nitrates/nitrites, nitrofurantoin, phenobarbital, phenytoin, quinine). Caution with other products containing local anesthetics; consider the amount absorbed from all formulations.

PREGNANCY: Category B, caution in nursing.

MECHANISM OF ACTION: Amide-type local anesthetic; provides dermal analgesia by releasing lidocaine and prilocaine into epidermal and dermal layers of skin and by accumulation in vicinity of dermal pain receptors and nerve endings. Also stabilizes neuronal membranes by inhibiting ionic fluxes required for initiation and conduction impulses, thereby effecting local anesthetic action.

PHARMACOKINETICS: Absorption: Lidocaine: (3 hrs 400cm²) C_{max}=0.12mcg/mL, T_{max}=4 hrs; (24 hrs 400cm²) C_{max}=0.28mcg/mL, T_{max}=10 hrs.

Prilocaine: (3 hrs 400cm²) C_{max}=0.07mcg/mL, T_{max}=4 hrs; (24 hrs 400 cm²) C_{max}=0.14mcg/mL, T_{max}=10 hrs. **Distribution:** V_d=1.5L/kg (lidocaine), 2.6L/kg (prilocaine); plasma protein binding 70% (lidocaine), 55% (prilocaine). Crosses placental and blood-brain barrier; found in breast milk. **Metabolism:** Lidocaine: Liver (rapid); monoethylglycinexylidide and glycinexylidide (active metabolites). Prilocaine: Liver and kidneys by amidases; *ortho*-toluidine and propylalanine (metabolites). **Elimination:** Lidocaine: Urine (>98%); $T_{1/2}$=110 min. Prilocaine: $T_{1/2}$=70 min.

NURSING CONSIDERATIONS

Assessment: Assess for congenital or idiopathic methemoglobinemia, G6PD deficiency, hepatic disease, open wounds, hepatic/renal impairment, acutely ill, debilitated/elderly patients, pregnancy/nursing status, and possible drug interactions.

Monitoring: Monitor neonates and infants ≤3 months for methemoglobinemia levels before, during, and after application of cream. Monitor ECG changes, cardiac effects, hepatic dysfunction, methemoglobinemia, and ototoxicity.

Patient Counseling: Advise to avoid inadvertent trauma to treated area. Instruct not to apply near eyes or on open wounds. Inform about potential risks/benefits of drug. Apply as directed by physician. Advise to notify physician if pregnant/nursing or planning to become pregnant. Do not use in premature infants or in infants <12 months who are receiving treatment with methemoglobin-inducing agents. Instruct to consult physician if child becomes very dizzy, excessively sleepy, or develops duskiness of the face or lips after applying drug.

Administration: Topical route. Not for ophthalmic use. **Storage:** 15-30°C (59-86°F); store in tight container.

EMSAM — RX

selegiline (Bristol-Myers Squibb)

Antidepressants increased the risk of suicidal thinking and behavior (suicidality) in short-term studies in children, adolescents and young adults with major depressive disorder and other psychiatric disorders. Selegiline transdermal system is not approved for use in pediatric patients.

THERAPEUTIC CLASS: Monoamine oxidase inhibitor (Type B)

INDICATIONS: Treatment of major depressive disorder.

DOSAGE: *Adults:* Apply to dry, intact skin on the upper torso, upper thigh, or outer surface of upper arm once every 24 hrs. Initial/Target Dose: 6mg/24hrs. Titrate: May increase in increments of 3mg/24hrs at intervals no less than 2 weeks. Max: 12mg/24hrs. Elderly: 6mg/24hrs. Increase dose cautiously and monitor closely.

HOW SUPPLIED: Patch: 6mg/24 hrs, 9mg/24 hrs, 12mg/24 hrs [30[s]]

CONTRAINDICATIONS: Pheochromocytoma. Concomitant SSRIs (eg, fluoxetine, sertraline, paroxetine), dual serotonin and norepinephrine reuptake inhibitors (eg, venlafaxine, duloxetine), TCAs (eg, imipramine, amitriptyline), bupropion, buspirone, meperidine, analgesic agents (eg, tramadol, methadone, and propoxyphene), dextromethorphan, St. John's wort, mirtazapine, cyclobenzaprine, carbamazepine, oxcarbazepine, sympathetic amines (including amphetamines), cold products and weight-reducing preparations that contain vasoconstrictors (eg, pseudoephedrine, phenylephrine, phenylpropanolamine, ephedrine), oral selegiline, other MAOIs (eg, isocarboxazid, phenelzine, tranylcypromine), general anesthesia agents, cocaine, or local anesthesia containing sympathomimetic vasoconstrictors. Dietary modifications required with 9mg/24hrs and 12mg/24hrs systems.

WARNINGS/PRECAUTIONS: Hypertensive crisis may occur with ingestion of foods with a high concentration of tyramine. Postural hypotension may occur; consider dosage adjustment with orthostatic symptoms. Activation of mania/hypomania may occur; caution with history of mania. Caution with disorders or conditions that can produce altered metabolism or hemodynamic responses. Avoid elective surgery requiring general anesthesia.

ADVERSE REACTIONS: Headache, diarrhea, dyspepsia, insomnia, dry mouth, pharyngitis, sinusitis, application site reaction, rash.

INTERACTIONS: Avoid alcohol. See Contraindications.

PREGNANCY: Category C, caution in nursing.

MECHANISM OF ACTION: MAOI; non-selectively inhibits monoamine oxidase.

PHARMACOKINETICS: Absorption: AUC=46.2ng•hr/mL. **Distribution**: Plasma protein binding (90%). **Metabolism**: Hepatic (N-dealkylation, N-depropargylation) via CYP2B6, 2C9, 3A4/5 (major), CYP2A6 (minor); N-desmethylselegiline, methamphetamine, amphetamine (metabolites). **Elimination**: Urine (0.1%); $T_{1/2}$=18-25 hrs.

E

NURSING CONSIDERATIONS

Assessment: Assess for risk of bipolar disorder, history of mania, possible drug interactions, pre-existing orthostasis, and disease/condition that alters metabolism or hemodynamic response.

Monitoring: Monitor for signs/symptoms of clinical worsening (suicidality, unusual changes in behavior), hypertensive crises (occipital headaches, neck stiffness, NV, sweating), postural hypotension, and cognitive and motor impairment.

Patient Counseling: Avoid concomitant use of alcohol, tyramine-containing foods/supplements/beverages (during and 2 weeks following d/c), and cough medicine containing dextromethorphan. Instruct to use only one patch at a time; do not cut patch into smaller portions. Wash hands with soap and water after applying patch. Seek medical attention for symptoms of hypertensive crises (occipital headaches, neck stiffness, NV, sweating), postural hypotension, mania, and clinical worsening (suicidal ideation, unusual changes in behavior). Caution may impair physical/mental abilities. Instruct to continue therapy as directed despite improvement. Avoid exposing application site to external sources of direct heat (heating pads, hot tubs). Advise to change position gradually if lightheaded, faint, or dizzy.

Administration: Transdermal. **Storage**: 20-25°C (68-77°F). Do not store outside sealed pouch or expose to direct heat.

EMTRIVA — RX

emtricitabine (Gilead)

Lactic acidosis and severe hepatomegaly with steatosis, including fatal cases, reported with nucleoside analogs alone or with concomitant antiretrovirals. Not indicated for the treatment of chronic HBV infection; severe acute exacerbations of hepatitis B reported in patients co-infected with HBV and HIV upon discontinuation of emtricitabine.

THERAPEUTIC CLASS: Nucleoside analogue

INDICATIONS: Treatment of HIV-1 infection in combination with other antivirals.

DOSAGE: *Adults:* ≥18 yrs: Cap: 200mg qd. CrCl 30-49mL/min: 200mg q48h. CrCl 15-29mL/min: 200mg q72h. CrCl <15mL/min (including hemodialysis): 200mg q96h. Sol: 240mg (24mL) qd. CrCl 30-49mL/min: 120mg (12mL) qd. CrCl 15-29mL/min: 80mg (8mL) qd. CrCl <15mL/min (including hemodialysis): 60mg (6mL) qd.
Pediatrics: 0-3 months: Sol: 3mg/kg qd. 3 months-17 yrs: Cap: >33kg: 200mg qd. Sol: 6mg/kg qd. Max: 240mg (24mL).

HOW SUPPLIED: Cap: 200mg; Sol: 10mg/mL [170mL]

WARNINGS/PRECAUTIONS: Test for chronic hepatitis B prior to initiation; post-treatment exacerbations reported. Monitor hepatic function for several months in patients who d/c the drug and are co-infected with HIV and HBV. Reduce dose with renal dysfunction. Monitor changes in fasting cholesterol, serum amylase, creatinine kinase, and neutrophil count. Redistribution/accumulation of body fat reported. Immune reconstitution syndrome reported.

ADVERSE REACTIONS: Headache, diarrhea, NV, rash, dyspepsia, asthenia, abdominal pain, dizziness, insomnia, neuropathy, paresthesia, increased cough, rhinitis.

INTERACTIONS: Avoid co-administration with Atripla, Truvada, or lamivudine-containing products.

PREGNANCY: Category B, not for use in nursing.

MECHANISM OF ACTION: Nucleoside analog of cytidine; inhibits the activity of HIV-1 reverse transcriptase by competing with the natural substrate deoxycytidine 5'-triphosphate and incorporating into nascent viral DNA, resulting in chain termination.

PHARMACOKINETICS: Absorption: Rapid and extensive. C_{max}=1.8mcg/mL, T_{max}=1-2 hrs, AUC=10.0mcg•hr/mL. (Cap) Absolute bioavailabilty (93%). (Sol) Absolute bioavailabilty (75%). **Distribution:** Plasma protein binding (<4%). **Metabolism:** Hepatic (conjugation and oxidation). Metabolites: 3'sulfoxide diastereomers and 2'O-glucuronide. **Elimination:** Urine (86%), feces (14%); $T_{1/2}$=10 hrs.

NURSING CONSIDERATIONS

Assessment: Assess for impaired renal/hepatic function, HBV co-infection, risk factors for lactic acidosis, and possible drug interactions.

Monitoring: Monitor for signs/symptoms of lactic acidosis, hepatotoxicity (hepatomegaly and steatosis), peripheral neuropathy, myopathy, exacerbations of hepatitis, immune reconstitution syndrome, redistribution/accumulation of body fat, and closely monitor hepatic/renal function.

Patient Counseling: Advise to seek medical attention if symptoms of lactic acidosis, hepatitis, myopathy, infections, and if fat redistribution/accumulation occur. Counsel to take with/without food. Inform to take with combination therapy as a regular dosing schedule and to avoid missing dose.

Administration: Oral route. **Storage:** (Cap): 25°C (77F°); excursions permitted to 15-30°C (59-86°F). (Sol): Refrigerated 2-8°C (36-46°F); if stored at 25°C (77°) should be used within 3 months; excursions permitted to 15-30°C (59-86°F).

ENABLEX — RX

darifenacin (Novartis)

THERAPEUTIC CLASS: Muscarinic antagonist

INDICATIONS: Treatment of overactive bladder with symptoms of urge urinary incontinence, urgency and frequency.

DOSAGE: *Adults:* Initial: 7.5mg qd with liquid. Titrate: May increase up to 15mg qd after 2 weeks. Max: 15mg qd. Moderate Hepatic Impairment/Concomitant Potent CYP3A4 Inhibitors: Do not exceed 7.5mg/d. Severe Hepatic Impairment: Avoid use. Swallow whole; do not chew, divide, or crush.

HOW SUPPLIED: Tab, Extended-Release: 7.5mg, 15mg

CONTRAINDICATIONS: Urinary retention, gastric retention, uncontrolled narrow-angle glaucoma.

WARNINGS/PRECAUTIONS: Risk of urinary retention; caution with significant bladder outflow obstruction. Risk of gastric retention; caution with GI obstructive disorders. May decrease GI motility; caution with severe constipation, ulcerative colitis, and myasthenia gravis. Caution with moderate hepatic impairment and narrow-angle glaucoma. Avoid use with severe hepatic impairment. May produce blurred vision or dizziness.

ADVERSE REACTIONS: Dry mouth, constipation, dyspepsia, abdominal pain, nausea, diarrhea, UTI, dizziness, asthenia, dry eyes, hypersensitivity reactions (eg, angioedema), confusion and hallucinations, and palpitations.

INTERACTIONS: Do not exceed 7.5mg/day with concomitant potent CYP3A4 inhibitors. Caution with medications metabolized by CYP2D6. Additive effects with other anticholinergic agents.

PREGNANCY: Category C, caution in nursing.

MECHANISM OF ACTION: Muscarinic receptor antagonist; inhibits cholinergic muscarinic receptors, which mediate contractions of urinary bladder smooth muscle, and stimulation of salivary secretions.

PHARMACOKINETICS: Absorption: (7.5mg) Bioavailability (15%); extensive metabolizers (EM): C_{max}=2.01ng/mL, T_{max}=6.49 hrs, AUC=29.24ng•hr/mL. Poor metabolizers (PM): C_{max}=4.27ng/mL, T_{max}=5.2 hrs, AUC=67.56ng•hr/mL. (15mg) Bioavailability (19%); EM: C_{max}=5.76ng/mL, T_{max}=7.61 hrs, AUC=88.9ng•hr/mL. PM: C_{max}=9.99ng/mL, T_{max}=6.71 hrs, AUC=157.71ng.h/mL. **Distribution:** V_d=163L; plasma protein binding (98%). **Metabolism:** CYP2D6, 3A4 (monohydroxylation, ring opening, N-dealkylation). **Elimination:** Urine (3%); $T_{1/2}$=13-19 hrs.

NURSING CONSIDERATIONS

Assessment: Assess for bladder outflow obstruction (urinary retention), GI obstructive disorders (gastric retention), narrow-angle glaucoma, possible drug interactions, severe constipation, ulcerative colitis, myasthenia gravis, and hepatic impairment.

Monitoring: Monitor for symptoms of urinary retention, gastric retention, hepatic impairment, and hypersensitivity reactions.

Patient Counseling: Advise may produce dizziness or blurred vision; caution may impair physical/mental abilities. Instruct take once daily with liquid, with/without food, swallow whole, do not chew, divide, or crush. Advise to seek medical attention if symptoms of constipation, retention, heat prostration (decreased sweating), or hypersensitivity reactions occur.

Administration: Oral route. **Storage:** 25°C (77°F); excursions permitted to 15-30°C (59-86°). Protect from light.

ENBREL

etanercept (Amgen) **RX**

Serious infections, including bacterial sepsis and TB, reported; d/c if severe infection develops. Evaluate for TB risk factors and test for latent TB infection prior to initiation.

THERAPEUTIC CLASS: TNF-receptor blocker

INDICATIONS: To reduce signs/symptoms, induce major clinical response, improve physical function, and inhibit progression of structural damage in moderate to severe rheumatoid arthritis (RA) (may be initiated in combination with methotrexate [MTX] or alone). To reduce signs/symptoms, inhibit progression of structural damage of active arthritis, and improve physical function in psoriatic arthritis (may be used with MTX in patients not responding to MTX alone). To reduce signs/symptoms of moderate to severe polyarticular-course juvenile rheumatoid arthritis (JRA) unresponsive to one or more DMARDs. To reduce signs/symptoms of active ankylosing spondylitis (AS). Chronic moderate to severe plaque psoriasis for candidates of systemic therapy or phototherapy.

DOSAGE: *Adults:* ≥18 yrs: RA/Psoriatic Arthritis/AS: 50mg SQ per week, given as one SQ injection. May continue MTX, glucocorticoids, salicylates, NSAIDs, or analgesics. Psoriasis: Initial: 50mg SQ twice weekly given 3 or 4 days apart for 3 months. May begin with 25-50mg/week. Maint: 50mg/week.
Pediatrics: 2-17 yrs: JRA: 0.8mg/kg SQ per week. Max: 50mg/week. May continue glucocorticoids, NSAIDs, or analgesics.

HOW SUPPLIED: Inj: (MDV) 25mg, (Syringe) 50mg/mL

CONTRAINDICATIONS: Sepsis.

WARNINGS/PRECAUTIONS: May cause autoimmune antibodies. Avoid with active infections. Monitor closely if new infection develops. Caution with pre-existing or recent onset CNS demyelinating disorders. Rare cases of pancytopenia including aplastic anemia reported; d/c if significant hematologic abnormalities occur. May cause reactivation of hepatitis B virus; evaluate prior to therapy initiation. Caution in patients with heart failure; monitor closely. JRA patients should be brought up to date with current immunization guidelines prior to initiating therapy. D/C temporarily with significant varicella virus exposure and consider prophylaxis. Avoid with Wegener's granulomatosis. Needle cap on prefilled syringe and autoinjector contains dry natural rubber; caution with latex allergy.

ADVERSE REACTIONS: (**Adults/Pediatrics**) Injection site reactions, infections, headache. (Pediatrics) Varicella, gastroenteritis, depression, cutaneous ulcer, esophagitis.

INTERACTIONS: Do not give live vaccines. Avoid with cyclophosphamide. May cause neutropenia with anakinra.

PREGNANCY: Category B, not for use in nursing.

MECHANISM OF ACTION: TNF-receptor blocker; binds specifically to tumor necrosis factor (TNF) and blocks its interaction with cell surface TNF-receptors.

PHARMACOKINETICS: Absorption: SQ administration of different doses resulted in different parameters.

NURSING CONSIDERATIONS

Assessment: Assess for sepsis or localized or chronic infection, history of recurring infection, predisposition to infection (eg, DM), preexisting or recent-onset CNS demyelinating disorders, history of significant hematological events, HBV infection, heart failure, pregnancy/nursing status, and possible drug interactions. Assess patients with JRA are up-to-date with immunizations.

Monitoring: Monitor for signs/symptoms of infections (including sepsis), CNS demyelinating disorders, hematological events (eg, aplastic anemia), lymphoma, HBV reactivation, allergic reactions (eg, anaphylactoid reaction), CHF, lupus-like syndrome, and autoimmune hepatitis.

Patient Counseling: Counsel about adverse events; seek immediate medical attention if signs/symptoms of infection or anaphylactic reaction develop. Inform that needle cap on prefilled syringe and on autoinjector contains dry natural rubber, a derivative of latex; use caution if there is sensitivity to latex. Instruct patient or caregiver of proper injection techniques, accurate measurement/administration of correct dose, proper syringe/needle disposal. Inform to avoid reuse of needles and syringes.

Administration: SQ route. Rotate sites for injection (thigh, abdomen, or upper arm). Avoid injecting into areas where skin is tender, bruised, red, or hard. Patient should not self-administer until proper training on how to prepare/administer correct dose is received. Before injection, medication may be allowed to reach room temperature. Multiple-use vial: 1) Reconstitute using 1 mL of Sterile Bacteriostatic Water for Inj, USP to solution of 1 mL containing 25mg of drug. **Storage**: Refrigerate at 2-8°C (36-46°F). Do not freeze. Keep in original carton; protect from light. Do not shake. Reconstituted: May be stored for up to 14 days if refrigerated at 2-8°C (36-46°F). Discard after 14 days. Keep out of reach of children.

ENGERIX-B — RX

hepatitis B (recombinant) (GlaxoSmithKline)

OTHER BRAND NAMES: Engerix-B Pediatric/Adolescent (GlaxoSmithKline)

THERAPEUTIC CLASS: Vaccine

INDICATIONS: Immunization against all known hepatitis B virus subtypes.

DOSAGE: *Adults:* >19 yrs: 20mcg IM in deltoid or thigh at 0, 1, 6 months. Hemodialysis: 40mcg IM at 0, 1, 2, 6 months. Booster: 20mcg IM. Hemodialysis Booster: 40mcg IM. May give SQ with risk of hemorrhage.
Pediatrics: ≤19 yrs: 10mcg/0.5mL IM at 0, 1, 6 months. Booster: ≤10 yrs: 10mcg IM. 11-19 yrs: 20mcg IM. See PI for special populations. May give SQ with risk of hemorrhage.

HOW SUPPLIED: Inj: 10mcg/0.5mL, 20mcg/mL

CONTRAINDICATIONS: Yeast hypersensitivity.

WARNINGS/PRECAUTIONS: Will not prevent hepatitis A, C, and E virus infection. Vaccine may be ineffective with unrecognized hepatitis. Delay vaccine with moderate or severe febrile illnesses. May exacerbate MS (rare). Suboptimal immune response may occur with immunosuppressed persons. Have epinephrine injection (1:1000) available.

ADVERSE REACTIONS: Injection-site soreness and induration, fatigue, erythema, swelling, fever, headache, dizziness.

E

INTERACTIONS: Suboptimal immune response may occur with immunosuppressants; defer vaccine ≥3 months after immunosuppressive therapy.

PREGNANCY: Category C, caution in nursing.

MECHANISM OF ACTION: Stimulates the immune system to induce antibodies that may protect against infection caused by all known subtypes of hepatitis B virus.

NURSING CONSIDERATIONS

Assessment: Assess presence of moderate or severe febrile illness and medical history, immunocompromised status, immunization history for possible vaccine sensitivity, previous vaccine-related adverse reactions, and possible drug interactions.

Monitoring: Monitor for local injection-site reactions (eg, induration, erythema, swelling) and general reactions (eg, fever, headache, dizziness).

Patient Counseling: Inform that expected immune response may not be obtained for immunosuppressed persons. Counsel on importance of completing vaccination series. Advise to report any adverse reactions to healthcare provider.

Administration: IM and SQ. Inject IM in deltoid muscle for adults; and anterolateral thigh in neonates and infants. Administer SQ in persons at risk of hemorrhage. **Storage:** Refrigerate between 2-8°C (36-46°F). Do not freeze; discard if frozen. Do not dilute to administer.

ENJUVIA RX

conjugated estrogens (Duramed)

Estrogens increase the risk of endometrial cancer. Estrogens and progestins should not be used for the prevention of cardiovascular disease or dementia. Increased risks of MI, stroke, invasive breast cancer, PE, and DVT in postmenopausal women (50 to 79 years of age) reported. Increased risk of developing probable dementia in postmenopausal women ≥65 yrs of age reported.

THERAPEUTIC CLASS: Estrogen

INDICATIONS: Treatment of moderate-severe vasomotor symptoms associated with menopause. Treatment of symptoms of vulvar and vaginal atrophy associated with menopause. Treatment of moderate-severe vaginal dryness and pain with intercourse; if used solely for this purpose, topical vaginal products should be considered.

DOSAGE: *Adults:* Individualize dosing. Initial: 0.3mg qd. Adjust dose based on response.

HOW SUPPLIED: Tab: 0.3mg, 0.45mg, 0.625mg, 0.9mg, 1.25mg

CONTRAINDICATIONS: Pregnancy, undiagnosed abnormal genital bleeding, breast cancer, estrogen-dependent neoplasia, DVT/PE, arterial thromboembolic disease (eg, stroke, MI), liver dysfunction.

WARNINGS/PRECAUTIONS: Increased risk of retinal vascular thrombosis, severe hypercalcemia in patients with breast cancer and bone metastases, gallbladder disease and breast and ovarian cancers. Elevated BP reported; monitor BP at regular intervals. May elevate plasma triglycerides resulting in pancreatitis. Caution in patients with impaired liver function or history of cholestatic jaundice. May increase TBG; monitor thyroid function of patients dependent on thyroid hormone replacement therapy and adjust dosage if needed. May cause fluid retention; caution with cardiac or renal dysfunction. Caution in individuals with severe hypocalcemia. May cause exacerbation of asthma, diabetes mellitus, epilepsy, migraine or porphyria, systemic lupus erythematosus, and hepatic hemangiomas.

ADVERSE REACTIONS: Abdominal pain, accidental injury, flu-syndrome, headache, pain, flatulence, nausea, dizziness, paresthesia, bronchitis, rhinitis, sinusitis, breast pain, dysmenorrhea, vaginitis.

INTERACTIONS: CYP3A4 inducers (eg, St. John's wort, phenobarbital, carbamazepine, rifampin) may decrease levels, which may decrease therapeutic effects and/or uterine bleeding profile. CYP3A4 inhibitors (eg, erythromycin, clarithromycin, ketoconazole, itraconazole, ritonavir, grapefruit juice) may increase levels, which may result in side effects.

PREGNANCY: Category X, caution in nursing.

MECHANISM OF ACTION: Estrogen; binds to nuclear receptors in estrogen-responsive tissues. Circulating estrogens modulate pituitary secretion of the gonadotrophins, luteinizing hormone and follicle stimulating hormone, through negative feedback mechanism. Reduces elevated levels of these hormones in postmenopusal women.

PHARMACOKINETICS: Absorption: Refer to package insert for conjugated and unconjugated estrogen parameters. **Distribution:** Largely bound to sex hormone binding globulin and albumin; found in breast milk. **Metabolism:** Liver to estrone (metabolite), estriol (major urinary metabolite); sulfate and glucuronide conjugation (liver); intestinal hydrolysis; CYP 3A4 (partial metabolism). **Elimination:** Urine (parent compound and metabolites); Conjugated estrone: $T_{1/2}$=14 hrs; Conjugated equilin: $T_{1/2}$=11 hrs.

NURSING CONSIDERATIONS

Assessment: Assess for undiagnosed abnormal genital bleeding, presence or history of breast cancer, DVT, PE, estrogen-dependent neoplasia, liver dysfunction, history of cholestatic jaundice, pregnancy/nursing status, age of patient (≥ 65 yrs), hypertriglyceridemia, hypothyroidism, hypocalcemia, asthma, DM, epilepsy, migraine, porphyria, SLE, and possible drug interactions. Assess need for progestin therapy in patients who have not had a hysterectomy.

Monitoring: Monitor for signs/symptoms of cardiovascular disorders (eg, stroke, coronary heart disease, venous thromboembolism), malignant neoplasms (eg, endometrial, breast, or ovarian cancer), dementia, gallbladder disease, hypercalcemia, visual abnormalities (eg, retinal vascular thrombosis), elevations in BP, fluid retention, elevations in serum triglycerides, pancreatitis, hypothyroidism, hypocalcemia, exacerbation of endometriosis and other conditions (eg, asthma, DM, epilepsy, migraine, SLE). Monitor BP levels. Monitor thyroid function in patients on thyroid replacement therapy. If undiagnosed, persistent, or recurring abnormal vaginal bleeding occurs, perform proper diagnostic testing (eg, endometrial sampling) to rule out malignancy. Perform annual breast exam. Perform periodic monitoring (every 3-6 months) to determine therapy need.

Patient Counseling: Inform medication increases risk for uterine cancer. Report breast lumps, unusual vaginal bleeding, dizziness or faintness, changes in speech, severe headaches, chest pain, SOB, leg pains, changes in vision, or vomiting. Inform phýsician if planning surgery or prolonged immobilization. Perform monthly breast self-exams. Take with/without food. If a dose is missed, take as soon as possible; if almost time for next dose, skip missed dose and return to normal dosing schedule.

Administration: Oral route. **Storage:** 20-25°C (68-77°F). Dispense in tight container with child-resistant closure.

ENTOCORT EC — RX

budesonide (Prometheus)

THERAPEUTIC CLASS: Corticosteroid

INDICATIONS: Treatment of mild to moderate active Crohn's disease involving the ileum and/or ascending colon. Maintenance of clinical remission of mild to moderate Crohn's disease involving the ileum and/or ascending colon for up to 3 months.

DOSAGE: *Adults:* Usual: 9mg qd, in the am for up to 8 weeks. Recurring Episodes: Repeat therapy for 8 weeks. Maint: 6mg qd for 3 months, then taper to complete cessation. Moderate to Severe Hepatic Insufficiency/Concomitant CYP3A4 Inhibitors: Reduce dose. Swallow whole; do not chew or break.

HOW SUPPLIED: Cap, Delayed-Release: 3mg

E

WARNINGS/PRECAUTIONS: May reduce response of HPA axis to stress. Supplement with systemic glucocorticosteroids if undergoing surgery or other stressful situations. Increased risk of infection avoid exposure to chickenpox and measles. Caution with TB, HTN, DM, osteoporosis, peptic ulcer, glaucoma, cirrhosis, cataracts, family history of DM or glaucoma. Replacement of systemic glucocorticosteroids may unmask allergies. Chronic use may cause hypercorticism and adrenal suppression.

ADVERSE REACTIONS: Headache, respiratory infection, NV, back pain, dyspepsia, dizziness, abdominal pain, diarrhea, flatulence, sinusitis, viral infection, arthralgia.

INTERACTIONS: Increased levels with CYP3A4 inhibitors (eg, ketoconazole, itraconazole, saquinavir, erythromycin, grapefruit, grapefruit juice); reduce budesonide dose.

PREGNANCY: Category C, not for use in nursing.

MECHANISM OF ACTION: Glucocorticosteroid.

PHARMACOKINETICS: Absorption: C_{max}=5nmol/L; T_{max}=30-600 min; AUC=30nmol•hr/L. **Distribution:** V_d=2.2-3.9L/kg; plasma protein binding (85-90%). **Metabolism:** Liver; CYP3A4. **Elimination:** Urine (60%); $T_{1/2}$=2-3.6 hrs.

NURSING CONSIDERATIONS

Assessment: Assess for liver disease, history of chickenpox or measles, TB, HTN, osteoporosis, peptic ulcers, cataracts, history and/or family history of DM or glaucoma and possible drug interactions. Obtain baseline LFTs.

Monitoring: Monitor LFTs periodically and for signs/symptoms of hypersensitivity reactions.

Patient Counseling: Advise to swallow whole; do not chew or break. Avoid consumption of grapefruit juice during therapy. Take particular care to avoid exposure to chickenpox or measles.

Administration: Oral route. **Storage:** 25° (77°F); excursions permitted to 15-30°C (59-86°F). Keep container tightly closed.

EPIDUO — RX

benzoyl peroxide - adapalene (Galderma)

THERAPEUTIC CLASS: Antibacterial/keratolytic

INDICATIONS: Topical treatment of acne vulgaris in patients ≥12 yrs.

DOSAGE: *Adults:* Apply a pea-sized amount to the affected areas of the face and/or trunk once qd after washing.
Pediatrics: ≥12 yrs: Apply a pea-sized amount to the affected areas of the face and/or trunk once qd after washing.

HOW SUPPLIED: Gel: (Adapalene-Benzoyl Peroxide) 0.1%-2.5% [45g]

WARNINGS/PRECAUTIONS: Not for oral, ophthalmic, or intravaginal use. Minimize exposure to sunlight and sunlamps. Extreme weather may increase skin irritation. Avoid contact with eyes, lips, mucous membranes, cuts, abrasions, eczematous or sunburned skin. Erythema, scaling, dryness, stinging/burning may be experienced. Avoid concomitant use with potentially irritating topical products (eg, medicated/abrasive soaps/cleansers).

ADVERSE REACTIONS: Erythema, dry skin, scaling, stinging, burning, dryness, contact dermatitis, application-site burning/irritation, and skin irritation.

INTERACTIONS: Caution with concomitant sulfur, resorcinol, salicylic acid preparations, and topical acne therapy (eg, peeling, desquamatizing, or abrasive agents).

PREGNANCY: Category C, caution in nursing.

MECHANISM OF ACTION: Adapalene: Napthoic acid derivative; not established; binds to specific retinoic acid nuclear receptors. Benzoyl peroxide: Oxidizing agent with bacteriocidal and keratolytic effects.

PHARMACOKINETICS: Absorption: (Adapalene) C_{max}=0.21ng/mL; AUC_{0-24h}=1.99ng•h/mL. **Excretion:** (Adapalene) Bile. (Benzoic acid) Urine.

E

NURSING CONSIDERATIONS

Assessment: Assess for sunburned skin, eczema, abrasion, skin cuts. Assess use in pregnancy/nursing patients and for possible drug interactions.

Monitoring: Monitor for sensitivity or chemical irritation, cutaneous signs/symptoms (eg, erythema, dryness, scaling, burning, stinging, application-site burning/irritation, and contact dermatitis).

Patient Counseling: Instruct to avoid exposure to sunlight and sunlamps; use sunscreen and protective clothing over treated areas when exposed. Medication may also cause skin irritation when exposed to wind or cold. Avoid contact with eyes, lips, and mucous membranes. Do not apply medication to cuts, abrasions, eczematous or sunburned skin.

Administration: Topical application. **Storage:** Store at 25°C; excursions permitted to 15-30°C (59-86°F). Protect from light. Keep away from heat. Keep tube tightly closed.

EpiPen

epinephrine (Dey)

RX

OTHER BRAND NAMES: EpiPen Jr. (Dey)

THERAPEUTIC CLASS: Sympathomimetic catecholamine

INDICATIONS: Emergency treatment of allergic reactions (anaphylaxis) to insect stings or bites, foods, drugs, other allergens, and idiopathic or exercise-induced anaphylaxis.

DOSAGE: *Adults:* 0.3mg IM in thigh. May repeat with severe anaphylaxis. *Pediatrics:* 0.15mg or 0.3mg (0.01mg/kg) IM in thigh. May repeat with severe anaphylaxis.

HOW SUPPLIED: Inj: (Epipen Jr) 0.5mg/mL, (Epipen) 1mg/mL

WARNINGS/PRECAUTIONS: Not for IV use. Contains sulfites. Extreme caution with heart disease. Anginal pain may be induced with coronary insufficiency. Increased risk of adverse reactions with hyperthyroidism, CVD, HTN, DM, elderly, pregnancy, pediatrics <30kg with Epipen and <15kg with Epipen Jr.

ADVERSE REACTIONS: Palpitations, tachycardia, sweating, nausea, vomiting, respiratory difficulty, pallor, dizziness, weakness, tremor, headache, apprehension, anxiety.

INTERACTIONS: Potentiated by TCAs and MAOIs. Increased risk of arrhythmias with digitalis, mercurial diuretics, or quinidine. Pressor effects may be counteracted by rapidly acting vasodilators.

PREGNANCY: Category C, safety in nursing not known.

MECHANISM OF ACTION: Sympathomimetic drug; acts on both α and β receptors.

NURSING CONSIDERATIONS

Assessment: Assess for heart disease, coronary insufficiency, hyperthyroidism, HTN, DM, pregnancy, and drug interactions (eg, digitalis or MAOIs).

Monitoring: Monitor for anginal pain, arrhythmia, BP, and cerebral hemorrhage in overdosage or inadvertent intravascular injection.

Patient Counseling: Advise to go to the nearest emergency room if accidental injection into hands or feet; may result in loss of blood flow to affected area. Never inject into buttock or IV route.

Administration: IM or SQ into the anterolateral aspect of thigh. **Storage:** 25°C (77°F); excursions permitted to 15-30°C (59-86°F). Light sensitive; store in the tube provided. Do not refrigerate.

EPIVIR — RX

lamivudine (GlaxoSmithKline)

Lactic acidosis and severe hepatomegaly with steatosis, including fatal cases, reported. Epivir tablets and solution, used to treat HIV, contain higher dose of lamivudine than Epivir-HBV, used to treat hepatitis B; only use appropriate dosing forms for HIV treatment. Severe acute exacerbations of hepatitis B reported in patients coinfected with hepatitis B virus and HIV who discontinued therapy; monitor hepatic function closely.

THERAPEUTIC CLASS: Nucleoside analogue

INDICATIONS: Treatment of HIV infection in combination with other antiretrovirals.

DOSAGE: *Adults:* >16 yrs: 150mg bid or 300mg qd, concomitantly with other antiretrovirals. CrCl 30-49mL/min: 150mg qd. CrCl 15-29mL/min: 150mg first dose, then 100mg qd. CrCl 5-14mL/min: 150mg first dose, then 50mg qd. CrCl <5mL/min: 50mg first dose, then 25mg qd.
Pediatrics: Sol: 3 months-16 yrs: 4mg/kg bid, concomitantly with other antiretrovirals. Max: 150mg bid. Scored Tab: 14-21kg: 1/2 tab (75mg) in am and 1/2 tab (75mg) in pm. 21-30kg: 1/2 tab (75mg) in am and 1 tab (150mg) in pm. ≥30kg: 1 tab (150mg) in am and 1 tab (150mg) in pm. Adolescents: CrCl 30-49mL/min: 150mg qd. CrCl 15-29mL/min: 150mg first dose, then 100mg qd. CrCl 5-14mL/min: 150mg 1st dose, then 50mg qd. CrCl <5mL/min: 50mg 1st dose, then 25mg qd.

HOW SUPPLIED: Sol: 10mg/mL [240mL]; Tab: 150mg, 300mg

WARNINGS/PRECAUTIONS: Caution in pediatrics with history of prior antiretroviral nucleoside exposure, history of pancreatitis, or other significant risk factors for developing pancreatitis. D/C if pancreatitis develops. Post-treatment exacerbations of hepatitis reported. Hepatic decompensation occured when used with interferon-α w/ or w/o ribavirin. Suspend therapy if lactic acidosis or pronounced hepatotoxicity occurs. Reduce dose in renal dysfunction. Possible redistribution or accumulation of body fat. Immune reconstitution syndrome reported.

ADVERSE REACTIONS: Headache, malaise, fatigue, fever, chills, NV, diarrhea, anorexia, abdominal pain, neuropathy, dizziness, skin rash, musculoskeletal pain, cough.

INTERACTIONS: TMP/SMX increases levels of lamivudine. Avoid with zalcitabine, zidovudine, and fixed-dose combinations of abacavir, lamivudine, and zidovudine. Also avoid emtricitabine and fixed-dose combinations of emtricitabine, efavirenz, and tenofovir.

PREGNANCY: Category C, not for use in nursing.

MECHANISM OF ACTION: Nucleoside analogue; inhibits HIV-1 reverse transcriptase via DNA chain termination after incorporation into viral DNA.

PHARMACOKINETICS: Absorption: Rapid; (Tab) Absolute bioavailability (86%). (Sol) Absolute bioavailability (87%); C_{max}=1.5mcg/mL (HIV); T_{max}=0.9 hrs. **Distribution:** V_d=1.3L/kg; plasma protein binding (<36%). **Metabolism:** Hepatic (minor); trans-sulfoxide (metabolite). **Elimination:** Urine (unchanged); $T_{1/2}$=5-7 hrs.

NURSING CONSIDERATIONS

Assessment: Assess for impaired hepatic/renal function, risk factors for lactic acidosis, history of pancreatitis, HBV coinfection, DM, and possible drug interactions.

Monitoring: Monitor for signs/symptoms of pancreatitis, immune reconstitution syndrome, fat redistribution, lactic acidosis, hepatitis B exacerbation, hepatic/renal dysfunction.

Patient Counseling: Instruct to take with combination therapy on regular dosing schedule; avoid missing doses. Advise to seek medical attention if symptoms of pancreatitis, hepatitis, exacerbation of HBV, infection, or fat redistribution occur. Inform diabetics that oral solution contains sucrose. Counsel that therapy does not reduce risk of HIV transmission through sexual contact or blood contamination.

Administration: Oral route. **Storage:** 25°C (77°F); excursions permitted to 15-30°C (59-86°F).

EPIVIR-HBV

RX

lamivudine (GlaxoSmithKline)

Lactic acidosis and severe, possibly fatal, hepatomegaly reported. If prescribed for patients with unrecognized or untreated HIV infection, rapid emergence of HIV resistance is likely; Epivir-HBV contains a lower dose of lamiviudine than Epivir which is used to treat HIV. Severe acute exacerbations of hepatitis B reported upon discontinuation of therapy; follow-up liver function monitoring required.

THERAPEUTIC CLASS: Nucleoside analogue

INDICATIONS: Treatment of chronic hepatitis B associated with viral replication and active liver inflammation.

DOSAGE: *Adults:* 100mg qd. CrCl 30-49mL/min: 100mg Day 1, then 50mg qd. CrCl: 15-29mL/min: 100mg Day 1, then 25mg qd. CrCl 5-14mL/min: 35mg Day 1, then 15mg qd. CrCl <5mL/min: 35mg Day 1, then 10mg qd. *Pediatrics:* 2-17 yrs: 3mg/kg qd. Max: 100mg/day.

HOW SUPPLIED: Sol: 5mg/mL [240mL]; Tab: 100mg

WARNINGS/PRECAUTIONS: Reduce dose in renal dysfunction. Caution in elderly. This formulation is not appropriate in both HBV and HIV infections. Post-treatment exacerbations of hepatitis reported. Pancreatitis reported, especially in HIV-infected pediatrics with prior nucleoside exposure. Monitor patient regularly during treatment. Safety and efficacy of treatment after 1 yr is not known. Suspend therapy if lactic acidosis or pronounced hepatotoxicity develops. Emergence of resistance-associated HBV mutations.

ADVERSE REACTIONS: Pancreatitis, lactic acidosis, severe hepatomegaly, GI complaints, sore throat, infections, elevated LFTs, arthralgia.

INTERACTIONS: TMP/SMX may increase lamivudine levels. Avoid with zalcitabine.

PREGNANCY: Category C, not for use in nursing.

MECHANISM OF ACTION: Nucleoside analogue; phosphorylated to active 5'-triphosphate metabolite intracellularly; incorporation of monophosphate form into viral DNA by HBV reverse transcriptase results in DNA termination.

PHARMACOKINETICS: Absorption: Rapid; C_{max}=1.28mcg/mL (HBV), C_{max}=1.05mcg/mL (healthy); T_{max}=0.5-2.0 hrs; AUC=4.3mcg•h/mL (HBV), AUC=4.7mcg•h/mL (healthy). Tab: Absolute bioavailability (86%). Sol: Absolute bioavailability (87%). **Distribution:** Plasma protein binding (<36%); V_d=1.3L/kg. **Metabolism:** Hepatic (minor); trans-sulfoxide (metabolite). **Elimination:** Urine (unchanged); $T_{1/2}$=5-7 hrs.

NURSING CONSIDERATIONS

Assessment: Assess for HIV infection, impaired liver/renal function, history of pancreatitis, risk factors for lactic acidosis, and possible drug interactions.

Monitoring: Monitor signs/symptoms of pancreatitis, lactic acidosis, renal dysfunction, hepatic decompensation/dysfunction (LFTs), exacerbations of hepatitis B, and fat redistribution.

Patient Counseling: Advise to promptly report symptoms of pancreatitis, lactic acidosis, worsening of disease/emergence of resistant HBV, or fat redistribution/accumulation. Counsel on importance of HIV testing to avoid inappropriate therapy and development of resistant HIV. Offer HIV counseling and testing prior to initiation. Inform that therapy does not reduce risk of transmission of HBV through sexual contact or blood contamination. Inform diabetics that each 20mL of oral solution contains 4g of sucrose. Counsel to take with/without food at same time each day. Do not skip doses; if dose is missed, take immediately, but not 2 doses at once.

Administration: Oral route. **Storage:** Tab: 25°C (77°F); excursions permitted to 15-30°C (59-86°F). Sol: 20-25°C (68-77°F); store in tightly closed bottles.

EPOGEN RX

epoetin alfa (Amgen)

Increased mortality, serious cardiovascular/thromboembolic events, and increased risk of tumor progression or recurrence. (Renal Failure) Patients experienced greater risks for death and serious cardiovascular events when administered erythropoiesis-stimulating agents (ESAs) to target higher vs lower Hgb levels (13.5 vs 11.3 g/dL; 14 vs 10 g/dL) in 2 clinical studies. Individualize dosing to achieve and maintain Hgb levels within range of 10-12g/dL. (Cancer) ESAs shortened overall survival and/or increased risk of tumor progression or recurrence in clinical studies in patients with breast, non-small cell lung, head and neck, lymphoid, and cervical cancers. To decrease these risks, as well as risk of serious cardio- and thrombovascular events, use lowest dose needed to avoid RBC transfusions. Use ESAs only for treatment of anemia due to concomitant myelosuppressive chemotherapy. ESAs are not indicated for patients receiving myelosuppressive therapy when anticipated outcome is cure. D/C following completion of chemotherapy course. (Perisurgery) Epoetin alfa increased the rate of DVT in patients not receiving prophylactic anticoagulation. Consider DVT prophylaxis.

THERAPEUTIC CLASS: Erythropoiesis stimulator

INDICATIONS: Treatment of anemia of chronic renal failure (CRF), anemia related to zidovudine in HIV (serum erythropoietin ≤500 mU/mL and zidovudine ≤4200mg/week), chemotherapy-induced anemia in patients with non-myeloid malignancies, and reduction of allogeneic blood transfusions in anemic (Hgb ≤13 to >10 g/dL) patients scheduled for elective, noncardiac, nonvascular surgery.

DOSAGE: *Adults:* CRF: Initial: 50-100 U/kg IV/SQ 3x/week. IV is preferred route in dialysis patients. Maint: Individually titrate. Reduce dose by 25% when Hgb approaches 12g/dL or increases >1g/dL in any 2 week period. Increase dose by 25% if Hgb is <10g/dL and has not increased by 1g/dL after 4 weeks of therapy. Zidovudine-Treated HIV Patients: If serum erythropoietin ≤500 mU/mL and zidovudine ≤4200mg/week give100 U/kg IV/SQ 3x/week for 8 weeks. Titrate: Increase by 50-100 U/kg 3x/week after 8 weeks if necessary. Max: 300 U/kg 3x/week Maint: if Hgb >12g/dL, d/c until Hgb <11g/dL, then reduce dose by 25% when resume therapy. Chemotherapy-Induced Anemia: Initial: 150 U/kg SQ 3x/week. Titrate: Reduce by 25% when Hgb approaches 12g/dL or Hgb increases >1g/dL in any 2-week period. If Hgb >12g/dL, withhold and then restart at 25% below previous dose. May increase to 300 U/kg 3x/week if no response after 8 weeks of therapy. Max: 300 U/kg 3x/week. Weekly Dosing: 40,000 U SQ weekly. Titrate: If Hgb not increased by ≥1g/dL after 4 weeks, increase to 60,000 U weekly. If Hgb >12g/dL, withhold and then restart at 25% below previous dose. Reduce dose by 25% if very rapid Hgb response (eg, increase >1g/dL in any 2-week period. Max: 60,000 U weekly. Surgery: 300 U/kg/day SQ for 10 days before, on day of, and 4 days after surgery; or 600 U/kg SQ once weekly on 21, 14, and 7 days before surgery, and a 4th dose on day of surgery.
Pediatrics: CRF: Initial: 50 U/kg 3x/week IV/SQ. Maint: Individually titrate. Reduce dose by 25% when Hgb approaches 12g/dL or increases >1g/dL in any 2 week period. Increase dose by 25% if Hgb is <10g/dL and has not increased by 1g/dL after 4 weeks of therapy. Chemotherapy Induced Anemia: Initial: 600 U/kg IV weekly. Titrate: If Hgb not increased by ≥1g/dL after 4 weeks, increase to 900 U/kg IV weekly. If Hgb >12g/dL, withhold and then restart at 25% below previous dose. Reduce dose by 25% if very rapid Hgb response (eg, increase >1g/dL in any 2-week period. Max: 60,000 U weekly.

HOW SUPPLIED: Inj: 2000 U/mL, 3000 U/mL, 4000 U/mL, 10,000 U/mL, 20,000 U/mL, 40,000 U/mL

CONTRAINDICATIONS: Uncontrolled HTN. Hypersensitivity to mammalian cell-derived products and Albumin (human).

WARNINGS/PRECAUTIONS: Pure red cell aplasia and severe anemia (with or without other cytopenias) may occur. Caution with porphyria, HTN or a history of seizures. Evaluate iron stores prior to and during therapy. Most patients need iron supplementation. Monitor Hct, BP, iron levels, serum chemistry, and CBC. Menses may resume. Multidose formulation contains benzyl alcohol. Increased mortality, cardiovascular, and thromboembolic events in patients with CRF reported. ESAs shortened the time to tumor progression in patients with advanced head and neck cancer receiving radiation therapy. Dose should be carefully adjusted in patients with CRF or CHF.

ADVERSE REACTIONS: HTN, headache, fatigue, arthralgias, nausea, vomiting, diarrhea, edema, rash, pyrexia, clotted vascular access, respiratory congestion, dyspnea, asthenia, dizziness, seizures, thrombotic events.

INTERACTIONS: Adjust anticoagulant dose in dialysis patients.

PREGNANCY: Category C, caution in nursing.

MECHANISM OF ACTION: Erythropoiesis stimulator.

PHARMACOKINETICS: Absorption: (SC) T_{max}=5-24 hrs. **Elimination:** (IV) $T_{1/2}$=4-13 hrs.

NURSING CONSIDERATIONS

Assessment: Assess for uncontrolled HTN, porphyria, cardiovascular disease (ischemic heart disease, CHF), renal failure, possible drug interactions, hypersensitivity to mammalian cell-derived products and albumin. Obtain baseline BP measurements and iron status (transferrin saturation, serum ferritin).

Monitoring: Monitor BP, CBC with differential and platelet count, iron status (transferrin saturation, serum ferritin) regularly. CRF: Serum chemistries (BUN, uric acid, creatinine, phosphorus, K^+) regulary, Hgb twice weekly. HIV and cancer: Hgb once weekly. Monitor for signs/symptoms of CV events (MI, stroke, CHF), pure red cell aplasia, severe anemia, viral diseases, seizures, lack/loss of response to therapy, and hypersensitivity reactions.

Patient Counseling: Caution may impair physical/mental abilities. Advise to seek medical attention if symptoms of CV events, anemia, infections, seizures, or hypersensitivity reactions occur.

Administration: IV, SC route. **Storage:** 2-8°C (36-46°F). Do not freeze or shake.

EPZICOM — RX

abacavir sulfate - lamivudine (GlaxoSmithKline)

Fatal hypersensitivity reactions reported with abacavir sulfate; discontinue if hypersensitivity reaction suspected and do not restart. Lactic acidosis and severe hepatomegaly with steatosis, including fatal cases, have been reported with nucleoside analogs alone or in combination with other antivirals. Severe acute exacerbations of hepatitis B reported in patients co-infected with HBV and HIV and who have discontinued lamivudine.

THERAPEUTIC CLASS: Nucleoside analog combination

INDICATIONS: Treatment of HIV infection in combination with other antiretrovirals.

DOSAGE: *Adults:* ≥18 yrs: CrCl >50mL/min: 1 tab qd.

HOW SUPPLIED: Tab: (Abacavir Sulfate-Lamivudine) 600mg-300mg

CONTRAINDICATIONS: Hepatic impairment.

WARNINGS/PRECAUTIONS: Serious hypersensitivity reactions reported. Register abacavir hypersensitive patients at 1-800-270-0425. Suspend therapy if lactic acidosis or pronounced hepatotoxicity develops. Avoid with CrCl <50mL/min. Redistribution/accumulation of body fat reported. Hepatic decompensation has occurred in HIV/HCV co-infected patients receiving combination antiretroviral therapy for HIV and interferon alfa with or without ribavir. Immune reconstitution syndrome has been reported.

ADVERSE REACTIONS: Hypersensitivity, insomnia, depression, headache, fatigue, dizziness, nausea, diarrhea, rash, pyrexia, abdominal pain, abnormal dreams, anxiety.

INTERACTIONS: May increase methadone clearance. Decreased elimination with ethanol. TMP/SMX and/or nelfinavir may increase lamivudine exposure. Avoid with zalcitabine.

PREGNANCY: Category C, not for use in nursing.

MECHANISM OF ACTION: Abacavir: Carbocyclic nucleoside analogue. Inhibits HIV-1 reverse transcriptase (RT) by competing with natural substrate dGTP and incorporating into viral DNA. Lamivudine: Nucleoside analogue. Inhibits RT via DNA chain termination.

PHARMACOKINETICS: Absorption: Abacavir: Rapid, bioavailability (86%); C_{max}=4.26mcg/mL, AUC=11.95mcg•hr/mL. Lamivudine: Rapid, bioavailability (86%); C_{max}=2.04mcg/mL, AUC=8.87mcg•hr/mL. **Distribution:** Abacavir: V_d=0.86L/kg, plasma protein binding (50%). Lamivudine: V_d=1.3L/kg, plasma protein binding (70%). **Metabolism:** Abacavir: Via alcohol dehydrogenase. Lamivudine: Metabolite (trans-sulfoxide). **Elimination:** Abacavir: $T_{1/2}$=1.45 hrs. Lamivudine: (IV): Urine (70%); $T_{1/2}$=5-7 hrs.

NURSING CONSIDERATIONS

Assessment: Assess for hepatic/renal impairment, risk factors for lactic acidosis, acute respiratory disease, and possible drug interactions.

Monitoring: Monitor for signs/symptoms of lactic acidosis (eg, vomiting, diarrhea, abdominal pain), hepatic dysfunction (eg, decompensation, failure), immune reconstitution syndrome, fat redistribution, respiratory disorder (eg, dyspnea, cough), hypersensitivity reactions, and exacerbation of HBV. Monitor hepatic/renal function closely; observe for lab abnormalities (elevated LFTs, elevated CPK, elevated Cr, lymphopenia). Follow-up LFTs for several months after d/c therapy.

Patient Counseling: Inform if treatment is interrupted, do not restart or replace with any drug containing abacavir to avoid more serious symptoms (life-threatening hypotension) and possibly death. Advise to seek medical attention if symptoms of lactic acidosis (eg, vomiting, diarrhea, abdominal pain) hepatic dysfunction (eg, decompensation, failure), immune reconstitution syndrome, fat redistribution, respiratory disorder (eg, dyspnea, cough), hypersensitivity reactions (eg, fever, rash, NV), and exacerbation of HBV occur.

Administration: Oral route. **Storage:** 25°C (77°F); excursions permitted to 15-30°C (59-86°F).

EQUAGESIC **CIV**

meprobamate - aspirin (Wyeth/Women First)

THERAPEUTIC CLASS: Carbamate derivative/salicylate

INDICATIONS: Adjunct in short-term treatment of pain accompanied by tension and/or anxiety in patients with musculoskeletal disease.

DOSAGE: *Adults:* 1-2 tabs tid-qid prn. Elderly/Debilitated: Use lowest effective dose.

Pediatrics: ≥12 yrs: 1-2 tabs tid-qid prn.

HOW SUPPLIED: Tab: (Meprobamate-ASA) 200mg-325mg* *scored

CONTRAINDICATIONS: Acute intermittent porphyria.

WARNINGS/PRECAUTIONS: Extreme caution with peptic ulcer, asthma, coagulation abnormalities, hypoprothrombinemia, or vitamin K deficiency. Abuse, physical and psychological dependence reported. Abrupt withdrawal after prolonged and excessive use may precipitate recurrence of pre-existing symptoms. May impair mental and physical abilities. Caution with hepatic or kidney dysfunction. May precipitate seizures in epileptic patients. Prescribe cautiously and in small amounts to suicidal patients.

ADVERSE REACTIONS: Epigastric discomfort, NV, drowsiness, ataxia, dizziness, slurred speech, headache, vertigo, weakness.

INTERACTIONS: Additive CNS suppression with alcohol or other psychotropic drugs. May antagonize uricosuric activity of probenecid and sulfinpyrazone. Extreme caution with anticoagulants. May enhance hypoglycemic effects of sulfonylureas.

PREGNANCY: Safety in pregnancy or nursing not known.

MECHANISM OF ACTION: Meprobamate: Carbamate derivative; affects multiple sites in CNS. ASA: Salicylate (non-narcotic analgesic); antipyretic and anti-inflammatory effects.

NURSING CONSIDERATIONS

Assessment: Assess for history of peptic ulcer, abdominal conditions, Addison's disease, intracranial pressure, head injury, hypothyroidism, prostatic hypertrophy, uretheral stricture, acute intermittent porphyria, syndrome of asthma, rhinitis, and nasal polyps, viral infections, pregnancy status, suicidal tendencies, alcohol use, epilepsy, possible drug interactions, renal/hepatic impairment.

Monitoring: Monitor for GI ulceration and bleeding, Reye's syndrome, and hypersensitivity reactions.

Patient Counseling: Inform of pregnancy risks. Caution may impair physical/mental abilities. Seek medical attention if symptoms of GI bleeding or ulceration, Reye's syndrome, or hypersensitivity reactions occur.

Administration: Oral route. **Storage:** 20-25°C (68-77°F). Protect from moisture and light.

EQUETRO — RX

carbamazepine (Validus)

Serious and fatal dermatologic reactions, including toxic epidermal necrolysis (TEN), Stevens-Johnson syndrome (SJS), and presence of HLA-B*1502 allele reported. Aplastic anemia and agranulocytosis reported. Obtain complete pretreatment hematological testing as baseline. D/C if evidence of bone marrow depression develops.

THERAPEUTIC CLASS: Carboxamide

INDICATIONS: Treatment of acute manic and mixed episodes associated with bipolar I disorder.

DOSAGE: *Adults:* Initial: 400mg/day, given in divided doses, bid. Titrate: 200mg qd. Max: 1600mg/day. Do not crush or chew.

HOW SUPPLIED: Cap, Extended-Release: 100mg, 200mg, 300mg

CONTRAINDICATIONS: Avoid in patients with a history of previous bone marrow depression, hypersensitivity to the drug, or known sensitivity to any of the tricyclic compounds. Use of MAOIs is not recommended and MAOIs should be discontinued for a minimum of 14 days prior to use.

WARNINGS/PRECAUTIONS: Monitor blood levels. Avoid use with any other medication containing carbamazepine. May cause fetal harm during pregnancy. Severe dermatologic reactions, including toxic epidermal necrolysis (Lyell's syndrome), Stevens-Johnson syndrome, and presence of HLA-B*1502 allele reported with carbamazepine. Avoid abrupt discontinuation with seizure disorder. Carbamazepine has mild anticholinergic activity; observe closely with increased IOP. Caution in patients with a history of cardiac, hepatic, or renal damage; adverse hematologic reaction to other drugs may be at risk of bone marrow depression; or interrupted courses of therapy with carbamazepine. Closely monitor patients at high-risk for suicide attempts. May cause activate latent psychosis. May cause confusion/agitation in elderly. Perform eye exam and monitor LFTs and renal function at baseline and periodically.

ADVERSE REACTIONS: Dizziness, somnolence, NV, ataxia, headache, infection, pain, rash, diarrhea, dyspepsia, asthenia, amnesia, toxic epidermal necrolysis, Stevens-Johnson syndrome.

INTERACTIONS: See Contraindications. CYP3A4 inhibitors may increase plasma levels. CYP3A4 inducers may decrease plasma levels. May induce CYP1A2 and CYP3A4; may interact with any agent metabolized by these enzymes. May increase plasma levels of clomipramine, phenytoin, and primidone. May increase risk of neurotoxic side effects of lithium. Decreases levels of trazodone with concomitant administration. Anti-malarial drugs may antagonize the activity of carbamazepine. Caution with other centrally acting drugs and/or alcohol. Co-administration with delavirdine may lead to loss of virologic response and possible resistance to non-nucleoside reverse transcriptase inhibitors.

PREGNANCY: Category D, not for use in nursing.

E

MECHANISM OF ACTION: Carboxamide; mechanism not established. Suspected to modulate sodium and calcium ion channels, receptor-mediated neurotransmitters, and intracellular signaling pathways.

PHARMACOKINETICS: Absorption: C_{max}=1.9mcg/mL (single dose), 11.0mcg/mL (multiple doses); T_{max}=19 hrs (single dose), 5.9 hrs (multiple doses). **Distribution:** Plasma protein binding (76%); found in breast milk. **Metabolism:** Liver, via CYP3A4; carbamazepine-10,11-epoxide (metabolite). **Elimination:** Urine 72% (3% unchanged), feces (28%); $T_{1/2}$=35-40 hrs (single dose), 12-17 hrs (multiple doses).

NURSING CONSIDERATIONS

Assessment: Perform detailed physical exam prior to treatment. Assess use in patients with history of cardiac, hepatic/renal damage and in patients who had previous hematological reaction to other medications. Assess history of bone marrow depression, sensitivity to any tricyclic compounds, or concurrent MAOIs. Assess for HLA-B*1502 allele in suspected patient populations. Obtain baseline CBC (reticulocyte count), serum iron levels, LFTs, urinalysis, BUN, and eye exam.

Monitoring: Monitor for serious dermatological reactions (eg, toxic epidermal necrolysis, Stevens-Johnson syndrome), aplastic anemia, agranulocytosis, increased IOP, and suicidal ideation. Periodically monitor serum drug levels, CBC, urinalysis, BUN, total cholesterol levels, LDL, HDL, and periodic eye exams.

Patient Counseling: Instruct to immediately report signs/symptoms of hematologic disorders. Caution against performing hazardous tasks (operating machinery/driving). Inform that, if necessary, caps may be opened and contents sprinkled over food; do not crush or chew.

Administration: Oral route. **Storage:** 25°C (77°F); excursions permitted to 15-30°C (59-86°F). Protect from light and moisture.

ERAXIS RX

anidulafungin (Pfizer)

THERAPEUTIC CLASS: Echinocandin

INDICATIONS: Treatment of candidemia and other forms of *Candida* infections (intra-abdominal abscess and peritonitis); esophageal candidiasis.

DOSAGE: *Adults:* Candidemia/*Candida* Infections: LD: 200mg on Day 1. Follow with 100mg qd thereafter. Continue therapy for at least 14 days after last positive culture. Esophageal Candidiasis: LD: 100mg on Day 1. Follow with 50mg qd thereafter. Treat for minimum of 14 days and for at least 7 days after symptoms resolve.

HOW SUPPLIED: Inj: 50mg, 100mg

WARNINGS/PRECAUTIONS: Hepatic abnormalities may occur; monitor hepatic function if abnormal LFTs develop during therapy.

ADVERSE REACTIONS: Diarrhea, nausea, rash, hypokalemia, headache, increased LFTs, neutropenia.

INTERACTIONS: Slightly increased levels with cyclosporine.

PREGNANCY: Category C, caution in nursing.

MECHANISM OF ACTION: Antifungal; inhibits synthesis of 1, 3-β-D-glucan, an essential component of fungal cell walls.

PHARMACOKINETICS: Absorption: IV infusion of variable doses resulted in different parameters. **Distribution:** V_d=30-50L; plasma protein binding (>99%). **Elimination:** Urine, feces; $T_{1/2}$=40-50 hrs.

NURSING CONSIDERATIONS

Assessment: Assess cultures and other lab studies prior to therapy to properly identify causative organisms.

Monitoring: Monitor LFTs for possible hepatic dysfunction, hepatitis or worsening of hepatic failure, possible drug interactions, serum electrolytes (K^+), and signs of histamine-related reactions.

Patient Counseling: Inform of possible histamine-mediated symptoms including rash, urticaria, flushing, pruritus, dyspnea, and hypotension. Notify about signs/symptoms of hepatic dysfunction.

Administration: IV route. Rate of infusion should not exceed 1.1mg/min. 1) Reconstitute 50mg vial: Add 15mL of companion diluent. 100mg vial: Add 30mL of companion diluent. Reconstituted vial must be further diluted. Further Dilution: 2) Transfer the contents of reconstituted vial into the appropriately sized IV bag (or bottle) containing either 5% dextrose or 0.9% NS.

Storage: Unreconstituted vials and companion diluent vials should be stored at 25°C (77°F); excursions permitted to 15-30°C (59-86°F). Do not refrigerate or freeze. Reconstituted vials: 25°C (77°F). Excursions permitted to 15-30°C (59-86°F). Do not refrigerate or freeze. Use within 24 hrs. Diluted Product: 25°C (77°F); excursions permitted to 15-30°C (59-86°F). Do not refrigerate or freeze.

ERBITUX RX

cetuximab (Bristol-Myers Squibb)

Severe infusion reactions have occurred; immediately interrupt and permanently d/c infusion if these reactions occur. Cardiopulmonary arrest and/or sudden death have occurred with squamous cell carcinoma of the head and neck treated with radiation therapy and cetuximab; closely monitor serum electrolytes during and after therapy.

THERAPEUTIC CLASS: Epidermal growth factor receptor (EGFR) antagonist

INDICATIONS: In combination with irinotecan for the treatment of epidermal growth factor receptor (EGFR)-expressing, metastatic colorectal carcinoma in patients who are refractory to irinotecan-based chemotherapy. As monotherapy, for the treatment of EGFR-expressing, metastatic colorectal carcinoma in patients after failure of both irinotecan- and oxaliplatin-based regimens. In combination with radiation therapy for the treatment of locally or regionally advanced squamous cell carcinoma of the head and neck. As monotherapy, for the treatment of patients with recurrent or metastatic squamous cell carcinoma of the head and neck for whom prior platinum-based therapy has failed.

DOSAGE: *Adults:* Premedication with H_1 antagonist (eg, diphenhydramine 50mg) IV 30-60 min prior to 1st dose is recommended. Colorectal Cancer: LD: 400mg/m² IV infusion over 120 min. Maint: 250mg/m² IV infusion over 60 min once weekly. Max Infusion Rate: 10mg/min. Squamous Cell Carcinoma of Head and Neck: Combination Therapy: Initial: 400mg/m² IV over 120 min 1 week prior to initiation of a course of radiation treatment. Maint: 250mg/m² over 60 min weekly for duration of radiation therapy. Max Infusion Rate: 10mg/min. Recurrent/Metastatic Squamous Cell Carcinoma of Head and Neck: Monotherapy: Initial: 400mg/m². Maint: 250mg/m² until disease progression or unacceptable toxicity. Mild-Moderate (Grade 1 or 2) Infusion Reactions: Reduce rate by 50%. Severe (Grade 3 or 4) Infusion Reactions: D/C. Development of Severe Acneform Rash: Delay infusion 1-2 weeks for 1st three occurrences. 1st Occurrence: If improvement, continue at 250mg/m². 2nd Occurrence: If improvement, reduce dose to 200mg/m². 3rd Occurrence: If improvement, reduce dose to 150mg/m². 4th Occurrence/No Improvement After Delaying Therapy: D/C therapy.

HOW SUPPLIED: Inj: 2mg/mL

WARNINGS/PRECAUTIONS: Infusion reactions reported; observe closely for 1 hr following infusion. Permanently d/c therapy if serious infusion reactions develop. Dermatologic (eg, acneform rash, skin drying/fissuring, paronychial inflammation, and infectious sequelae) or pulmonary toxicities may occur. D/C if interstitial lung disease confirmed. Adjust dose in cases of severe acneform rash. Apply sunscreen and limit sun exposure. Caution with hypersensitivity to murine proteins. Potential for immunogenicity. Caution with radiation therapy and cisplatin therapy. Monitor for hypomagnesemia, hypocalcemia, and hypokalemia, during and for at least 8 weeks following completion of therapy.

ADVERSE REACTIONS: Acneform rash, mucositis, asthenia/malaise, diarrhea, NV, abdominal pain, fatigue, fever, constipation, infusion reactions, dermatologic toxicities, infection, headache, anorexia, dyspnea, insomnia.

PREGNANCY: Category C, not for use in nursing.

MECHANISM OF ACTION: Epidermal growth factor receptor antagonist; binds specifically to EGFR on normal and tumor cells and inhibits binding of epidermal growth factor and other ligands, such as transforming growth factor-α.

PHARMACOKINETICS: Absorption: C_{max}=168-235µg/mL. **Distribution:** V_d=2-3L/m². **Elimination:** $T_{1/2}$=112 hrs.

NURSING CONSIDERATIONS

Assessment: Assess prior history of CAD, MI, CHF, arrhythmias, pregnancy/nursing status, and possible drug interactions. Obtain baseline serum electrolyte levels (Mg^{2+}, K^+, Ca^{2+}).

Monitoring: Monitor electrolytes (Mg^{2+}, K^+, Ca^{2+}) during and 8 weeks after drug administration. Monitor for signs/symptoms of hypomagnesemia, hypocalcemia, hypokalemia, acute onset or worsening of pulmonary symptoms, infusion reaction, dermatologic toxicities, and infectious sequelae.

Patient Counseling: Inform of pregnancy/nursing risks; advise to use effective contraceptive methods during and 6 months after therapy for both sexes. Advise to d/c nursing and limit sun exposure during and 2 months after therapy. Instruct to seek medical attention if symptoms of infusion reaction (fever, chills, breathing problems), electrolyte imbalances, dermatologic toxicities (acneform rash, skin drying), infectious sequelae (cellulitis, abscess formation), acute onset or worsening of pulmonary symptoms occur.

Administration: IV infusion. Do not administer as IV push or bolus. Administer through low protein binding 0.22-µm in-line filter. **Storage:** (Vials): Refrigerate; 2-8°C (36-46°F). Do not freeze. Stable for 12 hrs at 2-8°C (36-46°F), 8 hrs at 20-25°C (68-77°F). Do not shake or dilute.

ERYC **RX**

erythromycin (Warner Chilcott)

THERAPEUTIC CLASS: Macrolide

INDICATIONS: Treatment of mild to moderate upper/lower respiratory tract and skin and soft tissue infections, pertussis, diphtheria, erythrasma, intestinal amebiasis, acute pelvic inflammatory disease (PID) (*N. gonorrhoeae*), listeriosis, primary syphilis (if PCN allergy), Legionnaires' disease, chlamydial infections (eg, newborn conjunctivitis, pneumonia of infancy, urogenital infections during pregnancy, or urethral, endocervical, or rectal, infections in adults when tetracyclines are contraindicated or not tolerated), and nongonococcal urethritis caused by susceptible strains of microorganisms. Prophylaxis of initial or recurrent attacks of rheumatic fever if PCN allergy.

DOSAGE: *Adults:* Usual: 250mg q6h or 500mg q12h. Max: 4g/day. Do not take bid when dose is >1g/day. Treat strep infections for at least 10 days. Streptococcal Infection Prophylaxis with Rheumatic Heart Disease: 250mg bid. Chlamydial Urogenital Infection During Pregnancy: 500mg qid for at least 7 days or 250mg qid for 14 days. Urethral/Endocervical/Rectal Chlamydial Infections: 500mg qid for at least 7 days. Primary Syphilis: 30-40g in divided doses for 10-15 days. Acute PID: 500mg (erythromycin lactobionate) IV q6h for 3 days, then 250mg PO q6h for 7 days. Intestinal Amebiasis: 250mg qid

for 10-14 days. Pertussis: 40-50mg/kg/day in divided doses for 5-14 days. Legionnaires' Disease: 1-4g/day in divided doses. Nongonococcal Urethritis: 500mg PO qid for at least 7 days.
Pediatrics: Usual: 30-50mg/kg/day in divided doses. Severe Infections: 60-100mg/kg/day in divided doses. Treat strep infections for at least 10 days. Streptococcal Infection Prophylaxis with Rheumatic Heart Disease: 250mg bid. Intestinal Amebiasis: 30-50mg/kg/day in divided doses for 10-14 days.

HOW SUPPLIED: Cap, Delayed-Release: 250mg

CONTRAINDICATIONS: Concomitant terfenadine or astemizole.

WARNINGS/PRECAUTIONS: *Clostridium difficile*-associated diarrhea, hepatic dysfunction, and prolonged QT syndrome reported. Caution with impaired hepatic function. May aggravate weakness of patients with myasthenia gravis.

ADVERSE REACTIONS: NV, abdominal pain, diarrhea, anorexia, abnormal LFTs, allergic reaction, superinfection (prolonged use).

INTERACTIONS: See Contraindications. May increase levels of theophylline, digoxin, drugs metabolized by CYP450 (eg, carbamazepine, cyclosporine, phenytoin, tacrolimus, hexobarbital). May increase effects of oral anticoagulants and triazolam. Risk of acute ergot toxicity with ergotamine or dihydroergotamine.

PREGNANCY: Category B, caution in nursing.

MECHANISM OF ACTION: Macrolide; inhibits protein synthesis by binding 50*S* ribosomal subunits of susceptible organisms.

PHARMACOKINETICS: Absorption: Readily absorbed; C_{max}=1.13-1.68mcg/mL; T_{max}=3 hrs. **Distribution:** Largely bound to plasma proteins. Crosses blood-brain barrier, placenta, breast milk. Diffuses into most body fluids. **Elimination:** Bile, urine (≤5%).

NURSING CONSIDERATIONS

Assessment: Assess for history of impaired hepatic function, myasthenia gravis, hearing loss, arrhythmias. Note other diseases/conditions and drug therapies (eg, lovastatin).

Monitoring: Monitor LFTs, renal function tests, creatinine kinase and serum transaminase levels, CDAD, convulsions, arrhythmias, hypersensitivity reactions.

Patient Counseling: Inform therapy treats bacterial, not viral, infections. Take exactly as directed; complete entire course of therapy, do not skip doses. Advise to report adverse effects, lack of response, prolonged/persistent diarrhea. Inform can be taken without regard to meals.

Administration: Oral route. **Storage:** 15-30°C (59-86°F).

ERY-TAB

erythromycin (Abbott)

RX

THERAPEUTIC CLASS: Macrolide

INDICATIONS: Treatment of mild to moderate upper/lower respiratory tract and skin and skin structure infections, listeriosis, pertussis, diphtheria, erythrasma, intestinal amebiasis, acute pelvic inflammatory disease (PID) (*N.gonorrhoeae*), primary syphilis (if PCN allergy), Legionnaires' disease, chlamydial infections (eg, newborn conjunctivitis, pneumonia of infancy, urogenital infections during pregnancy, or urethral, endocervical, or rectal infections when tetracyclines are contraindicated or not tolerated), and nongonococcal urethritis caused by susceptible strains of microorganisms. Prophylaxis of initial and recurrent attacks of rheumatic fever if PCN allergy.

DOSAGE: *Adults:* Usual: 250mg qid, 333mg q8h or 500mg q12h. Max: 4g/day. Do not take bid when dose is >1g/day. Treat strep infections for at least 10 days. Streptococcal Infection Long-Term Prophylaxis with Rheumatic Fever: 250mg bid. Chlamydial Urogenital Infection During Pregnancy: 500mg qid or 666mg q8h for at least 7 days, or 500mg q12h, 333mg q8h or 250mg qid for at least 14 days. Urethral/Endocervical/Rectal Chlamydial Infections

and Nongonococcal Urethritis: 500mg qid or 666mg q8h for at least 7 days. Primary Syphilis: 30-40g in divided doses for 10-15 days. Acute PID: 500mg (erythromycin lactobionate) IV q6h for 3 days, then 500mg PO q12h or 333mg q8h for 7 days. Intestinal Amebiasis: 500mg q12h, 333mg q8h or 250mg q6h for 10-14 days. Pertussis: 40-50mg/kg/day in divided doses for 5-14 days. Legionnaires' Disease: 1-4g/day in divided doses.
Pediatrics: Usual: 30-50mg/kg/day in divided doses. Severe Infections: May double dose. Max: 4g/day. Treat strep infections for at least 10 days. Streptococcal Infection Long-Term Prophylaxis with Rheumatic Fever: 250mg bid. Chlamydial Conjunctivitis of Newborns/Chlamydial Pneumonia in Infancy: 12.5mg/kg qid for 2 weeks and 3 weeks, respectively. Intestinal Amebiasis: 30-50mg/kg/day in divided doses for 10-14 days.

HOW SUPPLIED: Tab, Delayed-Release: 250mg, 333mg, 500mg

CONTRAINDICATIONS: Concomitant terfenadine, astemizole, pimozide, or cisapride.

WARNINGS/PRECAUTIONS: Pseudomembranous colitis, hepatic dysfunction reported. Caution with impaired hepatic function. May aggravate weakness of patients with myasthenia gravis. Erythromycin does not reach adequate concentrations in fetus to prevent congenital syphilis.

ADVERSE REACTIONS: NV, abdominal pain, diarrhea, anorexia, abnormal LFTs, allergic reactions, superinfection (prolonged use).

INTERACTIONS: See Contraindications. Rhabdomyolysis reported with lovastatin. May increase levels of theophylline, digoxin, drugs metabolized by CYP450 (eg, carbamazepine, cyclosporine, phenytoin, alfentanil, disopyramide, lovastatin, bromocriptine, valproate, etc). Increases effects of oral anticoagulants, triazolam, midazolam. Risk of acute ergot toxicity with ergotamine or dihydroergotamine. May increase AUC of sildenafil; consider dose reduction of sildenafil.

PREGNANCY: Category B, caution in nursing.

MECHANISM OF ACTION: Macrolide antibiotic; inhibits protein synthesis by binding 50*S* ribosomal subunits of susceptible organisms.

PHARMACOKINETICS: Absorption: (PO) readily absorbed. **Distribution:** Largely bound to plasma proteins. Crosses blood-brain barrier, placenta, and breast milk. Diffuses into most bodily fluids. **Elimination:** Biliary and urinary excretion (<5%).

NURSING CONSIDERATIONS

Assessment: Assess history of impaired hepatic function, myasthenia gravis, hearing loss, arrhythmias. Note other diseases/conditions and drug therapies.

Monitoring: Monitor LFTs, renal function, CDAD, hearing loss, pancreatitis, arrhythmias, infantile hypertrophic pyloric stenosis, and hypersensitivity reactions.

Patient Counseling: Inform to take exactly as directed and to complete entire course of therapy. Instruct to take on empty stomach. Advise to report any adverse effects, lack of response, and prolonged/persistent diarrhea.

Administration: Oral route. **Storage:** 30°C (86°F).

ERYTHROCIN — RX

erythromycin stearate (Abbott)

THERAPEUTIC CLASS: Macrolide

INDICATIONS: Treatment of mild to moderate upper/lower respiratory tract, and skin and skin structure infections, listeriosis, pertussis, diphtheria, erythrasma, intestinal amebiasis, acute pelvic inflammatory disease (PID) (*N.gonorrhoeae*), primary syphilis (if PCN allergy), Legionnaires' disease, chlamydial infections (eg, newborn conjunctivitis, pneumonia of infancy, urogenital infections during pregnancy or urethral, endocervical, or rectal infections when tetracyclines are contraindicated or not tolerated), and nongonococcal urethritis caused by susceptible strains of microorganisms. Prophylaxis of initial and recurrent attacks of rheumatic fever if PCN allergy.

DOSAGE: *Adults:* Usual: 250mg q6h or 500mg q12h without food. Max: 4g/day. Treat strep infections for at least 10 days. Streptococcal Infection Long-Term Prophylaxis in Rheumatic Fever: 250mg bid. Chlamydial Urogenital Infection During Pregnancy: 500mg qid or 666mg q8h for at least 7 days or 500mg q12h, 333mg q8h, or 250mg qid for at least 14 days. Urethral/ Endocervical/Rectal Chlamydial Infections and Nongonococcal Urethritis: 500mg qid or 666mg q8h for at least 7 days. Primary Syphilis: 30-40g in divided doses over 10-15 days. Acute PID: 500mg (erythromycin lactobionate) IV q6h for 3 days, then 500mg PO q12h or 333mg PO q8h for 7 days. Intestinal Amebiasis: 500mg q12h, 333mg q8h, or 250mg q6h for 10-14 days. Pertussis: 40-50mg/kg/day in divided doses for 5-14 days. Legionnaires' Disease: 1-4g/day in divided doses.
Pediatrics: Usual: 30-50mg/kg/day in divided doses without food. Severe Infections: May double dose. Max: 4g/day. Treat strep infections for at least 10 days. Chlamydial Conjunctivitis of Newborns/Chlamydial Pneumonia in Infancy: (Sus) 12.5mg/kg qid for 2 weeks and 3 weeks, respectively. Intestinal Amebiasis: 30-50mg/kg/day in divided doses for 10-14 days.

HOW SUPPLIED: Tab: 250mg, 500mg

CONTRAINDICATIONS: Concomitant terfenadine, astemizole, pimozide, or cisapride.

WARNINGS/PRECAUTIONS: Hepatic dysfunction, pseudomembranous colitis reported. Caution with impaired hepatic function.

ADVERSE REACTIONS: Abdominal pain, N/V, diarrhea, anorexia, abnormal LFTs, superinfection (prolonged use).

INTERACTIONS: See Contraindications. Rhabdomyolysis reported with lovastatin. May increase levels of theophylline, digoxin, drugs metabolized by CYP450 (eg, carbamazepine, cyclosporine, phenytoin, etc). Increases effects of oral anticoagulants, triazolam. Risk of acute ergot toxicity with ergotamine or dihydroergotamine. May increase AUC of sildenafil; consider dose reduction of sildenafil.

PREGNANCY: Category B, caution in nursing.

MECHANISM OF ACTION: Macrolide; inhibits protein synthesis by binding 50S ribosomal subunits of susceptible organisms.

PHARMACOKINETICS: Absorption: (PO) Readily absorbed. **Distribution:** Largely bound to plasma proteins; crosses placenta, blood-brain barrier, and is excreted in breast milk. **Metabolism:** Liver via CYP3A. **Elimination:** Bile and urine (<5% unchanged).

NURSING CONSIDERATIONS

Assessment: Assess for history of impaired hepatic function, myasthenia gravis, hearing loss, arrhythmias. Note other diseases/conditions and drug therapies.

Monitoring: Monitor LFTs, renal function, CK, CDAD, hearing loss, pancreatitis, arryhthmias, infantile hypertrophic pyloric stenosis, hypersensitivity reactions.

Patient Counseling: Inform to take as directed and to complete entire prescription. Take on empty stomach. Report adverse effects, lack of response, and prolonged/persistent diarrhea.

Administration: Oral route. **Storage:** 30°C (≤86°F).

Erythromycin Base — RX

erythromycin (Various)

THERAPEUTIC CLASS: Macrolide

INDICATIONS: Treatment of mild to moderate upper/lower respiratory tract and skin and skin structure infections, listeriosis, pertussis, diphtheria, erythrasma, intestinal amebiasis, acute pelvic inflammatory disease (PID)

(*N.gonorrhoeae*), primary syphilis (if PCN allergy), Legionnaires' disease, chlamydial infections (eg, newborn conjunctivitis, pneumonia of infancy, urogenital infections during pregnancy or urethral, endocervical, or rectal infections when tetracyclines are contraindicated or not tolerated), and nongonococcal urethritis caused by susceptible strains of microorganisms. Prophylaxis of initial and recurrent attacks of rheumatic fever if PCN allergy.

DOSAGE: *Adults:* Usual: 250mg qid or 500mg q12h without food. Max: 4g/day. Treat strep infections for at least 10 days. Streptococcal Infection Long-Term Prophylaxis of Rheumatic Fever: 250mg bid. Chlamydial Urogenital Infection During Pregnancy: 500mg qid for at least 7 days or 500mg q12h or 250mg qid for at least 14 days. Urethral/Endocervical/Rectal Chlamydial Infections and Nongonococcal Urethritis: 500mg qid for at least 7 days. Primary Syphilis: 30-40g in divided doses over 10-15 days. Acute PID: 500mg (erythromycin lactobionate) IV q6h for 3 days, then 500mg PO q12h for 7 days. Intestinal Amebiasis: 500mg q12h or 250mg q6h for 10-14 days. Pertussis: 40-50mg/kg/day in divided doses for 5-14 days. Legionnaires' Disease: 1-4g/day in divided doses.
Pediatrics: Usual: 30-50mg/kg/day in divided doses without food. Severe Infections: May double dose. Max: 4g/day. Treat strep infections for at least 10 days. Streptococcal Infection Long-Term Prophylaxis of Rheumatic Fever: 250mg bid. Chlamydial Conjunctivitis of Newborns/Chlamydial Pneumonia in Infancy: (Sus) 12.5mg/kg qid for 2 weeks and 3 weeks, respectively. Intestinal Amebiasis: 30-50mg/kg/day in divided doses for 10-14 days.

HOW SUPPLIED: Tab: 250mg, 500mg

CONTRAINDICATIONS: Concomitant terfenadine, astemizole, pimozide, or cisapride.

WARNINGS/PRECAUTIONS: Pseudomembranous colitis, hepatic dysfunction reported. Caution with impaired hepatic function. May aggravate weakness of patients with myasthenia gravis.

ADVERSE REACTIONS: Abdominal pain, N/V, diarrhea, anorexia, abnormal LFTs, allergic reactions, superinfection (prolonged use).

INTERACTIONS: See Contraindications. Rhabdomyolysis reported with lovastatin. May increase levels of theophylline, digoxin, drugs metabolized by CYP450 (eg, carbamazepine, cyclosporine, phenytoin, etc). Increases effects of oral anticoagulants, triazolam. Risk of acute ergot toxicity with ergotamine or dihydroergotamine. May increase AUC of sildenafil; consider dose reduction of sildenafil.

PREGNANCY: Category B, caution in nursing.

MECHANISM OF ACTION: Macrolide; inhibits protein synthesis by binding 50S ribosomal subunits of susceptible organisms.

PHARMACOKINETICS: Absorption: (PO) readily absorbed. **Distribution:** Largely bound to plasma proteins. Crosses blood-brain barrier, placenta, breast milk. Diffuses into most body fluids. **Elimination:** Bile, urine (<5% unchanged).

NURSING CONSIDERATIONS

Assessment: Assess for history of impaired hepatic function, myasthenia gravis, hearing loss, arryhthmias. Note other diseases/conditions and drug therapies.

Monitoring: Monitor LFTs, renal function tests, CK, *C.difficile*-associated diarrhea, hearing loss, pancreatitis, arrhythmias, infantile hypertrophic pyloric stenosis, and hypersensitivity reactions.

Patient Counseling: Inform that therapy only treats bacterial infections. Instruct to take exactly as directed and to complete entire course of therapy. Take on an empty stomach. Advise to report any adverse effects, lack of response, or prolonged/persistent diarrhea.

Administration: Oral route. **Storage:** Below 30°C (86°F). Keep tightly closed.

E

ERYTHROMYCIN DELAYED-RELEASE RX

erythromycin (Various)

THERAPEUTIC CLASS: Macrolide

INDICATIONS: Treatment of mild to moderate upper/lower respiratory tract and skin and skin structure infections, listeriosis, pertussis, diphtheria, erythrasma, intestinal amebiasis, acute pelvic inflammatory disease (PID) (*N.gonorrhoeae*), primary syphilis (if PCN allergy), Legionnaires' disease, chlamydial infections (eg, newborn conjunctivitis, pneumonia of infancy, urogenital infections during pregnancy, or urethral, endocervical, or rectal infections when tetracyclines are contraindicated or not tolerated), and nongonococcal urethritis caused by susceptible strains of microorganisms. Prophylaxis of initial and recurrent attacks of rheumatic fever if PCN allergy.

DOSAGE: *Adults:* Usual: 250mg q6h or 500mg q12h without food. Max: 4g/day. Treat strep infections for 10 days. Streptococcal Infection Prophylaxis with Rheumatic Heart Disease: 250mg bid. Primary Syphilis: 30-40g in divided doses over 10-15 days. Intestinal Amebiasis: 250mg q6h for 10-14 days. Legionnaires' Disease: 1-4g/day in divided doses. Chlamydial Urogenital Infection During Pregnancy: 500mg qid for 7 days or 250mg qid for 14 days. Urethral/Endocervical/Rectal Chlamydial Infections and Nongonococcal Urethritis: 500mg qid for at least 7 days. Pertussis: 40-50mg/kg/day in divided doses for 5-14 days. Acute PID: 500mg (erythromycin lactobionate) IV q6h for 3 days, then 250mg PO q6h for 7 days.
Pediatrics: Usual: 30-50mg/kg/day in divided doses without food. Severe Infections: May double dose. Max: 4g/day. Treat strep infections for 10 days. Streptococcal Infection Prophylaxis with Rheumatic Heart Disease: 250mg bid. Intestinal Amebiasis: 30-50mg/kg/day in divided doses for 10-14 days.

HOW SUPPLIED: Cap, Delayed-Release: 250mg

CONTRAINDICATIONS: Concomitant terfenadine, astemizole, pimozide, or cisapride.

WARNINGS/PRECAUTIONS: Hepatic dysfunction and pseudomembranous colitis reported. May aggravate weakness of patients with myasthenia gravis.

ADVERSE REACTIONS: Abdominal pain, N/V, diarrhea, anorexia, hepatic dysfunction, abnormal LFTs, superinfection (prolonged use).

INTERACTIONS: See Contraindications. Rhabdomyolysis reported with lovastatin. May increase levels of theophylline, digoxin, drugs metabolized by CYP450 (eg, carbamazepine, cyclosporine, phenytoin, etc). Increases effects of oral anticoagulants, triazolam. Risk of acute ergot toxicity with ergotamine or dihydroergotamine. Extreme caution with terfenadine.

PREGNANCY: Category B, caution in nursing.

MECHANISM OF ACTION: Macrolide; inhibits protein synthesis by binding 50S ribosomal subunits of susceptible organisms.

PHARMACOKINETICS: Absorption: (PO) readily absorbed; C_{max}=1.13-1.68mcg/mL; T_{max}=3 hrs. **Distribution:** Largely bound to plasma proteins; diffuses into most bodily fluids; crosses blood-brain barrier, placenta, and breast milk. **Elimination:** Bile, urine (<5% unchanged).

NURSING CONSIDERATIONS

Assessment: Assess for history of impaired hepatic function, myasthenia gravis, hearing loss, arrhythmias. Note other diseases/conditions and drug therapies.

Monitoring: Monitor LFTs, renal function, CK, CDAD, hearing loss, pancreatitis, arrhythmias, infantile hypertrophic pyloric stenosis, and hypersensitivity reactions.

Patient Counseling: Inform therapy treats bacterial, not viral, infections. Take exactly as directed; complete entire course of therapy. Take medication on empty stomach. Advise to report adverse effects, lack of response, and prolonged/persistent diarrhea.

Administration: Oral route. **Storage:** Below 30°C (86°F). Protect from moisture and excessive heat.

ESCLIM — RX

estradiol (Women First)

Estrogens increase risk of endometrial cancer in postmenopausal women. Avoid during pregnancy.

E

THERAPEUTIC CLASS: Estrogen

INDICATIONS: Treatment of moderate to severe vasomotor symptoms associated with menopause and/or vulvar/vaginal atrophy. Treatment of hypoestrogenism due to hypogonadism, castration, or primary ovarian failure.

DOSAGE: *Adults:* Initial: 0.025mg twice weekly (q3-4 days). Titrate: Increase/decrease dose depending upon clinical response. Apply to clean, dry area of skin on buttocks, femoral triangle (upper inner thigh), or upper arm; avoid breasts and waistline. Rotate sites; allow 1 week between same site. Discontinue or taper at 3-6 month intervals. Wait 1 week after withdrawal of oral therapy before initiating therapy. Give continuously without intact uterus and cyclically (3 weeks on, 1 week off) with intact uterus.

HOW SUPPLIED: Patch: 0.025mg/24 hrs, 0.0375mg/24hrs, 0.05mg/24 hrs, 0.075mg/24 hrs, 0.1mg/24 hrs [8[s]]

CONTRAINDICATIONS: Pregnancy, undiagnosed abnormal genital bleeding, breast cancer except in appropriately selected patients being treated for metastatic disease, estrogen-dependent neoplasia, thrombophlebitis, thromboembolic disorders.

WARNINGS/PRECAUTIONS: Risk of gallbladder disease, breast and endometrial cancer, elevated BP. Possible risk of cardiovascular disease. Caution with liver dysfunction, asthma, epilepsy, migraine, and cardiac or renal dysfunction. Increase in HDL, triglycerides, thyroid binding globulin. Acceleration of PT, PTT. Impaired glucose tolerance. Consider adding progestin in patient with intact uterus. Risk of fetal congenital reproductive tract disorder, hypercalcemia with breast cancer and bone metastases; hypercoagulability effects. Uterine bleeding and mastodynia reported.

ADVERSE REACTIONS: Breast pain, headache, infection, anxiety, emotional lability, pruritus, abdominal pain, monilia vagina, nausea, sinusitis, asthenia, diarrhea, leukorrhea.

PREGNANCY: Category X, caution in nursing.

MECHANISM OF ACTION: Estrogen; circulating estrogens modulate pituitary secretion of the gonadotrophins, luteinizing hormone and follicle stimulating hormone, through negative feedback mechanism. Reduces elevated levels of these hormones in postmenopausal women.

PHARMACOKINETICS: Absorption: T_{max}=27 hrs; (0.05mg) C_{max}=62pg/mL; (0.1 mg) C_{max}=124pg/mL. **Distribution:** Mainly bound to sex hormone binding globulin and, to a lesser extent, albumin. **Metabolism:** Liver to estrone and estriol (major urinary metabolite); sulfate and glucuronide conjugation (liver), gut hydrolysis. **Elimination:** Urine (parent compound and metabolites).

NURSING CONSIDERATIONS

Assessment: Assess for pregnancy/nursing status, undiagnosed abnormal genital bleeding, presence of breast cancer, estrogen-dependent neoplasia, active thrombophlebitis or thromboembolic disorders, hyperlipidemia, and liver impairment. Assess need for progestin therapy. Prior to therapy, obtain a complete medical and family history.

Monitoring: Monitor for signs/symptoms of malignant neoplasm (eg, breast, endometrial cancer), gallbladder disease, cardiovascular disease (eg, MI, pulmonary embolism, thrombophlebitis), elevations in BP levels, hypercalcemia, fluid retention, hypercoagulability, elevations in plasma triglycerides, pancreatitis, uterine bleeding, and mastodynia. Perform regular breast exams. If undiagnosed, persistent, or recurring abnormal vaginal bleeding occurs, perform proper diagnostic measures (eg, endometrial sampling) to rule out malignancy. Perform periodic evaluation (every 3-6 months) to determine therapy need.

Patient Counseling: Instruct not to take medication if pregnant. Place medication on clean, dry skin on buttocks, femoral triangle (upper inner thigh), or upper arm; do not apply to breast or other parts of body. Area applied to should not be oily, damaged, or irritated. Apply immediately after removal from protective pouch; if medication system falls off, reapply same system. If necessary, apply new medication system; continue original treatment schedule. Perform self breast exams; report adverse events.

Administration: Transdermal route. **Storage:** 25°C (77°F); excursions permitted to 15-30°C (59-86°F). Do not store unpouched.

E

Esgic — RX

acetaminophen - caffeine - butalbital (Forest)

THERAPEUTIC CLASS: Barbiturate/analgesic

INDICATIONS: Tension or muscle contraction headaches.

DOSAGE: *Adults:* 1-2 caps/tabs q4h prn. Max: 6 caps/tabs/day.
Pediatrics: ≥12 yrs: 1-2 caps/tabs q4h prn. Max: 6 caps/tabs/day.

HOW SUPPLIED: Cap/Tab: (Butalbital-APAP-Caffeine) 50mg-325mg-40mg*
*scored

CONTRAINDICATIONS: Porphyria.

WARNINGS/PRECAUTIONS: May be habit-forming; potential for abuse. Not for long-term use. Caution in elderly, debilitated, severe renal or hepatic impairment, acute abdominal conditions, suicidal tendencies, history of drug abuse.

ADVERSE REACTIONS: Drowsiness, lightheadedness, dizziness, sedation, SOB, NV, abdominal pain, intoxicated feeling.

INTERACTIONS: Enhanced CNS effects with MAOIs. May enhance CNS depressant effects of other narcotic analgesics, alcohol, general anesthetics, tranquilizers, sedative hypnotics, or other CNS depressants.

PREGNANCY: Category C, not for use in nursing.

MECHANISM OF ACTION: Butalbital: Short- to intermediate-acting barbiturate. Acetaminophen: Nonopiate, nonsalicylate analgesic, antipyretic. Caffeine: CNS stimulant.

PHARMACOKINETICS: Absorption: APAP, caffeine: Rapid. **Distribution:** Butalbital: Plasma protein binding (45%); crosses placenta, found in breast milk. Caffeine: Found in breast milk. **Metabolism:** APAP: Conjugation. Caffeine: Biotransformation. **Elimination:** Butalbital: Urine (3.6%); $T_{1/2}$=35 hrs. APAP: Urine; $T_{1/2}$=1.25-3 hrs. Caffeine: Urine (3%); $T_{1/2}$=3 hrs.

NURSING CONSIDERATIONS

Assessment: Assess for porphyria, possible drug interactions, history of drug abuse/dependence, acute abdominal conditions, renal/hepatic impairment.

Monitoring: Monitor LFTs and renal function periodically. Monitor for hypersensitivity reactions, abuse/dependence, renal/hepatic dysfunction.

Patient Counseling: Instruct to take as prescribed (amount, frequency); avoid alcohol use. Caution may impair physical/mental abilities. Seek medical attention if hypersensitivity reactions occur.

Administration: Oral route. **Storage:** 15-30°C (59-86°F).

Esgic-Plus — RX

acetaminophen - caffeine - butalbital (Forest)

THERAPEUTIC CLASS: Barbiturate/analgesic

INDICATIONS: Tension or muscle contraction headaches.

DOSAGE: *Adults:* 1 cap/tab q4h prn. Max: 6 caps/tabs/day.
Pediatrics: ≥12 yrs: 1 cap/tab q4h prn. Max: 6 caps/tabs/day.

HOW SUPPLIED: Cap/Tab: (Butalbital-APAP-Caffeine) 50mg-500mg-40mg* *scored

CONTRAINDICATIONS: Porphyria.

WARNINGS/PRECAUTIONS: May be habit-forming; potential for abuse. Not for long-term use. Caution in elderly, debilitated, severe renal or hepatic impairment, acute abdominal conditions, suicidal tendencies, history of drug abuse.

E

ADVERSE REACTIONS: Drowsiness, lightheadedness, dizziness, sedation, SOB, NV, abdominal pain, intoxicated feeling.

INTERACTIONS: Enhanced CNS effects with MAOIs. May enhance CNS depressant effects of other narcotic analgesics, alcohol, general anesthetics, tranquilizers, sedative hypnotics, or other CNS depressants.

PREGNANCY: Category C, not for use in nursing.

MECHANISM OF ACTION: Butalbital: Short- to intermediate-acting barbiturate. Acetaminophen: Nonopiate, nonsalicylate analgesic, antipyretic. Caffeine: CNS stimulant.

PHARMACOKINETICS: Absorption: APAP, caffeine: Rapid. **Distribution:** Butalbital: Plasma protein binding (45%); crosses placenta; found in breast milk. Caffeine: Found in breast milk. **Metabolism:** APAP: Conjugation. Caffeine: Biotransformation. **Elimination:** Butalbital: Urine (3.6%); $T_{1/2}$=35 hrs. APAP: Urine; $T_{1/2}$=1.25-3 hrs. Caffeine: Urine (3%); $T_{1/2}$=3 hrs.

NURSING CONSIDERATIONS

Assessment: Assess for porphyria, possible drug interactions, history of drug abuse/dependence, acute abdominal conditions, renal/hepatic impairment.

Monitoring: Monitor LFTs and renal function periodically. Monitor for hypersensitivity reactions, abuse/dependence, renal/hepatic dysfunction.

Patient Counseling: Instruct to take as prescribed (amount, frequency); avoid alcohol use. Caution may impair physical/mental abilities. Seek medical attention if hypersensitivity reactions occur.

Administration: Oral route. **Storage:** 15-30°C (59-86°F).

ESKALITH — RX

lithium carbonate (GlaxoSmithKline)

Lithium toxicity is related to serum levels, and can occur at doses close to therapeutic levels.

OTHER BRAND NAMES: Eskalith CR (GlaxoSmithKline)

THERAPEUTIC CLASS: Antimanic agent

INDICATIONS: Treatment of manic episodes of manic-depressive illness.

DOSAGE: *Adults:* (Cap) 300mg tid-qid. (Tab, Extended-Release) 450mg q12h. Monitor every 1-2 weeks and adjust dose if needed. When stable, monitor every 2 months to achieve levels of 0.6-1.2mEq/L. Maint: 900-1200mg/day. Acute Mania: 1800mg/day in divided doses. Monitor levels twice weekly to achieve 1-1.5mEq/L. When switching to extended-release tabs, give same total daily dose when possible.
Pediatrics: ≥12 yrs: (Cap) 300mg tid-qid. (Tab, Extended-Release) 450mg q12h. Monitor every 1-2 weeks and adjust dose if needed. When stable, monitor every 2 months to achieve levels of 0.6-1.2 mEq/L. Maint: 900-1200mg/day. Acute Mania: 1800mg/day in divided doses. Monitor levels twice weekly to achieve 1-1.5mEq/L. When switching to extended-release tabs, give same total daily dose when possible.

HOW SUPPLIED: Cap: (Eskalith) 300mg; Tab, Extended-Release: (Eskalith CR) 450mg* *scored

WARNINGS/PRECAUTIONS: Avoid with significant renal or cardiovascular disease, severe debilitation, dehydration, or sodium depletion. Risk of encephalopathic syndrome (eg, weakness, lethargy, fever, tremulousness, confusion, EPS); d/c therapy. Maintain normal diet, adequate salt/fluid intake. Reduce dose or d/c with sweating, diarrhea, infection with elevated temperatures. Caution with hypothyroidism; may need supplemental therapy. Chronic therapy associated with diminution of renal concentrating ability, glomerular and interstitial fibrosis, and nephron atrophy.

ADVERSE REACTIONS: Fine hand tremor, polyuria, mild thirst, nausea, general discomfort, diarrhea, vomiting, drowsiness, muscular weakness.

INTERACTIONS: Increased risk of neurotoxicity with CCBs. Increased risk of toxicity with diuretics, metronidazole. Increased plasma levels with indomethacin, piroxicam, other NSAIDs, COX-2 inhibitors, ACE inhibitors, angiotensin II receptor antagonists. Caution with SSRIs. Decreased levels with acetazolamide, urea, xanthine agents, alkalinizing agents. Interacts with methyldopa, phenytoin, carbamazepine. May prolong effects of neuromuscular blockers.

PREGNANCY: Safety in pregnancy not known, not for use in nursing.

MECHANISM OF ACTION: Not established; suspected to alter sodium transport in nerve and muscle cells and effect a shift toward intraneuronal metabolism of catecholamines.

PHARMACOKINETICS: Distribution: Found in breast milk. **Elimination:** Urine (primary), feces (insignificant); $T_{1/2}$=24 hrs.

NURSING CONSIDERATIONS

Assessment: Assess for renal function/impairment, cardiovascular disorders, severe debilitation or dehydration, or sodium depletion prior to therapy with lithium. If these parameters exist, and therapy is still necessary, then perform initial lithium administration in hospital setting. Assess patient has access to facilities to obtain serum lithium levels while on therapy. Assess for possible drug interactions.

Monitoring: Monitor for signs/symptoms of lithium toxicity (eg, diarrhea, vomiting, tremor, muscle weakness). Monitor serum lithium levels. Levels should be taken just prior to administration of next dose. Perform periodic renal function tests (urinalysis, serum creatine) while on therapy. Monitor for diminution of renal concentrating ability associated with chronic lithium use, glomerular and interstitial fibrosis, nephron atrophy while on lithium, for encephalopathic syndrome in patients taking lithium plus a neuroleptic. Monitor effects of neuromuscular agents when given in combination with lithium. If patient develops protracted sweating or diarrhea, administer proper supplemental fluids and/or sodium under medical supervision and reduce or suspend lithium dosing. Monitor for development of concomitant infection with elevated temperatures. If present, lithium dosing may need to be reduced or suspended. Monitor thyroid levels in patients with a history of thyroid disease.

Patient Counseling: Counsel about signs/symptoms of lithium toxicity. Advise therapy may impair mental/physical abilities. Patients should be cautious in activities requiring alertness (operating machinery/driving). Lithium may decrease sodium levels in the body; maintain a normal diet, including proper sodium and fluid intake (2,500mL to 3,000mL), especially when beginning treatment.

Administration: Oral. **Storage:** 25°C (77°F); excursions permitted to 15-30°C (59-86°F).

ESTRACE — RX

estradiol (Warner Chilcott)

Estrogens increase risk of endometrial cancer in postmenopausal women. Avoid during pregnancy.

THERAPEUTIC CLASS: Estrogen

INDICATIONS: (Cre/Tab) Treatment of vulval and vaginal atrophy. (Tab) Treatment of moderate to severe vasomotor symptoms associated with menopause. Treatment of hypoestrogenism due to hypogonadism, castration, or primary ovarian failure. Palliative treatment of metastatic breast cancer and advanced androgen-dependent prostate carcinoma. Prevention of osteoporosis.

DOSAGE: *Adults:* (Cre) Vulval/Vaginal Atrophy: Initial: 2-4g/day for 1-2 weeks, then decrease to 1-2g/day for 1-2 weeks. Maint: 1g, 1-3x/week. Discontinue or taper at 3-6 month intervals. (Tab) Vasomotor Symptoms/Vulval/Vaginal Atrophy: Initial: 1-2mg/day (3 weeks on, 1 week off). Maint: Minimum effective dose. Discontinue or taper at 3-6 month intervals. Hypoestrogenism: 1-2mg/day. Maint: Minimum effective dose. Metastatic Breast Cancer: 10mg tid for at least 3 months. Prostate Carcinoma: 1-2mg tid. Osteoporosis Prevention: 0.5mg qd cyclically (23 days on and 5 days off).

E

HOW SUPPLIED: Cre, Vaginal: 0.1mg/g [12g, 42.5g]; Tab: 0.5mg*, 1mg*, 2mg* *scored

CONTRAINDICATIONS: Pregnancy, undiagnosed abnormal genital bleeding, breast cancer unless being treated for metastatic disease, estrogen-dependent neoplasia, thrombophlebitis, or thromboembolic disorders.

WARNINGS/PRECAUTIONS: Risk of gallbladder disease, cardiovascular disease, endometrial and breast carcinoma, fetal congenital reproductive tract disorder, elevated BP, and hypercalcemia with breast cancer and bone metastases. Caution in liver dysfunction, asthma, epilepsy, migraine, and cardiac or renal dysfunction. Increase in HDL, triglycerides, thyroid binding globulin. Acceleration of PT, PTT. Hypercoagulability effects. Impaired glucose tolerance. Consider adding progestin in patient with intact uterus.

ADVERSE REACTIONS: Altered vaginal bleeding, vaginal candidiasis, breast tenderness/enlargement, GI effects, melasma, CNS effects, weight changes, edema, altered libido.

PREGNANCY: Category X, caution in nursing.

MECHANISM OF ACTION: Estrogen; binds to nuclear receptors in estrogen-responsive tissue. Circulating estrogens modulate pituitary secretion of gonadotropins, luteinizing hormone, and follicle stimulating hormone, through negative feedback mechanism. Reduces elevated levels of these hormones in postmenopausal women.

PHARMACOKINETICS: Absorption: (Cre) Absorbed through skin, mucous membranes, and GI tract. **Distribution**: Largely bound to sex hormone-binding globulin and albumin; found in breast milk. **Metabolism**: Liver to estrone (metabolite), estriol (major urinary metabolite); sulfate and glucuronide conjugation (liver); gut hydrolysis; CYP3A4 (partial metabolism). **Elimination**: Urine (parent compound and metabolites).

NURSING CONSIDERATIONS

Assessment: Assess for undiagnosed abnormal genital bleeding, presence or history of breast cancer, DVT, PE, estrogen-dependent neoplasia, active or recent (within past yr) arterial thromboembolic disease (eg, stroke, MI), hepatic impairment, history of cholestatic jaundice, age (≥65 yrs old), hypertriglyceridemia, hypothyroidism, hypocalcemia, asthma, DM, epilepsy, migraine or porphyria, SLE, pregnancy/nursing status, and possible drug interactions. Assess need for progestin therapy in women who have not had a hysterectomy.

Monitoring: Monitor for signs/symptoms of cardiovascular disorders (eg, MI, stroke, venous thrombosis, pulmonary embolism), malignant neoplasms (eg, endometrial, breast, ovarian cancer), dementia, gallbladder disease, hypercalcemia, visual abnormalities (eg, retinal vascular thrombosis), elevations in BP, elevations in plasma triglycerides, pancreatitis, hypothyroidism, fluid retention, exacerbation of endometriosis and other conditions (eg, asthma, DM, epilepsy, migraine, SLE). For tablet formulation, monitor for hypersensitivity reactions. Monitor thyroid function in patients on thyroid replacement therapy. Monitor BP at regular intervals. If undiagnosed, persistent, or recurring abnormal vaginal bleeding occurs, perform proper diagnostic measures (eg, endometrial sampling) to rule out malignancy. Perform periodic monitoring (eg, every 3-6 months) to determine if treatment still required.

Patient Counseling: Inform medication increases chances of uterine cancer. Notify physician of upcoming surgery or need for prolonged bed rest. Contact physician if breast lumps, unusual vaginal bleeding, dizziness and faintness, changes in speech, severe headaches, chest pain, SOB, leg pains, changes in vision, or vomiting occur. Not for use during pregnancy. Perform monthly self breast exams.

Administration: Tab: Oral route. Cre: Intravaginal route. **Storage**: Tab: 20-25°C (68-77°F); dispense with child-resistant closure in a tight, light-resistant container. Cre: Store at room temperature; protect from temperatures >40°C (104°F). Keep out of reach of children.

ESTRADERM RX

estradiol (Novartis)

Estrogens increase the risk of endometrial cancer. Estrogens, with or without progestins, should not be used for the prevention of cardiovascular disease or dementia. Increased risks of MI, stroke, invasive breast cancer, PE, and DVT in postmenopausal women (50-79 yrs of age) reported. Increased risk of developing probable dementia in postmenopausal women ≥65 yrs of age reported.

THERAPEUTIC CLASS: Estrogen

INDICATIONS: Treatment of moderate-to-severe vasomotor symptoms and/or vulvar/vaginal atrophy associated with menopause. Treatment of hypoestrogenism due to hypogonadism, castration, or primary ovarian failure. Prevention of postmenopausal osteoporosis.

DOSAGE: *Adults:* Apply to clean, dry area on trunk of body. Do not apply to breast or waistline. Replace twice weekly. Rotate application sites. May give continuously without intact uterus. May give cyclically (3 weeks on, 1 week off) with intact uterus. Vasomotor Symptoms/Vulvar/Vaginal Atrophy: Initial: Apply 0.05mg/day twice weekly. Discontinue/Taper at 3-6 month intervals. Start 1 week after discontinuing oral hormone therapy. Osteoporosis Prevention: Initial: 0.05mg/day.

HOW SUPPLIED: Patch: 0.05mg/24 hrs, 0.1mg/24 hrs [8[s], 24[s]]

CONTRAINDICATIONS: Pregnancy, undiagnosed abnormal genital bleeding, breast cancer unless being treated for metastatic disease, estrogen-dependent neoplasia, DVT/PE, active or recent (eg, within past year) arterial thromboembolic disease (eg, stroke, MI), liver dysfunction or disease.

WARNINGS/PRECAUTIONS: May increase risk of cardiovascular events (eg, MI, stroke), venous thrombosis, and PE; d/c immediately if any of these events occur or are suspected. May increase risk of breast/endometrial cancer, and gallbladder disease. May lead to severe hypercalcemia with breast cancer and bone metastases; monitor and d/c if hypercalcemia occurs. Retinal vascular thrombosis reported; monitor and d/c if papilledema or retinal vascular lesions occur. Consider addition of a progestin if no hysterectomy. May elevate BP; monitor at regular intervals. May cause elevations of plasma triglycerides with pre-existing hypertriglyceridemia. Caution with history of cholestatic jaundice associated with past estrogen use or with pregnancy; d/c with recurrence. May lead to increased thyroid-binding globulin levels; monitor thyroid function. May cause fluid retention; caution with cardiac/renal dysfunction. Caution with severe hypocalcemia. May increase risk of ovarian cancer. May exacerbate endometriosis, asthma, DM, epilepsy, migraine, porphyria, SLE, and hepatic hemangiomas; use with caution.

ADVERSE REACTIONS: Redness/irritation at application site, altered vaginal bleeding, vaginal candidiasis, breast tenderness/enlargement, GI effects, melasma, CNS effects, retinal vascular thrombosis, weight changes, edema, altered libido.

INTERACTIONS: CYP3A4 inducers (eg, St. John's wort, phenobarbital, carbamazepine, rifampin) may decrease levels resulting in decreased therapeutic effects and/or changes in uterine bleeding profile. CYP3A4 inhibitors (eg, erythromycin, clarithromycin, ketoconazole, itraconazole, ritonavir, grapefruit juice) may increase levels and result in side effects.

PREGNANCY: Category X, caution in nursing.

MECHANISM OF ACTION: Estrogen; binds to nuclear receptors in estrogen-responsive tissues. Modulates pituitary secretion of gonadotropins, luteinizing hormone and follicle stimulating hormone, through negative feedback mechanism. Reduces elevated levels of these hormones in postmenopausal women,

PHARMACOKINETICS: Distribution: Largely bound to sex hormone binding globulin and albumin; found in breast milk. **Metabolism**: Liver to estrone (metabolite) and estriol (major urinary metabolite); sulfate and glucuronide conjugation (liver), gut hydrolysis; CYP3A4 (partial metabolism). **Elimination**: Urine (parent compound and metabolites); $T_{1/2}$=1 hr.

NURSING CONSIDERATIONS

Assessment: Assess for undiagnosed abnormal genital bleeding, presence or history of breast cancer, DVT, PE, estrogen-dependent neoplasia, active or recent (within past yr) arterial thromboembolic disease (eg, stroke, MI), pregnancy/nursing status, age of patient (≥65 yrs), hypertriglyceridemia, impaired liver function or history of cholestatic jaundice, hypothyroidism, hypocalcemia, asthma, DM, epilepsy, migraines or porphyria, SLE, and possible drug interactions. Assess need for progestin therapy in women who have not had a hysterectomy.

Monitoring: Monitor for signs/symptoms of cardiovascular events (eg, MI, stroke, venous thrombosis, PE), malignant neoplasms (eg, endometrial, breast, ovarian cancer), dementia, gallbladder disease, hypercalcemia, visual disorders (eg, retinal vascular thrombosis), elevations in BP, elevations in plasma triglycerides, pancreatitis, hypothyroidism, fluid retention, exacerbation of endometriosis and other conditions (eg, asthma, DM, epilepsy, migraines, SLE). Monitor thyroid function in patients on thyroid replacement therapy. Perform regular monitoring of BP levels, annual breast exam, and periodic evalution (every 3-6 months) to determine need for therapy. If undiagnosed, persistent, or recurring bleeding occurs, perform proper diagnostic testing (eg, endometrial sampling) to rule out malignancy.

Patient Counseling: Inform drug increases risk for uterine cancer. Report breast lumps, unusual vaginal bleeding, dizziness or faintness, changes in speech, severe headaches, chest pain, SOB, leg pains, changes in vision, or vomiting. Instruct to place medication system on clean, dry skin on the trunk (including buttocks and abdomen); site should not be exposed to sunlight; area should not be oily, damaged, or irritated; do not apply to breasts. Rotate application sites. Apply immediately after opening pouch. If medication system falls off, reapply same system; if not able to, apply new system; continue with original treatment schedule. Notify physician if planning surgery or prolonged immobilization. Advise to perform monthly self breast exams.

Administration: Transdermal route. **Storage**: Do not store above 30°C (86°F). Do not store unpouched.

ESTRASORB — RX

estradiol (Esprit)

Estrogens increase the risk of endometrial cancer. Estrogens, with or without progestins, should not be used for the prevention of cardiovascular disease or dementia. Increased risks of MI, stroke, invasive breast cancer, PE, and DVT in postmenopausal women (50-79 yrs of age) reported. Increased risk of developing probable dementia in postmenopausal women ≥65 yrs of age reported.

THERAPEUTIC CLASS: Estrogen

INDICATIONS: Treatment of moderate to severe vasomotor symptoms associated with menopause.

DOSAGE: *Adults:* Apply 2 pouches (0.05mg/day) qam. Apply one pouch to each leg from the upper thigh to the calf. Rub in for 3 min.

HOW SUPPLIED: Emulsion, Topical: 2.5mg/g

CONTRAINDICATIONS: Undiagnosed abnormal genital bleeding, breast cancer (unless being treated for metastatic disease), estrogen-dependent neoplasia, DVT/PE, active or recent (eg, within 1 year) arterial thromboembolic disease (eg, stroke, MI), liver dysfunction or disease, pregnancy.

WARNINGS/PRECAUTIONS: Limit use to the shortest duration consistent with goals and risks; re-evaluate periodically. Increased risk of cardiovascular events (eg, MI, stroke, venous thromboembolism, pulmonary embolism), gallbladder disease, breast and endometrial cancer. D/C 4-6 weeks before surgery associated with an increased risk of thromboembolism or during prolonged immobilization. Possible increased risk of ovarian cancer. May lead to severe hypercalcemia in patients with breast cancer and bone metastases. Consider adding progestin in patients with intact uterus to avoid endometrial hyperplasia. Increased thyroid-binding globulin levels (may need higher doses of thyroid hormone). May cause fluid retention; caution in cardiac or renal dysfunction. Retinal vascular thrombosis and elevated BP reported. May lead to severe hypercalcemia with breast cancer and bone metastases; monitor and d/c if hypercalcemia occurs. May exacerbate endometriosis, asthma, diabetes mellitus, epilepsy, migraine, porphyria, systemic lupus erythematosus (SLE), or hepatic hemangiomas; use with caution. Avoid use in close proximity to sunscreen application; may increase absorption. Potential for estradiol transfer through physical contact; wash application site 8 hours post-application. May cause elevations of plasma triglycerides with pre-existing hypertriglyceridemia. Caution with history of cholestatic jaundice associated with past estrogen use or with pregnancy; d/c with recurrence.

ADVERSE REACTIONS: Headache, infection, sinusitis, pruritus, breast pain, endometrial disorder.

INTERACTIONS: CYP3A4 inducers (eg, St. John's wort, phenobarbital, carbamazepine, rifampin) may decrease levels which may decrease therapeutic effects and/or change uterine bleeding profile. CYP3A4 inhibitors (eg, erythromycin, clarithromycin, ketoconazole, itraconazole, ritonavir, grapefruit juice) may increase levels which may result in side effects.

PREGNANCY: Contraindicated in pregnancy, caution in nursing.

MECHANISM OF ACTION: Estrogen; binds to nuclear receptors in estrogen-responsive tissues. Circulating estrogens modulate pituitary secretion of gonadotrophins, luteinizing hormone and follicle stimulating hormone, through negative feedback mechanism. Reduces elevated levels of these hormones in postmenopausal women.

PHARMACOKINETICS: Distribution: Largely bound to sex hormone binding globulin and albumin; found in breast milk. **Metabolism:** Liver to estrone (metabolite), estriol (major urinary metabolite); sulfate and glucuronide conjugation (liver), gut hydrolysis; CYP 3A4 (partial metabolism). **Excretion:** Urine (parent compound and metabolites).

NURSING CONSIDERATIONS

Assessment: Assess for undiagnosed abnormal genital bleeding, presence or history of breast cancer, DVT, PE, estrogen-dependent neoplasia, active or recent (within past yr) arterial thromboembolic disease (eg, MI, stroke), liver dysfunction, pregnancy/nursing status, familial hyperlipoproteinemia, age (≥65 yrs), hypothyroidism, hypocalcemia, asthma, DM, epilepsy, migraine, porphyria, SLE, and possible drug interactions. Assess need for progestin therapy in women who have not had a hysterectomy.

Monitoring: Monitor for signs/symptoms of cardiovascular events (eg, MI, stroke, venous thrombosis, PE), malignant neoplasms (eg, endometrial, breast, ovarian cancer), dementia, gallbladder disease, hypercalcemia, visual abnormalities (retinal vascular thrombosis), elevations in BP, elevations in plasma triglycerides, pancreatitis, hypothyroidism, fluid retention, exacerbation of endometriosis, and exacerbation of other conditions (eg, asthma, DM, epilepsy, migraines, SLE). Perform annual breast exam. Monitor thyroid function in patients on thyroid replacement therapy. Monitor BP levels at regular intervals. Perform proper diagnostic testing (eg, endometrial sampling) for abnormal, undiagnosed, persistent or recurring vaginal bleeding to rule out malignancy. Perform periodic evaluation (every 3-6 months) to determine need for therapy.

Patient Counseling: Inform estrogens increase chances of developing uterine cancer. Contact physician if breast lumps, unusual vaginal bleeding, dizziness or faintness, changes in speech, severe headaches, chest pain, SOB, leg pains, changes in vision, or vomiting occur. Advise to open medication pouches just prior to use; apply mornings to clean, dry skin of both thighs and calves. Avoid applying medication to irritated or red skin. Sunscreen should not be applied to treatment area at same time; may interact with medication.

Administration: Topical route. **Storage:** 20-25°C (68-77°F); excursions permitted to 15-30°C (59-86°F).

ESTRATEST RX

esterified estrogens - methyltestosterone (Solvay)

Estrogens increase risk of endometrial cancer in postmenopausal women. Avoid during pregnancy. Estrogens, with or without progestins, should not be used for the prevention of cardiovascular disease. Increased risks of MI, stroke, invasive breast cancer, PE, and DVT in postmenopausal women reported.

OTHER BRAND NAMES: Estratest H.S. (Solvay)

THERAPEUTIC CLASS: Estrogen/androgen combination

INDICATIONS: Treatment of moderate-severe vasomotor symptoms associated with menopause, when not improved by estrogens alone.

DOSAGE: *Adults:* Vasomotor Symptoms: 0.625-1.25mg or 1.25-2.5mg qd cyclically (3 weeks on, 1 week off). Discontinue/taper at 3-6 month intervals.

HOW SUPPLIED: Tab: (Esterified Estrogens-Methyltestosterone) (Estratest HS) 0.625-1.25mg;(Estratest) 1.25-2.5mg

CONTRAINDICATIONS: Pregnancy, nursing, severe liver damage, undiagnosed abnormal genital bleeding, breast cancer except in selected patients treated for metastatic disease, estrogen-dependent neoplasia, and thrombophlebitis or thromboembolic disease (active disease or past history associated with estrogen use, except when used in treatment of breast malignancy).

WARNINGS/PRECAUTIONS: Risk of gallbladder disease, endometrial carcinoma, thromboembolic disease, hepatic dysfunction/adenoma/neoplasm, peliosis hepatis, elevated BP, impaired glucose tolerance, hypercalcemia with breast cancer and bone metastases. Caution with metabolic bone disease associated with hypercalcemia or renal insufficiency. May increase size of pre-existing uterine leiomyomata. Caution in liver dysfunction, family history of breast cancer, breast nodules, fibrocystic disease, abnormal mammograms, diabetes, asthma, epilepsy, migraine, depression, and cardiac or renal dysfunction. D/C if cholestatic hepatitis and/or jaundice occurs, or if LFTs are abnormal. D/C 4 weeks prior to surgery if prolonged immobilization required. Increased risk of jaundice with history of jaundice during pregnancy. May effect epiphyseal closure; caution in young patients. D/C if virilization occurs. Increase in triglycerides, thyroid binding globulin, PT.

ADVERSE REACTIONS: Breakthrough bleeding, amenorrhea, virilization, inhibition of gonadotropin secretion, breast tenderness and enlargement, nausea, hirsutism, abdominal cramps, bloating, altered libido, cholestatic jaundice, weight gain, edema.

INTERACTIONS: May decrease insulin and anticoagulant requirements. May increase levels of oxyphenbutazone.

PREGNANCY: Category X, contraindicated in nursing.

MECHANISM OF ACTION: Esterified estrogen: Binds to nuclear receptors in estrogen-responsive tissues. Circulating estrogens modulate pituitary secretion of gonadotrophins, luteinizing hormone and follicle stimulating hormone, through negative feedback mechanism. Reduces elevated levels of these hormones in postmenopausal women. Methyltestosterone: An androgen; responsible for the normal growth and development of male sex hormones and for maintenance of secondary sex characteristics.

PHARMACOKINETICS: Distribution: Esterified estrogen: Largely bound to sex hormone-binding globulin and albumin; found in breast milk. Methyl testosterone: Bound to testosterone estradiol binding globulin (98%). **Metabolism:** Esterified estrogen: Liver to estrone (metabolite) and estriol (major urinary metabolite); sulfate and glucuronide conjugation (liver);

gut hydrolysis, CYP3A4 (partial metabolism). Methyl testosterone: Liver. **Elimination:** Esterified estrogen: Urine (parent compound and metabolites). Methyltestosterone: Urine (90%), feces (6%); $T_{1/2}$=10-100 min.

NURSING CONSIDERATIONS

Assessment: Assess for undiagnosed abnormal genital bleeding, presence or history of breast cancer, DVT or PE, estrogen-dependent neoplasia, active or recent (within past yr) arterial thromboembolic disease, liver disease, pregnancy/nursing status, age (≥65 yrs), DM, hypertriglyceridemia, hypothyroidism, asthma, epilepsy, migraines or porphyria, SLE, and possible drug interactions. Assess need for progestin therapy in females who have not had a hysterectomy. Assess for possible drug interactions.

Monitoring: Monitor for signs/symptoms of cardiovascular events (eg, MI, stroke, venous thrombosis, PE), malignant neoplasms (eg, breast, endometrial, ovarian cancer), dementia, gallbladder disease, glucose tolerance, hypercalcemia, visual abnormalities (eg, retinal vascular thrombosis), peliosis hepatitis, hepatic neoplasms, elevated BP, elevations in plasma triglycerides, hypothyroidism, fluid retention, exacerbation of endometriosis and other conditions (eg, asthma, DM, epilepsy, migraines, SLE), virilization, hypersensitivity reactions, and decreases in protein bound iodine. Perform annual breast exam. Monitor glucose levels with DM and thyroid function in patients on thyroid replacement therapy. Perform regular monitoring of BP levels and periodic LFTs. In females with disseminated breast carcinoma, perform frequent determinations of urine and serum calcium levels during course of androgen therapy. In patients on high doses of androgens, monitor for polycythemia by checking Hgb and Hct periodically. Monitor for undiagnosed persistent or recurring abnormal vaginal bleeding; perform adequate diagnostic testing (eg, endometrial sampling). Perform periodic evaluation (every 3-6 months) to determine need for therapy.

Patient Counseling: Inform drug increases chances of uterine cancer. Report any breast lumps, unusual vaginal bleeding, dizziness or faintness, changes in speech, severe headaches, chest pain, SOB, leg pains, changes in vision, vomiting, acne, changes in menstrual periods, increased facial hair, skin color changes, or ankle swelling. Counsel to perform self breast exams.

Administration: Oral route. **Storage:** 15-30°C (59-86°F). Keep out of reach of children.

ESTRING RX

estradiol (Pharmacia & Upjohn)

Estrogens increase risk of endometrial cancer in postmenopausal women. Estrogens with or without progestins should not be used for prevention of cardiovascular disease or dementia. Increased risk of stroke and DVT in postmenopausal women (50-79 yrs).

THERAPEUTIC CLASS: Estrogen

INDICATIONS: Treatment of urogenital symptoms associated with postmenopausal atrophy of vagina or lower urinary tract.

DOSAGE: *Adults:* Insert ring deeply into upper 1/3 of vaginal vault. Remove and replace after 90 days. Reassess at 3 or 6 month intervals.

HOW SUPPLIED: Vaginal Ring: 0.0075mg/24 hrs

CONTRAINDICATIONS: Pregnancy, undiagnosed abnormal vaginal bleeding, breast cancer, estrogen-dependent neoplasia, DVT or pulmonary embolism, arterial thromboembolic disease (eg, stroke, MI), liver dysfunction/disease.

WARNINGS/PRECAUTIONS: Increased risk of endometrial, breast, and ovarian cancer, dementia, gallbladder disease, visual abnormalities, hypercalcemia reported. Abnormal uterine bleeding, mastodynia reported. Caution with hepatic impairment, hypertriglyceridemia, hypothyroidism, hypocalcemia, vaginal stenosis, narrow vagina, prolapse, or vaginal infections. Expulsions from vagina reported. Hypercoagulation, hyperlipidemia, and fluid retention may occur.

ADVERSE REACTIONS: Headache, leukorrhea, back pain, genital moniliasis, sinusitis, vaginitis, vaginal discomfort, vaginal hemorrhage, arthralgia, insomnia, abdominal pain.

INTERACTIONS: Remove during treatment with other vaginally administered agents. CYP3A4 inhibitors (eg, erythromycin, clarithromycin, ketoconazole, itraconazole, ritonavir, grapefruit juice) may increase concentrations. CYP3A4 inducers (eg, St. John's wort, phenobarbital, carbamazepine, rifampin) may decrease concentrations.

PREGNANCY: Not for use in pregnancy or nursing.

MECHANISM OF ACTION: Estrogen; binds to nuclear receptors in estrogen-responsive tissue. Circulating estrogens modulate pituitary secretion of the gonadotropins, luteinizing hormone and follicle stimulating hormone, through negative feedback mechanism. Reduces elevated levels of these hormones in postmenopausal women.

PHARMACOKINETICS: Absorption: Well absorbed; C_{max}=63.2pg/mL; T_{max}=0.5-1 hr. **Distribution:** Largely bound to sex hormone binding globulin and albumin; found in breast milk. **Metabolism:** Liver to estrone (metabolite) and estriol (major urinary metabolite); sulfate and glucuronide conjugation (liver); intestinal hydrolysis; CYP3A4 (partial metabolism). **Elimination:** Urine (parent compound and metabolites).

NURSING CONSIDERATIONS

Assessment: Assess for undiagnosed abnormal genital bleeding, presence or history of breast cancer, estrogen-dependent neoplasia, active DVT or PE, active or recent (within past yr) arterial thromboembolic disease (eg, stroke, MI), liver dysfunction, pregnancy/nursing status, age (≥65 yrs), hypertriglyceridemia, hypothyroidism, hypocalcemia, asthma, DM, epilepsy, migraines or porphyria, SLE, and possible drug interactions. Assess need of progestin in women who have not had a hysterectomy.

Monitoring: Monitor for signs/symptoms of cardiovascular events (eg, stroke, DVT, MI, PE), malignant neoplasms (eg, endometrial, breast, ovarian cancer), dementia, gallbladder disease, hypercalcemia, visual abnormalities (eg, retinal vascular thrombosis), elevations in BP, elevations in serum triglycerides, pancreatitis, hypothyroidism, fluid retention, exacerbation of endometriosis and other conditions (eg, asthma, DM, epilepsy, migraines, SLE). Monitor BP levels regularly. Perform annual breast exam. Monitor thyroid function in patients on thyroid replacement therapy. If undiagnosed, persistent, or recurring abnormal vaginal bleeding occurs, perform adequate diagnostic measures (eg, endometrial sampling) to rule out malignancy.

Patient Counseling: Inform drug increases risk for uterine cancer. Report breast lumps, unusual vaginal bleeding, dizziness and faintness, changes in speech, severe headaches, chest pain, SOB, leg pains, vision changes, or vomiting. Perform monthly self breast exams. Wash and dry hands prior to handling medication. Remove medication ring from pouch and hold between thumb and index finger; press opposite sides of medication ring together and gently push compressed medication ring as far as possible, into upper one third of vagina. Should not feel anything once medication ring is properly in place. If there is discomfort, medication ring probably not far enough inside; push further into vagina. Medication ring should remain in place for 90 days.

Administration: Intravaginal route. **Storage:** 15-30°C (59-86°F). Keep out of reach of children.

ESTROGEL — RX

estradiol (Solvay)

Estrogens increase the risk of endometrial cancer. Estrogens, with or without progestins, should not be used for the prevention of cardiovascular disease. Increased risks of MI, stroke, invasive breast cancer, PE, and DVT in postmenopausal women reported.

THERAPEUTIC CLASS: Estrogen

INDICATIONS: Moderate to severe vasomotor symptoms and/or vulvar/vaginal atrophy associated with menopause.

DOSAGE: *Adults:* Apply one compression (1.25g) to one arm from wrist to shoulder once daily. Re-evaluate periodically.

HOW SUPPLIED: Gel: 0.06% (1.25g (0.75mg estradiol) of gel per compression) [93g]

CONTRAINDICATIONS: Undiagnosed abnormal genital bleeding, breast cancer, estrogen-dependent neoplasia, DVT or PE, active or recent (within 1 year) arterial thromboembolic disease (eg, stroke, MI), liver dysfunction or disease, pregnancy.

WARNINGS/PRECAUTIONS: May increase risk of cardiovascular events (eg, MI, stroke), venous thrombosis, and PE; d/c immediately if any of these events occur or are suspected. May increase risk of breast/endometrial cancer, and gallbladder disease. May lead to severe hypercalcemia with breast cancer and bone metastases; monitor and d/c if hypercalcemia occurs. Retinal vascular thrombosis reported; monitor and d/c if papilledema or retinal vascular lesions occur. Consider addition of a progestin if no hysterectomy. May elevate BP; monitor at regular intervals. May cause elevations of plasma triglycerides with pre-existing hypertriglyceridemia. Caution with history of cholestatic jaundice associated with past estrogen use or with pregnancy; d/c with recurrence. May lead to increased thyroid-binding globulin levels; monitor thyroid function. May cause fluid retention; caution with cardiac/renal dysfunction. Caution with severe hypocalcemia. May increase risk of ovarian cancer. May exacerbate endometriosis, asthma, DM, epilepsy, migraine, porphyria, SLE, and hepatic hemangiomas; use with caution. Alcohol-based gels are flammable; avoid fire, flame, or smoking until the gel dries.

ADVERSE REACTIONS: Headache, infection, breast pain, vaginitis, abdominal pain, rash, nausea, pruritus, diarrhea.

INTERACTIONS: CYP3A4 inducers (eg, St. John's wort, phenobarbital, carbamazepine, rifampin) may decrease levels which may decrease therapeutic effects and/or change uterine bleeding profile. CYP3A4 inhibitors (eg, erythromycin, clarithromycin, ketoconazole, itraconazole, ritonavir, grapefruit juice) may increase levels which may result in side effects. May require higher doses of thyroid hormone.

PREGNANCY: Contraindicated in pregnancy, caution in nursing.

MECHANISM OF ACTION: Estrogen; binds to nuclear receptors in estrogen-responsive tissues. Circulating estrogens modulate pituitary secretion of the gonadotrophins, luteinizing hormone and follicle stimulating hormone, through negative feedback mechanism. Reduces elevated levels of these hormones in postmenopausal women

PHARMACOKINETICS: Absorption: C_{max}=46.4pg/mL. **Distribution:** Largely bound to sex hormone binding globulin and albumin; found in breast milk. **Metabolism:** Liver to estrone (metabolite) and estriol (major urinary metabolite); sulfate and glucuronide conjugation (liver); gut hydrolysis; CYP 3A4 (partial metabolism). **Elimination:** Urine (parent compound and metabolites); $T_{1/2}$=36 hrs.

NURSING CONSIDERATIONS

Assessment: Assess for undiagnosed abnormal genital bleeding, presence or history of breast cancer, DVT or PE, estrogen-dependent neoplasia, active or recent (within past yr) arterial thromboembolic disease (eg, stroke, MI), liver dysfunction, history of cholestatic jaundice, pregnancy/nursing status, age (≥65 yrs), gallbladder disease, hypertriglyceridemia, hypothyroidism, hypocalcemia, asthma, DM, epilepsy, migraines, porphyria, SLE, and possible drug interactions. Assess need for progestin therapy in women who have not had a hysterectomy.

Monitoring: Monitor for signs/symptoms of cardiovascular disorders (eg, MI, stroke, venous thrombosis, PE), malignant neoplasms (eg, endometrial, breast, ovarian cancer), dementia, gallbladder disease, hypercalcemia, visual abnormalities (eg, retinal vascular thrombosis), elevations in BP, elevations in plasma triglycerides, pancreatitis, hypothyroidism, fluid retention, exacerbation of endometriosis and other conditions (eg, asthma, DM, epilepsy, migraines, SLE). Monitor BP levels regularly and thyroid function in patients on thyroid replacement therapy. Perform annual breast exam. If undiagnosed persistent or recurring abnormal vaginal bleeding occurs, perform adequate diagnostic measures (eg, endometrial sampling) to rule out malignancy. Periodically evaluate (every 3-6 months) to determine therapy need.

Patient Counseling: Inform estrogens increase risk for uterine cancer. Report if breast lumps, unusual vaginal bleeding, dizziness and faintness, changes in speech, severe headaches, chest pain, SOB, leg pain, vision changes, or vomiting occur. Notify physician if planning surgery or prolonged bed rest. Instruct to perform monthly self breast exams and have annual gynecologic exam. Before using medication for first time, pump must be primed; fully depress pump 2 (90g medication pump) or 3 times (50g or 25g medication pump); discard unused medication. Apply at same time daily to clean, dry, unbroken skin. Apply to one arm, spreading medication as thinly as possible over entire area on inside and outside of arm, from wrist to shoulder. Do not apply to breast. Allow 5 min to dry before dressing; wash hands following application. Medication is alcohol-based and flammable; avoid fire, flame, or smoking until dry. Instruct if dose is missed and next dose is <12 hrs away, wait to apply medication at normal dosing time; if >12 hrs away until next dose, apply missed dose, and return to normal dosing schedule.

Administration: Topical route. **Storage:** 20-25°C (68-77°F); excursions permitted to 15-30°C (59-86°F).

ESTROSTEP FE — RX

norethindrone acetate - ethinyl estradiol (Warner Chilcott)

THERAPEUTIC CLASS: Estrogen/progestogen combination

INDICATIONS: Prevention of pregnancy. Treatment of acne vulgaris in females ≥15 yrs who want contraception (for at least 6 months), have achieved menarche, and are unresponsive to topical acne agents.

DOSAGE: *Adults:* Contraception/Acne: 1 tab qd for 28 days, then repeat. Start 1st Sunday after menses begin or the 1st day of menses.
Pediatrics: ≥15 yrs: Contraception (Postpubertal Adolescents)/Acne: 1 tab qd for 28 days, then repeat. Start 1st Sunday after menses begins or the 1st day of menses.

HOW SUPPLIED: Tab: (Ethinyl Estradiol-Norethindrone) 0.035mg-1mg, 0.030mg-1mg, 0.020mg-1mg and 75mg ferrous fumarate

CONTRAINDICATIONS: Thrombophlebitis, history of DVT, active or history of thromboembolic disorders, pregnancy, cerebrovascular disease, CAD, undiagnosed abnormal genital bleeding, cholestatic jaundice of pregnancy, jaundice with prior pill use, hepatic adenoma or carcinoma, breast carcinoma, endometrium or other estrogen-dependent neoplasia.

WARNINGS/PRECAUTIONS: Cigarette smoking increases risk of serious cardiovascular side effects. This risk increases with age (especially >35 yrs) and heavy smoking. Increased risk of MI, vascular disease, thromboembolism, stroke, and gallbladder disease. Retinal thrombosis, hepatic neoplasia reported. May cause glucose intolerance. May increase BP, elevate LDL levels or cause other lipid changes, fluid retention, breakthrough bleeding, and spotting. May cause or exacerbate migraine. May develop visual changes with contact lenses. Increased risk of MI with HTN, hyperlipidemia, obesity, and diabetes. D/C if jaundice, significant depression, or ophthalmic irregularities develop. Perform annual physical exam. Use before menarche is not indicated. May affect certain endocrine, LFTs, and blood components.

ADVERSE REACTIONS: NV, breakthrough bleeding, spotting, amenorrhea, migraine, depression, vaginal candidiasis, edema, weight changes.

INTERACTIONS: Reduced effects, increased breakthrough bleeding, and menstrual irregularities with rifampin, barbiturates, phenylbutazone, phenytoin, carbamazepine, St. John's wort, and possibly with griseofulvin, ampicillin, and tetracyclines. Increased plasma levels with atorvastatin. Ascorbic acid and APAP may increase plasma levels. Decreased plasma levels of APAP.

Increased clearance of temazepam, salicylic acid, morphine, and clofibric acid. Increased plasma levels of cyclosporine, prednisolone, and theophylline.

PREGNANCY: Category X, not for use in nursing.

MECHANISM OF ACTION: Estrogen/progestogen oral contraceptive; acts by suppressing gonadotropins, inhibiting ovulation, and causing other alterations, including changes in the cervical mucus (increasing difficulty of sperm entry into uterus) and the endometrium (reducing likelihood of implantation).

PHARMACOKINETICS: Absorption: Rapid and complete. Absolute bioavailability: Norethindrone (64%), ethinyl estradiol (43%); T_{max}=1-2 hrs. **Distribution:** V_d=2-4L/kg; plasma protein binding (>95%). **Metabolism:** Norethindrone: Extensive; reduction, sulfate/glucuronide conjugation. Ethinyl estradiol: CYP3A4; oxidation, conjugation. **Elimination:** Norethindrone: $T_{1/2}$=13 hrs. Ethinyl estradiol: Urine, feces; $T_{1/2}$=19 hrs.

NURSING CONSIDERATIONS

Assessment: Assess for current or history of thrombophlebitis or thromboembolic disorders, cerebrovascular or coronary artery disease, known or suspected carcinoma of the breast, endometrium or other known or suspected estrogen-dependent neoplasia, undiagnosed abnormal genital bleeding, history of cholestatic jaundice of pregnancy or jaundice with previous pill use, hepatic adenomas or carcinomas, known or suspected pregnancy. Assess for possible drug interactions.

Monitoring: Monitor for development of MI, thromboembolism, stroke, hepatic neoplasia, carcinoma of the reproductive organs and breasts, and gallbladder disease, signs/symptoms of hepatotoxicity (eg, jaundice), ocular lesions, visual changes in patients who wear contact lenses, blood glucose levels in prediabetic and diabetic patients, signs/symptoms of HTN, fluid retention, signs of worsening depression with a history, onset or exacerbation of migraines or development of headaches, cholesterol levels with a history of hyperlipidemia, and bleeding irregularities.

Patient Counseling: Counsel about possible side effects. Inform that medication does not protect against HIV and other STDs. Counsel to avoid smoking while on medication. Advise to take at the same time every day; if a dose is missed, take as soon as possible, then take next dose at regular time. Advise if spotting, light bleeding, or nausea develops during first 1-3 packs of pills, to continue taking medication, and to notify physician if symptoms do not subside. If NV or diarrhea occurs, instruct use of backup birth control method until physician is contacted. Counsel to go for an annual physical.

Administration: Oral route. **Storage:** Do not store above 25°C (77°F). Protect from light. Store tablets inside pouch when not in use.

ETODOLAC RX

etodolac (Various)

NSAIDs may cause an increased risk of serious cardiovascular thrombotic events, MI, stroke and serious GI adverse events including bleeding, ulceration, and perforation of the stomach or intestines. Contraindicated for the treatment of perioperative pain in the setting of coronary artery bypass graft (CABG) surgery.

THERAPEUTIC CLASS: NSAID

INDICATIONS: Management of osteoarthritis (OA), rheumatoid arthritis (RA), and pain.

DOSAGE: *Adults:* ≥18 yrs: Acute Pain: Usual: 200-400mg q6-8h. Max: 1200mg/day. OA/RA: Usual: 300mg bid-tid, or 400-500mg bid. Max: 1200mg/day.

HOW SUPPLIED: Cap: 200mg, 300mg; Tab: 400mg, 500mg

CONTRAINDICATIONS: ASA or other NSAID allergy that precipitates asthma, urticaria or other allergic type reactions. Treatment of perioperative pain in the setting of CABG surgery.

WARNINGS/PRECAUTIONS: May lead to onset of new HTN or worsening of pre-existing HTN; monitor BP closely. Fluid retention and edema reported; caution with fluid retention or heart failure. Renal papillary necrosis and other renal injury reported after long-term use. Not recommended for use with advanced renal disease; if therapy must be initiated, monitor renal function. Anaphylactoid reactions may occur. May cause serious skin adverse events (eg, exfoliative dermatitis, Stevens-Johnson syndrome, and toxic epidermal necrolysis). Avoid in late pregnancy; may cause premature closure of ductus arteriosis. May cause elevations of LFTs; d/c if liver disease develops or systemic manifestations occur. Caution in elderly. Anemia may occur; with long-term use, monitor Hgb/Hct if signs or symptoms of anemia develop. May inhibit platelet aggregation and prolong bleeding time; monitor with coagulation disorders. Caution with asthma and avoid with ASA-sensitive asthma. Risk of GI ulceration, bleeding, and perforation.

ADVERSE REACTIONS: Dyspepsia, abdominal pain, diarrhea, flatulence, nausea, constipation, gastritis, asthenia, malaise, dizziness, increased bleeding time, GI ulcers, GI bleeding/perforation, heartburn, abnormal renal function.

INTERACTIONS: May elevate digoxin, lithium, and methotrexate serum levels. May enhance nephrotoxicity associated with cyclosporine. Avoid with phenylbutazone and ASA. Increased adverse effect potential with ASA. Caution with warfarin. Diuretics may increase risk of renal toxicity. May diminish antihypertensive effects of ACE inhibitors.

PREGNANCY: Category C, not for use in nursing.

MECHANISM OF ACTION: NSAID; suspected to inhibit prostaglandin synthetase, exerts anti-inflammatory, analgesic, and antipyretic actions.

PHARMACOKINETICS: Absorption: Well absorbed. Bioavailability (100%); C_{max}=14-37mcg/mL, T_{max}=80 min. **Distribution:** V_d=390mL/kg; plasma protein binding (99%). **Elimination:** Urine, feces; $T_{1/2}$=6.4 hrs.

NURSING CONSIDERATIONS

Assessment: Assess LFTs, renal function, CBC and coagulation profile. Assess for history of CABG surgery, asthma and allergic reactions to aspirin or other NSAIDs, active ulceration or chronic inflammation of GI tract, CVD, asthma, pregnancy status. Note other diseases/conditions and drug therapies.

Monitoring: Monitor for hypersensitivity reactions, cardiac complications, stroke, GI bleeding, asthma, skin side effects. Monitor BP, LFTs, renal function, CBC with differential and platelet count, coagulation profile, ocular effects and Reye's syndrome.

Patient Counseling: Counsel about side effects; seek medical attention if any occur. Tablet should be swallowed; not chewed or crushed. Advise to take as prescribed. Caution women against using medication late in pregnancy.

Administration: Oral route. **Storage:** 25-30°C (68-77°F). Protect from excessive heat and humidity.

ETODOLAC EXTENDED-RELEASE — RX

etodolac (Various)

NSAIDs may cause an increased risk of serious cardiovascular thrombotic events, MI, stroke and serious GI adverse events including bleeding, ulceration, and perforation of the stomach or intestines. Contraindicated for the treatment of perioperative pain in the setting of coronary artery bypass graft (CABG) surgery.

THERAPEUTIC CLASS: NSAID

INDICATIONS: Relief of signs and symptoms of osteoarthritis (OA), rheumatoid arthritis (RA), and juvenile rheumatoid arthritis (JRA).

DOSAGE: *Adults:* Usual: 400-1000mg qd. Max: 1200mg/day.
Pediatrics: 6-16 yrs: JRA: >60kg: 1000mg/day. 46-60kg: 800mg/day. 31-45kg: 600mg/day. 20-30kg: 400mg/day.

HOW SUPPLIED: Tab, Extended-Release: 400mg, 500mg, 600mg

CONTRAINDICATIONS: ASA or other NSAID allergy that precipitates asthma, urticaria, or allergic reaction. Treatment of perioperative pain in the setting of CABG surgery.

WARNINGS/PRECAUTIONS: May lead to onset of new HTN or worsening of pre-existing HTN; monitor BP closely. Fluid retention and edema reported; caution with fluid retention or heart failure. Renal papillary necrosis and other renal injury reported after long-term use. Not recommended for use with advanced renal disease; if therapy must be initiated, monitor renal function. Anaphylactoid reactions may occur. May cause serious skin adverse events (eg, exfoliative dermatitis, Stevens-Johnson syndrome, and toxic epidermal necrolysis). Avoid in late pregnancy; may cause premature closure of ductus arteriosus. May cause elevations of LFTs; d/c if liver disease develops or systemic manifestations occur. Caution in elderly. Anemia may occur; with long-term use, monitor Hgb/Hct if signs or symptoms of anemia develop. May inhibit platelet aggregation and prolong bleeding time; monitor with coagulation disorders. Caution with asthma and avoid with ASA-sensitive asthma.

E

ADVERSE REACTIONS: Dyspepsia, abdominal pain, diarrhea, flatulence, NV, constipation, GI ulcers, gross bleeding/perforation.

INTERACTIONS: May elevate digoxin, lithium, and methotrexate serum levels. May enhance nephrotoxicity associated with cyclosporine. Avoid with phenylbutazone. Increased adverse effect potential with ASA. Caution with warfarin. May decrease antihypertensive effects with ACE inhibitors. May reduce natriuretic effect of furosemide and thiazides.

PREGNANCY: Category C, not for use in nursing.

MECHANISM OF ACTION: NSAID; inhibits prostaglandin synthetase; exhibits anti-inflammatory, analgesic, and antipyretic activities.

PHARMACOKINETICS: Absorption: T_{max}=6 hrs. **Distribution:** V_d=566mL/kg; plasma protein binding (99%). **Metabolism:** Hydroxylation, glucuronidation. **Elimination:** Urine, feces; $T_{1/2}$=8.4 hrs.

NURSING CONSIDERATIONS

Assessment: Assess LFTs, renal function, CBC and coagulation profile. Assess for history of CABG surgery, asthma and allergic reactions to aspirin or other NSAIDs, active ulceration or chronic inflammation of GI tract, CVD, pregnancy status, and for possible drug interactions.

Monitoring: Monitor for hypersensitivity reactions, cardiac complications, stroke, GI bleeding, asthma, skin side effects. Monitor BP, LFTs, renal function, CBC with differential and platelet count, and coagulation profile.

Patient Counseling: Counsel about potential side effects; seek medical attention if any occur. Instruct to take as prescribed. Caution women against using late in pregnancy. Advise to avoid alcohol and smoking during therapy.

Administration: Oral route. **Storage:** 25-30°C (68-77°F). Protect from excessive heat and humidity.

ETOPOPHOS — RX

etoposide phosphate (Bristol-Myers Squibb)

Administer under supervision of qualified physician experienced in use of cancer chemotherapeutic agents. Severe myelosuppression with resulting infection or bleeding may occur.

THERAPEUTIC CLASS: Podophyllotoxin derivative

INDICATIONS: Adjunct therapy for management of refractory testicular tumors. First-line combination therapy for management of small cell lung cancer (SCLC).

DOSAGE: *Adults:* Testicular Cancer: Range: 50-100mg/m²/day on Days 1-5 to 100mg/m²/day on Days 1, 3, and 5. SCLC: Range: 35mg/m²/day for 4 days to 50mg/m²/day for 5 days. After adequate recovery from toxicity, repeat course for either therapy at 3-4 week intervals. CrCl 15-50mL/min: 75% of dose.

HOW SUPPLIED: Inj: 100mg

WARNINGS/PRECAUTIONS: Observe for myelosuppression during and after therapy. Risk of anaphylactic reaction manifested by chills, fever, tachycardia, bronchospasm, dyspnea, and hypotension. Increased risk of toxicity with a low serum albumin. Perform CBC before each dose, during, and after therapy. May cause fetal harm in pregnancy. Caution with low serum albumin.

ADVERSE REACTIONS: Myelosuppression, leukopenia, neutropenia, thrombocytopenia, anemia, NV, anaphylactic-like reactions, BP changes, alopecia, anorexia, asthenia/malaise, chills, fever.

INTERACTIONS: Caution with drugs known to inhibit phosphatase activities (eg, levamisole). High-dose oral cyclosporine reduces clearance.

PREGNANCY: Category D, not for use in nursing.

MECHANISM OF ACTION: Podophyllotoxin derivative; induces DNA strand breaks by interacting with DNA-topoisomerase II or formation of free radicals.

PHARMACOKINETICS: Absorption: Rapid, complete; Etopophos 150mg/m²: AUC=168.3µg•hr/mL, C_{max}=20µg/mL. **Distribution:** VePesid: V_d=7-17L/m²; plasma protein binding (97%). **Metabolism:** VePesid: Liver via CYP3A4 (O-demethylation); hydroxy acid (metabolite). **Elimination:** VePesid: Biliary excretion, feces, urine; $T_{1/2}$=4-11 hrs.

NURSING CONSIDERATIONS

Assessment: Assess for impaired renal function, pregnancy status, decreased serum albumin, and possible drug interactions. Obtain platelet, Hgb, and WBC with differential at start of therapy and before each cycle.

Monitoring: Monitor CBC and renal function periodically, for signs/symptoms of anaphylactic reaction, severe myelosuppression, and renal dysfunction.

Patient Counseling: Inform of pregnancy risks; avoid pregnancy. Advise to seek medical attention if symptoms of severe myelosuppression (infection or bleeding) or anaphylactic reaction (chills, fever, tachycardia, bronchospasm, dyspnea, hypotension) occur.

Administration: IV infusion. **Storage:** 2-8°C (36-46°F); refrigerate and protect from light. Reconstituted and diluted vials stable for 7 days refrigerated or 24 hrs at room temperature, 20-25°C (68-77°F).

EUFLEXXA — RX

sodium hyaluronate (Ferring)

THERAPEUTIC CLASS: Hyaluronan

INDICATIONS: Treatment of pain in osteoarthritis of the knee in patients who have failed to respond adequately to conservative non-pharmacologic therapy and simple analgesics (eg, APAP).

DOSAGE: *Adults:* Inject 2mL intra-articularly into affected knee at weekly intervals for 3 weeks, for a total of 3 injections. Use strict aseptic injection procedures.

HOW SUPPLIED: Inj: 1% [2mL]

CONTRAINDICATIONS: Avoid with knee joint infections, infections or skin diseases in area of injection site.

WARNINGS/PRECAUTIONS: Avoid mixing with quaternary ammonium salts (eg, benzalkonium chloride); may result in formation of a precipitate. Avoid injecting intravascularly. Patients having repeated exposure have the potential for an immune response. Safety and effectiveness in joints other than the knee or in conjunction with other intra-articular injectables have not been established. Remove any joint effusion before injecting. Transient pain and/or swelling of the injected joint may occur. Avoid any strenuous activities or prolonged (eg, more than 1 hour) weight-bearing activities within 48 hours following injection. Safety and effectiveness have not been demonstrated in children.

ADVERSE REACTIONS: Arthralgia, nausea, back pain, rhinitis, BP increase, joint effusion/swelling, tendonitis, knee pain, skin irritation, headache, paresthesia.

PREGNANCY: Safety in pregnancy and nursing not known.

NURSING CONSIDERATIONS

Assessment: Assess for knee joint infections, skin infections, or disease in the injection-site area.

Monitoring: Monitor for knee pain or swelling of joint.

Patient Counseling: Inform that drug may cause transient pain/swelling of injected joint. Avoid strenuous activities or prolonged weight-bearing activities (jogging, tennis) within 48 hrs following injection.

Administration: Intra-articular injection. **Storage:** 2-25°C (36-77°F). Protect from light. Remove from refrigeration at least 20-30 min before use. Do not freeze.

EVISTA RX

raloxifene HCl (Lilly)

Increased risk of DVT and PE reported. Avoid use in women with active or past history of venous thromboembolism. Increased risk of death due to stroke in postmenopausal women with documented coronary heart disease or at increased risk for major coronary events.

THERAPEUTIC CLASS: Selective estrogen receptor modulator

INDICATIONS: Treatment and prevention of osteoporosis in postmenopausal women. Reduction in risk of invasive breast cancer in postmenopausal women with osteoporosis or at high risk for invasive breast cancer.

DOSAGE: *Adults:* 60mg qd.

HOW SUPPLIED: Tab: 60mg

CONTRAINDICATIONS: Nursing, pregnancy, venous thromboembolic events (eg, DVT, PE, retinal vein thrombosis).

WARNINGS/PRECAUTIONS: May increase risk of DVT, PE, and retinal vein thrombosis; d/c 72 hrs prior to and during prolonged immobilization. May increase risk of death due to stroke in postmenopausal women with documented coronary heart disease or in women at increased risk for coronary events. Should not be used for primary or secondary prevention of CV disease. May increase levels of triglycerides with pre-existing hypertriglyceridemia. Not for use in premenopausal women or with systemic estrogens. Caution with hepatic impairment or with moderate or severe renal impairment. Venous thromboembolism reported.

ADVERSE REACTIONS: Hot flashes, leg cramps, abdominal pain, vaginal bleeding, arthralgia, rhinitis, headache.

INTERACTIONS: Avoid concomitant use with anion exchange resins; cholestyramine decreases absorption. Monitor PT/INR with warfarin and other anticoagulants. Caution with other highly protein-bound drugs (eg, diazepam, diazoxide, lidocaine). Avoid concomitant use with other systemic estrogens.

PREGNANCY: Category X, contraindicated in nursing.

MECHANISM OF ACTION: Selective estrogen receptor modulator; binds to estrogen receptors. Results in activation of estrogenic pathways in some tissues and blockade of estrogenic pathways in others. Actions depend on extent of recruitment of coactivators and corepressors to estrogen receptor target gene promotors. Acts as an estrogen agonist in bone. Decreases bone resorption and bone turnover, increases bone mineral density, and decreases fracture incidence.

PHARMACOKINETICS: Absorption: Rapid; Absolute bioavailability (2%); Single dose: C_{max}=0.5(ng/mL)/(mg/kg); AUC=27.2(ng•hr/mL)/(mg/kg). Multiple doses: C_{max}=1.36(ng/mL)/(mg/kg); AUC=24.2(ng•hr/mL)/(mg/kg). **Distribution:** Single dose: V_d=2348L/kg; Multiple doses: V_d=2853L/kg. Plasma protein binding (95%). **Metabolism:** Extensive; glucuronidation. **Elimination:** Feces (primary), urine (<0.2% unchanged). Single dose: $T_{1/2}$=27.7 hrs; Multiple doses: $T_{1/2}$=32.5 hr.

NURSING CONSIDERATIONS

Assessment: Assess for active or history of thromboembolism (eg, DVT, PE, retinal vein thrombosis), CVD, pregnancy/nursing status, prolonged immobilization, renal/hepatic impairment. Assess if postmenopausal, for presence of hypertriglyceridemia, history of breast cancer, and for possible drug interactions. Perform baseline breast exam and mammography.

Monitoring: Monitor for signs/symptoms of VTE, stroke, hypertriglyceridemia, uterine bleeding, and breast abnormalities. Monitor serum TG with history of hypertriglyceridemia. Perform regular breast exams and mammography.

Patient Counseling: For osteoporosis treatment/prevention, instruct to take supplemental calcium and/or vitamin D if intake is inadequate. Instruct to consider weight-bearing exercise and behavioral modification factors (eg, smoking, excessive alcohol consumption). Advise to d/c therapy at least 72 hrs prior to and during prolonged immobilization. Advise to avoid prolonged restrictions of movement during travel. Counsel drug may increase incidence of hot flashes or hot flashes may occur upon initiation of therapy. Inform regular breast exams and mammography are required while on therapy.

Administration: Oral route. **Storage:** 20-25°C (68-77°F); excursions permitted to 15-30°C (59-86°F).

EXELON RX

rivastigmine tartrate (Novartis)

THERAPEUTIC CLASS: Acetylcholinesterase inhibitor

INDICATIONS: Treatment of mild to moderate dementia of the Alzheimer's type and mild to moderate dementia associated with Parkinson's disease.

DOSAGE: *Adults:* Alzheimer's Dementia: Initial: 1.5mg bid. Titrate: May increase by 1.5mg bid every 2 weeks. Max: 12mg/day. If not tolerating, suspend therapy for several doses and restart at same or next lower dose. If interrupted longer than several days, reinitiate with lowest daily dose and titrate as above. Dementia Associated with Parkinson's Disease: Initial: 1.5mg bid. Titrate: May increase by 1.5mg every 4 weeks. Max: 12mg/day. Take with food in am and pm. May mix solution with water, cold fruit juice, or soda. Patch: Alzheimer's Dementia/Dementia Associated with Parkinson's Disease: Initial: Apply 4.6mg/24 hrs patch qd to clean, dry, hairless intact skin. Maint: Increase dose after 4 weeks. Max: 9.5mg/24 hrs if well tolerated. Switching from Capsules/Oral Sol: Total Oral Daily Dose <6mg: Switch to 4.6mg/24 hrs patch. Total Oral Daily Dose 6-12mg: Switch to 9.5mg/24 hrs patch. Apply 1st patch on day following last oral dose.

HOW SUPPLIED: Cap: 1.5mg, 3mg, 4.5mg, 6mg; Patch: 4.6mg/24 hrs, 9.5mg/24 hrs [30^s]; Sol: 2mg/mL [120mL]

CONTRAINDICATIONS: Hypersensitivity to carbamate derivatives.

WARNINGS/PRECAUTIONS: Significant GI intolerance (eg, nausea, vomiting, anorexia, and weight loss); always follow dosing guidelines. Vagotonic effect on HR (bradycardia), especially in "sick sinus syndrome" or supraventricular conduction abnormalities. May cause urinary obstruction and seizures. Monitor for peptic ulcers/GI bleeds. Caution in asthma and COPD. May exacerbate or induce extrapyramidal symptoms. (Patch) May impair mental/physical capabilities. Titrate dose with caution in patients with body weight below 50kg.

ADVERSE REACTIONS: NV, abdominal pain, dyspepsia, constipation, somnolence, anorexia, asthenia, headache, dizziness, fatigue, diarrhea, tremor, depression.

INTERACTIONS: May block effects of anticholinergics. May be synergistic with succinylcholine, similar neuromuscular blockers, or cholinergic agonists (eg, bethanechol). May exaggerate succinylcholine-type muscle relaxation during anesthesia.

PREGNANCY: Category B, not for use in nursing.

MECHANISM OF ACTION: Reversible cholinesterase inhibitor; not fully established, suspected to enhance cholinergic function by increasing concentration of acetylcholine through reversible inhibition of its hydrolysis by cholinesterase.

PHARMACOKINETICS: Absorption: Patch: T_{max}=10-16 hrs. Cap, Sol: Rapid, complete; absolute bioavailability (36%); T_{max}=1 hr. **Distribution:** V_d=1.8-2.7L/kg; plasma protein binding (40%). **Metabolism:** Cholinesterase-mediated hydrolysis. **Elimination:** Urine (97%), feces (0.4%); $T_{1/2}$=1.5 hrs.

NURSING CONSIDERATIONS

Assessment: Assess for history of ulcer disease, sick sinus syndrome, conduction defects, asthma or COPD, urinary obstruction, body weight, seizures, and possible drug interactions.

Monitoring: Monitor body weight and mental status; signs/symptoms of active or occult GI bleeding, extrapyramidal symptoms (EPS), and hypersensitivity reactions.

Patient Counseling: Inform to monitor for loss of weight or appetite, NV, anorexia, or diarrhea; may exacerbate or induce EPS. (Sol) Instruct to use provided syringe to withdraw prescribed amount. (Patch) Instruct to wash hands after application, and avoid contact with eyes; do not rub in or apply to area that is red, irritated, cut or to areas where cream, lotion, powder has recently been applied; replace every 24 hrs and consistent time of day; do not apply new patch to same spot for at least 14 days; can be used while bathing but avoid exposure to external heat sources (eg, excess sunlight, saunas, solariums). If dose is missed, apply new patch immediately, then continue scheduled dosage; do not apply 2 patches at once.

Administration: Oral, transdermal route. (Sol) Swallow directly from syringe or mix with small glass of water, juice or soda; stir before drinking. (Patch) Apply at upper or lower back. **Storage:** 25°C (77°F); excursions permitted to 15-30°C (59-86°F). Sol: Store in upright position and protect from freezing. Patch: Keep in sealed pouch until use.

EXFORGE — RX

amlodipine besylate - valsartan (Novartis)

When used in pregnancy, drugs that act directly on the renin-angiotensin system can cause injury and even death to the developing fetus. D/C therapy when pregnancy is detected.

THERAPEUTIC CLASS: ARB/Calcium channel blocker (dihydropyridine)

INDICATIONS: Treatment of hypertension. May be used in patients whose BP is not adequately controlled on either monotherapy. May also be used as initial therapy in patients likely to need multiple drugs to achieve their BP goals.

DOSAGE: *Adults:* Initial Therapy: 5mg-160mg qd. Add-On/Replacement Therapy: May be substituted for titrated components. Titrate: If inadequate control, may increase after 1-2 weeks of therapy. Max: 10mg-320mg qd. Elderly: Initial: 2.5mg amlodipine.

HOW SUPPLIED: Tab: (Amlodipine-Valsartan) 5mg-160mg, 10mg-160mg, 5mg-320mg, 10mg-320mg

WARNINGS/PRECAUTIONS: May cause excessive hypotension. May increase risk of angina and MI in patients with severe obstructive CAD. Caution with CHF, severe hepatic impairment, renal dysfunction, or renal artery stenosis.

ADVERSE REACTIONS: Peripheral edema, vertigo, nasopharyngitis, upper respiratory tract infection, dizziness.

INTERACTIONS: K^+ supplements, K^+-sparing diuretics (eg, spironolactone, triamterene, amiloride), or salt substitutes containing K^+ may increase serum K^+ and SrCr in heart failure patients.

PREGNANCY: Category D, not for use in nursing.

MECHANISM OF ACTION: Amlodipine: Calcium channel blocker (dihydropyridine); inhibits transmembrane influx of calcium ions into vascular smooth muscle and cardiac muscle. Valsartan: Angiotensin II receptor blocker; blocks vasoconstrictor and aldosterone-secreting effects of angiotensin II by selectively blocking binding of angiotensin II to AT_1 receptor.

PHARMACOKINETICS: Absorption: Amlodipine: Absolute bioavailability (64-90%); T_{max}=6-12 hrs. Valsartan: Absolute bioavailability (25%); T_{max}=2-4 hrs. **Distribution:** Amlodipine: V_d=21L; plasma protein binding (93%). Valsartan: V_d=17L (IV); plasma protein binding (95%). **Metabolism:** Amlodipine: Liver (90%). Valsartan: Valeryl 4-hydroxy valsartan (metabolite). **Elimination:** Amlodipine: Urine (10%); $T_{1/2}$=30-50 hrs. Valsartan: Feces, urine; $T_{1/2}$=6 hrs.

NURSING CONSIDERATIONS

Assessment: Assess severe obstructive CAD, CHF, recent MI, severe aortic stenosis, pregnancy status, possible drug interactions, renal/hepatic impairment.

Monitoring: Monitor for signs/symptoms of hypotension, hypersensitivity reactions, renal/hepatic dysfunction, symptoms of angina or MI after dosage initiation or increase.

Patient Counseling: Inform of pregnancy risks. Advise to seek medical attention if symptoms of hypotension or hypersensitivity reactions occur.

Administration: Oral route. **Storage:** 25°C (77°F); excursions permitted to 15-30°C (59-86°F). Protect from moisture.

EXJADE **RX**

deferasirox (Novartis)

THERAPEUTIC CLASS: Iron-chelating agent

INDICATIONS: Treatment of chronic iron overload due to blood transfusions (transfusional hemosiderosis).

DOSAGE: *Adults:* Initial: 20mg/kg/day. Titrate: May increase 5-10mg/kg q 3-6 months. Max: 30mg/kg/day. Take on empty stomach at least 30 min before food at same time each day. Tabs should be completely dispersed in 3.5oz of liquid if dose <1g or in 7oz if dose >1g. If serum ferritin falls below 500µg/L, consider interrupting therapy.
Pediatrics: ≥2 yrs: Initial: 20mg/kg/day. Titrate: May increase 5-10mg/kg q 3-6 months. Max: 30mg/kg/day. Take on empty stomach at least 30 min before food at same time each day. Tabs should be completely dispersed in 3.5oz of liquid if dose <1g or in 7oz if dose >1g. If serum ferritin falls below 500µg/L, consider interrupting therapy.

HOW SUPPLIED: Tab: 125mg, 250mg, 500mg

WARNINGS/PRECAUTIONS: Assess SCr before therapy and monitor monthly therafter; reduce dose, interrupt or d/c therapy if necessary. Intermittent proteinuria reported; monitor closely. Acute renal failure and cytopenias reported. Use caution and monitor SCr in those at risk of complications, having preexisting renal or comorbid conditions, receiving medicinal products that depress renal function, or elderly. Caution with pre-existing hematologic disorders; monitor CBC regularly. Hepatic abnormalities, increased transaminases reported; monitor LFTs monthly; modify dose for severe or persistent elevations. Reports of auditory (high frequency hearing loss, decreased hearing) and ocular disturbances (lens opacities, cataracts, elevated IOP, retinal disorders); initial and yearly auditory and ophthalmic testing recommended. Reports of skin rashes; d/c if severe, may reinitiate with short period of oral steroid.

ADVERSE REACTIONS: Diarrhea, NV, headache, abdominal pain, pyrexia, cough, increased SCr, rash, b-thalassemia, rare anemias, sicke cell disease.

INTERACTIONS: Avoid with aluminum-containing antacids or other iron chelator therapies.

PREGNANCY: Category B, caution in nursing.

MECHANISM OF ACTION: Iron chelating agent.

PHARMACOKINETICS: Absorption: T_{max}=1.5-4 hrs. **Distribution:** V_d=14.37; plasma protein binding (99%). **Metabolism:** Glucuronidation, deconjugation. **Elimination:** Feces (84%), urine (8%); $T_{1/2}$=8-16 hrs.

NURSING CONSIDERATIONS

Assessment: Assess LFTs, CBC, renal function, serum ferritin. Note other diseases/conditions and drug therapy.

Monitoring: Monitor for serum ferritin levels, acute renal failure, LFTs, CBC with platelet and differential count, hypersensitivity reactions, auditory and ocular disturbances, skin rashes.

Patient Counseling: Advise to take once daily on empty stomach at least 30 mins prior to food, preferably at same time every day. Instruct not to chew or swallow whole. Caution not to take drug and aluminum-containing antacids simultaneously. Patient should have auditory and ophthalmic testing before starting treatment and thereafter at regular intervals. Patient experiencing dizziness should exercise caution when operating machinery/driving.

Administration: Oral route. Disperse tab in water, orange juice, or apple juice; immediately drink resulting suspension. After swallowing suspension, resuspend any residue in small volume of liquid and swallow. **Storage:** 25°C (77°F). Excursions permitted to 15-30°C (59-86°F). Protect from moisture.

EXTINA — RX

ketoconazole (Stiefel)

THERAPEUTIC CLASS: Azole antifungal

INDICATIONS: Topical treatment of seborrheic dermatitis in immunocompetent patients ≥12 yrs of age.

DOSAGE: *Adults:* Apply to affected area(s) bid for 4 weeks.
Pediatrics: ≥12 yrs: Apply to affected area(s) bid for 4 weeks.

HOW SUPPLIED: Foam: 2% [50g, 100g]

WARNINGS/PRECAUTIONS: Contact sensitization, including photoallergenicity. Contents are flammable.

ADVERSE REACTIONS: Application site burning, dryness, erythema, irritation, paresthesia, pruritus, rash, warmth, contact sensitization.

PREGNANCY: Category C, caution in nursing.

MECHANISM OF ACTION: Antifungal agent; not established. Inhibits the synthesis of ergosterol, a key sterol in the cell membrane of *Malassezia furfur*.

NURSING CONSIDERATIONS

Assessment: Assess use in pregnancy/nursing.

Monitoring: Monitor for contact sensitization reactions, including photoallergenicity.

Patient Counseling: Counsel to notify physician if any type of skin irritation or contact sensitization reaction develops; or if no improvement in 4 weeks of treatment. Inform medication is flammable; do not administer near fire, open flame, or direct heat. Instruct to wash hands well following administration.

Administration: Topical application. Spray medication into cap of can or other cool surface prior to administration. Do not spray directly onto affected skin or hands because foam will melt immediately when it touches the skin. If hands are warm prior to administration, rinse them in cold water first and dry them prior to application. If can is warm, run it under cold water prior to use. **Storage:** Room temperature 20-25°C (68-77°F). Do not store under refrigerated conditions or in direct sunlight. Do not expose containers to heat or store at temperatures above 49°C (120°F). Keep out of reach of children.

FACTIVE
gemifloxacin mesylate (Oscient)

RX

Fluoroquinolones are associated with an increased risk of tendinitis and tendon rupture in all ages. Risk further increased in patients >60 yrs, patients taking corticosteroid drugs, and patients with kidney, heart or lung transplants.

F

THERAPEUTIC CLASS: Fluoroquinolone

INDICATIONS: Treatment of community-acquired pneumonia (CAP), including multi-drug resistant *Streptococcus pneumoniae* (MDRSP), and acute bacterial exacerbation of chronic bronchitis (ABECB).

DOSAGE: *Adults:* ≥18 yrs: ABECB: 320mg qd for 5 days. CAP: 320mg qd for 5 days (*S.pneumoniae, H.influenzae, M.pneumoniae*, or *C.pneumoniae*) or 7 days (MDRSP, *K.pneumoniae*, or *M.catarrhalis*). Renal Impairment: CrCl ≤40mL/min or Dialysis: 160mg qd. Take with fluids.

HOW SUPPLIED: Tab: 320mg

WARNINGS/PRECAUTIONS: May prolong QT interval; avoid in patients with a history of prolonged QTc interval, uncontrolled electrolyte disorders. Caution with proarrhythmic conditions, epilepsy, or if predisposed to convulsions. D/C at 1st sign of hypersensitivity (eg, rash). CNS effects, photosensitivity reactions, hypersensitivity reactions (some fatal) reported; d/c if any of these occur. *Clostridium difficile*-associated diarrhea, achilles and other tendon rupture reported. D/C therapy if rash, pain, inflammation, or ruptured tendon occurs. Caution in elderly patients taking corticosteroids. Avoid excessive sunlight and UV light. Maintain hydration. Increases of International Normalized Ratio (INR), or prothrombin time (PT), and/or clinical episodes of bleeding have been noted with concurrent administration with warfarin or derivatives.

ADVERSE REACTIONS: Diarrhea, rash, nausea, headache, abdominal pain, vomiting, dizziness.

INTERACTIONS: Magnesium- or aluminum-containing antacids, Videx® (didanosine) chewable/buffered tablets or pediatric powder, and products containing iron, and zinc, or other metal cations decrease absorption, space doses at least 3 hrs before or 2 hrs after administration. Space dosing of sucralfate by 2 hrs. Potentiated by probenecid. Monitor PT. Avoid Class IA (eg, quinidine, procainamide) or III (eg, amiodarone, sotalol) antiarrhythmics. Caution with drugs that prolong the QTc interval (eg, erythromycin, antipsychotics, TCAs).

PREGNANCY: Category C, not for use in nursing.

MECHANISM OF ACTION: Fluoroquinolone; synthetic broad-spectrum antimicrobial agent; inhibits enzymes topoisomerase II (DNA gyrase) and topoisomerase IV, which are required for bacterial DNA replication.

PHARMACOKINETICS: Absorption: Rapid; absolute bioavailability (71%); T_{max}=0.5-2 hrs; C_{max}=1.61µg/mL, AUC=8.36µg•hr/mL (respiratory infection, UTI). **Distribution:** V_d=4.18L/kg; plasma protein binding (55%-73%). **Metabolism:** Liver. **Elimination:** Feces (61%), urine (36%).

NURSING CONSIDERATIONS

Assessment: Assess renal function, LFTs, pregnancy status, prolonged QT interval, history of seizures. Note other diseases/conditions and drug therapies.

Monitoring: Monitor for cardiac arrest, seizure, status epilepticus, respiratory failure, angioedema, hypersensitivity reactions, dermatological reactions (Stevens-Johnson syndrome), CDAD, LFTs, renal function, CBC with platelet and differential count, tendon rupture, peripheral neuropathy.

Patient Counseling: Notify healthcare provider if symptoms of pain, swelling, or inflammation of a tendon, or weakness or inability to move joints; rest and refrain from exercise; and d/c therapy. Inform that drug treats bacterial, not viral, infections. Take exactly as directed; skipping doses or not completing full course may decrease effectiveness and increase resistance. Inform to take with or without food, and to drink fluids. Inform about potential benefits/risks. D/C and notify physician if skin rash, other allergic reaction, and watery and bloody stools (with or without stomach cramps and fever) occur. Notify if pregnant/nursing or taking antacids or sucralfate. Use caution in activities requiring mental alertness and coordination. Avoid sun exposure. Take full course as prescribed. Instruct to swallow tablet whole.

Administration: PO. **Storage:** 15-30°C (59-86°F); protect from light.

FAMVIR

famciclovir (Novartis) **RX**

THERAPEUTIC CLASS: Nucleoside analogue

INDICATIONS: Treatment of acute herpes zoster (shingles). Treatment or suppression of recurrent genital herpes; or treatment of recurrent herpes labialis (cold sores) in immunocompetent patients. Treatment of recurrent mucocutaneous herpes simplex infections in HIV-infected patients;

DOSAGE: *Adults:* ≥18 yrs: Herpes Zoster: Usual: 500mg q8h for 7 days; start within 72 hrs after rash onset. CrCl 40-59mL/min: 500mg q12h. CrCl 20-39mL/min: 500mg q24h. CrCl <20mL/min: 250mg q24h. Hemodialysis: 250mg following dialysis. Recurrent Genital Herpes: 1000mg bid for 1 day; start within 6 hrs of onset of symptom. CrCl 40-59mL/min: 500mg q12h; CrCl 20-39mL/min 500mg as single dose; CrCl <20mL/min 250mg as a single dose; Hemodialysis: 250mg following dialysis. Suppression of Recurrent Genital Herpes: 250mg bid for up to 1 yr. CrCl 20-39mL/min: 125mg q12h. CrCl <20mL/min: 125mg q24h. Hemodialysis: 125mg following dialysis. Recurrent Orolabial or Genital Herpes in HIV: 500mg bid for 7 days. CrCl <20mL/min: 250mg q24h. Hemodialysis: 250mg following dialysis. Recurrent Herpes Labialis: 1500mg as a single dose; CrCl 40-59mL/min: 750mg single dose; CrCl 20-39mL/min: 500mg single dose; CrCl <20mL/min: 20mg single dose; Hemodialysis: 250mg following dialysis

HOW SUPPLIED: Tab: 125mg, 250mg, 500mg

CONTRAINDICATIONS: Hypersensitivity to penciclovir cream.

WARNINGS/PRECAUTIONS: Prodrug of penciclovir. Dose adjustment in renal disease. Not indicated for initial episode of genital herpes infection, ophthalmic zoster, disseminated zoster or in immunocompromised patients with herpes zoster.

ADVERSE REACTIONS: Headache, migraine, NV, diarrhea, fatigue, urticaria, hallucinations, confusion.

INTERACTIONS: Increased plasma levels of penciclovir with probenecid and other drugs significantly eliminated by active renal tubular secretion. Potential interaction with drugs metabolized by aldehyde oxidase.

PREGNANCY: Category B, safety not known in nursing.

MECHANISM OF ACTION: Nucleoside analogue; inhibits HSV-2 DNA polymerase competitively with deoxyguanosine triphosphate, inhibiting herpes viral DNA synthesis and replication.

PHARMACOKINETICS: Absorption: Penciclovir: Absolute bioavailability (77%). **Distribution:** Penciclovir (IV) V_d=1.08L/kg; plasma protein binding (<20%) **Metabolism**: Hepatic; deacetylation and oxidation; famciclovir (prodrug) converted to penciclovir. **Elimination:** Urine (73%), feces (27%). Penciclovir: Urine (94%); $T_{1/2}$=2-3 hrs.

NURSING CONSIDERATIONS

Assessment: Assess for hepatic/renal dysfunction, galactose intolerance, severe lactase deficiency, or glucose-galactose malabsorption.

Monitoring: Monitor LFTs, total bilirubin, serum creatinine, CBC, amylase and lipase.

Patient Counseling: Avoid contact with lesions or intercourse when lesions and/or symptoms are present to avoid infecting partners. Caution may impair physical/mental abilities in patients with symptoms of CNS disturbances (dizziness, somnolence). Counsel to take without regard to meals.

Administration: Oral route. **Storage:** 25°C (77°F); excursions permitted to 15-30°C (59-86°F).

FASLODEX

fulvestrant (AstraZeneca)

RX

THERAPEUTIC CLASS: Estrogen receptor antagonist

INDICATIONS: Treatment of hormone receptor positive metastatic breast cancer in postmenopausal women with disease progression following antiestrogen therapy.

DOSAGE: *Adults:* 250mg IM into buttock once monthly as either a single 5mL injection or two concurrent 2.5mL injections. Administer slowly.

HOW SUPPLIED: Inj: 50mg/mL [2.5mL, 5mL]

CONTRAINDICATIONS: Pregnancy.

WARNINGS/PRECAUTIONS: May cause fetal harm during pregnancy; women of childbearing age should be advised not to become pregnant and pregnancy should be ruled out prior to initiating therapy. Avoid in patients with bleeding diatheses or thrombocytopenia. Safety and efficacy have not been studied in patients with moderate or severe hepatic impairment.

ADVERSE REACTIONS: NV, constipation, diarrhea, abdominal pain, headache, back pain, vasodilatation (hot flushes), pharyngitis, injection-site reactions, asthenia, pain, dyspnea, increased cough.

INTERACTIONS: Avoid with concurrent anticoagulants.

PREGNANCY: Category D, not for use in nursing.

MECHANISM OF ACTION: Estrogen receptor antagonist; binds to estrogen receptor and downregulates estrogen receptor protein in human breast cancer cells.

PHARMACOKINETICS: Absorption: C_{max}=8.5ng/mL; T_{max}=7 days; AUC=131ng•d/mL. **Distribution:** V_d=3-5L/kg; plasma protein binding (99%). **Metabolism:** CYP3A4; oxidation, aromatic hydroxylation, conjugation. **Elimination:** Feces (90%), urine (<1%); $T_{1/2}$=40 days.

NURSING CONSIDERATIONS

Assessment: Assess for hypersensitivity, hepatic impairment, bleeding diatheses, thrombocytopenia, pregnancy/nursing status, and possible drug interactions.

Monitoring: Monitor for NV, constipation/diarrhea, abdominal pain, headache, back pain, hot flushes, pharyngitis, vasodilation, anemia, hypersensitivity reactions, bleeding diatheses, women of childbearing potential, and hepatic dysfunction.

Patient Counseling: Counsel about pregnancy/nursing risks; avoid pregnancy. Seek immediate medical attention if NV, constipation/diarrhea, abdominal pain, headache, back pain, hot flushes, pharyngitis, vasodilation, anemia, hypersensitivity reactions, or bleeding diatheses develops.

Administration: IM route. Refer to PI for full instructions. **Storage:** 2-8°C (36-46°F). Protect from light. Store in original carton until time of use.

FAZACLO

clozapine (Avanir)

RX

Risk of agranulocytosis, seizures, myocarditis, and other cardiovascular and respiratory effects. Obtain baseline WBC and ANC before initiation of therapy, regularly during treatment, and for 4 weeks after discontinuation. Increased mortality in elderly patients with dementia-related psychosis.

THERAPEUTIC CLASS: Dibenzapine derivative

INDICATIONS: Management of severe schizophrenia when response to standard schizophrenia treatment fails.

DOSAGE: *Adults:* Initial: 12.5mg qd-bid. Titrate: Increase by 25-50mg/day, up to 300-450mg/day by end of 2 weeks, then increase weekly or bi-weekly by increments up to 100mg. Usual 100-900mg/day given tid. Max: 900mg/day. To d/c, gradually reduce dose over 1-2 weeks. Monitor for psychotic symptoms if abrupt discontinuation warranted (eg, leukopenia).

HOW SUPPLIED: Tab, Disintegrating: 12.5mg, 25mg*, 50mg, 100mg* *scored

CONTRAINDICATIONS: Myeloproliferative disorders, uncontrolled epilepsy, history of clozapine-induced agranulocytosis or severe granulocytopenia, severe CNS depression, coma, or with other agents with potential to cause agranulocytosis or suppress bone marrow function.

F

WARNINGS/PRECAUTIONS: Reserve treatment for severely ill patients unresponsive to other schizophrenia therapies. Monitor for hyperglycemia, worsening of glucose control with DM and FBG levels with diabetes risk. Significant risk of orthostatic hypotension and tachycardia. May impair alertness with initial doses. May cause high fever or pulmonary embolism. Cardiomyopathy reported; d/c unless benefit outweighs risk. Caution with prostatic enlargement, narrow angle glaucoma and renal, hepatic, or cardiac/pulmonary disease. NMS, tardive dyskinesias, impaired intestinal peristalsis and ECG changes reported. Obtain WBC and ANC at baseline, then weekly for 1st six months of therapy, then every 2 weeks for next 6 months, and then every 4 weeks thereafter if counts are acceptable. Avoid treatment if WBCs $<3500/mm^3$ or ANC $<2000/mm^3$, history of myeloproliferative disorder, previous clozapine-induced agranulocytosis, or granulocytopenia. D/C treatment if WBCs $<3000/mm^3$, ANC $<1500/mm^3$, eosinophils $>4000/mm^3$, or if myocarditis develops. D/C over 1-2 weeks.

ADVERSE REACTIONS: Drowsiness, vertigo, headache, tremor, salivation, sweating, dry mouth, visual disturbances, tachycardia, hypotension, syncope, constipation, nausea, fever.

INTERACTIONS: Avoid with other bone marrow suppressants, epinephrine, and carbamazepine. Caution with CNS-active drugs, anesthesia, alcohol, paroxetine, fluoxetine, fluvoxamine, sertraline, benzodiazepines, other psychotropics, or inhibitors/inducers of CYP1A2, 2D6, 3A4. Dosage reduction may be needed with drugs metabolized by CYP2D6 (eg, antidepressants, phenothiazines, carbamazepine, Type 1C antiarrhythmics). May potentiate hypotensive effects of antihypertensives and anticholinergic effects of atropine-type drugs. Caution with general anesthesia. CYP450 inducers (eg, phenytoin, nicotine, carbamazepine, rifampin) may decrease plasma levels. CYP450 inhibitors (eg, cimetidine, caffeine, fluvoxamine, erythromycin) may increase plasma levels.

PREGNANCY: Category B, not for use in nursing.

MECHANISM OF ACTION: Atypical antipsychotic agent. Interferes with the binding of dopamine specifically at the D_1 and D_4 receptors. Also acts as an antagonist at the adrenergic, cholinergic, histaminergic, and serotonergic receptors.

PHARMACOKINETICS: Absorption: C_{max}=413ng/mL, T_{max}=2.3 hrs. **Metabolism:** CYP1A2, 2D6; demethylation, hydroxylation. **Distribution:** Plasma protein binding (97%). **Elimination:** Urine (50%), feces (30%); $T_{1/2}$=8 hrs (initial dose), 12 hrs (multiple doses).

NURSING CONSIDERATIONS

Assessment: Assess previous course of standard therapy prior to treatment. Assess for history of myeloproliferative disorders, uncontrolled epilepsy, paralytic epilepsy, clozapine-induced agranulocytosis, severe granulocytopenia, or severe CNS depression prior to therapy. Assess risk of seizure, dementia related psychosis, narrow-angle glaucoma, male patients with prostrate enlargement, patients with concomitant illnesses (renal or cardiac disease), and patients undergoing general anesthesia. Perform baseline WBC count and ANC prior to treatment. Obtain baseline fasting blood glucose levels in patients at risk for hyperglycemia.

Monitoring: Monitor for clinical response to treatment, WBC counts and ANC while on therapy and for at least 4 weeks following discontinuation. Monitor for agranulocytosis, cardiovascular effects (myocarditis), severe respiratory effects, seizures, fever, pulmonary embolism, NMS, TD, and intestinal paralysis, signs/symptoms of hyperglycemia and check periodic fasting blood glucose levels in patients at risk for hyperglycemia, and for signs/symptoms of hepatitis while on therapy. Obtain LFTs if patient develops NV and/or anorexia.

Patient Counseling: Counsel can be taken with/without food. Inform about signs/symptoms of agranulocytosis; advise to immediately report lethargy, weakness, fever, sore throat. Inform phenylketonuric patients drug contains phenylalanine. Medication may cause cognitive/motor impairment. Avoid hazardous activities (operating machinery/driving) alcohol use, and advise females to avoid nursing while on medication. If a dose is missed for more than 2 days, consult physician before restarting medication. Advise if tablets are received in a blister, to keep unopened until immediately prior to use. If tablets are split, remaining half tablet must be discarded.

Administration: Oral route. **Storage:** 25°C (77°F); excursions permitted to 15-30°C (59-86°F). Protect from moisture.

FELBATOL RX
felbamate (Meda)

Associated with aplastic anemia and fatal hepatic failure. Monitor blood, LFTs. Avoid in history of hepatic dysfunction.

THERAPEUTIC CLASS: Dicarbamate anticonvulsant

INDICATIONS: Not for first line therapy. Monotherapy or adjunct therapy in partial seizures with and without generalization in adults. Adjunct therapy for partial and generalized seizures with Lennox-Gastaut syndrome in children.

DOSAGE: *Adults:* Initial Monotherapy: 300mg qid or 400mg tid. Titrate: Increase by 600mg every 2 weeks to 2.4g/day. Max: 3.6g/day. Initial Monotherapy Conversion/Adjunct Therapy: 300mg qid or 400mg tid while reducing present AED (see literature). Titrate: For conversion, increase at week 2 to 2.4g/day, at week 3 up to 3.6g/day. Adjunct Therapy: Increase by 1.2g/day every week up to 3.6mg/day. Renal Dysfunction: May need to reduce dose with concomitant AEDs.
Pediatrics: ≥14 yrs: Initial Monotherapy: 300mg qid or 400mg tid. Titrate: Increase by 600mg every 2 weeks to 2.4g/day. Max: 3.6g/day. Initial Monotherapy Conversion/Adjunct Therapy: 300mg qid or 400mg tid while reducing present AED (see literature). Titrate: For conversion, increase at week 2 to 2.4g/day, at week 3 up to 3.6g/day. Adjunct Therapy: Increase by 1.2g/day every week up to 3.6mg/day. 2-14 yrs: Lennox-Gastaut Adjunct Therapy: Initial: 15mg/kg/day in 3-4 divided doses. Titrate: Increase by 15mg/kg/day every week to 45mg/kg/day. Renal Dysfunction: May need to reduce dose with concomitant AEDs.

HOW SUPPLIED: Sus: 600mg/5mL [240mL, 960mL]; Tab: 400mg*, 600mg* *scored

CONTRAINDICATIONS: History of blood dyscrasias, hepatic dysfunction.

WARNINGS/PRECAUTIONS: Avoid abrupt discontinuation. Caution with renal dysfunction. Obtain written, informed consent. Obtain full hematologic evaluations and LFTs before, during, and after discontinuation. D/C if bone marrow depression or liver abnormalities occur.

ADVERSE REACTIONS: Anorexia, NV, insomnia, headache, anemias, hepatic failure.

INTERACTIONS: Increases plasma levels of phenytoin, valproate, active carbamazepine metabolite and phenobarbital. Decreases carbamazepine levels. Decreased felbamate levels with phenytoin, carbamazepine, and phenobarbital. Caution with OCs.

PREGNANCY: Category C, safety in nursing not known.

MECHANISM OF ACTION: Anticonvulsant; weak inhibitory effects on GABA-receptor binding and benzodiazepine receptor binding. Acts as an antagonist at the strychnine-insensitive glycine recognition site of the NMDA receptor-ionophore complex.

PHARMACOKINETICS: Absorption: Well-absorbed. **Distribution:** V_d=756mL/kg; plasma protein binding (22-25%). **Metabolism:** Parahydroxyfelbamate, 2-hydroxyfelbamate, felbamatemonocarbamate (metabolites, little activity). **Elimination:** Urine (40-50% unchanged); $T_{1/2}$=20-23 hrs.

NURSING CONSIDERATIONS

Assessment: Assess if patient has history of any blood dyscrasias or hepatic dysfunction. Assess renal function prior to therapy. Obtain baseline CBC (reticulocytes, platelets) and baseline LFTs.

Monitoring: Monitor for signs/symptoms of hepatic failure, aplastic anemia (signs of infection, bleeding, anemia), and bone marrow depression. Monitor LFTs, CBC (platelets, reticulocytes) while on therapy and following treatment. Monitor for occurrence of seizures in abrupt withdrawal.

Patient Counseling: Advise if signs of aplastic anemia (infection, bleeding, anemia) or liver dysfunction (jaundice, anorexia, gastrointestinal complaints and malaise) occur to contact physician immediately. Inform not to abruptly d/c medication and that there is still risk for hematological/hepatic complications following d/c; continuing monitoring of CBC and LFTs required.

Administration: Oral route. Shake oral suspension well before using. **Storage:** Store at controlled room temperature 20-25°C (68-77°F).

F

FEMARA

RX

letrozole (Novartis)

THERAPEUTIC CLASS: Nonsteroidal aromatase inhibitor

INDICATIONS: First-line treatment of hormone-receptor positive or hormone-receptor unknown locally advanced or metastatic breast cancer in postmenopausal women. Treatment of advanced breast cancer with disease progression following antiestrogen therapy in postmenopausal women. Extended adjuvant treatment of early breast cancer in postmenopausal women who have received 5 yrs of adjuvant tamoxifen therapy. Adjuvant treatment of postmenopausal women with hormone-receptor positive early breast cancer.

DOSAGE: *Adults:* 2.5mg qd. Continue until tumor progression is evident. Cirrhosis/Severe Liver Dysfunction: 2.5mg every other day.

HOW SUPPLIED: Tab: 2.5mg

CONTRAINDICATIONS: Women of premenopausal endocrine status.

WARNINGS/PRECAUTIONS: May cause fetal harm in pregnancy. May elevate LFTs and total cholesterol. May decrease bone density; monitor bone mineral density. Reduce dose in cirrhosis and severe liver dysfunction. May cause fatigue and dizziness; caution when driving or using machinery.

ADVERSE REACTIONS: Bone pain, back pain, NV, arthralgia, dyspnea, fatigue, chest pain, decreased weight, hot flushes, peripheral edema, HTN, constipation, diarrhea, musculoskeletal pain, insomnia, cough, alopecia.

INTERACTIONS: Coadministration with tamoxifen may reduce letrozole plasma levels; if coadministered, give letrozole immediately after tamoxifen.

PREGNANCY: Category D, caution in nursing.

MECHANISM OF ACTION: Nonsteroidal aromatase inhibitor; inhibits conversion of androgens to estrogens and competitively binds to the heme of cytochrome P450 subunit of the enzyme, resulting in a reduction of estrogen biosynthesis in all tissues.

PHARMACOKINETICS: Absorption: Rapid and complete (GI tract). **Distribution:** V_d=1.9L/kg; weakly protein bound. **Metabolism:** Liver via CYP450 isoenzymes: 3A4, 2A6. **Elimination:** Urine (90%, 6% unchanged); $T_{1/2}$=2 days.

NURSING CONSIDERATIONS

Assessment: Assess for premenopausal endocrine status, hepatic impairment, baseline bone mineral density, drug administrations.

Monitoring: Monitor LFTs, bone mineral density, hot flashes, cardiovascular complications, second malignancies.

Patient Counseling: Advise may cause fatigue, dizziness, and somnolence. Caution against operating machinery/driving. Counsel about side effects; seek medical attention if any develop.

Administration: Oral route. **Storage:** 25°C (77°F); excursions permitted to 15-30°C (59-86°F).

FEMHRT — RX

norethindrone acetate - ethinyl estradiol (Warner Chilcott)

Estrogens and progestins should not be used for prevention of cardiovascular disease or dementia. Increased risks of MI, stroke, invasive breast cancer, PE, and DVT in postmenopausal women (50-79 yrs of age) reported. Increased risk of developing probable dementia in postmenopausal women ≥65 yrs of age reported.

THERAPEUTIC CLASS: Estrogen/progestogen combination

INDICATIONS: In women with an intact uterus, treatment of moderate to severe vasomotor symptoms associated with menopause and prevention of postmenopausal osteoporosis.

DOSAGE: *Adults:* Vasomotor Symptoms: 1 tab qd. Re-evaluate at 3-6 month intervals. Osteoporosis Prevention: 1 tab qd. Assess response by measuring bone mineral density.

HOW SUPPLIED: Tab: (Ethinyl Estradiol-Norethindrone) 2.5mcg-0.5mg, 5mcg-1mg

CONTRAINDICATIONS: Pregnancy, undiagnosed abnormal genital bleeding, breast cancer, estrogen-dependent neoplasia, DVT/PE, thrombophlebitis, thromboembolic disorders, active or recent (eg, within past year) arterial thromboembolic disease (eg, stroke, MI).

WARNINGS/PRECAUTIONS: Risk of gallbladder disease, endometrial and breast carcinoma, elevated BP, visual disturbances, thromboembolism, and hypercalcemia with breast cancer or bone metastases. Possible risk of cardiovascular disease, ovarian cancer. Caution with liver dysfunction, asthma, epilepsy, migraine, depression, and cardiac or renal dysfunction. Increase in HDL, triglycerides, thyroxine binding globulin. Hypercoagulability effects. Impaired glucose tolerance. D/C if sudden onset of visual abnormalities or migraine. May exacerbate endometriosis.

ADVERSE REACTIONS: Headache, back pain, abdominal pain, NV, breast pain, nervousness, depression, rhinitis, sinusitis, UTI, vaginitis.

INTERACTIONS: Increases plasma levels of cyclosporine, prednisolone, and theophylline. May decrease plasma levels of acetaminophen. May increase clearance of temazapam, salicylic acid, morphine, and clofibric acid. CYP3A4 inducers (eg, St. John's wort, phenobarbital, carbamazepine, rifampin) may decrease levels which may decrease therapeutic effects and/or change uterine bleeding profile. CYP3A4 inhibitors (eg, erythromycin, clarithromycin, ketoconazole, itraconazole, ritonavir, grapefruit juice) may increase levels which may result in side effects. Reduced response to metyrapone test.

PREGNANCY: Contraindicated in pregnancy, caution in nursing.

MECHANISM OF ACTION: Ethinyl estradiol: Estrogen; binds to nuclear receptors in estrogen-responsive tissues. Circulating estrogens modulate pituitary secretion of the gonadotrophins, luteinizing hormone and follicle stimulating hormone, through negative feedback mechanism. Reduces elevated levels of these hormones in postmenopausal women. Norethindrone: Progestin; binds to specific progesterone receptors that interact with progesterone response elements in target genes. Enhances cellular differentiation and opposing the actions of estrogens by decreasing estrogen receptor levels, increasing local metabolism of estrogens to less active metabolites, or inducing gene products that blunt cellular response to estrogen.

PHARMACOKINETICS: Absorption: Ethinyl estradiol, Norethindrone: Rapidly absorbed; T_{max}=1-2 hrs; Norethindrone: Absolute bioavailability (64%); Ethinyl estradiol: Absolute bioavailability (55%). **Distribution:** V_d=2-4L/kg; plasma protein binding (>95%); found in breast milk. **Metabolism:** Norethindrone: Extensive via reduction; sulfate and glucuronide conjugation. Ethinyl estradiol: Liver to estrone (metabolite) and estriol (major urinary metabolite); oxidation and conjugation with sulfate and glucuronide (extensive); CYP3A4 to 2-hydroxyethinyl estradiol (primary oxidative metabolite). **Elimination:** Norethindrone: Urine, feces; $T_{1/2}$=13 hrs. Ethinyl estradiol: Urine, feces; $T_{1/2}$=24 hrs.

NURSING CONSIDERATIONS

Assessment: Assess for undiagnosed abnormal genital bleeding, presence or history of breast cancer, estrogen-dependent neoplasia, DVT or PE, active or recent (within past yr) arterial thromboembolic disease (eg, stroke, MI), liver dysfunction, pregnancy/nursing status, age (≥65 yrs), hypertriglyceridemia, hypothyroidism, hypocalcemia, asthma, DM, epilepsy, migraines or porphyria, SLE, and possible drug interactions.

Monitoring: Monitor for signs/symptoms of cardiovascular events (eg, MI, stroke, venous thrombosis, pulmonary embolism), malignant neoplasms (eg, breast, endometrial, ovarian cancer), dementia, gallbladder disease, hypercalcemia, visual abnormalities (eg, retinal vascular thrombosis), elevations in BP, elevations in plasma triglycerides, hypothyroidism, fluid retention, exacerbation of endometriosis and other conditions (eg, asthma, DM, epilepsy, migraines, SLE). Perform annual breast exam. If undiagnosed persistent or recurring abnormal vaginal bleeding occurs, perform adequate diagnostic measures (eg, endometrial sampling) to rule out malignancy. Monitor BP levels regularly. Monitor thyroid function in patients on thyroid replacement therapy. Perform periodic evaluation (every 3-6 months) to determine if treatment is still necessary.

Patient Counseling: Inform that medication may increase risk for heart attack, stroke, breast cancer, and blood clots. Report breast lumps, unusual vaginal bleeding, dizziness and faintness, changes in speech, severe headaches, chest pain, or SOB. Have annual breast exam and mammography; perform monthly self breast exams. Notify physician if planning surgery or bed rest. Take medication at same time every day.

Administration: Oral route. **Storage:** 25°C (77°F); excursions permitted to 15-30°C (59-86°F). Keep out of reach of children.

FENTORA

CII

fentanyl citrate (Cephalon)

Abuse liability. May cause life-threatening respiratory depression in opioid non-tolerant patients. Contraindicated in the management of acute or postoperative pain. Do not use in opioid non-tolerant patients. Adjust dose appropriately when converting from other oral fentanyl products. See Indications.

THERAPEUTIC CLASS: Opioid analgesic

INDICATIONS: Management of breakthrough pain in patients with cancer who are already receiving and who are tolerant to opioid therapy for their underlying persistent cancer pain.

DOSAGE: *Adults:* Initial: Breakthrough Pain: 100mcg. Repeat once (30 min after starting dose) during a single pain episode. Titration Above 100mcg: Use two 100mcg tabs (one on each side of buccal cavity), if not controlled use two 100mcg tabs on each side (total four 100mcg tabs). Titration Above 400mcg: Use 200mcg tab increments. Max: Not more than 4 tabs simultaneously. Re-evaluate maintenance (around-the-clock) opioid dose if >4 episodes of breakthrough pain per day occur. Do not chew, crush, swallow, or dissolve; consume over 14-25 min. Please see the PI for more information on conversion of dosage.

HOW SUPPLIED: Tab, Buccal: 100mcg, 200mcg, 400mcg, 600mcg, 800mcg

CONTRAINDICATIONS: Opioid non-tolerant patients and management of acute or postoperative pain.

WARNINGS/PRECAUTIONS: Caution with concomitant use of other CNS depressants may cause hypoventilation, hypotension, and profound sedation. Caution wtih COPD, bradyarrhythmias, and hepatic or renal impairment. May cause physical dependence, respiratory depression. Extreme caution with evidence of increased intracranial pressure or impaired consciousness. May cause paresthesia, ulceration, or bleeding at application site.

ADVERSE REACTIONS: Respiratory depression, circulatory depression, headache, hypotension, shock, NV, constipation, dizziness, dyspnea, anxiety, somnolence.

INTERACTIONS: Dangerous increases in plasma concentration with potent inhibitors of CYP3A4 (eg, ketoconazole, itraconazole, clarithromycin, nelfinavir, nefazadone, ritonavir), moderate inhibitors of CYP3A4 (eg, amprenavir, diltiazem, fluconazole). CYP3A4 inducers may reduce efficacy. Increased depressant effects with other CNS depressants, including opioids, sedatives, hypnotics, general anesthetics, phenothiazines, tranquilizers, skeletal muscle relaxants, sedating antihistamines. Avoid within 14 days of MAOIs.

PREGNANCY: Category C, not for use in nursing.

MECHANISM OF ACTION: Pure opioid agonist; produces analgesia. Precise analgesic action not established; known to be μ opioid receptor agonist. Specific CNS opioid receptors for endogenous compounds with opioid-like activity are found throughout the brain and spinal cord and are involved in producing analgesic effects.

PHARMACOKINETICS: Absorption: Absolute bioavailability (65%). **Distribution:** V_d=25.4 L/kg; plasma protein binding (80-85%); found in breast milk. **Metabolism:** Liver and intestinal mucosa via CYP3A4; norfentanyl (metabolite). **Elimination:** Urine (<7% unchanged), feces.

NURSING CONSIDERATIONS

Assessment: Assess pain intensity, opioid tolerance, respiratory disorders (eg, COPD), age of patient, drug abuse potential, presence of increased intracranial pressure or impaired consciousness, bradyarrhythmia, renal/hepatic impairment, pregnancy/nursing status, and possible drug interactions.

Monitoring: Monitor for signs/symptoms of respiratory depression, drug abuse, physical dependence, application-site reactions, and bradycardia.

Patient Counseling: Advise to notify physician if signs/symptoms of respiratory depression develop. Keep out of reach of children. Do not swallow whole; will reduce effectiveness. Contact physician if breakthrough pain is not alleviated or worsens. Counsel to avoid using concomitant therapy with other CNS depressants and alcohol. May cause mental/physical impairment; use caution during hazardous tasks (eg, operating machinery/driving). Advise to avoid abrupt withdrawal. Medication has potential for abuse. Counsel to dispose of unused medication via toilet.

Administration: Oral route. Do not substitute for other fentanyl products. Do not open blister package until ready for use. Do not attempt to push tablet through blister card. 1) Place tablet in buccal cavity (above a rear molar, between the upper cheek and gum). Do not attempt to split tablet. 2) Do not suck, chew or swallow. 3) Leave tablet between cheek and gum until disintegrated. 4) After 30 min, swallow remnants with glass of water. **Storage:** 20-25°C (68-77°F); excursions permitted to 15-30°C (59-86°F). Protect from freezing and moisture. Do not use if blister package has been tampered with.

FERRLECIT — RX

sodium ferric gluconate complex (Watson)

THERAPEUTIC CLASS: Hematinic

INDICATIONS: Treatment of iron deficiency anemia in patients ≥6 yrs old undergoing chronic hemodialysis and receiving supplemental epoetin therapy.

DOSAGE: *Adults:* 10mL (125mg) as IV infusion (diluted) over 1 hr or as slow IV injection (undiluted) at a rate of up to 12.5mg/min. Minimum Cumulative Dose: 1g elemental iron over 8 sequential dialysis sessions.

Pediatrics: ≥6 yrs: 0.12mL/kg (1.5mg/kg) as IV infusion over 1 hr at 8 sequential dialysis sessions. Max: 125mg/dose.

HOW SUPPLIED: Inj: 62.5mg elemental iron/5mL

CONTRAINDICATIONS: Anemia not associated with iron deficiency. Evidence of iron overload.

WARNINGS/PRECAUTIONS: Hypersensitivity reactions and hypotension reported. Iron overload is more common in patients with hemoglobinopathies and other refractory anemia. Should not be administered to patients with iron overload. Contains benzyl alcohol; avoid in neonates.

ADVERSE REACTIONS: Injection site reactions, chest pain, pain, asthenia, headache, abdominal pain, cramps, dizziness, dyspnea, hypotension, HTN, nausea, vomiting, diarrhea, leg cramps, pruritus, abnormal erythrocytes.

F

PREGNANCY: Category B, caution in nursing.

MECHANISM OF ACTION: Hematinic; used to replete the total body content of iron, which is critical for normal Hgb synthesis to maintain oxygen transport.

PHARMACOKINETICS: Absorption: Adults: Parameters varied by different dosage. (62.5mg) AUC=17.5mg-h/L; (125mg) C_{max}=19mg/L; T_{max}=7 min; AUC=35.6mg-h/L. **Pediatrics:** (1.5mg/kg) C_{max}=12.9mg/L; T_{max}=2 hrs; AUC=95mg•h/L. (3mg/kg) C_{max}=22.8mg/L; T_{max}=2.5 hrs; AUC=170.9mg•h/L. **Distribution:** V_d=6L. **Elimination:** $T_{1/2}$=1 hr.

NURSING CONSIDERATIONS

Assessment: Assess for evidence of iron overload, anemia, and possible drug interactions.

Monitoring: Monitor for hypersensitivity reactions, iatrogenic hemosiderosis, and hypotension.

Patient Counseling: Advise to seek medical attention if symptoms of hypersensitivity reaction, hypotension (light-headedness, malaise, fatigue, weakness), or hemosiderosis occurs.

Administration: IV. **Storage:** 20-25°C (68-77°F); excursions permitted to 15-30° (59-86°F). Do not freeze.

FINACEA — RX

azelaic acid (Intendis)

THERAPEUTIC CLASS: Dicarboxylic acid antimicrobial

INDICATIONS: Topical treatment of inflammatory papules and pustules of mild to moderate rosacea.

DOSAGE: *Adults:* Wash and dry skin. Massage gently into affected area bid (am and pm) for up to 12 weeks.

HOW SUPPLIED: Gel: 15% [30g]

CONTRAINDICATIONS: Hypersensitivity to propylene glycol.

WARNINGS/PRECAUTIONS: Avoid mouth, eyes, mucous membranes, occlusive dressings, or wrappings. Hypopigmentation reported. D/C if sensitivity or severe irritation occurs. Use only very mild soap or soapless cleansing lotion for facial cleansing. Avoid foods and beverages (eg, spicy foods, alcohol, thermally hot drinks) that may provoke erythema, flushing, and/or blushing.

ADVERSE REACTIONS: Burning, stinging, tingling, pruritus, scaling, dry skin.

INTERACTIONS: Avoid alcoholic cleansers, tinctures, astringents, abrasives and peeling agents.

PREGNANCY: Category B, caution in nursing.

MECHANISM OF ACTION: Dicarboxylic acid antimicrobial; not established.

PHARMACOKINETICS: Absorption: C_{max}=24.0-90.5ng/mL. **Elimination:** Urine (mainly unchanged).

NURSING CONSIDERATIONS

Assessment: Assess use in nursing patients. Assess for possible drug interactions.

Monitoring: Monitor for hypopigmentation and signs/symptoms of skin irritation (eg, pruritus, burning, or stinging).

Patient Counseling: Instruct medication is for external use only; avoid contact with eyes, mouth, and other mucous membranes. If contact with eyes occurs, wash with large amounts of water; consult physician if eye irritation persists. Cleanse affected areas with mild soap or soapless cleansing lotion and pat dry before applying medication. Wash hands following administration of medication. Avoid occlusive dressings or wrappings on treatment site. Cosmetics can be applied to treatment area after medication has dried. Skin irritation (eg, pruritus, burning, stinging) may occur during first few weeks of treatment. If it worsens or persists, instruct to d/c therapy and contact physician. Avoid any foods and beverages that may provoke erythema, flushing, and blushing (eg, spicy food, alcoholic beverage, and thermally hot drinks). Contact physician if abnormal changes in skin color occur.

Administration: Topical administration. **Storage:** 25°C (77°F); excursions permitted to 15-30°C (59-86°F).

FIORICET — RX

acetaminophen - caffeine - butalbital (Watson)

THERAPEUTIC CLASS: Barbiturate/analgesic

INDICATIONS: Tension or muscle contraction headaches.

DOSAGE: *Adults:* 1-2 tabs q4h prn. Max: 6 tabs/day. Not for extended use. *Pediatrics:* ≥12 yrs: 1-2 tabs q4h prn. Max: 6 tabs/day. Not for extended use.

HOW SUPPLIED: Tab: (Butalbital-APAP-Caffeine) 50mg-325mg-40mg

CONTRAINDICATIONS: Porphyria.

WARNINGS/PRECAUTIONS: May be habit-forming. Not for long-term use. Caution in elderly, debilitated, severe renal or hepatic impairment, acute abdominal conditions. Caution in mentally depressed and those with suicidal tendencies, history of drug abuse.

ADVERSE REACTIONS: Drowsiness, lightheadedness, dizziness, sedation, SOB, NV, abdominal pain, intoxicated feeling.

INTERACTIONS: Enhanced CNS effects with MAOIs. May enhance CNS depressant effects of other narcotic analgesics, alcohol, general anesthetics, tranquilizers, sedative hypnotics, or other CNS depressants.

PREGNANCY: Category C, not for use in nursing.

MECHANISM OF ACTION: Butalbital: Short- to intermediate-acting barbiturate. APAP: Nonopiate, nonsalicylate analgesic, antipyretic. Caffeine: CNS stimulant.

PHARMACOKINETICS: Absorption: Well absorbed (butalbital), rapid (APAP, caffeine). **Distribution:** Butalbital: Plasma protein binding (45%); found in breast milk; crosses placenta. Caffeine: Found in CNS, placenta, and breast milk. **Metabolism:** APAP: Liver (conjugation). Caffeine: Hepatic; 1-methylxanthine, 1-methyluric acid. **Elimination:** Butalbital: Urine (59-88% unchanged or metabolite); $T_{1/2}$=35 hrs. APAP: Urine (85% metabolite, unchanged); $T_{1/2}$=1.25-3 hrs. Caffeine: Urine 70% (3% unchanged); $T_{1/2}$=3 hrs.

NURSING CONSIDERATIONS

Assessment: Assess for porphyria, elderly/debilitated patients, renal/hepatic impairment, acute abdominal condition, alcohol intake, and possible drug interactions (eg, MAOIs).

Monitoring: Monitor for drug abuse/dependence. Monitor LFTs , renal function, false (+) test for urinary 5-hydroxyindoleacetic acid.

Patient Counseling: Advise to use caution during hazardous tasks (eg, operating machinery/driving). Instruct not to take with alcohol/other CNS depressants. Advise to take as directed. Inform drug may be habit-forming. Instruct to notify physician if pregnant/nursing.

Administration: Oral route. **Storage:** 30°C (86°F); tight container.

FIORICET WITH CODEINE CIII

codeine phosphate - acetaminophen - caffeine - butalbital (Watson)

THERAPEUTIC CLASS: Barbiturate/analgesic

INDICATIONS: Tension or muscle contraction headaches.

DOSAGE: *Adults:* 1-2 caps q4h prn. Max: 6 caps/day. Not for extended use.

HOW SUPPLIED: Cap: (Butalbital-APAP-Caffeine-Codeine) 50mg-325mg-40mg-30mg

CONTRAINDICATIONS: Porphyria.

WARNINGS/PRECAUTIONS: May be habit forming. Not for extended use. Respiratory depression and CSF pressure enhanced with head injury or intracranial lesions. Caution in elderly, debilitated, severe renal or hepatic impairment, hypothyroidism, urethral stricture, Addison's disease, BPH, and history of drug abuse. May mask signs of acute abdominal conditions.

ADVERSE REACTIONS: Drowsiness, lightheadedness, dizziness, sedation, SOB, NV, abdominal pain, intoxicated feeling.

INTERACTIONS: Enhanced CNS effects with MAOIs. May enhance CNS depressant effects of other narcotic analgesics, alcohol, general anesthetics, tranquilizers, sedative hypnotics, or other CNS depressants.

PREGNANCY: Category C, not for use in nursing.

MECHANISM OF ACTION: Codeine: Narcotic analgesic and antitussive. Butalbital: Short- to intermediate-acting barbiturate. Caffeine: CNS stimulant. APAP: Nonopiate, nonsalicylate analgesic and antipyretic. The role each component plays in relief of complex of symptoms known as tension headache is incompletely understood.

PHARMACOKINETICS: Absorption: Butalbital: Well absorbed. Codeine, caffeine, acetaminophen: Rapid. **Distribution:** Codeine: Crosses blood-brain barrier, found in fetal tissue, breast milk. Butalbital: Plasma protein binding (45%); found in breast milk; crosses placental barrier. Caffeine: Found in fetal tissue, CNS, breast milk. **Metabolism:** Caffeine: Hepatic biotransformation to 1-methylxanthine, 1-methyluric acid. APAP: Liver (conjugation). **Elimination:** Codeine: Urine (90%), feces; $T_{1/2}$=2.9 hrs. Butalbital: Urine (59-88% unchanged or metabolites); $T_{1/2}$=35 hrs. Caffeine: Urine (70%, only 3% unchanged); $T_{1/2}$=3 hrs. APAP: Urine (85% unchanged, conjugates); $T_{1/2}$=1.25-3 hrs.

NURSING CONSIDERATIONS

Assessment: Assess for porphyria, renal/hepatic impairment, head injuries or other intracranial lesions, elevated intracranial pressure, acute abdominal conditions, elderly/debilitated patients, hypothyroidism, urethral stricture, Addison's disease, prostatic hypertrophy, pregnancy/nursing status, alcohol intake, individual with ultra-rapid metabolizers, and possible drug interactions.

Monitoring: Serial monitoring of LFTs, renal function. Monitor serum amylase levels, false (+) test results for urinary 5-hydroxyindoleacetic acid, drug abuse/dependence, CSF, and signs of CNS depression (eg, drowsiness, confusion, or shallow breathing).

Patient Counseling: Advise to use caution during hazardous tasks (eg, driving/operating machinery). Instruct not to take with other CNS depressants or alcohol. Advise to take as prescribed. Instruct to notify physician if pregnant/nursing or planning to become pregnant. Counsel that drug may be habit-forming.

Administration: Oral route. **Storage**: 30°C (86°F); tight container.

FIORINAL

CIII

caffeine - aspirin - butalbital (Watson)

THERAPEUTIC CLASS: Barbiturate/analgesic

INDICATIONS: Tension or muscle contraction headache.

DOSAGE: *Adults:* 1-2 caps q4h prn. Max: 6 caps/day. Not for extended use.

HOW SUPPLIED: Cap: (Butalbital-ASA-Caffeine) 50mg-325mg-40mg

CONTRAINDICATIONS: Porphyria, peptic ulcer disease, serious GI lesions, hemorrhagic diathesis. Syndrome of nasal polyps, angioedema, and bronchospastic reactivity to ASA or NSAIDs.

F

WARNINGS/PRECAUTIONS: May be habit-forming. Not for extended use. Caution in elderly, debilitated, severe renal or hepatic impairment, hypothyroidism, urethral stricture, head injuries, elevated ICP, acute abdominal conditions, Addison's disease, prostatic hypertrophy, peptic ulcer, coagulation disorders. Avoid with ASA allergy. Risk of ASA hypersensitivity with nasal polyps and asthma. Caution in children with chickenpox or flu. Preoperative ASA may prolong bleeding time.

ADVERSE REACTIONS: Drowsiness, lightheadedness, dizziness, sedation, nausea, vomiting, flatulence.

INTERACTIONS: CNS effects enhanced by MAOIs. Additive CNS depression with alcohol, other narcotic analgesics, general anesthetics, tranquilizers (eg, chloral hydrate), sedatives/hypnotics, other CNS depressants. May enhance effects of anticoagulants. May cause hypoglycemia with oral antidiabetic agents and insulin. May cause bone marrow toxicity and blood dyscrasias with 6-MP and methotrexate. Increased risk of peptic ulceration and bleeding with NSAIDs. Decreased effects of uricosuric agents (eg, probenecid, sulfinpyrazone). Withdrawal of corticosteroids may cause salicylism with chronic ASA use.

PREGNANCY: Category C, not for use in nursing.

MECHANISM OF ACTION: Combines analgesic properties of ASA with anxiolytic and muscle relaxant properties of butalbital.

PHARMACOKINETICS: Absorption: ASA: T_{max}=40 min, C_{max}=8.8mcg/mL. Butalbital: Well-absorbed; C_{max}=202ng/mL, T_{max}=1.5 hrs. Caffeine: Rapid; C_{max}=1660ng/mL, $T_{max} \leq 1$ hr. **Distribution:** ASA: Found in fetal tissue, breast milk, CNS; Plasma protein binding (50-80%). Butalbital: Crosses placenta, found in breast milk; Plasma protein binding (45%). Caffeine: Found in placenta, breast milk, CNS. **Metabolism:** ASA: Liver; salicyluric acid, phenolic/acyl glucuronides of salicylate, and gentisic and gentisuric acid (major metabolites). Caffeine: Liver; 1-methylxanthine and 1-methyluric acid (metabolites). **Elimination:** ASA: Urine; $T_{1/2}$=12 min (ASA), 3 hrs (salicylic acid/total salicylates). Butalbital: Urine (59-88%); $T_{1/2}$=35 hrs. Caffeine: Urine 70% (3% unchanged); $T_{1/2}$=3 hrs.

NURSING CONSIDERATIONS

Assessment: Assess for hemorrhagic diathesis (eg, hemophilia, hypoprothrombinemia, von Willebrand's disease, thrombocytopenia, thrombasthenia and other ill-defined hereditary platelet dysfunctions, severe vitamin K deficiency and severe liver damage), syndrome of nasal polyps, angioedema and bronchospastic reactivity to aspirin and other NSAIDs, peptic ulcer, asthma, porphyria, renal/hepatic impairment, children with chickenpox or flu, head injuries, hypothyroidism, urethral stricture, elevated ICP, acute abdominal conditions, Addison's disease, prostatic hypertrophy, pregnancy/nursing status, and possible drug interactions.

Monitoring: Serial monitoring of LFTs and renal function. Monitor for anaphylactoid reactions, drug abuse/dependence, bleeding, prolongation of bleeding time, PT, urinary (glucose, 5-hydroxyindoleactic acid, Gerhardt ketone, VMA, uric acid, diacetic acid, spectrophotometric detection of barbiturates), Reye's syndrome, serum amylase, FBG, cholesterol, protein, and uric acid.

Patient Counseling: Advise not to take with ASA allergy. Instruct to take exactly as prescribed; do not take with alcohol or other CNS depressants.

Advise to use caution during hazardous tasks (eg, operating machinery/driving). Counsel that drug may be habit-forming. Advise to notify physician if pregnant, nursing, or planning to become pregnant.

Administration: Oral route. **Storage:** 77°F (25°C); tight container.

FIORINAL WITH CODEINE CIII

codeine phosphate - caffeine - aspirin - butalbital (Watson)

THERAPEUTIC CLASS: Barbiturate/analgesic

INDICATIONS: Tension or muscle contraction headache.

DOSAGE: *Adults:* 1-2 caps q4h prn. Max: 6 caps/day. Not for extended use.

HOW SUPPLIED: Cap: (Butalbital-ASA-Caffeine-Codeine) 50mg-325mg-40mg-30mg

CONTRAINDICATIONS: Porphyria, peptic ulcer disease, serious GI lesions, hemorrhagic diathesis. Syndrome of nasal polyps, angioedema and bronchospastic reactivity to ASA or NSAIDs.

WARNINGS/PRECAUTIONS: May be habit-forming. Not for extended use. Respiratory depression and CSF pressure may be enhanced with head injury or intracranial lesions. Caution in elderly, debilitated, severe renal or hepatic impairment, hypothyroidism, urethral stricture, head injuries, elevated ICP, acute abdominal conditions, Addison's disease, prostatic hypertrophy, peptic ulcer, coagulation disorders. Caution in children with chickenpox or flu. May obscure acute abdominal conditions. Preoperative ASA may prolong bleeding time. Avoid with ASA allergy. Risk of ASA hypersensitivity with nasal polyps and asthma.

ADVERSE REACTIONS: Drowsiness, lightheadedness, dizziness, sedation, SOB, NV, abdominal pain, intoxicated feeling.

INTERACTIONS: CNS effects enhanced by MAOIs. Additive CNS depression with alcohol, other narcotic analgesics, general anesthetics, tranquilizers (eg, chloral hydrate), sedatives/hypnotics, other CNS depressants. May enhance effects of anticoagulants. May cause hypoglycemia with oral antidiabetic agents, insulin. May cause bone marrow toxicity, blood dyscrasias with 6-MP and methotrexate. Increased risk of peptic ulceration, bleeding with NSAIDs. Decreased effects of uricosuric agents (eg, probenecid, sulfinpyrazone). Withdrawal of corticosteroids may cause salicylism with chronic ASA use.

PREGNANCY: Category C, not for use in nursing.

MECHANISM OF ACTION: Butalbital: Short to intermediate acting barbiturate. ASA: Analgesic, antipyretic, and anti-inflammatory. Caffeine: Stimulates CNS. Codeine: Narcotic analgesic and antitussive. Role each component plays in relief of complex of symptoms known as tension headache is incompletely understood.

PHARMACOKINETICS: Absorption: Codeine: Rapid; C_{max}=198ng/mL, T_{max}=1 hr. Butalbital: Well-absorbed; C_{max}=2020ng/mL, T_{max}=1.5 hrs. Caffeine: Rapid; C_{max}=1660ng/mL, T_{max}≤1 hr. **Distribution:** ASA: Plasma protein binding (50-80%); found in fetal tissue, breast milk, CNS. Codeine: Crosses BBB, placenta, and breast milk. Butalbital: Plasma protein binding (45%); crosses placenta and breast milk. Caffeine: Fetal tissue, breast milk and CNS. **Metabolism:** ASA: Liver; salicyluric acid, phenolic/acyl glucuronides of salicylate, and gentisic and gentisuric acid (major metabolites). Codeine: Glucuronidation. Caffeine: Liver; 1-methylxanthine and 1-methyluric acid. **Elimination:** ASA: Urine; $T_{1/2}$=12 min (ASA), 3 hrs (salicylic acid/total salicylate). Codeine: Urine (90%), feces; $T_{1/2}$=2.9 hrs. Butalbital: Urine (59-88%); $T_{1/2}$=35 hrs. Caffeine: Urine 70% (3% unchanged); $T_{1/2}$=3 hrs.

NURSING CONSIDERATIONS

Assessment: Assess for hemorrhagic diathesis (eg, hemophilia, hypoprothrombinemia, von Willebrand's disease, thrombocytopenia, thrombasthenia and other ill-defined hereditary platelet dysfunctions, severe vitamin K deficiency and severe liver damage), anticoagulant therapy, asthma, syndrome of nasal polyps, angioedema and bronchospastic reactivity to NSAIDs, peptic ulcer, porphyria, renal/hepatic impairment, hypothyroidism, urethral stricture, head injuries, elevated ICP, acute abdominal conditions, Addison's disease, prostatic hypertrophy, pregnancy/nursing status, children with chickenpox or flu, individuals with ultra-rapid metabolizers, alcohol intake, and possible drug interactions.

Monitoring: Serial monitoring of LFTs, renal function tests. Monitor for anaphylactoid reactions, symptoms of CNS depression (eg, drowsiness, confusion, shallow breathing), drug abuse/dependence, bleeding, prolongation of bleeding time, PT, urinary (glucose, 5-hydroxyindoleactic acid, Gerhardt ketone, VMA, uric acid, diacetic acid, spectrophotometric detection of barbiturates), Reye's syndrome, serum amylase, FBG, cholesterol, protein, and uric acid.

Patient Counseling: Advise not to take if patient has aspirin allergy. Take as prescribed; do not take with alcohol or other CNS depressants. Caution during hazardous tasks (eg, operating machinery/driving). Potential psychological dependence and for abuse. Notify if pregnant/nursing or planning to become pregnant. Inform about risks/benefits and to report any adverse reactions to physician.

Administration: Oral route. **Storage:** <25°C (77°F); tight container.

FLAGYL — RX

metronidazole (G.D. Searle)

> **Metronidazole has been shown to be carcinogenic in mice and rats. Unnecessary use of the drug should be avoided.**

THERAPEUTIC CLASS: Nitroimidazole

INDICATIONS: Treatment of symptomatic/asymptomatic trichomoniasis, asymptomatic consorts, acute intestinal amebiasis, amebic liver abscess, and anaerobic bacterial infections (following IV metronidazole therapy for serious infections) caused by susceptible strains of microorganisms. Treatment of intra-abdominal, skin and skin structure, bone/joint, CNS, lower respiratory tract, and gynecologic infections, septicemia, and endocarditis caused by susceptible strains of microorganisms.

DOSAGE: *Adults:* Trichomoniasis (Female/Male Sex Partner): Seven-Day Treatment: (Cap/Tab) 375mg bid or 250mg tid for 7 days. One-Day Therapy: (Tab) 2g as single dose or in two divided doses of 1g each given in the same day. If repeat course needed, reconfirm diagnosis and allow 4-6 weeks between courses. Acute Intestinal Amebiasis: 750mg PO tid for 5-10 days. Amebic Liver Abscess: 500mg or 750mg PO tid for 5-10 days. Anaerobic Bacterial Infection: Usually IV therapy initially if serious. 7.5mg/kg PO q6h for 7-10 days or longer. Max: 4g/24 hrs. Elderly: Adjust dose based on serum levels. Hepatic Disease: Give lower dose cautiously; monitor levels. *Pediatrics:* Amebiasis: 35-50mg/kg/24 hrs given tid for 10 days.

HOW SUPPLIED: Cap: 375mg; Tab: 250mg, 500mg

CONTRAINDICATIONS: Treatment during 1st trimester of pregnancy.

WARNINGS/PRECAUTIONS: Seizures and peripheral neuropathy reported. D/C if abnormal neurological signs occur. Caution with severe hepatic impairment, blood dyscrasias, or CNS diseases. Monitor leukocytes before and after therapy.

ADVERSE REACTIONS: Seizures, peripheral neuropathy, NV, headache, anorexia, urticaria, rash, metallic taste, dysuria, vaginal candidiasis, dizziness, leukopenia.

INTERACTIONS: Avoid alcohol during and for 3 days after use. Avoid within 2 weeks of disulfiram use; increased possibility of psychotic reactions. May potentiate anticoagulant effects of warfarin; monitor PT. Increased elimination with phenytoin, phenobarbital and other hepatic enzyme inducers. May impair phenytoin clearance. Potentiated by cimetidine and other hepatic enzyme inhibitors. May increase lithium levels.

PREGNANCY: Category B, not for use in nursing.

MECHANISM OF ACTION: Nitroimidazole antibacterial; exerts effect in anaerobic environment. Possesses bactericidal, amebicidal, and trichomonacidal activity.

PHARMACOKINETICS: Absorption: (PO) Well absorbed. PO administration of variable doses resulted in different parameters. **Distribution:** Plasma protein binding (<20%); excreted in breast milk. **Metabolism:** Side-chain oxidation and glucuronide conjugation. **Elimination:** Urine (60-80%), feces (6-15%); $T_{1/2}$=8 hrs.

NURSING CONSIDERATIONS

Assessment: Assess for history of convulsions, peripheral neuropathy, candidiasis, renal function tests, LFTs, pregnancy status, and possible drug interactions.

Monitoring: Monitor CBC with differential count, LFTs, seizures, hypersensitivity reactions, peripheral neuropathy, candidiasis.

Patient Counseling: Instruct to avoid alcohol during therapy and for at least 3 days afterward. Counsel to take as directed and to complete entire prescription. Take with food to reduce GI upset; may cause metallic taste. Exercise caution while driving or operating machinery. During treatment for trichomoniasis, treat partner also and use condoms to prevent reinfection.

Administration: Oral route. **Storage:** Below 25°C (77°F). Protect from light.

F

FLAGYL ER — RX

metronidazole (Pharmacia & Upjohn)

Metronidazole has been shown to be carcinogenic in mice and rats. Unnecessary use of the drug should be avoided.

THERAPEUTIC CLASS: Nitroimidazole

INDICATIONS: Treatment of bacterial vaginosis.

DOSAGE: *Adults:* 750mg qd for 7 days. Take 1 hr before or 2 hrs after meals. Elderly: Adjust dose based on serum levels. Hepatic Disease: Give lower dose cautiously; monitor levels.

HOW SUPPLIED: Tab, Extended-Release: 750mg

CONTRAINDICATIONS: Treatment during 1st trimester of pregnancy.

WARNINGS/PRECAUTIONS: Seizures and peripheral neuropathy reported. D/C if abnormal neurological signs occur. Caution with severe hepatic impairment, blood dyscrasias, or CNS diseases. Monitor leukocytes before and after therapy.

ADVERSE REACTIONS: Headache, vaginitis, NV, metallic taste, dizziness, seizures, peripheral neuropathy, leukopenia, urticaria, rash, dysuria, vaginal candidiasis.

INTERACTIONS: Avoid alcohol during and for 3 days after use. Avoid within 2 weeks of disulfiram; increased possibility of psychotic reactions. Potentiates anticoagulant effects of warfarin; monitor PT. Increased elimination with phenytoin, phenobarbital. May impair phenytoin clearance. Potentiated by cimetidine. Increased lithium levels.

PREGNANCY: Category B, not for use in nursing.

MECHANISM OF ACTION: Nitroimidazole antibacterial; exerts effect in anaerobic environment. Possesses bactericidal, amebicidal, and trichomonacidal activity.

PHARMACOKINETICS: Absorption: C_{max}=19.4µg/mL (fed), 12.5µg/mL (fasting); T_{max}=4 hrs (fed), 6.8 hrs (fasting); AUC=211µg/mL (fed), 198µg/mL (fasting). **Distribution:** Plasma protein binding (<20%). **Metabolism:** Side-chain oxidation and glucuronide conjugation. **Elimination:** Urine (60-80%), feces (6-15%); $T_{1/2}$=8 hrs.

NURSING CONSIDERATIONS

Assessment: Assess for history of convulsions, peripheral neuropathy, candidiasis, hepatic/renal function, pregnancy status, and possible drug interactions.

Monitoring: Monitor CBC with differential, LFTs, seizures, hypersensitivity reactions, peripheral neuropathy, candidial proliferation.

Patient Counseling: Inform to avoid alcohol during therapy and for at least 3 days after. Counsel to take as directed and complete entire prescription. Take with food to reduce GI upset; may cause metallic taste. Exercise caution while driving or operating machinery. During treatment for trichomoniasis, treat partner also and use condoms to prevent reinfection.

Administration: Oral route. **Storage:** Dry place at 25°C (77°F); excursions permitted to 15-86°C (59-86°F). Dispense in a well-closed container.

FLAGYL IV

RX

metronidazole HCl (Various)

Metronidazole has been shown to be carcinogenic in mice and rats. Unnecessary use of the drug should be avoided.

THERAPEUTIC CLASS: Nitroimidazole

INDICATIONS: Treatment of serious infections caused by susceptible anaerobic bacteria. Treatment of intra-abdominal, skin and skin structure, gynecologic, bone and joint, CNS, and lower respiratory tract infections; bacterial septicemia; and endocarditis caused by susceptible microorganisms. Prophylaxis of infection in contaminated or potentially contaminated colorectal surgery.

DOSAGE: *Adults:* Anaerobic Infections: LD: 15mg/kg IV. Maint: 7.5mg/kg IV q6h, starting 6 hrs after LD. Usual duration is 7-10 days or longer. Max: 4g/24 hrs. Surgical Prophylaxis: 15mg/kg given 1 hr before surgery, then 7.5mg/kg given 6 hrs and 12 hrs after initial dose.

HOW SUPPLIED: Inj: 500mg/100mL

WARNINGS/PRECAUTIONS: Seizures and peripheral neuropathy reported. D/C if abnormal neurological signs occur. Caution with severe hepatic impairment, blood dyscrasias, or CNS disease. Monitor leukocytes before and after therapy. Metronidazole IV is effective in *B.fragilis* infections resistant to clindamycin, chloramphenicol, or PCN.

ADVERSE REACTIONS: Convulsive seizures, peripheral neuropathy, NV, headache, leukopenia, rash, vaginal candidiasis, thrombophlebitis.

INTERACTIONS: Avoid alcohol during and for 3 days after use. Avoid within 2 weeks of disulfiram; increased possibility of psychotic reactions. Potentiates warfarin. Increased elimination with phenytoin, phenobarbital. May impair phenytoin clearance. Potentiated by cimetidine. Increased lithium levels.

PREGNANCY: Category B, not for use in nursing.

MECHANISM OF ACTION: Nitroimidazole antibacterial; exerts effect in anaerobic environment. Possesses bactericidal, amebicidal, and trichomonacidal activity.

PHARMACOKINETICS: Distribution: Plasma protein binding (<20%); found in breast milk. **Metabolism:** Liver via side-chain oxidation and glucuronide conjugation. **Elimination:** Urine (60-80%), feces (6-15%); $T_{1/2}$=8 hrs.

NURSING CONSIDERATIONS

Assessment: Assess LFTs, renal function, peripheral neuropathy, history of convulsions, candidiasis, pregnancy status, and possible drug interactions.

Monitoring: Monitor CBC with differential, LFTs, renal function, seizures, hypersensitivity reactions, peripheral neuropathy, candidial proliferation.

Patient Counseling: Instruct to take as directed and complete entire prescription. May cause metallic taste. Report any symptoms of CNS toxicity or adverse side effects.

Administration: IV route; via slow infusion (continuous or intermittent).
Storage: 15-30°C (59-86°F).

FLECTOR RX
diclofenac epolamine (Alpharma)

NSAIDs may cause an increased risk of serious cardiovascular thrombotic events, MI, stroke and serious GI adverse events including bleeding, ulceration, and perforation of the stomach or intestines. Contraindicated for the treatment of perioperative pain in the setting of coronary artery bypass graft (CABG) surgery.

F

THERAPEUTIC CLASS: NSAID

INDICATIONS: Topical treatment of acute pain due to minor strains, sprains, and contusions.

DOSAGE: *Adults:* Apply 1 patch to most painful area bid.

HOW SUPPLIED: Patch: 180mg [5[s]]

CONTRAINDICATIONS: ASA or other NSAID allergy that precipitates asthma, urticaria, or allergic-type reactions. Treatment of perioperative pain in the setting of CABG surgery. Application to non-intact or damaged skin (eg, exudative dermatitis, eczema, infected lesion, burns or wounds).

WARNINGS/PRECAUTIONS: May lead to onset of new HTN or worsening of pre-existing HTN; monitor BP closely. Fluid retention and edema reported; caution with fluid retention or heart failure. Renal papillary necrosis and other renal injury reported after long-term use. Not recommended for use with advanced renal disease; if therapy must be initiated, monitor renal function. Anaphylactoid reactions may occur. May cause serious skin adverse events (eg, exfoliative dermatitis, Stevens-Johnson syndrome, and toxic epidermal necrolysis). Avoid in late pregnancy; may cause premature closure of ductus arteriosus. May cause elevations of LFTs; d/c if liver disease develops or systemic manifestations occur. Rare cases of severe hepatic reactions (eg, jaundice, fatal fulminant hepatitis, liver necrosis, hepatic failure) reported. Anemia may occur; with long-term use, monitor Hgb/Hct if signs or symptoms of anemia develop. May inhibit platelet aggregation and prolong bleeding time; monitor with coagulation disorders. Caution with asthma and avoid with ASA-sensitive asthma. Wash hands after applying, handling, or removing patch. Avoid contact with eye and mucosa.

ADVERSE REACTIONS: Pruritus, dermatitis, burning, nausea, dysgeusia, dyspepsia, headache, paresthesia, somnolence.

INTERACTIONS: May diminish the antihypertensive effect of ACE inhibitors. Increased adverse effects with ASA; avoid use. May reduce natriuretic effect of furosemide and thiazides; monitor for renal failure. May enhance lithium and methotrexate toxicity; caution when co-administering. Synergistic effects on GI bleeding with warfarin.

PREGNANCY: Category C, not for use in nursing.

MECHANISM OF ACTION: NSAID; not established, suspected to inhibit prostaglandin synthetase.

PHARMACOKINETICS: Absorption: C_{max}=0.7-6ng/mL, T_{max}=10-20 hrs. **Ditribution:** Plasma protein binding (>99%). **Elimination:** Urine, bile; $T_{1/2}$=12 hrs.

NURSING CONSIDERATIONS

Assessment: Assess for history of asthma, cardiovascular disease (pre-existing HTN, CHF) or risk factors for disease, fluid retention, edema, exudative dermatitis, eczema, infected lesions, burns, wounds, pregnancy status, risk factors for GI events (bleeding, ulceration, perforation), possible drug interactions, renal/hepatic impairment.

Monitoring: Monitor CBC, LFTs, renal function and chemistries periodically. Monitor for signs/symptoms of GI events (bleeding, ulceration, perforation), CV thrombotic events, CHF, HTN, salt depletion, hypersensitivity reactions, renal/hepatic dysfunction.

Patient Counseling: Instruct only to use on intact skin (wash hands after handling). Avoid contact with eyes; do not wear when bathing or showering. Seek medical attention if experience symptoms of hepatotoxicity (nausea, fatigue, pruritis), anaphylactic reaction (difficulty breathing, swelling of face/throat), hypersensitivity reaction (rash), CV events (chest pain, SOB, weakness, slurring of speech), GI ulceration and bleeding (epigastric pain, dyspepsia, melena, hematemesis), bronchospasm (wheezing, SOB), weight gain or edema. Inform of pregnancy risks.

Administration: Transdermal route. **Storage**: 25°C (77°F) excursions permitted to 15-30°C (59-86°F). Keep sealed at all times when not in use.

F

FLEXERIL RX

cyclobenzaprine HCl (McNeil Consumer)

THERAPEUTIC CLASS: Skeletal muscle relaxant (central-acting)

INDICATIONS: Relief of muscle spasm associated with acute, painful musculoskeletal conditions.

DOSAGE: *Adults:* Usual: 5mg tid. Titrate: May increase to 10mg tid. Mild Hepatic Dysfunction/Elderly: Initial: 5mg qd, then slowly increase. Moderate/Severe Hepatic Dysfunction: Avoid use. Treatment should not exceed 2-3 weeks.
Pediatrics: ≥15 yrs: Usual: 5mg tid. Titrate: May increase to 10mg tid. Mild Hepatic Dysfunction/Elderly: Initial: 5mg qd, then slowly increase. Moderate/Severe Hepatic Dysfunction: Avoid use. Treatment should not exceed 2-3 weeks.

HOW SUPPLIED: Tab: 5mg, 10mg

CONTRAINDICATIONS: Acute recovery phase of MI, arrhythmias, heart block or conduction disturbances, CHF, hyperthyroidism, MAOI use during or within 14 days.

WARNINGS/PRECAUTIONS: Caution with history of urinary retention, angle-closure glaucoma, increased IOP, hepatic dysfunction. Caution in elderly due to increased risk of CNS effects. May produce arrhythmias, sinus tachycardia and conduction time prolongation. May impair mental/physical abilities.

ADVERSE REACTIONS: Drowsiness, dry mouth, headache, fatigue.

INTERACTIONS: Enhances effects of alcohol, barbiturates, and other CNS depressants. May block antihypertensive action of guanethidine and similar compounds. May enhance seizure risk with tramadol. Contraindicated with MAOIs. Caution with anticholinergic medication.

PREGNANCY: Category B, caution in nursing.

MECHANISM OF ACTION: Centrally acting skeletal muscle relaxant; relieves skeletal muscle spasm of local origin without interfering with muscle function; reduces tonic somatic motor activity by influencing both gamma and α motor systems.

PHARMACOKINETICS: Absorption: Oral bioavailability (33-55%); C_{max}=25.9ng/mL; AUC=177ng•hr/mL. **Metabolism**: Extensive; through N-demethylation pathway. Via CYP3A4, 1A2, and 2D6. **Elimination**: Urine (glucuronides); $T_{1/2}$=18 hrs.

NURSING CONSIDERATIONS

Assessment: Assess for hepatic impairment, seizures, hyperthyroidism, urinary retention, angle-closure glaucoma, IOP, recent MI, arrhythmias, heart block, CHF, alcohol intake, pregnancy/nursing status, and possible drug interactions (eg, MAOIs if concomitant use or within 14 days after d/c, and anticholinergic medications).

Monitoring: Monitor for cardiac arrhythmias, sinus tachycardia, MI, increased seizure risk, stroke, IOP, CBC, and LFTs.

Patient Counseling: Caution while performing hazardous tasks (eg, operating machinery/driving). Avoid alcohol or other CNS depressants. Notify if pregnant/nursing.

Administration: Oral route. **Storage**: 25°C (77°F); excursions permitted to 15-30°C (59-86°F).

FLOMAX RX
tamsulosin HCl (Boehringer Ingelheim)

THERAPEUTIC CLASS: Alpha$_{1a}$-antagonist

INDICATIONS: Treatment of signs and symptoms of benign prostatic hyperplasia.

DOSAGE: *Adults:* Initial: 0.4mg qd, 1/2 hr after same meal each day. Titrate: May increase to 0.8mg qd after 2-4 weeks. If therapy is interrupted, restart with 0.4mg qd.

F

HOW SUPPLIED: Cap: 0.4mg

WARNINGS/PRECAUTIONS: Rule out prostate cancer. Orthostasis/syncope may occur. May cause priapism (rare). Intraoperative Floppy Iris Syndrome (IFIS) has been observed during cataract surgery. Do not crush, chew, or open capsules. Use with caution if sulfa allergy present.

ADVERSE REACTIONS: Headache, dizziness, somnolence, diarrhea, asthenia, back pain, pharyngitis, rhinitis, abnormal ejaculation.

INTERACTIONS: Avoid use with other α-blockers. Decreased clearance with cimetidine; caution with concomitant use, especially with doses higher than 0.4mg. Caution with warfarin. Concomitant administration of Flomax with moderate or strong inhibitor of CYP2D6 or CYP3A4 may lead to increased Flomax plasma exposure.

PREGNANCY: Category B, not for use in women.

MECHANISM OF ACTION: α_{1A} adrenoreceptor antagonist.

PHARMACOKINETICS: Absorption: Complete, (0.4mg) C_{max}=10ng/mL, T_{max}=6 hrs, AUC=151ng•hr/mL. (0.8 mg) C_{max}=29.8ng/mL, T_{max}=7 hrs, AUC=440ng•hr/mL. Refer to PI for parameters in high-fat breakfast/fasted states. **Distribution:** V_d=16L, plasma protein binding (94-99%). **Metabolism:** CYP450. **Elimination:** Urine (<10%), feces; $T_{1/2}$=14-15 hrs.

NURSING CONSIDERATIONS

Assessment: Assess for sulfa allergy and possible drug interactions. Rule out prostate cancer.

Monitoring: Monitor for signs/symptoms of orthostasis and allergic reactions.

Patient Counseling: Advise about possible occurrence of symptoms related to postural hypotension; caution may impair physical/mental abilities. Avoid situations where injury could result if syncope occurs. Do not crush, chew, or open capsule. Advise if considering cataract surgery to inform ophthalmologist of drug use.

Administration: Oral route. **Storage:** 25°C (77°F); excursions permitted to 15-30°C (59-86°F).

FLONASE RX
fluticasone propionate (GlaxoSmithKline)

THERAPEUTIC CLASS: Corticosteroid

INDICATIONS: Management of the nasal symptoms of seasonal and perennial allergic rhinitis, and nonallergic rhinitis.

DOSAGE: *Adults:* Initial: 2 sprays per nostril qd or 1 spray per nostril bid. Maint: 1 spray per nostril qd. May dose as 2 sprays per nostril qd as needed for seasonal allergic rhinitis.
Pediatrics: ≥4 yrs: Initial: 1 sprays per nostril qd. If inadequate response, may increase to 2 sprays per nostril. Maint: 1 spray per nostril qd. Max: 2 sprays per nostril/day. ≥12 yrs: May dose as 2 sprays per nostril qd as needed for seasonal allergic rhinitis.

HOW SUPPLIED: Spray: 50mcg/spray [16g]

WARNINGS/PRECAUTIONS: Risk of adrenal insufficiency and withdrawal symptoms when replacing systemic corticosteroids with topical corticosteroids. Caution with active or quiescent TB, ocular herpes simplex, or untreated bacterial, fungal and systemic viral infections. Avoid with recent nasal trauma, surgery or septum ulcers. Risk for more severe/fatal course of infections (eg, chickenpox, measles); avoid exposure in patients who have not had disease or been properly immunized. *Candida* infection of nose and pharynx reported (rare). Potential for reduced growth velocity in pediatrics. Excessive use may cause signs of hypercorticism or HPA suppression.

ADVERSE REACTIONS: Headache, pharyngitis, epistaxis, nasal burning/irritation, asthma symptoms, nausea/vomiting, cough.

INTERACTIONS: Caution with ketoconazole or other potent CYP3A4 inhibitors, may increase serum fluticasone levels. Concomitant inhaled corticosteroids increase risk of hypercorticism and/or HPA axis suppression. Increased levels with ritonavir; avoid use.

PREGNANCY: Category C, caution in nursing.

MECHANISM OF ACTION: Glucocorticosteroid; not established. Acts as anti-inflammatory agent with wide range of effects on multiple cell types (eg, mast cells, eosinophils, macrophages, and lymphocytes) and mediators (eg, histamine, eicosanoids, leukotrienes, and cytokines) involved in inflammation.

PHARMACOKINETICS: Absorption: Absolute bioavailability (<2%), C_{max}=50pg/mL.

NURSING CONSIDERATIONS

Assessment: Assess for drug hypersensitivity, active or quiescent TB, untreated localized or systemic infections (eg, fungal, bacterial, systemic viral, parasitic), ocular herpes simplex, history of recent nasal septal ulcers, nasal surgery/trauma, concomitant use with other inhaled or systemic corticosteroids, and possible drug interactions.

Monitoring: Monitor acute adrenal insufficiency, hypercorticism and/or HPA-axis suppression, disseminated infections, chickenpox and measles, nasal or pharyngeal *Candida* infections, supression of growth velocity in children, hypersensitivity reactions or contact dermatitis, wheezing, nasal septum perforation, cataracts, glaucoma, and increased IOP.

Patient Counseling: Instruct to take as directed at regular intervals and to avoid exposure to chickenpox or measles and, consult physician immediately if exposed. Do not spray into eyes.

Administration: Intranasal route. **Storage:** 4-30°C (39-86°F).

FLOVENT HFA RX

fluticasone propionate (GlaxoSmithKline)

THERAPEUTIC CLASS: Corticosteroid

INDICATIONS: Maintenance treatment of asthma as prophylactic therapy in patients ≥4 years; to reduce or eliminate the need for oral corticosteroidal therapy.

DOSAGE: *Adults:* Previous Bronchodilator Only: Initial: 88mcg bid. Max: 440mcg bid. Previous Inhaled Corticosteroids: Initial: 88-220mcg bid. Max: 440mcg bid. Previous Oral Corticosteroids: Initial: 440mcg bid. Max: 880mcg bid. Reduce PO prednisone no faster than 2.5 to 5mg/day weekly, beginning at least 1 week after starting fluticasone. Rinse mouth after use.
Pediatrics: ≥12 yrs: Previous Bronchodilator Only: Initial: 88mcg bid. Max: 440mcg bid. Previous Inhaled Corticosteroids: Initial: 88-220mcg bid. Max: 440mcg bid. Previous Oral Corticosteroids: Initial: 440mcg bid. Max: 880mcg bid. 4-11 yrs: Initial/Max: 88mcg bid. Reduce PO prednisone no faster than 2.5 to 5mg/day weekly, beginning at least 1 week after starting fluticasone. Rinse mouth after use.

HOW SUPPLIED: MDI: 44mcg/inh [10.6g], 110mcg/inh [12g], 220mcg/inh [12g]

CONTRAINDICATIONS: Primary treatment of status asthmaticus or other acute asthma attacks.

WARNINGS/PRECAUTIONS: Deaths due to adrenal insufficiency have occurred with transfer from systemic corticosteroids to inhaled corticosteroids. Resume oral corticosteroids during stress or severe asthma attack. Wean slowly from systemic corticosteroid therapy. Observe for adrenal insufficiency, systemic corticosteroid withdrawal effects, hypercorticism, adrenal suppression (including adrenal crisis), reduction in growth velocity (children and adolescents). May increase susceptibility to infections. Not for acute bronchospasm. D/C if bronchospasm occurs after dosing. Caution with TB of respiratory tract; untreated systemic fungal, bacterial, viral or parasitic infections; or ocular herpes simplex. *Candida* infection of mouth and pharynx reported. Glaucoma, increased IOP and cataracts reported. Rare cases of eosinophilic conditions.

ADVERSE REACTIONS: Upper respiratory tract infection, headache, throat irritation, sinusitis/sinus infection, candidiasis (mouth/throat and non-site specific), and cough.

INTERACTIONS: Increased levels with ritonavir; avoid use. Caution with ketoconazole and other potent CYP3A4 inhibitors; may increase serum fluticasone levels and reduced plasma cortisol AUC.

PREGNANCY: Category C, caution in nursing.

MECHANISM OF ACTION: Synthetic trifluorinated corticosteroid; possesses potent anti-inflammatory activity and inhibits multiple cell types involved in asthmatic response.

PHARMACOKINETICS: Absorption: Acts locally in lung. **Distribution:** V_d=4.2 L/kg; plasma protein binding (99%). **Metabolism:** Liver via CYP3A4. **Elimination:** Feces (primary), urine (<5%); $T_{1/2}$=7.8 hrs.

NURSING CONSIDERATIONS

Assessment: Assess for primary treatment of status asthmaticus or other acute asthma attacks, lung function, adrenal insufficiency (eg, anorexia, nausea, weakness, fatigue, hypotension, hypoglycemia) in patients changing from systemic corticosteroids to inhaled corticosteroids, during initial therapy, and during times of stress.

Monitoring: Monitor respiratory status and lung sounds, withdrawal symptoms (eg, joint/muscular pain, lassitude, depression) during withdrawal from oral corticosteroids, growth rate in children, serum and urine glucose concentrations, adrenal function tests to assess degree of hypothalamic-pituitary-adrenal axis suppression in chronic therapy, and eosinophilic conditions.

Patient Counseling: Counsel patients to use drugs at regular intervals as directed. Notify physician if pregnant or intend to become pregnant, and nursing. Avoid exposure to chickenpox or measles and should consult physician immediately once exposed. Technique for administering drug to children should be similar to adult.

Administration: 1) Prime inhaler before using for first time by releasing 4 test sprays into air, away from face, shaking well for 5 seconds before each spray. If inhaler has not been used for >7 days, or when it has been dropped, prime inhaler again by shaking well before each spray and releasing 2 test sprays into air, away from face. 2) After inhalation, rinse mouth with water and spit out; do not swallow. Clean inhaler at least once a week after evening dose. Use only with actuator supplied with product. 3) Discard inhaler after 120 sprays have been used. **Storage:** 25°C (77°F); excursions permitted to 15-30°C (59-86°F). Store inhaler with mouthpiece down.

FLOXIN

RX

ofloxacin (Ortho-McNeil)

Fluoroquinolones are associated with an increased risk of tendinitis and tendon rupture in all ages. Risk further increased in patients >60 yrs, patients taking corticosteroid drugs, and patients with kidney, heart or lung transplants.

F

THERAPEUTIC CLASS: Fluoroquinolone

INDICATIONS: Treatment of complicated urinary tract infections (UTI), uncomplicated skin and skin structure infections (SSSI), acute bacterial exacerbation of chronic bronchitis (ABECB), community-acquired pneumonia (CAP), acute uncomplicated urethral and cervical gonorrhea, nongonococcal urethritis and cervicitis, mixed infections of urethra and cervix, acute pelvic inflammatory disease (PID), uncomplicated cystitis, and prostatitis caused by susceptible strains of microorganisms.

DOSAGE: *Adults:* ≥18 yrs: ABECB/CAP/SSSI: 400mg q12h for 10 days. Cervicitis/Urethritis: 300mg q12h for 7 days. Gonorrhea: 400mg single dose. PID: 400mg q12h for 10-14 days. Uncomplicated Cystitis: 200mg q12h for 3 days (*E.coli* or *K.pneumoniae*) or 7 days (other pathogens). Complicated UTI: 200mg q12h for 10 days. Prostatitis: *(E.coli)* 300mg q12h for 6 weeks. CrCl 20-50mL/min: Dose q24h. CrCl <20mL/min: After regular initial dose, give 50% of normal dose q24h. Severe Hepatic Impairment: Max: 400mg/day.

HOW SUPPLIED: Tab: 200mg, 300mg, 400mg

WARNINGS/PRECAUTIONS: Convulsions, increased ICP, toxic psychosis, CNS stimulation, and serious, sometimes fatal, hypersensitivity reactions reported; d/c if any occur. *Clostridium difficile*-associated diarrhea and ruptures of shoulder, hand, and Achilles tendon reported. Not shown to be effective for syphilis. Safety and efficacy unknown in patients <18 yrs old, pregnancy, and nursing. Maintain adequate hydration. Caution with renal or hepatic dysfunction, risk for seizures, CNS disorder with predisposition to seizures. Avoid excessive sunlight. Monitor blood, renal and hepatic function with prolonged therapy. Tendon ruptures reported. D/C immediately at the first appearance of skin rash, jaundice, or any other sign of hypersensitivity and supportive measures instituted. Drug therapy should be d/c if photosensitivity/phototoxicity occurs. Medications should be avoided in patients with known prolongation of the QT interval, patients with uncorrected hypokalemia, and patients receiving Class IA (quinidine, procainamide), or Class III (amiodarone, sotalol) antiarrhythmic agents. Caution in elderly taking corticosteroids.

ADVERSE REACTIONS: NV, insomnia, headache, dizziness, diarrhea, external genital pruritus in women, vaginitis.

INTERACTIONS: Decreased absorption with antacids, sucralfate, multivitamins, zinc, didanosine; separate dosing by 2 hrs. NSAIDs may increase risk of seizures. May potentiate theophylline, warfarin. May potentiate insulin, oral hypoglycemics; d/c if hypoglycemia occurs. May increase half-life of drugs metabolized by CYP450. Severe tendon disorder risks are increased with concomitant corticosteroid therapy.

PREGNANCY: Category C, not for use in nursing.

MECHANISM OF ACTION: Fluoroquinolone; synthetic broad-spectrum antimicrobial agent; inhibits topoisomerase II (DNA gyrase) and topoisomerase IV, which are required for bacterial DNA replication, transcription, repair, and recombination.

PHARMACOKINETICS: Absorption: Oral administration of variable doses resulted in different parameters; T_{max}=1-2 hrs; bioavailability (98%). **Elimination:** Biphasic ($T_{1/2}$=4-5 hrs, 20-25 hrs), renal.

NURSING CONSIDERATIONS

Assessment: Assess renal function, LFTs, pregnancy/nursing status, history of seizures, QTc prolongation, and possible drug interactions.

Monitoring: Monitor for QTc prolongation, hematologic manifestations, glucosuria, hematuria, pulmonary edema, hypo/hyperglycemia, cardiac arrest, seizure, status epilepticus, respiratory arrest, CDAD, renal function, LFTs, CBC, tendon rupture, peripheral neuropathy, hypersensitivity reactions (toxic epidermal necrolysis, Stevens-Johnson syndrome).

Patient Counseling: Notify healthcare provider if symptoms of pain, swelling, or inflammation of a tendon, or weakness or inability to move joints; rest and refrain from excercise; and d/c therapy. Inform that drug treats bacterial, not viral, infections. Take exactly as directed; skipping doses or not completing full course may decrease effectiveness and increase resistance. Inform about potential benefits/risks. D/C and notify physician if skin rash, other allergic reaction, and watery and bloody stools (with or without stomach cramps, and fever) occur. Use caution in activities requiring mental alertness and coordination. Advise diabetic patients to use caution; hypoglycemia may develop during therapy. Inform to take with or without meals, and to drink fluids. Avoid sun exposure. Take full course as prescribed.

Administration: Oral route. **Storage**: 25°C (77°F), excursions permitted to 15-30°C (59-86°F).

F

FLOXIN OTIC — RX

ofloxacin (Daiichi Sankyo)

OTHER BRAND NAMES: Floxin Otic Singles (Daiichi Sankyo)

THERAPEUTIC CLASS: Fluoroquinolone

INDICATIONS: Otitis externa in patients ≥6 months. Chronic suppurative otitis media in patients ≥12 yrs with perforated tympanic membranes. Acute otitis media in patients ≥1 yr with tympanostomy tubes.

DOSAGE: *Adults:* Otitis Externa: 10 drops or 2 single-dispensing containers (SDCs) once daily for 7 days. Chronic Suppurative Otitis Media with Perforated Tympanic Membrane: 10 drops or 2 SDCs bid for 14 days. *Pediatrics:* Otitis Externa: 6 mos-13 yrs: 5 drops or 1 single-dispensing container (SDC) once daily for 7 days. ≥13 yrs: 10 drops or 2 SDCs once daily for 7 days. Chronic Suppurative Otitis Media with Perforated Tympanic Membrane: ≥12 yrs: 10 drops or 2 SDCs bid for 14 days. Acute Otitis Media with Tympanostomy Tubes: 1-12 yrs: 5 drops or 1 SDC bid for 10 days.

HOW SUPPLIED: Sol: 0.3% [5mL, 10mL], (Singles) 0.3% [20^{s}]

WARNINGS/PRECAUTIONS: D/C if hypersensitivity reaction occurs. Re-evaluate if no improvement after one week.

ADVERSE REACTIONS: Pruritus, application site reaction, taste perversion.

PREGNANCY: Category C, not for use in nursing.

MECHANISM OF ACTION: Fluoroquinilone; exerts antibacterial activity; inhibits DNA gyrase (a bacterial topoisomerase), an essential enzyme which controls DNA topology and assists in DNA replication, repair, deactivation, and transcription.

PHARMACOKINETICS: Absorption: Perforated tympanic membrane; C_{max}=10ng/ml.

NURSING CONSIDERATIONS

Assessment: Assess for drug hypersensitivity, pre-existing cholesteatoma, foreign body or tumor.

Monitoring: Monitor for anaphylactic reactions, cardiovascular collapse, loss of consciousness, angioedema, airway obstruction, dyspnea, urticaria and itching, overgrowth of non-susceptible organisms (fungi), erosions or lesions of cartilage of weight-bearing joints, signs of arthropathy, and for improvment/persistence of otorrhea.

Patient Counseling: Counsel to avoid touching applicator tip to fingers or other surfaces to avoid contamination. D/C and contact physician if signs of allergy occur. Not for ophthalmic use, nor for injection.

Administration: Otic route. Warm bottle by holding for 1-2 min, to avoid dizziness. **Storage:** 25°C (77°F); excursions permitted to 15-30°C (59-86°F).

FLUDROCORTISONE RX

fludrocortisone acetate (Various)

THERAPEUTIC CLASS: Corticosteroid

INDICATIONS: Partial replacement therapy for adrenocortical insufficiency in Addison's disease. Treatment of salt-losing adrenogenital syndrome.

DOSAGE: *Adults:* Addison's Disease: Usual: 0.1mg/day with concomitant cortisone 10-37.5mg/day or hydrocortisone 10-30mg/day in divided doses. Dose Range: 0.1mg three times weekly to 0.2mg/day. If HTN develops, reduce to 0.05mg/day. Salt-Losing Adrenogenital Syndrome: 0.1-0.2mg/day.

F

HOW SUPPLIED: Tab: 0.1mg* *scored

CONTRAINDICATIONS: Systemic fungal infections.

WARNINGS/PRECAUTIONS: May increase dose before, during, and after stressful situations. Caution with hypothyroidism, cirrhosis, ocular herpes simplex, HTN, ulcerative colitis, diverticulitis, peptic ulcer, osteoporosis, myasthenia gravis, renal impairment, and elderly. May mask signs of infection or cause new infection. Avoid exposure to chickenpox or measles. Marked effect on sodium retention; monitor electrolytes. May need salt restriction and potassium supplements. Monitor for psychic disturbances. Risk of glaucoma, cataracts, and eye infections. Avoid abrupt withdrawal.

ADVERSE REACTIONS: HTN, CHF, edema, convulsions, hypokalemia, hypokalemic alkalosis, muscle weakness, impaired wound healing, menstrual irregularities, cataracts, suppression of growth, hyperglycemia, HPA-suppression, acne, rash.

INTERACTIONS: Decreases serum salicylate levels. Enhanced hypokalemia with amphotericin B and potassium-depleting diuretics (eg, furosemide, ethacrynic acid). Increased risk of digitalis toxicity and arrhythmias with hypokalemia. Decreased effects with rifampin, barbiturates, and hydantoins. Monitor PT with oral anticoagulants. Decreases effects of oral hypoglycemics, insulin. Enhanced edema with other anabolic steroids (eg, oxymethalone, norethandrolone). Adjust dose with initiation or termination of estrogen. Avoid live virus vaccines (including smallpox) and other immunizations. Caution with ASA.

PREGNANCY: Category C, caution in nursing.

MECHANISM OF ACTION: Synthetic adrenocortical steroid; acts on electrolyte balance and carbohydrate metabolism and on distal tubules of kidney to enhance reabsorption of sodium ions from tubular fluid into the plasma. Increases urinary excretion of both K^+ and hydrogen ions.

PHARMACOKINETICS: Distribution: Found in breast milk. **Metabolism:** Liver. **Elimination**: $T_{1/2}$=3.5 hrs (Plasma), 18-36 hr (Biological).

NURSING CONSIDERATIONS

Assessment: Assess for hypersensitivity reactions to drug, systemic fungal infections, other current infections, active TB, vaccination, HTN, heart disease, renal/hepatic impairment, unusual stress, psychotic tendencies, thyroid function, hypoprothrombinemia, osteoporosis, myasthenia gravis, peptic ulcers with/without impending perforation, fresh intestinal anastomosis, diverticulitis/ulcerative colitis and possible drug/lab test interactions (eg, nitrobluetetrazolium test for bacterial infection).

Monitoring: Monitor for occurrence of infections, edema, weight gain, psychic derangement, cataracts, and frequent measuring of serum electrolytes, TSH, LFTs, glucose, IOP, and BP.

Patient Counseling: Inform drug increases susceptibility to infections. Instruct to avoid exposure to chickenpox or measles. Counsel to carry supply of medication for emergency use. Advise on the importance of regular follow-up visits and to use medication exactly as directed. Advise to notify physician of dizziness, severe or continuing headaches, swelling of feet or lower legs, or unusual weight gain. Not to be used while nursing.

Administration: Oral route. **Storage**: 15-30°C (59-86°F).

FluLaval **RX**

influenza virus vaccine (GlaxoSmithKline)

THERAPEUTIC CLASS: Vaccine

INDICATIONS: Active immunization of adults (≥18 yrs) against influenza disease caused by influenza virus subtypes A and type B contained in the vaccine.

DOSAGE: *Adults:* ≥18 yrs: 0.5mL IM in deltoid muscle.

HOW SUPPLIED: Inj: 45mcg/0.5mL [5mL]

CONTRAINDICATIONS: Hypersenstivity reactions to egg proteins (eg, eggs, egg products), chicken proteins, or life-threatening reaction to previous administration of any influenza vaccine. Immunization should be delayed in patients with acute, evolving neurologic disorder.

WARNINGS/PRECAUTIONS: Caution if Guillain-Barre syndrome has occured within 6 weeks of receipt of prior influenza vaccine. Avoid with bleeding disorders or concomitant anticoagulants. May reduce immune response in immunocompromised. Have epinephrine injection (1:1000) available. May not protect all susceptible individuals.

ADVERSE REACTIONS: Pain, redness, and/or swelling at injection site, headache, fatigue, myalgia, low-grade fever, malaise.

INTERACTIONS: Do not mix with any other vaccine in same syringe or vial; administer other vaccines at different injection sites. May increase blood levels of warfarin, theophylline, phenytoin. Immunosuppressive therapies (eg, irradiation, antimetabolites, alkylating agents, cytotoxic drugs, corticosteroids used in greater than physiologic doses) may reduce effectiveness.

PREGNANCY: Category C, caution in nursing.

MECHANISM OF ACTION: Vaccine; elicits the formation of antibodies that may protect against influenza virus subtypes A and B.

NURSING CONSIDERATIONS

Assessment: Assess immune status, possible drug interactions, known hypersensitivity reactions to egg and chicken proteins, bleeding and neurologic disorders, or current anticoagulation therapy. Assess potential benefits and risks if Guillain-Barre syndrome occurred with previous influenza vaccination.

Monitoring: Monitor hypersensitivity reactions, local injection-site reactions (eg, pain, redness, swelling), systemic adverse events (eg, headache, fatigue, myalgia, low-grade fever, malaise), bleeding tendencies, and neuropathic events.

Patient Counseling: Inform recipients and caregivers that vaccine provides protection against illness due to influenza viruses only and not against all respiratory diseases. Advise that annual revaccination is recommended. Instruct to report any severe or unusual adverse reactions.

Administration: IM. Administer at the deltoid muscle of the upper arm. Use ≥1 inch needle length. Shake multidose vial vigorously each time before withdrawing a dose of vaccine. Inspect visually for particulate matter and discoloration; do not use if present. **Storage:** 2-8°C (36-46°F). Do not freeze.

FluMist **RX**

influenza virus vaccine live (MedImmune)

THERAPEUTIC CLASS: Vaccine

INDICATIONS: Active immunization of individuals 2-49 yrs of age against influenza disease caused by influenza virus subtypes A and type B contained in the vaccine.

DOSAGE: *Adults:* ≤49 yrs: One 0.2mL (0.1mL per nostril) dose.
Pediatrics: ≥9 yrs: One 0.2mL (0.1mL per nostril) dose. 2-8 yrs: Not Previously Vaccinated With Influenza Vaccine: 0.2mL (0.1mL per nostril) for 2 doses at

least 1 month apart. Previously Vaccinated With Influenza Vaccine: One 0.2mL (0.1mL per nostril) dose.

HOW SUPPLIED: Nasal Spray: 0.2mL [10s]

CONTRAINDICATIONS: Parenteral use. Hypersensitivity to eggs or egg products, gentamicin, gelatin, arginine. Children and adolescents 5-17 yrs of age receiving ASA or ASA-containing therapy.

WARNINGS/PRECAUTIONS: Avoid with history of asthma, active wheezing or children <5 yrs of age with recurrent wheezing. Have epinephrine available. Caution in individuals if Guillain-Barre syndrome has occurred within 6 weeks of any prior influenza vaccination, immunocompromised persons and those with underlying medical conditions predisposing to influenza complications.

ADVERSE REACTIONS: Runny nose, congestion, cough, irritability, headache, sore throat, fever, chills, muscle aches, vomiting, tiredness/weakness.

INTERACTIONS: See Contraindications. Avoid concurrent use with other vaccines and within 48 hrs after cessation of antiviral therapy; antiviral agents until 2 weeks after vaccination unless medically indicated; ASA or ASA-containing products in children and adolescents 5-17 yrs.

PREGNANCY: Category C, caution in nursing.

MECHANISM OF ACTION: Stimulates the immune system to produce antibodies (influenza-specific T cells) that may protect against influenza virus infection.

NURSING CONSIDERATIONS

Assessment: Assess immune and current health status, history of asthma/recurrent wheezing, sensitivity to influenza vaccine, and possible drug interactions.

Monitoring: Monitor for anaphylactic reaction, wheezing, runny nose, fever, headache, myalagia, irritability, insomnia, otitis media, and GI or respiratory infections.

Patient Counseling: Inform patient or caregivers of benefits/risks. Report adverse reactions to physician. Inform that annual influenza vaccination is recommended.

Administration: Intranasal. **Storage:** 2-8°C (35-46°F). Do not freeze.

FLUNISOLIDE NASAL SPRAY — RX

flunisolide (Various)

THERAPEUTIC CLASS: Corticosteroid

INDICATIONS: Relief of seasonal or perennial rhinitis.

DOSAGE: *Adults:* Initial: 2 sprays per nostril bid. Titrate: May increase to 2 sprays per nostril tid. Max: 8 sprays per nostril/day.
Pediatrics: 6-14 yrs: Initial: 1 spray per nostril tid or 2 sprays per nostril bid. Max: 4 sprays per nostril/day.

HOW SUPPLIED: Spray: 25mcg/spray [25mL]

CONTRAINDICATIONS: Untreated localized infection of the nasal mucosa.

WARNINGS/PRECAUTIONS: Risk of adrenal insufficiency and withdrawal symptoms when replacing systemic corticosteroids with topical corticosteroids. Caution with active or quiescent TB, ocular herpes simplex, or untreated bacterial, fungal and systemic viral infections. Avoid with recent nasal trauma, surgery or septum ulcers. Risk for more severe/fatal course of infections (eg, chickenpox, measles) and for *Candida* infections of the nose and pharynx.

ADVERSE REACTIONS: Nasal congestion, sneezing, epistaxis, bloody mucous, nasal irritation, watery eyes, sore throat, NV, headache.

INTERACTIONS: Concomitant systemic corticosteroids increases risk of hypercorticism and/or HPA axis suppression.

PREGNANCY: Category C, caution in nursing.

MECHANISM OF ACTION: Glucocorticosteroid; not established, acts as anti-inflammatory agent with potent glucocorticoid and weak mineralocorticoid activity.

PHARMACOKINETICS: Absorption: Well absorbed. **Metabolism:** Liver. **Elimination:** Urine (65-70%, metabolites), feces; $T_{1/2}$=1-2 hrs.

NURSING CONSIDERATIONS

Assessment: Assess for active or quiescent TB, untreated localized or systemic viral, fungal or bacterial infections, history of glaucoma or cataracts, history of nasal polyps, recent nasal septal ulcers, nasal surgery/trauma, and possible drug interactions.

Monitoring: Monitor for acute adrenal insufficiency, hypercorticism and/or HPA-axis suppression, nasal or pharyngeal *Candida* infections, suppression of growth velocity in children, hypersensitivity reactions or contact dermatitis, wheezing, nasal septum perforation, changes of vision, increased IOP.

Patient Counseling: Take as directed at regular intervals and do not increase prescribed dosage to increase effectiveness. Avoid exposure to chickenpox or measles; consult physician immediately if exposed or if experience episodes of epistaxis. Contact physician if symptoms don't improve or condition worsens. Avoid spraying into eyes.

Administration: Intranasal route. **Storage:** 20-25°(68-77°F).

FLUOROURACIL — RX

fluorouracil (Various)

Hospitalize patient during initial therapy due to possible severe toxic reactions.

THERAPEUTIC CLASS: Antimetabolite

INDICATIONS: Palliative management of colon, rectum, breast, stomach, and pancreatic carcinomas.

DOSAGE: *Adults:* 12mg/kg IV qd for 4 days. Max: 800mg/day. If no toxicity, give 6mg/kg IV on 6th, 8th, 10th, and 12th days. Skip Days 5, 7, 9, and 11. Inadequate Nutritional State: 6mg/kg IV for 3 days. If no toxicity, give 3mg/kg IV on 5th, 7th, and 9th days. Max: 400mg/day. Skip Days 4, 6, and 8. Maint (Use Schedule 1 or Schedule 2): Schedule 1: If no toxicity, repeat 1st course every 30 days after last day of previous course. Schedule 2: When toxic signs from initial course subside, give 10-15mg/kg/week IV single dose; do not exceed 1g/week.

HOW SUPPLIED: Inj: 50mg/mL [10mL, 50mL, 100mL]

CONTRAINDICATIONS: Poor nutritional state, depressed bone marrow function, potentially serious infection.

WARNINGS/PRECAUTIONS: Extreme caution in poor risk patients with history of high-dose irradiation, previous use of alkylating agents, hepatic/renal dysfunction, widespread bone marrow involvement by metastatic tumors. Dipyrimidine dehydrogenase deficiency prolongs 5-FU clearance; can cause severe toxicity. May cause fetal harm in pregnancy. Other therapy interfering with nutrition or depressing bone marrow function increases toxicity. D/C with stomatitis, esophagopharyngitis, leukopenia, intractable vomiting, diarrhea, GI ulceration or bleeding, thrombocytopenia, or hemorrhage from any site. Palmar-plantar erythrodysesthesia syndrome (hand-foot syndrome) reported. Perform WBC with differential before each dose. Narrow margin of safety; monitor patients very closely.

ADVERSE REACTIONS: Stomatitis, esophagopharyngitis, diarrhea, anorexia, nausea, emesis, leukopenia, alopecia, dermatitis.

INTERACTIONS: Leucovorin calcium may enhance toxicity.

PREGNANCY: Category D, not for use in nursing.

MECHANISM OF ACTION: Antineoplastic antimetabolite; interferes with the synthesis of DNA and to a lesser extent inhibits the formation of RNA, which are essential for cell division and growth.

PHARMACOKINETICS: Distribution: Found in tumors, intestinal mucosa, bone marrow, liver; crosses the blood-brain barrier and found in brain tissue and cerebrospinal fluid. **Metabolism:** Liver. **Elimination:** Urine (7-20% unchanged); $T_{1/2}$=16 min.

NURSING CONSIDERATIONS

Assessment: Assess nutritional state, bone marrow function or involvement of bone marrow by metastatic tumors, presence of serious infections, history of high-dose pelvic irradiation, previous use of alkylating agents, hepatic or renal impairment, dipyrimidine dehydrogenase deficiency, pregnancy/nursing status, and possible drug interactions. Assess WBC counts with differential before each dose.

F

Monitoring: Monitor for signs and symptoms of stomatitis, esophagopharyngitis, leukopenia (WBC count <3500), intractable vomiting, diarrhea, GI ulceration or bleeding, thrombocytopenia (platelet count <100,000), hemorrhage from any site, palmar-plantar erythrodysesthesia syndrome (eg, tingling sensation in hands and feet), alopecia, and dermatitis.

Patient Counseling: Counsel about possible effects of medication including NV and alopecia. Alopecia is usually a transient effect. Advise about risks of medication during pregnancy.

Administration: IV route; no dilution required. Should only be administered under the supervision of a physician experienced in cancer chemotherapy. Patient should be hospitalized during initial course of therapy. Avoid extravasation. **Storage:** 15-30°C (59-86°F). Protect from light. Retain in carton until time of use.

FLUVOXAMINE — RX

fluvoxamine maleate (Various)

Antidepressants increased the risk of suicidal thinking and behavior (suicidality) in short-term studies in children, adolescents, and young adults with major depressive disorder (MDD) and other psychiatric disorders. Fluvoxamine is not approved for use in pediatric patients except for pateints with obsessive compulsive disorder (OCD).

THERAPEUTIC CLASS: Selective serotonin reuptake inhibitor

INDICATIONS: Treatment of OCD.

DOSAGE: *Adults:* Initial: 50mg qhs. Titrate: Increase by 50mg every 4-7 days. Maint: 100-300mg/day. Give bid if total dose >100mg daily. Max: 300mg/day. Elderly/Hepatic Impairment: Modify initial dose and titration.
Pediatrics: 8-17 yrs: Initial: 25mg qhs. Titrate: Increase by 25mg every 4-7 days. Maint: 50-200mg/day. Max: 8-11 yrs: 200mg/day. Adolescents: 300mg/day. Give bid if total dose >50mg daily.

HOW SUPPLIED: Tab: 25mg, 50mg*, 100mg* *scored

CONTRAINDICATIONS: Co-administration of thioridazine, terfenadine, astemizole, cisapride, pimozide, alosetron, tizanidine.

WARNINGS/PRECAUTIONS: Activation of mania/hypomania, SIADH, and hyponatremia reported. Close supervision with high risk suicide patients. Caution with history of seizures, hepatic dysfunction, with conditions altering metabolism or hemodynamic responses. Smoking increases metabolism.

ADVERSE REACTIONS: Headache, asthenia, NV, diarrhea, anorexia, dyspepsia, insomnia, somnolence, nervousness, agitation, dizziness, anxiety, dry mouth, sweating, tremor, abnormal ejaculation.

INTERACTIONS: See Contraindications. May potentiate metoprolol, propranolol. Avoid alcohol, diazepam, terfenadine, astemizole, cisapride, primozide. Increases serum levels of theophylline, warfarin, clozapine, carbamazepine, methadone. Bradycardia with diltiazem. Potential for serious, fatal interactions with MAOIs. Lithium may increase serotonergic effects. Reduces clearance of mexiletine and benzodiazepines metabolized by hepatic oxidation (eg, alprazolam, midazolam, triazolam). Caution with sumatriptan, TCAs, tryptophan. Avoid thioridazine; produces dose-related QTc interval prolongation. Increases tacrine serum levels.

PREGNANCY: Category C, not for use in nursing.

MECHANISM OF ACTION: SSRI; inhibits neuronal uptake of serotonin.

PHARMACOKINETICS: Absorption: Absolute bioavailability (53%). Administration of variable doses resulted in different parameters; T_{max}=3-8 hrs. **Distribution:** V_d=25L/kg; plasma protein binding (80%). **Metabolism:** Hepatic (oxidative demethylation and deamination). **Elimination:** Urine; $T_{1/2}$=15.6 hrs.

NURSING CONSIDERATIONS

Assessment: Assess for risk for bipolar disorder, history of mania, possible drug interactions, history of seizures, disease/condition that alters metabolism or hemodynamic response, and hepatic impairment.

Monitoring: Monitor for signs/symptoms of clinical worsening (suicidality, unusual changes in behavior), serotonin syndrome, NMS (muscle rigidity, hyperthermia, mental status changes), abnormal bleeding, hyponatremia, seizures, hepatic dysfunction, cognitive and motor impairment. If d/c therapy (particularly if abrupt), monitor for symptoms of dysphoric mood, irritability, agitation, dizziness, sensory disturbances, anxiety, confusion, headache, lethargy, emotional lability, insomnia, and hypomania.

Patient Counseling: Advise to avoid alcohol. Seek medical attention for symptoms of serotonin syndrome (mental status changes, tachycardia, hyperthermia, NV, diarrhea, incoordination), NMS (muscle rigidity, hyperthermia, mental status changes), allergic reactions (rash, hives), abnormal bleeding (particularly if using NSAIDs or ASA), hyponatremia, activation of mania, seizures, clinical worsening (suicidal ideation, unusual changes in behavior) and discontinuation symptoms (irritability, agitation, dizziness, anxiety, headache, insomnia). Caution may impair physical/mental abilities.

Administration: Oral route. **Storage:** 15-30°C (59-86°F). Protect from high humidity. Dispense in tight, light-resistant container with child-resistant closure.

FLUZONE RX

influenza virus vaccine (Sanofi Pasteur)

THERAPEUTIC CLASS: Vaccine

INDICATIONS: Active immunization in persons ≥6 months of age against influenza disease caused by influenza virus subtypes A and type B contained in the vaccine.

DOSAGE: *Adults:* 0.5mL IM in deltoid muscle.
Pediatrics: 6-35 months: 0.25mL IM. 3-8 yrs: 0.5mL IM. ≥9 yrs: 0.5mL IM. Children <9 yrs who have not previously been vaccinated should receive two doses of vaccine ≥1 month apart. Administer in deltoid muscle for children >36 months and anterolateral aspect of thigh for children ≤36 months.

HOW SUPPLIED: Inj: 0.25mL, 0.5mL, 5mL

CONTRAINDICATIONS: Hypersensitivity reactions to egg proteins or life-threatening reactions after previous administration of any influenza vaccine.

WARNINGS/PRECAUTIONS: Caution with history of Guillain-Barre syndrome. Immunosuppressed patients may not obtain expected antibody response. May not protect all patients. Have epinephrine injection (1:1000) available.

ADVERSE REACTIONS: Local: soreness, pain, swelling. Systemic: fever, malaise, myalgia.

INTERACTIONS: Immunosuppressive therapies may reduce immune response. Do not mix with any other vaccine in the same syringe or vial; administer concomitant vaccines at different injection sites.

PREGNANCY: Category C, caution in nursing.

MECHANISM OF ACTION: Stimulates the immune system to produce antibodies that may protect against influenza virus.

NURSING CONSIDERATIONS

Assessment: Assess immunity and health/medical status, history of bleeding disorders, previous hypersensitivity or vaccination events (Guillain-Barre syndrome or active progressive neurological disorder), and possible drug interaction (eg, long-term use of ASA therapy).

Monitoring: Monitor for hypersensitivity reactions, injection-site swelling or pain, fever, headache, myalgia, irritability, insomnia, and neurological complications.

Patient Counseling: Inform patients or caregivers of benefits/risks ratio; report any adverse reactions to physician.

Administration: IM. **Storage:** 2-8°C (35-46°F). Do not freeze.

FML

fluorometholone (Allergan)

RX

OTHER BRAND NAMES: FML Forte (Allergan)

THERAPEUTIC CLASS: Corticosteroid

INDICATIONS: Treatment of inflammation of the palpebral and bulbar conjunctiva, cornea, and anterior segment of the globe.

DOSAGE: *Adults:* (Sus) 1 drop bid-qid or (Oint) apply 1/2 inch qd-tid. May give 0.1% q4h during initial 24-48 hrs. Re-evaluate after 2 days if no improvement. *Pediatrics:* ≥2 yrs: (Sus) 1 drop bid-qid or (Oint) apply 1/2 inch qd-tid. May give 0.1% q4h during initial 24-48 hrs. Re-evaluate after 2 days if no improvement.

HOW SUPPLIED: Oint: (S.O.P.) 0.1% [3.5g]; Sus: 0.1% [5mL, 10mL, 15mL]; (Forte) 0.25% [2mL, 5mL, 10mL, 15mL]

CONTRAINDICATIONS: Viral diseases of the cornea and conjunctiva including epithelial herpes simplex keratitis, vaccinia, and varicella. Mycobacterial infection and fungal diseases of the eye.

WARNINGS/PRECAUTIONS: Caution with glaucoma, herpes simplex, diseases causing thinning of cornea/sclera and other ocular viral infections. Prolonged use can cause glaucoma or secondary ocular infections (eg, fungal). Monitor IOP after 10 days of therapy. Re-evaluate if no response after 2 days. Ointment may retard corneal healing. May delay healing and increase incidence of bleb formation after cataract surgery. Avoid abrupt withdrawal with chronic use.

ADVERSE REACTIONS: Elevation of IOP, glaucoma, infrequent optic nerve damage, posterior subcapsular cataract formation, delayed wound healing, burning/stinging upon instillation, ocular irritation, taste perversion, visual disturbance.

PREGNANCY: Category C, not for use in nursing.

MECHANISM OF ACTION: Corticosteroid; suspected to act by induction of phospholipase A_2 inhibitory proteins called lipocortins, which control the biosynthesis of potent inflammation mediators (eg, prostaglandins, leukotrienes) by inhibiting release of their precursor, arachidonic acid.

NURSING CONSIDERATIONS

Assessment: Assess for viral diseases of cornea and conjunctiva, dendritic keratitis, vaccinia, varicella, mycobacterial infection of eye, fungal disease of ocular structures, glaucoma, mustard gas keratitis, Sjogren's keratoconjuctivitis, thinning of corneal/scleral epithelium, hypersensitivity, and for cataract surgery.

Monitoring: Frequent measuring of IOP and slit lamp microscopy exam when appropriate, fluorescein staining for monitoring of glaucoma with damage to the optic nerve (with defects in visual acuity and fields of vision), posterior subcapsular cataract, delayed corneal healing, thinning of cornea and sclera, ulceration, perforation, and secondary ocular infections or masking of existing infections.

Patient Counseling: Advise to d/c and notify physician if symptoms persist or worsen. Instruct to wait 15 min after instillation to wear soft contact lenses. Counsel to avoid touching bottle tip to eyelids or any other surface.

Administration: Ocular route. **Storage:** Store between 2-25°C (36-77°F); protect from freezing.

FML-S

RX

sulfacetamide sodium - fluorometholone (Allergan)

THERAPEUTIC CLASS: Sulfonamide/corticosteroid

INDICATIONS: Ocular inflammation associated with infection or risk of infection.

DOSAGE: *Adults:* 1 drop qid. Max: 20mL for initial prescription. Re-evaluate before refill.

HOW SUPPLIED: Sus: (Sulfacetamide-Fluorometholone) 10%-0.1% [5mL, 10mL]

CONTRAINDICATIONS: Viral diseases of the cornea and conjunctiva including epithelial herpes simplex keratitis, vaccinia, and varicella. Mycobacterial infection and fungal diseases of the eye.

WARNINGS/PRECAUTIONS: Caution with glaucoma, herpes simplex, diseases causing thinning of cornea/sclera and other ocular viral infections. Prolonged use can cause glaucoma or secondary ocular infections (eg, fungal). Monitor IOP after 10 days of therapy. Fatalities reported due to severe reactions to sulfonamides. Re-evaluate before renew prescription.

ADVERSE REACTIONS: Secondary infection, elevated IOP, delayed wound healing, allergic sensitization.

INTERACTIONS: Sulfacetamide preparations are incompatible with silver preparations.

PREGNANCY: Category C, not for use in nursing.

MECHANISM OF ACTION: Sulfonamide/corticosteroid. Fluorometholone: Corticosteroid; inhibits edema, fibrin deposition, capillary dilation, leukocyte migration, capillary proliferation, fibroblast proliferation, deposition of collagen, and scar formation associated with inflammation. May also inhibit body's defense mechanism against infection. Sulfacetamide: Anti-infective; provides activity against susceptible microorganisms.

NURSING CONSIDERATIONS

Assessment: Assess proper diagnosis of patient (eg, slit lamp biomicroscopy, fluorescein staining). Assess patient does not have viral diseases of cornea and conjunctiva (epithelial herpes simplex keratitis, dendritic keratitis, vaccinia and varicella). Assess patient does not have mycobacterial infection of the eye or fungal disease of the ocular structures. Assess for hypersensitivity to sulfonamides and other corticosteroids. Assess use in pregnant/nursing females, patients with glaucoma, patients who underwent recent cataract surgery, and in patients with a history of herpes simplex.

Monitoring: Monitor for masking of acute purulent infections, Stevens-Johnson syndrome, toxic epidermal necrolysis, fulminant hepatic necrosis, agranulocytosis, aplastic anemia, and other blood dyscrasias. In patients on prolonged therapy, monitor for glaucoma with damage to the optic nerve, defects in visual acuity and fields of vision, posterior subcapsular cataract formation, secondary ocular infections (eg, fungal), and corneal and scleral thinning. In patients on therapy for 10 days or longer, monitor IOP. In patients with a history of herpes simplex, perform frequent slit lamp microscopy.

Patient Counseling: Instruct to notify physician if pain or inflammation persists for longer than 48 hrs. Instruct to avoid touching bottle tip to eyelids or any other surface to prevent contamination.

Administration: Ocular route. Shake well before use. **Storage:** 15-30°C (59-86°F). Protect from freezing and light. Keep out of reach of children.

FOCALIN

dexmethylphenidate HCl (Novartis)

CII

THERAPEUTIC CLASS: Sympathomimetic amine

INDICATIONS: Treatment of attention deficit hyperactivity disorder (ADHD).

DOSAGE: *Adults:* Take bid at least 4 hrs apart. Methylphenidate Naive: Initial: 2.5mg bid. Titrate: Increase weekly by 2.5-5mg/day. Max: 20mg/day. Currently on Methylphenidate: Initial: Take 1/2 of methylphenidate dose. Max: 20mg/day. Reduce or d/c if paradoxical aggravation of symptoms. D/C if no improvement after appropriate dosage adjustments over 1 month.
Pediatrics: ≥6 yrs: Take bid at least 4 hrs apart. Methylphenidate Naive: Initial: 2.5mg bid. Titrate: Increase weekly by 2.5-5mg/day. Max: 20mg/day. Currently on Methylphenidate: Initial: Take 1/2 of methylphenidate dose. Max: 20mg/day. Reduce or d/c if paradoxical aggravation of symptoms. D/C if no improvement after appropriate dosage adjustments over 1 month.

HOW SUPPLIED: Tab: 2.5mg, 5mg, 10mg

CONTRAINDICATIONS: Marked anxiety, tension, and agitation; glaucoma; motor tics or family history or diagnosis of Tourette's syndrome; during or within 14 days of MAOI use.

WARNINGS/PRECAUTIONS: Caution in drug dependence or alcoholism. Avoid with known serious structural cardiac abnormalities, cardiomyopathy, serious heart rhythm abnormalities, CAD, or other serious cardiac problems. May cause modest increase in BP; caution with HTN, heart failure, recent MI, or ventricular arrhythmia. May exacerbate symptoms of behavior disturbance and thought disorder with pre-existing psychotic disorder. Caution when using stimulants to treat patients with comorbid bipolar disorder because of concern for possible induction of mixed/manic episodes in such patients. Stimulants at usual doses may cause treatment-emergent psychotic or manic symptoms (eg, hallucinations, delusional thinking, mania) in children and adolescents without prior history of psychotic illness or mania. Aggressive behavior or hostility reported in clinical trials and the postmarketing experience of some medications indicated for the treatment of ADHD. Suppression of growth reported with long-term use; monitor growth. May lower convulsive threshold; d/c in the presence of seizures. Visual disturbances reported. Monitor CBC, differential, and platelets with prolonged therapy.

ADVERSE REACTIONS: Abdominal pain, fever, anorexia, nausea, nervousness, insomnia. (Pediatrics) Loss of appetite, weight loss, tachycardia.

INTERACTIONS: See Contraindications. May decrease the effectiveness of antihypertensives. Caution with pressor agents. May inhibit metabolism of coumarin anticoagulants, anticonvulsants, and some antidepressants; adjust dose. Adverse events reported with clonidine.

PREGNANCY: Category C, caution in nursing.

MECHANISM OF ACTION: Sympathomimetic amine; blocks the reuptake of norepinephrine and dopamine into the presynaptic neuron and increases release of these monoamines into extraneuronal space.

PHARMACOKINETICS: Absorption: Readily absorbed; T_{max}=2.9 hrs (fed), 1.5 hrs (fasting). **Metabolism:** Via de-esterification (d-ritalinic acid; primary metabolite). **Elimination:** Urine (approximately 90%); $T_{1/2}$=2.2 hrs.

NURSING CONSIDERATIONS

Assessment: Assess for agitation, glaucoma, tics, family history of Tourette's syndrome, cardiovascular conditions (eg, severe HTN, angina pectoris, cardiac structural abnormalities, arrhythmias, heart failure, recent MI), hyperthyroidism or thyrotoxicosis, bipolar disorder, seizures, LFTs, renal function, history of drug dependence or alcoholism, possible drug interactions.

Monitoring: Monitor for cardiac abnormalities, exacerbations of behavior disturbances and thought disorder, bipolar disorder, aggression, seizures, and visual disturbances. Periodically monitor CBC, differential and platelet count, LFTs. Height and weight follow-up in children.

Patient Counseling: Inform about risks of treatment, appropriate use, drug abuse/dependence. Counsel about potential side effects and advise to report any.

Administration: Oral route. **Storage:** 25°C (77°F); excursions permitted to 15-30°C (59-86°F). Protect from light and moisture.

FOCALIN XR

dexmethylphenidate HCl (Novartis)

CII

Give cautiously to patients with a history of drug dependence or alcoholism. Chronic abusive use may lead to marked tolerance and psychological dependence with varying degrees of abnormal behavior.

THERAPEUTIC CLASS: Sympathomimetic amine

INDICATIONS: Treatment of attention deficit hyperactivity disorder (ADHD) in patients aged ≥6 yrs.

DOSAGE: *Adults:* Individualize dose: Methylphenidate Naive: Initial: 10mg/day. Titrate: May adjust weekly by 10mg-20mg qd. Max: 20mg/day. Currently on Methylphenidate: Initial: Take 1/2 of methylphenidate dose. Max: 20mg/day. Currently on Dexmethylphenidate Immediate Release: Switch to same daily dose of XR. Max: 20mg/day. Reduce or d/c if paradoxical aggravation of symptoms. Swallow capsule whole or sprinkle contents on applesauce. Contents should not be crushed, chewed or divided. D/C if no improvement after appropriate dosage adjustments over 1 month.
Pediatrics: ≥6 yrs: Individualize dose: Methylphenidate Naive: Initial: 5mg/day. Titrate: May adjust weekly by 5mg/day. Max: 20mg/day. Currently on Methylphenidate: Initial: Take 1/2 of methylphenidate dose. Max: 20mg/day. Currently on Dexmethylphenidate Immediate Release: Switch to same daily dose of XR. Max: 20mg/day. Reduce or d/c if paradoxical aggravation of symptoms. Swallow capsule whole or sprinkle contents on applesauce; contents should not be crushed, chewed or divided. D/C if no improvement after appropriate dosage adjustments over 1 month.

HOW SUPPLIED: Cap, Extended-Release: 5mg, 10mg, 15mg, 20mg

CONTRAINDICATIONS: Marked anxiety, tension, and agitation; glaucoma; motor tics or family history or diagnosis of Tourette's syndrome; during or within 14 days of MAOI use.

WARNINGS/PRECAUTIONS: Avoid with known serious structural cardiac abnormalities, cardiomyopathy, serious heart rhythm abnormalities, CAD, or other serious cardiac problems. May cause modest increase in BP; caution with HTN, heart failure, recent MI, or ventricular arrhythmia. May exacerbate symptoms of behavior disturbance and thought disorder with pre-existing psychotic disorder. Caution when using stimulants to treat patients with co-morbid bipolar disorder because of concern for possible induction of mixed/manic episodes in such patients. Stimulants at usual doses may cause treatment-emergent psychotic or manic symptoms (eg, hallucinations, delusional thinking, mania) in children and adolescents without prior history of psychotic illness or mania. Aggressive behavior or hostility reported in clinical trials and the postmarketing experience of some medications indicated for the treatment of ADHD. Suppression of growth reported with long-term use; monitor growth. May lower convulsive threshold; d/c in the presence of seizures. Visual disturbances reported. Monitor CBC, differential, and platelets with prolonged therapy.

ADVERSE REACTIONS: Dyspepsia, headache, anxiety. (Adults) dry mouth, pharyngolaryngeal pain, feeling jittery, dizziness. (Pediatrics) decreased appetite, nausea.

INTERACTIONS: See Contraindications. May decrease the effectiveness of antihypertensives. Caution with pressor agents. May inhibit metabolism of coumarin anticoagulants, anticonvulsants, and tricyclic drugs; adjust dose. Adverse events reported with clonidine. Antacids or acid supressants could alter the release of dexmethylphenidate.

PREGNANCY: Category C, caution in nursing.

MECHANISM OF ACTION: Sympathomimetic amine; CNS stimulant. Blocks reuptake of norepinephrine and dopamine into presynaptic neuron and increases release of these monoamines into extraneuronal space.

PHARMACOKINETICS: Absorption: Bimodal plasma concentration. T_{max}=1-4 hrs (first peak), 4-5.7 hrs (second peak). **Distribution:** V_d=2.65L/kg. **Metabolism:** Metabolized via de-esterification; d-ritalinic acid (metabolite). **Elimination:** Urine (90%); $T_{1/2}$=2-4.5 hrs.

NURSING CONSIDERATIONS

F

Assessment: Assess for agitation, glaucoma, tics, family history of Tourette's syndrome, cardiovascular conditions (eg, severe HTN, angina pectoris, cardiac arrhythmias, heart failure, recent MI), hyperthyroidism or thyrotoxicosis, bipolar disorder, history of drug dependence or alcoholism.

Monitoring: Monitor for cardiac abnormalities, exacerbations of behavior disturbances and thought disorder, bipolar disorder, aggression, seizures, and visual disturbances. Periodic monitoring of CBC, differential and platelet counts, and LFTs. Height and weight follow-up in children.

Patient Counseling: Inform about risks of therapy, appropriate use, drug abuse/dependence. Swallow tablet; never crush or chew. If unable to swallow, sprinkle over applesauce and swallow without chewing.

Administration: Oral route. **Storage:** 25°C (77°F), excursions permitted to 15-30° (59-86°F).

FOLGARD RX 2.2 RX

vitamin B12 - vitamin B6 - folic acid (Upsher-Smith)

THERAPEUTIC CLASS: Folic acid/vitamin combination

INDICATIONS: For nutritional support and folic acid supplementation.

DOSAGE: *Adults:* 1 tab qd.

HOW SUPPLIED: Tab: Folic Acid 2.2mg-Vitamin B_6 25mg-Vitamin B_{12} 0.5mg*
*scored

WARNINGS/PRECAUTIONS: Folic acid >0.1mg/day may obscure pernicious anemia.

ADVERSE REACTIONS: Allergic sensitization.

PREGNANCY: Safety in pregnancy and nursing is not known.

MECHANISM OF ACTION: Folic acid/vitamin combination.

NURSING CONSIDERATIONS

Assessment: Assess for pernicious anemia.

Monitoring: Monitor hematological parameters and for hypersensitivity reactions.

Patient Counseling: Report hypersensitivity reactions.

Administration: Oral route. **Storage:** 15-30°C (59-86°F). Protect from light and moisture. Dispense in tight container with child-resistant closure.

FOLIC ACID RX

folic acid (Various)

THERAPEUTIC CLASS: Erythropoiesis agent

INDICATIONS: Treatment of megaloblastic anemia due to folic acid deficiency and in anemias of nutritional origin, pregnancy, infancy or childhood.

DOSAGE: *Adults:* Usual: Up to 1mg/day. Maint: 0.4mg qd. Pregnancy/Nursing: Maint: 0.8mg qd. Max: 1mg/day. Increase maintenance dose with alcoholism, hemolytic anemia, anticonvulsant therapy, chronic infection.
Pediatrics: Usual: Up to 1mg/day. Maint: Infants: 0.1mg qd. <4 yrs: 0.3mg qd. ≥4 yrs: 0.4mg qd.

HOW SUPPLIED: Inj: 5mg/mL; Tab: (OTC) 0.4mg, 0.8mg, (RX) 1mg

WARNINGS/PRECAUTIONS: Not for monotherapy in pernicious anemia and other megaloblastic anemias with B_{12} deficiency. May obscure pernicious anemia in dosage >0.1 mg/day. Decreased B_{12} serum levels with prolonged therapy.

ADVERSE REACTIONS: Allergic sensitization.

INTERACTIONS: Antagonizes phenytoin effects. Methotrexate, phenytoin, primidone, barbiturates, alcohol, alcoholic cirrhosis, nitrofurantoin, and pyrimethamine increase loss of folate. Increased seizures with phenytoin, primidone and phenobarbital reported. Tetracycline may cause false low serum and red cell folate due to suppression of *Lactobacillus casei*.

F

PREGNANCY: Category A, requirement increases during nursing.

MECHANISM OF ACTION: Acts as cofactor for transformylation reactions in biosynthesis of purines and thymidylates of nucleic acids; acts on megaloblastic bone marrow to produce normo-blastic marrow; required for nucleo-protein synthesis and maintenance of normal erythropoiesis.

PHARMACOKINETICS: Absorption: Rapid (small intestine); T_{max}=1 hr. **Distribution:** Excreted in breast milk. **Metabolism:** Liver via reduced diphospho-pyridine nucleotide and folate reductase. **Elimination:** Urine, feces.

NURSING CONSIDERATIONS

Assessment: Assess for alcoholism, chronic infection, and pernicious, megaloblastic, and hemolytic anemias, and for possible drug interactions.

Monitoring: Monitor for allergic/hypersensitivity reactions.

Patient Counseling: Advise to seek medical attention if symptoms of allergic/hypersensitivity reaction occurs.

Administration: Oral route. **Storage**: 20-25°C (68-77°F).

Foltx

RX

vitamin B12 - vitamin B6 - folic acid (PamLab)

THERAPEUTIC CLASS: Folic acid/vitamin combination

INDICATIONS: To supply nutritional requirements for those with end stage renal failure, dialysis, hyperhomocysteinemia, homocystinuria, nutrient malabsorption.

DOSAGE: *Adults:* 1-2 tabs qd.

HOW SUPPLIED: Tab: Folic Acid 2.5mg-Vitamin B_6 25mg-Vitamin B_{12} 2mg

WARNINGS/PRECAUTIONS: Folic acid >0.1mg/day may obscure pernicious anemia (may be alleviated by B_{12} component).

ADVERSE REACTIONS: Allergic sensitization, paresthesia, somnolence, mild diarrhea, polycythemia vera, peripheral vascular thrombosis, itching, transitory exanthema, feeling of body swelling.

INTERACTIONS: Pyridoxine may antagonize levodopa; avoid concomitant use. May be used with carbidopa/levodopa. Decreases effect of phenytoin.

MECHANISM OF ACTION: Folic acid/vitamin combination.

NURSING CONSIDERATIONS

Assessment: Assess for Leber's optic atrophy, pernicious anemia, and hyperhomocysteinemia. Note other diseases/conditions and drug therapies.

Monitoring: Monitor for polycythemia vera, headache, paresthesia, and hypersensitivity reactions.

Patient Counseling: Counsel about adverse effects; immediately report if any occur. Take as directed by physician.

Administration: Oral route. **Storage:** Room temperature, 15-30°C (59-86°F). Protect from light and moisture. Dispense in original light-resistant container with child-resistant closure.

FORADIL

formoterol fumarate (Schering)

RX

Long-acting β_2-agonists may increase the risk of asthma-related death.

F

THERAPEUTIC CLASS: Beta$_2$-agonist

INDICATIONS: Long-term maintenance treatment of asthma and prevention of bronchospasm with reversible obstructive airway disease (including nocturnal asthma) in patients who require regular treatment with inhaled short acting β_2-agonists. Maintenance treatment of bronchoconstriction in chronic obstructive pulmonary disease (COPD). Acute prevention of excercise-induced bronchospasm (EIB).

DOSAGE: *Adults:* Do not swallow cap; give only by inhalation with Aerolizer Inhaler. Asthma/COPD: 12mcg q12h. Max: 24mcg/day. EIB: 12mcg 15 min before exercise (do not give added dose if already on q12h dose).
Pediatrics: ≥5 yrs: Do not swallow cap; give only by inhalation with Aerolizer™ Inhaler. Asthma/COPD: 12mcg q12h. Max: 24mcg/day. ≥12 yrs: EIB: 12mcg 15 min before exercise (do not give added dose if already on q12h dose).

HOW SUPPLIED: Cap (Inhalation): 12mcg [12^s, 60^s]

WARNINGS/PRECAUTIONS: Do not d/c inhaled corticosteroids. Only use short-acting β_2-agonist inhaler for acute symptoms. D/C if paradoxical bronchospasm occurs. D/C if ECG changes, QT interval increases, or ST depression occurs. Caution with cardiovascular disorders (eg, HTN, arrhythmias), thyrotoxicosis and convulsive disorders. Anaphylactic and other allergic reactions reported. Not for use in acute asthmatic conditions. Should not be used with other long-acting β_2-agonist medications. May cause hypokalemia.

ADVERSE REACTIONS: Viral infection, dyspnea, chest pain, tremor, HTN, hypotension, tachycardia, arrhythmias, headache, nausea, vomiting, fatigue, hypokalemia, hyperglycemia, exacerbation of asthma.

INTERACTIONS: Potentiates other sympathomimetics. Hypokalemia potentiated by xanthine derivatives (eg, theophylline), steroids and non-potassium sparing diuretics. Extreme caution with MAOIs, TCAs, and drugs known to prolong QT interval. Antagonized effect with β-blockers.

PREGNANCY: Category C, caution in nursing.

MECHANISM OF ACTION: Long-acting selective β_2-adrenergic receptor agonist; acts as a bronchodilator, activates adenyl cyclase on airway smooth muscles and increases the intracellular concentration of cyclic AMP. Increased cAMP levels are associated with relaxation of bronchial smooth muscle and inhibition of release of mediators of immediate hypersensitivity.

PHARMACOKINETICS: Absorption: Healthy: C_{max}=92pg/mL, T_{max}=5 min. COPD patient: (12mcg) C_{max}=4.0-8.8, 8, 17.3pg/mL at 10 min, 2 hrs, 6 hrs, respectively. **Distribution:** Plasma protein binding (61-64%), serum albumin binding (31-38%). **Metabolism:** Glucuronidation, O-methylation via CYP450 enzymes 2D6, 2C19, 2CP, 2A6. **Elimination:** Healthy: Urine (59-62%), feces (32-34%). With asthma: Urine (10% unchanged). COPD: Urine (7%). $T_{1/2}$=10 hrs.

NURSING CONSIDERATIONS

Assessment: Assess for convulsive disorders, hyperthyroidism, DM, CVD, and possible drug interactions.

Monitoring: Monitor pulse rate, BP, and ECG change, and for paradoxical bronchospasm and hypokalemia, hypersensitivity reactions, deterioration of asthma.

Patient Counseling: Inform that long-acting β_2-agonist may increase risk of asthma-related death. Take as directed. Report lack of response or adverse side effects. Capsule should not be swallowed.

Administration: Oral inhalation route. 1) Pull off aerolizer inhaler cover. 2) Twist mouthpiece in the direction of the arrow to open. 3) Make sure 4 pins can be seen in the capsule well. 4) Place capsule in capsule chamber and twist mouthpiece back to closed position. 5) Hold mouthpiece of inhaler upright and press both buttons at the same time. Only press once. A click should be heard as the capsule is being pierced. 6) Release the button and exhale. 7) Place the mouthpiece in mouth and breathe in quickly and deeply. 8) Remove inhaler from mouth and hold breath as long as possible and then exhale. 9) Open the inhaler to see if any powder is still in the capsule. If drug remains, repeat steps 7&8. 10) After use, open the inhaler, remove and discard the empty capsule. Close the mouthpiece and replace the cover. **Storage:** Prior to dispensing: 2-8°C (36-46°F). After dispensing: 20-25°C (68-77°F). Protect from heat and moisture. Capsule should always be stored in blister and only removed from blister before use.

FORTAMET

metformin HCl (Sciele)

RX

F

THERAPEUTIC CLASS: Biguanide

INDICATIONS: Adjunct to diet and exercise, to improve glycemic control in type 2 diabetes mellitus.

DOSAGE: *Adults:* ≥17 yrs: Take with evening meal. Initial: 500-1000mg qd. With Insulin: Initial: 500mg qd. Titrate: May increase by 500mg/week. Max: 2500mg/day. Decrease insulin dose by 10-25% if FPG <120mg/dL. Elderly/Debilitated/Malnourished: Conservative dosing; do not titrate to max.

HOW SUPPLIED: Tab, Extended-Release: 500mg, 1000mg

CONTRAINDICATIONS: Renal disease/dysfunction (SrCr ≥1.5mg/dL [males], ≥1.4mg/dL [females], or abnormal CrCl), acute or chronic metabolic acidosis, including diabetic ketoacidosis. D/C temporarily (48 hrs) for radiologic studies with intravascular iodinated contrast materials.

WARNINGS/PRECAUTIONS: Lactic acidosis (rare) reported; may occur with pathophysiologic conditions, including DM, hypoperfusion, and hypoxemia. Increased risk with renal insufficiency (both intrinsic renal disease and renal hypoperfusion), CHF, and patient's age. Avoid use in patients ≥80 yrs unless renal function is not reduced. Should be promptly withheld with hypoxemia, dehydration, or sepsis. Caution against excessive alcohol intake. Lactic acidosis may be suspected in diabetic patient with metabolic acidosis lacking evidence of ketoacidosis (ketonuria and ketonemia). Immediately d/c with lactic acidosis; prompt hemodialysis is recommended to correct the acidosis and remove the accumulated metformin. Caution using concomitant medications that may affect renal function, or result in significant hemodynamic change, or interfere with the disposition of metformin (eg, cationic drugs eliminated by renal tubular secretion). Temporarily d/c prior to surgery (due to restricted food intake) and procedures requiring intravascular iodinated contrast materials. D/C in hypoxic states (eg, shock, CHF, acute MI). Avoid in patients with hepatic impairment. May decrease vitamin B_{12} levels. Increased risk of hypoglycemia in elderly, debilitated/malnourished, adrenal or pituitary insufficiency, or alcohol intoxication. If loss of glycemic control occurs due to stress, temporarily withhold metformin and administer insulin. Reinstitute metformin after acute episode is resolved.

ADVERSE REACTIONS: Infection, diarrhea, nausea, accidental injury, headache, dyspepsia, and rhinitis.

INTERACTIONS: Furosemide, nifedipine, cimetidine, cationic drugs (eg, digoxin, amiloride, procainamide, quinidine, quinine, ranitidine, trimethoprim, vancomycin, triamterene, morphine) may increase metformin levels. Thiazides, other diuretics, corticosteroids, phenothiazines, thyroid products, estrogens, oral contraceptives, phenytoin, nicotinic acid, sympathomimetics, CCBs, and isoniazid may cause hyperglycemia. Risk of hypoglycemia with alcohol. Excess alcohol may increase potential for lactic acidosis. May decrease furosemide levels.

PREGNANCY: Category B, not for use in pregnancy or nursing.

MECHANISM OF ACTION: Biguanide; decreases hepatic glucose production, decreases intestinal absorption of glucose, and improves insulin sensitivity by increasing peripheral glucose uptake and utilization.

PHARMACOKINETICS: Absorption: C_{max}=2849ng/mL, T_{max}=6 hrs, AUC=26811ng•hr/mL. **Elimination:** Urine (90%); $T_{1/2}$=6.2 hrs (plasma), 17.6 hrs (blood).

NURSING CONSIDERATIONS

Assessment: Assess for renal FPG, HbA_{1c}, renal function, LFTs, and CBC. Assess for CHF, septicemia, acute or chronic metabolic acidosis, adrenal or pituitary insufficiency, alcoholism, pregnancy status. Evaluate for other medical/surgical conditions and for possible drug interactions.

Monitoring: Monitor for infection, diarrhea, nausea, accidental injury, headache, dyspepsia, and rhinitis.

F

Patient Counseling: Inform of the potential risks and benefits of Fortamet and of alternative modes of therapy. Inform drug is adjunct to diet and exercise, and necessity of regular testing of blood glucose, glycosylated hemoglobin, renal function, and hematologic parameters. Temporarily d/c therapy prior to intravascular radiocontrast study or surgery. Report unexplained hyperventilation, myalgia, malaise, unusual somnolence, or other nonspecific symptoms. Counsel patient to avoid excessive alcohol intake, either acute or chronic. Drug alone does not cause hypoglycemia but can occur in conjunction with oral sulfonylureas and insulin. Instruct drug must be swallowed whole with a full glass of water and should not be chewed, cut, or crushed. Inactive ingredients may be eliminated in the feces as a soft mass.

Administration: Oral route. Must swallow whole with a full glass of water; do not crush or chew. **Storage:** 20-25°C (68-77°F); excursions permitted to 15-30°C (59-86°F). Keep tightly closed. Protect from light.

FORTAZ RX

ceftazidime (GlaxoSmithKline)

THERAPEUTIC CLASS: Cephalosporin (3rd generation)

INDICATIONS: Treatment of lower respiratory tract (eg, pneumonia), skin and skin structure (SSSI), bone/joint, gynecologic, CNS (eg, meningitis), intra-abdominal, and urinary tract infections (UTI); and septicemia caused by susceptible strains of microorganisms. Treatment of sepsis.

DOSAGE: *Adults:* Usual: 1g IM/IV q8-12h. Uncomplicated UTI: 250mg IM/IV q12h. Complicated UTI: 500mg IM/IV q8-12h. Bone and Joint Infection: 2g IV q12h. Uncomplicated Pneumonia/SSSI: 500mg-1g IM/IV q8h. Gynecological/Intra-Abdominal/Meningitis/Severe Life-Threatening Infection: 2g IV q8h. Lung Infection Caused by *Pseudomonas* spp. in Cystic Fibrosis (Normal Renal Function): 30-50mg/kg IV q8h. Max: 6g/day. CrCl 31-50mL/min: 1g q12h. CrCl 16-30mL/min: 1g q24h. CrCl 6-15mL/min: 500mg q24h. CrCl <5mL/min: 500mg q48h. For severe infections (6g/day), increase renal impairment dose by 50% or increase dosing interval. Apply reduced dosage recommendations after initial 1g LD is given. Hemodialysis: Give 1g before, then 1g after each hemodialysis. Intra-Peritoneal Dialysis/Continuous Ambulatory Peritoneal Dialysis: Give 1g followed by 500mg q24h, or add to fluid at 250mg/2L. *Pediatrics:* 1 month-12 yrs: 30-50mg/kg IV q8h. Max: 6g/day. Neonates (0-4 weeks): 30mg/kg IV q12h. Higher doses for cystic fibrosis or meningitis. CrCl 31-50mL/min: 1g q12h. CrCl 16-30mL/min: 1g q24h. CrCl 6-15mL/min: 500mg q24h. CrCl <5mL/min: 500mg q48h. For severe infections (6g/day), increase renal impairment dose by 50% or increase dosing interval. Apply reduced dosage recommendations after initial 1g LD is given. Hemodialysis: Give 1g before, then 1g after each hemodialysis. Intra-Peritoneal Dialysis/Continuous Ambulatory Peritoneal Dialysis: Give 1g followed by 500mg q24h, or add to fluid at 250mg/2L.

HOW SUPPLIED: Inj: 500mg, 1g, 1g/50mL, 2g, 2g/50mL, 6g

WARNINGS/PRECAUTIONS: Monitor renal function; potential for nephrotoxicity. Prolonged use may result in overgrowth of nonsusceptible organisms. Possible cross-sensitivity between PCNs, cephalosporins, and other β-lactam antibiotics. *Clostridium difficile*-associated diarrhea reported and may range in severity from mild diarrhea to fatal colitis. Elevated levels with renal insufficiency can lead to seizures, encephalopathy, coma, asterixis, and neuromuscular excitability. Possible decrease in PT; caution with renal/hepatic impairment, poor nutritional state; monitor PT and give vitamin K if needed. Caution with colitis, other GI diseases, and elderly. Distal necrosis may occur after inadvertent intra-arterial administration. Continue therapy for 2 days after the signs and symptoms of infection have disappeared, but in complicated infections longer therapy may be required. False (+) for urine glucose with Benedict's solution, Fehling's solution, and Clinitest tabs.

ADVERSE REACTIONS: Phlebitis and inflammation at injection site, pruritus, rash, fever, diarrhea.

INTERACTIONS: Nephrotoxicity reported with aminoglycosides or potent diuretics (eg, furosemide). Avoid with chloramphenicol; may decrease effect of β-lactam antibiotics. Possible decrease in PT; caution with a protracted course of antimicrobial therapy; monitor PT and give vitamin K if needed. May reduce efficacy of oral contraceptives.

PREGNANCY: Category B, caution in nursing.

MECHANISM OF ACTION: 3rd-generation cephalosporin; bactericidal, inhibits cell-wall synthesis.

PHARMACOKINETICS: Absorption: (IV) Administration of variable doses resulted in different parameters. **Distribution:** Plasma protein binding (≤10%). **Elimination:** Urine (unchanged, 80-90%).

NURSING CONSIDERATIONS

Assessment: Assess for history of hypersensitivity to cephalosporins/PCNs, pregnancy status, possible drug interactions, renal impairment. Document indications for therapy, culture and susceptibility testing. Incision and drainage should be performed in conjunction with antibiotic therapy when indicated.

Monitoring: Monitor for signs and symptoms of hypersensitivity reactions (anaphylaxis), CDAD, seizures, LDH, LFTs, renal function, PT, hemolytic anemia, superinfection.

Patient Counseling: Inform therapy only treats bacterial, not viral, infections. Take exactly as directed; skipping doses or not completing full course may decrease effectiveness and increase resistance. May experience diarrhea; notify physician if watery/bloody stools, superinfection, or hypersensitivity reactions occur.

Administration: IM/IV route. For direct intermittent IV administration, slowly inject into vein over period of 3-5 min or give through tubing of administration set while patient also receives compatible IV fluid. **Storage:** In dry state, store between 15-30°C (59-86°F) and protect from light. Frozen as premixed solution should not be stored above -20°C.

FORTEO — RX

teriparatide (Lilly)

Increased incidence of osteosarcoma seen in rats. Only prescribe when benefits outweigh risks. Not for those at increased baseline risk for osteosarcoma, including Paget's disease or unexplained alkaline phosphatase elevations, open epiphyses, or prior radiation therapy involving the skeleton.

THERAPEUTIC CLASS: Recombinant human parathyroid hormone

INDICATIONS: Treatment of postmenopausal women with osteoporosis who are at high risk for fracture. To increase bone mass in men with primary or hypogonadal osteoporosis who are at high risk for fracture.

DOSAGE: *Adults:* 20mcg qd SQ into thigh or abdominal wall. Administer initially under circumstances where patient can sit or lie down if symptoms of orthostatic hypotension occur. Discard pen after 28 days. Use for >2 yrs is not recommended.

HOW SUPPLIED: Inj: 250mcg/mL [3mL pen]

WARNINGS/PRECAUTIONS: Avoid in Paget's disease of the bone, pediatrics, prior external beam or implant radiation therapy, or with bone metastases, or history of skeletal malignancies, metabolic bone diseases other than osteoporosis, or pre-existing hypercalcemia (eg, primary hyperparathyroidism). Potential exacerbation of active or recent urolithiasis. Transient episodes of symptomatic orthostatic hypotension observed infrequently. Increases serum uric acid levels. Transient calcium increases.

ADVERSE REACTIONS: Pain, arthralgia, asthenia, nausea, rhinitis, dizziness, headache, HTN, increased cough, pharyngitis, constipation, diarrhea, dyspepsia.

INTERACTIONS: Hypercalcemia may predispose to digitalis toxicity; caution with concomitant use.

PREGNANCY: Category C; not for use in nursing.

MECHANISM OF ACTION: Recombinant human parathyroid hormone; binds to specific high-affinity cell-surface receptors. Stimulates new bone formation on trabecular and cortical bone surfaces by preferential stimulation of osteoblastic activity over osteoclastic activity. Produces an increase in skeletal mass, an increase in markers of bone formation and resorption, and an increase in bone strength.

PHARMACOKINETICS: Absorption: Extensive; absolute bioavailability (95%); T_{max}=30 min. **Distribution:** (IV) V_d=0.12L/kg. **Metabolism:** Liver (nonspecific enzymatic mechanism). **Elimination:** Kidney; (IV) $T_{1/2}$=5 min; (SQ) $T_{1/2}$=1 hr.

NURSING CONSIDERATIONS

Assessment: Assess for Paget's disease of bone (eg, unexplained elevations in alkaline phosphatase), age of patient or presence of open epiphyses, history of external beam or implant radiation therapy, bone metastases or history of skeletal malignancies, metabolic bone disease other than osteoporosis, pre-existing hypercalcemia, active or recent urolithiasis, pregnancy/nursing status, and possible drug interactions. If active urolithiasis or hypercalciuria is present, measure urinary calcium excretion.

Monitoring: Monitor for signs/symptoms of osteosarcoma, orthostatic hypotension, hypercalcemia (eg, NV, constipation, muscle weakness).

Patient Counseling: Inform medication has been shown to cause osteosarcomas in animals (rats). Counsel to sit or lie down if lightheaded or develop palpitations following injection; if symptoms persist or worsen, contact physician before continuing treatment. Instruct to contact physician if develop signs of hypercalcemia (eg, NV, constipation, muscle weakness). Counsel how to properly use delivery device, properly dispose of needles, and to avoid sharing injection pens. Inform each injection pen can be used for up to 28 days; discard after 28 days. Counsel not to use medication more than 2 years. Advise about the roles of supplemental calcium and/or vitamin D, weight-bearing exercise, and behavior modification factors (eg, smoking/alcohol consumption).

Administration: SQ route, into thigh or abdominal wall. **Storage:** 2-8°C (36-46°F). Recap pen when not in use to protect cartridge from physical damage and light. Minimize time out of refrigerator. Do not freeze; do not use if frozen.

FORTICAL — RX

calcitonin-salmon (rdna origin) (Upsher-Smith)

THERAPEUTIC CLASS: Hormonal bone resorption inhibitor

INDICATIONS: Treatment of postmenopausal osteoporosis in females >5 yrs postmenopause in conjunction with an adequate calcium and vitamin D intake.

DOSAGE: *Adults:* 200 IU qd intranasally. Alternate nostrils daily.

HOW SUPPLIED: Nasal Spray: 200 IU/inh

CONTRAINDICATIONS: Clinical allergy to calcitonin-salmon.

WARNINGS/PRECAUTIONS: Possibility of systemic allergic reactions. Consider skin testing if sensitivity suspected. If nasal mucosa ulceration occurs, d/c until healed. D/C if severe ulceration of nasal mucosa occurs.

Perform periodic nasal exams. Incidence of rhinitis, irritation, erythema, and excoriation higher in geriatric patients.

ADVERSE REACTIONS: Rhinitis, nasal symptoms, back pain, arthralgia, epistaxis, headache

PREGNANCY: Category C, not for use in nursing.

MECHANISM OF ACTION: Hormonal bone resorption inhibitor; not established. Calcitonin receptors are found in osteoclasts and osteoblasts. Single use produces transient inhibition of bone resorptive process; persistent use causes smaller decreases in rate of bone resorption. Inhibits osteoclast function with loss of ruffled osteoclast border.

PHARMACOKINETICS: Absorption: Rapid.

NURSING CONSIDERATIONS

Assessment: Assess for sensitivity to calcitonin; perform skin testing if sensitivity suspected. Assess pregnancy/nursing status.

Monitoring: Monitor for signs/symptoms of allergic reaction (eg, anaphylactic shock, broncospasm, swelling of tongue or throat), nasal mucosal alterations, rhinitis, epitaxis, and sinusitis. Perform periodic nasal exams of nasal mucosa, turbinates, septum, and mucosal blood vessels. Perform periodic monitoring of urine sediment. Measure lumbar vertebral bone mass periodically to monitor for efficacy.

Patient Counseling: Counsel to notify physician of significant nasal irritation. Advise to store new, unassembled medication in refrigerator; do not freeze. Instruct that before priming pump and using new medication, allow to reach room temperature. Inform that after opening, store at room temperature, in upright position; discard unused medication 30 days after 1st use.

Administration: Intranasal route. **Storage:** Unopened: 2-8°C (36-46°F). Protect from freezing. Opened: 20-25°C (68-77°F); excursions permitted to 15-30°C (59-86°F). Store in upright position. Discard 30 days after 1st use.

FOSAMAX — RX

alendronate sodium (Merck)

THERAPEUTIC CLASS: Bisphosphonate

INDICATIONS: Treatment and prevention of osteoporosis in postmenopausal women. Treatment to increase bone mass in men with osteoporosis. Treatment of glucocorticoid-induced osteoporosis. Treatment of Paget's disease.

DOSAGE: *Adults:* Osteoporosis: Treatment: 70mg once weekly or 10mg qd. Prevention: 35mg once weekly or 5mg qd. Glucocorticoid-Induced: 5mg qd; 10mg qd for postmenopausal women not on estrogen. Paget's Disease: 40mg qd for 6 months. Take at least 30 min before the first food, beverage (other than water), or medication (Take tabs with 6-8 oz plain water or 2oz with oral sol). Do not lie down for at least 30 min and until after 1st food of day.

HOW SUPPLIED: Sol: 70mg [75mL]; Tab: 5mg, 10mg, 35mg, 40mg, 70mg

CONTRAINDICATIONS: Esophagus abnormalities which delay esophageal emptying such as stricture or achalasia; inability to stand or sit upright for at least 30 min; hypocalcemia.

WARNINGS/PRECAUTIONS: Caution with active upper GI problems. May cause local irritation of the upper GI mucosa. Correct hypocalcemia or other mineral metabolism disturbances before initiating therapy. Supplement calcium and vitamin D if needed. Not recommended with renal insufficiency (CrCl <35mL/min). D/C if symptoms of esophageal disease develop. When combined with glucocorticoids, perform BMD test at initiation and 6-12 months later. Reports of severe, incapacitating bone, joint, and/or muscle pain.

ADVERSE REACTIONS: Abdominal pain, nausea, dyspepsia, constipation, diarrhea, flatulence, acid regurgitation, musculoskeletal pain, gastric ulcers, joint swelling, asthenia, dizziness/vertigo, and rarely peripheral edema.

INTERACTIONS: Calcium supplements, antacids, other oral medications may interfere with absorption; dose at least one-half hour after alendronate. Increased GI irritation with ASA and alendronate >10mg. Caution with NSAIDs, other GI irritants.

PREGNANCY: Category C, caution in nursing.

MECHANISM OF ACTION: Bisphosphonate; binds to hydroxyapatite, a component of bone. Specific inhibitor of osteoclast-mediated bone resorption.

PHARMACOKINETICS: Distribution: V_d=28L; plasma protein binding (78%). **Excretion:** Urine (50%), feces (little or none); $T_{1/2}$>10 yrs.

NURSING CONSIDERATIONS

Assessment: Assess for esophageal abnormalities (eg, stricture, achalasia) or other upper GI disorders (eg, dysphagia, gastritis, duodenitis, ulcers), ability to stand or sit upright for at least 30 min, risk of aspiration, hypocalcemia, vitamin D deficiency, risk of osteonecrosis of the jaw, renal insufficiencies (eg, CrCl <35 mL/min), pregnancy/nursing status, and possible drug interactions. Assess for causes of osteoporosis other than estrogen deficiency, aging, and glucocorticoid use. Assess hormonal status and consider replacement therapy. If on concomitant therapy with glucocorticoids, obtain baseline bone mineral density measurement.

Monitoring: Monitor for signs/symptoms of upper GI mucosal irritation, esophageal complications (eg, esophagitis, esophageal ulcers, esophageal erosions, esophageal stricture or perforation), gastric and duodenal ulcers, musculoskeletal pain, and osteonecrosis of the jaw. With history of hypocalcemia, monitor calcium levels and for signs/symptoms of hypocalcemia. If on concomitant therapy with glucocorticoids, monitor bone mineral density every 6-12 months.

Patient Counseling: Instruct to take supplemental calcium and vitamin D if daily dietary intake is inadequate. Counsel to consider weight-bearing exercise as well as modification of certain behavioral factors (eg, cigarette smoking, excessive alcohol consumption). Take medication with plain water in the morning (at least 30 min before the first food, beverage, or medication). Swallow with a full glass of water. If taking oral solution formulation, advise to take with at least 2 oz of water following administration of medication. Avoid lying down for at least 30 min following administration and until after first food of the day. Avoid chewing or sucking on medication. Counsel not to take at bedtime or before rising for the day. Advise to d/c and contact physician if symptoms of esophageal disease (eg, difficulty swallowing, new or worsening heartburn) develop. Advise if the once a week dose is missed, take the following morning and return to taking dose on regularly scheduled day. Counsel to separate administration 30 min from other oral medications.

Administration: Oral route. **Storage:** Tab: 15-30°C (59-86°F); Oral sol: 25°C (77°F); excursions permitted to 15-30°C (59-86°F). Do not freeze.

FOSAMAX PLUS D — RX

alendronate sodium - cholecalciferol (Merck)

THERAPEUTIC CLASS: Bisphosphonate/vitamin D analog

INDICATIONS: Treatment of osteoporosis in postmenopausal women. Treatment to increase bone mass in men with osteoporosis.

DOSAGE: *Adults:* 1 tab (70mg/5600 IU or 70mg/2800 IU) once weekly. Take at least 30 min before 1st food, beverage (other than water), or medication. Do not lie down for at least 30 min and until after 1st food of day.

HOW SUPPLIED: Tab: (Alendronate Sodium-Cholecalciferol) 70mg-2800 IU, 70mg-5600 IU

CONTRAINDICATIONS: Esophagus abnormalities which delay esophageal emptying such as stricture or achalasia; inability to stand or sit upright for at least 30 min; hypocalcemia.

WARNINGS/PRECAUTIONS: Caution with active upper GI problems. May cause local irritation of the upper GI mucosa. Correct hypocalcemia or other mineral metabolism disturbances before initiating therapy. Do not use to treat vitamin D deficiency. May worsen hypercalcemia and/or hypercalciuria. Supplement calcium if needed. Not recommended with renal insufficiency (CrCl <35mL/min). D/C if symptoms of esophageal disease develop. Reports of severe, incapacitating bone, joint, and/or muscle pain.

ADVERSE REACTIONS: Abdominal pain, nausea, dyspepsia, constipation, diarrhea, flatulence, acid regurgitation, musculoskeletal pain, gastric ulcers, joint swelling, asthenia, dizziness/vertigo, and rarely peripheral edema.

INTERACTIONS: Calcium supplements, antacids, other oral medications may interfere with absorption; dose at least one-half hour after alendronate. Caution with NSAIDs, other GI irritants. Olestra, mineral oils, orlistat, bile acid sequestrants may impair absorption. Anticonvulsants, cimetidine, thiazides may increase catabolism.

PREGNANCY: Category C, caution in nursing.

MECHANISM OF ACTION: Alendronate: Bisphosphonate; binds to hydroxyapatite found in bone. Specific inhibitor of osteoclast-mediated bone resorption. Cholecalciferol: Vitamin D analog; increases intestinal absorption of calcium and phosphate; regulates excretion of serum calcium, renal calcium and phosphate, bone formation, and bone resorption.

PHARMACOKINETICS: Absorption: Cholecalciferol: C_{max}=4.0ng/mL; T_{max}=10.6 hrs; AUC=120.7ng•hr/mL. **Distribution:** Alendronate: V_d=28L; plasma protein binding (78%). Cholecalciferol: Found in breast milk. **Metabolism:** Cholecalciferol: Liver (rapid) (hydroxylation) to 25-hydroxyvitamin D_3 (major storage form metabolite); kidney to 1,25-dihydroxyvitamin D_3 (active metabolite). **Elimination:** Alendronate: Urine (50%), feces (little or none); $T_{1/2}$>10 years. Cholecalceferol: Urine (2.4%), feces (4.9%); $T_{1/2}$=14 hrs.

NURSING CONSIDERATIONS

Assessment: Assess for esophageal abnormalities (eg, stricture, achalasia) or upper GI disorders (eg, dysphagia, gastritis, duodenitis, ulcers), GI malabsorption syndrome, ability to stand or sit upright for at least 30 min, hypocalcemia and other disorders affecting mineral metabolism (eg, vitamin D deficiency), risk of osteonecrosis of the jaw, renal insufficiencies (eg, CrCl<35mL/min), pregnancy/nursing status, and possible drug interactions.

Monitoring: Monitor for signs/symptoms of local upper GI mucosa irritation, esophageal complications (eg, esophagitis, esophageal ulcers, esophageal erosions), musculoskeletal pain, and osteonecrosis of the jaw. If patients have unregulated overproduction of 1,25 dihydroxyvitamin D (eg, leukemia, lymphoma), monitor urine and serum calcium levels. With history of hypocalcemia, monitor serum calcium levels and for signs/symptoms of hypocalcemia.

Patient Counseling: Instruct to take supplemental calcium if intake is inadequate. Instruct to take additional vitamin D if at risk for vitamin D deficiency (eg, >70 yrs, nursing home-bound, chronically ill); vitamin D needs increase with GI malabsorption syndromes. Counsel to consider weight-bearing exercise, behavioral modification (eg, cigarette smoking, excessive alcohol consumption). Take with full glass of water first thing in the morning (at least 30 min before first food/beverage or medication). Avoid lying down for 30 min following administration. Avoid chewing or sucking on medication; avoid taking medication at bedtime or before rising for the day. Advise to d/c and contact physician if signs of esophageal disease (eg, difficulty swallowing, new or worsening heartburn) develop. If a dose is missed, take the following morning; return to taking on regularly scheduled day.

Administration: Oral route. **Storage:** 20-25°C (68-77°F); excursions permitted to 15-30°C (59-86°F). Protect from moisture and light. Store in original blister package until use.

FOSRENOL — RX

lanthanum carbonate (Shire)

THERAPEUTIC CLASS: Phosphate Binder

INDICATIONS: Reduction of serum phosphate in patients with end-stage renal disease.

DOSAGE: *Adults:* Initial: 750-1500mg/day in divided doses. Titrate: Every 2-3 weeks in increments of 750mg/day until acceptable serum phosphate level is reached. Take with meals and chew tablets completely before swallowing. Usual range: 1500-3000mg/day. Usual max: 3750mg/day.

HOW SUPPLIED: Tab, Chewable: 250mg, 500mg, 750mg, 1000mg

WARNINGS/PRECAUTIONS: Caution with acute peptic ulcer, ulcerative colitis, Crohn's disease or bowel obstruction.

ADVERSE REACTIONS: Nausea, vomiting, dialysis graft occulsion, abdominal pain.

F

INTERACTIONS: Should not be taken within 2 hrs of antacids.

PREGNANCY: Category C, caution in nursing.

MECHANISM OF ACTION: Inhibits absorption of phosphate by forming highly insoluble lanthanum phosphate complexes, consequently reducing both serum phosphate and calcium product.

PHARMACOKINETICS: Absorption: C_{max}=1.0ng/mL. **Distribution:** Plasma protein binding (>99%). **Metabolism:** Not metabolized. **Elimination:** $T_{1/2}$=53 hrs, ($T_{1/2}$=2-3.6 yrs, from bone).

NURSING CONSIDERATIONS

Assessment: Assess for acute peptic ulcer, ulcerative colitis, Crohn's disease, bowel obstruction, and pregnancy/nursing status.

Monitoring: Monitor for GI events and NV. Drug may appear as imaging agent in abdominal x-rays.

Patient Counseling: Take with or immediately after meals. Chew completely before swallowing. Do not swallow intact tablets.

Administration: Oral route. **Storage:** 25°C (77°F); excursions permitted to 15-30°C (59-86°F).

FRAGMIN — RX

dalteparin sodium (Eisai)

Risk of paralysis by spinal/epidural hematoma with neuraxial anesthesia or spinal puncture. Increased risk with indwelling epidural catheters for analgesia, drugs affecting hemostasis (eg, NSAIDs, platelet inhibitors, anticoagulants), and traumatic or repeated epidural or spinal puncture. Frequently monitor for signs and symptoms of neurological impairment.

THERAPEUTIC CLASS: Low molecular weight heparin

INDICATIONS: Prevention of ischemic complications in unstable angina and non-Q-wave MI with concurrent ASA therapy. Prophylaxis of DVT in hip replacement surgery, abdominal surgery in patients who are at high risk for thromboembolic complications, and for those at risk for thromboembolic complications due to severely restricted mobility during acute illness. Extended treatment of symptomatic VTE (proximal DVT and/or PE), to reduce the recurrence of VTE in patients with cancer.

DOSAGE: *Adults:* Administer SQ. Unstable Angina/Non-Q-Wave MI: 120 IU/kg up to 10,000 IU q12h with ASA (75-165mg/day) for 5-8 days. Hip Surgery: Pre-Op Start: Initial (if start 2 hrs pre-op): 2500 IU within 2 hrs pre-op, then 2500 IU 4-8 hrs post-op. Initial (if start 10-14 hrs pre-op): 5000 IU 10-14 hrs pre-op, then 5000 IU 4-8 hrs post-op. Maint (for either initial dose): 5000 IU SQ qd for 5-10 days post-op (up to 14 days). Post-Op Start: 2500 IU 4-8 hrs post-op. Maint: 5000 IU qd. Abdominal Surgery: 2500 IU 1-2 hrs pre-op. Maint: 2500 IU qd for 5-10 days post-op. Abdominal Surgery with High Risk: 5000 IU evening before surgery. Maint: 5000 IU qd for 5-10 days post-op. Abdominal Surgery with Malignancy: Initial: 2500 IU 1-2 hrs pre-op, then 2500 IU 12 hrs later. Maint: 5000 IU qd for 5-10 days post-op. Severely Restricted Mobility During Acute Illness: 5000 IU qd for 12-14 days. Symptomatic VTE in Cancer Patients: 200 IU/kg qd for first 30 days, then 150 IU/kg qd for months 2-6. Max: 18,000 IU/day. Platelet Count 50,000-100,000/mm^3: Reduce dose by 2500 IU until platelet count ≥100,000/mm³. Platelet Count <50,000/mm³: D/C therapy until platelet count >50,000/mm³. Renal Impairment (CrCl <30mL/min): Monitor anti-Xa levels to determine appropriate dose.

HOW SUPPLIED: Inj: (Syringe) 2500 IU/0.2mL, 5000 IU/0.2mL, 7500 IU/0.3mL, 10,000 IU/0.4mL, 10,000 IU/1mL, 12,500 IU/0.5mL, 15,000 IU/0.6mL, 18,000 IU/0.72mL; (MDV) 10,000 IU/mL [9.5mL], 25,000 IU/mL [3.8mL]

CONTRAINDICATIONS: Heparin or pork allergy, regional anesthesia with unstable angina, non-Q-wave MI or patients with cancer, active major bleeding, thrombocytopenia with a positive in vitro test for antiplatelet antibody.

WARNINGS/PRECAUTIONS: Not for IM injection. Cannot use interchangeably unit for unit with heparin or other low molecular weight heparins. Extreme caution with HIT, conditions with increased risk of hemorrhage (eg, bacterial endocarditis, hemorrhagic stroke, etc). Hemorrhage, thrombocytopenia, HIT may occur. May increase risk of thrombocytopenia with cancer or acute venous thromboembolism. Caution with bleeding diathesis, platelet defects, severe hepatic/kidney dysfunction, hypertensive or diabetic retinopathy, recent GI bleeding or in elderly with low body weight (<45kg) and predisposed to decreased renal function. D/C if thromboembolic event occurs. Perform periodic CBC, platelets, stool occult blood test. May increase LFTs. Multiple dose vial contains benzyl alcohol. Do not mix with other injections or infusions unless compatibility data available.

ADVERSE REACTIONS: Hemorrhage, injection-site pain, allergic reactions, thrombocytopenia.

INTERACTIONS: Caution with oral anticoagulants, platelet inhibitors, thrombolytic agents due to increased risk of bleeding.

PREGNANCY: Category B, caution in nursing.

MECHANISM OF ACTION: Low molecular weight heparin; antithrombotic properties. Enhances inhibition of Factor Xa and thrombin by antithrombin.

PHARMACOKINETICS: Absorption: Absolute bioavailability (87%). (2500 IU) C_{max}=0.19 IU/mL. (5000 IU) C_{max}= 0.41 IU/mL. (10,000 IU) C_{max}=0.82 IU/mL; T_{max}=4 hrs. **Distribution:** V_d=40-60mL/kg. **Elimination:** (40 IU/kg) (IV) $T_{1/2}$=2.1 hrs. (60 IU/kg) (IV) $T_{1/2}$=2.3 hrs; (SQ) $T_{1/2}$=3-5 hrs.

NURSING CONSIDERATIONS

Assessment: Assess for active major bleeding, thrombocytopenia, history of heparin-induced thrombocytopenia, risk of hemorrhage (eg, severe uncontrolled HTN, bacterial endocarditis, congenital/acquired bleeding disorders, active ulceration, angiodysplastic GI disease), presence of regional anesthesia, pregnancy/nursing status, known hypersensitivity to heparin or pork products, and drug interactions. Assess use with bleeding diathesis, severe hepatic/renal insufficiencies, and hypertensive or diabetic retinopathy.

Monitoring: Monitor for signs/symptoms of hemorrhage, thrombocytopenia, and allergic reactions. Monitor for signs/symptoms of spinal or epidural hematomas in patients on concomitant therapy with neuraxial anesthesia or spinal puncture. Perform periodic monitoring of CBC (platelet count), blood chemistry, and stool occult blood tests. In patients with severe renal impairment (CrCl <30mL/min); monitor anti-Xa levels.

Patient Counseling: Instruct to contact physician if any type of unusual bleeding or allergic reactions develop. Inform that periodic lab monitoring is required during medication. If pregnant, instruct to use preservative-free formulation.

Administration: SQ route. Not for IM injection. Do not mix with other injections or infusions. Patient should be sitting or lying down. Inj may be administered in U-shaped area around navel, upper outer side of thigh, or upper outer quadrangle of buttock. Vary inj site daily. 1) If area around navel or thigh is used, using thumb and forefinger, lift up fold of skin while giving inj. 2) Insert at 45-90 degree angle. **Storage:** 20-25°C (68-77°F).

FROVA RX

frovatriptan succinate (Endo)

THERAPEUTIC CLASS: 5-$HT_{1B/1D}$ agonist

INDICATIONS: Acute treatment of migraine with or without aura.

DOSAGE: *Adults:* ≥18 yrs: 2.5mg with fluids. If headache recurs after initial relief, may repeat after 2 hrs. Max: 7.5mg/day. Safety of treating >4 headaches/30 days not known.

HOW SUPPLIED: Tab: 2.5mg

F

CONTRAINDICATIONS: Ischemic heart disease, coronary artery vasospasm (eg, Prinzmetal's angina), significant cardiovascular disease, cerebrovascular syndromes, peripheral vascular disease, uncontrolled HTN, hemiplegic or basilar migraine, use within 24 hrs of treatment with another 5-HT_1 agonist or ergot-type agent.

WARNINGS/PRECAUTIONS: Confirm diagnosis. Supervise 1st dose and monitor cardiac function in those at risk of CAD (eg, HTN, hypercholesterolemia, smoker, obesity, diabetes, CAD family history, postmenopausal women, males >40 yrs). Serious adverse cardiac events, cerebrovascular events, vasospastic reactions reported with 5-HT_1 agonists. May bind to melanin in the eye; possibility of long-term effects. Serotonin syndrome symptoms (eg, mental status changes, autonomic instability, neuromuscular aberrations, and GI symptoms) reported.

ADVERSE REACTIONS: Dizziness, headache, paresthesia, dry mouth, dyspepsia, fatigue, hot or cold sensation, chest pain, skeletal pain, flushing.

INTERACTIONS: Prolonged vasospastic reactions reported with ergot-containing drugs; avoid use within 24 hours. Avoid within 24 hours of other 5-$HT_{1B/1D}$ agonists. Weakness, hyperreflexia, and incoordination reported with SSRIs (rare). Serotonin syndrome reported with combined use of SSRI or SNRI.

PREGNANCY: Category C, caution in nursing.

MECHANISM OF ACTION: Selective 5-HT_1 receptor agonist; binds with high affinity to 5-$HT_{1B/1D}$ receptors. Believed to act on extracerebral, intracranial blood vessels, and to inhibit excessive dilation of these vessels in migraine.

PHARMACOKINETICS: Absorption: Absolute bioavailability: (20%) male, (30%) female; T_{max}=2-4 hrs. **Distribution:** V_d=4.2L/kg (male), 3L/kg (female); plasma protein binding (15%). **Metabolism:** CYP1A2. **Elimination:** Feces (62%), urine (32%); $T_{1/2}$=26 hrs.

NURSING CONSIDERATIONS

Assessment: Confirm diagnosis of migraine before initiating therapy. Assess for IHD (eg, angina pectoris, Prinzmetal's variant angina, MI or documented silent MI), HTN, hemiplegic/or basilar migraine, cerebrovascular syndromes (eg, stroke, TIAs), PVD, presence of risk factors of CAD (eg, hypercholesterolemia, smoking, obesity, DM, strong family history of CAD, female with surgical or physiological menopause, or male >49 yrs), ECG changes, hepatic/renal impairment, pregnancy/nursing status, and possible drug interactions.

Monitoring: Administration of 1st dose should be in physician's office or medically staffed and equipped facility as cardiac ischemia may occur in absence of clinical symptoms; ECG should be obtained immediately during interval in those with risk factors. Monitor for signs/symptoms of cardiac events (eg, coronary vasospasm, acute MI, arrhythmia, ECG changes, follow-up coronary angiography), cerebrovascular events (eg, hemorrhage, stroke, TIAs), peripheral vascular ischemia, colonic ischemia with bloody diarrhea and abdominal pain, serotonin syndrome (eg, mental status changes, autonomic instability, neuromuscular aberrations and/or GI symptoms), ophthalmic effects, and increased BP.

Patient Counseling: Instruct to read PI before taking drug. Inform about potential risks (eg, serotonin syndrome manifestations), especially if taken with SSRIs or SNRIs. Report adverse reactions to physician. Advise to take as directed. Instruct to notify physician if pregnant/nursing or planning to become pregnant.

Administration: Oral route. **Storage**: 25°C (77°F); excursion permitted to 15-30°C (59-86°F).

FUROSEMIDE RX

furosemide (Various)

Can lead to profound water and electrolyte depletion with excessive use.

F

OTHER BRAND NAMES: Lasix (Sanofi-Aventis)

THERAPEUTIC CLASS: Loop diuretic

INDICATIONS: (Inj, PO) Treatment of edema associated with CHF, liver cirrhosis, and renal disease including nephrotic syndrome. (PO) Treatment of hypertension. (Inj) Adjunct therapy for acute pulmonary edema.

DOSAGE: *Adults:* (PO) HTN: Initial: 40mg bid. Edema: Initial: 20-80mg PO. May repeat or increase by 20-40mg after 6-8 hrs. Max: 600mg/day. Alternative Regimen: Dose on 2-4 consecutive days each week. Closely monitor if on >80mg/day. (Inj) Edema: Initial: 20-40mg IV/IM. May repeat or increase by 20mg after 2 hrs. Acute Pulmonary Edema: Initial: 40mg IV. May increase to 80mg IV after 1 hr.
Pediatrics: Edema: (PO) Initial: 2mg/kg single dose. May increase by 1-2mg/kg after 6-8 hrs. Max: 6mg/kg. (Inj) Initial: 1mg/kg IV/IM single dose. May increase by 1mg/kg IV/IM after 2 hrs. Max: 6mg/kg.

HOW SUPPLIED: Inj: 10mg/mL; Sol: 10mg/mL, 40mg/5mL; Tab: 20mg, 40mg*, 80mg *scored

CONTRAINDICATIONS: Anuria.

WARNINGS/PRECAUTIONS: Monitor for fluid/electrolyte imbalance (eg, hypokalemia), renal or hepatic dysfunction. Initiate in hospital with hepatic cirrhosis and ascites. Tinnitus, hearing impairment, hyperglycemia, hyperuricemia reported. May activate SLE. Cross-sensitivity with sulfonamide allergy. Avoid excessive diuresis, especially in elderly.

ADVERSE REACTIONS: Pancreatitis, jaundice, anorexia, paresthesias, ototoxicity, blood dyscrasias, dizziness, rash, urticaria, photosensitivity, fever, thrombophlebitis, restlessness.

INTERACTIONS: Ototoxicity with aminoglycosides, ethacrynic acid. Caution with high-dose salicylates. Lithium toxicity. Antagonizes tubocurarine. Potentiates antihypertensives, succinylcholine, ganglionic or peripheral adrenergic blockers. Decreases arterial response to norepinephrine. Separate sucralfate dose by 2 hrs. Indomethacin may decrease effects. Hypokalemia with ACTH, corticosteroids. Renal changes with NSAIDs. Orthostatic hypotension may be aggravated by alcohol, barbiturates, or narcotics.

PREGNANCY: Category C, caution in nursing.

MECHANISM OF ACTION: Anthranilic acid derivative (diuretic); primarily inhibits reabsorption of Na^+ and Cl^- in proximal and distal tubules and in loop of Henle.

PHARMACOKINETICS: Distribution: Plasma protein binding (91-99%). **Metabolism:** Biotransformation. Furosemide glucuronide (major metabolite). **Elimination:** Urine; $T_{1/2}$=2 hrs.

NURSING CONSIDERATIONS

Assessment: Assess for anuria, sulfonamide hypersensitivity, DM, possible drug interactions, hepatic/renal impairment. Obtain baseline serum electrolytes, renal function, urine, and blood glucose.

Monitoring: Monitor serum electrolytes frequently in first few months, then periodically; renal function, urine, and blood glucose periodically. Monitor for signs/symptoms of electrolyte imbalance, blood dyscrasias, hyperglycemia, hyperuricemia or precipitation of gout, hypotension, ototoxicity, persistent PDA, and hypersensitivity reactions.

Patient Counseling: Advise to seek medical attention if symptoms of electrolyte imbalance (dry mouth, thirst, weakness), hypotension, ototoxicity (tinnitus, hearing impairment), or hypersensitivity reactions occur.

Administration: Oral, IV route. **Storage**: Tab, Sol: 25°C (77°F); excursions permitted to 15-30°C (59-86°F). IV: 15-30°C (59-86°F). Protect from light.

FUZEON RX

enfuvirtide (Roche Labs)

F

THERAPEUTIC CLASS: Fusion inhibitor

INDICATIONS: Treatment of HIV-1 infection in combination with other antiretroviral agents in treatment-experienced patients with evidence of HIV-1 replication despite ongoing antiretroviral therapy.

DOSAGE: *Adults:* 90mg SQ bid. Inject SQ into upper arm, anterior thigh, or abdomen. Do not inject into moles, scar tissue, bruises, the navel, or near any blood vessels. Rotate sites; do not give if injection site reaction occurred from an earlier dose.
Pediatrics: 6-16 yrs: 2mg/kg SQ bid. Max: 90mg bid. 11-15.5kg: 27mg bid. 15.6-20.0kg: 36mg bid. 20.1-24.5kg: 45mg bid. 24.6-29.0kg: 54mg bid. 29.1-33.5kg: 63mg bid. 33.6-38.0kg: 72mg bid. 38.1-42.5kg: 81mg bid. ≥ 42.6kg: 90mg bid. Inject SQ into upper arm, anterior thigh, or abdomen. Do not inject into moles, scar tissue, bruises, or the navel. Rotate sites; do not give if injection site reaction occurred from an earlier dose.

HOW SUPPLIED: Inj: 90mg [60^s]

WARNINGS/PRECAUTIONS: Monitor for signs and symptoms of pneumonia, cellulitis, or local infection. D/C if hypersensitivity reactions occur. Theoretically may lead to production of anti-enfuvirtide antibodies; may result in false positive HIV test with an ELISA assay. Immune reconstitution syndrome reported. Increased risk of bleeding or bruising in patients with coagulation disorders.

ADVERSE REACTIONS: Diarrhea, nausea, fatigue, local injection site reactions, peripheral neuropathy, insomnia, depression, anxiety, cough, sinusitis, herpes simplex, decreased weight/appetite, pancreatitis, asthenia, pruritus, myalgia, nerve pain, bruising, hematomas.

PREGNANCY: Category B, not for use in nursing.

MECHANISM OF ACTION: Fusion inhibitor; inhibits the fusion of HIV-1 with $CD4^+$ cells by interfering with entry of HIV-1 into cells.

PHARMACOKINETICS: Absorption: (SQ) C_{max}=4.59µg/mL; T_{max}=8 hrs; AUC=55.8µg•hr/mL. (IV) Absolute bioavailabilty (84.3%). Values obtained from different parameters are different when combined with other antiretroviral agents. **Distribution:**V_d=5.5L; plasma protein binding (92%). **Metabolism:** Hepatic (hydrolysis); metabolite (M_3). **Elimination:** (SQ) $T_{1/2}$=3.8 hrs.

NURSING CONSIDERATIONS

Assessment: Assess for risk factors for pneumonia (history of lung disease, decreased $CD4^+$ cell count, increased viral load, IV drug use, smoking), infections, hemophilia, history of coagulation disorders, pregnancy/nursing status, and possible drug interactions.

Monitoring: Monitor for signs/symptoms of cellulitis or local infection, bacterial pneumonia, immune reconstitution syndrome, post-injection bleeding, and hypersensitivity.

Patient Counseling: Instruct on proper administration (reconstitute with 1.1 mL sterile water for Inj, tap for 10 secs and then gently roll to prevent foaming; let stand for 45 mins, until dissolved; then draw up correct dose and inject). Inject in the upper arm, abdomen, or anterior thigh; rotate inj sites (avoid injecting at the same site for 2 consecutive doses). Advise to seek medical attention for symptoms of pneumonia (cough with fever, rapid breathing, SOB), systemic hypersensitivity (rash, fever, NV, chills, rigors, hypotension), post-injection bleeding, cellulitis or local infection (pain, discomfort, induration, erythema), and nerve pain (paresthesia) occur. Inform of pregnancy/nursing risks. Instruct not to change dosage or schedule, or to stop drug without consulting physician. Caution may impair physical/mental abilities if dizziness occurs.

Administration: SQ route. **Storage:** 25°C (77°F); excursions permitted to 15-30°C (59-86°F). Reconstituted solutions should be stored refrigerated at 2-8°C (36-46°F) and used within 24 hrs.

GABITRIL
tiagabine HCl (Cephalon)

RX

THERAPEUTIC CLASS: Nipecotic acid derivative

INDICATIONS: Adjunctive therapy in the treatment of partial seizures.

DOSAGE: *Adults:* Initial: 4mg qd. Titrate: May increase weekly by 4-8mg until clinical response. Max: 56mg/day given bid-qid. Take with food.
Pediatrics: ≥12 yo: Initial: 4mg qd. Titrate: May increase to 8mg qd at beginning of Week 2, then increase weekly by 4-8mg until clinical response. Max: 32mg/day. Take with food.

HOW SUPPLIED: Tab: 2mg, 4mg, 12mg, 16mg

WARNINGS/PRECAUTIONS: Reports of new-onset seizure or status epilepticus in patients without epilepsy. D/C and evaluate for underlying seizure disorder. Avoid abrupt withdrawal. Monitor during initial titration for impaired concentration, speech problem, somnolence, fatigue; may require hospitalization if reaction is severe. May exacerbate EEG abnormalities; adjust dose. Status epilepticus and sudden death reported. Reduce dose or d/c if generalized weakness occurs. Reduce dose with hepatic impairment. Serious skin rash reported.

ADVERSE REACTIONS: Dizziness, asthenia, somnolence, NV, nervousness, tremor, abdominal pain, abnormal thinking, depression, confusion, pharyngitis, rash.

INTERACTIONS: May reduce valproate levels. Diminished effects with carbamazepine, phenytoin. Additive CNS depression with alcohol, triazolam, CNS depressants.

PREGNANCY: Category C, caution in nursing.

MECHANISM OF ACTION: Antiepileptic; not established. May enhance activity of gamma aminobutytic acid (GABA), the major inhibitory neurotransmitter in the CNS. Binds to recognition sites associated with the GABA uptake carrier, thereby blocking GABA uptake into presynaptic neurons, permitting more GABA to be available for receptor binding on the surface of post-synaptic cells.

PHARMACOKINETICS: Absorption: Absolute bioavailability (90%). T_{max}=2.5 hrs (fed), T_{max}=45 min (fasting). **Distribution:** Plasma protein binding (96%). **Metabolism:** Hepatic via oxidation and glucuronidation, CYP3A. **Elimination:** Urine (25%), feces (63%); $T_{1/2}$=7-9 hrs. For pediatric parameters refer to full PI.

NURSING CONSIDERATIONS

Assessment: Assess use of medication in patients who are not on at least 1 concomitant enzyme-inducing epilepsy drug. Assess hepatic function prior to therapy and for possible drug interactions.

Monitoring: Monitor for occurrence of new-onset seizures and status epilepticus in patients without a previous history of epilepsy, occurrence of seizures with abrupt discontinuation, cognitive and neuropsychiatric events (effects on thought processes, effects on levels of consciousness), EEG changes, rash (Stevens-Johnson syndrome), generalized weakness, and ophthalmologic changes.

Patient Counseling: Inform may cause CNS depression; avoid operating machinery/driving until adjusted to effects. Advise to contact physician if signs of rash develop. Instruct to take with food; not to abruptly d/c medication. If multiple doses are missed, contact physician before restarting.

Administration: Oral route. Titrate regimen. **Storage:** Controlled temperature, between 20-25°C (68-77°F). Protect from light and moisture.

GARDASIL RX
human papillomavirus recombinant vaccine, quadrivalent (Merck)

THERAPEUTIC CLASS: Vaccine

INDICATIONS: Vaccination of girls and women 9-26 yrs old for the prevention of cervical, vulvar, and vaginal cancer caused by human papillomavirus (HPV) types 16 and 18, genital warts (condyloma acuminata) caused by HPV types 6 and 11, cervical intraepithelial neoplasia (CIN) grades 2 and 3, cervical adenocarcinoma in situ (AIS), cervical intraepithelial neoplasia (CIN) grade 1, vulvar intraepithelial neoplasia (VIN) grades 2 and 3, and vaginal intraepithelial neoplasia (VaIN) grades 2 and 3 caused by HPV types 6, 11, 16, and 18.

DOSAGE: *Adults:* Give 3 separate 0.5mL IM doses in the deltoid region of upper arm or higher anterolateral area of the thigh. First dose: At elected date; second dose: 2 months after first dose; third dose: 6 months after first dose. *Pediatrics:* ≥9 yrs: Give 3 separate 0.5mL IM doses in the deltoid region of upper arm or higher anterolateral area of the thigh. First dose: At elected date; second dose: 2 months after first dose; third dose: 6 months after first dose.

HOW SUPPLIED: Inj: Vial/Syringe: 0.5mL

WARNINGS/PRECAUTIONS: Patients with impaired immune responsiveness may have reduced antibody response to active immunization. Medical treatment should be readily available in case of rare anaphylactic reactions. Does not protect against genital diseases not caused by HPV. Vaccination may not result in protection in all vaccine recipients.

ADVERSE REACTIONS: Local site reactions, fever, pyrexia, nausea, nasopharyngitis, dizziness, diarrhea, syncope, and headache.

INTERACTIONS: Immunosuppressive therapies, including irradiation, antimetabolites, alkylating agents, cytotoxic drugs, and corticosteroids (used in greater than physiologic doses) may reduce the immune responses to vaccines. May be administered concomitantly with Recombivax HB hepatitis B vaccine at a separate injection site.

PREGNANCY: Category B, caution in nursing.

MECHANISM OF ACTION: Develops humoral immune response that may protect against human papillomavirus types 6,11,16, and 18 (animal study).

NURSING CONSIDERATIONS

Assessment: Assess current health and immune status, history of bleeding disorders, and possible drug interactions.

Monitoring: Monitor for possible anaphylactic reactions, injection site for swelling, pain, erythema, fever, nausea, nasopharyngitis, dizziness, diarrhea, headache, local site reactions, syncope, and pyrexia.

Patient Counseling: Inform patient or caregiver of benefits/risks ratio; report any adverse reactions to physician. Syncope may follow vaccination. Does not substitute for routine cervical cancer screening and may not offer 100% protection. Not recommended during pregnancy.

Administration: IM in the deltoid region or anterolateral area of the thigh. **Storage:** 2-8°C (36-46°F). Do not freeze. Protect from light.

GEMZAR RX
gemcitabine HCl (Lilly)

THERAPEUTIC CLASS: Nucleoside analogue antimetabolite

INDICATIONS: Adjunct with cisplatin for 1st-line treatment of inoperable, locally advanced (Stage IIIA or IIIB) or metastatic (Stage IV) non-small cell lung cancer. If previously treated with 5-FU, 1st-line treatment of locally advanced (nonresectable Stage II or Stage III) or metastatic (Stage IV) pancreatic adenocarcinoma. Adjunct with paclitaxel for 1st-line treatment of metastatic breast cancer after failure of prior anthracycline-containing adjuvant chemotherapy, unless anthracyclines were clinically contraindicated. Combination with carboplatin for the treatment of advanced ovarian cancer that has relapsed at least 6 months after completion of platinum-based therapy.

DOSAGE: *Adults:* Pancreatic Cancer: $1000mg/m^2$ IV weekly up to 7 weeks, then 1 week off. Give subsequent cycles as weekly infusions for 3 out of every 4 weeks. Lung Cancer: 4-Week Cycle: $1000mg/m^2$ IV on Days 1, 8, and 15 of each 28-day cycle. Give cisplatin $100mg/m^2$ IV on Day 1 after gemcitabine infusion. 3-Week Cycle: $1250mg/m^2$ on Days 1 and 8 of each 21-day cycle. Give cisplatin $100mg/m^2$ IV on Day 1 after gemcitabine infusion. Breast Cancer: $1250mg/m^2$ IV on Days 1 and 8 of each 21-day cycle. Give paclitaxel $175mg/m^2$ IV on Day 1 before gemcitabine. Ovarian Cancer: $1000mg/m^2$ IV on Days 1 and 8 of each 21-day cycle. Give carboplatin AUC 4 on Day 1 after gemcitabine. Adjust dose based on hematologic toxicity. Infuse IV over 30 min.

G

HOW SUPPLIED: Inj: 200mg, 1g

WARNINGS/PRECAUTIONS: Increased toxicity with infusion time >60 min and more than once weekly dosing. Hemolytic-uremic syndrome, hepatotoxicity, pulmonary toxicity, renal failure, leukopenia, thrombocytopenia, and anemia reported. Myelosuppression is dose-limiting toxicity. D/C if severe lung toxicity occurs. Caution with significant renal or hepatic impairment. Pattern of tissue injury typically associated with radiation toxicity reported with concurrent and nonconcurrent use. Greater tendency for older women not to proceed to next cycle and to experience Grade 3/4 neutropenia and thrombocytopenia. Perform CBC, differential, and platelets before each dose. Decreased clearance in women and elderly.

ADVERSE REACTIONS: Myelosuppression, NV, diarrhea, stomatitis, elevated serum transaminases, proteinuria, hematuria, fever, rash, dyspnea, edema, flu syndrome, infection, alopecia, paresthesia.

INTERACTIONS: Monitor serum creatinine, K^+, calcium, and magnesium with cisplatin. Serious hepatotoxicity reported with hepatotoxic drugs.

PREGNANCY: Category D, not for use in nursing.

MECHANISM OF ACTION: Nucleoside analogue antimetabolite; exhibits cell cycle specificity, primarily killing cells undergoing DNA synthesis (S-phase); also blocks progression of cells through the G1/S-phase boundary.

PHARMACOKINETICS: Absorption: IV administration of variable doses resulted in different parameters. **Distribution:** Plasma protein binding (negligible). V_d=50L/m^2 (short-infusion), V_d=370L/m^2 (long-infusion). **Metabolism**: Intracellular by nucleoside kinases to the active diphosphate (dFdCDP) and triphosphate (dFdCTP). **Elimination:** Urine; $T_{1/2}$(short infusion, long infusion)=42-94 min, 245-638 min.

NURSING CONSIDERATIONS

Assessment: Assess renal/hepatic functions, CBC, pregnancy status. Note other diseases/conditions and drug therapies.

Monitoring: Monitor CBC with differential and platelet count, LFTs, renal failure, hemolytic uremic syndrome, pulmonary toxicity like ARDS, pulmonary edema, cardiovascular complications.

Patient Counseling: Inform drug can suppress bone marrow function manifested by leukopenia, thrombocytopenia, and anemia. Counsel about potential side effects; instruct to d/c drug and seek medical attention for adverse effects.

Administration: IV route. Reconstitute 5mL of 0.9% NaCl Inj (200mg vial) and 25mL of 0.9 NaCl Inj (1g vial). **Storage:** 20-25°C (68-77°F); excursions permitted to 15-30°C (59-86°F). Do not refrigerate.

GEODON RX

ziprasidone HCl (Pfizer)

Elderly patients with dementia-related psychosis treated with atypical antipsychotic drugs are at an increased risk of death; most appeared to be cardiovascular (eg, heart failure, sudden death) or infectious (eg, pneumonia) in nature. Ziprasidone is not approved for the treatment of patients with dementia-related psychosis.

OTHER BRAND NAMES: Geodon for Injection (Pfizer)

THERAPEUTIC CLASS: Benzisoxazole derivative

INDICATIONS: Treatment of schizophrenia. Treatment of acute manic or mixed episodes associated with bipolar disorder, with or without psychotic features. (Inj) Treatment of acute agitation in schizophrenic patients who need IM medication for rapid control of agitation.

DOSAGE: *Adults:* Schizophrenia: (Cap) Initial: 20mg bid with food. Titrate: May increase up to 80mg bid; adjust dose at intervals of not less than 2 days. Maint: 20-80mg bid for up to 52 weeks. (Inj) 10-20mg IM up to max 40mg/day. May give 10mg q2h or 20mg q4h up to 40mg/day for 3 days. Bipolar Mania: (Cap) Initial: 40mg bid with food. Titrate: Increase to 60-80mg bid on 2nd day of treatment. Maint: 40-80mg bid.

HOW SUPPLIED: Cap: (HCl) 20mg, 40mg, 60mg, 80mg; Inj: (Mesylate) 20mg/mL

CONTRAINDICATIONS: Concomitant dofetilide, sotalol, quinidine, Class Ia/III antiarrhythmics, mesoridazine, thioridazine, chlorpromazine, droperidol, pimozide, sparfloxacin, gatifloxacin, moxifloxacin, halofantrine, mefloquine, pentamidine, arsenic trioxide, levomethadyl acetate, dolasetron, probucol, tacrolimus, and drugs that prolong QT interval. History of QT prolongation, recent acute MI, uncompensated heart failure.

WARNINGS/PRECAUTIONS: D/C if persistent QTc measurements >500 msec, NMS, tardive dyskinesia occurs. Monitor for hyperglycemia in patients with DM or at risk for DM. Avoid with congenital long QT syndrome, history of arrhythmia. Caution in history of seizures. Esophageal dysmotility and aspiration reported. May elevate prolactin levels. Orthostatic hypotension reported; caution with cardiovascular or cerebrovascular disease, conditions predisposed to hypotension (eg, dehydration, hypovolemia). Caution with IM use in renal dysfunction.

ADVERSE REACTIONS: Asthenia, NV, constipation, dyspepsia, diarrhea, dry mouth, rash, somnolence, akathisia, dizziness, EPS, dystonia, hypertonia, respiratory disorder, upper respiratory infection, headache, injection site pain, swollen tongue, facial droop, tardive dyskinesia, enuresis, urinary incontinence.

INTERACTIONS: See Contraindications. Avoid drugs that prolong QTc intervals. Caution with centrally acting drugs. May enhance effects of antihypertensives. May antagonize effects of levodopa and dopamine agonists. Carbamazepine may decrease levels. CYP3A4 inhibitors may increase levels.

PREGNANCY: Category C, not for use in nursing.

MECHANISM OF ACTION: Benzisoxazole derivative; psychotropic agent; mechanism not established. Actions are mediated through a combination of dopamine type 2 (D_2) and serotonin type 2 (5HT2) antagonism.

PHARMACOKINETICS: Absorption: Well absorbed orally. Absolute bioavailability (60%); (PO) T_{max}=6-8 hrs, (IM) T_{max}=60 min. **Distribution:** V_d=1.5L/Kg; plasma protein binding (99%). **Metabolism:** Liver (extensive) via methylation and oxidation; CYP3A4 (major), 1A2 (minor). **Elimination:** Urine (20%, <1% unchanged), feces (66%, <4% unchanged); (PO) $T_{1/2}$=7 hrs; (IM) $T_{1/2}$=2-5 hrs.

NURSING CONSIDERATIONS

Assessment: Assess use in patients with known histories of QT prolongation (congenital long QT syndrome), recent MI, uncompensated heart failure, cardiac arrhythmias, and dementia-related psychosis. Assess baseline serum electrolytes (K, Mg) in patients at risk for QT prolongation. Replete serum electrolytes prior to treatment.

Monitoring: Monitor for QT prolongation, torsade de pointes, neuroleptic malignant syndrome, suicidal ideation, extrapyramidal symptoms, weight gain, and respiratory tract infections while on therapy. Monitor serum electrolytes (K^+, Mg) in patients taking concomitant diuretic therapy.

Patient Counseling: Counsel to take with food, avoid alcohol, and avoid high temperatures or humidity; drug may interfere with body's ability to adjust.

Administration: Oral, IM route. For IM preparation 1) Add 1.2mL of sterile water for injection to the vial and shake vigorously until dissolved. (Each mL of reconstituted solution contains 20mg ziprasodine. 2) To administer a 10mg dose, draw up 0.5mL of the reconstituted solution. 3) To administer a 20mg dose, draw up 1.0mL of the reconstituted solution. **Storage:** Capsules: 25°C (77°F), excursions permitted to 15-30°C (59-86°F). Inj: 25°C (77°F), excursions permitted to 15-30°C(59-86°F) for up to 24 hrs protected from light, or refrigerated at 2-8°C (36-46°F) for up to 7 days.

G

GLEEVEC — RX

imatinib mesylate (Novartis)

THERAPEUTIC CLASS: Protein-tyrosine kinase inhibitor

INDICATIONS: (Adults) Treatment of newly diagnosed adult patients with Philadelphia chromosome positive (Ph+) chronic myeloid leukemia (CML) in chronic phase. Treatment of Ph+ CML in blast crisis, accelerated phase, or in chronic phase after failure of interferon-alpha therapy. Treatment of relapsed or refractory Ph+ acute lympoblastic leukemia (ALL). Treatment of myelodysplastic/myeloproliferative diseases (MDS/MPD) associated with platelet-derived growth factor receptor (PDGFR) gene re-arrangements. Treatment of aggressive systemic mastocytosis (ASM) patients without the D816V c-Kit mutation or with unknown cKit mutational status. Treatment of hypereosinophilic syndrome (HES) and/or chronic eosinophilic leukemia (CEL) patients who have the FIP1L1-PDGFRα fusion kinase (mutational analysis or FISH demonstration of CHIC2 allele deletion) and for patients with HES and/or CEL who are FIP1L1-PDGFRα fusion kinase negative or unknown. Treatment of patients with unresectable, recurrent, and/or metastatic dermatofibrosarcoma protuberans (DFSP). Treatment of patients with Kit (CD117) positive unresectable and/or metastatic malignant gastrointestinal stromal tumors (GIST). Adjuvant treatment of patients following complete resection of Kit (CD117) positive GIST. (Pediatrics) Treatment of patients with Ph+ chronic phase CML in chronic phase who are newly diagnosed or whose disease has recurred after stem cell transplant or who are resistant to interferon-alpha therapy.

DOSAGE: *Adults:* CML: Chronic Phase: 400mg/d, may increase to 600mg qd. Accelerated Phase/Blast Crisis: 600mg/d, may increase to 400mg bid. Relapsed/Refractory Ph+ ALL: 600mg/d. MDS or MPD/ASM/HES and/or CEL: 400mg/d. ASM with eosinophilia/HES or CEL with FIP1L1-PDGFRα: Initial: 100mg/d. Titrate: May increase up to 400mg/d in the absence of adverse reactions and insufficient response. DFSP: 800mg/d. GIST (unresectable or metastatic/malignant): 400mg/d. Titrate: May increase up to 800mg (as 400mg bid) if clear signs/symptoms of disease progression and in the absence of adverse reactions. Severe Hepatic Impairment: Reduce dose by 25%. Co-administration with Strong CYP3A4 Inducers: Increase dose by at least 50% and monitor carefully. Hepatotoxicity/Non-Hematologic Adverse Reaction: If bilirubin >3x ULN or transaminases >5x ULN, hold drug until bilirubin <1.5x ULN and transaminases <2.5x ULN. Continue at reduced dose. Neutropenia/Thrombocytopenia: See PI for dosage adjustments. Take with food and plenty of water.

Pediatrics: CML: Newly Diagnosed: 340mg/m²/d. Chronic Phase: 260mg/m²/day given qd or split into 2 doses (morning and evening). Severe Hepatic Impairment: Reduce dose by 25%. Co-administration with Strong CYP3A4 Inducers: Increase dose by at least 50% and monitor carefully. Hepatotoxicity/Non-Hematologic Adverse Reaction: If bilirubin >3x ULN or transaminases >5x ULN, hold drug until bilirubin <1.5x ULN and transaminases <2.5x ULN.

Continue at reduced dose. Neutropenia/Thrombocytopenia: See PI for dosage adjustments. Take with food and plenty of water.

HOW SUPPLIED: Tab: 100mg, 400mg

WARNINGS/PRECAUTIONS: Fluid retention/edema (pleural effusion, pericardial effusion, pulmonary edema and ascites) reported; monitor weight. Anemia/neutropenia/thrombocytopenia reported; monitor CBC weekly during 1st month, biweekly during 2nd month, and periodically thereafter. In pediatric patients, the most frequent toxicities observed were grade 3 and 4 cytopenias. May be hepatotoxic; monitor LFTs at baseline, then monthly or as needed. Avoid becoming pregnant. Interrupt treatment if severe non-hematologic adverse reaction develops (eg, severe hepatotoxicity, severe fluid retention); resume if appropriate. GI bleeds reported. Severe CHF and left ventricular dysfunction. Hypereosinophilic cardiac toxicity. Stevens-Johnson syndrome reported. Hypothyroidism reported; monitor thyroid stimulating hormone (TSH) levels.

ADVERSE REACTIONS: NV, fluid retention, neutropenia, thrombocytopenia, diarrhea, hemorrhage, pyrexia, rash, headache, fatigue, abdominal pain, elevated transaminases or bilirubin, edema, muscle cramps, musculoskeletal pain, flatulence, nasopharyngitis, insomnia, anemia, anorexia, rhinitis.

INTERACTIONS: Increased levels with CYP3A4 inhibitors (eg, ketoconazole, atazanavir, indinavir, nefazodone, nelfinavir, ritonavir, saquinavir, telithromycin, voriconazole, clarithromycin, itraconazole). Grapefruit juice may increase levels. Decreased levels with CYP3A4 inducers (eg, dexamethasone, phenytoin, carbamazepine, rifampin, phenobarbital, St. John's wort). Caution with CYP3A4 substrates with narrow therapeutic windows (eg, alfentanil, cyclosporine, diergotamine, ergotamine, fentanyl, quinidine, sirolimus, tacrolimus, cyclosporine, pimozide). Increases levels of drugs metabolized by CYP3A4 (eg, dihydropyridines, triazolo-benzodiazepines, HMG-CoA reductase inhibitors). Switch patients on warfarin to low molecular weight or standard heparin.

PREGNANCY: Category D, not for nursing.

MECHANISM OF ACTION: Protein-tyrosine kinase inhibitor; inhibits the bcr-abl tyrosine kinase.

PHARMACOKINETICS: Absorption: Absolute bioavailability (98%); T_{max}=2-4 hrs. **Distribution:** Plasma protein binding (95%). **Metabolism:** Liver. N-demethyl derivative (major active metabolite). CYP3A4. **Elimination:** Urine and feces (predominant).

NURSING CONSIDERATIONS

Assessment: Assess for renal/hepatic functions, hypereosinophilic syndrome, cardiac disease, pregnancy status, GI bleeding. Note other diseases/conditions and drug therapies.

Monitoring: Monitor for fluid retention, edema, CBC with platelets and differential count, TSH levels, CHF, hepatotoxicity, hypereosinophilic cardiac toxicity, hemorrhage, upper respiratory infections, joint pain.

Patient Counseling: Take with a meal and large glass of water. Notify if pregnant or possibly pregnant. Do not breastfeed while taking drug. Inform of adverse effects; immediately report if any develop.

Administration: Oral route. **Storage:** 25°C (77°F); excursions permitted to 15-30°C (59-86°F). Dispense in tight container.

GLIPIZIDE — RX

glipizide (Various)

OTHER BRAND NAMES: Glucotrol (Pfizer)

THERAPEUTIC CLASS: Sulfonylurea (2nd generation)

INDICATIONS: Adjunct to diet and exercise to improve glycemic control in type 2 diabetes mellitus.

DOSAGE: *Adults*: Take 30 min before meals. Initial: 5mg qd before breakfast. Geriatric/Hepatic Impairment: 2.5mg qd. Titrate: Increase by 2.5-5mg after several days. Max: 40mg/day. Doses >15mg should be divided. Switch From Insulin: If ≤20 U/day: Stop insulin and start Glucotrol 5mg qd. If >20 U/day, decrease dose by 50% with 5mg qd. Further insulin reductions depend on response. Elderly/Debilitated/Malnourished/Renal or Hepatic Impairment: Dose conservatively.

HOW SUPPLIED: Tab: (Glipizide) 2.5mg, 5mg, 10mg; (Glucotrol) 5mg*, 10mg* *scored

CONTRAINDICATIONS: Diabetic ketoacidosis.

WARNINGS/PRECAUTIONS: Increased risk of hypoglycemia with the elderly, debilitated, malnourished, renal and hepatic disease, adrenal or pituitary insufficiency. Increased risk of cardiovascular mortality reported. Loss of blood glucose control when exposed to stress (fever, trauma, infection, or surgery); d/c therapy and start insulin. Secondary failure can occur over period of time.

G

ADVERSE REACTIONS: Hypoglycemia, GI disturbances, allergic skin reactions, hematologic disturbances, disulfiram-like reactions, hyponatremia, SIADH, dizziness, drowsiness, headache.

INTERACTIONS: Potentiated hypoglycemia with alcohol, NSAIDs, some azoles (eg, miconazole, fluconazole), highly protein-bound drugs, salicylates, sulfonamides, chloramphenicol, probenecid, coumarins, MAOIs, and β-blockers. Risk of hyperglycemia with diuretics, corticosteroids, phenothiazines, thyroid products, estrogens, oral contraceptives, phenytoin, nicotinic acid, sympathomimetics, CCBs, and isoniazid. β-blockers may mask signs of hypoglycemia.

PREGNANCY: Category C, not for use in nursing.

MECHANISM OF ACTION: Sulfonylurea; lowers blood glucose acutely by stimulating the release of insulin from the pancreas.

PHARMACOKINETICS: Absorption: Rapid and complete; T_{max}=1-3 hrs. **Distribution:** V_d=11L; plasma protein binding (98-99%). **Metabolism**: Liver. **Elimination**: Urine; $T_{1/2}$=2-4 hrs.

NURSING CONSIDERATIONS

Assessment: Assess FPG, HbA_{1c}, renal function, LFTs, type 1 DM, ketoacidosis, GI disease, pregnancy status, and possible drug interactions.

Monitoring: Monitor for hypoglycemia, FPG, HbA_{1c}, renal function, LFTs, diabetic ketoacidosis, asthenia, tremors, nervousness, CBC with differential and platelet count, porphyrias, metabolic reactions, syndrome of inappropriate antidiuretic hormone, rashes.

Patient Counseling: Advise to take 30 min before meals. Inform of the importance of adhering to dietary instructions, a regular exercise program, and regular testing of urine and/or blood glucose. Counsel about the increased risk of cardiovascular mortality and signs/symptoms of hypoglycemia.

Administration: Oral route. **Storage**: 15-30°C (59-86°F).

GLUCAGON RX

glucagon (Lilly)

THERAPEUTIC CLASS: Glucagon

INDICATIONS: Treatment for severe hypoglycemia. Diagnostic aid for radiologic examination of the stomach, duodenum, small bowel, and colon.

DOSAGE: *Adults:* Severe Hypoglycemia: 1mg (1 U) SQ/IM/IV. May give another dose after 15 min if patient does not respond, but IV glucose would be a better alternative. Use immediately after reconstitution; discard unused portion. After patient responds, give supplemental carbohydrate. Diagnostic Aid: Duodenum/Small Bowel: 0.25-0.5mg (0.25-0.5 U) IV, or 1mg (1 U) IM, or 2mg (2 U) IV/IM before procedure. Stomach: 0.5mg (0.5 U) IV or 2mg (2 U) IM before procedure. Colon: 2mg (2 U) IM 10 min before procedure.
Pediatrics: Severe Hypoglycemia: ≥20kg: 1mg (1 U) SQ/IM/IV. <20kg: 0.5mg (0.5 U) or 20-30mcg/kg. May give another dose after 15 min if patient does

not respond, but IV glucose would be a better alternative. Use immediately after reconstitution; discard unused portion. After patient responds, give supplemental carbohydrate.

HOW SUPPLIED: Inj: 1mg

CONTRAINDICATIONS: Pheochromocytoma.

WARNINGS/PRECAUTIONS: Caution with history suggestive of insulinoma and/or pheochromocytoma. Glucagon can cause pheochromocytoma tumor to release catecholamines, which may result in a sudden and marked increase in BP. Effective in treating hypoglycemia only if sufficient liver glycogen is present. Glucagon is not effective in states of starvation, adrenal insufficiency, or chronic hypoglycemia; use glucose to treat instead.

ADVERSE REACTIONS: NV, allergic reactions, urticaria, respiratory distress, hypotension.

PREGNANCY: Category B, caution in nursing.

MECHANISM OF ACTION: Anti-hypoglycemic agent; polypeptide hormone that increases blood glucose levels. Acts on liver glycogen, converting it to glucose. Relaxes smooth muscle of GI tract.

PHARMACOKINETICS: Absorption: C_{max}=7.9mg/mL (SC), 6.9ng/mL (IM); T_{max}=20 min (SC), 13 min (IM). **Distribution:** V_d=0.25L/kg; found in breast milk. **Metabolism:** Extensively degraded in liver, kidneys, plasma. **Elimination:** Urine; $T_{1/2}$=8-18 min.

NURSING CONSIDERATIONS

Assessment: Assess use with insulinoma and/or pheochromocytoma prior to treatment. Assess prior to therapy, if patient is in state of starvation, has adrenal insufficiencies, or chronic hypoglycemia.

Monitoring: Monitor for signs/symptoms of hypoglycemia or HTN and treat accordingly. Monitor for occurrence of allergic reactions (eg, uticaria, respiratory distress, and hypotension). Monitor blood glucose levels with hypoglycemia until asymptomatic.

Patient Counseling: Instruct, in event of emergency, how to properly prepare and administer glucagon. Inform about measures to prevent hypoglycemia. This includes following a uniform regimen on a regular basis, careful adjustment of insulin program, frequent testing of blood or urine for glucose, and routine carrying of hyperglycemic agents that will quickly elevate blood glucose levels (sugar, candy, or readily absorbed carbohydrates). Inform about symptoms of hypoglycemia and how to treat it appropriately. Inform caregivers that if patient is hypoglycemic, patient should be kept alert and hypoglycemia should be treated as quickly as possible to prevent CNS damage. Advise to inform physician when hypoglycemia occurs.

Administration: IM/IV/SQ routes. Accompanying diluent should be used only for parental injection. Glucagon should not be used in concentrations ≥1mg/mL (1 U/mL). Use reconstituted solution immediately and discard any unused portion. Severe hypoglycemia should be treated initially with IV glucose. If not available, then dissolve lyophilized glucagon using accompanying diluent solution. 1) Wipe rubber stopper on bottle. Do not remove plastic clip from syringe. 2) Swirl gently until dissolves completely. Do not use unless solution is clear and water-like consistency. 3) Hold bottle upside down, making sure needle tip remains in solution, gently withdrawing all of solution (1mg mark on syringe). 4) Cleanse injection site. 5) Insert needle into loose tissue. Apply light pressure at injection site, and withdraw needle. Press alcohol swab against injection site. **Storage:** 20-25°C (68-77°F).

GLUCOPHAGE XR — RX

metformin HCl (Bristol-Myers Squibb)

OTHER BRAND NAMES: Riomet (Ranbaxy) - Glucophage (Bristol-Myers Squibb)

THERAPEUTIC CLASS: Biguanide

INDICATIONS: Adjunct to diet and exercise or with a sulfonylurea or insulin, to improve glycemic control in type 2 diabetes mellitus.

DOSAGE: *Adults:* (Sol, Tab) Initial: 500mg bid or 850mg qd with meals. Titrate: Increase by 500mg/week, or 850mg every 2 weeks, or may increase from 500mg bid to 850mg bid after 2 weeks. Max: 2550mg/day. Give in 3 divided doses with meals if dose is >2g/day. (Tab, Extended-Release) Initial: ≥17 yrs: 500mg qd with evening meal. Titrate: Increase by 500mg/week. Max: 2000mg/day. With Insulin: Initial: 500mg qd. Titrate: Increase by 500mg/week. Max: 2500mg/day and 2000mg/day (XR). Decrease insulin dose by 10-25% when FPG <120mg/dL. Swallow whole; do not crush or chew. Elderly/Debilitated/Malnourished: Conservative dosing; do not titrate to max. *Pediatrics:* 10-16 yrs: (Sol, Tab) Initial: 500mg bid with meals. Titrate: Increase by 500mg/week. Max: 2000mg/day.

HOW SUPPLIED: Sol: (Riomet) 500mg/5mL; Tab: 500mg, 850mg, 1000mg*; Tab, Extended-Release: 500mg, 750mg *scored

G

CONTRAINDICATIONS: Renal disease/dysfunction (SrCr ≥1.5mg/dL [males], ≥1.4mg/dL [females], or abnormal CrCl), CHF, metabolic acidosis, diabetic ketoacidosis. D/C temporarily (48 hrs) for radiologic studies with intravascular iodinated contrast materials.

WARNINGS/PRECAUTIONS: Lactic acidosis reported (rare); increased risk with renal dysfunction, increased age, DM, CHF, and other conditions with risk of hypoperfusion and hypoxemia. Avoid use in patients ≥80 yrs unless renal function is normal. Monitor renal function and for ketoacidosis and metabolic acidosis. Avoid in renal/hepatic impairment. D/C in hypoxic states (eg, CHF, shock, acute MI), loss of blood glucose control due to stress (give insulin), acidosis, dehydration, sepsis. Temporarily d/c prior to surgery (due to restricted food intake) and procedures requiring intravascular iodinated contrast materials. May decrease serum vitamin B_{12} levels. Increased risk of hypoglycemia in elderly, debilitated/malnourished, adrenal or pituitary insufficiency, or alcohol intoxication. Monitor renal function.

ADVERSE REACTIONS: Lactic acidosis, diarrhea, nausea, vomiting, flatulence, abdominal discomfort, abnormal stools, hypoglycemia, myalgia, dizziness, dyspnea, nail disorder, rash, sweating, taste disorder, chest discomfort, chills, flu syndrome, palpitations, asthenia, indigestion, headache.

INTERACTIONS: Furosemide, nifedipine, cimetidine, cationic drugs (eg, digoxin, amiloride, procainamide, quinidine, quinine, ranitidine, trimethoprim, vancomycin, triamterene, morphine) may increase metformin levels. Thiazides, other diuretics, corticosteroids, phenothiazines, thyroid products, estrogens, oral contraceptives, phenytoin, nicotinic acid, sympathomimetics, CCBs, isoniazid may cause hyperglycemia. Risk of hypoglycemia with alcohol. Excess alcohol may increase potential for lactic acidosis. May decrease furosemide levels.

PREGNANCY: Category B, not for use in nursing.

MECHANISM OF ACTION: Biguanide; decreases hepatic glucose production, decreases intestinal absorption of glucose, and improves insulin selectivity by increasing peripheral glucose uptake and utilization.

PHARMACOKINETICS: Absorption: Absolute bioavailability (50-60%); T_{max}=7 hrs. **Distribution:** V_d=654L. **Elimination:** Urine (90%); $T_{1/2}$=6.2 hrs (plasma), 17.6 hrs (blood).

NURSING CONSIDERATIONS

Assessment: Assess FPG, HbA_{1c}, renal function, LFTs, CBC. Assess for CHF, septicemia, acute or chronic metabolic acidosis, adrenal or pituitary insufficiency, alcoholism, pregnancy status. Evaluate for other medical/surgical conditions and for possible drug interactions.

Monitoring: Monitor for hypoglycemia, lactic acidosis, prerenal azotemia, CHF, CVD. Monitor FPG, HbA_{1c}, renal function, LFTs, CBC.

Patient Counseling: Inform drug is adjunct to diet and exercise. Temporarily d/c therapy prior to intravascular radiocontrast study or surgery. Advise that excessive alcohol intake increases hypoglycemia risk. Report unexplained hyperventilation, myalgia, malaise, NV, and somnolence. Not recommended for use during pregnancy. Counsel about adverse effects; seek medical attention if any develop. Regular follow up needed; take as prescribed with evening meals.

Administration: Oral route. Must swallow whole; do not crush or chew.
Storage: 20-25°C (68-77°F).

GLUCOTROL XL RX

glipizide (Pfizer)

OTHER BRAND NAMES: Glipizide ER (Various) - Glucotrol (Pfizer)

THERAPEUTIC CLASS: Sulfonylurea (2nd generation)

G

INDICATIONS: Adjunct to diet and exercise, to improve glycemic control in type 2 diabetes mellitus.

DOSAGE: *Adults:* (Glucotrol XL) Do not chew, divide, or crush. Initial: 5mg qd with breakfast. Use lower doses if sensitive to hypoglycemics. Usual: 5-10mg qd. Max: 20mg/day. Combination Therapy: Initial: 5mg qd. (Glucotrol): Initial: 5mg qd 30 min before breakfast. Geriatric/Hepatic Impairment: Initial 2.5mg qd. Titrate: Increase by 2.5-5mg after several days. Max: 40mg/day. Divide doses >15mg and give 30 min before a meal. (Glucotrol XL, Glucotrol) Switch From Insulin: If on ≤20 U/day: Stop insulin; start Glucotrol XL or Glucotrol 5mg qd. If on >20 U/day: Reduce insulin dose by 50% and add Glucotrol XL or Glucotrol 5mg qd. Further insulin reductions depend on response.

HOW SUPPLIED: Tab: (Glucotrol) 5mg*, 10mg*; Tab, Extended-Release: (XL) 2.5mg, 5mg, 10mg *scored

CONTRAINDICATIONS: Diabetic ketoacidosis with or without coma, type 1 diabetes mellitus.

WARNINGS/PRECAUTIONS: Increased risk of hypoglycemia with the elderly, debilitated, malnourished, renal and hepatic disease, adrenal or pituitary insufficiency. Increased risk of cardiovascular mortality. Loss of blood glucose control when exposed to stress (fever, trauma, infection, or surgery); d/c therapy and start insulin. Secondary failure can occur over a period of time. (XL) GI disease will reduce retention time of the drug. Caution with pre-existing severe GI narrowing.

ADVERSE REACTIONS: Hypoglycemia, asthenia, headache, dizziness, nervousness, tremor, diarrhea, and flatulence.

INTERACTIONS: Potentiated hypoglycemia with alcohol, NSAIDs, some azoles (eg, miconazole, fluconazole), highly-protein bound drugs, salicylates, sulfonamides, chloramphenicol, probenecid, coumarins, MAOIs, and β-blockers. Risk of hyperglycemia with diuretics, corticosteroids, phenothiazines, thyroid products, estrogens, oral contraceptives, phenytoin, nicotinic acid, sympathomimetics, CCBs, and isoniazid. β-blockers may mask signs of hypoglycemia.

PREGNANCY: Category C, not for use in nursing.

MECHANISM OF ACTION: Sulfonylurea; lowers blood glucose acutely by stimulating the release of insulin from the pancreas.

PHARMACOKINETICS: Absorption: Rapid and complete; bioavailability (100%); T_{max}=6-12 hrs. **Distribution:** V_d=10L; plasma protein binding (98-99%). **Metabolism**: Liver; aromatic hydroxylation. **Elimination**: Urine (80%), feces (10%); $T_{1/2}$=2-5 hrs.

NURSING CONSIDERATIONS

Assessment: Assess FPG, HbA_{1c}, renal function, LFTs, pregnancy status, type 1 DM, ketoacidosis, GI disease, and for possible drug interactions.

Monitoring: Monitor blood and urine glucose, HbA_{1c} every 3 months, renal function, LFTs, signs/symptoms of hypoglycemia, and for endocrine, metabolic, and hematologic reactions.

Patient Counseling: Counsel to swallow whole with breakfast, not to chew, divide, or crush. Inform about importance of adhering to dietary instructions, a regular exercise program, and regular testing of urine/blood glucose. Educate on risks/benefits of therapy; signs/symptoms, predisposing conditions, and treatment of hypoglycemia; primary and secondary failure.

Administration: Oral route. **Storage**: 15-30°C (59-86°F).

GLUCOVANCE RX

metformin HCl - glyburide (Bristol-Myers Squibb)

THERAPEUTIC CLASS: Sulfonylurea/biguanide

INDICATIONS: Adjunct to diet and exercise to improve glycemic control in adults with type 2 diabetes mellitus.

DOSAGE: *Adults:* Take with meals. Inadequate Glycemic Control on Diet/Exercise Alone: Initial: 1.25mg-250mg qd. If HbA_{1c} >9% or FPG >200mg/dL, give 1.25mg-250mg bid (with morning and evening meals). Titrate: Increase by 1.25mg-250mg/day every 2 weeks. Do not use 5mg-500mg tab for initial therapy. Inadequate Glycemic Control on Sulfonylurea or Metformin: Initial: 2.5mg-500mg or 5mg-500mg bid. Starting dose should not exceed daily doses of glyburide (or sulfonylurea equivalent) or metformin already being taken. Titrate: Increase by no more than 5mg-500mg/day. Max: 20mg-2000mg/day. With Concomitant TZD: Initiate and titrate TZD as recommended. If hypoglycemia occurs, reduce glyburide component. Elderly/Debilitated/Malnourished: Conservative dosing; do not titrate to max.

HOW SUPPLIED: Tab: (Glyburide-Metformin) 1.25mg-250mg, 2.5mg-500mg, 5mg-500mg

CONTRAINDICATIONS: Renal disease or dysfunction (SrCr ≥1.5mg/dL [males], ≥1.4mg/dL [females], or abnormal CrCl), metabolic acidosis, including diabetic ketoacidosis. D/C temporarily (48 hrs) for radiologic studies with intravascular iodinated contrast materials.

WARNINGS/PRECAUTIONS: Lactic acidosis reported (rare); increased risk with renal dysfunction, increased age, DM, CHF, and other conditions with risk of hypoperfusion and hypoxemia. Avoid use in patients ≥80 yrs unless renal function is normal. Increased risk of cardiovascular mortality. Increased risk of hypoglycemia in elderly, debilitated/malnourished, adrenal or pituitary insufficiency, or alcohol intoxication. D/C in hypoxic states (eg, CHF, shock, acute MI), loss of blood glucose control due to stress (give insulin), acidosis and prior to surgical procedures (due to restricted food intake). Monitor renal function and for ketoacidosis and metabolic acidosis. Avoid in renal/hepatic impairment. May decrease serum vitamin B_{12} levels. When used with a TZD, monitor LFTs and for wt gain. Withhold treatment with any condition associated with hypoxemia, dehydration, or sepsis.

ADVERSE REACTIONS: Hypoglycemia, nausea, vomiting, abdominal pain, upper respiratory infection, headache, dizziness, diarrhea.

INTERACTIONS: Furosemide, nifedipine, cimetidine and cationic drugs (eg, digoxin, amiloride, procainamide, quinidine, quinine, ranitidine, trimethoprim, vancomycin, triamterene, morphine) may increase metformin levels. Potentiated hypoglycemia with alcohol, ciprofloxacin, miconazole, NSAIDs, salicylates, sulfonamides, chloramphenicol, probenecid, coumarins, MAOIs, TZDs (eg, rosiglitazone), and β-blockers. Thiazides and other diuretics, corticosteroids, phenothiazines, thyroid products, estrogens, oral contraceptives, phenytoin, nicotinic acid, sympathomimetics, CCBs, and isoniazid may cause hyperglycemia. Excess alcohol may increase potential for lactic acidosis. May decrease furosemide levels.

PREGNANCY: Category B, not for use in pregnancy or nursing.

MECHANISM OF ACTION: Glyburide: Sulfonylurea; lowers blood glucose acutely by stimulating release of insulin from the pancreas. Metformin: Biguanide; decreases hepatic glucose production and intestinal absorption of glucose and improves insulin sensitivity by increasing peripheral glucose uptake.

PHARMACOKINETICS: Absorption: Glyburide: T_{max}=4 hrs. Metformin: absolute bioavailability (50-60%). **Distribution:** Glyburide: plasma protein binding (extensive). Metformin: V_d=654L. **Metabolism:** Glyburide: metabolites: 4-trans-hydroxy (major) and 3-cis hydroxyl derivatives. **Elimination:** Glyburide: bile, urine (approximately 50% each route); $T_{1/2}$=10 hrs. Metformin: renal excretion (approximately 90%); $T_{1/2}$=6.2 hrs (plasma), 17.6 hrs (blood).

NURSING CONSIDERATIONS

Assessment: Assess FPG, HbA_{1c}, renal function, LFTs, CBC. Assess for CHF, septicemia, acute or chronic metabolic acidosis, adrenal or pituitary insufficiency, alcoholism, pregnancy status. Evaluate for other medical/surgical conditions, and for possible drug interactions.

Monitoring: Monitor for hypoglycemia, lactic acidosis, prerenal azotemia, CHF, CVD. Monitor FPG, HbA_{1c}, renal function, LFTs, CBC.

Patient Counseling: Inform drug is adjunct to diet and exercise. Temporarily d/c therapy prior to intravascular radiocontrast study or surgery. Excessive alcohol intake increases hypoglycemia risk. Report unexplained hyperventilation, myalgia, malaise, NV, and somnolence. Not recommended for use during pregnancy. Counsel about adverse effects; seek medical attention if any develop. Regular follow-ups needed; take as prescribed with meals.

Administration: Oral route. **Storage:** 25°C (77°F). Dispense in light-resistant container.

GLUMETZA — RX

metformin HCl (Depomed)

THERAPEUTIC CLASS: Biguanide

INDICATIONS: Adjunct to diet and exercise or with a sulfonylurea or insulin, to improve glycemic control in type 2 diabetes mellitus.

DOSAGE: *Adults:* ≥18 yrs: Take with evening meal. Initial: 1000mg qd. With Insulin: Initial: 500mg qd. Titrate: May increase by 500mg/week. Max: 2000mg/day. Decrease insulin dose by 10-25% if FPG <120mg/dL. Elderly/Debilitated/Malnourished: Conservative dosing; do not titrate to max. Swallow whole; do not crush or chew.

HOW SUPPLIED: Tab, Extended-Release: 500mg, 1000mg

CONTRAINDICATIONS: Renal disease or dysfunction (SrCr ≥1.5mg/dL [males], ≥1.4mg/dL [females], or abnormal CrCl), CHF, metabolic acidosis, including diabetic ketoacidosis. D/C temporarily (48 hrs) for radiologic studies with intravascular iodinated contrast materials.

WARNINGS/PRECAUTIONS: Lactic acidosis reported (rare); increased risk with renal dysfunction, increased age, DM, CHF, and other conditions with risk of hypoperfusion and hypoxemia. Avoid use in patients ≥80 yrs unless renal function is normal. Monitor renal function and for ketoacidosis and metabolic acidosis. Avoid in renal/hepatic impairment. D/C in hypoxic states (eg, CHF, shock, acute MI), loss of blood glucose control due to stress (give insulin), acidosis, dehydration, sepsis. Temporarily d/c prior to surgery (due to restricted food/fluid intake) or procedures requiring intravascular iodinated contrast materials. May decrease serum vitamin B_{12} levels. Increased risk of hypoglycemia in elderly, debilitated/malnourished, adrenal or pituitary insufficiency, or alcohol intoxication.

ADVERSE REACTIONS: Hypoglycemia, diarrhea, nausea.

INTERACTIONS: Furosemide, nifedipine, cimetidine, cationic drugs (eg, digoxin, amiloride, procainamide, quinidine, quinine, ranitidine, trimethoprim, vancomycin, triamterene, morphine) may increase metformin levels. Thiazides, other diuretics, corticosteroids, phenothiazines, thyroid products, estrogens, oral contraceptives, phenytoin, nicotinic acid, sympathomimetics, CCBs, isoniazid may cause hyperglycemia. Risk of hypoglycemia with alcohol. Excess alcohol may increase potential for lactic acidosis. May decrease furosemide levels.

PREGNANCY: Category B, not for use in nursing.

MECHANISM OF ACTION: Biguanide; decreases hepatic glucose production, decreases intestinal absorption of glucose, and improves insulin selectivity by increasing peripheral glucose uptake and utilization.

PHARMACOKINETICS: Absorption: Administration of variable doses resulted in different absorption parameters. T_{max}=7-8 hrs. **Distribution:** V_d=654L. **Elimination:** Urine (90%); $T_{1/2}$=6.2 hrs (plasma), 17.6 hrs (blood).

NURSING CONSIDERATIONS

Assessment: Assess FPG, HbA_{1c}, renal function, LFTs, CBC. Assess for CHF, septicemia, acute or chronic metabolic acidosis, adrenal or pituitary insufficiency, alcoholism, pregnancy status. Evaluate for other medical/surgical conditions and for possible drug interactions.

Monitoring: Monitor for hypoglycemia, lactic acidosis, prerenal azotemia, CHF, CVD. Monitor FPG, HbA_{1c}, renal function, LFTs, CBC.

Patient Counseling: Inform drug is adjunct to diet and exercise. Temporarily d/c therapy prior to intravascular radiocontrast study or surgery. Advise that excessive alcohol intake increases hypoglycemia risk. Report unexplained hyperventilation, myalgia, malaise, NV, and somnolence. Not recommended for use during pregnancy. Counsel about adverse effects; seek medical attention if any develop. Regular follow-ups needed; take as prescribed with evening meals.

Administration: Oral route. Must swallow whole; do not crush or chew. **Storage:** 20-25°C (68-77°F). Excursions permitted to 15-30°C (59-86°F).

G

GLYNASE PRESTAB — RX

glyburide (Pharmacia & Upjohn)

THERAPEUTIC CLASS: Sulfonylurea (2nd generation)

INDICATIONS: Adjunct to diet and exercise, to improve glycemic control in type 2 diabetes mellitus. May use in combination with metformin.

DOSAGE: *Adults:* Initial: 1.5-3mg qd with breakfast or 1st main meal. Renal/Hepatic Disease/Elderly/Debilitated/Malnourished/Adrenal or Pituitary Insufficiency: Initial: 0.75mg qd. Titrate: Increase by no more than 1.5mg/day at weekly intervals. Maint: 0.75-12mg qd or in divided doses. Max: 12mg/day given qd or bid. Transfer from Other Sulfonylureas: Starting dose should not exceed 3mg/day. Switch from Insulin: If <20 U/day, substitute with 1.5-3mg qd. If 20-40 U/day, give 3mg qd. If >40 U/day, decrease insulin dose by 50% and give 3mg qd. Titrate: Progressive withdrawal of insulin and increase by 0.75-1.5mg every 2-10 days.

HOW SUPPLIED: Tab: 1.5mg*, 3mg*, 6mg* *scored

CONTRAINDICATIONS: Diabetic ketoacidosis, and as sole therapy of type 1 DM.

WARNINGS/PRECAUTIONS: Increased risk of cardiovascular mortality. Risk of hypoglycemia, especially with renal and hepatic disease, elderly, debilitated, malnourished, and adrenal or pituitary insufficiency. Loss of blood glucose control when exposed to stress (eg, fever, trauma, infection, or surgery); d/c therapy and start insulin. Secondary failure can occur over a period of time. D/C if cholestatic jaundice or hepatitis occur. Retitrate when transferring from other glyburide products.

ADVERSE REACTIONS: Hypoglycemia, nausea, epigastric fullness, heartburn, allergic skin reactions, disulfiram-like reactions (rarely), hyponatremia, LFT abnormalities, angioedema, arthralgia, myalgia, and vasculitis.

INTERACTIONS: Hypoglycemia potentiated by alcohol, NSAIDs, miconazole, ciprofloxacin, highly protein-bound drugs, salicylates, sulfonamides, chloramphenicol, probenecid, coumarins, MAOIs, and β-blockers. Risk of hyperglycemia with diuretics, corticosteroids, phenothiazines, thyroid products, estrogens, oral contraceptives, phenytoin, nicotinic acid, sympathomimetics, CCBs, and isoniazid. β-Blockers may mask hypoglycemia.

PREGNANCY: Category B, not for use in nursing.

MECHANISM OF ACTION: Sulfonylurea; lowers blood glucose acutely by stimulating the release of insulin from the pancreas.

PHARMACOKINETICS: Absorption: C_{max}=106ng/mL; T_{max}=2-3 hrs. **Distribution:** Plasma protein binding (extensive). **Metabolism:** 4-trans-hydroxy derivative (major metabolite). **Elimination:** Bile (50%), urine (50%); $T_{1/2}$=4 hrs.

NURSING CONSIDERATIONS

Assessment: Assess FPG, HbA_{1c}, renal function, LFTs, type 1 DM, ketoacidosis, GI disease, pregnancy status, and possible drug interactions.

Monitoring: Monitor for hypoglycemia, FPG, HbA_{1c}, renal function, LFTs, diabetic ketoacidosis, asthenia, tremors, nervousness, CBC with differential and platelet count, porphyrias, metabolic reactions, SIADH.

G

Patient Counseling: Instruct to take with breakfast or first main meal. Inform about the importance of adhering to dietary instructions, a regular exercise program, and regular testing of urine and/or blood glucose. Counsel about increased risk of cardiovascular mortality, and symptoms of hypoglycemia.

Administration: Oral route. **Storage:** 20-25°C (68-77°F). Keep container tightly closed.

GLYSET — RX

miglitol (Pharmacia & Upjohn)

THERAPEUTIC CLASS: Alpha-glucosidase inhibitor

INDICATIONS: Adjunct to diet and exercise, to improve glycemic control in type 2 diabetes mellitus. May use in combination with a sulfonylurea.

DOSAGE: *Adults:* Initial: 25mg tid. May give 25mg qd (to minimize GI side effects) and gradually increase to tid. Titrate: After 4-8 weeks, increase to 50mg tid. Maint: 50mg tid. After 3 months may increase to 100mg tid if needed. Max: 100mg tid. Take with first bite of each main meal.

HOW SUPPLIED: Tab: 25mg, 50mg, 100mg

CONTRAINDICATIONS: Ketoacidosis, inflammatory bowel disease, colonic ulceration, partial intestinal obstruction or if predisposed to intestinal obstruction. Chronic intestinal diseases with digestion or absorption disorders/conditions may deteriorate with increased gas formation in the intestine.

WARNINGS/PRECAUTIONS: Use glucose (dextrose) not sucrose (cane sugar) to treat mild-moderate hypoglycemia. Temporary insulin therapy may be necessary at times of stress such as fever, trauma, infection, or surgery. Not recommended with renal impairment (SrCr >2mg/dL).

ADVERSE REACTIONS: Flatulence, diarrhea, abdominal pain, skin rash, decreased serum iron.

INTERACTIONS: Intestinal absorbents (eg, charcoal) and digestive enzyme preparations (eg, amylase, pancreatin) may reduce effects. May reduce bioavailability of ranitidine and propranolol. May interact with glyburide, metformin, and digoxin.

PREGNANCY: Category B, not for use in nursing.

MECHANISM OF ACTION: α-glucosidase inhibitor; inhibits membrane-bound intestinal α-glucosidase hydrolase enzymes.

PHARMACOKINETICS: Absorption: Complete, T_{max}=2.3 hrs. **Distribution:** V_d=0.18 L/kg; plasma protein binding (≤4.0%). **Elimination**: Urine (unchanged); $T_{1/2}$=2 hrs.

NURSING CONSIDERATIONS

Assessment: Assess for diabetic ketoacidosis, inflammatory bowel disease, colonic ulceration, partial intestinal obstruction, chronic intestinal disease, renal function, pregnancy status.

Monitoring: Monitor for hypoglycemia, FPG, HbA_{1c}, renal function, diabetic ketoacidosis, GI symptoms, skin rash, serum iron.

Patient Counseling: Inform that drug is adjunct to diet and exercise. Counsel about adverse effects. Advise on need for regular follow-ups and to take drug as prescribed. During periods of stress (fever, trauma, infection, or surgery), medication requirements may change; patients should seek medical advice promptly.

Administration: Oral route. **Storage**: 25°C (77°F); excursions permitted to 15-30°C (59-86°F).

GRIFULVIN V — RX

griseofulvin (Ortho Neutrogena)

THERAPEUTIC CLASS: *Penicillium*-derived antifungal

INDICATIONS: Management of tinea capitis, tinea corporis, tinea pedis, tinea unguium, tinea barbae, and tinea cruris. Inhibits the growth of fungi that commonly cause ringworm infections of hair, skin, and nails.

G

DOSAGE: *Adults:* Tinea Capitis: 500mg qd for 4-6 weeks. Tinea Corporis: 500mg qd for 2-4 weeks. Tinea Pedis: 1g qd for 4-8 weeks. Tinea Cruris: 500mg qd. Tinea Unguium: 1g qd for at least 4 months (fingernail) or at least 6 months (toenails).
Pediatrics: Usual: 5mg/lb/day. 30-50lb: 125-250mg qd. >50lb: 250-500mg qd. Tinea Capitis: Treat for 4-6 weeks. Tinea Corporis: Treat for 2-4 weeks. Tinea Pedis: Treat for 4-8 weeks. Tinea Unguium: Treat for at least 4 months (fingernail) or at least 6 months (toenails).

HOW SUPPLIED: Sus: 125mg/5mL [120mL]; Tab: 250mg, 500mg

CONTRAINDICATIONS: Porphyria, hepatocellular failure, pregnancy.

WARNINGS/PRECAUTIONS: Confirm diagnosis. Not for prophylactic use. Monitor renal, hepatic, and hematopoietic functions periodically with prolonged therapy. Cross-sensitivity with PCN may exist. Photosensitivity reported. D/C if granulocytopenia occurs.

ADVERSE REACTIONS: Rash, urticaria, oral thrush, NV, epigastric distress, diarrhea, headache, dizziness, insomnia, mental confusion.

INTERACTIONS: Oral anticoagulants may need adjustment. Barbiturates decrease effects. Decreases effects of oral contraceptives; may increase incidence of breakthrough bleeding.

PREGNANCY: Not for use in pregnancy or nursing.

MECHANISM OF ACTION: Acts systemically to inhibit the growth of *Trichophyton, Microsporum*, and *Epidermophyton* genera of fungi. Fungistatic amounts deposit in keratin, which is gradually exfoliated and replaced by noninfected tissue.

PHARMACOKINETICS: Absorption: C_{max}=0.5g; T_{max}=4 hrs.

NURSING CONSIDERATIONS

Assessment: Assess for proper diagnosis of infecting fungi. Assess for possible drug interactions and drug allergies (possible PCN cross-sensitivity).

Monitoring: Monitor for photosensitivity reactions. Periodically monitor organ system function, including renal, hepatic, and hematopoietic. Monitor for signs/symptoms of lupus erythematosus.

Patient Counseling: Counsel females to use additional forms of contraception while taking medication and for 1 month following cessation of therapy. Counsel males to use contraception while on treatment and for 6 months following. Warn patients to avoid exposure to intense natural or artificial sunlight. Counsel females to avoid use during pregnancy.

Administration: Oral route. **Storage:** Store at room temperature.

GRIS-PEG RX
griseofulvin (Pedinol)

THERAPEUTIC CLASS: *Penicillium*-derived antifungal

INDICATIONS: Treatment of t.capitis, t.corporis, t.pedis, t.unguium, t.barbae, and t.cruris.

DOSAGE: *Adults:* T.capitis: 375mg qd in single or divided doses for 4-6 weeks. T.corporis: 375mg qd in single or divided doses for 2-4 weeks. T.pedis: 375mg bid for 4-8 weeks. T.cruris: 375mg qd in single or divided doses. T.unguium: 375mg bid for at least 4 months (fingernail) or at least 6 months (toenails). *Pediatrics:* Usual: 3.3mg/lb/day. 35-60lb: 125-187.5mg qd. >60lb: 187.5-375mg qd. T.capitis: Treat for 4-6 weeks. T.corporis: Treat for 2-4 weeks. T.pedis: Treat for 4-8 weeks. T.unguium: Treat for at least 4 months (fingernail) or at least 6 months (toenails).

G

HOW SUPPLIED: Tab: 125mg*, 250mg* *scored

CONTRAINDICATIONS: Porphyria, hepatocellular failure, pregnancy.

WARNINGS/PRECAUTIONS: Not for prophylactic use. Periodically monitor renal, hepatic, and hematopoietic functions in prolonged therapy. Cross-sensitivity with PCN may exist. Photosensitivity reported. D/C if granulocytopenia occurs.

ADVERSE REACTIONS: Rash, urticaria, oral thrush, NV, epigastric distress, diarrhea, headache, dizziness, insomnia, mental confusion.

INTERACTIONS: Oral anticoagulants may need dose adjustments. Decreased effects with barbiturates. Decreased effects of oral contraceptives. Increased alcohol effects.

PREGNANCY: Not for use in pregnancy and in nursing.

MECHANISM OF ACTION: Fungistatic agent. Active against various species of *Microsporum*, *Epidermophyton* and *Trichophyton*. Has greater affinity for depositing in keratin precursor cells of diseased tissue. Tightly binds to new keratin, which then becomes highly resistant to fungal invasions.

PHARMACOKINETICS: Absorption: C_{max}=600ng/mL; T_{max}=4 hrs; AUC=8618ng•hr/mL.

NURSING CONSIDERATIONS

Assessment: Assess for ID of fungi responsible for infection (eg, cultures, microscopic exam). Assess pregnancy status prior to therapy.

Monitoring: Periodic monitoring of renal, hepatic, and hematopoietic functions should be performed with sustained therapy. Monitor for hypersensitivity reactions (eg, skin rashes, urticaria, and erythema multiform-like reactions). Monitor for signs/symptoms of lupus erythematosus or lupus-like syndrome and possible drug interactions while on therapy.

Patient Counseling: Counsel to avoid intense natural or artificial sunlight while on medication. Avoid alcohol. Instruct to take proper hygienic precautions to prevent spread of infection. Inform that medication may be swallowed whole or crushed; sprinkled into 1 tbl. of applesauce and swallowed immediately without chewing. Counsel about signs/symptoms of agranulocytosis. Advise females drug may interfere with oral contraceptives and to avoid pregnancy while on medication.

Administration: Oral route. **Storage:** Store at controlled room temperature 15-30°C (59-86°F) in tight, light-resistant containers.

HALCION CIV
triazolam (Pharmacia & Upjohn)

THERAPEUTIC CLASS: Benzodiazepine

INDICATIONS: Short-term treatment of insomnia.

DOSAGE: *Adults:* 0.25mg qhs. Max: 0.5mg. Elderly/Debilitated: Initial: 0.125mg. Max: 0.25mg.

HOW SUPPLIED: Tab: 0.125mg, 0.25mg* *scored

CONTRAINDICATIONS: Pregnancy. With ketoconazole, itraconazole, nefazodone, medications that impair CYP3A.

WARNINGS/PRECAUTIONS: Worsening or failure of response after 7-10 days may indicate other medical conditions. Increased daytime anxiety, abnormal thinking, and behavioral changes have occurred. May impair mental/physical abilities. Anterograde amnesia reported with therapeutic doses. Caution with baseline depression, suicidal tendencies, history of drug dependence, elderly/debilitated, renal/hepatic impairment, chronic pulmonary insufficiency, and sleep apnea. Withdrawal symptoms after discontinuation; avoid abrupt withdrawal.

ADVERSE REACTIONS: Drowsiness, dizziness, lightheadedness, headache, NV, coordination disorders, ataxia.

INTERACTIONS: See Contraindications. Avoid the concomitant use with inhibitors of the CYP3A (eg, ketoconazole, itraconazole, all azole-type antifungals, nefazodone). Potentiated by the coadministration of isoniazid, OCs, grapefruit juice, ranitidine. Caution with fluvoxamine, diltiazem, verapamil, cimetidine, ergotamine, cyclosporine, amiodarone, nicardipine, nifedipine, sertraline, paroxetine, macrolides. Additive CNS depression with psychotropics, anticonvulsants, antihistamines, and alcohol.

PREGNANCY: Category X, not for use in nursing.

MECHANISM OF ACTION: Triazolobenzodiazepine hypnotic agent.

PHARMACOKINETICS: Absorption: C_{max}=1-6ng/mL, T_{max}=2 hrs. **Metabolism:** Hydroxylation via CYP3A. **Elimination:** Urine (79.9%), $T_{1/2}$=1.5-5.5 hrs.

NURSING CONSIDERATIONS

Assessment: Assess for primary psychiatric and/or medical illness, chronic pulmonary insufficiency (sleep apnea, COPD), renal/hepatic function, and possible drug interactions.

Monitoring: Monitor worsening of insomnia, suicidality, severe sedation, complex behaviors (sleep-driving), abnormal thinking/behavioral changes (aggressiveness, hallucinations, and bizzare behavior), anterograde amnesia, paradoxical reactions.

Patient Counseling: Inform of benefits/risks of therapy and potential for physical/psychological dependence. Caution against hazardous tasks (operating machinery/driving). Do not increase dose or d/c before consulting physician. Avoid alcohol consumption. Notify if pregnant or planning to become pregnant.

Administration: Oral route. **Storage:** 20-25°C (68-77°F).

HALFLYTELY — RX

polyethylene glycol 3350 - sodium bicarbonate - potassium chloride - sodium chloride - bisacodyl (Braintree)

THERAPEUTIC CLASS: Bowel cleanser/stimulant laxative

INDICATIONS: Bowel cleansing prior to colonoscopy.

DOSAGE: *Adults:* Consume only clear liquids on day of preparation. Swallow all 4 bisacodyl tabs at noon (do not chew or crush). After 1st bowel movement (or max of 6 hrs) begin drinking sol, 240mL every 10 min (approx. 8 glasses). Drink all sol.

HOW SUPPLIED: Kit: Tab, Delayed-Release: (Bisacodyl) 5mg [4[s]]. Sol: (Polyethylene Glycol 3350-Potassium Chloride-Sodium Bicarbonate-Sodium Chloride) 210g-0.74g-2.86g-5.60g [2000mL].

CONTRAINDICATIONS: Ileus, GI obstruction, gastric retention, bowel perforation, toxic colitis, toxic megacolon.

WARNINGS/PRECAUTIONS: Do not add additional ingredients (eg, flavorings). Caution with severe ulcerative colitis, ileus or gastric retention. Monitor with impaired gag reflex, prone to regurgitation or aspiration. Slow administration or temporarily d/c if severe bloating, distention, or abdominal pain develops. Avoid large quantities of water during or after preparation or colonoscopy. Monitor closely with impaired water handling. Generalized tonic-clonic seizures, hives and skin rashes reported.

ADVERSE REACTIONS: NV, abdominal fullness, cramping, overall discomfort.

INTERACTIONS: Oral medications taken within 1 hr of start of administration start may not be absorbed from GI tract. Avoid bisacodyl delayed release tablets within 1 hr of taking an antacid.

PREGNANCY: Category C, caution in nursing.

MECHANISM OF ACTION: Stimulant laxative that induces diarrhea.

PHARMACOKINETICS: Metabolism: Hydrolysis by intestinal brush border enzymes and colonic bacteria to form bis-(hydroxyphenyl) pyridyl-2 methane (active metabolite).

NURSING CONSIDERATIONS

Assessment: Assess for known allergy to polyethylene glycol, GI obstruction, bowel perforation, toxic colitis, toxic megacolon, renal impairment, and seizures.

Monitoring: Perform baseline and post-colonoscopy lab tests with known/suspected hyponatremia. D/C use if severe bloating, abdominal distention, or abdominal pain occur. Monitor for hypersensitivity reactions, aspiration, asystole, ischemic colitis, and seizures.

Patient Counseling: Do not drink large quantities of clear liquids. Oral medication administered within 1 hr of start of administration of sol may be flushed from GI tract, hence not absorbed. Instruct to take exactly as directed.

Administration: Oral route. **Storage:** 20-25°C (68-77°F); excursions permitted to 15-30°C (59-86°F). Use the reconstituted solution, which may be refrigerated, within 48 hrs.

HALOPERIDOL RX

haloperidol (Various)

Elderly patients with dementia-related psychosis treated with atypical antipsychotic drugs are at an increased risk of death; most appeared to be cardiovascular (eg, heart failure, sudden death) or infectious (eg, pneumonia) in nature. Haloperidol is not approved for the treatment of patients with dementia-related psychosis.

OTHER BRAND NAMES: Haldol (Ortho-McNeil) - Haldol Decanoate (Ortho-McNeil)

THERAPEUTIC CLASS: Butyrophenone

INDICATIONS: (Immediate-Release) Treatment of psychosis, Tourette's disorder, severe childhood behavioral problems. Short-term treatment of hyperactivity in children. (Decanoate) Prolonged management of psychosis.

DOSAGE: *Adults:* (Immediate-Release) PO: Moderate Symptoms/Elderly/Debilitated: 0.5-2mg bid-tid. Severe Symptoms/Resistant Patients: 3-5mg bid-tid. Max: 100mg/day. IM: Acute Agitation: 2-5mg every 4-8 hrs or hourly as needed for moderately severe or very severe symptoms. Max: 100mg/day. (Decanoate) For IM inj only. Give every 4 weeks or monthly. Initial:10-20 times daily oral dose up to 100mg. Give remainder of dose 3-7 days later if initial dose >100mg. Usual: 10-15 times daily oral dose. Max: 450mg/month. Elderly/Debilitated: Initial: 10-15 times daily oral dose.
Pediatrics: 3-12 yrs: (15-40kg): PO: Psychosis: Initial: 0.05-0.15mg/kg/day given bid-tid. Nonpsychotic Disorder/Tourette's: 0.05-0.075mg/kg/day given bid-tid. Max: 6mg/day.

HOW SUPPLIED: Inj: 5mg/mL; Inj: (Decanoate) 50mg/mL, 100mg/mL; Sol: 2mg/mL; Tab: 0.5mg*, 1mg*, 2mg*, 5mg*, 10mg*, 20mg** scored

CONTRAINDICATIONS: Comatose states, severe toxic CNS depression, Parkinson's disease.

WARNINGS/PRECAUTIONS: Risk of tardive dyskinesia, especially in elderly. NMS, hyperpyrexia, heat stroke, bronchopneumonia reported. Decreased cholesterol, cutaneous and/or ocular changes may occur. Neurotoxicity may occur with thyrotoxicosis. Caution with CV disease, seizures, EEG abnormalities, QT-prolonging conditions, elderly. Do not administer IV. Cases of sudden death and torsade de pointes reported.

ADVERSE REACTIONS: Extrapyramidal symptoms, tardive dyskinesia, tardive dystonia, ECG changes, QT prolongation, ventricular arrhythmias, tachycardia, hypotension, HTN, nausea, vomiting, constipation, diarrhea, dry mouth, blurred vision, urinary retention.

INTERACTIONS: Caution with rifampin, anticonvulsants, anticoagulants, anticholinergics, antiparkinson agents. May potentiate CNS depression with alcohol, opiates, anesthetics, and other CNS depressants. Antagonizes epinephrine. Monitor for neurological toxicity with lithium. Avoid concomitant alcohol use.

PREGNANCY: Category C, not for use in nursing.

MECHANISM OF ACTION: Butyrophenone; not established, suspected to block effects of dopamine and increase turnover rate.

PHARMACOKINETICS: Absorption: T_{max}=6 days (IM). **Elimination:** $T_{1/2}$=3 weeks (IM).

NURSING CONSIDERATIONS

Assessment: Assess for severe toxic CNS depression or Parkinson's disease prior to treatment. Assess use of haloperidol in patients who have severe cardiovascular disorders, are on anticonvulsant medications, with a history of seizures, on CNS depressants, and on concomitant lithium therapy.

Monitoring: Monitor for signs/symptoms of NMS, EPS, TD, and bronchopneumonia. Monitor for neurotoxicity in patients with thyrotoxicosis. Monitor for cardiovascular effects (eg, torsade de pointes, QT prolongation) after receiving IM formulation.

Patient Counseling: Drug may impair mental/physical abilities. Avoid alcohol use with drug due to possible additive effects and hypotension. Counsel not to abruptly d/c medication.

Administration: Oral route, IM. **Storage:** (Tab/Sus) 20-25°C (68-77°F), (Inj) 15-30°C (59-86°F). Do not freeze. Protect from light.

Havrix

RX

hepatitis A vaccine (inactivated) (GlaxoSmithKline)

THERAPEUTIC CLASS: Vaccine

INDICATIONS: Active immunization in persons ≥12 months against hepatitis A virus.

DOSAGE: *Adults:* ≥18 yrs: 1440 EL U IM (deltoid), then booster after 6-12 months.
Pediatrics: 1-18 yrs: 720 EL U IM (deltoid), then booster after 6-12 months.

HOW SUPPLIED: Inj: 720 EL U/0.5mL, 1440 EL U/mL

CONTRAINDICATIONS: Hypersensitivity to any component, including neomycin.

WARNINGS/PRECAUTIONS: Epinephrine should be available for anaphylaxis. Delay with febrile illness. Caution with thrombocytopenia or bleeding disorders. Immunosuppressed may show suboptimal response. May not prevent hepatitis A in patients already infected.

ADVERSE REACTIONS: Injection-site soreness, induration, redness, swelling, fever, fatigue, malaise, anorexia, nausea, headache.

INTERACTIONS: Caution with anticoagulant therapy and IM injection. Give immunoglobulins and other vaccines in different syringe and injection site.

Caution with immunosuppressants, corticosteroids, alkylating drugs, antimetabolites, or radiation.

PREGNANCY: Category C, caution in nursing.

MECHANISM OF ACTION: May produce immune response for protection against hepatitis A virus infection.

NURSING CONSIDERATIONS

Assessment: Assess hypersensitivity, health and immune status, medical and immunization history, and for possible drug interactions.

Monitoring: Monitor injection site for induration, redness and swelling, general reactions (eg, fever, headache, dizziness), and creatinine phosphokinase.

Patient Counseling: Inform that expected immune response may not be obtained for immunosuppressed persons. Counsel on importance of completing vaccination series. Educate on potential benefits/risks; report any adverse reactions to physician.

Administration: IM route. **Storage:** 2-8°C (36-46°F). Do not freeze.

HELIDAC RX

tetracycline HCl - bismuth subsalicylate - metronidazole (Prometheus)

THERAPEUTIC CLASS: Antimicrobial

INDICATIONS: In combination with an H_2 antagonist for eradication of *H.pylori* and for treatment of *H.pylori* infection and duodenal ulcer disease.

DOSAGE: *Adults:* (Bismuth) 2 tabs (525mg) qid + (Metronidazole) 250mg qid + (Tetracycline) 500mg qid, all for 14 days with an H_2 antagonist. Take with meals and hs. Take metronidazole and tetracycline with a full glass of water; swallow whole.

HOW SUPPLIED: Cap: (Tetracycline) 500mg; Tab: (Metronidazole) 250mg; Tab, Chewable: (Bismuth Subsalicylate) 262.4mg

CONTRAINDICATIONS: Pregnancy, nursing, pediatrics, nitroimidazole hypersensitivity, ASA or salicylate hypersensitivity, renal/hepatic impairment.

WARNINGS/PRECAUTIONS: Do not use to treat nausea and vomiting in children or teenagers who have or are recovering from chickenpox or flu. Rare reports of neurotoxicity with excessive bismuth doses. Seizures and peripheral neuropathy reported with metronidazole; caution with CNS disease; d/c with abnormal neurological signs. Caution with blood dyscrasias. Unrecognized candidiasis may be unmasked. Avoid exposure to sunlight/UV light. Caution in elderly.

ADVERSE REACTIONS: NV, diarrhea, abdominal pain, melena, constipation, anorexia, asthenia, discolored tongue, headache, dyspepsia, dizziness. Temporary, harmless darkening of tongue and black stool with bismuth. Tetracycline may cause permanent discoloration of teeth during tooth development, enamel hypoplasia, photosensitivity reactions, BUN increase, breakthrough bleeding, pseudotumor cerebri.

INTERACTIONS: Monitor anticoagulants; possible risk of bleeding and/or decreased prothrombin activity. Bismuth subsalicylate: Caution with antidiabetic agents, ASA, probenecid, and sulfinpyrazone. Tetracycline: Impaired absorption with antacids containing aluminum, calcium, magnesium; agents containing iron, zinc, sodium bicarbonate. Possible reduced absorption with dairy products, bismuth, or calcium carbonate. May interfere with bactericidal action of penicillin; avoid concomitant use. May antagonize oral contraceptive effects. Fatal renal toxicity with methoxyflurane reported. Metronidazole (MET): Decreased plasma clearance with drugs that decrease metabolism (eg, cimetidine). Increased elimination with drugs that induce metabolism (eg, phenytoin, phenobarbital). May impair phenytoin clearance. May increase lithium levels. Avoid alcohol during and at least 1 day after MET. Psychotic reactions reported in alcoholics with concomitant disulfiram and MET; space MET and disulfiram dosing by 2 weeks.

PREGNANCY: Category D, not for use in nursing.

MECHANISM OF ACTION: Combination therapy with activity against *H.pylori*. Refer to individual PI for specific mechanism of action of each component.

PHARMACOKINETICS: Absorption: Salicylic acid: C_{max}=13.1mcg/mL. Metronidazole: Well-absorbed; C_{max}=6mcg/mL; T_{max}=1-2 hrs. Tetracycline: Readily absorbed. **Distribution**: Bismuth: Plasma protein binding (>90%). Salicylic acid: V_d=170mL/kg; plasma protein binding (90%). Metronidazole: Plasma protein binding (<20%), appears in the CSF, saliva, breast milk. Tetracycline: Crosses placenta, found in fetal tissues, secreted in breast milk. **Metabolism**: Salicyclic acid: Extensive. Metronidazole: Oxidation, glucuronide conjugation; 2-hydroxymethyl metabolite. **Elimination**: Bismuth: Urine, bile; $T_{1/2}$=21-72 days. Salicylic: Urine (10% unchanged); $T_{1/2}$=2-5 hrs. Metronidazole: Urine (60-80%), feces (6-15%); $T_{1/2}$=8 hrs. Tetracycline: Urine, feces.

NURSING CONSIDERATIONS

Assessment: Assess for pregnancy/nursing status, age of patient, renal/hepatic impairment, hypersensitivity to salicylates or aspirin, CNS diseases, presence or history of blood dyscrasias, and possible drug interactions. If using in pediatrics, assess for symptoms of flu or chickenpox.

Monitoring: Monitor for signs/symptoms of seizures, peripheral neuropathy, photosensitivity reactions, increases in BUN, darkening of stool or tongue, leukopenia, candidiasis, overgrowth of nonsusceptible bacteria, superinfection, and pseudotumor cerebri.

Patient Counseling: Instruct to take 4 times a day, at meal times and bedtime. Chew and swallow bismuth subsalicylate; swallow tetracycline and metronidazole tablet with a full glass of water. Take medication with an adequate amount of fluid to help prevent esophageal irritation and ulceration. If miss a dose, continue normal dosing until medication is done, do not double up doses. Continue therapy for full treatment period to prevent development of bacterial resistance. Inform that if on concomitant therapy with aspirin, and ringing in the ears occurs, d/c aspirin therapy until treatment is complete. Medication may decrease effectiveness of oral contraceptives; use different or additional form of contraception. Contact physician if breakthrough bleeding occurs. Avoid alcohol while on medication and for 1 day after d/c. Avoid exposure to sun/sun lamps. Inform may develop darkening of tongue or stool. Avoid pregnancy/nursing during therapy.

Administration: Oral route. **Storage**: 20-25°C (68-77°F).

H

HEPARIN SODIUM — RX

heparin sodium (Various)

THERAPEUTIC CLASS: Glycosaminoglycan

INDICATIONS: Prophylaxis and treatment of venous thrombosis and its extension, PE in atrial fibrillation, and peripheral arterial embolism. Prevention of postoperative DVT and PE. Diagnosis and treatment of acute and chronic consumptive coagulopathies, for prevention of clotting in arterial and cardiac surgery.

DOSAGE: *Adults:* Based on 68kg: Initial: 5000 U IV, then 10,000-20,000 U SQ. Maint: 8000-10,000 U q8h or 15,000-20,000 U q12h. Intermittent IV Injection: Initial: 10,000 U. Maint: 5000-10,000 U q4-6h. Continuous IV Infusion: Initial: 5000U. Maint: 20,000-40,000 U/24 hrs. Adjust to coagulation test results. See PI for details in specific disease states.
Pediatrics: Initial: 50 U/kg IV drip. Maint: 100 U/kg IV drip q4h or 20,000 U/m^2/24 hrs continuously.

HOW SUPPLIED: Inj: 1000 U/mL, 2500 U/mL, 5000 U/mL, 7500 U/mL, 10,000 U/mL

CONTRAINDICATIONS: Severe thrombocytopenia, if cannot perform appropriate blood-coagulation tests (with full-dose heparin), uncontrollable active bleeding state (except in DIC).

WARNINGS/PRECAUTIONS: Not for IM use. Hemorrhage can occur at any site; caution with increased danger of hemorrhage (severe HTN, bacterial endocarditis, surgery, etc.). Monitor blood coagulation tests frequently. Thrombocytopenia reported; d/c if platelets <100,000mm³ or if recurrent thrombosis develops. Contains benzyl alcohol. "White-clot syndrome" reported. Monitor platelets, Hct, and occult blood in the stool. Increased heparin resistance with fever, thrombosis, thrombophlebitis, infections with thrombosing tendencies, MI, cancer, and post-op. Higher bleeding incidence in women >60 yrs.

ADVERSE REACTIONS: Hemorrhage, local irritation, erythema, mild pain, hematoma, chills, fever, urticaria.

INTERACTIONS: Wait ≥5 hrs after last IV dose or 24 hrs after last SQ dose before measure PT for dicumarol or warfarin. Platelet inhibitors (eg, acetylsalicylic acid, dextran, phenylbutazone, ibuprofen, indomethacin, dipyridamole, hydroxychloroquine) may induce bleeding. Digitalis, tetracyclines, nicotine, or antihistamines may counteract anticoagulant action.

PREGNANCY: Category C, safe in nursing.

H

MECHANISM OF ACTION: Glycosaminoglycan; inhibits reactions that lead to blood clotting and the formation of fibrin clots. Acts at multiple sites in the normal coagulation system.

PHARMACOKINETICS: Absorption: (SC) T_{max}=2-4 hrs. **Metabolism:** Liver and reticulo-endothelial system. **Elimination:** $T_{1/2}$=10 min.

NURSING CONSIDERATIONS

Assessment: Assess for severe thrombocytopenia, pregnancy status, and drug interactions. Assess use in disease states at risk for hemorrhage (eg, subacute bacterial endocarditis, severe HTN) and use in older patients (>60 yrs). Assess that suitable coagulation tests (eg, whole blood clotting time, partial thromboplastin time) can be performed at appropriate intervals in patients on full-dose heparin.

Monitoring: Monitor for signs/symptoms of hemorrhage, thrombocytopenia, White Clot Syndrome, heparin resistance, and hypersensitivity reactions. Perform periodic monitoring of platelet counts, Hct, and tests for occult blood in stool. If given therapeutically, perform frequent coagulation tests. If given by continuous IV infusion, monitor coagulation time every 4 hrs during early stages of treatment. If given intermittently by IV inj, monitor coagulation tests before each inj during the initial phase of treatment and then at appropriate intervals thereafter.

Patient Counseling: Counsel about increased risk of bleeding tendencies while on medication. Instruct to notify physician if any type of unusual bleeding or hypersensitivity reaction occurs. Advise that periodic lab monitoring is required during treatment.

Administration: IV/SQ routes. If added to infusion solution for continuous IV administration, container should be inverted 6 times to insure adequate mixing and prevention of heparin pooling in the solution. **Storage:** 20-25°C (68-77°F).

HEPSERA — RX

adefovir dipivoxil (Gilead Sciences)

Discontinuation may result in severe acute exacerbations of hepatitis. Chronic use may result in nephrotoxicity in patients at risk of or having underlying renal dysfunction. HIV resistance may occur with unrecognized or untreated HIV infection. May cause lactic acidosis and severe hepatomegaly with steatosis.

THERAPEUTIC CLASS: Acyclic nucleotide analog

INDICATIONS: Treatment of chronic hepatitis B in patients ≥12 yrs of age with evidence of active viral replication and either evidence of persistent elevations in serum aminotransferases (ALT or AST) or histologically active disease.

DOSAGE: *Adults:* 10mg qd. Renal Impairment: CrCl 30-49mL/min: 10mg q48h. CrCl 10-29mL/min: 10mg q72h. Hemodialysis Patients: 10mg every 7

days following dialysis.
Pediatrics: ≥12 yrs: 10mg qd.

HOW SUPPLIED: Tab: 10mg

WARNINGS/PRECAUTIONS: Monitor hepatic function at repeated intervals upon discontinuation. Monitor renal function in patients with pre-existing or risk factors for renal dysfunction; adjust dosage appropriately. May require HIV antibody testing prior to treatment. Suspend treatment if lactic acidosis and severe hepatomegaly are suspected.

ADVERSE REACTIONS: Asthenia, headache, abdominal pain, nausea, flatulence, diarrhea, dyspepsia, increased creatinine, hypophosphatemia.

INTERACTIONS: Coadministration with drugs that reduce renal function or compete for active tubular secretion may increase concentrations of adefovir or the coadministered drugs.

PREGNANCY: Category C, caution in nursing.

MECHANISM OF ACTION: Acyclic nucleotide analog; inhibits HBV DNA polymerase by competing with natural substrate deoxyadenosine triphosphate and by causing DNA chain termination after incorporation into viral DNA.

PHARMACOKINETICS: Absorption: Absolute bioavailability (59%); C_{max}=18.4ng/mL; T_{max}=1.75 hrs; AUC=220ng•h/mL. **Pediatrics:** C_{max}=23.3ng/mL; AUC=248.8ng•h/mL. **Distribution:** V_d=392mL/kg (1mg/kg/day), 352mL/kg (3mg/kg/day); plasma protein binding (≤4%). **Elimination:** Urine (45%); $T_{1/2}$=7.48 hrs.

NURSING CONSIDERATIONS

Assessment: Assess for possible drug interactions and renal impairment. Perform HIV testing prior to therapy.

Monitoring: Monitor renal function; LFTs periodically and for several months after d/c. Monitor for signs/symptoms of exacerbations of hepatitis, nephrotoxicity, lactic acidosis, severe hepatomegaly with steatosis, and hypersensitivity reactions.

Patient Counseling: Instruct to report any severe abdominal pain, muscle pain, yellowing of eyes, dark urine, pale stools, loss of appetite, or hypersensitivity reactions immediately. Inform if miss dose, do not double doses.

Administration: Oral route. **Storage:** 25°C (77°F); excursions permitted to 15-30°C (59-86°F).

HERCEPTIN — RX

trastuzumab (Genentech)

May result in cardiac failure manifesting as CHF and decreased left ventricular ejection fraction (LVEF). Increased incidence/severity of left ventricular cardiac dysfunction in combination with anthracycline-containing regimens. Evaluate LVEF prior to and during therapy; d/c with significant decrease in left ventricular function or cardiomyopathy. Serious infusion reactions and pulmonary toxicity may result. Interrupt infusion if dyspnea or clinically significant hypotension develops. D/C with anaphylaxis, angioedema, interstitial pneumonitis, or acute respiratory distress syndrome.

THERAPEUTIC CLASS: Monoclonal antibody/HER2-blocker

INDICATIONS: Part of treatment regimen consisting of doxorubicin, cyclophosphamide, and either paclitaxel or docetaxel and with docetaxel and carboplatin for adjuvant treatment of HER2-overexpressing node-positive or node-negative breast cancer. Single agent for adjuvant treatment of HER2-overexpressing node-negative or node-positive breast cancer, following multimodality anthracycline-based therapy. In combination with paclitaxel for first-line treatment of HER2-overexpressing metastatic breast cancer. Single agent for treatment of HER2-overexpressing breast cancer in patients who received 1 or more chemotherapy regimens for metastatic disease.

DOSAGE: *Adults:* Adjuvant Treatment: During and Following Paclitaxel, Docetaxel, or Docetaxel/Carboplatin for 52 Weeks: IV infusion: Initial: 4mg/kg over 90 min. Maint: 2mg/kg/week over 30 min for the first 12 weeks (paclitaxel or docetaxel) or 18 weeks (docetaxel/carboplatin). One Week Following the Last Weekly Dose: 6mg/kg IV over 30-60 min q3 weeks. Following Completion of Multimodality, Anthracycline-based Regimens: Initial: 8mg/kg IV over 90 min. Maint: 6mg/kg over 30 min q3 weeks. Metastatic Breast Cancer: IV Infusion: Alone or With Paclitaxel: Initial: 4mg/kg over 90 min. Maint: 2mg/kg/week over 30 min until disease progression.

HOW SUPPLIED: Inj: 440mg

WARNINGS/PRECAUTIONS: Left ventricular cardiac dysfunction, arrhythmias, HTN, disabling cardiac failure, cardiomyopathy, and cardiac death may occur. Obtain baseline cardiac assessment (eg, history, physical, LVEF). Monitor LVEF prior to initiation, every 3 months during, and every 6 months following completion for at least 2 yrs. Fatal pulmonary toxicity may result. May exacerbate chemotherapy-induced neutropenia. HER2 testing is necessary to detect HER2 protein overexpression, which is needed to select patients for trastuzumab therapy. May increase risk of neutropenia. May cause severe infusion reactions; interrupt infusion and d/c permanently.

ADVERSE REACTIONS: Pain, asthenia, fever, NV, chills, headache, increased cough, diarrhea, abdominal pain, back pain, dyspnea, infection, rash, tachycardia, anemia, peripheral edema.

INTERACTIONS: Paclitaxel may increase serum levels. Concomitant anthracyclines and cyclophosphamide may increase incidence/severity of cardiac dysfunction.

PREGNANCY: Category D, caution in nursing.

MECHANISM OF ACTION: Monoclonal antibody/HER-2 blocker; inhibits the proliferation of human tumor cells that overexpress HER-2.

PHARMACOKINETICS: Absorption: (500mg) C_{max}=337mcg/mL. **Distribution:** V_d=44mL/kg. **Elimination:** $T_{1/2}$=2 days (10mg), $T_{1/2}$=12 days (500mg). Mean half -life increased and clearance decreased with increasing dose level. Refer to PI for detailed information.

NURSING CONSIDERATIONS

Assessment: Assess cardiac function, history and physical exam, baseline LVEF by echocardiogram or MUGA scan, HER-2 testing, CBC with differential and platelets, pregnancy status. Note other diseases/conditions and drug therapies.

Monitoring: Monitor for cardiac failure, CHF, LVEF every 3 months during and upon completion of therapy and every 6 months for 2 yrs following completion. Monitor for cardiomyopathy, infusion reactions, pulmonary reactions/toxicity, exacerbation of chemotherapy-induced neutropenia, fatigue, anemia, myalgia, dyspnea, rash/desquamation, headache, diarrhea, infections.

Patient Counseling: Advise to report of new onset or worsening SOB, cough, swelling of ankles/legs or face, palpitations, weight gain of more than 5lbs in 24 hrs, dizziness, or loss of consciousness. Advise females to use effective contraceptive methods during and at least 6 months following therapy.

Administration: IV route. Reconstitute each 440mg vial with 20mL Bacteriostatic Water for Injection, containing 1.1% benzyl alcohol as preservative to yield multidose solution containing 21mg/mL. Use SWFI if known hypersensitivity to benzyl alcohol. **Storage:** 2-8°C (34-46°F) for more than 24 hrs prior to use.

HUMALOG — RX

insulin lispro (Lilly)

THERAPEUTIC CLASS: Insulin

INDICATIONS: To control hyperglycemia in diabetes.

DOSAGE: *Adults:* Individualize dose. Inject SQ within 15 min before or immediately after a meal. May use with external insulin pump; do not dilute or mix with other insulins when used with pump.
Pediatrics: ≥3 yrs: Individualize dose. Inject SQ within 15 min before or

immediately after a meal. May use with external insulin pump; do not dilute or mix with other insulins when used with pump.

HOW SUPPLIED: Cartridge: 100 U/mL; Inj: 100 U/mL; Pen: 100 U/mL

CONTRAINDICATIONS: Hypoglycemia.

WARNINGS/PRECAUTIONS: Any change of insulin should be made cautiously. Changes in strength, manufacturer, type or method of manufacture may result in the need for a change in dosage. Hypoglycemia may occur with taking too much insulin, missing or delaying meals, exercising or working more than usual. An infection or illness (especially with diarrhea or vomiting) may change insulin requirements. With type 1 DM a longer-acting insulin is usually required to maintain glucose control; not required with type 2 DM if regimen includes sulfonylureas. May be diluted with sterile diluent. Caution with potassium-lowering drugs or drugs sensitive to serum potassium levels.

ADVERSE REACTIONS: Hypoglycemia, hypokalemia, allergic reactions, injection-site reaction, lipodystrophy, pruritus, rash.

H

INTERACTIONS: Increased insulin requirements with corticosteroids, isoniazid, niacin, estrogens, oral contraceptives, phenothiazines, thyroid replacement therapy. Decreased insulin requirements with oral hypoglycemics, salicylates, sulfa antibiotics, MAOIs, ACEIs, ARBs, β-blockers, octreotide, and alcohol. β-blockers may mask symptoms of hypoglycemia.

PREGNANCY: Category B, caution in nursing.

MECHANISM OF ACTION: Insulin lispro (rDNA origin); regulates glucose metabolism.

PHARMACOKINETICS: Absorption: Absolute bioavailability (55-77%); T_{max}=30-90 min. **Distribution:** V_d=0.26-0.36L/kg. **Elimination:** $T_{1/2}$=1 hr.

NURSING CONSIDERATIONS

Assessment: Assess renal function, LFTs, FPG, HbA_{1c}, hypokalemia, pregnancy status, autonomic neuropathy, and possible drug interactions.

Monitoring: Monitor blood glucose, potassium levels, and HbA_{1c} levels regularly. Monitor for antibody production, allergic reactions (redness, swelling, or itching at injection site), SOB, wheezing, reduction in BP, rapid pulse or sweating, anaphylactic reactions, pruritus, lipodystrophy.

Patient Counseling: Infusion set (reservoir syringe, tubing, and catheter), Disetronic D-TRON or D-TRON plus cartridge adapter, and Humalog in the external insulin pump reservoir should be replaced and a new infusion site selected every 48 hrs or less. If solution is cloudy, contains particulate matter, is thickened or discolored, contents must not be injected. Inform of the importance of proper insulin storage, injecting techniques, timing of dosage, adherence to meal planning, regular physical activity, regular blood glucose monitoring, periodic HbA_{1c} testing, recognition and management of hypo/hyperglycemia, and periodic assessment for diabetes complications.

Administration: SQ route. When used as mealtime insulin, the dose should be given within 15 min before or immediately after meals. Should not be diluted or mixed with any other insulin when used in an external insulin pump. Must not be used after expiration date. Unrefrigerated below 36°C (86°F), vials, cartridges, Pens, and KwikPens must be used within 28 days or be discarded, even if they still contain medication. **Storage:** Refrigerate at 2-8°C (36-46°F). Do not freeze or expose to temperatures above 37°C (98.6°F). Protect from direct heat and sunlight.

HUMALOG MIX 75/25 — RX

insulin lispro protamine - insulin lispro (Lilly)

THERAPEUTIC CLASS: Insulin

INDICATIONS: To control hyperglycemia in diabetes.

DOSAGE: *Adults:* Individualize dose. Inject SQ within 15 min before a meal. May need to reduce/adjust dose with renal/hepatic impairment.

HOW SUPPLIED: (Insulin Lispro Protamine, Human-Insulin Lispro, Human) Inj: 75 U-25 U/mL; Pen: 75 U-25 U/mL

CONTRAINDICATIONS: Hypoglycemia.

WARNINGS/PRECAUTIONS: Any change of insulin should be made cautiously. Changes in strength, manufacturer, type or method of manufacture may result in the need for a change in dosage. Hypoglycemia may occur with taking too much insulin, missing or delaying meals, exercising or working more than usual. An infection or illness (especially with diarrhea or vomiting) may change insulin requirements.

ADVERSE REACTIONS: Hypoglycemia, hypokalemia, allergic reactions, injection site reaction, lipodystrophy, pruritus, rash.

INTERACTIONS: Increased insulin requirements with corticosteroids, isoniazid, niacin, estrogens, oral contraceptives, phenothiazines, thyroid replacement therapy. Decreased insulin requirements with oral hypoglycemics, salicylates, sulfa antibiotics, MAOIs, ACEIs, ARBs, β-blockers, octreotide, and alcohol. β-blockers may mask symptoms of hypoglycemia.

H

PREGNANCY: Category B, caution in nursing.

MECHANISM OF ACTION: Insulin; 75% lispro protamine (intermediate-acting), 25% insulin lispro (rapid-acting); helps in the maintenance of blood glucose at near normal levels.

PHARMACOKINETICS: Absorption: T_{max}=60 min.

NURSING CONSIDERATIONS

Assessment: Assess renal function, LFTs, FPG, HbA_{1c}, hypokalemia, pregnancy status, autonomic neuropathy, and possible drug interactions.

Monitoring: Monitor blood glucose, potassium levels, and HbA_{1c} levels regularly. Monitor for antibody production, allergic reactions (redness, swelling, or itching at injection site), SOB, wheezing, reduction in BP, rapid pulse or sweating, anaphylactic reactions, pruritus, lipodystrophy.

Patient Counseling: Inform of the importance of proper insulin storage, injection techniques, timing of dosage, adherence to meal planning, regular physical activity, regular blood glucose monitoring, periodic HbA_{1c} testing, recognition and management of hypo- and hyperglycemia, and periodic assessment for diabetes complications.

Administration: SQ route (15 min before meals). **Storage:** Refrigerate at 2-8°C (36-46°F). Do not freeze. Protect from direct heat and light.

Humatrope — RX

somatropin (Lilly)

THERAPEUTIC CLASS: Human growth hormone

INDICATIONS: Treatment of children with short stature or growth failure associated with growth hormone deficiency (GHD), Turner syndrome, idiopathic short stature, short stature homeobox-containing gene (SHOX) deficiency, and for growth failure in children born small for gestational age who fail to demonstrate catch-up growth by 2-4 yrs. Treatment of adults with either childhood- or adult-onset GHD.

DOSAGE: *Adults:* GHD: Non-Weight Based: Initial: 0.2mg/day. Titrate: Every 1-2 months in increments of 0.1-0.2mg/day until acceptable clinical response and serum insulin-like growth factor I (IGF-I) concentrations are reached. Usual range: 0.15-0.30mg/day. Weight Based: Initial: 0.006mg/kg/day. Titrate: Increase dose based on individual requirement. Dose adjustment based on clinical response, side effects, and determination of age- and gender-adjusted serum insulin-like growth factor I (IGF-I) concentrations. Max: 0.0125mg/kg/day.
Pediatrics: GHD: 0.026-0.043mg/kg/day (0.18-0.30mg/kg/week) SQ. Max: 0.043mg/kg/day (0.30mg/kg/week). Turner Syndrome: Up to 0.054mg/kg/day (0.375mg/kg/week). Idiopathic Short Syndrome: Up to 0.053mg/kg/day (0.37mg/kg/week). SHOX Deficiency: 0.050mg/kg/day

(0.35mg/kg/week). SGA: Up to 0.067mg/kg/day (0.47mg/kg/week). Calculated weekly dosage should be divided into equal doses given either 6 or 7 days/week.

HOW SUPPLIED: Inj: 5mg [vial], 6mg, 12mg, 24mg [cartridge]

CONTRAINDICATIONS: Pediatrics with closed epiphyses. Active proliferative or severe non-proliferative diabetic retinopathy. Active malignancy. Hypersensitivity to Metacresol or glycerin. Acute critical illness due to complications after open heart or abdominal surgery, multiple accidental trauma or acute respiratory failure. Prader-Willi syndrome with severe obesity or severe respiratory impairment.

WARNINGS/PRECAUTIONS: If sensitivity to diluent occurs, reconstitute with bacteriostatic (contains benzyl alcohol; avoid in newborns) or sterile water for injection. Monitor GHD secondary to intracranial lesion for progression/recurrence. Monitor gait, glucose intolerance, for malignant transformation of skin lesions, scoliosis progression, intracranial HTN (perform fundoscopic exam at start and periodically). Caution with DM, endocrine disorders, hypopituitarism, and hypothyroidism. With Turner syndrome monitor for otic or cardiovascular disorders, autoimmune thyroid disease. Increased risk of a second neoplasm in childhood cancer survivors reported. Fluid retention, slipped capital femoral epiphysis, and local or systemic allergic reactions may occur.

H

ADVERSE REACTIONS: Injection-site reactions, hypersensitivity to the diluent, and hypothyroidism, edema, arthralgia, myalgia, carpal tunnel syndrome, paraesthesias and hyperglycemia.

INTERACTIONS: Antagonized by glucocorticoids. May alter clearance of CYP450 substrates (eg, corticosteroids, sex steroids, anticonvulsants, antipyrine, cyclosporine). May require larger dose with oral estrogen replacement. Adjust dose of insulin and/or oral agent in diabetic patients.

PREGNANCY: Category C, caution in nursing.

MECHANISM OF ACTION: Human growth hormone; stimulates linear growth synthesis, metabolizes lipids, reduces body fat stores by increasing cellular protein, and increases plasma fatty acids.

PHARMACOKINETICS: Absorption: (SQ) Absolute bioavailabilty (75%). (IM) Absolute bioavailabilty (63%). **Distribution:** (IV) V_d=0.07L/kg. **Metabolism:** Liver and kidney (protein catabolism). **Elimination:** Urine: (IV) $T_{1/2}$=0.36 hrs. (SQ) $T_{1/2}$=3.8 hrs. (IM) $T_{1/2}$=4.9 hrs.

NURSING CONSIDERATIONS

Assessment: Assess for hypersensitivity to either Metacresol or glycerin, closed epiphyses (pediatric), proliferative diabetic retinopathy, active malignancy, acute critical illness (complications of surgery, multiple accidental trauma, or acute respiratory failure), pre-existing type 1, type 2 DM or impaired glucose tolerance, history of scoliosis, pre-existing papilledema, hypothyroidism, diagnostic imaging (rule out pituitary or intracranial tumor), hypopituitarism and possible drug interactions. Obtain baseline fundoscopic exam. Prader-Willi syndrome: Evaluate for signs of upper airway obstruction or sleep apnea before initiation. Turner syndrome: Evaluate for otitis media or other ear disorders, and for cardiovascular disorders before initiation.

Monitoring: Monitor fasting blood glucose and thyroid function tests periodically, periodic fundoscopic exam, weight control (Prader-Willi syndrome). Signs/symptoms of malignant transformation of skin lesions, intracranial HTN, slipped capital femoral epiphysis (onset of limp, hip or knee pain), hypersensitivity/allergic reactions, respiratory infections (Prader-Willi syndrome), otitis media or ear disorders (Turner syndrome), CV disorders (Turner syndrome), and progression of scoliosis.

Patient Counseling: Instruct that cartridges should be reconstituted only with supplied diluent and should only be used if allergic to Metacresol or glycerin. Instruct thoroughly as to proper usage, proper disposal, and caution against any reuse of needles and syringes. Seek medical attention if symptoms of slipped capital femoral epiphysis (onset of limp, hip or knee pain), hypersensitivity/allergic reactions, respiratory infections, otitis media or ear disorders, CV disorders, and progression of scoliosis occur.

Administration: SQ, IV, and IM route. Rotate injection site (SQ) to avoid tissue atrophy. **Storage:** Refrigerate at 2-8°C (36-46°F). Avoid freezing. (Reconstitution: Diluent or Bacteriostatic water): Refrigerate; stable up to 14 days. (Reconstitution: Sterile water): Refrigerate; use within 24 hrs (Cartridges: after reconstitution): Refrigerate; stable for 28 days.

HUMIRA — RX

adalimumab (Abbott)

Reports of TB, invasive fungal infections, and other opportunistic infections. Evaluate for latent TB and treat if necessary prior to initiation of therapy.

THERAPEUTIC CLASS: Monoclonal antibody/TNF-blocker

INDICATIONS: For reducing signs and symptoms, inducing major clinical response, inhibiting structural damage progression, and improving physical function in moderately to severely active rheumatoid arthritis (RA). For reducing signs and symptoms of moderately to severely active polyarticular juvenile idiopathic arthritis in patients ≥4 yrs. For reducing signs and symptoms of active arthritis, inhibiting the progression of structural damage, and improving physical function in patients with psoriatic arthritis (PA). For reducing signs and symptoms of active ankylosing spondylitis (AS). For reducing signs and symptoms and inducing and maintaining clinical remission of moderately to severely active Crohn's disease in patients who have had an inadequate response to conventional therapy. For reducing signs and symptoms and inducing clinical remission in patients who have lost response to or are intolerant to infliximab. For treating moderate to severe chronic plaque psoriasis in patients who are candidates for systemic therapy or phototherapy.

DOSAGE: *Adults:* (RA/PA/AS): 40mg SQ every other week. Some patients with RA not taking concomitant MTX may derive additional benefit from increasing the dosing frequency to 40mg every week. Crohn's Disease: Initial: 160mg (may be given as 4 injections on Day 1, or 2 injections/day for 2 consecutive days); then 80mg after 2 weeks (Day 15). Maint: 40mg every other week beginning at Week 4 (Day 29). Plaque Psoriasis: Initial: 80mg. Maint: 40mg every other week starting 1 week after initial dose.
Pediatrics: (4-17 yrs) 15kg-<30kg: 20mg every other week; ≥30kg: 40mg every other week.

HOW SUPPLIED: Inj: 20mg/0.4mL, 40mg/0.8mL

WARNINGS/PRECAUTIONS: Serious infections including sepsis and TB reported. Monitor for signs of infection during and after therapy; d/c if serious infection develops. Avoid with active infection. Monitor HBV carriers as reactivation may occur; if reactivation occurs, stop adalimumab and start antiviral therapy. Caution with history of recurrent infections or underlying conditions predisposing to infections or in areas where TB and histoplasmosis are endemic. Caution with pre-existing or recent-onset CNS demyelinating disorders. Lymphomas, allergic reactions observed. May affect host defenses against infections and malignancies. May result in autoantibody formation; d/c if lupus-like syndrome develops. Rare possibility of anaphylaxis and pancytopenia including aplastic anemia. May cause CHF or worsen pre-existing disease.

ADVERSE REACTIONS: URI, injection site pain/reactions, headache, rash, sinusitis, nausea, UTI, flu syndrome, abdominal pain, hyperlipidemia, hypercholesterolemia, back pain, hematuria, HTN, immunogenicity.

INTERACTIONS: Do not give concurrently with live vaccines. Reduced clearance with MTX. Do not use concurrently with anakinra due to increased risk of serious infections.

PREGNANCY: Category B, not for use in nursing.

MECHANISM OF ACTION: Monoclonal antibody/TNF-blocker; binds specifically to TNF-α and blocks its interaction with p55 and p75 cell surface TNF receptors. Lyses surface TNF-expressing cells in the presence of complement. Modulates biological responses that are induced or regulated by

H

TNF. In plaque psoriasis, reduces the epidermal thickness and infiltration of inflammatory cells.

PHARMACOKINETICS: Absorption: Absolute bioavailability (64%); C_{max}=4.7mcg/mL; T_{max}=131 hrs. **Distribution:** V_d=4.7-6.0L. **Elimination:** $T_{1/2}$=2 weeks.

NURSING CONSIDERATIONS

Assessment: Assess for active infection (eg, chronic or localized infection), history of recurrent infection, predisposition to infection (eg, disease states), TB risk factors, risk of reactivation of hepatitis B virus, demyelinating disease, CHF, pregnancy/nursing status, and possible drug interactions. Obtain test for latent TB.

Monitoring: Monitor for signs/symptoms of infections (eg, sepsis, TB, opportunistic infections), malignancies (eg, lymphoma), hypersensitivity reactions (eg, anaphylaxis, angioneurotic edema), hepatitis B virus reactivation, demyelinating disease, hematological reactions (eg, thrombocytopenia, leukopenia, aplastic anemia), worsening CHF, autoimmunity and lupus-like syndrome, immunosuppression.

Patient Counseling: Inform about risks/benefits of therapy. Medication may lower the ability of immune system to fight infection; instruct to contact physician if any symptoms of infection, including TB and reactivation of hepatitis B, occur. Counsel about risk of lymphoma and other malignancies while on therapy, and to seek immediate medical attention if signs of severe allergic reactions (eg, anaphylaxis) develop. Advise to report any new or worsening medical conditions (eg, heart disease, neurological disease, autoimmune disorder) or any symptoms suggestive of a cytopenia (eg, bleeding, bruising, or persistent fever). Counsel about proper injection technique.

Administration: SQ route. Rotate injection sites. Avoid injecting into areas where skin is tender, bruised, red, or hard. If using pen formulation or prefilled syringe, inject full amount of syringe. **Storage:** 2-8°C (36-46°F). Do not freeze. Protect prefilled syringe from exposure to light. Store in original carton until time of administration. Keep out of reach of children.

HUMULIN — OTC

insulin human, rdna origin - insulin, human isophane - insulin, human regular (Lilly)

OTHER BRAND NAMES: Humulin N (Lilly) - Humulin R (Lilly)

THERAPEUTIC CLASS: Insulin

INDICATIONS: To control hyperglycemia in diabetes.

DOSAGE: *Adults:* Individualize dose.
Pediatrics: Individualize dose.

HOW SUPPLIED: Inj: 100 U/mL (Humulin N, Humulin R), 500 U/mL (Humulin R U-500); Pen: 100 U/mL (Humulin N).

CONTRAINDICATIONS: Hypoglycemia.

WARNINGS/PRECAUTIONS: Human insulin differs from animal source insulin. Any change of insulin should be made cautiously. Changes in strength, manufacturer, type or method of manufacture may result in the need for a change in dosage. Hypoglycemia may occur with taking too much insulin, missing or delaying meals, exercising or working more than usual. An infection or illness (especially with diarrhea or vomiting) may change insulin requirements. Administration of insulin SQ can result in lipoatrophy.

ADVERSE REACTIONS: Hypoglycemia, sweating, dizziness, palpitations, tremor, hunger, restlessness, lightheadedness, inability to concentrate, headache, injection site reaction, allergic reaction.

INTERACTIONS: Increased insulin requirements with oral contraceptives, corticosteroids, or thyroid replacement therapy. Reduced insulin requirements with oral hypoglycemics, salicylates, sulfa antibiotics, and certain antidepressants. Alcoholic beverages may change insulin requirements. β-blockers may mask symptoms of hypoglycemia.

PREGNANCY: Pregnancy category is not known.

MECHANISM OF ACTION: Insulin; regular insulin human injection of rDNA origin that helps in maintenance of blood glucose at near normal level.

NURSING CONSIDERATIONS

Assessment: Assess FPG, HbA_{1c}, renal function, LFTs, pregnancy status, infections, alcohol consumption, exercise routines, travel plans, adrenal or thyroid or pituitary diseases, and possible drug interactions.

Monitoring: Monitor FPG, HbA_{1c}, renal function, diabetic ketoacidosis, lipodystrophy, allergic reactions like SOB, hypotension, tachycardia. Monitor for signs of hypoglycemia (sweating, palpitations, seizures, disorientation, tremors).

H

Patient Counseling: Advise to never share needles and syringes. Vial must be carefully shaken to completely mix the insulin; should look uniformly cloudy or milky before administration. Do not use if solid particles stick to the bottom or there are clumps in the insulin after mixing. Instruct to always carry a quick source of sugar (hard candy or glucose tablets). Local reactions may be expected (redness, swelling, itching at injection site that usually clears up in a few days). Counsel about signs/symptoms of hypoglycemia, importance of frequent monitoring of blood glucose levels, and need for eating a balanced diet and exercising regularly. Advise to keep extra/spare supply of syringes and needles on hand and always wear diabetic identification.

Administration: SQ route (abdomen, thigh, and arms). **Storage:** Bottle not in use. Refrigerate. Do not freeze. (In-use): Below 30°C (86°F), away from heat and light. Do not use after the stamped expiration date.

HUMULIN 70/30 — OTC

insulin human, rdna origin - insulin, human (isophane/regular) (Lilly)

OTHER BRAND NAMES: Humulin 50/50 (Lilly)

THERAPEUTIC CLASS: Insulin

INDICATIONS: To control hyperglycemia in diabetes.

DOSAGE: *Adults:* Individualize dose. Administer SQ.
Pediatrics: Individualize dose. Administer SQ.

HOW SUPPLIED: (Isophane-Regular) Inj: (Humulin 70/30) 70 U-30 U/mL, (Humulin 50/50) 50 U-50 U/mL

WARNINGS/PRECAUTIONS: Human insulin differs from animal source insulin. Make any change of insulin cautiously. Changes in strength, manufacturer, type, or method of manufacture may result in the need for a change in dosage. Hypoglycemia may occur with too much insulin, missing or delaying meals, exercising, or working more than usual. Infection or illness (especially with diarrhea or vomiting) may change insulin requirements. Administration of insulin SQ can result in lipoatrophy.

ADVERSE REACTIONS: Hypoglycemia, sweating, dizziness, palpitations, tremor, hunger, restlessness, lightheadedness, inability to concentrate, headache, injection site reaction, allergic reaction.

INTERACTIONS: Increased insulin requirements with oral contraceptives, corticosteroids, or thyroid replacement therapy. Reduced insulin requirements with oral hypoglycemics, salicylates, sulfa antibiotics, and certain antidepressants. Alcoholic beverages may change insulin requirements. β-blockers may mask symptoms of hypoglycemia.

PREGNANCY: Pregnancy category is not known.

MECHANISM OF ACTION: Insulin; lowers blood glucose levels by stimulating peripheral glucose uptake, especially by skeletal muscle and fat, and by inhibiting hepatic glucose production. Inhibits lipolysis and proteolysis, and enhances protein synthesis.

NURSING CONSIDERATIONS

Assessment: Assess FPG, HbA_{1c}, renal function, LFTs, pregnancy status, infections, alcohol consumption, exercise routines, travel plans, adrenal or thyroid or pituitary diseases, and for possible drug interactions.

Monitoring: Monitor FPG, HbA_{1c}, renal function, diabetic ketoacidosis, lipodystrophy, allergic reactions, hypotension, tachycardia. Monitor for signs of hypoglycemia (sweating, palpitation, seizures, disorientation, tremors).

Patient Counseling: Advise never to share needles or syringes. Vial must be carefully shaken to completely mix insulin; should look uniformly cloudy or milky before administration. Do not use if solid particles stick to bottom or there are clumps in insulin after mixing. Instruct to always carry a quick source of sugar (hard candy or glucose tablets). Counsel that local reactions may be expected (redness, swelling, itching at injection site) which usually clear up in a few days. Educate about signs/symptoms of hypoglycemia, importance of frequent monitoring of blood glucose levels, and need for eating a balanced diet and exercising regularly. Advise to keep an extra/spare supply of syringes and needles and to always wear diabetic identification.

H

Administration: SQ route (alternate sites: abdomen, thigh, arms). Use syringe marked for U-100 insulin. **Storage:** Refrigerate unopened bottles. Do not freeze. Keep unopened bottles unrefrigerated at 30°C (86°F). Protect from heat and light.

HYALGAN RX

sodium hyaluronate (Sanofi-Aventis)

THERAPEUTIC CLASS: Hyaluronan

INDICATIONS: Treatment of pain in osteoarthritis of the knee in patients who have failed to respond adequately to conservative nonpharmacologic therapy, and to simple analgesics (eg, APAP).

DOSAGE: *Adults:* Administer 2mL by intra-articular injection once a week for a total of 5 injections. Some patients may experience benefit with 3 injections given at weekly intervals. Use strict aseptic technique.

HOW SUPPLIED: Inj: 2mL

CONTRAINDICATIONS: Intra-articular injections are contraindicated in cases of infections or skin disease in the area of the injection site.

WARNINGS/PRECAUTIONS: Avoid disinfectants containing quaternary ammonium salts for skin preparation; hyaluronic acid can precipitate in their presence. Anaphylactoid and allergic reactions reported. Transient increases in inflammation in the injected knee in some patients with inflammatory arthritis such as rheumatoid arthritis or gouty arthritis have been reported. Safety and effectiveness in joints other than the knee or concomitantly with other intra-articular injectables have not been established. Caution in patients who are allergic to avian proteins, feathers, and egg products. Avoid any strenuous activities or prolonged (eg, more than 1 hour) weight-bearing activities within 48 hours following the intra-articular injection. Remove any joint effusion before injecting. Safety and effectiveness have not been demonstrated in children.

ADVERSE REACTIONS: GI complaints, injection site pain, headache, local skin reactions (rash, ecchymosis), local joint pain, pruritus (local), knee swelling/effusion.

PREGNANCY: Safety in pregnancy and nursing not known.

NURSING CONSIDERATIONS

Assessment: Assess for knee joint infection, skin infection, or disease around injection site.

Monitoring: Monitor for anaphylactic and allergic reactions, injection-site pain, local skin reaction, and joint swelling/effusion.

Patient Counseling: Inform that drug may cause transient pain/swelling of injected joint. Avoid strenuous activities or prolonged weight-bearing activities (jogging, tennis) within 48 hrs following injection.

Adminstration: Intra-articular injection. **Storage**: Below 25°C (77°F). Do not freeze.

HYDRALAZINE RX
hydralazine HCl (Various)

THERAPEUTIC CLASS: Vasodilator

INDICATIONS: Management of HTN.

DOSAGE: *Adults:* Initial: 10mg qid for 2-4 days. Titrate: Increase to 25mg qid for the rest of the week, then increase to 50mg qid. Maint: Use lowest effective dose. Resistant Patients: 300mg/day or titrate to lower dose combined with thiazide diuretic and/or reserpine, or β-blocker.
Pediatrics: Initial: 0.75mg/kg/day given qid. Titrate: Increase gradually over 3-4 weeks to a max of 7.5mg/kg/day or 200mg/day.

HOW SUPPLIED: Inj: 20mg/mL; Tab: 10mg, 25mg, 50mg, 100mg

CONTRAINDICATIONS: CAD and mitral valvular rheumatic heart disease.

WARNINGS/PRECAUTIONS: D/C if SLE symptoms occur. May cause angina and ECG changes of MI. Caution with suspected CAD, CVA, advanced renal impairment. May increase pulmonary artery pressure in mitral valvular disease. Postural hypotension reported. Add pyridoxine if peripheral neuritis develops. Monitor CBC and ANA titer before and periodically during therapy.

ADVERSE REACTIONS: Headache, anorexia, NV, diarrhea, tachycardia, angina.

INTERACTIONS: Caution with MAOIs. Profound hypotension with potent parenteral antihypertensives (eg, diazoxide). May reduce pressor response to epinephrine.

PREGNANCY: Category C, safety in nursing not known.

MECHANISM OF ACTION: Vasodilator; not established. Apparently lowers BP by direct relaxation of vascular smooth muscle; interferes with calcium movement within vascular smooth muscle responsible for initiating or maintaining contraction.

PHARMACOKINETICS: Absorption: Rapid; T_{max}=1-2 hrs. **Distribution:** Plasma protein binding (87%). **Metabolism:** Acetylation. **Elimination:** Urine; $T_{1/2}$=3-7 hrs.

NURSING CONSIDERATIONS

Assessment: Assess for CAD, mitral valvular rheumatic heart disease, cerebral vascular accidents, renal disease, and possible drug interactions. Obtain baseline CBC and ANA.

Monitoring: Monitor CBC and ANA periodically. Monitor for signs/symptoms of peripheral neuritis, hypotension, blood dyscrasias, SLE-like symptoms, and hypersensitivity reactions.

Patient Counseling: Advise to seek medical attention if symptoms of peripheral neuritis (paresthesia, numbness, tingling), hypotension, blood dyscrasias, SLE-like symptoms, or hypersensitivity reactions occur.

Administration: Oral route. **Storage:** 15-30°C (59-86°F).

HYDROCHLOROTHIAZIDE RX
hydrochlorothiazide (Various)

THERAPEUTIC CLASS: Thiazide diuretic

INDICATIONS: Adjunct therapy in edema associated with CHF, hepatic cirrhosis, corticosteroid and estrogen therapy, renal dysfunction. Management of HTN.

DOSAGE: *Adults:* Edema: 25-100mg qd or in divided doses. May give every other day or 3-5 days/week. HTN: Initial: 25mg qd. Titrate: May increase to 50mg/day.
Pediatrics: Diuresis/HTN: 1-2mg/kg/day given qd-bid. Max: Infants up to 2 yrs: 37.5mg/day. 2-12 yrs: 100mg/day. <6 months: Up to 1.5mg/kg bid may be required.

HOW SUPPLIED: Tab: 12.5mg, 25mg*, 50mg* *scored

CONTRAINDICATIONS: Anuria, sulfonamide hypersensitivity.

WARNINGS/PRECAUTIONS: Caution in severe renal disease, liver dysfunction, electrolyte/fluid imbalance. Monitor electrolytes. Hyperuricemia, hyperglycemia, hypokalemia, hyponatremia, hypomagnesemia, hypercalcemia may occur. Increases in cholesterol and triglyceride levels reported. May exacerbate SLE. Sensitivity reactions reported. D/C prior to parathyroid test. Enhanced effects in post-sympathectomy patients.

ADVERSE REACTIONS: Weakness, hypotension, pancreatitis, jaundice, diarrhea, vomiting, blood dyscrasias, rash, photosensitivity, electrolyte imbalance, impotence.

INTERACTIONS: May potentiate orthostatic hypotension with alcohol, barbiturates, narcotics. Adjust antidiabetic drugs. Possible decreased response to pressor amines. Corticosteroids, ACTH increase electrolyte depletion. May potentiate nondepolarizing skeletal muscle relaxants, antihypertensives. Lithium toxicity. NSAIDs decrease effects. Decreased PO absorption with cholestyramine, colestipol.

PREGNANCY: Category B, not for use in nursing.

MECHANISM OF ACTION: Thiazide diuretic; affects renal tubular mechanism of electrolyte reabsorption, increasing excretion of Na^+ and Cl^-.

PHARMACOKINETICS: Distribution: Crosses placenta; found in breast milk. **Elimination:** Kidneys (61%); $T_{1/2}$=5.6-14.8 hrs.

NURSING CONSIDERATIONS

Assessment: Assess for anuria, SLE, DM, sulfonamide hypersensitivity, history of allergy or bronchial asthma, possible drug interactions, hepatic/renal impairment.

Monitoring: Monitor serum electrolytes periodically. Monitor for signs/symptoms of electrolyte imbalance, exacerbation or activation of SLE, hyperglycemia, hyperuricemia or precipitation of gout, hypersensitivity reactions, renal/hepatic dysfunction.

Patient Counseling: Advise to seek medical attention if symptoms of electrolyte imbalance (dry mouth, thirst, weakness) or hypersensitivity reactions occur.

Administration: Oral route. **Storage:** 20-25°C (68-77°F).

HYDROXYZINE HCL — RX

hydroxyzine HCl (Various)

THERAPEUTIC CLASS: Piperazine antihistamine

INDICATIONS: (PO) Relief of anxiety associated with psychoneurosis and as adjunct in organic disease states with anxiety. As a sedative when used as premedication and following general anesthesia. Management of allergic pruritus. (Inj) Management of anxiety, tension, and psychomotor agitation in conditions of emotional stress. As pre-/postoperative and pre-/postpartum adjunctive medication to permit reduction in narcotic dosage, allay anxiety, and control emesis. To control nausea and vomiting, excluding pregnancy.

DOSAGE: *Adults:* PO: Anxiety: 50-100mg qid. Pruritus: 25mg tid-qid. Sedation: 50-100mg. IM: Nausea/Vomiting: 25-100mg. Pre-/Postoperative and Pre-/Postpartum Adjunct: 25-100mg. Psychiatric/Emotional Emergencies: 50-100mg q4-6h prn.
Pediatrics: PO: Anxiety/Pruritus: <6 yrs: 50mg/day in divided doses. ≥6 yrs:

50-100mg in divided doses. Sedation: 0.6mg/kg. IM: Nausea/Vomiting: 0.5mg/lb. Pre-/Postoperative Adjunct: 0.5mg/lb.

HOW SUPPLIED: Inj: 25mg/mL, 50mg/mL; Syrup: 10mg/5mL; Tab: 10mg, 25mg, 50mg, 100mg

CONTRAINDICATIONS: Early pregnancy. Injection is intended only for IM administration and should not, under any circumstances, be injected subcutaneously, intra-arterially, or IV.

WARNINGS/PRECAUTIONS: Caution in elderly. May impair mental/physical abilities. Effectiveness as an antianxiety agent for long term use (>4 months) has not been established.

ADVERSE REACTIONS: Dry mouth, drowsiness, involuntary motor activity.

INTERACTIONS: Potentiates CNS depression with other CNS depressants (eg, narcotics, non-narcotic analgesics, barbiturates, alcohol). May increase alcohol effects.

PREGNANCY: Not for use in pregnancy or nursing.

H

MECHANISM OF ACTION: Believed to suppress activity in key regions of subcortical area of CNS; shown to have primary skeletal muscle relaxation, bronchodilator, antihistaminic, and analgesic effects.

PHARMACOKINETICS: Absorption: Rapid (GIT).

NURSING CONSIDERATIONS

Assessment: Assess pregnancy/nursing status and possible drug interactions. Obtain baseline renal function.

Monitoring: Monitor for hypersensitivity reactions and renal dysfunction.

Patient Counseling: Caution may impair physical/mental abilities. Advise to avoid alcohol and other CNS depressants.

Administration: Oral route. **Storage:** 20-25°C (68-77°F). Dispense in a tight container.

Hydroxyzine Pamoate RX

hydroxyzine pamoate (Various)

OTHER BRAND NAMES: Vistaril (Pfizer)

THERAPEUTIC CLASS: Piperazine antihistamine

INDICATIONS: Relief of anxiety. Allergic pruritus. For sedation as premedication and following anesthesia.

DOSAGE: *Adults:* Anxiety: 50-100mg qid. Pruritus: 25mg tid-qid. Sedation: 50-100mg.
Pediatrics: Anxiety/Pruritus: >6 yrs: 50-100mg/day in divided doses. <6 yrs: 50mg/day in divided doses. Sedation: 0.6mg/kg.

HOW SUPPLIED: Cap: 25mg, 50mg, 100mg

CONTRAINDICATIONS: Early pregnancy.

WARNINGS/PRECAUTIONS: Caution in elderly. May impair mental/physical abilities. Effectiveness as an antianxiety agent for long-term use (>4 months) has not been established.

ADVERSE REACTIONS: Dry mouth, drowsiness, involuntary motor activity.

INTERACTIONS: Potentiated by CNS depressants (eg, narcotics, non-narcotic analgesics, barbiturates); reduce dose.

PREGNANCY: Safety unknown in pregnancy and is contraindicated in early pregnancy, not for use in nursing.

MECHANISM OF ACTION: Believed to suppress activity in key regions of subcortical area of CNS; shown to have primary skeletal muscle relaxation, bronchodilator, antihistaminic, and analgesic effects.

PHARMACOKINETICS: Absorption: Rapid.

NURSING CONSIDERATIONS

Assessment: Assess for pregnancy/nursing status and possible drug interactions. Obtain baseline renal function.

Monitoring: Monitor for hypersensitivity reactions and renal dysfunction.

Patient Counseling: Caution may impair physical/mental abilities. Advise to avoid alcohol and other CNS depressants; seek medical attention if hypersensitivity reactions occur.

Administration: Oral route. **Storage:** Cap: Below 30°C (86°F). Susp: Shake vigorously until resuspended.

HYOSCYAMINE SULFATE RX

hyoscyamine sulfate (Various)

THERAPEUTIC CLASS: Anticholinergic

INDICATIONS: Adjunct treatment of peptic ulcer, irritable bowel syndrome, neurogenic bladder, and neurogenic bowel disturbances. To reduce symptoms of functional intestinal disorders (eg, mild dysenteries, diverticulitis). To control gastric secretion, visceral spasm, and hypermotility in spastic colitis, spastic bladder, cystitis, pylorospasm, and associated abdominal cramps. Symptomatic relief of biliary and renal colic with concomitant morphine or other narcotics. "Drying agent" for symptomatic relief of acute rhinitis. To reduce rigidity and tremors of Parkinson's disease and control associated sialorrhea and hyperhidrosis. For anticholinesterase poisoning.

DOSAGE: *Adults:* 0.125-0.25mg q4h or prn. Max: 1.5mg/24hrs. Take with or without water.
Pediatrics: ≥12 yrs: 0.125-0.25mg q4h or prn. Max: 1.5mg/24hrs. 2 to <12 yrs: 0.0625-0.125mg q4h or prn. Max: 0.75mg/24hrs. Take with or without water.

HOW SUPPLIED: Tab, Disintegrating: 0.125mg

CONTRAINDICATIONS: Glaucoma, obstructive uropathy, GI tract obstruction, paralytic ileus; intestinal atony of elderly/debilitated, unstable cardiovascular status in acute hemorrhage, toxic megacolon complicating ulcerative colitis, myasthenia gravis.

WARNINGS/PRECAUTIONS: Risk of heat prostration with high environmental temperature. Avoid activities requiring mental alertness. Psychosis has been reported in sensitive patients. Caution with diarrhea, autonomic neuropathy, hyperthyroidism, coronary heart disease, CHF, arrhythmias/tachycardia, HTN, renal disease, and hiatal hernia associated with reflux esophagitis. Contains phenylalanine.

ADVERSE REACTIONS: Anticholinergic effects, drowsiness, headache, nervousness.

INTERACTIONS: Additive effects with other antimuscarinics, amantadine, haloperidol, phenothiazines, MAOIs, TCAs, and some antihistamines. Antacids interfere with absorption; take ac and antacids pc.

PREGNANCY: Category C, caution in nursing.

MECHANISM OF ACTION: Belladonna alkaloid; inhibits action of acetylcholine on structures innervated by postganglionic cholinergic nerves and on smooth muscle that respond to acetylcholine but lack cholinergic innervation, inhibiting GI propulsive motility, decreasing gastric acid secretion, and controlling excess pharyngeal, tracheal, and bronchial secretions.

PHARMACOKINETICS: Absorption: Complete. **Distribution:** Crosses placenta and BBB. **Metabolism:** Partial hydrolysis; tropic acid, tropine (metabolites). **Elimination:** Urine (primarily unchanged); $T_{1/2}$=2-3.5 hrs.

NURSING CONSIDERATIONS

Assessment: Assess for possible drug interactions, bladder neck obstruction, prostatic hypertrophy, achalasia, pyloroduodenal stenosis, paralytic ileus, intestinal atony, CV status, UC, myasthenia gravis, autonomic neuropathy, hyperthyroidism, CAD, CHF, PKU, HTN, arrhythmias, renal disease, hiatal hernia, and glaucoma.

Monitoring: Monitor for signs/symptoms of heat prostration, incomplete intestinal obstruction, psychosis, and hypersensitivity reactions.

Patient Counseling: Caution may impair physical/mental abilities; hot environments may cause heat prostration (fever and heat stroke) due to decreased sweating. If on antacids, take drug before meals and antacids after meals. Seek medical attention if symptoms of incomplete intestinal obstruction (diarrhea), psychosis (confusion, disorientation, memory loss), or hypersensitivity reactions occur. Inform phenylketonurics that orally disintegrating tablets contain 0.5mg of phenylalanine/tablet.

Administration: Oral route. **Storage:** 25°C (77°F); excursions permitted to 15-30°C (59-86°F). Protect from moisture.

HYTRIN — RX

terazosin HCl (Abbott)

H

THERAPEUTIC CLASS: Alpha$_1$-blocker (quinazoline)

INDICATIONS: Treatment of hypertension. Treatment of symptomatic benign prostatic hyperplasia.

DOSAGE: *Adults:* HTN: Initial: 1mg hs, then slowly increase dose. Usual: 1-5mg/day. Max: 20mg/day. If response is substantially diminished at 24 hrs, may increase dose or give in 2 divided doses. BPH: Initial: 1mg qhs. Titrate: Increase stepwise as needed. Usual: 10mg/day. May increase to 20mg/day after 4-6 weeks. Max: 20mg/day. If discontinued for several days, restart at initial dose.

HOW SUPPLIED: Cap: 1mg, 2mg, 5mg, 10mg

WARNINGS/PRECAUTIONS: Monitor for orthostatic hypotension and syncope initially and with dose increase. Rule out prostate cancer. Priapism (rare) reported. Possibility of hemodilution.

ADVERSE REACTIONS: Asthenia, postural hypotension, headache, dizziness, dyspnea, nasal congestion/rhinitis, somnolence, impotence, blurred vision, palpitations, nausea, peripheral edema, priapism, thrombocytopenia, atrial fibrillation.

INTERACTIONS: Increased levels with verapamil. Possibility of significant hypotension with other antihypertensives; may need dose reduction or retitration of either agent.

PREGNANCY: Category C, caution with nursing.

MECHANISM OF ACTION: α-1 adrenoceptor blocker; (BPH) blocks receptors in bladder neck and prostate, relaxing smooth muscle; (HTN) blocks receptors decreasing total peripheral vascular resistance, causing decreased BP.

PHARMACOKINETICS: Absorption: Complete; T_{max}=1 hr. **Elimination:** Feces (20%), urine (10%); $T_{1/2}$=12 hrs.

NURSING CONSIDERATIONS

Assessment: Assess for possible drug interactions. Rule out prostate cancer.

Monitoring: Monitor BP periodically. Monitor for signs/symptoms of hypotension, priapism.

Patient Counseling: Inform of possibility of syncopal and orthostatic symptoms, especially at initiation of therapy. Avoid driving or hazardous tasks for 24 hrs after first dose, dosage increase, or when resuming therapy after interruption. Avoid situations where injury could result should syncope occur. Advise to sit or lie down when symptoms of low BP occur. Inform possibility of priapism; advise to seek medical attention if it occurs.

Administration: Oral route. **Storage:** Below 30°C (86°F).

HYZAAR RX

losartan potassium - hydrochlorothiazide (Merck)

Can cause death/injury to developing fetus during 2nd and 3rd trimesters. D/C if pregnancy detected.

THERAPEUTIC CLASS: Angiotensin II receptor antagonist/thiazide diuretic

INDICATIONS: Treatment of hypertension. Initial treatment of severe hypertension only when the value of achieving prompt BP control exceeds the risk. To reduce risk of stroke in patients with hypertension and left ventricular hypertrophy (may not apply to African-American patients).

DOSAGE: *Adults:* HTN: If BP uncontrolled on losartan monotherapy, HCTZ alone or controlled with HCTZ 25mg/day but hypokalemic: 50mg-12.5mg tab qd. Titrate/Max: If uncontrolled after 3 weeks, increase to 2 tabs of 50mg-12.5mg qd or 1 tab of 100mg-25mg qd. If uncontrolled on losartan 100mg monotherapy, may switch to 100mg-12.5mg qd. Severe HTN: Initial: 50mg-12.5mg qd. Titrate/Max: If inadequate response after 2-4 weeks, increase to 1 tab of 100mg-25mg qd. HTN With Left Ventricular Hypertrophy: Initial: Losartan 50mg qd. If BP reduction inadequate, add HCTZ 12.5mg or substitute losartan/HCTZ 50mg-12.5mg. If additional BP reduction is needed, losartan 100mg and HCTZ 12.5mg or losartan/HCTZ 100mg-12.5mg may be substituted, followed by losartan 100mg and HCTZ 25mg or losartan/HCTZ 100mg-25mg.

HOW SUPPLIED: Tab: (Losartan-HCTZ) 50mg-12.5mg, 100mg-12.5mg, 100mg-25mg

CONTRAINDICATIONS: Anuria, sulfonamide hypersensitivity.

WARNINGS/PRECAUTIONS: Can cause fetal injury/death. Correct volume or salt depletion before therapy. Caution with hepatic or renal dysfunction, renal artery stenosis, severe CHF, history of allergies, asthma. May exacerbate or activate SLE. Monitor serum electrolytes. Avoid if CrCl ≤30mL/min. Observe for signs of fluid or electrolyte imbalance. May precipitate hyperuricemia or gout. Enhanced effects in post-sympathectomy patient. May increase cholesterol, TG levels. Angioedema reported. Not recommended with hepatic dysfunction requiring losartan titration.

ADVERSE REACTIONS: Dizziness, upper respiratory infection, back pain, cough.

INTERACTIONS: Decreased levels with rifampin. Increased levels with fluconazole. Avoid K^+-sparing diuretics (eg, spironolactone, triamterene, amiloride), K^+ supplements, K^+-containing salt substitutes. Potentiates orthostatic hypotension with alcohol, barbiturates, narcotics. Adjust insulin, antidiabetic drugs. Cholestyramine, colestipol impair absorption. Corticosteroids, ACTH deplete electrolytes. May decrease response to pressor amines (eg, norepinephrine). Potentiates other antihypertensives, skeletal muscle relaxants (eg, tubocurarine). Risk of lithium toxicity. NSAIDs, including COX-2 inhibitors, may decrease effects and may result in a further deterioration of renal function in the renally impaired.

PREGNANCY: Category C (1st trimester) and D (2nd and 3rd trimesters), not for use in nursing.

MECHANISM OF ACTION: Losartan: Angiotensin II receptor antagonist; blocks vasoconstrictor and aldosterone-secreting effects of angiotensin II by selectively blocking binding of angiotensin II to AT_1 receptor. HCTZ: Thiazide diuretic; affects renal tubular mechanism of electrolyte reabsorption, directly increasing excretion of Na^+ and Cl^- and indirectly reducing plasma volume.

PHARMACOKINETICS: Absorption: Losartan: Well absorbed, bioavailability (33%); T_{max}=1 hr, 3-4 hrs (active metabolite). **Distribution:** Losartan: V_d=34L,12L (active metabolite). HCTZ: Crosses placenta; found in breast milk. **Metabolism:** Losartan: CYP2C9, 3A4 (biotransformation), Carboxylic acid (active metabolite). **Elimination:** Losartan, metabolite: Urine (4%, 6%), $T_{1/2}$=2 hrs, 6-9 hrs. HCTZ: Kidney (61%), $T_{1/2}$=5.6-14.8 hrs.

NURSING CONSIDERATIONS

Assessment: Assess for pregnancy status, possible drug interactions, volume/salt depletion, SLE, DM, anuria, sulfonamide hypersensitivity, history of allergy or bronchial asthma, hepatic/renal impairment.

Monitoring: Monitor serum electrolytes and renal function periodically. Monitor for signs/symptoms of electrolyte imbalance, exacerbation or activation of SLE, hypotension, hyperglycemia, hyperuricemia or precipitation of gout, hypersensitivity reactions, hepatic/renal dysfunction.

Patient Counseling: Inform of pregnancy risks. Advise that inadequate fluid intake or loss of fluids may result in drop of BP, leading to lightheadedness or syncope. Instruct not to use K^+ supplements or salt substitutes without consulting physician. Advise to seek medical attention if syncope, symptoms of electrolyte imbalance (dry mouth, thirst, weakness, lethargy), or hypersensitivity reactions occur.

Administration: Oral route. **Storage:** 25°C (77°F); excursions permitted to 15-30°C (59-86°F). Keep tightly closed and protect from light.

I

IFEX — RX

ifosfamide (Bristol-Myers Squibb)

Risk of urotoxic side effects, especially hemorrhagic cystitis, and CNS toxicities (eg, confusion, coma); may require discontinuation of therapy. Severe myelosuppression reported. Administer only under supervision of a physician experienced in the use of antineoplastic agents.

OTHER BRAND NAMES: Ifex/Mesnex (Bristol-Myers Squibb)

THERAPEUTIC CLASS: Cyclophosphamide analog

INDICATIONS: Third line chemotherapy of germ cell testicular cancer. Use in combination with prophylactic agent for hemorrhagic cystitis (eg, mesna).

DOSAGE: *Adults:* 1.2g/m²/day slow IV infusion over a minimum of 30 min for 5 consecutive days. Repeat treatment every 3 weeks or after recovery from hematologic toxicity (platelets ≥100,000/µL, WBC ≥4000/µL). Give with extensive hydration (eg, 2L fluid/day) and protector (eg, mesna) to prevent bladder toxicity/hemorrhagic cystitis.

HOW SUPPLIED: Inj (Ifosfamide): 1g, 3g; (Ifosfamide-Mesna) 1g-1g; 3g-1g

CONTRAINDICATIONS: Severely depressed bone marrow function.

WARNINGS/PRECAUTIONS: Hemorrhagic cystitis reported; obtain urinalysis before each dose. Withhold dose until complete resolution of microscopic hematuria. Monitor WBCs, platelets, Hgb before each dose and at appropriate intervals. Avoid with WBC <2000/µL and/or platelets <50,000/µL. D/C if somnolence, confusion, hallucinations, and/or coma occur. Caution with impaired renal function, compromised bone marrow reserve, prior radiation therapy. May interfere with normal wound healing.

ADVERSE REACTIONS: Myelosuppression, alopecia, NV, hematuria, CNS toxicity, infection, renal impairment, liver dysfunction, increased liver enzymes/bilirubin.

INTERACTIONS: Severe myelosuppression with other chemotherapeutic agents. Caution with other cytotoxic agents.

PREGNANCY: Category D, not for use in nursing.

MECHANISM OF ACTION: Chemotherapeutic agent; requires metabolic activation by microsomal liver enzymes and produces active metabolites that interact with DNA.

PHARMACOKINETICS: Metabolism: Extensive; 4-carboxyifosfamide, thiodiacetic acid, cysteine conjugates of chloroacetic acid (major metabolites). **Elimination:** (3.8-5g/m²): Urine (61%), $T_{1/2}$=15 hrs. (1.6-2.4g/m²/day): Urine (12-18%), $T_{1/2}$=7 hrs.

NURSING CONSIDERATIONS

Assessment: Assess for severely depressed bone marrow function, leukopenia, granulocytopenia, extensive bone marrow metastases, prior radiation or cytotoxic agent therapy, renal dysfunction, and possible drug interactions. Obtain baseline WBC, platelet count, Hgb, and urinalysis.

Monitoring: Monitor WBC, platelet count, Hgb, and urinalysis prior to each dose and periodically throughout. Monitor for signs/symptoms of hemorrhagic cystitis, confusion, coma, severe myelosuppression, renal dysfunction, and hypersensitivity reaction.

Patient Counseling: Educate that alopecia may occur. Advise to keep well hydrated and to seek medical attention if symptoms of hemorrhagic cystitis, confusion, coma, severe myelosuppression, renal dysfunction, or hypersensitivity reaction occur.

Administration: IV infusion. **Storage:** 20-25°C (68-77°F). Protect from temperatures above 30°C (86°F). (Constituted/Diluted): Refrigerate; stable for 24 hrs.

IMDUR

isosorbide mononitrate (Schering) **RX**

THERAPEUTIC CLASS: Nitrate vasodilator

INDICATIONS: Prevention of angina pectoris. Not for acute attack.

DOSAGE: *Adults:* Initial: 30-60mg qd in am. Titrate: May increase after several days to 120mg/day. Swallow whole with fluids. Elderly: Start at lower end of dosing range.

HOW SUPPLIED: Tab, Extended-Release: 30mg*, 60mg*, 120mg *scored

WARNINGS/PRECAUTIONS: Not for use with acute MI or CHF. Severe hypotension may occur; caution with volume depletion and hypotension. Hypotension may increase angina pectoris. May aggravate angina caused by hypertrophic cardiomyopathy. Monitor for tolerance. May interfere with cholesterol test.

ADVERSE REACTIONS: Headache, dizziness, hypotension.

INTERACTIONS: Severe hypotension with sildenafil. Orthostatic hypotension with CCBs. Additive vasodilation with other vasodilators (eg, alcohol).

PREGNANCY: Category B, caution with nursing.

MECHANISM OF ACTION: Nitrate vasodilator; relaxes vascular smooth muscle, and consequent dilatation of peripheral arteries and veins, especially the latter. Dilatation of veins leads to reducing the left ventricular end diastolic pressure and pulmonary capillary wedge pressure (preload). Arteriolar relaxation reduces systemic vascular resistance, systolic arterial pressure, and mean arterial pressure (afterload). It also dilates the coronary artery.

PHARMACOKINETICS: Absorption: Imdur: (60mg) C_{max}=557-572ng/mL, T_{max}=2.9-4.2 hrs, AUC=6625-7555ng•hr/mL. (120mg) C_{max}=1151-1180ng/mL, T_{max}=3.1-3.2 hrs, AUC=14241-16800ng•hr/mL. Absolute bioavailability (100%). **Distribution:** V_d=0.6-0.7L/kg; plasma protein binding (5%). **Metabolism:** Liver. Cleared through denitration and glucuronidation pathways. **Elimination:** Urine (96%), feces (1%). (60mg) $T_{1/2}$=6.2-6.3 hrs. (120mg) $T_{1/2}$=6.2-6.4 hrs.

NURSING CONSIDERATIONS

Assessment: Assess for severe hypotension, volume-depleted patients, angina caused by hypertrophic cardiomyopathy, pregnancy status, alcohol intake, and possible drug interactions.

Monitoring: Careful clinical or hemodynamic monitoring for hypotension and tachycardia. Monitor for paradoxical bradycardia and increased angina pectoris, headaches and lightheadedness on standing, manifestation of true physical dependence (chest pain, acute MI). Monitor for the interference with Zlatkis-Zak color reaction, causing false low readings in cholesterol levels and for manifestations of methemoglobinemia.

Patient Counseling: Counsel to carefully follow dosing regimen. Inform about headaches (markers of drug activity) and lightheadedness on standing. Avoid alcohol consumption.

Administration: Oral route. Swallow tab with glass of water; do not crush or chew. **Storage:** 25°C (77°F); excursions permitted to 15-30°C (59-86°F).

IMITREX RX

sumatriptan (GlaxoSmithKline)

THERAPEUTIC CLASS: 5-HT_1-agonist

INDICATIONS: (Inj, Spray, Tab) Acute treatment of migraine with or without aura. (Inj) Acute treatment of cluster headaches.

DOSAGE: *Adults:* ≥18 yrs: (Inj) Initial: 6mg SQ; may repeat after 1 hr. Max: 12mg/24 hrs. (Spray) 5mg, 10mg, or 20mg single dose; may repeat after 2 hrs. Max: 40mg/24 hrs. (Tab) Initial: 25-100mg; may repeat after 2 hrs. Max: 200mg/24 hrs. May give up to 100mg/day of tabs after initial inj dose. Hepatic Disease: Max: 50mg/single dose. Safety of treating >4 headaches/30 days not known.

HOW SUPPLIED: Inj: 6mg/0.5mL; Nasal Spray: 5mg, 20mg [0.1mL 6[s]]; Tab: 25mg, 50mg, 100mg [9[s]]

CONTRAINDICATIONS: History, symptoms, or signs of ischemic cardiac, cerebrovascular, or peripheral vascular syndromes. Other significant CVD, uncontrolled HTN, hemiplegic or basilar migraine, severe hepatic impairment, MAOIs during or within 2 weeks of use, within 24 hrs of ergotamine-containing agents, ergot-type agents, or other 5-HT_1 agonists.

WARNINGS/PRECAUTIONS: Confirm diagnosis. Supervise first dose and monitor cardiac function in those at risk of CAD (eg, HTN, hypercholesterolemia, smoker, obesity, diabetes, CAD family history, postmenopausal women, males >40 yrs). Monitor cardiac function in intermittent long-term users with CAD risk factors. Serious adverse cardiac events, cerebrovascular events, vasospastic reactions reported. Serotonin syndrome may occur; symptoms may include mental status changes, autonomic instability, neuromuscular aberrations, and GI symptoms. Avoid in elderly. Caution with hepatic or renal impairment, history of seizures or brain lesions. Possible long-term ophthalmic effects. Reconsider diagnosis before 2nd dose.

ADVERSE REACTIONS: Tingling, burning sensation, flushing, chest/mouth/tongue discomfort, injection site reaction, numbness, weakness, neck pain/stiffness.

INTERACTIONS: Prolonged vasospastic reactions with ergot-containing drugs; avoid use within 24 hrs. Serotonin syndrome reported with combined use of an SSRI or SNRI. Avoid MAOIs and other 5-HT_1 agonists.

PREGNANCY: Category C, caution in nursing.

MECHANISM OF ACTION: Selective 5-HT_1 receptor subtype agonist; activates vascular 5-HT_1 receptors, which are located on cranial arteries, on the basilar artery, and in the vasculature of human dura matter. Responsible for mediating vasoconstriction.

PHARMACOKINETICS: Absorption: (Intranasal, 5mg) C_{max}=5ng/mL; (Intranasal, 20mg) C_{max}= 16ng/mL; (SQ, 6mg) C_{max}=74ng/mL, T_{max}=12 min; (PO, 25mg) C_{max}=18ng/mL; (PO, 100mg) C_{max}=51ng/mL. **Distribution:** (PO) V_d=2.4L/kg, (SQ) V_d=2.7L/kg; plasma protein binding (14-21%); found in breast milk following SQ administration. **Metabolism:** Via monoamine oxidase. **Elimination:** (SQ) Urine (22% unchanged and 38% as metabolites), $T_{1/2}$=115 min; (Nasal Spray) Urine (3% unchanged and 42% as metabolites), $T_{1/2}$=2 hrs. (Oral) Urine (60%), feces (40%), $T_{1/2}$=2.5 hrs.

NURSING CONSIDERATIONS

Assessment: Assess for presence/history of cardiac ischemic syndrome, cerebrovascular syndrome, or peripheral vascular syndrome, uncontrolled HTN, presence of hemiplegic or basilar migraines, hepatic or renal impairment, history of epilepsy, pregnancy/nursing status, and possible drug interactions. Assess proper diagnosis of migraine headaches.

Monitoring: Monitor for signs/symptoms of cardiac events (eg, MI, cardiac rhythm disturbances, peripheral vascular ischemia, hypertensive crisis, chest tightness), colonic ischemia, bloody diarrhea, serotonin syndrome (eg, mental status changes), hypersensitivity reactions, jaw/neck tightness, seizures, exacerbation of headache, ophthalmic changes (eg, corneal opacities), and clinical response. In patients on long-term therapy and in patients with CAD risk factors, perform periodic monitoring of cardiovascular function. If clinical response does not occur following administration of first dose, reassess diagnosis.

Patient Counseling: Inform about possible adverse events (eg, cardiovascular effects, serotonin syndrome); consult physician if symptoms (eg, chest tightness, abdominal pain, SOB, confusion, hallucinations, flushing) occur.

Administration: Oral, SQ, or nasal route. **Storage:** Injection: 2-30°C (36-86°F). Protect from light. Tab, Nasal Spray: 2-30°C (36-86°F).

IMURAN — RX

azathioprine (Prometheus)

Increased risk of neoplasia with chronic therapy. Mutagenic potential and possible hematologic toxicities.

THERAPEUTIC CLASS: Purine antagonist antimetabolite

INDICATIONS: Adjunct therapy for prevention of rejection in renal homotransplantation. Management of active rheumatoid arthritis (RA) to reduce signs and symptoms.

DOSAGE: *Adults:* Renal Homotransplantation: Initial: 3-5mg/kg/day, start at time of transplant. Maint: 1-3mg/kg/day. Rheumatoid Arthritis: Initial: 1mg/kg/day given qd-bid. Titrate: Increase by 0.5mg/kg/day after 6-8 weeks, then at 4-week intervals. Max: 2.5mg/kg/day. Maint: Lowest effective dose. Decrease by 0.5mg/kg/day or 25mg/day every 4 weeks. If no response by Week 12, then consider refractory. Renal Dysfunction: Lower dose.

HOW SUPPLIED: Tab: 50mg* *scored

CONTRAINDICATIONS: Pregnancy in RA treatment. Previous treatment of RA with alkylating agents (eg, cyclophosphamide, chlorambucil, melphalan) may increase risk of neoplasia.

WARNINGS/PRECAUTIONS: Dose-related leukopenia, thrombocytopenia, macrocytic anemia, pancytopenia, and severe bone marrow suppression may occur. Monitor CBCs, including platelets, weekly during the 1st month, twice monthly for the 2nd and 3rd months, then monthly or more frequently if dose/therapy changes. Monitor for infections. Gastrointestinal hypersensitivity reactions (severe nausea and vomiting) associated with diarrhea, rash, fever, malaise, myalgias, elevated livers enzymes, and hypotension may develop.

ADVERSE REACTIONS: Leukopenia, thrombocytopenia, infections, N/V, hepatotoxicity.

INTERACTIONS: Caution with concomitant aminosalicylates (eg, sulphasalazine, mesalazine, olsalazine); may inhibit TPMT. Reduce dose to approximately 1/3-1/4 of the usual dose with allopurinol. Drugs affecting leukocyte production (eg, co-trimoxazole) may exaggerate leukopenia. ACE inhibitors may induce anemia, leukopenia. Inhibits anticoagulant effects of warfarin.

PREGNANCY: Category D, not for use in nursing.

MECHANISM OF ACTION: Immunosuppressive antimetabolite; an imidazolyl derivative of 6-mercaptopurine (6-MP). In homograft survival, it suppresses hypersensitivities of the cell-mediated type and causes variable alterations in antibody production. Immunoinflammatory response mechanisms not established; suppresses disease manifestation and underlying pathology in autoimmune disease.

PHARMACOKINETICS: Absorption: (PO) Well absorbed; T_{max}=1-2 hrs. **Distribution:** Plasma protein binding (30%); crosses placenta; found in breast milk. **Metabolism:** Liver and erythrocytes (extensive); 6-MP activated to 6-thioguanine nucleotides (major metabolites); inactivated via thiol methylation by thiopurine S-methyltransferase (TPMT) and oxidation by xanthine oxidase. **Elimination:** Urine; $T_{1/2}$=5 hrs.

NURSING CONSIDERATIONS

Assessment: Assess renal/hepatic dysfunction, previous treatment of rheumatoid arthritis with alkylating agents, pregnancy/nursing status, and for possible drug interactions. Conduct TPMT genotyping/phenotyping to identify absent or reduced enzymatic activity; risk of myelotoxicity with reduced activity.

Monitoring: Monitor CBC, including platelet/leukocyte counts, signs of bone marrow suppression, malignancy/neoplasia of skin, reticulum cell and lymphoma, serious infections (eg, fungal, viral, bacterial, protozoal), GI events (eg, NV, diarrhea), rash, fever, elevation of liver enzymes, and hypotension.

Patient Counseling: Inform about necessity of periodic CBC while on therapy, and to report any unusual bleeding or bruising or signs of infections. Inform about risk of malignancy. Educate about careful dosage instructions, especially with impaired renal function or concomitant use with allopurinol. Advise not to take during pregnancy/nursing.

Administration: IV and oral routes. **Storage:** 15-25°C (59-77°F).

INDAPAMIDE RX

indapamide (Various)

THERAPEUTIC CLASS: Indoline diuretic

INDICATIONS: Treatment of hypertension and salt/fluid retention associated with congestive heart failure.

DOSAGE: *Adults:* HTN: 1.25mg qam. Titrate: May increase to 2.5mg qd after 4 weeks, then to 5mg qd after another 4 weeks. Max: 5mg/day. CHF: 2.5mg qam. Titrate: May increase to 5mg qd after 1 week. Max: 5mg/day.

HOW SUPPLIED: Tab: 1.25mg, 2.5mg

CONTRAINDICATIONS: Anuria, sulfonamide hypersensitivity.

WARNINGS/PRECAUTIONS: Caution in severe renal disease, liver dysfunction. May exacerbate or activate SLE. Monitor for fluid/electrolyte imbalance. Hyperuricemia, hypercalcemia, hypokalemia, hypophosphatemia, and hyperglycemia may occur. Monitor renal function, serum uric acid levels periodically. May precipitate gout. May manifest latent DM. Enhanced effects in post-sympathectomy patient.

ADVERSE REACTIONS: Headache, infection, pain, back pain, dizziness, rhinitis, fatigue, muscle cramps, nervousness, numbness of extremities, electrolyte imbalance, anxiety, agitation.

INTERACTIONS: May decrease arterial responsiveness to norepinephrine. May potentiate other antihypertensives. Risk of lithium toxicity. Increases risk of hypokalemia with ACTH, corticosteroids. Antidiabetic agents may need adjustment.

PREGNANCY: Category B, not for use in nursing.

MECHANISM OF ACTION: Indoline diuretic.

PHARMACOKINETICS: Absorption: (2.5mg) C_{max}=115ng/mL, T_{max}=2 hrs. (5mg) C_{max}=260ng/mL, T_{max}=2 hrs. **Distribution:** Plasma protein binding (71-79%). **Metabolism:** Extensive. **Elimination:** Urine (7%), $T_{1/2}$=14 hrs.

NURSING CONSIDERATIONS

Assessment: Assess for anuria, sulfonamide hypersensitivity, gout, DM, SLE, possible drug interactions, hepatic/renal impairment.

Monitoring: Monitor serum electrolytes, renal function, blood glucose, uric acid, and serum electrolytes routinely and periodically. Monitor for signs/symptoms of electrolyte imbalance, hyperuricemia, activation or exacerbation of SLE, and hypersensitivity reactions.

Patient Counseling: Advise to seek medical attention if symptoms of electrolyte imbalance (dry mouth, thirst, weakness), hyperuricemia, or hypersensitivity reactions occur.

Administration: Oral route. **Storage:** 20-25°C (68-77°F). Avoid excessive heat.

INDERAL
propranolol HCl (Wyeth)

RX

THERAPEUTIC CLASS: Nonselective beta-blocker

INDICATIONS: (Tab) Management of hypertension, angina pectoris, hypertrophic subaortic stenosis. Migraine prophylaxis. (Inj/Tab) For cardiac arrhythmias (supraventricular, ventricular tachycardia, tachyarrhythmia of digitalis intoxication, resistant tachyarrhythmia), reduction of cardiovascular mortality post-MI, essential tremor, and pheochromocytoma.

DOSAGE: *Adults:* HTN: (Tab) Initial: 40mg bid. Titrate: Increase gradually. Maint: 120-240mg/day. Angina: (Tab) 80-320mg/day, given bid-qid. Arrhythmia: (Inj) 1-3mg IV at 1 mg/min. (Tab) 10-30mg tid-qid ac and qhs. MI: (Tab) 180-240mg/day, given bid-tid. Migraine: (Tab) Initial: 80mg/day in divided doses. Usual: 160-240mg/day in divided doses. Tremor: (Tab) Initial: 40mg bid. Maint: 120mg/day. Max: 320mg/day. Hypertrophic Subaortic Stenosis: (Tab) 20-40mg tid-qid, ac and qhs. Pheochromocytoma: (Tab) 60mg/day in divided doses for 3 days before surgery with α-blocker. Inoperable Tumor: (Tab) 30mg/day in divided doses.
Pediatrics: HTN (Tab): Initial: 1mg/kg/day PO. Usual: 1-2mg/kg bid. Max: 16mg/kg/day.

HOW SUPPLIED: Inj: 1mg/mL; Tab: 10mg*, 20mg*, 40mg*, 60mg*, 80mg*
*scored

CONTRAINDICATIONS: Cardiogenic shock, sinus bradycardia and >1st-degree block, bronchial asthma, CHF (unless failure is secondary to tachyarrhythmia treatable with propranolol).

WARNINGS/PRECAUTIONS: Caution with well-compensated cardiac failure, nonallergic bronchospasm, Wolff-Parkinson-White (WPW) syndrome, hepatic or renal dysfunction. Withdrawal before surgery is controversial. May mask hypoglycemia or hyperthyroidism symptoms. Avoid abrupt discontinuation. May reduce IOP. Can cause cardiac failure. Both digitalis glycosides and β-blockers slow atrioventricular conduction and decrease HR. Concomitant use can increase risk of bradycardia.

ADVERSE REACTIONS: Bradycardia, CHF, hypotension, lightheadedness, mental depression, NV, allergic reactions, agranulocytosis.

INTERACTIONS: Increased propranolol levels/toxicity with CYP2D6 inhibitors (eg, amiodarone, cimetidine, fluoxetine, paroxetine, quinidine, ritonavir), CYP1A2 inhibitors (eg, imipramine, cimetidine, ciprofloxacin, fluvoxamine, isoniazid, ritonavir, theophylline, zileuton, zolmitriptan, rizatriptan), and CYP2C19 inhibitors (eg, fluconazole, cimetidine, fluoxetine, fluvoxamine, teniposide, tolbutamide). Decreased blood levels with hepatic enzyme inducers (eg, rifampin, ethanol, phenytoin, phenobarbital, cigarette smoking). Propafenone levels increased with concurrent administration. Lidocaine metabolism is inhibited with coadministration. Increased levels with concurrent nisoldipine and nicardipine. Zolmitriptan and rizatriptan concentrations increased with concurrent administration. Decreased theophylline clearance with concurrent administration. Increased concentrations of diazepam and its metabolites with coadministration. Increased thioridazine plasma concentrations with concurrent administration of doses ≥160mg/day. Increased plasma concentrations with chlorpromazine. Aluminum hydroxide gel may decrease plasma concentrations. Decreased plasma concentrations with coadministration of cholestyramine or colestipol. Concurrent administration increases warfarin levels and PT. Increased risk of bradycardia with concomitant digitalis glycosides.

PREGNANCY: Category C, caution in nursing. Intrauterine growth retardation, small placenta, and congenital abnormalities have been reported in neonates whose mothers received propranolol during pregnancy. Neonates whose mothers received propranolol at parturition have exhibited bradycardia, hypoglycemia, and/or respiratory depression.

MECHANISM OF ACTION: Nonselective β-adrenergic receptor blocker; not established, proposed to decrease cardiac output, inhibit renin release and lessen tonic sympathetic nerve outflow.

PHARMACOKINETICS: Absorption: T_{max}=1-4 hrs. **Distribution:** V_d=4 L/kg; plasma protein binding (90%). Crosses placenta; found in breast milk. **Metabolism:** CYP2D6 (hydroxylation), CYP1A2, 2D6 (oxidation), N-dealkylation, glucuronidation. Propranolol glucuronide, naphthyloxylactic acid, glucuronic acid, sulfate conjugates (major metabolites). **Elimination:** $T_{1/2}$=3-6 hrs.

NURSING CONSIDERATIONS

Assessment: Assess for bronchial asthma, sinus bradycardia, AV heart block, cardiogenic shock, CHF, bronchospastic disease, hyperthyroidism, DM, possible drug interactions, WPW syndrome, history of heart failure, hepatic/renal impairment.

Monitoring: Monitor for signs/symptoms of cardiac failure, hypoglycemia, decreased IOP, thyrotoxicosis, withdrawal symptoms (angina, MI), and hypersensitivity reactions.

Patient Counseling: Instruct not to interrupt or d/c therapy without consulting physician. Inform may interfere with glaucoma screening test. Drug may mask signs of thyrotoxicosis and hypoglycemia. Advise to contact physician if symptoms of heart failure, withdrawal (angina), or hypersensitivity reactions occur.

I

Administration: Oral route. **Storage:** 20-25°C (68-77°F); excursions permitted to 15-30°C (59-86°F).

INDERAL LA — RX

propranolol HCl (Wyeth)

THERAPEUTIC CLASS: Nonselective beta-blocker

INDICATIONS: Management of hypertension, angina pectoris, hypertrophic subaortic stenosis. Migraine prophylaxis.

DOSAGE: *Adults:* HTN: Initial: 80mg qd. Maint: 120-160mg qd. Angina: Initial: 80mg qd. Titrate: Increase gradually every 3-7 days. Maint: 160mg qd. Max: 320mg/day. Migraine: Initial: 80mg qd. Maint: 160-240mg qd. Discontinue gradually if no response within 4-6 weeks. Hypertrophic Subaortic Stenosis: 80-160mg qd.

HOW SUPPLIED: Cap, Extended-Release: 60mg, 80mg, 120mg, 160mg

CONTRAINDICATIONS: Cardiogenic shock, sinus bradycardia and >1st-degree block, bronchial asthma, CHF (unless failure is secondary to tachyarrhythmia treatable with propranolol).

WARNINGS/PRECAUTIONS: Caution with well-compensated cardiac failure, nonallergic bronchospasm, Wolff-Parkinson-White (WPW) syndrome, hepatic or renal dysfunction. Withdrawal before surgery is controversial. May mask hypoglycemia or hyperthyroidism symptoms. Avoid abrupt discontinuation. May reduce IOP. Can cause cardiac failure. Exacerbation of angina, in some cases myocardial reported. D/C if these occurred. Stevens-Johnson syndrome, toxic epidermal necrolysis, exfoliative dermatitis, erythema multiforme, and urticaria reported. Hypoglycemia and postural hypotension reported.

ADVERSE REACTIONS: Bradycardia, CHF, hypotension, lightheadedness, mental depression, NV, allergic reactions, agranulocytosis, dry eyes, alopecia, SLE-like reactions, male impotence, Peyronie's disease.

INTERACTIONS: Increased propranolol levels/toxicity with CYP2D6 inhibitors (eg, amiodarone, cimetidine, fluoxetine, paroxetine, quinidine, ritonavir), CYP1A2 inhibitors (eg, imipramine, cimetidine, ciprofloxacin, fluvoxamine, isoniazid, ritonavir, theophylline, zileuton, zolmitriptan, rizatriptan), and CYP2C19 inhibitors (eg, fluconazole, cimetidine, fluoxetine, fluvoxamine, teniposide, tolbutamide). Decreased blood levels with hepatic enzyme inducers (eg, rifampin, ethanol, phenytoin, phenobarbital, cigarette smoking). Propafenone levels increased with concurrent administration. Lidocaine metabolism is inhibited with coadministration. Increased levels with concurrent nisoldipine and nicardipine. Zolmitriptan and rizatriptan concentrations increased with concurrent administration. Decreased theophylline clearance with concurrent administration. Increased concentrations of diazepam and its metabolites with coadministration. Increased thioridazine plasma concentrations with concurrent administration of doses ≥160mg/day. Increased plasma concentrations with chlorpromazine. Aluminum hydroxide gel may decrease plasma concentrations. Decreased plasma concentrations with coadministration of cholestyramine or colestipol. Concurrent administration increases warfarin levels and PT.

PREGNANCY: Category C, caution in nursing.

MECHANISM OF ACTION: Nonselective β-adrenergic receptor blocker; not fully established. Proposed to decrease cardiac output, inhibit renin release, and lessen tonic sympathetic nerve outflow.

PHARMACOKINETICS: Absorption: T_{max}=6 hrs. **Distribution:** V_d=4L/kg; plasma protein binding (90%); crosses placenta; found in breast milk. **Metabolism:** CYP2D6 (hydroxylation), CYP1A2, 2D6 (oxidation), N-dealkylation, glucuronidation. Propranolol glucuronide, naphthyloxylactic acid, glucuronic acid, sulfate conjugates (major metabolites). **Elimination:** $T_{1/2}$=10 hrs.

NURSING CONSIDERATIONS

Assessment: Assess for sinus bradycardia, AV heart block, cardiogenic shock, overt CHF, bronchial asthma, bronchospastic disease, hyperthyroidism, DM, WPW syndrome, history of heart failure, possible drug interactions, hepatic/renal impairment.

Monitoring: Monitor for signs/symptoms of cardiac failure, hypoglycemia, decreased IOP, thyrotoxicosis, withdrawal symptoms (angina, MI), and hypersensitivity reactions.

Patient Counseling: Instruct not to interrupt or d/c therapy without consulting physician. Inform drug may mask signs of thyrotoxicosis and hypoglycemia. Inform may interfere with glaucoma screening test. Advise to contact physician if symptoms of heart failure, withdrawal (angina), or hypersensitivity reactions occur.

Administration: Oral route. **Storage:** 20-25°C (68-77°F); excursions permitted to 15-30°C (59-86°F). Protect from light, moisture, freezing, and excessive heat.

INDERIDE — RX

propranolol HCl - hydrochlorothiazide (Wyeth)

THERAPEUTIC CLASS: Nonselective beta-blocker/thiazide diuretic

INDICATIONS: Management of hypertension. Not for initial therapy.

DOSAGE: *Adults:* Initial: 80-160mg propranolol/day; 25-50mg HCTZ/day. Max: (propranolol-HCTZ) 160mg-50mg/day. Elderly: Start at low end of dosing range. Do not substitute mg-for-mg of extended-release cap for immediate-release tab plus HCTZ. Dose tab bid and extended-release cap qd.

HOW SUPPLIED: (Propranolol-HCTZ) Tab: (Inderide) 40mg-25mg*, 80mg-25mg* *scored

CONTRAINDICATIONS: Cardiogenic shock, sinus bradycardia and >1st-degree block, bronchial asthma, CHF (unless failure is secondary to tachyarrhythmia treatable with propranolol), anuria, sulfonamide hypersensitivity.

WARNINGS/PRECAUTIONS: Caution with well-compensated cardiac failure, nonallergic bronchospasm, Wolff-Parkinson-White syndrome, hepatic or renal dysfunction. Withdrawal before surgery is controversial. May mask hypoglycemia or hyperthyroidism symptoms. Avoid abrupt discontinuation. May reduce IOP. Can cause cardiac failure, hypokalemia, hyperuricemia, hypercalcemia, hypophosphatemia. May exacerbate or activate SLE. Monitor for fluid/electrolyte imbalance. May manifest latent DM. Enhanced effect in postsympathectomy patient. Concomitant use with alcohol may increase plasma levels of propranolol.

ADVERSE REACTIONS: Bradycardia, CHF, hypotension, lightheadedness, mental depression, N/V, allergic reactions, blood dyscrasias, pancreatitis.

INTERACTIONS: Bradycardia/hypotension with catecholamine-depleting drugs. Potentiated by chlorpromazine, cimetidine. Antagonized by NSAIDs, phenytoin, phenobarbital, rifampin. May increase cardiac effects of CCBs. Reduces clearance of antipyrine, lidocaine, and theophylline. Aluminum hydroxide gel reduces intestinal absorption. Alcohol decreases absorption rate. May block epinephrine, thyroxine effects. Hypotension and cardiac arrest reported with haloperidol. May increase response to tubocurarine. May decrease arterial response to norepinephrine. Insulin dose may need adjustment. Risk of hypokalemia with corticosteroids, ACTH. Alcohol, barbiturates, or narcotics may aggravate orthostatic hypotension. Monitor digoxin. Potentiation with ganglionic or peripheral adrenergic-blockers. Concomitant use with alcohol may increase plasma levels of propranolol.

PREGNANCY: Category C, not for use in nursing. Intrauterine growth retardation, small placenta, and congenital abnormalities have been reported in neonates whose mothers received propranolol during pregnancy. Neonates whose mothers received propranolol at parturition have exhibited bradycardia, hypoglycemia, and/or respiratory depression.

I

MECHANISM OF ACTION: Propranolol: Nonselective β-adrenergic receptor blocker; not established, proposed to decrease cardiac output, inhibit renin release, and lessen tonic sympathetic nerve outflow. HCTZ: Thiazide diuretic; not established, affects renal tubular mechanism of electrolyte reabsorption.

PHARMACOKINETICS: Absorption: Propranolol: T_{max}=1-1.5 hrs. **Metabolism:** Propranolol: Liver. **Elimination:** Propranolol: $T_{1/2}$=4 hrs. HCTZ: Kidney.

NURSING CONSIDERATIONS

Assessment: Assess for sinus bradycardia, AV heart block, cardiogenic shock, overt CHF, bronchospastic disease, hyperthyroidism, WPW syndrome, history of heart failure, SLE, DM, anuria, sulfonamide hypersensitivity, possible drug interactions, history of allergy or bronchial asthma, hepatic/renal impairment.

Monitoring: Monitor serum electrolytes and renal function periodically. Monitor for signs/symptoms of cardiac failure, hypoglycemia, decreased IOP, thyrotoxicosis, withdrawal (angina, MI), electrolyte imbalance, exacerbation or activation of SLE, hyperglycemia, hyperuricemia or precipitation of gout, hypersensitivity reactions, hepatic/renal dysfunction.

Patient Counseling: Instruct not to interrupt or d/c therapy without consulting physician. Inform may mask signs of thyrotoxicosis and hypoglycemia. Inform may interfere with glaucoma screening test. Advise to contact physician if symptoms of heart failure, withdrawal (angina), hypersensitivity reactions, or electrolyte imbalance (dry mouth, thirst, weakness) occur.

Administration: Oral route. **Storage:** 20-25°C (68-77°F); excursions permitted to 15-30°C (59-86°F). Protect from moisture, freezing, and excessive heat.

INDOCIN I.V. RX

indomethacin sodium trihydrate (Ovation)

THERAPEUTIC CLASS: NSAID

INDICATIONS: To close hemodynamically significant patent ductus arteriosus in premature infants weighing between 500-1750g after 48 hrs of ineffective medical management.

DOSAGE: *Pediatrics:* Neonates 500-1750g: Therapy includes 3 doses at 12-24 hr intervals. <48 hrs old: 0.2mg/kg IV followed by 0.1mg/kg IV then 0.1mg/kg IV. 2-7 days old: 0.2mg/kg IV for 3 doses. >7 days old: 0.2mg/kg IV followed by 0.25mg/kg IV then 0.25mg/kg IV. If anuria or marked oliguria (urinary output <0.6mL/kg/hr) occurs at scheduled time of 2nd or 3rd dose, hold doses until renal function normalizes. May repeat course if ductus arteriosus reopens. Surgery may be needed if unresponsive after 2 courses.

HOW SUPPLIED: Inj: 1mg

CONTRAINDICATIONS: Untreated infection, bleeding, thrombocytopenia, coagulation defects, necrotizing enterocolitis, significant renal impairment, congenital heart disease when patency of ductus arteriosus is necessary for pulmonary or systemic blood flow.

WARNINGS/PRECAUTIONS: Risk of minor GI bleeding, intraventricular bleeding. May reduce urine output, CrCl, glomerular filtration rate and may increase SrCr, BUN. May cause renal insufficiency, including acute renal failure; caution with extracellular volume depletion, CHF, sepsis, hepatic dysfunction. Monitor renal function and serum electrolytes. May mask signs of infection. D/C if liver disease develops. Avoid extravascular injection or leakage.

ADVERSE REACTIONS: Intracranial bleeding, GI bleeding, hyponatremia, elevated serum potassium, retrolental fibroplasia.

INTERACTIONS: May prolong half-life of digitalis; monitor ECG and serum digitalis levels. May elevate gentamicin and amikacin levels. May decrease natriuretic effect of furosemide. May reduce renal function; consider reducing dosage of medications that rely on adequate renal function for elimination. Increased risk of renal insufficiency with nephrotoxic drugs. Increased risk of bleeding with anticoagulants.

PREGNANCY: Safety in pregnancy or nursing not known.

MECHANISM OF ACTION: NSAID; not fully established, believed to inhibit prostaglandin synthesis.

PHARMACOKINETICS: Elimination: Renal, biliary; half-life varies with age and weight.

NURSING CONSIDERATIONS

Assessment: Assess for bleeding (active intracranial hemorrhage, GI bleeding), thrombocytopenia, necrotizing enterocolitis, renal impairment, infection, coagulation defects, congenital heart disease (patent ductus arteriosus), and possible drug interactions. Obtain baseline CBC, serum electrolytes, and renal function.

Monitoring: Monitor renal function, serum electrolytes, and CBC periodically. Monitor for signs/symptoms of infection, liver disease, bleeding (intraventricular hemorrhage), renal dysfunction, necrotizing enterocolitis, and hypersensitivity reactions.

Patient Counseling: Advise to seek medical attention if symptoms of infection, liver disease, renal impairment, bleeding, necrotizing enterocolitis, or hypersensitivity reactions occur.

Administration: IV route. **Storage:** Below 30°C (86°F). Protect from light.

INDOMETHACIN — RX

indomethacin (Various)

NSAIDs may cause an increased risk of serious cardiovascular thrombotic events, MI, stroke and serious GI adverse events including bleeding, ulceration, and perforation of the stomach or intestines. Contraindicated for the treatment of perioperative pain in the setting of coronary artery bypass graft (CABG) surgery.

OTHER BRAND NAMES: Indocin (Merck)

THERAPEUTIC CLASS: NSAID

INDICATIONS: Management of moderate to severe rheumatoid arthritis (RA), ankylosing spondylitis, osteoarthritis (OA), acute painful shoulder (bursitis and/or tendinitis) and/or acute gouty arthritis.

DOSAGE: *Adults:* RA/Ankylosing Spondylitis/OA: Initial: 25mg PO bid-tid. Titrate: May increase by 25-50mg/day at weekly intervals. Max: 200mg/day. Bursitis/Tendinitis: 75-150mg/day given tid-qid for 7-14 days. Acute Gouty Arthritis: 50mg PO tid until pain is tolerable, then d/c. Take with food. *Pediatrics:* ≥14 yrs: RA/Ankylosing Spondylitis/OA: Initial: 25mg PO bid-tid. Titrate: May increase by 25-50mg/day at weekly intervals. Max: 200mg/day. Bursitis/Tendinitis: 75-150mg/day given tid-qid for 7-14 days. Acute Gouty Arthritis: 50mg PO tid until pain is tolerable, then d/c. 2-14 yrs (safety and effectiveness not established): Initial: 1-2mg/kg/day in divided doses. Max: 3mg/kg/day or 150-200mg/day. Take with food.

HOW SUPPLIED: Cap: 25mg, 50mg; Sus: 25mg/5mL [237mL]

CONTRAINDICATIONS: ASA or other NSAID allergy that precipitates acute asthmatic attack, urticaria, or rhinitis. Do not give suppositories with history of proctitis or recent rectal bleeding. Treatment of perioperative pain in the setting of CABG surgery.

WARNINGS/PRECAUTIONS: May lead to onset of new HTN or worsening of pre-existing HTN; monitor BP closely. Fluid retention and edema reported; caution with fluid retention or heart failure. Renal papillary necrosis and other renal injury reported after long-term use. Not recommended for use with advanced renal disease; if therapy must be initiated, monitor renal function. Anaphylactoid reactions may occur. May cause serious skin adverse events (eg, exfoliative dermatitis, Stevens-Johnson syndrome, and toxic epidermal necrolysis). Avoid in late pregnancy; may cause premature closure of ductus arteriosis. May cause elevations of LFTs; d/c if liver disease develops or systemic manifestations occur. Caution in elderly. Anemia may occur; with long-term use, monitor Hgb/Hct if signs or symptoms of anemia develop. May inhibit platelet aggregation and prolong bleeding time; monitor with coagulation disorders. Caution with asthma and avoid with ASA-sensitive asthma. Corneal deposits and retinal disturbances reported with prolonged therapy; perform eye exams at periodic intervals during prolonged therapy. May aggravate depression or other psychiatric disturbances, epilepsy, and parkinsonism; use with caution. D/C if severe CNS adverse reactions develop. May impair mental/physical abilities.

ADVERSE REACTIONS: Headache, dizziness, NV, dyspepsia, diarrhea, abdominal pain, constipation, vertigo, somnolence, depression, fatigue.

INTERACTIONS: Avoid salicylates, diflunisal, other NSAIDs, and triamterene. Potassium-sparing diuretics may cause hyperkalemia. Increase toxicity of methotrexate, cyclosporine, lithium, and digoxin. Probenecid increases levels. Caution with antihypertensives and anticoagulants. May decrease effects of diuretics, β-blockers, captopril.

PREGNANCY: Category C, not for use in nursing.

MECHANISM OF ACTION: NSAID; not established; exhibits antipyretic, analgesic, and anti-inflammatory properties. Potent inhibitor of prostaglandin synthesis; decreases prostaglandins in peripheral tissues, suppresses inflammation in RA, and diminishes basal and CO_2-stimulated cerebral blood flow.

PHARMACOKINETICS: Absorption: Readily absorbed. Bioavailability (100%); C_{max}=1-2mcg/mL; T_{max}=2 hrs. **Distribution:** Plasma protein binding (99%); crosses blood-brain barrier and placenta; found in breast milk. **Metabolism:** Desmethyl, desbenzoyl, desmethyldesbenzoyl (metabolites). **Elimination:** Urine (60% as drug/metabolites), feces (33% as drug); $T_{1/2}$=4.5 hrs.

NURSING CONSIDERATIONS

Assessment: Assess for history of asthma, urticaria or allergic-type reaction after previous use of NSAIDs, perioperative pain in setting of CABG surgery, CVD or risk factors for CVD, HTN, fluid retention or HF, hyponatremia, ulcer disease or GI bleeding, coagulation disorders or anticoagulant therapy, renal/hepatic impairment, rhinitis with or without nasal polyps, pregnancy/nursing status, depression or other psychiatric disturbances, epilepsy, parkinsonism, and possible drug interactions.

Monitoring: Monitor BP during initiation of therapy and thereafter. Monitor platelet function, CBCs, LFTs, dexamethasone suppression tests, renal function, and chemistry profile. Monitor signs/symptoms of anaphylactic/anaphylactoid reactions, adverse skin events (eg, exfoliative dermatitis, Stevens-Johnson syndrome, toxic epidermal necrolysis), eosinophilia, rash, corneal deposits and retinal disturbances with periodic ophthalmic exam, CNS effects, aggravation of depression or other psychiatric disturbances, GI bleeding/ulceration and perforation, anemia, CV thrombotic events, MI, stroke, new or worsening HTN, renal toxicity, renal papillary necrosis, other renal injury, and hyperkalemia.

Patient Counseling: Inform about potential serious side effects (eg, CV side effects such as MI or stroke); seek medical attention if signs/symptoms of chest pain, SOB, weakness, slurred speech, skin rash, blisters or fever, GI effects, bleeding, ulceration and perforation, signs of anaphylactic/anaphylactoid reaction, or hepatic toxicity occurs. Caution while performing hazardous tasks (eg, operating machinery/driving). Advise to notify physician if pregnant, nursing, planning to become pregnant, or if weight gain/edema occurs.

Administration: Oral route. **Storage:** 20-25°C (68-77°F); tight, light-resistant container.

INFERGEN RX
interferon alfacon-1 (Valeant)

May cause or aggravate fatal or life-threatening neuropsychiatric, autoimmune, ischemic, and infectious disorders. Monitor closely with periodic clinical and laboratory evaluations.

THERAPEUTIC CLASS: Biological response modifier

INDICATIONS: Treatment of chronic hepatitis C virus (HCV) with compensated liver disease in patients with anti-HCV antibodies and/or presence of HCV RNA.

DOSAGE: *Adults:* ≥18 yrs: 9mcg 3x/week (TIW) SQ for 24 weeks, wait 48 hrs between doses. If No Response or Relapse: 15mcg TIW for up to 48 weeks. Hold dose temporarily in severe adverse effects and reduce to 7.5mcg.

HOW SUPPLIED: Inj: 9mcg/0.3mL, 15mcg/0.5mL

CONTRAINDICATIONS: Decompensated hepatic disease, autoimmune hepatitis.

WARNINGS/PRECAUTIONS: Severe psychiatric adverse events (eg, depression, suicidal ideation, suicide attempt) may occur. Avoid in decompensated hepatic disease. Monitor CBC, platelets, and clinical chemistry tests before therapy and periodically thereafter. D/C if severe decrease in neutrophils or platelets, or serious hypersensitivity reaction occurs. Caution with cardiac disease, history of endocrine disorders, or low peripheral blood cell counts. Decrease/loss of vision and retinopathy reported; perform eye examination at baseline, if any ocular symptoms develop, and periodically with pre-existing disorder. May exacerbate autoimmune disorders. Neutropenia, thrombocytopenia, hypertriglyceridemia, and thyroid disorders reported. Caution in elderly. Pancreatitis, pneumonia, interstitial pneumonitis, colitis reported; d/c when signs and symptoms develop.

ADVERSE REACTIONS: Flu-like symptoms, depression, leukopenia, granulocytopenia, hot flushes, malaise, insomnia, dizziness, headache, myalgia, abdominal pain, NV, diarrhea, anorexia, thrombocytopenia, nervousness.

INTERACTIONS: Caution with agents that cause myelosuppression or are metabolized by CYP450.

PREGNANCY: Category C, caution in nursing.

MECHANISM OF ACTION: Type-I interferon; binds interferon to the cell-surface receptor, leading to the production of several interferon-stimulated gene products.

NURSING CONSIDERATIONS

Assessment: Assess for neuropsychiatric, autoimmune disease (ITP, RA, psoriasis), liver dysfunction (autoimmune hepatitis, decompensation, HBV), renal dysfunction, ophthalmologic disorders, endocrine disorders (thyroidism, DM), history of pulmonary disease, bone marrow suppression, immunocompromised, history of cardiac disease and possible drug interactions. Obtain baseline CBC, ANC, SrCr, LFTs, triglycerides, TFTs, Hgb, Hct, and eye exam.

Monitoring: Periodic monitoring of LFTs, CrCl, CBC, Hgb, platelet count, TFTs (baseline, 2 weeks after, and during therapy). Monitor for signs/symptoms of depression (suicidal ideation), cardiovascular and cerebrovascular events, ophthalmologic toxicity, pancreatitis, colitis, bone marrow toxicities, hyperglycemia, exacerbation of autoimmune disorders, renal impairment, worsening of liver disease/failure, respiratory, and hypersensitivity reactions.

Patient Counseling: Warn not to change brands of interferon or reduce dosage without consulting physician. Seek medical attention for symptoms of depression (suicidal ideation), chest pain, ocular symptoms, pancreatitis, colitis, fever, worsening of liver disease/failure (jaundice), respiratory, hyperglycemia and hypersensitivity reactions.

Administration: SQ route. **Storage:** In refrigerator, 2-8°C (36-46°F). Do not freeze; avoid vigorous shaking and exposure to direct sunlight.

INFUMORPH

CII

morphine sulfate (Baxter)

THERAPEUTIC CLASS: Opioid analgesic

INDICATIONS: Treatment of intractable chronic pain in microinfusion devices.

DOSAGE: *Adults:* Lumbar Intrathecal: Opioid Intolerant: 0.2-1mg/day. Opioid Tolerant: 1-10mg/day. Max: Must be individualized. Caution with >20mg/day. Epidural: Opioid Intolerant: 3.5-7.5mg/day. Opioid tolerant: 4.5-10mg/day. May increase to 20-30mg/day. Max: Must be individualized. Starting dose must be based on in-hospital evaluation of response to serial single-dose intrathecal/epidural bolus injections of regular morphine sulfate.

I

HOW SUPPLIED: Inj: 10mg/mL (200mg), 25mg/mL (500mg)

CONTRAINDICATIONS: For neuraxial analgesia: Infection at injection site, anticoagulants, uncontrolled bleeding diathesis, any therapy or condition that may render intrathecal or epidural administration hazardous.

WARNINGS/PRECAUTIONS: Have resuscitation equipment, oxygen, and antidote (eg, naloxone) available; severe respiratory depression may occur. Use only if less invasive means of controlling pain fail. Not for single-dose IV, IM, or SQ administration. May be habit-forming. Observe patient for 24 hours following test dose, and for 1st several days after catheter implantation. Caution with determining refill frequency. Make sure needle is properly placed in the filling port of device. Myoclonic-like spasm of the lower extremities reported if dose >20mg/day; may need detoxification. Caution with head injury, increased ICP, decreased respiratory reserve, hepatic/renal dysfunction (epidural injection), elderly. Avoid with chronic asthma, upper airway obstruction, other chronic pulmonary disorders. Biliary colic reported. May cause micturition disturbances especially with BPH. Increased risk of orthostatic hypotension with reduced circulating blood volume and impaired myocardial function. Avoid abrupt withdrawal. Risk of withdrawal in patients maintained on parenteral/oral narcotics. Not for routine use in obstetric labor/delivery.

ADVERSE REACTIONS: Respiratory depression, myoclonus convulsions, dysphoric reactions, pruritus, urinary retention, constipation, lumbar puncture-type headache, peripheral edema, orthostatic hypotension.

INTERACTIONS: Depressant effect may be potentiated by CNS depressants (eg, alcohol, sedatives, antihistamines, psychotropics). Increased risk of respiratory depression with neuroleptics. Contraindicated with anticoagulants. Risk of withdrawal with narcotic antagonists. Increased risk of orthostatic hypotension with sympatholytic drugs.

PREGNANCY: Category C, safety in nursing not known.

MECHANISM OF ACTION: Opioid analgesic; analgesic effects are produced via at least 3 areas of the CNS: the periaqueductal-periventricular gray matter, the ventromedial medulla, and the spinal cord. Interacts predominantly with μ-receptors which are found distributed in the brain, spinal cord, and in the trigeminal nerve.

PHARMACOKINETICS: Absorption: (Epidural): Rapid absorption; C_{max}=33-40ng/mL, T_{max}=10-15 min; (Intrathecal): C_{max}≤1-7.8ng/mL, T_{max}=5-10 mins. **Distribution:** Plasma protein binding (36%); Muscle tissue binding (54%). Readily passes into fetal circulation, found in breast milk. (IV):V_d=1.0-4.7L/kg. **Metabolism:** Hepatic glucuronidation. **Elimination:** Kidneys (major), urine (2-12% unchanged), feces (10%); $T_{1/2}$=1.5-4.5 hrs.

NURSING CONSIDERATIONS

Assessment: Assess for acute bronchial asthma, upper airway obstruction, hypotension, infection at injection site, bleeding diathesis, seizure disorder, presence of head injury or increased intracranial pressure, age of patient, hepatic/renal dysfunction, biliary tract disorders or recent biliary surgery, urinary system disorders, impaired myocardial function, hypotension, pregnancy/nursing status, and possible drug interactions.

Monitoring: Monitor for signs/symptoms of respiratory depression and/or respiratory arrest, myoclonic events, seizures, dysphoric reactions, toxic psychoses, biliary colic, urinary retention, drug abuse and dependence. If administered intrathecally or via epidural, closely monitor for 24 hrs for signs/symptoms of respiratory depression.

Patient Counseling: Counsel to notify physician immediately if develop signs/symptoms of respiratory depression. Advise to avoid using other CNS depressants and alcohol during therapy. Medication has potential for abuse and dependence. Avoid abrupt withdrawal of medication; withdrawal symptoms may occur. Instruct that if accidental skin contact occurs, wash affected area with water.

Administration: IV, epidural, or intrathecal route. Proper placement of needle or catheter should be verified before epidural injection. **Storage:** 20-25°C (68-77°F); excursions permitted to 15-30°C (59-86°F). Protect from light. Do not freeze.

I

INNOHEP — RX

tinzaparin sodium (Pharmion)

Risk of paralysis by spinal/epidural hematoma with neuraxial anesthesia or spinal puncture. Increased risk with indwelling epidural catheters for analgesia, drugs affecting hemostasis (eg, NSAIDs, platelet inhibitors, anticoagulants), and traumatic or repeated epidural or spinal puncture.

THERAPEUTIC CLASS: Low molecular weight heparin

INDICATIONS: Treatment of acute symptomatic DVT with or without PE with concomitant warfarin.

DOSAGE: *Adults:* 175 anti-Xa IU/kg SQ qd for at least 6 days and until anticoagulated with warfarin (INR is at least 2 for 2 days). Begin warfarin within 1-3 days of therapy.

HOW SUPPLIED: Inj: 20,000 anti-Xa IU/mL

CONTRAINDICATIONS: Heparin, sulfite, benzoyl alcohol, or pork allergy. Active major bleeding, with or history of heparin-induced thrombocytopenia (HIT).

WARNINGS/PRECAUTIONS: Not for IM injection. Cannot use interchangeably unit for unit with heparin or other low molecular weight heparins. Extreme caution in conditions with an increased risk of hemorrhage (eg, bacterial endocarditis, hemorrhagic stroke, etc). Bleeding can occur at any site during therapy. D/C if severe hemorrhage occurs. Perform periodic CBC, platelets, and stool occult blood test. Asymptomatic increase in AST and ALT. Priapism reported (rare). Thrombocytopenia can occur; d/c if platelets $<100,000/mm^3$. Multiple dose vial contains benzyl alcohol. Contains sodium metabisulfite. Caution with bleeding diathesis, uncontrolled arterial HTN, recent GI ulceration, diabetic retinopathy, hemorrhage. Reduced elimination with elderly or in renal dysfunction; use with caution. Increased risk for death in elderly patients with renal insufficiency.

ADVERSE REACTIONS: Bleeding, and urinary tract infection.

INTERACTIONS: Increased risk of bleeding with anticoagulants, platelet inhibitors (eg, salicylates, dipyridamole, sulfinpyrazone, dextran, NSAIDs, ticlopidine, clopidogrel), and thrombolytics; monitor closely if co-administered.

PREGNANCY: Category B, caution use in nursing.

MECHANISM OF ACTION: Low molecular-weight heparin with antithrombotic properties; inhibits reactions that lead to blood clotting including the formation of fibrin clots. Acts as a potent co-inhibitor of several activated coagulation factors, including Factors Xa and IIa (thrombin). Primary inhibitory activity mediated through plasma protease inhibitor, antithrombin.

PHARMACOKINETICS: Absorption: (4,500 IU, Single Dose) C_{max}=0.25 IU/ mL, T_{max}=3.7 hrs, AUC=2.0 IU•hr/mL. (175 IU/kg, Day 1) C_{max}=0.87 IU/mL, T_{max}=4.4 hrs, AUC=9.0 IU•hr/mL. (175 IU/kg, Day 5) C_{max}=0.93 IU/mL, T_{max}=4.6 hrs, AUC=9.7 IU•hr/mL; absolute bioavailability (86.7%). **Distribution:** V_d=3.1-5.0L. **Metabolism:** Partially metabolized by desulphation and depolymerization. **Elimination:** Renal; $T_{1/2}$=3-4 hrs.

NURSING CONSIDERATIONS

Assessment: Assess for signs of active major bleeding; presence or history of heparin-induced thrombocytopenia; severe renal impairment; hypersensitivity to heparin, sulfites, benzyl alcohol or pork products; pregnancy/nursing status, and drug interactions. Assess use in conditions with increased risk of hemorrhage (eg, bacterial endocarditis, severe uncontrolled HTN, congenital or acquired bleeding disorders) and in presence of spinal/epidural anesthesia or spinal puncture.

I

Monitoring: Monitor for signs/symptoms of bleeding (eg, decreases in Hct, Hgb, BP), thrombocytopenia, hypersensitivity reactions, and priapism. If concomitant therapy with neuraxial anesthesia, monitor for epidural or spinal hematomas and for neurological impairment. Perform periodic monitoring of CBC including platelet count, Hgb, Hct, and stool test for occult blood.

Patient Counseling: Advise about increased risk of bleeding during therapy. Instruct to notify physician if unusual bleeding or hypersensitivity reaction occurs. During pregnancy, advise risk of "Gasping Syndrome".

Administration: SQ route. Patients should be lying down or sitting when administering SQ Injection. Alternate between left and right anterolateral and posterolateral abdominal wall. 1) Hold skin fold between thumb and forefinger; insert whole length of needle into skin. To minimize bruising, do not rub injection site after administration. **Storage:** Store at 25°C (77°F); excursions permitted to 15-30°C (59-86°F).

INNOPRAN XL RX

propranolol HCl (GlaxoSmithKline)

THERAPEUTIC CLASS: Nonselective beta-blocker

INDICATIONS: For the management of hypertension.

DOSAGE: *Adults:* Initial: 80mg qhs (approximately 10 PM) consistently either on empty stomach or with food. Titrate: Based on response may titrate to dose of 120mg.

HOW SUPPLIED: Cap, Extended-Release: 80mg, 120mg

CONTRAINDICATIONS: Cardiogenic shock, sinus bradycardia and >1st-degree block, bronchial asthma.

WARNINGS/PRECAUTIONS: Caution with well-compensated cardiac failure, nonallergic bronchospasm (eg, chronic bronchitis, emphysema), Wolff-Parkinson-White syndrome, hepatic or renal dysfunction, or with history of severe anaphylactic reactions. Withdrawal before surgery is controversial. May mask hypoglycemia or hyperthyroidism symptoms. Avoid abrupt discontinuation. May reduce IOP. Can cause cardiac failure. Caution in patients with impaired hepatic or renal function. Not for treatment of hypertensive emergencies.

ADVERSE REACTIONS: Fatigue, dizziness (except vertigo), constipation.

INTERACTIONS: Caution with drugs that effect CYP2D6, 1A2, or 2C19 or that slow down AV conduction (eg, digitalis, lidocaine, CCBs). ACE inhibitors can cause hypotension and certain ACE inhibitors may increase bronchial hyperactivity. May antagonize clonidine effects; caution when withdrawing from clonidine. Potentiated by α-blockers (eg, prazosin, terazosin, doxazosin), antiarrhythmics (eg, propafenone, quinidine, amiodarone), CYP2D6 substrates or inhibitors (eg, cimetidine, delavudin, fluoxetine, paroxetine, quinidine, ritonavir), CYP1A2 substrates or inhibitors (eg, imipramine, cimetidine, ciprofloxacin, fluvoxamine, isoniazid, theophylline, zileuton, zolmitriptan, rizatriptan), CYP2C19 substrates or inhibitors (eg, fluconazole, fluoxetine, fluvoxamine, teniposide, tolbutamide). Severe bradycardia, asystole, and heart failure associated with concomitant disopyramide. Decreases clearance of lidocaine and theophylline. Uncontrolled HTN may develop with concurrent epinephrine. Closely monitor for excessive reduction of resting sympathetic nervous activity (eg, hypotension, bradycardia, vertigo, orthostatic hypotension, syncope) with concurrent reserpine; reserpine may also potentiate depression. Anesthetics (eg, methoxyflurane, trichloroethylene) may depress myocardial contractility. Effects may be reversed by β-agonists (eg, dobutamine, isoproterenol). May exacerbate hypotensive effects of MAOIs or TCAs. Hypotension and cardiac arrest reported with haloperidol. Antagonized by NSAIDs. May result in lower than expected T_3 level with concomitant thyroxine. Increases level of warfarin, diazepam, zolmitriptan, rizatriptan, thioridazine. Decreased levels with aluminum hydroxide gel (1200mg), cholestyramine, colestipol, rifampin, ethanol, and cigarette smoking. Co-administration with chlorpromazine may increase levels of both drugs. Decreases levels of lovastatin and pravastatin.

PREGNANCY: Category C; caution in nursing.

MECHANISM OF ACTION: β-adrenergic receptor blocker; not established, proposed to decrease cardiac output, inhibit renin, and diminute tonic sympathetic nerve outflow.

PHARMACOKINETICS: Absorption: T_{max}=12-14 hrs. **Distribution:** V_d=4L; plasma protein binding (90%). **Metabolism:** CYP2D6 (hydroxylation), CYP1A2, 2D6 (oxidation), N-dealkylation, glucuronidation. Propranolol glucuronide, napthyloxylactic acid, glucuronic acid, sulfate conjugates (major metabolites). **Elimination:** $T_{1/2}$=8 hrs.

NURSING CONSIDERATIONS

Assessment: Assess for sinus bronchial asthma, bradycardia, AV heart block, cardiogenic shock, overt CHF, bronchospastic disease, hyperthyroidism, DM, possible drug interactions, WPW syndrome, history of heart failure, hepatic/renal impairment.

Monitoring: Monitor for signs/symptoms of cardiac failure, hypoglycemia, decreased IOP, thyrotoxicosis, withdrawal symptoms (angina, MI), and hypersensitivity reactions.

Patient Counseling: Instruct not to interrupt or d/c therapy without consulting physician. Inform may mask signs of thyrotoxicosis and hypoglycemia. Drug may interfere with glaucoma screening test. Advise to contact physician if symptoms of heart failure, withdrawal (angina), or hypersensitivity reactions occur.

Administration: Oral route. **Storage:** 25°C (77°F), excursions permitted to 15-30°C (59-86°F).

INSPRA

eplerenone (Pfizer) **RX**

THERAPEUTIC CLASS: Aldosterone blocker

INDICATIONS: To improve survival with left ventricular systolic dysfunction and congestive heart failure (CHF) post-MI. Treatment of hypertension, alone or with other antihypertensives.

DOSAGE: *Adults:* CHF Post-MI: Initial: 25mg qd. Titrate: To 50mg qd within 4 weeks. Maint: 50mg qd. Adjust dose based on K^+ level: See PI. HTN: Initial: 50mg qd. May increase to 50mg bid if inadequate effect on BP. Max: 100mg/day. With Weak CYP3A4 Inhibitors: Initial: 25mg qd.

HOW SUPPLIED: Tab: 25mg, 50mg

CONTRAINDICATIONS: All: Serum K^+ >5.5mgEq/L at initiation, CrCl ≤30mL/min, with potent CYP3A4 inhibitors (eg, ketoconazole, itraconazole, nefazodone, troleandomycin, clarithromycin, ritonavir, nelfinavir). When treating

HTN: Type 2 diabetes with microalbuminuria, SCr >2mg/dL (males) or >1.8mg/dL (females), CrCl <50mg/min, with K^+ supplements or K^+-sparing diuretics (eg, amiloride, spironolactone, triamterene).

WARNINGS/PRECAUTIONS: Risk of hyperkalemia (>5.5mEq/L); monitor periodically. With CHF post-MI use caution with SCr >2mg/dL (males) or >1.8mg/dL (females), CrCl ≤50mL/min, and in diabetics (also with proteinuria).

ADVERSE REACTIONS: Headache, dizziness, hyperkalemia, increased SCr/triglycerides/GGT, angina/MI.

INTERACTIONS: Avoid with potent CYP3A4 inhibitors (eg, ketoconazole, itraconazole, nefazodone, troleandomycin, clarithromycin, ritonavir, nelfinavir). Increased levels with other CYP3A4 inhibitors (eg, erythromycin, verapamil, saquinavir, fluconazole). In HTN, use caution, with ACE inhibitors and angiotensin II receptor antagonists; increased risk of hyperkalemia especially with diabetics with microalbuminuria. Monitor lithium levels. Monitor antihypertensive effect with NSAIDs.

PREGNANCY: Category B, not for use in nursing.

MECHANISM OF ACTION: Aldosterone blocker; binds to mineralocorticoid receptor and blocks binding of aldosterone.

I

PHARMACOKINETICS: Absorption: T_{max}=1.5 hrs. **Distribution:** V_d=43-90L; plasma protein binding (50%). **Metabolism:** CYP3A4. **Elimination:** Urine, feces; $T_{1/2}$=4-6 hrs.

NURSING CONSIDERATIONS

Assessment: Assess serum K^+, serum creatinine. Assess for type 2 DM with microalbuminuria, proteinuria, impaired renal function, and possible drug interactions.

Monitoring: Monitor serum K^+ and renal function tests periodically. Monitor for signs/symptoms of hyperkalemia and hypersensitivity reactions.

Patient Counseling: Inform not to use K^+ supplements or salt substitutes containing K^+. Advise to seek medical attention if symptoms of hyperkalemia or hypersensitivity reactions occur.

Administration: Oral route. **Storage:** 25°C (77°F); excursions permitted to 15-30°C (59-86°F).

INTEGRILIN — RX

eptifibatide (Schering)

THERAPEUTIC CLASS: Glycoprotein IIb/IIIa inhibitor

INDICATIONS: Treatment of acute coronary syndrome (ACS) in patients being medically managed or undergoing percutaneous coronary intervention (PCI) including intracoronary stenting.

DOSAGE: *Adults:* ACS: 180mcg/kg IV bolus, then 2mcg/kg/min IV infusion until discharge, initiation of CABG, or up to 72 hrs. If undergoing PCI, continue until discharge or 18-24 hrs post-PCI. CrCl <50mL/min: 180mcg/kg IV bolus, then 1mcg/kg/min IV infusion. PCI: 180mcg/kg IV bolus immediately before PCI, then 2mcg/kg/min IV infusion. Give 2nd bolus of 180mcg/kg 10 min after 1st bolus. Continue until discharge or 18-24 hrs post-PCI. CrCl <50mL/min: 180mcg/kg IV bolus immediately before PCI, then 1mcg/kg/min IV infusion. Give 2nd bolus of 180mcg/kg 10 min after 1st bolus. See PI for concomitant ASA and heparin doses.

HOW SUPPLIED: Sol: 0.75mg/mL, 2mg/mL

CONTRAINDICATIONS: Active abnormal bleeding, history of bleeding diathesis, or stroke within past 30 days. Severe HTN uncontrolled with antihypertensives, major surgery within preceding 6 weeks, history of hemorrhagic stroke, concomitant parenteral glycoprotein IIb/IIIa inhibitor, renal dialysis dependency.

WARNINGS/PRECAUTIONS: Bleeding reported. Caution with renal dysfunction, platelets <100,000mm^3, femoral access site in PCI. Minimize vascular and other trauma. D/C if thrombocytopenia occurs. Monitor Hct, Hgb, platelets,

SrCr, and PT/aPTT before therapy (and activated clotting time before PCI). D/C before CABG surgery.

ADVERSE REACTIONS: Bleeding, thrombocytopenia, hypotension.

INTERACTIONS: Caution with other drugs that affect hemostasis (eg, thrombolytics, anticoagulants, NSAIDs, dipyridamole). Avoid other glycoprotein IIb/IIIa inhibitors. Cerebral, pulmonary, GI hemorrhage reported with ASA and heparin.

PREGNANCY: Category B, caution in nursing.

MECHANISM OF ACTION: Glycoprotein IIb/IIIa inhibitor; reversibly inhibits platelet aggregation by preventing the binding of fibrinogen, von Willebrand factor, and other adhesive ligands to glycoprotein IIb/IIIa.

PHARMACOKINETICS: Absorption: T_{max}=4-6 hrs. **Distribution:** Plasma protein binding (25%). **Elimination:** Urine; $T_{1/2}$=2.5 hrs.

NURSING CONSIDERATIONS

Assessment: Assess for history of bleeding diathesis, evidence of bleeding within previous 30 days, severe HTN, major surgery within the previous 6 weeks, history of any stroke, concomitant use of another GP IIb/IIIa inhibitor, dependency on renal dialysis, and for drug interactions. Assess use if platelet count is <100,000/mm³. Obtain baseline Hgb, Hct, platelet count, SrCr, and PT/aPTT. In patients undergoing PCI, obtain activated clotting time (ACT).

Monitoring: Monitor for signs/symptoms of bleeding (eg, intracranial bleeding), and thrombocytopenia (eg, platelet count <100,000/mm³). Periodically monitor aPTT and ACT.

Patient Counseling: Inform about bleeding tendency during therapy and instruct to contact physician if signs of unusual bleeding develop.

Administration: IV route. Do not administer in same line with furosemide.
Storage: Vial: 2-8°C (36-46°F); may be transferred to room temperature storage 25°C (77°F) with excursions permitted to 15-30°C (59-86°F); do not store at room temperature for longer than 2 months.

INTELENCE RX

etravirine (Tibotec)

THERAPEUTIC CLASS: Non-nucleoside reverse transcriptase inhibitor

INDICATIONS: In combination with other antiretrovirals for treatment of HIV-1 infection in antiretroviral treatment-experienced adult patients, who have evidence of viral replication and HIV-1 strains resistant to a non-nucleoside reverse transcriptase inhibitor (NNRTI) and other antiretrovirals.

DOSAGE: *Adults:* 200mg (two 100mg tabs) bid following a meal.

HOW SUPPLIED: Tab: 100mg

WARNINGS/PRECAUTIONS: Severe and life-threatening skin reactions (eg, Stevens-Johnson syndrome, hypersensitivity reaction, and erythema multiforme) reported; d/c use and treat accordingly if severe rash develops. May cause body fat redistribution or accumulation. Immune reconstitution syndrome reported with combination therapy.

ADVERSE REACTIONS: Rash, NV, abdominal pain, fatigue, diarrhea, peripheral neuropathy, HTN, headache.

INTERACTIONS: Coadministration of drugs that induce, inhibit or are substrates of CYP3A4, CYP2C9 and CYP2C19 may alter therapeutic effect and adverse reaction profile. Concomitant use with NNRTIs (eg, efavirenz, nevirapine, delavirdine) and protease inhibitors administered without low-dose ritonavir (eg, atazanavir, fosamprenavir, nelfinavir, indinavir) are not recommended. Ritonavir 600mg bid decreases plasma levels and should not be coadministered. Do not co-administer with tipranavir/ritonavir, fosamprenavi/ritonavir, atazanavir/ritonavir. Caution with saquinavir/ritonavir. May decrease levels of antiarrhythmics; monitor drug levels. May increase warfarin concentration; monitor INR. Do not use in combination with CYP450 inducers (eg, carbamazepine, phenobarbital, phenytoin, rifampin, rifapentine, rifabutin).

Adjust dose with antifungals. Consider alternatives to clarithromycin for treatment of MAC. May decrease levels of lovastatin and simvastatin. May increase levels of fluvastatin. Caution with immunosuppressants (eg, cyclosporine, sirolimus, tacrolimus). Monitor for withdrawal symptoms when coadministered with methadone. May need to alter sildenafil dose.

PREGNANCY: Category B, not for use in nursing.

MECHANISM OF ACTION: Non-nucleoside reverse transcriptase inhibitor of HIV-1; binds directly to reverse transcriptase and blocks the RNA dependent and DNA dependent DNA polymerase activities by causing a disruption of the enzyme's catalytic site.

PHARMACOKINETICS: Absorption: T_{max}=2.5-4 hrs. **Distribution:** Plasma protein binding (99.9%). **Metabolism:** Liver via CYP3A4, CYP2C9 and CYP2C19; (methyl hydroxylation). **Elimination:** Feces (93.7%); urine (1.2%); $T_{1/2}$=41 hrs.

NURSING CONSIDERATIONS

Assessment: Assess treatment history, pregnancy/nursing status, and possible drug interactions. Perform resistance testing.

Monitoring: Monitor for signs/symptoms of severe skin reactions (eg, Stevens-Johnson syndrome, hypersensitivity reactions, erythema multiforme); if severe rash develops, d/c treatment. Monitor for clinical response (eg, viral load, CD4 count), fat redistribution (eg, central obesity, dorsocervical peripheral wasting, facial wasting), and immune reconstitution syndrome.

Patient Counseling: Counsel that medication does not cure HIV and may continue to develop opportunistic infections and other complications of HIV disease. Medication does not reduce risk of HIV transmission to others; take precaution to avoid transmission (eg, safe sex practices). Take following a meal, twice a day as prescribed; swallow whole. If unable to swallow, disperse medication into glass of water; mix well and drink immediately; rinse glass several times with water; swallow each rinse to ensure full dose is taken. Avoid altering or stopping therapy without consulting physician. If a dose is missed within 6 hrs of time usually taken, take as soon as possible with a meal; if scheduled time exceeds 6 hrs, do not take missed dose; resume normal dosing schedule. Notify physician of all Rx or nonprescription medications and herbal products currently taking. D/C and notify if severe rash develops. Inform females to avoid nursing to reduce risk of transmission.

Administration: Oral route. **Storage:** 25°C (77°F); excursions permitted to 15-30° C (59-86°F). Keep bottle tightly closed to protect from moisture. Do not remove desiccant pouches.

INTRON A — RX

interferon alfa-2b (Schering)

May cause or aggravate fatal or life-threatening neuropsychiatric, autoimmune, ischemic, and infectious disorders. Monitor closely with periodic clinical and laboratory evaluations.

THERAPEUTIC CLASS: Biological response modifier

INDICATIONS: Treatment of hairy cell leukemia, malignant melanoma, follicular lymphoma, condylomata acuminata, AIDS-related Kaposi's sarcoma, chronic hepatitis C and B.

DOSAGE: *Adults:* ≥18 yrs: Hairy Cell Leukemia: 2 MIU/m² IM/SQ 3x/week up to 6 months. Reduce dose by 50% or stop therapy with severe reactions. Malignant Melanoma: Initial: 20 MIU/m² IV for 5 consecutive days/week for 4 weeks. Maint: 10 MIU/m² SQ 3x/week for 48 weeks. Follicular Lymphoma: 5 MIU SQ 3x/week up to 18 months. Condylomata Acuminata: 1 MIU into lesion 3x/week alternating days for 3 weeks. Max: 5 lesions/course. Kaposi's Sarcoma: 30 MIU/m² 3x/week IM/SQ. Hepatitis C: 3 MIU IM/SQ 3x/week for 18-24 months. Hepatitis B: IM/SC: 5 MIU qd or 10 MIU IM/SQ 3x/week for 16 weeks. Dose adjust according to severe adverse reactions and laboratory abnormalities (See PI for more information).
Pediatrics: ≥1 yr: Hepatitis B: 3 MIU/m² SQ 3x/week for 1 week, then 6 MIU/m² 3x/week for total therapy of 16-24 weeks. Max: 10 MIU/m² 3x/week. Reduce

dose by 50% or stop therapy with severe reactions. Adjust based on WBC, granulocyte, and/or platelet counts. Dose adjust according to severe adverse reactions and laboratory abnormalities (See PI for more information).

HOW SUPPLIED: Inj: 10 MIU, 18 MIU, 50 MIU, 10 MIU/mL, 3 MIU/0.2mL, 5 MIU/0.2mL, 10 MIU/0.2mL

CONTRAINDICATIONS: Autoimmune hepatitis, decompensated liver disease.

WARNINGS/PRECAUTIONS: Do not give IM if platelet count is less than 50,000 cells/mm^3. Hepatotoxicity, retinal hemorrhages, autoimmune diseases, pulmonary infiltrates, pneumonitis, thyroid abnormalities and pneumonia reported. Avoid with immunosuppressed transplant, autoimmune disorders, decompensated liver disease. Caution with cardiac disease, coagulation disorders, severe myelosuppression, pulmonary disease, thyroid disorders, or DM prone to ketoacidosis. Avoid with pre-existing psychiatric condition; depression, suicidal behavior, and aggressive behavior; monitor during treatment and in the 6 month follow-up period. D/C if psychiatric symptoms worsen or suicidal ideation is identified. Cases of encephalopathy observed in elderly treated with higher doses. Dental and periodontal disorders have been reported with ribavirin and interferon combination therapy. May exacerbate psoriasis or sarcoidosis. Do not interchange brands.

ADVERSE REACTIONS: Fever, headache, chills, fatigue, myalgia, GI disturbances, alopecia, dyspnea, depression.

INTERACTIONS: Increases theophylline levels by 100%. Caution with myelosuppressive agents (eg, zidovudine). Antidiabetics and thyroid agents may need adjustments. Increased risk of hemolytic anemia when coadministered with ribavirin. Risk of aplastic anemia and pure red cell aplasia with Rebetol.

PREGNANCY: Category C, Category X when used with ribavirin, not for use in nursing.

MECHANISM OF ACTION: α-interferon; binds to specific membrane receptors on cell surface initiating induction of enzymes, suppression of cell proliferation, immunomodulating activities, and inhibition of virus replication.

PHARMACOKINETICS: Absorption: (IM, SQ) C_{max}=18-116 IU/mL, T_{max}=3-12 hrs; (IV) C_{max}=135-273 IU/mL, T_{max}=30 min. **Elimination:** (IM, SQ) $T_{1/2}$=2-3 hrs; (IV) $T_{1/2}$=2 hrs.

NURSING CONSIDERATIONS

Assessment: Assess for neuropsychiatric conditions, autoimmune disease (psoriasis), liver dysfunction, ischemic, ophthalmologic and infectious disorders, preexisting thyroid abnormalities, hemoglobinopathies (thalassemia major, sickle cell anemia), DM, history of pulmonary disease (eg, COPD, sarcoidosis), coagulation disorders (thrombophlebitis, PE), severe myelosuppression, history of cardiovascular disease (MI, arrhythmic disorder), and possible drug interactions. Obtain baseline CBC and platelet counts, LFTs, electrolytes, TSH, Hgb, Hct, ECG, CXR.

Monitoring: Periodic monitoring of LFTs, CrCl, CBC, Hgb, platelet count, PT, alkaline phosphatase, albumin, bilirubin, TSH, ECG, CXR. CBC and platelet count should be repeated 1-2 weeks following initiation of therapy, and monthly thereafter. Serum ALT should be evaluated at approximately 3-month intervals to assess response to therapy. Monitor for signs/symptoms of depression (suicidal ideation), cardiovascular and cerebrovascular events, ophthalmologic toxicity pancreatitis, colitis, cytopenia, worsening of liver disease/failure, respiratory, and hypersensitivity reactions.

Patient Counseling: Instruct on proper use of product. Seek medical attention for symptoms of depression (suicidal ideation), cardiovascular (chest pain) and cerebrovascular events, ophthalmologic toxicity (eg, decreased/loss of vision), pancreatitis and colitis (eg, abdominal pain, NV), cytopenia (eg, fever, bruising, dyspnea), worsening of liver disease/failure (eg, jaundice), respiratory (eg, fever, cough, dyspnea), and hypersensitivity reactions. Keep well hydrated.

Administration: IM, SQ, IV, and intralesional administration. **Storage:** 2-8°C (36-46°F). After reconstitution use immediately, store up to 24 hrs.

INVANZ RX

ertapenem sodium (Merck)

THERAPEUTIC CLASS: Carbapenem

INDICATIONS: Treatment of complicated intra-abdominal infections; complicated skin and skin structure infections (cSSSI), including diabetic foot infections without osteomyelitis; community-acquired pneumonia (CAP); complicated urinary tract infections (UTI), including pyelonephritis; acute pelvic infections, including postpartum endomyometritis, septic abortion, and post-surgical gynecologic infections caused by susceptible strains of microorganisms. Prophylaxis of surgical site infection following elective colorectal surgery.

DOSAGE: *Adults:* 1g IM/IV qd. Treatment Duration: Intra-Abdominal Infections: 5-14 days. cSSSI: 7-14 days. CAP/UTI: 10-14 days. Acute Pelvic Infections: 3-10 days. May give IV for up to 14 days and IM for up to 7 days. Prophylaxis Following Colorectal Surgery: 1g IV as single dose given 1 hr prior to surgical incision. CrCl ≤30mL/min/1.73m²: 500mg IM/IV qd. Hemodialysis: Give 150mg IM/IV after dialysis only if 500mg dose was given within 6 hrs prior to dialysis. *Pediatrics:* ≥13 yrs: 1g IM/IV qd. 3 months-12 yrs: 15mg/kg IM/IV bid (Max: 1g/day). Treatment Duration: Intra-Abdominal Infections: 5-14 days. SSSI: 7-14 days. CAP/UTI: 10-14 days. Pelvic Infections: 3-10 days. May administer IV for up to 14 days and IM for up to 7 days.

HOW SUPPLIED: Inj: 1g (IM, IV)

CONTRAINDICATIONS: Anaphylactic reactions to β-lactams, hypersensitivity to local anesthetics of the amide type (due to lidocaine diluent).

WARNINGS/PRECAUTIONS: Serious, sometimes fatal, hypersensitivity reported with β-lactam therapy. *Clostridium difficile*-associated diarrhea (CDAD) reported. D/C if CDAD confirmed. Seizures and CNS adverse experiences reported. Increased risk of seizures with CNS disorders and/or compromised renal function. Use lidocaine HCl as diluent for IM use. Monitor renal, hepatic, hematopoietic functions during prolonged therapy. Do not inject into blood vessel.

ADVERSE REACTIONS: Diarrhea, infused vein complication, NV, headache, edema/swelling, fever, abdominal pain, constipation, altered mental status, headache, insomnia, rash, pruritis, vaginitis, phlebitis/thrombophlebitis.

INTERACTIONS: Decreased clearance with probenecid. Do not mix or co-infuse with other drugs. May decrease serum levels of valproic acid when coadministered.

PREGNANCY: Category B, caution in nursing.

MECHANISM OF ACTION: Broad-spectrum carbapenem; penetrates bacterial cells and interferes with synthesis of vital cell wall components, resulting in cell death.

PHARMACOKINETICS: Absorption: Administration of different doses resulted in different parameters. (IM): Absolute bioavailability (90%); T_{max}=2.3 hrs. **Distribution:** V_d=0.12L/kg (adult); 0.2L/kg (3 months-12 yrs); 0.16L/kg (13-17 yrs). Plasma protein binding (95%); found in breast milk. **Metabolism:** Liver via hydrolysis of the β-lactam ring. **Elimination:** (Adults, 13-17 yrs old) $T_{1/2}$=4 hrs. (3 months-12 years old) $T_{1/2}$=2.5 hrs; Urine (38% unchanged, 37% metabolite), feces (10%).

NURSING CONSIDERATIONS

Assessment: Assess for β-lactam/amide hypersensitivity, history of seizure or brain lesions, bacterial meningitis, renal impairment, and possible drug interactions.

Monitoring: Monitor for signs/symptoms of anaphylactoid or hypersensitivity reactions, CDAD, superinfections, and seizures.

Patient Counseling: Inform drug only treats bacterial, not viral, infections. Instruct to take as directed; skipping doses or not completing full course may decrease effectiveness and increase resistance. May experience diarrhea;

notify physician if watery/bloody stools, hypersensitivity reactions, infection, or seizures occur.

Administration: IV and IM routes. Reconstitute with normal saline. Refer to labeling for administration procedures. **Storage:** Before reconstitution: Do not store above 25°C (77°F). Reconstituted and infusion solutions: Room temperature (25°C) and used within 6 hrs, or stored for 24 hrs under refrigeration (5°C) and used within 4 hrs after removal from refrigeration. Do not freeze.

INVEGA — RX

paliperidone (Janssen)

Elderly patients with dementia-related psychosis treated with atypical antipsychotic drugs are at an increased risk of death; most appeared to be cardiovascular (eg, heart failure, sudden death) or infectious (eg, pneumonia) in nature. Paliperidone is not approved for the treatment of patients with dementia-related psychosis.

THERAPEUTIC CLASS: Benzisoxazole derivative

INDICATIONS: Acute and maintenance treatment of schizophrenia.

DOSAGE: *Adults:* 6mg qd in am. Range: 3-12mg/day. Titrate: May increase by 3mg/day at intervals of >5 days. Max: 12mg/day. Swallow whole; do not chew, divide, or crush. Mild Renal Impairment (CrCl ≥50 to <80mL/min): Initial: 3mg qd. Max: 6mg/day. Moderate To Severe Renal Impairment (CrCl ≥10 to <50mL/min): Initial: 1.5mg qd. Max: 3mg/day. Evaluate periodically for long-term use.

HOW SUPPLIED: Tab, Extended-Release: 1.5mg, 3mg, 6mg, 9mg

WARNINGS/PRECAUTIONS: May increase QTc interval; avoid with congenital long QT syndrome and with a history of cardiac arrhythmias. Neuroleptic malignant syndrome (NMS) and tardive dyskinesia (TD) may occur. Monitor for hyperglycemia; perform fasting blood glucose testing if symptoms develop or with risk factors for DM. Avoid with pre-existing severe GI narrowing. Cerebrovascular events (eg, stroke, TIA) reported in elderly with dementia-related psychosis. Not approved for the treatment of dementia-related psychosis. May induce priapism. May induce orthostatic hypotension and syncope; monitor closely in those vulnerable to hypotension. Caution with history of seizures or other conditions that may lower seizure threshold. May elevate prolactin levels. May cause esophageal dysmotility and aspiration; caution in those at risk for aspiration pneumonia. May disrupt body's ability to reduce core body temperature; caution in those who may experience conditions that may contribute to an elevation in core body temperature. Caution with known suicidal tendencies, cardiovascular disease, elderly, and renal impairment. May impair mental/physical abilities. Re-evaluate periodically.

ADVERSE REACTIONS: Tachycardia, nausea, akathisia, dizziness, extrapyramidal disorder, headache, somnolence, anxiety, parkinsonism, dyskinesia, and hyperkinesia.

INTERACTIONS: Caution with other CNS drugs, alcohol. May antagonize the effect of levodopa and other dopamine agonists. Because of its potential for inducing orthostatic hypotension, additive effect may be observed when administered with other agents that have this potential. Avoid in combination with other drugs known to prolong QTc interval including Class 1A (eg, quinidine, procainamide) or Class III (eg, amiodarone, sotalol) antiarrhythmics, antipsychotic medications (eg, chlopromazine, thioridazine), antibiotics (eg, gatifloxacin, moxifloxacin), or any other class of drugs known to prolong the QTc interval. Concomitant use with carbamazepine may decrease levels; re-evaluate and increase dosage if necessary.

PREGNANCY: Category C, caution in nursing.

MECHANISM OF ACTION: Benzisoxazole derivative; not established. Proposed to be mediated through a combination of central dopamine type 2 (D_2) and serotonin type 2 ($5HT_{2A}$) receptor antagonism.

PHARMACOKINETICS: Absorption: Absolute bioavailability (28%); T_{max}=24 hrs. **Distribution**: V_d=487L; plasma protein binding (74%); found in breast milk. **Metabolism**: Dealkylation, hydroxylation, dehydrogenation, benzisoxazole scission; CYP2D6, 3A4. **Elimination**: Urine (59% unchanged), feces (11%); $T_{1/2}$=23 hrs.

NURSING CONSIDERATIONS

Assessment: Assess for dementia-related psychosis, Parkinson's disease, and dementia prior to initiation. Assess use in patients with pre-existing severe GI narrowing, cardiovascular disease, history of seizures, known drug allergy to risperidone, renal function prior to administration, fasting blood glucose levels in patients at risk for hyperglycemia, and possible drug interactions.

Monitoring: Monitor for cerebrovascular adverse events in the elderly population, signs/symptoms of NMS, EPS, QT prolongation, TD, hyperglycemia, hyperprolactinemia, GI obstructions, orthostatic hypotension, seizures, attempted suicide, priapism, and thrombotic thrombocytopenia purpura. Perform periodic monitoring of fasting blood glucose levels in patients with DM.

Patient Counseling: Caution about operating machinery/driving. Avoid concomitant use of alcohol. Instruct to inform physician if taking, or plan to take, any prescription or over-the-counter drugs. Instruct to notify physician if patient becomes pregnant or intends to become pregnant. Inform medication may impair body's ability to regulate temperatures; take appropriate measures when exposed to increased temperatures. Medication must be swallowed whole with the aid of liquids; do not chew, divide, or crush. Tablet shell along with insoluble core components may be found in stool.

Administration: Oral route. **Storage**: 25°C (77°F); excursions permitted to 15-30°C (59-86°F). Protect from moisture. Keep out of reach of children.

INVIRASE RX

saquinavir mesylate (Roche Labs)

Not interchangeable with Fortovase.

THERAPEUTIC CLASS: Protease inhibitor

INDICATIONS: Treatment of HIV infection in combination with other antiretrovirals.

DOSAGE: *Adults:* 1000mg bid with ritonavir 100mg bid. Take within 2 hrs after a full meal.
Pediatrics: >16 yrs: 1000mg bid with ritonavir 100mg bid. Take within 2 hrs after a full meal.

HOW SUPPLIED: Cap: 200mg; Tab: 500mg

CONTRAINDICATIONS: Concomitant amiodarone, bepridil, flecainide, propafenone, quinidine, rifampin, pimozide, terfenadine, cisapride, astemizole, triazolam, midazolam, ergot derivatives.

WARNINGS/PRECAUTIONS: New onset DM, exacerbation of pre-existing DM, hyperglycemia may occur. Exacerbation of chronic liver dysfunction reported with hepatitis or cirrhosis. Spontaneous bleeding may occur with hemophilia A, B. Possible redistribution or accumulation of body fat. Caution with hepatic dysfunction. Interrupt therapy if serious toxicity occurs.

ADVERSE REACTIONS: Diarrhea, abdominal discomfort, NV, dyspepsia, mucosa damage, headache, paresthesia, extremity numbness, asthenia, myalgia, fatigue, pneumonia, lipodystrophy.

INTERACTIONS: See contraindications. Avoid lovastatin, simvastatin, St. John's wort, garlic capsules, tipranavir, trazodone, fluticasone. Decreased plasma levels with nevirapine. Consider alternatives to CYP3A4 inducers (eg, phenobarbital, phenytoin, dexamethasone, carbamazepine). Ritonavir increases adverse effects. Risk of toxicity with substrates of CYP3A4 substrates (eg, calcium CCBs, clindamycin, dapsone, quinidine, triazolam). Delavirdine increases plasma levels; monitor LFTs frequently. Saquinavir/ritonavir increases digoxin levels; monitor digoxin serum concentration and reduce dose if needed.

PREGNANCY: Category B, not for use in nursing.

MECHANISM OF ACTION: HIV protease inhibitor; binds to the protease active site and inhibits activity of the enzyme, preventing cleavage of the viral polyproteins and resulting in formation of immature, noninfectious virus particles.

PHARMACOKINETICS: Absorption: Administration of variable doses and combinations resulted in different parameters. **Distribution:** Plasma protein binding (98%). (IV): V_d=700L. **Metabolism:** Hepatic via CYP3A4. **Elimination:** (PO): Urine (1%), feces (88%). (IV): Urine (3%), feces (81%).

NURSING CONSIDERATIONS

Assessment: Assess for renal/hepatic impairment, history of DM, hemophilia, lipid disorder, and possible drug interactions. Perform clinical chemistry tests, viral load, and CD4 count prior to therapy.

Monitoring: Periodically monitor triglyceride levels. Monitor for signs/symptoms of hyperlipidemia, spontaneous bleeding, immune reconstitution syndrome, fat redistribution/accumulation, hyperglycemia, infections, hepatic/renal function.

Patient Counseling: Advise to report use of other Rx, OTC, or herbal products (eg, St. John's wort). Instruct to use in combination with ritonavir. Take drug within 2 hrs pc; do not alter or d/c therapy without consulting physician. If miss dose, take as soon as possible; do not double next dose. Seek medical attention if symptoms of hyperlipidemia, spontaneous bleeding, immune reconstitution syndrome, fat redistribution/accumulation, hyperglycemia, infections, hepatic/renal dysfunction occur.

Administration: Oral route. **Storage:** 25°C (77°F); excursions permitted to 15-30°C (59-86°F). Dispense in tightly closed bottles.

IQUIX

levofloxacin (Vistakon)

RX

THERAPEUTIC CLASS: Fluoroquinolone

INDICATIONS: Bacterial corneal ulcer.

DOSAGE: *Adults:* Days 1-3: 1-2 drops q30min-2h while awake and 4-6 hrs after retiring. Days 4-completion: 1-2 drops q1-4h while awake.
Pediatrics: ≥6 yrs: Days 1-3: 1-2 drops q30min-2h while awake and 4-6 hrs after retiring. Days 4-completion: 1-2 drops q1-4h while awake.

HOW SUPPLIED: Sol: 1.5% [5mL]

WARNINGS/PRECAUTIONS: D/C if hypersensitivity or superinfection occurs. Avoid contact lenses with corneal ulcer.

ADVERSE REACTIONS: Headache, taste disturbance.

INTERACTIONS: Systemic quinolone therapy increases theophylline levels, interferes with caffeine metabolism, enhances warfarin effects, and may elevate SCr with cyclosporine.

PREGNANCY: Category C, caution in nursing.

MECHANISM OF ACTION: Fluoroquinolone; antibacterial active against a broad spectrum of gram-positive and gram-negative ocular pathogens. Responsible for inhibition of bacterial topoisomerase IV and DNA gyrase, enzymes required for DNA replication, transcription, repair, and recombination.

PHARMACOKINETICS: Absorption: C_{max}=3.22ng/mL (initial dose), 10.9ng/mL (multiple doses).

NURSING CONSIDERATIONS

Assessment: Assess proper diagnosis (eg, slit lamp biomicroscopy, fluorescein staining), hypersensitivity to other quinolones, and for possible drug interactions. Assess use in pregnant/nursing females.

Monitoring: Monitor for signs/symptoms of hypersensitivity or anaphylactic reactions (eg, cardiovascular collapse, loss of consciousness, angioedema, airway obstruction, dyspnea, urticaria, and itching). In patients on prolonged therapy, monitor for overgrowth of non-susceptible organisms (eg, fungi), and for the development of superinfection. Perform periodic monitoring of patient using the aid of magnification (eg, slit-lamp biomicroscopy, fluorescein staining).

Patient Counseling: Instruct to avoid contaminating applicator tip with material from the eye, fingers, or other sources. Caution not to wear contact lenses if there are signs/symptoms of a corneal ulcer. Advise to d/c medication and contact physician if any signs/symptoms of a hypersensitivity reaction (eg, rash) develop.

Administration: Ocular route. Do not inject subconjunctivally or introduce directly into anterior chamber of eye. **Storage:** 15-25°C (59-77°F).

ISENTRESS RX

raltegravir potassium (Merck)

THERAPEUTIC CLASS: HIV-integrase strand transfer inhibitor

INDICATIONS: For use in combination with other antiretroviral agents for treatment of HIV-1 infection in treatment-experienced adults who have evidence of viral replication and HIV-1 strains resistant to multiple antiretroviral agents.

DOSAGE: *Adults:* 400mg bid.

HOW SUPPLIED: Tab: 400mg

WARNINGS/PRECAUTIONS: Monitor for immune reconstitution syndrome.

ADVERSE REACTIONS: Diarrhea, nausea, headache, pyrexia.

INTERACTIONS: Strong inducers of uridine diphosphate glucuronosyltransferase (UGT) 1A1 (eg, rifampin) may reduce plasma levels; use with caution.

PREGNANCY: Category C, not for use in nursing.

MECHANISM OF ACTION: HIV integrase strand transfer inhibitor; inhibits the catalytic activity of HIV-1 intergrase by preventing formation of HIV-1 provirus.

PHARMACOKINETICS: Absorption: T_{max}=3 hrs (fasting); variable doses resulted in different parameters. **Distribution:** Plasma protein binding (83%). **Metabolism:** Glucuronidation via UGT1A1. **Elimination:** Urine (32%), feces (51%); $T_{1/2}$=9 hrs.

NURSING CONSIDERATIONS

Assessment: Assess pregnancy/nursing status and for possible drug interactions.

Monitoring: Monitor for immune reconstitution syndrome, serum creatinine kinase, lab parameters, signs of myopathy and rhabdomyolysis.

Patient Counseling: Inform that drug does not cure, only helps control, HIV infection or AIDS. Advise to practice safe sex by using latex, polyurethane condoms, or other barrier methods. If a dose is missed, take as soon as remembered; if not remembered until next dose, instruct to skip missed dose and go back to regular schedule; do not take two tablets at same time.

Administration: Oral route. **Storage:** Store in a controlled room temperature 20-25°C (68-77°F). Excursions permitted to 15-30°C (59-86°F).

ISONIAZID RX

isoniazid (Various)

Severe, fatal hepatitis may develop. Monitor LFTs monthly.

OTHER BRAND NAMES: Nydrazid (Sandoz)

THERAPEUTIC CLASS: Isonicotinic acid hydrazide

INDICATIONS: Prevention and treatment of TB.

DOSAGE: *Adults:* Active TB: 5mg/kg as a single dose. Max: 300mg/day or 15mg/kg 2 to 3 times/week. Max: 900mg/day. Use with other antituberculosis agents. Prevention: 300mg qd single dose.
Pediatrics: Active TB: 10-15mg/kg as a single dose. Max: 300mg qd or 20-

40mg/kg 2 to 3 times/week. Max: 900mg/day. Use with other antituberculosis agents. Prevention: 10mg/kg qd single dose. Max: 300mg qd.

HOW SUPPLIED: Inj: 100mg/mL; Syrup: 50mg/5mL; Tab: 100mg, 300mg

CONTRAINDICATIONS: Severe hypersensitivity reactions including drug-induced hepatitis, previous INH-associated hepatic injury, severe adverse effects to INH (eg, drug fever, chills, arthritis), acute liver disease.

WARNINGS/PRECAUTIONS: D/C if hypersensitivity occurs. Monitor closely with liver or renal disease. Take with vitamin B_6 in malnourished and those predisposed to neuropathy.

ADVERSE REACTIONS: Peripheral neuropathy, NV, epigastric distress, elevated serum transaminases, bilirubinemia, jaundice, hepatitis, skin eruptions, pyridoxine deficiency.

INTERACTIONS: Alcohol is associated with hepatitis. May increase phenytoin, theophylline, and valproate serum levels. Do not take with food. Severe acetaminophen toxicity reported. Decreases carbamazepine metabolism and AUC of ketoconazole. Avoid tyramine- and histamine-containing foods.

PREGNANCY: Category C, caution in nursing.

MECHANISM OF ACTION: Inhibits mycoloic acid synthesis and acts against actively growing tuberculosis bacilli.

PHARMACOKINETICS: Distribution: Passes through placental barrier and into milk. **Metabolism**: Acetylation and dehydrazination. **Elimination**: Urine (50-70%).

NURSING CONSIDERATIONS

Assessment: Assess for previous isoniazid-associated hepatic injury, acute liver disease, HIV status, pregnancy status, and drug interactions. Document reasons for therapy, culture and susceptibility.

Monitoring: Prior to therapy and periodically thereafter, measure hepatic enzymes (AST, ALT). D/C at first sign of hypersensitivity reaction. Monitor for peripheral neuropathy, convulsions, NV, agranulocytosis, hemolytic anemia, SLE-like syndrome, metabolic and endocrine reactions (hyperglycemia, pyridoxine deficiency, pellagra).

Patient Counseling: Immediately report signs/symptoms consistent with liver damage or other adverse events (unexplained anorexia, NV, dark urine, icterus, rash, persistent paresthesias of the hands and feet, persistent fatigue, weakness or fever of >3 days duration and/or abdominal tenderness). Drug should not be taken with food and take as prescribed. Take pyridoxine tablets if peripheral neuropathy develops.

Administration: Oral and IM route. **Storage**: Store tab at 20-25°C (68-77°F) and syr at 15-30°C (59-86°F). Protect from light and moisture. Dispense in tight, light-resistant container with child-resistant closure. Store inj at 20-25°C (68-77°F). Protect from light. If vial contents crystallize, warm vial to room temperature to redissolve crystals before use.

ISOSORBIDE DINITRATE — RX

isosorbide dinitrate (Various)

OTHER BRAND NAMES: Isordil Titradose (Biovail) - Isordil (Biovail)

THERAPEUTIC CLASS: Nitrate vasodilator

INDICATIONS: Prevention of angina pectoris due to coronary artery disease.

DOSAGE: *Adults:* Prevention: Initial: 5-20mg bid-tid. Maint: 10-40mg bid-tid. Allow a dose-free interval of at least 14 hrs for both formulations. Elderly: Start at low end of dosing range.

HOW SUPPLIED: Tab: 5mg*, 10mg*, 20mg*, 30mg*; Tab, Extended-Release: 40mg; Tab, Sublingual: 2.5mg *scored

WARNINGS/PRECAUTIONS: Not for use with acute MI or CHF. Severe hypotension may occur. May aggravate angina caused by hypertrophic cardiomyopathy. Caution with volume depletion, hypotension, elderly. Monitor for tolerance.

ADVERSE REACTIONS: Headache, lightheadedness, hypotension, syncope, rebound HTN.

INTERACTIONS: Severe hypotension with sildenafil. Additive vasodilation with other vasodilators (eg, alcohol).

PREGNANCY: Category C, caution in nursing.

MECHANISM OF ACTION: Nitrate vasodilator; relaxes vascular smooth muscle, dilates peripheral arteries and veins, especially the latter. Dilatation of veins reduces left ventricular end diastolic pressure and pulmonary capillary wedge pressure (preload). Arteriolar relaxation reduces systemic vascular resistance, systolic arterial pressure, and mean arterial pressure (afterload). It also dilates the coronary artery.

PHARMACOKINETICS: Absorption: T_{max}=1 hr. **Distribution:** V_d=2-4L/kg. **Metabolism:** Liver; extensive first-pass metabolism; 2-mononitrate, 5-mononitrate (active metabolites). **Elimination:** $T_{1/2}$=5 hrs (5-mononitrate), 2 hrs (2-mononitrate).

I

NURSING CONSIDERATIONS

Assessment: Assess for severe hypotension, volume-depleted patients, angina caused by hypertrophic cardiomyopathy, alcohol intake, and possible drug interactions.

Monitoring: Careful clinical or hemodynamic monitoring for hypotension and tachycardia. Monitor for paradoxical bradycardia, increased angina pectoris, hemodynamic rebound, decreased exercise tolerance, headaches, lightheadedness on standing, manifestation of true physical dependence (chest pain, acute MI) and methemoglobinemia.

Patient Counseling: Counsel carefully follow dosing regimen. Inform about headaches (markers of drug activity) and lightheadedness on standing. Avoid alcohol consumption.

Administration: Oral route. **Storage:** 25°C (77°F).

IXEMPRA — RX

ixabepilone (Bristol-Myers Squibb)

Contraindicated in combination with capecitabine in patients with AST/ALT >2.5x ULN or bilirubin >1x ULN due to increased toxicity and neutropenia-related death.

THERAPEUTIC CLASS: Antimicrotubule agent

INDICATIONS: In combination with capecitabine for treatment of patients with metastatic or locally advanced breast cancer resistant to treatment with an anthracycline and a taxane, or whose cancer is taxane resistant and for whom further anthracycline therapy is contraindicated. As monotherapy for treatment of metastatic or locally advanced breast cancer in patients whose tumors are resistant or refractory to anthracyclines, taxanes, and capecitabine.

DOSAGE: *Adults:* 40mg/m² IV infusion over 3 hrs every 3 weeks. Adjust dose based on toxicities (see PI). Premedicate with H_1-antagonist (eg, diphenhydramine 50mg PO) and H_2-antagonist (eg, ranitidine 150-300mg PO) approximately 1 hr before infusion. Also premedicate with corticosteroid (eg, dexamethasone 20mg, IV 30 min before infusion or PO 60 min before infusion) if prior hypersensitivity reaction to ixabepilone. Hepatic Impairment: Monotherapy: Mild: AST and ALT ≤2.5x ULN and Bilirubin ≤1x ULN: 40mg/m². AST or ALT ≤10x ULN and Bilirubin ≤1x ULN: 32mg/m². Moderate (AST and ALT ≤10x ULN and Bilirubin >1.5 to ≤3x ULN): 20-30mg/m². Strong CYP3A4 Inhibitors: Avoid or reduce dose to 20mg/m².

HOW SUPPLIED: Inj: 15mg, 45mg

CONTRAINDICATIONS: Baseline neutrophil count <1500cells/mm³ or platelet count <100,000cells/mm³. In combination with capecitabine, AST or ALT >2.5x ULN or bilirubin >1x ULN. History of severe (CTC Grade 3/4) hypersensitivity reaction to Cremophor EL or derivatives (eg, polyoxyethylated castor oil).

WARNINGS/PRECAUTIONS: Peripheral neuropathy may occur; monitor for symptoms and manage by dose adjustment and delays. Myelosuppression, primarily neutropenia, may occur and is dose-dependent; monitor with frequent peripheral blood cell counts and adjust dose as needed. Hypersensitivity reactions may occur; premedicate all patients with H_1- and H_2-antagonists 1 hr before treatment. Caution with history of cardiac disease. Consider discontinuation of therapy if cardiac ischemia or impaired cardiac function develops. Avoid monotherapy if AST or ALT >10x ULN or bilirubin >3x ULN and use caution if AST or ALT >5x ULN.

ADVERSE REACTIONS: Peripheral neuropathy, fatigue/asthenia, myalgia/arthralgia, alopecia, NV, stomatitis/mucositis, diarrhea, musculoskeletal pain, palmar-plantar erythrodysesthesia (hand-foot) syndrome, anorexia, abdominal pain, nail disorder, constipation, neutropenia, leukopenia, anemia, thrombocytopenia.

INTERACTIONS: CYP3A4 inhibitors may increase levels; avoid or reduce dose with strong CYP3A4 inhibitors (eg, ketoconazole, itraconazole, clarithromycin, atazanavir, nefazodone, saquinavir, telithromycin, ritonavir, amprenavir, indinavir, nelfinavir, delavirdine, voriconazole), use caution with mild/moderate CYP3A4 inhibitors (eg, erythromycin, fluconazole, verapamil), and monitor all patients closely for acute toxicities. Strong CYP3A4 inducers (eg, dexamethasone, phenytoin, carbamazepine, rifampin, rifampicin, rifabutin, phenobarbital) may decrease levels; consider alternative agents. St. John's wort may decrease levels and should be avoided.

PREGNANCY: Category D, not for use in nursing.

MECHANISM OF ACTION: Microtubule inhibitor; binds directly to β-tubulin subunits on microtubules, leading to suppression of microtubule dynamics.

PHARMACOKINETICS: Absorption: C_{max}=252ng/mL; T_{max}=3 hrs; AUC=2143ng•hr/mL. **Distribution:** V_d=1000L. **Metabolism:** Liver (oxidation) via CYP3A4. **Elimination:** Urine (1.6%), feces (5.6%); $T_{1/2}$=52 hrs.

NURSING CONSIDERATIONS

Assessment: Assess for hypersensitivity to Cremophor EL or polyoxyethylated castor oil, history of cardiac disease, renal dysfunction, pregnancy/nursing status, and possible drug interactions. Obtain baseline LFTs and peripheral blood cell count.

Monitoring: Monitor LFTs and peripheral blood cell count periodically, for signs/symptoms of neuropathy, myelosuppression, fever/neutropenia, and hypersensitivity reactions.

Patient Counseling: Caution may impair mental/physical abilities. Instruct not to drink grapefruit juice. Inform of pregnancy/nursing risks; advise to use effective contraceptive methods and not to nurse. Advise to seek medical attention if symptoms of peripheral neuropathy (numbness, tingling in hands or feet), fever/neutropenia (chills, cough, burning or pain urinating), hypersensitivity reaction (urticaria, pruritis, rash, flushing, swelling, chest tightness, dyspnea), or cardiac events (chest pain, difficulty breathing, palpitations, unusual weight gain) occur.

Administration: IV infusion. **Storage**: Refrigerate; 2-8°C (36-46°F). Protect from light. (Constituted) Store for maximum 1 hr at room temperature and room light. (Diluted) Stable at room temperature and room light for maximum of 6 hrs.

JANUMET RX

metformin HCl - sitagliptin (Merck)

Lactic acidosis may occur due to metformin accumulation. If acidosis is suspected, d/c drug and hospitalize patient immediately.

THERAPEUTIC CLASS: Dipeptidyl peptidase-4 inhibitor/biguanide

INDICATIONS: Adjunct to diet and exercise to improve glycemic control in adult patients with type 2 diabetes mellitus who are not adequately controlled on metformin or sitagliptin alone or in patients already being treated with the combination of sitagliptin and metformin. Not for use in patients with type 1 diabetes or for treatment of diabetic ketoacidosis.

DOSAGE: *Adults:* Individualize dosing. Patient Not Controlled on Metformin Monotherapy: Initial: 100mg/day (50mg bid) of sitagliptin + metformin dose. Patient on Metformin 850mg BID: Initial: 50mg-1000mg tab bid. Patient Not Controlled on Sitagliptin Monotherapy: Initial: 50mg-500mg tab bid. Titrate: Gradual increase to 50mg-1000mg tab bid. Max: 100mg of sitagliptin and 2000mg of metformin. Take with meals.

HOW SUPPLIED: Tab: (Sitagliptin-Metformin) 50mg-500mg, 50mg-1000mg

CONTRAINDICATIONS: Renal disease (SrCr ≥1.5mg/dL [males], ≥1.4mg/dL [females], or abnormal CrCl), metabolic acidosis, including diabetic ketoacidosis. D/C for 48 hrs in patients undergoing radiologic studies with intravascular iodinated contrast materials.

WARNINGS/PRECAUTIONS: Lactic acidosis reported (rare), increased risk with renal dysfunction. Assess renal function prior to initiation and during treatment; caution in elderly. Avoid in renal/hepatic impairment. May decrease vitamin B_{12} levels; monitor hematologic parameters. May cause hypoglycemia in elderly, debilitated/malnourished, adrenal or pituitary insufficiency, or alcohol intoxication. D/C in hypoxic states (eg, CHF, shock, acute MI), prior to surgical procedures (due to restricted food and fluid intake), and procedures requiring use of intravascular iodinated contrast materials.

J

ADVERSE REACTIONS: (Metformin) Diarrhea, NV, flatulence, abdominal discomfort, indigestion, asthenia, and headache. (Sitagliptin) Nasopharyngitis.

INTERACTIONS: Furosemide, nifedipine, and cationic drugs (eg, digoxin, amiloride, procainamide, quinidine, quinine, ranitidine, trimethoprim, vancomycin, triamterene, morphine) may increase metformin levels. Caution with concomitant medications affecting renal function or metformin disposition. Thiazides and other diuretics, corticosteroids, phenothiazines, thyroid products, estrogens, oral contraceptives, phenytoin, nicotinic acid, sympathomimetics, CCBs, and isoniazid may cause hyperglycemia. Alcohol may potentiate effect of metformin on lactate metabolism; avoid excessive alcohol intake. May decrease furosemide levels. Monitor digoxin levels.

PREGNANCY: Category B, caution in nursing.

MECHANISM OF ACTION: Sitagliptin: Dipeptidyl peptidase-4 inhibitor; acts by slowing the inactivation of incretin hormones. Metformin: Biguanide; decreases hepatic glucose production, decreases intestinal absorption of glucose, and improves insulin selectivity by increasing peripheral glucose uptake and utilization.

PHARMACOKINETICS: Absorption: Sitagliptin: Absolute bioavailability (87%). Metformin: Absolute bioavailability (50-60%). **Distribution**: Sitagliptin: V_d=198L. Metformin: V_d=654L; plasma protein binding (38%). **Metabolism:** Sitagliptin: CYP3A4 and CYP2C8. **Elimination**: Sitagliptin: Feces (13%), urine (87%); $T_{1/2}$=12.4 hrs. Metformin: Urine (90%); $T_{1/2}$=6.2 hrs (plasma), 17.6 hrs (blood).

NURSING CONSIDERATIONS

Assessment: Assess FPG, HbA_{1c}, renal function, LFTs, CBC. Assess for CHF, septicemia, acute or chronic metabolic acidosis, adrenal or pituitary insufficiency, alcoholism, pregnancy status. Evaluate for other medical/surgical conditions and for possible drug interactions.

Monitoring: Monitor for hypoglycemia, lactic acidosis, prerenal azotemia, CHF, CVD. Monitor FPG, HbA_{1c}, renal function, LFTs, CBC, hypersensitivity reactions (eg, anaphylaxis), angioedema, exfoliative skin conditions (eg, Stevens-Johnson syndrome).

Patient Counseling: Inform drug is adjunct to diet and exercise; take as prescribed with meals. During periods of stress (eg, fever, trauma, infection, surgery), medication requirements may change; seek medical advice promptly. Advise that excessive alcohol intake increases the risk of hypoglycemia.

Report unexplained hyperventilation, myalgia, malaise, NV, and somnolence. Not recommended for use during pregnancy. Counsel about adverse effects; seek medical attention if any develop. Regular follow-ups needed.

Administration: Oral route. **Storage:** 20-25°C (68-77°F); excursions permitted to 15-30°C (59-86°F).

JANUVIA RX

sitagliptin phosphate (Merck)

THERAPEUTIC CLASS: Dipeptidyl peptidase-4 inhibitor

INDICATIONS: Monotherapy/Combination Therapy: Adjunct to diet and exercise to improve glycemic control in patients with type 2 diabetes mellitus. Avoid use in patients with type I diabetes or for treatment of diabetic ketoacidosis. Not studied in combination with insulin.

DOSAGE: *Adults:* 100mg qd. CrCl ≥30 to <50mL/min: 50mg qd. CrCl: <30mL/min: 25mg qd.

HOW SUPPLIED: Tab: 25mg, 50mg, 100mg

CONTRAINDICATIONS: Anaphylaxis or angioedema.

WARNINGS/PRECAUTIONS: Assess renal function prior to initiation of treatment. May cause hypoglycemia when used in combination with a sulfonylurea. Anaphylaxis, angioedema, and exfoliative skin conditions reported.

ADVERSE REACTIONS: (Monotherapy/Combination therapy) Upper respiratory tract infection, nasopharyngitis, headache. (Combination therapy) hypoglycemia.

INTERACTIONS: May slightly increase digoxin levels; monitor appropriately. May require lower dose of sulfonylurea to reduce risk of hypoglycemia.

PREGNANCY: Category B, caution in nursing.

MECHANISM OF ACTION: Dipeptidyl peptidase-4 inhibitor; suspected to exert action by slowing the inactivation of incretin hormones.

PHARMACOKINETICS: Absorption: Rapidly absorbed; absolute bioavailability (87%); T_{max}=1-4 hrs; AUC=8.52µM•hr; C_{max}=950nM. **Distribution:** V_d=198L; plasma protein binding (38%). **Metabolism:** Via CYP3A4 and CYP2C8 (minor). **Elimination:** Feces (13%), urine (87%); $T_{1/2}$=12.4 hrs.

NURSING CONSIDERATIONS

Assessment: Assess FPG, HbA_{1c}, renal function, ESRD, pregnancy status, type 1 DM. Evaluate for other medical/surgical conditions and for possible drug interactions.

Monitoring: Monitor for hypoglycemia, FPG, HbA_{1c}, renal function, diabetic ketoacidosis, URTI, nasopharyngitis, hypersensitivity reactions (eg, anaphylaxis, angioedema, exfoliative skin conditions, including Stevens-Johnson syndrome).

Patient Counseling: Inform drug is adjunct to diet and exercise. Counsel about adverse effects; seek medical attention if any develop. Regular follow-ups needed; take as prescribed. During periods of stress (eg, fever, trauma, infection, surgery), medication requirements may change; seek medical advice promptly.

Administration: Oral route. **Storage:** 20-25°C (68-77°F); excursions permitted to 15-30°C (59-86°F).

KADIAN

CII

morphine sulfate (Alpharma)

Contains morphine sulfate, an opioid agonist and Schedule II controlled substance, with an abuse liability similar to other opioid analgesics. Indicated for management of moderate-to-severe pain when a continuous, around-the-clock opioid analgesic is needed for an extended period of time. Not for use as a prn analgesic. The 100mg and 200mg capsules are for use in opioid-tolerant patients only. Swallow capsules whole or sprinkle contents on apple sauce. Do not crush, chew, or dissolve pellets in capsules.

THERAPEUTIC CLASS: Opioid analgesic

INDICATIONS: Management of moderate to severe pain.

DOSAGE: *Adults:* Individualize dose. Conversion from other Oral Morphine: Give 50% of daily oral morphine dose q12h or give 100% oral morphine dose q24h. Do not give more frequently than q12h. Conversion from Parenteral Morphine: Oral morphine 3x the daily parenteral morphine dose may be sufficient in chronic use settings. Conversion from Other Parenteral or Oral Opioids: Initial: Give 50% of estimated daily morphine demand and supplement with immediate-release morphine. May sprinkle contents on small amount of applesauce or in water for gastrostomy tube. Do not chew, crush or dissolve pellets. Avoid administration through NG-tube.

HOW SUPPLIED: Cap, Extended-Release: 10mg, 20mg, 30mg, 50mg, 60mg, 80mg, 100mg, 200mg

K

CONTRAINDICATIONS: Respiratory depression in the absence of resuscitative equipment, acute or severe bronchial asthma, paralytic ileus.

WARNINGS/PRECAUTIONS: Respiratory depression possible; caution in COPD, cor pulmonale, decreased respiratory reserve. May obscure neurologic signs in head injuries, intracranial lesions, or a pre-existing increase in ICP. May cause severe hypotension. Avoid with GI obstruction. Caution in biliary tract disease, elderly, debilitated, renal/hepatic insufficiency, Addison's disease, myxedema, hypothyroidism, prostatic hypertrophy, urethral stricture, CNS depression, toxic psychosis, acute alcoholism, delirium tremens, and convulsive disorders. Depresses cough reflex. Decreases gastric, biliary, and pancreatic secretions. D/C 24 hrs before procedure that interrupts pain transmission pathways (eg, cordotomy); give short-acting parenteral opioid.

ADVERSE REACTIONS: Drowsiness, dizziness, constipation, nausea, anxiety.

INTERACTIONS: Increased risk of respiratory depression, hypotension, profound sedation or coma with CNS depressants (eg, sedatives, hypnotics, general anesthetics, antiemetics, phenothiazines, tranquilizers, alcohol); reduce initial dose of one or both agents by 50%. May enhance neuromuscular blocking action of skeletal relaxants. Mixed agonist/antagonist analgesics may reduce analgesic effects or precipitate withdrawal symptoms. Avoid MAOIs during or within 14 days of use. May reduce diuretic effects.

PREGNANCY: Category C, not for use in nursing.

MECHANISM OF ACTION: Opioid analgesic; principle actions are analgesia and sedation. Precise mechanism of analgesic effects not established. Acts as a pure agonist, binding with and activating opioid receptors at sites in the peri-aqueductal and periventricular gray matter, the ventromedial medulla, and the spinal cord to produce analgesia.

PHARMACOKINETICS: Absorption: Various doses resulted in different parameters. **Distribution:** V_d=3-4 L/kg; plasma protein binding (30-35%); distributed to skeletal muscle, kidneys, liver, intestinal tract, lungs, spleen, brain; crosses the blood brain barrier (small amount); crosses placental membranes; found in breast milk. **Metabolism:** Liver (conjugation) to glucuronide metabolites; morphine-3-glucuronide (major metabolite), morphine-6-glucuronide (active metabolite). **Elimination:** Urine (major) (metabolites, 10% unchanged); bile (small amount); feces (7-10%); $T_{1/2}$=2-4 hrs.

NURSING CONSIDERATIONS

Assessment: Assess for opioid tolerance, pain levels, abuse potential, severe bronchial asthma, COPD, circulatory shock, GI obstruction (paralytic ileus), presence of debilitation (elderly), hepatic/renal impairment, presence of head injury or other intracranial lesions, increased intracranial pressure, adrenocortical insufficiency (eg, Addison's disease), CNS depression or coma, toxic psychosis, prostatic hypertrophy or urtheral stricture, acute alcoholism, delirium tremens, kyphoscoliosis, convulsive disorders, biliary tract disease (acute pancreatitis), pregnancy/nursing status, and drug interactions.

Monitoring: Monitor for signs/symptoms of respiratory depression, hypotension, anaphylaxis, convulsions, tolerance and physical dependence (eg, withdrawal symptoms), and signs of medication misuse or abuse. Monitor serum amylase levels.

Patient Counseling: Swallow medication whole (do not chew, crush, or dissolve) or open and sprinkle contents of capsule on small amount of applesauce; applesauce should be at room temperature or cooler. Instruct to rinse mouth after taking dose to ensure all pellets have been swallowed. Capsule may be administered through a French 16 gastrostomy tube if there is difficulty swallowing. Do not adjust dosing without physician's consent. Inform drug may impair mental/physical abilities; use caution when performing hazardous tasks (eg, operating machinery/driving). Avoid alcohol and other CNS depressants. Do not abruptly d/c medication. May develop severe constipation during therapy; appropriate concomitant therapy should be given at start of treatment. Medication has potential for abuse. Instruct to keep out of reach of children. If treatment is complete, dispose unused capsules via toilet.

Administration: Oral route. **Storage:** 25°C (77°F); excursions permitted to 15-30°C (59-86°F). Protect from light and moisture. Dispense in a sealed tamper-evident, childproof, light-resistant container.

K

KALETRA — RX

ritonavir - lopinavir (Abbott)

THERAPEUTIC CLASS: Protease inhibitor

INDICATIONS: Treatment of HIV infection in combination with other antiretrovirals.

DOSAGE: *Adults:* Therapy-Naive: 400/100mg (2 tabs or 5mL) bid or 800/200mg qd (4 tabs or 10mL). Therapy-Experienced: 400/100mg (2 tabs or 5mL) bid. Once daily administration not recommended. Concomitant Efavirenz, Nevirapine, Fosamprenavir, Nelfinavir: Therapy-Naive: 400/100mg (2 tabs) bid. Concomitant Efavirenz, Nevirapine, Amprenavir or Nelfinavir: 533/133mg (6.5mL) bid. Concomitant Efavirenz, Nevirapine, Fosamprenavir without Ritonavir, or Nelfinavir: Treatment-Experienced with Decreased Susceptibility to Lopinavir: 600/150mg (3 tabs) bid. Tabs can be taken with or without food. Oral solution must be taken with food.
Pediatrics: >12 yrs: Therapy-Naive: 400/100mg (2 tabs or 5mL) bid or 800/200mg qd (4 tabs or 10mL). Therapy-Experienced: 400/100mg (2 tabs or 5mL) bid. Once daily administration not recommended. Concomitant Efavirenz, Nevirapine, Fosamprenavir, Nelfinavir: Therapy-Naive: 400/100mg (2 tabs) bid. Concomitant Efavirenz, Nevirapine, Amprenavir or Nelfinavir: 533/133mg (6.5mL) bid. Concomitant Efavirenz, Nevirapine, Fosamprenavir without Ritonavir, or Nelfinavir: Treatment-Experienced with Decreased Susceptibility to Lopinavir: 600/150mg (3 tabs) bid. 6 months-12 yrs: >40kg: 400/100mg (4 tabs 100/25 mg, 2 tabs 200/50 mg or 5 mL) bid. 15-40kg: (Tab,Sol) 10/2.5mg/kg bid. 7-<15kg: (Sol) 12/3mg/kg bid. Concomitant Efavirenz, Nevirapine, (Fos)amprenavir: >45kg: 533/133mg (4 tabs 100/25 mg, 2 tabs 200/50 mg, or 6.5mL) bid. 15-45kg: (Tab,Sol) 11/2.75mg/kg bid. 7-<15kg: (Sol) 13/3.25mg/kg bid. Tabs can be taken with or without food. Oral solution must be taken with food.

HOW SUPPLIED: Tab: (Lopinavir-Ritonavir) 200mg-50mg, 100mg-25mg; Sol: 80mg-20mg/mL [160mL]

CONTRAINDICATIONS: Concomitant drugs dependent on CYP3A or CYP2D6 for clearance (eg, rifampin, St John's wort, lovastatin, simvastatin, dihydroergotamine, ergonovine, ergotamine, methylergonovine, cisapride, pimozide, midazolam, triazolam).

WARNINGS/PRECAUTIONS: May elevate triglyceride and total cholesterol levels; monitor levels at baseline then periodically. Possible redistribution or accumulation of body fat. D/C if symptoms of pancreatitis occur. May exacerbate DM or cause hyperglycemia. Caution in hepatic impairment. Increased bleeding may occur with hemophilia A and B. Risk of further transaminase elevation or hepatic decompensation in patients with underlying hepatitis B or C or marked transaminase elevation prior to treatment; monitor ALT/AST more frequently during first several months of therapy. Hepatic dysfunction reported.

ADVERSE REACTIONS: Abdominal pain, asthenia, headache, diarrhea, NV, dyspepsia, flatulence, insomnia, hepatotoxicity, pancreatitis.

INTERACTIONS: See Contraindications. Avoid use with rifampin, St. John's wort; may cause loss of virologic response and resistance. Avoid use with lovastatin and simvastatin; risk of myopathy and rhabdomyolysis. May increase levels of antiarrhythmics (eg, amiodarone, bepridil, systemic lidocaine, quinidine), dihydropyridine CCBs (eg, felodipine, nifedipine, nicardipine), immunosuppressants (eg, cyclosporine, tacrolimus, rapamycin); monitoring recommended. May increase levels of trazodone; use with caution and consider lower trazodone dose. May increase levels of fluticasone; coadministration not recommended. CYP3A inducers may decrease lopinavir levels. CYP3A inhibitors may increase lopinavir levels. May increase levels of drugs primarily metabolized by CYP3A. May increase levels of amprenavir, indinavir, saquinavir. May increase levels of clarithromycin with renal impairment; reduce clarithromycin dose by 50% if CrCl 30-60mL/min and by 75% if CrCl <30mL/min. Decreased effect with dexamethasone, carbamazepine, phenobarbital, phenytoin. Monitor PT/INR with warfarin. Space dosing with didanosine; give 1 hr before or 2 hrs after lopinavir/ritonavir. Increased levels with delavirdine. Efavirenz, nevirapine, and tipranavir may decrease levels; adjust dose. May increase levels of ketoconazole or itraconazole; avoid ketoconazole or itraconazole doses >200mg/day. May increase rifabutin levels; reduce usual rifabutin dose by 75%. Decreases atovaquone levels. Oral solution contains alcohol; disulfiram reaction may occur with disulfiram or metronidazole. May increase sildenafil, tadalafil, vardenafil levels; reduce dose of sildenafil (eg, 25mg q48h); reduce dose of tadalafil (eg, 10mg q72h); reduce dose of vardenafil (eg, 2.5mg q72h). May decrease methadone levels; may need to increase methadone dose. May decrease ethinyl estradiol levels; use alternate/additional contraception. Increased atorvastatin levels; use lowest atorvastatin or rosuvastatin dose or consider alternate HMG-CoA reductase inhibitors (eg, pravastatin, fluvastatin). Increases tenofovir levels. May increase nelfinavir levels; dosage adjustments needed. Do not administer with tipranivir coadministered with ritonavir.

K

PREGNANCY: Category C, not for use in nursing.

MECHANISM OF ACTION: Lopinavir: HIV-1 protease inhibitor; prevents cleavage of the Gag-Pol polyprotein, resulting in the production of immature, noninfectious viral particles. Ritonavir: CYP3A inhibitor; inhibits metabolism of lopinavir, increasing its plasma levels.

PHARMACOKINETICS: Absorption: Lopinavir: C_{max}=9.8mcg/mL, T_{max}=4 hrs, AUC=92.6mcg•h/mL. **Distribution:** Lopinavir: Plasma protein binding (98-99%). **Metabolism:** Lopinavir: Hepatic via CYP3A. Ritonavir: Induces own metabolism. **Elimination:** Urine (2.2%), feces (19.8%).

NURSING CONSIDERATIONS

Assessment: Assess for HBV, HCV, DM, hemophilia, renal/hepatic impairment, history of pancreatitis, and possible drug interactions.

Monitoring: Monitor liver function, total cholesterol, triglyceride, transaminase elevation, glucose, total bilirubin, AST, ALT, GGT, amylase. Monitor for signs/symptoms of pancreatitis, hyperglycemia, hepatoxicity, infections, and fat redistribution.

Patient Counseling: Instruct that tablet may be taken with/without food, swallowed whole and solution must be taken with food. If missed dose, take dose as soon as possible and return to normal schedule; do not double next dose. Seek medical attention if symptoms of pancreatitis (NV, abdominal pain), hyperglycemia, or fat redistribution occur.

Administration: Oral route. **Storage:** (Tab): 20-25°C (68-77°F); excursions permitted to 15-30°C (59-86°F). (Sol): 2-8°C (36-46°F). Avoid exposure to excessive heat.

KAPIDEX RX
dexlansoprazole (Takeda)

THERAPEUTIC CLASS: Proton pump inhibitor

INDICATIONS: Healing of all grades of erosive esophagitis (EE) for up to 8 weeks. Maintain healing of EE for up to 6 months. Treatment of heartburn associated with nonerosive gastroesophageal reflux disease (GERD) for 4 weeks.

DOSAGE: *Adults:* EE: 60mg qd for up to 8 weeks. Maint: 30mg qd for 6 months. Symptomatic Nonerosive GERD: 30mg qd for 4 weeks. Moderate Hepatic Impairment (Child-Pugh Class B): 30mg qd. Swallow whole. Can open cap and sprinkle intact granules on 1 tbl of applesauce; swallow immediately.

HOW SUPPLIED: Cap, Delayed-Release: 30mg, 60mg

WARNINGS/PRECAUTIONS: Symptomatic response does not preclude the presence of gastric malignancy.

ADVERSE REACTIONS: Diarrhea, abdominal pain, NV, upper respiratory tract infection, and flatulence.

INTERACTIONS: May reduce plasma levels of atazanavir; avoid concurrent use. May alter absorption of pH-dependent drugs (eg, ampicillin esters, digoxin, iron salts, ketoconazole). Concomitant use with warfarin may increase INR and PT.

PREGNANCY: Category B, not for use in nursing.

MECHANISM OF ACTION: Proton pump inhibitor; suppressess gastric acid secretion by specific inhibition of the (H^+,K^+) -ATPase in the gastric parietal cell.

PHARMACOKINETICS: Absorption: T_{max}= 1-2 hrs (1st peak) and 4-5 hrs (2nd peak). (60mg) C_{max}=1397ng/mL, AUC_{24}=6529ng•h/mL. (30mg) C_{max}=658ng/mL, AUC_{24}=3275ng•h/mL. **Distribution:** V_d=40.3L; plasma protein binding (98.8%). **Metabolism:** Liver (extensive) via CYP3A4 and CYP2C19. **Elimination:** Urine, feces (47.6%); $T_{1/2}$=1-2 hrs.

NURSING CONSIDERATIONS

Assessment: Assess for hepatic/renal impairment, pregnancy/nursing status, and possible drug interactions. Assess INR and PT.

Monitoring: Monitor for LFTs, INR, PT, hypersensitivity reactions, and hepatic impairment.

Patient Counseling: Instruct to swallow whole without regard to food. May add or sprinkle intact granules into one tablespoon of applesauce if cannot swallow whole. Notify physician if pregnant or intend to become pregnant, breastfeeding, or have liver problems.

Administration: Oral route. **Storage:** Store at 25°C (77°F); excursions permitted to 15-30°C (59-86°F).

KAYEXALATE RX
sodium polystyrene sulfonate (Sanofi-Aventis)

THERAPEUTIC CLASS: Cation-exchange resin

INDICATIONS: Treatment of hyperkalemia.

DOSAGE: *Adults:* PO: 15g qd-qid. Rectal Enema: 30-50g q6h. *Pediatrics:* Use 1g per 1mEq of K^+ as basis of calculation. Avoid PO administration in neonates.

HOW SUPPLIED: Sus: 15g/60mL

CONTRAINDICATIONS: Hypokalemia, obstructive bowel disease, neonates with reduced gut motility (post-op or drug-induced), oral administration in neonates.

WARNINGS/PRECAUTIONS: Hypokalemia may occur. May be insufficient for emergency correction of hyperkalemia. Monitor for electrolyte disturbances. Caution in those intolerant to sodium increases (eg, severe CHF or HTN, or marked edema).

ADVERSE REACTIONS: Anorexia, NV, constipation, hypokalemia, hypocalcemia, sodium retention, diarrhea, (elderly) fecal impaction.

INTERACTIONS: Avoid nonabsorbable cation-donating antacids and laxatives; systemic alkalosis may occur (eg, magnesium hydroxide, aluminum carbonate). Hypokalemia exaggerates toxic effects of digitalis. Intestinal obstruction reported with aluminum hydroxide. May decrease absorption of lithium and thyroxine. Avoid sorbitol.

PREGNANCY: Category C, caution in nursing.

MECHANISM OF ACTION: Cation exchange resin; partially releases sodium ions and replaced by K^+ ions.

NURSING CONSIDERATIONS

Assessment: Assess for hypokalemia, obstructive bowel disease, neonates with reduced gut motility, CHF, HTN, marked edema, and possible drug interactions.

Monitoring: Monitor for hypersensitivity reactions, hypokalemia, cardiac arrhythmias, electrolyte disturbances, systemic alkalosis, and constipation.

Patient Counseling: Counsel about potential side effects and advise to seek medical attention if signs/symptoms develop.

Administration: Oral/Rectal routes. **Storage:** 25°C (77°F); excursions permitted to 15-30°C (59-86°F).

K-DUR

RX

potassium chloride (Schering)

THERAPEUTIC CLASS: K^+ supplement

INDICATIONS: (For those unable to tolerate liquid or effervescent potassium preparations). Treatment and prevention of hypokalemia with or without metabolic alkalosis. Treatment of digitalis intoxication and hypokalemic familial periodic paralysis.

DOSAGE: *Adults:* Prevention: 20mEq/day. Hypokalemia: 40-100mEq/day. Divide dose if >20mEq. Take with meals and a full glass of water or liquid. Tab can be broken in half or dissolved in water.

HOW SUPPLIED: Tab, Extended-Release: 10mEq, 20mEq* *scored

CONTRAINDICATIONS: Hyperkalemia, esophageal ulceration, delay in GI passage (from structural, pathological, pharmacologic causes), cardiac patients with esophageal compression due to enlarged left atrium.

WARNINGS/PRECAUTIONS: Potentially fatal hyperkalemia may occur. Extreme caution with acidosis, cardiac and renal disease; monitor ECG and electrolytes. Hypokalemia with metabolic acidosis should be treated with an alkalinizing potassium salt (eg, potassium bicarbonate, potassium citrate). May produce ulcerative or stenotic GI lesions.

ADVERSE REACTIONS: Hyperkalemia, GI effects (obstruction, bleeding, ulceration), nausea, vomiting, abdominal pain, flatulence, diarrhea.

INTERACTIONS: Risk of hyperkalemia with ACE inhibitors (eg, captopril, enalapril), K^+-sparing diuretics and K^+ supplements. Contraindicated with anticholinergic agents due to possible delay in tablet passage through GI tract.

PREGNANCY: Category C, safe for use in nursing.

MECHANISM OF ACTION: K^+ supplement (electrolyte replenisher); potassium ions participate in maintenance of intracellular tonicity, transmission of nerve impulses, contraction of cardiac, skeletal, and smooth muscle, and maintenance of normal renal function.

NURSING CONSIDERATIONS

Assessment: Assess for chronic renal disease, conditions which impair K^+ excretion, esophageal compression due to enlarged left atrium, structural/pathologic cause for arrest/delay in passing through GI (diabetic gastroparesis), and possible drug interactions. Obtain baseline serum K^+ levels and renal function test.

Monitoring: Monitor serum K^+ levels, renal function, ECG, and acid-base balance. Monitor for hyperkalemia, signs of acute metabolic acidosis, acute dehydration, GI ulcerations, and hypersensitivity reactions.

Patient Counseling: Instruct to report symptoms of GI bleeding (tarry stools), ulcerations/perforations (severe vomiting, abdominal pain, distention), trouble swallowing, or tablet sticking in throat. Take with meals and full glass of water; swallow whole, do not crush, chew, or suck. If difficulty swallowing whole tablet; break tablet in half. Take each half separately with glass of water or place whole tab in 1/2 glass of water and allow 2 min to disintegrate, stir for half min after disintegration, swirl suspension and drink content. Add another 1oz of water, swirl, and drink immediately and repeat once more.

Administration: Oral route. **Storage:** 25°C (77°F); excursions permitted to 15-30°C (59-86°F). Keep tightly closed.

KENALOG — RX

triamcinolone acetonide (Apothecon)

K

THERAPEUTIC CLASS: Corticosteroid

INDICATIONS: Corticosteroid responsive dermatoses.

DOSAGE: *Adults:* (Cre, Lot, Oint) Apply 0.025% bid-qid. Apply 0.1% or 0.5% bid-tid. (Spray) Apply tid-qid. May use occlusive dressings for psoriasis or recalcitrant conditions. D/C dressings if infection develops.

HOW SUPPLIED: Cre: 0.1% [15g, 60g, 80g], 0.5% [20g]; Lot: 0.025%, 0.1% [60mL]; Oint: 0.1% [15g, 60g]; Spray: 0.147mg/g [63g]

WARNINGS/PRECAUTIONS: May produce reversible HPA axis suppression, manifestations of Cushing's syndrome, hyperglycemia, and glucosuria. D/C if irritation occurs. Pediatrics may be more susceptible to systemic toxicity. Monitor for HPA suppression if applied to large surface areas or under occlusive dressings. Avoid eyes.

ADVERSE REACTIONS: Burning, itching, irritation, dryness, folliculitis, hypertrichosis, acneiform eruptions, hypopigmentation, perioral dermatitis, allergic contact dermatitis.

PREGNANCY: Category C, caution in nursing.

MECHANISM OF ACTION: Corticosteroid; possesses anti-inflammatory, antipruritic, and vasoconstrictive actions. Anti-inflammatory action not established.

PHARMACOKINETICS: Absorption: Percutaneous; inflammation, other disease states, and use of occlusive dressings may increase absorption. **Distribution:** Systemically administered corticosteroids found in breast milk. **Metabolism:** Liver. **Excretion:** Kidneys, bile.

NURSING CONSIDERATIONS

Assessment: Assess pregnancy/nursing status.

Monitoring: Monitor for signs/symptoms of reversible HPA-axis suppression, Cushing's syndrome, hyperglycemia, glucosuria, thermal homeostasis impairment, treatment-site irritation, sensitivity reactions, and presence of dermatological infections (eg, fungal, bacterial). Monitor for withdrawal symptoms following d/c of therapy. If applying high doses of medication to large surface area or if using occlusive dressings, monitor for HPA-axis suppression by using urinary free cortisol and ACTH stimulation tests. (Pediatrics) Monitor for signs/symptoms of systemic toxicity, HPA-axis suppression (eg, linear growth retardation, delayed weight gain), Cushing's syndrome, and intracranial HTN.

Patient Counseling: Instruct to use externally and exactly as directed; avoid contact with eyes. Counsel not to bandage or wrap treated skin areas unless directed by physician. Advise to report any local adverse reactions. Advise caregivers of pediatric patients to avoid using tight fitting diapers or plastic pants on treatment area.

Administration: Topical route. **Storage:** Room temperature; avoid freezing.

KEPIVANCE — RX
palifermin (Amgen)

THERAPEUTIC CLASS: Keratinocyte growth factor

INDICATIONS: Decrease the incidence and duration of severe oral mucositis in patients with hematologic malignancies receiving myelotoxic therapy requiring hematopoietic stem cell support.

DOSAGE: *Adults:* 60mcg/kg/day IV bolus 3 consecutive days before and after myelotoxic therapy for a total of 6 doses.

HOW SUPPLIED: Inj: 6.25mg

CONTRAINDICATIONS: Known hypersensitivity to *E.coli*-derived proteins, palifermin, or any other component of the product.

K

WARNINGS/PRECAUTIONS: Potential for stimulation of tumor growth. Safety and efficacy have not been established in patients with non-hematologic malignancies.

ADVERSE REACTIONS: Rash, erythema, edema, fever, pruritus, dysesthesia, tongue discoloration, tongue thickening, alteration of taste, pain arthralgias.

INTERACTIONS: Do not administer 24 hrs before, during infusion, or 24 hrs after administration of myelotoxic chemotherapy due to risk of increased severity and duration of oral mucositis. If heparin is used to maintain IV line, use saline to rinse prior to and after administration.

PREGNANCY: Category C, caution in nursing.

MECHANISM OF ACTION: Keratinocyte growth factor; binds to the KGF receptor which results in proliferation, differentiation, and migration of the epithelial cells.

PHARMACOKINETICS: Elimination: $T_{1/2}$=4.5 hrs.

NURSING CONSIDERATIONS

Assessment: Assess for hepatic/renal functions, hypersensitivity to *E. coli*-derived proteins, or any other components of the drug.

Monitoring: Monitor for rash, erythema, edema, pruritis, oral/perioral dysthesia, tongue discoloration or thickening, alteration of taste.

Patient Counseling: Counsel about potential side effects; seek medical attention if any develop.

Administration: IV bolus for 3 consecutive days before and after myelotoxic therapy. **Storage:** 2-8°C (36-46°F) for up to 24 hrs. Do not freeze. Protect from light.

KEPPRA — RX
levetiracetam (UCB)

THERAPEUTIC CLASS: Pyrrolidine derivative

INDICATIONS: (PO) Adjunctive therapy for partial onset seizures in adults and children ≥4 yrs. Adjunctive therapy in the treatment of myoclonic seizures in adults and children ≥12 yrs with juvenile myoclonic epilepsy (JME). Adjunctive therapy in the treatment of primary generalized tonic-clonic (PGTC) seizures in adults and children ≥6 yrs with idiopathic generalized epilepsy. (Inj) Adjunctive therapy for partial onset seizures in adults with epilepsy.

Adjunctive therapy for myoclonic seizures in adults with JME. Alternative for adults (≥16 yrs) when oral administration is temporarily not feasible.

DOSAGE: *Adults:* Inj/PO: Initial: 500mg bid. Titrate: Increase by 1000mg/day every 2 weeks. Max: 3000mg/day. Inj: Replacement Therapy: Initial total daily dosage and frequency should equal total daily dosage and frequency of oral therapy. Dilute injection in 100mL of compatible diluent and give as 15-min IV infusion. Individualize dose: CrCl >80mL/min: 500mg-1500mg q12h. CrCl 50-80mL/min: 500mg-1000mg q12h.CrCl 30-50mL/min: 250mg-750mg q12h. CrCl <30mL/min: 250mg-500mg q12h. ESRD with Dialysis: 500-1000mg q24h. A supplemental dose of 250mg-500mg after dialysis is recommended. *Pediatrics:* PO: Partial Onset Seizures/PGTC: ≥16 yrs or JME: ≥12 yrs: Initial: 500mg bid. Titrate: Increase by 1000mg/day every 2 weeks. Max: 3000mg/day. Partial Onset Seizures: 4 to <16 yrs or PGTC: 6-16 yrs: Initial: 10mg/kg bid: Titrate: Increase by 20mg/kg/day every 2 weeks. Max: 60mg/kg/day. (Inj): Partial Onset Seizures: Initial: 500mg bid. Titrate: Increase by 1000mg/day every 2 weeks. Max: 3000mg/day. Replacement Therapy: Initial total daily dosage and frequency should equal total daily dosage and frequency of oral therapy. Dilute injection in 100mL of compatible diluent and give as 15-min IV infusion. CrCl >80mL/min: 500mg-1500mg q12h. CrCl 50-80mL/min: 500mg-1000mg q12h. CrCl 30-50mL/min: 250mg-750mg q12h. CrCl <30mL/min: 250mg-500mg q12h. ESRD with Dialysis: 500mg-1000mg q24h. A supplemental dose of 250mg-500mg after dialysis is recommended.

HOW SUPPLIED: Inj: 500mg/5mL; Sol: 100mg/mL; Tab: 250mg*, 500mg*, 750mg*, 1000mg* *scored

WARNINGS/PRECAUTIONS: Associated with somnolence, fatigue, coordination difficulties, and behavioral abnormalities (eg, psychotic symptoms, suicide ideation, and other abnormalities). Avoid abrupt withdrawal. Hematologic abnormalities reported. Caution in renal dysfunction. Myoclonic seizures reported.

ADVERSE REACTIONS: Somnolence, asthenia, headache, infection, pain, anorexia, dizziness, nervousness, vertigo, ataxia, pharyngitis, rhinitis, irritability, hepatic failure.

PREGNANCY: Category C, not for use in nursing.

MECHANISM OF ACTION: Antiepileptic drug; not established, proposed to inhibit burst firing without affecting normal neuronal excitability, suggesting that it may selectively prevent hypersynchronization of epileptiform burst firing and propagation of seizure activity.

PHARMACOKINETICS: Absorption: Rapid; complete. **Distribution:** Plasma protein binding (<10%); excreted in breast milk. **Metabolism:** Enzymatic hydrolysis (not extensive). Metabolite: Ucb L057. **Elimination:** Renal; urine (66%); $T_{1/2}$=6-8 hrs. Refer to PI for pediatric parameters.

NURSING CONSIDERATIONS

Assessment: Assess renal function, pregnancy status, and possible drug interactions prior to therapy.

Monitoring: Monitor for CNS adverse effects such as somnolence, fatigue, coordination difficulties (ataxia, incoordination), behavioral abnormalities (agitation, anger, emotional lability), suicide ideation. Monitor for hematological changes (RBCs, WBCs).

Patient Counseling: Instruct to take drug exactly as directed. Advise not to drive or operate heavy machinery until accustomed to the effects of medication. Monitor for changes in behavior (eg, aggression, anxiety, apathy, depression, irritability), psychotic symptoms and/or suicidal ideation. Notify if pregnant or intend to become pregnant.

Administration: Oral/IV route. Injection must be diluted prior to administration. Dilute in 100mL of compatible diluent. Refer to PI for further dilution information. IV to Oral Conversion: May switch to oral administration at the equivalent daily IV dosage and frequency. Oral to IV Conversion: The initial daily IV dose should be equivalent to the total daily dosage and frequency of the oral dosing. **Storage:** 25°C (77°F); excursions permitted to 15-30°C (59-86°F). Following IV dilution: Stable for 24 hrs at controlled room temperature 15-30°C (59-86°F).

Keppra XR

levetiracetam (UCB)

RX

THERAPEUTIC CLASS: Pyrrolidine derivative

INDICATIONS: Adjunct therapy for the treatment of partial onset seizures in patients ≥16 years with epilepsy.

DOSAGE: *Adults:* ≥16 yrs: Initial: 1000mg qd. Titrate: Dose adjusted in increments of 1000mg q 2 weeks. Max: 3000mg. CrCl >80mL/min: 1000-3000mg q24h. CrCl 50-80mL/min: 1000-2000mg q24h. CrCl 30-50mL/min: 500-1500mg q24h. CrCl <30mL/min: 500-1000 q24h. Swallow whole; do not chew, break, or crush.

HOW SUPPLIED: Tab, Extended-Release: 500mg, 750mg

WARNINGS/PRECAUTIONS: Associated with somnolence, fatigue, coordination difficulties, and behavioral abnormalities (eg, psychotic symptoms, suicide ideation, and other abnormalities). Withdraw gradually to minimize the potential of increased seizure frequency.

ADVERSE REACTIONS: Somnolence, influenza, nasopharyngitis, irritability, dizziness, and nausea.

PREGNANCY: Category C, not for use in nursing.

MECHANISM OF ACTION: Antiepileptic drug; not established, proposed to inhibit burst firing without affecting normal neuronal excitability, suggesting that it may selectively prevent hypersynchronization of epileptiform burst firing and propagation of seizure activity.

PHARMACOKINETICS: Absorption: Rapid; complete. **Distribution:** Plasma protein binding (<10%); excreted in breast milk. **Metabolism:** Enzymatic hydrolysis (not extensive). Metabolite: UcbL057. **Elimination:** Renal; urine (66%); $T_{1/2}$=7 hrs.

NURSING CONSIDERATIONS

Assessment: Assess renal function, pregnancy/nursing status, and possible drug interactions prior to therapy.

Monitoring: Monitor for CNS adverse effects such as somnolence, fatigue, coordination difficulties (ataxia, incoordination), behavioral abnormalities (agitation, anger, emotional lability), suicide ideation. Monitor for hematological changes (RBCs, WBCs).

Patient Counseling: Instruct to take drug exactly as directed. Advise not to drive or operate heavy machinery until accustomed to the effects of medication. Monitor for changes in behavior (eg, aggression, anxiety, apathy, depression, irritability), psychotic symptoms and/or suicidal ideation. Notify if pregnant or intend to become pregnant.

Administration: Oral route. **Storage:** Store at 25°C (77°F); excursions permitted to 15-30°C (59-86°F).

Ketek

telithromycin (Sanofi-Aventis)

RX

Contraindicated with myasthenia gravis.

THERAPEUTIC CLASS: Ketolide antibiotic

INDICATIONS: Treatment of mild to moderate community-acquired pneumonia (CAP) due to susceptible strains of microorganisms.

DOSAGE: *Adults:* 800mg qd for 7-10 days. Severe Renal Impairment (CrCl <30mL/min): 600mg qd. Hemodialysis: Give after dialysis session on dialysis days. Severe Renal Impairment (CrCl <30mL/min) with Hepatic Impairment: 400mg qd.

HOW SUPPLIED: Tab: 300mg, 400mg [Ketek Pak, 20[s]]

CONTRAINDICATIONS: Myasthenia gravis. History of hepatitis and/or jaundice associated with use of telithromycin or any macrolide antibiotic. Hypersensitivity to macrolide antibiotics; concomitant use with cisapride or pimozide.

WARNINGS/PRECAUTIONS: Acute hepatic failure and severe liver injury, including fulminant hepatitis and hepatic necrosis reported; monitor closely and d/c if any signs/symptoms of hepatitis occur. Visual disturbances and loss of consciousness reported; minimize hazardous activities such as driving and operating heavy machinery. May prolong QTc interval; avoid with congenital prolongation, ongoing proarrhythmic conditions (eg, uncorrected hypokalemia or hypomagnesemia), significant bradycardia. Torsades de pointes reported. *Clostridium difficile*-associated diarrhea reported. Reduce dose with severe renal impairment.

ADVERSE REACTIONS: Diarrhea, NV, headache, dizziness, visual disturbances.

INTERACTIONS: See Contraindications. Increases levels of drugs metabolized by the CYP450 system (eg, carbamazepine, cyclosporine, tacrolimus, sirolimus, hexobarbital, phenytoin, triazolam, metoprolol), especially CYP3A4. Avoid cisapride, pimozide, simvastatin, lovastatin, atorvastatin, rifampin, ergot alkaloid derivatives, Class IA (eg, quinidine, procainamide) or Class III (eg, dofetilide) antiarrhythmics. Increased levels with itraconazole, ketoconazole. Monitor with midazolam, digoxin. Decreased effects with CYP3A4 inducers (eg, phenytoin, carbamazepine, phenobarbital). Decreases levels of sotalol. Space dosing of theophylline by 1 hr to reduce GI effects. Concomitant administration with oral anticoagulants may potentiate effects of the oral anticoagulants.

K

PREGNANCY: Category C, caution in nursing.

MECHANISM OF ACTION: Ketolide; blocks protein synthesis by binding to domains II and V of 23S rRNA of 50S ribosomal subunit. May also inhibit assembly of nascent ribosomal units.

PHARMACOKINETICS: Absorption: Absolute bioavailability (57%); C_{max}=2mcg/mL; T_{max}=1hr. **Distribution:** V_d=2.9L/kg; plasma protein binding (60-70%). **Metabolism:** Metabolized via CYP3A4 dependent and independent pathways. **Elimination:** Urine (13% unchanged); feces (7% unchanged); $T_{1/2}$=10 hrs.

NURSING CONSIDERATIONS

Assessment: Assess for myasthenia gravis, LFTs, QTc prolongation, possible drug interactions. Document indications for therapy, culture and susceptibility testing.

Monitoring: Monitor LFTs, ECG, QTc prolongation, visual disturbances including blurred vision, difficulty focusing, diplopia, loss of consciousness associated with vagal syndrome, renal impairment, *C. difficile*-associated diarrhea, pancreatitis, allergic reactions (angioedema, anaphylaxis).

Patient Counseling: Inform therapy treats bacterial, not viral, infections. Take as directed; skipping doses or not completing full course may decrease effectiveness and increase resistance. Inform may experience diarrhea; notify physician if watery/bloody stools, superinfection, or hypersensitivity reactions occur. Counsel about signs/symptoms of hepatic failure (jaundice, malaise, anorexia), loss of consciousness, and advise to d/c medication. Exercise caution while operating machinery or driving.

Administration: Oral route. Can be given with/without food. Swallow tablet whole. **Storage:** Store at 25°C (77°F); excursions permitted to 15-30°C (59-86°F). Keep out of reach of children.

KETOCONAZOLE TOPICAL RX

ketoconazole (Various)

THERAPEUTIC CLASS: Azole antifungal

INDICATIONS: (Cre) Tinea corporis, tinea cruris, tinea pedis, tinea versicolor, cutaneous candidiasis, seborrheic dermatitis. (Shampoo) Tinea versicolor.

DOSAGE: *Adults:* (Cre) Cutaneous candidiasis, t.corporis, t.cruris, t.versicolor: Apply qd for 2 weeks. T.pedis: Apply qd for 6 weeks. Seborrheic Dermatitis: Apply bid for up to 4 weeks. Re-evaluate if no improvement after treatment period. (Shampoo) Apply to damp skin and lather. Rinse with water after 5 min. One application should be sufficient.

HOW SUPPLIED: Cre: 2% [15g, 30g, 60g]; Shampoo: 2% [120mL]

WARNINGS/PRECAUTIONS: Cre contains sulfites. Shampoo may remove curl from permanently waved hair. Avoid eyes.

ADVERSE REACTIONS: (Cre) Irritation, pruritus, stinging. (Shampoo) Abnormal hair texture, scalp pustules, mild skin dryness, pruritus, increase in normal hair loss, oily or dry scalp and hair.

PREGNANCY: Category C, (Cre) not for use in nursing, (Shampoo) caution in nursing.

MECHANISM OF ACTION: Azole antifungal; impairs synthesis of ergosterol, vital component of fungal cell membranes. Broad spectrum antifungal.

NURSING CONSIDERATIONS

Assessment: Assess for sulfite hypersensitivity. Assess use in pregnant/nursing patients.

K

Monitoring: Monitor for signs/symptoms of sensitivity reactions or chemical irritation and for clinical response following treatment end. Reassess diagnosis if no response.

Patient Counseling: Instruct to report sensitivity or chemical irritation. Counsel that ketoconazole shampoo may irritate mucous membranes of the eyes; avoid contact. Ketoconazole shampoo may remove curls from permanently waved hair.

Administration: Topical route. **Storage:** Store below 25°C (77°F). Protect from light.

KETOROLAC — RX

ketorolac tromethamine (Various)

For short-term use only (≤5 days). Contraindicated with peptic ulcer disease, GI bleeding/perforation, perioperative pain in coronary artery bypass graft (CABG) surgery, advanced renal impairment, risk of renal failure due to volume depletion, CV bleeding, hemorrhagic diathesis, incomplete hemostasis, high-risk of bleeding, intraoperatively when hemostasis is critical, intrathecal/epidural use, L&D, nursing, and with ASA, NSAIDs, or probenecid. Caution greater risk of GI events with elderly patients. NSAIDs may cause an increased risk of CV thrombotic events (MI, stroke). (PO) Contraindicated in pediatric patients and in minor or chronic painful conditions.

OTHER BRAND NAMES: Toradol (Roche Labs)

THERAPEUTIC CLASS: NSAID

INDICATIONS: Short-term (≤5 days) management of moderately severe, acute pain as continuation therapy from IV/IM.

DOSAGE: Adults: >16 yrs to <65 yrs: Single-Dose: 60mg IM or 30mg IV. Multiple-Dose: 30mg IM/IV q6h. Max: 120mg/day. Transition from IM/IV to PO: 20mg PO single dose, then 10mg PO q4-6h. Max: 40mg/24 hrs. ≥65 yrs/Renal Impairment/<50kg: Single-Dose: 30mg IM or 15mg IV. Multiple-Dose: 15mg IM/IV q6h. Max: 60mg/day. Transition from IM/IV to PO: 10mg PO q4-6h. Max: 40mg/24 hrs.

Pediatrics: 2-16 yrs: Single-Dose: IM: 1mg/kg. Max: 30mg. IV: 0.5mg/kg. Max: 15mg.

HOW SUPPLIED: Inj: 15mg/mL, 30mg/mL; Tab: 10mg

CONTRAINDICATIONS: Active or history of peptic ulcer, GI bleeding, perioperative pain in CABG surgery, advanced renal impairment or risk of renal failure due to volume depletion, labor/delivery, nursing mothers, ASA or NSAID allergy, preoperatively or intraoperatively when hemostasis is critical, cerebrovascular bleeding, hemorrhagic diathesis, incomplete hemostasis, high risk of bleeding, neuraxial (epidural or intrathecal) administration, and concomitant ASA, NSAIDs, probenecid, or pentoxifylline.

WARNINGS/PRECAUTIONS: Do not exceed 5 days of therapy. Risk of GI ulcerations, bleeding, and perforation. Caution with renal/hepatic dysfunction, dehydration, HTN, CHF, coagulation disorders, debilitated and elderly, pre-existing asthma. Preoperative use prolongs bleeding. CV thrombotic events, fluid retention, edema, NaCl retention, oliguria, anaphylactic reactions, elevated BUN and SrCr, anemia reported. Correct hypovolemia before therapy.

ADVERSE REACTIONS: Nausea, dyspepsia, GI pain, diarrhea, edema, headache, drowsiness, dizziness.

INTERACTIONS: May increase risk of bleeding with anticoagulants. May reduce diuretic response to furosemide. Increased serum levels with salicylates. Avoid ASA, NSAIDs, and probenecid. Increased lithium and methotrexate levels. May increase risk of renal impairment with ACE-inhibitors. May increase seizures with phenytoin and carbamazepine. Hallucinations reported with fluoxetine, thiothixene, and alprazolam. Do not mix in the same syringe as morphine. May have adverse effects with nondepolarizing muscle relaxants.

PREGNANCY: Category C, not for use in nursing.

MECHANISM OF ACTION: NSAID; suspected to inhibit prostaglandin synthetase; exerts anti-inflammatory, analgesic, and antipyretic actions.

PHARMACOKINETICS: Absorption: Absolute bioavailability (100%). **Distribution:** V_d=13L; plasma protein binding (99%); enters breast milk. **Metabolism:** Liver; hydroxylation, conjugation. **Elimination:** Urine (92%; 40% metabolites, 60% unchanged), feces (6%); $T_{1/2}$=5-6 hrs.

K

NURSING CONSIDERATIONS

Assessment: Assess LFTs, renal function, CBC and coagulation profile. Assess for history of CABG surgery, asthma and allergic reactions to aspirin or other NSAIDs, active ulceration or chronic inflammation of GI tract, CVD, pregnancy status. Note other diseases/conditions and drug therapies.

Monitoring: Monitor for hypersensitivity reactions, cardiac complications, stroke, GI bleeding, asthma, dermatological side effects. Monitor BP, LFTs, renal function, CBC with differential and platelet count, coagulation profile, and ophthalmic exams.

Patient Counseling: Counsel about side effects; seek medical attention if any occur. Avoid alcohol and smoking during treatment. Advise to take exactly as prescribed. Caution women against using late in pregnancy. Inform that drug is used as continuation treatment following IM or IV dosing and should not exceed 5 days.

Administration: IM/IV/Oral routes. **Storage:** 15-30°C (59-86°F).

KINERET — RX

anakinra (Amgen)

THERAPEUTIC CLASS: Interleukin-1 receptor antagonist

INDICATIONS: As sole or adjunct therapy with DMARDs (except TNF blockers) to reduce the signs/symptoms and slow the progression of moderate to severe rheumatoid arthritis unresponsive to one or more DMARDs.

DOSAGE: *Adults:* ≥18 yrs: 100mg SQ qd at approximately same time every day. CrCl <30mL/min: 100mg SQ qod.

HOW SUPPLIED: Inj: 100mg/0.67mL

WARNINGS/PRECAUTIONS: Increased incidence of serious infections alone and with coadministration with etanercept. D/C if serious infection or hypersensitivity reaction occurs. Do not initiate with active infection. Obtain neutrophil count before therapy, monthly for 3 months, quarterly thereafter for up to one yr.

ADVERSE REACTIONS: Injection site reactions, headache, nausea, diarrhea, infections, abdominal pain, arthralgia, flu-like symptoms.

INTERACTIONS: Neutropenia and higher rate of infections reported with etanercept. Vaccines may be ineffective; avoid live vaccines. Concurrent therapy with etanercept is not recommended.

PREGNANCY: Category B, caution in nursing.

MECHANISM OF ACTION: Interleukin-1 receptor antagonist; blocks biologic activity of IL-1 by competitively inhibiting IL-1 binding to the interleukin-1 type I receptor (IL-1RI), which is expressed in a wide variety of tissues and organs.

PHARMACOKINETICS: Absorption: Absolute bioavailability (95%); T_{max}=3-7 hrs. **Elimination:** $T_{1/2}$=4-6 hrs.

NURSING CONSIDERATIONS

Assessment: Assess for known hypersensitivity to *Escherichia coli*-derived proteins, active infection, immunosuppression, severe renal insufficiency or end-stage renal disease, pregnancy/nursing status, and possible drug interactions. Obtain neutrophil count prior to treatment.

Monitoring: Monitor for signs/symptoms of serious infections (eg, cellulitis, pneumonia, bone and joint infections), hypersensitivity reactions, neutropenia, and malignancies (eg, lymphomas). Monitor neutrophil count monthly for 3 months, and quarterly thereafter for up to a year.

Patient Counseling: Advise to avoid receiving live vaccines while on therapy. Counsel about proper dosage and administration of medication, proper disposal of medication; caution against reuse of needles, syringes, and drug product. Medication should not be given in combination with TNF-blocking agents. Counsel about signs/symptoms of allergic and adverse drug reactions. If severe hypersensitivity reaction occurs, d/c medication and start appropriate therapy. Advise that needle cover of prefilled syringe contains dry natural rubber, which may cause allergic reactions in latex-sensitive individuals.

Administration: SQ route. **Storage:** 2-8°C (36-46°F). Do not freeze or shake. Protect from light.

KLONOPIN

CIV

clonazepam (Roche Labs)

OTHER BRAND NAMES: Klonopin Wafers (Roche Labs)

THERAPEUTIC CLASS: Benzodiazepine

INDICATIONS: Adjunct or monotherapy in Lennox-Gastaut syndrome, akinetic and myoclonic seizures. Absence seizures refractory to succinimides. Panic disorder with or without agoraphobia.

DOSAGE: *Adults:* Seizure Disorders: Initial: Not to exceed 1.5mg/day given tid. Titrate: May increase by 0.5-1mg every 3 days. Max: 20mg qd. Panic Disorder: Initial: 0.25mg bid. Titrate: Increase to 1mg/day after 3 days, then may increase by 0.125-0.25mg bid every 3 days. Max: 4mg/day. Wafer: Dissolve in mouth with or without water.

Pediatrics: <10 yrs or 30kg: Seizure Disorders: Initial: 0.01-0.03mg/kg/day up to 0.05mg/kg/day given bid-tid. Titrate: Increase by no more than 0.25-0.5mg every 3 days. Maint: 0.1-0.2mg/kg/day given tid. Wafer: Dissolve in mouth with or without water.

HOW SUPPLIED: Tab: 0.5mg*, 1mg, 2mg; Tab, Disintegrating (Wafer): 0.125mg, 0.25mg, 0.5mg, 1mg, 2mg *scored

CONTRAINDICATIONS: Significant liver disease, acute narrow-angle glaucoma, untreated open-angle glaucoma.

WARNINGS/PRECAUTIONS: May increase incidence of generalized tonic-clonic seizures. Monitor blood counts and LFTs periodically with long-term therapy. Caution with renal dysfunction, chronic respiratory depression. Increased fetal risks during pregnancy. Avoid abrupt withdrawal. Hypersalivation reported. Caution may alter mental alertness.

ADVERSE REACTIONS: Somnolence, depression, ataxia, CNS depression, upper respiratory tract infection, fatigue, dizziness, sinusitis, colpitis.

INTERACTIONS: Decreased serum levels with CYP450 inducers (eg, phenytoin, carbamazepine, phenobarbital). Caution with CYP3A inhibitors (eg, oral antifungals). Alcohol, narcotics, barbiturates, nonbarbiturate hypnotics, antianxiety agents, phenothiazines, thioxanthene and butyrophenone antipsychotics, MAOIs, TCAs and other anticonvulsant drugs potentiate CNS-depressant effects.

PREGNANCY: Category D, not for use in nursing.

MECHANISM OF ACTION: Benzodiazepine; not established, suspected to enhance activity of GABA, the major inhibitory neurotransmitter in the CNS.

PHARMACOKINETICS: Absorption: Rapid and complete. Absolute bioavailability (90%), T_{max}=1-4 hrs. **Distribution:** Plasma protein binding (85%). **Metabolism:** Hepatic via acetylation, hydroxylation, and glucuronidation, CYP450. **Elimination:** Renal. Urine (<2% unchanged); $T_{1/2}$=30-40 hrs.

NURSING CONSIDERATIONS

Assessment: Assess renal/hepatic function prior to therapy, significant liver disease, acute narrow-angle glaucoma, and possible drug interactions. Assess use with open-angle glaucoma and chronic respiratory diseases.

Monitoring: Monitor periodic blood counts and LFTs with prolonged therapy. Monitor for worsening of seizures, status epilepticus with abrupt withdrawal, and renal function with a history of renal impairment.

Patient Counseling: Advise medication may cause CNS depression; avoid operating machinery/driving. Avoid abrupt withdrawal, alcohol use, and the use of other CNS depressants. Take at bedtime to avoid somnolence. Counsel females about possible risks if used during pregnancy.

Administration: Oral route. Disintegrating Tablet: 1) After opening pouch, peel back foil on blister. Do not push tablet through foil. 2) Using dry hands, place tablet in mouth. **Storage:** 25°C (77°F); excursions permitted to 15-30°C (59-86°F).

K

K-LOR RX

potassium chloride (Abbott)

THERAPEUTIC CLASS: K^+ supplement

INDICATIONS: Treatment and prevention of hypokalemia with or without metabolic alkalosis. Treatment of digitalis intoxication and hypokalemic familial periodic paralysis.

DOSAGE: *Adults:* Prevention: 20mEq/day. Hypokalemia: 40-100mEq/day. Divide dose if >20mEq. Dissolve each 20mEq in 4oz of cold water or juice.

HOW SUPPLIED: Pow: 20mEq

CONTRAINDICATIONS: Hyperkalemia.

WARNINGS/PRECAUTIONS: Potentially fatal hyperkalemia may occur. Extreme caution with acidosis, cardiac and renal disease; monitor ECG and electrolytes. Hypokalemia with metabolic acidosis should be treated with an alkalinizing potassium salt (eg, potassium bicarbonate, potassium citrate).

ADVERSE REACTIONS: Hyperkalemia, NV, flatulence, abdominal pain, diarrhea.

INTERACTIONS: Risk of hyperkalemia with ACE inhibitors (eg, captopril, enalapril), K^+-sparing diuretics and K^+ supplements.

PREGNANCY: Category C, safe for use in nursing.

MECHANISM OF ACTION: K^+ supplement (electrolyte replenisher); helps in maintenance of intracellular tonicity, transmission of nerve impulses, contraction of cardiac, skeletal, and smooth muscles, and maintenance of normal renal function.

NURSING CONSIDERATIONS

Assessment: Assess for chronic renal disease, conditions which impair K^+ excretion, and possible drug interactions. Obtain baseline serum K^+ levels and renal function test.

Monitoring: Monitor serum K^+ levels, renal function, ECG, and acid-base balance. Monitor for hyperkalemia, signs of acute metabolic acidosis, acute dehydration, and hypersensitivity reactions.

Patient Counseling: Instruct to report any adverse reactions. Dissolve in 1/2 glass of cold water or juice; take after a meal.

Administration: Oral route. **Storage:** Below 30°C (86°F).

Klor-Con M RX

potassium chloride (Upsher-Smith)

OTHER BRAND NAMES: Klor-Con (Upsher-Smith)

THERAPEUTIC CLASS: K^+ supplement

INDICATIONS: (For those unable to tolerate liquid or effervescent potassium preparations). Treatment of hypokalemia with or without metabolic alkalosis, in digitalis intoxication and with hypokalemic familial periodic paralysis. Prevention of hypokalemia in patients at risk (eg, digitalized, cardiac arrhythmias).

K

DOSAGE: *Adults:* Prevention: 20mEq/day. Hypokalemia: 40-100mEq/day. Divide dose if >20mEq. Take with meals and fluids. Swallow tabs whole; may break Klor-Con M in half or mix with 4 ounces of water.

HOW SUPPLIED: (Klor-Con M) Tab, Extended Release: 10mEq, 15mEq, 20mEq; (Klor-Con) Pow: 20mEq, 25mEq; Tab, Extended Release: 8mEq, 10mEq

CONTRAINDICATIONS: Hyperkalemia, esophageal ulceration, delay in GI passage (from structural, pathological, pharmacologic causes), cardiac patients with esophageal compression due to enlarged left atrium.

WARNINGS/PRECAUTIONS: Potentially fatal hyperkalemia may occur. Extreme caution with acidosis, cardiac, and renal disease; monitor ECG and electrolytes. Hypokalemia with metabolic acidosis should be treated with an alkalinizing potassium salt (eg, potassium bicarbonate, potassium citrate). May produce ulcerative or stenotic GI lesions.

ADVERSE REACTIONS: Hyperkalemia, GI effects (obstruction, bleeding, ulceration), nausea, vomiting, abdominal pain, flatulence, diarrhea.

INTERACTIONS: Risk of hyperkalemia with ACE inhibitors (eg, captopril, enalapril), K^+-sparing diuretics, and K^+ supplements. Contraindicated with anticholinergics or other agents that decrease GI motility.

PREGNANCY: Category C, safe for use in nursing.

MECHANISM OF ACTION: K^+ supplement (electrolyte replenisher); intended to provide extended-release of K^+ from matrix to minimize likelihood of high localized concentrations of K^+ within GI tract.

PHARMACOKINETICS: Absorption: T_{max}=4-8 hrs, GI tract. **Elimination:** Urine and feces.

NURSING CONSIDERATIONS

Assessment: Assess for chronic renal disease, conditions that impair K^+ excretion, esophageal compression due to enlarged left atrium, structural/pathologic cause for arrest/delay in passing through GI tract (diabetic gastroparesis), and possible drug interactions. Obtain baseline serum K^+ levels and renal function test.

Monitoring: Monitor serum K^+ levels, renal function, ECG and acid-base balance. Monitor for hyperkalemia, signs of acute metabolic acidosis, acute dehydration, GI ulcerations, and hypersensitivity reactions.

Patient Counseling: Instruct to report symptoms of GI bleeding (tarry stools), ulcerations/perforations (severe vomiting, abdominal pain, distention), trouble swallowing, or tablet sticking in throat. Take with meals and full glass of water; swallow whole, do not crush, chew, or suck.

Administration: Oral route. **Storage:** 15-30°C (59-86°F). Protect from light and moisture.

KRISTALOSE RX
lactulose (Cumberland)

THERAPEUTIC CLASS: Osmotic laxative

INDICATIONS: Treatment of constipation.

DOSAGE: *Adults:* 10-20g/day. Max 40g/day. Dissolve pkt contents in 4oz of water.

HOW SUPPLIED: Powder (crystals for suspension): 10g/pkt, 20g/pkt [1[s], 30[s]]

CONTRAINDICATIONS: Patients who require a low galactose diet.

WARNINGS/PRECAUTIONS: Caution in DM due to galactose and lactose content. Monitor electrolytes periodically in elderly or debilitated if used for >6 months. Potential for explosive reaction with electrocautery procedures during proctoscopy or colonoscopy.

ADVERSE REACTIONS: Flatulence, intestinal cramps, diarrhea, NV.

INTERACTIONS: Nonabsorbable antacids may decrease effects.

PREGNANCY: Category B, caution in nursing.

MECHANISM OF ACTION: Osmotic laxative; increases osmotic pressure and slight acidification of the colonic contents.

PHARMACOKINETICS: Absorption: Poorly absorbed from GI tract. **Elimination:** Urine (≤3%).

NURSING CONSIDERATIONS

Assessment: Assess for DM, patients requiring a low-galactose diet.

Monitoring: Monitor serum electrolytes (potassium, sodium, chloride, carbon dioxide), diarrhea, vomiting.

Patient Counseling: May be diluted with fruit juice, water, or milk. Report any potential adverse effects.

Administration: Oral route. Dissolve contents of packet in 4 ounces of water. **Storage:** Store 15-30°C (59-86°F).

K-TAB RX
potassium chloride (Abbott)

OTHER BRAND NAMES: Klotrix (Apothecon)

THERAPEUTIC CLASS: K^+ supplement

INDICATIONS: (For those unable to tolerate liquid or effervescent potassium preparations). Treatment and prevention of hypokalemia with or without metabolic alkalosis. Treatment of digitalis intoxication and hypokalemic familial periodic paralysis.

DOSAGE: *Adults:* Prevention: 20mEq/day. Hypokalemia: 40-100mEq/day. Divide dose if >20mEq. Take with meals and full glass of water or liquid. Do not cut, crush or chew tab.

HOW SUPPLIED: Tab, Extended-Release: 10mEq

CONTRAINDICATIONS: Hyperkalemia, esophageal ulceration, delay in GI passage (from structural, pathological, pharmacologic causes), cardiac patients with esophageal compression due to enlarged left atrium.

WARNINGS/PRECAUTIONS: Potentially fatal hyperkalemia may occur. Extreme caution with acidosis, cardiac and renal disease; monitor ECG and electrolytes. Hypokalemia with metabolic acidosis should be treated with an alkalinizing potassium salt (eg, potassium bicarbonate, potassium citrate).

May produce ulcerative or stenotic GI lesions. Use with caution in elderly due to decreased renal function, start dose at low end of dosing range.

ADVERSE REACTIONS: Hyperkalemia, GI effects (obstruction, bleeding, ulceration), nausea, vomiting, abdominal pain, flatulence, diarrhea.

INTERACTIONS: Risk of hyperkalemia with ACE inhibitors (eg, captopril, enalapril), potassium-sparing diuretics and potassium supplements. Contraindicated with anticholinergic agents due to possible delay in tablet passage through GI tract.

PREGNANCY: Category C, safe for use in nursing.

MECHANISM OF ACTION: K^+ supplement (electrolyte replenisher). Slows release of K^+, so likelihood of high localized concentrations of K^+ within GI is reduced.

NURSING CONSIDERATIONS

Assessment: Assess for chronic renal disease, conditions that impair K^+ excretion, esophageal compression due to enlarged left atrium, structural/pathologic cause for arrest/delay in passing through GI tract (eg, diabetic gastroparesis), and possible drug interactions. Obtain baseline serum K^+ levels and renal function test.

Monitoring: Monitor serum K^+ levels, renal function, ECG, and acid-base balance. Monitor for hyperkalemia, signs of acute metabolic acidosis, acute dehydration, GI ulcerations, and hypersensitivity reactions.

K

Patient Counseling: Instruct to report symptoms of GI bleeding (tarry stools), ulcerations/perforations (severe vomiting, abdominal pain, distention), trouble swallowing, or tablet sticking in throat. Take with meals and full glass of water. Swallow whole; do not crush, chew, or suck.

Administration: Oral route. **Storage:** Below 30°C (86°F).

KYTRIL RX

granisetron HCl (Roche Labs)

THERAPEUTIC CLASS: 5-HT_3 receptor antagonist

INDICATIONS: (Inj, Sol, Tab) Prevention of nausea and vomiting associated with chemotherapy. (Sol, Tab) Prevention of nausea and vomiting associated with radiation. (Inj) Prevention and treatment of post-op nausea and vomiting.

DOSAGE: *Adults:* Prevention with Chemotherapy: (PO) 2mg qd up to 1 hr before chemotherapy or 1mg bid (up to 1 hr before chemotherapy and 12 hrs later). (IV) 10mcg/kg within 30 min before chemotherapy. Prevention with Radiation: (PO) 2mg within 1 hr of radiation. Post-Op Prevention: (IV) Administer 1mg over 30 sec before induction of anesthesia or immediately before anesthesia reversal. Post-Op Treatment: (IV) Administer 1mg over 30 sec. *Pediatrics:* 2-16 yrs: Prevention with Chemotherapy: 10mcg/kg IV within 30 min before chemotherapy.

HOW SUPPLIED: Inj: 0.1mg/mL, 1mg/mL; Sol: 2mg/10mL [30mL]; Tab: 1mg

WARNINGS/PRECAUTIONS: (Inj) Does not stimulate gastric or intestinal peristalsis. Do not use instead of nasogastric suction. May mask progressive ileus or gastric distension.

ADVERSE REACTIONS: Headache, asthenia, somnolence, diarrhea, constipation, abdominal pain, dizziness, insomnia, increased hepatic enzymes.

INTERACTIONS: Hepatic CYP450 enzyme inducers or inhibitors may alter clearance.

PREGNANCY: Category B, caution in nursing.

MECHANISM OF ACTION: 5-HT_3 receptor antagonist; blocks serotonin stimulation on vagal nerve terminals and in chemoreceptor trigger zone and subsequent vomiting after emetogenic stimuli.

PHARMACOKINETICS: Absorption: (IV, 40mcg/kg) C_{max}=63.8 ng/mL. (PO,1mg) C_{max}=3.63ng/mL. **Distribution:** Plasma protein binding (65%). (IV) V_d=3.07L/kg; (PO) V_d=3.94L/kg. **Metabolism:** CYP3A4; N-demethylation, oxidation, conjugation. **Elimination:** PO: Urine (11% unchanged), feces. Inj: Urine (12% unchanged), feces; (IV, PO) $T_{1/2}$=8.95 hrs, 6.23 hrs.

NURSING CONSIDERATIONS

Assessment: Assess for possible drug interactions.

Monitoring: Monitor for signs/symptoms of hypersensitivity reactions, progressive ileus, and gastric distention.

Patient Counseling: Advise to seek medical attention if symptoms of hypersensitivity reactions, progressive ileus, or gastric distention occur.

Administration: Oral, IV route. **Storage:** Tab: 15-30°C (59-86°F). Protect from light. Sol, Inj: 25°C (77°F); excursions permitted to 15-30°C (59-86°F). Sol: Store upright, protect from light. Inj: Do not freeze.

LABETALOL — RX

labetalol HCl (Various)

THERAPEUTIC CLASS: Nonselective beta-blocker/$alpha_1$ blocker

INDICATIONS: (Tab) Management of hypertension. (Inj) Management of severe hypertension.

DOSAGE: *Adults:* (Tab) HTN: Initial: 100mg bid. Titrate: 100mg bid every 2-3 days. Maint: 200-400mg bid. Severe HTN: 1200-2400mg/day given bid-tid. Increments should not exceed 200mg bid for titration. (Inj) Severe HTN: Administer in supine position. Repeated IV Infusion: Initial: 20mg over 2 min. Titrate: Give additional 40-80mg at 10 min intervals if needed. Max: 300mg. Slow Continuous Infusion: 200mg at rate of 2mg/min. May adjust dose according to BP. Switch to tabs when BP is stable while in hospital. Initial: 200mg, then 200-400mg 6-12 hrs later on Day 1. Titrate: May increase at 1-day interval.

HOW SUPPLIED: Inj: 5mg/mL; Tab: 100mg*, 200mg*, 300mg *scored

CONTRAINDICATIONS: Bronchial asthma, obstructive airway disease, overt cardiac failure, >1st-degree heart block, cardiogenic shock, severe bradycardia, other conditions associated with severe and prolonged hypotension.

WARNINGS/PRECAUTIONS: Severe hepatocellular injury reported; caution with hepatic dysfunction. Monitor LFTs periodically; d/c at 1st sign of hepatic injury. Caution with well-compensated heart failure. Can cause heart failure. Exacerbation of ischemic heart disease with abrupt withdrawal. Caution in nonallergic bronchospasm patients refractory to or intolerant to other antihypertensives. May mask hypoglycemia symptoms. Withdrawal before surgery is controversial. Paradoxical HTN may occur with pheochromocytoma. Death reported during surgery. Avoid injection with low cardiac indices and elevated systemic vascular resistance.

ADVERSE REACTIONS: Fatigue, dizziness, dyspepsia, nausea, nasal stuffiness.

INTERACTIONS: Increased tremors with TCAs. Potentiated by cimetidine. Blunts reflex tachycardia of NTG without preventing hypotensive effect. Caution with calcium antagonists. Antagonizes bronchodilator effect of β-agonists. Antidiabetic agents may need dose adjustment. May block epinephrine effects. (Inj) Synergistic with halothane; do not use ≥3% halothane.

PREGNANCY: Category C, caution in nursing.

MECHANISM OF ACTION: α-1 and nonselective β-adrenergic receptor blocker; produces dose-related falls in BP without reflex tachycardia and significant reduction in heart rate.

PHARMACOKINETICS: Absorption: Complete; T_{max}=1-2 hrs. **Distribution:** Plasma protein binding (50%); crosses placenta. **Metabolism:** Conjugation. **Elimination**: Urine, feces; (Tab) $T_{1/2}$=6-8 hrs, (IV) $T_{1/2}$=5.5 hrs.

NURSING CONSIDERATIONS

Assessment: Assess for bronchial asthma, bronchospastic disease, AV block, severe bradycardia, cardiogenic shock, overt CHF, DM, pheochromocytoma, possible drug interactions, hepatic impairment, severe or prolonged hypotension, history of obstructive airway disease, and history of heart failure.

Monitoring: Monitor LFTs periodically. Monitor for signs/symptoms of cardiac failure, hypoglycemia, withdrawal symptoms (angina, MI), hypersensitivity reactions, and hepatic dysfunction.

Patient Counseling: Instruct not to d/c or interrupt therapy without consulting physician. Inform of possible transient tingling of scalp. Advise to seek medical attention if symptoms of cardiac failure, hepatic dysfunction (pruritis, dark urine, anorexia, jaundice), or hypersensitivity reactions occur.

Administration: Oral, IV route. **Storage**: Tab: 15-30°C (59-86°F). IV: 2-30°C (36-86°F). Protect from light and freezing.

LACTULOSE — RX

lactulose (Various)

OTHER BRAND NAMES: Constulose (Actavis) - Generlac (Morton Grove) - Enulose (Alpharma)

THERAPEUTIC CLASS: Osmotic laxative

INDICATIONS: Treatment of constipation. Prevention and treatment of portal-systemic encephalopathy, including stages of hepatic pre-coma and coma.

DOSAGE: *Adults:* Constipation: 15-30mL qd. Max 60mL/day. May mix with fruit juice, water, or milk. Portal-Systemic Encephalopathy: 30-45mL tid-qid. Adjust dose every 1 or 2 days to produce 2-3 soft stools daily. Rectal Use: Reversal of Coma: Mix 300mL with 700mL of water or saline and retain for 30-60 min. May repeat q4-6h. Oral doses should be started before completely stopping enema.
Pediatrics: Portal-Systemic Encephalopathy: Older Children/Adolescents: 40-90mL/day divided tid-qid adjusted to produce 2-3 soft stools daily. *Infants:* 2.5-10mL in divided doses to produce 2-3 soft stools daily.

HOW SUPPLIED: Sol: 10g/15mL

CONTRAINDICATIONS: Patients who require a low galactose diet.

WARNINGS/PRECAUTIONS: Caution in DM due to galactose and lactose content. Monitor electrolytes periodically in elderly or debilitated if used >6 months. Potential for explosive reaction with electrocautery procedures during proctoscopy or colonoscopy.

ADVERSE REACTIONS: Flatulence, intestinal cramps, diarrhea, NV.

INTERACTIONS: Decreased effect with nonabsorbable antacids.

PREGNANCY: Category B, caution in nursing.

MECHANISM OF ACTION: Synthetic disaccharide; broken down primarily to lactic acid, by the action of colonic bacteria, resulting in increased osmotic pressure and slight acidification of colonic content, causing an increase in stool water content and softens the stool. In portal-systemic encephalopathy, acidification of colonic contents results in retention of ammonia in colon as ammonium ion; ammonia then migrates from blood into colon to form ammonium ion, which traps and prevents absorption of ammonia; finally, laxative actions expels trapped ammonium ion from colon.

PHARMACOKINETICS: Absorption: Poor. **Elimination:** Urine (≤3%).

NURSING CONSIDERATIONS

Assessment: Assess for DM. Assess patients requiring a low-galactose diet and those requiring electrocautery procedures.

Monitoring: Monitor serum electrolytes (potassium, sodium, chloride, carbon dioxide) periodically, diarrhea, vomiting.

Patient Counseling: Drug may be diluted with fruit juice, water, or milk. Report potential adverse effects.

Administration: Oral route. **Storage:** 25°C (77°F); excursions permitted to 15-30°C (59-86°F). Dispense in tight, light-resistant container with child-resistant closure.

LAMICTAL

lamotrigine (GlaxoSmithKline)

RX

Serious life-threatening rash, including Stevens-Johnson syndrome and toxic epidermal necrolysis, reported. Occurs more often in pediatrics than adults. D/C at 1st sign of rash.

OTHER BRAND NAMES: Lamictal CD (GlaxoSmithKline)

THERAPEUTIC CLASS: Phenyltriazine

INDICATIONS: Adjunctive therapy in patients (≥2 yrs) with partial seizures and for generalized seizures of Lennox-Gastaut syndrome. For conversion to monotherapy in adults (≥16 yrs) with partial seizures receiving a single enzyme-inducing antiepileptic drug (EIAED) or valproate (VPA). Maintenance treatment of bipolar I disorder to delay the time to occurrence of mood episodes (depression, mania, hypomania, mixed episodes) in patients treated for acute mood episodes with standard therapy.

DOSAGE: *Adults:* Epilepsy: Concomitant AEDs with valproate (VPA): Weeks 1 and 2: 25mg every other day. Weeks 3 and 4: 25mg qd. Titrate: Increase every 1-2 weeks by 25-50mg/day. Maint: 100-400mg/day, given qd or bid; 100-200mg/day when added to VPA alone. Concomitant EIAEDs without VPA: Weeks 1 and 2: 50mg qd. Weeks 3 and 4: 50mg bid. Titrate: Increase every 1-2 weeks by 100mg/day. Maint: 150-250mg bid. Conversion to Monotherapy From Single EIAED: ≥16 yrs: Weeks 1 and 2: 50mg qd. Weeks 3 and 4: 50mg bid. Titrate: Increase every 1-2 weeks by 100mg/day. Maint: 250mg bid. Withdraw EIAED over 4 weeks. Conversion to Monotherapy From VPA: ≥16 yrs: Step 1: Follow Concomitant AEDs with VPA dosing regimen to achieve Lamictal dose of 200mg/day. Maintain previous VPA dose. Step 2: Maintain Lamictal 200mg/day. Decrease VPA to 500mg/day by decrements of ≤500mg/day per week. Maintain VPA 500mg/day for 1 week. Step 3: Increase to Lamictal 300mg/day for 1 week. Decrease VPA simultaneously to 250mg/day for 1 week. Step 4: D/C VPA. Increase Lamictal 100mg/day every week to maint dose of 500mg/day. Bipolar Disorder: Patients not taking carbamazepine, other enzyme-inducing drugs (EIDs) or VPA: Weeks 1 and 2: 25mg qd. Weeks 3 and 4: 50mg qd. Week 5: 100mg qd. Weeks 6 and 7: 200mg qd. Patients taking VPA: Weeks 1 and 2: 25mg every other day. Weeks 3 and 4: 25mg qd. Week 5: 50mg qd. Weeks 6 and 7: 100mg qd. Patients taking carbamazepine (or other EIDs) and not taking VPA: Weeks 1 and 2: 50mg qd. Weeks 3 and 4: 100mg qd (divided doses). Week 5: 200mg qd (divided doses). Week 6: 300mg qd (divided doses). Week 7: up to 400mg qd (divided doses). After d/c of psychotropic drugs excluding VPA, carbamazepine, or other EIDs: Maintain current dose. After d/c of VPA and current lamotrigine dose of 100mg qd: Week 1: 150mg qd. Week 2 and onward: 200mg qd. After d/c of carbamazepine or other EIDs and current lamotrigine dose of 400mg qd: Week 1: 400mg qd. Week 2: 300mg qd. Week 3 and Onward: 200mg qd. Concomitant or starting estrogen-containing oral contraceptives: not taking carbamazepine, phenytoin, phenobarbital, primidone, or rifampin, lamotrigine should be increased by as much as 2-fold over the recommended target maintenance dose; the dose increase should start at the same time as the initiation and continuation of contraceptives. Stopping estrogen-containing oral contraceptives: may decrease lamotrigine by as much as 50%. Hepatic Impairment: Initial/Titrate/Maint: Reduce by 50% for moderate (Child-Pugh Grade B) and 75% for severe (Child-Pugh Grade C) impairment. Significant Renal Impairment: Maint: Reduce dose. Elderly: Start at low end of dosing range.

Pediatrics: Round dose down to nearest whole tab. 2-12 yrs: ≥6.7kg: Lennox-Gastaut/Partial Seizures: Concomitant AEDs with VPA: Weeks 1 and 2: 0.15mg/kg/day given qd-bid. Weeks 3 and 4: 0.3mg/kg/day given qd or bid. Titrate: Increase every 1-2 weeks by 0.3mg/kg/day. Maint: 1-5mg/kg/day given qd or bid; 1-3mg/kg/day when added to VPA alone. Max: 200mg/day. Concomitant EIAEDs without VPA: Weeks 1 and 2: 0.3mg/kg bid. Weeks 3 and 4: 0.6mg/kg bid. Titrate: Increase every 1-2 weeks by 1.2mg/kg/day. Maint: 2.5-7.5mg/kg bid. Max: 400mg/day. >12 yrs: Concomitant AEDs with VPA: Weeks 1 and 2: 25mg every other day. Weeks 3 and 4: 25mg qd. Titrate:

L

Increase every 1-2 weeks by 25-50mg/day. Maint: 100-400mg/day, given qd or bid; 100-200mg/day when added to VPA alone. Concomitant EIAEDs without VPA: Weeks 1 and 2: 50mg qd. Weeks 3 and 4: 50mg bid. Titrate: Increase every 1-2 weeks by 100mg/day. Maint: 150-250mg bid. Hepatic Impairment: Initial/Titrate/Maint: Reduce by 50% for moderate (Child-Pugh Grade B) and 75% for severe (Child-Pugh Grade C) impairment. Significant Renal Impairment: Maint: Reduce dose.

HOW SUPPLIED: Tab: 25mg*, 100mg*, 150mg*, 200mg*; Tab, Chewable: (Lamictal CD) 2mg, 5mg, 25mg *scored

WARNINGS/PRECAUTIONS: Risk of serious life-threatening rash; d/c if rash occurs. Multiorgan failure, sudden unexplained death, hypersensitivity reactions, and pure red cell aplasia reported. Avoid abrupt withdrawal. Caution with renal, hepatic, or cardiac functional impairment. May cause ophthalmic toxicity. Do not exceed recommended initial dose and dose escalations. Caution in elderly. Chewable tabs may be swallowed whole, chewed (with water/diluted fruit juice) or dispersed in water/diluted fruit juice; do administer partial quantities.

ADVERSE REACTIONS: Serious rash, dizziness, ataxia, somnolence, headache, diplopia, blurred vision, NV, insomnia, back/abdominal pain, fatigue, xerostomia, rhinitis.

INTERACTIONS: Decreased levels with phenytoin, carbamazepine, phenobarbital, primidone, rifampin, estrogen-containing oral contraceptives. Risk of life-threatening rash with valproic acid. Lamotrigine decreases valproic acid levels; valproic acid increases lamotrigine levels. Inhibits dihydrofolate reductase; may potentiate folate inhibitors.

L

PREGNANCY: Category C, not for use in nursing.

MECHANISM OF ACTION: Phenyltriazine; mechanism not established. Suspected to inhibit voltage-sensitive sodium channels, thereby stabilizing neuronal membranes and consequently modulating presynaptic transmitter release of excitatory amino acids.

PHARMACOKINETICS: Absorption: Rapid and complete. Absolute bioavailability (98%), T_{max}=1.4-4.8 hrs. **Distribution:** V_d=0.9-1.3L/kg; plasma protein binding (55%); found in breast milk. **Metabolism:** Liver via glucuronic acid conjugation, 2-N-glucuronide conjugate (major metabolite, inactive). **Elimination:** Renal, urine (94%), feces (2%). Refer to full PI for pediatric parameters.

NURSING CONSIDERATIONS

Assessment: Assess renal/hepatic function prior to therapy. Assess use in patients with concomitant illnesses (renal/hepatic or cardiac impairment). Evaluate use in pediatric patients who have a history of major depressive disorder or other psychiatric disorder. Assess for possible drug interactions.

Monitoring: Monitor for signs/symptoms of rash (eg, Stevens-Johnson syndrome, toxic epidermal necrosis), hypersensitivity reaction, multiorgan failure, blood dyscrasias, status epilepticus, and opththalmological changes. Monitor for worsening depressive symptoms and symptoms of suicidal ideation in patients with bipolar disorder, occurrence of seizures in patients who abruptly d/c medication. Monitor drug levels with concomitant medications or if dosage adjustments are being made.

Patient Counseling: Instruct to notify physician immediately if rash, signs/symptoms of hypersensitivity reaction, blood dyscrasias, multi-organ failure, worsening depression, or suicide ideation occur. Inform CNS depression may occur; avoid operating machinery/driving until adjusted to effects. Advise females to notify physician if plan to start or stop oral contraceptives or other hormonal preparations, if they become pregnant, or experience changes in menstrual pattern. Do not abruptly d/c therapy; if therapy is stopped, notify physician before restarting.

Administration: Oral route. Chewable dispersible tablets may be swallowed whole, chewed, dispersed in water, or diluted in fruit juice. If tablets are chewed, consume a small amount of water or diluted fruit juice to aid in swallowing. When dispersing in water or diluted fruit juice, add tablets to small amount of liquid (1 teaspoon, or enough to cover tablets) and approximately

1 min later, swirl solution and consume entire quantity immediately. **Storage:** 25°C (77°F); excursions permitted to 15-30°C (59-86°F), in a dry place, protected from light.

LAMISIL **RX**

terbinafine HCl (Novartis)

THERAPEUTIC CLASS: Allylamine antifungal

INDICATIONS: (Granules) Treatment of tinea capitis in patients ≥4 yrs. (Tabs) Treatment of onychomycosis of toenail or fingernail due to dermatophytes (tinea unguium).

DOSAGE: *Adults:* Tabs: Fingernail: 250mg qd for 6 weeks. Toenail: 250mg qd for 12 weeks. Granules: Take qd with food for 6 weeks. <25 kg: 125mg/day. 25-35kg: 187.5mg/day. >35kg: 250mg/day.
Pediatrics: ≥4 yrs: Granules: Take qd with food for 6 weeks. <25 kg: 125mg/day. 25-35kg: 187.5mg/day. >35kg: 250mg/day.

HOW SUPPLIED: Granules: 125mg/pkt, 187.5mg/pkt; Tab: 250mg

WARNINGS/PRECAUTIONS: Liver disease and serious skin reactions reported; d/c therapy if these develop. Avoid with liver disease or renal impairment (CrCl ≤50 mL/min). Check serum transaminases before therapy. Monitor CBC if immunocompromised and taking terbinafine >6 weeks. Severe neutropenia reported; d/c therapy if neutrophil count ≤1,000 cells/mm^3. Changes in ocular lens and retina reported (unknown significance).

ADVERSE REACTIONS: (Granules) Nasopharyngitis, headache, pyrexia, cough, vomiting, upper respiratory tract infection, upper abdominal pain, diarrhea, liver enzyme abnormalities, rash. (Tabs) Headache, diarrhea, dyspepsia, abdominal pain, liver enzyme abnormalities, rash.

INTERACTIONS: Increased clearance of cyclosporine. May potentiate levels of drugs metabolized by CYP2D6 (eg, TCAs, β-blockers, SSRIs, MAOIs-type B). Decreased clearance of IV caffeine. Clearance increased by rifampin and decreased by cimetidine.

PREGNANCY: Category B, not for use in nursing.

MECHANISM OF ACTION: Allylamine antifungal; acts by inhibiting squalene epoxidase, thus blocking biosynthesis of ergosterol, an essential component of fungal-cell membranes.

PHARMACOKINETICS: Absorption: (Tab) Well-absorbed (>70%), absolute bioavailability (40%); (250mg) C_{max}=1mcg/mL; T_{max}=2 hrs; AUC =4.56mcg.h/mL. **Distribution:** Plasma protein binding (>99%). **Metabolism:** Extensive, CYP2D6. **Elimination:** Urine (70%); $T_{1/2}$=200-400 hrs.

NURSING CONSIDERATIONS

Assessment: Prior to treatment, conduct LFTs and obtain appropriate nail specimens for lab testing (KOH preparation, fungal culture, or nail biopsy) to diagnose onychomycosis. Assess for pre-existing liver disease.

Monitoring: Monitor for signs of hepatotoxicity, occurrence of progressive skin rash (Stevens-Johnson syndrome), and signs/symptoms of lupus erythematosus. Perform CBC, LFTs, and renal function tests (CrCl) during therapy.

Patient Counseling: Inform that taste disturbances may occur while on medication. Counsel females to avoid nursing.

Administration: Oral route. **Storage**: Below 25°C (77°F). Dispense in a tight, light-resistant container.

LANOXIN **RX**

digoxin (GlaxoSmithKline)

OTHER BRAND NAMES: Digitek (Mylan Bertek) - Lanoxicaps (GlaxoSmithKline)

THERAPEUTIC CLASS: Cardiac glycoside

L

INDICATIONS: Treatment of mild to moderate heart failure and to control ventricular response rate with chronic atrial fibrillation.

DOSAGE: *Adults:* Rapid Digitalization: LD: (Cap/Inj) 0.4-0.6mg PO/IV or (Tab) 0.5-0.75mg PO, may give additional (Cap/Inj) 0.1-0.3mg or (Tab) 0.125-0.375mg at 6-8 hr intervals until clinical effect. Maint: (Tab) 0.125-0.5mg qd. Elderly (>70 yrs)/Renal Dysfunction: Initial: 0.125mg qd. Marked Renal Dysfunction: Initial: 0.0625mg qd. Titrate: Increase every 2 weeks based on response. A-Fib: Titrate to minimum effective dose for desired response. *Pediatrics:* (Ped Sol) Oral Digitalizing Dose: Premature Infants: 20-30mcg/kg. Full-Term Infants: 25-35mcg/kg. 1-24 months: 35-60mcg/kg. 2-5 yrs: 30-40mcg/kg. 5-10 yrs: 20-35mcg/kg. >10 yrs: 10-15mcg/kg. Maint: Premature Infants: 20-30% of PO digitalizing dose/day. Full-Term Infants to >10 yrs: 25-35% of PO digitalizing dose. (Ped Inj) IV Digitalizing Dose: Premature Infants: 15-25mcg/kg. Full-Term Infants: 20-30mcg/kg. 1-24 months: 30-50mcg/kg. 2-5 yrs: 25-35mcg/kg. 5-10 yrs: 15-30mcg/kg. >10 yrs: 8-12mcg/kg. Maint: Premature Infants: 20-30% of IV digitalizing dose. Full-Term Infants to >10 yrs: 25-35% of IV digitalizing dose/day. (Cap) Oral Digitalizing Dose: 2-5 yrs: 25-35mcg/kg. 5-10 yrs: 15-30mcg/kg. >10 yrs: 8-12mcg/kg. Maint: ≥2 yrs: 25-25% of PO or IV digitalizing dose. (Tab) Maint: 2-5 yrs: 10-15mcg/kg. 5-10 yrs: 7-10mcg/kg. >10 yrs: 3-5mcg/kg. A-Fib: Titrate to minimum effective dose for desired response.

HOW SUPPLIED: Cap: (Lanoxicaps) 0.1mg, 0.2mg; Inj: (Pediatric Inj) 0.1mg/mL, 0.25mg/mL; Sol: (Pediatric Sol) 0.05mg/mL [60mL]; Tab: 0.125mg*, 0.25mg* *scored

CONTRAINDICATIONS: Ventricular fibrillation, digitalis hypersensitivity.

L

WARNINGS/PRECAUTIONS: May cause severe sinus bradycardia or sinoatrial block with pre-existing sinus node disease. May cause advanced or complete heart block with pre-existing incomplete AV block. May cause very rapid ventricular response or ventricular fibrillation. Caution with thyroid disorders, AMI, hypermetabolic states, restrictive cardiomyopathy, constrictive pericarditis, amyloid heart disease, elderly, acute cor pulmonale, and idiopathic hypertrophic subaortic stenosis. Caution with renal dysfunction; high risk for toxicity. Caution with hypokalemia, hypomagnesemia, or hypercalcemia; toxicity may occur. Hypocalcemia can nullify effects of digoxin. Monitor electrolytes and renal function periodically. Risk of ventricular arrhythmia with electrical cardioversion. Bioavailability is different between dosage forms.

ADVERSE REACTIONS: Heart block, rhythm disturbances, anorexia, NV, diarrhea, visual disturbances, headache, weakness, dizziness, mental disturbances.

INTERACTIONS: Risk of toxicity with K^+-depleting diuretics. Increased risk of arrhythmias with calcium, sympathomimetics, and succinylcholine. Increased serum levels with quinidine, verapamil, amiodarone, propafenone, indomethacin, itraconazole, alprazolam, and spironolactone; monitor for toxicity. Increased absorption with propantheline, diphenoxylate, macrolides, and tetracycline; monitor for toxicity. Decreased intestinal absorption with antacids, kaolin-pectin, sulfasalazine, neomycin, cholestyramine, certain anticancer drugs, and metoclopramide. Decreased serum levels with rifampin. Increased digoxin dose requirement with thyroid supplements. Additive effects on AV node conduction with β-blockers or CCBs. Caution with drugs that deteriorate renal function.

PREGNANCY: Category C, caution in nursing.

MECHANISM OF ACTION: Cardiac glycoside; inhibits Na^+-K^+ ATPase, leading to increase in intracellular concentration of Ca^+.

PHARMACOKINETICS: Absorption: (Tab) Absolute bioavailability (60%-80%), T_{max}=1-3 hrs. (Sol) Absolute bioavailability (70-85%). (Lanoxicaps) Absolute bioavailability (90-100%). (Inj) Absolute bioavailability (100%). **Distribution:** Plasma protein binding (25%), crosses placenta. **Metabolism:** Hydrolysis, oxidation, and conjugation. **Elimination:** Urine (50%-70%); $T_{1/2}$=1.5-2 days.

NURSING CONSIDERATIONS

Assessment: Assess for possible drug interactions, thyroid and electrolyte disorders, hypermetabolic states, sinus node disease, incomplete AV block, renal impairment, ventricular fibrillation, atrial fibrillation/flutter with accessory AV pathway (WPW syndrome), restrictive cardiomyopathy, constrictive pericarditis, amyloid heart disease, acute cor pulmonale, and IHSS.

Monitoring: Monitor serum electrolytes and renal function periodically. Monitor for signs/symptoms of sinoatrial block, severe sinus bradycardia, complete AV block, electrolyte imbalances, and hypersensitivity reactions.

Patient Counseling: Advise to seek medical attention if symptoms of hypersensitivity, electrolyte imbalance, or CV events occur.

Administration: Oral, IV route. **Storage:** 25°C (77°F); excursions permitted to 15-30°C (59-86°F). Store in dry place and protect from light.

LANTUS RX

insulin glargine, human (Sanofi-Aventis)

THERAPEUTIC CLASS: Insulin

INDICATIONS: Treatment of adults and pediatrics with type 1 diabetes mellitus. Treatment of adults with type 2 diabetes mellitus who require basal (long-acting) insulin.

DOSAGE: *Adults:* Individualize dose. For SQ injection only. Administer qd at same time each day. Insulin naive patients on oral antidiabetic drugs, start with 10 U qd. Switching from once-daily NPH or Ultralente does not require initial dose change. Switching from bid NPH, reduce initial dose by 20%. Maint: 2-100 U/day.
Pediatrics: ≥6 yrs: Individualize dose. For SQ injection only. Administer qd at same time each day. Insulin naive patients on oral antidiabetic drugs, start with 10 U qd. Switching from once-daily NPH or Ultralente does not require initial dose change. Switching from bid NPH, reduce initial dose by 20%. Maint: 2-100 U/day.

HOW SUPPLIED: Inj: 100 U/mL; OptiClik: 100 U/mL

WARNINGS/PRECAUTIONS: Human insulin differs from animal source insulin. Any change of insulin should be made cautiously. Changes in strength, manufacturer, type or method of manufacture may result in the need for a change in dosage. Hypoglycemia may occur with taking too much insulin, missing or delaying meals, exercising or working more than usual. An infection or illness (especially with diarrhea or vomiting) may change insulin requirements. Administration of insulin SQ can result in lipodystrophy. Not for IV use. Do not mix with other insulins. May cause sodium retention and edema. Caution in patients with renal and hepatic dysfunction.

ADVERSE REACTIONS: Hypoglycemia, allergic reactions, injection site reactions, lipodystrophy, pruritus, rash.

INTERACTIONS: Increased glucose lowering effects with ACE inhibitors, disopyramide, fibrates, fluoxetine, MAOIs, propoxyphene, salicylates, somatostatin analog, sulfonamide antibiotics, and other antidiabetic agents. Decreased blood glucose lowering effects with corticosteroids, danazol, diuretics, sympathomimetic amines, isoniazid, phenothiazine derivatives, somatropin, thyroid hormones, estrogens, progestogens, protease inhibitors, and atypical antipsychotics. Pentamidine may cause hypoglycemia, followed by hyperglycemia. β-blockers, clonidine, lithium salts, and alcohol may potentiate or weaken glucose lowering effect. β-blockers, clonidine, guanethidine, and reserpine may reduce or mask signs of hypoglycemia.

PREGNANCY: Category C, caution in nursing.

MECHANISM OF ACTION: Insulin glargine (rDNA origin); regulates glucose metabolism by stimulating peripheral glucose uptake by skeletal muscle and fat, inhibits hepatic glucose production, lipolysis in the adipocyte, proteolysis, and enhances protein synthesis.

PHARMACOKINETICS: Absorption: Slow, prolonged, and relatively constant. **Metabolism:** Partly metabolized into 2 active metabolites [M1 (21^A-Gly-insulin) and M2 (21^A-Gly-des-30^B-Thr-insulin)].

NURSING CONSIDERATIONS

Assessment: Assess FPG, HbA_{1c}, renal function, LFTs, pregnancy status, infections, alcohol consumption, exercise routines, and possible drug interactions.

Monitoring: Monitor FPG, HbA_{1c}, renal function, diabetic ketoacidosis, lipodystrophy, allergic reactions. Monitor for signs of hypoglycemia (sweating, palpitations, seizures, disorientation, tremors).

Patient Counseling: Use only if the solution is clear and colorless, with no visible particles. Do not dilute or mix with other insulins or solutions. Counsel about signs/symptoms of hypoglycemia, hyperglycemia, diabetic ketoacidosis, the importance of frequent monitoring of blood glucose levels, the need for eating a balanced diet and exercising regularly. Advise to avoid excessive alcohol. During periods of stress (eg, trauma, infection, surgery), insulin requirements may be changed; advise patients to seek prompt medical advice. Counsel on proper administration techniques.

Administration: SQ route only. 1) Inspect solution for particles and discoloration before administration. 2) Do not mix with other solutions. 3) Alternate injection sites (upper arm, thigh, abdomen). 4) Leave needle in skin for 10 seconds after injection. The number in the dose window should read zero. 5) Gently press the spot injected; do not rub the area. **Storage:** Unopened: 2-8°C (36-46°F). Do not freeze. In-use: Below 30°C (86°F).

Lescol XL RX

fluvastatin sodium (Novartis)

L

OTHER BRAND NAMES: Lescol (Novartis)

THERAPEUTIC CLASS: HMG-CoA reductase inhibitor

INDICATIONS: Adjunct to diet, to reduce elevated total cholesterol (Total-C), LDL-C, TG, and Apo B levels, and to increase HDL-C in primary hypercholesterolemia and mixed dyslipidemia (Types IIa and IIb) when response to nonpharmacological measures is inadequate. To slow coronary atherosclerosis progression in coronary heart disease by lowering Total-C and LDL-C. To reduce risk of undergoing coronary revascularization procedures in patients with coronary heart disease. Adjunct to diet, to reduce Total-C, LDL-C, and Apo B levels in adolescent boys and girls who are at least 1 yr post-menarche, 10-16 yrs of age, with heterozygous familial hypercholesterolemia when response to dietary restriction is inadequate and LDL-C remains ≥190mg/dL, or if LDL-C remains ≥160mg/dL and there is positive family history of premature CV disease, or 2 or more other CV disease risk factors are present.

DOSAGE: *Adults:* ≥18 yrs: (For LDL-C reduction of ≥25%) Initial: 40mg cap qpm or 80mg XL tab at any time of day or 40mg cap bid. (For LDL-C reduction of <25%) Initial: 20mg cap qpm. Range: 20-80mg/day. Severe Renal Impairment: Caution with dose >40mg/day. Take 2 hrs after bile-acid resins qhs.

Pediatrics: Heterozygous Familial Hypercholesterolemia: 10-16 yrs (≥1 yr post-menarche): Individualize dose: Initial: One 20mg cap. Titrate: Adjust dose at 6-week intervals. Max: 40mg cap bid or 80mg XL tab qd.

HOW SUPPLIED: Cap: (Lescol) 20mg, 40mg; Tab, Extended-Release: (Lescol XL) 80mg

CONTRAINDICATIONS: Active liver disease or unexplained, persistent elevations of serum transaminases, pregnancy, nursing mothers.

WARNINGS/PRECAUTIONS: Monitor LFTs prior to therapy, at 12 weeks, or with dose elevation. D/C if AST or ALT ≥3x ULN on 2 consecutive occasions. Risk of myopathy and/or rhabdomyolysis reported. D/C if markedly elevated CPK levels occur, if myopathy is diagnosed or suspected, or if predisposition to renal failure secondary to rhabdomyolysis. Less effective with homozygous familial hypercholesterolemia. Caution with heavy alcohol use and/or history of hepatic disease. Evaluate if endocrine dysfunction develops.

ADVERSE REACTIONS: Dyspepsia, abdominal pain, headache, nausea, diarrhea, abnormal LFTs, myalgia, flu-like symptoms.

INTERACTIONS: Rifampicin significantly decreases serum levels. Increases levels of glyburide, diclofenac, and phenytoin. Increased serum levels with glyburide, phenytoin, cimetidine, ranitidine, and omeprazole. Caution with drugs that decrease levels of endogenous steroid hormones (eg, ketoconazole, spironolactone, cimetidine). Avoid fibrates. Cyclosporine, colchicine, gemfibrozil, erythromycin, or niacin may increase risk of myopathy/rhabdomyolysis. Cholestyramine given within 4 hrs decreases serum levels but has additive effects when given 4 hrs after fluvastatin (immediate-release). Monitor digoxin, anticoagulants.

PREGNANCY: Category X, not for use in nursing.

MECHANISM OF ACTION: Competitive inhibition of HMG-CoA reductase; inhibits conversion of HMG-CoA to mevalonate (precursor of sterols, including cholesterol). Inhibition of cholesterol biosynthesis reduces cholesterol in hepatic cells, which stimulates the synthesis of LDL receptors, thereby increasing uptake of LDL particles, resulting in reduction of plasma cholesterol concentration.

PHARMACOKINETICS: Absorption: Rapid and complete, bioavailability (29%); T_{max}=3 hrs (fasting). **Distribution:** V_d=0.35L/kg, plasma protein binding (98%); found in breast milk. **Metabolism:** Liver via CYP2C9, 2C8 and 3A4 through N-dealkylation, β-oxidation pathways. **Elimination:** Feces (90% metabolites, <2% unchanged), urine (5%); $T_{1/2}$=9 hrs.

NURSING CONSIDERATIONS

Assessment: Assess for active liver disease or unexplained, persistent elevations in serum transaminase, pregnancy/nursing status, alcohol intake, homozygous familial hypercholestrolemia, renal impairment, DM, and possible drug interactions. Perform LFTs prior to therapy and at 12 weeks thereafter. Control hypercholesterolemia through appropriate diet, exercise, and weight reduction prior to therapy.

Monitoring: Monitor LFTs, CPK, thyroid functions. Monitor for signs/symptoms of myopathy (eg, diffuse muscle pain, tenderness or weakness, and fever or malaise), rhabdomyolysis, renal failure, endocrine dysfunction, and CNS toxicity or CNS vascular lesions (eg, hemorrhage and edema).

Patient Counseling: Inform about potential risks/benefits of therapy. Report promptly unexplained muscle pain, tenderness, or weakness, and malaise or fever. Notify physician if pregnant/nursing or planning to become pregnant.

Administration: Oral route. **Storage:** 25°C (77°F); 15-30°C (15-86°F).

LETAIRIS RX

ambrisentan (Gilead)

Potential liver injury and contraindicated in pregnancy. Available only through the Letairis Education and Access Program (LEAP), by calling 1-866-664-LEAP (5327).

THERAPEUTIC CLASS: Endothelin receptor antagonist

INDICATIONS: Treatment of pulmonary arterial hypertension (WHO Group 1) in patients with WHO class II or III symptoms to improve exercise capacity and delay clinical worsening.

DOSAGE: *Adults:* Initial: 5mg qd. May increase to 10mg qd if 5mg tolerated. Max: 10mg qd. Do not split, crush, or chew.

HOW SUPPLIED: Tab: 5mg, 10mg

CONTRAINDICATIONS: Pregnancy.

WARNINGS/PRECAUTIONS: Monitor liver chemistries before therapy and at least every month thereafter. Avoid therapy if elevated aminotransferase levels (>3x ULN) at baseline. If aminotransferase level is >3x ULN and ≤5x ULN, reduce daily dose or interrupt treatment and continue to monitor every 2 weeks until levels are <3x ULN. If aminotransferase elevations >5x ULN and ≤8x ULN, d/c and continue monitoring until levels are <3x ULN; may then re-initiate with more frequent monitoring of aminotransferase levels. If aminotransferase elevations >8x ULN, d/c and avoid re-initiation. May cause peripheral edema; if clinically significant, with or without weight gain, further evaluate to determine cause, such as heart failure and possible need for treatment. May decrease Hgb and Hct; measure Hgb prior to initiation, at 1 month, then periodically thereafter.

ADVERSE REACTIONS: Peripheral edema, headache, nasal congestion, palpitations, flushing, constipation, dyspnea, sinusitis, nasopharyngitis, abdominal pain.

INTERACTIONS: Cyclosporine-A may increase levels; caution when co-administering. Also use caution with strong CYP3A4 inhibitors (eg, ketoconazole), CYP2C19 inhibitors (eg, omeprazole), inducers of P-gp, CYPs, and UGTs.

PREGNANCY: Category X, not for use in nursing.

MECHANISM OF ACTION: Endothelin receptor antagonist; not established.

PHARMACOKINETICS: Absorption: Rapid, T_{max}=2 hrs. **Distribution:** Plasma protein binding (99%). **Elimination:** $T_{1/2}$=15 hrs.

NURSING CONSIDERATIONS

Assessment: Assess for hepatic impairment, pregnancy status, and possible drug interactions. Obtain baseline LFT, Hgb, Hct, and pregnancy test.

Monitoring: Monitor LFT, Hgb, Hct, and pregnancy test monthly. Monitor for signs/symptoms of hepatotoxicity, peripheral edema, and hypersensitivity reactions.

Patient Counseling: Instruct of pregnancy risks and to use 2 forms of contraception during therapy and 1 month after d/c. If IUD or tubal sterilization is used, second contraception not needed. Advise if dose is missed, take as soon as remembered; take next dose at regular time (do not double dose). Take whole; do not split, crush, or chew. Seek medical attention if symptoms of liver injury (eg, NV, fever, malaise, itching), peripheral edema, or hypersensitivity reactions occur.

Administration: Oral route. **Storage:** 25°C (77°F); excursions permitted to 15-30°C (59-86°F).

LEUKERAN — RX

chlorambucil (GlaxoSmithKline)

Risk of severe bone marrow suppression. Potentially carcinogenic, mutagenic, and teratogenic. Produces human infertility.

THERAPEUTIC CLASS: Nitrogen mustard alkylating agent

INDICATIONS: Treatment of chronic lymphatic (lymphocytic) leukemia (CLL), malignant lymphomas, and Hodgkin's disease.

DOSAGE: *Adults:* Usual: 0.1-0.2mg/kg qd for 3-6 weeks. Adjust according to response; reduce with abrupt WBC decline. Lymphocytic Infiltration of Bone Marrow/Hypoplastic Bone Marrow: Max: 0.1mg/kg/day. Caution within 4 weeks of full course of radiation or chemotherapy.

HOW SUPPLIED: Tab: 2mg

CONTRAINDICATIONS: Prior resistance to therapy.

WARNINGS/PRECAUTIONS: Convulsions, infertility, leukemia and secondary malignancies observed. Shown to cause chromatid or chromosome damage and sterility. Skin rash progressing to erythema multiforme, toxic epidermal necrolysis, or Stevens-Johnson syndrome reported. Avoid becoming pregnant. Lymphopenia reported, usually returns to normal upon completion. Monitor Hgb, leukocyte count and differential, platelet counts weekly. Avoid live vaccines in the immunocompromised.

ADVERSE REACTIONS: Bone marrow suppression, NV, diarrhea, tremors, muscular twitching, confusion, agitation, ataxia, urticaria, angioneurotic syndrome, pulmonary fibrosis, hepatotoxicity, jaundice.

INTERACTIONS: Cross-hypersensitivity may occur with other alkylating agents.

PREGNANCY: Category D, not for use in nursing.

MECHANISM OF ACTION: Nitrogen mustard alkylating agent.

PHARMACOKINETICS: Absorption: Rapid and complete. (0.6-1.2 mg/kg) T_{max}=1 hr; (0.2mg/kg) C_{max}=492ng/mL, T_{max}=0.83 hrs, AUC=883ng•h/mL; (Phenylacetic acid mustard) C_{max}=306ng/mL, T_{max}=1.9 hrs; AUC=1204ng•h/mL. **Distribution:** Plasma protein binding (99%); crosses placenta. **Metabolism:** Liver (rapid). Phenylacetic acid mustard (major metabolite). **Elimination:** Low urinary excretion; $T_{1/2}$=1.5 hrs (0.6-1.2mg/kg); $T_{1/2}$=1.3 hrs (0.2mg/kg); $T_{1/2}$=1.8 hrs (phenylacetic acid mustard).

NURSING CONSIDERATIONS

Assessment: Assess for prior resistance, history of seizure disorder or head trauma, and possible drug interactions. Obtain baseline WBC and platelet count.

Monitoring: Monitor Hgb, WBC with differential and platelet count weekly. During first 3-6 weeks of therapy, obtain WBC levels 3 or 4 days after each weekly blood count. Monitor for signs/symptoms of myelosuppression, hypersensitivity reaction, secondary malignancies, and skin reactions.

Patient Counseling: Inform of pregnancy risks; avoid pregnancy. Advise to avoid vaccinations with live vaccines. Inform that major toxicities are related to hypersensitivity, drug fever, myelosuppression, hepatotoxicity, infertility, seizures, GI toxicity, and secondary malignancies. Instruct not to take without medical supervision; consult physician if skin rash, bleeding, fever, jaundice, persistent cough, seizures, or unusual lumps/masses occur.

Administration: Oral route. **Storage:** Refrigerate; 2-8°C (36-46°F).

LEUKINE

RX

L

sargramostim (Berlex)

THERAPEUTIC CLASS: Granulocyte-macrophage colony stimulating factor

INDICATIONS: Acute myelogenous leukemia (AML) following induction chemotherapy in older adults (≥55 yrs) to shorten time to neutrophil recovery and to reduce incidence of severe and life-threatening infections and infections resulting in death. For mobilization of hematopoietic progenitor cells into peripheral blood for collection by leukopheresis. Myeloid recovery after autologous bone marrow transplantation (BMT) in non-Hodgkin's lymphoma (NHL), acute lymphoblastic leukemia (ALL), and Hodgkin's disease. Myeloid recovery after allogeneic BMT. BMT (allogeneic or autologous) failure or engraftment delay.

DOSAGE: *Adults:* ≥55 yrs: Neutrophil Recovery Post-Chemo in AML: Hypoplastic Bone Marrow with <5% Blasts: 250mcg/m^2/day IV over 4 hrs starting on day 11 or 4 days after completion of induction chemo. If 2nd cycle of induction chemo needed, give 4 days after completion of chemo. Continue until ANC >1500 cells/mm^3 for 3 consecutive days or max of 42 days. D/C immediately if leukemic regrowth occurs; reduce dose by 50% or temporarily d/c if severe adverse reaction occurs. Mobilization of Peripheral Blood Progenitor Cells (PBPC): 250mcg/m^2/day IV over 24 hrs or SC once daily. Continue through PBPC collection period. Reduce dose by 50% if WBC >50,000 cells/mm^3. Post Peripheral Blood Progenitor Cell Transplant: 250mcg/m^2/day IV over 24 hrs or SC once daily. Begin immediately after infusion of progenitor cells and continue until ANC >1500 cells/mm^3 for 3 consecutive days. Myeloid Reconstitution After BMT: 250mcg/m^2/day IV over 2 hrs 2-4 hrs post bone marrow infusion and not less than 24 hrs after last dose of chemo- or radiotherapy. Do not give until ANC <500 cells/mm^3. Continue until ANC >1500 cells/mm^3 for 3 consecutive days. May reduce dose by 50% or temporarily d/c if severe adverse reaction occurs. D/C immediately if blast cells appear or disease progression occurs. BMT Failure/Engraftment Delay: 250mcg/m^2/day IV over 2 hrs for 14 days. May repeat after 7 days if needed. Give 3rd course after another 7 days of 500mcg/m^2/day IV for 14 days if needed. May reduce dose by 50% or temporarily d/c if severe adverse reaction occurs. D/C immediately if blast cells appear or disease progression occurs. Reduce dose by 50% or interrupt treatment if ANC >20,000 cells/mm^3.

HOW SUPPLIED: Inj: 250mcg/vial, 500mcg/mL

CONTRAINDICATIONS: Excessive leukemic myeloid blasts in bone marrow or peripheral blood (≥10%), concomitant chemotherapy or radiotherapy.

WARNINGS/PRECAUTIONS: Contains benzyl alcohol; avoid use in neonates. Caution with pre-existing fluid retention, pulmonary infiltrate, CHF, hypoxia, cardiac disease, renal/hepatic dysfunction, or myeloid malignancies. Monitor CBC twice weekly and renal/hepatic function every other week with pre-existing dysfunction.

ADVERSE REACTIONS: Fever, NV, diarrhea, alopecia, rash, headache, stomatitis, anorexia, mucous membrane disorder, asthenia, malaise, abdominal pain, edema, HTN.

INTERACTIONS: Caution with drugs that may potentiate myeloproliferative effects (eg, lithium, corticosteroids).

PREGNANCY: Category C, caution in nursing.

MECHANISM OF ACTION: Recombinant human granulocyte-macrophage colony stimulating factor (GM-CSF); stimulates proliferation and differentiation of hematopoietic progenitor cells.

PHARMACOKINETICS: Absorption: IV: (liquid) C_{max}=5ng/mL, AUC=640ng/mL•min; (lyophilized) C_{max}=5.4ng/mL, AUC=677ng/mL•min. SC: C_{max}=1.5ng/mL, T_{max}=1-3 hrs; (liquid) AUC=549ng/mL•min; (lyophilized) AUC=501ng/mL•min. **Elimination:** $T_{1/2}$=60 min (IV); 162 min (SC).

NURSING CONSIDERATIONS

L

Assessment: Assess for excessive leukemic myeloid blasts in bone marrow or peripheral blood (≥10%), hypersensitivity to yeast, chemotherapy and radiotherapy use, pre-existing fluid retention, pulmonary infiltrates, CHF, lung disease, hypoxia, pre-existing pleural or pericardial effusion, malignancy with myeloid characteristics, pre-existing cardiac disease (arrhythmias), renal/hepatic dysfunction, pregnancy status, and possible drug interactions. Obtain baseline renal function, CBC with differential, body weight, and LFTs.

Monitoring: Monitor CBC with differential and exam for blast cells twice weekly; LFTs and renal function once every other week; body weight and hydration status periodically. Monitor for signs/symptoms of edema, capillary leak syndrome, hypersensitivity reactions, pleural/pericardial effusion, dyspnea or other respiratory symptoms, transient supraventricular arrhythmias, and syndrome characterized by respiratory distress, flushing, hypoxia, hypotension, syncope, and tachycardia.

Patient Counseling: Inform of pregnancy risks. Advise to seek medical attention for symptoms of hypersensitivity reactions, effusion, arrhythmias, dyspnea or other respiratory symptoms.

Administration: IV/SQ routes. Refer to PI for preparation. **Storage:** 2-8°C (36-46°F). Do not freeze or shake.

LEVAQUIN — RX

levofloxacin (Ortho-McNeil)

Fluoroquinolones are associated with an increased risk of tendinitis and tendon rupture in all ages. Risk further increased in patients >60 yrs, patients taking corticosteroid drugs, and patients with kidney, heart or lung transplants.

THERAPEUTIC CLASS: Fluoroquinolone

INDICATIONS: Uncomplicated and complicated skin and skin structure (SSSI), and urinary tract infections (UTI), acute bacterial sinusitis, acute bacterial exacerbation of chronic bronchitis (ABECB), community-acquired pneumonia (CAP), including multi-drug resistant *Streptococcus pneumoniae*, nosocomial pneumonia, chronic bacterial prostatitis (CBP), and acute pyelonephritis caused by susceptible strains of microorganisms. To reduce the incidence or progression of disease of inhalational anthrax following exposure to *Bacillus anthracis* in adults and pediatric patients ≥6 months.

DOSAGE: *Adults:* ≥18 yrs: IV/PO: ABECB: 500mg qd for 7 days. CAP: 500mg qd for 7-14 days or 750mg qd for 5 days. Sinusitis: 500mg qd for 10-14 days or 750mg qd for 5 days. CBP: 500mg qd for 28 days. Uncomplicated SSSI: 500mg qd for 7-10 days. Complicated SSSI/Nosocomial Pneumonia: 750mg qd for 7-14 days. Inhalational Anthrax: 500mg qd for 60 days. Complicated SSSI/Nosocomial Pneumonia/CAP/Sinusitis: CrCl 20-49mL/min: 750mg, then 750mg q48h. CrCl 10-19mL/min/Hemodialysis/CAPD: 750mg, then 500mg q48h. ABECB/CAP/Sinusitis/Uncomplicated SSSI/CBP/Inhalational Anthrax: CrCl 20-49mL/min: 500mg, then 250mg q24h. CrCl 10-19mL/min/Hemodialysis/CAPD: 500mg, then 250mg q48h. Complicated UTI/Acute Pyelonephritis: 250mg qd for 10 days or 750mg qd for 5 days. CrCl 10-19mL/min: 250mg, then 250mg q48h or 750mg, then 500mg q48h. Hemodialysis: 750mg, then 500mg q48h. Uncomplicated UTI: 250mg qd for 3 days. Take oral solution 1 hr before or 2 hrs after eating.
Pediatrics: ≥ 6 months: >50kg: 500mg q24h for 60 days. <50kg: 8mg/kg (not to exceed 250mg per dose) q12h for 60 days.

HOW SUPPLIED: Inj: 5mg/mL, 25mg/mL; Sol: 25mg/mL; Tab: 250mg, 500mg, 750mg [Leva-pak, 5[s]]

WARNINGS/PRECAUTIONS: Only administer injection via IV infusion over period of not less than 60 or 90 min, depending on dosage. Convulsions, toxic psychoses, increased ICP, CNS stimulation reported; d/c if any occur. Caution with CNS disorders that may predispose to seizures/lower seizure threshold (eg, epilepsy, renal insufficiency, drug therapy). Moderate to severe phototoxicity can occur. Serious/fatal hypersensitivity reactions; d/c at first sign of rash. Colitis reported. May permit overgrowth of Clostridia. *Clostridium difficile*-associated diarrhea reported. Liver, hematologic (including agranulocytosis, thrombocytopenia) and renal toxicities may occur after multiple doses. Caution in renal insufficiency. Severe hepatotoxicity (eg, acute hepatitis) reported; d/c if signs and symptoms of hepatitis occur. Prolongation of QT interval and torsades de pointes reported; caution with any factors that may predispose to QTc prolongation or proarrhythmic conditions. Peripheral neuropathy, Stevens-Johnson syndrome reported. Causes musculoskeletal disorder in pediatrics and arthropathic effects in animals. More susceptible to QT interval prolongation and caution in elderly taking corticosteroids.

ADVERSE REACTIONS: Nausea, diarrhea, headache, insomnia, constipation, pain, swelling, tendon tears.

INTERACTIONS: Decreased levels with antacids, sucralfate, didanosine, metal cations (eg, iron), and multivitamins with zinc; separate dosing by 2 hrs with PO dosing. Concomitant NSAIDs may increase seizure risk and CNS stimulation. Blood glucose changes with concomitant antidiabetic agents. May increase theophylline levels; monitor closely. Increases PT with warfarin; monitor closely. Severe tendon disorders are increased with concomitant corticosteroid therapy. Caution with concomitant drugs that may result in prolongation of the QT interval. Hyperglycemia or hypoglycemia may occur with insulin or oral hypoglycemics.

PREGNANCY: Category C, not for use in nursing.

MECHANISM OF ACTION: Synthetic broad-spectrum antimicrobial agent; inhibits topoisomearase II (DNA gyrase) and topoisomerase IV, which are required for bacterial DNA replication, transcription, repair, and recombination.

PHARMACOKINETICS: Absorption: Rapid and complete; T_{max}=1-2 hrs. **Distribution:** V_d=74-112L; plasma protein binding (approximately 24-38%). **Metabolism:** Limited. **Elimination:** Urine, $T_{1/2}$=6-8 hrs.

NURSING CONSIDERATIONS

Assessment: Assess renal function, LFTs, pregnancy status, history of seizures, QTc prolongation, history of tendon or joint-related problems, and possible drug interactions.

Monitoring: Monitor for QTc prolongation, hematologic manifestations, glucosuria, hematuria, pulmonary edema, hypo/hyperglycemia, cardiac arrest, seizure, status epilepticus, respiratory arrest, CDAD, renal function, LFTs, CBC, tendon rupture, peripheral neuropathy, hypersensitivity reactions (toxic epidermal necrolysis, Stevens-Johnson syndrome).

Patient Counseling: Notify healthcare provider if symptoms of pain, swelling, or inflammation of a tendon, or weakness or inability to move joints; rest and refrain from excercise; and d/c therapy. Inform that drug treats bacterial, not viral, infections. Take exactly as directed; skipping doses or not completing full course may decrease effectiveness and increase resistance. Inform about potential benefits/risks. D/C and notify physician if allergic reaction, skin rash, and watery and bloody stools (with or without stomach cramps and fever) occur. Notify if pregnant/nursing or taking antiarrhythmics, OTC drugs, multivitamins, antacids, or sucralfate. Use caution in activities requiring mental alertness and coordination. Avoid excessive sun exposure. Advise diabetic patients to use caution; hypoglycemia may develop during therapy. Instruct to drink liberal amounts of fluids.

Administration: IV, oral route. **Storage:** 25°C (77°F).

LEVBID RX

hyoscyamine sulfate (Alaven)

OTHER BRAND NAMES: Levsinex (Alaven) - Levsin (Alaven)

THERAPEUTIC CLASS: Anticholinergic

INDICATIONS: Adjunct treatment of peptic ulcer, irritable bowel syndrome, neurogenic bladder, and neurogenic bowel disturbances. Management of functional intestinal disorders (eg, mild dysenteries, diverticulitis). To control gastric secretion, visceral spasm, and hypermotility in spastic colitis, spastic bladder, cystitis, pylorospasm, and associated abdominal cramps. Symptomatic relief of biliary and renal colic with concomitant morphine or other narcotics. Drying agent for symptomatic relief of acute rhinitis. To reduce rigidity and tremors of Parkinson's disease and control associated sialorrhea and hyperhidrosis. For anticholinesterase poisoning. To reduce pain and hypersecretion in pancreatitis. For certain cases of partial heart block associated with vagal activity. (Elixir, Drops) Treatment of infant colic. (Inj) Facilitates GI diagnostic procedures. Reduces pain and hypersecretion in pancreatitis, in cases of partial heart block associated with vagal activity, and as antidote for anticholinesterase poisoning. In anesthesia as a pre-op antimuscarinic. In urology to improve radiologic visibility of kidneys.

DOSAGE: *Adults:* May also chew or swallow SL tab. (Drops, Elixir, Tab, and Tab, SL) 0.125-0.25mg q4h or prn. Max: 1.5mg/24 hrs. (Cap and Tab, Extended-Release) 0.375-0.75mg q12h; or 1 cap q8h. Max: 1.5mg/24 hrs. Do not crush or chew. (Inj) GI Disorders: 0.25-0.5mg IM/IV/SQ as single dose or up to qid at 4-hr intervals. Diagnostic Procedures: 0.25-0.5mg IV 5-10 min before procedure. Anesthesia: 5mcg/kg IM/IV/SQ 30-60 min before anesthesia or with narcotic/sedative administration. GI Disorders: 0.25-0.5mg IM/IV/SQ as single dose; may require bid-qid administration at 4-hr intervals. Diagnostic Procedures: 0.25-0.5mg IV 5-10 min prior. Drug-Induced Bradycardia (Surgery): Increments of 0.25mL IV; repeat prn. Neuromuscular Blockade Reversal: 0.2mg for every 1mg neostigmine or equal dose of physostigmine or pyridostigmine.

Pediatrics: May also chew or swallow SL tab. ≥12 yrs: (Drops, Elixir, Tab, and Tab, SL) 0.125-0.25mg q4h or prn. Max: 1.5mg/24 hrs. (Cap and Tab, Extended-Release) 0.375-0.75mg q12h; or 1 cap may be given q8h. Max: 1.5mg/24 hrs. Do not crush or chew. 2 to <12 yrs: (Tab and Tab, SL) 0.0625-0.125mg q4h or prn. Max: 0.75mg/24 hrs. (Elixir) Give q4h or prn. 10kg: 1.25mL. 20kg: 2.5mL. 40kg: 3.75mL. 50kg: 5mL. Max: 30mL/24 hrs. (Drops) 0.25-1mL q4h or prn. Max: 6mL/24 hrs. <2 yrs: (Drops) Give q4h or prn. 3.4kg: 4 drops. Max: 24 drops/24 hrs. 5kg: 5 drops. Max: 30 drops/24 hrs. 7kg: 6 drops. Max: 36 drops/24 hrs. 10kg: 8 drops. Max: 48 drops/24 hrs. >2 yrs: Anesthesia: (Inj) 5mcg/kg IM/IV/SQ 30-60 min before anesthesia or with narcotic/sedative administration.

HOW SUPPLIED: (Levbid) Tab, Extended-Release: 0.375mg. (Levsin) Drops: 0.125mg/mL [15mL]; Elixir: 0.125mg/5mL [473mL]; Inj: 0.5mg/mL; Tab: 0.125mg*; Tab, SL: 0.125mg*. (Levsinex) Cap, Extended-Release: 0.375mg
*scored

CONTRAINDICATIONS: Glaucoma, obstructive uropathy, GI tract obstruction, paralytic ileus; intestinal atony of elderly/debilitated, unstable CV status in acute hemorrhage, toxic megacolon complicating ulcerative colitis, myasthenia gravis.

WARNINGS/PRECAUTIONS: Risk of heat prostration with high environmental temperature. Avoid activities requiring mental alertness. Psychosis has been reported. Caution with diarrhea, autonomic neuropathy, hyperthyroidism, coronary heart disease, CHF, arrhythmias/tachycardia, HTN, renal disease, and hiatal hernia associated with reflux esophagitis. D/C if diarrhea occurs.

ADVERSE REACTIONS: Anticholinergic effects, drowsiness, headache, nervousness.

INTERACTIONS: Additive effects with other antimuscarinics, amantadine, haloperidol, phenothiazines, MAOIs, TCAs, and some antihistamines. Antacids interfere with absorption; take ac and antacids pc.

PREGNANCY: Category C, caution in nursing.

MECHANISM OF ACTION: Anticholinergic/antipasmodic; inhibits specifically the actions of acetylcholine on structures innervated by postganglionic cholinergic nerves and on smooth muscles that respond to acetylcholine but lack cholinergic innervation.

PHARMACOKINETICS: Absorption: Complete. **Distribution:** Crosses blood-brain barrier and placental barrier. **Metabolism:** Hydrolyzed partially to tropic acid. **Elimination:** Urine (unchanged); $T_{1/2}$=2-3.5 hrs.

NURSING CONSIDERATIONS

Assessment: Assess for glaucoma, obstructive uropathy, GI obstruction, paralytic ileus, intestinal atony, unstable CV status in acute hemorrhage, severe ulcerative colitis, toxic megacolon complicating ulcerative colitis, myasthenia gravis, and possible drug interactions.

Monitoring: Monitor for diarrhea, drowsiness, dizziness or blurred vision, psychosis, and CNS signs/symptoms including confusion, disorientation, short-term memory loss, hallucinations, dysarthria, ataxia, euphoria, anxiety, fatigue, insomnia, agitation, and unusual mannerisms.

Patient Counseling: Warn not to engage in activities requiring mental alertness (eg, operating a motor vehicle or other machinery), or to perform hazardous work while on treatment. Inform that decreased sweating resulting in heat prostration, fever or heat stroke may occur; caution if febrile, or exposed to high environmental temperatures. Counsel that extended-release tab/cap may not completely disintegrate and may be excreted.

Administration: Oral, IV, IM, SQ routes. **Storage:** 15-30°C (59-86°F).

LEVEMIR RX

insulin detemir, rdna origin (Novo Nordisk)

THERAPEUTIC CLASS: Insulin

INDICATIONS: Treatment of adults and pediatrics with type 1 diabetes or adults with type 2 diabetes who require basal (long-acting) insulin for the control of hyperglycemia.

DOSAGE: *Adults:* Individualize dose. Administer SQ qd or bid. Once-Daily Dosing: Administer with evening meal or bedtime. Twice-Daily Dosing: Administer evening dose with evening meal, at bedtime, or 12 hrs after morning dose. Type 1/Type 2 Diabetes on Basal-Bolus Treatment or Patients Only on Basal Insulin: Change on a unit-to-unit basis. Insulin-Naive with Type 2 Diabetes Inadequately Controlled on Oral Antidiabetics: Initial: 0.1-0.2 U/kg in evening or 10 U qd or bid.
Pediatrics: Individualize dose. Administer SQ qd or bid. Once-Daily Dosing: Administer with evening meal or bedtime. Twice-Daily Dosing: Administer evening dose with evening meal, at bedtime, or 12 hrs after morning dose. Type 1 Diabetes on Basal-Bolus Treatment or Patients Only on Basal Insulin: Change on a unit-to-unit basis.

HOW SUPPLIED: Inj: 100 U/mL [3mL, 10mL]

WARNINGS/PRECAUTIONS: Monitor glucose; may cause hypoglycemia. Not for use in an insulin infusion pump. Should not be diluted or mixed with any other insulin preparations. May cause lipodystrophy or hypersensitivity. Dose adjustment may be needed in renal or hepatic impairment and during intercurrent conditions such as illness, emotional disturbances, or other stresses.

ADVERSE REACTIONS: Allergic reactions, inj site reactions, lipodystrophy, pruritus, rash, hypoglycemia, wt gain.

INTERACTIONS: Avoid mixing with other insulins. Increased glucose lowering effects with ACE inhibitors, disopyramide, fibrates, fluoxetine, MAOIs, propoxyphene, salicylates, somatostatin analog, sulfonamide antibiotics, and other antidiabetic agents. Decreased blood glucose lowering effects with corticosteroids, danazol, diuretics, sympathomimetic agents, isoniazid, phenothiazine derivatives, somatotropin, thyroid hormones, estrogens, progestogens. Pentamidine may cause hypoglycemia, followed by hyperglycemia. β-blockers, clonidine, lithium salts, and alcohol may potentiate or weaken glucose lowering effect. β-blockers, clonidine, guanethidine, and reserpine may reduce or mask signs of hypoglycemia.

PREGNANCY: Category C, caution in nursing.

MECHANISM OF ACTION: Insulin detemir (rDNA origin); regulates glucose metabolism and lowers blood glucose by facilitating cellular uptake and inhibiting the glucose output from the liver.

PHARMACOKINETICS: Absorption: Slow, prolonged; absolute bioavailability (60%); T_{max}=6-8 hrs. **Distribution:** V_d=0.1L/kg; plasma protein binding (≥98%). **Metabolism:** Liver. **Elimination:** $T_{1/2}$=5-7 hrs.

L

NURSING CONSIDERATIONS

Assessment: Assess FPG, HbA_{1c}, renal function, LFTs, pregnancy status, infections, alcohol consumption, exercise routines, and possible drug interactions.

Monitoring: Monitor FPG, HbA_{1c}, hypokalemia, renal function, diabetic ketoacidosis, vision changes, lipodystrophy, allergic reactions. Monitor for signs of hypoglycemia (sweating, palpitations, seizures, disorientation, tremors).

Patient Counseling: Use only if the solution is clear and colorless with no visible particles. Do not dilute or mix with other insulins or solutions. Counsel about signs/symptoms of hypoglycemia, hyperglycemia, diabetic ketoacidosis, the importance of frequent monitoring of blood glucose levels, the need for eating a balanced diet and exercising regularly. Advise to avoid excessive alcohol. During periods of stress (eg, trauma, infection, surgery), insulin requirements may be changed; advise patients to seek prompt medical advice. Counsel on proper administration techniques.

Administration: SQ route (thigh, abdominal wall, or upper arm). **Storage:** 2-8°C (36-46°F). Do not use if frozen.

LEVITRA — RX

vardenafil HCl (Schering)

THERAPEUTIC CLASS: Phosphodiesterase type 5 inhibitor

INDICATIONS: Treatment of erectile dysfunction (ED).

DOSAGE: *Adults:* Initial: 10mg one hour prior to sexual activity at frequency of up to once daily. Titrate: May decrease to 5mg or increase to max of 20mg based on response. Elderly: ≥65 yrs: Initial: 5mg. Moderate Hepatic Impairment: Initial: 5mg; Max: 10mg. Concomitant Ritonavir: Max: 2.5mg/72 hrs. Concomitant Indinavir/Saquinavir/Atazanavir/Clarithromycin/Ketoconazole 400mg daily/Itraconazole 400mg daily: Max: 2.5mg/24 hrs. Concomitant Ketoconazole 200mg daily/Itraconazole 200mg daily/Erythromycin: Max: 5mg/24 hrs.

HOW SUPPLIED: Tab: 2.5mg, 5mg, 10mg, 20mg

CONTRAINDICATIONS: Concomitant nitrates or nitric oxide donors.

WARNINGS/PRECAUTIONS: Avoid when sexual activity is inadvisable due to underlying CV status. Increased sensitivity to vasodilation effects with left ventricular outflow obstruction. Decrease in supine BP reported. Avoid with unstable angina, hypotension (SBP<90 mmHg), uncontrolled HTN(>170/100 mmHg), recent history of stroke, life-threatening arrhythmia, MI (within last 6 months), severe cardiac failure, severe hepatic impairment (Child-Pugh C), end-stage renal disease requiring dialysis, hereditary degenerative retinal disorders including retinitis pigmentosa, congenital QT prolongation. Caution with bleeding disorders, peptic ulcers, anatomical deformation of the penis, or predisposition to priapism. Rare reports of non-arteritic anterior ischemic optic neuropathy (NAION) with PDE5 inhibitors. Sudden decrease or loss of hearing accompanied by tinnitus and dizziness reported.

ADVERSE REACTIONS: Headache, flushing, rhinitis, dyspepsia, sinusitis, flu syndrome, sudden decrease or loss of hearing, tinnitus.

INTERACTIONS: See Contraindications. Avoid use with α-blockers, nitrates, Class IA (eg, quinidine, procainamide) or Class III (eg, amiodarone, sotalol) antiarrhythmics, and other agents for ED. Increased levels with ritonavir, indinavir, saquinavir, atazanavir, ketoconazole, clarithromycin, erythromycin. May have additive hypotensive effect with nifedipine. Increased levels with CYP3A4 inhibitors.

PREGNANCY: Category B, not for use in nursing.

MECHANISM OF ACTION: Phosphodiesterase type 5 inhibitor; enhances the effect of nitric oxide by inhibiting phosphodiesterase type 5, which is responsible for the degradation of cGMP in the corpus cavernosum.

PHARMACOKINETICS: Absorption: Rapid, absolute bioavailability (15%); T_{max}=30 min-2 hrs. **Distribution:** V_d=208L; plasma protein binding (95%). **Metabolism:** Via CYP3A4, CYP3A5, CYP2C. M1 (major metabolite). **Elimination:** Feces (91-95%), urine (2-6%); $T_{1/2}$=4-5 hrs.

NURSING CONSIDERATIONS

Assessment: Assess for CVD, long QT syndrome, retinitis pigmentosa, bleeding disorders, active peptic ulceration, anatomical deformation of the penis, renal/hepatic impairment. Assess potential underlying causes of erectile dysfunction and for possible drug interactions.

Monitoring: Monitor potential for cardiac risk due to sexual activity, postural hypotension, color vision changes, hypersensitivity reactions, stomach ulcers. Monitor therapeutic effect when used in combination with other drugs.

Patient Counseling: Seek medical assistance if erection persists >4 hrs. Advise of potential BP-lowering effect of α-blockers and antihypertensive medications, and cardiac risk of sexual activity. Counsel about protective measures necessary to guard against STDs, including HIV. D/C and inform doctor if sudden loss of vision, color vision, or hearing occur. Counsel to take as prescribed.

Administration: Oral route. **Storage:** 25°C (77°F); excursions permitted to 15-30° (59-86°F).

LEVOTHROID — RX

levothyroxine sodium (Forest)

THERAPEUTIC CLASS: Thyroid replacement hormone

INDICATIONS: Hypothyroidism. As a pituitary TSH suppressant for nonendemic goiter and for chronic lymphocytic thyroiditis. Diagnostic agent in suppression tests to differentiate mild hyperthyroidism or thyroid gland autonomy. Adjunct therapy with antithyroid drugs to treat thyrotoxicosis. Adjunct to surgery and radioiodine therapy for TSH-dependent thyroid cancer.

DOSAGE: *Adults:* Hypothyroidism: Usual: 100-200mcg/day. Endocrine/Cardiovascular Complications: Initial: 50mcg/day. Titrate: Increase by 50mcg/day every 2-4 weeks until euthyroid. Hypothyroid with Angina: Initial: 25mcg/day. Titrate: Increase by 25-50mcg every 2-4 weeks until euthyroid. *Pediatrics:* Hypothyroidism: >12 yrs: Usual: 100-200mcg/day. 6-12 yrs:

4-5mcg/kg/day. 1-5 yrs: 5-6mcg/kg/day. 6-12 months: 6-8mcg/kg/day. 0-6 months: 10-15mcg/kg/day. May crush tab and sprinkle over food (applesauce) or mix with 5-10mL water, formula (non-soy), or breast milk.

HOW SUPPLIED: Tab: 25mcg*, 50mcg*, 75mcg*, 88mcg*, 100mcg*, 112mcg*, 125mcg*, 137mcg*, 150mcg*, 175mcg*, 200mcg*, 300mcg* *scored

CONTRAINDICATIONS: Untreated thyrotoxicosis, acute MI, and uncorrected adrenal insufficiency.

WARNINGS/PRECAUTIONS: Do not use in the treatment of obesity; larger doses in euthyroid patients can cause serious or even life-threatening toxicity. Caution with cardiovascular disease, HTN. May aggravate diabetes mellitus or insipidus and adrenal cortical insufficiency. Excessive doses in infants may produce craniosynostosis. Add glucocorticoid with myxedema coma.

ADVERSE REACTIONS: Lactose hypersensitivity, transient partial hair loss in children.

INTERACTIONS: Monitor insulin and oral hypoglycemic requirements. May potentiate anticoagulant effects of warfarin; adjust warfarin dose and monitor PT/INR. Increased adrenergic effects of catecholamines; caution with CAD. Decreased absorption with cholestyramine and colestipol; space dosing by 4-5 hrs. Estrogens increase thyroxine-binding globulin; increase in thyroid dose may be needed. Large dose may cause life-threatening toxicities with sympathomimetic amines. Avoid mixing crushed tabs with foods/formula with large amounts of iron, soybean or fiber.

PREGNANCY: Category A, caution in nursing.

MECHANISM OF ACTION: Thyroid hormone; not understood, suspected to control DNA transcription and protein synthesis. Regulates multiple metabolic processes.

L

PHARMACOKINETICS: Distribution: Plasma protein binding (99%). **Metabolism:** Deiodination (major pathway), conjugation (minor pathway) in liver (mainly), kidneys, and other tissues. **Elimination:** Urine; T_4 (feces 20% unchanged); $T_{1/2}$=6-7 days; $T_{1/2}$=≤2 days (T_3).

NURSING CONSIDERATIONS

Assessment: Assess for drug hypersensitivity, CV disease, angina pectoris, acute MI, suppressed serum TSH level with normal T_3 and T_4 levels, overt thyrotoxicosis, DM, clotting disorder, adrenal/pituitary gland problems, malabsorption, autoimmune polyglandular syndrome, undergoing surgery, and possible drug and test interactions. Assess infants with congenital hypothyroidism for other congenital anomalies.

Monitoring: Requires frequent lab tests and clinical evaluation of thyroid function by TSH levels, and also glucose/lipid metabolism, urinary glucose in diabetics, and clotting status. Monitor for CV signs such as arrhythmia and coronary insufficiency, growth/development, bone metabolism, cognitive function, emotional state, GI function, reproductive function, partial hair loss in children, and signs/symptoms of thyrotoxicosis.

Patient Counseling: Counsel to take 1 hr before breakfast, and not to to use as part of weight control regimen. Inform that replacement therapy is essential for life, except in cases of transient hypothyroidism. Advise to notify physician if pregnant/nursing or intend to become pregnant. Advise to notify if taking any other drugs. Counsel to not d/c or change dosage. Instruct to report signs/symptoms of thyroid toxicity.

Administration: Oral route. **Storage:** 25°C (77°F); excursions permitted to 15-30°C (59-86°F). Protect from light and moisture.

Levoxyl — RX

levothyroxine sodium (King)

THERAPEUTIC CLASS: Thyroid replacement hormone

INDICATIONS: Hypothyroidism. As a pituitary TSH suppressant in the treatment and prevention of euthyroid goiters, including thyroid nodules, lymphocytic thyroiditis, and multinodular goiter. Adjunct to surgery and radioiodine therapy for thyrotropin-dependent well-differentiated thyroid cancer.

DOSAGE: *Adults:* Take in the AM at least one-half hour before food. Hypothyroid: Usual: 1.7mcg/kg/day. >200mcg/day (seldom). >50 yrs/<50 yrs with Cardiac Disease: Initial: 25-50mcg/day. Titrate: Increase by 12.5-25mcg/day every 6-8 weeks until euthyroid. Elderly with Cardiac Disease: Initial: 12.5-25mcg/day. Titrate: Increase by 12.5-25mcg/day every 4-6 weeks until euthyroid. Severe Hypothyroidism: Initial: 12.5-25mcg/day. Titrate: Increase by 25mcg/day every 2-4 weeks until euthyroid. Pregnancy: May increase dose requirements. Subclinical Hypothyroidism: Lower doses required. *Pediatrics:* Take in the AM at least one-half hour before food. Hypothyroidism: 0-3 months: 10-15mcg/kg/day. 3-6 months: 8-10mcg/kg/day. 6-12 months: 6-8mcg/kg/day. 1-5 yrs: 5-6mcg/kg/day. 6-12 yrs: 4-5mcg/kg/day. >12 yrs: 2-3mcg/kg/day. Growth/Puberty Complete: 1.7mcg/kg/day. Cardiac Risk: Initial: Use lower dose. Titrate: Increase dose every 4-6 weeks until euthyroid. Infants with Serum T_4 <5mcg/dL: Initial: 50mcg/day. Chronic/Severe Hypothyroidism: Children: Initial: 25mcg/day. Titrate: Increase by 25mcg/day every 2-4 weeks until desired effect. Minimize Hyperactivity in Older Children: Initial: Give 1/4 of full replacement dose. Titrate: Increase by same amount weekly until full dose achieved. May crush tab and mix with 5-10mL water.

HOW SUPPLIED: Tab: 25mcg*, 50mcg*, 75mcg*, 88mcg*, 100mcg*, 112mcg*, 125mcg*, 137mcg*, 150mcg*, 175mcg*, 200mcg* *scored

CONTRAINDICATIONS: Untreated thyrotoxicosis, acute MI, and uncorrected adrenal insufficiency.

WARNINGS/PRECAUTIONS: Do not use in the treatment of obesity; larger doses in euthyroid patients can cause serious or even life threatening toxicity. Caution with cardiovascular disease, CAD, adrenal insufficiency, and the elderly with risk of occult cardiac disease. Carefully titrate dose to avoid over or under treatment. Decreased bone mineral density with long term use. Caution with nontoxic diffuse goiter or nodular thyroid disease. With adrenal insufficiency supplement with glucocorticoids before therapy.

L

ADVERSE REACTIONS: Pseudotumor cerebri in children reported. Seizures (rare), hypersensitivity reactions, dysphagia, choking, gagging, hyperthyroidism (increased appetite, weight loss, heat intolerance, hyperactivity, tremors, palpitations, tachycardia, diarrhea, vomiting, hair loss).

INTERACTIONS: Sympathomimetics may increase risk of coronary insufficiency with CAD. Upward dose adjustments needed for insulin and oral hypoglycemic agents. Decreased absorption with soybean flour (infant formula), cottonseed meal, walnuts, and fiber. May potentiate oral anticoagulant effects; adjust dose and monitor PT/INR. May decrease levels and effects of digitalis glycosides. Cholestyramine, colestipol, ferrous sulfate, aluminum hydroxide, sodium polystyrene, soybean flour, sucralfate may decrease absorption. Reduced TSH secretion with dopamine/dopamine agonists, glucocorticoids, octreotide. Decreased thyroid hormone secretion with aminoglutethimide, amiodarone, iodine (including iodine-containing radiographic contrast agents), lithium, methimazole, PTU, sulfonamides, tolbutamide. Increased thyroid hormone secretion with amiodarone, iodide (including iodine-containing radiographic contrast agents). Decreased T_4 absorption with antacids (aluminum & magnesium hydroxides), simethicone, bile acid sequestrants (cholestyramine, colestipol), calcium carbonate, cation exchange resins (kayexalate), ferrous sulfate, sucralfate. Increased serum TBG concentration with clofibrate, estrogens, heroin/methadone, 5-FU, mitotane, tamoxifen. Decreased serum TBG concentration with androgens/anabolic steroids, asparaginase, glucocorticoids, nicotinic acid (slow-release). Protein-binding site displacement with furosemide, heparin, hydantoins, NSAIDs, salicylates. Increased hepatic metabolism with carbamazepine, hydantoins, phenobarbital, rifampin. Decreased conversion of T_4 to T_3 levels with amiodarone, β-adrenergic antagonists (propranolol >160mg/day), glucocorticoids (dexamethasone >4mg/day), PTU. Additive effects of both agents with antidepressants. Interferon-(alpha) may cause development of antithyroid microsomal antibodies causing transient hypothyroidism, hyperthyroidism, or both. Interleukin-2 has been associated with transient painless thyroiditis.

Excessive use with growth hormones may accelerate epiphyseal closure. Ketamine use may produce marked HTN and tachycardia. May reduce uptake of iodine-containing radiographic contrast agents. Altered levels of thyroid hormone and/or TSH level with choral hydrate, diazepam, ethionamide, lovastatin, metoclopramide, 6-mercaptopurine, nitroprusside, para-aminosalicylate sodium, perphenazine, resorcinol (excessive topical use), thiazide diuretics.

PREGNANCY: Category A, caution in nursing.

MECHANISM OF ACTION: Thyroid hormone; not understood, suspected to control DNA transcription and protein synthesis.

PHARMACOKINETICS: Distribution: Plasma protein binding (99%); found in breast milk. **Metabolism:** Deiodination (major pathway) and conjugation in liver (mainly), kidneys, other tissues. **Elimination:** Urine, feces (20% unchanged); (T_4) $T_{1/2}$=6-7days; (T_3) $T_{1/2}$≤2 days.

NURSING CONSIDERATIONS

Assessment: Assess for suppressed serum TSH level with normal T_3, T_4 levels, or overt thyrotoxicosis, thyroid diseases (nontoxic diffuse or nodular goiter), endocrine disorders (eg, hypothalamic/pituitary hormone deficiencies and/or autoimmune polyglandular disorders), cardiovascular diseases (eg, angina pectoris, acute MI), DM, clotting status, upcoming surgery, hypersensitivity history, and possible drug/lab test interactions. Assess infants for associated congenital anomalies.

Monitoring: Perform frequent lab tests and clinical evaluation of thyroid functions (TSH and free T_4 levels), lipid metabolism, blood and/or urinary glucose in DM and clotting parameters, cardiovascular signs (eg, arrhythmias, coronary insufficiency), growth/development, bone metabolism, cognitive function, emotional status, GI function, reproductive functions, partial hair loss in infants and signs/symptoms of thyroid toxicity.

Patient Counseling: Inform that drug is to be taken for life; not to be taken for treatment of obesity or for weight loss. Instruct to take on empty stomach 1/2 hr to 1 hr before breakfast with full glass of water. Notify physician if pregnant/nursing or planning to become pregnant. Notify if taking any other drugs. Instruct to not d/c or change dose unless directed by physician. Advise to report any signs/symptoms of thyroid toxicity.

Administration: Oral route. **Storage:** Store at 25°C (77°F); excursions permitted to 15-30°C (59-86°F). Protect from light and moisture.

LEXAPRO — RX

escitalopram oxalate (Forest)

Antidepressants increased the risk of suicidal thinking and behavior (suicidality) in short-term studies in children, adolescents, and young adults with major depressive disorder (MDD) and other psychiatric disorders. Escitalopram is not approved for use in pediatric patients.

THERAPEUTIC CLASS: Selective serotonin reuptake inhibitor

INDICATIONS: Acute and maintenance treatment of Major Depressive Disorder (MDD) in adults and adolescents aged 12-17 years. Acute treatment of generalized anxiety disorder (GAD) in adults.

DOSAGE: *Adults:* MDD: Initial: 10mg qd, in am or pm. Titrate: May increase to 20mg after 1 week. Max: 20mg qd. GAD: Initial: 10mg qd, in am or pm. Titrate: May increase to 20mg after 1 week. Elderly/Hepatic Impairment: 10mg qd. Re-evaluate periodically.

Pediatrics: 12-17 yrs: MDD: Initial: 10mg qd, in am or pm. Titrate: May increase to 20mg after 3 weeks. Max: 20mg qd. Re-evaluate periodically.

HOW SUPPLIED: Sol: 5mg/5mL [240mL]; Tab: 5mg, 10mg*, 20mg* *scored

CONTRAINDICATIONS: Concomitant use of MAOI or pimozide therapy.

WARNINGS/PRECAUTIONS: Avoid abrupt withdrawal. May increase the risk of bleeding events. Activation of mania/hypomania, hyponatremia reported. SIADH reported with citalopram. Caution with history of mania or seizures, hepatic impairment, severe renal impairment, and conditions that alter metabolism or hemodynamic responses. May impair mental/physical abilities. Serotonin syndrome or NMS like reactions reported. Manage with immediate discontinuation and monitor.

ADVERSE REACTIONS: Nausea, insomnia, ejaculation disorder, increased sweating, somnolence, fatigue, diarrhea.

INTERACTIONS: See Contraindications. Avoid alcohol, citalopram, or within 14 days of MAOI therapy. Caution with other CNS drugs, lithium, carbamazepine, cimetidine, drugs metabolized by CYP2D6 (eg, desipramine). Increased risk of bleeding with NSAIDs, ASA, warfarin. May increase metoprolol levels which leads to decreased cardioselectivity. Rare reports of weakness, hyperreflexia, incoordination with an SSRI and sumatriptan. Serotonin syndrome reported with linezolid.

PREGNANCY: Category C, not for use in nursing.

MECHANISM OF ACTION: SSRI; inhibits CNS neuronal reuptake of serotonin.

PHARMACOKINETICS: Absorption: T_{max}=5 hrs. **Distribution:** Plasma protein binding (56%). **Metabolism:** Hepatic (biotransformation: N-demethylation) via CYP3A4, 2C19. **Elimination:** Urine (8%); $T_{1/2}$=27-36 hrs.

NURSING CONSIDERATIONS

Assessment: Assess for risk of bipolar disorder, history of mania, possible drug interactions, history of seizures, disease/condition that alters metabolism or hemodynamic response, hepatic/renal impairment.

Monitoring: Monitor for signs/symptoms of clinical worsening (suicidality, unusual changes in behavior), serotonin syndrome, abnormal bleeding, hyponatremia, seizures, cognitive and motor impairment, and hepatic/renal dysfunction. If abruptly d/c therapy, monitor for symptoms of dysphoric mood, irritability, agitation, dizziness, sensory disturbances, anxiety, confusion, headache, lethargy, emotional lability, insomnia, and hypomania. Monitor for serotonin syndrome and NMS.

Patient Counseling: Advise to avoid alcohol. Seek medical attention for symptoms of serotonin syndrome (mental status changes, tachycardia, hyperthermia, NV, diarrhea, incoordination), abnormal bleeding (particularly if using NSAIDs or ASA), hyponatremia, activation of mania, seizures, clinical worsening (suicidal ideation, unusual changes in behavior) and discontinuation symptoms (irritability, agitation, dizziness, anxiety, headache, insomnia). Caution against operating hazardous machinery, including automobiles, until they are reasonably certain that Lexapro therapy does not affect their ability to engage in such activities. Inform may notice improvement in 1-4 weeks; continue therapy as directed.

Administration: Oral route. **Storage:** 25°C (77°F); excursions permitted to 15-30°C (59-86°F).

LEXIVA — RX

fosamprenavir calcium (GlaxoSmithKline)

THERAPEUTIC CLASS: Protease inhibitor

INDICATIONS: Treatment of HIV infection in combination with other antiretrovirals.

DOSAGE: *Adults:* Therapy-naive: 1400mg bid OR 1400mg qd + ritonavir 200mg qd OR 700mg bid + ritonavir 100mg bid. PI-Experienced: 700mg bid + ritonavir 100mg bid. Mild/Moderate Hepatic Impairment (without ritonavir): 700mg bid. Mild Hepatic Impairment: 700mg bid + ritonavir 100mg qd. Moderate Hepatic Impairment: 450mg bid + ritonavir 100mg qd. Severe Hepatic Impairment: 350mg bid (without ritonavir).
Pediatrics: 2-5 yrs: Therapy-naive: 30mg/kg bid, do not exceed 1,400mg bid; Therapy-naive ≥6 yrs: : 30mg/kg bid, not to exceed 1,400mg bid. or 18mg/kg + ritonovir 3mg/kg bid, not to exceed 700mg + ritonovir 100mg bid. Therapy-experienced: ≥6 yrs: 18 mg/kg + ritonovir 3 mg/kg, not to exceed 700 mg + ritonovir 100 mg bid. For patients weighing >47 kg use adult Lexiva monotherapy. When administered in combination with ritonovir, Lexiva tabs may

be used in patients weighing >39 kg and ritonovir caps for patients weighing >33 kg.

HOW SUPPLIED: Tab: 700mg; Sus: 50mg/mL [225mL]

CONTRAINDICATIONS: Concomitant drugs dependent on CYP3A4 for clearance (eg, flecainide, propafenone, rifampin, delavirdine, lovastatin, simvastatin, dihydroergotamine, ergonovine, ergotamine, methylergonovine, cisapride, pimozide, midazolam, triazolam). If used with ritonavir, refer to ritonavir monograph.

WARNINGS/PRECAUTIONS: Severe and life-threatening skin reactions (including Stevens-Johnson syndrome), hemolytic anemia, new onset, or exacerbation of, DM, hyperglycemia, diabetic ketoacidosis, and immune reconstitution syndrome reported. Caution with known sulfonamide allergy. Reduce dose and use caution in hepatic impairment. Caution with underlying hepatitis B or C or marked elevations in transaminases; monitor LFTs prior to and during therapy. Spontaneous bleeding reported with hemophilia A and B. Redistribution/accumulation of body fat observed. Increased triglycerides may occur.

ADVERSE REACTIONS: Diarrhea, NV, headache, rash, severe skin reactions, AST increased, ALT increased.

INTERACTIONS: See Contraindications. Concurrent nevirapine without ritonavir not recommended. Indinavir and nelfinavir may increase levels. Decreased levels with efavirenz (add additional 100mg/day ritonavir), nevirapine, lopinavir/ritonavir (also decreases lopinavir), saquinavir, carbamazepine, phenobarbital, phenytoin, dexamethasone, H_2 antagonists. May decrease levels of methadone (consider dose increase) and paroxetine. May increase levels of oral contraceptives (use alternate non-hormonal methods), amiodarone, lidocaine (systemic), quinidine, bepridil, ketoconazole/itraconazole (reduce dose with >400mg/day; avoid >200mg/day with concurrent ritonavir), rifabutin (reduce dose by at least 50% or 75% with ritonavir; monitor CBCs weekly), benzodiazepines, CCBs, atorvastatin, rosuvastatin (use lowest possible dose), cyclosporine, tacrolimus, rapamycin, fluticasone (use with caution and avoid with ritonavir), sildenafil/tadalafil/vardenafil (reduce dose), amitriptyline, imipramine, trazodone. May affect warfarin levels; monitor INR.

PREGNANCY: Category C, not for use in nursing.

MECHANISM OF ACTION: HIV protease inhibitor; hydrolyzed to prodrug (amprenavir) which binds to HIV-1 protease active site and prevents the processing of viral Gag and Gag-Pol polyprotein precursors; forms immature infectious viral particles.

PHARMACOKINETICS: Absorption: Oral administration of variable doses resulted in different parameters. **Distribution:** Amprenavir: Plasma protein binding (90%). **Metabolism:** Fosamprenavir: Hepatic (hydrolyzation). Amprenavir: Hepatic via CYP3A4. **Elimination**: Amprenavir: Urine (1%); $T_{1/2}$=7.7 hrs.

NURSING CONSIDERATIONS

Assessment: Assess for sulfonamide allergy, liver/kidney problems, DM, hemophilia, and possible drug interactions.

Monitoring: Periodically monitor TG, lipase, ALT, AST, and glucose levels. Observe for symptoms of skin reactions, HBV or HCV, marked elevations in transaminase, exacerbation of pre-existing DM and hyperglycemia, inflammatory response to opportunistic infections, redistribution/accumulation of body fat, acute hemolytic anemia, hemophilia (spontaneous bleeding) and lipid elevations.

Patient Counseling: Inform that drug does not reduce the risk of transmitting HIV to others. Advise to complete prescribed course unless directed. If miss dose by fewer than 4 hrs, take missed dose right away. Seek medical attention for symptoms of skin reactions, hepatic dysfunction, exacerbation of pre-existing DM and hyperglycemia, inflammatory response to opportunistic infection, redistribution/accumulation of body fat, acute hemolytic anemia, hemophilia (spontaneous bleeding) and lipid elevations. (Sus): Shake vigorously; adults and pediatrics take without food.

Administration: Oral route. **Storage:** (Tab): 25°C (77°F); excursions permitted to 15-30°C (59-86°F). Keep tightly closed. (Sus): 5-30°C (41-86°F). Do not freeze.

LIALDA

mesalamine (Shire) RX

THERAPEUTIC CLASS: Anti-inflammatory Agent

INDICATIONS: Induction of remission in adult patients with active, mild to moderate ulcerative colitis.

DOSAGE: *Adults:* 2-4 tabs qd with meals for up to 8 weeks. Max: 2.4g or 4.8g per day.

HOW SUPPLIED: Tab, Delayed-Release: 1.2g

WARNINGS/PRECAUTIONS: Prolonged gastric retention with pyloric stenosis, delaying mesalamine release in the colon. Caution with sulfasalazine allergy. May cause acute intolerance syndrome, if suspected prompt withdrawal is required. Caution with cardiac hypersensitivity reactions, myocarditis and pericarditis reported. Renal impairment, including minimal change nephropathy, and acute or chronic interstitial nephritis reported; caution with known renal dysfunction. Monitor renal function prior to therapy and periodically after.

ADVERSE REACTIONS: Headache, flatulence.

INTERACTIONS: Concurrent use with nephrotoxic agents (eg, NSAIDs) may increase risk of renal reactions. Concurrent azathioprine or 6-mercaptopurine can increase potential for blood disorders.

PREGNANCY: Category B, caution in nursing.

MECHANISM OF ACTION: Not established; suspected to diminish inflammation by blocking cyclooxygenase and inhibiting prostaglandin production in colon.

PHARMACOKINETICS: Absorption: PO administration of variable doses resulted in different parameters. **Distribution:** Plasma protein binding (43%). **Metabolism:** Liver and intestinal mucosa (acetylation), N-acetyl-5-aminosalicylic acid (metabolite). **Elimination:** Urine (≤8%); (2.4g) $T_{1/2}$=7-9 hrs; (4.8g) $T_{1/2}$=8-12 hrs

NURSING CONSIDERATIONS

Assessment: Assess for pyloric stenosis, history of sulfa allergy, renal dysfunction, hepatic impairment, possible drug interactions, conditions predisposing to development of myo- and pericarditis. Obtain baseline renal function, cardiac function and LFTs.

Monitoring: Monitor renal function periodically. Monitor for signs/symptoms of acute intolerance syndrome (cramping, acute abdominal pain, bloody diarrhea), prolonged gastric retention (pyloric stenosis), hypersensitivity, and allergic reactions.

Patient Counseling: Instruct to swallow whole, do not break outer coating. Seek medical attention if symptoms of acute intolerance syndrome (cramping, acute abdominal pain, bloody diarrhea), prolonged gastric retention (pyloric stenosis), hypersensitivity and allergic reactions occur.

Administration: Oral route. **Storage:** 15-25°C (59-77°F); excursions permitted to 30°C (86°F).

LIBRAX

chlordiazepoxide HCl - clidinium bromide (Valeant) CIV

THERAPEUTIC CLASS: Benzodiazepine/anticholinergic

INDICATIONS: Adjunct treatment of irritable bowel syndrome (IBS), acute enterocolitis, and peptic ulcer.

DOSAGE: *Adults:* Usual/Maint: 1-2 caps tid-qid ac and hs. Elderly/Debilitated: Initial: 2 caps/day and increase gradually, if needed.

HOW SUPPLIED: Cap: (Chlordiazepoxide-Clidinium) 5mg-2.5mg

CONTRAINDICATIONS: Glaucoma, prostatic hypertrophy, benign bladder neck obstruction.

WARNINGS/PRECAUTIONS: Risk of congenital malformations during first trimester of pregnancy; avoid use. Avoid abrubt withdrawal. Paradoxical reactions reported in psychiatric patients. Caution with depression, renal or hepatic dysfunction, the elderly. Inhibition of lactation may occur.

ADVERSE REACTIONS: Drowsiness, ataxia, confusion, skin eruptions, extrapyramidal symptoms, dry mouth, nausea, constipation, altered libido, blood dyscrasias, jaundice, hepatic dysfunction.

INTERACTIONS: Avoid with other psychotropics; if combination is indicated, use caution especially with MAOIs and phenothiazines. Caution with alcohol, other CNS depressants. Altered coagulation effects with oral anticoagulants.

PREGNANCY: Not for use in pregnancy; safety in nursing is not known.

MECHANISM OF ACTION: Anticholinergic/spasmolytic and antianxiety agent.

NURSING CONSIDERATIONS

Assessment: Assess for glaucoma, prostatic hypertrophy, benign bladder neck obstruction, renal/hepatic dysfunction, alcohol intake, and for possible drug interactions (eg, MAOIs).

Monitoring: Monitor for ataxia, oversedation, confusion, paradoxical reactions (eg, excitement, stimulation, acute rage), and for possible physical and psychological dependence.

L

Patient Counseling: Inform that psychological and physical dependence may develop, to avoid performing hazardous tasks (eg, operating machinery/driving), and to consult physician before increasing dose or abruptly d/c.

Administration: Oral route.

LIBRIUM

CIV

chlordiazepoxide HCl (Valeant)

THERAPEUTIC CLASS: Benzodiazepine

INDICATIONS: Management of anxiety disorders and short-term relief of anxiety symptoms, withdrawal symptoms of acute alcoholism, and preoperative apprehension and anxiety.

DOSAGE: *Adults:* Mild-Moderate Anxiety: 5-10mg tid-qid. Severe Anxiety: 20-25mg tid-qid. Alcohol Withdrawal: 50-100mg; repeat until agitation controlled. Max: 300mg/day. Preoperative Anxiety: 5-10mg PO tid-qid on days prior to surgery. Elderly/Debilitated: 5mg bid-qid.
Pediatrics: ≥6 yrs: 5mg bid-qid. May increase to 10mg bid-tid.

HOW SUPPLIED: Cap: 5mg, 10mg, 25mg

WARNINGS/PRECAUTIONS: Avoid in pregnancy. Paradoxical reactions reported in psychiatric patients and in hyperactive aggressive pediatrics. Caution with porphyria, renal or hepatic dysfunction. Reduce dose in elderly, debilitated. Avoid abrupt withdrawal after extended therapy. May impair mental/physical abilities.

ADVERSE REACTIONS: Drowsiness, ataxia, confusion, skin eruptions, edema, nausea, constipation, extrapyramidal symptoms, libido changes, EEG changes.

INTERACTIONS: Additive effects with CNS depressants and alcohol. Avoid other psychotropic agents.

PREGNANCY: Not for use in pregnancy, safety in nursing not known.

MECHANISM OF ACTION: Not established; has antianxiety, sedative, appetite stimulating, and weak analgesic actions; suspected to block EEG arousal from stimulation of brain stem reticular formation.

PHARMACOKINETICS: Elimination: Urine (1-2% unchaged, 3-6% as conjugates); $T_{1/2}$=24-48 hrs.

NURSING CONSIDERATIONS

Assessment: Assess for pregnancy status, hepatic/renal function, and possible drug interactions.

Monitoring: Monitor geriatric patients for ataxia and oversedation, drowsiness, confusion; paradoxical reactions in psychiatric patients and in hyperactive aggressive pediatric patients. Periodic blood counts and LFTs are advisable when treatment is protracted.

Patient Counseling: Inform that psychological/physical dependence may result; consult physician before increasing dose or abruptly d/c drug. May impair mental/physical abilities; caution while operating machinery/driving. May impair mental alertness in children. Avoid alcohol and other CNS depressant drugs.

Administration: Oral route. **Storage:** 25°C (77°F); excursions permitted to15-30°C (59-86°F).

LIDOCAINE OINTMENT RX

lidocaine (Fougera)

THERAPEUTIC CLASS: Acetamide local anesthetic

INDICATIONS: Topical anesthesia of the oropharynx. Anesthetic lubricant for intubation. Temporary relief of pain associated with minor burns, abrasions, and insect bites.

DOSAGE: *Adults:* Apply up to 5g (6 inches)/application. Max: 17-20g/day. *Pediatrics:* Determine dose by age and weight. Max: 4.5mg/kg.

HOW SUPPLIED: Oint: 5% [35g]

WARNINGS/PRECAUTIONS: Reduce dose in elderly, debilitated, acutely ill, and children. Avoid excessive dosage or too frequent administration; may result in serious adverse effects requiring resuscitative measures. Caution with heart block and severe shock. Extreme caution if mucosa is traumatized or sepsis is present in the area of application; risk of rapid systemic absorption.

ADVERSE REACTIONS: Lightheadedness, nervousness, confusion, euphoria, dizziness, drowsiness, blurred vision, tremors, convulsions, respiratory depression, bradycardia, hypotension, urticaria, edema, anaphylactoid reactions.

PREGNANCY: Category B, caution in nursing.

MECHANISM OF ACTION: Local anesthetic; stabilizes neuronal membrane by inhibiting ionic fluxes required for the initiation and conduction of impulses.

PHARMACOKINETICS: Absorption: Rapid (after intratracheal administration). **Distribution:** Plasma protein binding (60-80%); crosses placenta. **Metabolism:** Hepatic (biotransformation). **Elimination:** Urine. (IV): $T_{1/2}$=1.5-2 hrs.

NURSING CONSIDERATIONS

Assessment: Assess for special population, severe shock, heart block, acidosis, possible drug interactions, hepatic/renal function.

Monitoring: Monitor renal/hepatic function and for signs/symptoms of malignant hyperthermia (eg, tachycardia, tachypnea, labile BP).

Patient Counseling: Inform that drug may impair swallowing and enhance danger of aspiration. Food should not be ingested for 60 min following use of preparation in mouth or throat area, particularly in children. Numbness of tongue or buccal mucosa may increase danger of biting trauma. Avoid chewing gum. Instruct to strictly follow recommended dosage and administration. Seek medical attention if symptoms of malignant hyperthermia (tachycardia, tachypnea) occur.

Administration: Topical route. **Storage:** 15-30°C (59-86° F).

L

LIDODERM PATCH — RX
lidocaine (Endo)

THERAPEUTIC CLASS: Acetamide local anesthetic

INDICATIONS: Relief of pain associated with post-herpetic neuralgia.

DOSAGE: *Adults:* Apply to intact skin, cover most painful area. Apply up to 3 patches, once for up to 12 hrs within 24-hr period. May cut patches into smaller sizes before removal of the release liner. Debilitated/Impaired Elimination: Treat smaller areas. Remove if irritation or burning occurs; may reapply when irritation subsides.

HOW SUPPLIED: Patch: 5% [30^{s}]

WARNINGS/PRECAUTIONS: Serious adverse events may occur in children or pets if ingested. Increased risk of toxicity in severe hepatic disease. Avoid broken or inflamed skin, eye contact, larger area or longer duration than recommended. Increased levels with application of >3 patches, small patients.

ADVERSE REACTIONS: Application site reactions such as: erythema, edema, bruising, papules, vesicles, discoloration, depigmentation, burning sensation, pruritus, dermatitis, petechia, blisters, exfoliation, abnormal sensation, irritation, allergic reactions (rare).

INTERACTIONS: Additive toxic effects with concomitant Class I antiarrhythmics (eg, tocainide, mexiletine). Consider total amount absorbed from all formulations with other local anesthetics.

PREGNANCY: Category B, caution in nursing.

L

MECHANISM OF ACTION: Local anesthetic; stabilizes neuronal membranes by inhibiting ionic fluxes required for initiation and conduction of impulses.

PHARMACOKINETICS: Absorption: C_{max}=0.13mcg/mL; T_{max}=11 hrs. **Distribution:** V_d=1.5L/kg; plasma protein binding (70%); crosses placenta. **Metabolism:** Hepatic, monoethylglycinexylidide, glycinexylidide (metabolites). **Elimination:** Kidneys; $T_{1/2}$=81-149 min.

NURSING CONSIDERATIONS

Assessment: Assess for hepatic disease and possible drug interactions.

Monitoring: Monitor liver function, pain intensity, and pain relief scores periodically for 12 hrs.

Patient Counseling: Instruct if irritation or burning sensation occurs during application, to remove patch and not to reapply until irritation subsides. If eye contact occurs, immediately wash with water or saline and protect eye until sensation returns.

Administration: Transdermal route. **Storage:** Store at 25°C (77°F); excursions permitted to 15-30°C (59-86°F).

LIMBREL — RX
flavocoxid (Primus)

THERAPEUTIC CLASS: Flavonoid

INDICATIONS: Clinical dietary management of the metabolic processes of osteoarthritis (OA).

DOSAGE: *Adults*: 250-500mg q12h for total daily dose of 500-1000mg/day. May increase to 2 or more caps q12h under physician supervision.

HOW SUPPLIED: Cap: 250mg, 500mg

CONTRAINDICATIONS: Hypersensitivity to flavocoxid or flavonoids (eg, colored fruits and vegetables, dark chocolate, tea, red wine, Brazil nuts).

ADVERSE REACTIONS: Varicose veins, HTN, fluid accumulation in knee, psoriasis, NV, rash, itching, synovitis, joint pain, fever.

PREGNANCY: Not recommended for pregnant or lactating patients.

MECHANISM OF ACTION: Flavonoid; acts on COX-1, COX-2 and 5-LOX pathways; restores and maintains the balance of fatty acids in OA and also acts as a strong antioxidant.

PHARMACOKINETICS: Metabolism: Liver via CYP450 enzymes (glucuronidation and sulfation).

NURSING CONSIDERATIONS

Assessment: Assess for history of gastric ulcer, hepatic impairment, pregnancy/nursing status, and possible drug interactions.

Monitoring: Monitor for GI ulcer.

Patient Counseling: Take drug under physician supervision and as prescribed; 1 hr before or 2 hrs after meals. Notify if pregnant/nursing.

Administration: Oral route. **Storage:** 15-30°C (59-86°F); light-resistant container.

LINDANE — RX

lindane (Alpharma)

Only for patients who are intolerant or have failed first-line therapy with safer agents. Seizures and deaths reported with repeat or prolonged use. Caution in infants, children, elderly, those with other skin conditions, and those <50kg due to increased risk of neurotoxicity. Contraindicated in premature infants or those with uncontrolled seizure disorders. Instruct patients on proper use and inform that itching occurs after successful killing of scabies or lice.

THERAPEUTIC CLASS: Ectoparasiticide/ovicide

INDICATIONS: (Lot) Treatment of *Sarcoptes scabiei* (scabies) resistant to other therapies. (Shampoo) Treatment of head and pubic lice resistant to or if intolerant to other therapies.

DOSAGE: *Adults:* (Lot) Apply 1-2oz to dry skin; rub in thoroughly. Apply to whole body from neck down. Wash off after 8-12 hrs. Apply only once. (Shampoo) Wash and dry hair with regular shampoo. Apply to hair without water. Add water after 4 min; lather then rinse immediately. Towel briskly. Remove nits with comb or tweezers. Use 1oz for short hair, 1.5oz for medium length hair, and 2oz for long hair. Max: 2oz/application. Retreat if lice remain after 7 days.
Pediatrics: (Lot) Apply (≥6 yrs) 1-2oz or 1oz (<6 yrs) to dry skin; rub in thoroughly. Apply to whole body from neck down. Wash off after 8-12 hrs. Apply only once. (Shampoo) Wash and dry hair with regular shampoo. Apply to hair without water. Add water after 4 min; lather then rinse immediately. Towel briskly. Remove nits with comb or tweezers. Use 1oz for short hair, 1.5oz for medium length hair, and 2oz for long hair. Max: 2oz/application. Retreat if lice remain after 7 days.

HOW SUPPLIED: Lot, Shampoo: 1% [60mL, 480mL]

CONTRAINDICATIONS: Premature infants, Norwegian (crusted) scabies, skin conditions (eg, atopic dermatitis, psoriasis) that increase systemic absorption of the drug, uncontrolled seizure disorders.

WARNINGS/PRECAUTIONS: Adverse events with serious outcomes reported. Caution in those at increased risk of seizure (eg, HIV, head trauma, prior seizure, CNS tumor, severe hepatic cirrhosis, excessive alcohol use, abrupt alchol or sedative withdrawal). Give Medication Guide to each patient when dispensing. Avoid eyes and mouth. Do not use with open wounds, cuts, or sores. Use rubber gloves to apply.

ADVERSE REACTIONS: CNS stimulation, dizziness, convulsions.

INTERACTIONS: Avoid creams, ointments, oils, oil-based hair dressings or conditioners; may enhance absorption. Caution with drugs that may lower seizure threshold (eg, antipsychotics, antidepressants, theophylline, cyclosporine, mycophenolate, tacrolimus, penicillins, imipenem, quinolones, chloroquine sulfate, pyrimethamine, isoniazid, meperidine, radiographic contrast agents, centrally active anticholinesterases, methocarbamol).

PREGNANCY: Category C, not for use in nursing.

MECHANISM OF ACTION: Ectoparasiticide/ovicide; exerts action by being directly absorbed into parasites and their ova.

PHARMACOKINETICS: Absorption: C_{max}=28ng/mL, T_{max}=6 hrs (infants and children). **Distribution:** Found in breast milk.

NURSING CONSIDERATIONS

Assessment: Assess for current infestation with live lice, and other therapies that were not tolerated or have failed. Assess for uncontrolled seizure disorder, crusted (Norwegian) scabies or other skin conditions (eg, atopic dermatitis, psoriasis). Assess use in patients <110 lbs (50kg), elderly, increased risk for seizures (eg, HIV infection, CNS tumors, severe hepatic cirrhosis, consumption of excessive amounts of alcohol, abrupt withdrawal from alcohol or CNS depressants), pregnancy/nursing, and possible drug interactions.

Monitoring: Monitor for signs/symptoms of seizures and neurotoxicity.

Patient Counseling: Medication can be poisonous if misused, itching may occur after lice have been killed and is not necessarily an indication for retreatment. Do not apply medication to open wounds or sores unless directed by physician. Inform the individual who is applying the treatment to wear gloves made of nitrile, latex with neoprene, or sheer vinyl, and to thoroughly clean hands after applying medication. Do not cover hair with anything that does not breathe (eg, shower cap, towel) following administration. Avoid using oil treatments, oil-based hair dressings or conditioners immediately before and after applying the shampoo. Wash all recently worn clothing, underwear, pajamas, hats, sheets, pillow cases, and towels in hot water or dry-clean.

Administration: Administered topically as shampoo. Shake well before using.
Storage: 15-30°C (59-86°F).

LIPITOR — RX

atorvastatin calcium (Parke-Davis/Pfizer)

THERAPEUTIC CLASS: HMG-CoA reductase inhibitor

INDICATIONS: Adjunct to diet, to reduce total cholesterol (total-C), LDL-C, TG, and Apo B levels, and to increase HDL-C in primary hypercholesterolemia (heterozygous familial and nonfamilial) and mixed dyslipidemia (Types IIa and IIb). Adjunct to diet for elevated serum TG levels (Type IV). Treatment of primary dysbetalipoproteinemia (Type III) inadequately responding to diet. Adjunct to other lipid-lowering treatments or if treatments are unavailable, to reduce total-C and LDL-C in homozygous familial hypercholesterolemia. Adjunct to diet to lower total-C, LDL-C and apolipoprotein B in postmenarchal adolescents with heterozygous familial hypercholesterolemia. To reduce the risk of MI, revascularization procedures, and angina in adults without clinically evident CHD but with multiple risk factors for CHD. To reduce the risk of MI and stroke in patients with Type II DM, and without clinically evident CHD, but with multiple risk factors for CHD. In patients with clinically evident CHD to reduce the risk of non-fatal MI, fatal and non-fatal stroke, revascularization procedures, hospitalization for CHF, and angina.

DOSAGE: *Adults:* Hypercholesterolemia/Mixed Dyslipidemia: Initial: 10-20mg qd (or 40mg qd for LDL-C reduction >45%). Titrate: Adjust dose if needed at 2-4 week intervals. Usual: 10-80mg qd. Homozygous Familial Hypercholesterolemia: 10-80mg qd.
Pediatrics: Heterozygous Familial Hypercholesterolemia: 10-17 yrs (post-menarchal): Initial: 10mg/day. Titrate: Adjust dose if needed at intervals of ≥4 weeks. Max: 20mg/day.

HOW SUPPLIED: Tab: 10mg, 20mg, 40mg, 80mg

CONTRAINDICATIONS: Active liver disease, unexplained persistent elevations of serum transaminases, pregnancy, nursing mothers.

WARNINGS/PRECAUTIONS: Monitor LFTs prior to therapy, at 12 weeks or with dose elevation, and periodically thereafter. Reduce dose or withdraw if AST or ALT ≥3x ULN persists. Caution with heavy alcohol use and/or history of hepatic disease. D/C if markedly elevated CPK levels occur, if myopathy is diagnosed or suspected, or if predisposition to renal failure secondary to rhabdomyolysis. Caution in patients with recent stroke or TIA. Rare cases of rhabdomyolysis reported.

ADVERSE REACTIONS: Constipation, flatulence, dyspepsia, abdominal pain, transaminase and CK elevation in higher doses.

INTERACTIONS: Increases levels with erythromycin. Increases levels of oral contraceptives (norethindrone, ethinyl estradiol), digoxin. Monitor digoxin. Cyclosporine, fibric acid derivatives, niacin, erythromycin, and azole antifungals may increase risk of myopathy. Caution with drugs that decrease levels or activity of endogenous steroid hormones (eg, ketoconazole, spironolactone, cimetidine). Decreases levels with Maalox® TC, but LDL-C reduction not altered. Colestipol decreases levels when coadministered, but greater LDL-C reduction with coadministration than when each given alone. Avoid fibrates.

PREGNANCY: Category X, not for use in nursing.

MECHANISM OF ACTION: Competitive inhibitor of HMG-CoA reductase; inhibits conversion of HMG-CoA to mevalonate (precursor of sterols, including cholesterol).

PHARMACOKINETICS: Absorption: Rapid; absolute bioavailability (14%); T_{max}=1-2 hrs. **Distribution:** V_d=381L; plasma protein binding (≥98%); found in breast milk. **Metabolism:** Extensive; via CYP3A4 to ortho- and parahydroxylated derivatives, and various β-oxidation products. **Elimination:** Bile (drug, metabolites), urine (<2%); $T_{1/2}$=14 hrs.

NURSING CONSIDERATIONS

Assessment: Assess for active liver disease or unexplained and persistent elevations in serum transaminase, pregnancy/nursing status, alcohol intake, renal impairment, and possible drug interactions. Perform LFTs prior to therapy and at 12 weeks thereafter. Try to control hypercholesterolemia through appropriate diet, exercise, and weight reduction prior to therapy.

Monitoring: Monitor LFTs, CPK, signs/symptoms of myopathy (eg, diffuse muscle pain, tenderness or weakness, and fever or malaise), rhabdomyolysis, acute renal failure, endocrine dysfunction, and CNS toxicity or CNS vascular lesions (eg, hemorrhage and edema).

Patient Counseling: Inform about potential risks/benefits. Report promptly any signs of myopathy (eg, unexplained muscle pain, tenderness, or weakness, and malaise or fever). Follow standard cholesterol-lowering diet prior to and during therapy. Notify if pregnant/nursing or planning to become pregnant.

Administration: Oral route. **Storage:** 20-25°C (68-77°F).

L

LITHIUM CARBONATE RX

lithium carbonate (Roxane)

Lithium toxicity is related to serum lithium levels and can occur at doses close to therapeutic levels.

THERAPEUTIC CLASS: Antimanic agent

INDICATIONS: Treatment of manic episodes of bipolar disorder and maintenance treatment of bipolar disorder.

DOSAGE: *Adults:* Acute Mania: 600mg tid to achieve effective serum levels of 1-1.5mEq/L; monitor levels twice a week until stabilized. Maint: 300mg tid-qid to maintain serum levels of 0.6-1.2 mEq/L; monitor levels every 2 months. Elderly: Reduce dose.
Pediatrics: ≥12 yrs: Acute Mania: 600mg tid. Effective serum levels are 1-1.5mEq/L; monitor levels twice a week until stabilized. Maint: 300mg tid-qid to maintain serum levels of 0.6-1.2mEq/L; monitor levels every 2 months.

HOW SUPPLIED: Cap: 150mg, 300mg, 600mg; Tab: 300mg

CONTRAINDICATIONS: Renal or cardiovascular disease, severe debilitation or dehydration, sodium depletion, and diuretic use.

WARNINGS/PRECAUTIONS: May cause fetal harm; if possible withdraw for at least the 1st trimester of pregnancy. Caution in the elderly. Maintain normal diet, adequate salt/fluid intake. Assess kidney function prior to and during therapy. May impair mental/physical abilities. Reduce dose or d/c with sweating, diarrhea, infection with elevated temperatures. Caution with thyroid disorders; monitor thyroid function. Chronic therapy associated with diminution of renal concentrating ability (eg, diabetes insipidus), glomerular and interstitial fibrosis, and nephron atrophy.

ADVERSE REACTIONS: Fine hand tremor, polyuria, mild thirst, nausea, incoordination, diarrhea, vomiting, drowsiness, muscular weakness.

INTERACTIONS: Risk of encephalopathic syndrome (eg, weakness, lethargy, fever, tremulousness, confusion, EPS) with haloperidol and other antipsychotics; discontinue therapy if such signs occur. May prolong effects of neuromuscular blockers. Increased levels with indomethacin, piroxicam and other NSAIDs. Increased risk of toxicity due to decreased clearance with diuretics and ACE inhibitors; contraindicated with diuretics.

PREGNANCY: Category D, not for use in nursing.

MECHANISM OF ACTION: Mood-stabilizing agent; mechanism not established. Suspected to alter sodium transport in nerve and muscle cells and effect a shift toward intraneuronal metabolism of catecholamines.

PHARMACOKINETICS: Distribution: Found in breast milk. **Elimination**: Urine (primary), feces; $T_{1/2}$=24 hrs.

NURSING CONSIDERATIONS

L

Assessment: Assess use with significant renal or cardiovascular disease, severe debilitation or dehydration, sodium depletion, diuretics, drug interactions (eg, neuromuscular blocking agents), pregnancy status, baseline renal function (SrCr, urinalysis), and thyroid function.

Monitoring: Monitor for diminution of renal concentrating ability (eg, nephrogenic diabetes insipidus), glomerular and interstitial fibrosis and nephron atrophy, renal function and thyroid function while on therapy. Monitor serum lithium levels twice weekly during acute phase and until serum lithium level and condition of patient stabilized. Monitor for signs/symptoms of lithium toxicity (eg, diarrhea, vomiting, tremor, mild ataxia, drowsiness, muscular weakness).

Patient Counseling: Counsel about early signs of lithium toxicity (eg, diarrhea, vomiting, tremor, mild ataxia, drowsiness, muscle weakness) and activities requiring mental alertness. Counsel females to avoid pregnancy/nursing while on medication. Advise to maintain normal diet, including salt, and adequate fluid intake (2500-3000mL), at least during initial stabilization period. Counsel to contact physician if diarrhea or concomitant infection with elevated temperatures develop; may require change in dosing.

Administration: Oral route. **Storage**: 25°C (77°F); excursions permitted to 15-30°C (59-86°F). Protect from moisture. Dispense in a tight container.

LITHOBID

RX

lithium carbonate (JDS)

Lithium toxicity is related to serum levels, and can occur at doses close to therapeutic levels.

THERAPEUTIC CLASS: Antimanic agent

INDICATIONS: Treatment of manic episodes of manic-depressive illness.

DOSAGE: *Adults:* Acute Mania: Initial: 900mg bid or 600mg tid to achieve effective serum levels of 1-1.5mEq/L; monitor levels twice weekly until stabilized. Maint: 900-1200mg/day, given bid-tid to maintain serum levels of 0.6-1.2mEq/L; monitor levels every 2 months.
Pediatrics: ≥12 yrs: Acute Mania: Initial: 900mg bid or 600mg tid to achieve effective serum levels of 1-1.5mEq/L; monitor levels twice weekly until stabilized. Maint: 900-1200mg/day, given bid-tid to maintain serum levels of 0.6-1.2 mEq/L; monitor levels every 2 months.

HOW SUPPLIED: Tab, Extended-Release: 300mg

WARNINGS/PRECAUTIONS: Avoid with significant renal or cardiovascular disease, severe debilitation, dehydration, or sodium depletion. Assess kidney function prior to and during therapy. Risk of encephalopathic syndrome (eg, weakness, lethargy, fever, tremulousness, confusion, EPS); d/c therapy. May impair mental/physical abilities. Reduce dose or d/c with sweating, diarrhea, infection with elevated temperatures. Caution with hypothyroidism; may need supplemental therapy. Chronic therapy associated with diminution of renal concentrating ability, glomerular and interstitial fibrosis, and nephron atrophy.

ADVERSE REACTIONS: Fine hand tremor, polyuria, mild thirst, nausea, general discomfort, diarrhea, vomiting, drowsiness, muscular weakness.

INTERACTIONS: Avoid diuretics and ACE inhibitors; risk of lithium toxicity due to reduced renal clearance. May prolong effects of neuromuscular blockers. Decreased levels with acetazolamide, urea, xanthine preparations, and alkalinizing agents. May produce hypothyroidism with iodide preparations. Increased plasma levels with indomethacin, piroxicam, other NSAIDs. Increased risk of neurotoxic effects with carbamazepine and CCBs. Reduced renal clearance with metronidazole. Fluoxetine may increase and/or decrease lithium levels.

PREGNANCY: Category D, not for use in nursing.

MECHANISM OF ACTION: Not established; suspected to alter sodium transport in nerve and muscle cells and effects a shift toward intraneuronal metabolism of catecholamines.

PHARMACOKINETICS: Elimination: Urine (primary), feces (insignificant); $T_{1/2}$=24 hrs.

L

NURSING CONSIDERATIONS

Assessment: Assess use with significant renal dysfunction, cardiovascular disease, severe debilitation, dehydration, sodium depletion, concomitant therapy with either ACE inhibitors or diuretics. Assess renal function (urinalysis, SrCr) prior to therapy. Assess thyroid function with history of thyroid disease.

Monitoring: Monitor for diminution of renal concentrating ability (eg, nephrogenic diabetes insipidus), glomerular and interstitial fibrosis, and nephron atrophy in patients on long-term therapy, encephalopathic syndrome, renal function while on therapy, thyroid function in patients with a history of hypothyroidism, serum lithium levels, signs of lithium toxicity (eg, diarrhea, vomiting, tremor).

Patient Counseling: Instruct to maintain a normal diet, including proper sodium and fluid intake (2500mL-3500mL). Instruct to notify physician if protracted sweating or diarrhea, or concomitant infection with elevated temperatures develops; may require dose adjustment. Counsel to d/c therapy and notify physician if clinical signs of lithium toxicity (eg, diarrhea, vomiting, tremor, muscular weakness) occur. Inform may impair mental/physical abilities; use caution with activities requiring alertness.

Administration: Oral route. **Storage:** 15-30°C (59-86°C). Protect from moisture. Dispense in tight, light- and child-resistant containers.

Lo/Ovral — RX

norgestrel - ethinyl estradiol (Wyeth)

OTHER BRAND NAMES: Cryselle (Duramed) - Low-Ogestrel (Watson)

THERAPEUTIC CLASS: Estrogen/progestogen combination

INDICATIONS: Prevention of pregnancy.

DOSAGE: *Adults:* Start 1st Sunday after menses begins or the 1st day of menses. *21-day:* 1 tab qd for 21 days, stop 7 days, then repeat. *28-day:* 1 tab qd for 28 days, then repeat.

HOW SUPPLIED: Tab: (Ethinyl Estradiol-Norgestrel) 0.03mg-0.3mg

CONTRAINDICATIONS: Thrombophlebitis, DVT or thromboembolic disorders, pregnancy, cerebrovascular or coronary artery disease, undiagnosed abnormal genital bleeding, cholestatic jaundice of pregnancy or jaundice with prior pill use, hepatic adenomas or carcinomas, breast cancer or other estrogen-dependent neoplasia, thrombogenic valvulopathies, thrombogenic rhythm disorders, diabetes with vascular involvement, uncontrolled HTN, endometrium carcinoma, active liver disease if liver function has not returned to normal.

WARNINGS/PRECAUTIONS: Cigarette smoking increases risk of serious cardiovascular side effects; risk increases with age (especially >35 yrs) and heavy smoking. Increased risk of MI, vascular disease, thromboembolism, stroke and gallbladder disease. Retinal thrombosis, hepatic neoplasia reported. May cause glucose intolerance. May increase BP, elevate LDL levels or cause other lipid changes, fluid retention, breakthrough bleeding, and spotting. May cause or exacerbate migraine. May develop visual changes with contact lens. Increased risk of MI with HTN, hyperlipidemia, obesity, and diabetes. D/C if jaundice, significant depression or ophthalmic irregularities develop. Perform annual physical exam. Use before menarche is not indicated. May affect certain endocrine, LFTs and blood components.

ADVERSE REACTIONS: NV, breakthrough bleeding, spotting, amenorrhea, migraine, depression, vaginal candidiasis, edema, weight changes.

INTERACTIONS: Reduced effects, increased breakthrough bleeding, and menstrual irregularities with rifampin, rifabutin, barbiturates, phenylbutazone, phenytoin, griseofulvin, topiramate, some protease inhibitors, modafinil and possibly with St. John's wort, some penicillins, ampicillin and tetracylines. Increased levels with ascorbic acid and acetaminophen, indinavir, fluconazole, troleandomycin, and atorvastatin. May affect cyclosporine, theophylline and corticosteroid levels.

L

PREGNANCY: Category X, not for use in nursing.

MECHANISM OF ACTION: Estrogen/progestogen combination oral contraceptive; acts by suppressing gonadotropins. Primarily acts by inhibiting ovulation. Also responsible for causing changes in cervical mucus (increases difficulty of sperm entry into uterus) and in endometrium (reduces likelihood of implantation).

NURSING CONSIDERATIONS

Assessment: Assess for current or history of thrombophlebitis or thromboembolic disorders, CVD or CAD, thrombogenic valvulopathies, thrombogenic rhythm disorders, major surgery with prolonged immobilization, DM with vascular involvement, headaches with focal neurological symptoms, uncontrolled HTN, known/suspected or history of carcinoma of breast, endometrium or other known/suspected estrogen-dependent neoplasia, undiagnosed abnormal genital bleeding, cholestatic jaundice of pregnancy or jaundice with prior pill use, hepatic adenomas or carcinomas, active liver disease with abnormal liver function, and known/suspected pregnancy. Assess use with HTN, hyperlipidemia, obesity, DM, women >35 yrs who smoke ≥15 cigarettes/day, or for possible drug interactions.

Monitoring: Monitor for venous and arterial thrombotic and thromboembolic events (eg, MI, stroke), hepatic neoplasia, gallbladder disease, and HTN, signs of fluid retention, onset or exacerbation of migraines or headaches, bleeding irregularities, development of ocular lesions. Monitor serum glucose levels in DM or prediabetic patients, lipid levels with history of hyperlipidemia, BP with history of HTN. Refer patients with contact lenses to ophthalmologist if visual changes occur. Monitor liver function, signs of depression with previous history, and signs of GI upset (eg, diarrhea, vomiting). Perform annual physical exam while on therapy.

Patient Counseling: Counsel about possible adverse effects of drug. Advise to avoid smoking while on medication. Inform that drug does not protect against HIV infection and other STDs. Instruct women to use additional method of birth control until after first 7 days of administration in initial cycle. Instruct to take medication at same time every day and at intervals not exceeding 24 hrs. Inform that if dose missed, take next pill as soon as possible, then take next dose at regular time. If patient skips 2 or more doses, advise to use another method of contraception until patient has taken medication for 7 consecutive days. Counsel that if spotting or breakthrough bleeding occurs, continue taking medication; notify physician if bleeding is persistent or prolonged.

Administration: Oral route. **Storage:** Store at controlled room temperature 20-25°C (68-77°F).

Locoid RX

hydrocortisone butyrate (Ferndale)

THERAPEUTIC CLASS: Corticosteroid

INDICATIONS: (Cre, Oint) Corticosteroid-responsive dermatoses. (Sol) Seborrheic dermatitis.

DOSAGE: *Adults:* (Cre, Oint) Apply bid-tid. May use occlusive dressings for psoriasis or recalcitrant conditions. D/C dressings if infection develops. (Sol) Apply bid-tid.
Pediatrics: (Cre, Oint) Apply bid-tid. May use occlusive dressings for psoriasis or recalcitrant conditions. D/C dressings if infection develops. (Sol) Apply bid-tid.

HOW SUPPLIED: Cre, Oint: 0.1% [15g, 45g]; Sol: 0.1% [20mL, 60mL]

WARNINGS/PRECAUTIONS: May produce reversible HPA axis suppression, manifestations of Cushing's syndrome, hyperglycemia, and glucosuria. D/C if irritation occurs. Use appropriate antifungal or antibacterial agent with dermatological infections. Peds may be more susceptible to systemic toxicity. Caution when applied to large surface areas. Avoid contact with eyes. Limit to least amount compatible with an effective therapeutic regimen. Chronic corticosteroid therapy may interfere with the growth and development of children.

ADVERSE REACTIONS: Burning, itching, irritation, dryness, folliculitis, hypertrichosis, acneiform eruptions, hypopigmentation, perioral dermatitis, allergic dermatitis, skin maceration, secondary infection, skin atrophy, striae, miliaria.

PREGNANCY: Category C, caution in nursing.

MECHANISM OF ACTION: Corticosteroid; possesses anti-inflammatory, anti-pruritic, and vasoconstrictive properties. Anti-inflammatory actions not established.

PHARMACOKINETICS: Absorption: Percutaneous; inflammation, other disease states, and occlusive dressings may increase absorption. **Distribution:** Bound to plasma proteins to varying degrees. Systemically administered corticosteroids found in breast milk. **Metabolism:** Liver. **Elimination:** Renal (major), bile.

NURSING CONSIDERATIONS

Assessment: Assess use in pregnant/nursing patients.

Monitoring: Monitor for signs/symptoms of reversible HPA-axis suppression, Cushing's syndrome, hyperglycemia, glucosuria, dermatological infections (eg, fungal, bacterial), and steroid withdrawal. For patients on large doses or in patients using occlusive dressings, perform periodic monitoring for HPA-axis suppression using urinary free cortisol and ACTH stimulation tests. (Pediatrics) Monitor for signs/symptoms of systemic toxicity, HPA-axis suppression (eg, linear growth retardation, delayed weight gain), Cushing's syndrome, and intracranial HTN.

Patient Counseling: Counsel to use externally and exactly as directed; avoid contact with eyes. Report signs of adverse reactions; do not bandage, cover or wrap treated skin area. Inform caregivers of pediatric patients to avoid using tight-fitting diapers or plastic pants on treatment area.

Administration: Topical route. **Storage:** Cream: 15-25°C (59-77°F), Ointment: 2-30°C (36-86°F), Solution: 5-25°C (41-77°F).

LOESTRIN RX

norethindrone acetate - ethinyl estradiol - ferrous fumarate (Duramed/Warner Chilcott)

OTHER BRAND NAMES: Junel 1.5/30 (Barr) - Junel 1/20 (Barr) - Junel Fe 1/20 (Barr) - Junel Fe 1.5/30 (Barr) - Microgestin Fe 1/20 (Watson) - Microgestin Fe 1.5/30 (Watson) - Loestrin Fe 1.5/30 (Duramed/Warner Chilcott) - Loestrin Fe 1/20 (Duramed/Warner Chilcott) - Loestrin 1.5/30 (Duramed/Warner Chilcott) - Loestrin 1/20 (Duramed/Warner Chilcott)

THERAPEUTIC CLASS: Estrogen/progestogen combination

INDICATIONS: Prevention of pregnancy.

DOSAGE: *Adults:* Start 1st Sunday after menses begin or the 1st day of menses. *21-day:* 1 tab qd for 21 days, stop 7 days, then repeat. *28-day:* 1 tab qd for 28 days, then repeat.

HOW SUPPLIED: Tab:(Ethinyl Estradiol-Norethindrone) (1/20) 20mcg-1mg, (1.5/30) 30mcg-1.5mg; (Fe 1/20) 20mcg-1mg and 75mg ferrous fumarate, (Fe 1.5/30) 30mcg-1.5mg and 75mg ferrous fumarate

CONTRAINDICATIONS: Thrombophlebitis, DVT or thromboembolic disorders, pregnancy, cerebrovascular or coronary artery disease, undiagnosed abnormal genital bleeding, cholestatic jaundice of pregnancy or jaundice with prior pill use, hepatic adenomas or carcinomas, breast cancer or other estrogen-dependent neoplasia.

L

WARNINGS/PRECAUTIONS: Cigarette smoking increases risk of serious cardiovascular side effects. This risk increases with age (especially >35 yrs) and heavy smoking. Increased risk of MI, vascular disease, thromboembolism, stroke, and gallbladder disease. Retinal thrombosis, hepatic neoplasia, carcinoma of breast and reproductive organs reported. May cause glucose intolerance. May increase BP, elevate LDL levels or cause other lipid changes, fluid retention, breakthrough bleeding, and spotting. May cause or exacerbate migraine. May develop visual changes with contact lens. Increased risk of MI with HTN, hyperlipidemia, obesity, and diabetes. D/C if jaundice, significant depression or ophthalmic irregularities develop. Perform annual physical exam. Use before menarche is not indicated. May affect certain endocrine, LFTs, and blood components.

ADVERSE REACTIONS: NV, breakthrough bleeding, spotting, amenorrhea, migraine, depression, vaginal candidiasis, edema, weight changes.

INTERACTIONS: Reduced effects, increased breakthrough bleeding, and menstrual irregularities with rifampin, barbiturates, phenylbutazone, phenytoin, carbamazepine, and possibly with griseofulvin, ampicillin, and tetracyclines. Increased levels with atorvastatin, ascorbic acid, and APAP. Increased plasma levels of cyclosporine, prednisolone, and theophylline. Decreased levels of APAP. Increased clearance of temazepam, salicylic acid, morphine, and clofibric acid. Troglitazone reduces plasma levels of hormones.

PREGNANCY: Category X, not for use in nursing.

MECHANISM OF ACTION: Estrogen/progestogen combination oral contraceptive; acts by suppression of gonadotropins. Primarily inhibits ovulation. Causes changes in cervical mucus (increasing difficulty of sperm entry into uterus) and endometrium (reducing likelihood of implantation).

PHARMACOKINETICS: Absorption: Rapid and complete. Norethindrone Acetate: Absolute bioavailability (64%); Single dose: C_{max}=8420pg/mL, T_{max}=1.0 hr, AUC=33390pg/mL•hr; Multiple doses: C_{max}=16400pg/mL, T_{max}=1.3 hrs, AUC=88160pg/mL•hr. Ethinyl Estradiol: Absolute bioavailability (43%); Single dose: C_{max}=64.5pg/mL, T_{max}=1.3 hrs, AUC=465.4pg/mL•hr. Multiple doses: C_{max}=81.9pg/mL, T_{max}=1.7 hrs, AUC=701.3pg/mL•hr. **Distribution:** V_d=2-4L/kg; plasma protein binding (≥95%). **Metabolism:** Norethindrone: Reduction, (sulfate-glucuronide conjugation). Ethinyl Estradiol: 1st-pass metabolism, CYP3A4 (oxidation). **Elimination:** Urine, feces. Norethindrone: $T_{1/2}$=8 hrs. Ethinyl Estradiol: $T_{1/2}$=14 hrs.

NURSING CONSIDERATIONS

Assessment: Assess current or history of thrombophlebitis or thromboembolic disorder, CVD or CAD, valvular heart disease with thrombogenic complications, severe HTN, DM with vascular involvement, headaches with focal neurological symptoms, major surgery with prolonged immobilization, known/suspected carcinoma of breast, endometrium or other known or suspected estrogen-dependent neoplasia, undiagnosed abnormal genital bleeding, cholestatic jaundice of pregnancy or jaundice with prior pill use, hepatic adenomas or carcinomas, active liver disease, or known/suspected pregnancy. Assess use in women ≥35 yrs who smoke ≥15 cigarettes/day, and for possible drug interactions.

Monitoring: Monitor for venous and arterial thrombotic and thromboembolic events (eg, MI, stroke), hepatic neoplasia, gallbladder disease, ocular lesions, HTN, fluid retention, onset or exacerbation of migraines or headaches, bleeding irregularities (eg, breakthrough bleeding, spotting). Monitor blood glucose levels in DM and prediabetic women, BP with history of HTN, lipid levels with history of hyperlipidemia, for signs/symptoms of hepatotoxicity (eg, jaundice), and for signs of worsening depression with previous history. Refer patients with contact lenses to opthalmologist if visual changes develop. Perform annual physical exam while on therapy.

Patient Counseling: Counsel about potential adverse effects. Inform that drug does not protect against HIV infection and other STDs. Instruct to use additional method of birth control for first 7 days of administration. Instruct to take exactly as directed and at intervals not exceeding 24 hrs. Advise that if dose missed, take as soon as remembered, then take next dose at regularly scheduled time. Counsel to take with/without food. Advise to continue regimen if spotting or breakthrough bleeding occurs; notify physician if prolonged or persists. Instruct to avoid smoking while on medication.

Administration: Oral route. **Storage:** Store at 25°C (77°F); excursions permitted to 15-30°C (59-86°F).

LOFIBRA
fenofibrate (Gate)

RX

THERAPEUTIC CLASS: Fibric acid derivative

INDICATIONS: Adjunct to diet, for treatment of hypertriglyceridemia (Types IV and V). Adjunct to diet, for reduction of total-C, LDL-C, Apo B, and TG in primary hypercholesterolemia or mixed dyslipidemia (Types IIa and IIb).

DOSAGE: *Adults:* Hypercholesterolemia/Mixed Dyslipidemia: Initial: Cap: 200mg qd. Hypercholesterolemia/Mixed Hyperlipidemia: Tab: 160mg qd. Hypertriglyceridemia: Initial: Cap: 67-200mg/day. Tab: 54-160mg qd. Titrate: Adjust if needed after repeat lipid levels at 4-8 week intervals. Max: Cap: 200mg/day. Tab: 160mg/day. Renal Dysfunction/Elderly: Initial: Cap: 67mg/day. Tab: 54mg/day. Take with meals.

HOW SUPPLIED: Cap: 67mg, 134mg, 200mg; Tab: 54mg, 160mg

CONTRAINDICATIONS: Pre-existing gallbladder disease, unexplained persistent hepatic function abnormality, hepatic or severe renal dysfunction (including primary biliary cirrhosis).

WARNINGS/PRECAUTIONS: Monitor LFTs regularly; d/c if >3x ULN. May cause cholelithiasis; d/c if gallstones found. D/C if myopathy or marked CPK elevation occurs. Decreased Hgb, Hct, WBCs, thrombocytopenia, and agranulocytosis reported; monitor CBCs during first 12 months of therapy. Acute hypersensitivity reactions (rare) and pancreatitis reported. Monitor lipids periodically initially, d/c if inadequate response after 2 months on 200mg/day. Minimize dose in severe renal impairment. Caution in elderly.

ADVERSE REACTIONS: Abdominal pain, back pain, headache, abnormal LFTs, increased creatine phosphokinase, respiratory disorder.

INTERACTIONS: May potentiate coumarin anticoagulants; reduce anticoagulant dose and monitor PT/INR. Avoid HMG-CoA reductase inhibitors unless benefits outweigh risks. Bile acid sequestrants may impede absorption; take at least 1 hr before or 4-6 hrs after the resin. Evaluate benefits/risks with immunosuppressants (eg, cyclosporine) and other nephrotoxic agents.

PREGNANCY: Category C, not for use in nursing.

MECHANISM OF ACTION: Fenofibric acid derivative; activates peroxisome proliferator receptor alpha (PPRα); increases lipolysis and elimination of triglyceride-rich particles from plasma by activating lipoprotein lipase and reducing production of apoprotein C-III. Reduces serum uric acid levels by increasing urinary excretion of uric acid.

PHARMACOKINETICS: Absorption: Well absorbed; T_{max}=6-8 hrs. **Distribution:** Plasma protein binding (99%). **Metabolism:** Via esterases through hydrolysis and glucuronidation. **Elimination:** Urine (60%), feces (25%); $T_{1/2}$=20 hrs.

NURSING CONSIDERATIONS

Assessment: Assess for hepatic/renal dysfunction, primary biliary cirrhosis, persistent, unexplained liver function abnormality, persistent elevation of lipid levels, hypothyroidism, pre-existing gallbladder disease, pregnancy/nursing status, DM, and possible drug interactions (eg, anticoagulants). Control serum lipid levels with appropriate diet, exercise, and weight reduction in obese patients prior to therapy.

Monitoring: Periodically monitor lipids and LFTs, CPK, PT, INR, CBC. Monitor for signs of myopathy (eg, unexplained muscle pain, tenderness, or weakness with fever or malaise), cholelithiasis/cholecystitis, pancreatitis, hepatocellular, chronic active and cholestatic hepatitis, liver cirrhosis, malignancy, and severe skin rash.

L

Patient Counseling: Inform about potential risks/benefits of therapy. Report promptly unexplained muscle pain, tenderness, or weakness, with malaise or fever. Notify physician if pregnant/nursing or planning to become pregnant. Follow standard cholesterol-lowering diet prior to and during therapy.

Administration: Oral route. **Storage:** 20-25°C (68-77°F).

LOMOTIL

CV

diphenoxylate HCl - atropine sulfate (Pharmacia & Upjohn)

OTHER BRAND NAMES: Lonox (Sandoz)

THERAPEUTIC CLASS: Opioid/anticholinergic

INDICATIONS: Adjunctive therapy for management of diarrhea.

DOSAGE: *Adults:* Initial: 2 tabs or 10mL qid. Titrate: Reduce dose after symptoms are controlled. Maint: 2 tabs or 10mL qd. Max: 20mg/day diphenoxylate. D/C if symptoms not controlled after 10 days at max dose of 20mg/day (diphenoxylate).

Pediatrics: 2-12 yrs: Initial: 0.3-0.4mg/kg/day of solution given qid. 13-16 yrs: Initial: 2 tabs or 10mL tid. Titrate: Reduce dose after symptoms are controlled. Maint: 25% of initial dose. D/C if no improvement within 48 hrs.

HOW SUPPLIED: (Diphenoxylate-Atropine) Sol: 2.5mg-0.025/5mL [60mL]; Tab: 2.5mg-0.025mg

CONTRAINDICATIONS: Obstructive jaundice, diarrhea associated with pseudomembranous enterocolitis or enterotoxin-producing bacteria.

WARNINGS/PRECAUTIONS: May induce toxic megacolon in ulcerative colitis; d/c if abdominal distention occurs. May cause intestinal fluid retention. Avoid with diarrhea associated with organisms that penetrate the intestinal mucosa, and with pseudomembranous enterocolitis. Caution in pediatrics, especially with Down's syndrome. Extreme caution advanced hepatorenal disease and liver dysfunction. Do not use with severe dehydration or electrolyte imbalance until corrective therapy is initiated.

ADVERSE REACTIONS: Numbness of extremities, dizziness, anaphylaxis, hyperthermia, tachycardia, urinary retention, flushing, drowsiness, toxic megacolon, nausea, vomiting.

INTERACTIONS: May potentiate barbiturates, tranquilizers and alcohol. MAOIs may precipitate hypertensive crisis.

PREGNANCY: Category C, caution in nursing.

MECHANISM OF ACTION: Diphenoxylate: Antidiarrheal. Atropine: Anticholinergic.

PHARMACOKINETICS: Absorption: (4 tabs): C_{max}=163ng/mL; T_{max}=2 hrs. **Metabolism:** Rapid and extensive metabolism through ester hydrolysis to diphenoxylic acid (major metabolite). **Elimination:** Urine (14%, 6% conjugate), feces (49%). $T_{1/2}$=12-14 hrs (diphenoxylic acid).

NURSING CONSIDERATIONS

Assessment: Assess renal function test, LFTs, ulcerative colitis, Down's syndrome, diarrhea caused by *E coli*, salmonella, shigella, obstructive jaundice, pseudomembranous enterocolitis.

Monitoring: Monitor for severe dehydration and electrolyte imbalance, LFTs, renal function test, toxic megacolon in ulcerative colitis, pancreatitis.

Patient Counseling: Take as directed. Dosing to be accompanied by adequate fluids and electrolytes. Exercise caution while operating machinery/driving. Should not be used in children under 2 years. Report lack of response or adverse effects. Avoid alcohol and other CNS depressants.

Administration: Oral route. Plastic dropper should be used when measuring liquid for administration to children. **Storage:** Dispense liquids in original container.

LOPID

gemfibrozil (Parke-Davis)

RX

L

THERAPEUTIC CLASS: Fibric acid derivative

INDICATIONS: Types IV and V hyperlipidemia with risk of pancreatitis not responding to dietary management (usually TG >2000mg/dL). May consider therapy if TG 1000-2000mg/dL with history of pancreatitis or recurrent abdominal pain typical of pancreatitis. Risk reduction of CAD in Type IIb patients without history or symptoms of existing coronary heart disease inadequately responding to weight loss, dietary therapy, exercise, other pharmacologic agents; with triad of low HDL, and elevated LDL and TG levels.

DOSAGE: *Adults:* 600mg bid. Give 30 min before morning and evening meals.

HOW SUPPLIED: Tab: 600mg* *scored

CONTRAINDICATIONS: Hepatic or severe renal dysfunction, including primary biliary cirrhosis; pre-existing gallbladder disease, concomitant cerivastatin.

WARNINGS/PRECAUTIONS: Abnormal LFTs reported; monitor periodically. Only use if indicated and d/c if significant lipid response not obtained. Associated with myositis. D/C if suspect or diagnose myositis, if abnormal LFTs persist, or gallstones develop. Cholelithiasis reported. Monitor blood counts periodically during first 12 months. May worsen renal insufficiency.

ADVERSE REACTIONS: Dyspepsia, abdominal pain, diarrhea, fatigue, bacterial and viral infections, musculoskeletal symptoms, abnormal LFTs, hematologic changes, hypesthesia, paresthesia, taste perversion.

INTERACTIONS: Caution with anticoagulants; reduce dose and monitor PT. Increased risk of myopathy and rhabdomyolysis with HMG-CoA reductase inhibitors. Benefit with concomitant HMG-CoA reductase inhibitors does not outweigh risks. Avoid initiating therapy with repaglinide. If already on repaglinide therapy, monitor levels and adjust repaglinide dose. Avoid itraconazole in patients taking gemfibrozil and repaglinide.

PREGNANCY: Category C, not for use in nursing.

MECHANISM OF ACTION: Lipid regulating agent; decreases serum TG and VLDL cholesterol and increases HDL cholesterol. Not established; shown to inhibit peripheral lipolysis, decrease hepatic extraction of free fatty acids, thus reducing hepatic TG production and inhibiting synthesis and increasing clearance of VLDL carrier apolipoprotein B, leading to decreased VLDL production.

PHARMACOKINETICS: Absorption: Complete; T_{max}=1-2 hr. **Metabolism:** Oxidation to hydroxymethyl and carboxyl metabolites. **Elimination:** Urine (70% glucoronide conjugate) (2% unchanged), feces (6%).

NURSING CONSIDERATIONS

Assessment: Assess for hepatic/renal dysfunction, primary biliary cirrhosis, persistent abnormal levels of lipids, gallbladder disease, DM, hypothyroidism, pregnancy/nursing status, coronary heart disease, and possible drug interactions (eg, anticoagulants). Control serum lipids with appropriate diet, exercise, and weight loss in obese patients prior to therapy.

Monitoring: Monitor lipids periodically and for LFTs, CPK, CBC, creatinine, INR, PT. Monitor for signs of myopathy (eg, unexplained muscle pain, weakness, or tenderness with fever or malaise), cholelithiasis, cataracts, malignancy, abdominal pain leading to appendectomy, and noncoronary mortality.

Patient Counseling: Inform about potential risks/benefits of therapy. Report signs of myopathy (eg, unexplained muscle pain, tenderness, or weakness with fever or malaise). Notify physician if pregnant/nursing or planning to become pregnant.

Administration: Oral route. **Storage:** 20-25°C (68-77°F).

LOPRESSOR — RX

metoprolol tartrate (Novartis)

THERAPEUTIC CLASS: Selective $beta_1$-blocker

INDICATIONS: Treatment of hypertension. Long-term treatment of angina pectoris. To reduce cardiovascular mortality in hemodynamically stable patients with definite or suspected AMI.

DOSAGE: *Adults:* HTN: Initial: 100mg/day in single or divided doses. Titrate: May increase at weekly (or longer) intervals. Usual: 100-450mg/day. Max: 450mg/day. Angina: Initial: 50mg bid. Titrate: May increase weekly. Usual: 100-400mg/day. Max: 400mg/day. MI (Early Phase): 5mg IV every 2 min for 3 doses (monitor BP, HR, and ECG). If tolerated, give 50mg PO q6h for 48 hrs. If not tolerated, give 25-50mg PO q6h. Initiate PO dose 15 min after last IV dose. MI (Late Phase): 100mg bid for at least 3 months. Take PO with or immediately following meals.

HOW SUPPLIED: Inj: 1mg/mL; Tab: 50mg*, 100mg* *scored

CONTRAINDICATIONS: (HTN, Angina) Sinus bradycardia, >1st-degree heart block, cardiogenic shock, overt cardiac failure, sick-sinus syndrome, severe peripheral arterial circulatory disorders, pheochromocytoma. (MI) HR <45 beats/min, 2nd- and 3rd-degree heart block, significant 1st-degree heart block, SBP <100mmHg, moderate to severe cardiac failure.

WARNINGS/PRECAUTIONS: Caution with ischemic heart disease, avoid abrupt withdrawal; taper over 1-2 weeks. Withdrawal before surgery is controversial. May mask hyperthyroidism and hypoglycemia symptoms. May exacerbate cardiac failure. Caution with hepatic dysfunction, CHF controlled by digitalis. Avoid in bronchospastic disease. May decrease sinus HR and/or slow AV conduction. D/C if heart block or hypotension occurs.

ADVERSE REACTIONS: Bradycardia, SOB, fatigue, dizziness, depression, diarrhea, pruritus, rash, heart block, hypotension.

INTERACTIONS: Additive effects with catecholamine-depleting drugs (eg, reserpine). May block epinephrine effects. Caution with digitalis; both agents slow AV conduction. Potent CYP2D6 inhibitors may increase levels. Stop metoprolol several days before clonidine discontinuation when both agents given concurrently.

PREGNANCY: Category C, caution in nursing.

MECHANISM OF ACTION: β-adrenergic receptor blocker; not established, proposed to competitively antagonize catecholamines at peripheral adrenergic-neuronal sites; have central effect leading to reduced sympathetic outflow to periphery and suppression of renin activity.

PHARMACOKINETICS: Absorption: Rapid and complete. **Distribution:** Serum albumin binding (12%). **Metabolism:** CYP2D6 (oxidation). **Elimination:** Urine (<5%); $T_{1/2}$=2.8 hrs (extensive metabolizers); $T_{1/2}$=7.5 hrs (poor metabolizers). IV: Urine (10%).

NURSING CONSIDERATIONS

Assessment: Assess for sinus bradycardia, AV heart block, cardiogenic shock, overt CHF, bronchospastic disease, hyperthyroidism, DM, possible drug interactions, sick sinus syndrome, severe peripheral arterial circulatory disorders, pheochromocytoma, history of CHF, and hepatic impairment.

Monitoring: Monitor hemodynamic status periodically. Monitor for signs/symptoms of cardiac failure, hypoglycemia, thyrotoxicosis, withdrawal symptoms (angina, MI), hypotension, and hypersensitivity reactions.

Patient Counseling: Instruct to take regularly and continuously, as directed, with or immediately following meals. If dose missed, take next dose at scheduled time (without doubling). Do not d/c without consulting physician. Caution may impair physical/mental abilities. Advise to contact physician before any surgery, or if symptoms of heart failure (difficulty breathing), withdrawal (angina), or hypersensitivity reactions occur. Inform may mask signs of thyrotoxicosis and hypoglycemia.

Administration: Oral, IV route. **Storage:** 25°C (77°F); excursions permitted to 15-30°C (59-86°F). Protect from moisture.

LOPRESSOR HCT — RX

metoprolol tartrate - hydrochlorothiazide (Novartis)

L

THERAPEUTIC CLASS: Selective $beta_1$-blocker/thiazide diuretic

INDICATIONS: Management of hypertension. Not for initial therapy.

DOSAGE: *Adults:* Usual: 100-450mg metoprolol/day and 12.5-50mg HCTZ/day. Max: 50mg HCTZ/day.

HOW SUPPLIED: Tab: (Metoprolol-HCTZ) 50mg-25mg*, 100-25mg*, 100mg-50mg* *scored

CONTRAINDICATIONS: Sinus bradycardia, >1st-degree heart block, cardiogenic shock, overt cardiac failure, sick-sinus syndrome, severe peripheral arterial circulatory disorders, pheochromocytoma, anuria, sulfonamide hypersensitivity.

WARNINGS/PRECAUTIONS: Avoid abrupt withdrawal; taper over 1-2 weeks. Withdrawal before surgery is controversial. May mask hyperthyroidism and hypoglycemia symptoms. May cause cardiac failure. Caution with hepatic dysfunction, CHF controlled by digitalis, severe renal disease, allergy or asthma history. Avoid in bronchospastic disease. Monitor for fluid/electrolyte imbalance. May manifest latent DM. Hypokalemia, hyperuricemia, hypercalcemia, hypophosphatemia, and hypomagnesemia may occur. May exacerbate SLE. Enhanced effects in post-sympathectomy patient.

ADVERSE REACTIONS: Fatigue, dizziness, flu syndrome, drowsiness, hypokalemia, headache, bradycardia.

INTERACTIONS: Additive effects with catecholamine-depleting drugs (eg, reserpine). May block epinephrine effects. Caution with digitalis; both agents slow AV conduction. Potent CYP2D6 inhibitors may increase levels. Stop metoprolol several days before clonidine discontinuation when both agents given concurrently. Corticosteroids, ACTH may increase risk of hypokalemia. Risk of lithium toxicity. NSAIDs may reduce diuretic effects. Insulin may need adjustment. Impaired absorption with cholestyramine, colestipol. Additive effects with other antihypertensives. May increase responsiveness to tubocurarine. Alcohol, barbiturates, or narcotics may potentiate orthostatic hypotension. May decrease arterial responsiveness to norepinephrine.

PREGNANCY: Category C, not for use in nursing.

MECHANISM OF ACTION: Metoprolol: β-adrenergic receptor blocker; not established, proposed to competitively antagonize catecholamines at peripheral adrenergic-neuronal sites, have central effect leading to reduced sympathetic outflow to periphery and suppression of renin activity. HCTZ: Thiazide diuretic; affects renal tubular mechanism of electrolyte reabsorption.

PHARMACOKINETICS: Absorption: Metoprolol: Rapid and complete. HCTZ: Rapid; T_{max}=1-2.5 hrs. **Distribution:** Metoprolol: Plasma protein binding (12%). HCTZ: V_d=3.6-7.8L/kg; plasma protein binding (67.9%). **Metabolism:** Metoprolol: CYP2D6 (oxidation). **Elimination:** Metoprolol: Urine (<5%); $T_{1/2}$=2.8 hrs (extensive metabolizers), 7.5 hrs (poor metabolizers). HCTZ: Urine (72-97%); $T_{1/2}$=10-17 hrs.

NURSING CONSIDERATIONS

Assessment: Assess for history of allergy or bronchial asthma, sinus bradycardia, AV block, cardiogenic shock, overt CHF, bronchospastic disease, SLE, hyperthyroidism, DM, possible drug interactions, sick sinus syndrome, severe peripheral arterial circulatory disorders, pheochromocytoma, history of CHF, anuria, sulfonamide hypersensitivity, hepatic/renal impairment. Obtain baseline serum electrolyte levels.

Monitoring: Monitor serum electrolytes periodically. Monitor for signs/symptoms of electrolyte imbalance, hypoglycemia, thyrotoxicosis, withdrawal (angina, MI), cardiac failure, hypersensitivity reactions, exacerbation or activation of SLE, hyperuricemia or precipitation of gout, renal/hepatic dysfunction.

Patient Counseling: Instruct to take regularly and continuously, as directed, with or immediately following meals. If dose is missed, take next dose at scheduled time (without doubling); do not d/c without consulting physician. Caution may impair physical/mental abilities. Advise to contact physician before any surgery, or if symptoms of heart failure (difficulty breathing), hypersensitivity reactions, withdrawal (angina), or electrolyte imbalance (dry mouth, thirst, weakness) occur. Inform may mask signs of thyrotoxicosis and hypoglycemia.

L

Administration: Oral route. **Storage:** 25°C (77°F); excursions permitted to 15-30°C (59-86°F). Protect from moisture.

LOPROX — RX

ciclopirox (Medicis)

OTHER BRAND NAMES: Loprox TS (Medicis)

THERAPEUTIC CLASS: Broad-spectrum antifungal

INDICATIONS: (Cre/Sus) Treatment of dermal infections of tinea pedis, tinea cruris, tinea corporis, cutaneous candidiasis and tinea versicolor. (Gel) Treatment of interdigital tinea pedis and tinea corporis. (Gel/Shampoo) Treatment of seborrheic dermatitis of the scalp.

DOSAGE: *Adults:* (Cre/Gel/Sus) Massage affected and surrounding areas bid (am and pm) up to 4 weeks. (Shampoo) Apply about 5mL (up to 10mL for long hair) to wet scalp. Lather and rinse off after 3 min. Repeat twice weekly for 4 weeks, at least 3 days apart.

Pediatrics: ≥10 yrs: (Cre/Sus) Massage affected and surrounding areas bid (am and pm) up to 4 weeks. Gel or shampoo not recommended in pediatrics <16 yrs.

HOW SUPPLIED: Cre: 0.77% [15g, 30g, 90g]; Gel: 0.77% [30g, 45g, 100g]; Shampoo: 1% [120mL]; Sus: (Loprox TS) 0.77% [30mL, 60mL]

WARNINGS/PRECAUTIONS: Avoid eyes, mucous membranes, occlusive wrappings or dressings. D/C if sensitization or chemical irritation occurs. Hair discoloration reported in patients with lighter hair color.

ADVERSE REACTIONS: Contact dermatitis, pruritus, burning.

PREGNANCY: Pregnancy B, caution in nursing.

MECHANISM OF ACTION: Broad-spectrum antifungal; acts by chelation of polyvalent cations (Fe^{3+}or Al^{3+}) resulting in the inhibition of the metal-dependent enzymes that are responsible for degradation of peroxides in the fungal cell wall. Inhibits the growth of pathogenic dermatophytes, yeasts, and *Malassezia furfur*.

PHARMACOKINETICS: Elimination: Renal and feces; $T_{1/2}$= 5.5 hrs.

NURSING CONSIDERATIONS

Assessment: Assess proper diagnosis of causative organisms. Assess use in pregnant/nursing patients.

Monitoring: Monitor for signs/symptoms of sensitivity or chemical irritation reactions.

Patient Counseling: Counsel to continue therapy for the full treatment time even if symptoms improve. Instruct to notify physician if there are no signs of improvement after 4 weeks of therapy or if signs of increased irritation (eg, redness, itching, blistering, oozing) develop at the application site. Instruct to avoid occlusive wrappings or dressings. Advise that burning or itching may occur when using the gel formulation at the scalp site. Advise patients with lighter hair color who are using the shampoo formulation that medication may discolor hair.

Administration: Topical route. **Storage:** 15-30°C (59-86°F).

LORCET

CIII

hydrocodone bitartrate - acetaminophen (Forest)

OTHER BRAND NAMES: Lorcet 10/650 (Forest) - Lorcet HD (Forest) - Lorcet Plus (Forest)

L

THERAPEUTIC CLASS: Opioid analgesic

INDICATIONS: Relief of moderate to moderately severe pain.

DOSAGE: *Adults:* (Plus, 10/650) Usual: 1 cap/tab q4-6h prn pain. Max: 6 tabs or caps/day. (HD) 1-2 caps q4-6h prn pain. Max: 8 caps/day.

HOW SUPPLIED: (Hydrocodone-APAP) Cap: (HD) 5mg-500mg; Tab: (Plus) 7.5mg-650mg*, (10/650) 10mg-650mg* *scored

WARNINGS/PRECAUTIONS: May produce dose-related respiratory depression. May obscure acute abdominal conditions or head injuries. Caution in elderly, debilitated, severe hepatic or renal dysfunction, hypothyroidism, Addison's disease, prostatic hypertrophy, urethral stricture, pulmonary disease and postoperative use. May be habit-forming. Suppresses cough reflex.

ADVERSE REACTIONS: Dizziness, drowsiness, NV, dysphoria, urinary retention, urethral spasm, dyspnea, SOB, rash.

INTERACTIONS: May potentiate CNS depression with narcotics, alcohol, antianxiety agents, antihistamines, antipsychotics, other CNS depressants. Increased effect of antidepressant or hydrocodone with MAOIs or TCAs.

PREGNANCY: Category C, not for use in nursing.

MECHANISM OF ACTION: Hydrocodone: Narcotic analgesic; not established. Suspected to be related to existence of opiate receptors in the CNS. APAP: Nonopiate, nonsalicylate analgesic and antipyretic. Mechanism of analgesic actions not established; involves peripheral influences. Antipyretic activity is mediated through hypothalamic heat regulating centers. Inhibits prostaglandin synthetase.

PHARMACOKINETICS: Absorption: Hydrocodone: C_{max}=23.6ng/mL; T_{max}=1.3 hrs. APAP: Rapidly absorbed. **Distribution:** APAP: Found in breast milk. **Metabolism**: Hydrocodone: O-demethylation, N-demethylation, and 6-keto reduction. APAP: Liver (conjugation). **Elimination**: Hydrocodone: $T_{1/2}$=3.8 hrs. APAP: Urine (85%); $T_{1/2}$=1.25-3 hrs.

NURSING CONSIDERATIONS

Assessment: Assess for impaired hepatic/renal function, presence of head injury or other intracranial lesions, elevations in ICP, acute abdominal conditions, presence of debilitation (elderly), hypothyroidism, Addison's disease, prostatic hypertrophy or urethral stricture, pulmonary disease, pregnancy/nursing status, and possible drug interactions.

Monitoring: Monitor for signs/symptoms of respiratory depression, elevated CSF pressure, dependence on medication, and abuse. Monitor serial hepatic/renal function tests in with severe hepatic/renal disease.

Patient Counseling: Advise that medication may impair mental/physical abilities; use caution when performing hazardous tasks (eg, operating machinery/driving). Advise to avoid using alcohol and other CNS depressants during therapy. Inform that medication may be habit-forming; counsel to take only as long as prescribed, in amounts prescribed, and not more frequently than prescribed.

Administration: Oral route. **Storage:** 20-25°(68-77°); excursions permitted to 15-30°C (59-86°F). Dispense in tight, light-resistant container.

LORTAB **CIII**

hydrocodone bitartrate - acetaminophen (UCB)

THERAPEUTIC CLASS: Opioid analgesic

INDICATIONS: Relief of moderate to moderately severe pain.

DOSAGE: *Adults:* (2.5/500, 5/500) 1-2 tabs q4-6h prn. Max: 8 tabs/day. (7.5/500, 10/500) 1 tab q4-6h prn. Max: 6 tabs/day. (Sol) 15mL q4-6h prn. Max: 90mL/day.
Pediatrics: ≥2 yrs: (Sol) 12-15kg: 3.75mL. 16-22kg: 5mL. 23-31kg: 7.5mL. 32-45kg: 10mL. ≥46kg: 15mL. May repeat q4-6h prn.

HOW SUPPLIED: (Hydrocodone-APAP) Sol: 7.5mg-500mg/15mL; Tab: 2.5mg-500mg*, 5mg-500mg*, 7.5mg-500mg*, 10mg-500mg* *scored

L

WARNINGS/PRECAUTIONS: May produce dose-related respiratory depression. May obscure acute abdominal conditions or head injuries. Caution in elderly, debilitated, severe hepatic or renal dysfunction, hypothyroidism, Addison's disease, prostatic hypertrophy, urethral stricture, pulmonary disease, postoperative use. May be habit-forming. Suppresses cough reflex.

ADVERSE REACTIONS: Lightheadedness, dizziness, sedation, NV.

INTERACTIONS: Additive CNS depression with other narcotics, antihistamines, antipsychotics, antianxiety agents, alcohol, CNS depressants. Increased effect of antidepressant or hydrocodone with MAOIs or TCAs.

PREGNANCY: Category C, not for use in nursing.

MECHANISM OF ACTION: Hydrocodone: Narcotic analgesic and antitussive; not established. Suspected to be related to existence of opiate receptors in CNS. APAP: Nonopioid, nonsalicylate analgesic, and antipyretic. Analgesic action involves peripheral influences; specific mechanism not established. Antipyretic activity is mediated through hypothalamic heat-regulating centers. Inhibits prostaglandin synthetase.

PHARMACOKINETICS: Administration: Hydrocodone: C_{max}=23.6ng/mL; T_{max}=1.3 hrs. APAP: Rapidly absorbed. **Distribution:** Hydrocodone: Crosses placental barrier. APAP: Found in breast milk. **Metabolism:** Hydrocodone: O-demethylation, N-demethylation and 6-keto reduction. APAP: Liver (conjugation). **Elimination:** Hydrocodone: $T_{1/2}$=3.8 hrs; APAP: Urine (85%); $T_{1/2}$=1.25-3 hrs.

NURSING CONSIDERATIONS

Assessment: Assess for pulmonary disease, renal/hepatic impairment, presence of debilitation (elderly), hypothyroidism, Addison's disease, prostatic hypertrophy or urethral stricture, presence of acute abdominal conditions, head injury or other intracranial lesions, increased ICP, pregnancy/nursing status, and possible drug interactions.

Monitoring: Monitor for signs/symptoms of respiratory depression, elevations in CSF pressure, drug dependence, and drug abuse. Monitor serial hepatic/renal function tests in patients with severe hepatic/renal disease.

Patient Counseling: Inform that medication may impair mental/physical abilities; use caution when performing hazardous tasks (eg, operating machinery/driving). Avoid the use of alcohol and other CNS depressants while on medication. Inform that medication may be habit forming; instruct to only take amount prescribed for duration of time prescribed.

Administration: Oral route. **Storage:** (2.5mg/500mg): 15-30°C (59-86°F); (5 mg/500mg, 10mg/500mg, 7.5mg/500mg, (Sol) 7.5mg-500mg/15mL): 20-25°C (68-77°F). Dispense in tight, light-resistant container with child-resistant closure.

LOTEMAX RX

loteprednol etabonate (Bausch & Lomb)

THERAPEUTIC CLASS: Corticosteroid

INDICATIONS: Treatment of inflammation of the palpebral and bulbar conjunctiva, cornea and anterior segment of the globe. Management of post-operative inflammation.

DOSAGE: *Adults:* Steroid-Responsive Disease: 1-2 drops qid, may increase up to 1 drop every hr within the 1st week of treatment. Re-evaluate after 2 days if no improvement. Postoperative: 1-2 drops qid starting 24 hrs post-op and continue for 2 weeks.

HOW SUPPLIED: Sus: 0.5% [2.5mL, 5mL, 10mL, 15mL]

CONTRAINDICATIONS: Viral diseases of the cornea and conjunctiva including epithelial herpes simplex keratitis, vaccinia, and varicella. Mycobacterial infection and fungal diseases of the eye.

WARNINGS/PRECAUTIONS: Caution with glaucoma, history of herpes simplex, and diseases causing thinning of cornea/sclera. Prolonged use can cause glaucoma, optic nerve damage, defects in visual acuity and fields of vision, cataracts, or secondary ocular infections (eg, fungal). Monitor IOP after 10 days of therapy. Re-evaluate if no response after 2 days. May delay healing and increase incidence of bleb formation after cataract surgery. May mask or enhance existing infection in acute, purulent conditions.

ADVERSE REACTIONS: Elevated IOP, abnormal vision, chemosis, discharge, dry eyes, burning on instillation, epiphora, itching, photophobia, foreign body sensation, optic nerve damage, visual field defects.

PREGNANCY: Category C, caution in nursing.

MECHANISM OF ACTION: Glucocorticoid; anti-inflammatory agent, no accepted explanation for MOA; suspected to inhibit edema, fibrin deposition, capillary dilation and deposition of collagen and scar formation by the induction of phospholipase A_2 inhibitory proteins, lipocortins.

NURSING CONSIDERATIONS

Assessment: Assess for viral diseases of cornea and conjunctiva, dendritic keratitis, vaccinia, varicella, mycobacterial infection, fungal disease of ocular structures, glaucoma, thinning of corneal/scleral epithelium, hypersensitivity, cataract surgery.

Monitoring: Frequent measuring of IOP and slit lamp microscopy exam where appropriate, fluorescein staining for monitoring of glaucoma with damage to optic nerve with defects in visual acuity and fields of vision, posterior subscapsular cataract, delayed corneal healing, thinning of cornea and sclera, ulceration, perforation, secondary ocular infections or masking of existing infections.

Patient Counseling: Advise to d/c drug and notify physician if symptoms persist or worsen. Instruct to not wear soft contact lenses during treatment. Counsel to avoid touching bottle tip to eyelids or any other surface.

Administration: Ocular route. Shake vigorously before using. **Storage:** 15-25°C (59-77°F). Do not freeze.

LOTENSIN RX

benazepril HCl (Novartis)

When used in pregnancy, ACE inhibitors can cause injury and even death to the developing fetus. D/C therapy when pregnancy detected.

THERAPEUTIC CLASS: ACE inhibitor

INDICATIONS: Treatment of hypertension. May be used alone or with thiazide diuretics.

DOSAGE: *Adults:* If possible, d/c diuretic 2-3 days prior to initiation of therapy. Initial: 10mg qd or 5mg with concomitant diuretic. Maint: 20-40mg/day given qd-bid. Resume diuretic if BP not controlled. Max: 80mg/day. CrCl <30mL/min/1.73m^2: Initial: 5mg qd. Max: 40mg/day.
Pediatrics: ≥6 yrs: Initial: 0.2mg/kg qd. Max: 0.6mg/kg.

HOW SUPPLIED: Tab: 5mg, 10mg, 20mg, 40mg

WARNINGS/PRECAUTIONS: D/C if angioedema, jaundice, or if marked LFT elevation occurs. Risk of hyperkalemia with DM, renal dysfunction. Persistent nonproductive cough reported. Monitor WBCs in renal and collagen vascular disease. Anaphylactoid reactions reported. Fetal/neonatal morbidity and death reported. Monitor for hypotension in high-risk patients (eg, surgery/anesthesia, prolonged diuretic therapy, heart failure, volume and/or salt depletion, etc). Caution with CHF, renal dysfunction, and renal artery stenosis. Less effective on BP in blacks and more reports of angioedema than nonblacks.

ADVERSE REACTIONS: Cough, dizziness, headache, fatigue, somnolence, postural dizziness, nausea.

INTERACTIONS: May increase lithium levels. Hypotension risk with diuretics. Increased risk of hyperkalemia with K^+-sparing diuretics, K^+-containing salt substitutes, or K^+ supplements.

PREGNANCY: Category D, not for use in nursing.

MECHANISM OF ACTION: ACE inhibitor; not established, effects appear to result from suppression of renin-angiotensin-aldosterone system.

PHARMACOKINETICS: Absorption: Absolute bioavailability (≥37%); T_{max}=0.5-1 hr, 1-4 hrs (metabolite). **Distribution:** Parent, metabolite: Plasma protein binding (96.7%, 95.3%). **Metabolism:** Cleavage of ester group; benazeprilat (active metabolite). **Elimination:** Urine (7%). Benazeprilat: Urine (20%), biliary (11-12%); $T_{1/2}$=10-11 hrs (adults), 5 hrs (pediatrics).

NURSING CONSIDERATIONS

Assessment: Assess for pregnancy status, volume/salt depletion, collagen vascular disease (SLE, scleroderma), CHF, DM, possible drug interactions, renal/hepatic impairment.

Monitoring: Monitor renal function for 1st few weeks, WBC (collagen vascular disease), and serum electrolytes periodically. Monitor for signs/symptoms of hypotension, anaphylactoid or hypersensitivity reactions, head/neck and intestinal angioedema, agranulocytosis, hyperkalemia, renal/hepatic dysfunction.

Patient Counseling: Inform of pregnancy risks. Inform that inadequate fluid intake or fluid loss may lead to drop in BP resulting in lightheadedness or syncope; avoid K^+ supplements or salt substitutes. Advise to seek medical attention if symptoms of hypotension (syncope), anaphylactoid or hypersensitivity reactions, angioedema (head/neck; abdominal pain with/without NV), infection (sore throat, fever), hyperkalemia, or hepatic dysfunction occur.

Administration: Oral route. **Storage:** Below 30°C (86°F). Protect from moisture.

LOTENSIN HCT

RX

benazepril HCl - hydrochlorothiazide (Novartis)

When used in pregnancy, ACE inhibitors can cause injury and even death to the developing fetus. D/C therapy when pregnancy detected.

THERAPEUTIC CLASS: ACE inhibitor/thiazide diuretic

INDICATIONS: Treatment of hypertension. Not for initial therapy.

DOSAGE: *Adults:* Initial (if not controlled on benazepril monotherapy): 10mg-12.5mg or 20mg-12.5mg. Titrate: May increase after 2-3 weeks. Initial (if controlled on 25mg HCTZ/day with hypokalemia): 5mg-6.25mg. Replacement Therapy: Substitute combination for titrated components.

HOW SUPPLIED: Tab: (Benazepril-HCTZ) 5mg-6.25mg*, 10mg-12.5mg*, 20mg-12.5mg*, 20mg-25mg* *scored

CONTRAINDICATIONS: Anuria, sulfonamide hypersensitivity.

WARNINGS/PRECAUTIONS: Avoid if CrCl ≤30mL/min/1.73m². D/C if angioedema, jaundice, or marked LFT elevation occur. Risk of hyperkalemia with DM, renal dysfunction. May cause persistent nonproductive cough, hypokalemia, hyperuricemia, hypomagnesemia, hypercalcemia, hypophosphatemia. Monitor WBCs in renal and collagen vascular disease. Anaphylactoid reactions reported. Fetal/neonatal morbidity and death reported. Monitor for hypotension in high-risk patients (eg, surgery/anesthesia, prolonged diuretic therapy, heart failure, volume and/or salt depletion, etc). Caution with CHF, renal dysfunction, and renal artery stenosis. More reports of angioedema in blacks than nonblacks. Monitor for fluid/electrolyte imbalance. May increase cholesterol and TG levels. May exacerbate/activate SLE.

L

ADVERSE REACTIONS: Cough, dizziness/postural dizziness, headache, fatigue.

INTERACTIONS: Increased risk of hyperkalemia with K^+ supplements, K^+-sparing diuretics, or K^+-containing salt substitutes. Risk of lithium toxicity. May increase responsiveness to tubocurarine. NSAIDs reduce effects. Cholestyramine, colestipol decrease absorption. Insulin may need adjustment. May decrease arterial responsiveness to norepinephrine.

PREGNANCY: Category D, not for use in nursing.

MECHANISM OF ACTION: Benazepril: ACE inhibitor; not established, effects appear to result from suppression of renin-angiotensin-aldosterone system. HCTZ: Thiazide diuretic; affects renal tubular mechanisms of electrolyte reabsorption, directly increasing excretion of Na^+ and Cl^-, and indirectly reducing plasma volume.

PHARMACOKINETICS: Absorption: Benazepril: T_{max} = 0.5-1 hr, 1-4 hrs (metabolite); absolute bioavailability: (≥37%). **Distribution:** Benazepril, metabolite: plasma protein binding (96.7%, 95.3%). HCTZ: Plasma protein binding (67.9%); V_d= 3.6-7.8 L/Kg; crosses placenta. **Metabolism**: Benazepril: Cleavage of ester group; benazeprilat (active metabolite). **Elimination:** Benazepril: Urine (trace). Benazeprilat: Urine (20%), biliary (11-12%); $T_{1/2}$= 10-11 hrs. HCTZ: Kidney; $T_{1/2}$= 5-15 hrs.

NURSING CONSIDERATIONS

Assessment: Assess for pregnancy status, volume/salt depletion, collagen vascular disease (SLE, scleroderma), CHF, DM, possible drug interactions, unilateral or bilateral renal artery stenosis, anuria, sulfonamide hypersensitivity, history of allergy or bronchial asthma, renal and hepatic impairment. Obtain baseline electrolyte levels and renal function.

Monitoring: Monitor renal function for 1st few weeks, WBC (collagen vascular disease), and serum electrolytes periodically. Monitor for signs and symptoms of hypotension, anaphylactoid or hypersensitivity reactions, head/neck and intestinal angioedema, agranulocytosis, hyperkalemia, electrolyte imbalance, gout, exacerbation or activation of SLE, renal/hepatic dysfunction.

Patient Counseling: Inform of pregnancy risks. Instruct that inadequate fluid intake or fluid loss may lead to drop in BP resulting in lightheadedness or syncope; avoid K^+ supplements or salt substitutes. Advise to seek medical attention if symptoms of hypotension (syncope), anaphylactoid or hypersensitivity reactions, angioedema (head/neck; abdominal pain with/without NV), infection (sore throat, fever), hyperkalemia, or hepatic dysfunction occur.

Administration: Oral route. **Storage**: Below 30°C (86°F).

LOTREL — RX

benazepril HCl - amlodipine besylate (Novartis)

When used in pregnancy, ACE inhibitors can cause injury and even death to the developing fetus. D/C therapy when pregnancy detected.

THERAPEUTIC CLASS: Calcium channel blocker (dihydropyridine)/ACE inhibitor

INDICATIONS: Treatment of hypertension. Not for initial therapy.

DOSAGE: *Adults:* Usual: 2.5-10mg amlodipine and 10-80mg benazepril per day. Small/Elderly/Frail/Hepatic Impairment: Initial: 2.5mg amlodipine.

HOW SUPPLIED: Cap: (Amlodipine-Benazepril) 2.5mg-10mg, 5mg-10mg, 5mg-20mg, 5mg-40mg, 10mg-20mg, 10mg-40mg

WARNINGS/PRECAUTIONS: D/C if angioedema, jaundice, or if marked LFT elevation occurs. Risk of hyperkalemia with DM, renal dysfunction. Persistent nonproductive cough reported. Monitor WBCs in collagen vascular disease. Anaphylactoid reactions reported. Fetal/neonatal morbidity and death reported. Monitor for hypotension in high-risk patients (heart failure, surgery/anesthesia, volume and/or salt depletion, etc). Caution with CHF, severe hepatic or renal dysfunction, and renal artery stenosis. Avoid if CrCl ≤30mL/min.

L

ADVERSE REACTIONS: Cough, headache, dizziness, edema.

INTERACTIONS: May increase lithium levels. Hypotension risk with diuretics. Increased risk of hyperkalemia with K^+-sparing diuretics, K^+ supplements, or K^+-containing salt substitutes. Caution with other peripheral vasodilators.

PREGNANCY: Category D, not for use in nursing.

MECHANISM OF ACTION: Benazepril: ACE inhibitor; not established, effects appear to result from suppression of renin-angiotensin-aldosterone system. Amlodipine: Ca^{2+} channel blocker (dihydropyridine); inhibits transmembrane influx of Ca^{2+} ions into vascular smooth muscle and cardiac muscle.

PHARMACOKINETICS: Absorption: Amlodipine: Absolute bioavailability (64-90%); T_{max}=6-12 hrs. Benazepril: Absolute bioavailability (≥37%); T_{max}=0.5-2 hrs, 1.5-4 hrs (metabolite). **Distribution:** Amlodipine: V_d=21 L/kg; plasma protein binding (93%). Benazepril: V_d=0.7 L/kg. **Metabolism:** Amlodipine: Liver. Benazepril: Cleavage of ester group; benazeprilat (active metabolite). **Elimination:** Amlodipine: Urine (10%); $T_{1/2}$=2 days. Benazepril: Urine (trace), biliary (11-12%). Benazeprilat: Urine (20%); $T_{1/2}$=10-11 hrs.

NURSING CONSIDERATIONS

Assessment: Assess for severe aortic stenosis, CHF, severe obstructive CAD, pregnancy status, volume/salt depletion, collagen vascular disease (SLE, scleroderma), DM, unilateral or bilateral renal artery stenosis, possible drug interactions, hepatic/renal impairment.

Monitoring: Monitor renal function for 1st few weeks (renal artery stenosis), WBC (collagen vascular disease), and serum electrolytes periodically. Monitor for signs/symptoms of hypotension, anaphylactoid or hypersensitivity reactions, head/neck and intestinal angioedema, agranulocytosis, hyperkalemia, renal/hepatic dysfunction. Monitor for symptoms of angina or MI after dosage initiation or increase.

Patient Counseling: Inform of pregnancy risks. Advise to seek medical attention if symptoms of hypotension, anaphylactoid or hypersensitivity reactions, angioedema (head/neck; abdominal pain with/without NV), infection, hyperkalemia, or hepatic dysfunction occur.

Administration: Oral route. **Storage:** 25°C (77°F); excursions permitted to 15-30°C (59-86°F). Protect from moisture.

LOTRISONE

RX

betamethasone dipropionate - clotrimazole (Schering)

THERAPEUTIC CLASS: Corticosteroid/azole antifungal

INDICATIONS: Topical treatment of tinea pedis, tinea cruris, and tinea corporis caused by *Trichophyton rubrum*, *Trichophyton mentagrophytes*, and *Epidermophyton floccosum*.

DOSAGE: *Adults:* ≥17 yrs: Massage sufficient amount bid (am and pm) to area for 2 weeks for t.cruris and t.corporis and 4 weeks for t.pedis. D/C if condition persists after 2 weeks for t.cruris and t.corporis, or after 4 weeks for t.pedis.

HOW SUPPLIED: (Betamethasone-Clotrimazole) Cre: 0.05-1% [15g, 45g]; Lot: 0.05-1% [30mL]

WARNINGS/PRECAUTIONS: May produce reversible HPA axis suppression, Cushing's syndrome, hyperglycemia, and glucosuria. D/C if irritation develops. Pediatrics may be more susceptible to systemic toxicity. Not for use with occlusive dressing.

ADVERSE REACTIONS: Paresthesia, rash, edema, secondary infection.

PREGNANCY: Category C, caution in nursing.

MECHANISM OF ACTION: Corticosteroid/azole antifungal agent. Clotrimazole: Antifungal; inhibits 14-α-demethylation of lanosterol in fungi by binding to 1 of the cytochrome P-450 enzymes. Leads to accumulation of 14-α-methylsterols and reduced concentrations of ergosterol, a sterol essential for a normal fungal cytoplasmic membrane. The methylsterols may affect the electron transport system, thereby inhibiting growth of fungi. Betamethasone: Corticosteroid; possesses anti-inflammatory, antipruritic, and vasoconstrictive properties.

PHARMACOKINETICS: Absorption: Percutaneous. Inflammation, other disease states, or occlusive dressings may increase absorption. **Metabolism:** Liver. **Elimination:** Renal, biliary.

NURSING CONSIDERATIONS

Assessment: Assess for hypersensitivity to other corticosteroids or imidazoles. Assess use in pediatric patients and in pregnant/nursing females.

Monitoring: Monitor for signs/symptoms of HPA-axis suppression, Cushing's syndrome, hyperglycemia, glucosuria, glucocorticosteroid insufficiencies, and skin irritation. When used on large surface areas and/or with occlusive dressings, perform periodic monitoring for HPA-axis suppression using ACTH test, morning plasma cortisol test, and urinary free-cortisol level test. (Pediatrics) Monitor for systemic toxicity, HPA-axis suppression, Cushing's syndrome, delayed weight gain, and intracranial HTN.

Patient Counseling: Counsel to use exactly as directed for fully prescribed treatment period. Inform to contact physician if no improvement after 1 week of treatment of tinea cruris or tinea corporis, or 2 weeks with tinea pedis. Instruct to avoid using occlusive dressings or tight-fitting clothing on treated areas and not to use with other corticosteroids.

Administration: Topical route. Shake lotion well before each use. **Storage:** 25C°(77°F), upright position only; excursions permitted to 15-30°C (59-86°F).

LOTRONEX

RX

alosetron HCl (Prometheus)

Serious GI adverse events, some fatal, reported (eg, ischemic colitis, serious constipation complications). Physicians must enroll in the Prescribing Program for Lotronex and patients must sign the Patient-Physician Agreement. Discontinue immediately if constipation or symptoms of ischemic colitis develop (rectal bleeding, bloody diarrhea, abdominal pain); do not resume therapy.

THERAPEUTIC CLASS: 5-HT_3 receptor antagonist

INDICATIONS: Treatment for women with severe diarrhea-predominant IBS who have chronic symptoms (>6 months), exclusion of anatomic or biochemical abnormalities of GI tract, failure to respond to conventional therapy, frequent and severe abdominal pain/discomfort, frequent bowel urgency/fecal incontinence, and disability/restriction of daily activities due to IBS.

DOSAGE: *Adults:* Initial: 1mg qd for 4 weeks. Titrate: If tolerated and IBS symptoms not controlled, may increase to 1mg bid. Discontinue after 4 weeks if symptoms not controlled on 1mg bid.

HOW SUPPLIED: Tab: 0.5mg, 1mg

CONTRAINDICATIONS: Current constipation. History of chronic/severe constipation or sequelae of constipation, intestinal obstruction/stricture, toxic megacolon, GI perforation/adhesions, ischemic colitis, impaired intestinal circulation, thrombophlebitis, hypercoagulable state, Crohn's disease, ulcerative colitis, diverticulitis, severe hepatic impairment. Inability to understand/comply with Patient-Physician Agreement.

L

WARNINGS/PRECAUTIONS: Increased risk of constipation and ischemic colitis. Caution with mild or moderate hepatic impairment.

ADVERSE REACTIONS: Constipation, abdominal discomfort/pain, nausea, GI discomfort/pain.

INTERACTIONS: Increased risk of constipation with medications that decrease GI motility. Inducers and inhibitors of hepatic CYP drug-metabolizing enzymes may change the clearance of alosetron. Fluvoxamine increases AUC, concomitant administration is contraindicated. Avoid with quinolone antibiotics and cimetidine. Caution with ketoconazole, clarithromycin, telithromycin, protease inhibitors, voriconazole, itraconazole.

PREGNANCY: Category B, caution in nursing.

MECHANISM OF ACTION: 5-HT_3 receptor antagonist.

PHARMACOKINETICS: Absorption: Rapidly absorbed, absolute bioavailability (50-60%), C_{max}=5ng/mL (male), 9ng/mL (female); T_{max}=1 hr. **Distribution:** V_d=65-95L, plasma protein binding (82%). **Metabolism:** Extensively metabolized. **Elimination:** Urine (73%), feces (24%); $T_{1/2}$=1.5 hrs.

NURSING CONSIDERATIONS

Assessment: Assess history of chronic or severe constipation, intestinal obstruction, stricture, toxic megacolon, GI perforation or adhesion, ischemic colitis, impaired intestinal circulation, thrombophlebitis or hypercoagulable state, Crohn's disease, ulcerative colitis, diverticulitis, severe hepatic impairment.

Monitoring: Monitor LFTs, signs/symptoms of ischemic colitis and serious complications of constipation, hypersensitivity reactions.

Patient Counseling: Review side effects and advise to report if any develop. Inform that tab may be taken with or without meals. Instruct to d/c treatment and seek medical attention if no response after 4 weeks.

Administration: Oral route. **Storage:** 25°C (77°F); excursions permitted to 15-30°C (59-86°F). Protect from light and moisture.

LOVAZA
omega-3-acid ethyl esters (GlaxoSmithKline) **RX**

THERAPEUTIC CLASS: Lipid-regulating agent

INDICATIONS: Adjunct to diet to reduce very high (≥ 500mg/dL) triglyceride levels in adult patients.

DOSAGE: *Adults:* 4g qd. Given as single 4-g dose (4 caps) or as two 2-g doses (2 caps bid).

HOW SUPPLIED: Cap: 1g

WARNINGS/PRECAUTIONS: Caution in patients with diabetes, hypothyroidism, hepatic or pancreatic problems, or known sensitivity or allergy to fish. Lower alcohol use. Lose weight if you are overweight. Possible increases in alanine aminotransferase levels without a concurrent increase in aspartate aminotransferase levels. Possible increased low-density lipoprotein cholesterol levels.

ADVERSE REACTIONS: Eructation, infection, flu-syndrome, dyspepsia.

INTERACTIONS: Possible prolongation of bleeding time with concomitant anticoagulants (aspirin, warfarin, coumarin, clopidogrel).

PREGNANCY: Category C, caution in nursing.

MECHANISM OF ACTION: Lipid-regulating agent; not completely understood; inhibits acyl CoA:1,2-diacylglycerol acyltransferase, increases mitochondrial, peroxisomal β-oxidation in the liver and decreases lipogenesis in the liver, and increases plasma lipoprotein lipase activity.

NURSING CONSIDERATIONS

Assessment: Assess for persistent abnormal TG levels, DM, thyroid conditions, pregnancy or nursing status, and for possible drug interactions (eg, anticoagulants). Attempt to control serum TG levels with appropriate diet, exercise, and weight loss in obese patients before instituting therapy.

Monitoring: Periodic monitoring of TG, LFTs, LDL-C, PT, and INR.

Patient Counseling: Notify physician if allergic to fish. Counsel about the importance of adhering to diet during therapy.

Administration: Oral route. **Storage:** 15-30°C (59-86°F). Do not freeze.

LOVENOX
enoxaparin sodium (Sanofi-Aventis) **RX**

Risk of paralysis by spinal/epidural hematoma with neuraxial anesthesia or spinal puncture. Increased risk with indwelling epidural catheters for analgesia, drugs affecting hemostasis (eg, NSAIDs, platelet inhibitors, anticoagulants), and traumatic or repeated epidural or spinal puncture.

THERAPEUTIC CLASS: Low molecular weight heparin

INDICATIONS: Prevention of DVT in hip or knee replacement surgery, abdominal surgery, or with severely restricted mobility during acute illness. With concomitant warfarin, inpatient treatment of acute DVT with or without PE and outpatient treatment of DVT without PE. Prevention of ischemic complications in unstable angina and non-Q-wave MI with concurrent ASA therapy. Treatment of acute ST-segment elevation MI (STEMI) in patients receiving thrombolysis and being managed medically or with percutaneous coronary intervention (PCI).

DOSAGE: *Adults:* Hip/Knee Surgery: 30mg SQ q12h, starting 12-24 hrs post-op, for 7-10 days (up to 14days) or 40mg SQ qd starting 12 hrs pre-op for hip surgery for 3 weeks. Abdominal Surgery: 40mg SQ qd, starting 2 hrs pre-op, for 7-10 days (up to 12 days). DVT with or without PE treatment: (inpatient/outpatient) 1mg/kg SQ q12h or (inpatient) 1.5mg/kg qd with warfarin (start within 72 hrs) for 7 days (up to 17 days). Acute Illness: 40mg SQ qd for 6-11 days (up to 14 days). Unstable Angina/Non-Q-Wave MI: 1mg/kg SQ q12h with

100-325mg/day of ASA for 2-8 days (up to 12.5 days). Acute STEMI (<75 yrs): 30mg single IV bolus plus a 1mg/kg SQ dose followed by 1mg/kg SQ q12h with ASA. Max: 100mg for 1st 2 doses only. Acute STEMI (≥75 yrs): 0.75mg/kg SQ q12h (no initial bolus) with ASA. Max: 75mg for 1st 2 doses only. When given with thrombolytic, give enoxaparin dose between 15 min before and 30 min after start of fibrinolytic therapy. With PCI, if last enoxaparin SQ dose was given >8 hrs before balloon inflation, an IV bolus of 0.3mg/kg of enoxaparin should be given. CrCl <30mL/min: Surgery/Acute Illness: 30mg SQ qd. DVT with or without PE treatment (inpatient/outpatient)/Unstable Angina/Non-Q-Wave MI: 1mg/kg SQ qd. Acute STEMI: <75 yrs: 30mg single IV bolus plus a 1mg/kg SQ dose followed by 1mg/kg SQ qd. ≥75 yrs: 1mg/kg SQ qd (no initial bolus).

HOW SUPPLIED: Inj: (MDV) 300mg/3mL; (Syringe) 30mg/0.3mL, 40mg/0.4mL, 60mg/0.6mL, 80mg/0.8mL, 100mg/mL, 120mg/0.8mL, 150mg/mL

CONTRAINDICATIONS: Heparin or pork allergy, active major bleeding, thrombocytopenia with a positive in vitro test for anti-platelet antibody. Hypersensitivity to benzyl alcohol (multi-dose formulation).

WARNINGS/PRECAUTIONS: Not for IM injection. Cannot use interchangeably unit for unit with heparin or other low molecular weight heparins. Extreme caution with HIT, conditions with an increased risk of hemorrhage (eg, bacterial endocarditis, hemorrhagic stroke, etc). Major hemorrhages (eg, retroperitoneal, intracranial), thrombocytopenia reported. D/C if platelets <100,000/mm^3. Perform periodic CBC, platelets, and stool occult blood test. Caution with bleeding diathesis, uncontrolled arterial HTN, recent GI ulceration, diabetic retinopathy, hemorrhage. Delayed elimination with elderly or in renal dysfunction. Monitor elderly with low body weight (<45 kg) and predisposition to decreased renal function. Higher risk of thromboembolism in pregnant women with prosthetic heart valves. Not for thromboprophylaxis in prosthetic heart valve patients. Achieve homeostasis at puncture site before sheath removal after PCI. Caution in hepatic impairment.

ADVERSE REACTIONS: Hemorrhage, thrombocytopenia, local reactions (ecchymosis, erythema), anemia, elevation of aminotransferases.

INTERACTIONS: D/C agents that increase risk of hemorrhage (eg, anticoagulants, acetylsalicylic acid, salicylates, NSAIDs, ketorolac, dipyridamole, sulfinpyrazone), unless really needed; monitor closely if co-administered.

PREGNANCY: Category B, caution in nursing.

MECHANISM OF ACTION: Low molecular-weight heparin with antithrombotic properties.

PHARMACOKINETICS: Absorption: (1mg/kg bid) C_{max}=1.2 IU/mL. **Distribution:** V_d=4.3L. **Metabolism:** Liver. **Elimination:** Urine; $T_{1/2}$=4.5 hrs (single dose); 7 hrs (multiple doses).

NURSING CONSIDERATIONS

Assessment: Assess for risk of hemorrhage (eg, bacterial endocarditis, congenital or acquired bleeding disorders, active ulcerative and angiodysplastic GI disease), active major bleeding, known hypersensitivity to heparin or pork products, hypersensitivity to benzyl alcohol, history of heparin-induced thrombocytopenia, nursing/pregnancy status, renal/hepatic impairment, presence of neuraxial anesthesia or spinal puncture, and drug interactions.

Monitoring: Monitor for signs/symptoms of hemorrhage and thrombocytopenia. Monitor for epidural or spinal hematomas, and for neurological impairment if used concomitantly with spinal/epidural anesthesia or spinal puncture. Periodically monitor CBC including platelet count, stool occult blood tests. If bleeding occurs, monitor anti-factor Xa.

Patient Counseling: Advise that bleeding time may be extended during therapy and bruising and bleeding may occur more easily. Instruct to report any unusual bleeding or scheduled surgery to physician. Advise pregnant females about risk of "Gasping Syndrome" with use of multiple-dose vials.

Administration: SC or IV (bolus) injection route. SC: Lie down during administration. If using prefilled syringe, do not expel air bubble before injection.

Alternate administration sites between left and right anterolateral and posterolateral abdominal wall. The entire length of the needle should be introduced into skin fold held between thumb and forefinger; skin fold should be held throughout injection. To minimize bruising, do not rub injection site. **Storage:** 25°C (77°F); excursions permitted to 15-30° (59-86°F). Do not store multiple-dose vials for >28 days after first use.

LUCENTIS

ranibizumab (Genentech) **RX**

THERAPEUTIC CLASS: Monoclonal antibody/VEGF-A blocker

INDICATIONS: Treatment of patients with neovascular (wet) age-related macular degeneration.

DOSAGE: *Adults:* Administer 0.5mg (0.05mL) by intravitreal injection once a month. May reduce to 1 injection every 3 months after the first 4 injections if monthly injections not feasible.

HOW SUPPLIED: Inj: 10mg/mL

CONTRAINDICATIONS: Ocular or periocular infections.

WARNINGS/PRECAUTIONS: Intravitreal injections have been associated with endophthalmitis and retinal detachments. Increased IOP noted within 60 min of intravitreal injection. Arterial thromboembolic events were observed.

ADVERSE REACTIONS: Conjunctival hemorrhage, eye pain, vitreous floaters, increased IOP, intraocular inflammation.

INTERACTIONS: May develop serious intraocular inflammation when used adjunctively with Verteporfin photodynamic therapy.

PREGNANCY: Category C, caution in nursing.

MECHANISM OF ACTION: Monoclonal antibody/VEGF-A blocker; responsible for binding to VEGF-A, which prevents the interaction of VEGF-A with its receptors (VEGFR1 and VEGFR2) on the surface of endothelial cells. This reduces endothelial cell proliferation, vascular leakage, and new blood vessel formation.

PHARMACOKINETICS: Absorption: C_{max}=1.5ng/mL; T_{max}=1 day. **Elimination:** $T_{1/2}$=9 days.

NURSING CONSIDERATIONS

Assessment: Prior to therapy, assess patient for ocular or periocular infections. Assess use in pregnant/nursing females.

Monitoring: Monitor for signs/symptoms of endophthalmitis, retinal detachment, elevated IOP, and arterial thromboembolic events. Following the intravitreal injection, check the perfusion of the optic nerve. Perform tonometry 30 min following injection and biomicroscopy between 2 and 7 days after injection.

Patient Counseling: Inform about risks of developing endophthalmitis following administration of the injection. Instruct that if eye becomes red, sensitive to light, painful, or a change in vision develops, to seek immediate care from an ophthalmologist.

Administration: Ophthalmic intravitreal injection. Procedure should be carried out under controlled aseptic conditions, which include the use of sterile gloves, sterile drape, and a sterile eyelid speculum. Adequate anesthesia and a broad-spectrum microbicide should be given prior to injection. Each vial should only be used for the treatment of a single eye. **Storage:** 2-8°C (36-46°F). Do not freeze. Protect from light and store in the original carton until time of use.

LUMIGAN

bimatoprost (Allergan) **RX**

THERAPEUTIC CLASS: Prostaglandin analog

L

INDICATIONS: Reduction of elevated IOP in open-angle glaucoma. Ocular hypertension if intolerant or unresponsive to other IOP therapies.

DOSAGE: *Adults:* 1 drop qd in pm. Max: Once daily dosing. Space dosing other ophthalmic drugs by 5 min.

HOW SUPPLIED: Sol: 0.03% [2.5mL, 5mL]

WARNINGS/PRECAUTIONS: Changes to pigmented tissues, growth of eyelashes, and macular edema reported. May change eye color and eyelashes. Do not administer with contact lenses. Caution with intraocular inflammation, renal or hepatic impairment. Caution with active intraocular inflammation, aphakic patients, pseudophakic patients with a torn posterior lens capsule, patients at risk of macular edema, and renal or hepatic impairment. Not for the treatment of angle closure, inflammatory, or neovascular glaucoma.

ADVERSE REACTIONS: Conjunctival hyperemia, ocular pruritus, growth of eyelashes, ocular dryness, visual disturbances, eye burning, foreign body sensation, eye pain, periocular skin pigmentation, blepharitis, cataract, eyelid erythema, eyelash darkening, superficial punctate keratitis.

INTERACTIONS: Space dosing of other eye drops by 5 min.

PREGNANCY: Category C, caution in nursing.

MECHANISM OF ACTION: Prostaglandin analog: selectively mimics the effects of naturally occuring substances, prostamides. Believed to lower intraocular pressure (IOP) by increasing outflow of aqueous humor through both the trabecular meshwork and uveoscleral routes.

PHARMACOKINETICS: Absorption: C_{max}=0.08ng/mL; T_{max}=10 min; AUC=0.09ng•hr/mL. **Distribution:** V_d=0.67L/kg. **Metabolism:** Via oxidation, N-de-ethylation and glucuronidation. **Elimination:** Urine (67%), feces (25%); $T_{1/2}$=45 min.

L

NURSING CONSIDERATIONS

Assessment: Assess use in aphakic patients, pseudophakic patients with a torn posterior lens capsule, patients at risk for macular edema, pregnant/nursing females, and patients with angle-closure, inflammatory, with neovascular glaucoma.

Monitoring: Monitor for increased iris pigmentation, changes in the periorbital tissue (eyelid), changes in eyelashes or growth of eyelashes, macular edema (eg, cystoid macular edema), and bacterial keratitis.

Patient Counseling: Counsel medication may cause permanent increase in brown pigmentation of the iris, eyelid skin darkening which may be reversible, changes in the eyelashes and vellus hair. Instruct to avoid touching container tip to the eye, surrounding structures, fingers, or any other surface to avoid contamination. Inform to contact physician if an intercurrent ocular condition (eg, trauma or infection), any type of ocular reactions (eg, conjunctivitis, eyelid reaction) develop while on medication. Instruct to remove contact lenses prior to instillation; reinsert 15 mins after administration. Inform that if more than 1 topical ophthalmic medication is used, separate administration by at least 5 min.

Administration: Ocular route. **Storage:** Store in original container at 2-25°C (36-77°F).

LUNESTA

eszopiclone (Sepracor) **CIV**

THERAPEUTIC CLASS: Nonbenzodiazepine hypnotic agent

INDICATIONS: Treatment of insomnia.

DOSAGE: *Adults:* Initial: 2mg qhs. Max: 3mg qhs. Elderly: Difficulty Falling Asleep: Initial: 1mg qhs. Max: 2mg qhs. Difficulty Staying Asleep: Initial/Max: 2mg qhs. Avoid high-fat meal.

HOW SUPPLIED: Tab: 1mg, 2mg, 3mg

WARNINGS/PRECAUTIONS: Abnormal thinking and behavioral changes reported. Amnesia and other neuropsychiatric symptoms may occur. Worsening of depression including suicidal thinking reported in primarily depressed patients. Avoid rapid dose decrease or abrupt discontinuation. Should only be taken immediately prior to bed or after going to bed and experiencing difficulty falling asleep. Avoid hazardous occupations. Caution in elderly, debilitated, or conditions affecting metabolism or hemodynamic responses. Reduce dose with severe hepatic impairment or concurrent use of potent CYP3A4 inhibitors. Caution with signs and symptoms of depression or suicidal tendencies.

ADVERSE REACTIONS: Headache, unpleasant taste, somnolence, dry mouth, dizziness, infection, rash, chest pain, peripheral edema, migraine.

INTERACTIONS: Possible additive effect on psychomotor performance with ethanol. Coadministration with olanzapine produced a decrease in DSST score. Strong inhibitors of CYP3A4 may significantly increase the AUC of eszopiclone.

PREGNANCY: Category C, caution in nursing.

MECHANISM OF ACTION: Not established. Pyrrolopyrazine derivative; suspected to interact with GABA-receptor complexes at binding domains located close to or allosterically coupled to benzodiazepine receptor.

PHARMACOKINETICS: Absorption: Rapidly absorbed; T_{max}=1 hr. **Distribution:** Plasma protein binding (52-59%). **Metabolism:** Liver (extensive); oxidation and demethylation pathways via CYP3A4 and CYP2E1. Primary metabolites: (S)-zopiclone-N-oxide and (S)-N-desmethyl zopiclone. **Elimination:** Urine (75% metabolite), (<10% parent drug); $T_{1/2}$=6 hrs, 9 hrs (elderly).

NURSING CONSIDERATIONS

Assessment: Assess for psychiatric or physical illness, diseases/conditions that could affect metabolism or hemodynamic response. Assess for depression, suicidal ideations, respiratory function, hepatic/renal impairment, hypersensitivity reactions, drug interactions (eg, other CNS depressants), and pregnancy/nursing status.

Monitoring: Anaphylactic/anaphylactoid reactions, insomnia, severe sedation, memory disorders, abnormal thinking/behavioral changes (eg, aggressiveness or extraversion that seem out of character), complex/bizarre behavior (eg, hallucinations, agitation, sleep-driving), worsening of depression including suicidal thoughts, physical/psychological dependence, respiratory depression, motor or cognitive performance in elderly, withdrawal-emergent anxiety, and rebound insomnia.

Patient Counseling: Inform about potential benefits/risks of drug and possibility of physical/psychological dependence. Counsel to take immediately before bed when patient can dedicate 8 hrs to sleep. Do not take with alcohol or other sedating drugs; notify physician if pregnant. Avoid hazardous tasks (eg, operating machinery/driving).

Administration: Oral route. **Storage:** 25°C (77°F), excursions permitted to 15-30°C (59-86°F).

LUPRON — RX

leuprolide acetate (TAP)

THERAPEUTIC CLASS: Synthetic gonadotropin releasing hormone analog

INDICATIONS: Palliative treatment of advanced prostate cancer.

DOSAGE: *Adults:* 1mg SQ qd. Rotate injection sites.

HOW SUPPLIED: Inj: 5mg/mL

CONTRAINDICATIONS: Pregnancy.

WARNINGS/PRECAUTIONS: Transient worsening of symptoms may occur during 1st few weeks of therapy. Closely monitor patients with metastatic vertebral lesions and/or urinary tract obstruction during 1st few weeks of therapy; may cause neurological problems or increase obstruction. Monitor serum testosterone, acid phosphatase levels. Contains benzyl alcohol.

L

ADVERSE REACTIONS: General pain, headache, hot flashes, urinary disorders, dizziness/vertigo, ECG changes/ischemia, peripheral edema, HTN, asthenia, constipation, anorexia, insomnia, myocardial infarction, diabetes, respiratory problems.

PREGNANCY: Category X, not for use in nursing.

MECHANISM OF ACTION: LH-RH agonist; acts as a potent inhibitor of gonadotropin secretion resulting in suppression of testicular and ovarian steroidogenesis.

PHARMACOKINETICS: Absorption: (M-1): T_{max}=2-6 hrs. **Distribution:** V_d=27L, plasma protein binding (43-49%). **Metabolism:** M-I (major metabolite). **Elimination:** Urine (<5%); $T_{1/2}$=3 hrs.

NURSING CONSIDERATIONS

Assessment: Assess pregnancy status, metastatic vertebral lesions, urinary tract obstruction, and possible drug interactions. Obtain baseline serum testosterone and PSA levels.

Monitoring: Monitor serum testosterone and PSA levels periodically and for signs/symptoms of anaphylactoid reactions, transient worsening of symptoms, and injection-site reaction.

Patient Counseling: Inform of pregnancy risks. Advise not to d/c therapy even if feeling better. If need alternative syringe, may use low-dose insulin syringes. Advise not to attempt to get every last drop in vial. Seek medical attention if symptoms of hot flushes, transient worsening of symptoms (bone pain, increased difficulty in urinating, onset or aggravation of nerve symptoms), injection-site reaction (burning, itching, swelling), or anaphylactoid reactions occur.

Administration: SQ route. **Storage:** 25°C (77°F). Do not freeze. Protect from light.

Lupron Depot (GYN) RX

leuprolide acetate (TAP)

OTHER BRAND NAMES: Lupron Depot 3.75 mg (TAP) - Lupron Depot-3 Month 11.25mg (TAP)

THERAPEUTIC CLASS: Synthetic gonadotropin releasing hormone analog

INDICATIONS: Management of endometriosis alone or with norethindrone acetate 5mg, including pain relief and reduction of endometriotic lesions. Retreatment of endometriosis with norethindrone acetate 5mg daily. Adjunct with iron for preoperative hematologic improvement of anemia caused by uterine leiomyomata.

DOSAGE: *Adults:* Endometriosis: 11.25mg IM every 3 months or 3.75mg IM monthly, alone or with norethindrone acetate 5mg/day. Max: 6 months of therapy. If symptoms recur after course of therapy, may retreat with the combination (leuprolide + norethindrone) up to 6 months. Uterine Leiomyomata: 11.25mg IM single dose or 3.75mg IM monthly up to 3 months. Assess bone density before retreatment.

HOW SUPPLIED: Inj: (1 month) 3.75mg, (3 month) 11.25mg

CONTRAINDICATIONS: Undiagnosed abnormal vaginal bleeding, pregnancy, nursing.

WARNINGS/PRECAUTIONS: Exclude pregnancy before therapy. Use nonhormonal methods of contraception. D/C if pregnancy occurs. Retreatment is not recommended with endometriosis. Limit to 6 months of therapy. Use if require hormonal suppression for at least 3 months. Transient worsening of symptoms may occur during initial days of therapy. Breakthrough bleeding with skipped doses. May develop or worsen depression and cause memory disorders.

ADVERSE REACTIONS: Hot flashes, sweating, dizziness, headache, vaginitis, depression, emotional lability, general pain, asthenia, decreased libido, joint disorder, breast tenderness/pain, GI upset, edema, bone density loss.

PREGNANCY: Category X, not for use in nursing.

MECHANISM OF ACTION: GnRH analog; suppresses pituitary gonadotropins.

PHARMACOKINETICS: Absorption: (3.5mg): C_{max}=4.6-10.2 ng/mL, T_{max}=4 hrs. **Distribution:** Plasma protein binding (43-49%), V_d=27L (IV). **Elimination:** $T_{1/2}$=3 hrs.

NURSING CONSIDERATIONS

Assessment: Assess risk factors for CVD, loss of bone mineral content (chronic alcohol use, tobacco use, family history), abnormal vaginal bleeding, possible drug interaction, and pregnancy/nursing status.

Monitoring: Monitor for signs/symptoms of abnormal vaginal bleeding, development or worsening of depression, and hypersensitivity reactions.

Patient Counseling: Inform of pregnancy risks; instruct to use non-hormonal method of contraception. Counsel on possibility of development or worsening of depression and occurrence of memory disorders. Instruct to notify physician if regular menstruation persists.

Administration: IM route. **Storage:** 25°C (77°F); excursions permitted to 15-30°C (59-86°F).

LUPRON DEPOT (ONCOLOGY) RX

leuprolide acetate (TAP)

OTHER BRAND NAMES: Lupron Depot 7.5mg (TAP) - Lupron Depot 3-Month 22.5 mg (TAP) - Lupron Depot 4-Month (TAP)

THERAPEUTIC CLASS: Synthetic gonadotropin releasing hormone analog

INDICATIONS: Palliative treatment of advanced prostate cancer.

DOSAGE: *Adults:* 7.5mg IM as single dose monthly, 22.5mg IM single dose every 3 months, or 30mg IM single dose every 4 months. Rotate injection site.

HOW SUPPLIED: Inj: (1-month) 7.5mg, (3-month) 22.5mg, (4-month) 30mg

CONTRAINDICATIONS: Pregnancy.

WARNINGS/PRECAUTIONS: Transient worsening of symptoms may occur during 1st few weeks of therapy. Closely monitor patients with metastatic vertebral lesions and/or urinary tract obstruction during 1st few weeks of therapy. Monitor serum testosterone, PSA. (7.5mg, 30mg) Temporary increase in bone pain. Ureteral obstruction and spinal cord compression reported; may initiate with SQ formulation for 1st 2 weeks to facilitate withdrawal if needed.

ADVERSE REACTIONS: Injection site reactions, general pain, headache, hot flashes, sweating, edema, urinary disorders, dizziness/vertigo, asthenia, GI disorders, impotence.

PREGNANCY: Category X, safety in nursing not known.

MECHANISM OF ACTION: LH-RH agonist; acts as a potent inhibitor of gonadotropin secretion resulting in suppression of testicular and ovarian steroidogenesis.

PHARMACOKINETICS: Absorption: (7.5mg, 22.5mg, 30mg): C_{max}=20ng/mL, 48.9ng/mL, 59.3ng/mL T_{max}=4 hrs; (M-1) T_{max}=2-6hrs. **Distribution:** V_d=27L, plasma protein binding (43-49%). **Metabolism:** M-I (Major metabolite). **Elimination:** Urine (<5%); $T_{1/2}$=3 hrs.

NURSING CONSIDERATIONS

Assessment: Assess pregnancy status, metastatic vertebral lesions, urinary tract obstruction, and possible drug interactions. Obtain baseline serum testosterone and PSA levels.

Monitoring: Monitor serum testosterone and PSA levels periodically and for signs/symptoms of anaphylactoid reactions, transient worsening of symptoms, and injection-site reactions.

Patient Counseling: Inform of pregnancy risks. Advise not to d/c therapy even if feeling better. Seek medical attention if symptoms of hot flushes, transient worsening of symptoms (bone pain, increased difficulty in urinating, onset or aggravation of nerve symptoms), injection-site reaction (burning, itching, swelling), or anaphylactoid reactions occur.

Administration: IM route. **Storage:** 25°C (77°F); excursions permitted to 15-30°C (59-86°F).

Lupron Pediatric RX

leuprolide acetate (TAP)

OTHER BRAND NAMES: Lupron Depot-Ped (TAP)

THERAPEUTIC CLASS: Synthetic gonadotropin releasing hormone analog

INDICATIONS: Treatment of central precocious puberty.

DOSAGE: *Pediatrics:* Initial: 50mcg/kg/d as single SQ dose or (depot) 0.3mg/kg every 4 weeks (minimum 7.5mg) as single IM dose. Depot Start Dose: ≤25kg: 7.5mg; >25-37.5kg: 11.25mg; >37.5kg: 15mg. Titrate: Increase by 10 mcg/kg/day SQ or (depot) 3.75mg IM every 4 weeks if downregulation not achieved. Maint: Dose that produces adequate downregulation. Verify adequate downregulation with significant weight increase.

HOW SUPPLIED: Inj: 5mg/mL, (Depot) 7.5mg, 11.25mg, 15mg

CONTRAINDICATIONS: Pregnancy.

WARNINGS/PRECAUTIONS: Monitor hormonal effects after 1-2 months of therapy. Measure bone age every 6-12 months. Increase in clinical signs and symptoms may occur in early phase of therapy due to rise in gonadotropins and sex steroids. D/C before age 11 in females and age 12 in males.

L

ADVERSE REACTIONS: Initial exacerbation of signs and symptoms, injection site reactions, pain, acne/seborrhea, rash, urogenital bleeding/discharge, vaginitis.

PREGNANCY: Category X, not for use in nursing.

MECHANISM OF ACTION: A GnRH agonist; initially stimulates gonadotropins. Chronic stimulation results in reversible suppression of ovarian and testicular steroidogenesis.

PHARMACOKINETICS: Absorption: C_{max}=20ng/mL; T_{max}=4 hrs. **Distribution:** V_d=27L, plasma protein binding (43-49%). **Metabolism:** M-I (major metabolite). **Elimination:** Urine (<5% parent and metabolite); $T_{1/2}$=3 hrs.

NURSING CONSIDERATIONS

Assessment: Assess pregnancy status prior to therapy.

Monitoring: Monitor GnRH stimulation test, sex steroid levels, pituitary gonadotropic and gonadal functions and Tanner staging. GnRH stimulation tests and sex steroid levels should be monitored 1-2 months following initiation of therapy. Monitor measurements of bone age for advancement every 6-12 months.

Patient Counseling: Counsel about importance of adherence to 4-week drug administration schedule. Inform females that menses or spotting may occur during first 2 months of therapy. Report any irritation at injection site and any unusual signs/symptoms immediately. D/C of medication should be considered before age 11 in females and age 12 for males.

Administration: IM route. 1) Visually inspect powder. 2) Gently mix powder thoroughly to form uniform suspension. 3) Administered IM. Discard suspension if unused. **Storage:** 25°C (77°F); excursions permitted to 15-30°C (59-86°F).

Luvox CR RX

fluvoxamine maleate (Jazz Pharmaceuticals, Inc.)

Antidepressants increased the risk of suicidal thinking and behavior (suicidality) in short-term studies in children, adolescents, and young adults with major depressive disorder (MDD) and other psychiatric disorders. Fluvoxamine is not approved for use in pediatric patients.

THERAPEUTIC CLASS: Selective serotonin reuptake inhibitor

INDICATIONS: Treatment of social anxiety disorder and obsessive compulsive disorder.

DOSAGE: *Adults:* Initial: 100mg qhs. Titrate: May increase by 50mg every week. Maint: 100-300mg/day. Max: 300mg/day. Elderly/Hepatic Impairment: Titrate slowly following initial dose.

HOW SUPPLIED: Cap, Extended Release: 100mg, 150mg

CONTRAINDICATIONS: Co-administration of alosetron, tizanidine, thioridazine, or pimozide. Concurrent use of MAOIs or MAOI usage within 14 days of discontinuing treatment with Luvox CR.

WARNINGS/PRECAUTIONS: May experience worsening of depression and/or emergence of suicidal behavior. Close supervision with high-risk suicide patients. Activation of mania/hypomania, seizures, and hyponatremia reported. Serious discontinuation symptoms reported. Caution with history of MI or unstable heart disease, liver dysfunction, or conditions altering metabolism or hemodynamic responses. Interference with cognitive or motor performance. Serotonin syndrome reported with concomitant use of triptans and MAOIs. Reduce dose gradually and do not d/c abruptly. May increase risk of bleeding events with ASA, NSAIDs and other anticoagulants. Neuroleptic malignant syndrome (NMS) or NMS-like events may occur with concomitant antipsychotics. Smoking increases metabolism.

ADVERSE REACTIONS: Headache, asthenia, nausea, diarrhea, vomiting, anorexia, dyspepsia, insomnia, somnolence, nervousness, dizziness, anxiety, dry mouth, tremor, abnormal ejaculation.

INTERACTIONS: See Contraindications. Increases serum levels of theophylline, warfarin, clozapine, carbamazepine, methadone, tacrine, propranolol and other β-blockers. Bradycardia with diltiazem. Potential for serious, fatal interactions with MAOIs. Lithium may increase serotonergic effects. Reduces clearance of mexiletine and benzodiazepines metabolized by hepatic oxidation (eg, alprazolam, midazolam, triazolam). Caution with sumatriptan, TCAs, tryptophan, NSAIDs, ASA, linezolid, tramadol, St. John's wort. Avoid ramelteon.

PREGNANCY: Category C, not for use in nursing.

MECHANISM OF ACTION: SSRI: inhibits neuronal uptake of serotonin.

PHARMACOKINETICS: Absorption: C_{max} (at doses 100mg, 200mg, 300mg) =47ng/mL, 161ng/mL, 319ng/mL. **Distribution:** V_d=25L/kg. Plasma protein binding (80%). **Metabolism:** Extensive via liver. **Elimination:** Urine (94%), $T_{1/2}$ =16.3 hrs.

NURSING CONSIDERATIONS

Assessment: Assess for risk for bipolar disorder, history of mania, possible drug interactions, history of seizures, disease/condition that alters metabolism or hemodynamic response, and hepatic impairment .

Monitoring: Monitor for signs/symptoms of clinical worsening (suicidality, unusual changes in behavior), serotonin syndrome, NMS (muscle rigidity, hyperthermia, mental status changes), abnormal bleeding, hyponatremia, seizures, hepatic dysfunction, cognitive and motor impairment. If d/c therapy (particularly if abrupt), monitor for symptoms of dysphoric mood, irritability, agitation, dizziness, sensory disturbances, anxiety, confusion, headache, lethargy, emotional lability, insomnia, and hypomania.

Patient Counseling: Advise to avoid alcohol. Instruct to seek medical attention for symptoms of serotonin syndrome (eg, mental status changes, tachycardia, hyperthermia, N/V, diarrhea, incoordination), NMS (eg, muscle rigidity, hyperthermia, mental status changes), allergic reactions (eg, rash, hives), abnormal bleeding (particularly if using NSAIDs or ASA), hyponatremia, activation of mania, seizures, clinical worsening (eg, suicidal ideation, unusual changes in behavior) and discontinuation symptoms (eg, irritability, agitation, dizziness, anxiety, headache, insomnia). Caution that physical/mental abilities may be impaired.

Administration: Oral route. **Storage:** 15-30°C (59-86°F). Protect from high humidity.

Luxiq
RX

betamethasone valerate (Stiefel)

THERAPEUTIC CLASS: Corticosteroid

INDICATIONS: Corticosteroid-responsive dermatoses of the scalp.

DOSAGE: *Adults:* Place foam onto saucer or other cool surface first, then apply in small amounts to scalp. Gently massage into affected area bid (am and pm) until foam disappears. Reassess if no improvement after 2 weeks.

HOW SUPPLIED: Foam: 0.12% [50g, 100g]

WARNINGS/PRECAUTIONS: May produce reversible HPA axis suppression, manifestations of Cushing's syndrome, hyperglycemia, and glucosuria. Caution when applied to large surface areas, for prolonged use, or under occlusive dressings. Use appropriate antifungal or antibacterial agent with dermatological infections; d/c if infection does not clear. Pediatrics may be more susceptible to systemic toxicity. Avoid eyes. D/C if irritation occurs.

ADVERSE REACTIONS: Burning, stinging, pruritus, paresthesia, acne, alopecia, conjunctivitis.

PREGNANCY: Category C, caution in nursing.

MECHANISM OF ACTION: Corticosteroid; possesses anti-inflammatory, antipruritic, and vasoconstrictive properties. Anti-inflammatory mechanism not established. Suspected to induce phospholipase A_2 inhibitory proteins, lipocortins. Lipocortins control biosynthesis of potent mediators of inflammation (eg, prostaglandins, leukotrienes) by inhibiting release of their precursor, arachidonic acid.

L

PHARMACOKINETICS: Absorption: Percutaneous. Occlusion, inflammation, and other disease states may increase absorption. **Distribution:** Systemically administered corticosteroids are found in breast milk. **Metabolism:** Liver. **Elimination:** Renal (major), bile.

NURSING CONSIDERATIONS

Assessment: Assess for hypersensitivity to other corticosteroids. Assess use in pregnant/nursing patients.

Monitoring: Monitor for signs/symptoms of reversible HPA-axis suppression, Cushing's syndrome, hyperglycemia, glucosuria, local skin irritation, allergic contact dermatitis (eg, failure to heal), and for the development of dermatological infections (eg, fungal, bacterial). Monitor for signs of glucocorticoid insufficiency following withdrawal from treatment. In patients on high doses or using occlusive dressings, perform periodic monitoring for HPA-axis suppression using ACTH stimulation, A.M plasma cortisol, and urinary free cortisol tests. In pediatric patients, monitor for signs/symptoms of systemic toxicity, HPA-axis suppression, Cushing's syndrome, linear growth retardation, delayed weight gain, and intracranial HTN.

Patient Counseling: Inform to use exactly as directed; avoid contact with eyes. Instruct not to bandage, cover, or wrap treated scalp area unless directed by physician. Contact physician if no improvement within 2 weeks of starting therapy or if adverse reactions develop. Avoid contact with fire, flames, or smoking during and immediately following drug application.

Administration: Administered topically on scalp. Invert can for proper dispensing of foam. **Storage:** 20-25°C (68-77°F). Do not expose to heat or store at temperatures above 49°C (120°F). Do not puncture or incinerate container. Contents under pressure.

Lybrel
RX

ethinyl estradiol - levonorgestrel (Wyeth)

THERAPEUTIC CLASS: Estrogen/progestogen combination

INDICATIONS: Prevention of pregnancy.

DOSAGE: *Adults:* 1 tab qd. Start Day: No Current Contraceptive Therapy: Day 1 of menstrual cycle. 21- or 28-day Regimen: Day 1 of withdrawal bleed (at the latest 7 days after last active tablet). Progestin-Only Pill: Day after taking progestin-only pill. Implant: Day of implant removal. Inj: Day next inj due. Use nonhormonal back-up method of birth control for 1st 7 days of Lybrel therapy when initiating after progestin-only pill, implant, or inj.

HOW SUPPLIED: Tab: (Ethinyl Estradiol-Levonorgestrel) 0.02mg-0.09mg

CONTRAINDICATIONS: Thrombophlebitis, DVT or thromboembolic disorders, cerebrovascular or CAD, valvular heart disease with thrombogenic complications, thrombogenic rhythm disorders, hereditary or acquired thrombophilias, major surgery with prolonged immobilization, DM with vascular involvement, headaches with focal neurological symptoms, uncontrolled HTN, breast cancer, endometrial carcinoma or other estrogen-dependent neoplasia, undiagnosed abnormal genital bleeding, cholestatic jaundice of pregnancy or jaundice with prior pill use, hepatic adenomas or carcinomas, active liver disease, pregnancy.

WARNINGS/PRECAUTIONS: Cigarette smoking increases risk of serious CV side effects; risk increases with age (especially >35 yrs) and extent of smoking. Increased risk of venous and arterial thrombotic and thromboembolic events (eg, MI, thromboembolism, stroke, TIA), hepatic neoplasia, gallbladder disease, and HTN. May increase risk of breast and cervical cancer. Retinal thrombosis reported; d/c if unexplained loss of vision. May worsen existing gallbladder disease. May cause glucose tolerance; monitor prediabetic and diabetic women. May cause fluid retention and increase BP; monitor closely with HTN and d/c if significant elevation of BP occurs. May cause onset or development of migraine or development of headache. Weigh benefit of fewer planned menses against inconvenience of unscheduled breakthrough bleeding and spotting. Ectopic or intrauterine pregnancy may occur. Monitor closely with hyperlipidemias. D/C if jaundice develops. Monitor closely with depression and d/c if depression recurs to serious degree. Perform annual physical exam. Use before menarche is not indicated.

ADVERSE REACTIONS: NV, spotting, amenorrhea, edema, weight or appetite (increase or decrease), spotting, dizziness, GI symptoms (eg, abdominal pain, cramps, bloating), nervousness, vaginitis, including candidiasis.

INTERACTIONS: Reduced effects, increased breakthrough bleeding with rifampin, rifabutin, barbiturates, phenylbutazone, primidone, dexamethasone, phenytoin, carbamazepine, felbamate, oxcarbazepine, griseofulvin, topiramate, St. Johns wort, modafinil, and possibily with ampicillin and tetracyclines. Atorvastatin, ascorbic acid, acetaminophen, CYP3A4 inhibitors (eg, itraconazole, ketoconazole) may increase hormones levels. Protease inhibitors may increase or decrease levels. May increase levels of cyclosporine, prednisolone, theophylline. May decrease levels of acetaminophen and lamotrigine. Increases clearance of temazepam, salicylic acid, morphine, clofibric acid.

PREGNANCY: Category X, not for use in nursing

MECHANISM OF ACTION: Estrogen/progesterone combination oral contraceptive. Acts by suppression of gonadotropins. Primarily inhibits ovulation. Also responsible for changes in cervical mucus (increasing difficulty of sperm entry into uterus) and in endometrium (reducing likelihood of implantation).

PHARMACOKINETICS: Absorption: Oral administration of variable days resulted in different parameters. Levonorgestrel: Rapid and completely absorbed, absolute bioavailability (100%); Ethinyl estradiol: Rapid and completely absorbed, absolute bioavailability (38-48%). **Distribution:** Levonorgestrel: Plasma protein binding (97%). **Metabolism:** Levonorgestrel: Reduction, hydroxylation and conjugation. Ethinyl Estradiol: Hepatic via CYP3A4 (hydroxylation). **Elimination:** Levonorgestrel: Urine (40-68%), feces (16-48%); $T_{1/2}$=36 hrs. Ethinyl Estradiol: Urine, feces; $T_{1/2}$=21 hrs.

NURSING CONSIDERATIONS

Assessment: Assess for current/past history of thrombophlebitis or thromboembolic disorders, CVD, CAD, valvular heart disease with thrombogenic complications, thrombogenic rhythm disorder, hereditary or acquired thrombophilias, major surgery with prolonged immobilization, DM with vascular involvement, headache with focal neurological symptoms, uncontrolled HTN, known/suspected carcinoma (breast, endometrium or other known/suspected estrogen-dependent neoplasia), abnormal genital bleeding, cholestatic jaundice of pregnancy or jaundice with prior pill use, hepatic adenomas or carcinomas, and known/suspected pregnancy. Assess for possible drug interactions, use in patients >35 years old who smoke ≥15 cigarettes/day.

Monitoring: Monitor for venous and arterial thrombotic and thromboembolic events (eg, MI, stroke), hepatic neoplasia, gallbladder disease, ocular lesions, HTN, fluid retention, bleeding irregularities, and onset or exacerbation of headaches or migraines. Monitor blood glucose levels with history of DM or in prediabetic patients, BP with history of HTN, lipid levels with a history of hyperlipidemia. Monitor for signs/symptoms of liver toxicity (eg, jaundice), GI upset (eg, diarrhea, vomiting), and signs of worsening depression with previous history. Refer patients with contact lenses to ophthalmologist if ocular changes develop. Perform annual physical exam.

Patient Counseling: Instruct that medication does not protect against HIV infection and other STDs. Inform may experience spotting/bleeding; continue therapy and notify physician if persists. Advise to avoid smoking. Intruct to take pill at same time every day. Inform that if 1 pill missed, take as soon as remembered; take next pill at next regular scheduled time. Advise that pregnancy can occur if patient has sexual intercourse during 7 days after restarting pills; use nonhormonal birth control method during that time.

Administration: Oral route. **Storage:** 25°C (77°F); excursions permitted to 15-30°C (59-86°F).

LYRICA

pregabalin (Pfizer)

CV

THERAPEUTIC CLASS: GABA analog

INDICATIONS: Adjunct therapy for adult patients with partial onset seizures. Management of neuropathic pain associated with diabetic peripheral neuropathy. Management of post-herpetic neuralgia and fibromyalgia.

DOSAGE: *Adults:* Neuropathic Pain: Initial: 50mg tid (150mg/day). Titrate: May increase to 300mg/day within 1 week. Max: 100mg tid (300mg/day). Post-Herpetic Neuralgia: Initial: 150mg/day divided bid or tid. Max: 600mg/day divided bid or tid. Epilepsy: Initial: 150mg/day divided bid-tid. Max: 600mg/day. Fibromyalgia: Initial: 75mg bid (150mg/day). Titrate: May increase to 150mg bid (300mg/day) within 1 week based on efficacy and tolerability. May further increase to 225mg bid (450mg/day) if needed. Max: 450mg/day. Renal Impairment: CrCl 30-60 mL/min: 75-300mg/day divided bid or tid. CrCl 15-30 mL/min: 25-150mg/day divided qd or bid. CrCl <15mL/min: 25-75mg/day given qd. Give supplemental dose (25-150mg) immediately after every 4-hr hemodialysis treatment. Refer to prescribing information for further details. D/C: Taper over minimum of 1 week.

HOW SUPPLIED: Cap: 25mg, 50mg, 75mg, 100mg, 150mg, 200mg, 225mg, 300mg

WARNINGS/PRECAUTIONS: Avoid abrupt withdrawal. Gradually taper over 1 week. Possible tumorigenic potential. May impair physical/mental abilities. May cause weight gain; blurred vision, monitor for ophthalmic changes; peripheral edema, caution in heart failure; elevated creatine kinase, d/c if myopathy or markedly elevated creatine kinase levels occur; decreased platelet count; and mild PR-interval prolongation. Angioedema reported in initial and chronic treatment.

ADVERSE REACTIONS: Somnolence, dizziness, dry mouth, edema, blurred vision, weight gain, abnormal thinking (difficulty with concentration/attention), headache, nausea, diarrhea.

INTERACTIONS: Additive CNS side effects with CNS depressants (eg, opiates, benzodiazepines). May potentiate the impairment of motor skills and sedation of alcohol; avoid consumption of alcohol during therapy.

PREGNANCY: Category C, not for use in nursing.

MECHANISM OF ACTION: Gamma-aminobutyric acid derivative; not fully established. Suspected to bind to α-2-delta receptors in CNS tissues. In vitro, shown to reduce calcium-dependent release of several neurotransmitters, possibly by modulation of calcium channel function. Produces antinociceptive and antiseizure effects.

PHARMACOKINETICS: Absorption: T_{max}=1.5 hrs; bioavailability (≥90%). **Distribution:** V_d=0.5L/kg; crosses placenta and blood-brain barrier, found in milk. **Metabolism:** N-methylated derivative (major metabolite). **Elimination:** Urine (90% unchanged); $T_{1/2}$=6.3 hrs.

NURSING CONSIDERATIONS

Assessment: Assess impaired renal function, history of drug abuse, previous episode of angioedema or seizure.

Monitoring: Monitor creatinine kinase, platelet count, and renal function. Monitor for angioedema, hypersensitivity reactions, weight gain, peripheral edema, ophthalmic changes, myopathy, seizures, dizziness, somnolence, and possible drug interactions. Monitor for PR interval prolongation and possible seizures when withdrawing therapy.

Patient Counseling: Inform may cause mental impairment; use caution when operating machinery/driving. Instruct to report unexplained muscle pain, tenderness, or weakness, particularly if these symptoms are accompanied by malaise or fever. Avoid consuming alcohol. Inform about signs/symptoms of angioedema, and not to abruptly d/c; taper dose over a week. Take with/without food.

Administration: Oral route. **Storage:** 25°C (77°F); excursions permitted to 15-30°C (59-86°F).

MACROBID — RX

nitrofurantoin monohydrate (Procter & Gamble)

M

THERAPEUTIC CLASS: Imidazolidinedione antibacterial

INDICATIONS: Treatment of acute uncomplicated urinary tract infections (acute cystitis).

DOSAGE: *Adults:* 100mg q12h for 7 days. Take with food.
Pediatrics: >12 yrs: 100mg q12h for 7 days. Take with food.

HOW SUPPLIED: Cap: 100mg

CONTRAINDICATIONS: Anuria, oliguria, CrCl <60mL/min, pregnancy at term (38-42 weeks gestation), labor and delivery, and neonates <1 month of age, history of cholestatic jaundice or hepatic dysfunction.

WARNINGS/PRECAUTIONS: Acute, subacute, or chronic pulmonary reactions have occurred. Anemia, diabetes mellitus, renal dysfunction, electrolyte imbalance, vitamin B deficiency, and debilitating disease enhance occurrence of peripheral neuropathy. Stop therapy with acute and chronic pulmonary reactions, hepatic disorders, hemolysis, or peripheral neuropathy. Monitor renal function, LFTs, and pulmonary function periodically during long-term therapy. Optic neuritis and hepatic reactions reported. *Clostridium difficile*-associated diarrhea has been reported. Cases of hemolytic anemia reported. D/C if hepatitis occur.

ADVERSE REACTIONS: Pulmonary disorders, hepatic damage, peripheral neuropathy, nausea, headache, flatulence, diarrhea, dizziness, alopecia, exfoliative dermatitis, Stevens-Johnson syndrome, anaphylaxis, aplastic anemia.

INTERACTIONS: Antacids, especially magnesium trisilicate, decrease rate and extent of absorption. Uricosuric drugs (eg, probenecid and sulfinpyrazone) increase nitrofurantoin levels.

PREGNANCY: Category B, not for use in nursing.

MECHANISM OF ACTION: Imidazolidinedione antibacterial; inhibits protein synthesis, aerobic energy metabolism, DNA, RNA, and cell-wall synthesis.

PHARMACOKINETICS: Absorption: C_{max} ≤1mcg/mL. **Elimination:** Urine (20-25% unchanged).

NURSING CONSIDERATIONS

Assessment: Assess for anuria, oliguria, renal impairment (CrCl <60mL/min or significant SrCr elevation), glucose 6 phosphate dehydrogenase deficiency, DM, anemia, hypersensitivity, and drug interactions.

Monitoring: Monitor for acute/chronic pulmonary reactions (eg, diffuse interstitial pneumonitis, fibrosis), hepatic reactions (eg, hepatitis, cholestatic jaundice, chronic active hepatitis, and hepatic necrosis), peripheral neuropathy, optic neuritis, hematologic manifestations, CDAD, renal function, LFTs, benign intracranial HTN, Stevens-Johnson syndrome, cyanosis (methemoglobinemia).

Patient Counseling: Advise to take with food to enhance tolerance and improve drug absorption. Advise not to use antacids containing magnesium trisilicate and uricosuric drugs. Inform that therapy treats bacterial, not viral, infections. Take exactly as directed; skipping doses or not completing full course may decrease effectiveness and increase resistance. Inform may experience diarrhea; notify physician if watery/bloody stools, hypersensitivity reactions, or benign intracranial HTN develops. Instruct to complete full course of therapy. Advise to contact their physician if unusual symptoms occur.

Administration: Oral route. **Storage:** 15-30°C (59-86°F).

MACRODANTIN — RX

nitrofurantoin macrocrystals (Procter & Gamble)

THERAPEUTIC CLASS: Imidazolidinedione antibacterial

INDICATIONS: Treatment of urinary tract infection.

DOSAGE: *Adults:* 50-100mg qid for at least 7 days. Take with food. Long-term Suppressive Use: 50-100mg at bedtime.
Pediatrics: ≥1 month: 5-7mg/kg/day given qid for at least 7 days. Take with food. Long-term Suppressive Use: 1mg/kg/day given qd-bid.

M

HOW SUPPLIED: Cap: 25mg, 50mg, 100mg

CONTRAINDICATIONS: Anuria, oliguria, CrCl <60mL/min, pregnancy at term (38-42 weeks gestation), labor and delivery, neonates <1 month of age.

WARNINGS/PRECAUTIONS: Acute, subacute or chronic pulmonary reactions have occurred. Anemia, diabetes mellitus, renal dysfunction, electrolyte imbalance, vitamin B deficiency, and debilitating disease enhance occurrence of peripheral neuropathy. Stop therapy with acute and chronic pulmonary reactions, hepatic disorders, hemolysis, or peripheral neuropathy. Monitor renal function, LFTs and pulmonary function periodically during long-term therapy. Optic neuritis and hepatic reactions reported. False (+) reaction for glucose in urine may occur with Benedict's and Fehling's solution.

ADVERSE REACTIONS: Pulmonary disorders, hepatic damage, peripheral neuropathy, nausea, emesis, anorexia, dizziness, alopecia, exfoliative dermatitis, Stevens-Johnson syndrome, anaphylaxis, headache, drowsiness, asthenia, vertigo.

INTERACTIONS: Antacids, especially magnesium trisilicate, decrease rate and extent of absorption. Uricosuric drugs (eg, probenecid and sulfinpyrazone) increase nitrofurantoin levels.

PREGNANCY: Category B, not for use in nursing

MECHANISM OF ACTION: Imidazolidinedione antibacterial; inhibits protein synthesis, aerobic energy metabolism, DNA, RNA, and cell-wall synthesis.

NURSING CONSIDERATIONS

Assessment: Assess for anuria, oliguria, renal impairment (CrCl <60mL/min, significant SrCr elevation), glucose 6 phosphate dehydrogenase deficiency, DM, anemia, hypersensitivity, and drug interactions.

Monitoring: Monitor for acute/chronic pulmonary reactions (eg, diffuse interstitial pneumonitis or fibrosis), hepatic reactions (eg, hepatitis, cholestatic jaundice, chronic active hepatitis, and hepatic necrosis), peripheral neuropathy, optic neuritis, hematologic manifestations, CDAD, renal function, LFTs, benign intracranial HTN, Stevens-Johnson syndrome, cyanosis (methemoglobinemia).

Patient Counseling: Advise to take with food to enhance tolerance and improve drug absorption. Advise not to use antacids containing magnesium trisilicate and uricosuric drugs. Inform that therapy treats bacterial, not viral, infections. Take exactly as directed; skipping doses or not completing full course may decrease effectiveness and increase resistance. Inform may experience diarrhea; notify physician if watery/bloody stools, hypersensitivity reactions, or benign intracranial HTN develops.

Administration: Oral route.

Macugen

pegaptanib sodium (Eyetech/Pfizer)

RX

THERAPEUTIC CLASS: Vascular endothelial growth factor (VEGF) inhibitor

INDICATIONS: Treatment of neovascular (wet) age-related macular degeneration.

DOSAGE: *Adults*: 0.3mg by intravitreous injection once every 6 weeks.

HOW SUPPLIED: Inj: 0.3mg

CONTRAINDICATIONS: Ocular or periocular infections.

WARNINGS/PRECAUTIONS: Rare post-marketing cases of anaphylaxis/anaphylactoid reactions, including angioedema, reported. Endophthalmitis associated with intravitreous injections. Use proper aseptic injection technique. Monitor for increased IOP. For ophthalmic intravitreal injection only.

ADVERSE REACTIONS: Anterior chamber inflammation, blurred vision, cataract, conjunctival hemorrhage, corneal edema, eye discharge, eye irritation, eye pain, HTN, increased IOP, ocular discomfort, punctate keratitis, reduced visual acuity, visual disturbance, vitreous floaters, and vitreous opacities.

PREGNANCY: Category B, caution in nursing.

MECHANISM OF ACTION: Selective vascular endothelial growth factor (VEGF) antagonist; inhibits VEGF, which is responsible for inducing angiogenesis, increasing vascular permeability and inflammation. VEGF has also been implicated in blood retinal barrier breakdown and pathological ocular neovascularization.

PHARMACOKINETICS: Absorption: Slowly into circulation from eye. **Distribution:** Vitreous fluid, retina, aqueous fluid. Metabolism: Via endo- and exonucleases. **Elimination:** Urine; $T_{1/2}$=10 days.

NURSING CONSIDERATIONS

Assessment: Prior to therapy, assess for ocular or periocular infections. Assess medical history for hypersensitivity reactions.

Monitoring: Monitor for signs/symptoms of elevated IOP, endophthalmitis, anaphylaxis reactions (eg, angioedema), retinal detachment, and iatrogenic traumatic cataract. Monitor perfusion of optic nerve immediately, perform tonometry within 30 min and biomicroscopy between 2 and 7 days following injection.

Patient Counseling: Advise about risk of developing endophthalmitis following administration. Instruct to seek immediate care with ophthalmologist if eye becomes red, sensitive to light, painful, or if change in vision develops.

Administration: Ophthalmic intravitreal injection. Injection procedure should be carried out under controlled aseptic conditions, including sterile gloves, sterile drape, and sterile eyelid speculum. Adequate anesthesia and a broad-spectrum microbicide should be given prior to injection. **Storage:** 2-8°C (36-46°F). Do not freeze or shake vigorously.

MALARONE — RX

proguanil HCl - atovaquone (GlaxoSmithKline)

OTHER BRAND NAMES: Malarone Pediatric (GlaxoSmithKline)

THERAPEUTIC CLASS: Pyrimidine synthesis inhibitor

INDICATIONS: Prophylaxis or treatment of malaria caused by *P.falciparum*.

DOSAGE: *Adults:* Prevention: Begin 1-2 days before entering endemic area, continue during stay and for 7 days after return. 1 tab qd. Treatment: 4 tabs qd for 3 days. Repeat dose if vomiting occurs within 1 hr after dosing. Take as single dose with food or milky drink.
Pediatrics: Prevention: Begin 1-2 days before entering endemic area, continue during stay and for 7 days after return. 11-20kg: 1 pediatric tab qd. 21-30kg: 2 pediatric tabs qd. 31-40kg: 3 pediatric tabs qd. >40kg: Dose as adult. Treatment: Treat for 2 consecutive days. 5-8kg: 2 pediatric tabs qd. 9-10kg: 3 pediatric tabs. 11-20kg: 1 tab qd. 21-30kg: 2 tabs qd. 31-40kg: 3 tabs. >40kg: Dose as adult. Repeat dose if vomiting occurs within 1 hr after dosing. Take as single dose with food or milky drink.

HOW SUPPLIED: (Atovaquone-Proguanil) Tab: 250mg-100mg; Tab, Pediatric: 62.5mg-25mg

CONTRAINDICATIONS: For prophylaxis in severe renal impairment (CrCl <30mL/min).

WARNINGS/PRECAUTIONS: Not for cerebral malaria. Patients with severe malaria are not candidates for PO therapy. Rare cases of anaphylaxis reported.

ADVERSE REACTIONS: Vomiting, pruritus, elevation of LFTs.

M

INTERACTIONS: Rifampin, rifabutin may decrease levels; concomitant use is not recommended. Reduced bioavailability with metoclopramide and tetracycline.

PREGNANCY: Category C, caution in nursing.

MECHANISM OF ACTION: Pyramidine synthesis inhibitor. Atovaquone: Antiparasitic agent that acts as a selective inhibitor of parasite mitochondrial electron transport. Proguanil: Antiparasitic agent that acts on the metabolite cycloguanil, which inhibits dihydrofolate reductase in the malaria parasite, resulting in disruption of deoxythymidylate synthesis.

PHARMACOKINETICS: Absorption: Atovaquone: Absolute bioavailability (23%). Proguanil: Extensively absorbed. **Distribution:** Atovaquone: V_d=8.8L/kg; plasma protein binding (≥99%). Proguanil: V_d=1617-2502L (adult and pediatric patients ≥15 yrs with body weight 31-110kg), V_d=462-966L (pediatric patients ≤15 yrs with body weight 11-56kg). Plasma protein binding (75%). **Metabolism:** Proguanil: CYP2C19. **Elimination:** Atovaquone: Feces (unchanged), urine (≤0.6%). $T_{1/2}$=2-3 days (adult). Proguanil: Via hepatic biotransformation and renal excretion; urine (40-60%); $T_{1/2}$=12-21 hrs (adult and pediatric patients).

NURSING CONSIDERATIONS

Assessment: Assess for uncomplicated *P.falciparum* malaria, renal impairment, cerebral malaria, hyperparasitemia, pulmonary edema, diarrhea, vomiting, decreased hepatic/renal function, pregnancy status. Note other diseases/conditions and drug therapies.

Monitoring: Monitor for parasitemia and parasite relapse. Monitor for adverse reactions including abdominal pain, NV, headache, diarrhea, asthenia, anorexia, dizziness, and pruritus.

Patient Counseling: Take tablet at the same time each day with food or a milky drink; repeat dose if vomiting occurs within 1 hr after dosing. If dose is missed, take as soon as possible and then return to normal dosing schedule. Do not double dose if dose is skipped. Use protective clothing, insect repellant, and bednets for malaria prophylaxis. Consult physician for any febrile illness that occurs during or after return from a malaria-endemic area.

Pregnant/nursing women anticipating travel to malarious areas should inform physician.

Administration: Oral route. **Storage:** 25°C (77°F); excursions permitted to 15-30°C (59-86°F).

MARINOL

dronabinol (Unimed)

CIII

THERAPEUTIC CLASS: Cannabinoid

INDICATIONS: Treatment of anorexia associated with weight loss in AIDS patients and nausea and vomiting associated with chemotherapy when conventional treatment has failed.

DOSAGE: *Adults:* Appetite Stimulation: Initial: 2.5mg bid before lunch and supper or 2.5mg qpm or qhs if 5mg/day is intolerable. Max: 20mg/day in divided doses. Antiemetic: Initial: 5mg/m^2 given 1-3 hrs before chemotherapy, then q2-4h after chemotherapy, up to 4-6 doses/day. Titrate: May increase by 2.5mg/m^2 increments. Max: 15mg/m^2/dose.

HOW SUPPLIED: Cap: 2.5mg, 5mg, 10mg

CONTRAINDICATIONS: Hypersensitivity to sesame oil and cannabinoids.

WARNINGS/PRECAUTIONS: Do not engage in any hazardous activity until ability to tolerate drug is established. Caution with cardiac disorders due to possible HTN/hypotension, syncope, tachycardia. Caution with history of substance abuse. Monitor with mania, depression, schizophrenia; may exacerbate illness. Caution in elderly due to increased sensitivity to the psychoactive, neurological, and postural hypotensive effects. Initial dose and adjustments should be supervised by responsible adult. Caution with history of seizure disorders, may lower seizure threshold.

ADVERSE REACTIONS: Euphoria, dizziness, paranoid reaction, somnolence, abnormal thinking, abdominal pain, NV, diarrhea, conjunctivitis, hypotension, flushing.

INTERACTIONS: Highly protein-bound drugs may require dosage changes. Additive effects with alcohol, sedatives, hypnotics, or other psychoactive drugs. Additive HTN, tachycardia, and possible cardiotoxicity with amphetamines, cocaine, and sympathomimetics. Increased tachycardia, and drowsiness with anticholinergic agents. Potentiates effects of TCAs and CNS depressants. Decreases clearance of antipyrine and barbiturates.

PREGNANCY: Category C, not for use in nursing.

MECHANISM OF ACTION: Cannabinoid; has complex effects on the CNS, including central sympathomimetic activity.

PHARMACOKINETICS: Absorption: Complete (90-95%); (2.5mg bid) C_{max}=1.32ng/mL, T_{max}=1 hr, AUC=2.88ng•hr/mL; (5mg bid) C_{max}=2.96ng/mL, T_{max}=2.5 hr, AUC=6.16ng•hr/mL; (10mg bid) C_{max}=7.88ng/mL, T_{max}=1.5 hr, AUC=15.2ng•hr/mL. **Distribution:** V_d=10L/kg; plasma protein binding (97%). Found in breast milk. **Metabolism:** Liver via microsomal hydroxylation; 11-OH-delta-9-THC (active metabolite). **Elimination:** Urine (10-15%), and feces (<5%, unchanged); $T_{1/2}$=25-36 hrs.

NURSING CONSIDERATIONS

Assessment: Assess for hypersensitivity, especially to sesame oil, seizure/cardiac disorders, history of substance abuse (including alcohol abuse/dependence), mania, depression, schizophrenia, pregnancy/nursing status, hepatic/renal impairment, and possible drug interactions.

Monitoring: Monitor for psychiatric illness exacerbation, abdominal pain, NV, dizziness, euphoria, paranoid reaction, somnolence, abnormal thinking, hypotension or HTN, syncope, tachycardia, and for psychological and physiological dependence.

Patient Counseling: Do not drink alcohol or take other CNS depressants. Use caution while performing hazardous tasks (eg,operating machinery/driving) until well tolerated. Inform of mood changes and other behavioral effects that may occur during therapy. Must be under constant supervision during initial use. Immediately report any adverse effects to physician.

Adminisration: Oral route. **Storage:** 8-15°C (46-59°F). Avoid freezing.

MAVIK RX

trandolapril (Abbott)

ACE inhibitors can cause death/injury to developing fetus during 2nd and 3rd trimesters. Stop therapy if pregnancy detected.

THERAPEUTIC CLASS: ACE inhibitor

INDICATIONS: Treatment of hypertension. To decrease risk of hospitalization and mortality in stable patients with signs of left-ventricular systolic dysfunction or CHF post-MI.

DOSAGE: *Adults:* HTN: If possible, d/c diuretic 2-3 days before therapy. Initial: 1mg qd in nonblack patients; 2mg qd in black patients; 0.5mg with concomitant diuretic. Titrate: Adjust at 1-week intervals. Usual: 2-4mg qd. Resume diuretic if not controlled. Max: 8mg/day. Post-MI: Initial: 1mg qd. Titrate: Increase to target dose of 4mg qd as tolerated. CrCl <30mL/min/Hepatic Cirrhosis for HTN or Post-MI: Initial: 0.5mg qd.

HOW SUPPLIED: Tab: 1mg*, 2mg, 4mg *scored

CONTRAINDICATIONS: History of ACE inhibitor-associated angioedema.

WARNINGS/PRECAUTIONS: D/C if angioedema or jaundice occurs. Risk of hyperkalemia with DM, renal dysfunction. Persistent nonproductive cough reported. Monitor WBCs in renal impairment and/or collagen vascular disease. Anaphylactoid reactions reported. Fetal/neonatal morbidity and death reported. Monitor for hypotension in high-risk patients (heart failure, surgery/anesthesia, prolonged diuretic therapy, volume and/or salt depletion, etc). Caution with CHF, renal dysfunction, and renal artery stenosis. More reports of angioedema in blacks than nonblacks.

M

ADVERSE REACTIONS: Cough, dizziness, hypotension, elevated serum uric acid, elevated BUN, elevated creatinine, asthenia, syncope, myalgia, gastritis, hypocalcemia, hyperkalemia, dyspepsia.

INTERACTIONS: May increase lithium levels. Hypotension risk with diuretics. Increase risk of hyperkalemia with K^+-sparing diuretics, K^+-containing salt substitutes, or K^+ supplements.

PREGNANCY: Category C (1st trimester) and D (2nd and 3rd trimesters), not for use in nursing.

MECHANISM OF ACTION: ACE inhibitor; inhibits ACE activity, reducing angiotensin II formation, decreasing vasoconstriction and aldosterone secretion and increasing plasma renin.

PHARMACOKINETICS: Absorption: Parent, metabolite: Absolute bioavailability (10%, 70%); T_{max}=1 hr, 4-10 hrs. **Distribution:** V_d=18L; plasma protein binding (80%). **Metabolism:** Cleavage of ester group; trandolaprilat (metabolite). **Elimination:** Urine, feces; $T_{1/2}$=6 hrs, 10 hrs (metabolite).

NURSING CONSIDERATIONS

Assessment: Assess for pregnancy status, volume/salt depletion, collagen vascular disease (SLE, scleroderma), CHF, DM, possible drug interactions, ischemic heart disease, aortic stenosis, cerebrovascular disease, renal/hepatic impairment.

Monitoring: Monitor renal function for 1st few weeks; WBC (collagen vascular disease) periodically. Monitor for signs/symptoms of hypotension, anaphylactoid or hypersensitivity reactions, head/neck and intestinal angioedema, agranulocytosis, hyperkalemia, renal/hepatic dysfunction.

Patient Counseling: Inform of pregnancy risks. Inform that inadequate fluid intake or fluid loss may lead to drop in BP resulting in lightheadedness or syncope; avoid K^+ supplements or salt substitutes. Advise to seek medical attention if symptoms of hypotension (syncope), anaphylactoid or hypersensitivity reactions, angioedema (head/neck; abdominal pain with/without NV), infection (sore throat, fever), hyperkalemia, or hepatic dysfunction occur.

Administration: Oral route. **Storage:** 20-25°C (68-77°F).

MAXAIR RX
pirbuterol acetate (Graceway)

OTHER BRAND NAMES: Maxair Autohaler (Graceway)

THERAPEUTIC CLASS: $Beta_2$-agonist

INDICATIONS: Prevention and reversal of bronchospasm in reversible bronchospasm (eg, asthma).

DOSAGE: *Adults:* 1-2 inh q4-6h. Max: 12 inh/day.
Pediatrics: ≥12 yrs: 1-2 inh q4-6h. Max: 12 inh/day.

HOW SUPPLIED: Autohaler: 0.2mg/inh [14g, 25.6g]; MDI: 0.2mg/inh [14g]

WARNINGS/PRECAUTIONS: Caution with cardiovascular disorders, (eg, ischemic heart disease, HTN, arrhythmias), hyperthyroidism, diabetes, convulsive disorders. Fatalities reported with excessive use. Can produce paradoxical bronchospasm. Monitor BP.

ADVERSE REACTIONS: Nervousness, tremor, headache, dizziness, palpitations, tachycardia, cough, nausea.

INTERACTIONS: Avoid other aerosol β_2 agonists. Vascular effects may be potentiated by MAOIs, TCAs, and sympathomimetics. ECG changes and/or hypokalemia may occur with non-potassium sparing diuretics. Decreased effect with β-blockers.

PREGNANCY: Category C, caution in nursing.

MECHANISM OF ACTION: β_2-adrenergic bronchodilator; activates adenyl cyclase on airway smooth muscles and increases intracellular concentration of cyclic AMP. Increased cAMP levels are associated with relaxation of bronchial smooth muscle and inhibition of release of mediators of immediate hypersensitivity.

PHARMACOKINETICS: Elimination: Urine; $T_{1/2}$=2 hrs.

NURSING CONSIDERATIONS

Assessment: Assess for history of hypersensitivity to drug. Assess for convulsive disorders, hyperthyroidism, DM, CVD, and possible drug interactions.

Monitoring: Monitor pulse rate, BP, ECG changes, for paradoxical bronchospasm and hypokalemia, hypersensitivity reactions, deterioration of asthma.

Patient Counseling: Take as directed. Report lack of response or adverse side effects.

Administration: Oral inhalation administration. **Storage:** 15-30°C (59-86°F). Shake well before use. Do not puncture. Do not use or store near heat or open flame. Keep out of reach of children.

MAXALT RX
rizatriptan benzoate (Merck)

OTHER BRAND NAMES: Maxalt-MLT (Merck)

THERAPEUTIC CLASS: $5\text{-}HT_{1B/1D}$ agonist

INDICATIONS: Acute treatment of migraine attacks with or without aura.

DOSAGE: *Adults:* ≥18 yrs: 5-10mg, may repeat q2h. Max: 30mg/24 hrs. Safety of treating >4 headaches/30 days not known. MLT: Dissolve on tongue without water. Concomitant Propranolol: 5mg, up to 3 doses/24 hrs.

HOW SUPPLIED: Tab: 5mg, 10mg; Tab, Disintegrating: (MLT) 5mg, 10mg

CONTRAINDICATIONS: Ischemic heart disease, coronary artery vasospasm (eg, Prinzmetal's angina), uncontrolled HTN, significant cardiovascular

M

disease, hemiplegic or basilar migraine, MAOI use within 14 days, other 5-HT_1 agonist or ergot-type agent use within 24 hrs.

WARNINGS/PRECAUTIONS: Confirm diagnosis. Supervise 1st dose and monitor cardiac function in those at risk of CAD (eg, HTN, hypercholesterolemia, smoker, obesity, diabetes, CAD family history, postmenopausal women, males >40 yrs). Serious adverse cardiac events, cerebrovascular events, vasospastic reactions, hypertensive crisis, and fatalities reported with 5-HT_1 agonists. Disintegrating tabs contain phenylalanine. Caution with renal dialysis and hepatic dysfunction. Serotonin syndrome may occur; symptoms may include mental status changes, autonomic instability, neuromuscular aberrations, and GI symptoms.

ADVERSE REACTIONS: Paresthesia, dry mouth, nausea, dizziness, somnolence, asthenia/fatigue.

INTERACTIONS: Increased plasma levels with propranolol. Prolonged vasospastic reactions with ergot-type agents and other 5-HT_1 agonists. Serotonin syndrome reported with combined use of an SSRI or SNRI. Avoid MAOIs during or within 14 days.

PREGNANCY: Category C, caution in nursing.

MECHANISM OF ACTION: 5-$HT_{1B/1D}$ receptor agonist; binds with high affinity to 5-$HT_{1B/1D}$ receptors on the extracerebral, intracranial blood vessels that become dilated during migraine attack; activation of these receptors results in cranial vessel constriction, inhibition of neuropeptide release, and reduced transmission in trigeminal pain pathways.

PHARMACOKINETICS: Absorption: Complete; absolute bioavailability (45%); T_{max}=1-1.5 hrs. **Distribution:** V_d=140L (male), 110L (female); plasma protein binding (14%). **Metabolism:** Oxidative deamination via MAO-A. N-monodesmethyl-rizatriptan (active metabolite). **Elimination:** Urine (82%), (14% unchanged, 51% indole acetic acid metabolite), feces (12%); $T_{1/2}$=2-3 hrs.

NURSING CONSIDERATIONS

Assessment: Confirm the diagnosis of migraine before instituting therapy. Assess for history of IHD (eg, angina pectoris, MI or documented silent ischemia), coronary artery vasospasm (eg, Prinzmetal's variant angina), HTN, hemiplegic or basilar migraine, presence of risk factors for CAD (eg, HTN, hypercholesterolemia, smoker, obesity, DM, strong family history of CAD, female with surgical or physiological menopause, or male >40 years of age), hepatic/renal impairment, phenylketonuria, pregnancy/nursing status, ECG changes, and possible drug interactions.

Monitoring: Administration of first dose should be in physician's office or medically staffed and equipped facility as cardiac ischemia may occur in absence of clinical symptoms; ECG should be obtained immediately during interval in those with risk factors. Monitor for signs/symptoms of cardiac events (eg, coronary vasospasm, acute MI, arrhythmia, ECG changes, follow-up coronary angiography), cerebrovascular events (eg, hemorrhage, stroke, TIAs), peripheral vascular ischemia, colonic ischemia with bloody diarrhea and abdominal pain, serotonin syndrome (eg, mental status changes, autonomic instability, neuromuscular aberrations and/or GI symptoms), ophthalmic effects, and increased BP.

Patient Counseling: Caution during hazardous tasks (eg, operating machinery/driving). Warn of risk of serotonin syndrome, especially if combined with SSRIs or SNRIs. Instruct to read patient package insert before taking. Notify physician if pregnant/nursing or planning to become pregnant.

Administration: Oral route. Disintegrating Tabs: Just prior to dosing, remove blister from outer pouch with dry hands, place on tongue to be dissolved and swallow. **Storage:** 15-30°C (59-86°F); tight container.

MAXAQUIN — RX

lomefloxacin HCl (G.D. Searle)

THERAPEUTIC CLASS: Fluoroquinolone

INDICATIONS: Treatment of acute bacterial exacerbation of chronic bronchitis (ABECB) and uncomplicated/complicated urinary tract infections (UTI). Preoperatively for the prevention of infections from transrectal prostate biopsy (TRPB) and in transurethral surgical procedures (TUSP).

DOSAGE: *Adults:* ≥18 yrs: ABECB: 400mg qd for 10 days. Uncomplicated Cystitis: 400mg qd for 3 days (*E.coli*) or 10 days (*K.pneumoniae, P.mirabilis,* or *S.saprophyticus*). Complicated UTI: 400mg qd for 14 days. Hemodialysis/ CrCl >10 to <40mL/min: LD: 400mg. Maint: 200mg qd. Preoperative Prevention: TRPB: 400mg single dose 1-6 hrs before procedure. TUSP: 400mg single dose 2-6 hrs before procedure.

HOW SUPPLIED: Tab: 400mg* *scored

WARNINGS/PRECAUTIONS: Rare cases of torsades de pointes have been reported; avoid with known prolongation of the QT interval, uncorrected hypokalemia, concomitant treatment with Class IA (quinidine, procainamide) or class III (amiodarone, sotalol) antiarrhythmic agents. Moderate to severe phototoxicity, convulsions, pseudomembranous colitis, serious fatal hypersensitivity reactions reported. Avoid in pregnancy and nursing. Not for empiric treatment of *Pseudomonas* bacteremia or ABECB caused by *S.pneumoniae*. Caution with CNS disorder or those predisposed to seizures. Adjust dose in renal impairment. D/C if pain, inflammation, or tendon rupture occurs. Increased risk of tendon rupture in patients receiving concomitant corticosteriods. Maintain adequate hydration. Rare cases of sensory or sensorimotor axonal polyneuropathy reported; d/c if symptoms of neuropathy occur.

ADVERSE REACTIONS: Headache, nausea, photosensitivity, dizziness, diarrhea, abdominal pain.

INTERACTIONS: Decreased bioavailability with sucralfate, divalent or trivalent cations (didanosine), and magnesium- or aluminum-containing antacids; take 4 hrs before or 2 hrs after lomefloxacin. Cimetidine may increase effects. Probenecid slows the renal elimination. May enhance cyclosporine, warfarin effects.

M

PREGNANCY: Category C, not for use in nursing.

MECHANISM OF ACTION: Fluoroquinolone; synthetic broad-spectrum antimicrobial agent; inhibits topoisomearase II (DNA gyrase) and topoisomerase IV, which are required for bacterial DNA replication, transcription, repair, and recombination.

PHARMACOKINETICS: Absorption: Rapid, bioavailability (95%-98%); C_{max}(400mg)=2.8mcg/mL, T_{max}=1.5 hrs; AUC=25.9mcg•h/mL. **Elimination:** Urine (65% unchanged); $T_{1/2}$(400mg)=7.75 hrs.

NURSING CONSIDERATIONS

Assessment: Assess renal function, LFTs, pregnancy status, history of seizures, QTc prolongation, and possible drug interactions.

Monitoring: Monitor for QTc prolongation, hematologic manifestations, glucosuria, hematuria, pulmonary edema, hypo/hyperglycemia, cardiac arrest, seizure, status epilepticus, respiratory arrest, CDAD, renal function, LFTs, CBC, tendon rupture, peripheral neuropathy, hypersensitivity reactions (toxic epidermal necrolysis, Stevens-Johnson syndrome).

Patient Counseling: Counsel to use caution in activities requiring mental alertness and coordination. Report adverse side effects, persistent tendon/ joint pain, diarrhea and avoid sun exposure. Counsel therapy treats bacterial, not viral, infections. Take as directed; skipping doses or not completing full course may decrease effectiveness and increase resistance. Advise diabetic patients to use caution; hypoglycemia may develop during therapy. Instruct to drink liberal amounts of fluids.

Administration: PO. **Storage:** 59-77°F (15-25°C).

MAXIPIME — RX

cefepime HCl (Elan)

THERAPEUTIC CLASS: Cephalosporin (4th generation)

INDICATIONS: Treatment of uncomplicated/complicated urinary tract (UTI), uncomplicated skin and skin structure (SSSI), and complicated intra-abdominal infections, and pneumonia caused by susceptible strains of microorganisms. Emperic therapy for febrile neutropenia.

DOSAGE: *Adults:* Moderate-Severe Pneumonia: 1-2g IV q12h for 10 days. Febrile Neutropenia Emperic Therapy: 2g IV q8h for 7 days or until neutropenia resolved. Mild-Moderate UTI: 0.5-1g IM/IV q12h for 7-10 days. Severe UTI/ Moderate-Severe SSSI: 2g IV q12h for 10 days. Complicated Intra-Abdominal Infections: 2g IV q12h for 7-10 days. Renal Impairment: Initial: Normal dose. Maint: CrCl >60mL/min: Normal dose. CrCl 30-60mL/min: 500mg-2g q24h or 2g q12h. CrCl 11-29mL/min: 500mg-2g q24h. CrCl <11mL/min: 250mg-1g q24h. CAPD: 500mg-2g q48h. Hemodialysis: 1g on Day 1, then 500mg q24h. *Pediatrics:* 2 months-16 yrs: ≤40kg: UTI/SSSI/Pneumonia: 50mg/kg IV q12h. Febrile Neutropenia: 50mg/kg IV q8h. Max: Do not exceed adult dose.

HOW SUPPLIED: Inj: 500mg, 1g, 2g

WARNINGS/PRECAUTIONS: Caution with PCN sensitivity; cross hypersensitivity may occur. *Clostridium difficile*-associated diarrhea reported. Treatment may result in overgrowth of nonsusceptible organisms. Caution with renal impairment or history of GI disease especially colitis. Encephalopathy, myoclonus, seizures, and/or renal failure reported. D/C if seizure occurs. Associated with a fall in PT; monitor PT with renal or hepatic impairment, poor nutritional state, and protracted course of antimicrobials; give vitamin K as indicated. Associated with (+) direct Coombs' test.

ADVERSE REACTIONS: Local reactions (eg, phlebitis) rash, diarrhea.

INTERACTIONS: Increased risk of nephrotoxicity and ototoxicity with aminoglycosides. Risk of nephrotoxicity with potent diuretics (eg, furosemide).

PREGNANCY: Category B, caution in nursing.

M

MECHANISM OF ACTION: Cephalosporin; bactericidal due to inhibition of cell-wall synthesis.

PHARMACOKINETICS: Absorption: IV administration of variable doses resulted in different parameters. **Distribution:** V_d=18L; plasma protein binding (20%). **Metabolism:** Metabolized to N-methylpyrrolidine, which is rapidly converted to N-oxide. **Elimination:** Urine; $T_{1/2}$=2hrs.

NURSING CONSIDERATIONS

Assessment: Assess for history of hypersensitivity to cephalosporins/PCNs, pregnancy status, possible drug interactions, renal impairment. Document indications for therapy, culture, and susceptibility testing.

Monitoring: Monitor for signs/symptoms of hypersensitivity reactions (anaphylaxis), CDAD, seizures, encephalopathy, renal functions, PT, superinfection.

Patient Counseling: Inform that therapy only treats bacterial, not viral, infections. Take as directed; skipping doses or not completing full course may decrease effectiveness and increase resistance. Inform may experience diarrhea; Notify physician if watery/bloody stools, superinfection, or hypersensitivity reactions occur.

Administration: IV/IM routes. **Storage:** 2-25°C (36-77°F). Protect from light. Store in dry state.

MAXZIDE **RX**

triamterene - hydrochlorothiazide (Mylan Bertek)

OTHER BRAND NAMES: Maxzide-25 (Mylan Bertek)

THERAPEUTIC CLASS: K^+-sparing diuretic/thiazide diuretic

INDICATIONS: For hypertension or edema if hypokalemia occurs on HCTZ alone, or when a thiazide diuretic is required and cannot risk hypokalemia.

DOSAGE: *Adults:* (37.5mg-25mg tab) 1-2 tabs qd. (75mg-50mg tab) 1 tab qd.

HOW SUPPLIED: (Triamterene-HCTZ) Tab: (Maxzide) 75mg-50mg*, (Maxzide-25) 37.5mg-25mg* *scored

CONTRAINDICATIONS: Hyperkalemia, anuria, acute or chronic renal insufficiency, sulfonamide hypersensitivity, diabetic neuropathy, K^+-sparing agents (eg, diuretics), K^+ supplements, K^+ salt substitutes, K^+-rich diet.

WARNINGS/PRECAUTIONS: Risk of hyperkalemia (≥5.5mEq/L) especially with renal impairment, elderly, DM or severely ill; monitor levels frequently. Check ECG if hyperkalemia occurs. Caution with history of renal lithiasis, hepatic dysfunction. Monitor BUN and creatinine periodically. D/C if azotemia increases. May contribute to megaloblastosis in folic acid deficiency. Hyperuricemia, hypercalcemia, hypophosphatemia, hypokalemia may occur. May manifest latent DM. May decrease serum PBI levels. Monitor for fluid/electrolyte imbalance.

ADVERSE REACTIONS: Jaundice, pancreatitis, NV, taste alteration, drowsiness, dry mouth, depression, anxiety, tachycardia, blood dyscrasias, electrolyte disturbances.

INTERACTIONS: May potentiate other antihypertensives. Risk of lithium toxicity. Indomethacin may cause renal failure; caution with NSAIDs. Increased risk of hyperkalemia with ACE inhibitors. May increase responsiveness to tubocurarine. May decrease arterial responsiveness to norepinephrine. May alter insulin requirements. Alcohol, barbiturates, or narcotics may potentiate orthostatic hypotension.

PREGNANCY: Category C, not for use in nursing.

MECHANISM OF ACTION: HCTZ: Thiazide diuretic; blocks renal tubular absorption of Na^+ and Cl^- ions. This natriuresis and diuresis is accompanied by a secondary loss of K^+ and bicarbonate. Triamterene: Potassium-sparing diuretic; acts on the distal renal tubule to inhibit the reabsorption of Na^+ in exchange for K^+ and H^+, thus increases Na^+ excretion and reduces excessive loss of K^+ and H^+ associated with HCTZ.

PHARMACOKINETICS: Absorption: HCTZ: T_{max}=2 hrs. Triamterene: Rapid, T_{max}=1 hr. **Metabolism:** Triamterene: Liver; sulfate conjugation; hydroxytriamterene (metabolite). **Elimination**: HCTZ: Urine (unchanged).

M

NURSING CONSIDERATIONS

Assessment: Assess for hyperkalemia, anuria, acute or chronic renal insufficiency, hepatic impairment or progressive liver disease, diabetic neuropathy, DM, risk for respiratory or metabolic acidosis, history of renal lithiasis, SLE, history of allergy or bronchial asthma, and possible drug interactions.

Monitoring: Monitor serum potassium levels, ECG, serum and urine electrolytes, folic acid levels, parathyroid function, BUN, creatinine (frequent intervals), signs of hyperkalemia (eg, paresthesias, muscular weakness, fatigue, flaccid paralysis of the extremities, bradycardia, and shock), electrolyte imbalance (eg, dry mouth, thirst, drowsiness, restlessness, oliguria, tachycardia, GI disturbance), folic acid deficiency or megaloblastosis, renal stone formation, hyperuricemia or acute gout, metabolic and endocrine effects, dilutional hyponatremia, hypokalemia, pathological changes in the parathyroid gland with hypercalcemia/hypophosphatemia and hepatic coma.

Patient Counseling: Inform about warning signs of hyperkalemia, and importance of periodic monitoring of serum potassium levels and ECG. Notify if pregnant/nursing.

Administration: Oral route. **Storage:** 20-25°C (68-77°F); in tight, light-resistant container.

MEDROL

RX

methylprednisolone (Pharmacia & Upjohn)

OTHER BRAND NAMES: Medrol Dose Pack (Pharmacia & Upjohn)

THERAPEUTIC CLASS: Glucocorticoid

INDICATIONS: Steroid-responsive disorders.

DOSAGE: *Adults:* Initial: 4-48mg/day depending on disease and response. Maint: Decrease dose by small amounts to lowest effective dose. MS: Initial:

160mg/day for 1 week. Maint: 64mg every other day for 1 month. Alternate Day Therapy: Twice the usual dose every other day for long-term therapy. *Pediatrics:* Initial: 4-48mg/day depending on disease and response. Maint: Decrease dose by small amounts to lowest effective dose. MS: Initial: 160mg/day for 1 week. Maint: 64mg every other day for 1 month. Alternate Day Therapy: Twice the usual dose every other day for long-term therapy.

HOW SUPPLIED: Tab: 2mg*, 4mg*, 8mg*, 16mg*, 32mg*; (Dose-Pak) 4mg* [21s] *scored

CONTRAINDICATIONS: Systemic fungal infections.

WARNINGS/PRECAUTIONS: May need to increase dose before, during, and after stressful situations. May mask signs of infection or cause new infections. Prolonged use may produce glaucoma, optic nerve damage, secondary ocular infections. Increases BP, salt/water retention, potassium excretion. More severe/fatal course of infections reported with chickenpox, measles. Caution with Strongyloides, latent TB, hypothyroidism, cirrhosis, ocular herpes simplex, HTN, diverticulitis, fresh intestinal anastomoses, ulcerative colitis, osteoporosis, myasthenia gravis, renal insufficiency, peptic ulcer disease. Kaposi's sarcoma reported. Growth and development of children on prolonged therapy should be monitored. Monitor for psychic disturbances. Avoid abrupt withdrawal. The 24mg tabs contain tartrazine; caution with tartrazine sensitivity.

ADVERSE REACTIONS: Fluid and electrolyte disturbances, HTN, osteoporosis, muscle weakness, cushingoid state, menstrual irregularities, nervousness, insomnia, impaired wound healing, DM, ulcerative esophagitis, excessive sweating, increased ICP, carbohydrate intolerance, glaucoma, cataracts, weight gain, nausea, malaise.

INTERACTIONS: Reduced efficacy with hepatic enzyme inducers (eg, phenobarbital, phenytoin, and rifampin). Increases clearance of chronic high-dose ASA. Caution with ASA in hypoprothrombinemia. Effects on oral anticoagulants are variable; monitor PT. Increased insulin and oral hypoglycemic requirements in DM. Avoid live vaccines with immunosuppressive doses. Possible decreased vaccine response with killed or inactivated vaccines with immunosuppressive doses. Mutual inhibition of metabolism with cyclosporine; convulsions reported. Potentiated by ketoconazole and troleandomycin.

M

PREGNANCY: Safety in pregnancy and nursing not known.

MECHANISM OF ACTION: Anti-inflammatory glucocorticoid; causes profound and varied metabolic effects and modifies the body's immune responses to diverse stimuli.

PHARMACOKINETICS: Absorption: Readily absorbed from GI tract.

NURSING CONSIDERATIONS

Assessment: Assess for systemic fungal infections, current infections, active TB, vaccination history, ulcerative colitis, diverticulitis, peptic ulcer with impending perforation, renal/hepatic insufficiency, septic arthritis/unstable joint, HTN, osteoporosis, myasthenia gravis, thyroid status, psychotic tendencies, and possible drug interactions.

Monitoring: Monitor for adrenocortical insufficiency, occurrence of infection, psychic derangement, cataracts, acute myopathy, Kaposi's sarcoma, fluid retention, measurement of serum electrolytes, TSH, LFTs, IOP, and BP. Monitor urinalysis, blood sugar, weight, chest X-ray, and upper GI X-ray (if ulcer history) regularly during prolonged therapy.

Patient Counseling: Inform that susceptibility to infections may increase. Avoid exposure to chickenpox or measles; report immediately if exposed. Dietary salt restriction and supplementation of K^+ is advised.

Administration: Oral route. **Storage:** 20-25°C (68-77°F).

MEGACE ES — RX

megestrol acetate (Par)

OTHER BRAND NAMES: Megace Suspension (Bristol-Myers Squibb)

THERAPEUTIC CLASS: Progesterone

INDICATIONS: Management of anorexia, cachexia, or unexplained significant weight loss in AIDS patients.

DOSAGE: *Adults:* (Megace) Initial: 800mg/day (20mL/day). Usual: 400-800mg/day. Shake well before use. Elderly: Start at lower end of dosing range. (Megace ES) Initial/Usual: 625mg/day (5mL/day).

HOW SUPPLIED: Sus: 40mg/mL [240mL], (ES) 125mg/mL [150mL]

CONTRAINDICATIONS: Pregnancy.

WARNINGS/PRECAUTIONS: May cause fetal harm; avoid in pregnancy. New onset or exacerbation of diabetes or Cushing's syndrome reported. Risk of adrenal suppression if taking or withdrawing from chronic therapy; monitor for hypotension, nausea, vomiting, dizziness, or weakness. Caution with history of thromboembolic diseases. Use in HIV-infected women has been limited. Do not use as prophylactic to avoid weight loss.

ADVERSE REACTIONS: Diarrhea, impotence, rash, flatulence, HTN, asthenia, insomnia, nausea, anemia, fever, decreased libido, dyspepsia, headache, hyperglycemia, vomiting, pneumonia.

INTERACTIONS: May increase insulin requirements. Decrease in pharmacokinetic parameters of indinavir; higher dose should be considered.

PREGNANCY: Category X, not for use in nursing.

MECHANISM OF ACTION: Progesterone; not established; has appetite-enhancing property.

PHARMACOKINETICS: Absorption: PO administration of variable doses resulted in different parameters. **Elimination:** Urine (major), feces.

NURSING CONSIDERATIONS

Assessment: Assess for pre-existing DM, history of thromboembolic disease, renal dysfunction, treatable causes of weight loss, pregnancy status, and possible drug interactions.

Monitoring: Monitor for adrenal insufficiency, hypoadrenalism (NV, dizziness, hypotension, weakness), breakthrough bleeding, renal function, and hypersensitivity reactions.

Patient Counseling: Inform of pregnancy risks; avoid becoming pregnant. Advise to seek medical attention if symptoms of adrenal insufficiency, hypoadrenalism (NV, dizziness, hypotension, weakness), breakthrough bleeding, or hypersensitivity reactions occur.

Administration: Oral route. **Storage:** 15-25°C (59-77°F). Protect from heat.

MEPERIDINE/PROMETHAZINE CII

meperidine HCl - promethazine HCl (Ethex)

OTHER BRAND NAMES: Meprozine (Vintage)

THERAPEUTIC CLASS: Opioid analgesic/phenothiazine

INDICATIONS: Management of moderate pain and sedation for postoperative and postpartum use, and pain associated with malignancies.

DOSAGE: *Adults:* 1 cap q4-6h prn.

HOW SUPPLIED: Cap: (Meperidine-Promethazine) 50mg-25mg

CONTRAINDICATIONS: During or within 14 days of MAOIs.

WARNINGS/PRECAUTIONS: May cause tolerance and dependence; potential for abuse. Extreme caution with head injury, increased ICP, intracranial lesions, acute asthma, COPD, cor pulmonale, decreased respiratory reserve, respiratory depression, hypoxia, hypercapnia. Severe hypotension may occur with depleted blood volume. Orthostatic hypotension may occur. Caution with atrial flutter and other supraventricular tachycardias. May obscure diagnosis or clinical course of acute abdominal conditions. Reduce initial dose in elderly, debilitated, severe hepatic or renal dysfunction, hypothyroidism, Addison's disease, prostatic hypertrophy, urethral stricture. May aggravate seizure disorders. Not for use in pregnant women prior to labor.

ADVERSE REACTIONS: Lightheadedness, dizziness, sedation, NV, sweating.

INTERACTIONS: See Contraindications. Additive sedative effects with CNS depressants (eg, narcotics, anesthetics, phenothiazines, tranquilizers, sedative-hypnotics, TCAs, alcohol). Reduce analgesic depressant dose by 25-50% and dose of barbiturates by 50%. Severe hypotension possible with concurrent phenothiazines, certain anesthetics.

PREGNANCY: Safety in pregnancy and nursing not known.

MECHANISM OF ACTION: Meperidine: Narcotic analgesic. Promethazine: Phenothiazine derivative; has antiemetic, sedative, antihistaminic actions.

NURSING CONSIDERATIONS

Assessment: Assess for hypothyroidism, Addison's disease, seizure disorder, urethral stricture, prostatic hypertrophy, acute abdominal conditions, increased ICP, head injury, intracranial lesions, asthma, COPD, cor pulmonale, decreased respiratory reserve, respiratory depression, hypoxia, hypercapnia, atrial flutter, SVT, possible drug interactions, renal/hepatic impairment.

Monitoring: Monitor for signs/symptoms of seizures, respiratory depression, hypotension, tachycardia, and hypersensitivity reactions.

Patient Counseling: Caution may impair physical/mental abilities. Advise to seek medical attention if symptoms of seizures, respiratory depression, hypotension, tachycardia, or hypersensitivity reactions occur.

Administration: Oral route. **Storage:** 25°C (77°F). Protect from light.

MEPRON RX

atovaquone (GlaxoSmithKline)

THERAPEUTIC CLASS: Napthoquinone antiprotozoal

INDICATIONS: Prevention and treatment of mild to moderate *Pneumocystis carinii* pneumonia (PCP) in those intolerant to trimethoprim-sulfamethoxazole.

DOSAGE: *Adults:* Take with food. Prevention: 1500mg qd. Treatment: 750mg bid for 21 days.
Pediatrics: 13-16 yrs: Take with food. Prevention: 1500mg qd. Treatment: 750mg bid for 21 days.

HOW SUPPLIED: Sus: 750mg/5mL [5mL, 42[s]; 210mL]

WARNINGS/PRECAUTIONS: Monitor with severe hepatic impairment. Absorption significantly increased with food.

ADVERSE REACTIONS: Rash, nausea, GI effects, cough increased, rhinitis, asthenia, infection, dyspnea, insomnia, asthenia, pruritus.

INTERACTIONS: Significantly decreased plasma levels with rifampin. Caution with other highly protein-bound drugs.

PREGNANCY: Category C, caution in nursing.

MECHANISM OF ACTION: Naphthoquinone antiprotozoal; site of action appears to be cytochrome bc_1 complex which is linked to mitochondrial electron transport. Inhibition of electron transport by atovaquone will result in indirect inhibition of these enzymes, resulting in nucleic acid and ATP synthesis inhibition.

PHARMACOKINETICS: Absorption: Absolute bioavailability (47%); PO administration of variable doses resulted in different parameters. **Distribution:** V_d=0.6L/kg; plasma protein binding (99.9%). **Elimination:** Feces (≥94%, unchanged), urine (≤0.6%).

NURSING CONSIDERATIONS

Assessment: Assess CBC with differential and platelets, renal/hepatic functions. Note other diseases/conditions and drug therapies.

Monitoring: Monitor for hypersensitivity reactions (eg, rash, fever, allergic reaction), GI events (eg, NV, diarrhea), bronchospasm. Monitory lab tests such as CBC, LFTs (ALT, AST, alkaline phosphatase, amylase), BUN, creatinine, and serum electrolytes.

Patient Counseling: Instruct to take as prescribed, daily, with meals. Counsel about potential side effects; seek medical attention if any develop.

Administration: Oral route. **Storage:** 15-25°C (59-77°F). Do not freeze.

MERIDIA

CIV

sibutramine HCl monohydrate (Abbott)

THERAPEUTIC CLASS: Dopamine/norepinephrine/serotonin reuptake inhibitor

INDICATIONS: Management of obesity, including weight loss and maintenance of weight loss, and should be used in conjunction with a reduced calorie diet. Recommended for obese patients with an initial BMI ≥30kg/m² or ≥27kg/m² with risk factors (eg, HTN, diabetes, dyslipidemia).

DOSAGE: *Adults:* Initial: 10mg qd. Titrate: May increase after 4 weeks to 15mg qd. Max: 15mg/day. Use 5mg/day in patients unable to tolerate 10mg/day. May continue for up to 2 yrs.

Pediatrics: ≥16 yrs: Initial: 10mg qd. Titrate: May increase after 4 weeks to 15mg qd. Use 5mg/day in patients unable to tolerate 10mg/day. Max: 15mg/day. May continue for up to 2 yrs.

HOW SUPPLIED: Cap: 5mg, 10mg, 15mg

CONTRAINDICATIONS: Concomitant use of MAOIs or centrally-acting weight loss drugs, eating disorders (eg, anorexia/bulimia nervosa).

WARNINGS/PRECAUTIONS: May increase BP and/or pulse. Avoid with uncontrolled or poorly controlled HTN, CAD, CHF, arrhythmias, stroke, severe hepatic or renal dysfunction. Monitor BP and pulse before therapy and regularly thereafter. Caution with narrow angle glaucoma, mild to moderate renal impairment, and if predisposed to bleeding, and history of HTN. D/C if seizures develop. Exclude organic causes of obesity. Gallstones precipitated with weight loss. Caution in elderly.

ADVERSE REACTIONS: Anorexia, constipation, increased appetite, nausea, dyspepsia, dry mouth, insomnia, dizziness, nervousness, HTN, tachycardia, dysmenorrhea, and headache.

INTERACTIONS: Avoid excess alcohol, CNS-active drugs, other serotonergic agents (eg, SSRIs, migraine therapy agents, certain opioids), within 14 days of MAOI use. Caution with drugs affecting hemostasis or platelet function; ephedrine, pseudoephedrine; and other agents that increase BP, heart rate. Possible decreased metabolism with ketoconazole and erythromycin.

PREGNANCY: Category C, not for use in nursing.

MECHANISM OF ACTION: Inhibits norepinephrine, serotonin, and dopamine reuptake.

PHARMACOKINETICS: Absorption: Rapid; T_{max}=1.2 hrs; (15mg Dose, M_1, M_2) C_{max}=4ng/mL, 6.4ng/mL; T_{max}=3.6 hrs, 3.5 hrs; AUC=25.5ng•h/mL, 92.1ng•h/mL. **Distribution:** Plasma protein binding (97%); M_1, M_2 (94%). **Metabolism:** Liver via CYP3A4; M_1 and M_2 (active metabolites). **Elimination:** Urine (77%), feces; $T_{1/2}$=1.1 hrs, 14 hrs (M_1), 16 hrs (M_2).

NURSING CONSIDERATIONS

Assessment: Assess for renal/hepatic impairment, anorexia nervosa, bulimia nervosa, history of HTN, history of CAD, CHF, arrhythmias, stroke, narrow-angle glaucoma, seizures, hypothyroidism, and possible drug interactions. Obtain baseline BP and pulse rate. Evaluate for history of drug abuse.

Monitoring: Monitor BP and pulse rate periodically. Monitor for signs/symptoms of mydriasis, HTN, seizures, bleeding events, gallstone formation, psychomotor or cognitive performance, serotonin syndrome, and hypersensitivity reactions. If ≥4 lbs not lost in first 4 weeks, consider reevaluation of therapy.

Patient Counseling: Advise to notify physician if taking any prescription (eg, lithium, sumatriptan, antidepressants, dihydroergotamine) or OTC drugs (eg, decongestants, cough suppressants), or if allergic reactions, seizures, bleeding events, signs/symptoms of serotonin syndrome or visual disturbances develop, and breast feeding in nursing mothers. Regular BP and pulse monitoring recommended.

Administration: Oral route. **Storage:** 25°C (77°F); excursions permitted to 15-30°C (59-86°F). Protect from heat and moisture.

MERREM RX

meropenem (AstraZeneca)

THERAPEUTIC CLASS: Carbapenem

INDICATIONS: Treatment of intra-abdominal infections, bacterial meningitis, and complicated skin and skin structure infections (cSSSI) caused by susceptible strains of microorganisms.

DOSAGE: *Adults:* IV: Intra-Abdominal: 1g q8h. CrCl 26-50mL/min: 1g q12h. CrCl 10-25mL/min: 500mg q12h. CrCl <10mL/min: 500mg q24h. cSSSI: 500mg q8h. CrCl 26-50mL/min: 500mg q12h. CrCl 10-25mL/min: 250mg q12h. CrCl <10mL/min: 250mg q24h.
Pediatrics: IV: ≥3 months: >50kg: Intra-Abdominal: 1g q8h. Meningitis: 2g q8h. cSSSI: 500mg q8h. ≤50kg: Intra-Abdominal: 20mg/kg q8h. Max: 1g q8h. Meningitis: 40mg/kg q8h. Max: 2g q8h. cSSSI: 10mg/kg q8h. Max: 500mg q8h.

HOW SUPPLIED: Inj: 500mg, 1g

CONTRAINDICATIONS: Hypersensitivity to β-lactams.

WARNINGS/PRECAUTIONS: Severe and fatal hypersensitivity reactions reported; increased risk with allergens and/or PCN sensitivity. *Clostridium difficile*-associated diarrhea reported; if CDAD suspected d/c therapy. Seizures and other CNS effects reported, particularly with pre-existing CNS disorders, bacterial meningitis, and renal dysfunction. Thrombocytopenia reported with severe renal impairment. Prolonged use may result in superinfection. Use as monotherapy for meningitis caused by penicillin nonsusceptible strains of *Streptococcus pneumoniae* has not been established.

ADVERSE REACTIONS: Headache, rash, local reactions, diarrhea, NV, constipation.

INTERACTIONS: Probenecid inhibits renal excretion; avoid concomitant use. May reduce valproic acid levels.

PREGNANCY: Category B, caution in nursing.

MECHANISM OF ACTION: Broad-spectrum carbapenem; penetrates bacterial cells and interferes with synthesis of vital cell wall components, resulting in cell death.

PHARMACOKINETICS: Absorption: 30 min infusion: C_{max}=23mcg/mL (500mg); 49mcg/mL (1g). 5-min bolus injection: C_{max}=45mcg/mL (500mg); 112mcg/mL (1g). **Distribution:** Plasma protein binding (2%). **Elimination:** Urine (70%); $T_{1/2}$=1 hr, 1.5 hrs (3mo-2yrs).

NURSING CONSIDERATIONS

Assessment: Assess for β-lactam hypersensitivity, history of seizure or brain lesions, bacterial meningitis, renal impairment, and possible drug interactions.

Monitoring: Monitor for signs/symptoms of anaphylactoid/hypersensitivity reactions, *C. difficile*-associated diarrhea, superinfections, and seizures.

Patient Counseling: Inform drug only treats bacterial, not viral, infections. Instruct to take as directed; skipping doses or not completing full course may decrease effectiveness and increase resistance. Inform may experience diarrhea; contact physician if watery/bloody stools, hypersensitivity reactions, infection, or seizures occur.

Administration: IV route. Refer to PI for preparation of solution and stability parameters. **Storage:** 20-25°C (68-77°F).

METADATE CD

methylphenidate HCl (UCB)

CII

THERAPEUTIC CLASS: Sympathomimetic amine

INDICATIONS: Treatment of attention deficit hyperactivity disorder (ADHD).

DOSAGE: *Pediatrics:* ≥6 yrs: Usual: 20mg qam before breakfast. Titrate: Increase weekly by 20mg depending on tolerability/efficacy. Max: 60mg/day. Reduce dose or discontinue if paradoxical aggravation of symptoms occur. D/C if no improvement after appropriate dose adjustments over 1 month. Swallow whole with liquids or open and sprinkle on 1 tbs applesauce followed by water. Do not crush, chew, or divide.

HOW SUPPLIED: Cap, Extended-Release: 10mg, 20mg, 30mg, 40mg, 50mg, 60mg

CONTRAINDICATIONS: Marked anxiety, tension, and agitation; glaucoma; motor tics, family history or diagnosis of Tourette's syndrome, severe HTN, angina pectoris, cardiac arrhythmias, heart failure, recent MI, hyperthyroidism or thyrotoxicosis; during or within 14 days of MAOI use.

WARNINGS/PRECAUTIONS: Monitor growth in children. Not for severe depression or fatigue. May exacerbate symptoms of behavior disturbance and thought disorder in psychotic patients. Caution when using stimulants to treat patients with comorbid bipolar disorder because of concern for possible induction of mixed/manic episode in such patients. Stimulants at usual doses can cause treatment emergent psychotic or manic symptoms (eg, hallucinations, delusional thinking, mania) in children and adolescents without prior history of psychotic illness. Aggressive behavior or hostility reported in clinical trials and postmarketing experience of some medications indicated for the treatment of ADHD. May lower seizure threshold, especially in known EEG abnormalities. Caution with HTN, conditions affected by BP or HR elevation, history of drug abuse or alcoholism. Monitor during withdrawal from abusive use. Visual disturbances may occur (rare). Monitor CBC, differential, and platelets with prolonged use. Avoid with serious structural cardiac abnormalities, cardiomyopathy, serious heart rhythm abnormalities, CAD, or other serious cardiac problems.

ADVERSE REACTIONS: Headache, abdominal pain, anorexia, insomnia.

INTERACTIONS: See Contraindications. Potentiates anticoagulants, anticonvulsants (eg, phenobarbital, phenytoin, primidone), TCAs, and SSRIs. Caution with α-agonist (eg, clonidine) and pressor agents.

PREGNANCY: Category C, caution in nursing.

MECHANISM OF ACTION: CNS stimulant; not established, thought to block reuptake of norepinephrine and dopamine into presynaptic neuron and increase release of these monoamines into extraneuronal space.

PHARMACOKINETICS: Absorption: (PO) Readily absorbed. Administration of variable doses resulted in different parameters. **Metabolism:** Via de-esterification. Metabolite: α-phenyl-piperidine acetic acid (ritalinic acid). **Elimination:** $T_{1/2}$=6.8 hrs.

NURSING CONSIDERATIONS

Assessment: Assess for agitation, glaucoma, tics, family history of Tourette's syndrome, cardiovascular conditions (eg, severe HTN, angina pectoris, cardiac abnormalities, arrhythmias, heart failure, recent MI), hyperthyroidism or thyrotoxicosis, bipolar illness, history of drug dependence or alcoholism.

Monitoring: Monitor for cardiac abnormalities, exacerbations of behavior disturbances and thought disorder, bipolar illness, aggression, seizures, and visual disturbances. Periodic monitoring of CBC, differential and platelet count, LFTs. Height and weight follow-up in children.

Patient Counseling: Inform about risks of therapy, appropriate use, and drug abuse/dependence. Must swallow tablet; never crush or chew. Take last dose before 6 pm to avoid insomnia.

Administration: Oral route. **Storage:** 25°C (77°F); excursions permitted to 15-30°C (59-86°F).

METADATE ER

methylphenidate HCl (UCB)

CII

THERAPEUTIC CLASS: Sympathomimetic amine

INDICATIONS: Treatment of attention deficit disorder and narcolepsy.

DOSAGE: *Adults:* (Immediate-Release Methylphenidate) 10-60mg/day given bid-tid 30-45 min ac. Take last dose before 6 pm if insomnia occurs. (Tab, Extended-Release) May use in place of immediate release tabs when the 8 hr dose corresponds to the titrated 8 hr immediate release dose. Swallow whole; do not chew or crush.

Pediatrics: ≥6 yrs: (Immediate-Release Methylphenidate) Initial: 5mg bid before breakfast and lunch. Titrate: Increase gradually by 5-10mg weekly. Max: 60mg/day. (Tab, Extended-Release) May use in place of immediate release tabs when the 8 hr dose corresponds to the titrated 8hr immediate release dose. Swallow whole; do not chew or crush. Reduce dose or discontinue if paradoxical aggravation of symptoms occur. Discontinue if no improvement after appropriate dose adjustment over 1 month.

HOW SUPPLIED: Tab, Extended-Release: 10mg, 20mg

CONTRAINDICATIONS: Marked anxiety, tension, and agitation; glaucoma; motor tics or family history or diagnosis of Tourette's syndrome; during or within 14 days of MAOI use.

WARNINGS/PRECAUTIONS: Caution with comorbid bipolar disorder. Monitor growth in children. Not for severe depression or fatigue. May exacerbate symptoms of behavior disturbance and thought disorder in psychotic children. Treatment emergent psychotic/manic symptoms in children and adolescents may occur. Aggressive behavior or hostility observed. May lower seizure threshold, especially in known EEG abnormalities. Caution with HTN, emotionally-unstable patients. Monitor during withdrawal. Visual disturbances may occur (rare). Monitor CBC, differential, and platelets with prolonged use. Periodically d/c to assess condition.

ADVERSE REACTIONS: Nervousness, insomnia, hypersensitivity reactions, anorexia, nausea, dizziness, palpitations, headache, dyskinesia, drowsiness, BP and pulse changes, tachycardia, angina, arrhythmia, abdominal pain.

INTERACTIONS: See Contraindications. May decrease hypotensive effect of guanethidine. Caution with pressor agents. Potentiates anticoagulants, anticonvulsants (eg, phenobarbital, phenytoin, primidone), phenylbutazone, TCAs (eg, imipramine, clomipramine, desipramine).

PREGNANCY: Safety in pregnancy and nursing not known.

MECHANISM OF ACTION: Not established, suspected to have sympathomimetic activity in the brain stem arousal system and cortex.

PHARMACOKINETICS: Absorption: Slowly absorbed. T_{max}=1.3-8.2 hrs (sustained-release tab), 0.3-4.4 hrs (immediate release tab).

NURSING CONSIDERATIONS

Assessment: Assess for agitation, hereditary problems of galactose intolerance, Lapp lactase deficiency or glucose-galactose malabsorption, glaucoma, tics, family history of Tourette's syndrome, cardiovascular conditions (severe HTN, angina pectoris, cardiac arrhythmias, heart failure, recent MI), hyperthyroidism or thyrotoxicosis, bipolar illness, history of drug dependence or alcoholism.

Monitoring: Monitor for cardiac abnormalities, exacerbations of behavior disturbances and thought disorder, bipolar illness, aggression, seizures, and visual disturbances. Periodic monitoring of CBC, differential and platelet count, LFTs. Height and weight follow-up in children.

Patient Counseling: Inform about potential risks of therapy, appropriate use, drug dependence/abuse. Must swallow, never crush or chew. Take last dose before 6 pm to avoid insomnia.

Administration: Administer PO, preferably 30-45 min before meals. **Storage:** 20-25°C (77°F); excursions permitted to 15-30°C (59-86°F). Keep tightly closed. Protect from moisture.

METAGLIP RX

metformin HCl - glipizide (Bristol-Myers Squibb)

THERAPEUTIC CLASS: Sulfonylurea/biguanide

INDICATIONS: Adjunct to diet and exercise to improve glycemic control in adults with type 2 diabetes mellitus.

DOSAGE: *Adults:* Inadequate Glycemic Control on Diet/Exercise Alone: Initial: 2.5mg-250mg qd. If FBG 280-320mg/dL, give 2.5mg-500mg bid. Titrate: Increase by 1 tab/day every 2 weeks. Max: 10mg-1g/day or 10mg-2g/day given in divided doses. Inadequate Glycemic Control on Sulfonylurea or Metformin: Initial: 2.5mg-500mg or 5mg-500mg bid (with morning and evening meals). Starting dose should not exceed daily dose of metformin or glipizide already being taken. Titrate: Increase by no more than 5mg-500mg/day. Max: 20mg-2g/day. Elderly/Debilitated/Malnourished: Do not titrate to max dose. Take with meals.

HOW SUPPLIED: Tab: (Glipizide-Metformin) 2.5mg-250mg, 2.5mg-500mg, 5mg-500mg

CONTRAINDICATIONS: Renal disease/dysfunction (SrCr ≥1.5mg/dL [males], ≥1.4mg/dL [females], abnormal CrCl), metabolic acidosis, diabetic ketoacidosis. D/C temporarily (48 hrs) for radiologic studies with intravascular iodinated contrast materials.

WARNINGS/PRECAUTIONS: Lactic acidosis reported (rare); increased risk with renal dysfunction, increased age, DM, CHF, and other conditions with risk of hypoperfusion and hypoxemia. Avoid use in patients ≥80 yrs unless renal function is normal. Increased risk of cardiovascular mortality. Increased risk of hypoglycemia in elderly, debilitated/malnourished, adrenal or pituitary insufficiency, or alcohol intoxication. D/C in hypoxic states (eg, CHF, shock, acute MI) and prior to surgical procedures (due to restricted food intake). Avoid in renal/hepatic impairment. May decrease serum vitamin B_{12} levels. Impaired renal and/or hepatic function may slow glipizide excretion. Withhold treatment with any condition associated with dehydration or sepsis. Monitor renal function.

ADVERSE REACTIONS: Upper respiratory tract infection, HTN, headache, diarrhea, dizziness, musculoskeletal pain, nausea, vomiting, abdominal pain.

INTERACTIONS: Furosemide, nifedipine, cimetidine and cationic drugs (eg, digoxin, amiloride, procainamide, quinidine, quinine, ranitidine, trimethoprim, vancomycin, triamterene, morphine) may increase metformin levels. Potentiated hypoglycemia with alcohol, NSAIDs, some azoles, and other highly protein bound drugs, salicylates, sulfonamides, chloramphenicol, probenecid, coumarins, MAOIs, and β-blockers. Severe hypoglycemia reported with concomitant oral miconazole. Thiazides and other diuretics, corticosteroids, phenothiazines, thyroid products, estrogens, oral contraceptives, phenytoin, nicotinic acid, sympathomimetics, CCBs, and isoniazid may cause hyperglycemia. Alcohol potentiates effect of metformin on lactate metabolism. May decrease furosemide levels.

PREGNANCY: Category C, not for use in pregnancy or nursing.

MECHANISM OF ACTION: Sulfonylurea; lowers blood glucose acutely by stimulating release of insulin from the pancreas. Biguanide; decreases hepatic glucose production and intestinal absorption of glucose and improves insulin sensitivity by increasing peripheral glucose uptake.

PHARMACOKINETICS: Absorption: Glipizide: Rapid, complete, T_{max}=1-3 hrs. Metformin: absolute bioavailability (50-60%). **Distribution:** Glipizide: plasma protein binding (98%); V_d=11L (IV). Metformin: V_d=654L. **Metabolism:** Glipizide:

M

liver (extensive) **Elimination:** Glipizide: urine; $T_{1/2}$=2-4 hrs. Metformin: renal excretion (approximately 90%); $T_{1/2}$=6.2hrs (plasma), 17.6 hrs (blood).

NURSING CONSIDERATIONS

Assessment: Assess FPG, HbA_{1c}, renal function, LFTs, CBC. Assess for CHF, septicemia, acute or chronic metabolic acidosis, adrenal or pituitary insufficiency, alcoholism, pregnancy status, other medical/surgical conditions, and possible drug interactions.

Monitoring: Monitor for hypoglycemia, lactic acidosis, prerenal azotemia, CHF, CVD. Monitor FPG, HbA_{1c}, renal function, LFTs, CBC.

Patient Counseling: Inform drug is adjunct to diet and exercise programs for type 2 diabetes. Temporarily d/c therapy prior to intravascular radiocontrast study or surgical procedure. Advise that excessive alcohol intake increases risk of hypoglycemia. Regular follow-ups needed; take as prescribed with meals. Counsel to report unexplained hyperventilation, myalgia, malaise, NV, and somnolence. Not recommended for use during pregnancy. Counsel about potential adverse effects and advise to seek medical attention if any develop.

Administration: Oral route. **Storage:** 20-25°C (68-77°F); excursions permitted to 15-30°C (59-86°F).

METHADOSE

CII

methadone HCl (Mallinckrodt)

Deaths, cardiac and respiratory, reported during initiation and conversion from other other opioid agonists. Respiratory depression and QT prolongation observed. Only certified/approved opioid treatment programs can dispense oral methadone for treatment of narcotic addiction. Use as analgesic should be initiated only if benefits outweigh risks.

M

THERAPEUTIC CLASS: Opioid analgesic

INDICATIONS: Detoxification and maintenance treatment of narcotic addiction (heroin or other morphine-like drugs) in conjunction with appropriate social and medical services.

DOSAGE: *Adults:* Detoxification: Initial/Induction: 20-30mg/day. Give 5-10mg 2-4 hrs later if needed. Max: 40mg on first day. Adjust dose to control withdrawl symptoms over 1st week. Stabilize for 2-3 days, then may decrease every 1-2 days depending on symptoms. Maintenance: Titrate to a dose at which symptoms prevented for 24 hrs. Usual: 80-120mg/day. Pain in Opioid Non-Tolerant: Usual: 2.5-10mg q8-12h, slowly titrated to effect. Conversion From Parenteral: Initial: Use a 1:2 dose ratio parenteral to oral. Switching From Other Chronic Opioids: Use caution; see PI for dosing details.

HOW SUPPLIED: Oral Concentrate: 10mg/mL; Tab: 5mg, 10mg, 40mg; Tab, Dispersible: 40mg

CONTRAINDICATIONS: Respiratory depression. Acute bronchial asthma or hypercarbia. Paralytic ileus.

WARNINGS/PRECAUTIONS: Do not inject agent. Extreme caution if use narcotic antagonists in patients physically dependent on narcotics. Can cause respiratory depression and elevate CSF pressure. Caution with head injuries, acute asthma attacks, COPD, cor pulmonale, decreased respiratory reserve, pre-existing respiratory depression, hypoxia, or hypercapnia. Reduce initial dose in elderly, debilitated, severe hepatic or renal impairment, hypothyroidism, Addison's disease, prostatic hypertrophy, or urethral stricture. Risk of tolerance, dependence, and abuse may occur. Impairs physical and mental abilities. Ineffective in relieving anxiety. May mask symptoms of acute abdominal conditions. May produce hypotension.

ADVERSE REACTIONS: Lightheadedness, dizziness, sedation, sweating, nausea, vomiting.

INTERACTIONS: Concurrent µ-agonists (eg, pentazocine, nalaxone, buprenorphine), or St. John's wort may precipitate withdrawal. Decreased levels with CYP3A4 inducers (eg, rifampin). Increased levels with CYP3A4 inhibitors (eg, ketoconazole). Caution and reduce dose with CNS depressants (eg, tranquilizers, sedative-hypnotics, phenothiazines, TCAs, alcohol). MAOIs may cause severe reactions.

PREGNANCY: Category C, not for use in nursing.

MECHANISM OF ACTION: Synthetic opioid analgesic; μ-agonist. Produces actions similiar to morphine; acts on CNS and organs composed of smooth muscle. May also act as N-methyl-D-aspartate (NMDA) receptor antagonist.

PHARMACOKINETICS: Absorption: Bioavailability (36-100%); C_{max}=124-1255ng/mL; T_{max}=1-7.5 hrs. **Distribution:** V_d=1-8 L/kg; bound to α_1-acid glycoprotein (85-90%); secreted in saliva, breast milk, amniotic fluid, and umbilical cord plasma. **Metabolism:** Hepatic N-demethylation; CYP3A4, 2B6, 2C19 (major); 2C9, 2D6 (minor)**. Elimination**: Urine, feces; $T_{1/2}$=7-59 hrs.

NURSING CONSIDERATIONS

Assessment: Assess for respiratory depression, acute bronchial asthma or hypercarbia, COPD, myxedema, kyphoscoliosis, CNS depression or coma, paralytic ileus, history of cardiac conduction abnormalities, hypokalemia, hypomagnesemia, head injury or other intracranial lesions, increased ICP, acute abdominal conditions, volume depletion, hepatic/renal impairment, presence of debilitation (eg, elderly), hypothyroidism, Addison's disease, prostatic hypertrophy or urethral stricture, pregnancy/nursing status, and possible drug interactions.

Monitoring: Monitor for signs/symptoms of respiratory depression, QT prolongation and arrhythmias (eg, torsade de pointes), misuse or abuse of medication, physical dependence and tolerance, elevations in CSF pressure, and hypotension.

Patient Counseling: Inform that medication may impair mental/physical abilities; use caution when performing hazardous tasks (eg, operating machinery/driving). Advise to avoid using alcohol and other CNS depressants. Instruct to seek immediate medical care if develop signs/symptoms of arrhythmia (eg, palpitations, dizziness, syncope) or if develop difficulty in breathing; orthostatic hypotension may occur. Instruct to keep out of reach of children. Advise to avoid abrupt withdrawal; taper dosing. Inform patients treated for opioid dependence that d/c may lead to relapse of illicit drug use. Educate on potential for abuse and to protect from theft.

Administration: Oral route. Not for injection. Initial dose should be carefully titrated. **Storage:** 20-25°C (68-77°F); dispense in tight container, protected from light.

M

METHOTREXATE — RX

methotrexate (Various)

Should only be used by physicians whose knowledge and experience includes the use of antimetabolite therapy. Only for life-threatening neoplastic diseases, or with severe, recalcitrant, disabling disease not adequately responsive to other forms of therapy. Fetal death/congenital anomalies reported. Elimination reduced with impaired renal function, ascites, or pleural effusions; monitor carefully. Severe, sometimes fatal, bone marrow suppression and GI toxicity reported with concomitant NSAIDs. May cause hepatotoxicity, fibrosis, and cirrhosis (usually after prolonged use). Lung disease, malignant melanomas, and potentially fatal opportunistic infections may occur. Interrupt therapy if diarrhea or ulcerative colitis occur. May induce tumor lysis syndrome. Severe, occasionally fatal, skin reactions reported. Concomitant radiotherapy may increase risk of soft tissue necrosis and osteonecrosis.

OTHER BRAND NAMES: Rheumatrex (Stada)

THERAPEUTIC CLASS: Dihydrofolic acid reductase inhibitor

INDICATIONS: (Inj/PO) Treatment of neoplastic diseases (eg, acute lymphocytic leukemia, gestational choriocarcinoma, chorioadenoma destruens, hydatidiform mole, breast cancer, epidermoid cancer of the head and neck, advanced mycosis fungoides, lung cancer, advanced stage non-Hodgkin's lymphomas). Prophylaxis and treatment of meningeal leukemia, and maintenance with other chemotherapeutics. For prolonging relapse-free survival in non-metastatic osteosarcoma followed by leucovorin. Symptomatic control of severe, recalcitrant, disabling psoriasis. (PO) Management of rheumatoid arthritis (RA) or polyarticular-course juvenile rheumatoid arthritis (JRA) unresponsive to other therapies.

DOSAGE: *Adults:* Choriocarcinoma/Trophoblastic Disease: 15-30mg qd PO/IM for 5 days. May repeat 3-5 times as required with rest period of ≥1 week. Leukemia: Induction: 3.3mg/m² with prednisone 60mg/m² qd. Remission Maintenance: 15mg/m² PO/IM twice weekly or 2.5mg/kg IV every 14 days. Burkitt's Tumor: Stages I-II: 10-25mg/day PO for 4-8 days. Administer several courses with rest periods of 7-10 days in between. Lymphosarcoma: Stage III: 0.625-2.5mg/kg/day with other antitumor agents. Mycosis Fungoides: 5-50mg once weekly. If poor response, give 15-37.5mg twice weekly. Adjust dose based on response and hematologic monitoring. Osteosarcoma: Initial: 12g/m² IV, increase to 15g/m² if peak serum levels of 1000 micromolar not reached at end of infusion. Meningeal Leukemia: Dilute preservative free MTX to 1mg/mL. Give 12mg intrathecally at 2-5 day intervals. Psoriasis: Initial: 10-25mg PO/IM/IV weekly until response or use divided oral dose schedule, 2.5mg at 12 hr intervals for 3 doses. Titrate: Increase gradually until optimal response. Maint: Reduce to lowest effective dose. Max: 30mg/week. Rheumatoid Arthritis: Initial: 7.5mg PO once weekly, or 2.5mg q12h for 3 doses given as a course once weekly. Titrate: Gradual increase. Max: 20mg weekly. After response, reduce dose to lowest effective amount of drug.
Pediatrics: Meningeal Leukemia: Dilute preservative free MTX to 1mg/mL. <1 yr: 6mg. 1 yr: 8mg. 2 yrs: 10mg. ≥3yrs: 12mg. Give intrathecally at 2-5 day intervals. JRA: 2-16 yrs: Initial: 10mg/m² once weekly. Adjust dose gradually to achieve optimal response.

HOW SUPPLIED: Inj: (Generic) (Methotrexate Sodium) 25mg/mL, 1g; Tab: (Generic) (Methotrexate) 2.5mg*; Tab: (Rheumatrex) (Methotrexate) 2.5mg* [Dose Pack 15mg, 4 x 6 tabs; 12.5mg, 4 x 5 tabs; 10mg, 4 x 4 tabs; 7.5mg, 4 x 3 tabs; 5mg, 4 x 2 tabs] *scored

CONTRAINDICATIONS: Pregnant women with psoriasis or RA (should be used in treatment of pregnant women with neoplastic diseases only when potential benefit outweighs risk), nursing mothers. Psoriasis or RA patients with alcoholism, alcoholic liver disease, chronic liver disease, immunodeficiency syndromes, and pre-existing blood dyscrasias (eg, bone marrow hypoplasia, leukopenia, thrombocytopenia, significant anemia).

WARNINGS/PRECAUTIONS: Monitor closely; toxicity may be related to dose and frequency of administration. When reactions do occur, doses should be reduced or discontinued and corrective measures should be taken. Avoid pregnancy if either partner is receiving therapy. Avoid intrathecal administration or high-dose therapy. Injection contains benzyl alcohol; avoid use in neonates (<1 month), may cause gasping syndrome.

ADVERSE REACTIONS: Ulcerative stomatitis, leukopenia, nausea, abdominal distress, malaise, fatigue, chills, fever, dizziness, decreased resistance to infection, anemia, photosensitivity, rash, pruritus, hepatotoxicity.

INTERACTIONS: See Black Box Warning. Avoid NSAIDs with high doses. Caution with nephrotoxic agents (eg, cisplatin), NSAIDs, probenecid, and highly protein bound drugs (eg, sulfonamides, phenytoin, phenylbutazone, salicylates). Oral antibiotics (eg, tetracycline, chloramphenicol) may decrease absorption or interfere with enterohepatic circulation. Penicillins may decrease clearance. Closely monitor with hepatotoxins (eg, azathioprine, retinoids, sulfasalazine). Folic acid may decrease response to MTX. TMP/SMZ may increase bone marrow suppression. May decrease theophylline clearance.

PREGNANCY: Category X, contraindicated in nursing.

MECHANISM OF ACTION: Dihydrofolic acid reductase inhibitor; interferes with DNA synthesis, repair, and cellular replication. MOA in rheumatoid arthritis not established; may affect immune function.

PHARMACOKINETICS: Absorption: (PO, Healthy) T_{max}=1-2 hrs. (IM) T_{max}=30-60 min. Oral administration resulted in different parameters according to disease state and dosing; refer to PI for further information. **Distribution:** (IV, Initial) V_d=0.18L/kg; (Steady state) V_d=0.4-0.8L/kg; plasma protein binding (50%); found in breast milk. **Metabolism:** Hepatic and intracellular; 7-hydroxymethotrexate (metabolite). **Elimination:** Renal (primary route), bile (≤10%).

(Psoriasis, rheumatoid arthritis, low-dose chemotherapy at <30mg/m²) $T_{1/2}$=3-10 hrs; (High dose) $T_{1/2}$=8-15 hrs.

NURSING CONSIDERATIONS

Assessment: Assess pregnancy/nursing status, alcoholism, alcoholic or other chronic liver disease, immunodeficiency, active infection, blood dyscrasias (eg, bone marrow hypoplasia, leukopenia, thrombocytopenia), impaired renal function, ascites, pleural effusions, debility, and possible drug interactions. Obtain baseline CBC with differential and platelet counts, hepatic enzymes, renal function tests, and chest X-ray.

Monitoring: Monitor for signs/symptoms of bone marrow suppression, hematological effects, GI toxicity (eg, vomiting, diarrhea, stomatitis), hepatotoxicity, fibrosis, cirrhosis, lung disease (eg, dry, nonproductive cough), malignant lymphomas, opportunistic infections, neurotoxicity (eg, seizures, leukoencephalopathy), nephrotoxicity, and skin reactions (eg, toxic epidermal necrolysis, Stevens-Johnson syndrome). Monitor for tumor lysis syndrome in patients with rapidly growing tumors. If given concomitantly with radiotherapy, monitor for soft-tissue necrosis and osteonecrosis. For psoriasis treatment, monitor CBC with differential and platelet counts monthly; renal/liver functions every 1-2 months. Perform more frequent monitoring of lab parameters during antineoplastic therapy. If drug-induced lung disease is suspected, perform pulmonary function tests. For psoriatic patients on long-term therapy, perform periodic liver biopsies.

Patient Counseling: Counsel about risks/benefits of therapy, effects on reproduction in both males and females. Advise about early signs/symptoms of toxicity; contact physician immediately. Periodic laboratory tests necessary during therapy. If taking oral dose for rheumatoid arthritis or psoriasis, dose is taken weekly.

Administration: Oral, IM, IV, intra-arterial, or intrathecal route. **Storage:** Tablet: 20-25°C (68-77°F); excursions permitted to 15-30°C (59-86°F), protect from light. Injection: 15-30°C (59-86°F), protect from light.

METHYLDOPA — RX

methyldopa (Various)

THERAPEUTIC CLASS: Central alpha-adrenergic agonist

INDICATIONS: Treatment of hypertension.

DOSAGE: *Adults:* Initial: 250mg bid-tid for 48 hrs. Adjust dose at intervals of not less than 2 days. Maint: 500mg-2g/day given bid-qid. Max: 3g/day. Concomitant Antihypertensives (other than thiazides): Initial: Limit to 500mg/day. Renal Impairment: May respond to lower doses.
Pediatrics: Initial: 10mg/kg/day given bid-qid. Max: 65mg/kg/day or 3g/day, whichever is less.

HOW SUPPLIED: Tab: 125mg, 250mg, 500mg

CONTRAINDICATIONS: Active hepatic disease, history of methyldopa associated liver disorder, concomitant MAOIs.

WARNINGS/PRECAUTIONS: Positive Coombs' test, hemolytic anemia, and liver disorders may occur. Fever reported within the first 3 weeks of therapy. HTN has recurred after dialysis. Caution with liver disease or dysfunction. D/C if signs of heart failure, or involuntary choreoathetotic movements develop. Edema and wt gain reported. Blood count, Coombs' test and LFTs prior to therapy and periodically thereafter.

ADVERSE REACTIONS: Sedation, headache, asthenia, edema/wt gain, hepatic disorders, vomiting, diarrhea, nausea, sore or "black" tongue, blood dyscrasias, BUN increase, gynecomastia, impotence.

INTERACTIONS: See Contraindications. May potentiate other antihypertensives. Anesthetics may need dose reduction. Monitor for lithium toxicity. Ferrous sulfate and ferrous gluconate may decrease bioavailability; avoid coadministration.

PREGNANCY: Category B, caution in nursing.

MECHANISM OF ACTION: Aromatic-aminoacid decarboxylase inhibitor; not established, antihypertensive effect probably due to metabolism to α-methylnorepinephrine, which lowers arterial pressure by stimulation of central inhibitory α-adrenergic receptors, false neurotransmission, and reduction of plasma renin activity.

PHARMACOKINETICS: Distribution: Crosses placenta, found in breast milk. **Metabolism:** Extensive. **Elimination:** Urine; $T_{1/2}$=105 min.

NURSING CONSIDERATIONS

Assessment: Assess for active hepatic disease (eg, acute hepatitis, active cirrhosis), other liver disorders, pheochromocytoma, severe bilateral cerebrovascular disease, and possible drug interactions. Obtain baseline blood count (Hct, Hgb, RBC), direct Coombs' test, and LFTs.

Monitoring: Monitor LFTs for 1st 6-12 weeks of therapy or if unexplained fever occurs; direct Coombs' test at 6 and 12 months after therapy, and blood count periodically. Monitor for signs/symptoms of hemolytic anemia, progressive edema, heart failure, hypersensitivity reactions, and hepatic dysfunction.

Patient Counseling: Advise to seek medical attention if symptoms of hemolytic anemia, progressive edema, heart failure, hypersensitivity reactions, or hepatic dysfunction occurs.

Administration: Oral route. **Storage:** 20-25°C (68-77°F). Protect from light.

METHYLDOPA/HCTZ RX

methyldopa - hydrochlorothiazide (Various)

Not for initial therapy of HTN.

M

THERAPEUTIC CLASS: Central alpha-adrenergic agonist/thiazide diuretic

INDICATIONS: Treatment of HTN. Not for initial treatment.

DOSAGE: *Adults:* Initial: 250mg-15mg tab bid-tid, 250mg-25mg tab bid, or 500mg-30mg qd. Max: 50mg HCTZ/day or 3g methyldopa/day.

HOW SUPPLIED: Tab: (HCTZ-Methyldopa) 15mg-250mg, 25mg-250mg

CONTRAINDICATIONS: Active hepatic disease, anuria, sulfonamide allergy, concomitant MAOIs, history of methyldopa associated liver disorder.

WARNINGS/PRECAUTIONS: Positive Coombs' test, hemolytic anemia, liver disorders, sensitivity reactions, hypokalemia, hyperuricemia, hyperglycemia, hypomagnesemia, hypercalcemia may occur. Fever reported within first 3 weeks of therapy. HTN has recurred after dialysis. Caution with liver disease or dysfunction, severe renal disease. D/C if signs of heart failure, progressive renal dysfunction, or involuntary choreoathetotic movements develop. Edema and wt gain reported. Blood count, Coombs' test, and LFTs before therapy and periodically thereafter. Monitor electrolytes. May exacerbate or activate SLE. May increase cholesterol and TG levels. Enhanced effects in postsympathectomy patient.

ADVERSE REACTIONS: Weakness, asthenia, headache, pancreatitis, diarrhea, NV, constipation, blood dyscrasias, rash, electrolyte imbalance, renal failure, impotence, vertigo.

INTERACTIONS: See Contraindications. Potentiates orthostatic hypotension with alcohol, barbiturates, narcotics. Lithium toxicity. Adjust antidiabetic drugs. NSAIDs decrease diuretic effects. Reduce dose of anesthetics. Ferrous sulfate and ferrous gluçonate may decrease bioavailability; avoid coadministration. May potentiate nondepolarizing skeletal muscle relaxants, antihypertensives. May decrease response to pressor amines. Corticosteroids, ACTH intensify electrolyte depletion. Impaired absorption with cholestyramine, colestipol.

PREGNANCY: Category C, not for use in nursing.

MECHANISM OF ACTION: Methyldopa: Central α-adrenergic agonist. Aromatic-amino-acid decarboxylase inhibitor; lowers arterial pressure by stimulating central inhibitory α-adrenergic receptor, false neurotransmission, and/or reduction of plasma renin activity. HCTZ: Thiazide diuretic; affects renal tubular mechanism of electrolyte reabsorption, directly increasing excretion of sodium salt and chloride.

PHARMACOKINETICS: Distribution: Methyldopa: Crosses placental barrier, appears in breast milk and cord blood. HCTZ: Crosses placenta, excreted in breast milk. **Metabolism:** Methyldopa: Extensive. **Elimination:** Methyldopa: Urine (70%); $T_{1/2}$=105 min; HCTZ: Urine (61% unchanged); $T_{1/2}$=5.6-14.8 hrs.

NURSING CONSIDERATIONS

Assessment: Assess LFTs, renal functions, CBC with platelet and differential count, Coombs' test, PT time, serum electrolytes. Assess for sulfite allergy, SLE, pregnancy status, bronchial asthma, and possible drug interactions.

Monitoring: Monitor BP, Hct, serum electrolytes, LFTs, bilirubin, PT time, Coombs' test, CBC with differential, BUN, lipid profile. Monitor for arrhythmias, pancreatitis, aggravation of angina, CHF, orthostatic hypotension, hyperprolactinemia, hyperuricemia, hyperglycemia, renal function, bone marrow depression, hypersensitivity (myocarditis, pericarditis, vasculitis), toxic epidermal necrolysis, xanthopsia.

Patient Counseling: Instruct that fixed combination drug not indicated for initial therapy of HTN and patient re-evaluation required as conditions warrant. Advise to contact physician if any adverse events occur.

Administration: Oral route. **Storage:** 15-30°C (59-86°F). Protect from light, moisture, freezing -20°C (-4°F). Keep container tightly closed.

METHYLIN

CII

methylphenidate HCl (Mallinckrodt)

M

OTHER BRAND NAMES: Methylin ER (Mallinckrodt)

THERAPEUTIC CLASS: Sympathomimetic amine

INDICATIONS: Treatment of attention deficit disorder and narcolepsy.

DOSAGE: *Adults:* (Sol/Tab/Tab, Chewable) 10-60mg/day given bid-tid 30-45 min ac. Take last dose before 6 pm if insomnia occurs. (Tab, Extended-Release) May use in place of immediate release tabs when 8 hr dose corresponds to titrated 8 hr immediate release dose. Swallow whole; do not chew or crush.

Pediatrics: ≥6 yrs: (Sol/Tab/Tab, Chewable) Initial: 5mg bid before breakfast and lunch. Titrate: Increase gradually by 5-10mg weekly. Max: 60mg/day. (Tab, Extended-Release) May be use in place of immediate release tabs when 8 hr dose corresponds to titrated 8 hr immediate release dose. Swallow whole; do not chew or crush. Reduce dose or d/c if paradoxical aggravation of symptoms occur. D/C if no improvement after appropriate dose adjustment over 1 month.

HOW SUPPLIED: Sol: 5mg/5mL [500mL], 10mg/5mL [500mL]; Tab: 5mg, 10mg, 20mg; Tab, Chewable: 2.5mg, 5mg, 10mg; Tab, Extended-Release: 10mg, 20mg

CONTRAINDICATIONS: Marked anxiety, tension, and agitation; glaucoma; motor tics or family history or diagnosis of Tourette's syndrome; during or within 14 days of MAOI use.

WARNINGS/PRECAUTIONS: Monitor growth in children. Not for severe depression or fatigue. May exacerbate symptoms of behavior disturbance or thought disorder in psychotic children. Caution when using stimulants to treat patients with comorbid bipolar disorder because of concern for possible induction of mixed/manic episode in such patients. Stimulants at usual doses can cause treatment emergent psychotic or manic symptoms (hallucinations, delusional thinking, mania) in children and adolescents without prior history of psychotic illness. Aggressive behavior or hostility has been reported in clinical trials and the postmarketing experience of some medications indicated for the treatment of ADHD. May lower seizure threshold, especially in known EEG abnormalities. Caution with HTN, heart failure, recent MI, ventricular arrhythmia, or emotionally-unstable patients. Monitor during withdrawal. Visual disturbances may occur (rare). Monitor CBC, differential, and platelets with prolonged use. Periodically d/c to assess condition. Avoid with serious structural cardiac abnormalities, cardiomyopathy, serious heart rhythm abnormalities, CAD, or other serious cardiac problems. Caution in emotionally unstable patients with history of drug dependence or alcoholism.

ADVERSE REACTIONS: Nervousness, insomnia, hypersensitivity reactions, anorexia, nausea, dizziness, palpitations, headache, dyskinesia, drowsiness, BP and pulse changes, tachycardia, angina, arrhythmia, abdominal pain.

INTERACTIONS: May decrease hypotensive effect of guanethidine. Caution with pressor agents. Avoid during or within 14 days of MAOI use. Potentiates anticoagulants, anticonvulsants (phenobarbital, diphenylhydantoin, primidone), phenylbutazone, TCAs (imipramine, clomipramine, desipramine). Caution with α_2-agonists (eg, clonidine); serious adverse reactions reported with concurrent use.

PREGNANCY: Category C, caution in nursing.

MECHANISM OF ACTION: CNS stimulant; activates the brain-stem arousal system and cortex to produce its stimulant effect. Blocks the reuptake of norepinephrine and dopamine into the presynaptic neuron and increases release of monoamines into extraneuronal space.

PHARMACOKINETICS: Absorption: (20mg, Sol) C_{max}=9ng/mL, T_{max}=1-2 hrs. **Metabolism:** Deesterification to α-phenyl-piperidine acetic acid. **Elimination:** Urine (90%), $T_{1/2}$=2.7 hrs (sol), 3 hrs (chewable).

NURSING CONSIDERATIONS

Assessment: Assess for agitation, glaucoma, tics, family history of Tourette's syndrome, cardiovascular conditions (eg, severe HTN, angina pectoris, cardiac arrhythmias, heart failure, recent MI), hyperthyroidism or thyrotoxicosis, bipolar illness, history of drug dependence or alcoholism.

Monitoring: Monitor for cardiac abnormalities, exacerbations of behavior disturbances and thought disorders, bipolar illness, aggression, seizures, and visual disturbances. Periodic monitoring of CBC, differential and platelet count, and LFTs. Height and weight follow-up in children.

Patient Counseling: Inform about risks of treatment, its appropriate use, drug abuse/dependence. Inform to take last dose before 6pm to avoid insomnia.

Administration: Oral route. **Storage:** 20-25°C (68-77°F)

METOCLOPRAMIDE RX

metoclopramide HCl (Various)

OTHER BRAND NAMES: Reglan Injection (Baxter) - Reglan (Schwarz)

THERAPEUTIC CLASS: Dopamine antagonist/prokinetic

INDICATIONS: (PO) Symptomatic treatment of gastroesophageal reflux in patients who fail to respond to conventional therapy. (Inj, PO) Symptomatic relief of diabetic gastroparesis. (Inj) Prevention of post-op or chemo-induced nausea/vomiting. Diagnostic aid during radiological examination and facilitates intubation of small intestine.

DOSAGE: *Adults:* GERD: PO: 10-15mg qid 30 min ac and hs. Elderly: 5 mg qid. Max: 12 weeks of therapy. Intermittent Symptoms: Up to 20mg as single dose prior to provoking situation. Gastroparesis: 10mg PO 30 min ac and hs for 2-8 weeks. Severe Gastroparesis: May give same doses IV/IM for up to 10 days if needed. Antiemetic: (Post-op) 10-20mg IM near end of surgery. (Chemotherapy-Induced) 1-2mg/kg 30 min before chemotherapy then q2h for 2 doses, then q3h for 3 doses. Give 2mg/kg for highly emetogenic drugs for initial 2 doses. Small Bowel Intubation/Radiological Exam: 10mg IV as single dose. CrCl <40mL/min: 50% of normal dose.
Pediatrics: Small Bowel Intubation: 6-14 yrs: 2.5-5mg IV single dose. <6 yrs: 0.1mg/kg IV single dose. CrCl <40mL/min: 50% of normal dose.

HOW SUPPLIED: Inj: 5mg/mL; Syr: 5mg/5mL; Tab: 5mg, 10mg* *scored

CONTRAINDICATIONS: Where GI mobility stimulation is dangerous (eg, perforation, obstruction, hemorrhage), pheochromocytoma, seizure disorder, concomitant drugs that cause EPS effects.

WARNINGS/PRECAUTIONS: Caution with HTN, Parkinson's disease, depression. EPS, tardive dyskinesia, Parkinsonian-like symptoms, neuroleptic malignant syndrome reported. Administer IV injection slowly. Risk of developing fluid retention and volume overload especially with cirrhosis or CHF; d/c if these occur. May increase pressure of suture lines.

ADVERSE REACTIONS: Restlessness, drowsiness, fatigue, EPS effects (acute dystonic reactions), galactorrhea, hyperprolactinemia, hypotension, arrhythmia, diarrhea, dizziness, urinary frequency.

INTERACTIONS: See Contraindications. May decrease gastric absorption of drugs (eg, digoxin) and increase intestinal absorption of drugs (eg, APAP, tetracycline, levodopa, ethanol, and cyclosporine). Additive sedation with alcohol, hypnotics, narcotics, or tranquilizers. Caution with MAOIs. Antagonized by anticholinergics, narcotics. Insulin dose or timing of dose may need adjustment to prevent hypoglycemia.

PREGNANCY: Category B, caution with nursing.

MECHANISM OF ACTION: Dopamine antagonist/promotility agent; not established, stimulates motility of upper GI tract, increases tone of gastric contractions, relaxes pyloric sphincter and duodenal bulb, increases peristalsis of duodenum and jejunum resulting in increased gastric emptying and intestinal transit, increases resting tone of LES, antagonizes central and peripheral dopamine receptors blocking stimulation of CTZ.

PHARMACOKINETICS: Absorption: Rapid; absolute bioavailability (80%). (Peds) C_{max} at tenth dose=56.8mcg/L, T_{max}=2.5 hrs. (Adults) T_{max}=1-2 hrs. **Distribution:** Plasma protein binding (30%); (adults)V_d=3.5L/kg; (peds) V_d =4.4L/kg. **Elimination:** Urine; (adults) $T_{1/2}$=5-6 hrs, (peds) $T_{1/2}$=4.1 hrs.

M

NURSING CONSIDERATIONS

Assessment: Assess for GI hemorrhage, mechanical obstruction or perforation, CHF, cirrhosis, pheochromocytoma, depression, Parkinson's disease, TD, epilepsy, and possible drug interactions.

Monitoring: Monitor for signs/symptoms of depression, EPS, NMS, TD, HTN, fluid retention, volume overload, exacerbation of Parkinson's, and hypersensitivity reactions.

Patient Counseling: Caution may impair physical/mental abilities. Seek medical attention if symptoms of depression, EPS (involuntary movements of limbs, facial grimacing, torticollis), TD, NMS (hyperthermia, muscle rigidity, altered consciousness), HTN, fluid retention, volume overload, or hypersensitivity reactions occur.

Administration: Oral, IV/IM route. Refer to PI for IV admixture compatibilities. **Storage:** Tab, Inj, Sol: 20-25°C (68-77°F). Inj: Protect from light. Diluted; stable for 24 hrs. Sol: Protect from freezing.

METROGEL — RX

metronidazole (Galderma)

OTHER BRAND NAMES: MetroLotion (Galderma) - MetroCream (Galderma)

THERAPEUTIC CLASS: Imidazole antibiotic

INDICATIONS: Treatment of inflammatory papules and pustules of rosacea.

DOSAGE: *Adults:* (Cre, Gel 0.75%, Lot) Wash affected area(s) then apply bid, am and pm. (Gel 1%) Wash affected area(s) then apply qd.

HOW SUPPLIED: Cre: 0.75% [45g]; Gel: 0.75%, 1% [45g]; Lot: 0.75% [59mL]

WARNINGS/PRECAUTIONS: Avoid eye contact. Decrease frequency or d/c if skin irritation occurs. Caution with blood dyscrasias.

ADVERSE REACTIONS: Burning, skin irritation, dryness, redness, metallic taste, tingling/numbness of extremities, nausea.

INTERACTIONS: Oral metronidazole may potentiate warfarin; unknown effect with topical formulation.

PREGNANCY: Category B, not for use in nursing.

MECHANISM OF ACTION: Imidazole antibiotic; not established. Suspected to have an anti-inflammatory effect.

PHARMACOKINETICS: Absorption: (1g of 1% Gel) C_{max}=32ng/mL; T_{max}=6-10 hrs; AUC_{0-24}=595ng•hr/mL. (1g of 0.75% Lot) C_{max}=96ng/mL; AUC_{0-24}=962ng•hr/mL.

NURSING CONSIDERATIONS

Assessment: Assess nursing status, use with evidence/history of blood dyscrasias, and for possible drug interactions.

Monitoring: Monitor for tearing of eyes and local skin irritation reactions.

Patient Counseling: Instruct to use medication exactly as directed (for external use only, avoid contact with eyes, and cleanse affected area(s) before applying). Advise to report adverse reactions, and use less frequently or d/c if local skin irritation develops. May use cosmetics following application.

Administration: Topical application only. Wash areas to be treated with mild cleanser before application. **Storage:** 20-25°C (68-77°F).

MetroGel-Vaginal RX

metronidazole (Graceway)

THERAPEUTIC CLASS: Imidazole antibacterial

INDICATIONS: Treatment of bacterial vaginosis.

DOSAGE: *Adults:* Insert 1 applicatorful intravaginally qd-bid for 5 days. For once daily dosing, administer hs.

HOW SUPPLIED: Gel: 0.75% [70g]

CONTRAINDICATIONS: Hypersensitivity to other nitroimidazole derivatives.

WARNINGS/PRECAUTIONS: Caution with CNS or severe hepatic disease. D/C if abnormal neurologic signs appear. Avoid vaginal intercourse during therapy. May develop *Candida* vaginitis. May interfere with lab tests (ALT, SGPT, AST, SGOT, LDH, triglycerides, and glucose hexokinase).

ADVERSE REACTIONS: *Candida* cervicitis/vaginitis, vaginal discharge, pelvic discomfort, nausea, vomiting, headache, vulva/vaginal irritation, GI discomfort, change in WBC count.

INTERACTIONS: May potentiate warfarin, other anticoagulants, and lithium. Cimetidine may potentiate metronidazole. Avoid alcohol; possible disulfiram-like reaction may occur. Do not administer gel within 2 weeks of discontinuing disulfiram therapy.

PREGNANCY: Category B, not for use in nursing.

MECHANISM OF ACTION: Antibacterial/antiprotozoal agent; not established, suspected that 5-nitro group of metronidazole is reduced by metabolically active anaerobes and the reduced form of the drug interacts with bacterial DNA.

PHARMACOKINETICS: Absorption: C_{max}=237ng/mL; T_{max}=6-12 hrs. **Distribution:** Found in breast milk and crosses placental barrier.

NURSING CONSIDERATIONS

Assessment: Assess for hypersensitivity to drug, hepatic impairment, CNS diseases, vaginal candidiasis, alcohol intake, for possible drug/lab test interactions (eg, disulfiram).

Monitoring: Monitor for convulsive seizures and peripheral neuropathy, psychotic reactions, disulfiram-like reaction, *Candida* vaginitis, lab tests for AST, ALT, LDH, TG, glucose hexokinase, and WBCs.

Patient Counseling: Instruct not to engage in vaginal intercourse or drink alcohol during treatment. Avoid contact with eyes; rinse with cool tap water if occurs.

Administration: Intravaginal route. Insert applicator into vagina, push plunger to deposit gel, and then withdraw applicator. **Storage:** 15-30°C (59-86°F). Protect from freezing.

MEVACOR RX

lovastatin (Merck)

THERAPEUTIC CLASS: HMG-CoA reductase inhibitor

INDICATIONS: To reduce risk of MI, unstable angina, and coronary revascularization procedures in patients without symptomatic coronary disease, average to moderately elevated total-C and LDL-C, and below average HDL-C. To slow coronary atherosclerosis progression in patients with coronary heart disease to reduce total-C and LDL-C. Adjunct to diet to lower total-C and LDL-C in primary hypercholesterolemia (Types IIa and IIb). Adjunct to diet to lower total-C, LDL-C, and apolipoprotein B in adolescents at least 1-yr postmenarchal with heterozygous familial hypercholesterolemia.

DOSAGE: *Adults:* Initial: 20mg qd at dinner (10mg/day if need LDL-C reduction <20%). Usual: 10-80mg/day given qd or bid. May adjust every 4 weeks. Max: 80mg/day. Concomitant Cyclosporine: Initial: 10mg/day. Max: 20mg/day. Fibrates/Niacin (≥1g/day): Max: 20mg/day. Concomitant Amiodarone/Verapamil: Max: 40mg/day. CrCl <30mL/min: Consider dose increase of >20mg/day carefully and implement cautiously.
Pediatrics: Heterozygous Familial Hypercholesterolemia: 10-17 yrs (at least 1-yr postmenarchal): Initial: If <20% LDL-C Reduction Needed: 10mg qd. If ≥20% LDL-C Reduction Needed: 20mg qd. May adjust every 4 weeks. Max: 40mg/day. Concomitant Cyclosporine: Initial: 10mg/day. Max: 20mg/day. Fibrates/Niacin (≥1g/day): Max: 20mg/day. Concomitant Amiodarone/Verapamil: Max: 40mg/day. CrCl <30mL/min: Consider dose increase of >20mg/day carefully and implement cautiously.

HOW SUPPLIED: Tab: 20mg, 40mg

CONTRAINDICATIONS: Active liver disease, unexplained persistent elevations of serum transaminases, pregnancy, nursing mothers.

WARNINGS/PRECAUTIONS: May increase serum transaminases and CPK levels; consider in differential diagnosis of chest pain. D/C if AST or ALT ≥3x ULN persists, or if myopathy diagnosed or suspected. Monitor LFTs prior to therapy, at 6 weeks, 12 weeks, then periodically or with dose elevation. Caution with heavy alcohol use and/or history of hepatic disease. Caution with dose escalation in renal insufficiency. Less effective with homozygous familial hypercholesterolemia. Rhabdomyolysis (rare), myopathy reported. D/C a few days before elective major surgery and when any major acute medical or surgical condition supervenes.

ADVERSE REACTIONS: Headache, constipation, flatulence, dizziness, rash, elevated transaminases or CK levels, GI upset, blurred vision.

INTERACTIONS: Increased risk of myopathy with CYP3A4 inhibitors (eg, cyclosporine, itraconazole, ketoconazole, erythromycin, clarithromycin, telithromycin, protease inhibitors, nefazodone, >1 quart/day of grapefruit juice), verapamil, amiodarone, fibrates (eg, gemfibrozil), danazol, and ≥1g/day of niacin. Monitor anticoagulants. Caution with drugs that diminish levels or activity of steroid hormones (eg, ketoconazole, spironolactone, cimetidine).

PREGNANCY: Category X, not for use in nursing.

MECHANISM OF ACTION: HMG-CoA reductase inhibitor; causes reduction of VLDL-C concentration and induction of LDL-receptor, leading to reduced production and/or increased catabolism of LDL-C. Also causes lowering of apolipoprotein B, component of LDL particles, consequently leading to reduction in concentration of circulating LDL.

PHARMACOKINETICS: Absorption: T_{max}=2-4 hrs. **Distribution:** Plasma protein binding (>95%). **Metabolism:** Liver (first pass); CYP450 3A4. β-hydroxyacid, 6'-hydroxy derivative (major active metabolites). **Elimination:** Urine (10%), feces (83%).

M

NURSING CONSIDERATIONS

Assessment: Assess for secondary causes of hypercholesterolemia (eg, poorly controlled DM, hypothyroidism, nephrotoxic syndrome, dysproteinemias, obstructive liver disease, other drug therapy, alcoholism), presence of active liver disease or unexplained elevations of serum transaminases, and pregnancy/nursing status. Assess lipid profile (total-C, HDL-C, and TG) and LFTs prior to therapy. Assess use in presence of homozygous familial hypercholesterolemia or renal insufficiencies and for possible drug interactions.

Monitoring: Monitor for signs/symptoms of myopathy (eg, muscle pain, tenderness, weakness), rhabdomyolysis, elevations of creatine kinase, liver dysfunction, endocrine dysfunction, and CNS toxicity (eg, optic nerve degeneration, CNS vascular lesions). Perform periodic monitoring of cholesterol levels, CK levels, and LFTs (eg, ALT, AST).

Patient Counseling: Inform about possible drug interactions and possible interaction with grapefruit juice. Advise to report any signs/symptoms of unexplained muscle pain, tenderness, or weakness immediately. Recommend a standard cholesterol-lowering diet. Inform that periodic blood testing is required to evaluate cholesterol levels and liver function. Counsel females about risks of use during pregnancy/nursing.

Administration: Oral route. **Storage:** 5-30°C (41-86°F). Protect from light.

MEXILETINE RX

mexiletine HCl (Various)

THERAPEUTIC CLASS: Class IB antiarrhythmic

INDICATIONS: Treatment of life-threatening ventricular arrhythmias.

M

DOSAGE: *Adults:* Initial: 200mg q8h when rapid control not essential. Titrate: Adjust by 50-100mg, not less than every 2-3 days. Usual: 200-300mg q8h. Max: 1200mg/day. If control with ≤300mg q8h, then may divide daily dose and give q12h. Max: 450mg q12h. For Rapid Control: LD: 400mg, then 200mg in 8 hrs. Transfer from Other Class I Oral Agents: Initial: 200mg and titrate as above, 6-12 hrs after last quinidine sulfate or disopyramide dose, 3-6 hrs after last procainamide dose, or 8-12 hrs after last tocainide dose. Severe Hepatic Disease: May need lower dose. Take with food or antacid.

HOW SUPPLIED: Cap: 150mg, 200mg, 250mg

CONTRAINDICATIONS: Cardiogenic shock, pre-existing 2nd- or 3rd-degree AV block (without pacemaker).

WARNINGS/PRECAUTIONS: Reserve for life-threatening arrhythmias. May treat patients with 2nd- or 3rd-degree AV block with a pacemaker; monitor continuously. Can worsen arrhythmias. Caution with hypotension, severe CHF, seizure disorder, hepatic impairment, sinus node dysfunction, or intraventricular conduction abnormalities. Leukopenia, agranulocytosis, and abnormal LFTs reported. Monitor ECG.

ADVERSE REACTIONS: GI distress, tremor, lightheadedness, coordination difficulties, NV, heartburn.

INTERACTIONS: Inhibition or induction of CYP2D6 and CYP1A2 enzymes may alter plasma levels. Slowly titrate dose of mexiletine to desired effect with concomitant fluvoxamine or propafenone. Avoid drugs or diet regimens that may alter urinary pH. Hepatic enzyme inducers (eg, rifampin, phenobarbital, phenytoin) may lower plasma levels. May increase theophylline levels. Decreases caffeine clearance. Cimetidine may alter plasma levels.

PREGNANCY: Category C, not for use in nursing.

MECHANISM OF ACTION: Class 1B antiarrhythmic; local anesthetic; inhibits inward Na^+ current, thus reducing the action potential rise rate, and decreases the effective refractory period in Purkinje fibers.

PHARMACOKINETICS: Absorption: Well absorbed; T_{max}=2-3 hrs. **Distribution:** V_d=5-7L/kg, plasma protein binding (50-60%), found in breast milk. **Metabolism:** Liver, through CYP2D6 and CYP1A2 metabolism, aromatic/aliphatic hydroxylation, dealkylation, deamination, N-oxidation, and glucuronidation pathways. P-hydroxymexiletine, hydroxy-methylmexiletine, and N-hydroxy-mexiletine (major metabolites). **Elimination:** Urine (10% unchanged); $T_{1/2}$=10-12hrs.

NURSING CONSIDERATIONS

Assessment: Assess for cardiogenic shock, pre-existing 2nd- or 3rd-degree AV block, life-threatening venticular arrhythmia (eg, sustained ventricular tachycardia, recent MI), liver impairment, hypotension, CHF, seizure, pregnancy/nursing status, blood dyscrasias, and possible drug/dietary regimen interactions.

Monitoring: Monitor LFTs, CBC, ANA, myelofibrosis, HR, BP, convulsions, worsening of arrhythmia, CHF, or hypotension.

Patient Counseling: Inform about risks/benefits; report adverse reactions. Notify if pregnant/nursing.

Administration: Oral route. Avoid dietary regimen or drugs that may alter urinary pH. **Storage:** 25°C (77°F); excursions permitted to 15-30°C (59-86°F).

MIACALCIN

RX

calcitonin-salmon (Novartis)

THERAPEUTIC CLASS: Hormonal bone resorption inhibitor

INDICATIONS: (Inj) Treatment of Paget's disease, hypercalcemia, and postmenopausal osteoporosis. (Spray) Treatment of postmenopausal osteoporosis in females >5 yrs postmenopause.

DOSAGE: *Adults:* (Inj) Paget's Disease: Usual: 100 IU IM/SQ qd. Hypercalcemia: Initial: 4 IU/kg IM/SQ q12h. Titrate: May increase to 8 IU/kg q12h after 1-2 days, then to 8 IU/kg q6h after 2 days if unsatisfactory response. Osteoporosis: (Inj) 100 IU IM/SQ every other day. If >2mL, use IM injection. (Spray) 200 IU qd intranasally. Alternate nostrils daily. Take with supplemental calcium and vitamin D for postmenopausal osteoporosis.

HOW SUPPLIED: Inj: 200 IU/mL; Nasal Spray: 200 IU/inh [2mL 2[s]]

WARNINGS/PRECAUTIONS: Possibility of systemic allergic reactions. Monitor urine sediment periodically with chronic use. If nasal mucosa ulceration occurs, d/c until healed. D/C if severe ulceration of the nasal mucosa occurs. Perform periodic nasal exams. Monitor drug effects.

ADVERSE REACTIONS: (Inj) NV, injection site inflammation, flushing of face or hands, nocturia, ear lobe pruritus, poor appetite, abdominal pain. (Spray) Nasal symptoms, back pain, headache, arthralgia, epistaxis.

INTERACTIONS: Prior diphosphonate use with Paget's disease may reduce anti-resorptive response.

PREGNANCY: Category C, not for use in nursing.

MECHANISM OF ACTION: Hormonal bone resorption inhibitor; actions on bone not fully established. Calcitonin receptors have been found in osteoclasts and osteoblasts. Initially causes a marked transient inhibition of the ongoing bone resorptive process. Prolonged use causes a smaller decrease in the rate of bone resorption. Thought to be associated with decrease in number of osteoclasts as well as decrease in resorptive activity.

PHARMACOKINETICS: Absorption: (Intranasal): Rapid, T_{max}=31-39 min; (Inj): T_{max}=16-25 min. **Elimination:** Urine; (Intranasal): $T_{1/2}$=43 min.

NURSING CONSIDERATIONS

Assessment: Assess for hypersensitivity to medication; consider skin testing. Assess pregnancy/nursing status. If using intranasal formulation, obtain baseline nasal exam (eg, visualization of the nasal mucosa, turbinates, septum, and mucosal blood vessel status). If using parenteral formulation and treating osteoporosis, obtain baseline measurement of bone resorption/turnover and bone mineral density.

Monitoring: Monitor for signs/symptoms of allergic reaction (eg, bronchospasm, swelling of tongue or throat, anaphylactic shock). Perform periodic

M

exams of urine sediment. If using intranasal formulation, monitor for nasal mucosal alterations, transient nasal conditions, and ulceration of nasal mucosa; perform periodic nasal exams. For intranasal formulation, perform periodic measurements of lumbar vertebral bone. If using parenteral formulation, monitor for hypocalcemic tetany. For parenteral administration in treatment of Paget's disease, perform periodic measurement of serum alkaline phosphatase and 24-hr urinary hydroxyproline. For parenteral administration in treatment of osteoporosis, monitor biochemical markers of bone resorption/turnover and bone mineral density.

Patient Counseling: Intranasal formulation: Instruct how to assemble and prime pump, and introduce medication in the nasal passages. Advise to contact physician if allergic reaction or nasal irritation occur. Inform that new, unassembled bottles should be refrigerated and protected from freezing. Allow medication to reach room temperature before priming pump and using a new bottle. Store opened bottle upright at room temperature for up to 35 days. Parenteral formulation: Advise to use sterile injection technique.

Administration: Intranasal/IM/SQ routes. **Storage:** Intranasal: Unopened: 2-8°C (36-46°F). Protect from freezing. Used: 15-30°C (59-86°F) in upright position for up to 35 days. Injection: 2-8°C (36-46°F).

MICARDIS RX

telmisartan (Boehringer Ingelheim)

Can cause death/injury to developing fetus during 2nd and 3rd trimesters. Stop therapy if pregancy detected.

M

THERAPEUTIC CLASS: Angiotensin II receptor antagonist

INDICATIONS: Treatment of hypertension, alone or with other antihypertensives.

DOSAGE: *Adults:* Initial: 40mg qd. Usual: 20-80mg/day. May add diuretic if need additional BP reduction after 80mg/day.

HOW SUPPLIED: Tab: 20mg, 40mg*, 80mg* *scored

WARNINGS/PRECAUTIONS: Can cause fetal injury/death. Correct volume or salt depletion before therapy. Changes in renal function may occur; caution with renal artery stenosis, severe CHF. Closely monitor with biliary obstructive disorders or hepatic dysfunction.

ADVERSE REACTIONS: Upper respiratory infection, back pain, sinusitis, diarrhea, bradycardia, eosinophilia, thrombocytopenia, increased uric acid, increased CPK, increased sweating, abnormal hepatic function/liver disorder, renal impairment including acute renal failure, anemia, edema, and cough.

INTERACTIONS: Increases digoxin levels. May alter warfarin levels.

PREGNANCY: Category C (1st trimester) and D (2nd and 3rd trimesters), not for use in nursing.

MECHANISM OF ACTION: Angiotensin II receptor antagonist; blocks vasoconstrictor and aldosterone-secreting effects of angiotensin II by selectively blocking binding of angiotensin II to AT_1 receptor.

PHARMACOKINETICS: Absorption: Absolute bioavailability (40mg, 160mg)=42%, 58%; T_{max}=0.5-1 hr. **Distribution:** V_d=500L; plasma protein binding (>99.5%). **Metabolism:** Conjugation. **Elimination**: Feces (>97%), urine; $T_{1/2}$=24 hrs.

NURSING CONSIDERATIONS

Assessment: Assess LFTs, renal function, BP, pregnancy status, and possible drug interactions.

Monitoring: Monitor BP, LFTs, renal function, CBC with platelet and differential count, serum potassium levels. Monitor for MI, CHF, angioneurotic edema, hypersensitivity reactions, diarrhea, sinusitis.

Patient Counseling: Counsel about signs/symptoms of adverse effects and advise to seek prompt medical attention. Inform about fetal risks if taken during pregnancy.

Administration: Oral route. **Storage:** Store at 25°C (77°F); excursions permitted to 15-30°C (59-86°F).

MICARDIS HCT

RX

telmisartan - hydrochlorothiazide (Boehringer Ingelheim)

Can cause death/injury to developing fetus during 2nd and 3rd trimesters. Stop therapy if pregnancy detected.

THERAPEUTIC CLASS: Angiotensin II receptor antagonist/thiazide diuretic

INDICATIONS: Treatment of hypertension. Not for initial therapy.

DOSAGE: *Adults:* If BP not controlled on 80mg telmisartan, or 25mg HCTZ/day, or controlled on 25mg HCTZ/day but serum K^+ decreased, 80mg-12.5mg tab qd. Titrate/Max: If uncontrolled after 2-4 weeks, increase to 160mg-25mg. Biliary Obstruction/Hepatic Dysfunction: Initial: 40mg-12.5mg tab qd; monitor closely.

HOW SUPPLIED: Tab: (HCTZ-Telmisartan) 12.5mg-40mg, 12.5mg-80mg, 25mg-80mg

CONTRAINDICATIONS: Anuria, sulfonamide hypersensitivity.

WARNINGS/PRECAUTIONS: Can cause fetal injury/death. Correct volume or salt depletion before therapy. Caution with hepatic or renal dysfunction, biliary obstructive disorders, renal artery stenosis, severe CHF, history of allergies, and asthma. May exacerbate or activate SLE. Monitor serum electrolytes. Avoid if CrCl ≤30mL/min. Hyperuricemia, hyperglycemia, hypokalemia, hypomagnesemia, hypercalcemia may occur. Enhanced effects in post-sympathectomy patient. May increase cholesterol and triglyceride levels.

ADVERSE REACTIONS: Dizziness, fatigue, sinusitis, upper respiratory infection, diarrhea, bradycardia, eosinophilia, thrombocytopenia, uric acid increased, abnormal hepatic function/liver disorder, renal impairment including acute renal failure, anemia, and increased CPK.

INTERACTIONS: Potentiates orthostatic hypotension with alcohol, barbiturates, and narcotics. Adjust insulin and antidiabetic drugs. Impaired absorption with cholestyramine, colestipol. Corticosteroids and ACTH deplete electrolytes. May decrease response to pressor amines. Potentiates other antihypertensives. May increase responsiveness to skeletal muscle relaxants. Risk of lithium toxicity. NSAIDs decrease diuretic effects. Increases digoxin levels. May alter warfarin levels.

PREGNANCY: Category C (1st trimester) and D (2nd and 3rd trimesters), not for use in nursing.

MECHANISM OF ACTION: Telmisartan: Angiotensin II receptor antagonist; blocks the vasoconstrictor and aldosterone-secreting effects of angiotensin II by selectively blocking the binding of angiotensin II to the AT_1 receptor in vascular smooth muscle and adrenal gland. HCTZ: Thiazide diuretic; affects renal tubular mechanism of electrolyte reabsorption, directly increasing excretion of sodium salt and chloride.

PHARMACOKINETICS: Absorption: Telmisartan: T_{max}=0.5-1 hr; Absolute bioavailability =42% (40mg), 58% (160mg). **Distribution:** Telmisartan: Plasma protein binding (≥99.5%); V_d= 500L. HCTZ: Crosses the placenta and excreted in breast milk. **Metabolism:** Telmisartan: Conjugation. **Elimination:** Telmisartan: $T_{1/2}$=24 hrs; feces (≥97%), urine. HCTZ: Urine (61%, unchanged); $T_{1/2}$=5.6-14.8 hrs.

NURSING CONSIDERATIONS

Assessment: Assess LFTs, renal function, BP, systemic lupus erythematosus, asthma, serum electrolytes, cirrhosis, pregnancy status, and possible drug interactions.

M

Monitoring: Monitor BP, LFTs, renal function, CBC with platelet count and differential count, serum electrolytes, hyperuricemia, lipid profile. Monitor for MI, CHF, angioneurotic edema, hypersensitivity reactions, upper respiratory tract infection, diarrhea, sinusitis, pancreatitis, Stevens-Johnson syndrome, xanthopsia.

Patient Counseling: Counsel about the signs and symptoms of potential adverse effects and advise to seek prompt medical attention. Inform about fetal risks if taken during pregnancy.

Administration: Oral route. **Storage:** 25°C (77°F); excursions permitted to 15-30°C (59-86°F).

MICRO-K — RX

potassium chloride (Ther-Rx)

THERAPEUTIC CLASS: K^+ supplement

INDICATIONS: (For those unable to tolerate liquid or effervescent potassium preparations). Treatment and prevention of hypokalemia with or without metabolic alkalosis. Treatment of digitalis intoxication and hypokalemic familial periodic paralysis.

DOSAGE: *Adults:* Prevention: 20mEq/day. Hypokalemia: 40-100mEq/day. Divide dose if >20mEq. Take with meal and full glass of water or liquid. May sprinkle on soft food; swallow without chewing.

HOW SUPPLIED: Cap, Extended-Release: 8mEq, 10mEq

CONTRAINDICATIONS: Hyperkalemia, esophageal ulceration, delay in GI passage (from structural, pathological, pharmacologic causes), cardiac patients with esophageal compression due to enlarged left atrium.

M

WARNINGS/PRECAUTIONS: Potentially fatal hyperkalemia may occur. Extreme caution with acidosis, cardiac and renal disease; monitor ECG and electrolytes. Hypokalemia with metabolic acidosis should be treated with an alkalinizing potassium salt (eg, potassium bicarbonate, potassium citrate). May produce ulcerative or stenotic GI lesions.

ADVERSE REACTIONS: Hyperkalemia, GI effects (obstruction, bleeding, ulceration), NV, abdominal pain, diarrhea.

INTERACTIONS: Risk of hyperkalemia with ACE inhibitors (eg, captopril, enalapril), K^+-sparing diuretics, and K^+ supplements. Contraindicated with anticholinergic agents due to possible delay in tablet passage through GI tract.

PREGNANCY: Category C, safe for use in nursing.

MECHANISM OF ACTION: K^+ supplement; helps in maintenance of intracellular tonicity, transmission of nerve impulses, contraction of cardiac, skeletal, and smooth muscle, and maintenance of normal renal function.

NURSING CONSIDERATIONS

Assessment: Assess for conditions that impair excretion of K^+, hyperkalemia, esophageal compression due to enlarged left atrium, conditions causing arrest or delay in passage through GI, renal insufficiency, DM, and possible drug interactions.

Monitoring: Monitor serum K^+ levels regularly; renal function, ECG, and acid-base balance. Monitor for GI ulceration/obstruction/perforation, hyperkalemia, renal dysfunction, and hypersensitivity reactions.

Patient Counseling: Instruct to take with meals; swallow with full glass of water or other suitable liquid. Do not crush, chew, or suck. Seek medical attention if symptoms of GI ulceration, obstruction, perforation (vomiting, abdominal pain, distention, GI bleeding), hyperkalemia, or hypersensitivity reactions occur.

Administration: Oral route. **Storage:** 20-25°C (68-77°F).

MICRONASE — RX

glyburide (Pharmacia & Upjohn)

THERAPEUTIC CLASS: Sulfonylurea (2nd generation)

INDICATIONS: Adjunct to diet and exercise, to improve glycemic control in type 2 diabetes mellitus.

DOSAGE: *Adults:* Initial: 2.5-5mg qd with breakfast or 1st main meal; give 1.25mg if sensitive to hypoglycemia. Titrate: Increase by no more than 2.5mg/day at weekly intervals. Maint: 1.25-20mg given qd or in divided doses. Max: 20mg/day. May give bid with >10mg/day. Renal or Hepatic Disease/Elderly/Debilitated/Malnourished/Adrenal or Pituitary Insufficiency: Initial: 1.25mg qd. Transfer From Other Oral Antidiabetic Agents: Initial: 2.5-5mg/day. Switch From Insulin: If <20 U/day: 2.5-5mg qd. If 20-40 U/day: 5mg qd. If >40 U/day, decrease dose by 50% and give 5mg qd. Titrate: Progressive withdrawal of insulin, and increase by 1.25-2.5mg/day every 2-10 days. Concomitant Metformin: Add glyburide gradually to max dose of metformin monotherapy after 4 weeks if needed.

HOW SUPPLIED: Tab: 1.25mg*, 2.5mg*, 5mg* *scored

CONTRAINDICATIONS: Diabetic ketoacidosis with or without coma and type 1 DM.

WARNINGS/PRECAUTIONS: Increased risk of cardiovascular mortality. Risk of hypoglycemia, especially with renal and hepatic disease, elderly, debilitated or malnourished patients, and those with adrenal or pituitary insufficiency. May need to d/c and give insulin with stress (eg, fever, trauma). Secondary failure may occur. D/C if jaundice, hepatitis, or persistent skin reaction occur. Hematologic reactions and hyponatremia reported.

ADVERSE REACTIONS: Hypoglycemia, nausea, epigastric fullness, heartburn, allergic skin reactions, hepatic porphyria and disulfiram-like reactions (rarely), hyponatremia, liver function abnormalities, photosensitivity reactions, angioedema, arthralgia, myalgia, vasculitis, leukopenia, and agranulocytosis.

M

INTERACTIONS: Hypoglycemia potentiated by alcohol, NSAIDs, miconazole, fluoroquinolones, highly protein-bound drugs, salicylates, sulfonamides, chloramphenicol, probenecid, coumarins, MAOIs, and β-blockers. Risk of hyperglycemia with diuretics, corticosteroids, phenothiazines, thyroid products, estrogens, oral contraceptives, phenytoin, nicotinic acid, sympathomimetics, CCBs, and INH. β-blockers may mask hypoglycemia. Disulfiram-like reactions (rarely) with alcohol.

PREGNANCY: Category B, not for use in nursing.

MECHANISM OF ACTION: Sulfonylurea; lowers blood glucose acutely by stimulating the release of insulin from the pancreas.

PHARMACOKINETICS: Absorption: T_{max}=4 hrs. **Distribution:** Serum protein binding (extensive). **Metabolism:** 4-trans-hydroxy derivative (major metabolite), 3-cishydroxy derivative (second metabolite). **Elimination:** Bile (50%), urine (50%); $T_{1/2}$=10 hrs.

NURSING CONSIDERATIONS

Assessment: Assess FPG, HbA_{1c}, renal function, LFTs, type 1 DM, ketoacidosis, GI disease, pregnancy status, and possible drug interactions.

Monitoring: Monitor hypoglycemia, diabetic ketoacidosis, asthenia, tremors, nervousness, metabolic reactions (eg, SIADH), and dermatologic reactions; FPG, HbA_{1c}, renal function tests, LFTs, CBC with differential and platelet count.

Patient Counseling: Counsel to take with breakfast or first main meal. Inform about importance of adhering to dietary instructions, regular exercise program, and regular testing of urine and blood glucose. Educate on signs/symptoms of hypoglycemia, its treatment, and predisposing conditions; primary and secondary failure; risks/benefits of therapy.

Administration: Oral route. **Storage:** 20-25°C (68-77°F). Dispense in well-closed containers with safety closures.

MICRONOR RX

norethindrone (Ortho-McNeil)

OTHER BRAND NAMES: Camila (Barr) - Errin (Barr)

THERAPEUTIC CLASS: Progestogen

INDICATIONS: Prevention of pregnancy.

DOSAGE: *Adults:* 1 tab qd without interruption (continuous regimen) on 1st day of menstrual period. If fully nursing, start 6 weeks postpartum. If partially nursing, start 3 weeks postpartum.

HOW SUPPLIED: Tab: 0.35mg

CONTRAINDICATIONS: Pregnancy, breast carcinoma, undiagnosed abnormal genital bleeding, benign or malignant liver tumors, acute liver disease.

WARNINGS/PRECAUTIONS: Avoid smoking. Perform annual physical exam. Not for use before menarche. May affect certain endocrine tests (eg, sex hormone binding globulin, thyroxine binding globulin). Monitor glucose tolerance in prediabetics and diabetics. May alter lipid metabolism. May increase risk of breast cancer and hepatic adenomas. May cause irregular menstrual patterns. Delayed follicular atresia/ovarian cysts and ectopic pregnancy may occur. D/C with recurrent migraines or severe headaches.

ADVERSE REACTIONS: Menstrual irregularities, frequent or irregular bleeding, headache, breast tenderness, nausea, dizziness, androgenic effects (rare).

INTERACTIONS: Reduced efficacy with hepatic enzyme inducers (eg, rifampin, phenytoin, carbamazepine, barbiturates).

PREGNANCY: Not for use in pregnancy, caution in nursing.

MECHANISM OF ACTION: Progestogen oral contraceptive; suppresses ovulation. Thickens cervical mucus to inhibit sperm penetration, lowers midcycle LH and FSH peaks, slows movement of ovum through fallopian tubes, and alters endometrium.

PHARMACOKINETICS: Absorption: T_{max}=2 hrs. **Distribution:** Rapid.

NURSING CONSIDERATIONS

Assessment: Assess for pregnancy, carcinoma of breast, undiagnosed abnormal genital bleeding, benign/malignant liver tumor, and acute liver disease. Assess use in smokers and for possible drug interactions.

Monitoring: Monitor for ectopic pregnancy, delayed follicular atresia, ovarian cysts, irregular genital bleeding, and hepatic neoplasias. Perform annual physical exam while on medication. Monitor serum glucose levels with DM and prediabetic patients, lipid levels while on medication, and for onset or exacerbation of migraine or development of severe headaches.

Patient Counseling: Counsel about possible adverse effects. Inform that drug does not protect against HIV infection (AIDS) or other STDs. Advise to avoid smoking while on medication. Instruct to take at same time daily. Instruct that if dose missed or taken 3 hrs past scheduled time, use backup form of contraception for next 48 hrs.

Administration: Oral route. **Storage:** 25°C (77°F); excursions permitted to 15-30°C (59-86°F). Keep out of reach of children.

MICROZIDE RX

hydrochlorothiazide (Watson)

THERAPEUTIC CLASS: Thiazide diuretic

INDICATIONS: Management of hypertension.

DOSAGE: *Adults:* Initial: 12.5mg qd. Max: 50mg/day.

HOW SUPPLIED: Cap: 12.5mg

CONTRAINDICATIONS: Anuria, sulfonamide hypersensitivity.

WARNINGS/PRECAUTIONS: Caution in severe renal disease, liver dysfunction, electrolyte/fluid imbalance. Monitor electrolytes. Hyperuricemia, hyperglycemia, hypokalemia, hyponatremia, hypomagnesemia, hypercalcemia may occur. Increases in cholesterol and triglyceride levels reported. May exacerbate SLE. Sensitivity reactions reported. D/C prior to parathyroid test. Enhanced effects in post-sympathectomy patient.

ADVERSE REACTIONS: Weakness, hypotension, pancreatitis, jaundice, diarrhea, vomiting, blood dyscrasias, rash, photosensitivity, electrolyte imbalance, impotence.

INTERACTIONS: May potentiate orthostatic hypotension with alcohol, barbiturates, narcotics. Adjust antidiabetic drugs. Possible decreased response to pressor amines. Corticosteroids, ACTH increase electrolyte depletion. May potentiate nondepolarizing skeletal muscle relaxants, antihypertensives. Lithium toxicity. NSAIDs decrease effects. Decreased PO absorption with cholestyramine, colestipol.

PREGNANCY: Category B, not for use in nursing.

MECHANISM OF ACTION: Thiazide diuretic; affects renal tubular mechanism of electrolyte reabsorption, directly increasing excretion of Na^+ and Cl^-.

PHARMACOKINETICS: Absorption: Well absorbed (65-75%); C_{max}=70-490ng/mL; T_{max}=1-5 hrs. **Distribution:** Plasma protein binding (40-68%). **Elimination:** Urine (unchanged), $T_{1/2}$=6-15 hrs.

NURSING CONSIDERATIONS

Assessment: Assess for anuria, known hypersensitivity to sulfonamide-derived drugs, DM, hypoglycemia, impaired renal/hepatic function, serum electrolytes, parathyroid disease, pregnancy status, and possible drug interactions.

Monitoring: Monitor BP, hyperuricemia or acute gout, signs/symptoms of electrolyte imbalance, serum glucose, lipid profile, pancreatitis, Stevens-Johnson syndrome, xanthopsia, impotence.

Patient Counseling: Counsel about signs/symptoms of electrolyte imbalance (dryness of mouth, thirst, weakness, lethargy, drowsiness, restlessness, muscle pains or cramps, muscular fatigue, hypotension, oliguria, tachycardia, and GI disturbance such as NV) and advise to seek prompt medical attention.

Administration: Oral route. **Storage:** 20-25°C (68-77°F). Protect from light, moisture, freezing -20°C (-4°F). Keep container tightly closed.

MIDAZOLAM INJECTION

CIV

midazolam HCl (Various)

Associated with respiratory depression and respiratory arrest especially when used for sedation in noncritical care settings. Do not administer by rapid injection to neonates. Continuous monitoring required.

THERAPEUTIC CLASS: Benzodiazepine

INDICATIONS: For sedation, anxiolysis, and amnesia induction pre-op, prior to or during diagnostic, therapeutic, or endoscopic procedures, either alone or in combination with other CNS depressants. For induction of general anesthesia. For sedation of intubated and ventilated patients.

DOSAGE: *Adults:* IV: Sedation/Anxiolysis/Amnesia Induction: <60 yrs: Initial: 1-2.5mg IV over 2 min. Max: 5mg. Titrate: In small increments at 2 min intervals if needed. Concomitant Narcotics/Other CNS Depressants: Reduce by 30%. ≥60 yrs/Debilitated/Chronically Ill: Initial: 1-1.5mg IV over 2 min. Max: 3.5mg. Titrate: In small increments at 2 min intervals if needed. Concomitant Narcotics/Other CNS Depressants. Reduce by 50%. Maint: 25% of sedation dose by slow titration. IM: Preoperative Sedation/Anxiolysis/Amnesia: <60 yrs: 0.07-0.08mg/kg IM up to 1 hr before surgery. ≥60 yrs/Debilitated: 1-3mg IM. Anesthesia Induction: Unpremedicated: <55 yrs: Initially: 0.3-0.35mg/kg IV over 20-30 seconds. May give additional doses of 25% of initial dose to complete induction. ≥55 yrs: Initial: 0.3mg/kg IV. Debilitated: Initial:

0.15-0.25mg/kg IV. Premedicated: <55 yrs: Initial: 0.25mg/kg IV over 20-30 seconds. ≥55 yrs: Initial: 0.2mg/kg IV. Debilitated: 0.15mg/kg IV. Maintenance Sedation: LD: 0.01-0.05mg/kg IV. May repeat dose at 10-15 min intervals until adequate sedation. Maint: 0.02-0.1mg/kg/hr. Titrate to desired level of sedation using 25-50% adjustments. Infusion rate should be decreased 10-25% every few hrs to find minimum effective infusion rate.
Pediatrics: Sedation/Anxiolysis/Amnesia Induction: IV: <6 months: Limited information; titrate with small increments and monitor. 6 months-5 yrs: Initial: 0.05-0.1mg/kg IV over 2-3 min, up to 0.6mg/kg if needed. Max: 6mg. 6-12 yrs: Initial: 0.025-0.05mg/kg IV over 2-3 min, up to 0.4mg/kg if needed. Max: 10mg. 12-16 yrs: 1-2.5mg IV over 2 min. Titrate: In small increments at 2 min intervals if needed. Max: 10mg. IM: 0.1-0.15mg/kg IM, up to 0.5mg/kg if needed. Max: 10mg. Sedation: LD: 0.05-0.2mg/kg IV infusion over 2-3 min. Maint: 0.06-0.12mg/kg/hr IV infusion. May adjust dose by 25%. Sedation in Critical Care: Neonatal Dose: <32 weeks: Initial: 0.03mg/kg/hr IV infusion. >32 weeks: Initial: 0.06mg/kg/hr IV infusion. Adjust to lowest effective dose.

HOW SUPPLIED: Inj: 1mg/mL, 5mg/mL

CONTRAINDICATIONS: Acute narrow-angle glaucoma, untreated open-angle glaucoma, intrathecal or epidural use.

WARNINGS/PRECAUTIONS: Agitation, involuntary movements, hyperactivity, and combativeness reported. Caution with CHF, chronic renal failure, pulmonary disease, uncompensated acute illnesses (eg, severe fluid or electrolyte disturbances), elderly or debilitated. Avoid use with shock or coma, or in acute alcohol intoxication with depression of vital signs. Contains benzyl alcohol. Administer IM or IV only.

ADVERSE REACTIONS: Decreased tidal volume and/or respiratory rate, BP/HR variations, apnea, hypotension, pain and local reactions at injection site, hiccoughs, nausea, vomiting.

M

INTERACTIONS: Prolonged sedation with CYP450 3A4 inhibitors (eg, erythromycin, diltiazem, verapamil, ketoconazole, itraconazole, saquinavir, cimetidine). Increased sedative effects with morphine, meperidine, fentanyl, secobarbital, droperidol or other CNS depressants. Avoid use with acute alcohol intoxication. May decrease concentration of halothane and thiopental required for anesthesia. May cause severe hypotension with concomitant use of fentanyl in neonates.

PREGNANCY: Category D, caution in nursing.

MECHANISM OF ACTION: Benzodiazepine; short-acting CNS depressant.

PHARMACOKINETICS: Absorption: (IM) Absolute bioavailability (>90%), C_{max}=90ng/mL, T_{max}=0.5 hr. (1-hydroxy-midazolam) C_{max}=8 ng/ml, T_{max}=1 hr. **Distribution:** Crosses placenta, found in breast milk and CSF. V_d=1.0-3.1L/kg; plasma protein binding (97%). **Metabolism:** Liver via CYP450-3A4;1-hydroxy-midazolam (major metabolite). **Elimination:** Urine; (0.5% unchanged 45%-57% as 4-hydroxy-midazolam); $T_{1/2}$=approximately 3 hrs.

NURSING CONSIDERATIONS

Assessment: Assess for primary psychiatric and/or medical illness, acute narrow-angle glaucoma, chronic pulmonary insufficiency (sleep apnea, COPD), renal/hepatic function, fluid electrolyte imbalances, and for possible drug interactions.

Monitoring: Monitor vital signs, cardiorespiratory complications, paradoxical reactions, CNS depression, air obstruction, apnea with pulse oximetry.

Patient Counseling: Inform of benefits/risks and potential for physical/psychological dependence. Caution while engaging in hazardous tasks (operating machinery/driving). Do not increase recommended dose or d/c before consulting physician. Avoid alcohol consumption; notify if pregnant or planning to become pregnant.

Administration: IM/IV route. **Storage:** 20-25°C (68-77°F).

MIDRIN

CIV

isometheptene mucate - dichloralphenazone - acetaminophen (Women First)

OTHER BRAND NAMES: Migrazone (Various) - Migquin (Qualitest) - Duradrin (Duramed) - Amidrine (Amide)

THERAPEUTIC CLASS: Analgesic/sedative/sympathomimetic

INDICATIONS: Relief of tension and vascular headaches. FDA has classified this agent as "possibly" effective in the treatment of migraine headache.

DOSAGE: *Adults:* Migraine: 2 caps, then 1 cap every hr until relieved. Max: 5 caps/12hrs. Tension Headache: 1-2 caps q4h. Max: 8 caps/day.

HOW SUPPLIED: Cap: (APAP-Dichloralphenazone-Isometheptene) 325mg-100mg-65mg

CONTRAINDICATIONS: Glaucoma, severe renal disease, HTN, organic heart disease, hepatic disease, concomitant MAOI therapy.

WARNINGS/PRECAUTIONS: Caution with HTN, peripheral vascular disease, or recent cardiovascular attacks.

ADVERSE REACTIONS: Transient dizziness, skin rash.

PREGNANCY: Safety in pregnancy and nursing are not known.

MECHANISM OF ACTION: Isometheptene: Sympathomimetic amine; acts by constricting dilated cranial and cerebral arterioles, reducing stimuli. Dichloralphenazone: Mild sedative; reduces emotional reaction to pain. Acetaminophen: Non-salicylate; raises threshold to painful stimuli exerting analgesic effect.

NURSING CONSIDERATIONS

Assessment: Assess for glaucoma, severe renal disease, HTN, organic heart disease, peripheral vascular disease, recent cardiovascular attack, hepatic disease, and possible drug interactions.

Monitoring: Monitor for hypersensitivity reaction.

Patient Counseling: Advise to reduce dose if hypersensitivity reaction (transient dizziness, skin rash) occurs.

Administration: Oral route. **Storage:** 15-30°C (59-86°F); protect from light and moisture.

MIGRANAL

RX

dihydroergotamine mesylate (Valeant)

Serious and life-threatening peripheral ischemia reported with potent CYP3A4 inhibitors (eg, protease inhibitors, macrolides). Elevated levels of dihydroergotamine increases risk of vasospasm leading to cerebral ischemia or ischemia of the extremities. Concomitant use with CYP3A4 inhibitors is contraindicated.

THERAPEUTIC CLASS: Ergot alkaloid

INDICATIONS: Acute treatment of migraine headache with or without aura.

DOSAGE: *Adults:* 1 spray per nostril, repeat in 15 min. Max: 6 sprays/24 hrs or 8 sprays/week.

HOW SUPPLIED: Nasal Spray: 0.5mg/spray [3.5mL]

CONTRAINDICATIONS: Ischemic heart disease (angina, history of MI, documented silent ischemia), coronary artery vasospasm (Prinzmetal's variant angina), uncontrolled HTN, known peripheral artery disease, sepsis, following vascular surgery, severe renal or hepatic dysfunction, hemiplegic or basilar migraine, pregnancy or nursing, with potent CYP3A4 inhibitors (eg, ritonavir, nelfinavir, indinavir, erythromycin, clarithromycin, troleandomycin, ketoconazole, itraconazole). Do not use with peripheral and central vasoconstrictors or within 24 hrs of 5-HT_1 agonists, ergot-type drugs, or methysergide.

WARNINGS/PRECAUTIONS: Confirm diagnosis. Monitor and consider ECG with 1st dose in patients with CAD risk factors (eg, HTN, hypercholesterolemia,

M

smoker, obesity, DM, strong family history, postmenopausal women, men >40 yrs). Risk of elevated BP, MI, and other adverse cardiac or vasospastic effects. Monitor cardiovascular function with intermittent long-term use. Fibrotic complications (eg, pleural and retroperitoneal fibrosis) reported.

ADVERSE REACTIONS: Rhinitis, altered taste, application site reactions, dizziness, NV, pharyngitis, somnolence.

INTERACTIONS: Potentiated BP elevation with peripheral and central vasoconstrictors. Additive coronary vasospastic effect with sumatriptan; avoid within 24 hrs of each other. Propranolol and nicotine may potentiate the vasoconstrictive action. Increased plasma levels and peripheral vasoconstriction with macrolides. Contraindicated with CYP3A4 inhibitors (eg, macrolides, protease inhibitors). Caution with less potent CYP3A4 inhibitors (eg, saquinavir, nefazodone, fluconazole, grapefruit juice, fluoxetine, fluvoxamine, zileuton, clotrimazole).

PREGNANCY: Category X, not for use in nursing.

MECHANISM OF ACTION: Ergotamine; binds with high affinity to 5-HT_{1D} receptors on intracranial blood vessels, causing vasoconstriction, or activates 5-HT_{1D} receptors on sensory nerve endings of trigeminal system, inhibiting proinflammatory neuropeptide release.

PHARMACOKINETICS: Absorption: Bioavailability (32%). **Distribution:** V_d=800L; plasma protein binding (93%). **Metabolism:** 8-β-hydroxydihydroergotamine (major metabolite). **Elimination:** Bile (major), urine (2%).

NURSING CONSIDERATIONS

Assessment: Assess for ischemic heart disease (angina pectoris, MI, silent ischemia), coronary artery vasospasm, Prinzmetal's variant angina, CAD or risk factors, HTN, peripheral arterial disease, sepsis, s/p vascular surgery, possible drug interaction, hemiplegic or basilar migraine, renal/hepatic impairment. Obtain baseline cardiac evaluation.

M

Monitoring: Perform periodic cardiac evaluations. Monitor for signs/symptoms of vasospasm, vasoconstriction, CV effects, and hypersensitivity reactions.

Patient Counseling: Once applicator prepared, discard after 8 hrs. Advise to seek medical attention immediately if numbness or tingling in fingers and toes, muscle pain in arms and legs, weakness in legs, chest pain, speeding or slowing of HR, swelling, or itching occur.

Administration: Intranasal. Prime (squeeze 4 times) before use. Spray once into each nostril; do not tilt back or sniff through nose while spraying or immediately after; wait 15 min; spray once again into each nostril. **Storage:** Below 25°C (77°F). Do not refrigerate, freeze, or keep opened vial for more than 8 hrs. Keep away from heat and light.

MINIPRESS RX

prazosin HCl (Pfizer)

THERAPEUTIC CLASS: $Alpha_1$-blocker (quinazoline)

INDICATIONS: Treatment of hypertension.

DOSAGE: *Adults:* Initial: 1mg bid-tid. Maint: 6-15mg/day in divided doses. Max: 40mg/day. Concomitant Diuretic/Antihypertensive: Reduce to 1-2mg tid, then retitrate.

HOW SUPPLIED: Cap: 1mg, 2mg, 5mg

WARNINGS/PRECAUTIONS: Syncope may occur, usually after initial dose or dose increase. Excessive postural hypotensive effects. Avoid driving for 24 hrs after 1st dose or dose increase. Always start on 1mg cap. False (+) for pheochromocytoma.

ADVERSE REACTIONS: Dizziness, headache, drowsiness, lack of energy, weakness, palpitations, nausea.

INTERACTIONS: Additive hypotensive effects with diuretics, β-blockers, or other antihypertensives. Dizziness or syncope may occur with alcohol.

PREGNANCY: Category C, caution in nursing.

MECHANISM OF ACTION: α_1 blocker; blockade of postsynaptic α-adrenoreceptors causes a reduction in total peripheral resistance.

PHARMACOKINETICS: Absorption: T_{max}=3 hrs. **Distribution:** Plasma protein binding (highly bound). **Metabolism:** Demethylation and conjugation. **Elimination:** Bile and feces; $T_{1/2}$=2-3 hrs.

NURSING CONSIDERATIONS

Assessment: Assess BP, LFTs, pregnancy status, and for possible drug interactions.

Monitoring: Monitor BP, LFTs, HR, ANA titer. Monitor for orthostatic hypotension, edema, epistaxis, lichen planus, angina pectoris.

Patient Counseling: Avoid driving or performing hazardous tasks for first 24 hrs; dizziness or drowsiness may occur. Avoid alcohol, standing for long periods, and exercising in hot weather. Counsel that getting up slowly may help prevent orthostatic hypotension.

Administration: Oral route.

MINOCIN RX

minocycline HCl (Triax)

THERAPEUTIC CLASS: Tetracycline derivative

INDICATIONS: Treatment of inclusion conjunctivitis, nongonococcal urethritis, and other infections (eg, respiratory tract, endocervical, rectal, urinary tract, skin and skin structure) caused by susceptible strains of microorganisms. Alternative treatment, when penicillin is contraindicated, in certain other infections (eg, urethritis, gonococcal, syphilis, anthrax). Adjunctive therapy in acute intestinal amebiasis and severe acne. Treatment of *Mycobacterium marinum* and asymptomatic carriers of *Neisseria meningitidis*.

DOSAGE: *Adults:* Usual: 200mg initially, then 100mg q12h; alternative is 100-200mg initially, then 50mg qid. Uncomplicated Gonococcal Infection (Men, other than urethritis and anorectal infections): 200mg initially, then 100mg q12h for minimum 4 days. Uncomplicated Gonococcal Urethritis (Men): 100mg q12h for 5 days. Syphilis: Administer usual dose for 10-15 days. Meningococcal Carrier State: 100mg q12h for 5 days. *Mycobacterium marinum:* 100mg q12h for 6-8 weeks. Uncomplicated Urethral, Endocervical, or Rectal Infection Caused by *Chlamydia trachomatis* or *Ureaplasma urealyticum*: 100mg q12h for at least 7 days. Gonorrhea in Patients Sensitive to PCN: 200mg initially, then 100mg q12h for at least 4 days, with post-therapy cultures within 2-3 days. Take with plenty of fluids. Renal Dysfunction: Max: 200mg/24 hrs. *Pediatrics:* >8 yrs: 4mg/kg initially followed by 2mg/kg q12h, not to exceed adult dose. Take with plenty of fluids. Renal Dysfunction: Max: 200mg/24 hrs.

HOW SUPPLIED: Cap: 50mg, 100mg; Inj: 100mg; Sus: 50mg/5mL [60mL]

WARNINGS/PRECAUTIONS: May cause fetal harm during pregnancy. Use during tooth development (last half of pregnancy, infancy, <8 yrs) may cause permanent discoloration of the teeth or enamel hypoplasia; avoid use during this period. Renal toxicity, hepatotoxicity, photosensitivity, increased BUN, superinfection, pseudotumor cerebri may occur; perform hematopoietic, renal, and hepatic monitoring. Caution with hepatic dysfunction. Caution in renal impairment; may lead to azotemia, hyperphosphatemia, and acidosis. Use alternate form of contraception other than oral contraceptives. May decrease bone growth in premature infants. If *Clostridium difficile*-associated diarrhea (CDAD) develops, appropriate therapy should be initiated.

ADVERSE REACTIONS: Anorexia, NV, diarrhea, dysphagia, enterocolitis, pancreatitis, increased LFTs, renal toxicity, rash, exfoliative dermatitis, Stevens-Johnson syndrome, skin and mucous membrane pigmentation, blood dyscrasias, headache, tooth discoloration.

INTERACTIONS: May require downward adjustments of anticoagulant dosage. May interfere with bactericidal action of penicillin; avoid concurrent use when possible. May decrease efficacy of oral contraceptives. Impaired absorption with antacids containing aluminum, calcium, or magnesium- and iron-containing products. Fatal renal toxicity with methoxyflurane has been reported. Avoid isotretinoin shortly before, during and after therapy. Caution with other hepatotoxic drugs. Risk of ergotism with ergot alkaloids.

PREGNANCY: Category D, not for use in nursing.

MECHANISM OF ACTION: Tetracycline; bacteriostatic, thought to inhibit protein synthesis.

PHARMACOKINETICS: Absorption: Rapid; C_{max}=3.5mcg/mL; T_{max}=2.1 hrs. **Elimination:** Urine, feces; $T_{1/2}$=15.5 hrs.

NURSING CONSIDERATIONS

Assessment: Assess for pregnancy status, possible drug interactions, hepatic/renal impairment.

Monitoring: Monitor renal function periodically and for signs/symptoms of hypersensitivity reactions, photosensitivity, superinfection, *C. difficile*-associated diarrhea, and pseudotumor cerebri.

Patient Counseling: Instruct to take at least 1 hr before or 2 hrs after meals; swallow whole and take with full glass of liquid. Inform of pregnancy risks and photosensitivity reactions (d/c at first sign of skin erythema). Inform therapy treats bacterial, not viral, infections. Take as directed; skipping doses or not completing full course may decrease effectiveness and increase resistance. Inform may experience diarrhea; notify physician if watery/bloody stools, hypersensitivity reactions, superinfection, photosensitivity, or pseudotumor cerebri (blurred vision, headache) occurs.

M

Administration: Oral route. **Storage:** 20-25°C (68-77°F). Protect from excess heat, moisture, and light.

MINOXIDIL RX

minoxidil (Par)

May cause pericardial effusion, occasionally progressing to tamponade, and angina pectoris may be exacerbated. Only for nonresponders to maximum therapeutic doses of two other antihypertensives and a diuretic. Administer under supervision with a β-blocker and diuretic. Monitor in hospital for a decrease in BP in those receiving guanethidine with malignant hypertension.

THERAPEUTIC CLASS: Peripheral vasodilator

INDICATIONS: Treatment of hypertension that is symptomatic or associated with target organ damage and is not manageable with maximum therapeutic doses of diuretic plus 2 other antihypertensive drugs.

DOSAGE: *Adults:* Initial: 5mg qd. Titrate: Increase by no less than 3 days; may increase every 6 hrs if closely monitored. Usual: 10-40mg/day. Max: 100mg/day. Frequency: Give qd if diastolic BP is reduced to <30mmHg and if reduced to >30mmHg give bid. Give with a diuretic (eg, HCTZ 50mg bid, furosemide 40mg bid) and a β-blocker (equivalent to propranolol 80-160mg/day) or methyldopa (250-750mg bid starting 24 hrs before therapy). Renal Failure/Dialysis: Reduce dose.

Pediatrics: >12 yrs: Initial: 5mg qd. Titrate: Increase by no less than 3 days; may increase every 6 hrs if closely monitored. Usual: 10-40mg/day. Max: 100mg/day. Frequency: Give qd if diastolic BP is reduced to <30mmHg and if reduced to >30mmHg give bid. Give with a diuretic (eg, HCTZ 50mg bid, furosemide 40mg bid) and a β-blocker (equivalent to propranolol 80-160mg/day) or methyldopa (250-750mg bid starting 24 hrs before therapy). <12 yrs: 0.2mg/kg qd. Titrate: May increase by 50-100% increments. Usual: 0.25-1mg/kg/day. Max: 50mg/day. Renal Failure/Dialysis: Reduce dose.

HOW SUPPLIED: Tab: 2.5mg*, 10mg* *scored

CONTRAINDICATIONS: Pheochromocytoma.

WARNINGS/PRECAUTIONS: Administer with a diuretic and β-blocker. Pericarditis, pericardial effusion and tamponade reported. With renal failure or dialysis, reduce dose to prevent renal failure exacerbation and precipitation of cardiac failure. Avoid rapid control with severe HTN. Monitor body wt, fluid and electrolyte balance. Extreme caution with post-MI. Hypersensitivity reactions reported.

ADVERSE REACTIONS: Salt and water retention, pericarditis, pericardial effusion, tamponade, hypertrichosis, NV, rash, ECG changes, hemodilution effects.

INTERACTIONS: Severe orthostatic hypotension with guanethidine.

PREGNANCY: Category C, not for use in nursing.

MECHANISM OF ACTION: Antihypertensive peripheral vasodilator; reduces systolic and diastolic BP by decreasing peripheral vascular resistance.

PHARMACOKINETICS: Absorption: Almost complete (90%); T_{max}=1 hr. **Metabolism:** Glucuronide conjugation. **Elimination:** Urine; $T_{1/2}$=4.2 hrs.

NURSING CONSIDERATIONS

Assessment: Assess for hypersensitivity, pheochromocytoma, MI, CHF, BP, pregnancy status, renal dysfunction, and possible drug interactions.

Monitoring: Monitor fluid and electrolyte balance, body weight, HR, BP, pericarditis, cerebrovascular episodes, orthostatic effects, hypertrichosis, Stevens-Johnson syndrome, renal functions, ECG, EKG, chest x-ray, urinalysis, for thrombocytopenia, leukopenia, and NV. Observe for signs/symptoms of pericardial effusion.

Patient Counseling: Instruct to take as directed; do not d/c without consulting physician. Do not skip doses. If dose is missed, wait until time for next dose and continue with regular schedule. Advise to immediately report any adverse effects (eg, NV, rash, change in HR or body weight, headache, fatigue, breast tenderness, chest pain, dizziness, difficulty breathing). Inform that body hair may grow darker or longer on certain parts of the body within 3-6 weeks from start and will disappear within 1-6 months after completion.

Administration: Oral route. **Storage:** 15-30°C (59-86°F). Dispense in tight, child-resistant container.

M

MIRALAX — OTC

polyethylene glycol 3350 (Schering-Plough)

THERAPEUTIC CLASS: Osmotic laxative

INDICATIONS: Treatment of occasional constipation.

DOSAGE: *Adults:* Stir and dissolve 17g in 4-8 oz of beverage and drink qd. Use no more than 7 days.
Pediatrics: ≥17 yrs: Stir and dissolve 17g in 4-8 oz of beverage and drink qd. Use no more than 7 days.

HOW SUPPLIED: Powder: 17g/dose [119g, 238g]

WARNINGS/PRECAUTIONS: Avoid in kidney disease.

MIRAPEX — RX

pramipexole dihydrochloride (Boehringer Ingelheim)

THERAPEUTIC CLASS: Non-ergot dopamine agonist

INDICATIONS: Treatment of signs and symptoms of idiopathic Parkinson's disease. Treatment of moderate-to-severe primary Restless Legs Syndrome (RLS).

DOSAGE: *Adults:* Parkinson's: Initial: 0.125mg tid. Titrate: May increase every 5-7 days (eg, Week 2: 0.25mg tid; Week 3: 0.5mg tid; Week 4: 0.75mg tid; Week 5: 1mg tid; Week 6: 1.25mg tid; Week 7: 1.5mg tid). Maint: 0.5-1.5mg tid. Max: 1.5mg tid. CrCl >60mL/min: Initial: 0.125mg tid. Max: 1.5mg tid. CrCl 35-59mL/min: Initial: 0.125mg bid. Max: 1.5mg bid. CrCl 15-34mL/min: Initial:

0.125mg qd. Max: 1.5mg qd. RLS: Initial: 0.125mg once daily, 2-3 hours before bedtime. Titrate: May double dose every 4-7 days up to 0.5mg/day.

HOW SUPPLIED: Tab: 0.125mg, 0.25mg*, 0.5mg*, 0.75mg, 1mg*, 1.5mg*
*scored

WARNINGS/PRECAUTIONS: Somnolence, symptomatic hypotension, hallucinations and rhabdomyolysis reported. Caution with renal insufficiency. May potentiate dyskinesia. May cause retinal pathology, fibrotic complications, withdrawal-emergent hyperpyrexia and confusion. Consider discontinuation if significant daytime sleepiness or sudden onset of sleep occurs during daily activities. Cases of pathological gambling, hypersexuality, and compulsive eating reported. Rebound and augmentation in RLS reported. Falling asleep during activities of daily living. Melanoma reported; monitor regularly.

ADVERSE REACTIONS: Nausea, dizziness, somnolence, insomnia, constipation, asthenia, hallucination, vision abnormalities, peripheral edema, arthritis, dry mouth, postural hypotension, chest pain, malaise.

INTERACTIONS: Cimetidine, ranitidine, diltiazem, triamterene, verapamil, quinidine, and quinine may decrease clearance. Dopamine antagonists (eg, phenothiazines, butyrophenones, thioxanthenes, metoclopramide) may decrease effects.

PREGNANCY: Category C, not for use in nursing.

MECHANISM OF ACTION: Non-ergot dopamine agonist; suspected to stimulate dopamine receptors on the striatum.

PHARMACOKINETICS: Absorption: Rapid, absolute bioavailability (>90%), T_{max}=2 hrs. **Distribution:** V_d=500L; plasma protein binding (15%). **Elimination:** Urine (90% unchanged); $T_{1/2}$=12hrs (elderly).

NURSING CONSIDERATIONS

M

Assessment: Assess for symptomatic hypotension, sleep disorders, renal function test, dyskinesia, retinal exam. Note other diseases/conditions and drug therapies.

Monitoring: Monitor BP, renal function test, signs/symptoms of rhabdomyolysis, NMS, melanomas, fibrotic complications, hallucinations, impulse control behaviors/compulsive behaviors.

Patient Counseling: Instruct to take with/without food. Caution while operating machinery/driving. Counsel about impulse control disorders/compulsive behaviors; avoid concomitant use of alcohol; report side effects. Notify physician if intense urge to gamble, increased sexual urges, and other intense urges occur.

Administration: Oral route. **Storage:** 25°C (77°F); excursions permitted to 15-30°C (59-86°F). Protect from light.

MIRCETTE — RX

desogestrel - ethinyl estradiol (Duramed)

OTHER BRAND NAMES: Kariva (Barr)

THERAPEUTIC CLASS: Estrogen/progestogen combination

INDICATIONS: Prevention of pregnancy.

DOSAGE: *Adults:* Start 1st Sunday after menses begin or 1st day of menses. 28-day: 1 tab qd for 28 days, then repeat.

HOW SUPPLIED: Tab: (Ethinyl Estradiol-Desogestrel) 0.02mg-0.15mg and 0.01mg-NA

CONTRAINDICATIONS: Thrombophlebitis, DVT or thromboembolic disorders, pregnancy, cerebrovascular or coronary artery disease, undiagnosed abnormal genital bleeding, cholestatic jaundice of pregnancy or jaundice with prior pill use, hepatic adenomas or carcinomas, breast cancer or other estrogen-dependent neoplasia.

WARNINGS/PRECAUTIONS: Cigarette smoking increases risk of serious cardiovascular side effects. This risk increases with age (especially >35 yrs)

and heavy smoking. Increased risk of MI, vascular disease, thromboembolism, stroke and gallbladder disease. Retinal thrombosis, hepatic neoplasia, carcinoma of breast and reproductive organs reported. May cause glucose intolerance. May increase BP, elevate LDL levels or cause other lipid changes, fluid retention, breakthrough bleeding, and spotting. May cause or exacerbate migraine. May develop visual changes with contact lens. Increased risk of MI with HTN, hyperlipidemia, obesity, and diabetes. D/C if jaundice, significant depression, or ophthalmic irregularities develop. Perform annual physical exam. Use before menarche is not indicated. May affect certain endocrine, LFTs and blood components.

ADVERSE REACTIONS: NV, breakthrough bleeding, spotting, amenorrhea, migraine, depression, vaginal candidiasis, edema, weight changes.

INTERACTIONS: Reduced effects, increased breakthrough bleeding, and menstrual irregularities with rifampin, barbiturates, phenylbutazone, phenytoin, carbamazepine, and possibly with griseofulvin, ampicillin, and tetracyclines.

PREGNANCY: Category X, not for use in nursing.

MECHANISM OF ACTION: Oral contraceptive combination; supresses gonadotropins, inhibits ovulation, increases difficulty of sperm entry into uterus, and reduces likelihood of implantation by producing changes in cervical mucus and endometrium, respectively.

PHARMACOKINETICS: Absorption: Desogestrel: Rapid, complete; relative bioavailability (100%). Ethinyl estradiol: Rapid, complete; absolute bioavailability (93-99%). **Distribution:** Desogestrel: Sex hormone-binding globulin (99%, metabolite). Ethinyl estradiol: Plasma protein binding (98.3%). **Metabolism:** Desogestrel: Hydroxylation in intestinal mucosa; etonogestrel (metabolite). Ethinyl estradiol: Conjugation. **Elimination:** Urine, bile, feces. Desogestrel: $T_{1/2}$=27.8 hrs (metabolite). Ethinyl estradiol: $T_{1/2}$=23.9 hrs.

M

NURSING CONSIDERATIONS

Assessment: Assess for history or recent DVT or thromboembolic disorders, thrombophlebitis, CVD, CAD, breast cancer, endometrium or other estrogen-dependent neoplasia, abnormal genital bleeding, cholestatic jaundice of pregnancy or jaundice with prior pill use, hepatic adenomas or carcinomas, and pregnancy. Obtain complete medical history and physical exam with special reference to BP, breasts, abdomen and pelvic organs, cervical cytology, and relevant lab tests.

Monitoring: Monitor for thromboembolic disorders and other vascular problems, malignant neoplasms, MI, stroke, hepatic neoplasia, jaundice, emotional disorders, ocular lesions, gallbladder disease, carbohydrate and lipid metabolic effects, elevated BP, bleeding irregularities, migraine headaches, lipid profile (HDL, LDL, TG), LFTs, PT, TBG, T_3 and T_4, blood glucose, and serum folate levels.

Patient Counseling: Strongly advise not to smoke; increases risk of cardiovascular side effects. Instruct to take daily at same time as directed. Counsel that light bleeding is possible. Inform that drug does not protect against HIV infections/AIDS and other STDs. Caution that some drugs decrease efficacy, and to consult with physician before use to determine appropriate back-up contraceptive method. Advise to immediately report sharp chest pains, coughing of blood, sudden SOB, pain in calf, severe headache and vomiting, dizziness or fainting, disturbances of vision or speech, severe pain or tenderness in stomach area, difficulty sleeping, weakness, changes in mood, and jaundice.

Administration: Oral route. **Storage:** 20-25°C (68-77°F).

MIRENA

RX

levonorgestrel (Bayer Healthcare)

THERAPEUTIC CLASS: Progestogen

INDICATIONS: For intrauterine contraception.

DOSAGE: *Adults:* Insert intravaginally for contraception. Initial insertion is recommended within 7 days of the onset of menses. Replacement may be done at any time in the cycle. May insert 6 weeks postpartum or until involution of uterus is complete, and immediately after 1st trimester abortion. Reexamine within 3 months after insertion. Replace every 5 yrs.

HOW SUPPLIED: Intrauterine Insert: 52mg

CONTRAINDICATIONS: Pregnancy, congenital or acquired uterine anomaly, acute or history of PID, postpartum endometriosis, infected abortion in the past 3 months, uterine or cervical neoplasia, abnormal Pap smear, genital bleeding of unknown etiology, untreated acute cervicitis or vaginitis, acute liver disease, liver tumor, women or partner with multiple sexual partners, conditions associated with increased susceptibility to microorganisms, genital actinomycosis, previously inserted IUD that is not removed, breast carcinoma, and predisposition to ectopic pregnancy.

WARNINGS/PRECAUTIONS: Risk of ectopic pregnancy, glucose intolerance. Pregnancy with IUD in place, increases risk of septic abortion, congenital anomalies, premature labor, miscarriage. Increased risk of PID, sepsis, ovarian cysts. Can alter bleeding patterns. Partial penetration or embedment in myometrium may decrease effectiveness. May perforate the uterus or cervix during insertion. Displacement may occur.

ADVERSE REACTIONS: Abdominal pain, leukorrhea, headache, vaginitis, back pain, breast pain, acne, depression, HTN, upper respiratory infection, nausea, dysmenorrhea, weight increase, skin disorder, decreased libido, abnormal pap smear.

INTERACTIONS: Enzyme inducers may decrease effectiveness.

PREGNANCY: Category X, not for use in nursing.

MECHANISM OF ACTION: Progestrone; not conclusively demonstrated. Thickening of cervical mucus preventing passage of sperm into uterus, inhibition of sperm capacitation or survival, and alteration of endometrium.

M

PHARMACOKINETICS: Absorption: C_{max}(20mcg/day)=150-200pg/mL. **Distribution:** Found in breast milk.

NURSING CONSIDERATIONS

Assessment: Perform complete medical and social history (including that of partner), pelvic exam, ultrasonography of uterus to assess patency of endocervical canal and congenital or acquired uterine anomalies (eg, fibroids and endometriosis), pap smear, tests for STDs, risk of pelvic inflammatory disease (PID), ectopic pregnancy or condition that would predispose to ectopic pregnancy, pregnancy status, previous infected abortion, cervical/uterine neoplasia, genital bleeding, cervicitis/vaginitis, genital actimycosis, hepatic diseases or tumors, cardiovascular diseases, coagulopathy/receiving anticoagulants, immune status, previous IUD insertion, product hypersensitivity, breast cancer, and possible drug interactions.

Monitoring: Monitor for ectopic pregnancy, intrauterine pregnancy, miscarriage, sepsis, premature labor, premature delivery, and congenital anomalies of baby, Group A streptococcal sepsis, PID, irregular bleeding/amenorrhea, partial penetration/embedment, perforation, ovarian cysts, and blood glucose in diabetics.

Patient Counseling: Advise that drug does not protect against HIV infection (AIDS) and other STDs. Inform of risks/benefits of the device. Advise to immediately report any symptoms of PID (eg, menstrual disorders, unusual vaginal discharge, abdominal/pelvic pain/tenderness, dyspareunia, chills, fever) and if partner becomes HIV-positive or acquires an STD.

Administration: Administered into the uterine cavity. **Storage**: 25°C (77°F); excursions permitted to 15-30°C (59-86°F).

M-M-R II RX

rubella vaccine live - measles vaccine live - mumps vaccine live (Merck)

THERAPEUTIC CLASS: Vaccine

INDICATIONS: Vaccination against measles, mumps, and rubella.

DOSAGE: *Adults:* 0.5mL SQ into outer aspect of upper arm.
Pediatrics: 12-15 months: 0.5mL SQ into outer aspect of upper arm. Repeat before entering elementary school. If vaccinated at 6-12 months due to measles outbreak, give another dose between 12-15 months and then before entering elementary school.

HOW SUPPLIED: Inj: 0.5mL

CONTRAINDICATIONS: Pregnant females and avoid pregnancy for 3 months after vaccine, anaphylactic reaction to neomycin, febrile/active respiratory illness, immunosuppressive therapy (except corticosteroids as replacement therapy), blood dyscrasias, leukemia, lymphoma, malignant neoplasms affecting bone marrow or lymphatic system, immunodeficiency states and family history of congenital or hereditary immunodeficiency.

WARNINGS/PRECAUTIONS: Caution with egg allergy, cerebral injury, and individual/family history of convulsions. Avoid conditions that cause stress due to fever. Defer vaccination for 3 months after blood or plasma transfusions or administration of human immune globulin. Avoid pregnancy for 3 months after vaccination. May worsen thrombocytopenia. Contains albumin, remote risk of viral infection transmission. Have epinephrine (1:1000) available.

ADVERSE REACTIONS: Atypical measles, fever, syncope, headache, dizziness, malaise, diarrhea, local reactions, vomiting, nausea, arthralgia, pneumonitis, sore throat, Stevens-Johnson syndrome.

INTERACTIONS: Do not give with immune globulin. May depress TB skin sensitivity, administer test either simultaneously or before. Do not give <1 month before or after other live viral vaccines. Do not give simultaneously with DTP or oral poliovirus vaccine.

PREGNANCY: Category C, caution in nursing.

MECHANISM OF ACTION: May induce antibodies that may protect against measles, mumps, and rubella.

NURSING CONSIDERATIONS

Assessment: Assess for immune and current health/medical status, history of blood dyscrasias, previous sensitivity/vaccination history, family history of neurological or immunodeficiency disorders, and possible drug interactions.

Monitoring: Monitor for anaphylactoid reactions, panniculitis, atypical measles, fever, syncope, headache, dizziness, malaise, irritability, vasculitis, pancreatitis, DM, diarrhea, NV, thrombocytopenia, encephalitis, optic neuritis, and orchitis.

Patient Counseling: Inform patients or caregivers of benefits/risks ratio; report any adverse reactions. Do not take during pregnancy or with active untreated TB.

Administration: SQ route. **Storage:** 2-8°C (36-46°F). Do not freeze.

MOBIC — RX

meloxicam (Boehringer Ingelheim)

NSAIDs may cause an increased risk of serious cardiovascular thrombotic events, MI, stroke and serious GI adverse events including bleeding, ulceration, and perforation of the stomach or intestines. Contraindicated for the treatment of perioperative pain in the setting of coronary artery bypass graft (CABG) surgery.

THERAPEUTIC CLASS: NSAID

INDICATIONS: Relief of signs and symptoms of osteoarthritis (OA) and rheumatoid arthritis (RA). Relief of the signs and symptoms of pauciarticular or polyarticular course juvenile rheumatoid arthritis (JRA) in patients ≥2 yrs.

DOSAGE: *Adults:* ≥18 yrs: OA/RA: Initial/Maint: 7.5mg qd. Max: 15mg/day.
Pediatrics: >2 yrs: JRA: 0.125mg/kg qd. Max: 7.5mg/day.

HOW SUPPLIED: Sus: 7.5mg/5mL; Tab: 7.5mg, 15mg

CONTRAINDICATIONS: ASA or other NSAID allergy that precipitates asthma, urticaria, or allergic-type reactions. Treatment of perioperative pain in the setting of CABG surgery.

WARNINGS/PRECAUTIONS: May lead to onset of new HTN or worsening of pre-existing HTN; monitor BP closely. Fluid retention and edema reported; caution with fluid retention, HTN, or heart failure. Renal papillary necrosis, renal insufficiency, acute renal failure, and other renal injury reported after long-term use. Not recommended for use with advanced renal disease; if therapy must be initiated, monitor renal function. Anaphylactoid reactions may occur. May cause serious skin adverse events (eg, exfoliative dermatitis, Stevens-Johnson syndrome, and toxic epidermal necrolysis). Avoid in late pregnancy; may cause premature closure of ductus arteriosis. May cause elevations of LFTs; d/c if liver disease develops or systemic manifestations occur. Caution with considerable dehydration and in elderly. Anemia may occur; with long-term use, monitor Hgb/Hct if signs or symptoms of anemia develop. May inhibit platelet aggregation and prolong bleeding time; monitor with coagulation disorders. Caution with asthma and avoid with ASA-sensitive asthma.

ADVERSE REACTIONS: Abdominal pain, constipation, diarrhea, dyspepsia, NV, headache, anemia, arthralgia, insomnia, upper respiratory tract infection, UTI.

INTERACTIONS: May decrease antihypertensive effects of ACE inhibitors. Potentiates GI bleeds with ASA; avoid concomitant use. Increased clearance with cholestyramine. May decrease natriuretic effects of furosemide, thiazides. Decreased lithium clearance/increased serum levels. Monitor PT/INR with warfarin. Caution with methotrexate.

PREGNANCY: Category C, not for use in nursing.

MECHANISM OF ACTION: NSAIDs; unknown, may inhibit prostaglandin synthetase.

M

PHARMACOKINETICS: Absorption: Absolute bioavailability (89%), C_{max}=1.05mcg/mL, T_{max}=4.9 hrs. **Distribution:** V_d=10 L/kg, plasma protein binding (99.4%). **Metabolism:** Hepatic (oxidation) via CYP2C9 (major), CYP3A4 (minor). **Elimination:** Urine (0.2%), feces (1.6%); $T_{1/2}$=20.1 hrs. Significant biliary and/or enteral secretion.

NURSING CONSIDERATIONS

Assessment: Assess for history of asthma, cardiovascular disease (pre-existing HTN, CHF) or risk factors for disease, fluid retention, edema, increased risk of serious cardiovascular thrombotic events, stroke, pregnancy status, risk factors for GI events (bleeding, ulceration, perforation), possible drug interactions, renal/hepatic dysfunction.

Monitoring: Monitor CBC, LFTs, renal function, and chemistries periodically. Monitor for signs/symptoms of GI events (bleeding, ulceration, perforation), CV thrombotic events, CHF, HTN, salt depletion, renal/liver dysfunction.

Patient Counseling: Seek medical attention if symptoms of hepatotoxicity (nausea, fatigue, pruritus), anaphylactic reaction (difficulty breathing, swelling of face/throat), hypersensitivity reaction (rash), CV events (chest pain, SOB, weakness, slurring of speech), GI ulceration and bleeding (epigastric pain, dyspepsia, melena, hematemesis), weight gain, or edema occur. Inform of pregnancy risks. Caution may impair physical/mental abilities if experience drowsiness, dizziness, vertigo, or depression during therapy.

Administration: Oral route. **Storage:** (Tab; Sus): 25°C (77°F); excursions permitted to 15-30°C (59-86°F).

MONODOX — RX

doxycycline monohydrate (Watson)

THERAPEUTIC CLASS: Tetracycline derivative

INDICATIONS: Treatment of rocky mountain spotted fever, typhus fever and the typhus group, Q fever, rickettsialpox, and ticks fever, respiratory tract, urinary tract, skin and skin structure, inclusion conjunctivitis, uncomplicated urethral/endocervical/rectal infection caused by *C.trachomatis*, nongonococcal urethritis caused by *C.trachomatis* and *U.urealyticum*, lymphogranuloma, psittacosis, trachoma, tularemia, campylobacter fetus, yaws, vincent's infection, actinomycosis, chancroid, plague, cholera, brucellosis. Treatment of uncomplicated gonorrhea, syphilis, listeriosis, anthrax, *Clostridium* species when PCN is contraindicated. Adjunct therapy for amebicides and severe acne.

DOSAGE: *Adults:* Usual: 100mg q12h or 50mg q6h for 1 day, then 100mg/day. Severe Infection: 100mg q12h. Uncomplicated Gonococcal Infections (except anorectal infections in men): 100mg bid for 7 days or 300mg stat, then repeat in 1 hr. Acute Epididymo-Orchitis caused by *N.gonorrhea* or *C.trachomatis:* 100mg bid for at least 10 days. Primary/Secondary Syphilis: 300mg/day in divided dose for at least 10 days. Uncomplicated Urethral/Endocervical/ Rectal Infection caused by *C.trachomatis:* 100mg bid for at least 7 days. Nongonococcal Urethritis caused by *C.trachomatis* and *U.urealyticum:* 100mg bid for at least 7 days. Take with full glass of water. Take with food if GI upset occurs. Inhalational Anthrax (post-exposure): 100mg bid for 60 days. *Pediatrics:* >8 yrs: ≤100 lbs: 2mg/lb divided in 2 doses for 1 day, then 1mg/ lb daily in single or 2 divided doses. Severe Infection: May use up to 2mg/lb/ day. >100 lbs: 100mg q12h or 50mg q6h for 1 day, then 100mg/day. Severe Infection: 100mg q12h. Take with full glass of water. Take with food if GI upset occurs.

HOW SUPPLIED: Cap: 50mg, 75mg, 100mg

WARNINGS/PRECAUTIONS: Avoid direct sunlight or UV light. May cause permanent tooth discoloration during tooth development (last half of pregnancy and children <8 years). Enamel hypoplasia reported. Monitor renal/ hepatic function, and blood with long-term therapy. May increase BUN. Photosensitivity, pseudotumor cerebri reported. D/C if superinfection occurs. Bulging fontanels in infants and intracranial HTN in adults reported. *Clostridium difficile*-associated diarrhea reported.

ADVERSE REACTIONS: GI effects, photosensitivity, rash, blood dyscrasias, hypersensitivity reactions.

INTERACTIONS: Carbamazepine, barbiturates, phenytoin decrease half-life of doxycycline. May decrease PT; adjust anticoagulants. May decrease bactericidal agents (eg, penicillin). May decrease effects of oral contraceptives. Take 1 hr before or 2 hrs after dairy products. Aluminum-, calcium-, iron-, and magnesium-containing products and bismuth subsalicylate impair absorption. Fatal renal toxicity may occur with methoxyflurane.

PREGNANCY: Category D, not for use in nursing.

MECHANISM OF ACTION: Tetracycline; bacteriostatic, thought to inhibit protein synthesis.

PHARMACOKINETICS: Absorption: C_{max}=3.61mcg/mL; T_{max}=2.6 hrs. **Elimination**: Urine, feces; $T_{1/2}$=16.33 hrs.

NURSING CONSIDERATIONS

Assessment: Assess for pregnancy status, possible drug interactions, and renal impairment.

Monitoring: Monitor for signs/symptoms of hypersensitivity reactions, photosensitivity, superinfection, *C. difficile*-associated diarrhea, vaginal candidiasis, and benign intracranial HTN.

Patient Counseling: Inform of pregnancy risks and photosensitivity reactions (d/c at 1st sign of skin erythema). Advise to avoid excessive sunlight/UV light and wear sunscreen or sunblock. Instruct to drink fluid liberally to reduce risk of esophageal irritation or ulceration. Inform therapy treats bacterial, not viral, infections. Take as directed; skipping doses or not completing full course may decrease effectiveness and increase resistance. Inform may experience diarrhea; notify physician if watery/bloody stools, hypersensitivity reactions, superinfections, photosensitivity, or benign intracranial HTN occur.

Administration: Oral route. **Storage**: 20-25°C (68-77°F).

MONOKET RX

isosorbide mononitrate (Schwarz)

THERAPEUTIC CLASS: Nitrate vasodilator

INDICATIONS: Prevention and treatment of angina pectoris. Not for acute attack.

DOSAGE: *Adults:* 20mg bid (space doses 7 hours apart). Small Stature Patients: Initial: 5mg per dose for 1 day, then increase to 10mg by 2nd or 3rd day.

HOW SUPPLIED: Tab: 10mg*, 20mg* *scored

WARNINGS/PRECAUTIONS: Not for use with acute MI or CHF. Severe hypotension may occur; caution with volume depletion or hypotension. May aggravate angina caused by hypertrophic cardiomyopathy. Monitor for tolerance.

ADVERSE REACTIONS: Headache, dizziness, fatigue, GI upset.

INTERACTIONS: Severe hypotension with sildenafil. Marked orthostatic hypotension with CCBs. Additive vasodilation with other vasodilators (eg, alcohol).

PREGNANCY: Category B, caution with nursing.

MECHANISM OF ACTION: Nitrate vasodilator; relaxes vascular smooth muscle, and consequent dilatation of peripheral arteries and veins, especially the latter. Dilatation of veins leads to reducing the left ventricular end-diastolic pressure and pulmonary capillary wedge pressure (preload). Arteriolar relaxation reduces systemic vascular resistance, systolic arterial pressure, and mean arterial pressure (afterload). It also dilates the coronary artery.

M

PHARMACOKINETICS: Absorption: (Tab, 60mg) C_{max}=557-572ng/mL, T_{max}=2.9-4.2 hrs, AUC=6625-7555ng•hr/mL. (120mg) C_{max}=1151-1180ng/mL, T_{max}=3.1-3.2 hrs, AUC=14241-16800ng•hr/mL. **Distribution:** V_d=0.6-0.7L/kg, plasma protein binding (5%). **Metabolism:** Liver. Cleared through glucuronidation pathways. **Elimination:** Urine (96%), feces (1%); (60mg) $T_{1/2}$=6.2-6.3 hrs; (120mg) $T_{1/2}$=6.2-6.4 hrs.

NURSING CONSIDERATIONS

Assessment: Assess for severe hypotension or volume-depleted patients, angina caused by hypertrophic cardiomyopathy, pregnancy status, alcohol intake, and possible drug interactions.

Monitoring: Careful clinical or hemodynamic monitoring for hypotension and tachycardia. Monitor for paradoxical bradycardia and increased angina pectoris, headaches and lightheadedness on standing, manifestation of true physical dependence (chest pain, acute MI). Monitor for the interference with Zlatkis-Zak color reaction, causing false low readings in cholesterol levels and for manifestations of methemoglobinemia.

Patient Counseling: Counsel to carefully follow dosing regimen. Inform about headaches (markers of drug activity) and lightheadedness on standing. Avoid alcohol consumption.

Administration: Oral route. **Storage:** 20-25°C (68-77°F).

MONOPRIL RX

fosinopril sodium (Bristol-Myers Squibb)

ACE inhibitors can cause death/injury to developing fetus during 2nd and 3rd trimesters. Stop therapy if pregnancy detected.

THERAPEUTIC CLASS: ACE inhibitor

INDICATIONS: Treatment of hypertension. Adjunct therapy for heart failure.

DOSAGE: *Adults:* If possible, d/c diuretic 2-3 days before therapy. Initial: 10mg qd, monitor carefully if cannot d/c diuretic. Maint: 20-40mg/day. Resume diuretic if BP not controlled. Max: 80mg/day. Heart Failure: Initial: 10mg qd, 5mg with moderate to severe renal failure or vigorous diuresis. Titrate: Increase over several weeks. Maint: 20-40mg qd. Max: 40mg qd. Elderly: Start at low end of dosing range.

HOW SUPPLIED: Tab: 10mg*, 20mg, 40mg *scored

CONTRAINDICATIONS: History of ACE inhibitor associated angioedema.

WARNINGS/PRECAUTIONS: D/C if angioedema, jaundice, or if marked LFT elevation occur. Risk of hyperkalemia with DM, renal dysfunction. Persistent non-productive cough reported. Monitor WBCs in renal and collagen vascular disease. Anaphylactoid reactions reported. Fetal/neonatal morbidity and death reported. Monitor for hypotension in high-risk patients (heart failure, volume and/or salt depletion, surgery/anesthesia, etc.). Less effective on BP in blacks and more reports of angioedema than nonblacks. Caution with CHF, renal or hepatic dysfunction, renal artery stenosis. May cause false low measurement of serum digoxin level.

ADVERSE REACTIONS: Dizziness, cough, hypotension, musculoskeletal pain.

INTERACTIONS: May increase lithium levels. Hypotension risk with diuretics. Increased risk of hyperkalemia with K^+-sparing diuretics, K^+-containing salt substitutes, or K^+ supplements. Decreased absorption with antacids; space dosing by 2 hrs.

PREGNANCY: Category C (1st trimester) and D (2nd and 3rd trimesters), not for use in nursing.

MECHANISM OF ACTION: ACE inhibitor; inhibition results in decreased plasma angiotensin II, which leads to decreased vasopressor activity and decreased aldosterone secretion.

PHARMACOKINETICS: Absorption: Slow; T_{max}=3 hrs. **Distribution**: Plasma protein binding (99.4%). **Metabolism:** Hepatic, glucuronidation. **Elimination:** Renal; $T_{1/2}$=11.5 hrs.

M

NURSING CONSIDERATIONS

Assessment: Assess BP, LFTs, renal function, CHF, renal artery stenosis, pregnancy status, and for possible drug interactions.

Monitoring: Monitor BP, LFTs, renal function, CBC with platelet and differential count, serum potassium levels. Monitor for MI, CHF, head/neck and intestinal angioedema, anaphylactoid reactions, hepatic failure, hypersensitivity reactions, cough, NV, and dizziness.

Patient Counseling: Counsel about fetal risks during pregnancy and signs/symptoms of angioedema (laryngeal edema, tongue edema, abdominal pain); advise to seek prompt medical attention if symptoms develop. Inform about potential adverse effects (anaphylaxis, cough, hypotension, hyperkalemia). Inform about need for periodic monitoring of electrolytes and blood counts. Caution that inadequate fluid intake, excessive perspiration, diarrhea, vomiting can lead to excessive fall in BP, resulting in lightheadedness and possible syncope.

Administration: Oral route. **Storage:** 25°C (77°F); excursions permitted to 15-30°C (59-86°F). Protect from moisture; keep bottle tightly closed.

MONOPRIL HCT RX

fosinopril sodium - hydrochlorothiazide (Bristol-Myers Squibb)

ACE inhibitors can cause death/injury to developing fetus during 2nd and 3rd trimesters. Stop therapy if pregnancy detected.

THERAPEUTIC CLASS: ACE inhibitor/thiazide diuretic

INDICATIONS: Hypertension. Not for initial therapy.

DOSAGE: *Adults:* Initial (if not controlled with fosinopril/HCTZ monotherapy): 12.5mg-10mg tab or 12.5mg-20mg tab qd.

HOW SUPPLIED: Tab: (Fosinopril-HCTZ) 10mg-12.5mg, 20mg-12.5mg

CONTRAINDICATIONS: Anuria, sulfonamide hypersensitivity.

WARNINGS/PRECAUTIONS: D/C if angioedema, jaundice, or marked LFT elevation occurs. Risk of hyperkalemia with DM, renal dysfunction. Persistent nonproductive cough reported. Monitor WBCs in renal and collagen vascular disease. Anaphylactoid reactions reported. Fetal/neonatal morbidity and death reported. Monitor for hypotension in high-risk patients (eg, surgery/anesthesia, volume/salt depletion). Caution with CHF, renal or hepatic dysfunction. More reports of angioedema in blacks than nonblacks. May exacerbate or activate SLE. Monitor electrolytes. Avoid if CrCl ≤30mL/min/1.7m². May increase cholesterol, TG. Hypercalcemia, hypomagnesemia, hyperuricemia may occur.

ADVERSE REACTIONS: Headache, cough, fatigue, dizziness, upper respiratory infection, musculoskeletal pain.

INTERACTIONS: Increased risk of hyperkalemia with K^+-sparing diuretics, K^+ supplements, or K^+-containing salt substitutes. Risk of lithium toxicity. Antacids may impair absorption; separate dose by 2 hrs. May alter insulin requirements. May increase responsiveness to tubocurarine. NSAIDs reduce effects. May decrease effects of methenamine. Reduced absorption with cholestyramine, colestipol. Caution with other antihypertensives. May decrease response to norepinephrine.

PREGNANCY: Category C (1st trimester) and D (2nd and 3rd trimesters), not for use in nursing.

MECHANISM OF ACTION: ACE inhibitor; inhibition results in decreased plasma angiotensin II, which leads to decreased vasopressor activity and decreased aldosterone secretion. Thiazide diuretic; affects renal tubular mechanism of electrolyte reabsorption directly increasing excretion of sodium salt and chloride.

PHARMACOKINETICS: Absorption: Fosinopril: Slow, T_{max}=3 hrs; HCTZ: T_{max}=1-2.5 hrs. **Distribution**: Fosinopril: Plasma protein binding (95%). HCTZ: V_d =3.6-7.8L; plasma protein binding (67.9%). **Metabolism:** Hepatic, glucuronidation. **Elimination:** Fosinopril: Renal, $T_{1/2}$=11.5 hrs. HCTZ: Renal; $T_{1/2}$=5-15 hrs.

M

NURSING CONSIDERATIONS

Assessment: Assess BP, LFTs, renal function, CHF, renal artery stenosis, SLE, serum electrolytes, pregnancy status, history of allergy to sulfonamides, bronchial asthma, parathyroid disorders, and for possible drug interactions.

Monitoring: Monitor BP, LFT, renal functions, CBC with platelet and differential count, serum electrolytes. Monitor for MI, CHF, angioedema of head/neck and intestines, anaphylactoid reactions, hepatic failure, hyperuricemia, hyperglycemia, hypersensitivity reactions, cough, NV, dizziness.

Patient Counseling: Inform about fetal risks if taken during pregnancy. Caution that inadequate fluid intake, excessive perspiration, diarrhea, or vomiting can lead to excessive fall in BP, with the same consequences of lightheadedness and possible syncope. Advise not to use salt or K^+ supplements. Counsel about signs/symptoms of neutropenia (infections), angioedema, electrolyte imbalance (thirst, weakness, lethargy), and other adverse effects; advise to seek prompt medical attention.

Administration: Oral route. **Storage:** 25°C (77°F); excursions permitted to 15-30°C (59-86°F). Protect from moisture by keeping bottle tightly closed.

MORPHINE SULFATE IMMEDIATE RELEASE CII

morphine sulfate (Various)

THERAPEUTIC CLASS: Opioid analgesic

INDICATIONS: Relief of severe pain.

DOSAGE: *Adults:* (Sol) 10-20mg q4h. (Tab) 15-30mg q4h.

HOW SUPPLIED: Sol: 10mg/5mL, 20mg/5mL [100mL, 500mL]; Tab: 15mg*, 30mg* *scored

CONTRAINDICATIONS: Respiratory insufficiency or depression; severe CNS depression; attack of bronchial asthma; heart failure secondary to chronic lung disease; cardiac arrhythmias; increased ICP or CSF pressure; head injuries; brain tumor; acute alcoholism; delirium tremens; convulsive disorders; after biliary tract surgery; suspected surgical abdomen; surgical anastomosis; concomitantly with MAOIs or within 14 days of such treatment.

WARNINGS/PRECAUTIONS: May cause tolerance, psychological/physical dependence; avoid abrupt withdrawal. Caution with head injury, increased ICP, acute asthma attack, chronic COPD or cor pulmonale, decreased respiratory reserve, pre-existing respiratory depression, hypoxia, hypercapnia, elderly, debilitated, severe hepatic/renal impairment, hypothyroidism, Addison's disease, prostatic hypertrophy, or urethral stricture. May cause severe hypotension. May obscure diagnosis or clinical course with abdominal conditions. May impair mental/physical abilities.

ADVERSE REACTIONS: Respiratory depression, lightheadedness, dizziness, sedation, NV, sweating.

INTERACTIONS: See Contraindications. Effects may be potentiated by alkalinizing agents and antagonized by acidifying agents. Analgesic effect may be potentiated by chlorpromazine and methocarbamol. Depressant effects may be enhanced by other CNS depressants (eg, anesthetics, sedatives, hypnotics, TCAs, barbiturates, phenothiazines, chloral hydrate, glutethimide, antihistamines, β-blockers (propranolol), alcohol, furazolidone, and other narcotic analgesics). May increase anticoagulant activity of coumarin and other anticoagulants.

PREGNANCY: Category C, caution in nursing.

MECHANISM OF ACTION: Opioid analgesic; binds to CNS opiate receptors, producing analgesic effects. Also produces respiratory depression by direct action on brain stem respiratory centers, and depresses cough reflex by direct action on cough center in the medulla.

PHARMACOKINETICS: Absorption: Bioavailability (40%). **Distribution:** V_d=4L/kg; skeletal muscle, kidneys, liver, intestinal tract, lungs, spleen, and brain; crosses placenta; found in breast milk. **Metabolism:** Gut wall and liver; morphine-3-glucuronide (inactive metabolite). **Elimination:** Urine, bile; $T_{1/2}$=2-4 hrs.

M

NURSING CONSIDERATIONS

Assessment: Assess for pre-existing respiratory depression, COPD, cor pulmonale, acute or severe bronchial asthma, paralytic ileus, severe hepatic/renal or pulmonary impairment, head injury, increased ICP, intracranial lesions, patients in circulatory shock, myxedema or hypothyroidism, adrenocortical insufficiency (eg, Addison's disease), CNS depression or coma, toxic psychosis, prostatic hypertrophy or urethral stricture, acute alcoholism, delirium tremens, kyphoscoliosis or inability to swallow, pre-existing convulsions, acute pancreatitis, undergoing biliary tract surgery or active biliary tract disease, pregnancy/nursing status, and for possible drug interactions.

Monitoring: Monitor for signs/symptoms of respiratory/CNS depression and development of psychological and physical dependence.

Patient Counseling: Inform that therapy may produce physical or psychological dependence. Caution against performing hazardous tasks (eg, operating machinery/driving). Avoid alcohol or CNS respiratory depressants during therapy. Notify physician if pregnant/nursing.

Administration: Oral route. **Storage:** 25°C (77°F); excursions permitted to 15-30°C (59-86°F); dispense in tight, light-resistant container.

MOTRIN — RX

ibuprofen (Pharmacia & Upjohn)

NSAIDs may cause an increased risk of serious cardiovascular thrombotic events, MI, stroke and serious GI adverse events including bleeding, ulceration, and perforation of the stomach or intestines. Contraindicated for the treatment of perioperative pain in the setting of coronary artery bypass graft (CABG) surgery.

THERAPEUTIC CLASS: NSAID

INDICATIONS: Adults: Relief of mild-to-moderate pain. Dysmenorrhea. Rheumatoid arthritis (RA) Osteoarthritis (OA). **Pediatrics:** Fever. Relief of mild to moderate pain. Juvenile arthritis (JA).

DOSAGE: *Adults:* Pain: 400mg q4-6h prn. Max: 2400mg/day. Dysmenorrhea: 400mg q4-6h prn. Max: 2400mg/day. RA/OA: 300mg qid or 400mg, 600mg or 800mg tid-qid. Max: 3200mg/day. Fever: 200-400mg q4-6h. Max: 1200mg/day. Take with meals/milk. Renal Impairment: Reduce dose. *Pediatrics:* Fever: 6 months-12 yrs: 5mg/kg for temp <102.5°F; 10mg/kg if temp ≥102.5°F q6-8h. Max: 40mg/kg/day. Pain: 6 months-12 yrs: 10mg/kg q6-8h. Max: 40mg/kg/day. JA: 30-40mg/kg/day divided into 3 or 4 doses. Milder disease may use 20mg/kg/day.

HOW SUPPLIED: Sus: 100mg/5mL; Tab: 400mg, 600mg, 800mg

CONTRAINDICATIONS: Syndrome of nasal polyps, angioedema, and bronchospastic reactions to ASA or other NSAIDs. Treatment of perioperative pain in the setting of CABG surgery.

WARNINGS/PRECAUTIONS: May lead to onset of new HTN or worsening of pre-existing HTN; monitor BP closely. Fluid retention and edema reported; caution with fluid retention or heart failure. Renal papillary necrosis and other renal injury reported after long-term use. Not recommended for use with advanced renal disease; if therapy must be initiated, monitor renal function. Anaphylactoid reactions may occur. May cause serious skin adverse events (eg, exfoliative dermatitis, Stevens-Johnson syndrome, and toxic epidermal necrolysis). Avoid in late pregnancy; may cause premature closure of ductus arteriosis. May cause elevations of LFTs; d/c if liver disease develops or systemic manifestations occur. Caution in elderly. Anemia may occur; with long-term use, monitor Hgb/Hct if signs or symptoms of anemia develop. May inhibit platelet aggregation and prolong bleeding time; monitor with coagulation disorders. Caution with asthma and avoid with ASA-sensitive asthma. D/C if visual disturbances occur. Aseptic meningitis with fever and coma reported.

ADVERSE REACTIONS: Nausea, epigastric pain, heartburn, dizziness, rash.

INTERACTIONS: Use caution with anticoagulants. May enhance methotrexate toxicity. May decrease natriuretic effects of furosemide or thiazides. Avoid use with ASA. May decrease lithium clearance; monitor for toxicity. May diminish antihypertensive effect of ACE inhibitors. Caution with concomitant warfarin use.

PREGNANCY: Category C, not for use in nursing.

MECHANISM OF ACTION: NSAIDs; unknown, suspected to inhibit prostaglandin synthetase.

PHARMACOKINETICS: Absorption: (Tab) Rapid. (Susp) **Adults:** C_{max}=19µg/mL; T_{max}=0.79 hrs; AUC=64µg•h/mL. Febrile children: C_{max}= 55µg/mL; T_{max}=0.97 hrs; AUC=155µg•h/mL. **Distribution:** (Susp): Plasma protein binding (>99%). **Adults:** V_d=0.12L/kg; febrile children: V_d=0.2L/kg. **Metabolism:** Hepatic. **Elimination:** (Tab): $T_{1/2}$=1.8-2 hrs. (Sus): Urine (1%); $T_{1/2}$=2 hrs.

NURSING CONSIDERATIONS

Assessment: Assess for history of asthma, cardiovascular disease (pre-existing HTN, CHF) or risk factors for CVD, fluid retention, edema, DM, SLE, connective tissue disease, pregnancy status, risk factors for GI events (bleeding, ulceration, perforation), possible drug interactions, renal/hepatic dysfunction.

Monitoring: Monitor CBC, LFTs, renal function, blood glucose, and chemistries periodically. Monitor for signs/symptoms of aseptic meningitis (SLE, connective tissue disease), GI events (bleeding, ulceration, perforation), CV thrombotic events, CHF, HTN, salt depletion, ophthalmic effects, renal/liver dysfunction.

Patient Counseling: Seek medical attention for symptoms of hepatotoxicity (nausea, fatigue, pruritus), anaphylactic reactions (difficulty breathing, swelling of face/throat), hypersensitivity reaction (rash), CV events (chest pain, SOB, weakness, slurring of speech), GI ulceration and bleeding (epigastric pain, dyspepsia, melena, hematemesis), weight gain, and edema. Inform of pregnancy risks.

Administration: Oral route. **Storage:** (Sus): 15-30°C (59-86°F). Shake before use. (Tab): 20-25°C (68-77°F).

MOVIPREP

RX

ascorbic acid - sodium ascorbate - polyethylene glycol 3350 - potassium chloride - sodium chloride - sodium sulfate (Salix)

THERAPEUTIC CLASS: Bowel cleanser

INDICATIONS: Colon cleansing as a preparation for colonoscopy in adults ≥18 yrs of age.

DOSAGE: *Adults:* ≥18 yrs: Split-Dose Regimen: 8oz every 15 min (first liter) followed by 0.5 liters of clear liquid the evening prior, then another liter over 1 hr followed by 0.5 liters of clear liquid in the morning at least 1 hr prior to colonoscopy. Evening-Only Regimen: Around 6 pm take 8oz every 15 min (first liter), then 1.5 hrs later take second liter over one hour, additionally take 1 liter of clear liquid.

HOW SUPPLIED: Pow: (PEG 3350-Sodium Sulfate-Sodium Chloride-Potassium Chloride-Ascorbic Acid-Sodium Ascorbate) 100g-7.5g-2.69g-1.015g-4.7g-5.9g

WARNINGS/PRECAUTIONS: Rare reports of generalized tonic-clonic seizures with use of PEG colon preparations. Caution with concomitant medications that increase risk of electrolyte abnormalities (eg, diuretics, ACEIs) or in patients with hyponatremia; consider baseline and post-colonoscopy lab tests (eg, sodium, potassium, calcium, creatinine, BUN).

ADVERSE REACTIONS: Abdominal distension, anal discomfort, thirst, NV, abdominal pain, sleep disorder, rigors, hunger, malaise, dizziness.

INTERACTIONS: Oral medications given within 1 hour of administration may be flushed from GI and may not be absorbed.

PREGNANCY: Category C, caution in nursing.

MECHANISM OF ACTION: Laxative/evacuant; produces watery stool leading to cleansing of colon.

NURSING CONSIDERATIONS

Assessment: Assess for electrolyte abnormalities, seizures, ileus, GI obstruction, gastric retention, bowel perforation, toxic colitis or toxic megacolon, severe ulcerative colitis, phenylalanine levels.

Monitoring: Perform baseline and post-colonoscopy lab tests with known or suspected hyponatremia. D/C use if severe bloating, abdominal distention, or abdominal pain. Monitor for hypersensitivity reactions. Exercise caution while administering to patients prone to aspirate.

Patient Counseling: Advise to adequately hydrate before, during, and after use. Inform that may have clear soup and/or plain yogurt for dinner, finishing evening meal at least 1 hr prior to start of treatment until after the colonoscopy. Advise that if severe abdominal discomfort occurs, stop drinking temporarily, or drink at longer intervals until symptoms disappear. Instruct to take exactly as directed.

Administration: Oral route. **Storage**: 25°C (77°F); excursions permitted to 15-30°C (59-86°F). When reconstituted, store upright and keep refrigerated. Use within 24 hrs.

MS CONTIN

CII

morphine sulfate (Purdue Pharma)

Contains morphine sulfate with an abuse liability similar to other opioid analgesics. Not intended for use as a prn analgesic. MS Contin 100mg and 200mg tablets are for use in opioid-tolerant patients only. Tablets are to be swallowed whole; do not break, crush, chew, or dissolve.

THERAPEUTIC CLASS: Opioid analgesic

M

INDICATIONS: Management of moderate to severe pain when a continuous, around-the-clock opioid analgesic is needed for an extended period of time.

DOSAGE: *Adults:* Conversion from Immediate-Release Oral Morphine: Give 1/2 of patient's 24 hr requirement as MS Contin q12h or give 1/3 of daily requirement as MS Contin q8h. Conversion from Parenteral Morphine: Initial: If daily morphine dose ≤120mg/day, give MS Contin 30mg. Titrate: Switch to 60mg or 100mg MS Contin. Swallow whole; do not crush, chew, or break. Taper dose; do not d/c abruptly.

HOW SUPPLIED: Tab, Extended-Release: 15mg, 30mg, 60mg, 100mg, 200mg

CONTRAINDICATIONS: Paralytic ileus, respiratory depression in the absence of resuscitative equipment, acute or severe bronchial asthma.

WARNINGS/PRECAUTIONS: Extreme caution with COPD, cor pulmonale, decreased respiratory reserve, hypoxia, hypercapnia, respiratory depression. Caution with elderly, debilitated, head injury, increased ICP, circulatory shock, severe hepatic/renal/pulmonary dysfunction, myxedema, hypothyroidism, adrenocortical insufficiency, CNS depression, coma, toxic psychosis, prostatic hypertrophy, urethral stricture, alcoholism, delirium tremens, kyphoscoliosis, inability to swallow, convulsive disorder, acute abdominal problems, biliary tract surgery, acute pancreatitis secondary to biliary tract disease. May cause hypotension and drug dependence. Reserve 200mg tabs for opioid-tolerant patients requiring ≥400mg/day of morphine. May cause neonatal withdrawal syndrome.

ADVERSE REACTIONS: Constipation, lightheadedness, dizziness, sedation, NV, sweating, dysphoria, euphoria, respiratory depression.

INTERACTIONS: Additive depressant effects with other CNS depressants (eg, sedatives, hypnotics, general anesthetics, phenothiazines, tranquilizers, alcohol). Enhances neuromuscular blocking effects and increases respiratory depression with skeletal muscle relaxants. Avoid agonist/antagonist analgesics (eg, pentazocine, nalbuphine, butorphanol, buprenorphine); may reduce analgesic effect or cause withdrawal symptoms. Risk of hypotension with phenothiazines or general anesthetics.

PREGNANCY: Category C, not for use in nursing.

MECHANISM OF ACTION: Opioid analgesic; pure opioid agonist whose principal therapeutic action is analgesia. Precise mechanism of analgesic action not established. Specific CNS opiate receptors for endogenous compounds with opioid like activity are found throughout the brain and spinal cord and are likely to play a role in analgesic effects.

PHARMACOKINETICS: Distribution: V_d = 4L/kg; found in skeletal muscle, kidneys, liver, intestinal tract, lungs, spleen, and brain; crosses placental membranes; found in breast milk. **Metabolism:** Liver to glucuronide metabolites, M3G (major metabolite), M6G (active metabolite). **Elimination:** Renal (primary), bile; (IV): $T_{1/2}$=2-4 hrs.

NURSING CONSIDERATIONS

Assessment: Assess for opioid tolerance, respiratory depression, acute or severe bronchial asthma or hypercabia, COPD, paralytic ileus, head injury or other intracranial lesions, presence of increased ICP, circulatory shock, presence of debilitation, hepatic/renal impairment, myxedema or hypothyroidism, adrenocortical insufficiency (eg, Addison's disease), CNS depression or coma, toxic psychosis, prostatic hypertrophy or urethral stricture, acute alcoholism, delerium tremens, kyphoscoliosis, acute abdominal conditions, biliary tract disease, acute pancreatitis, ability to swallow, pregnancy/nursing status, drug abuse potential, and possible drug interactions.

Monitoring: Monitor for signs/symptoms of respiratory depression, elevations in CSF pressure, hypotension, convulsions, tolerance and physical dependence, and misuse or abuse.

Patient Counseling: Instruct to swallow medication whole (do not break, chew, dissolve, or crush). Advise not to adjust dosing without consulting physician. Counsel to report episodes of breakthrough pain or adverse events (eg, respiratory depression). Advise that drug may cause mental/physical impairment; use caution if performing hazardous tasks (eg, operating machinery/

driving). Instruct to avoid alcohol or other CNS depressants. Avoid abrupt withdrawal if on medication more than few weeks; taper dosing. Advise medication has drug abuse potential; protect from theft. Inform patient may see empty matrix of tablet in stool. Keep out of reach of children.

Administration: Oral route. **Storage:** Store at 25°C (77°F); excursions permitted between 15-30°C (59-86°F).

MYCAMINE RX

micafungin sodium (Astellas)

THERAPEUTIC CLASS: Glucan synthesis inhibitor

INDICATIONS: Treatment of candidemia, acute disseminated candidiasis, *Candida* peritonitis, abscesses, and esophageal candidiasis. Prophylaxis of *Candida* infections in patients undergoing hematopoietic stem cell transplantation (HSCT).

DOSAGE: *Adults:* Candidemia/Acute Disseminated Candidiasis/*Candida* Peritonitis/Abscesses: 100mg IV qd (usual range 10-47 days). Esophageal Candidiasis: 150mg IV qd (usual range 10-30 days). *Candida* Infection Prophylaxis in HSCT: 50mg IV qd (usual range 6-51 days). Do not mix or co-infuse with other drugs.

HOW SUPPLIED: Inj: 50mg, 100mg

WARNINGS/PRECAUTIONS: Reports of serious hypersensitivity reactions (eg, anaphylaxis, anaphylactoid, shock); d/c drug and administer appropriate treatment. LFT abnormalities, monitor for evidence of worsening. Reports of significant renal dysfunction, acute renal failure, and elevations in BUN and creatinine. Reports of acute intravascular hemolysis, hemolytic anemia and hemoglobinuria.

ADVERSE REACTIONS: Hyperbilirubinemia, neutropenia, headache, rash, phlebitis, NV, diarrhea, pyrexia, hypokalemia, thrombocytopenia.

INTERACTIONS: Monitor for sirolimus, nifedipine, or itraconazole toxicity; reduce dose if toxicity occurs. May precipitate when mixed or co-infused with other drugs.

PREGNANCY: Category C, caution in nursing.

MECHANISM OF ACTION: Antifungal agent; inhibits the synthesis of 1,3-β-D-glucan, a component of fungal cell walls.

PHARMACOKINETICS: Absorption: IV infusion of variable doses resulted in different parameters. **Distribution:** V_d=0.39±0.11L/kg (terminal phase); plasma protein binding (≥99%). **Metabolism:** Metabolized to M-1 (catechol form) by arylsulfatase and further metabolized to M-2 (methoxy form) by catechol-O-methyltransferase. Catalyzed by CYP450 isoenzymes. **Elimination:** Urine and feces (major route).

NURSING CONSIDERATIONS

Assessment: Assess cultures and other diagnostic tests prior to therapy and for possible drug interactions.

Monitoring: Monitor for hypersensitivity and anaphylaxis reaction (shock), LFTs for possible hepatic dysfunction, hepatitis or hepatic failure, elevations in BUN and creatinine, and signs/symptoms of renal dysfunction or acute renal failure. Monitor for hematological effects (hemolysis, hemoglobinuria).

Patient Counseling: Instruct to notify physician if signs/symptoms of hypersensitivity or anaphylaxis reactions, hematological reactions, hepatic complications, or renal complications develop.

Administration: IV infusion. 1) Aseptically add 5mL of 0.9% NaCl Inj, USP (without bacteriostatic agent) to each 50mg or 100mg vial to yield a preparation containing 10mg, 20mg micafungin/mL. 2) To minimize foaming, gently dissolve the powder by swirling the vial. Do not vigorously shake vial. **Storage:** Unopened vial: Stored at room temperature, 25°C (77°F); excursions permitted to 15-30°C (59-86°F). Reconstitituted, diluted infusions: May be stored at room temperature 25°C (77°F) for up to 24 hrs.

M

MYCELEX TROCHE — RX
clotrimazole (Ortho-McNeil)

THERAPEUTIC CLASS: Azole antifungal

INDICATIONS: Local treatment of oropharyngeal candidiasis. Prophylactically to reduce the incidence of oropharyngeal candidiasis in immunocompromised conditions (eg, chemotherapy, radiotherapy, steroid therapy).

DOSAGE: *Adults:* Treatment: Slowly dissolve 1 troche in mouth 5 times/day for 14 days. Prophylaxis: Slowly dissolve 1 troche in mouth tid for duration of chemotherapy or until steroids reduced to maint levels.
Pediatrics: ≥3 yrs: Treatment: Slowly dissolve 1 troche in mouth 5 times/day for 14 days. Prophylaxis: Slowly dissolve 1 troche in mouth tid for duration of chemotherapy or until steroids reduced to maint levels.

HOW SUPPLIED: Tab: 10mg

WARNINGS/PRECAUTIONS: Not for systemic mycoses. May cause abnormal LFTs; monitor hepatic function. Only use in patients mentally and physically able to dissolve the troche. Confirm diagnosis by KOH smear and/or culture.

ADVERSE REACTIONS: Abnormal LFTs, NV, unpleasant mouth sensations, pruritus.

PREGNANCY: Category C, safety in nursing is not known.

MECHANISM OF ACTION: Broad-spectrum antifungal agent; inhibits growth of pathogenic yeasts by altering cell membrane permeability.

PHARMACOKINETICS: Absorption: C_{max}=4.98ng/mL (30 min), 3.23ng/mL (60 min).

NURSING CONSIDERATIONS

Assessment: Assess for proper diagnosis of oropharyngeal candidiasis prior to therapy (KOH smear or culture).

Monitoring: Periodically monitor for LFTs. Monitor for NV, pruritus, and unpleasant mouth sensations.

Patient Counseling: Counsel to allow lozenge to dissolve slowly in mouth; report adverse reactions.

Administration: Oral route. **Storage:** Store below 30°C (86°F). Avoid freezing.

M

MYFORTIC — RX
mycophenolic acid (Novartis)

Increased susceptibility to infection. Possible development of lymphoma and other neoplasms. Female users of childbearing potential must use contraception. Increased risk of pregnancy loss and congenital malformations.

THERAPEUTIC CLASS: Inosine monophosphate dehydrogenase inhibitor

INDICATIONS: Prophylaxis of organ rejection in patients receiving allogeneic renal transplants, administered in combination with cyclosporine and corticosteroids.

DOSAGE: *Adults:* 720mg bid on empty stomach, 1 hr before or 2 hrs after food intake.
Pediatrics: 400mg/m² bid. Max: 720mg bid. BSA 1.19-1.58m²: 540mg bid. BSA >1.58m²: 720mg bid. BSA <1.19m² cannot be accurately adminsitered with current formulations.

HOW SUPPLIED: Tab, Delayed-Release: 180mg, 360mg

WARNINGS/PRECAUTIONS: Risk of lymphomas and other malignancies, especially of skin. Avoid sunlight to decrease risk of skin cancer. May cause fetal harm during pregnancy. Must have negative serum/urine pregnancy test within 1 week before therapy. Two reliable forms of contraception required before and during therapy, and 6 weeks following discontinuation. Monitor for bone marrow suppression. Risk of GI ulceration, hemorrhage, and perforation; caution with active digestive system disease. Caution with delayed renal graft function post-transplant. Oral suspension contains phenylalanine; caution with phenylketonurics. Monitor CBC weekly during the 1st month, twice monthly for the 2nd and 3rd months, and then monthly through 1st year. Avoid with rare hereditary deficiency of hypoxanthine-guanine phosphoribosyltransferase (eg, Lesch-Nyhan and Kelley-Seegmiller syndrome). Female users of childbearing potential must use contraception. Increased risk of pregnancy loss and congenital malformations.

ADVERSE REACTIONS: Infections, diarrhea, leukopenia, sepsis, vomiting, GI bleeding, pain, abdominal pain, fever, headache, asthenia, chest pain, back pain, anemia, leukopenia, thrombocytopenia.

INTERACTIONS: Additive bone marrow suppression with azathioprine; avoid use. Reduced efficacy with drugs that interfere with enterohepatic recirculation (eg, cholestyramine). Efficacy/safety with other immunosuppressive agents not determined. Avoid live attenuated vaccines. Increased levels of both drugs with acyclovir, ganciclovir. Decreased levels with magnesium- and aluminum-containing antacids; space dosing. Decreased effects of oral contraceptives. Increased levels with probenecid. Other drugs that compete for renal tubular secretion may raise levels of both drugs.

PREGNANCY: Category D, not for use in nursing.

MECHANISM OF ACTION: Inosine monophosphate dehydrogenase inhibitor; inhibits the de novo pathway of guanosine nucleotide synthesis without incorporation to DNA.

PHARMACOKINETICS: Absorption: Absolute bioavailability (72%); T_{max}=1.5-2.75 hrs. **Distribution:** V_d=54L (steady state); plasma protein binding: ≥98% (mycophenolic acid (MPA), 82% (mycophenolic acid glucuronide (MPAG). **Metabolism:** (MPA) metabolized by glucuronyl transferase to MPAG (major metabolite). **Elimination:** Urine: >60% (MPAG), 3% (unchanged), and bile; $T_{1/2}$=8-16 hrs (MPA), 13-17 hrs (MPAG).

M

NURSING CONSIDERATIONS

Assessment: Assess for drug hypersensitivity, hepatic/renal impairment, pregnancy status, vaccination history, inherited deficiency of HGPRT such as Lesch-Nyhan and Kelley-Seegmiller syndromes, and possible drug interactions.

Monitoring: Monitor for signs of delayed graft rejection (eg, anemia, thrombocytopenia, and hyperkalemia), lymphomas, skin cancer, GI bleeding/perforation, infection or opportunistic infection (eg, herpes virus, fatal infection, sepsis). Monitor unexpected bruising, bleeding, or signs of bone marrow suppression with periodic CBCs.

Patient Counseling: Counsel to take on an empty stomach, to swallow tab whole; do not crush, chew, or cut. Instruct to avoid prolonged exposure to sunlight and UV light. Inform medication is not to be used by women who are pregnant/nursing or planning to become pregnant. Advise to follow dosage instructions and have periodic laboratory tests performed. Inform about increased risk for malignancies and infections.

Administration: Oral route. **Storage:** Store at 25°C (77°F); excursions permitted to 15-30°C (59-86°F).

MYLERAN — RX

busulfan (GlaxoSmithKline)

Do not use unless CML diagnosis is established. May induce severe bone marrow hypoplasia; reduce dose or d/c if unusual depression of bone marrow function occurs.

THERAPEUTIC CLASS: Alkylating agent

INDICATIONS: Palliative treatment of chronic myelogenous leukemia (CML).

DOSAGE: *Adults:* 60mcg/kg/day or 1.8mg/m²/day. Range: 4-8mg/day. Reserve dose >4mg/day for the most compelling symptoms.
Pediatrics: 60mcg/kg/day or 1.8mg/m²/day. Range: 4-8mg/day. Reserve dose >4mg/day for the most compelling symptoms.

HOW SUPPLIED: Tab: 2mg* *scored

CONTRAINDICATIONS: Lack of definitive diagnosis of CML.

WARNINGS/PRECAUTIONS: Induction of bone marrow failure resulting in severe pancytopenia reported. Bronchopulmonary dysplasia with pulmonary fibrosis, cellular dysplasia, malignant tumors, acute leukemias, hepatic veno-occlusive disease reported. Ovarian suppression and amenorrhea with menopausal symptoms have occurred. Cardiac tamponade in patients with thalassemia and seizures reported. Caution with compromised bone marrow reserve from prior irradiation/chemotherapy. Seizures reported.

ADVERSE REACTIONS: Myelosuppression, pulmonary fibrosis, cardiac tamponade, hyperpigmentation, weakness, fatigue, weight loss, nausea, vomiting, melanoderma, hyperuricemia, myasthenia gravis, hepatic veno-occlusive disease.

INTERACTIONS: Additive myelosuppression with myelosuppressive drugs. Additive pulmonary toxicity with myelotoxic drugs. Increased clearance of cyclophosphamide and busulfan with phenytoin pretreatment. Decreased clearance with concomitant cyclophosphamide alone. Reduced clearance with itraconazole; monitor for signs of toxicity. Concurrent thioguanine was associated with portal HTN and esophageal varices with abnormal LFTs; caution with long-term therapy.

PREGNANCY: Category D, not for use in nursing.

MECHANISM OF ACTION: Bifunctional alkylating agent.

PHARMACOKINETICS: Absorption: (IV, PO) Absolute bioavailability (adults 80%, children 68%); C_{max}(2mg, 4mg)=30ng/mL, 68ng/mL; T_{max}=0.9 hrs; AUC (4mg) =269ng•hr/mL **Distribution**: Plasma protein binding (32%); crosses blood-brain barrier. **Metabolism**: Liver (extensive); 3-hydroxytetrahydrothiopene-1, 1-dioxide (major metabolite). **Elimination**: Urine (>2% unchanged); $T_{1/2}$=2.69 hrs.

M

NURSING CONSIDERATIONS

Assessment: Assess for chronic myelogenous leukemia, history of seizure disorder, head trauma, if receiving other potentially epileptogenic drugs, pregnancy status. Note other diseases/conditions and drug therapies.

Monitoring: Periodically measure serum transaminases, alkaline phosphatase, and bilirubin for early detection of hepatotoxicity, and evaluate weekly Hgb/Hct, total WBC count and differential, quantitative platelet count, and bone marrow exam for evaluation of marrow status. Monitor for signs/symptoms of busulfan toxicity and bronchopulmonary dysplasia with pulmonary fibrosis, secondary malignancies, chromosomal aberrations.

Patient Counseling: Counsel about need for periodic blood counts and to report unusual bleeding, fever, breathing difficulty, anorexia, weight loss, or melanoderma.

Administration: Oral route. **Storage**: 25°C (77°F); excursions permitted to 15-30°C (59-86°F).

MYLOTARG — RX

gemtuzumab ozogamicin (Wyeth)

Only use as monotherapy. Severe myelosuppression, severe hypersensitivity reactions (eg, anaphylaxis, pulmonary events, infusion-related reactions) can occur. Hepatotoxicity, including severe hepatic veno-occlusive disease (VOD) reported.

THERAPEUTIC CLASS: IgG_4 kappa antibody/calicheamicin conjugate

INDICATIONS: Treatment of patients with CD33 positive acute myeloid leukemia (AML) in 1st relapse patients ≥60 yrs who are not candidates for chemotherapy.

DOSAGE: *Adults:* ≥60 yrs: 9mg/m² as 2 hr IV infusion, for 2 doses with 14 days between doses. Premedicate 1 hr prior with diphenhydramine 50mg and APAP 650-1000mg (may give additional APAP dose q4h for 2 doses as needed). Monitor vital signs during infusion and for 4 hrs after.

HOW SUPPLIED: Inj: 5mg

CONTRAINDICATIONS: Lactating mothers.

WARNINGS/PRECAUTIONS: Monitor CBC, LFTs, and electrolytes. Monitor vital signs during infusion and 4 hrs after. Interrupt infusion if dyspnea or significant hypotension develop. Consider discontinuing if anaphylaxis, pulmonary edema, or ARDS develop. Increased risk of severe VOD if used before or after hematopoietic stem-cell transplant, underlying hepatic disease or abnormal liver function, or with combination chemotherapy. Extra caution with hepatic impairment. Administer in appropriate facility. Tumor lysis syndrome may occur. Not for IV push or bolus use.

ADVERSE REACTIONS: Chills, fever, NV, headache, hypotension, HTN, hypoxia, dyspnea, hyperglycemia, antibody formation, myelosuppression, anemia, thrombocytopenia, sepsis, pneumonia, epistaxis, mucositis, hepatotoxicity, neutropenia.

PREGNANCY: Category D, not for use in nursing.

MECHANISM OF ACTION: IgG4 kappa antibody/calicheamicin conjugate; binds to CD33 antigen, resulting in formation of a complex that is internalized. Upon internalization, the calicheamicin derivative is released inside lysosomes of myeloid cell, which then binds to DNA in the minor groove, resulting in DNA double strand breaks and cell death.

PHARMACOKINETICS: Elimination: $T_{1/2}$=41 hrs (total), 143 hrs (conjugated).

NURSING CONSIDERATIONS

Assessment: Assess for history of liver disease or hematopoietic stem cell transplant (HSCT). Consider leukoreduction with hydroxyurea or leukapheresis to reduce peripheral WBC count to <30,000/uL.

Monitoring: Monitor for symptoms of hepatotoxicity, veno-occlusive disease (VOD), tumor lysis syndrome, hyperglycemia, infections, severe hypersensitivity reactions, and other infusion-related reactions including severe pulmonary events. Monitor vital signs (during infusion and 4 hrs following infusion), electrolytes, LFTs, CBC, with differential and platelet counts.

Patient Counseling: Not for use by lactating mothers. Advise women to avoid pregnancy while on therapy. Counsel about signs/symptoms of potential adverse effects; report if any develop.

Administration: IV, do not administer as an IV push or bolus. Do not co-administer other drugs through same infusion line. **Storage**: Refrigerate 2-8°C (36-46°F), protect from light.

NABUMETONE — RX

nabumetone (Various)

NSAIDs may cause an increased risk of serious cardiovascular thrombotic events, MI, stroke and serious GI adverse events including bleeding, ulceration, and perforation of the stomach or intestines. Contraindicated for the treatment of perioperative pain in the setting of coronary artery bypass graft (CABG) surgery.

THERAPEUTIC CLASS: NSAID

INDICATIONS: Relief of signs and symptoms of osteoarthritis and rheumatoid arthritis.

DOSAGE: *Adults:* Initial: 1000mg qd. Max: 2000mg/day.

HOW SUPPLIED: Tab: 500mg, 750mg

CONTRAINDICATIONS: Allergy to ASA or other NSAID that precipitates asthma, urticaria, or other allergic-type reaction. Treatment of perioperative pain in the setting of CABG surgery.

WARNINGS/PRECAUTIONS: May lead to onset of new HTN or worsening of pre-existing HTN; monitor BP closely. Fluid retention and edema reported; caution with fluid retention or heart failure. Renal papillary necrosis and other renal injury reported after long-term use. Not recommended for use with advanced renal disease; if therapy must be initiated, monitor renal function.

Anaphylactoid reactions may occur. May cause serious skin adverse events (eg, exfoliative dermatitis, Stevens-Johnson syndrome, and toxic epidermal necrolysis). Avoid in late pregnancy; may cause premature closure of ductus arteriosis. May cause elevations of LFTs; d/c if liver disease develops or systemic manifestations occur. Caution in elderly. Anemia may occur; with long-term use, monitor Hgb/Hct if signs or symptoms of anemia develop. May inhibit platelet aggregation and prolong bleeding time; monitor with coagulation disorders. Caution with asthma and avoid with ASA-sensitive asthma. May induce photosensitivity. Risk of GI ulceration, bleeding, and perforation.

ADVERSE REACTIONS: Diarrhea, dyspepsia, abdominal pain, constipation, flatulence, nausea, positive stool guaiac, dizziness, headache, pruritus, rash, tinnitus, edema.

INTERACTIONS: Caution with warfarin, other protein bound drugs. Nephrotoxicity risk with diuretics. May elevate lithium and methotrexate levels. May diminish antihypertensive effect of ACE inhibitors. Avoid concomitant ASA.

PREGNANCY: Category C, not for use in nursing.

MECHANISM OF ACTION: NSAID (napthylalkanone derivative); suspected to inhibit prostaglandin synthetase, exerts anti-inflammatory, analgesic, and antipyretic actions.

PHARMACOKINETICS: Absorption: Well-absorbed (GIT). PO administration of variable doses resulted in different parameters. **Distribution:** Plasma protein binding (≥99%). **Metabolism:** Liver (extensive biotransformation), 6-methoxy-2-naphthylacetic acid (active metabolite). **Elimination:** Urine (approximately 75%), feces; $T_{1/2}$=24 hrs.

NURSING CONSIDERATIONS

Assessment: Assess LFTs, renal function, CBC and coagulation profile. Assess for history of CABG surgery, asthma and allergic reactions to aspirin or other NSAIDs, active ulceration or chronic inflammation of GI tract, CVD, asthma, pregnancy status. Note other diseases/conditions and drug therapies.

N

Monitoring: Monitor for hypersensitivity reactions, cardiac complications, stroke, GI bleeding, asthma, skin adverse effects. Monitor BP, LFTs, renal function, CBC with differential and platelet count, coagulation profile, ocular effects, photosensitivity.

Patient Counseling: Counsel about potential side effects; seek medical attention if any develop. Take as prescribed. Advise women not to use late in pregnancy.

Administration: Oral route. **Storage:** Controlled room temperature 15-30°C (59-86°F). Dispense in tight, light-resistant container.

NADOLOL — RX

nadolol (Various)

OTHER BRAND NAMES: Corgard (King)

THERAPEUTIC CLASS: Nonselective beta-blocker

INDICATIONS: Long-term management of angina pectoris. Treatment of hypertension.

DOSAGE: *Adults:* Angina Pectoris: Initial: 40mg qd. Titrate: Increase by 40-80mg every 3-7 days. Usual: 40-80mg qd. Max: 240mg/day. HTN: Initial: 40mg qd. Titrate: Increase by 40-80mg. Max: 320mg/day. CrCl 31-50mL/min: Dose q24-36h. CrCl 10-30mL/min: Dose q24-48h. CrCl <10mL/min: Dose q40-60h.

HOW SUPPLIED: Tab: 20mg*, 40mg*, 80mg*, 120mg*, 160mg* *scored

CONTRAINDICATIONS: Bronchial asthma, sinus bradycardia and >1st-degree conduction block, cardiogenic shock, overt cardiac failure.

WARNINGS/PRECAUTIONS: Caution in well-compensated cardiac failure, nonallergic bronchospasm, renal dysfunction. Exacerbation of ischemic heart disease with abrupt withdrawal. Withdrawal before surgery is controversial.

May mask hyperthyroidism or hypoglycemia symptoms. Can cause cardiac failure.

ADVERSE REACTIONS: Bradycardia, peripheral vascular insufficiency, dizziness, fatigue.

INTERACTIONS: Additive hypotension and/or bradycardia with catecholamine-depleting drugs. Antidiabetic agents may need adjustment. General anesthetics may exaggerate hypotension. May block epinephrine effects.

PREGNANCY: Category C, not for use in nursing.

MECHANISM OF ACTION: Nonselective β-adrenergic receptor blocker; inhibits β_1 and β_2 receptors inhibiting chronotrophic, inotropic, and vasodilator responses to β-adrenergic stimulation.

PHARMACOKINETICS: Absorption: T_{max}=3-4 hrs. **Distribution:** Plasma protein binding (30%). **Elimination:** Kidney; $T_{1/2}$=20-40 hrs.

NURSING CONSIDERATIONS

Assessment: Assess for bronchial asthma, sinus bradycardia, AV block, cardiogenic shock, CHF, bronchospastic disease, CAD, hyperthyroidism, DM, possible drug interactions, and renal impairment.

Monitoring: Monitor renal function periodically. Monitor for signs/symptoms of cardiac failure, hypoglycemia, thyrotoxicosis, withdrawal symptoms, renal dysfunction, and hypersensitivity reactions.

Patient Counseling: Warn against interruption or d/c of therapy without consulting physician. Inform drug may mask signs of thyrotoxicosis and hypoglycemia. Advise to seek medical attention if symptoms of heart failure, withdrawal (angina, tremulousness, sweating, headache) or hypersensitivity reactions occur.

Administration: Oral route. **Storage:** Room temperature; avoid excessive heat. Protect from light.

NALOXONE

naloxone HCl (Various) **RX**

OTHER BRAND NAMES: Narcan (Endo)

THERAPEUTIC CLASS: Opioid antagonist

INDICATIONS: For complete or partial opioid depression reversal induced by natural and synthetic opioids. Diagnosis of suspected opioid tolerance or acute opioid overdose. Adjunct in management of septic shock to increase blood pressure.

DOSAGE: *Adults:* Opioid Overdose: Initial: 0.4-2mg IV every 2-3 minutes up to 10mg. IM/SQ if IV route not available. Post-op Opioid Depression: 0.1-0.2mg IV every 2-3 minutes to desired response. May repeat in 1-2 hr intervals. Supplemental IM doses last longer. Narcan Challenge Test: IV: 0.1-0.2mg, observe 30 secs for signs of withdrawal, then 0.6mg, observe for 20 min. SQ: 0.8mg, observe for 20 min.
Pediatrics: Opioid Overdose: Initial: 0.01mg/kg IV. Inadequate Response: repeat 0.1mg/kg once. IM/SQ in divided doses if IV route not available. Post-op Opioid Depression: 0.005-0.01mg IV every 2-3 min to desired response. May repeat in 1-2 hr intervals. Supplemental IM doses last longer. Neonates: Opioid-induced Depression: 0.01mg/kg IV/IM/SQ, may repeat every 2-3 min until desired response.

HOW SUPPLIED: Inj: 0.4mg/mL, 1mg/mL

WARNINGS/PRECAUTIONS: Caution in patients including newborns of mothers known or suspected of opioid physical dependence. May precipitate acute withdrawal syndrome. Have other resuscitative measures available. Caution with cardiac, renal, or hepatic disease. Monitor patients satisfactorily responding due to extended opioid duration of action. Abrupt postoperative opioid depression reversal may result in serious adverse effects leading to death.

ADVERSE REACTIONS: HTN, hypotension, ventricular tachycardia and fibrillation, dyspnea, pulmonary edema, cardiac arrest, NV, sweating, seizures, body aches, fever, nervousness.

INTERACTIONS: Caution using drugs with potential adverse cardiac effects. Reversal of buprenorphine-induced respiratory depression may be incomplete.

PREGNANCY: Category B, caution in nursing.

MECHANISM OF ACTION: Narcotic antagonist; prevents or reverses effects of opioids, including respiratory depression, sedation, and hypotension, by competing for same receptor sites. Also reverses psychotomimetic and dysphoric effects of agonist-antagonists (eg, pentazocine).

PHARMACOKINETICS: Distribution: Rapid; plasma protein binding (weak). **Metabolism:** Liver; via glucuronide conjugation; naloxone-3-glucuronide (major metabolite). **Elimination:** Urine (25-40%); $T_{1/2}$=30-80 min (adults), 3.1 hrs (neonates).

NURSING CONSIDERATIONS

Assessment: Assess for hypersensitivity, history of drug dependency, presence of resuscitative measures (eg, free airway, artificial ventilation, cardiac massage, vasopressors), hypo/hypertension, ventricular tachycardia and fibrillation, pulmonary edema, and cardiac arrest.

Monitoring: Monitor for signs/symptoms of opioid withdrawal (eg, body aches, diarrhea, tachycardia, fever, runny nose, sneezing, piloerection, sweating, yawning, NV, nervousness, restlessness, irritability, shivering or trembling, abdominal cramps, weakness, increase BP), and satisfactory response.

Administration: IM/IV/SQ routes. **Storage:** 20-25°C (68-77°F). Protect from light.

N

NAMENDA RX

memantine HCl (Forest)

THERAPEUTIC CLASS: NMDA receptor antagonist

INDICATIONS: Treatment of moderate to severe dementia of the Alzheimer's type.

DOSAGE: *Adults:* Initial: 5mg qd. Titrate: Increase at intervals of at least one week to 5mg bid, then 5mg and 10mg as separate doses, then to 10mg bid. Severe Renal Impairment:(5-29mL/min): Target Dose: 5mg bid.

HOW SUPPLIED: Sol: 2mg/mL; Tab: 5mg, 10mg; Titration-Pak: 5mg [28[s]], 10mg [21[s]].

WARNINGS/PRECAUTIONS: Use not evaluated with seizure disorders. Alkalinized urine (eg, renal tubular acidosis, severe urinary tract infections) may increase levels. Reduce dose with severe renal impairment. Should be administered with caution to patients with severe hepatic impairment.

ADVERSE REACTIONS: Dizziness, confusion, headache, constipation, coughing, HTN, pain, vomiting, somnolence, hallucinations.

INTERACTIONS: Caution with other NMDA antagonists (eg, amantadine, ketamine, dextromethorphan), urinary alkalinizers (eg, carbonic anhydrase inhibitors, sodium bicarbonate). Other renally-excreted drugs (eg, HCTZ, triamterene, metformin, cimetidine, ranitidine, quinidine, nicotine) may alter levels of both agents.

PREGNANCY: Category B, caution in nursing.

MECHANISM OF ACTION: NMDA receptor antagonist; postulated to exert effect by binding to NMDA receptor-operated cation channels.

PHARMACOKINETICS: Absorption: T_{max}=3-7 hrs. **Distribution:** V_d=9-11L/kg; plasma protein binding (45%). **Metabolism:** Hepatic (partial). **Elimination:** Urine (48%); $T_{1/2}$=60-80 hrs.

NURSING CONSIDERATIONS

Assessment: Assess for conditions that raise urine pH (carbonic anhydrase inhibitors, $NaHCO_3$, RTA, severe UTI), possible drug interactions, renal/hepatic function.

Monitoring: Monitor renal/hepatic function.

Patient Counseling: Inform can be taken with/without food.

Administration: Oral route. **Storage**: 25°C (77°F); excursions permitted to 15-30°C (59-86°F).

NAPRELAN

naproxen sodium (Elan)

RX

NSAIDs may cause an increased risk of serious cardiovascular thrombotic events, MI, stroke and serious GI adverse events including bleeding, ulceration, and perforation of the stomach or intestines. Contraindicated for the treatment of perioperative pain in the setting of coronary artery bypass graft (CABG) surgery.

THERAPEUTIC CLASS: NSAID

INDICATIONS: Treatment of rheumatoid arthritis (RA), osteoarthritis (OA), ankylosing spondylitis (AS), tendinitis, bursitis, primary dysmenorrhea and acute gout. Relief of mild to moderate pain.

DOSAGE: *Adults:* RA/OA/AS: Usual: 750mg-1g qd. Max: 1.5g/day. Pain/Primary Dysmenorrhea/Tendinitis/Bursitis: 1q/day or 1.5g for a limited period. Max: 1g/day thereafter. Acute Gout: 1-1.5g qd for 1 day, then 1g qd until attack subsides.

HOW SUPPLIED: Tab, Extended-Release: 375mg, 500mg

CONTRAINDICATIONS: History of angioedema, urticaria, bronchospastic reactivity, nasal polyps. NSAID allergy that precipitates asthma, nasal polyps, urticaria, and hypotension. Treatment of perioperative pain in the setting of CABG surgery.

N

WARNINGS/PRECAUTIONS: May lead to onset of new HTN or worsening of pre-existing HTN; monitor BP closely. Fluid retention and edema reported; caution with fluid retention or heart failure. Renal papillary necrosis and other renal injury reported after long-term use. Not recommended for use with advanced renal disease; if therapy must be initiated, monitor renal function. Anaphylactoid reactions may occur. May cause serious skin adverse events (eg, exfoliative dermatitis, Stevens-Johnson syndrome, and toxic epidermal necrolysis). Avoid in late pregnancy; may cause premature closure of ductus arteriosis. May cause elevations of LFTs; d/c if liver disease develops or systemic manifestations occur. Caution in elderly. Anemia may occur; with long-term use, monitor Hgb/Hct if signs or symptoms of anemia develop. May inhibit platelet aggregation and prolong bleeding time; monitor with coagulation disorders. Caution with asthma and avoid with ASA-sensitive asthma.

ADVERSE REACTIONS: Headache, dyspepsia, flu syndrome, pain, infection, nausea, diarrhea, constipation, abdominal pain, heartburn, drowsiness, edema, skin rash, ecchymoses.

INTERACTIONS: Avoid with other products containing naproxen. May inhibit natriuretic effect of furosemide. Probenecid increases plasma levels and extends its plasma half-life. May increase methotrexate toxicity. Avoid ASA. Caution with coumarin-type anticoagulants, hydantoins, sulfonamides or sulfonylureas; monitor for toxicity. ACE inhibitors may potentiate renal disease states. May displace albumin-bound drugs. May reduce antihypertensive effect of β-blockers. May increase lithium levels.

PREGNANCY: Category C, not for use in nursing.

MECHANISM OF ACTION: NSAID; not fully established, suspected to inhibit prostaglandin synthetase.

PHARMACOKINETICS: Absorption: Rapid, complete; bioavailability (95%); C_{max}=94mcg/mL; T_{max}=5 hrs; AUC=1448mcg•hr/mL. **Distribution:** V_d=0.16L/kg; plasma protein binding (>99%). **Metabolism:** Hepatic; 6-O-desmethyl naproxen (metabolite). **Elimination:** Urine, feces (≤5%); $T_{1/2}$=15 hrs.

NURSING CONSIDERATIONS

Assessment: Assess for CVD (HTN, CHF) or risk factors for disease, history of ulcer disease, asthma, pregnancy status, risk factors for GI events (bleeding, ulceration, perforation), possible drug interactions, renal and hepatic dysfunction.

Monitoring: Monitor BP, CBC, LFTs, renal function, and chemistries periodically. Monitor for signs/symptoms of GI events (bleeding, ulceration, perforation), hypersensitivity reaction (eosinophilia, rash), renal/liver dysfunction.

Patient Counseling: Advise to seek medical attention if symptoms of hepatotoxicity (nausea, fatigue, pruritus), anaphylactic reaction (difficulty breathing, swelling of face/throat), hypersensitivity reaction (rash), CV events (chest pain, SOB, weakness, slurring of speech), GI ulceration and bleeding (epigastric pain, dyspepsia, melena, hematemesis), weight gain, or edema occur. Inform of pregnancy risks.

Administration: Oral route. **Storage:** 20-25°C (68-77°F).

NAPROSYN RX

naproxen (Roche Labs)

NSAIDs may cause an increased risk of serious cardiovascular thrombotic events, MI, stroke and serious GI adverse events including bleeding, ulceration, and perforation of the stomach or intestines. Contraindicated for the treatment of perioperative pain in the setting of coronary artery bypass graft (CABG) surgery.

OTHER BRAND NAMES: EC-Naprosyn (Roche Labs)

THERAPEUTIC CLASS: NSAID

INDICATIONS: (Naprosyn, EC-Naprosyn) Relief of signs and symptoms of rheumatoid arthritis (RA), osteoarthritis (OA), ankylosing spondylitis, and juvenile arthritis (JA). (Naprosyn) Relief of signs and symtoms of tendinitis, bursitis, and acute gout. Management of pain and primary dysmenorrhea. EC-Naprosyn not recommended for initial treatment of acute pain.

N

DOSAGE: *Adults:* RA/OA/Ankylosing Spondylitis: Naprosyn: 250, 375, or 500mg bid; EC-Naprosyn: 375 or 500mg bid. Max: 1500mg/day. Acute Gout: Naprosyn: 750mg followed by 250mg q8h until attack subsides. Pain/Dysmenorrhea/Tendinitis/Bursitis: Naprosyn: 500mg followed by 500mg q12h or 250mg q6-8h prn. Max: 1250mg on Day 1, then 1000mg/day. EC-Naprosyn should not be chewed, crushed, or broken.
Pediatrics: ≥2 yrs: JA: (Sus) 5mg/kg bid. Max: 15mg/kg/day.

HOW SUPPLIED: (Naproxen) Sus: 25mg/mL; Tab: 250mg*, 375mg, 500mg*; Tab, Delayed-Release: (EC-Naprosyn) 375mg, 500mg *scored

CONTRAINDICATIONS: History of ASA or NSAID allergy that cause symptoms of asthma, rhinitis, nasal polyps, and hypotension. Treatment of perioperative pain in the setting of CABG surgery.

WARNINGS/PRECAUTIONS: May lead to onset of new HTN or worsening of pre-existing HTN; monitor BP closely. Fluid retention, edema, and peripheral edema reported; caution with fluid retention, HTN, or heart failure. Renal papillary necrosis and other renal injury reported after long-term use. Not recommended for use with advanced renal disease; if therapy must be initiated, monitor renal function. Anaphylactoid reactions may occur. May cause serious skin adverse events (eg, exfoliative dermatitis, Stevens-Johnson syndrome, and toxic epidermal necrolysis). Avoid in late pregnancy; may cause premature closure of ductus arteriosis. Monitor Hgb levels with long-term therapy if initial Hgb ≤10g. Monitor for visual changes or disturbances. May cause elevations of LFTs; d/c if liver disease develops or systemic manifestations occur. Caution with high doses in chronic alcoholic liver disease and elderly. Anemia may occur; with long-term use, monitor Hgb/Hct if signs or symptoms of anemia develop. May inhibit platelet aggregation and prolong bleeding time; monitor with coagulation disorders. Caution with asthma and avoid with ASA-sensitive asthma.

ADVERSE REACTIONS: Edema, drowsiness, dizziness, constipation, heartburn, abdominal pain, nausea, headache, tinnitus, dyspnea, pruritus, skin eruptions, ecchymoses.

INTERACTIONS: (Naprosyn, EC-Naprosyn) Avoid with other products containing naproxen. Decreased plasma levels with ASA. May reduce tubular secretion of methotrexate; monitor for toxicity. May increase nephrotoxicity of cyclosporine; caution when coadministering. May diminish antihypertensive effect and potentiate renal disease with ACE inhibitors. May reduce natriuretic effect of furosemide and thiazides; monitor for renal failure. May increase lithium levels; monitor for toxicity. Synergistic effects on GI bleeding with warfarin. Observe for dose adjustment with hydantoins, sulfonamides, or sulfonylureas. May reduce antihypertensive effects of propranolol and other β-blockers. Probenecid may increase half-life. (EC-Naprosyn) Avoid with H_2-blockers, sucralfate, or intensive antacid therapy.

PREGNANCY: Category C, not for use in nursing.

MECHANISM OF ACTION: NSAIDs; unknown, suspected to inhibit prostaglandin synthetase.

PHARMACOKINETICS: Absorption: Rapid and complete. Bioavailability (95%), C_{max}=97.4mcg/mL; T_{max}=1.9 hrs; AUC_{0-12h}=767mcg•hr/mL. (Tab, Delayed-Release) C_{max}=94.9mcg/mL; T_{max}=4 hrs; AUC_{0-12h}=845mcg•hr/mL. (Sus) T_{max}=1-4 hrs. **Distribution:** V_d=0.16L/kg; plasma protein binding (>99%); excreted in breast milk. **Metabolism:** Hepatic. Metabolite (6-O-desmethyl naproxen). **Elimination:** Urine (95%), feces (≤3%); $T_{1/2}$=12-17 hrs.

NURSING CONSIDERATIONS

Assessment: Assess for history of asthma, cardiovascular thrombotic events, CABG surgery, stroke, MI, cardiovascular disease (pre-existing HTN, CHF) or risk factors for disease, fluid retention, edema, pregnancy status, risk factors for GI events (bleeding, ulceration, perforation), possible drug interactions, renal/hepatic dysfunction.

Monitoring: Monitor BP, CBC, LFTs, renal function, and chemistries periodically. Monitor for signs/symptoms of GI events (bleeding, ulceration, perforation), CV thrombotic events, CHF, HTN, salt depletion, renal/liver dysfunction.

Patient Counseling: Seek medical attention if symptoms of hepatotoxicity (nausea, fatigue, pruritus), anaphylactic reaction (difficulty breathing, swelling of face/throat), hypersensitivity reaction (rash), CV events (chest pain, SOB, weakness, slurring of speech), GI ulceration and bleeding (epigastric pain, dyspepsia, melena, hematemesis), weight gain, and edema. Inform of pregnancy risks. Caution may impair physical/mental abilities if experience drowsiness, dizziness, vertigo or depression during therapy.

Administration: PO. **Storage:** (Sus): 15-30°C (59-86°); avoid excessive heat, above 40°C (104°F). Dispense in light-resistant containers. Shake before use. (Tab, Delayed-Release): 15-30° (59-86°F) in well closed containers; dispense in light-resistant containers. (Tab): 15-30°C (59-86°F) in well-closed containers.

N

NARDIL

RX

phenelzine sulfate (Parke-Davis)

Antidepressants increased the risk of suicidal thinking and behavior (suicidality) in short-term studies in children, adolescents, and young adults with major depressive disorder (MDD) and other psychiatric disorders. Phenelzine is not approved for use in pediatric patients.

THERAPEUTIC CLASS: Monoamine oxidase inhibitor

INDICATIONS: Treatment of atypical, nonendogenous or neurotic depression not responsive to other antidepressants.

DOSAGE: *Adults:* Initial: 15mg tid. Titrate: Increase to 60-90mg/day at a fairly rapid pace until maximum benefit. Maint: Reduce slowly over several weeks to 15mg qd or 15mg every other day.

HOW SUPPLIED: Tab: 15mg

CONTRAINDICATIONS: Pheochromocytoma, CHF, history of liver disease, abnormal LFTs, severe renal impairment or renal disease, meperidine, MAOIs, dextromethorphan, CNS depressants, alcohol, certain narcotics, sympathomimetic drugs (eg, amphetamines, cocaine, methylphenidate, dopamine, epinephrine, norepinephrine), or related compounds (eg, methyldopa, L-dopa, L-tryptophan, L-tyrosine, phenylalanine), high tyramine-containing food (eg, cheese, pickled herring, beer, wine, yeast extract, salami, yogurt), excessive caffeine and chocolate, dextromethorphan, CNS depressants, buspirone, serotoninergic agents (eg, dexfenfluramine, fluoxetine, fluvoxamine, paroxetine, sertraline, venlafaxine), bupropion, guanethidine.

WARNINGS/PRECAUTIONS: Hypertensive crisis, postural hypotension reported; monitor BP frequently. Caution with epilepsy, asthma, DM, or psychosis. D/C if palpitations or headache occur. Excessive stimulation in schizophrenics. D/C 10 days prior to elective surgery. Avoid abrupt withdrawal.

ADVERSE REACTIONS: Dizziness, headache, drowsiness, sleep disturbances, constipation, dry mouth, GI disturbances, elevated serum transaminases, weight gain, edema, sexual disturbances.

INTERACTIONS: See Contraindications. Hypertensive crisis with other MAOIs, sympathomimetics, high tyramine-containing foods. Allow 10 days between starting another MAOI, or antidepressant or buspirone. Serious reactions reported with serotoninergic agents. Allow 5 weeks after discontinuing fluoxetine before starting therapy. Allow 2 weeks after discontinuing therapy before starting bupropion. Avoid cocaine and local, general, and spinal anesthesia. Reduce dose of barbiturates. Caution with rauwolfia alkaloids. Exaggerated hypotensive effects with antihypertensives. Excitation, seizures, delirium, hyperpyrexia, circulatory collapse, coma, and death have been reported with meperidine.

PREGNANCY: Safety in pregnancy and nursing not known.

MECHANISM OF ACTION: MAOI; inhibits MAO activity.

PHARMACOKINETICS: Absorption: (30mg): C_{max}=19.8ng/mL, T_{max}=43 mins. **Metabolism:** Oxidation via MAO. Acetylation (minor). **Elimination:** (30mg): $T_{1/2}$=11.6 hrs.

N

NURSING CONSIDERATIONS

Assessment: Assess for DM, pheochromocytoma, CHF, history of liver disease, possible drug interactions, risk for bipolar disorder, history of mania or seizures or schizophrenia, pregnancy/nursing status, severe renal/hepatic impairment.

Monitoring: Monitor BP, renal/hepatic function, for signs/symptoms of clinical worsening (suicidality, unusual changes in behavior), hypertensive crises (occipital headaches, neck stiffness, NV, sweating), seizures, liver dysfunction, postural hypotension, hypoglycemia, increased psychosis, and activation of mania.

Patient Counseling: Instruct to avoid concomitant use of alcohol, tyramine-containing foods/supplements/beverages (during and 2 weeks following d/c), and any cough medicine containing dextromethorphan. Seek medical attention for symptoms of hypertensive crises (occipital headaches, neck stiffness, NV, sweating), hypoglycemia, increased psychosis, seizures, postural hypotension, mania, clinical worsening (suicidal ideation, unusual changes in behavior), and liver dysfunction. Advise to change position gradually if lightheaded, faint, or dizzy. Counsel about pregnancy risks.

Administration: Oral route. **Storage:** 15-30°C (59-86°F).

NAROPIN — RX

ropivacaine HCl (Abraxis)

THERAPEUTIC CLASS: Local anesthetic

INDICATIONS: Production of local or regional anesthesia in surgery. Management of acute pain.

DOSAGE: *Adults:* Dose may vary by procedure, area to be anesthetized, tissue vascularity, duration and depth of anesthesia needed. Administer test dose of 3-5mL before induction of complete block. Surgical: Lumbar Epidural: Usual: 75-200mg in 15-30mL. Thoracic Epidural for Surgery: 25-113mg in 5-15mL. Lumbar Epidural in Cesarean: 100-150mg in 15-30mL. Major Nerve Block: 75-300mg in 10-50mL. Field Block: 5-200mg in 1-40mL Labor: Lumbar Epidural: Initial: 20-40mg. Maint: 12-28mg/h. Postoperative: Lumbar/Thoracic Epidural: 12-28mg/hr. Infiltration: 2-200mg in 1-100mL.

HOW SUPPLIED: Inj: 2mg/mL, 5mg/mL, 7.5mg/mL, 10mg/mL

WARNINGS/PRECAUTIONS: Administer in incremental doses. High risk of arrhythmias, circulatory arrest, and death reported in pregnant patients. Not for production of obstetrical paracervical block, retrobulbar block, or spinal anesthesia. Use lowest effective dose. Perform syringe aspiration to avoid extravasation and subarachnoid injection. Administer test dose with epidural anesthesia. Anxiety, dizziness, blurred vision, tremors, depression, and tinnitus are early signs of CNS toxicity. Caution in hepatic impairment, cardiovascular disorders, hypotension, hypovolemia, heart block. Should cardiac arrest occur, prolonged resuscitative efforts may be required to improve the probability of a successful outcome.

ADVERSE REACTIONS: Hypotension, bradycardia, NV, paresthesia, back pain, fever, chills, headache, pain, urinary retention, dizziness, pruritus, HTN, anemia.

INTERACTIONS: Caution with other local anesthetics, amide-type anesthetics; additive toxic effects may occur. Caution with class III antiarrhythmics. Increased levels with inhibitors of CYP450 1A2 (eg, fluvoxamine) and CYP450 3A4 (eg, ketoconazole).

PREGNANCY: Category B, caution in nursing.

MECHANISM OF ACTION: Mono amide class of local anesthetic agent; blocks the generation and conduction of nerve impulses, presumably by increasing the threshold for electrical excitation in the nerve by slowing the propagation of the nerve impulse and by reducing the rate of rise of the action potential.

PHARMACOKINETICS: Absorption: Complete and biphasic absorption (epidural space). Systemic concentration of drug is dependent on total dose, concentration, and route of administration; refer to PI for more information. **Distribution:** V_d=41L (IV); plasma protein binding (94%); crosses placenta; excreted in breast milk. **Metabolism:** Liver (extensive); aromatic hydroxylation, CYP4501A; 3-hydroxyropivacaine. **Elimination:** Urine: IV (86%), (1% unchanged); $T_{1/2}$=1.8 hrs and 4.2 hrs (epidural).

NURSING CONSIDERATIONS

Assessment: Assess for drug hypersensitivity, hepatic disease, impaired cardiovascular function, hypotension, hypovolemia or heart block or taking class III antiarrhythmic drugs (eg, amiodarone), pregnancy/nursing status, and possible drug interactions.

Monitoring: Monitor HR, BP and ECG, for allergic reactions, test dose reactions (eg, palpitations, nervousness and circumoral pallor), signs of CNS toxicity (eg, anxiety, light headedness, blurred vision, dizziness, and tremors), signs of unintended intrathecal administration, cardiovascular/respiratory vital signs, state of consciousness, and malignant hyperthermia.

Patient Counseling: Informed may experience temporary loss of sensation and motor activity in the anesthetized part of the body.

Administration: Epidural, IV route. **Storage:** 20-25°C (68-77°F).

NASACORT AQ — RX

triamcinolone acetonide (Sanofi-Aventis)

THERAPEUTIC CLASS: Corticosteroid

INDICATIONS: Treatment of the nasal symptoms of seasonal and perennial allergic rhinitis symptoms in adults and children ≥2 yrs.

DOSAGE: *Adults:* Initial/Max: 2 sprays per nostril qd. With improvement, may reduce dose to 1 spray per nostril qd.
Pediatrics: ≥12 yrs: Initial/Max: 2 sprays per nostril qd. With improvement, may reduce dose to 1 spray per nostril qd. 6-12 yrs: Initial: 1 spray per nostril qd. Max: 2 sprays per nostril qd. 2-5 yrs: Initial/Max: 1 spray per nostril qd.

HOW SUPPLIED: Spray: 55mcg/spray [16.5g]

WARNINGS/PRECAUTIONS: Glaucoma and/or cataracts may occur. Risk of adrenal insufficiency and withdrawal symptoms when replacing systemic corticosteroid with topical corticosteroids. Caution with active or quiescent TB, ocular herpes simplex, or untreated bacterial, fungal and systemic viral infections. Avoid with recent nasal trauma, surgery or septum ulcers. Risk for more severe/fatal course of infections (eg, chickenpox, measles) and for *Candida* infections of nose and pharynx. Potential for reduced growth velocity in pediatrics. Epistaxis and nasal septal perforation reported.

ADVERSE REACTIONS: Pharyngitis, epistaxis, increased cough, flu syndrome, bronchitis, dyspepsia, tooth disorder, headache, pharyngolaryngeal pain, nasopharyngitis, upper abdominal pain, diarrhea, asthma, and rash.

PREGNANCY: Category C, caution in nursing.

MECHANISM OF ACTION: Corticosteroid; not established; anti-inflammatory action.

PHARMACOKINETICS: Absorption: C_{max}=0.5ng/mL; T_{max}=1.5 hrs; AUC (110mcg, 400mcg)=1.4ng•hr/mL, 4.7ng•hr/mL. **Distribution:** V_d=99.5L. **Elimination:** $T_{1/2}$=3.1 hrs.

NURSING CONSIDERATIONS

Assessment: Assess for hypersensitivity, active or quiescent TB, untreated local or systemic fungal or bacterial infections, systemic viral or parasitic infections, ocular herpes simplex, nasal polyps or recent nasal septal ulcers, nasal surgery/trauma, concomitant use with other inhaled or systemic corticosteroids, and possible drug interactions.

Monitoring: Monitor for acute adrenal insufficiency, withdrawal symptoms, joint and/or muscular pain, lassitude and depression, hypercorticism and/or HPA-axis suppression, disseminated infections (eg, chickenpox and measles), nasal or pharyngeal *Candida* infections, hypoadrenalism in infants whose mothers received corticosteroids during pregnancy, suppression of growth velocity in children, nasal septal perforation or nasal septum discomfort, epistaxis, glaucoma, and cataracts.

Patient Counseling: Instruct to take as directed at regular intervals. Avoid exposure to chickenpox or measles; immediately notify physician if exposed, if symptoms worsen or do not improve, or if sneezing or nasal irritation occurs. Avoid spraying into eyes.

Administration: Intranasal. **Storage:** 20-25°C (68-77°F).

NASAREL — RX
flunisolide (Ivax)

THERAPEUTIC CLASS: Corticosteroid

INDICATIONS: Relief of seasonal or perennial rhinitis.

DOSAGE: *Adults:* Initial: 2 sprays per nostril bid. Titrate: May increase to 2 sprays per nostril tid. Max: 8 sprays per nostril/day.
Pediatrics: 6-14 yrs: Initial: 1 spray per nostril tid or 2 sprays per nostril bid. Max: 4 sprays per nostril/day.

HOW SUPPLIED: Spray: 29mcg/spray [25mL]

CONTRAINDICATIONS: Untreated localized infection of the nasal mucosa.

WARNINGS/PRECAUTIONS: Risk of adrenal insufficiency and withdrawal symptoms when replacing systemic corticosteroids with topical corticosteroids. Caution with active or quiescent TB, ocular herpes simplex, or untreated bacterial, fungal and systemic viral infections. Avoid with recent nasal trauma, surgery or septum ulcers. Risk for more severe/fatal course of infections (eg, chickenpox, measles) and for *Candida* infections of nose and pharynx. Potential for reduced growth velocity in pediatrics.

ADVERSE REACTIONS: After taste, nasal burning/stinging, cough, epistaxis, nasal dryness, pharyngitis, sinusitis.

INTERACTIONS: Concomitant systemic corticosteroids increases risk of hypercorticism and/or HPA axis suppression.

PREGNANCY: Category C, caution in nursing.

MECHANISM OF ACTION: Glucocorticosteroid; anti-inflammatory agent with potent glucucorticoid and weak mineralocorticoid activity.

PHARMACOKINETICS: Absorption: Well absorbed. **Metabolism:** Liver (rapidly). **Elimination:** Urine (65-70%) primary metabolite, feces.

NURSING CONSIDERATIONS

Assessment: Assess for drug hypersensitivity, active or quiescent TB, untreated localized/systemic fungal or bacterial infection, systemic viral infection, ocular herpes simplex, history of glaucoma or cataracts, history of nasal polyps, recent nasal septal ulcers, nasal surgery/trauma, concomitant use with other inhaled or systemic corticosteroids, possible drug interactions.

Monitoring: Monitor for hypersensitivity reactions, adrenal insufficiency, withdrawal symptoms (joint/muscle pain, lassitude, depression), hypothalamic-pituitary-adrenal suppression, nasal septal perforation with temporary/permanent loss of smell/taste, retardation of growth velocity in children, nasal/pharyngeal candida infections, chickenpox or measles.

Patient Counseling: Counsel to take as directed at regular intervals. Avoid exposure to chicken pox or measles; immediately consult physician if exposed, symptoms worsen, or severe nasal irritation occurs. Avoid spraying into eyes.

Administration: Intranasal route. **Storage:** 15-30°C (59-86°F).

NASONEX

mometasone furoate monohydrate (Schering)

RX

N

THERAPEUTIC CLASS: Corticosteroid

INDICATIONS: Treatment of the nasal symptoms of seasonal and perennial allergic rhinitis. Prophylaxis of the nasal symptoms of seasonal allergic rhinitis. Treatment of nasal polyps in patients 18 years of age and older.

DOSAGE: *Adults:* Allergic Rhinitis: Treatment/Prophylaxis: 2 sprays per nostril qd. For prophylaxis, start 2-4 weeks before allergy season. Nasal Polyps: 2 sprays per nostril bid.
Pediatrics: ≥12 yrs: Treatment/Prophylaxis: 2 sprays per nostril qd. For prophylaxis, start 2-4 weeks before allergy season. 2-11 yrs: Treatment: 1 spray per nostril qd.

HOW SUPPLIED: Spray: 50mcg/spray [17g]

WARNINGS/PRECAUTIONS: Risk of adrenal insufficiency and withdrawal symptoms when replacing systemic corticosteroids with topical corticosteroids. Caution with active or quiescent TB, ocular herpes simplex, or untreated bacterial, fungal and systemic viral infections. Avoid with recent nasal trauma, surgery or septum ulcers. Risk for more severe/fatal course of infections (eg, chickenpox, measles) and for *Candida* infections of nose and pharynx. Potential for reduced growth velocity in pediatrics.

ADVERSE REACTIONS: Headache, viral infection, pharyngitis, epistaxis, cough, upper respiratory tract infection, dysmenorrhea, myalgia, sinusitis.

PREGNANCY: Category C, caution with nursing.

MECHANISM OF ACTION: Corticosteroid; not established; demonstrates anti-inflammatory properties, shown to have a wide range of effects on multiple cell types (eg, mast cells, eosinophils, neutrophils, macrophages, lymphocytes) and mediators (eg, histamine, eicosanoids, leukotrienes, cytokines) involved in inflammation.

PHARMACOKINETICS: Distribution: Plasma protein binding (98-99%). **Metabolism:** Liver (extensive) via CYP3A4. **Elimination:** Bile (as metabolites); $T_{1/2}$=5.8 hrs.

NURSING CONSIDERATIONS

Assessment: Assess for active or quiescent TB, untreated localized or systemic viral, fungal or bacterial infections, history of glaucoma or cataracts, history of nasal polyps, recent nasal septal ulcers, nasal surgery/trauma, and possible drug interactions.

Monitoring: Monitor for acute adrenal insufficiency, hypercorticism and/or HPA-axis suppression, nasal or pharyngeal *Candida* infections, suppression of growth velocity in children, hypersensitivity reactions or contact dermatitis, wheezing, nasal septum perforation, changes in vision, increased IOP.

Patient Counseling: Take as directed at regular intervals; do not increase prescribed dosage to increase effectiveness. Avoid exposure to chickenpox or measles; immediately consult physician if exposed or experience episodes of epistaxis. Contact physician if symptoms worsen or do not improve. Avoid spraying into eyes or directly onto nasal septum.

Administration: Intranasal route. **Storage:** 25°C (77°F); excursions permitted to 15-30°C.

NATRECOR RX

nesiritide (Scios Inc.)

THERAPEUTIC CLASS: Human B-type natriuretic peptide

INDICATIONS: Treatment of acutely decompensated congestive heart failure with dyspnea at rest or with minimal activity.

DOSAGE: *Adults:* 2mcg/kg IV bolus over 60 seconds, then 0.01mcg/kg/min IV infusion. Reduce dose or d/c if hypotension occurs.

HOW SUPPLIED: Inj: 1.5mg

CONTRAINDICATIONS: Primary therapy with cardiogenic shock or systolic BP <90mmHg.

WARNINGS/PRECAUTIONS: Avoid with low cardiac filling pressures. Use precautions for parenteral administration of protein pharmaceuticals or *E.coli*-derived products; may cause allergic reaction. Avoid when vasodilators are inappropriate (eg, significant valvular stenosis, restrictive/obstructive cardiomyopathy, constrictive pericarditis, pericardial tamponade, conditions where cardiac output is dependent on venous return). May affect renal function; azotemia reported. Monitor BP closely; hypotension reported. Caution with BP <100mmHg at baseline. Reduce dose or d/c if hypotension occurs.

ADVERSE REACTIONS: Hypotension, ventricular tachycardia, ventricular extrasystoles, headache, back pain, dizziness, anxiety, nausea, abdominal pain, insomnia

INTERACTIONS: Increased risk of hypotension with drugs that cause hypotension such as oral ACE inhibitors. Do not co-administer through the same IV catheter with heparin, insulin, ethacrynate sodium, bumetanide, enalaprilat, hydralazine, furosemide, or injectable drugs containing sodium metabisulfite. Flush catheter between uses with incompatible drugs.

PREGNANCY: Category C, caution in nursing.

MECHANISM OF ACTION: Human B-type natriuretic peptide; binds to the particulate guanylate cyclase receptor of vascular smooth muscle and endothelial cells, leading to increased intracellular concentrations of cGMP and smooth muscle relaxation.

PHARMACOKINETICS: Distribution: V_{ss}=0.19L/kg. **Elimination:** Renal; $T_{1/2}$=18 min.

NURSING CONSIDERATIONS

Assessment: Assess for cardiogenic shock or with SBP ≤90mmHg, significant valvular stenosis, restrictive or obstructive cardiomyopathy, constrictive pericarditis, pericardial tamponade, low cardiac filling pressure, and known hypersensitivity to drug and to any of its components.

Monitoring: Monitor renal function test, symptoms of hypotension, cardiac index/status, and hemodynamic monitoring, HR, VT, bradycardia, NV.

Patient Counseling: Counsel about potential adverse effects of drug.

Administration: (IV) Infusion bag preparation: 1) Reconstitute one 1.5mg vial by adding 5mL of diluent. 2) Do not shake the bottle. Rock the vial gently so that all surfaces, including the stopper, are in contact with the diluent to ensure complete reconstitution. 3) Withdraw the entire contents of the reconstituted vial and add to the 250mL plastic IV bag. The IV bag should be inverted several times to ensure complete mixing. 4) Use reconstituted solution within 24 hrs and store at 2-25°C (36-77°F). **Storage:** 25°C. Do not freeze. Keep vial in the outer carton to protect from light.

NAVANE

thiothixene (Pfizer)

RX

THERAPEUTIC CLASS: Thioxanthene

INDICATIONS: Management of schizophrenia.

DOSAGE: *Adults:* Mild Condition: Initial: 2mg tid. Titrate: May increase to 15mg/day. Severe Condition: Initial: 5mg bid. Usual: 20-30mg/day. Max: 60mg/day.
Pediatrics: ≥12 yrs: Mild Condition: Initial: 2mg tid. Titrate: May increase to 15mg/day. Severe Condition: Initial: 5mg bid. Usual: 20-30mg/day. Max: 60mg/day.

HOW SUPPLIED: Cap: 1mg, 2mg, 5mg, 10mg, 20mg

CONTRAINDICATIONS: Circulatory collapse, comatose states, CNS depression, blood dyscrasias.

WARNINGS/PRECAUTIONS: May develop tardive dyskinesia, NMS. May mask symptoms of overdose of toxic drugs. May obscure conditions such as intestinal obstruction and brain tumor. May lower seizure threshold. Monitor for pigmentary retinopathy and lenticular pigmentation. Caution with cardiovascular disease, extreme heat exposure, activities requiring alertness. May elevate prolactin levels.

ADVERSE REACTIONS: Tachycardia, hypotension, lightheadedness, syncope, drowsiness, agitation, insomnia, hyperreflexia, cerebral edema, pseudoparkinsonism, LFT elevation, blood dyscrasias, rash, photosensitivity, dry mouth, blurred vision.

INTERACTIONS: Possible additive effects including hypotension with CNS depressants, alcohol. Caution with atropine or related drugs. Paradoxical effects with pressor agents.

PREGNANCY: Safety in pregnancy and nursing not known.

MECHANISM OF ACTION: Thioxanthene derivative.

NURSING CONSIDERATIONS

Assessment: Assess for history of CV disorders, CNS depression or coma, blood dyscrasias, convulsive disorders, alcohol intake, and possible drug interactions.

Monitoring: Monitor for hypersensitivity reactions, TD, clinical manifestations of NMS, CV effects, visual disturbances, extrapyramidal symptoms. Monitor liver enzymes, bilirubin, CBC, prolactin, and blood glucose.

Patient Counseling: Advise about risk of chronic use of drug. Use caution when performing hazardous tasks (operating machinery/driving). Warn about possible additive effects (hypotension) when drug is combined with CNS depressants and/or alcohol.

Administration: Oral route.

NAVELBINE RX

vinorelbine tartrate (GlaxoSmithKline)

For IV use only; fatal if given intrathecally. Severe granulocytopenia may occur; granulocyte counts should be ≥1000cells/mm³ prior to administration. Use extreme caution to prevent extravasation (can cause local tissue necrosis); if this occurs, d/c and restart in another vein. Administer only under supervision of a physician experienced in the use of antineoplastic agents.

THERAPEUTIC CLASS: Vinca alkaloid

INDICATIONS: Single agent or in combination with cisplatin for 1st-line treatment of unresectable, advanced non-small cell lung cancer (NSCLC), including Stage IV NSCLC. For use in combination with cisplatin for Stage III NSCLC .

DOSAGE: *Adults:* Single-Agent: 30mg/m² IV weekly over 6-10 min. With Cisplatin: 25mg/m² weekly with cisplatin 100mg/m² every 4 weeks, or 30mg/m² weekly with cisplatin 120mg/m² on Days 1 and 29, then every 6 weeks. Adjustments Based on Granulocytes: If 1000-1499cells/mm³ give 50% starting dose. If <1000cells/mm³, hold dose and repeat count in 1 week. D/C if hold 3 consecutive weekly doses because granulocyte <1000cells/mm³. If fever and/or sepsis occurs while granulocytopenic or if hold 2 consecutive weekly doses due to granulocytopenia; give 75% of the starting dose if granulocytes ≥1500cells/mm³, and 37.5% of the starting dose if granulocytes 1000-1499cells/mm³. Hepatic Insufficiency: (bilirubin 2.1-3mg/dL) 50% of starting dose or (bilirubin >3mg/dL) 25% of starting dose. If both hematologic toxicity and hepatic insufficiency, use lowest dose. Neurotoxicity: D/C if Grade ≥2 develops.

HOW SUPPLIED: Inj: 10mg/mL

CONTRAINDICATIONS: Pretreatment granulocytes <1000cells/mm³.

WARNINGS/PRECAUTIONS: Monitor for myleosuppression during and after therapy, and for infection and/or fever with developing severe granulocytopenia. Interstitial pulmonary changes, ARDS, acute shortness of breath and severe bronchospasm reported. Extreme caution with compromised bone marrow reserve due to prior irradiation or chemotherapy. Radiation recall reactions may occur. Monitor for new or worsening signs/symptoms of neuropathy. D/C if moderate or severe neurotoxicity develops. Avoid contact with skin, mucosa, and eyes. Avoid pregnancy. May cause severe constipation, paralytic ileus, intestinal obstruction, necrosis, and/or perforation.

ADVERSE REACTIONS: Granulocytopenia, leukopenia, thrombocytopenia, anemia, asthenia, injection site reactions/pain, phlebitis, peripheral neuropathy, NV, diarrhea, severe constipation, paralytic ileus, intestinal obstruction, necrosis, and/or perforation, dyspnea, alopecia, chest pain, fatigue.

INTERACTIONS: Risk of acute pulmonary reactions with mitomycin. Increased incidence of granulocytopenia with cisplatin. Monitor for signs/symptoms of neuropathy with paclitaxel, either concomitantly or sequentially. Radiosensitizing effects may occur with prior or concomitant radiation therapy. Caution with CYP450 3A inhibitors, or with hepatic dysfunction; earlier onset and/or increased severity of side effects may occur.

PREGNANCY: Category D, not for use in nursing.

MECHANISM OF ACTION: Vinca alkaloid; antitumor activity thought to be due primarily to inhibition of mitosis at metaphase through its interaction with tubulin. Also interferes with amino acid, cyclic AMP, and glutathione metabolism; calmodulin-dependent Ca^{++}-transport ATPase activity; cellular respiration; and nucleic acid and lipid biosynthesis.

PHARMACOKINETICS: Distribution: V_d=25.4-40.1L/kg, plasma protein binding (79.6%-91.2%). **Metabolism**: CYP450, 3A4: deacetylvinorelbine (major metabolite), vinorelbine N-oxide. **Elimination**: Feces (46%), urine (18%); $T_{1/2}$=27.7-43.6 hrs.

NURSING CONSIDERATIONS

Assessment: Assess CBC with differential, LFTs, pulmonary function. Assess for history of prior irradiation or chemotherapy, neuropathy, CVD, pregnancy status.

Monitoring: Monitor CBC with differential, LFTs, pulmonary function, constipation, paralytic ileus, injection-site reactions, chest pain.

Patient Counseling: Inform about major acute toxicities (bone marrow toxicity, specifically granulocytopenia with increased susceptibility to infection). Immediately report fever or chills, SOB, cough, other new pulmonary symptoms, abdominal pain, or constipation. Advise women to avoid pregnancy. D/C nursing.

Administration: IV. Extremely important to properly position IV needle or catheter before injection. **Storage:** Refrigerate vials at 2-8°C (36-46°F) in the carton. Protect from light; do not freeze.

NEFAZODONE — RX

nefazodone HCl (Various)

Antidepressants increased the risk of suicidal thinking and behavior (suicidality) in short-term studies in children, adolescents, and young adults with major depressive disorder (MDD) and other psychiatric disorders. Nefazodone is not approved for use in pediatric patients. Life-threatening hepatic failure reported. Avoid with active liver disease or elevated serum transaminases. D/C and do not retreat if symptoms of hepatic disease develop or if ALT/AST ≥3x ULN.

THERAPEUTIC CLASS: Serotonin and norepinephrine reuptake inhibitor

INDICATIONS: Treatment of depression.

DOSAGE: *Adults:* Initial: 100mg bid. Usual: 300-600mg/day. Titrate: May increase by 100-200mg/day at intervals of no less than 1 week. Elderly/Debilitated: Initial: 50mg bid.

HOW SUPPLIED: Tab: 50mg, 100mg*, 150mg*, 200mg, 250mg *scored

CONTRAINDICATIONS: Coadministration of terfenadine, astemizole, cisapride, pimozide, carbamazepine, triazolam. Liver injury from previous treatment.

WARNINGS/PRECAUTIONS: May cause postural hypotension. Caution with cardiovascular or cerebrovascular disease that could be exacerbated by hypotension and conditions with predisposition to hypotension (eg, dehydration, hypotension). May activate mania/hypomania. Priapism reported. Caution with history of MI, unstable heart disease, seizures, liver cirrhosis. Avoid with active liver disease.

ADVERSE REACTIONS: Hepatic failure, somnolence, dry mouth, nausea, dizziness, insomnia, agitation, constipation, asthenia, lightheadedness, blurred vision, confusion, abnormal vision.

INTERACTIONS: Avoid MAOIs within 14 days of use. Avoid alcohol, terfenadine, astemizole, cisapride, pimozide. Reduce triazolam dose by 75% and avoid in elderly. Reduce alprazolam dose by 50%. Effects antagonized by carbamazepine. Caution with highly protein bound drugs, drugs metabolized by CYP3A4, CNS-active drugs. Discontinue prior to general anesthesia. Haloperidol may need dose adjustment. Increases plasma levels of cyclosporine, tacrolimus. Rhabdomyolysis (rare) reported with simvastatin and lovastatin. Monitor digoxin. Institute a wash-out period and lower doses if used after fluoxetine therapy. May increase buspirone levels; decrease buspirone dose to 2.5mg qd.

PREGNANCY: Category C, caution in nursing.

MECHANISM OF ACTION: 5-HT and NE reuptake inhibitor (phenylpiperazine); potentiates neurotransmitter activity of CNS by inhibiting neuronal serotonin and norephinephrine reuptake.

PHARMACOKINETICS: Absorption: Rapid; absolute bioavailability (20%), T_{max}=1 hr. **Distribution:** V_d=0.22-0.87L/kg; plasma protein binding (>99%). **Metabolism:** N-dealkylation and aliphatic and aromatic hydroxylation. **Elimination:** Urine (<1%); $T_{1/2}$=2-4 hrs.

NURSING CONSIDERATIONS

Assessment: Assess liver function, bipolar disorder risk, history of mania and seizures, possible drug interactions, CV and cerebrovascular diseases.

Monitoring: Monitor HR, BP, and LFTs. Monitor for signs/symptoms of clinical worsening (suicidality, unusual changes in behavior), allergic reactions (rash, hives), postural hypotension, visual disturbances (blurred vision, scotoma, visual trails), hepatic dysfunction (jaundice, anorexia, GI complaints, malaise), seizures, cognitive/motor impairment.

Patient Counseling: Advise to continue therapy even if symptoms improve. Avoid alcohol. Seek medical attention if symptoms of mania, allergic reaction (rash, hives), seizures, clinical worsening (suicidal ideation, unusual changes in behavior), postural hypotension, visual disturbances (blurred vision, scotoma, visual trails), and hepatic dysfunction (jaundice, anorexia, GI complaints, malaise) occur. Caution may impair physical/mental abilities.

Administration: Oral route. **Storage:** 20-25°C (68-77°F). Dispense in tight, light-resistant container with child-resistant closure.

NEOMYCIN/POLY B/HYDROCORTISONE OTIC RX

polymyxin B sulfate - hydrocortisone - neomycin (Various)

THERAPEUTIC CLASS: Antibacterial/corticosteroid combination

INDICATIONS: (Sol/Sus) Treatment of superficial bacterial infections of the external auditory canal. (Sus) Treatment of infections of mastoidectomy and fenestration cavities.

DOSAGE: *Adults:* Clean and dry ear canal. Dropper: 4 drops tid-qid for up to 10 days. Alternate Regimen: Insert cotton wick into ear canal, then saturate cotton. Repeat q4h to keep cotton moist. Replace wick q24h.
Pediatrics: Clean and dry ear canal. Dropper: 3 drops tid-qid for up to 10 days. Alternate Regimen: Insert cotton wick into ear canal, then saturate cotton. Repeat q4h to keep cotton moist. Replace wick q24h.

N

HOW SUPPLIED: Sol, Sus: (Neomycin-Hydrocortisone-Polymyxin B) 0.35%-1%-10,000 U/mL [10mL]

CONTRAINDICATIONS: Herpes simplex, vaccinia, and varicella infections.

WARNINGS/PRECAUTIONS: Caution with perforated eardrum, chronic otitis media. Prolonged use may result in secondary infection. Re-evaluate if no improvement after 1 week. D/C after 10 days. Solution contains sulfites. May cause cutaneous sensitization.

ADVERSE REACTIONS: Skin sensitization, burning, itching, irritation, dryness, folliculitis, hypertrichosis, acneiform eruptions, secondary infection.

PREGNANCY: Category C, caution in nursing.

MECHANISM OF ACTION: Neomycin, Polymyxin B: Anti-infective agents; provide antibacterial activity against susceptible organsims. Hydrocortisone: Corticosteroid; possesses anti-inflammatory activity and inhibits body's defense mechanism against infection.

NURSING CONSIDERATIONS

Assessment: Assess for drug hypersensitivity, external auditory canal disorder due to cutaneous viral infection, chronic otitis media, stasis dermatitis, asthmatic history, perforated tympanic membrane, and pregnancy/nursing status.

Monitoring: Monitor for hypersensitivity reactions or cutaneous sensitization (eg, chronic dermatoses, reddening with swelling, dry scaling and itching), auditory function, ototoxicity, overgowth of nonsusceptible organisms, lab monitoring of eosinophils, and urinary 17-hydroxycorticosteroids.

Patient Counseling: Instruct to avoid touching dropper to ear or other surface. For otic use only. D/C drug and contact physician if sensitization occurs.

Administration: Otic route. **Storage**: 15-25°C (59-77°F).

NEORAL

RX

cyclosporine (Novartis)

Increased susceptibility to infection, and development of neoplasia, HTN, nephrotoxicity. Monitor blood levels to avoid toxicity. Neoral is not bioequivalent to Sandimmune. Risk of skin malignancies if previously treated with PUVA, UVB, coal tar, radiation, MTX, or other immunosuppressives.

THERAPEUTIC CLASS: Cyclic polypeptide immunosuppressant

INDICATIONS: Organ rejection prophylaxis in kidney, liver, and heart allogeneic transplants. Treatment of severe active, rheumatoid arthritis (RA) unresponsive to methotrexate (MTX). Treatment of nonimmunocompromised adults with severe, recalcitrant, plaque psoriasis unresponsive to at least 1 systemic therapy (eg, PUVA, retinoids, MTX) or when other systemic therapies are contraindicated/not tolerated.

DOSAGE: *Adults:* Transplant: Give initial oral dose 4-12 hrs before transplant or post-op. Dose bid. Initial: Renal Transplant: 9 ± 3mg/kg/day. Liver Transplant: 8±4mg/kg/day. Heart Transplant: 7 ± 3mg/kg/day. Give with corticosteroids initially. Conversion from Sandimmune: 1:1 dose conversion. Adjust to trough levels. Monitor every 4-7 days. RA: Initial: 1.25mg/kg bid. Titrate: May increase by 0.5-0.75mg/kg/day after 8 weeks, again after 12 weeks. Max: 4mg/kg/day. Discontinue if no benefit by week 16. Psoriasis: Initial: 1.25mg/kg bid for 4 weeks. Titrate: May increase by 0.5mg/kg/day every 2 weeks. Max: 4mg/kg/day. Decrease dose by 25-50% to control adverse events. Take at the same time every day. Dilute sol in orange or apple juice that is room temp.

HOW SUPPLIED: Cap: 25mg, 100mg; Sol: 100mg/mL [50mL]

CONTRAINDICATIONS: Abnormal renal function, uncontrolled HTN, malignancies. PUVA or UVB therapy, MTX, other immunosuppressants, coal tar, or radiation in psoriasis patients.

WARNINGS/PRECAUTIONS: Risk of hepatotoxicity and nephrotoxicity. Caution in elderly. Hyperkalemia, hyperuricemia, thrombocytopenia, microangiopathic hemolytic anemia, and encephalopathy reported in transplant patients. Monitor CBC and LFTs monthly with MTX. Monitor BP and renal function before therapy, every 2 weeks during 1st 3 months, then monthly if stable with RA or psoriasis. Monitor SCr after initiation or increase NSAID dose in RA. Monitor CBC, uric acid, K^+, lipids, and magnesium every 2 weeks during 1st 3 months, then monthly if stable in RA. Monitor LFTs repeatedly. Monitor CBC, SCr with transplants.

ADVERSE REACTIONS: Renal dysfunction, HTN, hirsutism, muscle cramps, acne, tremor, headache, gingival hyperplasia, diarrhea, nausea, vomiting, paresthesia, flushing, dyspepsia, hypertrichosis, stomatitis, hypomagnesemia.

INTERACTIONS: Phenytoin, phenobarbital, rifampin, nafcillin, carbamazepine, orlistat, ticlopidine, octreotide, St. John's wort, oxcarbazepine, and bosentan decrease cyclosporine levels. Increases MTX levels. Potentiated by clarithromycin, diltiazem, fluconazole, erythromycin, itraconazole, ketoconazole, voriconazole, verapamil, nicardipine, quinupristin/dalfopristin, allopurinol, bromocriptine, danazol, metoclopramide, colchicine, amiodarone, grapefruit juice. Aminoglycosides, ciprofloxacin, vancomycin, SMZ/TMP, melphalan, ketoconazole, NSAIDs, colchicine, cimetidine, ranitidine, tacrolimus, amphotericin B, bezafibrate, fenofibrate, and methotrexate may potentiate renal dysfunction. Digitalis toxicity reported. Myotoxicity with statins, frequent gingival hyperplasia with nifedipine, and convulsions with high-dose methylprednisolone reported. Avoid potassium-sparing diuretics, grapefruit juice. Decreased clearance of prednisolone, digoxin, and lovastatin. Caution with HIV protease inhibitors, ACEIs, angiotensin II blockers. Decreased effects of vaccinations; avoid live attenuated vaccines.

PREGNANCY: Category C, not for use in nursing.

MECHANISM OF ACTION: Immunosuppressive agent; inhibits immunocompetent lymphocytes in the G_0-and G_1 phase of cell cycle, T-lymphocytes, T-helper and T-suppressor cells. Also inhibits lymphokine production and release, including interleukin-2.

N

PHARMACOKINETICS: Absorption: Incomplete; T_{max}=1.5-2 hrs. Pharmacokinetic parameters varied with different indications (renal, liver, rheumatoid arthritis and/or psoriasis). **Distribution:** V_d=3.5L/kg (IV); plasma protein binding (90%); found in breast milk. **Metabolism:** (extensive) Via CYP3A, in liver, GI tract, kidneys. Major metabolites (M1, M9, and M4N); oxidation and demethylation pathways. **Elimination:** Bile (primary), urine (6% unchanged and metabolites); $T_{1/2}$=8.4 hrs.

NURSING CONSIDERATIONS

Assessment: Baseline lab assessment for CBC, SrCr, BUN, BP, serum magnesium, K^+, uric acid, bilirubin, liver enzymes and lipids. Assess for occult infections, malignancies, skin lesions, RA/psoriasis and immunosuppressive agents, vaccination history, pregnancy/nursing status, and possible drug interactions.

Monitoring: Routinely monitor for cyclosporine blood concentrations, CBC, K^+, uric acid, lipids, bilirubin, liver enzymes, magnesium, microangiopathic hemolytic anemia, vasculopathy, BP, lymphomaproliferative and skin malignancies, convulsions, encephalopathy, impaired consciousness, graft-versus-host disease, infections, symptoms/signs of graft rejection or nephrotoxicity, kidney biopsies for renal tubular atrophy and interstitial fibrosis.

Patient Counseling: Counsel not to administer cyclosporine concurrently with PUVA or UVB, other radiation therapy/immunosuppressive agents. Inform of necessity for repeated lab tests. Instruct to take exactly as directed.

Administration: Oral route. (Dilute only with orange or apple juice, not grapefruit juice). **Storage:** 20-25°C (68-77°F).

NEOSPORIN OPHTHALMIC RX

bacitracin zinc - polymyxin B sulfate - neomycin sulfate (King)

N

THERAPEUTIC CLASS: Antibacterial combination

INDICATIONS: Superficial ocular infections including conjunctivitis, keratitis and keratoconjunctivitis, blepharitis and blepharoconjunctivitis.

DOSAGE: *Adults:* (Oint) Apply q3-4h for 7-10 days. (Sol) Instill 1-2 drops q4h for 7-10 days. Severe Infection: 2 drops q1h.

HOW SUPPLIED: Oint: (Bacitracin-Neomycin-Polymyxin B) 400U-3.5mg-10,000U/g [3.5g]; Sol: (Gramicidin-Neomycin-Polymyxin B) 0.025mg-1.75mg-10,000U/mL [10mL]

WARNINGS/PRECAUTIONS: May cause cutaneous sensitization. Ointment may retard corneal wound healing.

ADVERSE REACTIONS: Itching, swelling, conjunctival erythema, local irritation, superinfection.

PREGNANCY: Category C, caution in nursing.

MECHANISM OF ACTION: Antibacterial combination. Neomycin: Aminoglycoside antibiotic; inhibits protein synthesis by binding with ribosomal RNA and causing misreading of the bacterial genetic code. Polymyxin B: Increases permeability of the bacterial cell membrane by interacting with the phospholipid components of the membrane. Gramicidin: Increases permeability of bacterial cell membrane to inorganic cations by forming network of channels through normal lipid bilayer of membrane.

NURSING CONSIDERATIONS

Assessment: Assess for proper diagnosis of causative organisms and use in pregnant/nursing females.

Monitoring: Monitor for hypersensitivity reactions (rash), allergic cross-reactions, and cutaneous sensitization (eg, itching, reddening, edema of the conjunctiva or eyelid, failure to heal). For patients on sustained therapy, monitor for overgrowth of nonsusceptible organisms (eg, fungi) and development of superinfection. Monitor for signs of bacterial resistance (eg, purulent discharge, inflammation, pain). Monitor for bacterial keratitis in patients using multiple-dose containers.

Patient Counseling: Instruct to avoid allowing tip of dispensing container to contact eye, eyelid, fingers, or any other surfaces. To avoid spread of infection, do not share medication with other people. Instruct that ocular products, if handled improperly, can cause ocular infections. Advise if condition persists or gets worse, or if rash or allergic reaction occurs, to notify physician.

Administration: Ocular route. Do not inject into eye. **Storage:** 15-25°C (59-77°F). Protect from light.

NEULASTA RX
pegfilgrastim (Amgen)

THERAPEUTIC CLASS: Pegylated granulocyte colony stimulating factor

INDICATIONS: To decrease the incidence of infection, as manifested by febrile neutropenia, in patients with nonmyeloid malignancies receiving myelosuppressive anticancer drugs.

DOSAGE: *Adults:* 6mg SQ once per chemotherapy cycle. Do not administer in the period between 14 days before and 24 hrs after chemotherapy.

HOW SUPPLIED: Inj: 6mg/0.6mL

CONTRAINDICATIONS: Hypersensitivity to *E.coli*-derived proteins.

WARNINGS/PRECAUTIONS: Rare cases of splenic rupture reported, some fatal. Evaluate for enlarged spleen or splenic rupture if complaints of upper abdominal and/or shoulder tip pain. Acute respiratory distress syndrome (ARDS), allergic reactions (eg, anaphylaxis, rash) reported with filgrastim. Caution with sickle cell disease; monitor for sickle cell crises. Obtain CBC, platelets before chemotherapy. Monitor Hct, platelets regularly. Do not use in infants, children, and smaller adolescents <45kg.

ADVERSE REACTIONS: Bone pain, myalgia, arthralgia, peripheral edema, NV, fatigue, alopecia, diarrhea, constipation, fever, anorexia, headache.

INTERACTIONS: Lithium may potentiate release of neutrophils; monitor neutrophil counts. Increased hematopoietic activity of the bone marrow in response to growth factor therapy has been associated with transient positive bone-imaging changes. This should be considered when interpreting bone-imaging results.

PREGNANCY: Category C, caution in nursing.

MECHANISM OF ACTION: Pegylated granulocyte colony stimulating factor; acts on hematopoietic cells by binding to specific cell surface receptors, thereby stimulating proliferation, differentiation, commitment, and end cell functional activation.

PHARMACOKINETICS: Elimination: (SQ) $T_{1/2}$=80 hrs.

NURSING CONSIDERATIONS

Assessment: Assess for myeloid malignancies, myelodysplasia, history of chemotherapy/radiation therapy, history of hypersensitivity to *E.coli*-derived proteins, and possible drug interactions.

Monitoring: Monitor CBC with differential, platelet count. Perform annual bone marrow and cytogenetic evaluations throughout treatment on patients with congenital neutropenia. Monitor for hypersensitivity reactions, splenic rupture, ARDS, alveolar hemorrhage and hemoptysis, sickle cell crises (in patients with sickle cell disease), and Sweet's syndrome.

Patient Counseling: Discuss signs/symptoms of allergic drug reactions and advise appropriate actions. Counsel on importance of compliance with treatment, including regular monitoring of blood counts. Caution patient and caregivers against reuse of needles, syringes, or drug product, and thoroughly instruct in their proper disposal.

Administration: SQ route. **Storage:** Refrigerate at 2-8°C (36-46°F). Avoid freezing.

NEUMEGA

RX

oprelvekin (Wyeth)

Allergic or hypersensitivity reactions, including anaphylaxis, reported; permanently d/c if an allergic or hypersensitivity reaction develops.

THERAPEUTIC CLASS: Thrombopoietic agent

INDICATIONS: Prevention of severe thrombocytopenia and reduction of the need for platelet transfusions following myelosuppressive chemotherapy in nonmyeloid malignancy patients at high risk.

DOSAGE: *Adults:* 50mcg/kg qd SQ. Severe renal impairment (CrCl<30mL/min) 25mcg/kg qd SQ.Initiate 6-24 hrs after chemotherapy completion. Monitor platelets to assess optimal duration of therapy. Continue therapy until post-nadir platelets ≥50,000 cells/mcL. D/C at least 2 days before next chemotherapy cycle. Max: 21 days of therapy.

HOW SUPPLIED: Inj: 5mg

WARNINGS/PRECAUTIONS: Fluid retention reported; caution in CHF and patients receiving aggressive hydration. Capillary leak syndrome, pleural/pericardial effusion, renal failure, visual disturbances, papilledema, stroke, and rash reported. Monitor fluid and electrolyte balance with chronic diuretic therapy. Permanently d/c if significant allergic reactions occur. Moderate decreases in Hgb, Hct, and RBCs reported. Caution with history of atrial arrhythmias. May develop antibodies to therapy. Obtain CBC before therapy, then regularly. Monitor platelets during expected nadir time and until adequate recovery.

ADVERSE REACTIONS: Edema, dyspnea, tachycardia, conjunctival injection, palpitations, atrial arrhythmias, pleural effusions, syncope, pneumonia, neutropenic fever, headache, N/V, fever, mucositis, diarrhea.

PREGNANCY: Category C, not for use in nursing.

MECHANISM OF ACTION: Thrombopoietic agent; stimulates megakaryocytopoiesis and thrombopoiesis.

PHARMACOKINETICS: Absorption: Absolute bioavailability (>80%); C_{max}=17.4ng/mL; T_{max}=3.2 hrs. **Elimination:** Kidneys (animal studies); $T_{1/2}$=6.9 hrs.

NURSING CONSIDERATIONS

Assessment: Assess pregnancy status, bone marrow transplant, fluid retention or overload, capillary leak syndrome, pleural/pericardial effusion, CHF, aggressive hydration, history of papilledema or tumors of CNS, renal failure, prior myeloablative chemotherapy, history of atrial arrhythmias, and history of stroke or transient ischemic attack. Obtain baseline CBC including platelet count.

Monitoring: Periodically monitor CBC including platelet counts, fluid balance, fluid and electrolyte status (chronic diuretics). Monitor for signs/symptoms of hypersensitivity reactions, papilledema, fluid retention, pleural/pericardial effusion, atrial arrhythmias, and anemia.

Patient Counseling: Inform of pregnancy risks. Advise to seek medical attention if symptoms of hypersensitivity reactions (edema, SOB, wheezing, chest pain, hypotension), worsening of dyspnea (CHF, pleural effusion), atrial arrhythmias, anemia, or papilledema (blurred vision, blindness) occur.

Administration: SQ route; thigh, abdomen, or hip (upper arm if not self-injecting). **Storage:** 2-8°C (36-46°F). Protect from light; do not freeze. Reconstituted: 2-8°C (36-46°F) or room temperature, 25°C (77°F); stable for 3 hrs. Do not freeze or shake.

NEUPOGEN RX

filgrastim (Amgen)

THERAPEUTIC CLASS: Granulocyte colony stimulating factor

INDICATIONS: To decrease incidence of infection, as manifested by febrile neutropenia, in nonmyeloid malignancies with myelosuppressive anti-cancer drugs (eg, bone marrow transplants). To reduce duration of neutropenia and fever in adults after induction or consolidation chemotherapy with acute myeloid leukemia. For peripheral blood progenitor cell collection (PBPC) and therapy. For severe chronic neutropenia.

DOSAGE: *Adults:* Myelosuppressive Chemotherapy: Initial: 5mcg/kg qd SQ bolus, short IV infusion, or continuous SQ/IV infusion. Monitor CBCs and platelets before therapy, twice weekly during therapy. Titrate: Increase 5mcg/kg for each chemotherapy cycle according to duration and severity of ANC nadir. Avoid 24 hrs before through 24 hrs after cytotoxic chemotherapy. Perform CBC twice weekly during therapy. Continue therapy after chemotherapy until the post nadir ANC =10,000/mm^3. BMT: Following BMT, 10mcg/kg/day by IV infusion of 4 or 24 hrs, or by continuous 24-hr SQ infusion. First dose at least 24 hrs after chemotherapy and at least 24 hrs after bone marrow infusion. Dose Adjustment: If ANC >1000/mm^3 for 3 days, 5mcg/kg/day; increase to 10mcg/kg/day if ANC <1000/mm^3. If ANC >1000/mm^3 for 3 more days, stop therapy. If ANC drops to <1000/mm^3, resume 5mcg/kg/day. PBPC: 10mcg/kg/day bolus or continuous SQ 4 days before and for 6-7 days with leukapheresis on days 5, 6, and 7. Monitor neutrophils after 4 days and adjust if WBC >100,000/mm^3. Chronic Neutropenia: Congenital Neutropenia: Initial: 6mcg/kg SQ bid. Idiopathic or Cyclic Neutropenia: Initial: 5mcg/kg SQ qd. Adjust dose based on clinical course and ANC.

HOW SUPPLIED: Inj: 300mcg/0.5mL, 300mcg/mL, 480mcg/0.8mL, 480mcg/1.6mL [10^s]

CONTRAINDICATIONS: Hypersensitivity to *E. coli*-derived proteins.

WARNINGS/PRECAUTIONS: Allergic-type reactions may occur. Rare cases of splenic rupture reported, some fatal. Evaluate for enlarged spleen or splenic rupture if complaints of left upper abdominal and/or shoulder tip pain. Acute respiratory distress syndrome reported with sepsis; d/c until resolved. Sickle cell crisis reported with sickle cell disease; keep patient well hydrated. Potential for immunogenicity. The patient may be at greater risk of thrombocytopenia, anemia, and nonhematologic consequences due to the potential of receiving higher doses of chemotherapy. Regular monitoring of Hct and platelet count recommended. Alveolar hemorrhage manifesting as pulmonary infiltrates and hemoptysis requiring hospitalization reported.

ADVERSE REACTIONS: Bone pain, NV, rash, alopecia, diarrhea, neutropenic fever, mucositis, fatigue, anorexia, dyspnea.

INTERACTIONS: Caution with drugs that may potentiate the release of neutrophils (eg, lithium). Transient positive bone imaging changes have been associated with increased hematopoietic activity of the bone marrow in response to growth factor therapy. This should be considered when interpreting bone-imaging results.

PREGNANCY: Category C, caution in nursing.

MECHANISM OF ACTION: Granulocyte colony-stimulating factor (G-CSF); acts on hematopoietic cells by binding to specific cell surface receptors. Stimulates proliferation, differentiation commitment, and some end-cell functional activation.

PHARMACOKINETICS: Absorption: (IV, 20mcg/kg over 24 hrs): C_{max}=48ng/mL; (SQ, 3.45mcg/kg, 11.5mcg/kg): C_{max}=4ng/mL, 49ng/mL. **Distribution**: V_d=150mL/kg. **Elimination**: (IV) $T_{1/2}$=231 min (34.5mcg/kg). (SQ) $T_{1/2}$=210 min (3.45mcg/kg).

NURSING CONSIDERATIONS

Assessment: Assess for severe chronic neutropenia, history of chemotherapy/radiation therapy, history of hypersensitivity to *E. coli*-derived proteins, and possible drug interactions.

Monitoring: Monitor CBC with differential, platelet count. Perform annual bone marrow and cytogenetic evaluations throughout treatment for patients with congenital neutropenia. Monitor for hypersensitivity reactions, splenic rupture, ARDS, alveolar hemorrhage and hemoptysis, and sickle cell crises (in patients with sickle cell disease).

Patient Counseling: Counsel about potential adverse effects; seek medical attention if any develop. Advise to report any left upper abdominal or shoulder tip pain.

Administration: SQ/IV route. Refer to PI for details. **Storage:** Refrigerate at 2-8°C (36-46°F). Avoid shaking.

NEURONTIN — RX

gabapentin (Parke-Davis)

THERAPEUTIC CLASS: GABA analog

INDICATIONS: Adjunct therapy for partial seizures with or without secondary generalization in patients ≥12 yrs. Adjunct therapy for partial seizures in pediatrics 3-12 yrs. Management of postherpetic neuralgia (PHN).

DOSAGE: *Adults:* Epilepsy: Initial: 300mg tid. Titrate: Increase up to 1800mg/day. Max: 3600mg/day. PHN: 300mg single dose on Day 1, then 300mg bid on Day 2, and 300mg tid on Day 3. Increase further prn for pain. Max: 600mg tid. Renal Impairment: CrCl 30-59mL/min: 400-1400 mg/day. CrCl 15-29mL/min: 200-700 mg/day. CrCl 15mL/min: 100-300mg/day. CrCl <15 mL/min: Reduce dose in proportion to CrCl. Hemodialysis: Maint: Base on CrCl. Give supplemental dose (125-350mg) after 4 hrs of hemodialysis. Refer to prescribing information for dose adjustment.

N

Pediatrics: Epilepsy: >12 yrs: Initial: 300mg tid. Titrate: Increase up to 1800mg/day. Max: 3600mg/day. 3-12 yrs: Initial: 10-15mg/kg/day given tid. Titrate: Increase over 3 days. Usual: 3-4 yrs: 40mg/kg/day given tid. ≥5 yrs: 25-35mg/kg/day given tid. Max: 50mg/kg/day. Renal Impairment: ≥12 yrs: CrCl 30-59mL/min: 400-1400 mg/day. CrCl 15-29mL/min: 200-700 mg/day. CrCl 15mL/min: 100-300mg/day. CrCl <15 mL/min: Reduce dose in proportion to CrCl. Hemodialysis: Maint: Base on CrCl. Give supplemental dose (125-350 mg) after 4 hrs of hemodialysis. Refer to prescribing information for dose adjustment.

HOW SUPPLIED: Cap: 100mg, 300mg, 400mg; Sol: 250mg/5mL; Tab: 600mg*, 800mg* *scored

WARNINGS/PRECAUTIONS: Avoid abrupt withdrawal. Possible tumorigenic potential. Sudden and unexplained deaths reported. Neuropsychiatric adverse events in pediatrics (3-12 yrs).

ADVERSE REACTIONS: Somnolence, dizziness, ataxia, nystagmus, fatigue, tremor, rhinitis, weight gain, N/V, viral infection, fever, dysarthria, diplopia.

INTERACTIONS: Take 2 hrs after antacids. Increased levels with controlled-release morphine.

PREGNANCY: Category C, caution in nursing.

MECHANISM OF ACTION: Anticonvulsant; not established. Anticonvulsant activity: Suspected to bind to different areas of the brain including neocortex and hippocampus. Analgesic effects: Prevents allodynia and hyperalgesia.

PHARMACOKINETICS: Absorption: PO administration of variable doses resulted in different parameters. **Distribution:** V_d=58L; plasma protein binding (<3%); found in breast milk. **Metabolism:** Not appreciably metabolized. **Elimination:** Renal excretion (unchanged); $T_{1/2}$=5-7 hrs. Refer to PI for pediatric parameters.

NURSING CONSIDERATIONS

Assessment: Assess renal function and possible drug interactions prior to therapy.

Monitoring: Monitor for neuropsychiatric events (emotional lability, hostility, thought disorders, and hyperkinesia) in pediatric patients. Monitor for withdrawal-precipitated seizures, status epilepticus, and the emergence of tumors while on medication.

Patient Counseling: Instruct that medication may be taken with or without food. Caution against operating machinery/driving until accustomed to effects of medication. Counsel about signs/symptoms of CNS depression. Instruct not to abruptly d/c drug or skip doses. Counsel that if taking Maalox, separate dosing by 2 hrs.

Administration: Oral route. Advise that scored tabs can be broken in half. The remaining half tab should be administered at next dose. Discard half tabs after several days. **Storage:** Cap/Tab: Store at 25°C (77°F); excursions permitted to 15-30°C (59-86°F). Oral Solution: Store refrigerated. 2-8°C (36-46°F).

NEVANAC RX

nepafenac (Alcon)

THERAPEUTIC CLASS: NSAID

INDICATIONS: Treatment of pain and inflammation associated with cataract surgery.

DOSAGE: *Adults:* 1 drop tid, start 24 hrs prior to surgery, continue to 2 weeks post-op.

HOW SUPPLIED: Sus: 0.1% [3mL]

WARNINGS/PRECAUTIONS: Possible cross-sensitivity to acetylsalicylic acid, phenylacetic acid derivatives, and other NSAIDs. May cause increased bleeding of ocular tissue; slowed or delayed healing; keratitis. With continued use, may cause epithelial breakdown, corneal thinning, erosion, ulceration, perforation. Caution with bleeding tendencies and in complicated ocular surgeries, corneal denervation, corneal epithelial defects, diabetes mellitus, ocular surface diseases, rheumatoid arthritis, or repeat ocular surgeries.

ADVERSE REACTIONS: Capsular opacity, decreased visual acuity, foreign body sensation, increased IOP, and sticky sensation.

PREGNANCY: Category C, caution in nursing.

MECHANISM OF ACTION: NSAID; inhibits the cyclo-oxygenase that is essential for the biosynthesis of prostaglandins.

NURSING CONSIDERATIONS

Assessment: Assess for hypersensitivity or cross-sensitivity with some drugs (eg, acetylsalicylic acid), history of complicated or repeated ocular surgeries, corneal denervation, corneal epithelial defects, DM, ocular surface diseases (eg, dry eye syndrome), RA, bleeding tendencies, and history of concomitant use of medications that may prolong bleeding time or delay wound healing.

Monitoring: Monitor for hypersensitivity reactions, wound healing problems, keratitis, corneal thinning, corneal erosion, corneal ulceration or perforation, increased bleeding time, and bleeding of ocular tissues (hyphemas) in conjunction with ocular surgery.

Patient Counseling: Instruct not to administer suspension while wearing contact lenses.

Administration: Intraocular route. **Storage:** 2-25°C (36-77°F).

NEXAVAR RX

sorafenib (Bayer/Onyx)

THERAPEUTIC CLASS: Multikinase inhibitor

N

INDICATIONS: Treatment of advanced renal cell carcinoma or unresectable hepatocellular carcinoma.

DOSAGE: *Adults:* 400mg bid without food (1 hr before or 2 hrs after eating). Continue until no clinical benefit or unacceptable toxicity. Temporary interruption or dose reduction to 400mg qd or qod may be necessary if serious adverse events suspected.

HOW SUPPLIED: Tab: 200mg

WARNINGS/PRECAUTIONS: Risk of ischemia and/or infarction occured; temporary or permanent discontinuation may be necessary. Increased risk of bleeding may occur; consider discontinuation if bleeding necessitates medical intervention. HTN reported; monitor BP weekly during first 6 weeks and periodically thereafter. Hand-foot skin reaction and rash may occur; may require topical treatment, temporary treatment interruption, dose modification, or permanent discontinuation. D/C if GI perforation occurs. Temporary interruption of therapy recommended when undergoing surgical procedures. May cause fetal harm; women of childbearing potential should avoid becoming pregnant during therapy. Hepatic impairment may reduce plasma levels. Caution when co-administered with docetaxel and doxorubicin.

ADVERSE REACTIONS: HTN, fatigue, wt loss, rash/desquamation, hand-foot skin reaction, alopecia, pruritus, diarrhea, N/V, anorexia, constipation, hemorrhage, dyspnea, abdominal pain, liver dysfunction, cardiac ischemia.

INTERACTIONS: Caution with compounds metabolized/eliminated predominantly by the UGT1A1 pathway (eg, irinotecan); systemic exposure to substrates of UGT1A1 and UGT1A9 may increase with co-administration. May increase AUC of docetaxel and doxorubicin; co-administer with caution. May alter AUC of fluorouracil; co-administer with caution. Systemic exposure to substrates of CYP2B6 and CYP2C8 may increase with co-administration. CYP3A4 inducers may increase metabolism and decrease levels of sorafenib. May increase INR; monitor with concomitant warfarin.

PREGNANCY: Category D, not for use in nursing.

MECHANISM OF ACTION: Multikinase inhibitor; inhibits multiple intracellular and cell surface kinases which are thought to be involved in tumor cell signaling, angiogenesis, and apoptosis.

PHARMACOKINETICS: Absorption: Relative bioavailability (38-49%), T_{max}=3 hrs. **Distribution**: Plasma protein binding (99.5%). **Metabolism**: Liver via oxidation and glucuronidation; CYP3A4, UGT1A9: Pyridine N-oxide. **Elimination**: Feces (77%, 51% unchanged), urine (19% as glucuronidated metabolites); $T_{1/2}$=25-48 hrs.

NURSING CONSIDERATIONS

Assessment: Assess for CVD, bleeding problems, HTN, renal/hepatic dysfunction, pregnancy status. Note other diseases/conditions and drug therapies.

Monitoring: Monitor BP, changes in PT, INR, or clinical bleeding episodes. Monitor for risks of cardiac ischemia or infarction, hemorrhage, HTN, dermatologic toxicities, GI perforation, hypophosphatemia, LFTs, depression.

Patient Counseling: Counsel about possible side effects; report any episodes of chest pain, bleeding, or any other adverse effects. Both males and females should use effective birth control during treatment to avoid conception. Tablet should be swallowed and taken without food.

Administration: Oral route, taken without food (at least 1 hr before or 2 hrs after a meal). **Storage**: 25°C (77°F); excursions permitted to 15-30°C (59-86°F). Store in dry place. Keep out of reach of children.

NEXIUM — RX

esomeprazole magnesium (AstraZeneca)

THERAPEUTIC CLASS: Proton pump inhibitor

INDICATIONS: Symptomatic treatment of GERD; healing and maintenance treatment of erosive esophagitis. Reduction in occurrence of gastric ulcers associated with continuous NSAID therapy in patients at risk for developing gastric ulcers. Adjunct therapy (with amoxicillin and clarithromycin) for *H.pylori* eradication to reduce the risk of duodenal ulcer recurrence. Long-term treatment of pathological hypersecretory conditions including Zollinger-Ellison syndrome.

DOSAGE: *Adults:* Erosive Esophagitis: Healing: 20mg or 40mg qd for 4-8 weeks; may extend treatment for 4-8 weeks if not healed. Maint: 20mg qd for up to 6 months. Risk Reduction of NSAID-Associated Gastric Ulcer: 20mg or 40mg qd for up to 6 months. Symptomatic GERD: 20mg qd for 4 weeks; may extend treatment for 4 weeks if symptoms do not resolve. *H.pylori:* Triple Therapy: 40mg qd + amoxicillin 1000mg bid + clarithromycin 500mg bid, all for 10 days. Zollinger-Ellison Syndrome: 40mg bid. Severe Hepatic Dysfunction: Max: 20mg/day. Take 1 hr before meals. Swallow capsule whole. Contents may be mixed with soft food (eg, applesauce, yogurt) that does not require chewing.
Pediatrics: GERD: 12-17 yrs: 20mg or 40mg qd for up to 8 weeks. 1-11 yrs: 10mg qd for up to 8 weeks. Erosive Esophagitis: 1-11 yrs: ≥20kg: 10mg or 20mg qd for 8 weeks. <20kg: 10mg qd for 8 weeks. Severe Hepatic Dysfunction: Max: 20mg/day. Take 1 hr before meals. Swallow capsule whole. Contents may be mixed with soft food (eg, applesauce, yogurt) that does not require chewing.

HOW SUPPLIED: Cap, Delayed-Release: 20mg, 40mg; Sus, Delayed-Release: 10mg, 20mg, 40mg (granules/pkt).

CONTRAINDICATIONS: Hypersensitivity to substituted benzimidazoles.

WARNINGS/PRECAUTIONS: Atrophic gastritis may occur. Symptomatic response does not preclude gastric malignancy.

ADVERSE REACTIONS: Headache, diarrhea, abdominal pain, constipation, nausea, flatulence, dry mouth.

INTERACTIONS: Potentiates diazepam. May alter absorption of pH-dependent drugs (eg, ketoconazole, digoxin, iron salts). May reduce levels of atazanavir when used concomitantly. Increased levels with amoxicillin and clarithromycin. Clarithromycin is contraindicated with pimozide. Concomitant use with warfarin may increase INR and PT. Concomitant use with CYP2C19 and CYP3A4 (eg, voriconazole) may result in doubling of plasma exposure.

PREGNANCY: Category B, not for use in nursing.

MECHANISM OF ACTION: Proton pump inhibitor; suppresses gastric acid secretion by specific inhibition of the H^+/K^+-ATPase in the gastric parietal cell.

PHARMACOKINETICS: Absorption: (40 mg) C_{max}=4.7μmol/L; T_{max}=1.6 hrs; AUC=12.6μmol•hr/L. (20mg) C_{max}=2.1μmol/L; T_{max}=1.6 hrs; AUC=4.2μmol•hr/L. **Distribution:** V_d=16L; plasma protein binding (97%). **Metabolism:** Liver (extensive) via CYP2C19, CYP3A4. **Elimination:** Urine (80%), feces; $T_{1/2}$=1-1.5 hrs. For pediatric parameters, refer to full PI.

NURSING CONSIDERATIONS

Assessment: Assess for hypersensitivity to other proton pump inhibitors, presence of gastric malignancy, severe hepatic impairment, pregnancy/nursing status, and possible drug interactions.

Monitoring: Monitor for signs/symptoms of atrophic gastritis, and hypersensitivity reactions (eg, anaphylaxis, angioedema).

Patient Counseling: Counsel to contact physician if signs/symptoms of hypersensitivity reaction occur. May take antacids while on therapy. Advise to take 1 hr before meals and to swallow capsules whole. If difficulty swallowing, open capsules and empty granules into applesauce, which should not be warm. For oral suspension, empty packet of medication into container containing 1 tablespoon of water (15mL); stir contents, let stand for 2-3 min to thicken; drink solution within 15 min. If contents of solution remain, add more water, stir, and drink immediately.

Administration: Oral route. **Storage:** 25°C (77°F); excursions permitted to 15-30°C (59-86°F). Dispense in tightly closed container.

NEXIUM IV

RX

esomeprazole sodium (AstraZeneca)

THERAPEUTIC CLASS: Proton pump inhibitor

INDICATIONS: Short-term treatment (up to 10 days) of GERD with history of erosive esophagitis when oral therapy not possible or appropriate.

DOSAGE: *Adults:* 20mg or 40mg qd IV injection (no less than 3 min) or infusion (10-30 min). D/C as soon as patient able to resume oral therapy. Severe Hepatic Dysfunction: Max: 20mg/day.

HOW SUPPLIED: Inj: 20mg, 40mg

WARNINGS/PRECAUTIONS: Atrophic gastritis may occur. Symptomatic response does not preclude gastric malignancy. D/C and convert to oral therapy as soon as possible.

ADVERSE REACTIONS: Headache, flatulence, dyspepsia, nausea, abdominal pain, diarrhea, and dry mouth.

INTERACTIONS: Potentiates diazepam. May alter absorption of gastric pH-dependent drugs (eg, ketoconazole, iron salts, digoxin). Concomitant warfarin therapy may increase INR and PT. Avoid with nelfinavir and atazanavir. May reduce plasma levels of atazanavir. Concomitant CYP2C19 and CYP3A4 inhibitor (eg, voriconazole) may double plasma levels.

PREGNANCY: Category B, not for use in nursing.

MECHANISM OF ACTION: Proton pump inhibitor. Suppresses gastric acid secretion by specific inhibition of the H^+/K^+-ATPase in the gastric parietal cell.

PHARMACOKINETICS: Absorption: (20mg): AUC=5.11µmol•hr/L; C_{max}=3.86µmol/L; (40mg): AUC=16.21µmol•hr/L. **Distribution**: V_d= 16L; plasma protein binding (97%). **Metabolism:** Liver (extensive) via CYP2C19, 3A4. **Elimination**: Urine (primary), (<1% unchanged), feces; $T_{1/2}$=1.1-1.4 hrs.

N

NURSING CONSIDERATIONS

Assessment: Assess for hypersensitivity to other proton pump inhibitors, presence of gastric malignancy, severe hepatic insufficiency, pregnancy/nursing status, and possible drug interactions.

Monitoring: Monitor for signs/symptoms of atrophic gastritis.

Patient Counseling: Instruct to contact physician if any adverse events develop.

Administration: IV injection or infusion route. Injection: Reconstitute vial with 5mL of 0.9% NaCl and inject. Infusion: 1) Reconstitute vial with 5mL of compatible solution (eg, 0.9% NaCl, Lactated Ringer's, or 5% Dextrose). 2) Further dilute to final volume of 50mL. Should not be administered concomitantly with any other medications through same IV site or tubing. Always flush IV line both prior to and after administration. IV formulation should be switched to oral formulation as soon as possible. **Storage:** Vial: 25°C (77°F); excursions permitted to 15-30°C (59-86°F). Protect from light. Store in carton until time of use. Reconstituted: 30°C (86°F); administer within 12 hrs. Infusion: Up to 30°C (86°F); if reconstituted with 0.9% NaCl or Lactated Ringer's, use within 12 hrs; 5% Dextrose, use within 6 hrs.

NIASPAN

RX

niacin (Abbott)

THERAPEUTIC CLASS: Nicotinic acid

INDICATIONS: Adjunct to diet, to reduce total cholesterol (total-C), LDL-C, TG, and Apo B levels, and to increase HDL-C in primary hypercholesterolemia (heterozygous familial and nonfamilial) and mixed dyslipidemia (Types IIa and IIb). With concomitant lovastatin, to further reduce LDL-C and TG, or increase HDL-C in primary hypercholesterolemia (heterozygous familial and nonfamilial) and mixed dyslipidemia (Types IIa and IIb). To reduce risk of recurrent nonfatal MI with history of MI and hypercholesterolemia. With concomitant bile acid binding resin, to slow progression/promote regression of atherosclerotic disease with history of CAD and hypercholesterolemia. Adjunct to diet with concomitant bile acid binding resin to reduce total-C and LDL-C in primary hypercholesterolemia (Type IIa) inadequately responding to diet or diet plus monotherapy. Adjunct for very high TG levels (Type IV and Type V hyperlipidemia) with risk of pancreatitis, inadequately responding to diet.

DOSAGE: *Adults:* Take qhs after low-fat snack. Initial: 500mg qhs. Titrate: Increase by 500mg every 4 weeks. Maint: 1-2g qhs. Max: 2g/day. Take ASA or NSAIDs 30 min before to reduce flushing. Do not chew, crush, or break; swallow whole. Women may respond to lower doses than men.

HOW SUPPLIED: Tab, Extended-Release: 500mg, 750mg, 1000mg

CONTRAINDICATIONS: Unexplained or significant hepatic dysfunction, active peptic ulcer disease, arterial bleeding.

WARNINGS/PRECAUTIONS: Do not substitute with equivalent doses of immediate-release niacin (severe hepatic toxicity may occur). Associated with abnormal LFTs; monitor LFTs before therapy, every 6-12 weeks during 1st yr, then periodically thereafter. D/C if LFTs ≥3x ULN persists or develop signs of hepatotoxicity. Monitor for rhabdomyolysis. Observe closely with history of jaundice, hepatobiliary disease, and peptic ulcer; monitor LFTs and blood glucose frequently. Dose-related rise in glucose tolerance in diabetics. Caution with history of hepatic disease, heavy alcohol use, renal dysfunction, unstable angina, and acute phase of MI. Elevated uric acid levels reported. May reduce platelet and phosphorous levels.

ADVERSE REACTIONS: Flushing episodes (eg, warmth, redness, itching, tingling), dizziness, tachycardia, SOB, sweating, chills, edema, headache, diarrhea.

INTERACTIONS: Rhabdomyolysis may occur with HMG-CoA reductase inhibitors. May potentiate antihypertensives (eg, ganglionic blockers, vasoactive drugs). Separate dosing from bile acid resins by at least 4-6 hrs. Avoid concomitant alcohol or hot drinks; may increase flushing and pruritus. High-dose niacin or nicotinamide may potentiate adverse effects. Caution with anticoagulants. Antidiabetic agents may need adjustment.

PREGNANCY: Category C, not for use in nursing.

MECHANISM OF ACTION: Nicotinic acid; not established. May partially inhibit release of free fatty acids from adipose tissue, and increase lipoprotein lipase activity, which increases rate of chylomicron triglyceride removal from plasma. Decreases rate of hepatic synthesis of VLDL and LDL.

PHARMACOKINETICS: Absorption: Rapid and extensive. **Distribution:** Liver, kidney, adipose tissue; found in breast milk. **Metabolism:** Liver (extensive) to nicotinamide and other metabolites. **Elimination:** Urine; parent and metabolites (60-76%), (12% unchanged).

NURSING CONSIDERATIONS

Assessment: Prior to initiation, assess for secondary causes of hypercholesterolemia (eg, poorly controlled DM, hypothyroidism, nephrotic syndrome, dysproteinemias, obstructive liver disease, other drug therapy, alcoholism). Obtain baseline lipid profile (TC, HDL-C, TG) and LFTs. Assess history of liver disease, renal dysfunction, unstable angina, active peptic ulcer disease, arterial bleeding, pregnancy/nursing status, and for possible drug interactions.

Monitoring: Monitor for signs/symptoms of hepatotoxicity (eg, fulminant hepatic necrosis), rhabdomyolysis (eg, muscle pain, tenderness, weakness), decreases in platelet counts, and increases in prothrombin time. Monitor LFTs (eg, AST, ALT) every 6-12 weeks during first year and periodically every 6 months thereafter. Monitor blood glucose and cholesterol levels; serum creatine phosphokinase and potassium levels with combined HMG-CoA reductase inhibitor therapy; phosphorus levels with risk of hypophosphatemia.

Patient Counseling: Counsel to take at bedtime after a low-fat snack. Inform that flushing may occur but should subside after several weeks of therapy; taking aspirin or NSAIDs 30 min prior may minimize. Instruct to avoid ingestion of alcohol or hot drinks with administration to prevent flushing. Advise not to break, crush, or chew, and to swallow whole. Instruct to contact physician if discontinuing drug for extended period of time, taking vitamins, other nutritional supplements, or if dizziness occurs. Notify diabetics that changes in blood glucose levels may occur.

Administration: Oral route. **Storage:** 20-25°C (68-77°F).

NIFEDIPINE RX

nifedipine (Various)

OTHER BRAND NAMES: Procardia (Pfizer)

THERAPEUTIC CLASS: Calcium channel blocker (dihydropyridine)

INDICATIONS: Management of vasospastic angina and chronic stable angina.

DOSAGE: *Adults:* >18 yrs: Initial: 10mg tid. Usual: 10-20mg tid. Titrate: Increase dose every 3 days if needed. Usual: 20-30mg tid. Patients with Evidence of Coronary Artery Spasm: 20-30mg tid-qid. Doses above 120mg qd are rarely necessary. Max: 180mg/day.

HOW SUPPLIED: Cap: 10mg, 20mg

WARNINGS/PRECAUTIONS: May cause hypotension; monitor BP initially or with titration. May exacerbate angina from β-blocker withdrawal. CHF risk, especially with aortic stenosis or β-blockers. Peripheral edema reported. Not for acute reduction of BP or essential HTN. May increase angina or MI with severe obstructive CAD. Avoid with acute coronary syndrome or within 1-2 weeks of MI. Caution in elderly.

ADVERSE REACTIONS: Dizziness, lightheadedness, giddiness, flushing, muscle cramps, headache, weakness, nausea, peripheral edema, nervousness/mood changes.

INTERACTIONS: β-Blockers may increase risk of CHF, severe hypotension, or angina exacerbation. Possible hypotension with fentanyl. Potentiates digoxin. Monitor quinidine, coumarin. Potentiated by cimetidine and grapefruit juice. Avoid grapefruit juice.

N

PREGNANCY: Category C, unknown use in nursing.

MECHANISM OF ACTION: Calcium channel blocker; inhibits the transmembrane influx of calcium ions into cardiac muscle and smooth muscle. Angina: MOA not fully determined; believed to act by relaxation and prevention of coronary artery spasm, and reduction of oxygen utlilization.

PHARMACOKINETICS: Absorption: Rapid and full; T_{max}=30 min. **Distribution:** Plasma protein binding (92-98%). **Metabolism:** Liver, via biotransformation. **Elimination:** Urine (80%).

NURSING CONSIDERATIONS

Assessment: Assess for CHF, aortic stenosis, hepatic/renal impairment, essential HTN, recent MI, β-blocker withdrawal syndrome with increased angina, and possible drug interactions.

Monitoring: Monitor for hypotension and/or increased fluid volume requirements, increased angina and/or MI, HF, peripheral edema, allergic hepatitis, cholestatsis with/without jaundice. Monitor BP, alkaline phosphatase, CPK, LDH, SGOT, SGPT, BUN, SrCr, decreased platelet aggregation, increased bleeding time, positive direct Coombs' test with/without hemolytic anemia.

Patient Counseling: Not to be used for acute reduction of BP. Do not take with grapefruit juice. Inform about potential risks/benefits of drug.

Administration: Oral route. **Storage:** 15-25°C (59-77°F). Avoid freezing.

NILANDRON RX

nilutamide (Sanofi-Aventis)

Interstitial pneumonitis reported. Perform routine chest X-ray and baseline pulmonary function test before therapy. D/C if symptoms occur.

THERAPEUTIC CLASS: Nonsteroidal antiandrogen

INDICATIONS: Treatment of metastatic prostatic cancer (Stage D_2) in combination with surgical castration.

DOSAGE: *Adults:* Initial: 300mg/day for 30 days. Maint: 150mg qd. Begin on the same day or the day after surgical castration.

HOW SUPPLIED: Tab: 150mg

CONTRAINDICATIONS: Severe hepatic impairment, respiratory insufficiency.

WARNINGS/PRECAUTIONS: Hepatotoxicity, aplastic anemia reported. D/C if develop jaundice or ALT >2x ULN. Delay in adaptation to dark; caution with driving at night or in tunnels; wear tinted glasses to alleviate effect. Evaluate baseline hepatic enzymes before therapy, at regular intervals for 1st 4 months, and periodically thereafter.

ADVERSE REACTIONS: Hot flushes, decreased libido, abnormal vision, increased LFTs, dyspnea, GI effects, dry skin, sweating, dizziness, HTN, anemia, testicular atrophy, gynecomastia.

INTERACTIONS: May potentiate vitamin K antagonists, phenytoin, and theophylline. Intolerance to alcohol (eg, hypotension, malaise).

PREGNANCY: Category C, safety in nursing not known.

MECHANISM OF ACTION: Nonsteroidal antiandrogen; acts by blocking effects of testosterone at the androgen receptor sites.

PHARMACOKINETICS: Absorption: Rapid and complete. **Elimination**: Urine (62%), feces (1.4%-7%); $T_{1/2}$=38-59.1 hrs (100-300mg single dose).

NURSING CONSIDERATIONS

Assessment: Assess severe hepatic impairment and respiratory insufficiency. Note other diseases/conditions and drug therapies.

Monitoring: Prior to treatment and periodically thereafter, measure baseline hepatic enzymes, routine chest x-ray, pulmonary function tests, serum transaminase levels, and LFTs. Monitor for occurrence of interstitial pneumonitis, hepatotoxicity, hypersensitivity reactions.

Patient Counseling: Instruct to report new or worsening SOB, NV, abdominal pain, or jaundice. Inform to start on day of or day after surgical castration; do not interrupt or d/c dosing without consulting physician. Advise to avoid alcohol intake if intolerant (eg, facial flushes, malaise, hypotension). Instruct patients who experience delay in adaption to dark to wear tinted glasses when driving at night or through tunnels.

Administration: Oral route; with/without food. **Storage**: 25°C (77°F); excursions permitted to 15-30°C (59-86°F). Protect from light.

NIMODIPINE — RX

nimodipine (Various)

Do not administer IV or by other parenteral routes. Deaths and serious, life-threatening adverse events have occurred when contents of capsules injected parenterally.

OTHER BRAND NAMES: Nimotop (Bayer Healthcare)

THERAPEUTIC CLASS: Calcium channel blocker

INDICATIONS: Improvement of neurological outcome in patients with subarachnoid hemorrhage (SAH) from ruptured intracranial berry aneurysms regardless of their post-ictus neurological condition.

DOSAGE: *Adults:* 60mg q 4 hrs for 21 days, 1 hr before or 2 hrs after meals. Hepatic Cirrhosis: 30mg q 4 hrs for 21 days. Start therapy within 96 hrs of SAH. If cannot swallow cap, extract contents into syringe and empty into NG tube, then flush with 30mL of 0.9% NaCl.

HOW SUPPLIED: Cap: 30mg

WARNINGS/PRECAUTIONS: Carefully monitor BP. Monitor BP and HR closely with hepatic dysfunction. Do not administer IV or by other parenteral routes.

ADVERSE REACTIONS: Decreased BP, headache, rash, diarrhea, bradycardia, nausea, abnormal LFTs.

INTERACTIONS: May enhance cardiovascular effects of other CCBs. Increased serum levels with cimetidine. May intensify effects of antihypertensives.

PREGNANCY: Category C, not for use in nursing.

MECHANISM OF ACTION: Calcium channel blocker; not established; suspected to inhibit calcium ion transfer into smooth muscle cells, thereby inhibiting contractions of vascular smooth muscle.

PHARMACOKINETICS: Absorption: Rapid; T_{max}=1 hr. **Distribution:** Plasma protein binding (≥95%). Crosses blood-brain barrier. **Elimination:** Urine (≤1% unchanged); $T_{1/2}$=8-9 hrs.

NURSING CONSIDERATIONS

Assessment: Assess for hepatic impairment and possible drug interactions.

Monitoring: Carefully monitor BP and pulse rate. Monitor for serious adverse effects when administering IV (eg, death, cardiac arrest, cardiovascular collapse, hypotension, and bradycardia).

Patient Counseling: Inform about potential risks/benefits of drug. Do not take with grapefruit juice. Regular BP monitoring recommended.

Administration: Oral route. **Storage:** Store at 25°C (77°F); excursions permitted to 15-30°C (59-86°F). Avoid light and freezing.

NIRAVAM

CIV

alprazolam (Schwarz)

THERAPEUTIC CLASS: Benzodiazepine

INDICATIONS: Management of anxiety disorders and short-term relief of anxiety symptoms. Treatment of panic disorder with or without agoraphobia.

DOSAGE: *Adults:* Anxiety: Initial: 0.25-0.5mg tid. Titrate: May increase every 3-4 days. Max: 4mg/day. Panic Disorder: Initial: 0.5mg tid. Titrate: Increase by no more than 1mg/day every 3-4 days; slower titration if ≥4mg/day. Usual: 1-10mg/day. Decrease dose slowly (no more than 0.5mg every 3 days). Elderly/Advanced Liver Disease/Debilitated: Initial: 0.25mg bid-tid. Titrate: Increase gradually as tolerated.

HOW SUPPLIED: Tab, Orally Disintegrating: 0.25mg*, 0.5mg*, 1mg*, 2mg*
*scored

CONTRAINDICATIONS: Acute narrow-angle glaucoma, untreated open-angle glaucoma, concomitant ketoconazole or itraconazole.

WARNINGS/PRECAUTIONS: Risk of dependence. Withdrawal symptoms, including seizure, reported with dose reduction or abrupt discontinuation; avoid abrupt withdrawal. Risk of CNS depression and impaired performance. May cause fetal harm. Caution with impaired renal, hepatic, or pulmonary function, severe depression, obesity, elderly and debilitated. Hypomania/mania reported with depression. Weak uricosuric effect.

ADVERSE REACTIONS: Drowsiness, fatigue/tiredness, impaired coordination, irritability, memory impairment, cognitive disorder, dysarthria, decreased libido, confusional state, lightheadedness, dry mouth, hypotension, increased salivation.

INTERACTIONS: Avoid with potent CYP3A inhibitors (eg, azole antifungals). Potentiated by nefazodone, fluvoxamine, cimetidine, fluoxetine, oral contraceptives. Decreased plasma levels with propoxyphene and carbamazepine. Caution with diltiazem, isoniazid, macrolides, grapefruit juice, sertraline, paroxetine, ergotamine, cyclosporine, amiodarone, nicardipine, nifedipine and other CYP3A inhibitors. Increases levels of imipramine and desipramine. Additive CNS depressant effects with psychotropic agents, anticonvulsants, antihistamines, ethanol.

PREGNANCY: Category D, not for use in nursing.

MECHANISM OF ACTION: Benzodiazepine; not established, CNS depressant, believed to exert its effects by binding at stereo specific receptor at several sites within the CNS.

PHARMACOKINETICS: Absorption: Readily absorbed; C_{max}=8-37ng/mL; T_{max}=1.5-2 hrs. **Distribution:** Plasma protein binding (80%). **Metabolism:** Metabolized (extensively), hydroxylation, 4-hydroxyalprazolam and α-hydroxyalprazolam (major metabolites). **Elimination:** Urine, $T_{1/2}$=12.5 hrs.

NURSING CONSIDERATIONS

Assessment: Assess for known sensitivity to drug, open-angle and acute-closed glaucoma, renal/hepatic impairment, pulmonary function insufficiency, and possible drug interactions. Assess for risk of dependence among panic disorder patients.

Monitoring: Monitor early morning anxiety and emergence of anxiety symptoms, CNS depression, physical/psychological dependence, suicidality, mania/hypomania, uricosuric effects, acute renal failure, seizures and status epilepticus. Monitor blood counts, urinalysis, and blood chemistry analysis.

Patient Counseling: Inform of benefits/risks and possibilty of physical/psychological dependence. Caution against hazardous tasks (eg, operating machinery/driving). Avoid alcohol. Notify physician if pregnant or planning to become pregnant or before increasing dose or d/c the drug.

Administration: Oral route. Remove tablets from bottle just before dosing. Can be swallowed with/without water. **Storage:** 20-25°C (68-77°F); excursions permitted to 15-30°C (59-86°F). Protect from moisture. Dispense in tight container.

NITRO-BID — RX

nitroglycerin (Fougera)

THERAPEUTIC CLASS: Nitrate vasodilator

INDICATIONS: Prevention of angina pectoris. Not for acute attacks.

DOSAGE: *Adults:* Initial: Apply 0.5 inch bid (once in the am and 6 hrs later). Titrate: May increase to 1 inch bid, then to 2 inches bid. Should have 10-12 hr nitrate-free period.

HOW SUPPLIED: Oint: 2% (15mg/inch) [1g (48[s]), 30g, 60g]

WARNINGS/PRECAUTIONS: Monitor with acute MI or CHF. Severe hypotension may occur; caution with volume depletion and hypotension. May aggravate angina caused by hypertrophic cardiomyopathy. Tolerance to other nitrates may decrease effects. Topical use only. See Drug Interactions.

ADVERSE REACTIONS: Headache, lightheadedness, hypotension, flushing, syncope, rebound HTN.

INTERACTIONS: Additive vasodilating effects with other vasodilators (eg, alcohol). Severe hypotension with sildenafil. Marked orthostatic hypotension reported with CCBs.

PREGNANCY: Category C, caution in nursing.

MECHANISM OF ACTION: Nitrate vasodilator; relaxes vascular smooth muscle, and consequent dilatation of peripheral arteries and veins, especially the latter. Dilatation of veins leads to reduced left ventricular end-diastolic pressure and pulmonary capillary wedge pressure (preload). Arteriolar relaxation reduces systemic vascular resistance, systolic arterial pressure, and mean arterial pressure (afterload). It also dilates the coronary artery.

PHARMACOKINETICS: Distribution: V_d=3L/kg. **Metabolism:** Extrahepatic metabolism (RBC and vascular walls), inorganic nitrate and 1,2-and 1,3-dinitrogylcerin (metabolites). Dinitrates are metabolized to mononitrates, gycerol and CO_2. **Elimination:** $T_{1/2}$=3 min.

NURSING CONSIDERATIONS

Assessment: Assess for severe hypotension or volume-depleted patients, angina caused by hypertrophic cardiomyopathy, alcohol intake, and possible drug interactions.

Monitoring: Careful clinical or hemodynamic monitoring for hypotension and tachycardia. Monitor for paradoxical bradycardia and increased angina

N

pectoris, rebound and decreased exercise tolerance, headaches and lightheadedness on standing, manifestation of true physical dependence (chest pain, acute MI), and methemoglobinemia.

Patient Counseling: Counsel to carefully follow dosing regimen. Inform about headaches (markers of drug activity) and lightheadedness on standing. Avoid alcohol consumption. Topical use only.

Administration: Topical route. Place applicator on flat surface, printed side down. Squeeze necessary amount from tube onto applicator. Place applicator on desired area of skin and tape into place. **Storage:** 15-30°C (59-86°F).

NITRO-DUR RX

nitroglycerin (Schering)

OTHER BRAND NAMES: Nitrek (Mylan Bertek) - Minitran (Graceway)

THERAPEUTIC CLASS: Nitrate vasodilator

INDICATIONS: Prevention of angina pectoris. Not for acute attack.

DOSAGE: *Adults:* Initial: 0.2-0.4mg/hr for 12-14 hrs. Remove for 10-12 hrs.

HOW SUPPLIED: Patch: (Minitran) 0.1mg/hr, 0.2mg/hr, 0.4mg/hr, 0.6mg/hr [30s]; (Nitrek) 0.2mg/hr, 0.4mg/hr, 0.6mg/hr [30s]; (Nitro-Dur) 0.1mg/hr, 0.2mg/hr, 0.3mg/hr, 0.4mg/hr, 0.6mg/hr, 0.8mg/hr [30s]

CONTRAINDICATIONS: Allergy to adhesives in NTG patches.

WARNINGS/PRECAUTIONS: Severe hypotension may occur; caution with volume depletion or hypotension. Vasodilatory effects with phosphodiesterase inhibitors (eg, sildenafil) can result in severe hypotension. May aggravate angina caused by hypertrophic cardiomyopathy. Tolerance to other nitrate forms may decrease effects. Monitor with acute MI or CHF. Do not discharge defibrillator/cardioverter through the patch.

ADVERSE REACTIONS: Headache, lightheadedness, hypotension, syncope.

N

INTERACTIONS: Additive vasodilating effects with other vasodilators (eg, alcohol). Marked orthostatic hypotension reported with CCBs. Severe hypotension with sildenafil.

PREGNANCY: Category C, caution in nursing.

MECHANISM OF ACTION: Nitrate vasodilator; relaxes vascular smooth muscle, and consequent dilatation of peripheral arteries and veins, especially the latter. Dilatation of veins leads to reduced left ventricular end-diastolic pressure and pulmonary capillary wedge pressure (preload). Arteriolar relaxation reduces systemic vascular resistance, systolic arterial pressure, and mean arterial pressure (afterload). It also dilates the coronary artery.

PHARMACOKINETICS: Absorption: T_{max}=2 hrs. **Distribution:** V_d=3L/kg. **Metabolism:** Extrahepatic metabolism (RBC and vascular walls). Inorganic nitrate and the 1,2- and 1,3- dinitroglycerols. Dinitrates are metabolized to mononitrates and to glycerol and CO_2. **Elimination:** $T_{1/2}$=3 min.

NURSING CONSIDERATIONS

Assessment: Assess for severe hypotension or volume depleted patients, angina caused by hypertrophic cardiomyopathy, alcohol intake and possible drug interactions.

Monitoring: Careful clinical or hemodynamic monitoring for hypotension and tachycardia. Monitor for paradoxical bradycardia and increased angina pectoris, decreased exercise tolerance and hemodynamic rebound, headaches and lightheadedness on standing, manifestation of true physical dependence (chest pain, acute MI), and methemoglobinemia.

Patient Counseling: Counsel to carefully follow dosing regimen. Inform about headaches (markers of drug activity) and lightheadedness on standing. Avoid alcohol consumption.

Administration: Transdermal route. **Storage:** 15-30°C (59-86°F).

NITROLINGUAL SPRAY — RX

nitroglycerin (Sciele)

OTHER BRAND NAMES: NitroMist (NovaDel Pharma)

THERAPEUTIC CLASS: Nitrate vasodilator

INDICATIONS: For acute relief of angina attack. Prophylaxis of angina pectoris.

DOSAGE: *Adults:* Acute: 1-2 sprays at onset of attack onto or under tongue. Max: 3 sprays/15 min. Prophylaxis: 1-2 sprays onto or under tongue 5-10 min before activity that may cause acute attack. Do not expectorate medication or rinse mouth for 5-10 min after administration.

HOW SUPPLIED: Spray: 400mcg/spray

CONTRAINDICATIONS: Concomitant use with phosphodiesterase type 5 (PDE5) inhibitors such as sildenafil, vardenafil, and tadalafil.

WARNINGS/PRECAUTIONS: Severe hypotension may occur; caution with volume depletion or hypotension. May aggravate angina caused by hypertrophic cardiomyopathy. Tolerance and cross-tolerance to other nitrates/nitrites may occur. Monitor during early days of AMI.

ADVERSE REACTIONS: Headache, hypotension, flushing, dizziness, weakness, rash, exfoliative dermatitis.

INTERACTIONS: See Contraindications. Avoid PDE5 inhibitors (eg, sildenafil, vardenafil, tadalafil); severe hypotension may occur. Concomitant use with CCBs may cause orthostatic hypotension. Alcohol may cause hypotension. (NitroMist) Increased hypotensive effects with β-adrenergic blockers (eg, labetolol). ASA may increase levels. May decrease anticoagulant effect of heparin. Avoid ergotamine. Caution with tissue-type plasminogen activator.

PREGNANCY: Category C, caution in nursing.

MECHANISM OF ACTION: Nitrate vasodilator; activates guanylate cyclase, resulting in an increase cyclic GMP in smooth muscle and other tissues; leads to dephosphorylation of myosin light chains, which regulates the contractile state in smooth muscle and results in vasodilation.

PHARMACOKINETICS: Absorption: Rapid, C_{max}=0.8ng/mL, T_{max}=8 min. **Distribution:** V_d=3.3L/kg. **Metabolism:** Extrahepatic metabolism (red cells and vascular walls); 1,2-dinitroglycerin and 1,3-dinitroglycerin (major metabolites). **Elimination:** $T_{1/2}$=3 min (nitroglycerin), 10 min (1,2-dinitroglycerin), 11 min (1,3-dinitroglycerin).

NURSING CONSIDERATIONS

Assessment: Assess for hypotension, volume-depleted patients, severe anemia, increased intracranial pressure, angina caused by hypertrophic cardiomyopathy, and possible drug interactions (eg, with phosphodiasterase inhibitor such as sildenafil).

Monitoring: Monitor for tolerance development, hypotension, tachycardia, paradoxical bradycardia, increased angina pectoris, rash, flushing, exfoliative dermatitis and headache. Monitor for methemoglobinemia and signs of impaired oxygen delivery despite of adequate arterial PO_2.

Patient Counseling: Instruct not to take concomitantly with drugs used for erectile dysfunction, potential side effects (eg, headaches and lightheadedness). Do not forcibly open bottle or use near open flame. Do not use when liquid reaches the top to middle of the hole on the side. Avoid alcohol consumption.

Administration: Nitrolingual spray. Spray on or under the tongue. **Storage:** 25°C (77°F); excursions permitted to 15-30°C (59-85°F). Store upright.

N

NITROSTAT RX
nitroglycerin (Parke-Davis)

OTHER BRAND NAMES: Nitroquick (Ethex)

THERAPEUTIC CLASS: Nitrate vasodilator

INDICATIONS: For acute relief of angina attack. Prophylaxis of angina pectoris.

DOSAGE: *Adults:* Treatment: 1 tab SL or in buccal pouch at onset of attack. May repeat in 5 min. Max: 3 tabs in 15 min. Prophylaxis: Take 5-10 min before activity that may cause acute attack. Administer in sitting position.

HOW SUPPLIED: Tab, Sublingual: 0.3mg, 0.4mg, 0.6mg

CONTRAINDICATIONS: Early MI, severe anemia, increased ICP, concomitant sildenafil.

WARNINGS/PRECAUTIONS: Do not swallow tabs. Severe hypotension may occur; caution with volume depletion or hypotension. May aggravate angina caused by hypertrophic cardiomyopathy. D/C if develop blurred vision or dry mouth. May interfere with cholesterol test. Monitor with acute MI or CHF. Tolerance to other nitrate forms may decrease effects. Caution in elderly.

ADVERSE REACTIONS: Headache, vertigo, dizziness, weakness, palpitation, syncope, flushing, postural hypotension, drug rash, exfoliative dermatitis.

INTERACTIONS: Additive hypotension with alcohol, β-blockers, phenothiazines, CCBs, other antihypertensives. Avoid ergotamine (related drugs), sildenafil. Vasodilatory and hemodynamic effects potentiated by ASA. Caution with alteplase. TCAs, anticholinergics may make sublingual dissolution difficult. Long-acting nitrates may decrease effects.

PREGNANCY: Category C, caution in nursing.

MECHANISM OF ACTION: Nitrate vasodilator; relaxes the vascular smooth muscle; activates guanylate cyclase, resulting in an increase of guanosine 3'5' monophosphate in smooth muscle and other tissues, resulting in vasodilatation.

PHARMACOKINETICS: Absorption: (SL) rapid, absolute bioavailability (40%). (0.3mg) C_{max}=2.3ng/mL, T_{max}=6.4 min, AUC=14.9ng•mL/min; (0.6mg) C_{max}=2.1ng/mL, T_{max}=7.2 min, AUC=14.9ng•mL/min. **Distribution:** V_d=3.3 L/kg, plasma protein binding (60%). **Metabolism:** Liver via reductase, extrahepatic (red cells and vascular wall). 1,2- and 1,3-dinitroglycerin (major metabolites). **Elimination:** (0.3mg) $T_{1/2}$=2.8 min, (0.6mg) 2.6 min.

NURSING CONSIDERATIONS

Assessment: Assess for hypotension, volume depletion, severe anemia, angina caused by hypertrophic cardiomyopathy, and possible drug interactions.

Monitoring: Careful clinical or hemodynamic monitoring for hypotension and tachycardia. Monitor for paradoxical bradycardia, increased angina pectoris, headache and lightheadedness on standing, manifestation of true physical dependence (chest pain, acute MI), and methemoglobinemia.

Patient Counseling: Use smallest dose to relieve acute attacks to prevent developing dependence. Inform about side effects of drug (eg, headaches, lightheadedness on standing, burning or tingling sensation when administered SL). Avoid alcohol.

Administration: Sublingual route. **Storage:** 20-25°C (68-77°F).

NIZORAL RX
ketoconazole (Janssen)

Risk of fatal hepatotoxicity. Concomitant terfenadine, astemizole and cisapride are contraindicated due to serious cardiovascular adverse events.

THERAPEUTIC CLASS: Azole antifungal

N

INDICATIONS: Treatment of the following systemic fungal infections: candidiasis, chronic mucocutaneous candidiasis, oral thrush, candiduria, blastomycosis, coccidioidomycosis, histoplasmosis, chromomycosis, and paracoccidioidomycosis. Treatment of severe recalcitrant cutaneous dermatophyte infections not responsive to topical therapy or oral griseofulvin. Not for treatment of fungal meningitis.

DOSAGE: *Adults:* Initial: 200mg qd. Max: 400mg qd.
Pediatrics: >2 yrs: 3.3-6.6mg/kg/day.

HOW SUPPLIED: Tab: 200mg* *scored

CONTRAINDICATIONS: Concomitant terfenadine, astemizole, cisapride or oral triazolam.

WARNINGS/PRECAUTIONS: Hepatotoxicity reported. Monitor LFTs prior to therapy and periodically thereafter. Serum testosterone levels may be lowered. Hypersensitivity reactions reported. Tablets require acidity for dissolution. Not for use in children unless benefit outweighs risk.

ADVERSE REACTIONS: NV, abdominal pain, pruritus.

INTERACTIONS: See Contraindications. Give antacids, anticholinergics, and H_2 blockers 2 hrs after ketoconazole. May potentiate midazolam, triazolam, oral hypoglycemics. May enhance anticoagulant effect of coumarin-like drugs. Avoid rifampin, isoniazid. Monitor digoxin, phenytoin. May alter metabolism of cyclosporine, tacrolimus, methylprednisolone and drugs metabolized by CYP3A4.

PREGNANCY: Category C, not for use in nursing.

MECHANISM OF ACTION: Azole antifungal; impairs synthesis of ergosterol, a vital component of fungal cell membranes.

PHARMACOKINETICS: Absorption: C_{max}=3.5mcg/mL; T_{max}=1-2 hrs. **Distribution**: Plasma protein binding (99%). **Metabolism**: Via oxidation, degradation of imidazole and piperazine rings, oxidative dealkylation and aromatic hydroxylation. CYP3A4 inhibitor. **Elimination:** Biphasic. $T_{1/2}$=2 hrs (during first 10 hrs); $T_{1/2}$=8 hrs (thereafter); bile (major), urine (13%).

NURSING CONSIDERATIONS

Assessment: Assess for lab, as well as clinical, documentation of infection prior to therapy. Assess LFTs and possible drug interactions (eg, terfenadine, astemizole) prior to therapy.

Monitoring: Monitor LFTs, signs/symptoms of hepatotoxicity and anaphylaxis. Monitor for cardiovascular events if using concomitant therapy with terfenadine or astemizole.

Patient Counseling: Counsel females to avoid nursing while on medication. Advise to report any signs/symptoms of liver dysfunction (eg, fatigue, anorexia, NV, jaundice, dark urine, or pale stools). If concomitant antacids, anticholinergics and H_2-blockers are needed, give at least 2 hrs after administration of drug. Continue treatment until tests indicate infection subsided.

Administration: Oral route. In cases of achlorhydria, instruct to dissolve each tab in 4mL aqueous solution of 0.2 N HCl. Use drinking straw to avoid contact with teeth. Follow administration with cup of water. **Storage**: Oral; store at controlled room temperature 15-25°C (59-77°F). Protect from moisture. Keep out of reach of children.

NIZORAL SHAMPOO — RX

ketoconazole (McNeil Consumer)

THERAPEUTIC CLASS: Azole antifungal

INDICATIONS: Tinea versicolor.

DOSAGE: *Adults:* Apply to damp skin and lather. Rinse with water after 5 min. One application should be sufficient.

HOW SUPPLIED: Shampoo: 2% [4oz]

WARNINGS/PRECAUTIONS: Shampoo may remove curl from permanently waved hair. Avoid eyes. D/C if chemical irritation occurs. Do not use on broken or inflamed scalp.

ADVERSE REACTIONS: Abnormal hair texture, scalp pustules, mild skin dryness, pruritus, increase in normal hair loss, oily or dry scalp and hair.

PREGNANCY: Category C, caution in nursing.

MECHANISM OF ACTION: Azole antifungal; impairs synthesis of ergosterol, a vital component of fungal membranes.

NURSING CONSIDERATIONS

Assessment: Assess for drug hypersensitivity.

Monitoring: Monitor for sensitivity or chemical irritation and adverse reactions such as hair loss, abnormal hair texture, scalp pustules, mild dryness of skin and hair and scalp, itching, oiliness, hair discoloration.

Patient Counseling: Inform that shampoo may be irritating to mucous membranes of eyes; avoid contact with eyes. Advise that usage could remove curls from permanently waved hair. Exercise caution when administering to nursing women.

Administration: Topical application. Apply shampoo to damp skin of affected area and wide margin surrounding this area. Lather, leave in place for 5 min, then rinse off with water. **Storage:** Store at temperature no more than 25°C (77°F). Protect from light.

Norco

hydrocodone bitartrate - acetaminophen (Watson)

CIII

N

THERAPEUTIC CLASS: Opioid analgesic

INDICATIONS: Relief of moderate to moderately severe pain.

DOSAGE: *Adults:* Usual: (5/325) 1-2 tabs q4-6h prn pain. Usual: (7.5/325, 10/325) 1 tab q4-6h prn pain. Max: 6 tabs/day.

HOW SUPPLIED: Tab: (Hydrocodone-APAP) 5mg-325mg*, 7.5mg-325mg*, 10mg-325mg* *scored

WARNINGS/PRECAUTIONS: May produce dose-related respiratory depression. May obscure diagnosis of acute abdominal conditions or head injuries. Caution in elderly, debilitated, severe hepatic or renal dysfunction, hypothyroidism, Addison's disease, prostatic hypertrophy, urethral stricture, pulmonary disease and postoperative use. May be habit-forming. Suppresses cough reflex.

ADVERSE REACTIONS: Lightheadedness, dizziness, sedation, NV.

INTERACTIONS: Additive CNS depression with narcotics, antipsychotics, antihistamines, antianxiety agents, alcohol, or other CNS depressants. Increased effect of antidepressant or hydrocodone with MAOIs or TCAs.

PREGNANCY: Category C, not for use in nursing.

MECHANISM OF ACTION: Hydrocodone: Opioid analgesic; most effects involve the CNS and smooth muscles. Precise MOA not established; suspected to relate to existence of opiate receptors in the CNS. APAP: Nonopiate, nonsalicylate analgesic and antipyretic. Analgesic activity involves peripheral influences; mechanism not established. Antipyretic activity is mediated through hypothalmic heat regulating centers; inhibits prostaglandin synthetase.

PHARMACOKINETICS: Absorption: Hydrocodone: C_{max}=23.6ng/mL; T_{max}=1.3 hrs. APAP: Rapidly absorbed. **Distribution:** APAP: Excreted in breast milk. **Metabolism:** Hydrocodone: O-demethylation, N-demethylation and 6-ketoreduction; APAP: Liver via conjugation. **Elimination:** Hydrocodone: $T_{1/2}$=3.8 hrs; APAP: Urine (85%). $T_{1/2}$=1.25-3 hrs.

NURSING CONSIDERATIONS

Assessment: Assess for head injury, intracranial lesions, elevations in ICP, acute abdominal conditions, presence of debilitation (eg, elderly), hepatic/

renal impairment, hypothyroidism, Addison's disease, prostatic hypertrophy or urethral stricture, pulmonary disease, nursing/pregnancy status, and possible drug interactions.

Monitoring: Monitor for signs/symptoms of respiratory depression, elevations in CSF pressure, medication dependence or tolerance, and medication abuse or misuse. Monitor serial hepatic/renal function tests with severe hepatic/renal disease.

Patient Counseling: Inform that medication may impair mental/physical abilities; use caution if performing hazardous tasks (eg, operating machinery/driving). Advise to avoid alcohol and other CNS depressants. Inform that medication may be habit forming; only take for as long as prescribed; in amounts prescribed and no more frequently than prescribed.

Administration: Oral route. **Storage:** 15-30°C (59-86°F). Store in tight, light-resistant container with child-resistant closure.

NORDETTE-28 — RX

ethinyl estradiol - levonorgestrel (Duramed)

OTHER BRAND NAMES: Portia (Barr) - Levora (Watson)

THERAPEUTIC CLASS: Estrogen/progestogen combination

INDICATIONS: Prevention of pregnancy.

DOSAGE: *Adults:* 1 tab qd for 28 days, then repeat. Start 1st Sunday after menses begin.

HOW SUPPLIED: Tab: (Ethinyl Estradiol-Levonorgestrel) 0.03mg-0.15mg

CONTRAINDICATIONS: Thrombophlebitis, DVT or thromboembolic disorders, pregnancy, cerebrovascular or coronary artery disease, undiagnosed abnormal genital bleeding, cholestatic jaundice of pregnancy or jaundice with prior pill use, hepatic adenomas or carcinomas, breast cancer or other estrogen-dependent neoplasia.

WARNINGS/PRECAUTIONS: Cigarette smoking increases risk of serious cardiovascular side effects; risk increases with age (especially >35 yrs) and heavy smoking. Increased risk of MI, vascular disease, thromboembolism, stroke and gallbladder disease. Retinal thrombosis, hepatic neoplasia, carcinoma of breast and reproductive organs reported. May cause glucose intolerance. May increase BP, elevate LDL levels or cause other lipid changes, fluid retention, breakthrough bleeding, and spotting. May cause or exacerbate migraine. May develop visual changes with contact lens. Increased risk of MI with HTN, hyperlipidemia, obesity, and diabetes. D/C if jaundice, significant depression or ophthalmic irregularities develop. Perform annual physical exam. Use before menarche is not indicated. May affect certain endocrine, LFTs and blood components.

ADVERSE REACTIONS: NV, breakthrough bleeding, spotting, amenorrhea, migraine, depression, vaginal candidiasis, edema, weight changes.

INTERACTIONS: Reduced effects, increased breakthrough bleeding, and menstrual irregularities with rifampin, barbiturates, phenylbutazone, phenytoin, griseofulvin, topiramate, some protease inhibitors, modafinil, and possibly St. John's wort, penicillins, and tetracyclines. Increased plasma levels with ascorbic acid, APAP, indinavir, fluconazole, troleandomycin, and atorvastatin. May affect cyclosporine, theophylline, and corticosteroid levels.

PREGNANCY: Category X, not for use in nursing.

MECHANISM OF ACTION: Estrogen/progestogen oral contraceptive; acts by suppressing gonadotropins. Primarily responsible for inhibiting ovulation. Also causes changes in cervical mucus (increases difficulty of sperm entry into uterus) and endometrium (reduces likelihood of implantation).

PHARMACOKINETICS: Distribution: Found in breast milk.

NURSING CONSIDERATIONS

Assessment: Assess for current or history of thrombophlebitis or thromboembolic disorders, cerebrovascular or coronary artery disease, known/suspected carcinoma of the breast, endometrium, or other suspected estrogen-dependent neoplasia, undiagnosed abnormal genital bleeding, cholestatic jaundice of pregnancy or jaundice with prior pill use, hepatic adenomas, hepatic carcinomas, benign liver tumors, and known/suspected pregnancy. Assess use in patients ≥35 yrs who smoke ≥15 cigarettes/day. Assess use with history of HTN, DM, hyperlipidemias, hypercholesterolemia, increased age, obesity, and possible drug interactions.

Monitoring: Monitor for MI, thromboembolism, stroke, hepatic neoplasia, ocular lesions, onset or exacerbation of headaches or migraines, bleeding irregularities, fluid retention, and gallbladder disease. Monitor serum glucose levels with DM or prediabetic patients, lipid levels with history of hyperlipidemia, BP with history of HTN. Monitor for signs of liver toxicity (eg, jaundice) while on therapy and for signs of worsening depression with previous history. Refer patients with contact lenses to ophthalmologist if visual changes develop. Perform annual physical exam.

Patient Counseling: Inform that drug does not protect against HIV infection (AIDS) and other STDs. Advise to take exactly as directed at intervals not exceeding 24 hrs. Counsel to use an additional form of contraception until after first 7 days of administration in initial cycle of medication. Instruct if pill missed, take as soon as possible; take next dose at regularly scheduled time. Advise to continue to take medication if spotting or breakthrough bleeding occur; notify physician if it persists. Instruct not to smoke while on therapy.

Administration: Oral route. **Storage:** 15-25°C (59-77°F).

NORDITROPIN RX

somatropin (Novo Nordisk)

OTHER BRAND NAMES: Norditropin Nordiflex (Novo Nordisk)

THERAPEUTIC CLASS: Human growth hormone

N

INDICATIONS: (Adults) Replacement of endogenous growth hormone deficiency who meet either of the following criteria: (1) adult-onset patients with growth hormone deficiency, either alone or associated with multiple hormone deficiencies (hypopituitarism), as a result of pituitary disease, hypothalamic disease, surgery, radiation therapy, or trauma; or (2) childhood-onset patients who were growth hormone deficient during childhood should have growth hormone deficiency confirmed as an adult before replacement therapy is started. (Pediatrics) Long-term treatment of children with growth failure due to inadequate growth hormone secretion. Treatment of children with short stature associated with Noonan syndrome and Turner syndrome. Treatment of children with short stature born small for gestational age (SGA) with no catch-up growth by age 2-4 yrs.

DOSAGE: *Adults:* Initial: No more than 0.004mg/kg/day. Increase to no more than 0.016mg/kg/day after 6 weeks.
Pediatrics: Growth Hormone Deficiency: 0.024-0.034mg/kg SQ 6-7x/week. Noonan Syndrome: Dose up to 0.066mg/kg/day. Turner Syndrome/SGA: Dose up to 0.067mg/kg/day. <4 yrs (SGA): Initial: 0.033mg/kg/day. Titrate dose over time as needed.

HOW SUPPLIED: Inj: (Norditropin (cartridge) and Norditropin Nordiflex (prefilled pen) 5mg/1.5mL, 15mg/1.5mL, 10mg/1.5mL (prefilled pen)

CONTRAINDICATIONS: Presence of active neoplasia; acute critical illness due to complications following open heart or abdominal surgery, multiple accidental trauma or acute respiratory failure; proliferative or preproliferative diabetic retinopathy; closed epiphyses; and Prader-Willi syndrome with severe obesity or severe respiratory impairment.

WARNINGS/PRECAUTIONS: Monitor for recurrence or progression of underlying disease in growth hormone deficiency secondary to intracranial lesions. Hypothyroidism reported. May develop slipped capital epiphyses. Intracranial HTN with papilledema, visual changes, headache, nausea, and vomiting reported. Progression of scoliosis may occur in rapid growth. Monitor for any form of malignant skin lesion prior to and during therapy. May decrease insulin sensitivity; monitor blood sugar. Dose dependent/transient fluid retention may occur. Increased occurrence of otitis media in patients with Turner syndrome. Monitor closely for cardiovascular disorders (e.g., stroke, aortic aneurysm/dissection, hypertension).

ADVERSE REACTIONS: (Pediatrics) Headache, injection-site reaction, localized muscle pain, rash, weakness, mild hyperglycemia, glucosuria, arthralgia, leukemia. (Adults) Edema, arthralgia, myalgia, infection, parasthesia, skeletal pain, headache, bronchitis.

INTERACTIONS: Diminished effects with glucocorticoid therapy. Insulin resistance reported. May reduce plasma levels of oral estrogens.

PREGNANCY: Category C, caution in nursing.

MECHANISM OF ACTION: Human growth hormone; binds to dimeric GH receptor in cell membrane of target cells resulting in intracellular signal transduction.

PHARMACOKINETICS: Absorption: T_{max}=4-5 hrs; (4mg) C_{max}=13.8ng/mL; (8mg) C_{max}=17.1ng/mL. **Elimination**: $T_{1/2}$=7-10 hrs.

NURSING CONSIDERATIONS

Assessment: Assess for closed epiphyses (pediatric), proliferative diabetic retinopathy, active malignancy, acute critical illness, pre-existing type 1 or type 2 DM or impaired glucose tolerance, history of scoliosis, pre-existing papilledema, hypothyroidism, diagnostic imaging (rule out pituitary or intracranial tumor), hypopituitarism and possible drug interactions. Obtain baseline fundoscopic exam. Prader-Willi syndrome: Evaluate for signs of upper airway obstruction or sleep apnea before initiation. Turner Syndrome: Evaluate for otitis media or other ear disorders, and for cardiovascular disorders before initiation.

Monitoring: Monitor fasting blood glucose and thyroid function tests periodically, periodic fundoscopic exam, signs/symptoms of malignant transformation of skin lesions, intracranial HTN, slipped capital femoral epiphysis (onset of limp, hip or knee pain), hypersensitivity/allergic reactions, respiratory infections (Prader-Willi syndrome), otitis media or ear disorders, CV disorders (Turner syndrome), and progression of scoliosis.

Patient Counseling: Instruct thoroughly on proper usage, proper disposal, and caution against reuse of needles and syringes. Seek medical attention if symptoms of slipped capital femoral epiphysis (onset of limp, hip or knee pain), hypersensitivity/allergic reactions, respiratory infections, otitis media or ear disorders, CV disorders, and progression of scoliosis occur.

Administration: SC. **Storage**: After 1st injection, either refrigerate at 2-8°C (36-46°F) and use within 4 weeks or store for up to 3 weeks at no more than 25°C (77°F). Discard unused portion.

NORITATE RX

metronidazole (Dermik)

THERAPEUTIC CLASS: Imidazole antibiotic

INDICATIONS: Inflammatory lesions and erythema of rosacea.

DOSAGE: *Adults:* Apply thin film to clean area qd.

HOW SUPPLIED: Cre: 1% [30g, 60g]

WARNINGS/PRECAUTIONS: Conjunctivitis reported with use on face. Avoid eye contact. Caution with blood dyscrasias.

ADVERSE REACTIONS: Local irritation, condition aggravated.

INTERACTIONS: May potentiate anticoagulant effects of warfarin.

PREGNANCY: Category B, not for use in nursing.

MECHANISM OF ACTION: Imidazole antibiotic; not established. Suspected to reduce inflammatory lesions of rosacea.

PHARMACOKINETICS: Absorption: C_{max}=27.6ng/mL; T_{max}=8-12 hrs. **Distribution:** Crosses placental barrier; secreted in breast milk.

NURSING CONSIDERATIONS

Assessment: Assess for evidence or history of blood dyscrasia. Assess pregnancy/nursing status and possible drug interactions.

Monitoring: Monitor for signs/symptoms of local skin irritation, conjunctivitis, allergic reactions, and flare-up of comedonal acne or rosacea.

Patient Counseling: Use as directed, externally. Avoid contact with eyes. Instruct to cleanse affected area before applying and report any potential adverse reactions.

Administration: Topical. For external use only. **Storage:** 20-25°C (68-77°F).

NORPACE RX

disopyramide phosphate (Pharmacia & Upjohn)

OTHER BRAND NAMES: Norpace CR (Pharmacia & Upjohn)

THERAPEUTIC CLASS: Class I antiarrhythmic

INDICATIONS: Treatment of documented life-threatening ventricular arrhythmias.

DOSAGE: *Adults:* Usual: 400-800mg/day in divided dose. Recommended: 150mg q6h immediate-release (IR) or 300mg q12h extended-release (CR). Adjust dose with anticholinergic effects. Weight <110lbs/Moderate Hepatic or Renal Insufficiency (CrCl >40mL/min): 100mg q6h IR or 200mg q12h CR. Severe Renal Insufficiency (with or without initial 150mg LD): CrCl 30-40mL/min: 100mg q8h IR. CrCl 30-15mL/min: 100mg q12h IR. CrCl <15mL/min: 100mg q24h IR. Rapid Control of Ventricular Arrhythmia: LD: 300mg IR (200mg if <110lbs). Follow with maint dose. Cardiomyopathy/Cardiac Decompensation: Initial: 100mg q6-8h IR. Adjust gradually. See PI if no response or toxicity occurs. Elderly: Start at low end of dosing range. *Pediatrics:* <1 yr: 10-30mg/kg/day. 1-4 yrs: 10-20mg/kg/day. 4-12 yrs: 10-15mg/kg/day. 12-18 yrs: 6-15mg/kg/day. Give in equally divided doses q6h. Hospitalize patient during initial therapy. Start dose titration at lower end of range.

HOW SUPPLIED: Cap: (Norpace) 100mg, 150mg; Cap, Extended-Release: (Norpace CR) 100mg, 150mg

CONTRAINDICATIONS: Cardiogenic shock, 2nd- or 3rd-degree AV block (if no pacemaker present), congenital QT prolongation.

WARNINGS/PRECAUTIONS: Proarrhythmic; reserve for life-threatening ventricular arrhythmias. May cause or worsen CHF and produce hypotension due to negative inotropic properties. Reduce dose if 1st-degree heart block occurs. Avoid with urinary retention, glaucoma, and myasthenia gravis unless adequate overriding measures taken. Atrial flutter/fibrillation; digitalize first. Monitor closely or withdraw if QT prolongation >25% occurs and ectopy continues. D/C if QRS widening >25% occurs. Avoid LD with cardiomyopathy or cardiac decompensation. Correct K^+ abnormalities before therapy. Reduce dose with renal/hepatic dysfunction; monitor ECG. Avoid CR formulation with CrCl ≤40mL/min. Caution with sick sinus syndrome, Wolff-Parkinson-White syndrome, bundle branch block, or elderly. May significantly lower blood glucose.

ADVERSE REACTIONS: Dry mouth, urinary retention/frequency/urgency, constipation, blurred vision, GI effects, dizziness, fatigue, headache.

INTERACTIONS: Avoid type IA and IC antiarrhythmics, and propranolol except in unresponsive, life-threatening arrhythmias. Hepatic enzyme inducers may lower levels. Avoid within 48 hrs before or 24 hrs after verapamil. Possible fatal interactions with CYP3A4 inhibitors. Monitor blood glucose with β-blockers, alcohol.

PREGNANCY: Category C, not for use in nursing.

MECHANISM OF ACTION: Type I antiarrhythmic; decreases rate of diastolic depolarization in cells with augmented automaticity, decreases upstroke velocity, and increases action potential duration of normal cardiac cells.

N

Decreases disparity in refractoriness between infracted and adjacent normally perfused myocardium and has no effect on α- or β-adrenergic receptors.

PHARMACOKINETICS: Absorption: Rapid and complete; C_{max}=2.22mcg/mL, T_{max}=4.5 hrs. **Distribution:** Plasma protein binding (50-65%). **Metabolism:** Liver. **Elimination:** Urine (50% unchanged), (20% mono-N-dealkylated metabolite), (10% other metabolite); $T_{1/2}$=11.65 hrs.

NURSING CONSIDERATIONS

Assessment: Prior to therapy, patients with atrial flutter or AF should be digitalized and potassium abnormalities should be corrected. Assess for cardiogenic shock, pre-existing 2nd- or 3rd-degree HB, presence of functioning pacemaker, sick sinus syndrome (bradycardia/tachycardia syndrome), Wolff-Parkinson-White syndrome, bundle branch block, congenital QT prolongation, MI, life-threatening arrhythmia, CHF, cardiomyopathy or myocarditis, chronic malnutrition, hepatic/renal impairment, alcohol intake, glaucoma, myasthenia gravis, urinary retention or BPH, pregnancy/nursing status, and possible drug interactions.

Monitoring: Monitor for hypotension, HF, PR interval prolongation, widening of QRS, hypoglycemia, HB, urinary retention, and myasthenia crisis.

Patient Counseling: Inform about risks/benefits; report adverse reactions. Notify if pregnant/nursing.

Administration: Oral route. **Storage:** 25°C (77°F); excursions permitted to 15-30°C (59-86°F).

NORPLANT II — RX

levonorgestrel (Population Council)

OTHER BRAND NAMES: Jadelle (Population Council)

THERAPEUTIC CLASS: Progestogen

INDICATIONS: Long-term (up to 5 yrs) prevention of pregnancy.

DOSAGE: *Adults:* Implant 150mg (2 implants) in midportion of upper arm during 1st 7 days of onset of menses. Place in a "V" shape 30° apart. Replace by end of 5th year.

HOW SUPPLIED: Implant: 75mg

CONTRAINDICATIONS: Active thrombophlebitis or thromboembolic disorders, undiagnosed abnormal genital bleeding, pregnancy, acute live disease or liver tumors, carcinoma of the breast, and idiopathic intracranial HTN.

WARNINGS/PRECAUTIONS: Complications related to insertion and removal of capsules reported. Bleeding irregularities have occurred. Retinal thrombosis leading to partial or complete loss of vision, hepatic neoplasia, carcinoma of breast and reproductive organs reported. Risk of thromboembolic and thrombotic diseases, MI, ectopic pregnancy, ovarian cysts, breast cancer, gall bladder and autoimmune diseases, cerebrovascular diseases. Cigarette smoking increases risk of serious cardiovascular side effects; risk increases with age (especially >35 yrs) and the extent of smoking. Idiopathic intracranial HTN and increases in BP reported. Caution with fluid retention. Vision changes reported; caution with contact lenses. Weight gain, thrombosis, and thrombophlebitis reported. May worsen depression, increase LDL levels. If jaundice develops, remove implants. Altered glucose tolerance; monitor diabetics. Rare reports of congenital anomalies with use during early pregnancy.

ADVERSE REACTIONS: Menorrhagia, amenorrhea, oligomenorrhea, irregular bleeding, pain/itching or infection at implant site, headache, nervousness, GI effects, dizziness, rash, acne, weight gain, cervicitis.

INTERACTIONS: Not recommended with chronic phenytoin, carbamazepine, phenobarbital, or oxcarbazepine use; decreased effectiveness. Back-up method of contraception with short-term therapy with CYP450 inducers. Rifampicin and St. John's wort may decreases levels and effectiveness.

PREGNANCY: Use in pregnancy not known, caution in nursing.

MECHANISM OF ACTION: Progestin; inhibits ovulation and thickens cervical mucus.

PHARMACOKINETICS: Absorption: C_{max}=722pg/mL (day 2), T_{max}=2-3 days. **Distribution:** Highly bound to sex-hormone-binding globulin. **Metabolism:** β-hydroxylation. **Excretion:** Urine (40-68%), feces (16-48%); $T_{1/2}$=13-18 hrs

NURSING CONSIDERATIONS

Assessment: Perform physical exam of implant site, breast, abdomen, and pelvis. Assess cervical cytology and relevant lab tests, pregnancy status, breast cancer, vaginal bleeding, thromboembolic disorders/active thrombophlebitis and/or cerebrovascular diseases, osteoporosis, history of depression, DM, hepatic/renal impairment, CV disease, HTN, and possible drug/lab test interactions.

Monitoring: Monitor for insertion and removal complications, amenorrhea, menstrual irregularity, manifestations of thromboembolic disorders (eg, thrombophlebitis, PE, cerebrovascular disorders, retinal thrombosis), ocular disorders, manifestations of fluid retention, epilepsy, abdominal pain, weight changes. Lab monitoring of bone mineral density for osteoporosis/osteoporotic fractures, LFTs, TFTs, glucose, lipid profile, and coagulation tests.

Patient Counseling: Inform of potential benefits/risks of therapy and insertion/removal procedure. Inform drug does not protect against HIV infection/AIDS or other STDs. Advise to avoid smoking while on therapy.

Administration: Subdermal implantation. Refer to PI for full instructions on insertion/removal. **Storage:** 15-30°C (59-86°F).

NORVASC — RX

amlodipine besylate (Pfizer)

N

THERAPEUTIC CLASS: Calcium channel blocker (dihydropyridine)

INDICATIONS: Treatment of hypertension and Coronary Artery Disease (CAD) including chronic stable or vasospastic angina (Prinzmetal's or Variant Angina).

DOSAGE: *Adults:* HTN: Initial: 5mg qd. Titrate over 7-14 days. Max: 10mg qd. Small, Fragile, or Elderly/Hepatic Dysfunction/Concomitant Antihypertensive: Initial: 2.5mg qd. Angina: 5-10mg qd. Elderly/Hepatic Dysfunction: 5mg qd. CAD: 5-10mg qd.
Pediatrics: 6-17 yrs: HTN: 2.5-5mg qd.

HOW SUPPLIED: Tab: 2.5mg, 5mg, 10mg

WARNINGS/PRECAUTIONS: May increase angina or MI with severe obstructive CAD. Caution with severe aortic stenosis, CHF, severe hepatic impairment, and in elderly.

ADVERSE REACTIONS: Edema, flushing, palpitation, dizziness, headache, fatigue.

PREGNANCY: Category C, not for use in nursing.

MECHANISM OF ACTION: A dihydropyridine calcium antagonist (calcium ion antagonist or slow-channel blocker) that inhibits transmembrane influx or calcium ions into vascular smooth muscle and cardiac muscle. Binds to both dihydropyridine and nondihydropyridine binding sites, which results in peripheral arterial vasodilation and reduction in BP.

PHARMACOKINETICS: Absorption: Absolute bioavailability (64-90%); T_{max}=6-12 hrs. **Distribution:** Plasma protein binding (93%). **Metabolism:** Hepatic. **Elimination:** Urine, $T_{1/2}$=30-50 hrs.

NURSING CONSIDERATIONS

Assessment: Assess for CAD, severe aortic stenosis, CHF, LFTs, BP, and possible drug interactions.

Monitoring: Monitor BP, LFTs. Monitor for arrhythmias, chest pain, peripheral neuropathies, CHF, MI, dyspnea, epistaxis, CBC with platelets and differential count, migraine, sexual dysfunction, asthenia, rash.

Patient Counseling: Counsel about potential adverse effects; advise to seek medical attention if any develop. Instruct to take as prescribed.

Administration: Oral route. **Storage:** 15-30°C (59-86°F); store in tight, light-resistant container.

NORVIR

ritonavir (Abbott)

RX

Use with certain non-sedating antihistamines, sedative hypnotics, antiarrhythmics, or ergot alkaloids may result in life-threatening adverse events.

THERAPEUTIC CLASS: Protease inhibitor

INDICATIONS: Treatment of HIV infection in combination with other antiretrovirals.

DOSAGE: *Adults:* Initial: 300mg bid. Titrate: Increase every 2-3 days by 100mg bid. Maint: 600mg bid. If combined with saquinavir, adjust dose to 400mg bid. Elderly: Start at low end of dosing range. Take with meals if possible. *Pediatrics:* >1 month: Initial: 250mg/m² po bid. Titrate: Increase by 50mg/m² every 2-3 days. Maint: 350-400mg/m² po bid or highest tolerated dose. Max: 600mg bid.

HOW SUPPLIED: Cap: 100mg; Sol: 80mg/mL [240mL]

CONTRAINDICATIONS: Alfuzosin, amiodarone, bepridil, flecainide, propafenone, quinidine, voriconazole, astemizole, terfenadine, ergot derivatives, midazolam, triazolam, cisapride, pimozide, dihydroergotamine, ergonovine, ergotamine, methylergonovine, midazolam, triazolam.

WARNINGS/PRECAUTIONS: Allergic reactions (eg, urticaria, mild skin eruptions, bronchospasm, and angioedema), pancreatitis, new onset/exacerbation of pre-existing diabetes mellitus, hyperglycemia, immune reconstitution syndrome, hepatic transaminase elevations and hepatic dysfunction reported. Caution with moderate to severe hepatic impairment and in elderly. Monitor LFTs, especially 1st three months. Increased bleeding may occur with hemophilia A and B. Possible redistribution or accumulation of body fat. May increase total triglyceride and cholesterol levels. Cardiac and neurologic events reported.

ADVERSE REACTIONS: Diarrhea, anorexia, NV, abdominal pain, asthenia, headache, malaise, vasodilation, constipation, dizziness, taste perversion, peripheral paresthesia, circumoral, insomnia, and sweating.

INTERACTIONS: See Contraindications. Avoid use with rifampin, St. John's wort; may cause loss of virologic response and resistance. Avoid use with lovastatin and simvastatin; risk of myopathy and rhabdomyolysis. Neurologic and cardiac events reported with disopyramide, mexiletine, nefazodone, fluoxetine, and β-blockers. Concomitant use with tipranavir may cause hepatitis and hepatic decompensation. May increase levels of saquinavir, atazanavir, darunavir, fosamprenavir, desipramine, indinavir, rifabutin. May increase levels of clarithromycin with renal impairment; reduce clarithromycin dose by 50% if CrCl 30-60mL/min and by 75% if CrCl<30mL/min. May increase ketoconazole levels; avoid ketoconazole doses >200mg/day. May increase sildenafil levels; do not exceed sildenafil 25mg/48 hrs. May increase levels of tramadol, propoxyphene, disopyramide, lidocaine, mexilitene, carbamazepine, clonazepam, ethosuximide, bupropion, nefazodone, SSRIs, TCAs, dronabinol, itraconazole, quinine, metoprolol, timolol, diltiazem, nifedipine, verapamil, atorvastatin, rosuvastatin, cyclosporine, tacrolimus, sirolimus, perphenazine, risperidone, thioridazine, clorazepate, diazepam, estazolam, flurazepam, zolpidem, dexamethasone, fluticasone, prednisone, methamphetamine. May increase levels of trazodone; use with caution and consider lower trazodone dose. Decreases levels of theophylline, meperidine, methadone. May decrease levels of phenytoin, divalproex, lamotrigine, and atovaquone. Separate dosing with didanosine by 2.5 hrs. May increase plasma levels of drugs metabolized by CYP3A or CYP2D6. May decrease ethinyl estradiol levels; use alternative contraceptive measures. Monitor PT/INR with warfarin. Contains alcohol; may produce disulfiram-like reactions with disulfiram, metronidazole.

PREGNANCY: Category B, not for use in nursing.

MECHANISM OF ACTION: HIV protease inhibitor; renders enzyme incapable of processing *gag-pol* polyprotein precursor, which leads to production of non-infectious immature HIV particles.

PHARMACOKINETICS: Absorption: C_{max}=11.2mcg/mL; T_{max}=2 hrs (fasting), 4 hrs (fed); AUC=121.7mcg•h/mL (Cap), 129mcg•hr/mL (Sol). **Metabolism:** CYP3A, 2D6 (oxidation); isopropylthiazole (major metabolite). **Elimination:** Urine (3.5%), feces (33.8%); $T_{1/2}$=3-5 hrs.

NURSING CONSIDERATIONS

Assessment: Assess for pre-existing liver disease or impairment (enzyme abnormalities, hepatitis), DM, and possible drug interactions. Obtain baseline triglyceride/cholesterol panel.

Monitoring: Monitor LFTs periodically for first 3 months. Monitor for signs/symptoms of anaphylactoid/allergic reactions, new onset or exacerbation of DM, hyperglycemia, pancreatitis, immune reconstitution syndrome, fat redistribution or accumulation, and hepatic dysfunction.

Patient Counseling: Inform that drug does not cure HIV; may continue to develop opportunistic infections. Does not reduce risk of transmitting HIV. Instruct to take every day with food, if possible; do not alter dose or d/c without consulting physician. If miss dose, take next dose as soon as possible; do not double dose. Advise to report use of prescription and nonprescription medications and to seek medical attention if symptoms of allergic reactions, pancreatitis (NV, abdominal pain), infections, fat redistribution/accumulation occur.

Administration: Oral route. **Storage:** Cap: 2-8°C (36-46°F). Protect from light. Avoid exposure to excessive heat. Sol: 20-25°C (68-77°F). Do not refrigerate. Shake well before use. Avoid exposure to excessive heat.

N

NOVOLIN OTC

insulin human, rdna origin - insulin, human isophane - insulin, human regular (Novo Nordisk)

OTHER BRAND NAMES: Novolin R (Novo Nordisk) - Novolin N (Novo Nordisk)

THERAPEUTIC CLASS: Insulin

INDICATIONS: To control hyperglycemia in diabetes.

DOSAGE: *Adults:* Individualize dose.
Pediatrics: Individualize dose.

HOW SUPPLIED: Inj: 100 U/mL (Novolin N, Novolin R); PenFill: 100 U/mL (Novolin N, Novolin R); Prefilled: 100 U/mL (Novolin N, Novolin R)

WARNINGS/PRECAUTIONS: Human insulin differs from animal source insulin. Any change in insulin should be made cautiously. Changes in strength, manufacturer, type or method of manufacture may result in the need for a change in dosage. Hypoglycemia may occur with taking too much insulin, missing or delaying meals, exercising or working more than usual. An infection or illness (especially if accompanied by diarrhea or vomiting) may change insulin requirements. Administration of insulin SQ can result in lipoatrophy. Novolin R is not recommended for use in insulin pumps.

ADVERSE REACTIONS: Hypoglycemia, sweating, dizziness, palpitations, tremor, hunger, restlessness, lightheadedness, inability to concentrate, headache, injection-site reaction, allergic reaction.

INTERACTIONS: Increased insulin requirements with oral contraceptives, corticosteroids, or thyroid replacement therapy. Reduced insulin requirements with oral hypoglycemics, salicylates, sulfa antibiotics, and certain antidepressants. Alcoholic beverages may change insulin requirements. β-blockers may mask symptoms of hypoglycemia.

PREGNANCY: Pregnancy category is not known.

MECHANISM OF ACTION: Insulin (rDNA origin); regulates glucose metabolism, lowers blood glucose by facilitating cellular uptake of glucose and simultaneously inhibiting the glucose output from the liver.

NURSING CONSIDERATIONS

Assessment: Assess FPG, HbA_{1c}, renal function, LFTs, pregnancy status, infections, alcohol consumption, exercise routines, and for possible drug interactions.

Monitoring: Monitor FPG, HbA_{1c}, hypokalemia, renal function, diabetic ketoacidosis, vision changes, lipodystrophy, allergic reactions. Monitor for signs of hypoglycemia (sweating, palpitations, seizures, disorientation, tremors).

Patient Counseling: Use only if solution is clear and colorless with no visible particles. Counsel about signs/symptoms of hypoglycemia, hyperglycemia, diabetic ketoacidosis, the importance of frequent monitoring of blood glucose levels, eating a balanced diet and exercising regularly. Advise to avoid excessive alcohol. During periods of stress (eg, trauma, infection, surgery), insulin requirements may be changed; advise patients to seek prompt medical advice. Counsel on proper administration techniques.

Administration: SQ route. Refer to labeling for administration techniques.
Storage: Below 30°C (86°F). Do not freeze. Protect from light.

Novolin 70/30 — OTC

insulin human, rdna origin - insulin, human (isophane/regular) (Novo Nordisk)

THERAPEUTIC CLASS: Insulin

INDICATIONS: To control hyperglycemia in diabetes.

DOSAGE: *Adults:* Individualize dose. Administer SQ.
Pediatrics: Individualize dose. Administer SQ.

HOW SUPPLIED: (Isophane/Regular) Inj: 70 U-30 U/mL; PenFill: 70 U-30 U/mL; Prefilled: 70 U-30 U/mL

N

WARNINGS/PRECAUTIONS: Human insulin differs from animal source insulin. Any change of insulin should be made cautiously. Changes in strength, manufacturer, type or method of manufacture may result in the need for a change in dosage. Hypoglycemia may occur with taking too much insulin, missing or delaying meals, exercising or working more than usual. An infection or illness (especially with diarrhea or vomiting) may change insulin requirements. Caution with diseases of adrenal, pituitary, or thyroid glands, or progression of kidney or liver disease. Administration of insulin SQ can result in lipoatrophy.

ADVERSE REACTIONS: Hypoglycemia, sweating, dizziness, palpitation, tremor, hunger, restlessness, lightheadedness, inability to concentrate, headache, injection-site reaction, allergic reaction.

INTERACTIONS: Increased insulin requirements with oral contraceptives, corticosteroids, or thyroid replacement therapy. Reduced insulin requirements with oral hypoglycemics, salicylates, sulfa antibiotics, and certain antidepressants. Alcoholic beverages may change insulin requirements. β-blockers may mask symptoms of hypoglycemia.

PREGNANCY: Pregnancy category is not known.

MECHANISM OF ACTION: Insulin (rDNA origin); has 70% NPH human insulin isophane suspension and 30% regular human insulin. Regulates glucose metabolism, lowers blood glucose by facilitating cellular uptake of glucose and simultaneously inhibiting the glucose output from the liver.

NURSING CONSIDERATIONS

Assessment: Assess FPG, HbA_{1c}, renal function, LFTs, pregnancy status, infections, alcohol consumption, exercise routines, and for possible drug interactions.

Monitoring: Monitor FPG, HbA_{1c}, hypokalemia, renal function, diabetic ketoacidosis, vision changes, lipodystrophy, allergic reactions. Monitor for signs of hypoglycemia (sweating, palpitation, seizures, disorientation, tremors).

Patient Counseling: Use only if the solution is clear and colorless with no visible particles. Counsel about signs/symptoms of hypoglycemia, hyperglycemia, diabetic ketoacidosis, the importance of frequent monitoring of blood glucose levels, the need for eating a balanced diet and exercising regularly. Advise to avoid excessive alcohol. During periods of stress (eg, trauma, infection, surgery) insulin requirements may be changed; advise patients to seek prompt medical advice. Counsel on proper administration techniques.
Administration: SQ route. Refer to labeling for administration techniques.
Storage: Below 30°C (86°F). Do not freeze. Protect from light.

NOVOLOG — RX

insulin aspart (Novo Nordisk)

THERAPEUTIC CLASS: Insulin

INDICATIONS: To control hyperglycemia in diabetes.

DOSAGE: *Adults:* Individualize dose. Inject SQ within 5-10 min before a meal. Draw first when mixing with NPH human insulin; inject immediately. Do not mix with crystalline zinc insulins, animal source insulins, or other manufacturer insulins. (External Pump) Do not use or mix with any other insulin or diluent in pump.
Pediatrics: ≥4 yrs: Individualize dose. Inject SQ within 5-10 min before a meal. Draw first when mixing with NPH human insulin; inject immediately. Do not mix with crystalline zinc insulins, animal source insulins, or other manufacturer insulins. (External Pump) Do not use or mix with any other insulin or diluent in pump.

HOW SUPPLIED: Inj: 100 U/mL; PenFill: 100 U/mL; Prefilled: 100 U/mL

CONTRAINDICATIONS: Hypoglycemia.

WARNINGS/PRECAUTIONS: Any change of insulin should be made cautiously. Changes in strength, manufacturer, type, or method of manufacture may result in the need for a change in dosage. Hypoglycemia may occur with taking too much insulin, missing or delaying meals, exercising or working more than usual, diseases of adrenal, pituitary, or thyroid glands, or progression of kidney or liver disease. May cause hypokalemia. Dosage adjustments may be needed with hepatic or renal dysfunction, during any infection, illness (especially with diarrhea or vomiting) or pregnancy. A longer-acting insulin is usually required to maintain adequate glucose control. Infusion sets and the insulin in the infusion sets should be changed q48h or sooner. Do not use in quick-release infusion sets or cartridge adapters.

ADVERSE REACTIONS: Hypoglycemia, hypokalemia, lipodystrophy, hypersensitivity reaction, injection site reactions, pruritus, rash.

INTERACTIONS: Increased glucose lowering effects with ACE inhibitors, disopyramide, fibrates, fluoxetine, MAOIs, propoxyphene, salicylates, somatostatin analog, sulfonamide antibiotics and other antidiabetic agents. Decreased blood glucose lowering effects with corticosteroids, niacin, danazol, diuretics, sympathomimetic agents, isoniazid, phenothiazine derivatives, somatropin, thyroid hormones, estrogens, progestogens. Pentamidine may cause hypoglycemia followed by hyperglycemia. β-blockers, clonidine, lithium salts, and alcohol may potentiate or weaken glucose lowering effect. Masked or reduced hypoglycemic symptoms with β-blockers, clonidine, guanethidine, and reserpine.

PREGNANCY: Category B, caution in nursing.

MECHANISM OF ACTION: Insulin aspart (rDNA origin); regulates glucose metabolism, lowers blood glucose by facilitating cellular uptake of glucose and simultaneously inhibiting glucose output from the liver.

PHARMACOKINETICS: Absorption: C_{max}=82.1 mU/L; T_{max}=40-50 min. **Distribution:** Plasma protein binding (0-9%). **Elimination:** $T_{1/2}$=81 min.

NURSING CONSIDERATIONS

Assessment: Assess FPG, HbA_{1c}, renal function, LFTs, pregnancy status, infections, alcohol consumption, exercise routines, and possible drug interactions.

Monitoring: Monitor FPG, HbA_{1c}, hypokalemia, renal function, diabetic ketoacidosis, vision changes, lipodystrophy, allergic reactions. Monitor for signs of hypoglycemia (sweating, palpitations, seizures, disorientation, tremors).

Patient Counseling: Use only if the solution is clear and colorless with no visible particles. Counsel about signs/symptoms of hypoglycemia, hyperglycemia, diabetic ketoacidosis, the importance of frequent monitoring of blood glucose levels, the need for eating a balanced diet and exercising regularly. Advise to avoid excessive alcohol. During periods of stress (eg, trauma, infection, surgery), insulin requirements may be changed; advise to seek prompt medical advice. Counsel on proper administration techniques.

Administration: IV, SQ route in abdominal wall, thigh, or upper arm. Give immediately before a meal. Refer to labeling information for administration techniques. **Storage:** 2-8°C (36-46°F). Do not freeze. Insulin exposed to temperatures >37°C (98°F) should be discarded.

NovoLog Mix 70/30 RX

insulin aspart protamine - insulin aspart (Novo Nordisk)

THERAPEUTIC CLASS: Insulin

INDICATIONS: To control hyperglycemia in diabetes.

DOSAGE: *Adults:* Individualize dose. For SQ inj only. Inject SQ bid within 15 min before breakfast and dinner. Do not mix with other insulins or use in insulin pumps.

HOW SUPPLIED: (Insulin Aspart Protamine-Insulin Aspart) Inj: 70 U-30 U/mL; PenFill: 70 U-30 U/mL; Prefilled: 70 U-30 U/mL

CONTRAINDICATIONS: Hypoglycemia.

WARNINGS/PRECAUTIONS: Any change of insulin should be made cautiously. Changes in strength, manufacturer, type or method of manufacture may result in the need for a change in dosage. Hypoglycemia and hypokalemia may occur; caution with fasting and autonomic neuropathy. Illness, stress, change in meals and exercise may change insulin requirements. Smoking, temperature, and exercise affect insulin absorption. Caution with liver or kidney disease. Administration of insulin SQ can result in lipoatrophy.

ADVERSE REACTIONS: Hypoglycemia, hypokalemia, lipodystrophy, hypersensitivity reaction, injection-site reactions, pruritus, rash.

INTERACTIONS: Increased glucose lowering effects with ACE inhibitors, disopyramide, fibrates, fluoxetine, MAOIs, propoxyphene, salicylates, somatostatin analog, sulfonamide antibiotics, and oral antidiabetics. Decreased blood glucose lowering effects with corticosteroids, niacin, danazol, diuretics, sympathomimetics, isoniazid, phenothiazine derivatives, somatropin, thyroid hormones, estrogens, progestogens. β-blockers, clonidine, lithium salts, and alcohol may potentiate or weaken glucose lowering effect. β-blockers, clonidine, guanethidine, and reserpine may reduce or mask signs of hypoglycemia. Do not mix with other insulin products. Caution with potassium-lowering drugs or drugs sensitive to serum potassium levels. Pentamidine may cause hypoglycemia, followed by hyperglycemia.

PREGNANCY: Category C, safety in nursing not known.

MECHANISM OF ACTION: Insulin; regulates glucose metabolism. Lowers blood glucose by facilitating cellular uptake of glucose, simultaneously inhibiting output of glucose from liver.

PHARMACOKINETICS: Absorption: (0.2, 0.3 U/kg): C_{max}=23.4, 61.3m U/L; T_{max}=60, 85 min. **Distribution:** Plasma protein binding (0-9%). **Elimination:** $T_{1/2}$=8-9 hrs.

NURSING CONSIDERATIONS

Assessment: Assess FPG, HbA_{1c}, renal function, LFTs, pregnancy status, infections, alcohol consumption, exercise routines, and for possible drug interactions.

N

Monitoring: Monitor FPG, HbA_{1c}, hypokalemia, renal function, diabetic ketoacidosis, vision changes, lipodystrophy, allergic reactions. Monitor for signs and symptoms of hypoglycemia (eg, sweating, palpitation, seizures, disorientation, tremors).

Patient Counseling: Inform to use only if solution is clear and colorless with no visible particles, and not to dilute or mix with other insulins or solution. Counsel about the signs and symptoms of hypoglycemia, hyperglycemia, and diabetic ketoacidosis; importance of frequent monitoring of blood glucose levels, need for a balanced diet, and regular exercise. Advise to avoid excessive alcohol. Counsel that during periods of stress (eg, trauma, infection, surgery), insulin requirements may be changed; advise to seek prompt medical attention. Educate on proper administration techniques.

Administration: SQ route. Administer in abdominal wall, thigh, or upper arm. Give with meals. Refer to PI for administration techniques. **Storage**: 2-8°C (36-46°F). Do not freeze.

NOXAFIL RX

posaconazole (Schering)

THERAPEUTIC CLASS: Azole antifungal

INDICATIONS: Prophylaxis of invasive *Aspergillus* and *Candida* infections in patients ≥13 yrs who are at high risk of developing these infections due to being severely immunocompromised. Treatment of oropharyngeal candidiasis, including oropharyngeal candidiasis refractory to itraconazole and/or fluconazole.

DOSAGE: *Adults:* Prophylaxis of Invasive Fungal Infections: 200mg (5mL) tid. Base duration of therapy on recovery from neutropenia or immunosuppression. Oropharyngeal Candidiasis: LD: 100mg (2.5mL) bid on 1st day, then 100mg qd for 13 days. Oropharyngeal Candidiasis Refractory to Itraconazole and/or Fluconazole: 400mg (10mL) bid. Base duration of therapy on severity of underlying disease and clinical response. Give each dose with full meal or nutritional supplement.

Pediatrics: ≥13 yrs: Prophylaxis of Invasive Fungal Infections: 200mg (5mL) tid. Base duration of therapy on recovery from neutropenia or immunosuppression. Oropharyngeal Candidiasis: LD: 100mg (2.5mL) bid on 1st day, then 100mg qd for 13 days. Oropharyngeal Candidiasis Refractory to Itraconazole and/or Fluconazole: 400mg (10mL) bid. Base duration of therapy on severity of underlying disease and clinical response. Give each dose with full meal or nutritional supplement.

HOW SUPPLIED: Susp: 40mg/mL

CONTRAINDICATIONS: Concomitant ergot alkaloids, terfenadine, astemizole, cisapride, pimozide, halofantrine, quinidine or sirolimus.

WARNINGS/PRECAUTIONS: Hepatic reactions (eg, mild to moderate elevations in ALT, AST, alkaline phosphatase, total bilirubin, and/or clinical hepatitis) reported; monitor LFTs at start of and during therapy. Caution with hepatic impairment. Monitor closely with severe renal impairment. Prolongation of QT interval reported; caution with potentially proarrhythmic conditions.

ADVERSE REACTIONS: Fever, headache, rigors, HTN, anemia, neutropenia, diarrhea, NV, abdominal pain, constipation, hypokalemia, thrombocytopenia, coughing, dyspnea.

INTERACTIONS: See Contraindications. May elevate cyclosporine and tacrolimus levels; consider dose reduction and more frequent clinical monitoring of cyclosporine and tacrolimus when therapy is initiated. Avoid use with drugs that are known to prolong the QTc interval and are metabolized through CYP3A4. Avoid concurrent use of cimetidine, rifabutin, phenytoin, and efavirenz unless benefits outweigh risks. If concomitant phenytoin is required, monitor closely and consider phenytoin dose reduction. If concomitant rifabutin is required, monitor CBC and adverse events. Monitor adverse events with concomitant benzodiazepines metabolized by CYP3A4; consider dose reduction of these benzodiazepines during coadministration. May increase levels of vinca alkaloids; consider dose adjustment of vinca alkaloid. Consider dose reduction of concomitant HMG-CoA reductase inhibitors (statins). Monitor for adverse events and toxicity with concomitant CCBs; dose reduction of CCBs may be needed.

PREGNANCY: Category C, not for use in nursing.

MECHANISM OF ACTION: Antifungal agent; blocks synthesis of ergosterol, a key component of fungal cell membrane, through inhibition of the enzyme lanosterol 14α-demethylase and accumulation of methylated sterol precursors.

PHARMACOKINETICS: Administration: Oral administration of variable doses resulted in different parameters. **Distribution:** V_d=1774L, plasma protein binding (≥98%). **Metabolism:** Via UDP glucuronidation; CYP3A4 enzyme. **Elimination:** Feces (71%), urine (13%); $T_{1/2}$=35 hrs.

NURSING CONSIDERATIONS

Assessment: Assess for drug interactions (ergot alkaloids, CYP3A4 substrates, cylosporine, QT prolonging medications). Assess liver function (LFTs, bilirubin) prior to therapy. Assess use in patients with proarrhythmic conditions.

Monitoring: Monitor liver function (LFTs, bilirubin) while on therapy. Monitor for signs/symptoms of hepatic toxicity, QT prolongation, and arrhythmias.

Patient Counseling: Instruct to take medication with full meal or liquid nutritional supplement. Instruct to inform physician if severe diarrhea or vomiting develop. Inform physician of all medications being taken.

Administration: Oral. **Storage:** 25°C (77°F); excursions permitted to 15-30°C (59-86°F).

NUBAIN RX

nalbuphine HCl (Endo)

THERAPEUTIC CLASS: Agonist-antagonist analgesic

INDICATIONS: Relief of moderate to severe pain. Adjunct to balanced anesthesia for pre- and postoperative analgesia, and for obstetrical analgesia during labor and delivery.

DOSAGE: *Adults:* ≥18 yrs: Pain: Initial: 10mg/70kg IV/IM/SQ q3-6h prn. Adjust according to severity, physical status and concomitant agents. Max: 20mg/dose or 160mg/day. Anesthesia Adjunct: Induction: 0.3-3mg/kg IV over 10-15 min. Maint: 0.25-0.5mg/kg IV.

HOW SUPPLIED: Inj: 10mg/mL, 20mg/mL

WARNINGS/PRECAUTIONS: Increased risk of respiratory depression with head injury, intracranial lesions, or pre-existing increased ICP. Only for use by specifically trained persons. Naloxone, resuscitative and intubation equipment, and oxygen should be readily available. Caution with emotionally unstable patients, narcotic abuse, impaired respiration, MI with nausea and vomiting, biliary tract surgery. May impair ability to drive or operate machinery. Caution with renal or hepatic dysfunction; reduce dose. Caution during labor and delivery; monitor newborns for respiratory depression, apnea, bradycardia, and arrhythmias.

ADVERSE REACTIONS: Sedation, sweating, NV, dizziness/vertigo, dry mouth, headache, injection-site reactions.

INTERACTIONS: Possible additive effects with narcotic analgesics, general anesthetics, phenothiazines, tranquilizers, sedatives, hypnotics, or other CNS depressants. Incompatible with nafcillin and ketorolac.

PREGNANCY: Category B, caution in nursing.

MECHANISM OF ACTION: Opioid agonist-antagonist analgesic; kappa agonist/partial mu antagonist analgesic.

PHARMACOKINETICS: Metabolism: Liver. **Elimination:** Urine; $T_{1/2}$=5 hrs.

NURSING CONSIDERATIONS

Assessment: Assess for emotional instability, history of opioid abuse, head injury, intracranial lesions, increased ICP, possible drug interactions, respiratory, renal and hepatic impairment.

Monitoring: Monitor for signs/symptoms of respiratory depression, hypersensitivity reactions, increased ICP, and withdrawal symptoms.

Patient Counseling: May impair physical/mental abilities. Advise to seek medical attention if symptoms of respiratory depression, hypersensitivity reactions, increased ICP, or withdrawal symptoms (upon abrupt d/c) occur.

Administration: SC, IM, or IV. **Storage:** 25°C (77°F); excursions permitted to 15-30°C (59-86°F). Protect from excessive light.

NUTROPIN RX

somatropin (Genentech)

OTHER BRAND NAMES: Nutropin AQ (Genentech)

THERAPEUTIC CLASS: Human growth hormone

INDICATIONS: (Adults) Replacement of endogenous growth hormone (GH) in GH deficiency (GHD). (Pediatrics) Long-term treatment of growth failure due to lack of adequate endogenous GH secretion, in short stature associated with Turner syndrome, and in idiopathic short stature (ISS). Treatment of growth failure associated with chronic renal insufficiency (CRI) up to the time of renal transplantation.

DOSAGE: *Adults:* GHD: Initial: Up to 0.006mg/kg/day SQ. Max: <35 yrs: 0.025mg/kg/day. ≥35 yrs: 0.0125mg/kg/day. Alternatively may use 0.2mg/day (range: 0.15-0.30mg/day). Increase every 1-2 months by increments of 0.1-0.2mg/day.

Pediatrics: GHD: Usual: 0.3mg/kg/week divided into daily SQ doses. Pubertal Patients: Up to 0.7mg/kg/week divided into daily SQ doses. CRI: 0.35mg/kg/week divided into daily SQ doses. Continue until renal transplantation. Hemodialysis: Give qhs or 3-4 hrs post-dialysis. Chronic Cycling Peritoneal Dialysis: Give in am after dialysis. Chronic Ambulatory Peritoneal Dialysis: Give qhs during overnight exchange. Turner Syndrome: Up to 0.375mg/kg/week SQ in divided doses 3-7x/week. ISS: 0.3mg/kg/week divided into daily SQ doses.

HOW SUPPLIED: Inj: 5mg, 10mg, (AQ) 5mg/mL

CONTRAINDICATIONS: Acute critical illness after serious surgeries (eg, open heart or abdominal surgery, accidental trauma, acute respiratory failure), closed epiphyses in pediatrics, active proliferative or severe nonproliferative diabetic retinopathy, active neoplasia, evidence of recurrence or progression of an intracranial tumor. Prader-Willi syndrome (unless also diagnosed with GH deficiency) with severe obesity or respiratory impairment.

WARNINGS/PRECAUTIONS: Caution with epiphyseal closure in adults treated with GH-replacement therapy in childhood. Recurrence/progression reported with intracranial lesions. Renal osteodystrophy may occur with growth failure secondary to renal impairment. Scoliosis and slipped capital femoral epiphysis may develop in rapid growth. Caution with Turner syndrome and ISS. Intracranial hypertension with papilledema, visual changes, headache, nausea, and/or vomiting has been reported. Funduscopic exam should be done before and during treatment. Monitor for malignant transformation of skin lesions. Injecting SQ in same site over long period of time may cause tissue atrophy. May decrease insulin sensitivity; monitor blood sugar.

ADVERSE REACTIONS: Antibodies to the protein, leukemia, transient peripheral edema, arthralgia, carpal tunnel syndrome, malignant transformations, gynecomastia, pancreatitis.

INTERACTIONS: Decreased effects with glucocorticoids. May reduce insulin sensitivity; may need insulin adjustment. May need to increase dose in adult women on estrogen replacement.

PREGNANCY: Category C, caution in nursing.

MECHANISM OF ACTION: Human growth hormone; increases growth rate and serum insulin-like growth factor-I levels.

PHARMACOKINETICS: Absorption: (SQ) Absolute bioavailability (81%), C_{max}=71.1mcg/L, T_{max}=3.9 hrs, AUC=677 mcg•hr/L. **Distribution:** V_d=50mL/kg. **Metabolism:** Liver and kidneys. **Elimination:** (SQ) $T_{1/2}$=2.3 hrs. (IV) $T_{1/2}$=19.5 min.

NURSING CONSIDERATIONS

Assessment: Assess for closed epiphyses (pediatric), proliferative diabetic retinopathy, active malignancy, acute critical illness due to complications of surgery, multiple accidental trauma, or acute respiratory failure, pre-existing type 1 or type 2 DM or impaired glucose tolerance, history of scoliosis, pre-existing papilledema, hypothyroidism, diagnostic imaging (rule out pituitary or intracranial tumor), hypopituitarism and possible drug interactions. Obtain baseline funduscopic exam. Chronic renal insufficiency (pediatrics): Baseline x-ray of hips. Prader-Willi syndrome: Evaluate for signs of upper airway obstruction or sleep apnea before initiation. Turner syndrome: Evaluate for otitis media or other ear disorders, and for cardiovascular disorders before initiation.

Monitoring: Monitor fasting blood glucose, and thyroid function tests periodically, periodic funduscopic exam, weight control (Prader-Willi), signs/symptoms of malignant transformation of skin lesions, intracranial HTN, renal osteodystrophy, slipped capital femoral epiphysis (onset of limp, hip or knee pain), hypersensitivity/allergic reactions, respiratory infections (Prader-Willi), otitis media or ear disorders, CV disorders (Turner syndrome), and progression of scoliosis.

Patient Counseling: Instruct thoroughly on proper usage, proper disposal, and caution against reuse of needles and syringes. Seek medical attention if symptoms of slipped capital femoral epiphysis (onset of limp, hip or knee pain), hypersensitivity/allergic reactions, respiratory infections (Prader-Willi), otitis media or ear disorders, CV disorders (Turner syndrome), and progression of scoliosis occur.

Administration: SQ route. **Storage:** Before and after reconstitution: 2-8°C (36-46°F) (under refrigeration). Avoid freezing. (AQ): Stable for 28 days after initial use. Protect from light. (Nutropin): Stable 14 days after reconstitution.

NUVARING — RX

etonogestrel - ethinyl estradiol (Organon)

THERAPEUTIC CLASS: Estrogen/progestogen combination

INDICATIONS: Prevention of pregnancy.

DOSAGE: *Adults:* Insert ring vaginally on or before the 5th day of cycle. Remove ring after 3 consecutive weeks. Insert new ring 1 week later on same day of the week and same time of day.

HOW SUPPLIED: Vaginal ring: (Ethinyl estradiol-Etonogestrel) 0.015mg-0.120mg/day

CONTRAINDICATIONS: Thrombophlebitis, active or history of thromboembolic disorders, history of DVT, cerebrovascular or coronary artery disease, valvular heart disease with complications, severe HTN, diabetes with vascular complications, headaches with focal neurological symptoms, major surgery with prolonged immobilization, breast carcinoma, endometrial carcinoma or other estrogen-dependent neoplasia, undiagnosed abnormal genital bleeding, cholestatic jaundice of pregnancy or jaundice with prior hormonal contraceptive use, hepatic tumors, active liver disease, pregnancy, heavy smoking and >35 yrs.

WARNINGS/PRECAUTIONS: Cigarette smoking increases risk of serious cardiovascular side effects. This risk increases with age (especially >35 yrs) and heavy smoking. Increases risk of MI, thromboembolism, stroke, and gallbladder disease, and hypertension. Retinal thrombosis and benign hepatic adenomas reported. May decrease glucose tolerance. May increase BP, PT, sex hormone-binding globulins, thyroid hormone, or LDL levels. May cause other lipid changes, fluid retention, breakthrough bleeding and spotting, or exacerbate migraines. May develop visual changes with contact lens. D/C if jaundice, significant depression, severe headaches or migraines develop. Toxic shock syndrome with tampon use reported. Increased risk of morbidity and mortality in certain inherited thrombophilias, obesity, and diabetes. Older women who take hormonal contraceptive should take the lowest possible dose formulation that is effective.

ADVERSE REACTIONS: Vaginitis, headache, upper respiratory tract infection, leukorrhea, sinusitis, weight gain, nausea.

INTERACTIONS: Reduced effects with barbiturates, griseofulvin, rifampin, phenylbutazone, phenytoin, carbamazepine, felbamate, oxycarbazepine, topiramate, modafinil, St. John's wort, and possibly with ampicillin and tetracyclines. Increases levels of cyclosporine, prednisolone, and theophylline. Protease inhibitors may affect efficacy. Increased levels of ethinyl estradiol with atorvastatin, ascorbic acid, APAP, and CYP3A4 inhibitors (eg, ketoconazole, itraconazole). Increased levels of etonogestrel and ethinyl estradiol with vaginal miconazole nitrate. Decreases levels of APAP and increases clearance of temazepam, salicylic acid, morphine, and clofibric acid. Elevations of triglycerides leading to pancreatitis reported. D/C if depression observed and recurs to a serious degree.

PREGNANCY: Category X, not for use in nursing.

MECHANISM OF ACTION: Combination hormonal contraceptive; suppresses gonadotropins, leading to inhibition of ovulation, and increases difficulty of sperm entry into uterus and reduces likelihood of implantation by producing changes in cervical mucus and endometrium, respectively.

PHARMACOKINETICS: Absorption: Etonorgestrel: Rapid; bioavailability (100%); C_{max}=1716pg/mL; T_{max}=200.3 hrs. Ethinyl estradiol: Rapid; absolute bioavailability (56%); C_{max}=34.7pg/mL; T_{max}=59.3 hrs. **Distribution:** Etonorgestrel: Serum albumin binding (66%), sex hormone-binding globulin (32%). Ethinyl estradiol: Serum albumin binding (98.5%). **Metabolism:** Hepatic via CYP3A4. **Elimination:** Urine, bile, feces; Etonorgestrel: $T_{1/2}$=29.3 hrs; Ethinyl estradiol: $T_{1/2}$=44.7 hrs.

NURSING CONSIDERATIONS

Assessment: Assess for thrombophlebitis, thromboembolic disorder, DVT, MI, cerebrovascular or coronary disease, valvular heart disease, severe HTN, headaches with focal neurological symptoms, breast cancer, edometrium carcinoma or other estrogen-dependent neoplasia, abnormal genital bleeding, hepatic tumor or active liver disease, pregnancy/nursing, cholestatic jaundice of pregnancy or with contraceptives, hyperlipidemia, retinal thrombosis, depression, hypersensitivity reactions, and possible drug interactions.

Monitoring: Monitor for bleeding irregularities, amenorrhea, fluid retention, thromboembolic/thrombotic diseases, MI, cerebrovascular diseases, worsening of depression, toxic shock syndrome, ocular lesions, hepatic tumors, gallbadder disease, carcinoma of productive organs and breasts, and lab tests (PT, factors VII, VIII, IX, and X, TBG, protein-bound iodine, T_4, free T_3, sex hormone-binding globulins, serum glucose, serum folate, lipoproteins). Evaluate annual physical exam with special reference to BP, breasts, abdomen, pelvic organs, cervical cytology, and vagina.

Patient Counseling: Counsel that drug does not protect against HIV infection/AIDS or other STDs and to take as directed. Counsel about possibility of light spotting. Advise to avoid smoking to prevent cardiovascular side effects. Instruct to seek immediate medical attention if vaginitis, headache, upper respiratory tract infection, sinusitis, weight gain, nausea, or bleeding irregularities develop. Caution that some medications decrease efficacy and should not be used without physician instructions.

Administration: Intravaginal route. Refer to PI for specific instructions. **Storage:** 2-8°C (36-46°F). After dispensing store up to 4 months at 25°C (77°F). Avoid direct sunlight or above 30°C (86°F).

NUVIGIL CIV

armodafinil (Cephalon)

THERAPEUTIC CLASS: Wakefulness-promoting agent

INDICATIONS: To improve wakefulness in patients with excessive daytime sleepiness associated with narcolepsy, obstructive sleep apnea/hypopnea syndrome (OSAHS), shiftwork sleep disorder (SWSD). As adjunct to standard treatment for underlying obstruction in OSAHS.

DOSAGE: *Adults:* OSAHS/Narcolepsy: 150mg or 250mg qd in AM. SWSD: 150mg qd 1 hour prior to work shift. Hepatic Dysfunction: Reduce dose. Elderly: Consider dose reduction.

HOW SUPPLIED: Tab: 50mg, 150mg, 250mg

WARNINGS/PRECAUTIONS: May cause serious rash, including Stevens-Johnson syndrome, anaphylactoid reactions, angioedema, and multi-organ hypersensitivity. May impair mental/physical abilities. Psychiatric adverse experiences reported; consider discontinuing treatment if psychiatric symptoms develop and use caution with history of psychosis, depression, or mania. Caution with history of MI or unstable angina. Avoid with history of left ventricular hypertrophy, ischemic ECG changes, chest pain, arrhythmia, or other manifestations of mitral valve prolapse with CNS stimulants. Monitor hypertensive patients.

ADVERSE REACTIONS: Headache, nausea, dizziness, insomnia, diarrhea, dry mouth, anxiety, depression, rash.

INTERACTIONS: Potent CYP3A4/5 inducers, (eg, carbamazepine, phenobarbital, rifampin) or inhibitors, (eg, ketoconazole, erythromycin) may alter plasma levels. Effectiveness of CYP3A substrates (eg, cyclosporine, ethinyl estradiol, midazolam, triazolam) may be reduced. May cause moderate inhibition of CYP2C19 activity; dosage reduction may be required for some CYP2C19 substrates (eg, omeprazole, diazepam, phenytoin, propranolol). Methylphenidate or dextroamphetamine may delay absorption. Caution with MAOIs. Monitor PT/INR with warfarin. Effectiveness of steroidal contraceptives may be reduced during and for 1 month after discontinuation of therapy; alternate or concomitant methods of contraception are recommended.

PREGNANCY: Category C, caution in nursing.

MECHANISM OF ACTION: Not known; suspected to bind to the dopamine transporter and inhibit dopamine reuptake.

PHARMACOKINETICS: Absorption: Readily absorbed. T_{max}=2 hrs (fasted), 2-4 hrs (fed). **Distribution**: V_d=42L; plasma protein binding (60%). **Metabolism**: Liver via amide hydrolysis with sulfone formation by CYP450, 3A4, 3A5: R-modafinil acid, modafinil sulfone. **Elimination**: Feces, urine; $T_{1/2}$=15 hrs.

NURSING CONSIDERATIONS

Assessment: Perform complete evaluation of patient's excessive sleepiness, LFTs. Note other diseases/conditions and drug therapies.

Monitoring: Monitor for hypersensitivity reactions, psychiatric symptoms (depression, hallucination, suicidal ideations), cardiac abnormalities.

Patient Counseling: Avoid taking alcohol concurrently; exercise caution while driving, operating machinery, or performing other activities that require mental alertness. Potential increased risk of pregnancy when using steroidal contraceptives with drug and for 1 month after d/c therapy. Report adverse side effects, allergic reactions, psychiatric symptoms, chest pain.

Administration: Oral route. **Storage**: 20-25°C (68-77°F). Keep out of reach of children.

NYSTATIN ORAL RX

nystatin (Various)

THERAPEUTIC CLASS: Polyene antifungal

N

INDICATIONS: (Sus) Treatment of oral candidiasis. (Tab) Treatment of non-esophageal mucous membrane GI candidiasis.

DOSAGE: *Adults:* Oral Candidiasis: (Sus) 4-6mL qid. Retain in mouth as long as possible before swallowing. GI Candidiasis: (Tab) 500,000-1,000,000 U tid.
Pediatrics: Oral Candidiasis: (Sus) 4-6mL qid. Infants: 2mL qid. Retain in mouth as long as possible before swallowing.

HOW SUPPLIED: Sus: 100,000 U/mL [60mL, 480mL]; Tab: 500,000 U

WARNINGS/PRECAUTIONS: Not for systemic mycoses. D/C if irritation/hypersensitivity occurs. Confirm diagnosis with KOH smear and/or cultures if symptoms persist after course of therapy. Continue at least 48 hrs after clinical response.

ADVERSE REACTIONS: Diarrhea, NV, GI distress, rash, urticaria, Stevens-Johnson syndrome, oral irritation.

PREGNANCY: Category C, caution in nursing.

MECHANISM OF ACTION: Fungistatic and fungicidal agent; acts by binding to sterols in the cell membrane of susceptible *Candida* species with a resultant change in membrane permeability, allowing leakage of intracellular components.

PHARMACOKINETICS: Absorption: GI (insignificant). **Elimination:** Stool (unchanged).

NURSING CONSIDERATIONS

Assessment: Assess for proper diagnosis of oral candidiasis and pregnancy/nursing status.

Monitoring: Monitor for possible adverse reactions including oral irritation, sensitization, diarrhea, NV, GI upset/disturbance, and rash (eg, Stevens-Johnson syndrome).

Patient Counseling: Not for treatment of systemic mycoses. D/C medication if sensitization or irritation occurs. Notify physician if rash occurs.

N

Administration: Oral route. **Storage:** Store at controlled room temperature 15-30°C (59-86°F). Avoid freezing. Dispense in tight, light-resistant container.

NYSTATIN VAGINAL — RX

nystatin (Odyssey)

THERAPEUTIC CLASS: Polyene antifungal

INDICATIONS: Local treatment of vulvovaginal candidiasis.

DOSAGE: *Adults:* Insert 1 tablet vaginally qd for 2 weeks. Deposit tablets high in the vagina by means of the applicator.

HOW SUPPLIED: Tab, Vaginal: 100,000U [15[s]]

WARNINGS/PRECAUTIONS: D/C if sensitization or irritation occurs. Confirm diagnosis by KOH smears and/or cultures.

PREGNANCY: Category A, safety in nursing not known.

MECHANISM OF ACTION: Antimycotic polyene antibiotic; fungistatic and fungicidal against yeast and yeast-like fungi; acts by binding to sterols in the cell membrane of fungus with a resultant change in membrane permeability allowing leakage of intracellular components.

PHARMACOKINETICS: Absorption: None from intact skin or mucous membrane.

NURSING CONSIDERATIONS

Assessment: Assess for history of hypersensitivity, KOH smears, cultures, or other diagnostic method to rule out infection caused by other pathogens.

Monitoring: Monitor for possible allergic reaction, burning, itching, rash, eczema and pain, irritation or sensitization development; d/c and notify physician if occurs.

Patient Counseling: Instruct to use as directed; not for systemic, oral, or ophthalmic infections. Advise not to interrupt or d/c therapy until completed. Caution that therapeutic douches are unnecessary but may use cleansing douches if not pregnant. Counsel to promptly report any adverse effect (eg, irritation, sensitization) to physician.

Administration: Intravaginally. Refer to labeling for instruction on use.
Storage: 20-25°C (68-77°F). Avoid excessive heat.

NYSTOP RX
nystatin (Paddock)

THERAPEUTIC CLASS: Polyene antifungal

INDICATIONS: Treatment of cutaneous and mucocutaneous mycotic infections caused by susceptible *Candida* species.

DOSAGE: *Adults:* Apply to lesions bid-tid until healing is complete. For fungal infections of the feet, dust powder on feet and also in shoes.
Pediatrics: Neonates and Older: Apply to lesions bid-tid until healing is complete. For fungal infections of the feet, dust powder on feet and also in shoes.

HOW SUPPLIED: Powder, Topical: 100,000 U/g [15g, 30g, 60g]

WARNINGS/PRECAUTIONS: D/C if irritation or sensitization occurs. Confirm diagnosis. Not for systemic, oral, intravaginal, or ophthalmic use.

ADVERSE REACTIONS: Allergic reactions, burning, itching, rash, eczema, pain at application site.

PREGNANCY: Category C, caution in nursing.

MECHANISM OF ACTION: Polyene antifungal; binds sterols in the cell membrane of susceptible species causing a change in membrane permeability and subsequent leakage of intracellular components. Fungistatic and fungicidal.

PHARMACOKINETICS: Absorption: Not absorbed from intact skin or mucous membranes.

NURSING CONSIDERATIONS

Assessment: Assess proper diagnosis of cutaneous or mucocutaneous candidiasis through use of KOH smears, cultures, or other diagnostic methods. Assess use in pregnancy/nursing.

Monitoring: Monitor for irritation or sensitization and therapeutic response. If no therapeutic response, reassess diagnosis (eg, KOH smears, cultures, other diagnostic methods).

Patient Counseling: Instruct to use exactly as directed and not to interrupt or d/c therapy even if symptom relief occurs within first few days of treatment. Notify physician if skin irritation develops.

Administration: Topical route. **Storage:** 15-30°C (59-86°F); avoid excessive heat 40°C (104°F).

OCUFLOX RX
ofloxacin (Allergan)

THERAPEUTIC CLASS: Fluoroquinolone

INDICATIONS: Management of bacterial infections in conjunctivitis and corneal ulcers.

DOSAGE: *Adults:* Conjunctivitis: 1-2 drops q2-4h for 2 days, then 1-2 drops qid for 5 days. Corneal Ulcer: 1-2 drops every 30 min while awake and 1-2 drops 4-6 hrs after retiring for 2 days, then 1-2 drops q1h while awake for 5-7 days, then 1-2 drops qid for 2 days or until treatment completion.
Pediatrics: ≥1 yr: Conjunctivitis: 1-2 drops q2-4h for 2 days, then 1-2 drops qid for 5 days. Corneal Ulcer: 1-2 drops every 30 min while awake and 1-2 drops 4-6 hrs after retiring for 2 days, then 1-2 drops q1h while awake for 5-7 days, then 1-2 drops qid for 2 days or until treatment completion.

HOW SUPPLIED: Sol: 0.3% [5mL, 10mL]

WARNINGS/PRECAUTIONS: Not for injection into eye. Do not inject subconjunctivally nor into the eye's anterior chamber. Superinfection may result with prolonged use. Fatal hypersensitivity reactions reported after 1st dose of systemic quinolone therapy. Avoid allowing tip of container to contact fingers, eye or surrounding structures.

ADVERSE REACTIONS: Transient ocular burning or discomfort, stinging, redness, itching, keratitis, ocular periocular/facial edema, photophobia, blurred vision, tearing, dryness, eye pain.

INTERACTIONS: Systemic quinolone therapy may increase theophylline levels, interfere with caffeine metabolism, enhance warfarin effects, and elevate SrCr with cyclosporine.

PREGNANCY: Category C, not for use in nursing.

MECHANISM OF ACTION: Fluoroquinolone; exerts bactericidal effect on susceptible bacteria by inhibiting DNA gyrase, an essential bacterial enzyme that is a critical catalyst in duplication, transcription, and repair of bacterial DNA.

PHARMACOKINETICS: Absorption: C_{max}=1.1 ng/mL (Day 1, qid dosing), 1.9 ng/mL (Day 11, qid dosing). **Excretion:** Urine.

NURSING CONSIDERATIONS

Assessment: Assess for proper diagnosis of causative organisms (eg, slit lamp biomicroscopy, fluorescein staining), allergies to other quinolones, use in pregnant/nursing females, and possible drug interactions.

Monitoring: Monitor for signs/symptoms of serious hypersensitivity or anaphylactic reactions (eg, cardiovascular collapse, loss of consciousness, angioedema, airway obstruction, dyspnea, urticaria, and itching), Stevens-Johnson syndrome and toxic epidermal necrosis. For patients on sustained therapy, monitor for overgrowth of nonsusceptible organisms (eg, fungal) and for development of superinfection. Monitor creatinine levels in patients receiving cyclosporine concomitantly.

Patient Counseling: Advise to avoid contaminating applicator tip with material from eye, fingers, or other sources. Instruct to immediately report first sign of a rash or allergic reaction.

Administration: Ocular route. Do not inject into eye. **Storage:** 15-25°C (59-77°F).

OCUPRESS RX

carteolol HCl (Novartis Ophthalmics)

THERAPEUTIC CLASS: Nonselective beta-blocker

INDICATIONS: Reduction of intraocular pressure (IOP) in chronic open-angle glaucoma and intraocular hypertension.

DOSAGE: *Adults:* 1 drop bid.

HOW SUPPLIED: Sol: 1% [5mL, 10mL, 15mL]

CONTRAINDICATIONS: Bronchial asthma, severe COPD, sinus bradycardia, 2nd- and 3rd-degree AV block, overt cardiac failure, cardiogenic shock.

WARNINGS/PRECAUTIONS: May be absorbed systemically. Caution with cardiac failure, bronchospasm, diminished pulmonary function, and DM. May mask symptoms of hypoglycemia and hyperthyroidism. Not for use alone in angle-closure glaucoma. May potentiate muscle weakness. D/C if cardiac failure develops. Withdrawal before surgery is controversial.

ADVERSE REACTIONS: Eye irritation, burning, tearing, conjunctival hyperemia, conjunctival edema, photophobia, decreased night vision, ptosis, bradycardia, decreased BP, dyspnea, asthenia, headache, dizziness, taste perversion.

INTERACTIONS: May potentiate systemic effects with oral β-blockers. Possible hypotension and bradycardia with catecholamine-depleting drugs (eg, reserpine). May antagonize epinephrine.

PREGNANCY: Category C, caution in nursing.

MECHANISM OF ACTION: Nonselective β-adrenergic blocker; reduces normal and elevated levels of IOP. Exact mechanism of ocular hypotensive effect not definitely demonstrated. β-adrenergic blockers also associated with reducing cardiac output and increasing airway resistance in bronchi and bronchioles.

NURSING CONSIDERATIONS

Assessment: Prior to therapy, assess for presence or history of bronchial asthma, severe COPD, sinus bradycardia, AV-block, overt cardiac failure, and cardiogenic shock. Assess use with DM (or patients subject to episodes of spontaneous hypoglycemia), non-allergic bronchospasm (eg, chronic bronchitis, emphysema), hyperthyroidism, undergoing elective surgery, angle-closure glaucoma, use in pregnant/nursing, and possible drug interactions.

Monitoring: Monitor for severe respiratory or cardiac reactions (eg, cardiac failure), muscle weakness, anaphylactic reactions, symptoms of hypoglycemia in patients with DM, and development of thyroid storm in patients with thyrotoxicosis who abruptly d/c medication.

Patient Counseling: Instruct to immediately notify physician if any respiratory, cardiac, or anaphylaxic reaction develops. Avoid touching dropper tip to eyelids or surrounding areas to prevent contamination.

Administration: Ocular route. **Storage:** 15-25°C (59-77°F). Protect from light. Keep bottle tightly closed.

OGEN RX

estropipate (Pharmacia & Upjohn)

Estrogens increase the risk of endometrial cancer. Estrogens, with or without progestins, should not be used for the prevention of cardiovascular disease. Increased risks of MI, stroke, invasive breast cancer, PE, and DVT in postmenopausal women (50-79 yrs of age) reported. Increased risk of developing probable dementia in postmenopausal women ≥65 yrs of age reported.

THERAPEUTIC CLASS: Estrogen

INDICATIONS: Treatment of moderate to severe vasomotor symptoms and/or vulval/vaginal atrophy associated with menopause. Treatment of hypoestrogenism due to hypogonadism, castration, or primary ovarian failure. Prevention of postmenopausal osteoporosis.

O

DOSAGE: *Adults:* Vasomotor Symptoms: 0.75-6mg/day (as estropipate). Start cyclic administration arbitrarily if not menstruating, or on Day 5 of bleeding if menstruating. Vulval/Vaginal Atrophy: 0.75-6mg/day (as estropipate), administer cyclically. Discontinue/Taper over 3-6 month interval. Hypoestrogenism: 1.5-9mg/day (as estropipate) for 1st 3 weeks of cycle, then 8-10 days off. Maint: Lowest effective dose. For female hypogonadism, repeat dose if bleeding doesn't occur or add progestogen in 3rd week of cycle. Osteoporosis Prevention: 0.75mg (as estropipate) qd for 25 days of 31-day cycle.

HOW SUPPLIED: Tab: 0.625mg* (0.75mg estropipate), 1.25mg* (1.5mg estropipate), 2.5mg* (3mg estropipate) *scored

CONTRAINDICATIONS: Pregnancy, undiagnosed abnormal genital bleeding, breast cancer, estrogen-dependent neoplasia, DVT/PE, active or recent (eg, within past year) arterial thromboembolic disease (eg, stroke, MI), liver dysfunction or disease.

WARNINGS/PRECAUTIONS: May increase risk of cardiovascular events (eg, MI, stroke), venous thrombosis, and PE; d/c immediately if any of these events occur or are suspected. May increase risk of breast/endometrial cancer, and gallbladder disease. May lead to severe hypercalcemia with breast cancer and bone metastases; monitor and d/c if hypercalcemia occurs. Retinal vascular thrombosis reported; monitor and d/c if papilledema or retinal vascular lesions occur. Consider addition of a progestin if no hysterectomy. May elevate BP; monitor at regular intervals. May cause elevations of plasma triglycerides with pre-existing hypertriglyceridemia. Caution with history of cholestatic jaundice associated with past estrogen use or with pregnancy; d/c with recurrence. May lead to increased thyroid-binding globulin levels; monitor thyroid function. May cause fluid retention; caution with cardiac/renal dysfunction. Caution with severe hypocalcemia. May increase risk of ovarian cancer. May exacerbate endometriosis, asthma, DM, epilepsy, migraine, porphyria, SLE, and hepatic hemangiomas; use with caution.

ADVERSE REACTIONS: Altered vaginal bleeding, vaginal candidiasis, breast tenderness/enlargement, GI effects, melasma, CNS effects, weight changes, edema, altered libido.

INTERACTIONS: CYP3A4 inducers (eg, St. John's wort, phenobarbital, carbamazepine, rifampin) may decrease levels which may decrease therapeutic effects and/or change uterine bleeding profile. CYP3A4 inhibitors (eg, erythromycin, clarithromycin, ketoconazole, itraconazole, ritonavir, grapefruit juice) may increase levels which may result in side effects.

PREGNANCY: Contraindicated in pregnancy, caution in nursing

MECHANISM OF ACTION: Estrogen; binds to nuclear receptors in estrogen-responsive tissues. Circulating estrogens modulate pituitary secretion of the gonadotropins, luteinizing hormone and follicle stimulating hormone, through negative feedback mechanism. Reduces elevated levels of these hormones in postmenopausal women.

PHARMACOKINETICS: Absorption: Well-absorbed. **Distribution:** Largely bound to sex hormone binding globulin and albumin; found in breast milk. **Metabolism:** Liver, to estrone (metabolite) and estriol (major urinary metabolite); sulfate and glucuronide conjugation (liver). **Excretion:** Urine (parent drug and metabolites).

NURSING CONSIDERATIONS

Assessment: Assess for undiagnosed abnormal genital bleeding, presence or history of breast cancer, estrogen-dependent neoplasia, DVT or PE, active or recent (within past yr) arterial thromboembolic disease (eg, stroke, MI), liver dysfunction, history of cholestatic jaundice, pregnancy/nursing status, age (≥65 yrs old), hypertriglyceridemia, hypothyroidism, hypocalcemia, asthma, DM, epilepsy, migraines or porphyria, SLE, and possible drug interactions. Assess need for progestin therapy in females who have not had hysterectomy.

O

Monitoring: Monitor for signs/symptoms of cardiovascular disorders (eg, MI, stroke, venous thrombosis, PE), malignant neoplasms (eg, cancers of endometrium, breast, ovaries), dementia, gallbladder disease, hypercalcemia, visual abnormalities (eg, retinal vascular thrombosis), BP elevations, elevations in plasma triglycerides, pancreatitis, hypothyroidism, fluid retention, exacerbation of endometriosis and other conditions (eg, asthma, DM, epilepsy, migraines, SLE). Perform annual breast exam. Monitor BP levels regularly. Monitor thyroid function in patients on thyroid replacement therapy. Perform periodic evaluation (every 3-6 months) to determine treatment need. If undiagnosed persistent or recurring genital bleeding occurs, perform adequate diagnostic measures (eg, endometrial sampling) to rule out malignancy.

Patient Counseling: Inform that drug increases risk for uterine cancer, heart attack, stroke, breast cancer, and blood clots. Report any breast lumps, unusual vaginal bleeding, dizziness or faintness, changes in speech, severe headaches, chest pain, SOB, leg pains, changes in vision, or vomiting. Advise to notify physician if planning surgery or bedrest and to perform monthly self breast exams.

Administration: Oral route. **Storage:** Below 25°C (77°F).

OLUX — RX

clobetasol propionate (Stiefel)

THERAPEUTIC CLASS: Corticosteroid

INDICATIONS: Short-term treatment of inflammatory and pruritic manifestations of moderate to severe corticosteroid-responsive dermatoses of the scalp. Short-term treatment of mild to moderate plaque-type psoriasis of non-scalp regions excluding the face and intertriginous areas.

DOSAGE: *Adults:* Apply to affected area bid (am and pm). No more than 1.5 capfuls/application. Limit to 2 consecutive weeks. Avoid with occlusive dressings. Max 50g/week.
Pediatrics: ≥12 yrs: Apply to affected area bid (am and pm). No more than 1.5 capfuls/application. Limit to 2 consecutive weeks. Avoid with occlusive dressings. Max 50g/week.

HOW SUPPLIED: Foam: 0.05% [50g, 100g]

WARNINGS/PRECAUTIONS: May produce reversible HPA axis suppression, manifestations of Cushing's syndrome, hyperglycemia, and glucosuria. Caution when applied to large surface areas or under occlusive dressings. Use appropriate antifungal or antibacterial agent with dermatological infections; d/c if infection does not clear. Pediatrics may be more susceptible to systemic toxicity. Avoid eyes. D/C if irritation occurs.

ADVERSE REACTIONS: Burning/stinging, pruritus, irritation, erythema, folliculitis, cracking/fissuring of skin, numbness of fingers, telangiectasia, skin atrophy.

PREGNANCY: Category C, caution in nursing.

MECHANISM OF ACTION: Corticosteroid; possesses anti-inflammatory, antipruritic, and vasoconstrictive properties. Anti-inflammatory effects not established; suspected to act by induction of phospholipase A_2 inhibitory proteins, lipocortins. Lipocortins control biosynthesis of inflammation mediators (prostaglandins and leukotrienes) by inhibiting release of their common precursor, arachidonic acid.

PHARMACOKINETICS: Absorption: Percutaneous; occlusion, inflammation, and other disease states may increase absorption. **Distribution:** Systemically administered corticosteroids are found in breast milk. **Metabolism:** Liver. **Elimination**: Kidney (major), bile.

NURSING CONSIDERATIONS

Assessment: Assess use in pregnant/nursing and pediatric patients.

Monitoring: Monitor for signs/symptoms of reversible HPA-axis suppression, Cushing's syndrome, hyperglycemia, glucosuria, skin irritation, contact dermatitis (eg, failure to heal), and dermatological infections (eg, fungal, bacterial). In patients on high doses or using occlusive dressings, perform periodic monitoring for HPA-axis suppression using ACTH stimulation, A.M plasma cortisol, and urinary free cortisol tests. Following withdrawal from therapy, monitor for signs/symptoms of glucocorticosteroid insufficiencies. In pediatric patients, monitor for systemic toxicity, HPA-axis suppression, Cushing's syndrome, linear growth retardation, and intracranial HTN.

Patient Counseling: Counsel to use exactly as directed, externally, and not for >2 weeks. Propellant in this foam is flammable; avoid fire, flame, or smoking during and immediately following application. Advise not to bandage or wrap treated skin area, unless directed by physician. Avoid contact with eyes or other mucus membranes. Wash hands following use.

Administration: Topical. 1) Place small amount of medication into cap of medication container, onto a saucer, other cool surface, or directly onto affected skin area. Do not use more than 1 1/2 capfuls. Do not squirt medication directly into the hands (unless hands are the treatment area); medication will melt in contact with warm skin. If fingers are warm, rinse in cold water and dry prior to application. If can is warm, run under cold water prior to administration. 2) Using fingertips, massage medication into treatment area. **Storage:** Store at controlled room temperature, 20-25°C (68-77°F). Do not expose to heat or store above 49°C (120°F).

Olux-E

RX

clobetasol propionate (Stiefel)

THERAPEUTIC CLASS: Corticosteroid

INDICATIONS: Treatment of inflammatory and pruritic manifestations of corticosteroid-responsive dermatoses.

DOSAGE: *Adults:* Apply thin layer to affected area bid (am and pm). Limit to 2 consecutive weeks. Avoid with occlusive dressings. Max: 50g/week.
Pediatrics: ≥12 yrs: Apply thin layer to affected area bid (am and pm). Limit to 2 consecutive weeks. Avoid with occlusive dressings. Max: 50g/week.

HOW SUPPLIED: Foam: 0.05% [50g,100g]

WARNINGS/PRECAUTIONS: May produce reversible HPA axis suppression, manifestations of Cushing's syndrome, hyperglycemia, and glucosuria. Caution when applied to large surface area or under occlusive dressings. Use appropriate antifungal or antibacterial agent with dermatological infections; d/c if infection does not clear. Pediatrics may be more susceptible to systemic toxicity. D/C if irritation occurs. Should not be used to treat rosacea or perioral dermatitis. Avoid use on face, groin, axillae, or other intertriginous areas.

ADVERSE REACTIONS: Folliculitis, acneiform eruptions, hypopigmentation, perioral dermatitis, allergic contact dermatitis, secondary infection, irritation, striae, miliaria.

PREGNANCY: Category C, caution in nursing.

MECHANISM OF ACTION: Corticosteroid; possesses anti-inflammatory, antipruritic, and vasoconstrictive properties. Anti-inflammatory effect not established; suspected to act by induction of phospholipase A_2 inhibitory proteins called lipocortins. Lipocortins control biosynthesis of inflammation mediators (prostaglandins and leukotrienes) by inhibiting release of their common precursor, arachidonic acid.

PHARMACOKINETICS: Absorption: Percutaneous; occlusion, inflammation, and other disease states may increase absorption; C_{max}=59pg/mL; T_{max}=5 hrs. **Distribution:** Systemically administered corticosteroids are found in breast milk. **Metabolism:** Liver. **Elimination**: Kidneys, bile.

NURSING CONSIDERATIONS

Assessment: Assess pregnancy/nursing status and presence of concomitant skin infections. Assess that treatment is not for perioral dermatitis or rosacea.

Monitoring: Monitor for signs/symptoms of reversible adrenal suppression, Cushing's syndrome, hyperglycemia, glucosuria, treatment-site irritation, allergic contact dermatitis (eg, failure to heal), and development of skin infections (eg, fungal, bacterial). If applying to large surface area or areas under occlusion, monitor for HPA-axis suppression using cosyntropin (ACTH) stimulation test. Following d/c of therapy, monitor for glucocorticosteroid insufficiency. In pediatrics, monitor for signs/symptoms of systemic toxicity, HPA-axis suppression, Cushing's syndrome, and intracranial HTN.

Patient Counseling: Counsel to use externally and exactly as directed; avoid use on face, in skin folds (eg, underarms, groin), contact with eyes or other mucous membranes. Wash hands following adminstration. Advise not to bandage or wrap treatment area as to be occlusive, unless directed by physician. Counsel to contact physician if any local or systemic adverse events occur or if no improvement seen after 2 weeks. Inform that propellant in medication is flammable; avoid fire, flame, or smoking during and immediately following application.

Administration: Topical route. **Storage:** Controlled room temperature 20-25°C (68-77°F); keep away from children.

OMNARIS RX

ciclesonide (Sepracor)

THERAPEUTIC CLASS: Non-halogenated glucocorticoid

INDICATIONS: Treatment of nasal symptoms associated with seasonal allergic rhinitis in adults and children ≥6 yrs. Treatment of nasal symptoms associated with perennial allergic rhinitis in adults and adolescents ≥12 yrs.

DOSAGE: *Adults:* Seasonal Allergic Rhinitis/Perennial Allergic Rhinitis: 2 sprays (50mcg/spray) each nostril qd.
Pediatrics: Seasonal Allergic Rhinitis: ≥6 yrs: 2 sprays (50mcg/spray) each

nostril qd. Perennial Allergic Rhinitis: ≥12 yrs: 2 sprays (50mcg/spray) each nostril qd.

HOW SUPPLIED: Spray: 50mcg/spray [12.5g]

WARNINGS/PRECAUTIONS: Risk of acute adrenal insufficiency and withdrawal symptoms when replacing systemic corticosteroids with topical corticosteroids; monitor closely. Risk for more severe/fatal course of infections (eg, chickenpox, measles); avoid exposure in patients who have not had the disease or been properly immunized. May cause reduced growth velocity in pediatrics; routinely monitor growth of pediatrics. May impair wound healing; avoid in recent nasal septal ulcers, nasal surgery, or nasal trauma until healed. *Candida* infections of nose or pharynx may occur; examine periodically and treat accordingly. Caution with active or quiescent TB infections, untreated local or systemic fungal or bacterial infections, systemic viral or parasitic infections, or ocular herpes simplex. Taper dose if symptoms of hypercorticism occur. Caution with history of glaucoma and/or cataracts; monitor IOP accordingly.

ADVERSE REACTIONS: Headache, epistaxis, nasopharyngitis, ear pain, pharyngolaryngeal pain.

INTERACTIONS: Ketoconazole may increase levels of the pharmacologically active metabolite des-ciclesonide; co-administer with caution.

PREGNANCY: Category C, caution in nursing.

MECHANISM OF ACTION: Not established; glucocorticoid has anti-inflammatory effect and other effects on multiple cell types (eg, mast cells, eosinophils, macrophages, and lymphocytes) and mediators (eg, histamine, eicosanoids, leukotrienes, and cytokines) involved in allergic inflammation.

PHARMACOKINETICS: Absorption: (50-800mcg) C_{max}<30pg/mL (adults); (25-200mcg) C_{max}<45pg/mL (pediatrics). **Metabolism:** Nasal mucosa estrases to des-ciclesonide (active metabolite) followed by liver CYP3A4, 2D6.

NURSING CONSIDERATIONS

Assessment: Assess for drug hypersensitivity, active or quiescent TB, untreated localized or systemic fungal or bacterial infections, systemic viral infections, ocular herpes simplex, history of recent nasal septal ulcers, nasal surgery/trauma, concomitant use with other inhaled or systemic corticosteroids, withdrawal symptoms in event of replacing systemic with topical corticosteroids, and possible drug interactions.

Monitoring: Monitor for acute adrenal insufficiency, TB, local/systemic fungal or bacterial infections, systemic viral or parasitic infections, ocular herpes simplex, or other infections (chickenpox, measles). Monitor growth velocity in children, wound healing, hypercorticism (eg, menstrual irregularities, acneiform lesions, and cushingoid features), hypoadrenalism in infant born to mother receiving corticosteroids during pregnancy, hypersensitivity reactions, or contact dermatitis.

Patient Counseling: Avoid spraying in eyes or directly onto nasal septum. Counsel to take as directed at regular intervals; do not exceed prescribed dosage. Avoid exposure to chickenpox or measles; consult physician immediately if exposed or symptoms worsen.

Administration: Intranasal route, shake gently before use, spray tip into one nostril, and close other nostril with finger. **Storage:** 25°C (77°F); excursions permitted to 15-30°C (59-86°F). Do not freeze. Keep out of reach of children.

OMNICEF — RX

cefdinir (Abbott)

THERAPEUTIC CLASS: Cephalosporin (3rd generation)

INDICATIONS: Community-acquired pneumonia (CAP), acute exacerbations of chronic bronchitis (AECB), acute maxillary sinusitis, pharyngitis/tonsillitis, uncomplicated skin and skin structure infections (SSSI), and acute bacterial otitis media.

DOSAGE: *Adults:* (Cap) SSSI/CAP: 300mg q12h for 10 days. AECB/Pharyngitis/Tonsillitis: 300mg q12h for 5-10 days or 600mg q24h for 10 days. Sinusitis: 300mg q12h or 600mg q24h for 10 days. CrCl <30mL/min: 300mg qd. Hemodialysis: Initial: 300mg or 7mg/kg qod. Max: 600mg qd. *Pediatrics:* (Sus) 6 months-12 yrs: Otitis Media/Pharyngitis/Tonsillitis: 7mg/kg q12h for 5-10 days or 14mg/kg q24h for 10 days. Sinusitis: 7mg/kg q12h or 14mg/kg q24h for 10 days. SSSI: 7mg/kg q12h or 14mg/kg q24h for 10 days. (Cap) ≥13 yrs: CAP/SSSI: 300mg q12h for 10 days. AECB/Pharyngitis/Tonsillitis: 300mg q12h for 5-10 days or 600mg q24h for 10 days. Sinusitis: 300mg q12h or 600mg q24h for 10 days. CrCl <30mL/min/1.73m^2: 7mg/kg qd. Max: 300mg qd.

HOW SUPPLIED: Cap: 300mg; Sus: 125mg/5mL, 250mg/5mL [60mL, 100mL]

WARNINGS/PRECAUTIONS: Cross-sensitivity to PCNs and other cephalosporins may occur. *Clostridium difficile*-associated diarrhea has been reported. Positive direct Coombs' tests may occur. Caution with renal dysfunction, history of colitis. Sus contains 2.86g/5mL of sucrose; caution in diabetes. False (+) for urine glucose with Clinitest and Benedict's or Fehling's solution.

ADVERSE REACTIONS: Diarrhea, vaginal moniliasis, and nausea.

INTERACTIONS: Iron-fortified foods, iron supplements, and aluminum- or magnesium-containing antacids reduce absorption; separate doses by 2 hrs. Probenecid inhibits the renal excretion. Reddish stools reported with iron-containing products.

PREGNANCY: Category B, safe in nursing.

MECHANISM OF ACTION: Extended-spectrum cephalosporin; bactericidal activity from inhibition of cell-wall synthesis.

PHARMACOKINETICS: Absorption: Cap: (300mg) Bioavailability (21%), C_{max}=1.6µg/mL, T_{max}=2.9 hrs, AUC=7.05µg•h/mL. (600mg) Bioavailability (16%), C_{max}=2.87µg/mL, T_{max}=3 hrs, AUC=11.1µg•h/mL. Sus: (7mg/kg) Bioavailability (25%), C_{max}=2.3µg/mL, T_{max}=2.2 hrs, AUC=8.31µg•h/mL. (14mg/kg) C_{max}=3.86µg/mL, T_{max}=1.8 hrs, AUC=13.4µg•h/mL. **Distribution:** V_d=0.35L/kg (adults), 0.67L/kg (pediatrics); plasma protein binding (60-70%). **Elimination:** (300mg) Urine (18.4%); (600mg) Urine (11.6%); $T_{1/2}$=1.7 hrs.

NURSING CONSIDERATIONS

Assessment: Assess for history of colitis, possible drug interactions, and renal impairment.

Monitoring: Monitor for signs/symptoms of hypersensitivity reactions, *C. difficile*-associated diarrhea, and superinfections.

Patient Counseling: Instruct to take 2 hrs before or after antacid or iron supplements. Inform diabetics suspension contains sucrose. Counsel therapy treats bacterial, not viral, infections. Take as directed; skipping doses or not completing full course may decrease effectiveness and increase resistance. Inform may experience diarrhea; notify physician if watery/bloody stools, superinfection, or hypersensitivity reactions occur.

Administration: Oral route. **Storage:** 25°C (77°F); excursions permitted to 15-30°C (59-86°F). Reconstituted: Room temperature; stable for 10 days.

OMNITROPE — RX

somatropin (Sandoz)

THERAPEUTIC CLASS: Human growth hormone

INDICATIONS: Long-term treatment of pediatric patients who have growth failure due to an inadequate secretion of endogenous growth hormone. Long-term replacement therapy in adults with growth hormone deficiency (GHD) of either childhood- or adult-onset etiology.

DOSAGE: *Adults:* Individualize dose. GHD: ≤0.04mg/kg/week. May increase at 4-8 week intervals. Max: 0.08mg/kg/week. Divide dose into daily SQ injections (give preferably in the evening).

Pediatrics: Individualize dose. GHD: 0.16-0.24mg/kg/week. Divide dose into daily SQ injections (give preferably in the evening).

HOW SUPPLIED: Inj: 1.5mg, 5.8mg; Prefill: 5mg/1.5mL (15 IU), 10mg/1.5mL (30 IU)

CONTRAINDICATIONS: Evidence of neoplastic activity. Pediatrics with fused epiphyses. Acute critical illness due to complications after open heart or abdominal surgery, multiple accidental trauma, or with acute respiratory failure. Patients with Prader-Willi syndrome who are severely obese or have severe respiratory impairment.

WARNINGS/PRECAUTIONS: Contains benzyl alcohol; avoid use in newborns. Patients with GHD secondary to an intracranial lesion should be monitored closely for progression or recurrence of underlying disease process. Monitor closely for any malignant transformation of skin lesions, scoliosis progression, or gait abnormalities. Monitor closely with DM, glucose intolerance, hypopituitarism. Intracranial HTN reported. Funduscopic exam recommended at initiation, and periodically during course of therapy.

ADVERSE REACTIONS: Hypothyroidism, elevated HbA_{1c}, eosinophilia, hematoma, headache, hypertriglyceridemia, leg pain.

INTERACTIONS: Growth promoting effects may be inhibited by glucocorticoids. May alter clearance of CYP450 substrates (eg, corticosteroids, sex steroids, anticonvulsants, cyclosporine); monitor closely. May need insulin dose adjustment.

PREGNANCY: Category B, caution in nursing.

MECHANISM OF ACTION: Human growth hormone; binds to dimeric GH receptor in cell membrane of target cells resulting in intracellular signal transduction.

PHARMACOKINETICS: Absorption: C_{max}=72mcg/mL, T_{max}=4 hrs. **Elimination:** $T_{1/2}$=2.8 hrs.

NURSING CONSIDERATIONS

Assessment: Assess for closed epiphyses, proliferative diabetic retinopathy, active malignancy, acute critical illness due to complications of surgery or multiple accidental trauma, acute respiratory failure, Prader-Willi syndrome (severely obese or severe respiratory failure), preexisting type 1 or type 2 DM or impaired glucose tolerance, history of scoliosis, pre-existing papilledema, hypothyroidism, undernutrition, advanced bone age, diagnostic imaging (rule out pituitary or intracranial tumor), hypopituitarism and possible drug interactions.

Monitoring: Monitor fasting blood glucose and thyroid function tests periodically. Periodic funduscopic exam. Signs/symptoms of malignant transformation of skin lesions, intracranial HTN, slipped capital femoral epiphysis (onset of limp, hip or knee pain), hypersensitivity/allergic reactions, and progression of scoliosis.

Patient Counseling: Instruct thoroughly as to proper usage, proper disposal, and caution against any reuse of needles and syringes.

Administration: SQ route. **Storage:** 2-8°C (36-46°F). Protect from light. Do not freeze. After 1st injection: Refrigerate, discard after 21 days. (Reconstitution): Diluent without preservative: refrigerate up to 24 hrs. Diluent with preservative: Use within 3 weeks.

ONCASPAR — RX

pegaspargase (Enzon)

THERAPEUTIC CLASS: Protein synthesis inhibitor

INDICATIONS: Acute lymphoblastic leukemia in patients who have developed hypersensitivity to the native forms of L-asparaginase. May be given as monotherapy if multi-agent therapy is inappropriate.

DOSAGE: *Adults:* Usual: 2500 IU/m² IM or IV every 14 days.
Pediatrics: 1-9 yrs: 2500 IU/m² IM on Day 3 of 4-Week induction phase and on Day 3 of each of two 8-Week delayed intensifications phases.

HOW SUPPLIED: Inj: 750 IU/mL [5mL]

CONTRAINDICATIONS: Pancreatitis. History of pancreatitis, significant hemorrhagic events, or serious thrombosis with prior L-asparaginase therapy.

WARNINGS/PRECAUTIONS: May be a contact irritant. Avoid inhalation or contact with skin or mucous membranes. Serious allergic reaction, pancreatitis, or glucose intolerance can occur. Increased prothrombin time, partial thromboplastin time, and hypofibrinogenemia can occur; monitor coagulation parameters. May predispose to infections, bleeding, thrombosis. D/C in patients with serious thrombotic event including sagittal sinus thrombosis.

ADVERSE REACTIONS: Allergic reactions (including anaphylaxis), CNS thrombosis, coagulopathy, elevated transaminases, hyperbilirubinemia, hyperglycemia, pancreatitis.

INTERACTIONS: May increase toxicity of protein bound drugs. May interfere with the action of drugs that require cell replication for their lethal effects (eg, methotrexate), and the enzymatic detoxification of other drugs, particularly in the liver. Caution with concomitant anticoagulants (eg, coumadin, heparin, dipyridamole, ASA, or NSAIDs), hepatotoxic agents.

PREGNANCY: Category C, not for use in nursing.

MECHANISM OF ACTION: Protein synthesis inhibitor; selectively kills leukemic cells due to depletion of plasma asparagine.

PHARMACOKINETICS: Elimination: $T_{1/2}$=5.8 days.

NURSING CONSIDERATIONS

Assessment: Assess for history of serious allergic reactions to L-asparginase, thrombosis, pancreatitis, and serious hemorrhagic events.

Monitoring: Monitor coagulation parameters at baseline and periodically during and after treatment. Monitor for occurrence of anaphylaxis, thrombosis, pancreatitis, glucose intolerance, and coagulopathy.

Patient Counseling: Advise to immediately report swelling, SOB, severe headache, chest pain, severe abdominal pain, excessive thirst, or any increase in volume or frequency of urination.

Administration: IM or IV. When administered IM, the volume at a single injection site should be limited to 2mL. If the volume to be administered is greater than 2 mL, multiple inj sites should be used. When administered IV, should be given over period of 1-2 hrs in 100mL of NaCl or dextrose inj 5%, through an already running infusion. **Storage**: Refrigerate at 2-8°C (36-46°F).

Opana ER

CII

oxymorphone HCl (Endo)

(Tab, Extended-Release) Abuse liability and potential. For continuous analgesia only; not intended for prn use. To be swallowed whole; not to be broken, chewed, dissolved, or crushed. Must not be taken with alcohol.

OTHER BRAND NAMES: Opana (Endo)

THERAPEUTIC CLASS: Opioid analgesic

INDICATIONS: (Tab) Relief of moderate to severe acute pain. (Tab, Extended-Release) Relief of moderate to severe pain in patients requiring continuous, around-the-clock opioid treatment for extended period of time.

DOSAGE: *Adults:* Individualize dose. Opana: Opioid-Naive: Initial: 5-20mg q4-6h. Titrate based on response. Max: 20mg/dose. Conversion from Parenteral Oxymorphone: Give 10x total daily parenteral oxymorphone dose in 4 or 6 equally divided doses. Conversion from Other Oral Opioids: Give half of calculated total daily dose in 4-6 equally divided doses, q4-6h. Opana ER: Swallow whole; do not break, chew, crush, or dissolve. Opioid-Naive: Initial: 5mg q12h. Titrate based on response. Usual: Increase dose by 5-10mg q12h every 3-7 days. Conversion from Opana: Divide 24h Opana dose in half to obtain q12h dose. Conversion from Parenteral Oxymorphone: Give 10x total daily parenteral oxymorphone dose in 2 equally divided doses. Conversion from Other Oral Opioids: Divide calculated 24h Opana dose (refer to PI for conversion ratios) in half to obtain q12h dose. Mild Hepatic Impairment or Renal Impairment (CrCl <50mL/min): Start with lowest dose and titrate slowly while carefully monitoring side effects. With CNS Depressants: Start at 1/3 to 1/2 of usual dose. Elderly: Start at lower end of dosing range.

HOW SUPPLIED: Tab: (Opana) 5mg, 10mg; Tab, Extended-Release: (Opana ER) 5mg, 7.5mg, 10mg, 15mg, 20mg, 30mg, 40mg

CONTRAINDICATIONS: Respiratory depression (except in monitored settings with resuscitative equipment), acute/severe bronchial asthma or hypercarbia, paralytic ileus, moderate/severe hepatic impairment. (Opana ER) Not indicated for pain in immediate post-operative period (12-24 hrs following surgery) for patients not previously taking opioids or, if the pain is mild or not expected to persist for extended period of time.

WARNINGS/PRECAUTIONS: Schedule II controlled substance with abuse liability. May have additive effects in conjunction with alcohol, other opioids, or illicit drugs that cause CNS depression; respiratory depression, hypotension, and profound sedation or coma may result. Extreme caution with hypoxia, hypercapnia, or decreased respiratory reserve. With head injury, intracranial lesions or a pre-existing increase in ICP, possible respiratory depressant effects and potential to elevate CSF pressure may be markedly exaggerated; effects on pupillary response and consciousness may obscure neurologic signs of further increases in ICP with head injuries. May cause severe hypotension with compromised ability to maintain BP due to depleted blood volume. Caution in elderly or debilitated patients sensitive to CNS depressants. Caution with circulatory shock, acute alcoholism, adrenocortical insufficiency (eg, Addison's disease), CNS depression or coma, delirium tremens, kyphoscoliosis associated with respiratory depression, myxedema or hypothyroidism, prostatic hypertrophy or urethral stricture, severe impairment of pulmonary or renal function, mild/moderate hepatic impairment and toxic psychosis. May aggravate convulsions with convulsive disorders; may induce or aggravate seizures in some clinical settings. Monitor for decreased bowel motility in post-op patients. May cause spasm of the sphincter of Oddi; caution with biliary tract disease (including acute pancreatitis). May produce tolerance and dependence. Should not abruptly d/c, may cause abstinence syndrome in physically-dependent patients.

ADVERSE REACTIONS: Constipation, NV, pyrexia, somnolence, headache, dizziness, pruritus, increased sweating, xerostomia, sedation, diarrhea, insomnia, fatigue, tachycardia, miosis, biliary colic, hypotension.

INTERACTIONS: Additive CNS depression with other CNS depressants (eg, sedatives, hypnotics, tranquilizers, general anesthetics, phenothiazines, other opioids, alcohol); reduce dose of either/both agents. Caution with concomitant use of MAOIs; reduce dose of either/both agents. Anticholinergics may increase risk of urinary retention and/or severe constipation, which may lead to paralytic ileus. CNS toxicity (eg, confusion, disorientation, respiratory depression, apnea, seizures) reported with cimetidine. Avoid use with mixed agonist/antagonist opioid analgesics, may reduce effect and/or precipitate withdrawal symptoms.

PREGNANCY: Category C, caution with nursing.

MECHANISM OF ACTION: Opioid analgesic; an opioid agonist. Prescise action not established. However, specific CNS opioid receptors for endogenous compounds with opioid-like activity have been found throughout the brain and spinal cord and play a role in analgesic effects. Opioid receptors have also been found in the peripheral nervous system.

PHARMACOKINETICS: Absorption: Absolute bioavailability (10%); various doses led to altered parameters. **Distribution**: Plasma protein binding (10-12%); crosses placenta. **Metabolism:** Liver (conjugation) to form oxymorphone-3-glucuronide (major metabolite), 6-OH-oxymorphone (major active metabolite). **Elimination:** Urine (<1% unchanged), feces.

NURSING CONSIDERATIONS

Assessment: Assess type and severity of pain, respiratory depression, acute or severe bronchial asthma or hypercarbia, COPD, myxedema or hypothyroidism, kyphoscoliosis, CNS depression or coma, head injury or intracranial lesions, presence of increased ICP, intraparalytic ileus, circulatory shock, presence of debilitation (eg, elderly), hepatic/renal impairment, cardiovascular disease, prostatic hypertrophy or urethral stricture, toxic psychosis, acute abdominal conditions, convulsive disorders, biliary tract disease, acute pancreatitis, pregnancy/nursing status, drug abuse potential, and possible drug interactions.

Monitoring: Monitor for signs/symptoms of respiratory depression, presence of elevated CSF pressure, hypotension, convulsions, spasms of sphincter of Oddi, physical dependence and tolerance, and abuse or misuse of medication.

Patient Counseling: Advise to swallow medication whole; do not break, chew, dissolve, or crush. If broken or chewed, contents of tab may release all at once and cause fatal overdose. Instruct to take on empty stomach, at least 1 hr prior to or 2 hrs after eating. Drug may impair physical/mental abilities; use caution if performing hazardous tasks (eg, operating machinery/driving). Counsel to avoid alcohol (eg, beverages, medications containing alcohol) and other CNS depressants during therapy. Advise to contact physician if episodes of breakthrough pain or adverse events (eg, respiratory depression) develop. Instruct not to adjust dosing without consulting physician. Inform that medication has potential for abuse; protect from theft. Inform that if on therapy for a few days to weeks, avoid abrupt withdrawal; taper dosing. Instruct to keep out of reach of children.

Administration: Oral route. **Storage**: 25°C (77°F); excursions permitted to 15-30°C (59-86°F). Dispense in tight container with child-resistant closure.

OptiPranolol RX

metipranolol (Bausch & Lomb)

O

THERAPEUTIC CLASS: Nonselective beta-blocker

INDICATIONS: Treatment of elevated intraocular pressure (IOP) in ocular hypertension or open-angle glaucoma.

DOSAGE: *Adults:* 1 drop in affected eye bid.

HOW SUPPLIED: Sol: 0.3% [5mL, 10mL]

CONTRAINDICATIONS: Bronchial asthma, severe COPD, symptomatic sinus bradycardia, greater than 1st-degree AV block, cardiogenic shock, overt cardiac failure.

WARNINGS/PRECAUTIONS: May be absorbed systemically. Severe respiratory and cardiac reactions may occur. Caution with heart failure, DM, cerebrovascular insufficiency, and in those with a history of anaphylactic reactions. May mask signs of hyperthyroidism; abrupt withdrawal may precipitate a thyroid storm. May cause muscle weakness. Withdraw gradually before surgery. Avoid with COPD.

ADVERSE REACTIONS: Abnormal vision, blepharitis, photophobia, uveitis, conjunctivitis, eyelid dermatitis, allergic reactions.

INTERACTIONS: Additive systemic blockade with oral β-blockers. Additive hypotension or bradycardia with catecholamine-depleting agents (eg, reserpine). CCBs may precipitate left ventricular dysfunction and hypotension. Digoxin and CCBs may prolong AV conduction. Caution with adrenergic psychotropics. Effects can be reversed by β-agonists. Use with miotic agent in angle-closure glaucoma.

PREGNANCY: Category C, caution in nursing.

MECHANISM OF ACTION: Nonselective β-adrenoreceptor blocker; reduces elevated as well as normal IOP. Responsible for reducing aqueous humor production and possibly increasing the outflow of aqueous humor. β-adrenergic blockers, when administered orally, produce a reduction in cardiac output and an increase in bronchi and bronchioles airway resistance.

PHARMACOKINETICS: Absorption: T_{max}=2 hrs.

NURSING CONSIDERATIONS

Assessment: Assess for bronchial asthma (or previous history of it), severe COPD, symptomatic sinus bradycardia, greater than 1st-degree AV block, cardiogenic shock, or overt cardiac failure. Assess use of medication in patients with asthma, COPD (mild or moderate), a history of cardiac failure, patients undergoing elective surgery, hyperthyroidism, cerebrovascular insufficiencies, DM, angle-closure glaucoma, and in pregnant/nursing females. Assess for possible drug interactions.

Monitoring: Monitor for signs/symptoms of reduced cerebral blood flow, severe respiratory reactions (eg, bronchospasm), cardiac reactions (eg, cardiac failure), anaphylactic reactions; signs/symptoms of hyperthyroidism, muscle weakness, and acute hypoglycemia.

Patient Counseling: Inform to immediately notify physician if any respiratory, cardiac, or anaphylactic reaction develop. Inform patients at risk for hypoglycemia (eg, diabetics) that medication may mask symptoms of hypoglycemia. Instruct to avoid touching container tip to the eye or surrounding structures. Advise to remove contact lenses prior to administration; may be reinserted 15 min after.

Administration: Ocular route. **Storage:** 15-30°C (59-86°F). Replace cap immediately after use.

OPTIVAR — RX

azelastine HCl (Meda)

THERAPEUTIC CLASS: H_1-antagonist

INDICATIONS: Treatment of itching of the eye associated with allergic conjunctivitis.

DOSAGE: *Adults:* 1 drop bid.
Pediatrics: ≥3 yrs: 1 drop bid.

HOW SUPPLIED: Sol: 0.05% [6mL]

WARNINGS/PRECAUTIONS: Not for injection or oral use. Do not wear contact lens if the eye is red. Not for treatment of contact-lens irritation. Wait 10 min after instilling drops to insert contact lens.

ADVERSE REACTIONS: Transient eye burning/stinging, headaches, asthma, conjunctivitis, dyspnea, eye pain, fatigue, influenza-like symptoms, pharyngitis, pruritus, rhinitis, temporary blurring.

PREGNANCY: Category C, caution in nursing.

MECHANISM OF ACTION: Antihistaminic agent; relatively selective H_1-receptor antagonist; inhibits release of histamine and other mediators from cells (eg, mast cells) involved in the allergic response and decreases chemotaxis and activation of eosinophils.

PHARMACOKINETICS: Metabolism: N-desmethylazelastine (principle metabolite).

NURSING CONSIDERATIONS

Assessment: Assess for drug hypersensitivity.

Monitoring: Monitor for transient burning/stinging, headaches, and bitter taste.

Patient Counseling: Counsel not to wear contact lenses if the eye is red. Avoid touching tip of dropper to eye or any other surface to avoid contamination. Wait 10 min after instillation to wear soft-contact lenses.

Administration: Ocular route. **Storage:** Store upright at 2-25°C (36-77°F).

ORACEA RX

doxycycline (CollaGenex)

THERAPEUTIC CLASS: Tetracycline derivative

INDICATIONS: Treatment of only inflammatory lesions (papules and pustules) of rosacea.

DOSAGE: *Adults:* 40mg qd in am. Take on empty stomach.

HOW SUPPLIED: Cap: 40mg (30mg Immediate-Release and 10mg Delayed-Release beads)

WARNINGS/PRECAUTIONS: May cause fetal harm during pregnancy. Use during tooth development (last half of pregnancy, infancy, ≤8 yrs) may cause permanent discoloration of teeth or enamel hypoplasia. Pseudomembranous colitis reported. Caution in patients with renal impairment. May cause superinfection, photosensitivity, increase in BUN, bacterial resistance, autoimmune syndromes and hyperpigmentation. Bulging fontanels in infants and benign intracranial HTN in adults reported.

ADVERSE REACTIONS: Nasopharyngitis, sinusitis, fungal infection, influenza, diarrhea, HTN, pharyngolaryngeal pain, nasal congestion, abdominal pain, dry mouth, anxiety, sinus headache.

INTERACTIONS: May require downward adjustments of anticoagulant dosage. May interfere with bactericidal action of penicillin; avoid concurrent use when possible. Concomitant use with methoxyflurane may result in fatal renal toxicity. Bismuth subsalicylate, proton pump inhibitors, antacids containing aluminum, calcium or magnesium and iron-containing preparations may impair absorption. May interfere with the effectiveness of oral contraceptives. Avoid concurrent use with oral retinoids (eg, isotetinoin). False elevations of urinary catecholamine levels may occur.

PREGNANCY: Category D, not for use in nursing.

MECHANISM OF ACTION: Tetracycline derivative. Antibacterial agent; does not produce any long-term effects on bacterial flora in the oral cavity, skin, intestinal tract, or vagina.

O

PHARMACOKINETICS: Absorption: Single Dose: C_{max}=510ng/mL; T_{max}=3 hrs; AUC=9227ng•hr/mL. Multiple Doses: C_{max}=600ng/mL; T_{max}=2 hrs; AUC=7543ng•hr/mL. **Distribution**: Plasma protein binding (>90%), crosses the placenta, excreted in breast milk. **Elimination**: Urine, feces; $T_{1/2}$=21.2 hrs (single dose), 23.2 hrs (multiple doses).

NURSING CONSIDERATIONS

Assessment: Determine pregnancy/nursing status. Assess use in patients with renal impairment, history of or predisposition to candidiasis overgrowth, and those with gastric insufficiencies (eg, patients with gastrectomy, gastric bypass surgery, or in patients who are achlorhydric). Assess for possible drug interactions.

Monitoring: Monitor for signs/symptoms of pseudomembranous colitis, photosensitivity reactions, exfoliative dermatitis, maculopapular and erythematous rashes, hypersensitivity reactions, increased BUN levels, overgrowth of nonsusceptible organisms (eg, fungi) superinfection development, tissue hyperpigmentation, pseudotumor cerebri, autoimmune syndrome (eg, fever, rash, arthalgia, and malaise) and perform appropriate diagnostic tests (eg, LFTs, ANA, CBC). In patients with renal insufficiencies, monitor for signs/symptoms of azotemia, hyperphosphatemia, and acidosis. Perform periodic monitoring of drug serum levels in patients with renal impairment. In all patients, perform periodic monitoring of organ systems, including hematopoietic, renal, and hepatic studies.

Patient Counseling: Take medication 1 hr before or 2 hrs after meals with fluid. Minimize or avoid exposure to natural or artificial sunlight (eg, tanning beds). Wear loose fitting-clothes that protect skin from sun exposure. Counsel medication may cause autoimmune disorders; contact physician if arthalgia, fever, rash, or malaise develop. Advise drug may cause discoloration of skin, scars, teeth, or gums. Inform females drug may render oral contraceptives less effective, and to avoid if pregnant or nursing. Instruct to avoid use if planning to conceive.

Administration: Oral route. **Storage**: 15-30°C (59-86°F). Dispense in tight, light-resistant containers. Keep out of reach of children.

ORAMORPH SR

morphine sulfate (Xanodyne)

CII

This is a sustained-release tablet. Swallow tab whole; do not break in half, crush or chew.

THERAPEUTIC CLASS: Opioid analgesic

INDICATIONS: Relief of pain in patients who require opioid analgesics for more than a few days.

DOSAGE: *Adults:* Conversion from Parenteral or Immediate Release Oral Morphine: Daily dose determined by daily requirement of immediate-release formulation. Single dose is 1/2 of daily requirement given q12h. Initial: 30mg is recommended if daily morphine requirement is ≤120mg. Use 15mg for low daily morphine requirements. Titrate: Increase to 60mg or 100mg after stable dose reached.

HOW SUPPLIED: Tab, Extended-Release: 15mg, 30mg, 60mg, 100mg

CONTRAINDICATIONS: Respiratory depression in the absence of resuscitative equipment, acute or severe bronchial asthma, paralytic ileus.

WARNINGS/PRECAUTIONS: Not for initial treatment. Caution with hepatic and renal dysfunction, increased ICP or with head injury, decreased respiratory reserve (eg, emphysema, severe obesity, kyphoscoliosis, or paralysis of the phrenic nerve), chronic asthma, upper airway obstruction, or in other chronic pulmonary disorders. Tolerance, psychological and physical dependence may develop. Avoid abrupt discontinuation. Not for pediatrics or use in women during or immediately before labor.

ADVERSE REACTIONS: Constipation, NV, dizziness, sedation, dysphoria, euphoria, and sweating, respiratory depression.

INTERACTIONS: Potentiated depressant effects with CNS depressants, alcohol, sedatives, antihistaminics, or psychotropics. Increased risk of respiratory depression, hypotension, sedation and coma with neuroleptics. Mixed agonist/antagonist opioid analgesics (eg, pentazocine, nalbuphine, butorphanol, or buprenorphine) may alter effect or precipitate withdrawal symptoms.

PREGNANCY: Category C, not for use in nursing.

MECHANISM OF ACTION: Opioid analgesic; interacts predominantly with μ-receptor. μ binding sites are found distributed in the brain, spinal cord, and in trigeminal nerve. Primary actions are analgesia and sedation.

PHARMACOKINETICS: Absorption: Absolute bioavailability (40%), oral administration of variable doses resulted in different parameters. **Distribution:** V_d=4L/kg; crosses placental membrane; found in breast milk. **Metabolism:** Liver to glucuronide metabolites; morphine-3-glucuronide (major metabolite), morphine-6-glucuronide (active metabolite). **Elimination:** Kidneys (major), feces (10%), bile (small amount); $T_{1/2}$=2-4 hrs.

NURSING CONSIDERATIONS

Assessment: Assess for respiratory depression, acute or severe bronchial asthma, COPD, presence of debilitation (eg, elderly), paralytic ileus, ICP or head injury, hepatic/renal dysfunction, pregnancy/nursing status, and possible drug interactions.

Monitoring: Monitor for signs/symptoms of respiratory depression, elevations in CSF pressure, medication dependence and abuse.

Patient Counseling: Instruct to swallow medication whole; do not break, chew, or crush. Drug may cause psychological and/or physical dependence. Do not adjust dose without consulting physician. Avoid abrupt withdrawal of medication. Advise to avoid alcohol or other CNS depressants. Medication

O

may impair mental/physical abilities; use caution if performing hazardous tasks (eg, operating machinery/driving).

Administration: Oral route. **Storage:** 25°C (77°F); excursions permitted to 15-30°C (59-86°F).

ORAPRED RX

prednisolone sodium phosphate (Biomarin)

OTHER BRAND NAMES: Orapred ODT (Sciele)

THERAPEUTIC CLASS: Glucocorticoid

INDICATIONS: Steroid-responsive disorders.

DOSAGE: *Adults:* (Sol) Initial: 5-60mg/day depending on disease and response. (Tab) Initial: 10-60mg/day depending on disease and response. Maint: Decrease dose by small amounts to lowest effective dose. (Sol/Tab) MS Exacerbations: 200mg qd for 1 week, then 80mg every other day for 1 month. *Pediatrics:* (Sol/Tab) Initial: 0.14-2mg/kg/day, depending on disease and response, given tid-qid. Nephrotic Syndrome: $20mg/m^2$ tid for 4 weeks, then $40mg/m^2$ every other day for 4 weeks. Uncontrolled Asthma: 1-2mg/kg/day in single or divided doses until peak expiratory flow rate of 80% is achieved (usually 3-10 days).

HOW SUPPLIED: Sol: 15mg/5mL [237mL]; Tab, Orally Disintegrating: 10mg, 15mg, 30mg

CONTRAINDICATIONS: Systemic fungal infections.

WARNINGS/PRECAUTIONS: May produce reversible HPA axis suppression. Adjust dose during stress or change in thyroid status. May mask signs of infection or cause new infections. May activate latent amebiasis. Avoid with cerebral malaria. Avoid exposure to chickenpox or measles. Not for treatment of optic neuritis or active ocular herpes simplex. May cause elevation of BP or IOP, cataracts, glaucoma, optic nerve damage, Kaposi's sarcoma, psychic derangements, salt/water retention, increased excretion of potassium and/or calcium, osteoporosis, growth suppression in children, secondary ocular infections. Caution with strongyloides, CHF, diverticulitis, HTN, renal insufficiency, fresh intestinal anastomoses, active or latent peptic ulcer, ulcerative colitis. Enhanced effect in hypothyroidism or cirrhosis. Avoid abrupt withdrawal.

ADVERSE REACTIONS: Edema, fluid/electrolyte disturbances, osteoporosis, muscle weakness, pancreatitis, peptic ulcer, impaired wound healing, increased intracranial pressure, cushingoid state, hirsutism, menstrual irregularities, growth suppression in children, glaucoma, nausea, weight gain.

INTERACTIONS: Enhanced metabolism with barbiturates, phenytoin, ephedrine, and rifampin. Use with cyclosporine may increase activity of both drugs; convulsions reported with concomitant use. Decreased metabolism with estrogens or ketoconazole. May inhibit response to warfarin. Increased risk of GI side effects with ASA or other NSAIDs. May increase clearance of salicylates. High doses or concurrent neuromuscular drugs may cause acute myopathy. Enhanced possibility of hypokalemia when given with potassium-depleting agents. May produce severe weakness in myasthenia gravis patients on anticholinesterase agents. Avoid live vaccines with immunosuppressive doses. Possible diminished response with killed or inactivated vaccines. May increase blood glucose; adjust antidiabetic agents. May suppress reactions to skin tests.

PREGNANCY: Category C, caution in nursing.

MECHANISM OF ACTION: Synthetic adrenocorticoid steroid; promotes gluconeogenesis, increases deposition of glycogen in the liver, inhibits glucose utilization, increases catabolism of protein, lipolysis, glomerular filtration that leads to increased urinary excretion of urate and calcium.

PHARMACOKINETICS: Absorption: Readily absorbed from GI tract. **Distribution:** Plasma protein binding (70-90%); found in breast milk. **Metabolism:** Liver. **Elimination:** Urine (as sulfate and glucuronide conjugates), $T_{1/2}$=2-4 hrs.

NURSING CONSIDERATIONS

Assessment: Assess for systemic fungal infection, other current infections, active TB, HTN, CHF, renal insufficiency, ophthalmic disease, osteoporosis, thyroid status, hepatic impairment, nonspecific ulcerative colitis, and possible drug interactions.

Monitoring: Monitor for adrenocortical insufficiency, occurrence of infections, psychic derangement, cataracts, acute myopathy, Kaposi's sarcoma, fluid retention, measurement of serum electrolytes, TSH, LFTs, glucose, IOP, and BP.

Patient Counseling: Advise not to d/c abruptly or without medical supervision. Avoid exposure to chickenpox or measles; report immediately if exposed. ODT tablets should be placed on tongue and allowed to dissolve in mouth, with/without water. Do not cut, split, or break tablets. Do not use partial tablets.

Administration: Oral route. **Storage:** (Sol) 2-8°C (36-46°F); (Tab) 20-25°C (68-77°F); protect from moisture.

ORENCIA — RX

abatacept (Bristol-Myers Squibb)

THERAPEUTIC CLASS: Selective costimulation modulator

INDICATIONS: To reduce signs and symptoms, inducing major clinical response, inhibiting the progression of structural damage, and improving physical function in adult patients with moderately to severely active rheumatoid arthritis who have had an inadequate response to one or more disease-modifying, anti-rheumatic drugs (DMARDs) (eg, MTX, TNF antagonists). May be used as monotherapy or concomitantly with DMARDs other than TNF-antagonists. For reducing signs and symptoms in pediatric patients ≥6 yrs with moderately to severely active polyarticular juvenile idiopathic arthritis. May be used as monotherapy or concomitantly with MTX.

DOSAGE: *Adults:* Initial: <60kg: 500mg; 60-100kg: 750mg; >100kg: 1g IV over 30 min. Maint: Give at 2 and 4 weeks after initial infusion, then every 4 weeks thereafter.
Pediatrics: 6-17 yrs: >75 kg: Follow adult dosing regimen. Max: 1000mg; <75kg: Initial: 10mg/kg IV over 30 min. Maint: Give at 2 and 4 weeks after initial infusion, then every 4 weeks thereafter.

HOW SUPPLIED: Inj: 250mg

WARNINGS/PRECAUTIONS: Increased risk of infections and serious infections with concomitant TNF-antagonist therapy; concurrent use not recommended. Anaphylaxis or anaphylactoid reactions reported. Caution with history of recurrent infections; d/c if serious infections develop. Screen for latent TB prior to initiation. Avoid live vaccines. Caution with COPD. Concurrent use with anakinra is not recommended. Cases of lung cancer and lymphoma reported. Screening for viral hepatitis is recommended before initiation of therapy. Juvenile idiopathic arthritis patients should be brought up to date with all immunizations prior to therapy.

ADVERSE REACTIONS: Headache, nasopharyngitis, dizziness, cough, back pain, HTN, dyspepsia, UTI, rash, pain in extremities.

INTERACTIONS: See Warnings/Precautions.

PREGNANCY: Category C, not for use in nursing.

MECHANISM OF ACTION: Selective costimulation modulator; inhibits T cell activation by binding to CD80 and CD86, thereby blocking interaction with CD28.

PHARMACOKINETICS: Absorption: C_{max}=292mcg/mL. **Distribution:** V_d=0.09L/Kg. **Elimination:** $T_{1/2}$=16.7 days.

NURSING CONSIDERATIONS

Assessment: Assess for history of recurrent infections, chronic/latent/localized infections, disease states which may predispose to infection, COPD, preg-

O

nancy/nursing status, and possible drug interactions (eg, TNF antagonists). Screen for latent TB infection (eg, tuberculin skin test) and for viral hepatitis.

Monitoring: Monitor for signs/symptoms of hypersensitivity (eg, anaphylaxis), infection, immunosuppression, malignancies (eg, lymphoma), and hepatitis B reactivation. If COPD present, monitor for COPD exacerbation, cough, rhonchi, and dyspnea. Monitor overall health at each treatment visit.

Patient Counseling: Inform should not receive live vaccines during therapy or within 3 months following d/c. Immediately contact physician if hypersensitivity reaction (eg, anaphylaxis) occur. Discuss side effects (eg, infection, malignancies).

Administration: IV infusion route. Reconstitute: 1) Using silicone-free disposable syringe, inject 10mL of Sterile Water for Inj, USP into vial for concentration of 250mg/10mL. 2) Upon complete dissolution, vent vial with needle to dissipate any foam present. Further dilute to 100mL. 3) From infusion bag or bottle, withdraw a volume of 0.9% NaCl Inj, USP, equal to the volume of the reconstituted solution, using the same silicone-free disposable syringe. 4) Gently mix. Administer diluted solution over 30 min. Infusion must be completed within 24 hrs of reconstitution of vials. **Storage:** Lypholized powder: 2-8°C (36-46°F). Do not use after expiration date. Protect vials from light; store in original package until time of use. Diluted: Room temperature, or refrigerate at 2-8°C (36-46°F); use within 24 hrs.

ORTHO EVRA — RX

ethinyl estradiol - norelgestromin (Ortho-McNeil)

THERAPEUTIC CLASS: Estrogen/progestogen combination

INDICATIONS: Prevention of pregnancy.

DOSAGE: *Adults:* Start 1st Sunday after menses begin or 1st day of menses. Apply patch every week on same day for 3 weeks. Week 4 is patch-free. Apply to clean, dry intact skin on buttock, abdomen, upper arm, or upper torso.

HOW SUPPLIED: Patch: (Ethinyl Estradiol-Norelgestromin): 0.75mg-6mg [1[s], 3[s]]

O

CONTRAINDICATIONS: Thrombophlebitis, DVT, thromboembolic disorders, pregnancy, cerebrovascular or coronary artery disease, valvular heart disease with complications, undiagnosed abnormal genital bleeding, cholestatic jaundice of pregnancy or jaundice with prior pill use, hepatic adenomas or carcinomas, breast cancer or other estrogen-dependent neoplasia, severe HTN, diabetes with vascular involvement, headaches with focal neurological symptoms, major surgery with prolonged immobilization, acute/chronic hepatocellular disease with abnormal liver function.

WARNINGS/PRECAUTIONS: Cigarette smoking increases risk of serious cardiovascular side effects. This risk increases with age (especially >35 yrs) and heavy smoking. Increased risk of MI, vascular disease, thromboembolism, stroke, and gallbladder disease. Retinal thrombosis, hepatic neoplasia reported. May cause glucose intolerance. May increase BP, elevate LDL levels or cause other lipid changes, fluid retention, breakthrough bleeding, and spotting. May cause or exacerbate migraine. May develop visual changes with contact lens. Increased risk of MI with HTN, hyperlipidemia, and diabetes. D/C if jaundice or depression develops. Perform annual physical exam. Use before menarche is not indicated. May affect certain endocrine, LFTs, and blood components. May be less effective in women with body weight ≥198 lbs.

ADVERSE REACTIONS: Breast symptoms, headache, application site reaction, nausea, upper respiratory infection, menstrual cramps, abdominal pain.

INTERACTIONS: Reduced effects and increased breakthrough bleeding with rifampin, bosentan, barbiturates, phenytoin, carbamazepine, topiramate, St. John's wort, griseofulvin, felbamate, oxcarbazepine, possibly with ampicillin. Protease inhibitors alter levels. Increased levels with atorvastatin, ascorbic acid, acetaminophen, and CYP3A4 inhibitors (eg, itraconazole, ketoconazole). May increase levels of cyclosporine, prednisolone, theophylline. May decrease levels of acetaminophen and increase clearance of temazepam, salicylic acid, morphine, and clofibric acid.

PREGNANCY: Category X, not for use in nursing.

MECHANISM OF ACTION: Contraceptive; suppresses gonadotropin, inhibits ovulation, promotes changes in cervical mucus (which increases difficulty of sperm entry into uterus) and the endometrium (which reduce likelihood of implantation).

PHARMACOKINETICS: Absorption: Norelgestromin: C_{max}=0.305-1.53ng/mL, AUC_{0-168}=107ng•h/mL. Ethinyl estradiol: C_{max}=11.2-137pg/mL, AUC_{0-168}=6796pg•h/mL. **Distribution:** Norelgestromin: Serum protein binding (>97%). Ethinyl estradiol: Serum albumin binding (extensive). **Metabolism:** GI tract and/or liver (1st pass metabolism). **Elimination:** Norelgestromin: Urine, feces; $T_{1/2}$=28 hrs. Ethinyl estradiol: Urine, feces; $T_{1/2}$=17 hrs.

NURSING CONSIDERATIONS

Assessment: Assess for increased risk of thrombophlebitis or thromboembolic disorder, history of deep vein thrombophlebitis, cerebral vascular or coronary artery disease, valvular heart disease, severe HTN, local neurological symptoms, history of breast cancer, carcinoma of the endometrium or other known or suspected estrogen-dependent neoplasia, abnormal genital bleeding, abnormal liver function, suspected pregnancy. Assess patients who smoke (may increase risk of heart attack), hypercholesterolemia, glucose intolerance, obesity and DM, exacerbation of migraine or development of headache, hypersensitivity to any component, and any possible drug interactions. Assess for depression.

Monitoring: Monitor for PT, factors VII, VIII, IX, X, platelet count, TBG, sex hormone binding globulin, antithrombin 3, BP, thyroid hormone, PBI, T4, glucose tolerance, serum folate level, lipid and lipoprotein level, LDL. Monitor for vision, onset of proptosis or diplopia, papilledema, or retinal vascular. Periodic monitoring for vaginal bleeding and spotting, uncomfortable irritation on the patch site. Monitor if depression develops.

Patient Counseling: Inform that drug does not protect against HIV infection (AIDS) and other STDs. Advise to avoid smoking. Counsel that physical exam and follow-up required. Instruct to apply patch to clean, dry, intact healthy skin (on buttock, abdomen, upper outer arm or upper torso) where it will not be rubbed by tight clothing. Instruct not to place on red, irritated, or cut skin or on the breast.

Administration: Transdermal route. **Storage:** 25°C (77°F); excursions permitted to 15-30°C (59-86°F).

ORTHO TRI-CYCLEN — RX

ethinyl estradiol - norgestimate (Ortho-McNeil)

OTHER BRAND NAMES: Tri-Previfem (Teva) - Tri-Sprintec (Barr)

THERAPEUTIC CLASS: Estrogen/progestogen combination

INDICATIONS: Prevention of pregnancy. Treatment of acne vulgaris in females ≥15 yrs who want contraception, have achieved menarche and are unresponsive to topical acne agents.

DOSAGE: *Adults:* Contraception/Acne: 28-day: 1 tab qd for 28 days, then repeat. Start 1st Sunday after menses begin or 1st day of menses.
Pediatrics: Contraception (postpubertal adolescents)/Acne: 28-day: 1 tab qd for 28 days, then repeat. Start 1st Sunday after menses begin or 1st day of menses.

HOW SUPPLIED: Tab: (Ethinyl Estradiol-Norgestimate) 0.035mg-0.18mg, 0.035mg-0.215mg, 0.035mg-0.25mg

CONTRAINDICATIONS: Thrombophlebitis, deep vein thrombophlebitis, thromboembolic disorders, pregnancy, cerbrovascular or coronary artery disease, migraine with focal aura, acute or chronic hepatocellular disease with abnormal liver function, undiagnosed abnormal genital bleeding, cholestatic jaundice of pregnancy or jaundice with prior pill use, hepatic adenomas or carcinomas, breast cancer, endometrium carcinoma, or other estrogen-dependent neoplasia.

WARNINGS/PRECAUTIONS: Cigarette smoking increases risk of serious cardiovascular side effects. This risk increases with age (especially >35 yrs) and heavy smoking. Increased risk of MI, vascular disease, thromboembolism, stroke, and gallbladder disease. Retinal thrombosis, hepatic neoplasia, carcinoma of breast and reproductive organs reported. May cause glucose intolerance, fluid retention, breakthrough bleeding, and spotting. May increase BP, elevate LDL levels, or cause other lipid changes. May cause or exacerbate migraine. May develop visual changes with contact lens. Increased risk of morbidity and mortality with HTN, hyperlipidemia, obesity, and diabetes. D/C if jaundice, significant depression, or ophthalmic irregularities develop. Perform annual physical exam. Use before menarche is not indicated. May affect certain endocrine, LFTs, and blood components.

ADVERSE REACTIONS: NV, breakthrough bleeding, spotting, amenorrhea, migraine, depression, vaginal candidiasis, edema, weight changes.

INTERACTIONS: Reduced effects, increased breakthrough bleeding, and menstrual irregularities with rifampin, barbiturates, phenylbutazone, phenytoin, carbamazepine, griseofulvin, topiramate, St. John's wort, and possibly with ampicillin and tetracyclines.

PREGNANCY: Category X, not for use in nursing.

MECHANISM OF ACTION: Estrogen/progestogen oral contraceptive; acts by suppressing gonadotropin, inhibiting ovulation, and causing other alterations, including changes in cervical mucus (increases difficulty of sperm entry into uterus) and endometrium (reduces likehood of implantation).

PHARMACOKINETICS: Absorption: Rapid. Oral administration on various days during dosing led to altered parameters. **Distribution:** Norgestimate: Albumin binding (>97%). Ethinyl estradiol: Albumin binding (>97%). **Metabolism:** Norgestimate: GI tract and/or liver (1st pass mechanism). Norelgestromin (primary active metabolite): Hepatic, norgestrel (active metabolite). Ethinyl estradiol: Hydroxylated, glucuronide, sulfate conjugates. **Elimination:** Norgestimate: Urine (47%), feces (37%).

NURSING CONSIDERATIONS

Assessment: Assess for current or history of thrombophlebitis or thromboembolic disorder, cerebral vascular or coronary artery disease, valvular heart disease with complications, severe HTN, DM with vascular involvement, headaches with focal neurological symptoms, major surgery with prolonged immobilization, known/suspected or history of carcinoma of breast, endometrium or other known/suspected estrogen-dependent neoplasia. Assess use in patients ≥35 who smoke ≥15 cigarettes/day. Assess use with history of HTN, hyperlipidemias, obesity, and DM. Assess for possible drug interactions.

Monitoring: Monitor for signs/symptoms of MI, thromboembolism, stroke, hepatic neoplasia, breast cancer, ocular lesions, bleeding irregularities, fluid retention, onset or exacerbation of migraines or headache, gallbladder disease, and etopic pregnancy. Monitor serum glucose levels in DM and prediabetic patients. Monitor BP with history of HTN, lipid levels with history of hyperlipidemia, worsening depression with previous history. Refer patients with contact lenses to an ophthalmologist if ocular changes develop. Perform annual physical exam while on therapy. Monitor liver function and for signs of liver toxicity (eg, jaundice).

Patient Counseling: Inform that drug does not protect against HIV infection (AIDS) and other STDs. Advise to avoid smoking while on medication. Instruct to take medication at same time every day. Advise about risk of pregnancy if dose is missed. Instruct that if 1 dose missed, take as soon as possible, then take next dose at regularly scheduled time. Inform may have spotting, light bleeding, or nausea during first 1-3 packs of pills; advise not to d/c medication and if symptoms persist, contact physician.

Administration: Oral route. **Storage:** 25°C (77°F); excursions permitted to 15-30°C (59-86°F).

Ortho Tri-Cyclen Lo

RX

ethinyl estradiol - norgestimate (Ortho-McNeil)

THERAPEUTIC CLASS: Estrogen/progestogen combination

INDICATIONS: Prevention of pregnancy.

DOSAGE: *Adults:* 1 tab qd for 28 days, then repeat. Start 1st Sunday after menses begin or 1st day of menses.

HOW SUPPLIED: Tab: (Ethinyl Estradiol-Norgestimate) 0.025mg-0.18mg, 0.025mg-0.215mg, and 0.025mg-0.25mg

CONTRAINDICATIONS: Thrombophlebitis, deep vein thrombophlebitis, thromboembolic disorders, pregnancy, cerebrovascular or CAD, valvular heart disease with complications, severe HTN, DM with vascular involvement, headaches with focal neurological symptoms, major surgery with prolonged immobilization, undiagnosed abnormal genital bleeding, cholestatic jaundice of pregnancy or jaundice with prior pill use, hepatic adenomas or carcinomas, breast cancer, endometrial carcinoma or other estrogen-dependent neoplasia.

WARNINGS/PRECAUTIONS: Cigarette smoking increases risk of serious CV side effects; risk increases with age (especially >35 yrs) and heavy smoking. Increased risk of MI, vascular disease, thromboembolism, stroke, and gallbladder disease. Retinal thrombosis, hepatic neoplasia, carcinoma of breast and reproductive organs reported. May cause glucose intolerance, fluid retention, breakthrough bleeding, and spotting. May increase BP, elevate LDL levels or cause other lipid changes. May cause or exacerbate migraine. May develop visual changes with contact lens. Increased risk of morbidity and mortality with HTN, hyperlipidemia, obesity, and DM. D/C if jaundice, significant depression, or ophthalmic irregularities develop. Perform annual physical exam. Use before menarche is not indicated. May affect certain endocrine, LFTs, and blood components.

ADVERSE REACTIONS: NV, breakthrough bleeding, spotting, amenorrhea, migraine, depression, vaginal candidiasis, edema, weight changes.

INTERACTIONS: Reduced effects, increased breakthrough bleeding with rifampin, barbiturates, phenylbutazone, phenytoin, carbamazepine, felbamate, oxcarbazepine, griseofulvin, topiramate, St. John's wort, and possibly with ampicillin and tetracyclines. Atorvastatin, ascorbic acid, APAP, CYP3A4 inhibitors (eg, itraconazole, ketoconazole) may increase hormone levels. HIV protease inhibitors may increase or decrease levels. Increases levels of cyclosporine, prednisolone, theophylline. Decreases levels of APAP. Increases clearance of temazepam, salicylic acid, morphine, clofibric acid.

PREGNANCY: Category X, not for use in nursing.

MECHANISM OF ACTION: Estrogen/progestogen oral contraceptive; acts by suppressing gonadotropin, inhibiting ovulation, changes in cervical mucus (increases difficulty of sperm entry into uterus) and endometrium (reduces likehood of implantation).

PHARMACOKINETICS: Absorption: Rapidly absorbed. Oral administration on various days during dosing schedule led to altered parameters. **Distribution:** Found in breast milk. Norgestimate: Serum protein binding (>97%). Ethinyl Estradiol: Serum albumin binding (>97%). **Metabolism:** Norgestimate: 1st pass metabolism, GI tract and/or liver. norelgestromin (active major metabolite) norgestrel (active major metabolite). Norelgestromin: Hepatic. Ethinyl Estradiol: Hydroxylated, glucuronide and sulfate congugates. **Elimination:** Urine, feces; $T_{1/2}$=28.1 hrs (norelgestromin), 36.4 hrs (norgestrel), 17.7 hrs (ethinyl estradiol).

NURSING CONSIDERATIONS

Assessment: Assess for current or history of thrombophlebitis or thromboembolic disorder, cerebrovascular or coronary artery disease, valvular heart disease with complications, severe HTN, DM with vascular involvement, headaches with focal neurological symptoms, major surgery with prolonged immobilization, known/suspected or history of carcinoma of breast, endometrium

O

or other known or suspected estrogen-dependent neoplasia, abnormal genital bleeding, abnormal liver function, and known/suspected pregnancy. Assess use in patients ≥35 yrs who smoke ≥15 cigarettes/day. Assess use with HTN, hyperlipidemias, DM, obesity, and increased age. Assess for possible drug interactions.

Monitoring: Monitor for signs/symptoms of MI, thromboembolism, stroke, hepatic neoplasia, ocular lesions, bleeding irregularities, fluid retention, headache, gallbladder disease, and etopic pregnancy. Monitor serum glucose levels in DM or prediabetic patients, BP with history of HTN, lipid levels with history of hyperlipidemia, for signs/symptoms of liver dysfunction while on therapy (eg, jaundice), for signs of worsening depression with previous history. Refer patients with contact lenses to an ophthalmologist if ocular changes occur. Perform annual physical exam.

Patient Counseling: Inform that drug does not protect against HIV infection (AIDS) and other STDs. Advise to avoid smoking. Counsel about potential adverse effects. Instruct to take exactly as directed at intervals not exceeding 24 hrs. Instruct that if one dose missed, take as soon as possible; take next pill at regularly scheduled time. Inform may experience spotting, light bleeding, or nausea during first 1-3 packs of pills; advise not to d/c medication and if symptoms persist, notify physician.

Administration: Oral route. **Storage:** 25°C (77°F); excursions permitted to 15-30°C (59-86°F).

ORTHO-CEPT — RX

desogestrel - ethinyl estradiol (Ortho-McNeil)

THERAPEUTIC CLASS: Estrogen/progestogen combination

INDICATIONS: Prevention of pregnancy.

DOSAGE: *Adults:* 1 tab qd for 28 days, then repeat. Start 1st Sunday after menses begin or 1st day of menses.

HOW SUPPLIED: Tab: (Ethinyl Estradiol-Desogestrel) 0.03mg-0.15mg

O

CONTRAINDICATIONS: Thrombophlebitis, DVT or thromboembolic disorders, pregnancy, cerebrovascular or coronary artery disease, undiagnosed abnormal genital bleeding, cholestatic jaundice of pregnancy or jaundice with prior pill use, hepatic adenomas or carcinomas, breast cancer or other estrogen-dependent neoplasia.

WARNINGS/PRECAUTIONS: Cigarette smoking increases risk of serious cardiovascular side effects. This risk increases with age (especially >35 yrs) and heavy smoking. Increased risk of MI, vascular disease, thromboembolism, stroke, and gallbladder disease. Retinal thrombosis, hepatic neoplasia, carcinoma of breast and reproductive organs reported. May cause glucose intolerance. May increase BP, elevate LDL levels or cause other lipid changes, fluid retention, breakthrough bleeding, and spotting. May cause or exacerbate migraine. May develop visual changes with contact lens. Increased risk of MI with HTN, hyperlipidemia, obesity, and diabetes. D/C if jaundice, significant depression, or ophthalmic irregularities develop. Perform annual physical exam. Use before menarche is not indicated. May affect certain endocrine, LFTs, and blood components.

ADVERSE REACTIONS: NV, breakthrough bleeding, spotting, amenorrhea, migraine, depression, vaginal candidiasis, edema, weight changes.

INTERACTIONS: Reduced effects, increased breakthrough bleeding, and menstrual irregularities with rifampin, barbiturates, phenylbutazone, phenytoin, carbamazepine, griseofulvin, topiramate, St. John's wort, and possibly with ampicillin and tetracyclines.

PREGNANCY: Category X, not for use in nursing.

MECHANISM OF ACTION: Estrogen/progestogen combination oral contraceptive; responsible for suppressing gonadotropins. Primarily inhibits ovulation. Also causes changes in cervical mucus (increases difficulty of sperm entry into uterus) and endometrium (reduces likehood of implantation).

PHARMACOKINETICS: Absorption: Desogestrel: Rapid, C_{max}=2,805pg/mL (single dose), 5840 (multiple doses), T_{max}=1.4 hrs (single dose), 1.4 hrs (after multiple doses); AUC=33,858pg/mL•hr (single dose), 52,299pg/mL•hr (after multiple doses); Ethinyl estradiol: C_{max}=95pg/mL (single dose), 141pg/mL (multiple doses), T_{max}=1.5 hrs (single dose), 1.4 hrs (multiple doses) AUC=1471pg/mL•hr. **Distribution:** Found in breast milk. **Metabolism:** Desogestrel: 3-keto-desogestrel (major active metabolite), conjugation into sulfates and glucuronides. Ethinyl estradiol: Phase I metabolism: 2-OH-ethinyl estradiol, 2-methoxy-ethinyl-estradiol (major metabolites), hepatic conjugation. **Elimination:** 3-ketodesogestrel: $T_{1/2}$=38 hrs; Ethinyl estradiol: $T_{1/2}$=26 hrs.

NURSING CONSIDERATIONS

Assessment: Assess for current or history of thrombophlebitis or thromboembolic disorder, cerebrovascular or coronary artery disease, valvular heart disease with complications, severe HTN, DM with vascular involvement, headaches with focal neurological symptoms, major surgery with prolonged immobilization, known/suspected or history of breast cancer, carcinoma of endometrium or other known/suspected estrogen-dependent neoplasia, abnormal genital bleeding, cholestatic jaundice of pregnancy or jaundice with prior pill use, hepatic adenomas or carcinomas, and known/suspected pregnancy. Assess use in patients ≥35 yrs who smoke ≥15 cigarettes/day. Assess for possible drug interactions.

Monitoring: Monitor for MI, thromboembolism, stroke, hepatic neoplasia, gallbladder disease, headaches, bleeding irregularities, ocular lesions, hyperlipidemia, HTN, fluid retention, and ectopic pregnancy. Monitor blood glucose levels in DM or prediabetic patients, BP with history of HTN, lipid levels with history of hyperlipidemia, for signs of worsening depression with previous history, for signs/symptoms of liver dysfunction (eg, jaundice). Instruct patients with contact lenses to an ophthalmologist if ocular changes develop. Perform annual physical exam.

Patient Counseling: Inform that drug does not protect HIV infection (AIDS) and other STDs. Advise to avoid smoking while on drug. Instruct to take medication at same time daily. Inform that if dose missed, take as soon as possible; take next dose at regularly scheduled time. Inform may have spotting, light bleeding or nausea during first first 1-3 packs of pills; advise not to d/c medication and if symptoms persist, notify physician.

Administration: Oral route. **Storage:** 25°C (77°F); excursions permitted to 15-30°C (59-86°F).

ORTHO-CYCLEN — RX

ethinyl estradiol - norgestimate (Ortho-McNeil)

OTHER BRAND NAMES: MonoNessa (Watson) - Sprintec (Barr)

THERAPEUTIC CLASS: Estrogen/progestogen combination

INDICATIONS: Prevention of pregnancy.

DOSAGE: *Adults:* 1 tab qd for 28 days, then repeat. Start 1st Sunday after menses begin or 1st day of menses.

HOW SUPPLIED: Tab: (Ethinyl Estradiol-Norgestimate) 0.035mg-0.25mg

CONTRAINDICATIONS: Thrombophlebitis, deep vein thrombophlebitis, thromboembolic disorders, pregnancy, cerebrovascular or coronary artery disease, migraine with focal aura, acute or chronic hepatocellular disease with abnormal liver function, undiagnosed abnormal genital bleeding, cholestatic jaundice of pregnancy or jaundice with prior pill use, hepatic adenomas or carcinomas, breast cancer, endometrium carcinoma, or other estrogen-dependent neoplasia.

WARNINGS/PRECAUTIONS: Cigarette smoking increases risk of serious cardiovascular side effects; risk increases with age (especially >35 yrs) and heavy smoking. Increased risk of MI, vascular disease, thromboembolism, stroke, and gallbladder disease. Retinal thrombosis, hepatic neoplasia, carcinoma of breast and reproductive organs reported. May cause glucose intolerance. May increase BP, elevate LDL levels or cause other lipid changes, fluid retention, breakthrough bleeding, and spotting. May cause or exacerbate migraine. May develop visual changes with contact lens. Increased risk of MI with HTN, hyperlipidemia, obesity, and diabetes. D/C if jaundice, significant depression, or ophthalmic irregularities develop. Perform annual physical exam. Use before menarche is not indicated. May affect certain endocrine, LFTs, and blood components.

ADVERSE REACTIONS: NV, breakthrough bleeding, spotting, amenorrhea, migraine, depression, vaginal candidiasis, edema, weight changes.

INTERACTIONS: Reduced effects, increased breakthrough bleeding, and menstrual irregularities with rifampin, barbiturates, phenylbutazone, phenytoin, carbamazepine, griseofulvin, topiramate, St. John's wort, and possibly with ampicillin and tetracyclines.

PREGNANCY: Category X, not for use in nursing.

MECHANISM OF ACTION: Estrogen/progestogen combination oral contraceptive; acts by suppressing gonadotropins. Primarily inhibits ovulation. Also causes changes in cervical mucus (increases difficulty of sperm entry into uterus) and endometrium (reduces likehood of implantation).

PHARMACOKINETICS: Absorption: Rapid. Oral administration of various doses led to altered parameters. **Distribution:** Norgestimate: Albumin binding (>97%). Ethinyl estradiol: Albumin binding (>97%). **Metabolism:** Norgestimate: GI tract and/or liver (1st pass mechanism), hepatic. Norelgestromin (major active metabolite), norgestrel (major active metabolite) Ethinyl estradiol: Hydroxylated, glucuronide, and sulfate conjugates. **Elimination:** Norgestimate: Urine (47%), feces (37%).

NURSING CONSIDERATIONS

Assessment: Assess for current or history of thrombophlebitis or thromboembolic disorder, cerebrovascular or coronary artery disease, valvular heart disease with complications, severe HTN, DM with vascular involvement, headaches with focal neurological symptoms, major surgery with prolonged immobilization, known/suspected or history of carcinoma of the breast, endometrium, or other known or suspected estrogen-dependent neoplasia. Assess use in patients ≥35 who smoke ≥15 cigarettes/day. Assess use with history of HTN, hyperlipidemia, obesity, or DM. Assess for possible drug interactions.

Monitoring: Monitor for MI, thromboembolism, stroke, hepatic neoplasia, breast cancer, ocular lesions, bleeding irregularities, fluid retention, onset or exacerbation of migraines or headaches, gallbladder disease, and ectopic pregnancy. Monitor serum glucose levels in DM and prediabetic patients, BP with history of HTN, lipid levels with history of hyperlipidemia, for signs of worsening depression with previous history, liver function and for signs of liver toxicity (eg, jaundice). Refer patients to an ophthalmologist if ocular changes develop. Perform annual physical exam.

Patient Counseling: Inform that drug does not protect against HIV infection (AIDS) and other STDs. Advise to avoid smoking while on medication. Instruct to take medication at same time everyday. Advise about risk of pregnancy if dose is missed. Counsel that if dose missed, take as soon as possible; take next dose at regularly scheduled time. Inform may have spotting, light bleeding, or stomach sickness during first 1-3 packs of pills; advise not to d/c medication and if symptoms persist, contact physician.

Administration: Oral route. **Storage:** 25°C (77°F); excursions permitted to 15-30°C (59-86°F).

ORTHO-NOVUM 1/35 RX

ethinyl estradiol - norethindrone (Ortho-McNeil)

OTHER BRAND NAMES: Nortrel 1/35 (Barr) - Norinyl 1/35 (Watson) - Necon 1/35 (Watson)

THERAPEUTIC CLASS: Estrogen/progestogen combination

INDICATIONS: Prevention of pregnancy.

DOSAGE: *Adults:* 1 tab qd for 28 days, then repeat. Start 1st Sunday after menses begin or 1st day of menses.

HOW SUPPLIED: Tab: (Ethinyl Estradiol-Norethindrone) 0.035mg-1mg

CONTRAINDICATIONS: Thrombophlebitis, DVT or thromboembolic disorders, pregnancy, cerebrovascular or coronary artery disease, undiagnosed abnormal genital bleeding, cholestatic jaundice of pregnancy or jaundice with prior pill use, hepatic adenomas or carcinomas, breast cancer or other estrogen-dependent neoplasia.

WARNINGS/PRECAUTIONS: Cigarette smoking increases risk of serious cardiovascular side effects. This risk increases with age (especially >35 yrs) and heavy smoking. Increased risk of MI, vascular disease, thromboembolism, stroke and gallbladder disease. Retinal thrombosis, hepatic neoplasia, carcinoma of breast and reproductive organs reported. May cause glucose intolerance. May increase BP, elevate LDL levels or cause other lipid changes, fluid retention, breakthrough bleeding, and spotting. May cause or exacerbate migraine. May develop visual changes with contact lens. Increased risk of MI with HTN, hyperlipidemia, obesity, and diabetes. D/C if jaundice, significant depression, or ophthalmic irregularities develop. Perform annual physical exam. Use before menarche is not indicated. May affect certain endocrine, LFTs and blood components.

ADVERSE REACTIONS: NV, breakthrough bleeding, spotting, amenorrhea, migraine, depression, vaginal candidiasis, edema, weight changes.

INTERACTIONS: Reduced effects, increased breakthrough bleeding, and menstrual irregularities with rifampin, barbiturates, phenylbutazone, phenytoin, carbamazepine, griseofulvin, topiramate, St. John's wort, and possibly with ampicillin and tetracyclines.

PREGNANCY: Category X, not for use in nursing.

MECHANISM OF ACTION: Estrogen/progestogen combination oral contraceptive; acts by suppressing gonadotropins, primarily inhibiting ovulation, and causing changes in cervical mucus (increasing difficulty of sperm entry into uterus) and endometrium (reducing likelihood of implantation).

NURSING CONSIDERATIONS

Assessment: Assess for current/history of thrombophlebitis or thromboembolic disorders, cerebral vascular disorder, CAD, valvular heart disease with complications, severe HTN, DM with vascular involvement, headaches with focal neurological symptoms, major surgery with prolonged immobilization, known/suspected carcinoma of breast, endometrium, or other known/suspected estrogen dependent-neoplasia, undiagnosed abnormal genital bleeding, cholestatic jaundice of pregnancy or jaundice with prior pill use, acute or chronic hepatocellular disease with abnormal liver function, hepatic adenomas or carcinomas, and known/suspected pregnancy. Assess use in patients ≥35 yrs who smoke ≥15 cigarettes/day, with HTN, hyperlipidemia, obesity, DM, and for possible drug interactions.

Monitoring: Monitor for signs/symptoms of MI, thromboembolism, stroke, hepatic neoplasia, breast cancer, ocular lesions, bleeding irregularities, fluid retention, HTN, onset or exacerbation of migraines or headaches, gallbladder disease, and ectopic pregnancy. Monitor serum glucose levels in DM and prediabetic patients, BP with history of HTN, lipid levels with history of hyperlipidemias, signs of liver toxicity (eg, jaundice), and signs of worsening depression. Refer patients with contact lenses to ophthalmologist if ocular changes develop. Perform annual physical exam while on therapy.

Patient Counseling: Counsel about possible side effects. Inform that drug does not protect against HIV (AIDS) and other STDs. Instruct to take pill same time daily; if dose missed, take as soon as possible then take next dose at usual time. Inform may have spotting, light bleeding, or nausea during first 1-3 packs of pills; advise not to d/c medication and if symptoms persist, notify physician. Counsel that if develop vomiting/diarrhea or taking other medication (eg, antibiotics) efficacy may decrease; use backup method of contraception. Advise to avoid smoking while on therapy.

Administration: Oral route. **Storage:** 15-25°C (59-77°F).

Ortho-Novum 1/50 RX

norethindrone - mestranol (Ortho-McNeil)

OTHER BRAND NAMES: Brevicon (Watson) - Necon 1/50 (Watson) - Norinyl 1/50 (Watson)

THERAPEUTIC CLASS: Estrogen/progestogen combination

INDICATIONS: Prevention of pregnancy.

DOSAGE: *Adults:* 1 tab qd for 28 days, then repeat. Start 1st Sunday after menses begins or 1st day of menses.

HOW SUPPLIED: Tab: (Mestranol-Norethindrone) 0.05mg-1mg

CONTRAINDICATIONS: Thrombophlebitis, DVT or thromboembolic disorders, pregnancy, cerebrovascular or coronary artery disease, undiagnosed abnormal genital bleeding, cholestatic jaundice of pregnancy or jaundice with prior pill use, hepatic adenomas or carcinomas, breast cancer or other estrogen-dependent neoplasia.

WARNINGS/PRECAUTIONS: Cigarette smoking increases risk of serious cardiovascular side effects. This risk increases with age (especially >35 yrs) and heavy smoking. Increased risk of MI, vascular disease, thromboembolism, stroke, and gallbladder disease. Retinal thrombosis, hepatic neoplasia, carcinoma of breast and reproductive organs reported. May cause glucose intolerance. May increase BP, elevate LDL levels or cause other lipid changes, fluid retention, breakthrough bleeding, and spotting. May cause or exacerbate migraine. May develop visual changes with contact lens. Increased risk of MI with HTN, hyperlipidemia, obesity, and diabetes. D/C if jaundice, significant depression, or ophthalmic irregularities develop. Perform annual physical exam. Use before menarche is not indicated. May affect certain endocrine, LFTs, and blood components.

ADVERSE REACTIONS: NV, breakthrough bleeding, spotting, amenorrhea, migraine, depression, vaginal candidiasis, edema, weight changes.

INTERACTIONS: Reduced effects, increased breakthrough bleeding, and menstrual irregularities with rifampin, barbiturates, phenylbutazone, phenytoin, carbamazepine, griseofulvin, topiramate, St. John's wort, and possibly with ampicillin and tetracyclines.

PREGNANCY: Category X, not for use in nursing.

MECHANISM OF ACTION: Estrogen/progestogen combination oral contraceptive; acts by suppressing gonadotropin, inhibiting ovulation, causing changes in cervical mucus (increasing difficulty of sperm entry into uterus) and endometrium (reducing likehood of implantation).

PHARMACOKINETICS: Distribution: Found in breast milk.

NURSING CONSIDERATIONS

Assessment: Assess for current or history of thrombophlebitis or thromboembolic disorder, cerebrovascular disease, CAD, known/suspected carcinoma of breast, endometrium or other known/suspected estrogen-dependent neoplasia, undiagnosed abnormal genital bleeding, cholestatic jaundice of pregnancy or jaundice with prior pill use, hepatic adenomas or carcinomas, benign liver tumors, and known/suspected pregnancy. Assess use in patients with hyperlipidemia, hypercholesterolemia, HTN, obesity, DM, and in patients ≥35 yrs who smoke ≥15 cigarettes/day. Assess for possible drug interactions.

Monitoring: Monitor for MI, thromboembolism, stroke, hepatic neoplasia, ocular lesions, bleeding irregularities, fluid retention, onset or exacerbation of headaches or migraines, vascular disease, HTN, hypertriglyceridemia, and gallbladder disease. Monitor glucose levels in DM or prediabetic patients, BP with history of HTN, and lipid levels with history of hyperlipidemia, for signs of liver dysfunction (eg, jaundice), and signs of worsening depression with previous history. Perform annual physical exam while on therapy.

Patient Counseling: Inform that drug does not protect against HIV infection and other STDs. When initiating treatment, instruct to use additional form of contraception until after 7 days on therapy. Instruct to take 1 pill at same time daily at intervals not exceeding 24 hrs. If dose missed, take as soon as possible, then take next dose at regularly scheduled time. Instruct to continue medication if spotting or breakthrough bleeding occur; notify physician if symptoms persist. Inform that missing a pill can cause spotting or light bleeding. Advise not to smoke while on therapy.

Administration: Oral route. **Storage:** 15-25°C (59-77°F).

Ortho-Novum 10/11 RX

ethinyl estradiol - norethindrone (Ortho-McNeil)

OTHER BRAND NAMES: Necon 10/11 (Watson)

THERAPEUTIC CLASS: Estrogen/progestogen combination

INDICATIONS: Prevention of pregnancy.

DOSAGE: *Adults:* 1 tab qd for 28 days, then repeat. Start 1st Sunday after menses begin or 1st day of menses.

HOW SUPPLIED: Tab: (Ethinyl Estradiol-Norethindrone) 0.035mg-0.5mg and 0.035mg-1mg

CONTRAINDICATIONS: Thrombophlebitis, DVT or thromboembolic disorders, pregnancy, cerebrovascular or coronary artery disease, undiagnosed abnormal genital bleeding, cholestatic jaundice of pregnancy or jaundice with prior pill use, hepatic adenomas or carcinomas, breast cancer or other estrogen-dependent neoplasia.

WARNINGS/PRECAUTIONS: Cigarette smoking increases risk of serious cardiovascular side effects; risk increases with age (especially >35 yrs) and heavy smoking. Increased risk of MI, vascular disease, thromboembolism, stroke, and gallbladder disease. Retinal thrombosis, hepatic neoplasia reported. May cause glucose intolerance. May increase BP, elevate LDL levels or cause other lipid changes, fluid retention, breakthrough bleeding, and spotting. May cause or exacerbate migraine. May develop visual changes with contact lens. Morbidity and mortality risk increased with HTN, hyperlipidemia, obesity, and diabetes. D/C if jaundice, significant depression, or ophthalmic irregularities develop. Perform annual physical exam. Use before menarche is not indicated. May affect certain endocrine, LFTs, and blood components.

ADVERSE REACTIONS: NV, breakthrough bleeding, spotting, amenorrhea, migraine, depression, vaginal candidiasis, edema, weight changes.

INTERACTIONS: Reduced effects, increased breakthrough bleeding, and menstrual irregularities with rifampin, barbiturates, phenylbutazone, phenytoin, carbamazepine, and possibly with griseofulvin, ampicillin, and tetracyclines.

PREGNANCY: Category X, not for use in nursing.

MECHANISM OF ACTION: Estrogen/progestogen combination oral contraceptive; acts by suppressing gonadotropins. Primarily inhibits ovulation. Also causes changes in cervical mucus (increases difficulty of sperm entry into uterus) and endometrium (reduces likelihood of implantation).

PHARMACOKINETICS: Distribution: Found in breast milk.

NURSING CONSIDERATIONS

Assessment: Assess for current or history of thrombophlebitis or thromboembolic disorders, cerebrovascular disease, CAD, valvular heart disease with complications, severe HTN, DM with vascular involvement, headaches with focal neurological symptoms, major surgery with prolonged immobilization, known/suspected carcinoma of breast, endometrium or other known/suspected estrogen-dependent neoplasia, undiagnosed abnormal genital bleeding, cholestatic jaundice of pregnancy or jaundice with prior pill use, acute or chronic hepatocellular disease with abnormal liver function, hepatic adenoma or carcinoma, and known/suspected pregnancy. Assess use with HTN, hyperlipidemias, obesity, DM, or in patients ≥35 yrs who smoke ≥15 cigarettes/day). Assess for possible drug interactions.

Monitoring: Monitor for signs/symptoms of MI, thromboembolism, stroke, vascular disease, hepatic neoplasia, ocular lesions, bleeding irregularities, fluid retention, onset or exacerbation of migraines or headaches, gallbladder disease, hypertriglyceridemia, HTN, and ectopic pregnancy. Monitor serum glucose levels in DM and prediabetic patients, lipid levels with history of hyperlipidemia, for signs of liver dysfunction (eg, jaundice), for signs of worsening depression with previous history. Refer patients with contact lenses to ophthalmologist if ocular changes develop. Perform annual physical exam while on medication.

Patient Counseling: Inform that does not protect against HIV infection and other STDs. Advise to avoid smoking while on therapy. Instruct to take 1 pill at same time daily, at intervals not exceeding 24 hrs. Instruct if dose is missed, take as soon as possible, then take next dose at regularly scheduled time. Inform may have spotting, light bleeding, or stomach upset during first 1-3 packs of pills; advise not to d/c medication and notify physician if symptoms persist. Inform if vomiting, having diarrhea, or taking concomitant medications, efficacy of medication may be affected; use backup forms of contraception.

Administration: Oral route. **Storage:** 25°C (77°F); excursions permitted to 15-30°C (59-86°F).

Ortho-Novum 7/7/7 RX

ethinyl estradiol - norethindrone (Ortho-McNeil)

OTHER BRAND NAMES: Nortrel 7/7/7 (Barr)

THERAPEUTIC CLASS: Estrogen/progestogen combination

INDICATIONS: Prevention of pregnancy.

DOSAGE: *Adults:* 1 tab qd for 28 days, then repeat. Start 1st Sunday after menses begin or 1st day of menses.

HOW SUPPLIED: Tab: (Ethinyl Estradiol-Norethindrone) 0.035mg-0.5mg, 0.035mg-0.75mg and 0.035mg-1mg

CONTRAINDICATIONS: Thrombophlebitis, DVT or thromboembolic disorders, pregnancy, cerebrovascular or coronary artery disease, undiagnosed abnormal genital bleeding, cholestatic jaundice of pregnancy or jaundice with prior pill use, hepatic adenomas or carcinomas, breast cancer or other estrogen-dependent neoplasia.

WARNINGS/PRECAUTIONS: Cigarette smoking increases risk of serious cardiovascular side effects; risk increases with age (especially >35 yrs) and heavy smoking. Increased risk of MI, vascular disease, thromboembolism, stroke and gallbladder disease. Retinal thrombosis, hepatic neoplasia, carcinoma of breast and reproductive organs reported. May cause glucose intolerance. May increase BP, elevate LDL levels or cause other lipid changes, fluid retention, breakthrough bleeding, and spotting. May cause or exacerbate migraine. May develop visual changes with contact lens. Increased risk of MI with HTN, hyperlipidemia, obesity, and diabetes. D/C if jaundice, significant depression or ophthalmic irregularities develop. Perform annual physical exam. Use before menarche is not indicated. May affect certain endocrine, LFTs, and blood components.

ADVERSE REACTIONS: NV, breakthrough bleeding, spotting, amenorrhea, migraine, depression, vaginal candidiasis, edema, weight changes.

INTERACTIONS: Reduced effects, increased breakthrough bleeding, and menstrual irregularities with rifampin, barbiturates, phenylbutazone, phenytoin, carbamazepine, griseofulvin, topiramate, St. John's wort, and possibly with ampicillin and tetracyclines.

PREGNANCY: Category X, not for use in nursing.

MECHANISM OF ACTION: Estrogen/progestogen combination oral contraceptive; acts by suppression of gonadotropins. Primarily inhibits ovulation. Also causes changes in cervical mucus (increases difficulty of sperm entry into uterus) and endometrium (reduces likelihood of implantation).

PHARMACOKINETICS: Distribution: Found in breast milk.

NURSING CONSIDERATIONS

Assessment: Assess for current or history of thrombophlebitis or thromboembolic disorders, cerebrovascular disease, CAD, valvular heart disease with complications, severe HTN, DM with vascular involvement, headaches with focal neurological symptoms, major surgery with prolonged immobilization, known/suspected carcinoma of breast, endometrium or other known/suspected estrogen dependent neoplasia, undiagnosed abnormal genital bleeding, cholestatic jaundice of pregnancy or jaundice with prior pill use, acute or chronic hepatocellular disease with abnormal liver function, hepatic adenoma or carcinoma, and known/suspected pregnancy. Assess use in patients with HTN, hyperlipidemia, obesity, DM, in patient ≥35 yrs who smoke ≥15 cigarettes/day. Assess for possible drug interactions.

Monitoring: Monitor for MI, thromboembolism, stroke, vascular disease, hepatic neoplasia, ocular lesions, bleeding irregularities, fluid retention, onset or exacerbation of migraines or headaches, gallbladder disease, hypertriglyceridemia, HTN, and ectopic pregnancy. Monitor serum glucose levels in DM and prediabetic patients, lipid levels with history of hyperlipidemia, for signs of liver dysfunction (eg, jaundice), and signs of worsening depression with previous history. Refer patients with contact lenses to an ophthalmologist if ocular changes develop. Perform annual history and physical exam.

Patient Counseling: Inform that drug does not protect against HIV infection and other STDs. Advise not to smoke while on therapy. Instruct to take 1 pill at same time daily at intervals not exceeding 24 hrs. Counsel if dose missed, take as soon as possible; take next dose at regularly scheduled time. Inform may have spotting, light bleeding, or nausea during first 1-3 packs of pills; advise not to d/c medication and if symptoms persist, notify physician. Inform that if vomiting, diarrhea, or taking concomitant medications, efficacy of medication may be effected; use backup forms of contraception.

Administration: Oral route. **Storage**: 25°C (77°F); excursions permitted to 15-30°C (59-86°F).

OVACE

RX

sulfacetamide sodium (Healthpoint)

THERAPEUTIC CLASS: Sulfonamide

INDICATIONS: Topical application for seborrheic dermatitis, seborrhea sicca (dandruff). Treatment of secondary bacterial infections of the skin.

DOSAGE: *Adults:* Seborrheic Dermatitis/Dandruff: (Cre/Gel/Foam) Apply to affected area bid for 8-10 days. (Wash) Wash affected area bid for 8-10 days. To prevent recurrence, apply once or twice weekly, or every other week. Bacterial Infection: (Cre/Gel) Apply to affected area bid for 8-10 days. (Foam) Apply to affected area qd for 8-10 days. (Wash) Wash affected area qd for 8-10 days.

HOW SUPPLIED: Cre: 10% [30g, 60g]; Gel: 10% [30g, 60g]; Foam: 10% [50g, 100g]; Wash: 10% [170mL, 340mL]

CONTRAINDICATIONS: Hypersensitivity to sulfonamides.

WARNINGS/PRECAUTIONS: Stevens-Johnson syndrome in hypersensitive individuals, and systemic lupus erythematous reported with sulfonamides. May cause proliferation of nonsusceptible organisms. D/C if hypersensitivity or untoward reactions occur. Greater systemic absorption in application to large, infected, abraded, denuded or severely burned area.

ADVERSE REACTIONS: Irritation, hypersensitivity.

INTERACTIONS: Incompatible with silver preparations.

PREGNANCY: Category C, caution in nursing.

MECHANISM OF ACTION: Sulfonamide; exerts a bacteriostatic effect against susceptible gram-positive and gram-negative microorganisms. Acts by restricting the synthesis of folic acid required by bacteria for growth, through competition with paraminobenzoic acid (PABA).

NURSING CONSIDERATIONS

Assessment: Assess for sulfonamide hypersensitivity. Assess use in pregnant/nursing females. Assess for possible drug interactions.

Monitoring: Monitor for signs/symptoms of hypersensitivity reactions, Stevens-Johnson syndrome, drug-induced systemic lupus erythematosus, overgrowth of nonsusceptible organism (eg, fungi). In patients applying medication to a large, infected, abraded, denuded, or severely burned area, monitor for increased occurrence of adverse drug events.

Patient Counseling: Counsel to d/c therapy and notify physician if condition worsens or if rash develops. Instruct to contact physician if any signs of arthritis, fever, or sores of the mouth develop while on medication.

Administration: Topical route. **Storage**: 20-25°C (68-77°F). Do not freeze. Keep out of reach of children.

Ovcon-35 RX

ethinyl estradiol - norethindrone (Warner Chilcott)

OTHER BRAND NAMES: Balziva (Barr) - Ovcon-50 (Warner Chilcott)

THERAPEUTIC CLASS: Estrogen/progestogen combination

INDICATIONS: Prevention of pregnancy.

DOSAGE: *Adults:* 1 tab qd for 28 days, then repeat. Start 1st Sunday after menses begin or the 1st day of menses.

HOW SUPPLIED: Tab: (Ethinyl Estradiol-Norethindrone) (Ovcon 35, Balziva) 0.035mg-0.4mg; (Ovcon 50) 0.05mg-1mg

CONTRAINDICATIONS: Thrombophlebitis, DVT or thromboembolic disorders, pregnancy, cerebrovascular or coronary artery disease, valvular heart disease with thrombogenic complications, uncontrolled HTN, DM with vascular involvement, HA with focal neurological symptoms, major surgery with prolonged immobilization, undiagnosed abnormal genital bleeding, cholestatic jaundice of pregnancy or jaundice with prior pill use, hepatic adenomas or carcinomas, breast cancer, endometrial cancer or other estrogen-dependent neoplasia.

WARNINGS/PRECAUTIONS: Cigarette smoking increases risk of serious cardiovascular side effects. This risk increases with age (especially >35 yrs) and heavy smoking. Increased risk of MI, vascular disease, thromboembolism, stroke and gallbladder disease. Retinal thrombosis, hepatic neoplasia, carcinoma of breast and reproductive organs reported. May cause glucose intolerance. May increase BP, elevate LDL levels or cause other lipid changes, fluid retention, breakthrough bleeding, and spotting. May cause or exacerbate migraine. May develop visual changes with contact lens. Increased risk of MI with HTN, hyperlipidemia, obesity, and diabetes. D/C if develop jaundice, significant depression or ophthalmic irregularities. Perform annual physical exam. Use before menarche is not indicated. May affect certain endocrine, LFTs and blood components.

ADVERSE REACTIONS: NV, breakthrough bleeding, spotting, amenorrhea, migraine, depression, vaginal candidiasis, edema, weight changes.

INTERACTIONS: Reduced effects, increased breakthrough bleeding, and menstrual irregularities with rifampin, barbiturates, phenylbutazone, phenytoin, carbamazepine, felbamate, oxcarbazepine, topiramate, griseofulvin, ampicillin, and tetracyclines. Anti-HIV PIs may change (increase or decrease) the levels of OCs. Herbal products, such as St. John's wort may reduce the levels of OCs and result in breakthrough bleeding. Atorvastatin, ascorbic acid, acetaminophen, CYP3A4 inhibitors (itraconazole or ketoconazole) may increase the levels of ehinyl estradiol. Increased levels of cyclosporin, prednisolone, theophylline reported. Decreased levels of actaminophen and increased clearance of temazepam, salicylic acid, morphine, clofibric acid reported.

PREGNANCY: Category X, not for use in nursing.

MECHANISM OF ACTION: Estrogen/progestogen combination oral contraceptive; acts by suppressing gonadotropins, primarily inhibiting ovulation, and causing changes in cervical mucus (increasing difficulty of sperm entry into uterus) and endometrium (reducing likelihood of implantation).

PHARMACOKINETICS: Distribution: Found in breast milk.

NURSING CONSIDERATIONS

Assessment: Assess for current or history of thrombophlebitis or thromboembolic disorders, cerebrovascular disease, CAD, valvular heart disease with complications, severe HTN, DM with vascular involvement, headaches with focal neurological symptoms, major surgery with prolonged immobilization, known/suspected carcinoma of breast and endometrium or other known/suspected estrogen dependent-neoplasia, undiagnosed abnormal genital bleeding, cholestatic jaundice of pregnancy or jaundice with prior pill use, acute or chronic hepatocellular disease with abnormal liver function, hepatic adenomas or carcinomas, and known/suspected pregnancy. Assess use in patients ≥35 yrs who smoke ≥15 cigarettes/day, with HTN, hyperlipidemia, obesity, DM, and for possible drug interactions.

Monitoring: Monitor for MI, thromboembolism, stroke, hepatic neoplasia, breast cancer, ocular lesions, bleeding irregularities, fluid retention, HTN, onset or exacerbation of migraines or headaches, gallbladder disease, and ectopic pregnancy. Monitor serum glucose levels in DM and prediabetic patients, BP with history of HTN, lipid levels with history of hyperlipidemias, signs of liver toxicity (eg, jaundice), and signs of worsening depression. Refer patients with contact lenses to ophthalmologist if ocular changes develop. Perform annual physical exam while on therapy.

Patient Counseling: Counsel about possible serious side effects. Inform that medication does not protect against HIV/AIDS and other STDs. Advise to avoid smoking while on therapy. Instruct to take 1 pill at same time daily. If dose missed, take as soon as remembered; take next dose at usual time. If spotting, light bleeding, or nausea occurs during first 1-3 packs of pills, advise not to d/c medication and if symptoms persist, notify physician. Inform if vomiting, diarrhea or taking other medications, efficacy may decrease; use backup method of contraception.

Administration: Oral route. **Storage:** Below 30°C (86°F).

Ovcon-35 Fe — RX

ethinyl estradiol - ferrous fumarate - norethindrone (Warner Chilcott)

THERAPEUTIC CLASS: Estrogen/progestogen combination

INDICATIONS: Prevention of pregnancy.

DOSAGE: *Adults:* 1 tab qd for 28 days, then repeat. Start 1st Sunday after menses begin or the 1st day of menses.

HOW SUPPLIED: Tab, Chewable: (Ethinyl Estradiol-Norethindrone) 0.035mg-0.4mg [21[s]], (Ferrous Fumarate) 75mg [7[s]]

CONTRAINDICATIONS: Thrombophlebitis, DVT or thromboembolic disorders, pregnancy, cerebrovascular or coronary artery disease, valvular heart disease with thrombogenic complications, uncontrolled HTN, DM with vascular involvement, HA with focal neurological symptoms, major surgery with prolonged immobilization, undiagnosed abnormal genital bleeding, cholestatic jaundice of pregnancy or jaundice with prior pill use, hepatic adenomas or carcinomas, breast cancer, endometrial cancer or other estrogen-dependent neoplasia.

WARNINGS/PRECAUTIONS: Cigarette smoking increases risk of serious cardiovascular side effects; risk increases with age (especially >35 yrs) and heavy smoking. Increased risk of MI, vascular disease, thromboembolism, stroke and gallbladder disease. Retinal thrombosis, hepatic neoplasia, carcinoma of breast and reproductive organs reported. May cause glucose intolerance. May increase BP, elevate LDL levels or cause other lipid changes, fluid retention, breakthrough bleeding, and spotting. May cause or exacerbate migraine. May develop visual changes with contact lens. Increased risk of MI with HTN, hyperlipidemia, obesity, and diabetes. D/C if jaundice, significant depression, or ophthalmic irregularities develop. Perform annual physical exam. Use before menarche is not indicated. May affect certain endocrine, LFTs and blood components.

ADVERSE REACTIONS: NV, breakthrough bleeding, spotting, amenorrhea, migraine, depression, vaginal candidiasis, edema, weight changes.

INTERACTIONS: Reduced effects, increased breakthrough bleeding, and menstrual irregularities with rifampin, barbiturates, phenylbutazone, phenytoin, carbamazepine, felbamate, oxcarbazepine, topiramate, griseofulvin, ampicillin, and tetracyclines. Anti-HIV PIs may change (increase or decrease) the levels of OCs. Herbal products, such as St. John's wort may reduce the levels of OCs and result in breakthrough bleeding. Atorvastatin, ascorbic acid, acetaminophen, CYP3A4 inhibitors (itraconazole or ketoconazole) may increase the levels of ethinyl estradiol. Increased levels of cyclosporine, prednisolone, theophylline reported. Decreased levels of acetaminophen and increased clearance of temazepam, salicylic acid, morphine, clofibric acid reported.

PREGNANCY: Category X, not for use in nursing.

MECHANISM OF ACTION: Estrogen/progestogen combination oral contraceptive; acts by suppressing gonadotropins. Primarily inhibits ovulation. Also causes changes in cervical mucus (increases difficulty of sperm entry ino uterus) and endometrium (reduces likehood of implantation).

PHARMACOKINETICS: Absorption: Rapid. Norethindrone: Absolute bioavailability (65%), C_{max}=4210.6pg/mL, T_{max}=1.24 hr, AUC=18034.9pg•h/mL. Ethinyl estradiol: Absolute bioavailability (43%), C_{max}=131.4pg/mL, T_{max}=1.44 hrs, AUC=1065.8pg•h/mL. **Distribution:** V_d=2-4L/kg; Norethindone: Sex hormone-binding globulin binding (36%), albumin binding (61%). Ethinyl estradiol: Albumin binding (98.5%). **Metabolism:** Norethindone: Reduction, sulfate, glucuronide conjugation. Ethinyl estradiol: CYP3A4, via oxidation (conjugation with sulfate and glucuronide), 2-hydroxy-ethinyl estradiol (primary oxidative metabolite). **Elimination:** Norethindrone: Urine (50%), feces (20-40%); $T_{1/2}$=9 hrs. Ethinyl Estradiol: Urine, feces; $T_{1/2}$=17 hrs.

NURSING CONSIDERATIONS

Assessment: Assess for current or history of thrombophlebitis or thromboembolic disorder, cerebrovascular disease, CAD, valvular heart disease with thrombogenic complications, uncontrolled HTN, DM with vascular involvement, headaches with focal neurological problems, major surgery with prolonged immobilization, known/suspected carcinoma of breast, endometrium or other known/suspected estrogen-dependent neoplasia, abnormal genital bleeding, cholestatic jaundice, hepatic adenomas or carcinoma, and known/suspected pregnancy. Assess use with inherited thrombophilias, HTN, hyperlipidemias, obesity, DM, or in patients ≥35 yrs who smoke ≥15 cigarettes/day. Assess for possible drug/lab test interactions.

Monitoring: Monitor for venous and arterial thrombotic events (eg, MI, thromboembolism, stroke), hepatic neoplasias, ocular lesions, bleeding irregularities, fluid retention, onset or exacerbation of headaches or migraines, gallbladder disease, hypertriglyceridemia, and HTN. Monitor blood glucose levels in DM and prediabetic patients, BP with history of HTN, lipid levels with history of hyperlipidemia, for signs of liver dysfunction (eg, jaundice), and of worsening depression with previous history. Refer patients with contact lenses to an ophthalmologist if visual changes occur. Perform annual history and physical exam.

Patient Counseling: Advise about possible serious cardiovascular and respiratory effects. Inform that medication does not protect against HIV infection (AIDS) and other STDs. Advise to avoid smoking while on medication. Instruct to take medication at same time daily. Instruct if dose missed, take as soon as possible; take next pill at regularly scheduled time. Inform may have spotting, light bleeding, or stomach upset during first 1-3 packs of pills; advise not to d/c medication and if symptoms persist, notify physician. If vomiting, diarrhea, or taking other medications may alter efficacy; use backup forms of contraception. Perform regular physical exams.

Administration: Oral route. **Storage:** 25° (77°F); excursions permitted to 15-30°C (59-86°F).

OxyContin CII

oxycodone HCl (Purdue Pharma)

For continuous analgesia. Abuse potential. 80mg tabs only for opioid-tolerant patients. Swallow tabs whole.

THERAPEUTIC CLASS: Opioid analgesic

INDICATIONS: Management of moderate to severe pain when a continuous analgesic is needed for an extended period. Only for postoperative use in patients already receiving the drug before surgery or those expected to have moderate-severe postoperative pain for an extended period of time.

DOSAGE: *Adults:* ≥18 yrs: Opioid Naive: 10mg q12h. Titrate: May increase to 20mg q12h, then may increase the total daily dose by 25-50% of the current dose. Increase every 1-2 days. Conversion from Oxycodone: Divide 24 hr oxycodone dose in half to obtain q12h dose. Round down to appropriate tab strength. Opioid Tolerant Patients: May use 80mg tabs. D/C other around-the-clock opioids. With CNS Depressants: Reduce dose by 1/3 or 1/2. Swallow whole; do not break, crush, or chew.

HOW SUPPLIED: Tab, Extended-Release: 10mg, 20mg, 40mg, 80mg

CONTRAINDICATIONS: Significant respiratory depression, acute or severe bronchial asthma, hypercarbia, paralytic ileus.

WARNINGS/PRECAUTIONS: Do not break, chew, or crush tabs. Extreme caution with COPD, cor pulmonale, decreased respiratory reserve, hypoxia, hypercapnia, pre-existing respiratory depression. Caution with circulatory shock, delirium tremens, acute alcoholism, adrenocortical insufficiency, CNS depression, myxedema or hypothyroidism, BPH, severe hepatic/renal/pulmonary impairment, toxic psychosis, biliary tract disease, increased ICP or head injury, elderly or debilitated. May cause severe hypotension. May produce drug dependence; caution in known drug abuse. May aggravate convulsive disorders and mask abdominal disorders.

ADVERSE REACTIONS: Respiratory depression, constipation, NV, somnolence, dizziness, pruritus, headache, dry mouth, sweating, asthenia.

INTERACTIONS: Respiratory depression, hypotension and profound sedation with other CNS depressants (eg, sedatives, anesthetics, phenothiazines, alcohol). Mixed agonist/antagonist analgesics may reduce the analgesic effect and/or cause withdrawal. Risk of severe hypotension with phenothiazines, or other agents that compromise vasomotor tone. May enhance skeletal muscle relaxant effects and increase respiratory depression. May interact with CYP2D6 inhibitors (eg, amiodarone, quinidine, polycyclic antidepressants). Caution with MAOIs.

PREGNANCY: Category B, not for use in nursing.

MECHANISM OF ACTION: Opioid analgesic; pure agonist opioid whose principle therapeutic action is analgesia. Precise analgesic action not established. However, specific CNS opioid receptors for endogenous compounds with opioid-like activity have been found throughout the brain and spinal cord and play a role in analgesic effects.

PHARMACOKINETICS: Absorption: Well absorbed, various doses resulted in altered parameters. **Distribution:** V_d=2.6L/kg; plasma protein binding (45%); found in breast milk. **Metabolism:** Extensively to noroxycodone (major metabolite), CYP2D6 to oxymorphone (active metabolite). **Elimination:** Urine (major); $T_{1/2}$=4.5 hrs.

NURSING CONSIDERATIONS

Assessment: Assess for respiratory depression, type and level of pain, acute or severe bronchial asthma or hypercarbia, COPD or cor pulmonale, kyphoscoliosis, paralytic ileus, risk for drug misuse or abuse, head injury, intracranial lesions, increased ICP, circulatory shock, acute alcoholism, adrenocortical insufficiency (eg, Addison's disease), CNS depression or coma, delirium tremens, presence of debilitation (eg, elderly), myexedema or hypothyroidism, prostatic hypertrophy or urethral stricture, hepatic/renal impairment, presence of acute abdominal conditions, biliary tract disease, acute pancreatitis, toxic psychosis, convulsive seizures, pregnancy/nursing status, and possible drug interactions.

Monitoring: Monitor for signs/symptoms of respiratory depression, elevations in CSF pressure, hypotension, spasm of sphincter of Oddi, tolerance and physical dependence, and abuse/misuse of medication. Monitor serum amylase levels.

Patient Counseling: Instruct to swallow medication whole; do not break, chew, or crush. If broken or chewed, contents may release all at once and cause fatal overdose. Advise to report episodes of breakthough pain or adverse events (eg, respiratory depression). Do not adjust dosing without consulting physician. May impair mental/physical abilities; use caution if performing hazardous tasks (eg, operating machinery, driving). Avoid alcohol or other CNS depressants. Inform that medication has potential for abuse; protect from theft. Inform patient may pass empty matrix tablets via stool. If on medication for more than a few weeks, avoid abrupt withdrawal; taper dosing. Keep out of reach of children. Dispose any unused medication via toilet.

Administration: Oral route. **Storage:** 25°C (77°F); excursions permitted to15-30°C (59-86°F). Dispense in tight, light-resistant container.

OxyIR

CII

oxycodone HCl (Purdue Pharma)

THERAPEUTIC CLASS: Opioid analgesic

INDICATIONS: Moderate to moderately severe pain.

DOSAGE: *Adults:* Usual: 5mg q6h prn for pain. May add to 30mL of juice or other liquid, applesauce, pudding, or other semi-solid foods.

HOW SUPPLIED: Cap: 5mg

CONTRAINDICATIONS: Respiratory depression, acute or severe bronchial asthma, hypercarbia, paralytic ileus, situations where opioids are contraindicated.

WARNINGS/PRECAUTIONS: Extreme caution with COPD, cor pulmonale, decreased respiratory reserve, hypoxia, hypercapnia, pre-existing respiratory depression. Caution with circulatory shock, delirium tremens, acute alcoholism, adrenocortical insufficiency, CNS depression, myxedema or hypothyroidism, BPH, severe hepatic/renal/pulmonary impairment, toxic psychosis, biliary tract disease, increased ICP, or head injury, elderly or debilitated. May cause severe hypotension. May produce drug dependence; caution in known drug abuse. May aggravate convulsive disorders and mask abdominal disorders. May impair mental/physical abilities.

ADVERSE REACTIONS: Lightheadedness, dizziness, NV, sedation.

INTERACTIONS: Respiratory depression, hypotension and profound sedation with other CNS depressants (eg, sedatives, anesthetics, phenothiazines, alcohol). Mixed agonist/antagonist analgesics may reduce the analgesic effect and/or cause withdrawal. Risk of severe hypotension with phenothiazines, or other agents that compromise vasomotor tone. May enhance skeletal muscle relaxant effects and increase respiratory depression. May interact with CYP2D6 inhibitors (eg, amiodarone, quinidine, polycyclic antidepressants). Caution with MAOIs.

PREGNANCY: Category B, not for use in nursing.

MECHANISM OF ACTION: Opioid analgesic; pure agonist opioid whose principle therapeutic effect is analgesia. Precise action not established. However, specific CNS opioid receptors for endogenous compounds with opioid-like activity are found throughout the brain and spinal cord and play a role in analgesic effects.

PHARMACOKINETICS: Distribution: Found in breast milk. **Metabolism:** Via CYP2D6 to oxymorphone (metabolite).

NURSING CONSIDERATIONS

Assessment: Assess for respiratory depression, acute or severe bronchial asthma or hypercarbia, chronic obstructive pulmonary disease, paralytic ileus, circulatory shock, pregnancy/nursing status, acute alcoholism, adrenocortical insufficiency (eg, Addison's disease), CNS depression or coma, delirium tremens, presence of debilitation (eg, elderly), kyphoscoliosis associated with respiratory depression, myxedema or hypothyroidism, prostatic hypertrophy or urethral stricture, severe impairment of hepatic/renal function, toxic psychosis, convulsive disorders, biliary tract disease, acute pancreatitis, presence of head injury or other intracranial lesions, presence of increased ICP, acute abdominal condition, and possible drug interactions.

Monitoring: Monitor for signs/symptoms of respiratory depression, hypotension, convulsions, medication dependence and tolerance, medication abuse, sphincter of Oddi spasms, elevations in CSF pressure, and elevations in serum amylase levels.

Patient Counseling: Advise not to adjust dosing without consulting physician. Inform that medication may impair mental/physical abilities required for performing hazardous tasks (eg, operating machinery/driving). Counsel to avoid alcohol and other CNS depressants. Inform medication has potential for abuse; protect from theft. Advise not to abruptly d/c medication if on therapy for a few weeks; taper dosing.

Administration: Oral route. **Storage:** 25°C (77°F); excursions permitted to 15-30°C (59-86°F).

OXYTROL — RX

oxybutynin (Watson)

THERAPEUTIC CLASS: Anticholinergic

INDICATIONS: Treatment of overactive bladder with symptoms of urge urinary incontinence, urgency, and frequency.

DOSAGE: *Adults:* Apply to dry, intact skin on the abdomen, hip, or buttock twice weekly (every 3-4 days). Rotate sites.

HOW SUPPLIED: Patch: 3.9mg/day [8^s]

CONTRAINDICATIONS: Urinary retention, gastric retention, uncontrolled narrow-angle glaucoma, and in patients at risk for these conditions.

WARNINGS/PRECAUTIONS: Caution with hepatic or renal impairment, bladder outflow obstruction, GI obstructive disorders, ulcerative colitis, intestinal atony, myasthenia gravis, and gastroesophageal reflux. Heat prostration may occur when used in a hot environment.

ADVERSE REACTIONS: Application site reactions, dry mouth, diarrhea, constipation, drowsiness, dizziness, blurred vision.

INTERACTIONS: Increased adverse events with other anticholinergics. Alcohol may enhance drowsiness effect. Caution with bisphosphonates or other drugs that may exacerbate esophagitis. May alter GI absorption of other drugs due to GI motility effects.

PREGNANCY: Category B, caution in nursing.

MECHANISM OF ACTION: Antispasmodic, anticholinergic agent; acts as competitive antagonist of acetylcholine at postganglionic muscarinic receptor, resulting in relaxation of bladder smooth muscle.

PHARMACOKINETICS: Absorption: (Single dose) C_{max}=3-3.4ng/mL; T_{max}=36-48 hrs. (Multiple dose) C_{max}=4.2-6.6ng/mL; T_{max}=10-28 hrs. **Distribution:** V_d=193L. **Metabolism:** CYP3A4, N-desethyloxybutynin (active metabolite). **Elimination:** Urine (<0.1%); $T_{1/2}$=7-8 hrs.

NURSING CONSIDERATIONS

Assessment: Assess for bladder outflow obstruction (urinary retention), GI obstructive disorders (gastric retention), narrow-angle glaucoma, possible drug interactions, GERD, esophagitis, ulcerative colitis, intestinal atony, myasthenia gravis, renal/hepatic impairment.

Monitoring: Monitor for signs/symptoms of gastric retention, urinary retention, decreased gastric motility, hypersensitivity reactions, renal/hepatic dysfunction.

Patient Counseling: Inform heat prostration may occur in hot environment. Dizziness and blurred vision may also occur. Alcohol may enhance drowsiness. Apply to dry, intact skin on abdomen, hip, or buttocks. Avoid reapplication to same site for 7 days.

Administration: Transdermal route. **Storage:** 25°C (77°F); excursions permitted to 15-30°C (59-86°F). Protect from moisture and humidity. Do not store outside the sealed pouch.

PACERONE — RX

amiodarone HCl (Upsher-Smith)

THERAPEUTIC CLASS: Class III antiarrhythmic

INDICATIONS: Treatment of documented, life-threatening recurrent ventricular fibrillation and recurrent hemodynamically unstable ventricular tachycardia.

DOSAGE: *Adults:* Give LD in hospital. LD: 800-1600mg/day in divided doses for 1-3 weeks. After control is achieved, then 600-800mg/day for 1 month. Maint: 400mg/day; up to 600mg/day if needed. Use lowest effective dose. Take with meals. Elderly: Start at low end of dosing range.

HOW SUPPLIED: Tab: 100mg, 200mg*, 300mg*, 400mg* *scored

CONTRAINDICATIONS: Severe sinus-node dysfunction causing marked sinus bradycardia; 2nd- and 3rd-degree AV block; when episodes of bradycardia have caused syncope (except when used with a pacemaker).

P

WARNINGS/PRECAUTIONS: Only for life-threatening arrhythmias due to its substantial toxicity (eg, pulmonary toxicity, hepatic injury, arrhythmia exacerbation). Hospitalize when giving LD. May cause a clinical syndrome of cough and progressive dyspnea. D/C if LFTs are 3x the normal or if an elevated baseline doubles; monitor LFTs regularly. Optic neuropathy, optic neuritis reported. Fetal harm in pregnancy. May develop reversible corneal micro deposits (eg, visual halos, blurred vision), photosensitivity, peripheral neuropathy (rare). May decrease T_3 levels, increase thyroxine levels, increase inactive reverse T_3 levels and can cause hypo- or hyperthyroidism. Adult Respiratory Distress Syndrome reported with surgery. Correct K^+ or magnesium deficiency before therapy. Caution in elderly.

ADVERSE REACTIONS: Pulmonary toxicity (inflammation, fibrosis), arrhythmia exacerbation, hepatic injury, malaise, fatigue, tremor, poor coordination, paresthesis, NV, constipation, anorexia, ophthalmic abnormalities, photosensitivity.

INTERACTIONS: Risk of interactions after discontinuation due to long half-life. May increase sensitivity to myocardial depressant and conduction effects of halogenated inhalation anesthetics. Elevates cyclosporine plasma levels. D/C or reduce digoxin dose by 50%. D/C or decrease warfarin dose by 1/3-1/2. Caution with β-blockers, calcium channel blockers. May increase levels of quinidine, procainamide and phenytoin. Initiate added antiarrhythmic drug at lower than usual dose. D/C or decrease quinidine dose by 1/3-1/2. D/C or decrease procainamide dose by 1/3.

PREGNANCY: Category D, not for use in nursing.

MECHANISM OF ACTION: Class III antiarrhythmic; prolongs the myocardial cell-action potential duration and refractory period and noncompetitively inhibits α- and β-adrenergic receptors, which leads to decreased sinus rate, increased PR and QT interval, development of U-waves and changes in T-wave contour.

PHARMACOKINETICS: Absorption: Slow; bioavailability (50%); T_{max}=3-7 hrs. **Distribution:** V_d=60L/kg; protein binding (96%); found in breast milk. **Metabolism:** Liver via CYP3A4, 2C8; desethylamidarone (major metabolite). **Elimination:** Bile (major), urine.

NURSING CONSIDERATIONS

Assessment: Assess for cardiogenic shock, severe sinus-node dysfunction, bradycardia, second- or third-degree HB, syncope, presence of functioning pacemaker, liver impairment, thyroid function, hypokalemia or hypomagnesemia, pregnancy/nursing status, and possible drug interactions. Perform baseline chest X-ray and pulmonary function tests, including diffusion capacity.

Monitoring: Monitoring of history, physical exam, chest X-ray, and pulmonary function should be repeated every 3-6 months and evaluated. Monitor for pulmonary toxicities (eg, hypersensitivity pneumonitis or interstitial/alveolar pneumonitis), worsening of arrhythmia, induced hyperthyroidism/thyrotoxicosis, hepatic failure, optic neuritis/neuropathy, corneal microdeposits, loss of vision, neonatal hypo/hyperthyroidism, peripheral neuropathy, and photosensitivity. Monitor LFTs regularly, T4, T3, and reverse T3. Monitoring for hypotension and adult respiratory distress syndrome recommended with surgery.

Patient Counseling: Therapy should only be administered by physician experienced in treatment of life-threatening arrhythmia. Inform about risks/benefits; report adverse reactions. Avoid prolonged exposure to sunlight. Notify if pregnant/nursing.

Administration: Oral route. Do not take with grapefruit juice. **Storage:** 20-25°C (68-77°F). Protect from light.

PAMELOR RX

nortriptyline HCl (Mallinckrodt)

Antidepressants increased the risk of suicidal thinking and behavior (suicidality) in short-term studies in children, adolescents, and young adults with major depressive disorder (MDD) and other psychiatric disorders. Nortriptyline is not approved for use in pediatric patients.

THERAPEUTIC CLASS: Tricyclic antidepressant

INDICATIONS: Relief of symptoms of depression.

DOSAGE: *Adults:* 25mg tid-qid. Max: 150mg/day. Total daily dose may be given once a day. Monitor serum levels if dose >100mg/day. Elderly/Adolescents: 30-50mg/day in single or divided doses.

HOW SUPPLIED: Cap: 10mg, 25mg, 50mg, 75mg; Sol: 10mg/5mL

CONTRAINDICATIONS: MAOI use within 14 days, acute recovery period following MI.

WARNINGS/PRECAUTIONS: MI, arrhythmia, strokes have occurred. Caution with cardiovascular disease, glaucoma, history of urinary retention, hyperthyroidism. May lower seizure threshold, exacerbate psychosis or activate schizophrenia, cause symptoms of mania in bipolar disease, or alter glucose levels. D/C several days prior to elective surgery.

ADVERSE REACTIONS: Arrhythmias, hypotension, HTN, tachycardia, MI, heart block, stroke, confusion, hallucination, insomnia, tremors, ataxia, anxiety, dry mouth, blurred vision, skin rash, extrapyramidal symptoms, photosensitivity, SIADH, anorexia.

INTERACTIONS: See Contraindications. May block guanethidine effects. Arrhythmia risk with thyroid agents. Alcohol may potentiate effects. "Stimulating" effect with reserpine. Monitor with anticholinergic and sympathomimetic drugs. Increased plasma levels with cimetidine. Hypoglycemia reported with chlorpropamide. SSRIs, antidepressants, phenothiazines, propafenone, flecainide and CYP2D6 inhibitors (eg, quinidine) may potentiate effects. Decreased clearance with quinidine.

PREGNANCY: Safety during pregnancy and nursing not known.

MECHANISM OF ACTION: Tricyclic; inhibits activity of histamine, 5-hydroxytryptamine, and acetylcholine; increases pressor effect of NE, blocks pressor response of phenethylamine, and interferes with transport, release, and storage of catecholamine.

NURSING CONSIDERATIONS

Assessment: Assess if acute recovery period after MI, for bipolar disorder risk, history of mania, unrecognized/history of schizophrenia, possible drug interactions, history of seizures, CVD, hyperthyroidism, DM, glaucoma, urinary retention, and history of agitation or overactivity.

Monitoring: Periodically monitor thyroid function and blood glucose. Monitor for signs/symptoms of clinical worsening (suicidality, unusual changes in behavior), mania, cardiovascular events, increasing psychosis, increasing anxiety/agitation, mydriasis, hypo/hyperglycemia, seizures, cognitive/motor impairment.

Patient Counseling: Advise to avoid alcohol. Seek medical attention for symptoms of activation of mania, seizures, clinical worsening (suicidal ideation, unusual changes in behavior), cardiovascular events, increasing psychosis, increasing anxiety/agitation, mydriasis, and hypo/hyperglycemia. Caution may impair physical/mental abilities.

Administration: Oral route. **Storage:** 20-25°C (68-77°F).

PANAFIL — RX

chlorophyllin copper complex sodium - papain - urea (Healthpoint)

THERAPEUTIC CLASS: Proteolytic enzyme (debriding/healing agent)

INDICATIONS: Treatment of acute and chronic lesions such as varicose, diabetic and decubitus ulcers, burns, postoperative wounds, pilonidal cyst wounds, carbuncles and other traumatic or infected wounds.

DOSAGE: *Adults:* (Oint, Spray) Clean wound, then apply qd-bid. Cover with dressing.

HOW SUPPLIED: Oint: (Chlorophyllin-Papain-Urea) 0.5%-10%-10% [6g, 30g]; Spray: (Chlorophyllin-Papain-Urea) 0.5%-10%-10% [33mL]

WARNINGS/PRECAUTIONS: Not for ophthalmic use.

ADVERSE REACTIONS: Transient burning, skin irritation.

INTERACTIONS: May be inactivated by hydrogen peroxide, salts of heavy metals (eg, lead, silver, mercury).

PREGNANCY: Safety in pregnancy and nursing not known.

MECHANISM OF ACTION: Papain: Proteolytic enzyme; potent digestant of nonviable protein matter. Urea: Combines with papain to produce two chemical actions; 1) to expose activators of papain by solvent action, 2) denature the nonviable protein matter in lesions thereby rendering it more susceptible to enzymatic digestion. Chlorophyllin Copper Complex Sodium: Promotes healthy granulations, controls local inflammation, and reduces wound odors. Responsible for inhibiting the hemaglutinating and inflammatory properties of protein degradation products in the wound, including products of enzymatic digestion.

NURSING CONSIDERATIONS

Assessment: Assess pregnancy/nursing status and for possible drug interactions.

Monitoring: Monitor for signs/symptoms of irritation at treatment site.

Patient Counseling: Instruct to clean wound prior to application. Advise to avoid cleaning wound with hydrogen peroxide solution. Following application, instruct to cover treatment area with appropriate dressing and secure into place. Instruct to avoid contact with medications containing heavy metals (eg, lead, silver, mercury).

Administration: Topical route. **Storage**: 20-25°C (68-77°F).

PANDEL
hydrocortisone probutate (PharmaDerm)

RX

THERAPEUTIC CLASS: Corticosteroid

INDICATIONS: Relief of the inflammatory and pruritic manifestations of corticosteroid-responsive dermatoses in patients ≥18 yrs.

DOSAGE: *Adults:* Apply qd-bid depending on severity of condition. May use occlusive dressing for refractory lesions of psoriasis and other deep-seated dermatoses.

HOW SUPPLIED: Cre: 0.1% [15g, 45g, 80g]

WARNINGS/PRECAUTIONS: May produce reversible HPA axis suppression, manifestations of Cushing's syndrome, hyperglycemia, glucosuria. D/C if irritation occurs. Use appropriate antifungal or antibacterial agent with dermatological infections. Pediatrics may be more susceptible to systemic toxicity. Caution when applied to large surface areas. Avoid eyes.

ADVERSE REACTIONS: Burning, stinging, moderate paresthesia, itching, dryness, folliculitis, hypertrichosis, acneiform eruptions, hypopigmentation, perioral dermatitis, skin atrophy, secondary infections, striae, miliaria.

PREGNANCY: Category C, caution in nursing.

MECHANISM OF ACTION: Corticosteroid; posesses anti-inflammatory, anti-pruritic, and vasoconstrictive actions. Anti-inflammatory activity not established. Suspected to act by the induction of phospholipase A_2 inhibitory proteins, lipocortins. Lipocortins control the biosynthesis of potent mediators of inflammation (eg, prostaglandins, leukotrienes) by inhibiting the release of their common precursor, arachidonic acid.

PHARMACOKINETICS: Absorption: Percutaneous; inflammation, other disease states, or the use of occlusive dressings may increase absorption. Use of occlusive dressings ≤24 hrs does not increase penetration. Use of occlusive dressings ≥96 hrs markedly enhances penetration. **Distribution:** Systemically administered corticosteroids have been found in breast milk.

NURSING CONSIDERATIONS

Assessment: Assess use in pregnant/nursing females.

Monitoring: Monitor for signs/symptoms of reversible HPA-axis suppression, Cushing's syndrome, hyperglycemia, glucosuria, skin irritation, allergic contact dermatitis (eg, failure to heal), and for development of concomitant skin infections (eg, bacterial, fungal). In patients applying medication to a large body surface area or using occlusive dressings, perform periodic monitoring for HPA-axis suppression using ACTH stimulation, AM plasma cortisol, or urinary free cortisol tests. Monitor for glucocorticosteroid insufficiencies following withdrawal of medication.

Patient Counseling: Instruct to use externally and exactly as directed; avoid contact with eyes, use on face, underarms, or groin areas unless directed by physician. Advise not to bandage, cover, or wrap treated skin area. Instruct to contact physician if any signs of local adverse reactions (eg, burning, itching, irritation) develop or if no clinical improvement is seen within 2 weeks of initiating therapy.

Administration: Topical route. **Storage:** 15-30°C (59-86°F).

PARCOPA
levodopa - carbidopa (Schwarz)

RX

THERAPEUTIC CLASS: Dopa-decarboxylase inhibitor/dopamine precursor

INDICATIONS: Treatment of symptoms of idiopathic Parkinson's disease, postencephalitic parkinsonism, and symptomatic parkinsonism.

DOSAGE: *Adults:* ≥18yrs: 25mg-100mg tab: Initial: 1 tab tid. Titrate: Increase by 1 tab qd or qod until 8 tabs/day. 10mg-100mg tab: Initial: 1 tab tid-qid. Titrate: Increase 1 tab qd or qod until 2 tabs qid. 70-100mg/day carbidopa required. Max 200mg/day carbidopa. Levodopa must be discontinued 12 hrs before starting carbidopa-levodopa.

HOW SUPPLIED: Tab, Disintegrating: (Carbidopa-Levodopa) 10mg-100mg*, 25mg-100mg*, 25mg-250mg* *scored

CONTRAINDICATIONS: MAOIs during or within 14 days of use, narrow-angle glaucoma, suspicious, undiagnosed skin lesions, history of melanoma.

WARNINGS/PRECAUTIONS: Dyskinesias and mental disturbances may occur. Caution with severe cardiovascular or pulmonary disease, bronchial asthma, renal or hepatic disease, endocrine disease, chronic wide-angle glaucoma, peptic ulcer, and MI with residual arrhythmias. NMS reported during dose reduction or withdrawal. Dark color may appear in saliva, urine, or sweat. May cause false (+) ketonuria or false (-) glucosuria (glucose-oxidase method).

ADVERSE REACTIONS: Dyskinesias, choreiform, dystonic, other involuntary movements, nausea.

INTERACTIONS: See Contraindications. Risk of postural hypotension with antihypertensives, selegiline. HTN and dyskinesia may occur with TCAs. Reduced effects with dopamine D_2 antagonists (eg, phenothiazines, butyrophenones, risperidone), isoniazid. Antagonized by phenytoin, papaverine, metoclopramide. Reduced bioavailability with iron salts, high-protein diets.

PREGNANCY: Category C, caution in nursing

MECHANISM OF ACTION: Carbidopa: Inhibits decarboxylation of peripheral levodopa. Levodopa: Crosses blood-brain barrier, converting into dopamine and thereby increasing concentrations in the brain.

PHARMACOKINETICS: Absorption: Carbidopa: Bioavailability (99%). **Elimination:** Urine.

NURSING CONSIDERATIONS

Assessment: Assess LFTs, renal function, CBC, glaucoma, dyskinesia, psychosis, depression, cardiovascular complications, melanomas, asthma, phenyl alanine levels.

Monitoring: Monitor for cardiac, hepatic/renal functions during initial dosage adjustment period, depression and suicidal ideation, worsening of dyskinesia, rhabdomyolysis, diarrhea, hallucinations, fibrotic complications, hyperpyrexia, melanomas, IOP, and hypersensitivity reactions.

Patient Counseling: Instruct to take as prescribed. Caution while operating machinery/driving. Discoloration of body fluids may occur. High-protein diet, excessive acidity, and iron salts reduce clinical effectiveness. Wearing-off effect may be seen at end of dosing interval. Report any adverse effects. Place tablet on tongue and dissolve with saliva.

Administration: Oral route. **Storage:** 20-25°C (68-77°F); excursions permitted to 15-30°C (59-86°F).

PARLODEL RX

bromocriptine mesylate (Novartis)

THERAPEUTIC CLASS: Dopamine receptor agonist

INDICATIONS: Management of hyperprolactinemia including amenorrhea with or without galactorrhea, infertility, or hypogonadism. Treatment of prolactin-secreting adenomas, acromegaly, and symptoms of Parkinson's disease.

DOSAGE: *Adults:* Take with food. Parkinson's Disease: Initial: 1.25mg bid. Titrate: if needed, increase by 2.5mg/day every 2-4 weeks. Max: 100mg/day. Hyperprolactinemia: Initial: 1.25mg-2.5mg qd. Titrate: If needed, increase by 2.5mg every 2-7 days. Usual: 2.5-15mg/day. Acromegaly: Initial: 1.25-2.5mg qhs for 3 days. Titrate: Increase by 1.25-2.5mg every 3-7 days until optimal response. Usual: 20-30mg/day. Max: 100mg/day. Withdraw for 4-8 weeks every year in patients treated with pituitary irradiation.

Pediatrics: Take with food. 11-15 yrs: Prolactin-Secreting Pituitary Adenomas: Initial: 1.25-2.5mg/day. Titrate: Increase as tolerated. Usual: 2.5-10mg/day.

HOW SUPPLIED: Cap: 5mg; Tab: 2.5mg* *scored

CONTRAINDICATIONS: Uncontrolled HTN, ergot alkaloid sensitivity, postpartum with CVD unless withdrawal is medically contraindicated, pregnancy if treating hyperprolactinemia, HTN in pregnancy.

WARNINGS/PRECAUTIONS: Caution with renal or hepatic dysfunction, psychosis, CVD, peptic ulcer, dementia. D/C with macroadenomas associated with rapid regrowth of tumor and increased prolactin levels and if severe headache or HTN develops. Risk of pulmonary infiltrates, pleural effusion, thickening of pleura, and retroperitoneal fibrosis with long-term use. Not for prevention of physiological lactation. Monitor BP for symptomatic hypotension and HTN.

ADVERSE REACTIONS: Headache, dizziness, GI effects, orthostatic hypotension, fatigue, arrhythmia, insomnia, hallucinations, abnormal involuntary movements, depression, syncope.

INTERACTIONS: Decreased effects with dopamine antagonists (eg, butyrophenones, haloperidol, phenothiazines, pimozide, metoclopramide). Levodopa may cause hallucinations. Caution with antihypertensives. Alcohol may potentiate side effects. Not for use with other ergot alkaloids.

PREGNANCY: Category B, not for use in nursing.

MECHANISM OF ACTION: Dopamine receptor agonist; activates post-synaptic dopamine receptors and modulates prolactin secretion from anterior pituitary by secreting prolactin inhibitory factor.

PHARMACOKINETICS: Absorption: GI tract (28%); C_{max}=0.4652ng/mL (5mg); T_{max}=1-3 hrs. **Distribution:** Serum albumin binding (90-96%). **Metabolism:** Liver, via CYP3A and hydroxylation. **Elimination:** Liver and kidneys (6%); $T_{1/2}$=8-20 hrs.

NURSING CONSIDERATIONS

Assessment: Assess for HTN, history of CAD, pituitary tumors, dementia, unexplained pleuropulmonary disorder, history of psychosis, hereditary problems such as galactose intolerance, severe lactase deficiency or glucose malabsorption, and pregnancy status.

Monitoring: Monitor for somnolence, sudden sleep onset, confusion, mental disturbances, seizures, visual disturbances, pleuropulmonary disorders, constrictive pericarditis, retroperitoneal fibrosis, BP, prolactin level, LFTs, renal function, CBC, BP, and CNS toxicities.

Patient Counseling: Advise to use caution while operating machinery/driving. Instruct to take exactly as prescribed with meals. Counsel to report lack of response or adverse effects.

Administration: Oral route. **Storage:** Store below 25°C (77°F); tight, light-resistant container.

PARNATE RX

tranylcypromine sulfate (GlaxoSmithKline)

Antidepressants increased the risk of suicidal thinking and behavior (suicidality) in short-term studies in children, adolescents, and young adults with major depressive disorder and other psychiatric disorders. Tranylcypromine is not approved for use in pediatric patients.

THERAPEUTIC CLASS: Monoamine oxidase inhibitor

INDICATIONS: Treatment of major depressive episode without melancholia.

DOSAGE: *Adults:* Usual: 30mg/day in divided doses. Titrate: After 2 weeks, may increase by 10mg/day every 1-3 weeks depending on signs of improvement. Max: 60mg/day.

HOW SUPPLIED: Tab: 10mg

CONTRAINDICATIONS: Cardiovascular or cerebrovascular disorder, HTN, history of headache, pheochromocytoma. Concomitant MAOIs, dibenzazepine derivatives, sympathomimetics (including amphetamines), some CNS depressants (including narcotics and alcohol), antihypertensives, diuretics, antihistamines, sedatives, anesthetics, bupropion, buspirone, meperidine, SSRIs, dexfenfluramine, dextromethorphan, foods with high tyramine content (cheese) and excessive quantities of caffeine. Elective surgery requiring general anesthesia. History of liver disease or abnormal LFTs. Caution with anti-parkinsonism drugs.

WARNINGS/PRECAUTIONS: Use in patients who are resistant to other therapies. Hypotension reported. Drug dependency possible in doses excessive of the therapeutic range. May suppress anginal pain in myocardial ischemia. Caution with hyperthyroidism, renal dysfunction, diabetes, elderly. May aggravate depression symptoms. May lower seizure threshold. Inhibits MAO 10 days after discontinuation. D/C at least 10 days before elective surgery. D/C if palpitations or frequent headaches occur.

ADVERSE REACTIONS: Restlessness, insomnia, weakness, drowsiness, nausea, diarrhea, tachycardia, anorexia, edema, tinnitis, muscle spasm, overstimulation, dizziness, dry mouth, blood dyscrasias.

INTERACTIONS: See Contraindications. Caution with disulfiram. Additive hypotensive effects with phenothiazines. Tryptophan may precipitate disorientation, memory impairment and other neurological and behavioral signs. Avoid metrizamide; d/c 48 hrs before myelography and may resume 24 hrs post-procedure.

PREGNANCY: Safety in pregnancy and nursing not known.

MECHANISM OF ACTION: Non-hydrazine MAOI; inhibits monoamine oxidase, increasing concentration of epinephrine, norepinephrine, and serotonin in storage sites throughout nervous system.

NURSING CONSIDERATIONS

Assessment: Assess for DM, pheochromocytoma, HTN, history of headache, seizures, liver disease, possible drug interactions, risk for bipolar disorder, renal impairment, hyperthyroidism, Parkinson's disease, CV and cerebrovascular defects.

Monitoring: Monitor BP, renal function, and LFTs; signs/symptoms of clinical worsening (suicidality, unusual changes in behavior), hypertensive crises (occipital headaches, neck stiffness, NV, sweating), seizures, liver dysfunction, postural hypotension, and hypoglycemia.

Patient Counseling: Instruct to avoid concomitant use of alcohol, tyramine-containing foods/supplements/beverages (during and 2 weeks following d/c), and cough medicine containing dextromethorphan. Advise to seek medical attention if symptoms of hypertensive crises (occipital headaches, neck stiffness, NV, sweating), hypoglycemia, seizures, postural hypotension, clinical worsening (suicidal ideation, unusual changes in behavior), and liver dysfunction occur; change positions gradually if lightheaded, faint, or dizzy.

Administration: Oral route. **Storage:** 15-30°C (59-86°F).

PASER — RX

aminosalicylic acid (Jacobus)

THERAPEUTIC CLASS: Hydroxybenzoic acid derivative

INDICATIONS: Treatment of TB in combination with other agents.

DOSAGE: *Adults:* 4g tid. Sprinkle on applesauce, yogurt, or mix with tomato or orange juice.

Pediatrics: Use correspondingly smaller doses to the adult dose. Sprinkle on applesauce, yogurt, or mix with tomato or orange juice.

HOW SUPPLIED: Pkt: 4g

CONTRAINDICATIONS: Severe renal disease.

WARNINGS/PRECAUTIONS: Monitor for rash, or signs of intolerance during 1st 3 months. D/C if hypersensitivity occurs. Can desensitize by administering small, gradually increasing doses.

ADVERSE REACTIONS: Diarrhea, NV, abdominal pain, fever, dermatitis, lymphoma-like syndrome, agranulocytosis, thrombocytopenia, anemia, jaundice, hepatitis, hypoglycemia.

INTERACTIONS: Reduces acetylation of isoniazid, especially in rapid acetylators. Decreases vitamin B_{12} absorption; consider vitamin B_{12} maintenance treatment. Decreases digoxin levels.

PREGNANCY: Category C, safety in nursing not known.

MECHANISM OF ACTION: Bacteriostatic agent; believed to inhibit folic acid synthesis and/or inhibition of synthesis of the cell-wall component, mycobactin, thus reducing iron uptake by *M.tuberculosis.*

PHARMACOKINETICS: Absorption: C_{max}=20mcg/mL; T_{max}=6 hrs. **Distribution:** Plasma protein binding (50-60%), CSF penetration occurs only if the meninges is inflamed. **Metabolism:** Via acetylation. **Excretion:** Urine (80%); aminosalicylic acid (metabolite); $T_{1/2}$=26.4 min.

NURSING CONSIDERATIONS

Assessment: Assess renal function, LFTs, and possible drug interactions.

Monitoring: Monitor LFTs, renal functions, hepatomegaly, lymphadenopathy, diarrhea, leucocytosis, eosinophilia. Monitor for rash or signs of intolerance during first 3 months; desensitize by administering small, gradually increasing doses.

Patient Counseling: D/C if hypersensitivity (rash, fever, diarrhea) occurs. Inform that poor compliance in taking anti-TB drugs leads to treatment failure and resistance against organisms. Skeleton of the granules may be seen in stool. Sprinkle granules on acidic foods such as applesauce or yogurt or stir into a fruit drink and swirl to protect the coating from sinking. Store drug in refrigerator or freezer; do not use if the packets are swollen or the granules have lost their tan color and are dark brown or purple.

Administration: Oral route. **Storage:** Store below 15°C (59°F), refrigerate or freeze.

PATANOL RX

olopatadine HCl (Alcon)

P

THERAPEUTIC CLASS: H_1-antagonist and mast cell stabilizer

INDICATIONS: Allergic conjunctivitis.

DOSAGE: *Adults:* 1 drop bid, q6-8h.
Pediatrics: ≥3 yrs: 1 drop bid, q6-8h.

HOW SUPPLIED: Sol: 0.1% [5mL]

WARNINGS/PRECAUTIONS: May re-insert contact lens 10 min after dosing if eye is not red.

ADVERSE REACTIONS: Headache, asthenia, blurred vision, burning, stinging, cold syndrome, dry eye, foreign body sensation, hyperemia, hypersensitivity, keratitis, lid edema, nausea, pharyngitis, pruritus, rhinitis, sinusitis, taste perversion.

PREGNANCY: Category C, caution in nursing.

MECHANISM OF ACTION: Antihistaminic drug; relatively selective histamine H_1-antagonist; inhibits the type 1 immediate hypersensitivity reaction, including inhibition of histamine induced effects on human conjunctival epithelial cells.

PHARMACOKINETICS: Absorption: C_{max}=0.5-1.3ng/mL; T_{max}=2 hrs. **Metabolism:** Metabolites: Mono-desmethyl and N-oxide. **Elimination:** Urine (60-70% parent drug).

NURSING CONSIDERATIONS

Assessment: Assess for drug hypersensitivity.

Monitoring: Monitor for headache and other adverse reactions.

Patient Counseling: Counsel not to wear contact lenses if eye is red; wait at least 10 min after instillation to wear contact lenses. Instruct to avoid touching tip of container to eye or any other surface to avoid contamination.

Administration: Ocular route. **Storage:** 4-25°C (39-77°F). Keep bottle tightly closed.

PAXIL

RX

paroxetine HCl (GlaxoSmithKline)

Antidepressants increased the risk of suicidal thinking and behavior (suicidality) in short-term studies in children, adolescents, and young adults with major depressive disorder (MDD) and other psychiatric disorders. Paroxetine is not approved for use in pediatric patients.

THERAPEUTIC CLASS: Selective serotonin reuptake inhibitor

INDICATIONS: Treatment of major depressive disorder (MDD), panic disorder with or without agoraphobia. Treatment of obsessive compulsive disorder (OCD), social anxiety disorder (SAD), generalized anxiety disorder (GAD), and post-traumatic stress disorder (PTSD).

DOSAGE: *Adults:* Give qd, usually in the AM. MDD: Initial: 20mg/day. Max: 50mg/day. OCD: Initial: 20mg qd. Usual: 40mg qd. Max: 60mg/day. Panic Disorder: Initial: 10mg qd. Usual: 40mg/day. Max: 60mg/day. GAD: Initial: 20mg/day. Usual: 20-50mg/day. SAD: Initial/Usual: 20mg/day. Max: 60mg/day. PTSD: Initial: 20mg/day. Usual: 20-50mg/day. To titrate, may increase weekly by 10mg/day. Elderly/Debilitated/Severe Renal/Hepatic Impairment: Initial: 10mg qd. Max: 40mg/day.

HOW SUPPLIED: Sus: 10mg/5mL [250mL]; Tab: 10mg*, 20mg*, 30mg, 40mg *scored

CONTRAINDICATIONS: Concomitant MAOIs, thioridazine, or pimozide.

WARNINGS/PRECAUTIONS: Caution with history of mania or seizures, conditions that affect metabolism or hemodynamic responses, narrow angle glaucoma. D/C if seizures occur. Altered platelet function, hyponatremia, mydriasis reported. Avoid abrupt withdrawal. Re-evaluate periodically. Monitor for clinical worsening and/or suicidality, especially at initiation of therapy or dose changes.

ADVERSE REACTIONS: Somnolence, insomnia, nausea, asthenia, abnormal ejaculation, dry mouth, constipation, dizziness, diarrhea, decreased libido, sweating.

INTERACTIONS: See Contraindications. Avoid alcohol, tryptophan. May shift concentrations with plasma-bound drugs. Increased risk of bleeding with NSAIDs, aspirin, oral anticoagulants. May inhibit metabolism of TCAs. Rare reports of weakness, hyperreflexia, incoordination with an SSRI and sumatriptan. Caution with other agents that may affect serotonergic systems (eg, triptans, serotonin reuptake inhibitors, linezolid, lithium, tramadol, St. John's wort); increased risk of serotonin syndrome. Monitor theophylline. Increased levels with cimetidine. Reduce procyclidine dose if anticholinergic effects occur. Caution with diuretics, digoxin, lithium, cimetidine, warfarin, phenobarbital, phenytoin, drugs metabolized by CYP2D6 (eg, antidepressants, phenothiazines, Type 1C antiarrhythmics), or drugs that inhibit CYP2D6 (eg, quinidine). May increase levels of risperidone. May increase levels of atomoxetine; dosage adjustment of atomoxetine may be necessary and initiate atomoxetine at reduced dose. Fosamprenavir/ritonavir may decrease levels.

PREGNANCY: Category D, caution in nursing.

MECHANISM OF ACTION: SSRI; inhibits CNS neuronal reuptake of serotonin.

PHARMACOKINETICS: Absorption: Complete; C_{max}=61.7ng/mL; T_{max}=5.2 hrs. **Distribution:** Plasma protein binding (95%). **Metabolism:** Oxidation and methylation via CYP2D6. **Elimination:** Urine (2%), feces (<1%); $T_{1/2}$=21 hrs.

NURSING CONSIDERATIONS

Assessment: Assess for bipolar disorder risk, history of mania, possible drug interactions, history of seizures, narrow-angle glaucoma, disease/condition that alters metabolism or hemodynamic response, and hepatic/renal impairment.

Monitoring: Monitor for signs/symptoms of clinical worsening (suicidality, unusual changes in behavior), serotonin syndrome, abnormal bleeding, hyponatremia, activation of mania, mydriasis, akathisia, seizures, cognitive/motor impairment, hepatic/renal dysfunction. If d/c abruptly, monitor for symptoms of dysphoric mood, irritability, agitation, dizziness, sensory disturbances, anxiety, confusion, headache, lethargy, emotional lability, insomnia, and hypomania.

Patient Counseling: Counsel to swallow whole, not to chew or crush. Advise to avoid alcohol. Seek medical attention for symptoms of serotonin syndrome (mental status changes, tachycardia, hyperthermia, NV, diarrhea, incoordination), abnormal bleeding (particularly if using NSAIDs or ASA), akathisia, hyponatremia (headaches, unsteadiness), mydriasis, activation of mania, seizures, clinical worsening (suicidal ideation, unusual changes in behavior), or discontinuation symptoms (irritability, agitation, dizziness, anxiety, headache, insomnia). Caution may impair physical/mental abilities. Inform may notice improvement in 1-4 weeks; continue therapy as directed.

Administration: Oral route. **Storage:** (Tab): 15-30°C (59-86°F). (Sol): Below 25°C (77°F).

PAXIL CR — RX

paroxetine HCl (GlaxoSmithKline)

Antidepressants increased the risk of suicidal thinking and behavior (suicidality) in short-term studies in children, adolescents, and young adults with major depressive disorder (MDD) and other psychiatric disorders. Paroxetine is not approved for use in pediatric patients.

THERAPEUTIC CLASS: Selective serotonin reuptake inhibitor

INDICATIONS: Treatment of major depressive disorder (MDD), panic disorder with or without agoraphobia, social anxiety disorder (SAD), and premenstrual dysphoric disorder (PMDD).

DOSAGE: *Adults:* Give qd, usually in the AM. Swallow whole. MDD: Initial: 25mg/day. Titrate: May increase weekly by 12.5mg/day. Max: 62.5mg/day. Panic Disorder: Initial: 12.5mg/day. May increase weekly by 12.5mg/day. Max: 75mg/day. SAD: Initial: 12.5mg/day. May increase weekly by 12.5mg/day. Max: 37.5mg/day. PMDD: Initial: 12.5mg/day continuous or limited to luteal phase of cycle. May increase weekly by 12.5mg/day. Elderly/Debilitated/Severe Renal/Hepatic Impairment: Initial: 12.5mg/day. Max: 50mg/day.

HOW SUPPLIED: Tab, Controlled-Release: 12.5mg, 25mg, 37.5mg

CONTRAINDICATIONS: Concomitant MAOIs, thioridazine, or pimozide.

WARNINGS/PRECAUTIONS: Caution with history of mania or seizures, conditions that affect metabolism or hemodynamic responses, narrow-angle glaucoma. D/C if seizures occur. Hyponatremia, mydriasis reported. Avoid abrupt withdrawal. Re-evaluate periodically. Monitor for clinical worsening and/or suicidality, especially at initiation of therapy or dose changes.

ADVERSE REACTIONS: Somnolence, insomnia, nausea, asthenia, abnormal ejaculation, dry mouth, constipation, dizziness, diarrhea, decreased libido, sweating.

INTERACTIONS: See Contraindications. Avoid alcohol, tryptophan. May shift concentrations with plasma-bound drugs. May inhibit metabolism of TCAs. Rare reports of weakness, hyperreflexia, incoordination with an SSRI and sumatriptan. Caution with other drugs or agents that may affect the serotonergic neurotransmitter systems, such as tryptophan, triptans, serotonin reuptake inhibitors, linezolid, lithium, tramadol, or St. John's wort. Monitor theophylline. Increased risk of bleeding with NSAIDs, aspirin, oral anticoagulants. Reduce procyclidine dose if anticholinergic effects occur. Caution with TCAs, diuretics, digoxin, lithium, cimetidine, warfarin, phenobarbital, phenytoin, drugs metabolized by CYP2D6 (eg, antidepressants, phenothiazines, Type 1C antiarrhythmics), or drugs that inhibit CYP2D6 (eg, quinidine). May increase levels of risperidone. May increase levels of atomoxetine; dosage adjustment of atomoxetine may be necessary and initiate atomoxetine at reduced dose. Fosamprenavir/ritonavir may decrease levels.

PREGNANCY: Category C, caution in nursing.

MECHANISM OF ACTION: SSRI; inhibits CNS neuronal reuptake of serotonin.

PHARMACOKINETICS: Absorption: Complete; administration of variable doses resulted in different parameters; T_{max}=6-10 hrs. **Distribution:** Plasma protein binding (95%). **Metabolism:** Oxidation and methylation via CYP2D6. **Elimination:** Urine (2%), feces (<1%); $T_{1/2}$=15-20 hrs.

NURSING CONSIDERATIONS

Assessment: Assess bipolar disorder risk, history of mania, possible drug interactions, history of seizures, narrow-angle glaucoma, disease/condition that alters metabolism or hemodynamic response, hepatic/renal impairment.

Monitoring: Monitor for signs/symptoms of clinical worsening (suicidality, unusual changes in behavior), serotonin syndrome, abnormal bleeding, hyponatremia, activation of mania, mydriasis, akathisia, seizures, cognitive/motor impairment, hepatic/renal dysfunction. If d/c abruptly, monitor for symptoms of dysphoric mood, irritability, agitation, dizziness, sensory disturbances, anxiety, confusion, headache, lethargy, emotional lability, insomnia, and hypomania.

Patient Counseling: Counsel to swallow whole, not to chew or crush. Advise to avoid alcohol. Seek medical attention for symptoms of serotonin syndrome (mental status changes, tachycardia, hyperthermia, NV, diarrhea, incoordination), abnormal bleeding (particularly if using NSAIDs or ASA), akathisia, hyponatremia (headaches, unsteadiness), mydriasis, activation of mania, seizures, clinical worsening (suicidal ideation, unusual changes in behavior) or discontinuation symptoms (irritability, agitation, dizziness, anxiety, headache, insomnia). Caution may impair physical/mental abilities. Inform may notice improvement in 1-4 weeks; continue therapy as directed.

Administration: Oral route. **Storage:** At or below 25°C (77°F).

PCE

erythromycin (Abbott)

RX

THERAPEUTIC CLASS: Macrolide

INDICATIONS: Treatment of mild to moderate upper/lower respiratory tract and skin and skin structure infections, listeriosis, pertussis, diphtheria, erythrasma, intestinal amebiasis, acute pelvic inflammatory disease (PID) (*N.gonorrhoeae*), primary syphilis (if PCN allergy), Legionnaires' disease, chlamydial infections (eg, newborn conjunctivitis, pneumonia of infancy, urogenital infections during pregnancy or urethral, endocervical, or rectal infections when tetracyclines are contraindicated or not tolerated), and nongonococcal urethritis caused by susceptible strains of microorganisms. Prophylaxis of initial and recurrent attacks of rheumatic fever if PCN allergy.

DOSAGE: *Adults:* Usual: 333mg q8h or 500mg q12h without food. Max: 4g/day. Do not take bid when dose is ≥1g/day. Treat strep infections for at least 10 days. Streptococcal Infection Long-Term Prophylaxis of Rheumatic Fever: 250mg bid. Chlamydial Urogenital Infection During Pregnancy: 500mg qid or 666mg q8h for at least 7 days, or 500mg q12h, 333mg q8h, or 250mg qid for at least 14 days. Urethral/Endocervical/Rectal Chlamydial Infections and Nongonococcal Urethritis: 500mg qid or 666mg q8h for at least 7 days. Primary Syphilis: 30-40g in divided doses over 10-15 days. Acute PID: 500mg (erythromycin lactobionate) IV q6h for 3 days, then 500mg PO q12h or 333mg PO q8h for 7 days. Intestinal Amebiasis: 500mg q12h, 333mg q8h, or 250mg q6h for 10-14 days. Pertussis: 40-50mg/kg/day in divided doses for 5-14 days. Legionnaires' Disease: 1-4g/day in divided doses.
Pediatrics: Usual: 30-50mg/kg/day in divided doses without food. Severe Infections: May double dose. Max: 4g/day. Treat strep infections for at least 10 days. Streptococcal Infection Long-Term Prophylaxis of Rheumatic Fever: 250mg bid. Chlamydial Conjunctivitis of Newborns/Chlamydial Pneumonia in

Infancy: (Sus) 12.5mg/kg qid for 2 weeks and 3 weeks, respectively. Intestinal Amebiasis: 30-50mg/kg/day in divided doses for 10-14 days.

HOW SUPPLIED: Tab: 333mg, 500mg

CONTRAINDICATIONS: Concomitant terfenadine, astemizole, pimozide, or cisapride.

WARNINGS/PRECAUTIONS: *Clostridium difficile*-associated diarrhea, hepatic dysfunction reported. Caution with impaired hepatic function. May aggravate weakness of patients with myasthenia gravis. Erythromycin does not reach adequate concentrations in fetus to prevent congenital syphilis.

ADVERSE REACTIONS: Abdominal pain, N/V, diarrhea, anorexia, hepatic dysfunction, abnormal LFTs, allergic reactions, pseudomembranous colitis, QT prolongation, ventricular arrhythmias (eg, ventricular tachycardia, torsades de pointes), and reversible hearing loss (high dose and renal insufficiency).

INTERACTIONS: See Contraindications. Rhabdomyolysis reported with lovastatin. May increase levels of theophylline, digoxin, drugs metabolized by CYP450 (eg, carbamazepine, cyclosporine, phenytoin, alfentanil, disopyramide, lovastatin, bromocriptine, valproate, etc). Increases effects of oral anticoagulants, triazolam, midazolam. Risk of hypotension, bradyarrhythmias, and lactic acidosis with verapramil. Risk of acute ergot toxicity with ergotamine or dihydroergotamine. May increase AUC of sildenafil; consider dose reduction of sildenafil.

PREGNANCY: Category B, caution in nursing.

MECHANISM OF ACTION: Macrolide; inhibits protein synthesis by binding 50S ribosomal subunits of susceptible organisms.

PHARMACOKINETICS: Distribution: Crosses placenta, found in breast milk. **Elimination:** Biliary excretion, urine (<5%).

NURSING CONSIDERATIONS

Assessment: Assess for possible drug interactions, myasthenia gravis, and hepatic impairment.

Monitoring: Monitor for serum creatine kinase, transaminase levels, signs/symptoms of hepatic dysfunction, hypersensitivity reactions, *C. difficile*-associated diarrhea, aggravation of weakness in myasthenia gravis, superinfections, infantile hypertrophic pyloric stenosis (IHPS), pseudomembranous colitis, QT prolongation, ventricular arrhythmias, and hearing loss.

Patient Counseling: Instruct to take tab 30 min-2 hrs before meals. Inform therapy treats bacterial, not viral, infections. Take as directed; skipping doses or not completing full course may decrease effectiveness and increase resistance. Inform diarrhea may develop; notify physician if watery/bloody stools, superinfections, IHPS (vomiting or irritability with feeding), aggravation of myasthenia gravis, or hypersensitivity reactions occur.

Administration: Oral route. **Storage:** Below 30°C (86°F).

P

PEDIAPRED — RX

prednisolone sodium phosphate (Celltech)

THERAPEUTIC CLASS: Glucocorticoid

INDICATIONS: Steroid-responsive dermatoses.

DOSAGE: *Adults:* Initial: 5-60mg/day depending on disease and response. Maint: Decrease dose by small amounts to lowest effective dose. MS Exacerbations: 200mg qd for 1 week, then 80mg every other day for 1 month. *Pediatrics:* Initial: 0.14-2mg/kg/day given tid-qid. Nephrotic Syndrome: 20mg/m^2 tid for 4 weeks, then 40mg/m^2 every other day for 4 weeks. Uncontrolled Asthma: 1-2mg/kg/day in single or divided doses peak expiratory rate of 80% is achieved (usually 3-10 days).

HOW SUPPLIED: Sol: 5mg/5mL [120mL]

CONTRAINDICATIONS: Systemic fungal infections.

WARNINGS/PRECAUTIONS: May produce reversible HPA axis suppression. Adjust dose during stress or change in thyroid status. May mask signs of infection or cause new infections. May activate latent amebiasis. Avoid with cerebral malaria. Avoid exposure to chickenpox or measles. Not for treatment of optic neuritis or active ocular herpes simplex. May cause elevation of BP or IOP, cataracts, glaucoma, optic nerve damage, Kaposi's sarcoma, psychic derangements, salt/water retention, increased excretion of potassium and/or calcium, osteoporosis, growth suppression in children, secondary ocular infections. Caution with strongyloides, CHF, diverticulitis, HTN, renal insufficiency, fresh intestinal anastomoses, active or latent peptic ulcer, ulcerative colitis. Enhanced effect in hypothyroidism or cirrhosis. Avoid abrupt withdrawal. Use with caution in elderly, increased risk of corticosteroid-induced side effects; start at low end of dosing range; monitor bone mineral density.

ADVERSE REACTIONS: Edema, fluid/electrolyte disturbances, osteoporosis, muscle weakness, pancreatitis, peptic ulcer, impaired wound healing, increased intracranial pressure, cushingoid state, hirsutism, menstrual irregularities, growth suppression in children, glaucoma, nausea, weight gain.

INTERACTIONS: Enhanced metabolism with barbiturates, phenytoin, ephedrine, and rifampin. Use with cyclosporine may increase activity of both drugs; convulsions reported with concomitant use. Decreased metabolism with estrogens or ketoconazole. May inhibit response to warfarin. Increased risk of GI side effects with ASA or other NSAIDs. May increase clearance of salicylates. High doses or concurrent neuromuscular drugs may cause acute myopathy. Enhanced possibility of hypokalemia when given with potassium-depleting agents. May produce severe weakness in myasthenia gravis patients on anticholinesterase agents. Avoid live vaccines with immunosuppressive doses. Possible diminished response with killed or inactivated vaccines. May increase blood glucose; adjust antidiabetic agents. May suppress reactions to skin tests.

PREGNANCY: Category C, caution in nursing.

MECHANISM OF ACTION: Synthetic adrenocorticoid steroid; promotes gluconeogenesis, increases deposition of glycogen in the liver, inhibits glucose utilization, increases catabolism of protein, lipolysis, glomerular filtration that leads to increased urinary excretion of urate and calcium.

PHARMACOKINETICS: Absorption: Rapidly absorbed from GI tract. **Distribution:** Plasma protein binding (70-90%); found in breast milk. **Metabolism:** Liver. **Elimination:** Urine (as sulfate and glucuronide congugates); $T_{1/2}$=2-4 hrs.

NURSING CONSIDERATIONS

Assessment: Assess for systemic fungal/other infections, active TB, vaccination history, HTN, CHF, renal insufficiency, ophthalmic disease, osteoporosis, thyroid status, hepatic impairment, nonspecific ulcerative colitis, ulcers, and possible drug interactions.

Monitoring: Monitor for adrenocortical insufficiency, occurrence of infections, psychic derangement, cataracts, acute myopathy, Kaposi's sarcoma, fluid retention, and measurement of serum electrolytes, TSH, LFTs, glucose, IOP, and BP.

Patient Counseling: Advise not to d/c therapy abruptly or without medical supervision. Avoid exposure to chickenpox or measles; report immediately if exposed. Dietary salt restriction and K^+ supplementation is advised.

Administration: Oral route. **Storage:** 4-25°C (39-77°F).

PEDIARIX RX

pertussis vaccine, acellular - hepatitis B (recombinant) - poliovirus vaccine, inactivated - diphtheria toxoid - tetanus toxoid (GlaxoSmithKline)

THERAPEUTIC CLASS: Vaccine/toxoid combination

INDICATIONS: Active immunization against diphtheria, tetanus, pertussis, hepatitis B, and poliomyelitis (polioviruses Types 1, 2, and 3).

DOSAGE: *Pediatrics:* ≥6 weeks-up to 7 yrs: 3 doses of 0.5mL IM at 6-8 week intervals. Start at 2 months old or as early as 6 weeks old if necessary. May use to complete primary series in infants who have received 1 or 2 doses of Infanrix® or IPV or to complete a hepatitis B vaccine (Recombinant) series. Not recommended for completion of the first 3 doses of the DTaP vaccination series initiated with a DTaP vaccine from a different manufacturer.

HOW SUPPLIED: Inj: 0.5mL

CONTRAINDICATIONS: Hypersensitivity to yeast, neomycin, and polymyxin B. Anaphylaxis associated with previous dose or encephalopathy within 7 days of previous vaccine, progressive neurologic disorder (including infantile spasms, uncontrolled epilepsy, progressive encephalopathy).

WARNINGS/PRECAUTIONS: Higher rates of fever reported. Tip cap and plunger contains latex. Caution if within 48 hrs of previous whole-cell DTP or vaccine containing an acellular pertussis component, fever ≥105°F not due to another identifiable cause, collapse or shock-like state, or inconsolable crying lasting ≥3 hrs occurs, or if seizures occur within 3 days. Re-evaluate need if Guillain-Barre syndrome occurs within 6 weeks of receipt of tetanus toxoid-containing vaccine. Defer vaccination with moderate or severe illness, with or without fever. Administer antipyretic for initial 24 hrs for those with higher risk for seizures. Caution with bleeding disorders (eg, hemophilia, thrombocytopenia). Have epinephrine available. Suboptimal response may occur in immunocompromised patients.

ADVERSE REACTIONS: Local injection-site reactions, fever, fussiness.

INTERACTIONS: Avoid with anticoagulants unless benefit outweighs risk. Immunosuppressive therapy (eg, irradiation, antimetabolites, alkylating agents, cytotoxic drugs, large doses of corticosteroids) may decrease response. Do not mix with other vaccines in same syringe/vial. Tetanus immune globulin or diphtheria antitoxin should be given at separate site with separate needle/syringe.

PREGNANCY: Category C, safety in nursing not known.

MECHANISM OF ACTION: Vaccine/toxoid combination; stimulates immune system to elicit immune response, which produces antibodies that may protect against diphtheria, tetanus, pertussis, hepatitis B, and poliovirus infections.

NURSING CONSIDERATIONS

Assessment: Assess for hypersensitivity to yeast, neomycin, polymixin B, history of encephalopathy, progressive neurologic disorders (eg, infantile spasms, uncontrolled epilepsy, progressive encephalopathy), stable CNS disorders, hypersensitivity to latex, previous reactions to pertussis immunization (eg, temperature, collapse or shock-like state, persistent inconsolable crying, seizures), previous development of Guillain-Barre syndrome after vaccine administration, bleeding disorders (eg, hemophilia, thrombocytopenia), current health status and medical history, age of patient (eg, <7yrs old), and possible drug interactions.

Monitoring: Monitor for signs/symptoms of fever, seizures, hematoma, hypersensitivity reactions (eg, anaphylaxis), and local injection-site reactions (eg, pain, redness, swelling).

Patient Counseling: Inform about benefits/risks and importance of completing immunization series; report any adverse events. Advise that if at risk for developing seizures, an appropriate antipyretic should be taken at time of vaccination and for 24 hrs following administration.

Administration: IM route. Prior to administration, shake vial vigorously to obtain homogenous, turbid, white suspension. Do not use if resuspension does not occur with vigorous shaking. In children <1 yr, preferred site is anterolateral aspect of thigh; in older children, can administer via deltoid muscle. Do not inject in gluteal area or areas where there may be a major nerve trunk. Do not administer SQ or IV. Ephinephrine and other appropriate agents should be immediately available if acute anaphylactic reaction occurs. **Storage:** 2-8°C (36-46°F). Do not freeze; discard if frozen.

PEGASYS RX

peginterferon alfa-2a (Roche)

May cause or aggravate fatal or life-threatening neuropsychiatric, autoimmune, ischemic, and infectious disorders. Monitor closely with periodic clinical and laboratory evaluations. D/C with persistently severe or worsening signs or symptoms of these conditions. When used with ribavirin, refer to the individual monograph.

THERAPEUTIC CLASS: Pegylated virus proliferation inhibitor

INDICATIONS: Treatment of chronic hepatitis C, alone or in combination with Copegus, in adults with compensated liver disease not previously treated with interferon alfa. Treatment of adult patients with HBeAg positive and HBeAg negative chronic hepatitis B who have compensated liver disease and evidence of viral replication and liver inflammation.

DOSAGE: *Adults:* ≥18 yrs: HCV: Monotherapy: 180mcg SQ (in abdomen or thigh) once weekly for 48 weeks. Combination Therapy With Copegus: 180mcg SQ once weekly for 24 weeks with genotypes 2 and 3 or 48 weeks with genotypes 1 and 4. HCV w/ HIV: Monotherapy: 180mcg SQ once weekly for 48 weeks. Combination Therapy with Copegus: 180mcg SQ once weekly for 48 weeks, regardless of genotype. HBV: Monotherapy: 180mcg SQ once weekly for 48 weeks. Adjust dose based on hematological parameters and depression severity. (See PI for dose modifications).

HOW SUPPLIED: Inj: Prefilled syringe: 180mcg/0.5mL; Single Dose Vial: 180mcg/mL

CONTRAINDICATIONS: Autoimmune hepatitis, hepatic decompensation; neonates and infants (contains benzyl alcohol). When used with ribavirin, refer to the individual monograph.

WARNINGS/PRECAUTIONS: Life-threatening neuropsychiatric reactions may occur; extreme caution with history of depression. Risk of bone marrow suppression; obtain CBCs prior to initiation and routinely thereafter. HTN, arrhythmias, chest pain, and MI reported; caution with pre-existing cardiac disease. Decrease/loss of vision and retinopathy reported; perform eye exam at baseline (periodically with pre-existing disorder); d/c if patient develops new or worsening of ophthalmologic disorders. Monitor for signs/symptoms of toxicity with impaired renal function and caution with CrCl <50mL/min. Development or exacerbation of autoimmune disorders reported. Caution in elderly. May induce or aggravate dyspnea, pulmonary infiltrates, pneumonia, bronchiolitis obliterans, interstitial pneumonitis, and sarcoiditis; d/c if persistent or unexplained pulmonary infiltrates or pulmonary function impairment. Hypersensitivity reactions, hemorrhagic/ischemic colitis, and pancreatitis reported; d/c if any of these develop. May cause or aggravate hypothyroidism or hyperthyroidism. Hypoglycemia, hyperglycemia, and DM reported. Avoid if failed other alpha interferon treatments, liver or other organ transplant recipients, or with HIV or HBV coinfection. Monitor for severe viral, bacterial, fungal infections. Exacerbation of hepatitis B reported. Chronic hepatitis C patients with cirrhosis may be at risk for hepatic decompensation; monitor hepatic function and serum ALT's.

ADVERSE REACTIONS: Injection site reaction, fatigue/asthenia, pyrexia, rigors, NV, neutropenia, myalgia, headache, irritability/anxiety/nervousness, insomnia, depression, alopecia, pruritus, dermatitis, and rash.

INTERACTIONS: May inhibit CYP1A2 and increase theophylline AUC; monitor theophylline serum levels. Hepatic decompensation can occur with concomitant use of NRTIs and peginterferon alfa-2a/ribavirin. May increase methadone levels; monitor for methadone toxicity.

PREGNANCY: Category C (monotherapy) and Category X (with ribavirin), not for use in nursing.

MECHANISM OF ACTION: α-2a interferon; binds to specific receptors on the cell surface initiating intracellular signaling leading to rapid activation of gene transcription.

PHARMACOKINETICS: Absorption: T_{max}=72-96 hrs. **Elimination:** $T_{1/2}$=160 hrs (chronic HCV).

NURSING CONSIDERATIONS

Assessment: Assess for hepatic dysfunction (autoimmune hepatitis, decompensation, failure), history of depression, endocrine disorders, cardiac disease, autoimmune disorders, severe anemia, bone marrow suppression, pancreatitis, colitis, ophthalmologic disorders, renal impairment, and possible drug interactions. Obtain baseline CBC, SCr, TFTs, LFTs, $CD4^{+}$(HIV), Hgb, and Hct.

Monitoring: Monitor for signs/symptoms of neuropsychiatric, bone marrow toxicities, cardiovascular disorders (HTN, supraventricular arrhythmias, chest pain, MI), cerebrovascular disorder, infectious disorder (neutropenia, thrombocytopenia), hepatic failure, hypersensitivity reactions, endocrine disorder (thyroidism, DM), exacerbations of autoimmune disorders, pulmonary disorder, colitis, pancreatitis, and ophthalmologic disorders. Periodically monitor hematologic (week 2 and 4, or more if needed), biochemical (4 weeks), LFTs, TFTs, and eyes.

Patient Counseling: Instruct to remain well-hydrated. Advise to take with food. May impair physical/mental abilities if have symptoms of dizziness, confusion, somnolence, and fatigue. Seek medical attention if symptoms of depression (suicidal ideation), cardiovascular disorders (chest pain), infectious disorder (fever), hepatic failure, hypersensitivity reactions, hyper/hypoglycemia, exacerbation of autoimmune disorders, pulmonary disorder, colitis, pancreatitis, and ophthalmologic disorders occur. Should not be used during pregnancy. Instruct patient to practice effective contraception during and 6 months post-therapy. Advise risks of teratogenic/embryocidal.

Administration: SQ route. **Storage:** Refrigerate at 2-8°C (36-46°F). Do not freeze or shake. Protect from light.

PEG-INTRON RX

peginterferon alfa-2b (Schering)

May cause or aggravate fatal or life-threatening neuropsychiatric, autoimmune, ischemic, and infectious disorders. Monitor closely with periodic clinical and laboratory evaluations. D/C with severe or worsening signs or symptoms of these conditions. When used with Rebetol, refer to the individual monograph.

THERAPEUTIC CLASS: Pegylated virus proliferation inhibitor

INDICATIONS: Treatment of chronic hepatitis C (CHC) in combination with Rebetol® in patients ≥3 yrs with compensated liver disease. Treatment of chronic hepatitis C alone in patients ≥18 yrs with compensated liver disease not previously treated with interferon alpha.

DOSAGE: *Adults:* ≥18 yrs: Administer SQ once weekly for 1 yr. Monotherapy: 1mcg/kg/week. Combination Therapy With Rebetol: 1.5mcg/kg/week plus Rebetol 800-1400mg/day PO based on patients body weight for 48 weeks in genotype 1, and 24 weeks genotype 2 and 3 patients. CrCl <50mL/min: D/C therapy. Adjust dose based on hematological parameters and depression severity (see PI for dose modifications). Renal Impairment: CrCl 30-50mL/min: Reduce dose by 25%. CrCl 10-29mL/min: Reduce dose by 50%. D/C if renal function decreases, no 2 $\log_{10}$ drop or loss of HCV-RNA at 12 weeks, or HCV-RNA levels remain detectable after 24 weeks.

Pediatrics: 3-17 yrs: Combination Therapy With Rebetol: 60mcg/m^2/week SQ plus Rebetol 15mg/kg/day in 2 divided doses for 48 weeks in genotype 1, and 24 weeks in genotype 2 and 3 patients. CrCl <50mL/min: D/C therapy. Adjust dose based on hematological parameters and depression severity (see PI for dose modifications). Renal Impairment: CrCl 30-50mL/min: Reduce dose by 25%. CrCl 10-29mL/min: Reduce dose by 50%. D/C if renal function decreases, HCV-RNA dropped <2 $\log_{10}$ at 12 weeks, or HCV-RNA levels remain detectable after 24 weeks.

HOW SUPPLIED: Inj: 50mcg/0.5mL, 80mcg/0.5mL, 120mcg/0.5mL, 150mcg/0.5mL

CONTRAINDICATIONS: Known hypersensitivity reactions (eg, urticaria, angioedema, bronchoconstriction, anaphylaxis, Stevens-Johnson syndrome, and toxic epidermal necrolysis), autoimmune hepatitis, hepatic decompensation (Child-Pugh score >6 [class B and C]) in cirrhotic CHC patients. When used with Rebetol, refer to the individual monograph.

WARNINGS/PRECAUTIONS: Life-threatening neuropsychiatric reactions may occur; caution with history of depression or psychiatric symptoms/disorders. Risk of bone marrow suppression; monitor CBCs and blood chemistry at initiation and periodically thereafter. Hypotension, arrhythmia, tachycardia, angina pectoris, MI reported; caution with cardiovascular disease. Conduct baseline eye exam in all patients and periodical exams with pre-existing ophthalmologic disorders; d/c if new or worsening ophthalmologic disorders occur. Caution with CrCl <50mL/min, autoimmune disorders, and the elderly. D/C if persistent or unexplained pulmonary infiltrates, or pulmonary dysfunction, or hypersensitivity reaction occurs, or if hemorrhagic/ischemic colitis or pancreatitis, bone marrow toxicity (eg, severe decrease in neutrophil or platelet counts) develops. May cause or aggravate hypothyroidism/hyperthyroidism. Hyperglycemia and DM reported. Avoid if failed other alpha interferon treatments, liver or other organ transplant recipients, or with HIV or HBV co-infection. May elevate triglyceride levels. Monitor renal impairment for toxicity, including increase in serum creatinine levels. May cause severe decreases in neutrophil and platelet counts. Risk of hepatic decompensation and death in CHC patients with cirrhosis. Dental and periodontal disorders reported. Caution in elderly.

ADVERSE REACTIONS: Headache, fatigue, rigors, dizziness, NV, anorexia, depression, suicidal ideation, emotional lability/irritability, myalgia, injection site inflammation/reaction, abdominal pain, and neutropenia.

INTERACTIONS: Hemolytic anemia reported with ribavirin. May increase levels; monitor signs/symptoms of increased narcotic effect. Caution with medications metabolized by CYP2C8/9 (eg, warfarin and phenytoin) or CYP2D6 (eg, flecainide). Monitor treatment-associated toxicities (eg, hepatic decompenstion, anemia) with ribavirin and nucleoside reverse transcriptase inhibitors (NRTIs).

PREGNANCY: Category C (monotherapy) and X (combination therapy), not for use in nursing.

MECHANISM OF ACTION: α-2b interferon. Binds to and activates the human type 1 interferon receptor. Upon binding, the receptor subunits dimerize, and activate multiple intracellular signal transduction pathway.

P

PHARMACOKINETICS: Absorption: T_{max}=15-44 hrs. **Elimination:** $T_{1/2}$=approximately 40 hrs (HCV).

NURSING CONSIDERATIONS

Assessment: Assess for neuropsychiatric conditions, autoimmune disease, liver dysfunction (autoimmune hepatitis, decompensation), renal dysfunction, bone marrow suppression, ophthalmologic disorders, endocrine disorders (thryoidism, DM), colitis, pancreatitis, pulmonary function, history of CVD, and possible drug interactions. Obtain baseline CBC and platelet counts, LFTs, bilirubin, uric acid, TSH, Hgb, Hct, and ECG.

Monitoring: Monitor periodically CBC (hemoglobin, neutrophil and platelet count), LFTs, renal function (SrCr), bilirubin and uric acid, TSH level, HCV RNA, triglyceride levels, and complete eye exam. Signs/symptoms of autoimmune, ischemic, infectious disorders, neuropsychiatric events, bone marrow toxicity, hepatic failure, endocrine disorder, cardiovascular events, pulmonary disorders, colitis, pancreatitis, ophthalmic disorder, dental/periodontal disorders, and hypersensitivity.

Patient Counseling: Seek medical attention for symptoms of depression (suicidal ideation), cardiovascular (chest pain) and cerebrovascular events, ophthalmologic toxicity (decreased/loss of vision), pancreatitis and colitis (abdominal pain, NV), worsening of liver disease/failure (jaundice); respiratory (fever, cough, dyspnea), hyperglycemia, and hypersensitivity reactions. Keep well hydrated. Advise to brush teeth thoroughly twice a day and have regular dental examinations.

Administration: SQ **Storage:** (Redipen) 2-8°C (36-46°F). Do not freeze. (Vials) 25°C (77°F); excursions permitted to 15-30°C (59-86°F). After reconstitution, use solution immediately, but may store up to 24 hrs at 2-8°C (36-46°F). Do not freeze.

PENICILLIN VK — RX
penicillin V potassium (Various)

OTHER BRAND NAMES: Veetids (Sandoz)

THERAPEUTIC CLASS: Penicillin

INDICATIONS: Treatment of mild to moderately severe bacterial infections including conditions of the respiratory tract, oropharynx, skin and soft tissue caused by susceptible strains of microorganisms. Prevention of recurrence following rheumatic fever and/or chorea.

DOSAGE: *Adults:* Usual: Streptococcal Infections (Scarlet Fever/Erysipelas/Upper Respiratory Tract): 125-250mg q6-8h for 10 days. Pneumococcal Infections (Otitis Media/Respiratory Tract): 250-500mg q6h until afebrile for at least 2 days. Staphylococcus Infections (Skin/Soft Tissue): 250-500mg q6-8h. Fusospirochetosis Infections (Oropharnyx): 250-500mg q6-8h. Rheumatic Fever/Chorea Prevention: 125-250mg bid.
Pediatrics: ≥12 yrs: Usual: Streptococcal Infections (Scarlet Fever/Erysipelas/Upper Respiratory Tract): 125-250mg q6-8h for 10 days. Pneumococcal Infections (Otitis Media/Respiratory Tract): 250-500mg q6h until afebrile for at least 2 days. Staphylococcus Infections (Skin/Soft Tissue): 250-500mg q6-8h. Fusospirochetosis Infections (Oropharnyx): 250-500mg q6-8h. Rheumatic Fever/Chorea Prevention: 125-250mg bid.

HOW SUPPLIED: Sus: 125mg/5mL, 250mg/5mL [100mL, 200mL]; Tab: 250mg, 500mg

WARNINGS/PRECAUTIONS: Not for severe pneumonia, empyema, bacteremia, pericarditis, meningitis and arthritis during the acute stage. Serious, fatal anaphylactic reactions reported. Pseudomembranous colitis reported. Oral administration may not be effective with severe illnesses, nausea, vomiting, gastric dilation, cardiospasm, intestinal hypermotility. Cross-sensitivity with cephalosporins. Caution with asthma and allergies.

ADVERSE REACTIONS: Epigastric distress, N/V, diarrhea, hypersensitivity reactions, black hairy tongue, anaphylaxis, superinfection (prolonged use).

PREGNANCY: Category B, caution in nursing.

MECHANISM OF ACTION: Phenoxymethyl analog of penicillin G; exerts bactericidal action during stage of active multiplication by inhibiting biosynthesis of cell-wall mucopeptide.

PHARMACOKINETICS: Distribution: Plasma protein binding (80%). **Elimination:** Urine.

NURSING CONSIDERATIONS

Assessment: Assess for history of significant allergies or asthma, NV, gastric dilatation, severe illness, cardiospasm, intestinal hypermotility, and possible drug interactions.

Monitoring: Monitor for signs/symptoms of hypersensitivity reactions, *C. difficile*-associated diarrhea, and superinfections.

Patient Counseling: Inform drug only treats bacterial, not viral, infections. Instruct to take as directed; skipping doses or not completing full course may decrease effectiveness and increase resistance. May experience diarrhea; contact physician if watery and bloody stools or hypersensitivity reactions occur.

Administration: Oral route. **Storage:** 20-25°C (68-77°F).

PENLAC — RX
ciclopirox (Dermik)

THERAPEUTIC CLASS: Broad-spectrum antifungal

P

INDICATIONS: Mild to moderate onychomycosis of fingernails or toenails without lunula involvement due to *Trichophyton rubrum* (in immunocompetent patients).

DOSAGE: *Adults:* Apply qhs or 8 hrs before washing to nail bed, hyponychium, and under surface when it is free of nail bed. Apply daily over previous coat and remove with alcohol every 7 days. Repeat cycle up to 48 weeks.

HOW SUPPLIED: Sol: 8% [6.6mL]

WARNINGS/PRECAUTIONS: Only for use on nails and adjacent skin. Caution with removal of infected nail in insulin-dependent DM or diabetic neuropathy.

ADVERSE REACTIONS: Periungual erythema, erythema of proximal nail fold, nail shape change, nail irritation, ingrown toenail, nail discoloration.

INTERACTIONS: Avoid nail polish or other nail cosmetics on treated nails.

PREGNANCY: Category B, caution in nursing.

MECHANISM OF ACTION: Broad spectrum antifungal; acts by chelation of polyvalent cations (Fe^{+3} or Al^{+3}), resulting in the inhibition of the metal-dependent enzymes responsible for degradation of peroxides within fungal cell.

PHARMACOKINETICS: Absorption: Serum levels range from 12-80ng/mL following topical administration. **Elimination:** Urine (<5% of applied topical dose).

NURSING CONSIDERATIONS

Assessment: Assess use with insulin-dependent DM, diabetic neuropathy, and in pregnant/nursing females. Assess medication is only being used on nails or immediately adjacent skin.

Monitoring: Monitor for signs/symptoms of sensitivity reactions and chemical irritation. Perform frequent (eg, monthly) removal of unattached infected nails, trimming of onycholic nails, and filing of any excess horny material.

Patient Counseling: Advise to avoid bringing medication in contact with eyes and mucous membranes. Instruct to apply medication evenly over entire nail plate and 5mm of surrounding skin. Counsel to notify physician if signs of increased irritation at the application site develop (eg, redness, itching, burning, oozing, blistering). Inform to file away (with emery board) loose nail material and trim nails as required. Advise not to use nail polish or other nail cosmetic products on the treated nails. Instruct not to use medication near open flame. Inform that it may take up to 48 weeks of daily application of the medication (including monthly professional removal of unattached infected nails) before a clear or almost clear nail is seen.

P

Administration: Topical route. **Storage:** Between 15-30°C (59-86°F). Flammable; keep away from heat and flame.

PENTASA

mesalamine (Shire)

RX

THERAPEUTIC CLASS: Anti-inflammatory Agent

INDICATIONS: Induction of remission and for treatment of mild to moderate active ulcerative colitis.

DOSAGE: *Adults:* 1g qid. Can be given up to 8 weeks.

HOW SUPPLIED: Cap, Extended-Release: 250mg, 500mg

CONTRAINDICATIONS: Hypersensitivity to salicylates.

WARNINGS/PRECAUTIONS: Caution with hepatic and renal dysfunction; monitor closely. D/C if acute intolerance syndrome develops (eg, cramping, bloody diarrhea, abdominal pain, headache). If rechallenge is considered, perform under careful observation.

ADVERSE REACTIONS: Diarrhea, headache, nausea, abdominal pain.

PREGNANCY: Category B, caution in nursing.

MECHANISM OF ACTION: Unknown, suspected to act as anti-inflammatory agent for blocking cyclooxygenase and inhibiting prostaglandin in gastrointestinal use.

PHARMACOKINETICS: Absorption: C_{max}=1mcg/mL, T_{max}=3 hrs. (N-acetylmesalamine) C_{max}=1.8mcg/mL, T_{max}=3 hrs. **Metabolism:** N-acetylmesalamine (Metabolite). **Elimination:** Feces, N-acetylmesalamine: Urine (19-30%).

NURSING CONSIDERATIONS

Assessment: Assess for pre-existing renal disease, hepatic/renal impairment. Obtain baseline LFTs, BUN, creatinine, and urinalysis (protein).

Monitoring: Monitor LFTs, BUN, creatinine, and urinalysis (protein) periodically. Monitor signs/symptoms of hepatotoxicity, acute intolerance syndrome (cramping, acute abdominal pain, bloody diarrhea), hypersensitivity, and allergic reactions.

Patient Counseling: Seek medical attention if symptoms of hepatotoxicity, acute intolerance syndrome (cramping, acute abdominal pain, bloody diarrhea), hypersensitivity and allergic reactions occur.

Administration: Oral route. **Storage:** 25°C (77°F); excursions permitted to 15-30°C (59-86°F).

PEPCID — RX

famotidine (Merck)

OTHER BRAND NAMES: Pepcid RPD (Merck)

THERAPEUTIC CLASS: H_2-blocker

INDICATIONS: (PO/Inj) Short term treatment of active duodenal ulcer (DU), active benign gastric ulcer (GU), gastroesophageal reflux disease (GERD) and esophagitis due to GERD. Maintenance therapy for DU. Treatment of hypersecretory conditions (eg, Zollinger-Ellison syndrome). (Inj) For hospitalized patients with hypersecretory conditions or intractable ulcers. As an alternative in patients unable to take oral forms.

DOSAGE: *Adults:* (PO) Acute DU: 40mg qhs or 20mg bid for 4-8 weeks. Maint DU: 20mg qhs. GU: 40mg qhs. GERD: 20mg bid up to 6 weeks. GERD with Esophagitis: 20-40mg bid up to 12 weeks. Hypersecretory Conditions: Initial: 20mg q6h. Max: 160mg q6h. (Inj) 20mg IV q12h, hypersecretory conditions may require higher doses. CrCl <50mL/min: Reduce to 1/2 dose, or increase interval to q36-48h.

Pediatrics: 1-16 yrs: (PO) DU/GU: Usual: 0.5mg/kg/day qhs or divided bid. Max: 40mg/day. GERD With or Without Esophagitis: 0.5mg/kg PO bid. Max: 40mg bid. (Inj) 0.25mg/kg IV q12h up to 40mg/day. Base duration of therapy on clinical response, and/or pH, and endoscopy. (PO) GERD: 3 months-1yr: 0.5mg/kg bid for up to 8 weeks. <3 months: 0.5mg/kg qd for up to 8 weeks. CrCl <50mL/min: Reduce to 1/2 dose, or increase interval to q36-48h.

HOW SUPPLIED: Inj: 0.4mg/mL, 10mg/mL; Sus: 40mg/5mL [50mL]; Tab: 20mg, 40mg; Tab, Disintegrating: (RPD) 20mg, 40mg

CONTRAINDICATIONS: Hypersensitivity to other H_2 antagonists.

WARNINGS/PRECAUTIONS: CNS adverse effects reported with moderate to severe renal insufficiency; adjust dose. Disintegrating tabs contain phenylalanine; caution in phenylketonurics. Symptomatic response does not preclude the presence of gastric malignancy.

ADVERSE REACTIONS: Headache, dizziness, constipation, diarrhea, convulsions, interstitial pneumonia, Stevens-Johnson syndrome.

INTERACTIONS: May give with antacids.

PREGNANCY: Category B, not for use in nursing.

MECHANISM OF ACTION: Histamine H_2-receptor antagonist; inhibits both acid concentration and volume of gastric secretion.

PHARMACOKINETICS: Absorption: (Adults PO): Incompletely absorbed; T_{max}=1.3 hrs. (Adults, IV): T_{max}=20-30 min. **Distribution:** (Adult) Plasma protein binding (15-20%); excreted in breast milk. **Metabolism:** S-oxide (metabolite). **Elimination:** Renal (65-70%), (PO) 25-30% unchanged; (IV) 65-70%

P

unchanged. Metabolic (65-70%); (Adults) $T_{1/2}$=2.5-3.5 hrs. Refer to package insert for pediatric parameters.

NURSING CONSIDERATIONS

Assessment: Assess for hypersensitivity to other H_2 receptor antagonists, renal insufficiency, pregnancy/status.

Monitoring: If renal impairment present, monitor renal function. Monitor for signs/symptoms of hypersensitivity reactions (eg, anaphylaxis), GI effects (eg, constipation, diarrhea), and headache.

Patient Counseling: Instruct to contact physician if hypersensitivity or other adverse reactions develop. Inform may take antacids concomitantly. Avoid nursing while on medication.

Administration: Oral or IV route. **Storage:** Tablet: Controlled room temperature; preserve in well-closed, light-resistant containers. Injection: 2-8°C (36-46°F); if solution freezes, bring to room temperature; allow sufficient time to solubilize all components. Premixed: 25°C (77°F); avoid exposure of premixed product to excessive heat.

PERCOCET

CII

oxycodone HCl - acetaminophen (Endo)

OTHER BRAND NAMES: Endocet (Endo)

THERAPEUTIC CLASS: Opioid analgesic

INDICATIONS: Relief of moderate to moderately severe pain.

DOSAGE: *Adults:* (2.5/325): 1-2 tabs q6h. Max: 12 tabs/day. (5/325): 1 tab q6h prn. Max: 12 tabs/day. (7.5/500): 1 tab q6h prn. Max: 8 tabs/day. (10-650) 1 tab q6h prn. Max: 6 tabs/day. (7.5/325): 1 tab q6h prn. Max: 8 tabs/day. (10/325): 1 tab q6h prn. Max: 6 tabs/day. Do not exceed APAP 4g/day.

HOW SUPPLIED: Tab: (Oxycodone-APAP) 2.5mg-325mg, 5mg-325mg, 7.5mg-325mg, 7.5mg-500mg, 10mg-325mg, 10mg-650mg

WARNINGS/PRECAUTIONS: May cause drug dependence and tolerance; potential for abuse. Risk of respiratory depression. Capacity to elevate CSF pressure may be exaggerated with head injury, other intracranial lesions or a pre-existing increase in ICP. May obscure the diagnosis or clinical course with head injuries or with acute abdominal conditions. Caution with severe hepatic impairment, renal dysfunction, hypothyroidism, Addison's disease, prostatic hypertrophy, urethral stricture, the elderly or debilitated.

ADVERSE REACTIONS: Lightheadedness, dizziness, sedation, NV, euphoria, dysphoria, constipation, skin rash, pruritus.

INTERACTIONS: Potentiates CNS depression with other opioid analgesics, general anesthetics, phenothiazines, tranquilizers, sedative-hypnotics, alcohol and other CNS depressants. Risk of paralytic ileus with anticholinergics.

PREGNANCY: Category C, caution in nursing.

MECHANISM OF ACTION: Oxycodone: Opioid analgesic; semisynthetic pure opioid agonist whose principal therapeutic action is analgesia. Other pharmacological effects include anxiolysis, euphoria, and feelings of relaxation. Effects mediated by CNS receptors (eg, μ and kappa) for endogenous opioid-like compounds (eg, endorphins, enkephalins). APAP: Nonopiate, nonsalicyclic analgesic, and antipyretic. Site and mechanism of analgesic effect not established. Antipyretic effect produced through inhibition of endogenous pyrogen action on the hypothalmic heat-regulating centers.

PHARMACOKINETICS: Absorption: Oxycodone: Absolute bioavailability (87%). APAP: Rapid absorption. **Distribution:** Oxycodone: Plasma protein binding (45%); (IV):V_d= 211.9L; found in breast milk. APAP: Plasma protein binding (20-50%) (variable). **Metabolism:** Oxycodone: N-dealkylation to noroxycodone (metabolite); CYP2D6 (O-demethylation) to oxymorphone (metabolite). Acetaminophen: Liver via cytochrome P450 (conjugation), NAPQI (toxic metabolite). **Elimination:** Oxycodone: Urine (parent compound and metabolites); $T_{1/2}$=3.51 hrs. APAP: Urine (90-100%).

NURSING CONSIDERATIONS

Assessment: Assess for respiratory depression, acute or severe bronchial asthma or hypercarbia, chronic obstructive pulmonary disorder, paralytic ileus, potential for abuse, presence of debilitation (eg, elderly), head injury or other intracranial lesions, elevations in intracranial pressure, circulatory shock, acute abdominal condition, biliary tract disease, acute pancreatitis, hepatic/renal impairment, CNS depression, hypothyroidism, Addison's disease, prostatic hypertrophy, urethral stricture, acute alcoholism, delirium tremens, convulsive disorder, kyphoscoliosis with respiratory depression, myxedema, toxic psychosis, nursing/pregnancy status, medication abuse potential, and possible drug interactions.

Monitoring: Monitor for signs/symptoms of respiratory depression, elevations in CSF pressure, hypotension, hepatotoxicity, convulsions, anaphylactic reactions, decreased bowel motility, sphincter of Oddi spasms, increased serum amylase levels, tolerance and physical dependence, and medication abuse.

Patient Counseling: Instruct to keep out of reach of children. If accidental ingestion occurs, seek emergency medical care. Advise to flush unused medication down toilet. Counsel not to adjust dose without consulting physician. Inform drug may impair mental/physical abilities required to perform hazardous tasks (eg, operating machinery/driving). Advise to avoid alcohol or other CNS depressants. Instruct not to abruptly d/c if on for few weeks; taper dosing. Inform that medication has potential for abuse; protect from theft.

Administration: Oral route. **Storage:** 20-25°C (68-77°F). Dispense in tight, light-resistant container, with child-resistant closure.

PERCODAN

CII

oxycodone HCl - aspirin (Endo)

OTHER BRAND NAMES: Endodan (Endo)

THERAPEUTIC CLASS: Opioid analgesic

INDICATIONS: Relief of moderate to moderately severe pain.

DOSAGE: *Adults:* Usual: 1 tab q6h prn. Max: 12 tabs/day or ASA 4g/day.

HOW SUPPLIED: Tab: (Oxycodone HCl-ASA) 4.8355mg-325mg* *scored

WARNINGS/PRECAUTIONS: May cause drug dependence and tolerance; potential for abuse. Risk of respiratory depression. Capacity to elevate CSF pressure may be exaggerated with head injury, other intracranial lesions or a pre-existing increase in ICP. May obscure the diagnosis or clinical course with head injuries or with acute abdominal conditions. Caution with severe of hepatic impairment, renal dysfunction, hypothyroidism, Addison's disease, prostatic hypertrophy, urethral stricture, peptic ulcer, coagulation abnormalities, and the elderly or debilitated. May increase the risk of developing Reye's syndrome in children and teenagers. May impair mental/physical abilities.

ADVERSE REACTIONS: Lightheadedness, dizziness, sedation, NV, euphoria, dysphoria, constipation, pruritus.

INTERACTIONS: Additive CNS depression with other opioid analgesics, general anesthetics, phenothiazines, tranquilizers, sedative-hypnotics, or other CNS depressants (including alcohol). ASA may enhance effect of anticoagulants and inhibit effects of uricosuric agents.

PREGNANCY: Category B (Oxycodone) and D (ASA), not for use in nursing.

MECHANISM OF ACTION: Oxycodone: Semisynthetic pure opioid agonist. Principle therapeutic effect is analgesia. Other effects include anxiolysis, euphoria, and feelings of relaxation. Effects mediated by CNSb receptors (ex, μ, kappa) for endogenous opioid-like compounds (eg, endorphins, enkephalins). ASA: Inhibits prostaglandin production, including those involved in inflammation. (Prostaglandins cause pain sensation by stimulating muscle contractions and dilating blood vessels throughout body.) In CNS, works on hypothalamus heat-regulating center to reduce fever.

PHARMACOKINETICS: Absorption: Oxycodone: Absolute bioavailability (87%). ASA: Rapidly absorbed. **Distribution:** Oxycodone: Plasma protein binding (45%); found in breast milk; (IV) V_d=211.9L. ASA: Found in most body tissues, fluids (eg, fetal tissues, breast milk, CNS, liver, kidneys); variable serum protein binding. **Metabolism:** Oxycodone: N-dealkylation to noroxycodone (metabolite); CYP2D6 (O-demethylation) to oxymorphone (metabolite). ASA: Liver, hydrolysis to salicylate, salicyluric acid, salicyl phenolic glucuronide, salicyl acyl glucuronide, gentisic acid, gentisuric acid (major metabolites). **Elimination:** Oxycodone: Urine (parent compound and metabolites); $T_{1/2}$=3.51 hrs. ASA: Urine (parent compound and metabolites) (80-100%); $T_{1/2}$=2-3 hrs.

NURSING CONSIDERATIONS

Assessment: Assess for hemophilia, presence of viral infection if using in pediatrics, hypersensitivity to NSAIDS, asthma, rhinitis, nasal polyps, respiratory depression, hypercarbia, paralytic ileus, medication abuse potential, head injury or other intracranial lesions, presence of increased ICP, circulatory shock, inherited or acquired bleeding disorders (eg, hemophilia, vitamin K deficiency), active peptic ulcer disease, CNS depression, presence of debilitation (eg, elderly), hepatic/renal dysfunction, hypothyroidism, Addison's disease, prostatic hypertrophy, urethral stricture, acute alcoholism, delirium tremens, kyphoscoliosis with respiratory depression, myxedema, toxic psychosis, convulsive disorder, biliary tract disease, acute pancreatitis, pregnancy/nursing status, and possible drug interactions.

Monitoring: Monitor for signs/symptoms of respiratory depression, elevations in CSF pressure, hypotension, hemorrhage, GI effects (eg, stomach pain, heartburn, ulceration, GI bleeding), convulsions, anaphylactic reactions, decreased bowel motility, sphincter of Oddi spasms, tolerance, and physical dependence. Monitor for elevated hepatic enzymes, elevated BUN and SrCr, hyperkalemia, proteinuria, prolonged bleeding time, and increases in serum amylase levels. In pediatrics, monitor for Reye's syndrome.

Patient Counseling: Instruct to keep out of reach of children; if accidental ingestion occurs, seek medical attention. Advise to dispose of unused drug via toilet. Counsel to consult physician before adjusting dosing. Caution that drug may impair mental/physical abilities required for performing hazardous tasks (eg, operating machinery/driving). Instruct to avoid alcohol and other CNS depressants. Advise not to abruptly d/c if on medication for more than few weeks; taper dosing. Instruct to report adverse events (eg, respiratory depression). Inform that medication has potential for abuse; protect from theft.

Administration: Oral route. **Storage:** 25°C (77°F); excursions permitted to 15-30°C (59-86°F). Dispense in a tight, light-resistant container with child-resistant closure.

PERFOROMIST RX

formoterol fumarate (Dey)

Long-acting β_2-agonists may increase risk of asthma-related death.

THERAPEUTIC CLASS: Beta$_2$-agonist

INDICATIONS: Long-term maintenance treatment of bronchoconstriction in patients with chronic obstructive pulmonary disease (COPD), including chronic bronchitis and emphysema.

DOSAGE: *Adults:* 20mcg bid q12h. Administer by nebulizer.

HOW SUPPLIED: Sol, Inhalation: 20mcg/2mL [2.5mL, 60^s]

WARNINGS/PRECAUTIONS: Only use short-acting β_2-agonist inhaler for acute symptoms. Should not be used with other long acting β_2-agonist medications. D/C if paradoxical bronchospasm occurs. D/C if ECG changes, QT interval increases, or ST depression occurs. Caution with cardiovascular disorders (eg.coronary insufficiency, arrythmias, and HTN), convulsive disorders, thyrotoxicosis, and DM. May cause hypokalemia and hyperglycemia.

ADVERSE REACTIONS: Diarrhea, nausea, nasopharyngitis, dry mouth, angina, HTN, hypotension, tachycardia, arrythmias, nervousness, headache, tremor, muscle cramps, palpitations, dizziness.

INTERACTIONS: Adrenergic drugs may potentiate effects. Xanthine derivatives, steroids, diuretics, or non-potassium sparing diuretics may potentiate hypokalemia or ECG changes; use with caution. MAOIs, TCAs, and drugs known to prolong QTc interval may potentiate effect on cardiovascular system; use with extreme caution. β-blockers may decrease effectiveness; use with caution.

PREGNANCY: Category C, caution in nursing.

MECHANISM OF ACTION: Long acting β_2-agonist; acts as bronchodilator, stimulates intracellular adenyl cyclase, the enzyme that catalyzes the conversion of ATP to cAMP. Increased cAMP levels cause relaxation of bronchial smooth muscle and inhibition of release of mediators of immediated hypersensitivity from cells such as mast cells.

PHARMACOKINETICS: Absorption: C_{max}=72pg/mL; T_{max}=12 min. **Distribution:** Plasma protein binding (61-64%). **Metabolism:** Glucuronidation, O-demethylation; CYP2D6, 2C19, 2C19, 2A6. **Elimination:** Urine (unchanged); $T_{1/2}$=7 hrs.

NURSING CONSIDERATIONS

Assessment: Assess for acute COPD, asthma, acute bronchospasm, CVD (coronary insufficiency, cardiac arrhythmias, HTN), convulsive disorders, thyrotoxicosis, serum potassium level, DM, ketoacidosis, and possible drug interactions.

Monitoring: Monitor for serious asthma exacerbations, paradoxical bronchospasm, cardiovascular effects, hypokalemia, hyperglycemia, aggravation of DM, ketoacidosis, pulse rate, BP, and ECG changes (T-wave flattening, prolongation of QTc interval, ST segment depression).

Patient Counseling: Counsel to use as directed. Do not inhale more than prescribed. Excessive use may increase likelihood of cardiovascular side effects. Maximum daily dose is 1 vial twice daily. Use other inhaler (albuterol) only for acute symptoms, and consult with physician about use of other inhalers. Immediately report any side effects to physician (chest pain, rapid heart rate, headache, nervousness, dry mouth, muscle cramps, nausea, dizziness, fatigue, malaise, and BP changes). Always keep in foil patch, only remove for use, and discard container and top right after use.

Administration: Oral inhalation. Only administered via a standard jet nebulizer connected to an air compressor with adequate airflow and equipped with a facemask or mouthpiece. **Storage:** Prior to dispensing: 2-8°C (36-46°F). After dispensing: 2-25°C (36-77°F) for up to 3 months. Protect from heat.

P

PERSANTINE — RX

dipyridamole (Boehringer Ingelheim)

THERAPEUTIC CLASS: Platelet aggregation inhibitor

INDICATIONS: Adjunct to coumarin anticoagulants for prevention of postoperative thromboembolic complications of cardiac valve replacement.

DOSAGE: *Adults:* 75-100mg qid.

HOW SUPPLIED: Tab: 25mg, 50mg, 75mg

WARNINGS/PRECAUTIONS: Caution with hypotension or severe CAD (eg, unstable angina or recent MI); may aggravate chest pain. Elevated hepatic enzymes and hepatic failure reported.

ADVERSE REACTIONS: Dizziness, abdominal distress.

INTERACTIONS: Increases levels of adenosine. May counteract effects of cholinesterase inhibitors.

PREGNANCY: Category B, caution in nursing.

MECHANISM OF ACTION: Platelet inhibitor; inhibits uptake of adenosine into platelets, endothelial cells, and erythrocytes. Inhibition results in an increase in adenosine concentrations that act on the platelet A_2 receptor to stimulate platelet adenylate cyclase and increase platelet cyclic-3',5'-adenosine monophosphate (cAMP) levels. Platelet aggregation is thereby inhibited in response to various stimuli (eg, platelet activating factor (PAF), collagen, adenosine diphosphate). Also inhibits phosphodiesterase (PDE) in various tissues. Inhibits cyclic-3'5'-guanosine monophosphate-PDE (cGMP-PDE), which thereby augments the increase in cGMP produced by EDRF (endothelium-derived relaxing factor [nitric oxide]).

PHARMACOKINETICS: Absorption: T_{max}=75 min. **Distribution:** Highly bound to plasma proteins. Found in breast milk. **Metabolism:** Liver (conjugation). **Elimination:** Bile; $T_{1/2}$=40 min. (initial); $T_{1/2}$=10 hrs.

NURSING CONSIDERATIONS

Assessment: Assess for hepatic insufficiencies, hypotension, severe coronary artery disease (eg, unstable angina, recent MI), pregnancy/nursing status, and other drug interactions.

Monitoring: Monitor for elevations in hepatic enzymes (hepatic failure) and for signs/symptoms of chest pains in patients with CAD.

Patient Counseling: Advise to contact physician if any signs/symptoms of hepatic insufficiencies develop. Inform that aspirin should not be administered concomitantly with coumarin anticoagulants.

Administration: Oral route. **Storage:** 25°C (77°F); excursions permitted to 15-30°C (59-86°F). Keep out of reach of children.

PEXEVA — RX

paroxetine mesylate (Noven)

Antidepressants increased the risk of suicidal thinking and behavior (suicidality) in short-term studies in children, adolescents, and young adults with major depressive disorder (MDD) and other psychiatric disorders. Paroxetine is not approved for use in pediatric patients.

THERAPEUTIC CLASS: Selective serotonin reuptake inhibitor

INDICATIONS: Treatment of major depressive disorder (MDD), obsessive compulsive disorder (OCD), panic disorder with or without agoraphobia, and generalized anxiety disorder (GAD).

DOSAGE: *Adults:* MDD: Initial: 20mg/day. Max: 50mg/day. OCD: Initial: 20mg/day. Titrate: Increase by 10mg/day. Usual: 40mg/day. Max: 60mg/day. Panic Disorder: Initial: 10mg/day. Titrate: 10mg/day increments at intervals of at least 1 week. Max: 60mg/day. GAD: Initial: 20mg/day. Titrate: Increase by 10mg/day. Max: 50mg/day. Elderly/Debilitated/Severe Renal or Hepatic Impairment: Initial: 10mg qd. Max: 40mg/day.

P

HOW SUPPLIED: Tab: 10mg, 20mg, 30mg, 40mg

CONTRAINDICATIONS: Concomitant use of MAOIs, thioridazine, and pimozide.

WARNINGS/PRECAUTIONS: Avoid abrupt withdrawal. Re-evaluate periodically. May increase risk of bleeding events. Activation of mania/hypomania. Caution with history of mania, seizures, conditions that affect metabolism or hemodynamic responses, narrow-angle glaucoma. D/C if seizures occur. Altered platelet function, hyponatremia, mydriasis, and akathisia reported. Serotonin syndrome or neuroleptic malignant syndrome (NMS)-like reactions reported. Manage with immediate discontinuation and monitor. Monitor for clinical worsening and/or suicidality, especially at initiation of therapy or dose changes. Increase plasma concentrations may occur in patients with severe renal (CrCl <30mL/min) or severe hepatic impairment.

ADVERSE REACTIONS: Asthenia, sweating, nausea, decreased appetite, somnolence, dizziness, insomnia, tremor, nervousness, abnormal ejaculation, dry mouth, constipation, decreased libido, impotence, headache, tinnitus.

INTERACTIONS: See Contraindications. Avoid alcohol, tryptophan. May shift concentrations with plasma-bound drugs. Increased risk of bleeding with NSAIDS, aspirin, oral anticoagulants. May inhibit metabolism of TCAs. Caution with other agents that may affect serotonergic neurotransmitter systems (eg, triptans, linezolid, lithium, tramadol, St. John's wort). Serotonin syndrome or NMS-like reactions reported with serotonergic (eg, triptans), MAIOs, antipsychotics, or other dopamine antagonists. Monitor theophylline. Reduce procyclidine dose if anticholinergic effects occur. Increased levels with cimetidine. Caution with digoxin, lithium, warfarin, drugs metabolized by CYP2D6 (eg, antidepressants, phenothiazines, Type 1C antiarrhythmics), or drugs that inhibit CYP2D6 (eg,quinidine). Fosamprenavir/ritonavir may decrease levels. Concomitant with thioridazine may prolong QTc interval associated with serious ventricular arrhythmias (eg, torsade de pointes), sudden death, and may elevate thioridazine levels.

PREGNANCY: Category D, caution in nursing.

MECHANISM OF ACTION: SSRI; inhibits CNS neuronal reuptake of serotonin.

PHARMACOKINETICS: Absorption: Complete; C_{max}=81.3ng/mL; T_{max}=8.1 hr. **Distribution:** Plasma protein binding (95%). **Metabolism:** Oxidation and methylation via CYP2D6. **Elimination:** Urine (2%), feces (<1%); $T_{1/2}$=33.2 hrs.

NURSING CONSIDERATIONS

Assessment: Assess for bipolar disorder risk, history of mania, history of seizures, narrow-angle glaucoma, disease/condition that alters metabolism or hemodynamic response, hepatic/renal impairment, and possible drug interactions.

Monitoring: Monitor for signs/symptoms of clinical worsening (suicidality, unusual changes in behavior), serotonin syndrome/NMS-like reactions, abnormal bleeding, activation of mania, mydriasis, akathisia, hyponatremia, seizures, cognitive/motor impairment, hepatic/renal dysfunction. If abruptly d/c, monitor for symptoms of dysphoric mood, irritability, agitation, dizziness, sensory disturbances, anxiety, confusion, headache, lethargy, emotional lability, insomnia, and hypomania.

Patient Counseling: Instruct to swallow whole, not to chew or crush. Advise to avoid alcohol. Seek medical attention for symptoms of serotonin syndrome (mental status changes, tachycardia, hyperthermia, NV, diarrhea, incoordination), abnormal bleeding (particularly if using NSAIDs or ASA), akathisia, hyponatremia (headaches, unsteadiness), mydriasis, activation of mania, seizures, clinical worsening (suicidal ideation, unusual changes in behavior), or d/c symptoms (irritability, agitation, dizziness, anxiety, headache, insomnia). Caution against hazardous tasks (eg, operating machinery and driving). Inform may notice improvement in 1-4 weeks; continue therapy as directed. Notify physician if pregnant/intend to become pregnant, or breastfeeding. Counsel about benefits and risks of therapy. Inform physician if taking, or plan to take any over-the-counter prescriptions.

Administration: Oral route. **Storage:** 25°C (77°F); excursions permitted to 15-30°C (59-86°F). Protect from humidity.

PFIZERPEN RX

penicillin G potassium (Pfizer)

THERAPEUTIC CLASS: Penicillin

INDICATIONS: For therapy of severe infections when rapid and high blood levels of penicillin required. Management of streptococcal, pneumococcal, staphylococcal, clostridial, fusospirochetal, listeria, and gram negative bacillary, and pasteurella infections. For anthrax, actinomycosis, diphtheria, erysipeloid, meningitis, endocarditis, bacteremia, rat-bite fever, syphilis, and gonorrheal endocarditis and arthritis. With combined oral therapy, prophylaxis against endocarditis in patients with congenital heart disease, rheumatic, or other acquired valvular heart disease undergoing dental procedures or surgical procedures of upper respiratory tract.

DOSAGE: *Adults:* Anthrax/Gonorrheal Endocarditis/Severe Infections (Streptococci, Pneumococci, Staphylococci): Minimum of 5MU/day. Syphilis: Administer in hospital. Determine dose and duration based on age and wt. Meningococcic Meningitis: 1-2MU IM q2h or 20-30MU/day continuous IV. Actinomycosis: 1-6MU/day for cervicofacial cases; 10-20MU/day for thoracic and abdominal disease. Clostridial Infections: 20MU/day (adjunct to

antitoxin). Fusospirochetal Severe Infections: 5-10MU/day for oropharynx, lower respiratory tract, and genital area infection. Rat-bite Fever: 12-15MU/day for 3-4 weeks. Listeria Endocarditis: 15-20MU/day for 4 weeks. Pasteurella Bacteremia/Meningitis: 4-6MU/day for 2 weeks. Erysipeloid Endocarditis: 2-20MU/day for 4-6 weeks. Gram Negative Bacillary Bacteremia: 20-80MU/day. Diphtheria (carrier state): 0.3-0.4MU/day in divided doses for 10-12 days. Endocarditis Prophylaxis: 1MU IM mixed with 0.6MU procaine penicillin G 0.5-1 hr before procedure. Renal/Cardiac/Vascular Dysfunction: Consider dose reduction. For streptococcal infection, treat for minimum 10 days.
Pediatrics: Listeria Infections: Neonates: 0.5-1MU/day. Congenital Syphilis: Administer in hospital. Determine dose and duration based on age and wt. Endocarditis Prophylaxis: 30,000U/kg IM mixed with 0.6MU procaine penicillin G 0.5-1 hr before procedure. For streptococcal infection, treat for minimum 10 days.

HOW SUPPLIED: Inj: 1MU, 5MU, 20MU

WARNINGS/PRECAUTIONS: Serious, fatal anaphylactic reactions reported; increased risk with hypersensitivity to PCNs, cephalosporins, and other allergens. Avoid IV, intra-arterial administration, or injection into/near major peripheral nerves or blood vessels; may cause severe neurovascular damage. Take culture after therapy completion to determine streptococci eradication. Caution with history of significant allergies or asthma. May result in overgrowth of nonsusceptible organisms. Evaluate renal, hepatic and hematopoietic systems with prolonged therapy. Administer slowly to avoid electrolyte imbalance from potassium or sodium content; monitor electrolytes and consider dose reductions with renal, cardiac, or vascular dysfunction. Caution in newborns; evaluate organ system function frequently.

ADVERSE REACTIONS: Skin rash (eg, maculopapular eruption, exfoliative dermatitis) urticaria, chills, fever, edema, arthralgia, prostration, anaphylaxis, arrhythmias, cardiac arrest, Jarisch-Herxheimer reaction.

INTERACTIONS: Bacteriostatic agents (eg, tetracycline, erythromycin) may diminish effects. Prolonged levels with probenecid.

PREGNANCY: Category B, caution in nursing.

MECHANISM OF ACTION: Penicillin; exerts bactericidal action during stage of active multiplication by inhibiting biosynthesis of cell-wall mucopeptide.

PHARMACOKINETICS: Absorption: Rapid. **Distribution:** Found in breast milk. **Elimination:** Urine.

NURSING CONSIDERATIONS

Assessment: Assess for significant allergies or asthma and possible drug interactions. Obtain baseline serology and perform dark field exam (syphilis).

Monitoring: Monitor serum electrolytes, renal and hematopoietic function periodically, Coombs' test (after large doses), blood cultures after therapy (streptococci eradication), serologic tests monthly for ≥4 months during therapy and every 6 months for 2-3 yrs after therapy (syphilis). Monitor for signs/symptoms of superinfections, thrombophlebitis (IV), hypersensitivity, and anaphylactoid reactions.

Patient Counseling: Inform that therapy treats bacterial, not viral, infections. Take exactly as directed; skipping doses or not completing full course may decrease effectiveness and increase resistance. Advise to seek medical attention if symptoms of infection, thrombophlebitis, hypersensitivity, or anaphylactoid reactions occur.

Administration: IM/IV routes. **Storage:** Below 30°C (86°F).

PHENERGAN INJECTION — RX

promethazine HCl (Baxter)

THERAPEUTIC CLASS: Phenothiazine derivative

INDICATIONS: For blood or plasma allergic reactions, allergic reactions where oral therapy is not possible, sedation, and special surgical situations (eg, repeated bronchoscopy). Adjunct for anaphylactic reactions and postoperative pain. Treatment of motion sickness. Prevention and control of nausea and vomiting in surgery.

DOSAGE: *Adults:* (IM/IV) IM is preferred. Allergy: Initial: 25mg, may repeat within 2 hrs. Sedation: 25-50mg qhs. Nausea/Vomiting: 12.5-25mg q4h. Preoperative/Postoperative: 25-50mg. Obstetrics: 50mg in early labor, 25-75mg in established labor, may repeat once or twice q4h. Max: 100mg/24 hrs of labor. Do not give IV administration >25mg/mL and at a rate >25mg/min. *Pediatrics:* ≥2 yrs: Dose should not exceed half of adult dose. Premedication: Usual: 0.5mg/lb. Do not give IV administration >25mg/mL and at a rate >25mg/min.

HOW SUPPLIED: Inj: 25mg/mL, 50mg/mL

CONTRAINDICATIONS: Comatose states, intra-arterial or subcutaneous injection. Hypersensitivity to other phenothiazines.

WARNINGS/PRECAUTIONS: Caution in patients ≥2 yrs. Not recommended for uncomplicated vomiting in pediatrics. May cause marked drowsiness; caution with operating machinery. Fatal respiratory depression reported; avoid with respiratory dysfunction (eg, COPD, sleep apnea). Avoid prolonged sun exposure. May lower seizure threshold. Caution with bone marrow depression. NMS reported. Caution in acutely ill pediatric patients. Avoid in pediatrics with Reye's syndrome or hepatic disease. Avoid perivascular extravasation or inadvertent intra-arterial injection. Caution with narrow-angle glaucoma, prostatic hypertrophy, stenosing peptic ulcer, bladder-neck or pyloroduodenal obstruction, cardiovascular disease, hepatic dysfunction. Cholestatic jaundice reported. Alters HCG pregnancy test reading. May increase blood glucose.

ADVERSE REACTIONS: Drowsiness, dizziness, tinnitus, blurred vision, dry mouth, increased or decreased blood pressure, urticaria, NV, blood dyscrasia.

INTERACTIONS: Added sedative effects with CNS depressants (eg, alcohol, narcotics, narcotic analgesics, sedatives, hypnotics, general anesthetics, tranquilizers, TCAs); reduce dose or eliminate these agents. Reduce barbiturate dose by one-half and analgesic depressant dose by one-quarter to one-half. Caution with drugs that alter seizure threshold (eg, narcotics, local anesthetics). Do not use epinephrine for promethazine injection overdose. Caution with anticholinergics. Possible adverse reactions with MAOIs.

PREGNANCY: Category C, caution in nursing.

MECHANISM OF ACTION: Phenothiazine derivative/H_1 receptor antagonist; possesses antihistamine (does not block release of histamine), sedative, anti-motion sickness, antiemetic, and anticholinergic effects.

PHARMACOKINETICS: Metabolism: Liver; sulfoxides, N-desmethylpromethazine (metabolites). **Elimination:** Urine; $T_{1/2}$=9-16 hrs (IV), 9.8 hrs (IM).

P

NURSING CONSIDERATIONS

Assessment: Assess for seizure disorder, compromised respiratory function (COPD, sleep apnea), bone marrow depression, sulfite hypersensitivity, narrow-angle glaucoma, prostatic hypertrophy, stenosing peptic ulcer, pyloroduodenal obstruction, bladder-neck obstruction, CVD, hepatic impairment, and possible drug interactions.

Monitoring: Monitor for signs/symptoms of respiratory depression, seizures, leukopenia or agranulocytosis, NMS, injection site reaction, and hypersensitivity reactions.

Patient Counseling: Caution may impair physical/mental abilities. Warn to avoid prolonged exposure to sunlight. Seek medical attention if symptoms of respiratory depression, seizures, infections, NMS (hyperpyrexia, muscle rigidity, AMS), injection site reaction (burning, pain, erythema), or hypersensitivity reactions occur.

Administration: IV, IM route. **Storage:** 20-25°C (68-77°F). Protect from light.

PHENOBARBITAL

CIV

phenobarbital (Various)

THERAPEUTIC CLASS: Barbiturate

INDICATIONS: Treatment of generalized, tonic-clonic and cortical focal seizures. For relief of anxiety, tension and apprehension. Short-term treatment of insomnia.

DOSAGE: *Adults:* Sedation: 30-120mg/day given bid-tid. Max: 400mg/24h. Hypnotic: 100-200mg. Seizures: 60-200mg/day. Elderly/Debilitated/Renal or Hepatic Dysfunction: Reduce dosage.
Pediatrics: Seizures: 3-6mg/kg/day.

HOW SUPPLIED: Elixir: 20mg/5mL; Tab: 15mg, 30mg, 32.4mg, 60mg, 64.8mg, 100mg

CONTRAINDICATIONS: Respiratory disease with dyspnea or obstruction, porphyria, severe liver dysfunction. Large doses with nephritic patients.

WARNINGS/PRECAUTIONS: May be habit forming. Avoid abrupt withdrawal. Caution with acute or chronic pain; may mask symptoms or paradoxical excitement may occur. Cognitive deficits reported in children with febrile seizures. May cause excitement in children and excitement, depression or confusion in elderly, debilitated. Caution with hepatic dysfunction, borderline hypoadrenal function, depression.

ADVERSE REACTIONS: Drowsiness, residual sedation, lethargy, vertigo, somnolence, respiratory depression, hypersensitivity reactions, nausea, vomiting, headache.

INTERACTIONS: May be potentiated by MAOIs, antihistamines, alcohol, tranquilizers, sedative/hypnotics, other CNS depressants. Decreases effects of oral anticoagulants. Increases corticosteroid metabolism. Decreases effects of oral contraceptives. Decreases absorption of griseofulvin. Decreases half-life of doxycycline. May alter phenytoin metabolism. Increased levels with sodium valproate and valproic acid.

PREGNANCY: Category D, caution in nursing.

MECHANISM OF ACTION: Barbiturate; nonselective CNS depressant. Capable of producing all levels of CNS mood alteration. Responsible for depressing the sensory cortex, decreasing motor activity, altering cerebellar function, causing sedation and hypnosis.

PHARMACOKINETICS: Distribution: Distributed to all tissues and fluids. High concentrations found in the brain, liver, and kidneys. Found in breast milk. **Metabolism:** Hepatic. **Elimination:** Urine (primary), feces; $T_{1/2}$=79 hrs (adults), 110 hrs (children and newborns less than 48 hrs old).

NURSING CONSIDERATIONS

Assessment: Assess for history of manifest or latent porphyria, hepatic impairment, or respiratory disease with evidence of dyspnea or obstruction. Assess use in children, pregnant women, history of drug abuse, elderly or debilitated patients, acute or chronic pain, borderline hypoadrenal function, and history of depression or suicidal tendencies. Assess for possible drug interactions.

Monitoring: For patients on prolonged therapy, perform periodic evaluations of hematopoietic, renal/hepatic function. Monitor for signs of psychological/physical dependence, cognitive deficits in children, signs/symptoms of CNS depression, acute intoxication of medication (eg, unsteady gait, slurred speech), signs of chronic intoxication (eg, confusion, insomnia), and for exfoliative dermatitis (eg, Stevens-Johnson syndrome, toxic epidermal necrosis). Monitor for withdrawal symptoms (eg, anxiety, muscle twitching, weakness, convulsions, delirium) after d/c medication.

Patient Counseling: Inform psychological/physical dependence may result. Instruct not to increase dosage without consulting physician. Inform medication may impair mental/physical abilities; use caution when performing hazardous tasks. Avoid alcohol or other CNS depressants while on medication. Notify physician if any type of rash develops.

Administration: Oral route. **Storage:** Store at controlled room temperature, 15-30°C (59-86°F).

PHENYTEK — RX

phenytoin sodium (Mylan Bertek)

THERAPEUTIC CLASS: Hydantoin

INDICATIONS: Control of generalized tonic-clonic (grand mal) and complex partial (psychomotor, temporal lobe) seizures. Prevention and treatment of neurosurgically induced seizures.

DOSAGE: *Adults:* No Previous Treatment: Initial: 100mg extended phenytoin sodium capsule tid. Titrate: May increase at 7-10 day intervals. Usual: 100mg tid-qid. May increase up to 200mg Phenytek tid. Once Daily Dosing: 300mg Phenytek qd may replace 100mg extended phenytoin sodium capsule tid if seizures are controlled. LD (clinic/hospital): 1g in 3 divided doses (400mg, 300mg, 300mg) given 2 hrs apart. Start maintenance 24 hrs later. Avoid LD with renal and hepatic disease.
Pediatrics: Initial: 5mg/kg/day given bid-tid. Titrate: May increase at 7-10 day intervals. Maint: 4-8mg/kg/day. Max: 300mg/day. >6 yrs: May require the minimum adult dose (300mg/day).

HOW SUPPLIED: Cap, Extended-Release: 200mg, 300mg

WARNINGS/PRECAUTIONS: Avoid abrupt discontinuation. Caution with porphyria, hepatic dysfunction, elderly, diabetes, debilitated. D/C if rash occurs. Lymphadenopathy reported. Serum sickness may occur with lymph node involvement. Gingival hyperplasia reported; maintain proper dental hygiene. Hyperglycemia, birth defects, and osteomalacia reported. Monitor levels. Confusional states reported with toxic levels. Increased seizure frequency during pregnancy. Neonatal coagulation defects reported within first 24 hrs of birth; give vitamin K to mother before delivery and to neonate after birth. Avoid use with seizures due to hypoglycemia or other metabolic causes. Hemopoietic complications reported.

ADVERSE REACTIONS: Nystagmus, ataxia, slurred speech, decreased coordination, confusion, dizziness, insomnia, transient nervousness, motor twitchings, headaches, NV, constipation, rash, hypersensitivity reactions.

INTERACTIONS: Increased levels with acute alcohol intake, amiodarone, chloramphenicol, chlordiazepoxide, diazepam, dicumarol, disulfiram, estrogens, H_2-antagonists, halothane, isoniazid, methylphenidate, phenothiazines, phenylbutazone, salicylates, succinamides, sulfonamides, tolbutamide, trazodone. Decreased levels with chronic alcohol abuse, carbamazepine, reserpine, sucralfate. Decreases effects of corticosteroids, coumarin anticoagulants, digitoxin, doxycycline, estrogens, furosemide, oral contraceptives, quinidine, rifampin, theophylline, vitamin D. Phenobarbital, sodium valproate, valproic acid may increase or decrease levels. May increase or decrease levels of phenobarbital, sodium valproate, valproic acid. Calcium antacids decrease absorption; space dosing. Moban contains calcium ions that interfere with absorption. TCAs may precipitate seizures. Increased risk of phenytoin hypersensitivity with barbiturates, succinamides, oxazolidinediones.

PREGNANCY: Possibly teratogenic, weigh benefits versus risk; not for use in nursing.

MECHANISM OF ACTION: Inhibits spread of seizure activity; primary site of action appears to be the motor cortex. Possibly promotes sodium efflux from neurons, stabilizing the threshold against hyperexcitability caused by excessive stimulation or environmental changes capable of reducing membrane sodium gradient. Also reduces the posttetanic potentiation at synapses, which prevents cortical seizure foci from detonating adjacent cortical areas.

PHARMACOKINETICS: Absorption: T_{max}=4-12 hrs. **Metabolism:** Hepatic via hydroxylation. **Elimination:** Renal; bile (inactive metabolite) and urine; $T_{1/2}$=22 hrs.

P

NURSING CONSIDERATIONS

Assessment: Assess for impaired liver function, porphyria, seizures due to hypoglycemic or other metabolic causes and possible drug interactions.

Monitoring: Monitor serum phenytoin levels. Obtain levels to determine compliance and proper therapeutic efficacy just prior to patient's next scheduled dose. Monitor for skin rash (Stevens-Johnson syndrome), hyperglycemia, osteomalacia, phenytoin toxicity which may produce confusional states including delirium, psychosis, encephalopathy, development of lymphadenopathy.

Patient Counseling: Counsel to avoid alcohol while on medication. Instruct to notify physician if skin rash develops. Advise about importance of good dental hygiene to minimize development of gingival hyperplasia; importance of strictly adhering to prescribed dosage regimen, instruct not to abruptly d/c medication.

Administration: Oral. **Storage:** 20-25°C (68-77°F). Protect from light and moisture. Dispense in a tight, light-resistant container.

PhosLo — RX

calcium acetate (Fresenius)

THERAPEUTIC CLASS: Phosphate Binder

INDICATIONS: Control of hyperphosphatemia in end stage renal failure (ESRF). Does not promote aluminum absorption.

DOSAGE: *Adults:* Initial: 2 caps/tabs with each meal. Titrate: Increase gradually until serum phosphate <6mg/dL, as long as hypercalcemia does not develop. Maint: 3-4 caps/tabs with each meal.

HOW SUPPLIED: Cap: 667mg; Tab: 667mg

CONTRAINDICATIONS: Hypercalcemia.

WARNINGS/PRECAUTIONS: Increased risk of hypercalcemia when calcium given with meals in ESRF. Monitor serum calcium twice weekly during early dose adjustment period. If hypercalcemia develops, reduce dose or d/c depending on severity. Caution with arrhythmias.

ADVERSE REACTIONS: Hypercalcemia, constipation, anorexia, nausea, vomiting, confusion, delirium, stupor, coma.

INTERACTIONS: Decreased bioavailability of tetracyclines. Hypercalcemia may precipitate arrhythmia; avoid digitalis. Avoid other calcium supplements.

PREGNANCY: Category C, safety in nursing not known.

MECHANISM OF ACTION: Calcium acetate combines with dietary phosphate to form insoluble calcium phosphate, which is excreted in the feces.

NURSING CONSIDERATIONS

Assessment: Assess for hypercalcemia, patients taking digitalis, pregnancy status, and possible drug interaction.

Monitoring: Monitor serum calcium level twice weekly: (CaXP) product ≤66. X-ray suspect anatomical region to detect soft tissue calcification. Monitor for cardiac arrhythmia and vascular calcification.

Patient Counseling: Inform about compliance with dosage and diet instructions. Avoid use of nonprescription antacids. Inform about symptoms of hypercalcemia.

Administration: Oral route, taken with meal. **Storage:** 25°C (77°F); excursions permitted to 15-30°C (59-86°F).

Pilocarpine — RX

pilocarpine HCl (Various)

OTHER BRAND NAMES: Isopto Carpine (Alcon)

THERAPEUTIC CLASS: Cholinergic agent

INDICATIONS: To control IOP.

DOSAGE: *Adults:* 2 drops tid-qid or more if needed. Heavily pigmented irises may require higher strengths.

HOW SUPPLIED: Sol: 0.5%, 1%, 2%, 3%, 4%, 6% [15mL]

CONTRAINDICATIONS: Where constriction is undesirable (eg, acute iritis) or pupillary block glaucoma.

WARNINGS/PRECAUTIONS: Difficulty adapting in the dark. Caution while night driving and in poor illumination. Risk of retinal detachment.

ADVERSE REACTIONS: Local irritation, ciliary spasm, conjunctival vascular congestion, temporal or supraorbital headache, induced myopia, reduced visual acuity in poor illumination (elderly), lens opacity (prolonged use).

PREGNANCY: Category C, caution in nursing.

MECHANISM OF ACTION: Cholinergic agent; acts through direct stimulation of muscarinic neuroreceptors and smooth muscle such as iris and secretory glands. Produces miosis through contraction of iris sphincter, causing increased tension on scleral spur and opening of trabecular mesh work spaces to facilitate outflow of aqueous humor, thereby reducing outflow resistance and lowering IOP.

NURSING CONSIDERATIONS

Assessment: Prior to initiation, assess for acute iritis and pupillary block glaucoma. Assess pregnancy/nursing status.

Monitoring: Monitor for possible miosis, retinal detachment, and lens opacity with prolonged therapy.

Patient Counseling: Advise that visual difficulties in dark environments may occur; use caution performing hazardous activities in poor light. Do not touch dropper tip to any surface to avoid contamination.

Administration: Ocular route. **Storage:** 8-27°C (46-80°F).

PILOPINE HS — RX

pilocarpine HCl (Alcon)

THERAPEUTIC CLASS: Direct acting parasympathomimetic

INDICATIONS: To control IOP.

DOSAGE: *Adults:* Apply 1/2 inch into conjunctival sac hs.

HOW SUPPLIED: Gel: 4% [4g]

CONTRAINDICATIONS: Situations where constriction is undesirable (eg, acute iritis).

WARNINGS/PRECAUTIONS: For topical use only. May cause difficulty in dark adaptation; caution in night driving and situations in poor illumination.

ADVERSE REACTIONS: Lacrimation, burning, discomfort, headache, ciliary spasm, conjunctival vascular congestion, superficial keratitis, myopia.

PREGNANCY: Category C, caution in nursing.

MECHANISM OF ACTION: Cholinergic parasympathomimetic; stimulates muscarinic neuroreceptors and smooth muscle, producing miosis through contraction of iris sphincter, increasing tension of scleral spur, opening spaces to allow outflow of aqueous humor, reducing resistance and lowering IOP.

NURSING CONSIDERATIONS

Assessment: Assess for acute iritis and possible drug interactions.

Monitoring: Monitor for hypersensitivity reactions.

Patient Counseling: Advise may cause difficulty in adapting to dark; caution against hazardous occupations/driving in poor light. Advise not to touch tube tip to any surface to prevent contamination.

Administration: Ocular route. 1) Gently pull down lower eyelid to form pocket. 2) Gently squeeze and apply a continuous strip (1/2 inch) along pocket (wide as iris). 3) Grasp lower eyelid below lashes; lift lower eyelid and look down as close eyes. 4) Keep eye closed for 1 min. Repeat in other eye. **Storage:** 2-27°C (36-80°F). Avoid excessive heat. Do not freeze.

PINDOLOL — RX

pindolol (Various)

THERAPEUTIC CLASS: Nonselective beta-blocker

INDICATIONS: Management of hypertension.

DOSAGE: *Adults:* Initial: 5mg bid. Titrate: May increase by 10mg/day after 3-4 weeks. Max: 60mg/day.

HOW SUPPLIED: Tab: 5mg, 10mg

CONTRAINDICATIONS: Bronchial asthma, overt cardiac failure, cardiogenic shock, 2nd- and 3rd-degree heart block, severe bradycardia.

WARNINGS/PRECAUTIONS: Caution with well-compensated heart failure, nonallergic bronchospasm, renal or hepatic impairment. Can cause cardiac failure. Avoid abrupt withdrawal. Withdrawal before surgery is controversial. May mask hypoglycemia or hyperthyroidism symptoms.

ADVERSE REACTIONS: Dizziness, fatigue, insomnia, nervousness, dyspnea, edema, joint pain, muscle cramps/pain.

INTERACTIONS: Additive hypotension and/or bradycardia with catecholamine-depleting drugs. Both thioridazine and pindolol levels may increase when used concomitantly.

PREGNANCY: Category B, not for use in nursing.

MECHANISM OF ACTION: Nonselective β-blocker; inhibits β-andrenergic receptor with intrinsic sympathomimetic activity.

PHARMACOKINETICS: Absorption: Rapid; T_{max}=1 hr. **Distribution:** V_d=2L/Kg; plasma protein binding (40%). **Metabolism:** Metabolized to hydroxy-metabolites, which are excreted as glucoronides and ethereal sulfates. **Elimination:** Urine (35-40%), feces (6-9%); $T_{1/2}$=approximately 3-4 hrs, $T_{1/2}$=8 hrs (metabolites).

NURSING CONSIDERATIONS

P

Assessment: Assess for history of anaphylactic reaction, bronchial asthma, overt cardiac failure, cardiogenic shock, 2nd- or 3rd-degree heart block, severe bradycardia, bronchospastic disease, DM, thyrotoxicosis, LFTs, renal functions, pregnancy status, and possible drug interactions. D/C drug well before any surgeries.

Monitoring: Monitor for anaphylactic reactions, LFTs, dizziness, fatigue, edema, dyspnea, muscle pain, heart block, hypotension, claudication, visual disturbances, impotence, CBC with differential and platelet count, Peyronie's disease, CHF, bronchospasm.

Patient Counseling: Instruct not to interrupt or d/c therapy without consulting physician. Counsel about signs/symptoms of CHF, bronchospasm, and other adverse effects; seek prompt medical assistance if any develop.

Administration: Oral route. **Storage:** Below 30°C (86°F); tight, light-resistant container.

PIPERACILLIN — RX

piperacillin sodium (Various)

THERAPEUTIC CLASS: Broad-spectrum penicillin

INDICATIONS: Treatment of serious infections caused by susceptible strains of microorganisms in the following conditions: intra-abdominal, urinary tract, gynecologic, lower respiratory tract, skin and skin structure, bone/joint, and uncomplicated gonococcal urethritis, and septicemia. Perioperative surgical prophylaxis during certain procedures.

DOSAGE: *Adults:* Usual: 3-4g IM/IV q4-6h. Max: 24g/day; IM: 2g/site. Serious Infections: 200-300mg/kg/day IV divided q4-6h. Complicated UTI: 125-200mg/kg/day IV divided q6-8h. Uncomplicated UTI/CAP: 100-125mg/kg/day IM/IV divided q6-12h. Uncomplicated Gonorrhea: 2g IM single dose with 1g PO probenecid 1/2 hr before injection. Surgical Prophylaxis: 2g IV 20-30 min just prior to anesthesia (See PI for follow-up dosing). Renal Impairment: Uncomplicated/Complicated UTI: CrCl <20mL/min: 3g q12h. Complicated UTI: CrCl 20-40mL/min: 3g q8h. Serious Infection: CrCl 20-40mL/min: 4g q8h. CrCl <20mL/min: 4g q12h. Hemodialysis: Give 1g additional dose after each dialysis. Max: 2g q8h. Usual treatment is for 7-10 days; treat gynecologic infections for 3-10 days; treat *S.pyogenes* infections for at least 10 days.
Pediatrics: ≥12 yrs: Usual: 3-4g IM/IV q4-6h. Max: 24g/day; IM: 2g/site. Serious Infections: 200-300mg/kg/day IV divided q4-6h. Complicated UTI: 125-200mg/kg/day IV divided q6-8h. Uncomplicated UTI/CAP: 100-125mg/kg/day IM/IV divided q6-12h. Uncomplicated Gonorrhea: 2g IM single dose with 1g PO probenecid 1/2 hr before injection. Surgical Prophylaxis: 2g IV 20-30 min just prior to anesthesia (See PI for follow-up dosing). Renal Impairment: Uncomplicated/Complicated UTI: CrCl <20mL/min: 3g q12h. Complicated UTI: CrCl 20-40mL/min: 3g q8h. Serious Infection: CrCl 20-40mL/min: 4g q8h. CrCl <20mL/min: 4g q12h. Hemodialysis: Give 1g additional dose after each dialysis. Max: 2g q8h. Usual treatment is for 7-10 days; treat gynecologic infections for 3-10 days; treat *S.pyogenes* infections for at least 10 days.

HOW SUPPLIED: Inj: 2g, 3g, 4g

CONTRAINDICATIONS: Hypersensitivity to cephalosporins.

WARNINGS/PRECAUTIONS: Serious, sometimes fatal, hypersensitivity reactions reported with PCN therapy. *Clostridium difficile*-associated diarrhea reported. Cross-sensitivity to cephalosporins. Monitor renal, hepatic and hematopoietic functions with prolonged use. D/C if bleeding manifestations occur; increased risk with renal failure. Prolonged use may cause superinfections. May experience neuromuscular excitability or convulsions with higher than recommended doses. Contains 1.85mEq/g sodium; caution with salt restriction. Monitor electrolytes periodically with low potassium levels. Increased incidence of rash and fever in cystic fibrosis. Continue treatment for at least 48-72 hrs after patient becomes asymptomatic.

ADVERSE REACTIONS: Thrombophlebitis, erythema and pain at injection site, diarrhea, headache, dizziness, anaphylaxis, rash, superinfections.

INTERACTIONS: Do not mix with aminoglycoside in a syringe or infusion bottle; may cause inactivation of aminoglycoside. May prolong neuromuscular blockade of nondepolarizing muscle relaxants (eg, vecuronium). Increased risk of hypokalemia with cytotoxic therapy or diuretics. May reduce methotrexate clearance. Probenecid may increase levels. Monitor coagulation parameters closely with concomitant anticoagulants.

PREGNANCY: Category B, caution in nursing.

MECHANISM OF ACTION: Broad-spectrum penicillin; exerts bacterial activity by inhibiting both septum and cell wall synthesis; active against a variety of gram-positive and gram-negative aerobic and anaerobic bacteria.

PHARMACOKINETICS: Absorption: (2g) Rapid; C_{max}=36mcg/mL, T_{max}=30 min. **Distribution:** Plasma protein binding (16%). **Elimination:** Urine (60%-80%); (2g) $T_{1/2}$=54 min., (6g) 63 min.

NURSING CONSIDERATIONS

Assessment: Assess for history of allergic reaction to betalactams, renal impairment, CF, history of bleeding disorder, and possible drug interaction.

Monitoring: Monitor CBC, renal function and serum electrolytes periodically. Monitor for signs/symptoms of electrolyte imbalance (hypokalemia), hypersensitivity reactions, *C. difficile*-associated diarrhea, superinfections, leukopenia/neutropenia, bleeding maninfestations, neuromuscular excitability or convulsions, rash and fever in CF patients.

Patient Counseling: Inform drug only treats bacterial, not viral, infections. Take as directed; skipping doses or not completing full course may decrease effectiveness and increase resistance. May experience diarrhea; contact physician if develop watery/bloody stools or hypersensitivity reactions.

Administration: IM, IV. **Storage:** 20-25°C (68-77°F). Reconstituted: 20-25°C (68-77°F), stable for 24 hrs; refrigerated: 2-8°C (36-46°F), stable for 48 hrs.

PLAQUENIL RX

hydroxychloroquine sulfate (Sanofi-Aventis)

Be familiar with complete prescribing information before prescribing hydroxychloroquine.

THERAPEUTIC CLASS: Quinine derivative

INDICATIONS: Suppression and treatment of acute attacks of malaria in adults and children. Treatment of discoid and systemic lupus erythematosus and rheumatoid arthritis (RA) in adults.

DOSAGE: *Adults:* Malaria Suppression: 400mg weekly. Begin 2 weeks before exposure and continue for 8 weeks after leaving endemic area. Give 400mg q6h for 2 doses if therapy is not begun before exposure. Acute Attack: 800mg, then 400mg 6-8 hrs later, then 400mg for 2 more days. RA: Initial: 400-600mg qd with food or milk; increase until optimum response. Maint: After 4-12 weeks, 200-400mg qd with food or milk. Lupus Erythematosus: Initial: 400mg qd-bid for several weeks depending on response. Maint: 200-400mg/day.

Pediatrics: Malaria Suppression: 5mg/kg (base) weekly, max 400mg/dose. Begin 2 weeks before exposure and continue for 8 weeks after leaving endemic area. Acute Attack: 10mg base/kg, max 800mg/dose; then 5mg base/kg, max 400mg/dose at 6, 24 and 48 hrs after 1st dose.

HOW SUPPLIED: Tab: 200mg (200mg tab=155mg base)

CONTRAINDICATIONS: Long term therapy in children or if retinal/visual field changes due to 4-aminoquinoline compounds.

WARNINGS/PRECAUTIONS: Caution with hepatic disease, G6PD deficiency, alcoholism, psoriasis, and porphyria. Perform baseline and periodic (3 months) ophthalmologic exams and blood cell counts with prolonged therapy. Test periodically for muscle weakness. D/C if blood disorders occur. Avoid if possible in pregnancy. D/C after 6 months if no improvement in RA.

ADVERSE REACTIONS: Headache, dizziness, diarrhea, loss of appetite, muscle weakness, nausea, abdominal cramps, bleaching of hair, dermatitis, ocular toxicity, visual field defects.

INTERACTIONS: Caution with hepatotoxic drugs.

PREGNANCY: Safety in pregnancy and nursing not known.

MECHANISM OF ACTION: Quinine derivative; has antimalarial action. Precise mechanism not established.

NURSING CONSIDERATIONS

Assessment: Assess for retinal or visual field defects, psoriasis, hepatic disease, alcoholism, G-6-PD deficiency, chloroquine-resistant strains of *P. falciparum*, auditory damage, pregnancy status. Note other diseases/conditions and drug therapies.

Monitoring: Monitor CBC with differential and platelet count, dermatologic reactions, chloroquine retinopathy, psychosis, irritability, myopathy, abnormal nerve conduction, depression of deep tendon reflexes, and allergic reactions.

Patient Counseling: Counsel about adverse effects and to d/c drug and seek medical attention if any signs/symptoms develop. Advise about need for periodic follow-up.

Administration: Oral route. **Storage:** Room temperature up to 30°C (86°F).

PLAVIX — RX

clopidogrel bisulfate (Bristol-Myers Squibb/Sanofi-Aventis)

THERAPEUTIC CLASS: Platelet aggregation inhibitor

INDICATIONS: For reduction of thrombotic events in those with recent stroke or MI, established peripheral arterial disease (PAD); or with non-ST-segment elevation acute coronary syndrome (unstable angina/non-Q-wave MI); and patients with ST-segment elevation acute myocardial infarction (STEMI).

DOSAGE: *Adults:* MI/Stroke/PAD: 75mg qd. Acute Coronary Syndrome: Take with 75-325mg ASA qd. LD: 300mg. Maint: 75mg qd. STEMI: 75mg, with 75-325mg ASA, qd with or without LD.

HOW SUPPLIED: Tab: 75mg, 300mg

CONTRAINDICATIONS: Active pathological bleeding (eg, peptic ulcer, intracranial hemorrhage).

WARNINGS/PRECAUTIONS: Caution with risk of increased bleeding, ulcers or lesions with a propensity to bleed, severe hepatic or renal impairment. D/C 5 days before surgery if antiplatelet effect is not desired. Monitor blood cell count and other appropriate tests if symptoms of bleeding or undesirable hematological effects arise. Thrombotic thrombocytopenic purpura (TTP) reported (rare).

ADVERSE REACTIONS: Chest pain, influenza-like symptoms, pain, edema, HTN, headache, dizziness, abdominal pain, dyspepsia, diarrhea, arthralgia, purpura, upper respiratory tract infection, back pain, dyspnea.

INTERACTIONS: Potentiates effect of ASA on collagen-induced platelet aggregation. Caution with warfarin. Increased occult GI loss with NSAIDs. Inhibits CYP2C9; caution with phenytoin, tamoxifen, tolbutamide, warfarin, torsemide, fluvastatin, and many NSAIDs. Caution with drugs that may induce GI lesions.

PREGNANCY: Category B, not for use in nursing.

MECHANISM OF ACTION: Platelet aggregation inhibitor; selectively inhibits the binding of adenosine diphosphate (ADP) to its platelet receptor and subsequent ADP-mediated activation of the glycoprotein GIIb/IIIa complex. Platelet aggregation is thereby inhibited.

PHARMACOKINETICS: Absorption: Rapidly; C_{max}=3mg/L; T_{max}=1 hr. **Distribution:** Plasma protein binding (98%). **Metabolism:** Liver (hydrolysis); carboxylic acid derivative (major metabolite). **Elimination:** Urine (50%), feces (46%); $T_{1/2}$=8 hrs.

P

NURSING CONSIDERATIONS

Assessment: Assess for presence of active bleeding (eg, peptic ulcer, intracranial hemorrhage), hepatic impairment, nursing status, and drug interactions. Assess use in patients at risk for increased bleeding (eg, undergoing surgery, recent trauma).

Monitoring: Monitor for signs/symptoms of thrombotic thrombocytopenic purpura (eg, thrombocytopenia) and for bleeding (eg, GI bleeding). Perform CBC and other appropriate tests when bleeding is suspected.

Patient Counseling: Can be taken with/without food. Advise that medication may prolong bleeding time; contact physician if any unusual bleeding occurs. Advise to notify other physicians or dentists when taking or before scheduling surgery.

Administration: Oral route. **Storage:** 25°C (77°F); excursions permitted to 15-30°C (59-86°F).

PLENDIL — RX

felodipine (AstraZeneca)

THERAPEUTIC CLASS: Calcium channel blocker (dihydropyridine)

INDICATIONS: Treatment of hypertension.

DOSAGE: *Adults:* Initial: 5mg qd. Titrate: Adjust at no less than 2-week intervals. Maint: 2.5-10mg qd. Elderly: Initial: 2.5mg qd. Take without food or with a light meal. Swallow tab whole.

HOW SUPPLIED: Tab, Extended-Release: 2.5mg, 5mg, 10mg

WARNINGS/PRECAUTIONS: May cause hypotension and lead to reflex tachycardia with precipitation of angina. Caution with heart failure or ventricular dysfunction, especially with concomitant β-blockers. Monitor dose adjustment with hepatic dysfunction or elderly. Peripheral edema reported. Maintain good dental hygiene; gingival hyperplasia reported.

ADVERSE REACTIONS: Peripheral edema, headache, flushing, dizziness.

INTERACTIONS: CYP3A4 inhibitors (eg, itraconazole, ketoconazole, erythromycin, grapefruit juice, cimetidine) may increase plasma levels. Levels decreased with long-term anticonvulsant therapy. May increase metoprolol and tacrolimus levels.

PREGNANCY: Category C, not for use in nursing.

MECHANISM OF ACTION: Calcium channel blocker; reversibly competes with nitrendipine and/or other calcium channel blockers for dihydropyridine binding sites and blocks voltage-dependent calcium ion currents in vascular smooth muscle.

PHARMACOKINETICS: Absorption: Complete, systemic bioavailability (approximately 20%); T_{max}=2.5-5 hrs (oral). **Distribution:** V_d=10 L/kg; plasma protein binding (99%). **Elimination:** Urine (70%), feces (10%); $T_{1/2}$(immediate release)=11-16 hrs.

NURSING CONSIDERATIONS

Assessment: Assess for hypotension, CHF, LFTs, pregnancy status, and for possible drug interactions.

Monitoring: Monitor BP, LFT. Monitor for peripheral edema, CHF, CBC, palpitations, arrhythmias, angina.

Patient Counseling: Instruct to take tablet whole; do not crush or chew. Counsel about adverse side effects; notify physician if any develop.

Administration: Oral route. **Storage:** 30°C (86°F). Keep in tight, light-resistant container.

PLETAL — RX

cilostazol (Otsuka America)

Contraindicated with CHF of any severity due to possible decrease in survival.

THERAPEUTIC CLASS: Phosphodiesterase III inhibitor

INDICATIONS: Reduction of symptoms with intermittent claudication.

DOSAGE: *Adults:* 100mg bid, 1/2 hr before or 2 hrs after breakfast and dinner. Concomitant CYP3A4 and CYP2C19 Inhibitors: Consider 50mg bid.

HOW SUPPLIED: Tab: 50mg, 100mg

CONTRAINDICATIONS: CHF of any severity. Haemostatic disorders or active pathologic bleeding (eg, peptic ulcer, intracranial bleeding).

WARNINGS/PRECAUTIONS: Risks not known in patients with severe underlying heart disease, moderate or severe hepatic impairment, or with long-term use. Rare cases of thrombocytopenia or leukopenia reported.

ADVERSE REACTIONS: Headache, palpitation, tachycardia, abnormal stool, diarrhea, peripheral edema, dizziness, infection, rhinitis, blood pressure increase, aplastic anemia.

INTERACTIONS: Caution with CYP3A4 inhibitors (eg, ketoconazole, diltiazem, erythromycin) or CYP2C19 inhibitors (eg, omeprazole); may increase cilostazol levels. Avoid grapefruit juice.

PREGNANCY: Category C, not for use in nursing.

MECHANISM OF ACTION: Phosphodiesterase III inhibitor; not established. Inhibits phosphodiesterase activity and suppresses cyclic AMP (cAMP) degradation. Results in an increase of cAMP in platelets and blood vessels. Leads to reversible inhibition of platelet aggregation and produces vasodilation.

PHARMACOKINETICS: Distribution: Plasma protein binding (95-98%). **Metabolism:** Liver via CYP450 3A4 (primary), 2C19; 3,4-dehydro-cilostazol, 4'-trans-hydroxy-cilostazol (major active metabolites). **Elimination:** Urine (74%), feces (20%); $T_{1/2}$=11-13 hrs.

NURSING CONSIDERATIONS

Assessment: Assess for CHF, hemostatic disorders, presence of major bleeding (eg, peptic ulcer, intracranial bleeding), renal/hepatic function, pregnancy/nursing status, and drug interactions.

Monitoring: Monitor for signs/symptoms of thrombocytopenia, leukopenia, agranulocytosis, cardiovascular toxicity (eg, cardiovascular lesions), and headaches.

Patient Counseling: Advise to take at least 30 min before or 2 hours after food. Inform that benefits of medication may not be immediate; treatment required for up to 12 weeks before beneficial effect.

Administration: Oral route. **Storage:** 25°C (77°F); excursions permitted to 15-30°C (59-86°F).

PNEUMOVAX 23 — RX

pneumococcal vaccine (Merck)

THERAPEUTIC CLASS: Vaccine

INDICATIONS: Immunization against pneumococcal disease caused by those pneumococcal types included in the vaccine.

DOSAGE: *Adults:* Usual: 0.5mL SQ/IM in deltoid muscle or lateral mid-thigh. *Pediatrics:* ≥2 yrs: 0.5mL SQ/IM in deltoid muscle or lateral mid-thigh.

HOW SUPPLIED: Inj: 575mcg/0.5mL

WARNINGS/PRECAUTIONS: Vaccination timing is critical for chemotherapy or immunosuppressive therapy. Suboptimal response may occur in immunocompromised patients. Intradermal administration may cause severe local reactions. Caution with severely compromised cardiovascular or pulmonary function where systemic reaction would be a significant risk. Delay vaccine with febrile respiratory illness or other active infection. Do not revaccinate immunocompetent patients. Continue prophylaxis with pneumococcal antibiotics. May not prevent pneumococcal meningitis with chronic CSF leakage.

ADVERSE REACTIONS: Local injection-site reactions (eg, soreness, warmth, erythema, swelling, induration), fever (≤102°F).

PREGNANCY: Category C, caution use in nursing.

MECHANISM OF ACTION: Active immunization that may protect against pneumococcal infection.

NURSING CONSIDERATIONS

Assessment: Assess current health and previous vaccination history, immune status, history of cardiovascular and pulmonary function. Assess timing in chemotherapy and immunosuppressive therapy patients.

Monitoring: Monitor patients with compromised cardiovascular and pulmonary function. Monitor injection site for erythema, swelling, and induration.

Patient Counseling: May not offer 100% protection from pneumococcal infection. Inform of benefits/risks; report any serious adverse reactions.

Administration: IM (preferably in deltoid muscle or lateral mid-thigh) and SQ only. **Storage:** 2-8°C (36-46°F).

POLYTRIM — RX

polymyxin B sulfate - trimethoprim sulfate (Allergan)

THERAPEUTIC CLASS: Dihydrofolate reductase inhibitor/antibiotic

INDICATIONS: Surface ocular bacterial infections, including blepharoconjunctivitis, acute bacterial conjunctivitis.

DOSAGE: *Adults:* Mild-Moderate Infections: 1 drop q3h for 7-10 days. Max: 6 doses/day.
Pediatrics: ≥2 months: Mild-Moderate Infections: 1 drop q3h for 7-10 days. Max: 6 doses/day.

HOW SUPPLIED: Sol: (Trimethoprim-Polymyxin B) 1mg-10,000U/mL [10mL]

WARNINGS/PRECAUTIONS: Not indicated for the prophylaxis or treatment of ophthalmia neonatorum.

ADVERSE REACTIONS: Local irritation, lid edema, itching, increased redness, tearing, burning, stinging, circumocular rash, superinfection (prolonged use).

PREGNANCY: Category C, caution in nursing.

MECHANISM OF ACTION: Dihydrofolate reductase inhibitor/antibiotic. Polymyxin B: Increases permeability of bacterial cell membrane by interacting with phospholipid components of membrane. Trimethoprim: Blocks production of tetrahydrofolic acid from dihydrofolic acid by binding to and reversibly inhibiting the enzyme dihydrofolate reductase. Binding is stronger for bacterial enzyme than for corresponding mammalian enzyme, therefore selectively interferes with bacterial biosynthesis of nucleic acids and proteins.

PHARMACOKINETICS: Absorption: C_{max}=0.03mcg/mL (trimethoprim), 1 unit/mL (polymyxin B) (following two-time dosing of 2 drops of ophthalmic solution containing 1mg of trimethoprim and 10,000 units of polymyxin B).

NURSING CONSIDERATIONS

Assessment: Assess proper diagnosis of causative organisms, that medication is not being used as treatment for patients with ophthalmia neonatorum, and use in pregnant/nursing females.

Monitoring: Monitor for signs/symptoms of hypersensitivity reactions (eg, lid edema, itching, increased redness, tearing, and circumocular rash). For patients on prolonged therapy, monitor for overgrowth of nonsusceptible organisms (eg, fungi) and for the development of a superinfection.

P

Patient Counseling: Advise to avoid contaminating applicator tip with material from eye, fingers, or other sources. Instruct to d/c therapy if redness, irritation, swelling, or pain persists or worsens. Advise not to wear contact lenses if there are signs/symptoms of ocular bacterial infections.

Administration: Ocular route. Do not inject into eye. **Storage:** 15-25°C (59-77°F). Protect from light.

PONSTEL — RX

mefenamic acid (Sciele)

NSAIDs may cause an increased risk of serious cardiovascular thrombotic events, MI, stroke, and serious GI adverse events including bleeding, ulceration, and perforation of the stomach or intestines. Contraindicated for the treatment of perioperative pain in the setting of coronary artery bypass graft (CABG) surgery.

THERAPEUTIC CLASS: NSAID

INDICATIONS: Relief of mild to moderate pain in patients ≥14 yrs, when therapy will not exceed 7 days. Treatment of primary dysmenorrhea.

DOSAGE: *Adults:* Acute Pain: Usual: 500mg, then 250mg q6h prn up to 1 week. Primary Dysmenorrhea: Usual: 500mg, then 250mg q6h up to 3 days. Take with food.
Pediatrics: ≥14 yrs: Acute Pain: Usual: 500mg, then 250mg q6h prn up to 1

week. Primary Dysmenorrhea: Usual: 500mg, then 250mg q6h up to 3 days. Take with food.

HOW SUPPLIED: Cap: 250mg

CONTRAINDICATIONS: Pre-existing renal disease, active ulceration or chronic inflammation of the GI tract. Allergic-type reactions, including asthma and urticaria, after taking ASA or other NSAIDs. Treatment of perioperative pain in the setting of CABG surgery.

WARNINGS/PRECAUTIONS: May lead to onset of new HTN or worsening of pre-existing HTN; monitor BP closely. Fluid retention and edema reported; caution with fluid retention or heart failure. Renal papillary necrosis and other renal injury reported after long-term use. Not recommended for use with advanced renal disease. Anaphylactoid reactions may occur. May cause serious skin adverse events (eg, exfoliative dermatitis, Stevens-Johnson syndrome, and toxic epidermal necrolysis). Avoid in late pregnancy; may cause premature closure of ductus arteriosis. May cause elevations of LFTs; d/c if liver disease develops or systemic manifestations occur. Caution in elderly. Anemia may occur; with long-term use, monitor Hgb/Hct if signs or symptoms of anemia develop. May inhibit platelet aggregation and prolong bleeding time; monitor with coagulation disorders. Caution with asthma and avoid with ASA-sensitive asthma.

ADVERSE REACTIONS: Abdominal pain, constipation, diarrhea, dyspepsia, flatulence, gross bleeding/perforation, heartburn, nausea, GI ulcers, vomiting, abnormal renal function, anemia, dizziness, edema, elevated liver enzymes, headache, increased bleeding time, pruritus, rash, tinnitus.

INTERACTIONS: Caution with CYP2C9 inhibitors. ASA may increase adverse effects; avoid use. Warfarin may increase GI bleeding. May prolong PT with oral anticoagulants. May enhance methotrexate toxicity. Decreases effects of ACE inhibitors, furosemide, and thiazides; monitor for renal toxicity. Increases lithium levels. Magnesium hydroxide may increase mefenamic acid levels. Enhances methotrexate toxicity; caution with concomitant use.

PREGNANCY: Category C, not for use in nursing.

MECHANISM OF ACTION: NSAID (fenamate derivative); suspected to inhibit prostaglandin synthetase, exerts anti-inflammatory, analgesic, and antipyretic actions.

PHARMACOKINETICS: Absorption: Rapid; C_{max}=10-20mcg/mL[3], T_{max}=2-4 hrs. **Distribution:** V_d=1.06L/kg[2]; plasma protein binding (90%). **Metabolism**: Via CYP2C9. **Elimination:** Urine (52%), feces (20%); $T_{1/2}$=2 hrs.

NURSING CONSIDERATIONS

Assessment: Assess LFTs, renal function, CBC and coagulation profile. Assess for history of CABG surgery, asthma and allergic reactions to aspirin or other NSAIDs, active ulceration or chronic inflammation of GI tract, CVD, pregnancy status. Note other diseases/conditions and drug therapies.

Monitoring: Monitor for hypersensitivity reactions, cardiac complications, stroke, GI bleeding, asthma, skin side effects. Monitor BP, LFT, renal functions, CBC with differential and platelet count and coagulation profile, hyperglycemia.

Patient Counseling: Counsel about side effects; seek medical attention if any develop. Avoid alcohol and smoking during treatment. Take drug as prescribed. Caution women against using medication late in pregnancy.

Administration: Oral route. **Storage:** 20-25°C (68-77°F); excursions permitted to 15-30°C (59-86°F).

PRANDIMET — RX

metformin HCl - repaglinide (Novo Nordisk)

Lactic acidosis can occur due to metformin accumulation. If suspected, d/c drug and hospitalize patient.

THERAPEUTIC CLASS: Meglitinide/sulfonylurea

INDICATIONS: Adjunct to diet and exercise to improve glycemic control in adults with type 2 diabetes mellitus who are already treated with a meglitinide and metformin HCl or who have inadequate glycemic control on a meglitinide alone or metformin HCl alone.

DOSAGE: *Adults:* Individualize dose. Administer 2-3 times a day up to 4mg-1000mg/meal. Max Daily Dose: 10mg of repaglinide-2500mg of metformin. Patient Inadequately Controlled on Metformin Monotherapy: Initial: 1mg-500mg bid with meals. Titrate: Gradually escalate dose to reduce risk of hypoglycemia. Patient Inadequately Controlled with Meglitinide Monotherapy: Initial: 500mg of metformin bid. Titrate: Gradually escalate dose to reduce GI side effects. Concomitant use of Repaglinide/Metformin: Initiate at the dose of repaglinide and metformin HCl similar to (not exceeding) the current doses. Titrate to maximum daily dose as necessary.

HOW SUPPLIED: Tab: (Repaglinide-Metformin) 1mg-500mg, 2mg-500mg.

CONTRAINDICATIONS: Renal impairment (SrCr ≥1.5mg/dL [males], ≥1.4mg/dL [females], or abnormal CrCl). Acute or chronic metabolic acidosis, including diabetic ketoacidosis. Patients receiving both gemfibrozil and itraconazole.

WARNINGS/PRECAUTIONS: Lactic acidosis reported (rare), increased risk with sepsis, dehydration, excess alcohol intake, hepatic impairment, renal impairment, and acute congestive heart failure. Assess renal function prior to initiation and annually thereafter. Avoid in hepatic impairment and excess alcohol intake. D/C in hypoxic states (eg, acute CHF, shock, acute MI), prior to surgical procedures, procedures requiring use of intravascular iodinated contrast materials, and ketoacidosis. May cause vitamin B_{12} deficiency and hypoglycemia.

ADVERSE REACTIONS: Hypoglycemia, headache, diarrhea, nausea, and upper respiratory tract infection.

INTERACTIONS: Cationic drugs (eg, amiloride, digoxin, morphine, procainamide, quinidine, ranitidine, triamterene, trimethoprim, and vancomycin) may increase metformin levels. CYP2C8 inhibitors (gemfibrozil, trimethoprim), CYP3A4 inhibitors (itraconazole, ketaconazole), or CYP2C8/3A4 inducers (rifampin) may alter the pharmacokinetics and pharmacodynamics of repaglinide. Not for use in combination with NPH insulin.

PREGNANCY: Category C, not for use in nursing.

P

MECHANISM OF ACTION: Repaglinide: Meglitinide; lowers blood glucose levels by stimulating the release of insulin from functioning β-cells in the pancreas. **Metformin:** Biguanide; improves glucose tolerance, decreases hepatic glucose production, decreases intestinal absorption of glucose, and improves insulin sensitivity by increasing peripheral glucose uptake and utilization.

PHARMACOKINETICS: Absorption: Repaglinide: Absolute bioavailability (56%); T_{max}=1 hr. Metformin: Absolute bioavailabilty (50%-60%). **Distribution:** Repaglinide: V_d=31L; Plasma protein binding (>98%). Metformin: V_d=654L. **Metabolism:** Repaglinide: CYP2C8, 3A4 and direct conjugation; M2, M1, M7 (major metabolites). **Elimination:** Repaglinide: Feces (90%), urine (8%); $T_{1/2}$=1 hr. Metformin: Urine (90% unchanged); $T_{1/2}$=6.2 hrs (plasma), 17.6 hrs (blood).

NURSING CONSIDERATIONS

Assessment: Assess FPG, HbA_{1c}, renal function, LFTs, and CBCs. Assess for CHF, septicemia, acute or chronic metabolic acidosis, adrenal or pituitary insufficiency, and pregnancy status. Evaluate for other medical/surgical conditions, and for possible drug interactions.

Monitoring: Monitor for hypoglycemia, lactic acidosis, pre-renal azotemia, CHF, and CVD. Monitor FPG, HbA_{1c}, baseline, and annual renal function, LFTs, annual hematological parameters, hypersensitivity reactions (eg, anaphylaxis, angioedema, exfoliative skin conditions).

Patient Counseling: Inform that drug is an adjunct to diet and exercise and should be taken as prescribed with meals. Inform patient of importance of regular blood glucose, HbA_{1c}, renal function, and hematologic parameters testing. During periods of stress (eg, fever, trauma, infection, or surgery), medication requirements may change; patients should seek medical advice promptly. Inform about the risks of hypoglycemia, symptoms, treatment, and conditions that predispose development. Counsel to report unexplained hyperventilation, myalgia, malaise, and unusual somnolence. Not recommended for use during pregnancy. Counsel about adverse effects; advise patients to seek medical attention if adverse side effects develop. Counsel on the need for regular follow-ups.

Administration: Oral route. **Storage:** Not above 25°C (77°F).

PRANDIN — RX

repaglinide (Novo Nordisk)

THERAPEUTIC CLASS: Meglitinide

INDICATIONS: Adjunct to diet and exercise, to improve glycemic control in type 2 diabetes mellitus. May use in combination with metformin or thiazolidinediones (TZDs).

DOSAGE: *Adults:* Take within 15-30 min before meals. Skip dose if skipping meal and add dose if adding meal. Initial: Treatment-Naive or HbA_{1c} <8%: 0.5mg with each meal. Previous Oral Therapy/Combination Therapy and HbA_{1c} ≥8%: 1-2mg with each meal. Titrate: May double preprandial dose up to 4mg (bid-qid) at no less than 1 week intervals. Maint: 0.5-4mg with meals. Max: 16mg/day. If hypoglycemia with combination metformin or thiazolidinediones (TZDs) occurs, reduce repaglinide dose. Renal Dysfunction: CrCl 20-40mg/dL: Initial: 0.5mg with each meal; titrate carefully. Hepatic Dysfunction: Increase intervals between dose adjustments.

HOW SUPPLIED: Tab: 0.5mg, 1mg, 2mg

CONTRAINDICATIONS: Diabetic ketoacidosis and type 1 diabetes.

WARNINGS/PRECAUTIONS: Hypoglycemia risk especially with renal/hepatic insufficiency, elderly, malnourished, and adrenal/pituitary insufficiency. Loss of blood glucose control when exposed to stress (fever, trauma, infection, or surgery); d/c therapy and start insulin. Secondary failure can occur over a period of time. Caution with hepatic and renal dysfunction. Not indicated for use in combination with NPH insulin.

ADVERSE REACTIONS: Hyperglycemia, hypoglycemia, cardiovascular effects, respiratory infections, URI, bronchitis, sinusitis, rhinitis, paresthesia, N/V, diarrhea, constipation, dyspepsia, arthralgia, back pain, headache, chest pain.

INTERACTIONS: Increased metabolism with CYP3A4 inducers (eg, rifampin, barbiturates, carbamazepine). Ketoconazole, itraconazole, clarithromycin, and erythromycin (CYP3A4 inhibitors) and trimethoprim, gemfibrozil, and montelukast (CYP2C8 inhibitors) may inhibit metabolism. Increased levels with gemfibrozil; caution and monitor levels if already on both drugs, avoid initiation of concurrent use. Avoid itraconazole if already on gemfibrozil and repaglinide; synergistic effect may occur. Potentiated hypoglycemia with alcohol, β-blockers, NSAIDs, and other highly protein-bound drugs, salicylates, sulfonamides, chloramphenicol, coumarins, probenecid, MAOIs. Risk of hyperglycemia with diuretics, corticosteroids, phenothiazines, thyroid products, estrogens, phenytoin, nicotinic acid, sympathomimetics, CCBs, and isoniazid. β-blockers may mask hypoglycemia. Increased levels of repaglinide and levonorgestrel/ethinyl estradiol combination during coadminstration. Increased levels with simvastatin.

PREGNANCY: Category C, not for use in nursing.

MECHANISM OF ACTION: Meglitinide; lowers blood glucose levels by stimulating the release of insulin from the pancreas.

PHARMACOKINETICS: Absorption: Rapid and complete; bioavailability (56%); T_{max}=1 hr. **Distribution:** V_d=31L; plasma protein binding (98%). **Metabolism:** CYP2C8, 3A4; oxidation, glucuronidation. **Elimination:** Feces (90%), urine (8%); $T_{1/2}$=1 hr.

NURSING CONSIDERATIONS

Assessment: Assess FPG, HbA_{1c}, renal function, LFTs, pregnancy status, diabetic ketoacidosis, type 1 DM, cardiovascular risk factors, and for possible drug interactions.

Monitoring: Monitor blood glucose, HbA_{1c} every 3 months, hypo/hyperglycemia, and for severe adverse events.

Patient Counseling: Inform about importance of adherence to meal planning, regular physical activity, regular blood glucose monitoring, periodic HbA_{1c} testing, recognition and management of hypo/hyperglycemia, and periodic assessment of diabetes complications. Educate about risks/benefits of therapy and primary and secondary failure. During periods of stress (eg, trauma, infection, surgery), medication requirements may change; seek prompt medical advice. Instruct to take before meals.

Administration: Oral route. **Storage:** 25°C (77°F). Protect from moisture. Keep and dispense in tight containers with safety closures.

PRAVACHOL RX

pravastatin sodium (Bristol-Myers Squibb)

THERAPEUTIC CLASS: HMG-CoA reductase inhibitor

INDICATIONS: As adjunct to diet, to reduce elevated total-C, LDL-C, Apo B, TG levels, and to increase HDL-C in primary hypercholesterolemia and mixed dyslipidemia (Type IIa and IIb). Treatment of primary dysbetalipoproteinemia (Type III) and heterozygous familial hypercholesterolemia. To reduce elevated serum TG levels (Type IV). In hypercholesterolemic patients without coronary heart disease, to reduce risk of: MI, undergoing myocardial revascularization procedures, and cardiovascular mortality with no increase in death from noncardiovascular causes. In patients with coronary heart disease, to reduce risk of: mortality by reducing coronary death, undergoing myocardial revascularization procedures, MI, stroke, and TIA; and to slow progression of coronary atherosclerosis.

DOSAGE: *Adults:* ≥18 yrs: Initial: 40mg qd. Perform lipid tests within 4 weeks and adjust according to response and guidelines. Titrate: May increase to 80mg qd if needed. Significant Renal/Hepatic Dysfunction: Initial: 10mg qd. Concomitant Immunosuppressives (eg, cyclosporine): Initial:10mg qhs. Max: 20mg/day.

Pediatrics: Heterozygous Familial Hypercholesterolemia: 14-18 yrs: Initial: 40mg qd. 8-13 yrs: 20mg qd. Concomitant Immunosuppressives (eg, cyclosporine): Initial: 10mg qhs. Max: 20mg/day.

HOW SUPPLIED: Tab: 10mg, 20mg, 40mg, 80mg

CONTRAINDICATIONS: Active liver disease, unexplained persistent elevations of LFTs, pregnancy, nursing mothers.

WARNINGS/PRECAUTIONS: Perform LFTs before therapy, before dose increases, and if clinically indicated. Risk of myopathy, myalgia, and rhabdomyolysis. D/C if AST or ALT ≥3x ULN persists, if elevated CPK levels occur, or if myopathy diagnosed or suspected. Less effective with homozygous familial hypercholesterolemia. Monitor for endocrine dysfunction. Closely monitor with heavy alcohol use, recent history or signs of hepatic disease, or renal dysfunction.

ADVERSE REACTIONS: Rash, NV, diarrhea, headache, chest pain, influenza, abdominal pain, dizziness, increases ALT, AST, CPK.

INTERACTIONS: Risk of myopathy with fibrates, niacin, cyclosporine, erythromycin. Increased levels with gemfibrozil, itraconazole. Avoid fibrates unless benefit outweighs drug combination risk. Decreased levels with concomitant cholestyramine/colestipol; take 1 hr before or 4 hrs after resins. Caution with drugs that diminish levels or activity of steroid hormones (eg, ketoconazole, spironolactone, cimetidine).

PREGNANCY: Category X, not for use in nursing.

MECHANISM OF ACTION: HMG-CoA reductase inhibitor; causes increased number of LDL-receptors on cell surfaces and enhanced receptor mediated catabolism and clearance of circulating LDL. Inhibits LDL production by inhibiting hepatic synthesis of VLDL, LDL precursor.

PHARMACOKINETICS: Absorption: Rapid. Absolute bioavailability (17%); T_{max}=1-1.5 hrs. **Distribution:** Plasma protein binding (50%). **Metabolism:** Liver. **Elimination:** Feces (70%), urine (20%); $T_{1/2}$=77 hrs.

NURSING CONSIDERATIONS

Assessment: Prior to initiation, assess secondary causes of hypercholesterolemia (eg, poorly controlled DM, hypothyroidism, nephrotic syndrome, dysproteinemias, obstructive liver disease, other drug therapy, alcoholism), active liver disease, elevations in serum transaminases, pregnancy/nursing status, and possible drug interactions. Obtain baseline lipid profile and LFTs.

Monitoring: Monitor for signs/symptoms of active liver disease, rhabdomyolysis with acute renal failure, myoglobinuria, myopathies. Monitor CPK and LFTs periodically, and lipid levels every 4 weeks to evaluate response.

Patient Counseling: Advise to report signs/symptoms of unexplained muscle pain, tenderness, or weakness, particularly with malaise or fever. Recommend standard cholesterol-lowering diet prior to and during treatment. Educate about pregnancy/nursing risks. Counsel to take with/without food.

Administration: Oral route. **Storage:** 25°C (77°F); excursions permitted to 15-30°C (59-86°F). Protect from light.

PRECOSE

RX

acarbose (Bayer Healthcare)

THERAPEUTIC CLASS: Alpha-glucosidase inhibitor

INDICATIONS: Adjunct to diet and exercise, to improve glycemic control in type 2 diabetes mellitus. May use with insulin, metformin, or a sulfonylurea.

DOSAGE: *Adults:* Initial: 25mg tid with first bite of each main meal. To minimize GI effects: 25mg qd, increase gradually to 25mg tid. Titrate: After reaching 25mg tid, may increase at 4-8 week intervals. Maint: 50-100mg tid. Max: ≤60kg: 50mg tid. >60kg: 100mg tid. If no further reduction in post prandial or HbA_{1c} with 100mg tid, consider reducing dose.

HOW SUPPLIED: Tab: 25mg, 50mg, 100mg

CONTRAINDICATIONS: Diabetic ketoacidosis, cirrhosis, inflammatory bowel disease, colonic ulceration, partial or predisposition to intestinal obstruction, chronic intestinal disease with marked disorders of digestion or absorption, and conditions that may deteriorate from increased intestinal gas formation.

WARNINGS/PRECAUTIONS: Avoid with significant renal dysfunction (SrCr >2mg/dL). May need to d/c and give insulin with stress (eg, fever, trauma). Dose related elevated serum transaminase levels reported. Monitor serum transaminases every 3 months for first year then periodically. Reduce dose or d/c if elevated serum transaminases persist. Use glucose (dextrose) instead of sucrose (sugar cane) to treat mild to moderate hypoglycemia.

ADVERSE REACTIONS: Transient flatulence, diarrhea, abdominal pain.

INTERACTIONS: Risk of hyperglycemia with diuretics, corticosteroids, phenothiazines, thyroid products, estrogens, oral contraceptives, phenytoin, nicotinic acid, sympathomimetics, CCBs, and isoniazid. Reduced effect with intestinal adsorbents (eg, charcoal) and digestive enzymes containing carbohydrate-splitting enzymes (eg, amylase, pancreatin); avoid concomitant use. May affect digoxin bioavailability; may require dose adjustment of digoxin. Monitor for hypoglycemia with insulin or sulfonylureas.

PREGNANCY: Category B, not for use in nursing.

MECHANISM OF ACTION: α-glucosidase inhibitor; reversibly inhibits pancreatic α-amylase and membrane-bound intestinal α-glucoside hydrolase enzymes.

PHARMACOKINETICS: Absorption: Poor; T_{max}=1 hr. **Metabolism:** GI tract by intestinal bacteria or digestive enzymes; 4-methylpyrogallol derivatives (major metabolites). **Elimination:** Urine (unchanged); $T_{1/2}$=2 hrs.

NURSING CONSIDERATIONS

Assessment: Assess for renal dysfunction, cirrhosis, diabetic ketoacidosis, inflammatory bowel disease, colonic ulceration or partial intestinal obstruction, chronic intestinal disease, pregnancy status, and possible drug interactions.

Monitoring: Monitor for hypoglycemia, FPG, HbA_{1c}, LFTs, renal function, diabetic ketoacidosis, GI symptoms (eg, abdominal pain, diarrhea, flatulence), hypersensitivity reactions.

Patient Counseling: Instruct to take three times daily at the start of each meal. Counsel about signs/symptoms of hypoglycemia. Inform about importance of adhering to dietary instructions, a regular exercise program, and regular testing of urine and blood glucose.

Administration: Oral route. **Storage:** 25°C (77°F); protect from moisture; keep container tightly closed.

Pred Forte — RX

prednisolone acetate (Allergan)

THERAPEUTIC CLASS: Corticosteroid

INDICATIONS: Treatment of inflammation of the palpebral and bulbar conjunctiva, cornea and anterior segment of the globe.

DOSAGE: *Adults:* 1-2 drops bid-qid. May dose more frequently during initial 24-48 hrs. Re-evaluate after 2 days if no improvement.

HOW SUPPLIED: Sus: 1% [1mL, 5mL, 10mL, 15mL]

CONTRAINDICATIONS: Viral diseases of the cornea and conjunctiva including epithelial herpes simplex keratitis, vaccinia, and varicella. Mycobacterial infection and fungal diseases of the eye.

WARNINGS/PRECAUTIONS: Caution with glaucoma, herpes simplex, diseases causing thinning of cornea/sclera and other ocular viral infections. Prolonged use can cause glaucoma or secondary ocular infections (eg, fungal). Monitor IOP after 10 days of therapy. Re-evaluate if no response after 2 days. May delay healing and increase incidence of bleb formation after cataract surgery. Avoid abrupt withdrawal with chronic use. Contains sodium bisulfite.

ADVERSE REACTIONS: Elevation of IOP, glaucoma, infrequent optic nerve damage, posterior subcapsular cataract formation, delayed wound healing, burning/stinging upon instillation, ocular irritation, secondary infection, visual disturbance.

PREGNANCY: Category C, not for use in nursing.

MECHANISM OF ACTION: Glucocorticoid; anti-inflammatory agent; inhibitis edema, fibrin deposition, capillary dilation, deposition of collagen, and scar formation.

NURSING CONSIDERATIONS

Assessment: Assess for viral disease of cornea and conjunctiva, dendritic keratitis, vaccinia and varicella, mycobacterial infection and/or fungal disease of ocular structures, glaucoma, mustard gas keratitis, Sjogren's keratoconjuctivitis, thinning of corneal/scleral epithelium, hypersensitivity to sulfite, asthma, and cataract surgery.

Monitoring: Monitor for anaphylactic symptoms and asthma attacks. Frequent measuring of IOP and slit lamp microscopy exam where appropriate, fluorescein staining for monitoring of glaucoma with damage to the optic nerve with defects in visual acuity and fields of vision, posterior subcapsular cataract, delayed corneal healing, thinning of cornea and sclera, ulceration, perforation, and secondary ocular infections (or masking of existing infections).

Patient Counseling: Advise to d/c drug and consult physician if symptoms persist or worsen. Instruct to wait 15 min after instillation to wear soft contact lenses. Counsel to avoid touching bottle tip to eyelids or any other surface.

Administration: Ocular route. **Storage:** 25°C (77°F). Protect from freezing. Keep tightly closed.

PRED MILD — RX
prednisolone acetate (Allergan)

THERAPEUTIC CLASS: Corticosteroid

INDICATIONS: Treatment of noninfectious ocular inflammation.

DOSAGE: *Adults:* 1-2 drops bid-qid. May dose more frequently during initial 24-48 hrs. Re-evaluate after 2 days if no improvement.

HOW SUPPLIED: Sus: 0.12% [5mL, 10mL]

CONTRAINDICATIONS: Viral diseases of the cornea and conjunctiva including epithelial herpes simplex keratitis, vaccinia, and varicella. Mycobacterial infection and fungal diseases of the eye.

WARNINGS/PRECAUTIONS: Caution with glaucoma, herpes simplex, diseases causing thinning of cornea/sclera and other ocular viral infections. Prolonged use can cause glaucoma or secondary ocular infections (eg, fungal). Monitor IOP after 10 days of therapy. Re-evaluate if no response after 2 days. May delay healing and increase incidence of bleb formation after cataract surgery. Avoid abrupt withdrawal with chronic use. Contains sodium bisulfite.

ADVERSE REACTIONS: Elevation of IOP, glaucoma, infrequent optic nerve damage, posterior subcapsular cataract formation, delayed wound healing, burning/stinging upon instillation, ocular irritation, secondary infection, visual disturbance.

PREGNANCY: Category C, not for use in nursing.

MECHANISM OF ACTION: Glucocorticoid; inhibits edema, fibrin disposition, capillary dilation, and phagocytic migration of acute inflammatory response as well as capillary proliferation, deposition of collagen and scar formation.

NURSING CONSIDERATIONS

Assessment: Assess for viral diseases of the cornea and conjunctiva, dendritic keratitis, vaccinia, and varicella, mycobacterial infection and/or fungal diseases of ocular structures, and glaucoma.

Monitoring: Monitor for improvement of signs/symptoms; frequent measuring of IOP if using for >10 days.

Patient Counseling: Advise to d/c and notify physician if symptoms persist or worsen. Wait 15 min after instillation to wear soft contact lenses. Avoid touching bottle tip to eyelids or any other surface.

Administration: Intraocular route. **Storage:** 15-30°C (59-56°F). Protect from freezing. Keep tightly closed.

PRED-G — RX
prednisolone acetate - gentamicin sulfate (Allergan)

OTHER BRAND NAMES: Pred-G S.O.P. (Allergan)

THERAPEUTIC CLASS: Aminoglycoside/corticosteroid

INDICATIONS: Ocular inflammation associated with infection or risk of infection.

DOSAGE: *Adults:* (Sus) 1 drop bid-qid. May increase dose to every hour during initial 24-48 hrs. Max: 20mL for initial prescription. (Oint) Apply 1/2 inch in conjunctival sac qd-tid. Max: 8g for initial prescription.

HOW SUPPLIED: (Gentamicin-Prednisolone) Oint: (S.O.P.) 0.3%-0.6% [3.5g]; Sus: 0.3%-1% [2mL, 5mL, 10mL]

CONTRAINDICATIONS: Viral diseases of the cornea and conjunctiva including epithelial herpes simplex keratitis, vaccinia, and varicella. Mycobacterial infection and fungal diseases of the eye.

WARNINGS/PRECAUTIONS: Not for injection into eye. Caution with glaucoma, herpes simplex, diseases causing thinning of cornea/sclera and other ocular viral infections. Prolonged use can cause glaucoma or secondary ocular infections (eg, fungal). Monitor IOP after 10 days of therapy. Re-evaluate if no response after 2 days. May delay healing and increase incidence of bleb formation after cataract surgery. Ocular irritation and punctate keratitis reported. Cataract formation and optic nerve damage with prolonged use.

ADVERSE REACTIONS: Elevation of IOP, glaucoma, infrequent optic nerve damage, posterior subcapsular cataract formation, delayed wound healing, irritation upon instillation, ocular discomfort, secondary infection, allergic sensitization, burning, stinging, eye irritation.

PREGNANCY: Category C, not for use in nursing.

MECHANISM OF ACTION: Aminoglycoside/corticosteroid. Gentamicin: Anti-infective component that provides action against susceptible organisms. Prednisolone: Corticosteroid that suppresses the inflammatory response and delays or slows healing.

NURSING CONSIDERATIONS

Assessment: Prior to therapy, assess proper diagnosis of patient (eg, measurement of IOP, slit lamp biomicroscopy, fluorescein staining). Assess for hypersensitivity to other corticosteroids, viral diseases of the cornea and conjunctiva (eg, epithelial herpes simplex [dendritic keratitis], vaccina, and varicella), mycobacterial infection of the eye, and fungal diseases of the ocular structures. Assess use with glaucoma, history of herpes simplex, recent cataract surgery, and in pregnancy/nursing.

Monitoring: Monitor for masking of acute purulent infections, ocular irritation, and punctate keratitis. For patients on prolonged therapy, monitor for development of glaucoma with damage to the optic nerve, defects in visual acuity and fields of vision, posterior subcapsular cataract formation, corneal and scleral thinning, and secondary infections (eg, fungal, viral). Monitor IOP in patients on therapy for ≥10 days. Perform frequent slit lamp microscopy in patients with a history of herpes simplex.

P

Patient Counseling: Advise to d/c medication and consult physician if inflammation or pain persists longer than 48 hrs or becomes aggravated. Instruct to avoid touching bottle tip to the eyelids or other surfaces.

Administration: Ocular route. Do not inject into eye. Shake well before using.
Storage: 15-25°C (59-77°F). Avoid excessive heat, 40°C (104°F) and above. Protect from freezing.

PREDNISONE — RX

prednisone (Roxane)

OTHER BRAND NAMES: Deltasone (Pharmacia & Upjohn)

THERAPEUTIC CLASS: Glucocorticoid

INDICATIONS: Steroid-responsive disorders.

DOSAGE: *Adults:* Initial: 5-60mg/day depending on disease and response. Maint: Decrease dose by small amounts to lowest effective dose.
Pediatrics: Initial: 5-60mg/day depending on disease and response. Maint: Decrease dose by small amounts to lowest effective dose.

HOW SUPPLIED: Sol: 5mg/mL, 5mg/5mL; Tab: 1mg, 2.5mg*, 5mg*, 10mg*, 20mg*, 50mg* *scored

CONTRAINDICATIONS: Systemic fungal infections.

WARNINGS/PRECAUTIONS: May need to increase dose before, during, and after stressful situations. May mask signs of infection or cause new infections. Prolonged use may produce glaucoma, optic nerve damage, secondary ocular infections. Increases BP, salt/water retention, potassium excretion. More severe/fatal course of infections reported with chickenpox, measles. Caution with latent TB, hypothyroidism, cirrhosis, ocular herpes simplex, HTN, diverticulitis, fresh intestinal anastomosis, ulcerative colitis, osteoporosis, myasthenia gravis, renal insufficiency, peptic ulcer disease. Growth and development of children on prolonged therapy should be monitored. Monitor for psychic disturbances. Avoid abrupt withdrawal.

ADVERSE REACTIONS: Fluid and electrolyte disturbances, HTN, osteoporosis, muscle weakness, cushingoid state, menstrual irregularities, nervousness, insomnia, impaired wound healing, DM, ulcerative esophagitis, excessive sweating, increased ICP, carbohydrate intolerance, glaucoma, cataracts, weight gain, nausea, malaise.

INTERACTIONS: Increases clearance of high dose ASA; caution in hypoprothrombinemia. Increased insulin and oral hypoglycemic requirements in DM. Avoid smallpox vaccine, and live vaccines with immunosuppressive doses. Possible decreased vaccine response with killed or inactivated vaccines with immunosuppressive doses. Increased clearance with hepatic enzyme inducers. Decreased metabolism with troleandomycin, ketoconazole. Variable effect on oral anticoagulants.

PREGNANCY: Safety in pregnancy and nursing not known.

MECHANISM OF ACTION: Anti-inflammatory glucocorticoid; causes profound and varied metabolic effects and modifies the body's immune responses to diverse stimuli.

PHARMACOKINETICS: Absorption: Readily absorbed (GI tract).

NURSING CONSIDERATIONS

Assessment: Assess unusual stress, fungal/other current infections, active TB, thyroid status, vaccination status, hepatic/liver impairment, hypoprothrombinemia, psychiatric tendencies, ulcerative colitis, diverticulitis, peptic ulcer with/without impending perforation, intestinal anastamoses, HTN, osteoporosis, myasthenia gravis, pregnancy status.

Monitoring: In pediatrics, monitor for hypoadrenalism, growth and development. Monitor for psychiatric derangements, infection, cataracts, fluid retention, adrenocortical insufficiency, intestinal perforation/peritoneal irritation, serum electrolytes, TSH, glucose, LFTs, BP, IOP.

Patient Counseling: Avoid exposure to chickenpox or measles; report immediately if exposed. Advise regarding dietary salt restriction and K^+ supplementaion.

Administration: Oral route. **Storage:** 25°C (77°F); excursions permitted to 15-30°C.

PREFEST — RX

norgestimate - estradiol (King)

Estrogens and progestins should not be used for the prevention of cardiovascular disease. Increased risks of MI, stroke, invasive breast cancer, PE, and DVT in postmenopausal women (50-79 yrs of age) reported. Increased risk of developing probable dementia in postmenopausal women ≥65 yrs of age reported.

THERAPEUTIC CLASS: Estrogen/progestogen combination

INDICATIONS: In women with an intact uterus, treatment of moderate to severe vasomotor symptoms and/or vulvar/vaginal atrophy associated with menopause and prevention of postmenopausal osteoporosis.

DOSAGE: *Adults:* Vasomotor Symptoms/Vulvar/Vaginal Atrophy/ Osteoporosis Prevention: 1mg (estradiol) qd for 3 days followed by 1mg-0.09mg (estradiol-norgestimate) qd for 3 days. Repeat regimen continuously. Re-evaluate at 3-6 month intervals when treating menopausal symptoms.

HOW SUPPLIED: Tab: (Estradiol) 1mg and (Estradiol-Norgestimate) 1mg-0.09mg

CONTRAINDICATIONS: Pregnancy, undiagnosed abnormal genital bleeding, breast cancer, estrogen-dependent neoplasia, DVT/PE, active or recent (eg, within past year) arterial thromboembolic disease (eg, stroke, MI), liver dysfunction or disease.

WARNINGS/PRECAUTIONS: May increase risk of cardiovascular events (eg, MI, stroke), venous thrombosis, and PE; d/c immediately if any of these events occur or are suspected. May increase risk of breast/endometrial cancer, and gallbladder disease. May lead to severe hypercalcemia with breast cancer and bone metastases; monitor and d/c if hypercalcemia occurs. Retinal vascular thrombosis reported; monitor and d/c if papilledema or retinal vascular lesions occur. May elevate BP; monitor at regular intervals. May cause elevations of plasma triglycerides with pre-existing hypertriglyceridemia. Caution with history of cholestatic jaundice associated with past estrogen use or with pregnancy; d/c with recurrence. May lead to increased thyroid-binding globulin levels; monitor thyroid function. May cause fluid retention; caution with cardiac/renal dysfunction. Caution with severe hypocalcemia. May increase risk of ovarian cancer. May exacerbate endometriosis, asthma, DM, epilepsy, migraine, porphyria, SLE, and hepatic hemangiomas; use with caution.

ADVERSE REACTIONS: Altered vaginal bleeding, vaginal candidiasis, breast tenderness/enlargement, NV, melasma, headache, weight changes, edema, altered libido.

INTERACTIONS: CYP3A4 inducers (eg, St. John's wort, phenobarbital, carbamazepine, rifampin) may decrease levels which may decrease therapeutic effects and/or change uterine bleeding profile. CYP3A4 inhibitors (eg, erythromycin, clarithromycin, ketoconazole, itraconazole, ritonavir, grapefruit juice) may increase levels which may result in side effects.

PREGNANCY: Contraindicated in pregnancy, caution in nursing.

MECHANISM OF ACTION: Estradiol: Estrogen; binds to nuclear receptors in estrogen-responsive tissues and modulates pituitary secretion of the gonadotropins, luteinizing hormone and follicle stimulating hormone, through negative feedback mechanism. Reduces elevated levels of these hormones in postmenopausal women. Norgestimate: Progestin; binds to androgen and progestogen receptors. Counters estrogenic effects by decreasing number of estradiol receptors and suppressing epithelial DNA synthesis in endometrial tissue.

P

PHARMACOKINETICS: Absorption: Oral administration of variable doses resulted in different parameters. **Distribution:** Found in breast milk. Estradiol: Largely bound to sex hormone binding globulin and albumin. Norgestimate: (17-deacetylnorgestimate) (primary active metabolite): Plasma protein binding (99%). **Metabolism:** Estradiol: Liver to estrone (metabolite) and estriol (major urinary metabolite); sulfate and glucuronide conjugation (liver); gut hydrolysis; CYP3A4 (partial metabolism). Norgestimate: Extensively in GI tract and liver; 17-deacetylnorgestimate (primary active metabolite). **Elimination:** Estradiol: Urine (parent compound and metabolites); $T_{1/2}$=16 hrs. Norgestimate: Urine, feces; (Active metabolite): $T_{1/2}$=37 hrs.

NURSING CONSIDERATIONS

Assessment: Assess for undiagnosed abnormal genital bleeding, presence or history of breast cancer, estrogen-dependent neoplasia, DVT or PE, active or recent (within past yr) arterial thromboembolic disease (eg, stroke, MI), liver dysfunction, history of cholestatic jaundice, pregnancy/nursing status, age (≥65 yrs), hypertriglyceridemia, hypothyroidism, hypocalcemia, asthma, DM, epilepsy, migraines or porphyria, SLE, and possible drug interactions.

Monitoring: Monitor for signs/symptoms of cardiovascular disorders (eg, stroke, coronary heart disease, venous thromboembolism), malignant neoplasms (eg, endometrial, breast, ovarian cancer), dementia, gallbladder disease, hypercalcemia, visual abnormalities (eg, retinal vascular thrombosis), BP elevations, elevations in plasma triglycerides, pancreatitis, uterine bleeding, hypothyroidism, fluid retention, exacerbation of endometriosis and other conditions (eg, asthma, DM, epilepsy, migraines, SLE). Perform annual breast exam. Monitor BP levels regularly. Monitor thyroid function in patients on thyroid replacement therapy. Perform periodic evaluation (every 3-6 months) to determine treatment need. If undiagnosed persistent or recurring genital bleeding occurs, perform adequate diagnostic measures (eg, endometrial sampling) to rule out malignancy.

Patient Counseling: Inform that drug may increase risk for heart attack, stroke, breast cancer, blood clots, and dementia. Report any breast lumps, unusual vaginal bleeding, dizziness and faintness, changes in speech, severe headaches, chest pains, SOB, leg pains, changes in vision, or vomiting. Advise to notify physician if planning to undergo surgery or bed rest. Instruct to perform monthly self breast exams. Counsel if dose missed, take as soon as possible; if almost time for next dose, skip missed dose and go back to normal dosing schedule.

Administration: Oral route. **Storage:** 25°C (77°F); excursions permitted to 15-30°C (59-86°F). Keep out of reach of children.

PREMARIN IV

RX

conjugated estrogens (Wyeth)

Estrogens increase the risk of endometrial cancer. Estrogens, with or without progestins, should not be used for the prevention of CVD or dementia. Increased risks of MI, stroke, invasive breast cancer, PE, and DVT in postmenopausal women (50-79 yrs of age) reported. Increased risk of developing probable dementia in postmenopausal women ≥65 yrs of age reported.

THERAPEUTIC CLASS: Estrogen

INDICATIONS: Treatment of abnormal uterine bleeding due to hormonal imbalance in the absence of organic pathology.

DOSAGE: *Adults:* 25mg IV or IM. Repeat in 6-12 hrs if needed.

HOW SUPPLIED: Inj: 25mg

CONTRAINDICATIONS: Pregnancy, undiagnosed abnormal genital bleeding, breast cancer, estrogen-dependent neoplasia, DVT/PE, active or recent (eg, within past year) arterial thromboembolic disease (eg, stroke, MI), liver dysfunction or disease.

WARNINGS/PRECAUTIONS: May increase risk of cardiovascular events (eg, MI, stroke), venous thrombosis, and PE; d/c immediately if any of these events occur or are suspected. May increase risk of breast/endometrial cancer, and gallbladder disease. May lead to severe hypercalcemia with breast cancer and bone metastases; monitor and d/c if hypercalcemia occurs. Retinal vascular thrombosis reported; monitor and d/c if papilledema or retinal vascular lesions occur. Consider addition of a progestin if no hysterectomy. May elevate BP; monitor at regular intervals. May cause elevations of plasma triglycerides with pre-existing hypertriglyceridemia. Caution with history of cholestatic jaundice associated with past estrogen use or with pregnancy; d/c with recurrence. May lead to increased thyroid-binding globulin levels; monitor thyroid function. May cause fluid retention; caution with cardiac/renal dysfunction. Caution with severe hypocalcemia. May increase risk of ovarian cancer. May exacerbate endometriosis, asthma, DM, epilepsy, migraine, porphyria, SLE, and hepatic hemangiomas; use with caution.

ADVERSE REACTIONS: Abnormal vaginal bleeding, vaginal candidiasis, nausea, vomiting, abdominal cramps, bloating, breast pain/tenderness/enlargement, erythema multiforme, headache, dizziness, nervousness, weight changes, libido changes.

INTERACTIONS: CYP3A4 inducers (eg, St. John's wort, phenobarbital, carbamazepine, rifampin) may decrease levels which may decrease therapeutic effects and/or change uterine bleeding profile. CYP3A4 inhibitors (eg, erythromycin, clarithromycin, ketoconazole, itraconazole, ritonavir, grapefruit juice) may increase levels which may result in side effects.

PREGNANCY: Contraindicated in pregnancy, caution in nursing.

MECHANISM OF ACTION: Estradiol: Estrogen; responsible for development and maintenance of female reproductive system and secondary sexual characteristics by modulating pituitary secretion of gonadotropins, LH and FSH.

PHARMACOKINETICS: Absorption: Skin, mucous membranes, GI tract. **Metabolism:** Partial, via CYP3A4. Estrone (metabolite); estriol (major urinary metabolite). **Elimination:** Urine.

NURSING CONSIDERATIONS

Assessment: Assess for abnormal bleeding, breast or estrogen-dependent neoplasia, CAD, asthma, endometriosis, DM, epilepsy, migraine, porphyrias, SLE, hypothyroidism, pregnancy status, thromboembolic disease, hypocalcemia, and hepatic impairment.

Monitoring: Monitor BP regularly; thyroid function periodically. Breast exam by physician yearly and self-exam monthly; mammograms as required. Monitor for signs/symptoms of dementia, gallbladder disease, hypercalcemia, CV events (eg, MI, stroke), abnormal vaginal bleeding, thromboembolic disorders, fluid retention, visual abnormalities, hypersensitivity reactions, hepatic dysfunction, exacerbation of asthma, DM, epilepsy, SLE, migraines, and porphyria.

Patient Counseling: Inform of pregnancy risks. Advise to seek medical attention if symptoms of hepatic dysfunction (jaundice), hypercalcemia, visual disturbances (partial/complete loss of vision, diplopia), migraines, abnormal vaginal bleeding, hypersensitivity reactions, HTN, thromboembolic disorders, fluid retention, exacerbation of diseases, CV events, or dementia occur.

Administration: IV route. **Storage:** 2-8°C (36-46°F). Reconstitution: Stable for 60 days.

PREMARIN TABLETS RX

conjugated estrogens (Wyeth)

Estrogens increase the risk of endometrial cancer. Estrogens, with or without progestins, should not be used for the prevention of cardiovascular disease or dementia. Increased risks of MI, stroke, invasive breast cancer, PE, and DVT in postmenopausal women (50-79 yrs of age) reported. Increased risk of developing probable dementia in postmenopausal women ≥65 yrs of age reported.

THERAPEUTIC CLASS: Estrogen

P

INDICATIONS: Treatment of moderate to severe vasomotor symptoms and/or vulvar/vaginal atrophy associated with menopause. Treatment of hypoestrogenism due to hypogonadism, castration, or primary ovarian failure. Palliative treatment of breast cancer in patients with metastatic disease and/or advanced androgen-dependent carcinoma of the prostate. Prevention of postmenopausal osteoporosis.

DOSAGE: *Adults:* Vasomotor Symptoms/Vulvar/Vaginal Atrophy: 0.3mg qd continuously or cyclically (eg, 25 days on, 5 days off). Adjust dose based on response. Re-evaluate at 3-6 month intervals. Osteoporosis Prevention: 0.3mg qd continuously or cyclically (eg, 25 days on, 5 days off). Female Hypogonadism: 0.3-0.625mg qd cyclically (eg, 3 weeks on, 1 week off). Titrate at 6-12 month intervals. Female Castration/Ovarian Failure: 1.25mg qd cyclically. Breast Cancer (palliation): 10mg tid for minimum 3 months. Prostate Cancer (palliation): 1.25-2.5mg tid.

HOW SUPPLIED: Tab: 0.3mg, 0.45mg, 0.625mg, 0.9mg, 1.25mg

CONTRAINDICATIONS: Pregnancy, undiagnosed abnormal genital bleeding, breast cancer unless being treated for metastatic disease, estrogen-dependent neoplasia, DVT/PE, active or recent (eg, within past year) arterial thromboembolic disease (eg, stroke, MI), liver dysfunction or disease.

WARNINGS/PRECAUTIONS: May increase risk of cardiovascular events (eg, MI, stroke), venous thrombosis, and PE; d/c immediately if any of these events occur or are suspected. May increase risk of breast/endometrial cancer, and gallbladder disease. May lead to severe hypercalcemia with breast cancer and bone metastases; monitor and d/c if hypercalcemia occurs. Retinal vascular thrombosis reported; monitor and d/c if papilledema or retinal vascular lesions occur. Consider addition of a progestin if no hysterectomy. May elevate BP; monitor at regular intervals. May cause elevations of plasma triglycerides with pre-existing hypertriglyceridemia. Caution with history of cholestatic jaundice associated with past estrogen use or with pregnancy; d/c with recurrence. May lead to increased thyroid-binding globulin levels; monitor thyroid function. May cause fluid retention; caution with cardiac/renal dysfunction. Caution with severe hypocalcemia. May increase risk of ovarian cancer. May exacerbate endometriosis, asthma, DM, epilepsy, migraine, porphyria, SLE, and hepatic hemangiomas; use with caution.

ADVERSE REACTIONS: Abdominal pain, back pain, headache, infection, pain, arthralgia, leg cramps, breast pain, vaginal hemorrhage, vaginitis

INTERACTIONS: CYP3A4 inducers (eg, St. John's wort, phenobarbital, carbamazepine, rifampin) may decrease levels which may decrease therapeutic effects and/or change uterine bleeding profile. CYP3A4 inhibitors (eg, erythromycin, clarithromycin, ketoconazole, itraconazole, ritonavir, grapefruit juice) may increase levels which may result in side effects. Reduced response to metyrapone test.

PREGNANCY: Contraindicated in pregnancy, caution in nursing.

MECHANISM OF ACTION: Estrogen; binds to nuclear receptors in estrogen-responsive tissues. Circulating estrogens modulate pituitary secretion of the gonadotropins, luteinizing hormone and follicle stimulating hormone, through negative feedback mechanism. Reduces elevated levels of these hormones in postmenopausal women.

PHARMACOKINETICS: Absorption: Well absorbed; oral administration of variable doses resulted in different parameters. **Distribution:** Largely bound to sex hormone binding globulin and albumin; found in breast milk. **Metabolism:** Liver, to estrone (metabolite) and estriol (major urinary metabolite); sulfate and glucuronide conjugation (liver); gut hydrolysis; CYP3A4 (partial metabolism). **Elimination:** Urine (parent drug and metabolites).

NURSING CONSIDERATIONS

Assessment: Assess for undiagnosed abnormal genital bleeding, presence or history of breast cancer, estrogen-dependent neoplasia, DVT or PE, active or recent (within past yr) arterial thromboembolic disease (eg, stroke, MI), liver dysfunction, history of cholestatic jaundice, pregnancy/nursing status, age (≥65 yrs), hypertriglyceridemia, hypothyroidism, hypocalcemia, asthma, DM, epilepsy, migraines or porphyria, SLE, and possible drug interactions. Assess need for progestin therapy in women who have not had a hysterectomy.

Monitoring: Monitor for signs/symptoms of cardiovascular disorders (eg, stroke, coronary heart disease, venous thromboembolism), malignant neoplasms (eg, endometrial, breast, ovarian cancer), dementia, gallbladder disease, hypercalcemia, visual abnormalities (eg, retinal vascular thrombosis), BP elevations, elevations in plasma triglycerides, pancreatitis, hypothyroidism, fluid retention, exacerbation of endometriosis and other conditions (eg, asthma, DM, epilepsy, migraines, SLE). Perform annual breast exam. Monitor BP levels regularly and thyroid function in patients on thyroid replacement therapy. Perform periodic evaluation (every 3-6 months) to determine treatment need. If undiagnosed persistent or recurring genital bleeding occurs, perform adequate diagnostic measures (eg, endometrial sampling) to rule out malignancy.

Patient Counseling: Inform that drug increases risk for uterine cancer, heart attack, stroke, breast cancer, blood clots, and dementia. Report any breast lumps, unusual vaginal bleeding, dizziness and faintness, changes in speech, severe headaches, chest pain, SOB, leg pains, changes in vision, or vomiting. Advise to notify physician if planning surgery or bedrest. Instruct to take medication at same time daily and to perform monthly self breast exams. Counsel that if dose is missed, take as soon as possible; if almost time for next dose, skip dose, and go back to normal dosing schedule.

Administration: Oral route. **Storage:** 20-25°C (68-77°F); excursions permitted to 15-30°C (59-86°F); dispense in well-closed container.

PREMARIN VAGINAL RX

conjugated estrogens (Wyeth)

Estrogens increase risk of endometrial cancer. Estrogens, with or without progestins, should not be used for the prevention of cardiovascular disease or dementia. Increased risks of MI, stroke, invasive breast cancer, PE, and DVT in postmenopausal women (50-79 yrs of age) reported. Increased risk of developing probable dementia in postmenopausal women ≥65 yrs of age reported. Estrogens with or without progestins should be prescribed at the lowest effective dose and for the shortest duration consistent with treatment goals and risks for the individual woman.

THERAPEUTIC CLASS: Estrogen

INDICATIONS: Treatment of atrophic vaginitis, kraurosis vulvae, and moderate-to-severe dyspareunia.

DOSAGE: *Adults:* Atrophic Vaginitis/Kraurosis Vulvae: Usual: 0.5g intravaginally qd cyclically (3 weeks on, 1 week off). Titrate: 0.5-2g based on individual response. Moderate To Severe Dyspareunia: 0.5g intravaginally twice weekly (eg, Monday and Thursday) continuous regimen or qd cyclically (3 weeks on, 1 week off).

HOW SUPPLIED: Cre: 0.625mg/g [42.5g]

CONTRAINDICATIONS: Pregnancy, undiagnosed abnormal genital bleeding, breast cancer, estrogen-dependent neoplasia, DVT/PE, active or recent (eg, within past year) arterial thromboembolic disease (eg, stroke, MI), liver dysfunction or disease.

WARNINGS/PRECAUTIONS: May increase risk of breast/endometrial cancer, dementia and gallbladder disease. May lead to severe hypercalcemia with breast cancer and bone metastases; monitor and d/c if hypercalcemia occurs. Retinal vascular thrombosis reported; monitor and d/c if papilledema or retinal vascular lesions occur. Consider addition of a progestin if no hysterectomy. May elevate BP; monitor at regular intervals. May cause elevations of plasma triglycerides with pre-existing hypertriglyceridemia. Caution with history of cholestatic jaundice associated with past estrogen use or with pregnancy; d/c with recurrence. May lead to increased thyroid-binding globulin levels; monitor thyroid function. May cause fluid retention; caution with cardiac/renal dysfunction. Caution with severe hypocalcemia. May increase risk of ovarian cancer. May exacerbate endometriosis, asthma, DM, epilepsy, migraine, porphyria, SLE, and hepatic hemangiomas; use with caution. May weaken and contribute to the failure of condoms, diaphragms, or cervical caps made of latex or rubber.

ADVERSE REACTIONS: Breakthrough bleeding, vaginal candidiasis, change in cervical secretion, breast tenderness and enlargement, nausea, vomiting, abdominal cramps, bloating, chloasma, melasma, venous thromboembolism, pulmonary embolism, headache.

INTERACTIONS: CYP3A4 inducers (eg, St. John's wort, phenobarbital, carbamazepine, rifampin) may decrease levels, which may decrease therapeutic effects and/or change uterine bleeding profile. CYP3A4 inhibitors (eg, erythromycin, clarithromycin, ketoconazole, itraconazole, ritonavir, grapefruit juice) may increase levels, which may result in side effects.

PREGNANCY: Contraindicated in pregnancy, caution in nursing.

MECHANISM OF ACTION: Estrogen; binds to nuclear receptors in estrogen-responsive tissues. Circulating estrogens modulate pituitary secretion of the gonadotropins, luteinizing hormone and follicle stimulating hormone, through negative feedback mechanism. Reduces elevated levels of these hormones in postmenopausal women.

PHARMACOKINETICS: Absorption: Well-absorbed. **Distribution:** Largely bound to sex hormone binding globulin and albumin; found in breast milk. **Metabolism:** Liver to estrone (metabolite), estriol (major urinary metabolite); sulfate and glucuronide conjugation (liver); gut hydrolysis; CYP 3A4 (partial metabolism). **Elimination:** Urine (parent compound and metabolites).

NURSING CONSIDERATIONS

Assessment: Assess for undiagnosed abnormal genital bleeding, presence or history of breast cancer, DVT or PE, estrogen-dependent neoplasia, active or recent (within past yr) arterial thromboembolic disease (eg, stroke, MI), liver dysfunction or past history of cholestatic jaundice, pregnancy/nursing status, age (≥65 yrs), hypertriglyceridemia, hypothyroidism, hypocalcemia, asthma, DM, epilepsy, migraines or porphyria, SLE, and possible drug interactions. Assess need for progestin therapy in women who have not had a hysterectomy.

Monitoring: Monitor for signs/symptoms of cardiovascular disorders (eg, stroke, coronary heart disease, venous thromboembolism), malignant neoplasms (eg, endometrial, breast, ovarian cancer), dementia, gallbladder disease, hypercalcemia, visual abnormalities (eg, retinal vascular thrombosis), BP elevations, elevations in plasma triglycerides, pancreatitis, hypothyroidism, fluid retention, exacerbation of endometriosis and of other conditions (eg, asthma, DM, epilepsy, migraines, SLE). Perform annual breast exam. Monitor BP levels at regular intervals and thyroid function in patients on thyroid replacement therapy. Perform periodic evaluation (every 3-6 months) to determine treatment need. If undiagnosed persistent or recurring genital bleeding occurs, perform adequate diagnostic measures (eg, endometrial sampling) to rule out malignancy.

Patient Counseling: Inform that drug increases risk for uterine cancer, heart attack, stroke, breast cancer, blood clots, and dementia. Report any breast lumps, unusual vaginal bleeding, dizziness and faintness, changes in speech, severe headaches, chest pain, SOB, leg pain, changes in vision, and vomiting. Advise on proper administration of medication; applicator should be cleansed with mild soap and warm water following application; do not boil or use hot water. Instruct to perform monthly self breast exams. Inform that medication may weaken barrier contraceptives (eg, latex condoms, diaphragms, cervical caps).

Administration: Intravaginal route. Lie back with knees drawn up; insert applicator deeply into vagina; press plunger downward to its original position.
Storage: 20-25°C (68-77°F); excursions permitted to 15-30°C (59-86°F).

PREMPHASE RX

medroxyprogesterone acetate - conjugated estrogens (Wyeth)

Estrogens and progestins should not be used for prevention of cardiovascular disease or dementia. Increased risks of MI, stroke, invasive breast cancer, PE, and DVT in postmenopausal women (50-79 yrs of age) reported. Increased risk of developing probable dementia in postmenopausal women ≥65 yrs of age reported.

THERAPEUTIC CLASS: Estrogen/progestogen combination

INDICATIONS: In women with intact uterus, treatment of moderate to severe vasomotor symptoms and/or vulvar/vaginal atrophy associated with menopause and prevention of postmenopausal osteoporosis.

DOSAGE: *Adults:* Vasomotor Symptoms/Vulvar/Vaginal Atrophy/ Osteoporosis Prevention: 0.625mg tab qd on Days 1-14 and 0.625mg-5mg tab qd on Days 15-28. Re-evaluate after 3-6 months.

HOW SUPPLIED: Tab: 0.625mg (Estrogens, Conjugated) and 0.625mg-5mg (Estrogens, Conjugated-Medroxyprogesterone)

CONTRAINDICATIONS: Pregnancy, undiagnosed abnormal genital bleeding, breast cancer, estrogen dependent neoplasia, DVT/PE, active or recent (eg, within past year) arterial thromboembolic disease (eg, stroke, MI), liver dysfunction or disease.

WARNINGS/PRECAUTIONS: May increase risk of cardiovascular events (eg, MI, stroke), venous thrombosis, and PE; d/c immediately if any of these events occur or are suspected. May increase risk of breast/endometrial cancer, and gallbladder disease. May lead to severe hypercalcemia with breast cancer and bone metastases; monitor and d/c if hypercalcemia occurs. Retinal vascular thrombosis reported; monitor and d/c if papilledema or retinal vascular lesions occur. May elevate BP; monitor at regular intervals. May cause elevations of plasma triglycerides with pre-existing hypertriglyceridemia. Caution with history of cholestatic jaundice associated with past estrogen use or with pregnancy; d/c with recurrence. May lead to increased thyroid-binding globulin levels; monitor thyroid function. May cause fluid retention; caution with cardiac/renal dysfunction. Caution with severe hypocalcemia. May increase risk of ovarian cancer. May exacerbate endometriosis, asthma, DM, epilepsy, migraine, porphyria, SLE, and hepatic hemangiomas; use with caution.

ADVERSE REACTIONS: Abdominal pain, dysmenorrhea, vaginal moniliasis, breast pain, nausea, arthralgia, headache, depression, back pain, infection, pain, vaginal hemorrhage, vaginitis.

INTERACTIONS: CYP3A4 inducers (eg, St. John's wort, phenobarbital, carbamazepine, rifampin) may decrease levels which may decrease therapeutic effects and/or change uterine bleeding profile. CYP3A4 inhibitors (eg, erythromycin, clarithromycin, ketoconazole, itraconazole, ritonavir, grapefruit juice) may increase levels which may result in side effects.

PREGNANCY: Contraindicated in pregnancy, caution in nursing.

MECHANISM OF ACTION: Conjugated estrogens: Estrogen; binds to nuclear receptors in estrogen-responsive tissues. Circulating estrogens modulate pituitary secretion of gonadotropins, luteinizing hormone and follicle stimulating hormone. Medroxyprogesterone: Progesterone derivative; inhibits gonadotropin production which prevents follicular maturation and ovulation.

PHARMACOKINETICS: Absorption: Well-absorbed. Oral administration of various doses resulted in different parameters. **Distribution**: Found in breast milk. Conjugated Estrogen: Largely bound to sex hormone binding globulin and albumin. Medroxyprogesterone: Plasma protein binding (90%). **Metabolism**: Estrogen: Liver to estrone (metabolite) and estriol (major urinary metabolite); sulfate and glucuronide conjugation (liver); gut hydrolysis; CYP3A4 (partial metabolism). Medroxyprogesterone: Liver via hydroxylation, conjugation. **Elimination**: Estrogen: Urine (parent compound and metabolites); Medroxyprogesterone: Urine (metabolites).

NURSING CONSIDERATIONS

Assessment: Assess for undiagnosed abnormal genital bleeding, presence or history of breast cancer, DVT or PE, estrogen-dependent neoplasia, active or recent (within past yr) arterial thromboembolic disease (eg, stroke, MI), liver dysfunction, history of cholestatic jaundice, pregnancy/nursing status, age (≥65 yrs), hypertriglyceridemia, hypothyroidism, hypocalcemia, asthma, DM, epilepsy, migraines or porphyria, SLE, and possible drug interactions.

Monitoring: Monitor for signs/symptoms of cardiovascular disorders (eg, stroke, coronary heart disease, venous thromboembolism), malignant neoplasms (eg, endometrial, breast, ovarian cancer), dementia, gallbladder disease, hypercalcemia, visual abnormalities (eg, retinal vascular thrombosis), BP elevations, elevations in plasma triglycerides, pancreatitis, hypothyroidism, fluid retention, exacerbation of endometriosis and other conditions (eg, asthma, DM, epilepsy, migraines, SLE). Perform annual breast exam. Monitor BP levels at regular intervals and thyroid function if on thyroid replacement therapy. Perform periodic evaluation (every 3-6 months) to determine treatment need. If undiagnosed persistent or recurring genital bleeding occurs, perform adequate diagnostic measures (eg, endometrial sampling) to rule out malignancy.

Patient Counseling: Inform that drug may increase risk for heart attack, stroke, breast cancer, blood clots, and dementia. Report any breast lumps, unusual vaginal bleeding, dizziness and faintness, changes in speech, severe headaches, chest pain, SOB, leg pains, changes in vision, or vomiting. Advise to notify physician if planning surgery or prolonged immobilization. Counsel to perform monthly breast self-exams.

Administration: Oral route. **Storage**: 20-25°C (68-77°F); excursions permitted to 15-30°C (59-86°F).

PREMPRO

RX

medroxyprogesterone acetate - conjugated estrogens (Wyeth)

Estrogens and progestins should not be used for prevention of cardiovascular disease or dementia. Increased risks of MI, stroke, invasive breast cancer, PE, and DVT in postmenopausal women (50-79 yrs of age) reported. Increased risk of developing probable dementia in postmenopausal women ≥65 yrs of age reported.

THERAPEUTIC CLASS: Estrogen/progestogen combination

INDICATIONS: In women with intact uterus, treatment of moderate to severe vasomotor symptoms and/or vulvar/vaginal atrophy associated with menopause and prevention of postmenopausal osteoporosis.

DOSAGE: *Adults:* Vasomotor Symptoms/Vulvar/Vaginal Atrophy/ Osteoporosis Prevention: Initial: 0.3mg-1.5mg qd. Adjust dose based on response. Re-evaluate after 3-6 months.

HOW SUPPLIED: Tab: (Estrogens, Conjugated-Medroxyprogesterone) 0.3mg-1.5mg, 0.45mg-1.5mg, 0.625mg-2.5mg, 0.625mg-5mg

CONTRAINDICATIONS: Pregnancy, undiagnosed abnormal genital bleeding, breast cancer, estrogen dependent neoplasia, DVT/PE, active or recent (eg, within past year) arterial thromboembolic disease (eg, stroke, MI), liver dysfunction or disease.

WARNINGS/PRECAUTIONS: May increase risk of cardiovascular events (eg, MI, stroke), venous thrombosis, and PE; d/c immediately if any of these events occur or are suspected. May increase risk of breast/endometrial cancer, and gallbladder disease. May lead to severe hypercalcemia with breast cancer and bone metastases; monitor and d/c if hypercalcemia occurs. Retinal vascular thrombosis reported; monitor and d/c if papilledema or retinal vascular lesions occur. May elevate BP; monitor at regular intervals. May cause elevations of plasma triglycerides with pre-existing hypertriglyceridemia. Caution with history of cholestatic jaundice associated with past estrogen use or with pregnancy; d/c with recurrence. May lead to increased thyroid-binding globulin levels; monitor thyroid function. May cause fluid retention; caution with cardiac/renal dysfunction. Caution with severe hypocalcemia. May increase risk of ovarian cancer. May exacerbate endometriosis, asthma, DM, epilepsy, migraine, porphyria, SLE, and hepatic hemangiomas; use with caution.

ADVERSE REACTIONS: Abdominal pain, dysmenorrhea, vaginal moniliasis, breast pain, nausea, arthralgia, headache, depression, back pain, infection, pain, vaginal hemorrhage, vaginitis.

INTERACTIONS: CYP3A4 inducers (eg, St. John's wort, phenobarbital, carbamazepine, rifampin) may decrease levels which may decrease therapeutic effects and/or change uterine bleeding profile. CYP3A4 inhibitors (eg, erythromycin, clarithromycin, ketoconazole, itraconazole, ritonavir, grapefruit juice) may increase levels which may result in side effects. Reduced response to metyrapone test. Concomitant aminoglutethimide may significantly depress bioavailability of medroxyprogesterone.

PREGNANCY: Contraindicated in pregnancy, caution in nursing.

MECHANISM OF ACTION: Estrogen: Responsible for development and maintenance of female reproductive system, and secondary sexual characteristics by modulating pituitary secretion of gonadotropins, LH and FSH. Medroxyprogesterone (MPA): Progesterone derivative; decreases nuclear estrogen receptors and suppression of epithelial DNA synthesis in endometrial tissue.

PHARMACOKINETICS: Absorption: Oral administration of different doses resulted in different parameters. **Distribution**: MPA: Plasma protein binding (90%). **Metabolism**: Estrogen: Liver; Estrone (metabolite), estriol (major urinary metabolite). MPA: Hydroxylation, conjugation. **Elimination**: Estrogen: Urine. MPA: Urine.

NURSING CONSIDERATIONS

Assessment: Assess for abnormal bleeding, breast or estrogen-dependent neoplasia, CAD, asthma, endometriosis, DM, SLE, epilepsy, migraine, porphyria, hypothyroidism, pregnancy status, thromboembolic disorders, hypocalcemia, possible drug interactions, cardiac or renal/hepatic impairment.

Monitoring: Monitor BP regularly; TFTs periodically. Breast exam by physician yearly and self-exam monthly; mammogram as required. Monitor for signs/symptoms of dementia, gallbladder disease, hypercalcemia, CV events (eg, MI, stroke), abnormal vaginal bleeding, thromboembolic disorders, fluid retention, HTN, visual abnormalities, hypersensitivity reactions, hepatic dysfunction, exacerbation of asthma, DM, SLE, epilepsy, migraines, and porphyria.

Patient Counseling: Inform of pregnancy risks. Advise to seek medical attention if symptoms of hepatic dysfunction (jaundice), hypercalcemia, visual abnormalities (partial/complete loss of vision, diplopia), migraines, abnormal vaginal bleeding, hypersensitivity reactions, HTN, thromboembolic disorders, fluid retention, exacerbation of diseases, CV events, or dementia occur.

Administration: Oral route. **Storage**: 20-25°C (68-77°F); excursions permitted to 15-30°C (59-86°F).

PREVACID — RX

lansoprazole (TAP)

OTHER BRAND NAMES: Prevacid IV (TAP) - Prevacid Solutab (TAP)

THERAPEUTIC CLASS: Proton pump inhibitor

INDICATIONS: (PO) Treatment of active duodenal ulcer (DU), active benign gastric ulcer (GU), erosive esophagitis, symptomatic GERD. Maintain healing of erosive esophagitis and duodenal ulcers. Treatment of pathological hypersecretory conditions (eg, Zollinger-Ellison syndrome). Combination therapy with amoxicillin +/- clarithromycin for *H.pylori* eradication in duodenal ulcer disease, to reduce risk of ulcer recurrence. Treatment and risk reduction in NSAID induced gastric ulcer. (Inj) Short-term treatment of erosive esophagitis.

DOSAGE: *Adults:* >17 yrs: (PO) DU: 15mg qd for 4 weeks. Maint: 15mg qd. GU: 30mg qd up to 8 weeks. GERD: 15mg qd up to 8 weeks. Erosive Esophagitis: 30mg qd up to 8 weeks. May repeat for 8 weeks if needed. Maint: 15mg qd. NSAID-Induced GU: 30mg qd for 8 weeks. Reduce Risk of NSAID Induced GU: 15mg qd for 12 weeks. Hypersecretory Conditions: Initial: 60mg qd, then adjust. Max: 90mg bid. Divide dose if >120mg/day. *H.pylori*: Triple Therapy: 30mg + clarithromycin 500mg + amoxicillin 1000mg, all bid (q12h) for 10-14 days. Dual Therapy: 30mg + amoxicillin 1000mg both tid (q8h) for 14 days. Take before eating. Caps: Swallow whole or sprinkle cap contents on 1 tbsp of applesauce, ENSURE® pudding, cottage cheese, yogurt, strained pears, or in 60mL orange juice or tomato juice; swallow immediately. Sus: Do not chew or crush. Mix pkt with 30mL of water; stir well and drink immediately; not for use with NG tube. Solutab: Place on tongue with or without water. Oral Syringe: (SoluTab) Place 15mg tab in oral syringe and draw up 4mL of water, or 30mg tab in oral syringe and draw up 10mL of water. Shake contents and administer after tablet has dispersed within 15 mins. Refill syringe with 2mL (5mL for 30mg tab) of water, shake, and give any remaining contents. NG Tube: (Cap) Mix cap contents with 40mL apple juice and inject into NG tube; flush with additional juice to clear tube. (SoluTab) Place 15mg tab and draw up 4mL of water, or 30mg tab and draw up 10mL of water. Shake contents and after tablet has dispersed, inject through NG tube into stomach within 15 mins. Refill syringe with 5mL of water, shake, and flush NG tube. (Inj) Erosive Esophagitis: 30mg IV qd over 30 mins for 7 days. May switch to PO formulation for total of 6 to 8 weeks of therapy once patient is able to take oral medications. Severe Hepatic Impairment: Adjust dose.

Pediatrics: 12-17 yrs: Short-Term Symptomatic GERD: 15mg qd for up to 8 weeks. Erosive Esophagitis: 30mg qd for up to 8 weeks. 1-11 yrs: Short-Term Symptomatic GERD/Erosive Esophagitis: ≤30kg: 15mg qd for up to 12 weeks. >30kg: 30mg qd for up to 12 weeks. Titrate: May increase up to 30mg bid after 2 weeks if symptomatic. Severe Hepatic Impairment: Adjust dose. Take before eating. Caps: Swallow whole or sprinkle contents on 1 tbsp of applesauce, ENSURE® pudding, cottage cheese, yogurt, strained pears, or in 60mL orange juice or tomato juice; swallow immediately. Sus: Do not chew or crush. Mix pkt with 30mL water; stir well and drink immediately; not for use with NG tube. Solutab: Place on tongue with or without water. Oral Syringe: (SoluTab) Place 15mg tab in oral syringe and draw up 4mL of water, or 30mg tab in oral syringe and draw up 10mL of water. Shake contents and administer after tablet has dispersed within 15 mins. Refill syringe with 2mL (5mL for 30mg tab) of water, shake, and give any remaining contents. NG Tube: (Cap) Mix cap contents with 40mL apple juice and inject into NG tube; flush with additional juice to clear tube. (SoluTab) Place 15mg tab and draw up 4mL of water, or 30mg tab and draw up 10mL of water. Shake contents and after tablet has dispersed, inject through NG tube into stomach within 15 mins. Refill syringe with 5mL of water, shake, and flush NG tube.

HOW SUPPLIED: Cap, Delayed-Release: 15mg, 30mg; Inj: 30mg; Sus, Delayed-Release: 15mg, 30mg (granules/pkt); Tab, Disintegrating (SoluTab): 15mg, 30mg.

WARNINGS/PRECAUTIONS: Symptomatic response does not preclude the presence of gastric malignancy. Adjust dose with hepatic impairment.

ADVERSE REACTIONS: Abdominal pain, constipation, diarrhea, nausea, myositis, interstitial nephritis

INTERACTIONS: May alter absorption of pH-dependent drugs (eg, ketoconazole, ampicillin esters, digoxin, and iron salts). Give at least 30 minutes prior to sucralfate. Theophylline may need dose adjustment. Concomitant use with warfarin may increase INR and prothrombin time.

PREGNANCY: Category B, not for use in nursing.

MECHANISM OF ACTION: Proton pump inhibitor; suppresses gastric acid secretion by specific inhibition of the (H^+, K^+)-ATPase enzyme system at the secretory surface of the gastric parietal cell.

PHARMACOKINETICS: Absorption: (PO, adult) absolute bioavailability (>80%); T_{max}=1.7 hrs. (IV, adult) C_{max}=1705ng/mL; AUC=3192ng•hr/mL. **Distribution:** V_d=15.7L; plasma protein binding (97%). **Metabolism:** Liver (extensive) via CYP3A4 and CYP2C19. **Elimination:** Urine, feces; $T_{1/2}$≤2 hrs. Refer to package insert for pediatric parameters.

NURSING CONSIDERATIONS

Assessment: Assess for gastric malignancy, severe hepatic insufficiency, pregnancy/nursing status, and possible drug interactions. Oral formulation: Assess for hypersensitivity to phenylketonurics.

Monitoring: Monitor for signs/symptoms of GI effects (eg, diarrhea, dyspepsia).

Patient Counseling: Instruct to contact physician if adverse events occur. Oral formulation: Instruct to take before eating; swallow whole, do not crush or chew. If difficulty swallowing, open capsule and sprinkle granules onto tablespoon of applesauce, pudding, cottage cheese, yogurt, or strained pears or into apple/orange/tomato juice; rinse glass with two or more volumes of juice to ensure complete delivery of dose. Swallow completely.

Administration: Oral or IV route. **Storage:** 25°C (77°F); excursions permitted to 15-30°C (59-86°F). Protect injection vial from light.

PREVACID NAPRAPAC — RX

lansoprazole - naproxen (TAP)

NSAIDs may cause an increased risk of serious cardiovascular thrombotic events, MI, and stroke. Risk may increase with duration of use and in patients with cardiovascular disease or risk factors for cardiovascular disease. NSAIDs may cause an increased risk of serious GI events which may be fatal. Patients with history of gastric and/or duodenal ulcers (especially patients with history of bleeding or perforation) and geriatric patients are at greater risk for serious GI events. Contraindicated for the treatment of perioperative pain in the setting of coronary artery bypass graft (CABG) surgery.

THERAPEUTIC CLASS: NSAID/Proton Pump Inhibitor

INDICATIONS: To reduce the risk of NSAID-associated gastric ulcers in patients with a history of documented gastric ulcers who require the use of an NSAID for treatment of rheumatoid arthritis, osteoarthritis, and ankylosing spondylitis.

DOSAGE: *Adults:* Take am dose before eating. Lansoprazole 15mg qam + naproxen 500mg bid in am and pm. Max: 1000mg naproxen/day. Swallow lansoprazole whole.

HOW SUPPLIED: Cap, Delayed-Release: (Naproxen-Lansoprazole): 500mg-15mg [14 tabs naproxen + 7 caps lansoprazole/weekly blister card; 4 cards/pkg]

CONTRAINDICATIONS: Presence or history of NSAID/ASA-related asthma, urticaria, or allergic-type reactions. Perioperative pain in the setting of CABG surgery.

WARNINGS/PRECAUTIONS: Risk of GI ulceration, bleeding, and perforation. Monitor for visual disturbances, fluid retention/edema, Hgb levels (if initial ≤10g), and LFTs with chronic use. Acute interstitial nephritis, hematuria, proteinuria, nephrotic syndrome and severe hepatic reactions reported. Caution with impaired renal (CrCl <20mL/min) or hepatic function, elderly, heart failure, and high doses with chronic alcoholic liver disease. NSAIDs can lead to onset or worsening of pre-existing HTN; monitor BP closely. Naproxen can cause exfoliative dermatitis, Stevens-Johnson syndrome, toxic epidermal necrolysis.

ADVERSE REACTIONS: Nausea, abdominal pain, constipation, heartburn, headache, dizziness, drowsiness, pruritus, skin eruptions, ecchymoses, tinnitus, edema, dyspnea.

INTERACTIONS: Avoid other forms of naproxen, ASA. May potentiate renal disease with ACE inhibitors. Naproxen may displace other albumin-bound drugs. Caution with warfarin. Monitor for toxicity with hydantoin, sulfonamide, or sulfonylureas. Decreased plasma levels with ASA. May antagonize natriuretic effect of furosemide and thiazides. Decreases renal clearance of lithium and methotrexate. May decrease antihypertensive effects of propranolol and other β-blockers. Increased levels and half-life with probenecid. Take lansoprazole 30 min prior to sucralfate. Lansoprazole may alter absorption of pH-dependent drugs (eg, ketoconazole, ampicillin, iron, digoxin).

P

PREGNANCY: Category C, not for use in nursing.

MECHANISM OF ACTION: Naproxen: NSAID; inhibits prostaglandin synthetase. Lansoprazole: PPI; inhibits gastric acid secretion by blocking proton pumps.

PHARMACOKINETICS: Absorption: Naproxen: Rapid, complete; bioavailability (95%); T_{max}=2-4 hrs. Lansoprazole: Rapid; bioavailability (80%); T_{max}=1.7 hrs. **Distribution:** Naproxen: V_d=0.16 L/kg; plasma protein binding (≥99%); found in breast milk. Lansoprazole: Plasma protein binding (97%). **Metabolism:** Naproxen: Hepatic; 6-O-desmethyl naproxen (metobolite). Lansoprazole: Hepatic. **Elimination:** Naproxen: Kidney; urine (95%), feces (≤3%); $T_{1/2}$=12-17 hrs. Lansoprazole: Biliary; $T_{1/2}$≤2 hrs.

NURSING CONSIDERATIONS

Assessment: Assess for history of asthma, CVD (HTN, CHF) or risk factors for disease, fluid retention, edema, pregnancy status, risk factors for GI events (bleeding, ulceration, perforation), possible drug interactions, renal/hepatic dysfunction.

Monitoring: Monitor CBC, LFTs, renal function, and chemistries periodically. Monitor for signs/symptoms of GI events (bleeding, ulceration, perforation), CHF, HTN, salt depletion, renal/liver dysfunction.

Patient Counseling: Advise to seek medical attention if symptoms of hepatotoxicity (nausea, fatigue, pruritis), anaphylactic reaction (difficulty breathing, swelling of face/throat), hypersensitivity reaction (rash), CV events (chest pain, SOB, weakness, slurring of speech), GI ulceration and bleeding (epigastric pain, dyspepsia, melena, hematemesis), weight gain, or edema occurs.

Inform of pregnancy risks. Caution may impair physical/mental abilities if experience drowsiness, dizziness, vertigo, or depression during therapy.

Administration: Oral route. **Storage:** 25°C (77°F); excursions permitted to 15-30°C (59-86°F).

PREVNAR RX
pneumococcal vaccine, diphtheria conjugate (Wyeth)

THERAPEUTIC CLASS: Vaccine

INDICATIONS: Active immunization of children against invasive disease caused by *S.pneumoniae*. Active immunization of children against otitis media caused by serotypes included in the vaccine.

DOSAGE: *Pediatrics:* 6 weeks-2 months: 4 doses of 0.5mL IM. Give 3 doses at 2-month intervals and 4th dose at 12-15 months old. Unvaccinated Children: 7-11 months: 3 doses of 0.5mL IM. Give 1st 2 doses at least 4 weeks apart and 3rd dose after 1-yr birthday; separate from 2nd dose by at least 2 months. 12-23 months: 2 doses of 0.5mL IM at least 2 months apart. ≥24 months-9 yrs: 0.5mL IM single dose.

HOW SUPPLIED: Inj: 16mcg/0.5mL

CONTRAINDICATIONS: Hypersensitivity to any component.

WARNINGS/PRECAUTIONS: Avoid with thrombocytopenia or coagulation disorder. Avoid with acute severe febrile illness. Impaired immune responses may cause reduced response to active immunization. Not a substitute for diphtheria or 23-valent pneumococcal vaccinations. Do not give IV. Have epinephrine (1:1000) available. Caution with latex sensitivity; packaging contains dry natural rubber. Fever and rarely febrile seizures reported.

ADVERSE REACTIONS: Injection-site reactions, irritability, drowsiness, restless sleep, decreased appetite, vomiting, diarrhea, fever.

INTERACTIONS: Suboptimal response with immunosuppressants. Caution with anticoagulants.

PREGNANCY: Category C, not for use in nursing.

MECHANISM OF ACTION: Immunostimulant; elicits formation of antibodies that may protect against invasive pneumococcal disease and otitis media.

NURSING CONSIDERATIONS

Assessment: Assess health/immunity status, history of febrile convulsions, bleeding disorders, previous sensitivity/vaccination history, family history, and possibility of drug interactions.

Monitoring: Monitor hypersensitivity reactions, injection site for redness, tenderness, and induration, fever, irritability, drowsiness, restless sleep, anorexia, vomiting, and diarrhea.

Patient Counseling: Inform patient/guardian of benefits/risks ratio, the importance of completing the immunization series, and to report any adverse reactions to physician.

Administration: IM, at the anterolateral aspect of thigh (infants) or deltoid region (toddlers and young children). **Storage:** 2-8°C (36-46°F). Do not freeze.

PREVPAC RX
amoxicillin - clarithromycin - lansoprazole (TAP)

THERAPEUTIC CLASS: *H.pylori* treatment combination

INDICATIONS: Treatment of *H.pylori* infection associated with active duodenal ulcer and to reduce the risk of duodenal ulcer recurrence.

DOSAGE: *Adults:* 1g amoxicillin, 500mg clarithromycin and 30mg lansoprazole, all bid (am and pm) before meals for 10 or 14 days. Swallow each pill whole. Renal Impairment (with or without hepatic impairment): Decrease clarithromycin dose or prolong intervals. Avoid with CrCl <30mL/min.

HOW SUPPLIED: Cap: (Amoxicillin) 500mg, Tab: (Clarithromycin) 500mg, Cap, Delayed-Release: (Lansoprazole) 30mg

CONTRAINDICATIONS: Concomitant cisapride, pimozide, astemizole, terfenadine, ergotamine or dihydroergotamine. Hypersensitivity to prevacid, macrolide or penicillin antibiotics.

WARNINGS/PRECAUTIONS: Avoid if CrCl <30mL/min. Caution with cephalosporin/PCN allergy; anaphylactic reactions have been reported. Pseudomembranous colitis reported. Possibility of superinfections. Caution in elderly. Clarithromycin may increase colchicine; monitor for toxicity. Do not use clarithromycin during pregnancy. Symptomatic response to lansoprazole does not preclude the presence of gastric malignancy. *Clostridium difficile*-associated diarrhea (CDAD) reported. D/C if confirmed.

ADVERSE REACTIONS: Diarrhea, taste perversion, headache.

INTERACTIONS: Contraindicated with cisapride, pimozide, astemizole, terfenadine, ergotamine or dihydroergotamine. May interfere with absorption of drugs dependent on gastric pH for bioavailability (eg, atazanavir, ketoconazole, ampicillin esters, iron salts, digoxin). Clarithromycin increases plasma levels of carbamazepine, digoxin. Clarithromycin potentiates oral anticoagulants and may decrease triazolam clearance. Erythromycin or clarithromycin can cause acute ergot toxicity with ergotamine or dihydroergotamine. Clarithromycin increases levels of HMG CoA reductase inhibitors (eg, lovastatin, simvastatin). Theophylline may need dose adjustment. Take lansoprazole and other proton pump inhibitors 30 minutes before sucralfate. Caution with drugs metabolized by CYP450 (eg, cyclosporine, tacrolimus, phenytoin); monitor levels. QTc prolongation has occurred with coadministration of clarithromycin and antiarrhythmics (eg, quinidine, disopyramide). Concomitant clarithromycin and colchicine may lead to increased exposure to colchicine.

PREGNANCY: Category C, not for use in nursing.

MECHANISM OF ACTION: Lansoprazole: Substituted benzimidazole; inhibits gastric acid secretion. Amoxicillin: Semi-synthetic antibiotic; has broad spectrum of bactericidal activity against many gram-positive and gram-negative organisms. Clarithromycin: Semi-synthetic macrolide antibiotic.

PHARMACOKINETICS: Absorption: Lansoprazole: Rapidly absorbed; absolute bioavailability (80%); T_{max}=1.7 hrs. Amoxicillin: Rapidly absorbed. Clarithromycin: Rapidly absorbed; absolute bioavailability (50%); T_{max}=2-3 hrs. **Distribution:** Lansoprazole: Plasma protein binding (97%); found in breast milk. Amoxicillin: Plasma protein binding (approximately 20%). Clarithromycin: Found in breast milk. **Metabolism:** Lansoprazole: Liver (extensive). Clarithromycin: 14-OH clarithromycin (active metabolite). **Elimination:** Lansoprazole: Urine, feces; $T_{1/2}$=1.5 hrs. Amoxicillin: Urine (60%). Clarithromycin: Urine (30%); $T_{1/2}$=5-7 hrs; (metabolite); $T_{1/2}$=7-9 hrs.

NURSING CONSIDERATIONS

Assessment: Assess for hypersensitivity to other macrolides, PCNs, or cephalosporins. Assess for proper diagnosis of susceptible bacteria (eg, cultures), pregnancy/nursing status, renal impairment, gastric malignancy, presence of bacterial infection, and possible drug interactions.

Monitoring: Monitor for signs/symptoms of drug interactions (eg, cardiac arrhythmias), hypersensitivity reactions (eg, anaphylaxis), pseudomembranous colitis and *Clostridium difficile,* and development of superinfections.

Patient Counseling: Instruct to take each dose twice per day before eating; swallow pill whole. Advise to notify physician of all medications currently taking. Inform that drug treats bacterial, not viral, infections. Take exactly as directed; skipping doses may decrease effectiveness and increase resistance. Instruct to avoid pregnancy/nursing during therapy and contact physician if diarrhea occurs.

Administration: Oral route. **Storage:** 20-25°C (68-77°F); protect from light and moisture.

PREZISTA

RX

darunavir (Tibotec)

THERAPEUTIC CLASS: Protease inhibitor

INDICATIONS: For use with ritonavir, and other antiretroviral agents, for the treatment of HIV-1 infection in adult and pediatric (>6 yrs) patients.

DOSAGE: *Adults:* Treatment-Naive: 800mg (two 400mg tab) with ritonavir 100mg qd. Treatment-Experienced: 600mg (one 600mg or two 300mg tab) with ritonavir 100mg bid. Take with food.
Pediatrics: 6 to <18 yrs: ≥20-<30kg: 375mg with ritonavir 50mg bid. ≥30-<40kg: 450mg with ritonavir 60mg bid. ≥40kg: 600mg with ritonavir 100mg bid. Take with food.

HOW SUPPLIED: Tab: 75mg, 300mg, 400mg, 600mg

CONTRAINDICATIONS: Concomitant ergot derivatives (eg, dihydroergotamine, ergonovine, ergotamine, and methylergonovine), cisapride, pimozide, sedatives/hypnotics (eg, midazolam, triazolam), St. John's wort, HMG CoA reductase inhibitors (eg, lovastatin, simvastatin), and rifampin.

WARNINGS/PRECAUTIONS: Drug-induced hepatitis (eg, acute hepatitis, cytolytic hepatitis), including new or worsening liver dysfunction may occur; d/c therapy. Increased frequency of liver function abnormalities reported with pre-existing liver dysfunction, including chronic active hepatitis B or C. Severe skin rash, including erythema multiforme and Stevens-Johnson syndrome reported. Caution with sulfonamide allergy. New onset DM, exacerbation of pre-existing DM, and hyperglycemia reported. Redistribution/accumulation of body fat reported. Immune reconstitution syndrome may occur. Increased bleeding (eg, spontaneous skin hematomas and hemarthrosis) in hemophilia type A and B reported. Do not give in patients <3 yrs old.

ADVERSE REACTIONS: Diarrhea, NV, headache, abdominal pain, and rash.

INTERACTIONS: See Contraindications. Avoid with carbamazepine, phenobarbital, phenytoin, rifampin, St. John's wort; significant decreases in plasma concentrations may occur. Potential for serious reactions (eg, myopathy, rhabdomyolysis) with HMG-CoA reductase inhibitors. Concomitant darunavir/ritonavir and efavirenz may decrease darunavir and increase efavirenz levels; use with caution. Concentrations of antiarrhythmics (eg, bepridil, lidocaine, quinidine, amiodarone) may be increased with concomitant use; caution is warranted and therapeutic concentration monitoring recommended. Monitor INR with concomitant warfarin use. Trazadone concentrations may increase; use combination with caution. Therapeutic concentration monitoring recommended for concomitant immunosuppressants (eg, cyclosporine, tacrolimus, sirolimus). May decrease methadone concentrations. Alternative/additional measures of contraception should be used with concurrent use. Refer to Prescribing Information for a complete list of drug interactions.

PREGNANCY: Category C, not for use in nursing.

MECHANISM OF ACTION: Protease inhibitor; inhibits cleavage of HIV encoded Gag-Pol polyproteins in infected cells, preventing the formation of mature virus particles.

PHARMACOKINETICS: Absorption: Darunavir: Absolute bioavailability (37%). Darunavir/Ritonavir: Absolute bioavailability (82%). **Distribution:** Darunavir: Plasma protein binding (95%). **Metabolism:** Darunavir: Hepatic (oxidation) via CYP3A. **Elimination:** Darunavir: Urine (7.7%), feces (41.2%). Darunavir/Ritonavir: Urine (79.5%), feces (41.2%). Darunavir/Ritonavir: $T_{1/2}$=15 hrs.

NURSING CONSIDERATIONS

Assessment: Assess for sulfonamide allergy, liver dysfunction (chronic active hepatitis), endocrine disorders, hemophilia, possible drug interactions, and pregnancy/nursing status.

Monitoring: Monitor for signs/symptoms of severe skin reactions (eg, Stevens-Johnson syndrome), exacerbation of DM and hyperglycemia, LFT abnormalities, hemophilia, fat redistribution, immune reconstitution syndrome and lab abnormalities (biochemistry, hematology), and hepatic impairment.

P

Patient Counseling: Inform that drug does not cure HIV and may continue to develop opportunistic infections and other complications associated with HIV. Sustained decrease in plasma HIV RNA associated with a reduced risk of progression to AIDS and death. Advise to take with food qd, to swallow tab whole, and not to alter dose or d/c without consulting physician. If a dose is missed by 6 hrs, take next dose at regularly scheduled time; do not double next dose. Report use of any other Rx or OTC medication (eg, St. John's wort). Instruct to use alternative contraceptive measures to estrogen-based contraceptive during therapy. Seek medical attention if symptoms of severe skin reactions (eg, erythema multiforme, Stevens-Johnson syndrome), exacerbation of DM and hyperglycemia, liver dysfunction, bleeding (unexplained), fat redistribution, immune reconstitution syndrome occur.

Administration: Oral route. **Storage:** Store at 25°C (77°F); excursions permitted to 15-30°C (59-86°F).

PRIALT — RX

ziconotide acetate (Elan)

Severe psychiatric symptoms and neurological impairment may occur during treatment. Patients with a pre-existing history of psychosis should not be treated with ziconotide. Monitor patients for evidence of cognitive impairment, hallucinations, or changes in mood or consciousness. Therapy can be interrupted or discontinued abruptly without evidence of withdrawal effects in the event of serious neurological or psychiatric signs or symptoms.

THERAPEUTIC CLASS: N-type Calcium Channel Blocker

INDICATIONS: Management of severe chronic pain in patients for whom intrathecal (IT) therapy is warranted, and who are intolerant of or refractory to other treatment, such as systemic analgesics, adjunctive therapies, or IT morphine.

DOSAGE: *Adults*: Initial: No more than 2.4mcg/d IT (0.1mcg/hr). Titrate by 2.4mcg/d no more than 2-3x/week. Max: 19.2mcg/d (0.8mcg/hr) by Day 21.

HOW SUPPLIED: Sol: 25mcg/mL [20mL], 100mcg/mL [1mL, 2mL, 5mL]

CONTRAINDICATIONS: Pre-existing history of psychosis. Contraindications to the use of IT analgesia: presence of infection at the microinfusion injection site, uncontrolled bleeding diathesis, and spinal canal obstruction that impairs circulation of CSF.

P

WARNINGS/PRECAUTIONS: Caution against engaging in hazardous activity requiring complete mental alertness or motor coordination. Dosage adjustments may be necessary when combined with other CNS-depressants due to additive effects. Ziconotide is not an opiate and cannot prevent or relieve the symptoms associated with the withdrawal of opiates. Risk of meningitis due to inadvertent contamination of the microinfusion device. Monitor for signs and symptoms of meningitis. Reports of CNS-related adverse events: psychiatric symptoms, cognitive impairment, and decreased alertness/unresponsiveness. D/C if patient becomes unresponsive or stuporous. Monitor for elevations in serum creatine kinase levels.

ADVERSE REACTIONS: Dizziness, nausea, confusion, headache, somnolence, nystagmus, asthenia, pain, vertigo, blurred vision, constipation, dry mouth, anorexia.

INTERACTIONS: Coadministration with CNS depressants increases the risk of CNS adverse effects.

PREGNANCY: Category C, caution in nursing.

MECHANISM OF ACTION: Not established; suggested that it binds to N-type calcium channels, which leads to a blockade of excitatory neurotransmitter release from the primary afferent nerve terminals and antinociception.

PHARMACOKINETICS: Absorption: C_{max}=16.4-132ng/mL, T_{max}=1 hr, AUC=83.6-608ng•h/mL. **Distribution**: V_d=155mL; plasma protein binding (50%). **Metabolism:** Kidneys, liver, lungs, muscle via endopeptidases, exopeptidases and proteases. **Elimination**: $T_{1/2}$=4.6 hrs.

NURSING CONSIDERATIONS

Assessment: Assess for pre-exsisting history of psychosis, presence of infection at injection site, uncontrolled bleeding diathesis, spinal cord obstruction, immunocompromised patients, and possible drug interactions.

Monitoring: Monitor serum CK periodically; every other week for first month and monthly thereafter. Monitor signs/symptoms of serious infection or meningitis (eg, fever, headache, stiff neck, altered mental status), psychiatric symptoms, cognitive impairment, decreased alertness/unresponsiveness, reduced level of consciousness, hallucinations, changes in mood, paranoid reactions, elevated CK, EMG finding, myopathy, rhabdomyolysis, and acute renal failure.

Patient Counseling: Caution against engaging in hazardous activities (eg, operating machinery/driving). Do not take other CNS depressants. Inform about signs/symptoms of serious infection or meningitis; d/c and consult physician immediately if any occur. Consult physician immediately if experience change in mental status or mood, symptoms of depression or suicidal ideation, seizures, new or worsening muscle pain, soreness, and weakness with/without darkened urine occur.

Administration: IT route. **Storage**: 2-8°C (36-46°F). Refrigerate during transit. Do not freeze. Store at 2-8°C for 24 hrs if diluted.

PRILOSEC RX

omeprazole (AstraZeneca)

THERAPEUTIC CLASS: Proton pump inhibitor

INDICATIONS: Short-term treatment of active duodenal ulcer and active benign gastric ulcer in adults. Treatment of heartburn and other symptoms associated with GERD in adults and pediatrics. Short-term treatment of erosive esophagitis and to maintain healing of erosive esophagitis in adults and pediatrics. Long-term treatment of pathological hypersecretory conditions (eg, Zollinger-Ellison syndrome, multiple endocrine adenomas, systemic mastocytosis) in adults. Combination therapy with clarithromycin +/- amoxicillin for *H.pylori* eradication in duodenal ulcer disease, and to reduce risk of ulcer recurrence, in adults.

DOSAGE: *Adults:* Duodenal Ulcer: 20mg qd for 4-8 weeks. Gastric Ulcer: 40mg qd for 4-8 weeks. GERD: 20mg qd up to 4 weeks without esophageal lesions. Treatment Erosive Esophagitis with GERD: 20mg qd for 4-8 weeks. Maint: 20mg qd. Hypersecretory Conditions: Initial: 60mg qd, then adjust if needed. Divide dose if >80mg/day. Doses up to 120mg tid have been given. *H.pylori* Triple Therapy: 20mg + clarithromycin 500mg + amoxicillin 1g, all bid for 10 days. Give additional 18 days of omeprazole 20mg every morning if ulcer present initially. Dual Therapy: 40mg qd + clarithromycin 500mg tid for 14 days. Give additional 14 days of omeprazole 20mg every morning if ulcer present initially. Do not crush or chew. Take before eating. Can add contents of caps to applesauce if difficulty swallowing; swallow immediately without chewing.
Pediatrics: 1-16 yrs: GERD/Erosive Esophagitis: ≥20kg: 20mg qd. 10 to <20kg: 10mg qd. 5 to <10kg: 5mg qd. Do not crush or chew. Take before eating. Can add contents of caps to applesauce if difficulty swallowing; swallow immediately without chewing.

HOW SUPPLIED: Cap, Delayed-Release: 10mg, 20mg, 40mg; Sus, Delayed-Release: 2.5mg, 10mg granules/pkt

WARNINGS/PRECAUTIONS: Atrophic gastritis reported with long-term use. Symptomatic response does not preclude the presence of gastric malignancy.

ADVERSE REACTIONS: Headache, diarrhea, abdominal pain, flatulence, NV.

INTERACTIONS: May potentiate diazepam, warfarin, phenytoin, and drugs metabolized by oxidation. May alter absorption of pH-dependent drugs (eg, ketoconazole, ampicillin esters, iron salts). Monitor drugs metabolized by CYP450 (eg, cyclosporine, disulfiram, benzodiazepines). Increased levels with clarithromycin. Increases levels of clarithromycin. Voriconazole may increase levels. May reduce plasma levels of atazanavir. May increase levels of tacrolimus.

PREGNANCY: Category C, not for use in nursing.

MECHANISM OF ACTION: Proton pump inhibitor; suppresses gastric acid secretion by specific inhibition of the (H^+/K^+)-ATPase enzyme system at the secretory surface of the gastric parietal cell.

PHARMACOKINETICS: Absorption: Rapid; absolute bioavailability (30-40%); T_{max}=0.5-3.5 hrs. (Adult, single dose) C_{max}=668ng/mL; AUC=1220ng•hr/mL. (Children<20kg, 2-5yrs, 10mg single dose) C_{max}=288ng/mL; AUC=511ng•hr/mL. (Children >20kg, 6-16yrs, 20mg single dose) C_{max}=495ng/mL; AUC=1140ng•hr/mL. **Distribution:** Plasma protein binding (95%); found in breast milk. **Metabolism:** Hydroxyomeprazole and corresponding carboxylic acid (metabolites). **Elimination:** Urine (77%), feces; $T_{1/2}$=0.5-1 hr.

NURSING CONSIDERATIONS

Assessment: Assess for gastric malignancy, hepatic impairment, pregnancy/nursing status, and for possible drug interactions. Assess dosing in Asian patients.

Monitoring: Monitor for signs/symptoms of atrophic gastritis and other GI effects (eg, abdominal pain, diarrhea, nausea). Monitor INR and PT when given with warfarin.

Patient Counseling: Inform to take before eating; swallow whole, do not open, chew, or crush. May empty contents of capsule into one tablespoon of applesauce if cannot swallow whole. Mix with applesauce and swallow immediately with cool glass of water; do not chew or crush pellets.

Administration: Oral route. **Storage:** 15-30°C (59-86°F); protect from light and moisture.

PRIMAXIN I.M. RX

imipenem - cilastatin (Merck)

THERAPEUTIC CLASS: Thienamycin/dehydropeptidase I inhibitor

INDICATIONS: Treatment of lower respiratory tract (LRTI), skin and skin structure (SSSI), intra-abdominal, and gynecologic infections caused by susceptible strains of microorganisms. Not for severe or life-threatening infections.

P

DOSAGE: *Adults:* Dose according to imipenem. Mild to Moderate LRTI/SSSI/Gynecologic Infection: 500mg or 750mg IM q12h depending on severity. Intra-Abdominal Infection: 750mg IM q12h. Continue for at least 2 days after symptoms resolve. Elderly: Start at low end of dosing range. Continue for at least 2 days after symptoms resolve; do not treat >14 days. Max: 1500mg/day. Avoid if CrCl <20mL/min.

Pediatrics: ≥12 yrs: Dose according to imipenem. Mild to Moderate LRTI/SSSI/Gynecologic Infections: 500mg or 750mg IM q12h depending on severity. Intra-Abdominal Infection: 750mg IM q12h. Continue for at least 2 days after symptoms resolve; do not treat >14 days. Max: 1500mg/day. Avoid if CrCl <20mL/min.

HOW SUPPLIED: Inj: (Imipenem-Cilastatin) 500mg-500mg, 750mg-750mg

CONTRAINDICATIONS: Severe shock, heart block, hypersensitivity to local anesthetics of amide type (due to lidocaine diluent).

WARNINGS/PRECAUTIONS: Serious, sometimes fatal, hypersensitivity reactions reported with β-lactam therapy. *Clostridium difficile*-associated diarrhea reported. Prolonged use may result in overgrowth of nonsusceptible organisms. Avoid injection into blood vessel. Caution in elderly. CNS adverse events (eg, myoclonic activity, confusion, seizures) reported most commonly with CNS disorders and renal dysfunction; d/c if any occur. Positive Coombs test reported.

ADVERSE REACTIONS: Injection site pain, N/V, diarrhea, fever, rash, hypotension, seizures, dizziness, pruritus, urticaria, somnolence.

INTERACTIONS: Avoid probenecid. Do not mix or physically add with other antibiotics. May give concomitantly with other antibiotics. May decrease levels of valproic acid.

PREGNANCY: Category C, caution in nursing.

MECHANISM OF ACTION: Imipenem: Thienamycin; inhibits cell-wall synthesis. Cilastatin: Dehydropeptidase I inhibitor; prevents renal metabolism of parent drug.

PHARMACOKINETICS: Absorption: Imipenem: C_{max}=10mcg/mL (500mg), 12mcg/mL (750mg); T_{max}=2 hrs. Cilastatin: C_{max}=24mcg/mL (500mg), 33mcg/mL (750mg); T_{max}=1 hr. **Distribution:** Imipenem: Plasma protein binding (20%). Cilastatin: Plasma protein binding (40%). **Metabolism:** Imipenem: Kidneys. **Elimination:** Imipinem: Urine. Cilastatin: Urine.

NURSING CONSIDERATIONS

Assessment: Assess for severe shock, heart block, hypersensitivity to local anesthetics (amide), CNS disorders (brain lesions, history of seizures), and possible drug interactions.

Monitoring: Monitor for seizures, myoclonic activity, hypersensitivity reactions, *C. difficile*-associated diarrhea, and superinfections.

Patient Counseling: Inform therapy only treats bacterial, not viral, infections. Take as directed; skipping doses or not completing full course may decrease effectiveness and increase resistance. May experience diarrhea; notify physician if watery/bloody stools, hypersensitivity reactions, superinfections, seizures, or myoclonic activity occur.

Administration: IM route; use within 1 hr of reconstitution. **Storage:** Below 25°C (77°F).

PRIMAXIN I.V. RX

imipenem - cilastatin (Merck)

THERAPEUTIC CLASS: Thienamycin/dehydropeptidase I inhibitor

INDICATIONS: Treatment of serious lower respiratory tract, urinary tract (UTI), intra-abdominal, gynecologic, skin and skin structure, bone and joint, septicemia, endocarditis, and polymicrobic infections caused by susceptible strains of microorganisms.

P

DOSAGE: *Adults:* ≥70kg and CrCl >70mL/min: Dose based on imipenem component. Uncomplicated UTI: 250mg q6h. Complicated UTI: 500mg q6h. Mild Infection: 250-500mg q6h. Moderate Infection: 500mg q6-8h or 1g q8h. Severe, Life-Threatening Infection: 500mg-1g q6h or 1g q8h. Max: 50mg/kg/day or 4g/day, whichever lower. Renal Impairment and/or <70kg: Refer to PI. CrCl 6-20mL/min: 125-250mg q12h. CrCl ≤5mL/min: Administer hemodialysis within 48 hrs of dose.

Pediatrics: ≥3 months: Dose based on imipenem component. Non-CNS Infections: 15-25mg/kg q6h. Max: 2g/day if susceptible or 4g/day if moderately susceptible. May use up to 90mg/kg/day in older cystic fibrosis children. 4 weeks-3 months and ≥1500g: 25mg/kg q6h. 1-4 weeks and ≥1500g: 25mg/kg q8h. <1 week and ≥1500g: 25mg/kg q12h. Not recommended with CNS infection, and <30kg with impaired renal function.

HOW SUPPLIED: Inj: (Imipenem-Cilastatin) 250mg-250mg, 500mg-500mg

WARNINGS/PRECAUTIONS: Serious, sometimes fatal, hypersensitivity reactions reported with β-lactam therapy. *Clostridium difficile*-associated diarrhea reported. Prolonged use may result in overgrowth of nonsusceptible organisms. CNS adverse events (eg, myoclonic activity, confusion, seizures) reported most commonly with CNS disorders and renal dysfunction.

ADVERSE REACTIONS: Phlebitis/thrombophlebitis, N/V, diarrhea, rash, fever, hypotension, seizures, dizziness, pruritus, urticaria, somnolence, hepatitis (including fulminant hepatitis), hepatic failure.

INTERACTIONS: Seizures reported with ganciclovir; avoid concomitant use. Avoid probenecid. Do not mix or physically add to other antibiotics. May give concomitantly with other antibiotics. May decrease levels of valproic acid.

PREGNANCY: Category C, caution in nursing.

MECHANISM OF ACTION: Imipenem: Thienamycin; inhibits cell-wall synthesis. Cilastatin: Dehydropeptidase I inhibitor; prevents renal metabolism of parent drug.

PHARMACOKINETICS: Absorption: Variable doses resulted in different parameters. **Distribution:** Imipenem: Plasma protein binding (20%). Cilastatin: Plasma protein binding (40%). **Metabolism:** Imipenem: Kidneys. **Elimination:** Imipenem: Urine (70%). Cilastatin: Urine (70%).

NURSING CONSIDERATIONS

Assessment: Assess for CNS disorders (brain lesions, history of seizures), renal impairment, and possible drug interactions.

Monitoring: Monitor for seizures, myoclonic activity, confusional states, hypersensitivity reactions, *C. difficile*-associated diarrhea, and superinfections.

Patient Counseling: Inform therapy only treats bacterial, not viral, infections. Take as directed; skipping doses or not completing full course may decrease effectiveness and increase resistance. May experience diarrhea; notify physician if watery/bloody stools, hypersensitivity reactions, superinfections, seizures, myoclonic activity, or confusional states occur.

Administration: IV. **Storage:** Below 25°C (77°F). Reconstituted: refrigerate (5°C); stable for 24 hrs: room temperature; stable for 4 hrs.

PRIMSOL — RX

trimethoprim HCl (FSC Laboratories)

THERAPEUTIC CLASS: Tetrahydrofolic acid inhibitor

INDICATIONS: Treatment of acute otitis media in pediatrics and urinary tract infection (UTI) in adults due to susceptible microorganisms.

DOSAGE: *Adults:* UTI: Usual: 100mg q12h or 200mg q24h for 10 days. CrCl: 15-30mL/min: Give 50% of usual dose.
Pediatrics: Otitis Media: ≥6 months: 5mg/kg q12h for 10 days. CrCl: 15-30mL/min: Give 50% of usual dose.

HOW SUPPLIED: Sol: 50mg/5mL

CONTRAINDICATIONS: Megaloblastic anemia due to folate deficiency.

WARNINGS/PRECAUTIONS: May interfere with hematopoiesis. Serious blood disorders; monitor for sore throat, fever, pallor, and purpura. Caution with folate deficiency and renal/hepatic impairment, diarrhea, rash.

ADVERSE REACTIONS: Epigastric distress, NV, anemia, methemoglobinemia, hyperkalemia, hyponatremia, fever, elevation of serum transaminases and bilirubin, increases BUN and serum creatinine.

INTERACTIONS: May inhibit phenytoin metabolism.

PREGNANCY: Category C, caution in nursing.

MECHANISM OF ACTION: Dihydrofolate reductase inhibitor; blocks production of tetrahydrofolic acid from dihydrofolic acid by binding to and reversibly inhibiting dihydrofolate reductase.

PHARMACOKINETICS: Absorption: Rapid; C_{max}=1mcg/mL; T_{max}=1-4 hrs. **Distribution:** Crosses placenta; found in breast milk. **Metabolism:** Liver; 1- and 3-oxide, 3'- and 4'-hydroxy derivative (principal metabolites). **Elimination:** Urine; $T_{1/2}$=9 hrs.

NURSING CONSIDERATIONS

Assessment: Assess for megaloblastic anemia (folate deficiency), possible drug interactions, renal/hepatic impairment.

Monitoring: Monitor CBC and renal function periodically. Monitor for signs/symptoms of serious blood disorder and hypersensitivity reactions.

Patient Counseling: Advise to seek medical attention if symptoms of serious blood disorder (sore throat, fever, pallor, purpura) or hypersensitivity reactions occur.

Administration: Oral route. **Storage:** 15-25°C (59-77°F).

PRINIVIL
lisinopril (Merck)

RX

ACE inhibitors can cause death/injury to developing fetus during 2nd and 3rd trimesters. Stop therapy if pregnancy detected.

THERAPEUTIC CLASS: ACE inhibitor

INDICATIONS: Treatment of hypertension. Adjunct therapy in heart failure if inadequately controlled by diuretics and digitalis. Adjunct therapy in stable patients within 24 hrs of AMI to improve survival.

DOSAGE: *Adults:* HTN: If possible, d/c diuretic 2-3 days prior to therapy. Initial: 10mg qd; 5mg qd with diuretic. Usual: 20-40mg qd. Resume diuretic if BP not controlled. Max: 80mg/day. CrCl 10-30mL/min: Initial: 5mg/day. Max: 40mg/day. CrCl <10mL/min: Initial: 2.5mg/day. Max: 40mg/day. Heart Failure: Initial: 5mg qd. Usual: 5-20mg qd. Hyponatremia or CrCl ≤30mL/min: Initial: 2.5mg qd. AMI: Initial: 5mg within 24 hrs, then 5mg after 24 hrs, then 10mg after 48 hrs, then daily. Use 2.5mg during first 3 days with low systolic BP. Maint: 10mg qd for 6 weeks, 2.5-5mg with hypotension. D/C with prolonged hypotension. Elderly: Caution with dose adjustment.
Pediatrics: ≥6 yrs: HTN: Initial: 0.07mg/kg qd (up to 5mg total). Adjust dose based on BP response. Max: 0.61mg/kg qd (40mg/day).

HOW SUPPLIED: Tab: 5mg*, 10mg*, 20mg* *scored

CONTRAINDICATIONS: History of ACE inhibitor-associated angioedema and hereditary or idiopathic angioedema.

WARNINGS/PRECAUTIONS: Intestinal/head/neck angioedema reported. D/C if angioedema, jaundice, or if marked LFT elevation occurs. Risk of hyperkalemia with DM, renal dysfunction. Persistent nonproductive cough reported. Monitor WBCs in renal and collagen vascular disease. Anaphylactoid reactions reported. Fetal/neonatal morbidity and death reported. Monitor for hypotension in high-risk patients (eg, heart failure with systolic BP <100mmHg, surgery/anesthesia, hyponatremia, high-dose diuretic therapy, severe volume and/or salt depletion). Caution with renal artery stenosis, CHF, renal dysfunction, or if obstruction to left ventricle outflow tract. Less effective on BP in blacks and more reports of angioedema than nonblacks. Caution in hypoglycemia and leukopenia/neutropenia. Patients should report any indication of infection, which may be sign of leukopenia/neutropenia.

ADVERSE REACTIONS: Hypotension, diarrhea, headache, dizziness, cough, chest pain.

INTERACTIONS: May increase lithium levels. Hypotension risk with diuretics. May further decrease renal dysfunction with NSAIDs. Hyperkalemia with K^+-sparing diuretics, K^+-containing salt substitutes, or K^+ supplements. Nitritoid reactions have been reported rarely in patients on therapy with injectable gold and concomitant ACE inhibitor therapy. NSAIDs may diminish antihypertensive effects.

PREGNANCY: Category C (1st trimester) and D (2nd and 3rd trimesters), not for use in nursing.

MECHANISM OF ACTION: ACE inhibitor; inhibition results in decreased plasma angiotensin II, which leads to decreased vasopressor activity and aldosterone secretion.

PHARMACOKINETICS: Absorption: 25%; T_{max}=7 hrs. **Elimination:** Urine (unchanged); $T_{1/2}$=12 hrs.

P

NURSING CONSIDERATIONS

Assessment: Assess for aortic stenosis, hypertrophic cardiomyopathy, renal function, MI, CHF, LFTs, renal artery stenosis, HTN, pregnancy status, history of angioedema, DM, and possible drug interactions.

Monitoring: Monitor for head/neck and intestinal angioedema, anaphylactoid reactions, MI, CBC with platelet count and differential, serum K^+, hypoglycemia, LFTs, renal function.

Patient Counseling: Counsel about fetal risks during pregnancy, signs/symptoms of angioedema (eg, laryngeal edema, tongue edema, abdominal pain), adverse effects (eg, anaphylaxis, cough, hypotension, hyperkalemia). Infants with histories of in utero exposure should be closely observed for hypotension, oliguria, hyperkalemia. Inform that periodic monitoring of electrolytes and blood counts is required.

Administration: Oral route. **Storage:** 15-30°C (59-86°F); protect from moisture. Dispense in a tight container.

PRINZIDE RX

lisinopril - hydrochlorothiazide (Merck)

> **ACE inhibitors can cause death/injury to developing fetus during 2nd and 3rd trimesters. Stop therapy if pregnancy detected.**

THERAPEUTIC CLASS: ACE inhibitor/thiazide diuretic

INDICATIONS: Treatment of hypertension. Not for initial therapy.

DOSAGE: *Adults:* Initial (if not controlled with lisinopril/HCTZ monotherapy): 10mg-12.5mg tab or 20mg-12.5mg tab daily. Titrate: May increase after 2-3 weeks. Initial (if controlled on 25mg HCTZ/day with hypokalemia): 10mg-12.5mg tab. Replacement Therapy: Substitute combination for titrated components.

HOW SUPPLIED: Tab: (Lisinopril-HCTZ) 10mg-12.5mg, 20mg-12.5mg, 20mg-25mg

CONTRAINDICATIONS: History of ACE inhibitor associated angioedema and hereditary or idiopathic angioedema. Anuria, sulfonamide hypersensitivity.

WARNINGS/PRECAUTIONS: D/C if angioedema, jaundice, or if marked LFT elevation occurs. Risk of hyperkalemia with DM, renal dysfunction. Persistent nonproductive cough reported. Agranulocytosis and bone marrow depression in renal impairment, especially with collagen vascular disease; monitor WBCs in renal disease and collagen vascular disease. Anaphylactoid reactions reported. Fetal/neonatal morbidity and death reported. Monitor for hypotension in high-risk patients (eg, surgery/anesthesia, volume/salt depletion). Caution with CHF, renal or hepatic dysfunction, obstruction to left ventricle outflow tract, renal artery stenosis, elderly. More reports of angioedema in blacks than nonblacks. May exacerbate or activate SLE. Monitor electrolytes. Avoid if CrCl ≤30mL/min/1.73m². May increase cholesterol, TG. Hypercalcemia, hyperglycemia, hypomagnesemia, hyperuricemia may occur.

ADVERSE REACTIONS: Dizziness, cough, fatigue, orthostatic effects, diarrhea, nausea, muscle cramps, angioedema.

INTERACTIONS: Increase risk of hyperkalemia with K^+-sparing diuretics, K^+ supplements, or K^+-containing salt substitutes. Potentiates orthostatic hypotension with alcohol, barbiturates, and narcotics. Adjust antidiabetic drugs. Reduced absorption with cholestyramine, colestipol. Corticosteroids, ACTH deplete electrolytes. May decrease response to pressor amines. Potentiates other antihypertensives. May increase responsiveness to skeletal muscle relaxants. Risk of lithium toxicity. NSAIDs reduce effects and worsen renal dysfunction. Nitritoid reactions have been reported rarely in patients on therapy with injectable gold and concomitant ACE inhibitor therapy. Patients on diuretics may experience an excessive reduction of blood pressure.

PREGNANCY: Category C (1st trimester) and D (2nd and 3rd trimesters), not for use in nursing.

MECHANISM OF ACTION: Lisinopril: ACE inhibitor. Inhibition results in decreased plasma angiotensin II, which leads to decreased vasopressor activity and decreased aldosterone secretion. HCTZ: Thiazide diuretic; affects renal tubular mechanism of electrolyte reabsorption, directly increasing excretion of sodium salt and chloride.

PHARMACOKINETICS: Absorption: Lisinopril: T_{max}=7 hrs. **Distribution:** Lisinopril: Crosses blood-brain barrier. HCTZ: Crosses placental barrier. **Elimination:** Lisinopril: Urine (unchanged); $T_{1/2}$=12 hrs. HCTZ: Renal (61% unchanged); $T_{1/2}$=5.6-14.8 hrs.

NURSING CONSIDERATIONS

Assessment: Assess for aortic stenosis, hypertrophic cardiomyopathy, renal function, MI, CHF, LFTs, renal artery stenosis, HTN, pregnancy status, history of angioedema, serum electrolytes, DM, and possible drug interactions.

Monitoring: Monitor for angioedema (head/neck, intestinal), anaphylactoid reactions, MI, CBC with platelet count and differential, serum electrolytes, hypoglycemia, LFTs, renal function, hyperuricemia, hypersensitivity reactions.

Patient Counseling: Inform about fetal risks if taken during pregnancy. Caution that inadequate fluid intake, excessive perspiration, diarrhea, or vomiting may lead to excessive fall in BP, with same consequences of lightheadedness and possible syncope. Advise not to use K^+ supplements or salt substitutes containing K^+ without consulting physician. Counsel about signs/symptoms of neutropenia (eg, infections), angioedema, electrolyte imbalance (eg, thirst, weakness, lethargy), and other adverse effects and to seek prompt medical attention. Inform about importance for periodic monitoring of electrolytes and blood counts.

Administration: Oral route. **Storage:** 15-30°C (59-86°F). Protect from excessive light and humidity. Dispense in a well-closed container, if product package is subdivided.

PRISTIQ RX

desvenlafaxine (Wyeth)

> **Antidepressants increased the risk of suicidal thinking and behavior (suicidality) in short-term studies in children, adolescents, and young adults with major depressive disorder (MDD) and other psychiatric disorders. Desvenlafaxine is not approved for use in pediatric patients.**

P

THERAPEUTIC CLASS: Serotonin and norepinephrine reuptake inhibitor

INDICATIONS: Treatment of major depressive disorder (MDD).

DOSAGE: *Adults:* ≥18 yrs: 50mg qd. Renal Impairment (CrCl<30mL/min) or ESRD: 50mg every other day. Supplemental doses should not be given to patients after dialysis. Hepatic Impairment: Max: 100mg/day. Upon discontinuation: Gradually reduce dose (giving 50mg less frequently) rather than abrupt cessation. Do not divide, crush, chew or place in water.

HOW SUPPLIED: Tab, Extended-Release: 50mg, 100mg

CONTRAINDICATIONS: Concomitant MAOI or within 14 days of stopping.

WARNINGS/PRECAUTIONS: Worsening of depression and/or emergence of suicidal behavior may occur. Serotonin syndrome reported; caution with concomitant serotonergic drugs. May cause sustained increases in BP; monitor BP regularly. May increase risk of bleeding events. Monitor with increased IOP or if at risk of acute narrow-angle glaucoma. Activation of mania/hypomania reported. Caution with cardiovascular or cerebrovascular disease, recent MI, renal impairment, and seizure disorder. Cholesterol and triglyceride elevation may occur; consider monitoring. Discontinuation symptoms may occur; taper dose and monitor symptoms. Hyponatremia, interstitial lung disease and eosinophilic pneumonia may occur. Development of a potentially life-threatening serotonin syndrome or Neuroleptic Malignant Syndrome (NMS)-like reactions reported with SNRIs and SSRIs.

ADVERSE REACTIONS: Headache, N/V, dry mouth, diarrhea, dizziness, insomnia, somnolence, hyperhidrosis, fatigue, constipation, palpitations, anxiety, decreased appetite, specific male sexual disorders.

INTERACTIONS: See Contraindications. Avoid within 14 days of MAOI therapy. Upon discontinuation, wait at least 7 days before starting MAOI therapy. Caution with potent inhibitors of CYP3A4 and CYP2D6, CNS-active drugs (eg, triptans, SSRIs, lithium), and with serotonergic drugs (eg, tramadol, tryptophans, SNRIs). Aspirin, NSAIDs, warfarin, and other anticoagulants may increase the risk of bleeding. Avoid alcohol and products containing venlafaxine or desvenlafaxine.

PREGNANCY: Category C, not for use in nursing.

MECHANISM OF ACTION: Potent and selective serotonin and norepinephrine reuptake inhibitor; potentiates neurotransmitter activity of CNS activity by inhibiting neuronal serotonin and norephinephrine reuptake.

PHARMACOKINETICS: Absorption: Absolute oral bioavailability (80%); T_{max}=7.5 hrs. **Distribution:** Plasma protein binding (30%); V_d=3.4L/kg. **Metabolism:** Conjugation and via CYP3A4 mediated oxidation (minor). **Elimination:** Urine (45% unchanged).

NURSING CONSIDERATIONS

Assessment: Assess for risk for bipolar disorder, history of mania, possible drug interactions, hyperthyroidism, heart failure, recent MI, history of glaucoma, increased IOP, risk factors for acute-narrow angle glaucoma, preexisting HTN, history of seizures, disease/condition that alters metabolism or hemodynamic response, cholesterol levels, hepatic/renal impairment.

Monitoring: Monitor HR, BP, LFTs, renal function, serum cholesterol, serum TG and ECG changes. Monitor for signs and symptoms of clinical worsening (suicidality, unusual changes in behavior), serotonin syndrome, mydriasis, severe HTN, lung disease (progressive dyspnea, cough, chest discomfort), abnormal bleeding, allergic reactions (rash, hives), hyponatremia (headache, weakness, unsteadiness), seizures, cognitive and motor impairment. If d/c therapy (particularly if abrupt), monitor for symptoms of dysphoric mood, irritability, agitation, dizziness, sensory disturbances, anxiety, confusion, headache, lethargy, emotional lability, insomnia, and hypomania.

Patient Counseling: Take with or without food at same time each day; swallow whole. Advise to avoid alcohol. Seek medical attention for symptoms of serotonin syndrome (mental status changes, tachycardia, hyperthermia, N/V, diarrhea, uncoordination), abnormal bleeding (particularly if using NSAIDs, aspirin, warfarin, or other drugs affecting coagulation), hyponatremia (headache, weakness, unsteadiness), mydriasis, severe HTN, lung disease (progressive dyspnea, cough, chest discomfort), activation of mania/hypomania, allergic reaction (rash, hives), seizures, clinical worsening (suicidal ideation, unusual changes in behavior) and discontinuation symptoms (irritability, agitation, dizziness, anxiety, headache, insomnia). Caution may impair physical/mental abilities. May notice an inert matrix tablet passing in the stool or via colostomy.

Administration: Oral route. **Storage:** 20-25°C (68-77°F); excursions permitted to 15-30° (59-86°F). Store in dry place and well-closed container.

ProAir HFA — RX

albuterol sulfate (Teva)

THERAPEUTIC CLASS: $Beta_2$-agonist

INDICATIONS: Treatment or prevention of bronchospasm in patients ≥4 yrs with reversible obstructive airway disease. Prevention of exercise-induced bronchospasm (EIB) in patients ≥4 yrs.

DOSAGE: *Adults*: Treatment/Prevention of Bronchospasm: 2 inh q4-6h or 1 inh q4h. EIB: 2 inh 15-30 min before activity.
Pediatrics: ≥4 yrs: Treatment/Prevention of Bronchospasm: 2 inh q4-6h or 1 inh q4h. EIB: 2 inh 15-30 min before activity.

HOW SUPPLIED: MDI: 90mcg/inh [8.5g]

WARNINGS/PRECAUTIONS: May produce paradoxical bronchospasm; d/c therapy immediately. Monitor for worsening asthma. May produce clinically significant cardiovascular effects; caution with cardiovascular disorders, especially coronary insufficiency, cardiac arrhythmias, and HTN. Fatalities reported with excessive use. Immediate hypersensitivity reactions may occur. May need concomitant corticosteroids. Caution with convulsive disorders, hyperthyroidism, DM, and in patients unusually responsive to sympathomimetic amines. May cause significant hypokalemia and changes in blood glucose.

ADVERSE REACTIONS: Pharyngitis, headache, rhinitis, dizziness, pain, and tachycardia.

INTERACTIONS: Avoid use with other short-acting sympathomimetic aerosol bronchodilators. Caution with additional adrenergic drugs. Avoid β-blockers; if not possible, use cardioselective β-blockers with caution. Extreme caution with, or within 2 weeks of discontinuation of, MAOIs and TCAs. Monitor digoxin levels. May worsen ECG changes and/or hypokalemia with non-K^+-sparing diuretics; consider monitoring potassium levels.

PREGNANCY: Category C, not for use in nursing.

MECHANISM OF ACTION: β_2-adrenergic agonist; activates β_2-adrenergic receptors on airway smooth muscle. Activation of receptors leads to activation of adenylcyclase and increase in intracellular cyclic AMP (cAMP). Increased cAMP leads to activation of protein kinase A, which then leads to relaxation of smooth muscle of all airways, from the trachea to terminal bronchioles. Increased cAMP concentrations are also associated with inhibition of the release of mediators from mast cells in the airway.

PHARMACOKINETICS: Absorption: C_{max}=4100pg/mL; AUC=28,426pg•hr/mL. (Pediatrics) C_{max}=1100pg/mL; AUC=5120pg•hr/mL. **Metabolism:** GI tract by SULTIA3. **Elimination:** Renal excretion (80-100%), urine (unchanged), feces (<20%); $T_{1/2}$=6 hrs.(Pediatrics) $T_{1/2}$=166 min.

NURSING CONSIDERATIONS

Assessment: Assess for convulsive disorders, hyperthyroidism, DM, CVD, possible drug interactions, and pregnancy/nursing status. Assess use in patients unusually responsive to sympathomimetic amines.

Monitoring: Monitor HR, BP, ECG changes, blood glucose, paradoxical bronchospasm, hypokalemia, hypersensitivity reactions, and deterioration of asthma.

Patient Counseling: Instruct on how to properly prime, clean, and use inhaler. Inform to take as directed and to report lack of response or adverse side effects.

Administration: Oral inhalation route. Shake well before use. Avoid spraying in eyes. 1) Prime inhaler before using for 1st time or if inhaler has not been used for 2 weeks by releasing 3 test sprays into air, away from face. 2) Clean mouthpiece at least once a week. Use only with actuator supplied with product. 3) Discard inhaler after 200 sprays. **Storage:** 15-25°C (59-77°F). Protect from freezing and prolonged exposure to direct sunlight.

ProAmatine — RX

midodrine HCl (Shire)

Can cause marked elevation of supine BP. Clinical benefits of improving ability to carry out activities of daily living have not been verified.

THERAPEUTIC CLASS: $Alpha_1$-agonist

INDICATIONS: Treatment of symptomatic orthostatic hypotension.

DOSAGE: *Adults:* Initial: 10mg tid; at 3-4 hr intervals, while awake. Max: 30mg/day. To avoid supine HTN during sleep, do not give <4 hrs before bedtime or after evening meal. Renal Dysfunction: Initial: 2.5mg tid.

HOW SUPPLIED: Tab: 2.5mg*, 5mg*, 10mg *scored

CONTRAINDICATIONS: Severe organic heart disease, acute renal disease, urinary retention, pheochromocytoma, thyrotoxicosis, persistent and excessive HTN.

WARNINGS/PRECAUTIONS: Risk of supine HTN; monitor for symptoms (eg, pounding in ears, headache, blurred vision), supine and standing BP; d/c if supine HTN persists. Caution with urinary retention, diabetes, renal or hepatic dysfunction. Decreased HR due to vagal reflex.

ADVERSE REACTIONS: Supine and sitting HTN, paresthesia, scalp pruritus, goosebumps, chills, urinary urge/retention/frequency.

INTERACTIONS: Monitor BP with vasoconstrictors (eg, phenylephrine, ephedrine, dihydroergotamine, pseudoephedrine). Fludrocortisone may potentiate supine HTN due to salt-retaining properties. OTC cold and diet products may potentiate pressor effects. Antagonized by alpha-blockers (eg, prazosin, terazosin, doxazosin). Metformin, cimetidine, ranitidine, procainamide, triamterene, flecainide, and quinidine may increase clearance. Caution with cardiac glycosides, psychopharmacologics, and β-blockers.

PREGNANCY: Category C, caution in nursing.

MECHANISM OF ACTION: Desglymidodrine; (major metabolite); α_1-agonist; exerts its actions via activation of the α-adrenergic receptors of the arteriolar and venous vasculature, producing an increase in vascular tone and elevation of BP.

PHARMACOKINETICS: Absorption: Rapid; absolute bioavailability (93%), Midodrine; (prodrug); T_{max}=1/2 hr. Desglymidodrine; T_{max}=1-2 hrs. **Distribution:** Poorly, across blood-brain barrier. **Metabolism:** Liver via deglycination to desglymidodrine (major metabolite). **Elimination:** Urine; (metabolite 80%).

NURSING CONSIDERATIONS

Assessment: Assess for severe organic heart disease, acute renal impairment, urinary retention, hepatic impairment, pheochromocytoma or thyrotoxicosis, orthostatic hypotension with DM, history of visual problems, persistent/excessive supine/sitting HTN, pregnancy status and for possible drug interactions. Evaluate baseline renal and LFTs.

Monitoring: Monitor for signs/symptoms of supine HTN (eg, cardiac awareness, pounding in the ears, headache, and blurred vision), signs/symptoms of bradycardia (eg, pulse slowing, increased dizziness, syncope, cardiac awarness), supine and sitting BP, HR. Careful monitoring of renal/LFTs.

Patient Counseling: Caution about taking OTC products (eg, cold remedies and diet aids) can elevate BP and may potentiate the pressor effect of the drug. Inform about the signs/symptoms of supine HTN and bradycardia and to d/c drug if occur.

Administration: Oral route. Take during daytime, not to be taken after evening meals or <4 hrs before bedtime. **Storage:** 25°C (77°F); excursions permitted to 15-30°C (59-86°F).

PROBENECID RX

probenecid (Various)

THERAPEUTIC CLASS: Uricosuric

INDICATIONS: Treatment of hyperuricemia associated with gout and gouty arthritis. Adjunct to penicillin, ampicillin, methicillin, oxacillin, cloxacillin, or nafcillin for elevation and prolongation of plasma levels.

DOSAGE: *Adults:* Gout: Initial: 250mg bid for 1 week. Titrate: May increase by 500mg every 4 weeks. Maint: 500mg bid. Max: 2g/day. May reduce by 500mg every 6 months if acute attack has been absent ≥6 months and serum urate levels are normal. Renal Impairment: Usual: 1g/day. Adjunct Antibiotic Therapy: 500mg qid. Elderly/Renal Impairment: Reduce dose. Decrease dose with gastric intolerance. May not be effective if CrCl ≤30mL/min.
Pediatrics: 2-14 yrs: Adjunct Antibiotic Therapy: Initial: 25mg/kg. Maint: 10mg/kg qid. ≥50kg: 500mg qid.

HOW SUPPLIED: Tab: 500mg

CONTRAINDICATIONS: Blood dyscrasias, uric acid kidney stones and children <2 yrs. Do not use in acute gout attack.

WARNINGS/PRECAUTIONS: Initiate therapy when acute gout attack subsides. Exacerbation of gout may occur; treat with colchicine. Use APAP if analgesic needed. Severe allergic reactions and anaphylaxis reported. D/C if hypersensitivity occurs. Caution with peptic ulcer. Monitor for glycosuria. Maintain liberal fluid intake and alkalization of urine.

ADVERSE REACTIONS: Headache, acute gouty arthritis, dizziness, hepatic necrosis, vomiting, nausea, anorexia, sore gums, nephrotic syndrome, uric acid stones, renal colic, costovertebral pain, urinary frequency, anaphylaxis, fever, urticaria, pruritus, blood dyscrasias, dermatitis, alopecia, flushing.

INTERACTIONS: Probenecid increases plasma levels of penicillin and other β-lactams; psychic disturbances reported. Avoid use with penicillin in the presence of renal impairment. Salicylates and pyrazinamide antagonize uricosuric effects. Increased plasma levels of methotrexate, sulfonamides, sulfonylureas, thiopental or ketamine-induced anesthesia, some NSAIDs (eg, indomethacin, naproxen), lorazepam, APAP, and rifampin. Possible false high plasma levels of theophylline.

PREGNANCY: Safety in pregnancy and nursing is not known.

MECHANISM OF ACTION: Uricosuric/renal tubular blocking agent; inhibits tubular reabsorption of urate, increasing urinary excretion of uric acid and decreasing serum urate levels.

NURSING CONSIDERATIONS

Assessment: Assess for known blood dyscrasias, uric acid kidney stone, acute vs chronic attack, history of peptic ulcer, possible drug interactions, and renal impairment.

Monitoring: Monitor for signs/symptoms of gout exacerbation, allergic reactions, hematuria, renal colic, costovertebral pain, and uric acid stone formation.

Patient Counseling: Instruct on importance of liberal fluid intake. Advise to seek medical attention if symptoms of allergic reaction, hematuria, renal colic, or costovertebral pain occur.

Administration: Oral route. **Storage:** 20-25°C (68-77°F). Protect from light.

PROCARDIA XL — RX

nifedipine (Pfizer)

THERAPEUTIC CLASS: Calcium channel blocker (dihydropyridine)

INDICATIONS: Management of vasospastic angina and chronic stable angina. Treatment of hypertension.

DOSAGE: *Adults:* Angina/HTN: Initial: 30-60mg qd. Titrate over 7-14 days. Max: 120mg/day. Caution if dose >90mg with angina.

HOW SUPPLIED: Tab, Extended-Release: 30mg, 60mg, 90mg

WARNINGS/PRECAUTIONS: May cause hypotension; monitor BP initially or with titration. May exacerbate angina from β-blocker withdrawal. CHF risk, especially with aortic stenosis or β-blockers. Peripheral edema reported. May increase angina or MI with severe obstructive CAD. Caution in pre-existing severe GI narrowing.

ADVERSE REACTIONS: Dizziness, lightheadedness, giddiness, flushing, muscle cramps, headache, weakness, nausea, peripheral edema, nervousness/mood changes.

INTERACTIONS: β-Blockers may increase risk of CHF, severe hypotension, or angina exacerbation. Possible hypotension with fentanyl. Potentiates digoxin. Monitor quinidine, coumarin. Potentiated by cimetidine and grapefruit juice. Avoid grapefruit juice.

PREGNANCY: Category C, unknown use in nursing.

MECHANISM OF ACTION: Calcium channel blocker; inhibits calcium ion influx into cardiac muscle and smooth muscle.

PHARMACOKINETICS: Absorption: Complete. **Distribution:** Plasma protein binding (92-98%). **Metabolism:** Hepatic biotransformation. **Elimination:** Urine, feces; $T_{1/2}$=2 hrs.

NURSING CONSIDERATIONS

Assessment: Assess for aortic stenosis, CHF, hypotension, MI, angina (vasospastic, chronic stable), HTN, LFTs, GI narrowing, and possible drug interactions.

Monitoring: Monitor BP, left ventricular dysfunction, edema, GI obstructive symptoms, hypersensitivity reactions, hypotension, CHF, LFTs, bleeding time, Coombs' test, fatigue, dizziness.

Patient Counseling: Advise to take exactly as prescribed. Instruct to swallow tablet whole; do not crush or chew. Counsel about adverse effects; advise to report any.

Administration: Oral route. **Storage:** Below 30°C (86°F).

PROCHLORPERAZINE RX

prochlorperazine (Various)

THERAPEUTIC CLASS: Phenothiazine derivative

INDICATIONS: Control of severe nausea and vomiting. Management of psychotic disorders (eg, schizophrenia). Short-term treatment of generalized non-psychotic anxiety.

DOSAGE: *Adults:* Nausea/Vomiting: (Tab) Usual: 5-10mg tid-qid. Max: 40mg/day. (IM) 5-10mg IM q3-4h prn. Max: 40mg/day. (IV) 2.5-10mg IV (not bolus). Max: 10mg single dose and 40mg/day. Nausea/Vomiting with Surgery: 5-10mg IM 1-2 hrs or 5-10mg IV 15-30 min before anesthesia, or during or after surgery; repeat once if needed. Non-Psychotic Anxiety: (Tab) 5mg tid-qid; Psychosis: Mild/Outpatient: 5-10mg PO tid-qid. Moderate-Severe/Hospitalized: Initial: 10mg PO tid-qid. May increase in small increments every 2-3 days. Severe: (PO) 100-150mg/day. (IM) 10-20mg, may repeat q2-4 hrs if needed. Switch to oral after obtain control or if needed, 10-20mg IM q4-6h. Elderly: use lower dosing range and titrate more gradually.
Pediatrics: Nausea/Vomiting: >2 yrs and >20 lbs: (PO/PR) 20-29 lbs: Usual: 2.5mg qd-bid. Max: 7.5mg/day. 30-39 lbs: 2.5mg bid-tid. Max: 10mg/day. 40-85 lbs: 2.5mg tid or 5mg bid. Max: 15mg/day. (IM) 0.06mg/lb, usually single dose for control. Psychosis: (PO/PR) 2-12 yrs: Initial: 2.5mg bid-tid, up to 10mg/day on 1st day. Max: 2-5 yrs: 20mg/day. 6-12 yrs: 25mg/day. (IM) <12 yrs: 0.06mg/lb single dose. Switch to oral after obtain control.

HOW SUPPLIED: Inj: (Edisylate) 5mg/mL; Supp: 5mg, 25mg; Tab: (Maleate) 5mg, 10mg

CONTRAINDICATIONS: Comatose states, concomitant large dose CNS depressants (alcohol, barbiturates, narcotics), pediatric surgery, pediatrics <2 yrs or <20lbs.

WARNINGS/PRECAUTIONS: Secondary extrapyramidal symptoms can occur. Tardive dyskinesia, NMS may develop. Caution with activities requiring alertness. May mask symptoms of overdose of other drugs. May obscure diagnosis of intestinal obstruction, brain tumor, and Reye's syndrome. May interfere with thermoregulation. Caution with glaucoma, cardiac disorders. Caution in children with dehydration or acute illness and the elderly. D/C 48 hrs before myelography and may resume after 24 hrs post-procedure.

ADVERSE REACTIONS: Drowsiness, dizziness, amenorrhea, blurred vision, skin reactions, hypotension, NMS, cholestatic jaundice.

INTERACTIONS: May decrease oral anticoagulant effects. May potentiate α-adrenergic blockade. Thiazide diuretics potentiate orthostatic hypotension. Increased levels of both drugs with propranolol. Anticonvulsants may need adjustment. Risk of encephalopathic syndrome with lithium. May antagonize antihypertensive effects of guanethidine and related compounds.

PREGNANCY: Safety in pregnancy is not known; caution in nursing.

MECHANISM OF ACTION: Phenothiazine derivative; antiemetic and antipsychotic.

NURSING CONSIDERATIONS

Assessment: Assess for Reye's syndrome, TD, possible drug interactions, bone marrow depression, impaired CV system, and glaucoma.

Monitoring: Monitor for signs/symptoms of TD, NMS, hypotension, EPS, mydriasis, encephalopathic syndrome, and hypersensitivity reactions.

Patient Counseling: Caution may impair physical/mental abilities. Seek medical attention if symptoms of TD, NMS (hyperpyrexia, muscle rigidity, AMS), hypotension, mydriasis, encephalopathic syndrome (weakness, lethargy, fever), or hypersensitivity reactions occur.

Administration: IV, Oral route. **Storage:** Tab, inj: 20-25°C (68-77°F). Do not freeze. Protect from light.

PROCRIT

RX

epoetin alfa (Ortho Biotech)

Increased mortality, serious cardiovascular/thromboembolic events, and increased risk of tumor progression or recurrence. (Renal Failure) Patients experienced greater risks for death and serious cardiovascular events when administered erythropoiesis-stimulating agents (ESAs) to target higher vs lower Hgb levels (13.5 vs 11.3 g/dL; 14 vs 10 g/dL) in 2 clinical studies. Individualize dosing to achieve and maintain Hgb levels within range of 10-12g/dL. (Cancer) ESAs shortened overall survival and/or increased risk of tumor progression or recurrence in clinical studies in patients with breast, non-small cell lung, head and neck, lymphoid, and cervical cancers. To decrease these risks, as well as risk of serious cardio- and thrombovascular events, use lowest dose needed to avoid RBC transfusions. Use ESAs only for treatment of anemia due to concomitant myelosuppressive chemotherapy. ESAs are not indicated for patients receiving myelosuppressive therapy when anticipated outcome is cure. D/C following completion of chemotherapy course. (Perisurgery) Epoetin alfa increased the rate of DVT in patients not receiving prophylactic anticoagulation. Consider DVT prophylaxis.

THERAPEUTIC CLASS: Erythropoiesis stimulator

INDICATIONS: Treatment of anemia due to chronic renal failure (CRF), anemia related to zidovudine treatment of HIV, chemotherapy-induced anemia in non-myeloid malignancies, and reduction of allogeneic blood transfusions in anemic patients (>10 to ≤13g/dL) scheduled for elective, noncardiac, nonvascular surgery.

DOSAGE: *Adults:* CRF: Initial: 50-100 U/kg IV/SQ 3x/week. IV is preferred route in dialysis patients. Maint: Individually titrate. Reduce if Hgb approaches 12g/dL or if Hgb increases >1g/dL in any 2-week period. Increase when Hgb does not increase by 2g/dL after 8 weeks of therapy and Hgb is below target range (10-12g/dL). Zidovudine-Treated HIV Patients: If serum erythropoietin levels ≤500 mU/mL and zidovudine ≤4200mg/week, give 100 U/kg IV/SQ 3x/week for 8 weeks. Titrate: Increase by 50-100 U/kg 3x/week after 8 weeks if necessary. Max: 300 U/kg 3x/week. Maint: If Hgb >13g/dL, d/c until Hgb <12g/dL, then reduce dose by 25% when therapy resumes. Chemotherapy-Induced Anemia: Initial: 150 U/kg SQ 3x/week. Titrate: Reduce by 25% when Hgb approaches 12g/dL or Hgb increases >1g/dL in any 2-week period. If Hgb >13g/dL, withhold until Hgb <12g/dL then restart at 25% below previous dose. May increase to 300 U/kg 3x/week if no response after 8 weeks of therapy. Max: 300 U/kg 3x/week. Weekly Dosing: 40,000 U SQ weekly. Titrate: If Hgb not increased by ≥1g/dL after 4 weeks, increase to 60,000 U weekly. If Hgb >13g/dL, withhold until Hgb <12g/dL then restart with 25% dose reduction. Reduce dose by 25% if very rapid Hgb response (eg, increase >1g/dL in any 2-week period). Max: 60,000 U weekly. Surgery: 300 U/kg/day SQ for 10 days before surgery, on surgery day, and 4 days post-op or 600 U/kg SQ once weekly on 21, 14, and 7 days before surgery and a 4th dose on surgery day, with adequate iron supplement.

Pediatrics: CRF: Initial: 50 U/kg 3x/week IV/SQ. Titrate: Reduce if Hgb approaches 12g/dL or if Hgb increases by >1g/dL in any 2-week period. Increase

P

if Hgb does not increase by 2g/dL after 8 weeks of therapy and Hgb is below target range (10-12g/dL). Maint: Individually titrate. Chemotherapy Induced Anemia: Initial: 600 U/kg IV weekly. Titrate: If Hgb not increased by ≥1g/dL after 4 weeks, increase to 900 U/kg IV weekly. If Hgb >13g/dL, withhold until Hgb <12g/dL then restart with 25% dose reduction. Reduce dose by 25% if very rapid Hgb response (eg, increase >1g/dL in any 2-week period. Max: 60,000 U weekly.

HOW SUPPLIED: Inj: 2000 U/mL, 3000 U/mL, 4000 U/mL, 10,000 U/mL, 20,000 U/mL, 40,000 U/mL

CONTRAINDICATIONS: Uncontrolled HTN. Hypersensitivity to mammalian cell-derived products and albumin (human).

WARNINGS/PRECAUTIONS: Pure red cell aplasia and severe anemia (with or without other cytopenias) may occur. Caution with porphyria, HTN, or history of seizures. Monitor patients with pre-existing CV disease closely. Evaluate iron stores before and during therapy; most patients need iron supplementation. Monitor Hgb, BP, iron levels, serum chemistry, and CBC. Multidose formulation contains benzyl alcohol, which has been associated with an increased incidence of neurological and other complications in premature infants; these compilcations are sometimes fatal.

ADVERSE REACTIONS: HTN, headache, fatigue, arthralgias, nausea, vomiting, diarrhea, edema, rash, pyrexia, constipation, respiratory congestion, dyspnea, asthenia, skin reaction.

INTERACTIONS: Adjust anticoagulant dose in dialysis patients.

PREGNANCY: Category C, caution in nursing.

MECHANISM OF ACTION: Erythropoiesis stimulator.

PHARMACOKINETICS: Absorption: (SQ) T_{max}=5-24 hrs. **Elimination:** (IV) $T_{1/2}$=4-13 hrs.

NURSING CONSIDERATIONS

Assessment: Assess for uncontrolled HTN, porphyria, cardiovascular disease (ischemic heart disease, CHF), renal failure, possible drug interactions, hypersensitivity to mammalian cell-derived products and albumin. Obtain baseline BP measurements and iron status (transferrin saturation, serum ferritin).

Monitoring: Monitor BP, CBC with differential and platelet count, iron status (transferrin saturation, serum ferritin) regularly. CRF: Serum chemistries (BUN, uric acid, creatinine, phosphorus, K^+) regularly, Hgb twice weekly. HIV and cancer: Hgb once weekly. Monitor for signs/symptoms of CV events (MI, stroke, CHF), pure red cell aplasia, severe anemia, viral diseases, seizures, lack/loss of response to therapy, and hypersensitivity reactions.

P

Patient Counseling: Caution may impair physical/mental abilities. Seek medical attention if symptoms of CV events, anemia, infections, seizures, or hypersensitivity reactions occur.

Administration: IV, SC route. **Storage:** 2-8°C (36-46°F). Do not freeze or shake.

PROGRAF

RX

tacrolimus (Astellas)

Increased susceptibility to infection and development of lymphoma.

THERAPEUTIC CLASS: Macrolide immunosuppressant

INDICATIONS: Prophylaxis of organ rejection in allogenic liver, kidney, or heart transplants with concomitant adrenal corticosteroids. In heart transplant patients, azathioprine or mycophenolate mofetil coadministration is recommended.

DOSAGE: *Adults:* Initial (6 hrs after transplantation): 0.03-0.05mg/kg/day (liver, kidney) or 0.01mg/kg/day (heart) IV infusion if cannot tolerate PO. Hepatic Transplant: 0.05-0.075mg/kg PO q12h with grapefruit juice; start 8-12 hrs after last IV dose. Kidney Transplant: 0.1mg/kg PO q12h, 24 hrs after

transplant or until renal function recovered. Heart Transplant: 0.0375mg/kg PO q12h; start 8-12 hrs after last IV dose. Renal/Hepatic Impairment: Give lowest recommended dose. Severe Hepatic Impairment (Pugh ≥10): May require lower doses. Wait at least 48 hrs with post-op oliguria.
Pediatrics: Liver Transplant: Initial: 0.03-0.05mg/kg/day IV or 0.15-0.2mg/kg/day PO. Severe Hepatic Impairment (Pugh ≥10): May require lower doses.

HOW SUPPLIED: Cap: 0.5mg, 1mg, 5mg; Inj: 5mg/mL

CONTRAINDICATIONS: Hypersensitivity to HCO-60.

WARNINGS/PRECAUTIONS: Insulin-dependent post-transplant DM, HTN, myocardial hypertrophy, neurotoxicity, hyperkalemia, nephrotoxicity reported. Monitor drug levels frequently to prevent organ rejection and/or reduce potential toxicity. Monitor for anaphylaxis with infusion. Monitor levels closely with hepatic impairment.

ADVERSE REACTIONS: HTN, headache, insomnia, fever, pruritus, hyperglycemia, hyperkalemia, hypomagnesemia, diarrhea, nausea, vomiting, increased BUN, anorexia, constipation, tremor, rash, pleural effusion, gastroenteritis.

INTERACTIONS: CYP450 3A inducers (eg, carbamazepine, phenobarbital, phenytoin, rifabutin, caspofungin, rifampin, St. John's wort, sirolimus, etc.) may decrease plasma levels. Caution with other nephrotoxic drugs (eg, aminoglycosides, amphotericin B, cisplatin). May affect drugs metabolized by CYP450 3A. Avoid grapefruit juice. CYP450 3A inhibitors (eg, diltiazem, nicardipine, nifedipine, verapamil, azole antifungals, macrolides, cisapride, metoclopramide, etc.) may increase plasma levels. Vaccination may be less effective. Avoid live vaccines, cyclosporine (when switching to tacrolimus, wait at least 24 hrs after last cyclosporine dose), and K^+ -sparing diuretics.

PREGNANCY: Category C, not for use in nursing.

MECHANISM OF ACTION: Macrolide immunosuppressant; not established. Suspected to inhibit T-lymphocyte activation. Binds to intracellular protein (FKBP-12). Complex of tacrolimus-FKBP-12, calcium, calmodulin, and calcineurin is then formed and phosphatase activity of calcineurin inhibited. Effect may prevent dephosphorylation and translocation of nuclear factor of activated T cells (NF-AT), a nuclear component responsible for initiating gene transcription for the formation of lymphokines. Results in inhibition of T-lymphocyte activation.

PHARMACOKINETICS: Absorption: (PO) Incomplete and variable, absolute bioavailability (18%), C_{max}=29.7ng/mL, T_{max}=1.6 hrs, AUC=243ng•hr/mL; (IV) AUC=598ng•hr/mL. **Distribution:** Plasma protein binding (99%), appears in breast milk; (PO) V_d=1.94L/kg; (IV) V_d=1.91 L/kg. **Metabolism:** Hepatic, via CYP3A (demethylation and hydroxylation); 13-methyl tacrolimus (major metabolite); 31-demethyl (active metabolite). **Elimination:** (PO) Feces (92%), urine (2.3%); $T_{1/2}$=34.8 hrs. (IV) Feces (92.4%); $T_{1/2}$=34.2 hrs. Refer to PI for parameters in patients with renal, hepatic, and cardiac transplants.

P

NURSING CONSIDERATIONS

Assessment: Assess for hypersensitivity to HCO-60 (polyoxyl 60 hydrogenated castor oil), impaired hepatic/renal function, and possible drug interactions. Assess use in pregnant/nursing females.

Monitoring: Monitor for signs/symptoms of insulin dependent post-transplant DM, neurotoxicity, nephrotoxicity, hyperkalemia, lymphomas and other malignancies (eg, skin), lymphoproliferative disorder, anaphylactic reactions, HTN, and myocardial hypertrophy. Monitor with renal impairment for dose adjustments. Perform regular evaluation of SrCr, K^+, and fasting glucose. Monitor metabolic and hematologic systems as clinically warranted.

Patient Counseling: Inform that repeated lab testing required. Advise females about risks of use during pregnancy. Inform about increased risk of neoplasias and DM. Instruct to contact physician if frequent urination, increased hunger, or thirst occur. Counsel to wear protective clothing, use sunscreen, and avoid exposure to sunlight/UV light to reduce risk of malignant skin changes.

Administration: Oral/IV routes. IV: Must be diluted with 0.9% NS or D5W to concentration between 0.004mg/mL and 0.02 mg/mL. Patients receiving IV formulation should be under continuous observation for at least first 30 min following start of infusion and at frequent intervals thereafter. **Storage:** Cap: 25°C (77°F); excursions permitted to 15-30°C (59-86°F). Inj: 5-25°C (41-77°F). Store diluted infusion in glass or polyethylene containers and discarded after 24 hrs.

PROMETHAZINE RX

promethazine HCl (Various)

OTHER BRAND NAMES: Promethegan (G & W Labs) - Phenergan (Wyeth)

THERAPEUTIC CLASS: Phenothiazine derivative

INDICATIONS: Allergic and vasomotor rhinitis, allergic conjunctivitis, blood or plasma allergic reactions, dermographism, urticaria, angioedema. Pre- and postoperative sedation. Adjunct in anaphylaxis, postoperative pain. Prevention and control of nausea, vomiting, and motion sickness.

DOSAGE: *Adults:* Allergy: 25mg qhs or 12.5mg ac and hs. Motion Sickness: Initial: 25mg 30-60 min before travel, then 25mg 8-12 hrs later if needed. Maint: 25mg bid. Prevention/Control of Nausea/Vomiting: 25mg initially, then 12.5-25mg q4-6h prn. Sedation: 25-50mg qhs. Preoperative: 50mg night before surgery, then 50mg preoperatively. Postoperative: 25-50mg. *Pediatrics:* ≥2 yrs: Allergy: 25mg or 0.5mg/lb qhs or 6.25-12.5 tid. Motion Sickness: 12.5-25mg bid. Prevention/Control of Nausea/Vomiting: 25mg or 0.5mg/lb initially then 12.5-25mg or 0.5mg/lb q4-6h prn. Sedation: 12.5-25mg hs. Preoperative: 12.5-25mg night before surgery, then 0.5mg/lb preoperatively. Postoperative: 12.5-25mg.

HOW SUPPLIED: Sup: (Promethegan, Phenergan, Promethazine)12.5mg, 25mg, 50mg; Tab: (Phenergan, Promethazine)12.5mg*, 25mg*, 50mg *scored

CONTRAINDICATIONS: Treatment of lower respiratory tract symptoms (eg, asthma). Pediatric patients <2 yrs.

WARNINGS/PRECAUTIONS: Potential for fatal respiratory depression in pediatric patients <2 yrs. Caution in patients ≥2 yrs. Avoid with compromised respiratory function (eg, COPD, sleep apnea). Caution with bone marrow depression, narrow-angle glaucoma, stenosing peptic ulcer, bladder or pyloroduodenal obstruction, prostatic hypertrophy, CVD, hepatic dysfunction. Cholestatic jaundice reported. Alters HCG pregnancy tests. May lower seizure threshold, increase blood glucose, cause sun sensitivity. May impair mental/physical abilities.

P

ADVERSE REACTIONS: Drowsiness, sedation, blurred vision, dizziness, increased or decreased blood pressure, urticaria, dry mouth, nausea, vomiting.

INTERACTIONS: Additive sedative effects with CNS depressants (eg, alcohol, narcotic analgesics, sedatives, hypnotics, tranquilizers); reduce dose or eliminate these agents. Reduce barbiturate dose by one-half and analgesic depressant dose by one-quarter to one-half. Caution with drugs that alter seizure threshold (eg, narcotics, local anesthetics). Avoid sedatives and CNS depressants with sleep apnea.

PREGNANCY: Category C, not for use in nursing.

MECHANISM OF ACTION: Phenothiazine derivative; H_1 receptor-blocking agent. Also has sedative and antiemetic properties.

PHARMACOKINETICS: Absorption: GI tract (well absorbed). **Metabolism:** Liver. **Elimination:** Urine.

NURSING CONSIDERATIONS

Assessment: Assess for compromised respiratory depression, bone-marrow depression, seizure, LFTs, narrow-angle glaucoma, prostatic hypertrophy, stenosing peptic ulcer, pyloroduodenal obstruction, bladder-neck obstruction, and cardiovascular disease. Note other diseases/conditions and drug therapies.

Monitoring: Monitor respiratory function, LFTs, CBC with differential and platelet count, renal function, blood glucose, BP, temperature and EKG.

Monitor for neuroleptic malignant syndrome, raised intraocular pressure, and seizures.

Patient Counseling: Inform drug can cause drowsiness and impair mental or physical abilities required to perform potentially hazardous tasks (eg, operating machinery/driving). Counsel about side effects and to seek medical attention if any develop. Advise to avoid concomitant use of alcohol and other CNS depressants.

Administration: Oral route and rectal administration. **Storage:** (Tab) 20-25°C (68-77°F). Protect from light. Keep tightly closed. Dispense in light-resistant container. (Sup) Refrigerate 2-8°C (36-46°F).

PROMETHAZINE DM — RX

dextromethorphan hbr - promethazine HCl (Various)

THERAPEUTIC CLASS: Phenothiazine derivative/antitussive

INDICATIONS: Temporary relief of coughs and upper respiratory symptoms associated with allergy or the common cold.

DOSAGE: *Adults:* 5mL q4-6h. Max: 30mL/24 hr.
Pediatrics: ≥12 yrs: 5mL q4-6h. Max: 30mL/24hr. 6-11 yrs: 2.5-5mL q4-6h. Max: 20mL/24hr. 2-5 yrs: 1.25-2.5mL q4-6h. Max: 10mL/24hr.

HOW SUPPLIED: Syrup: (Promethazine-Dextromethorphan) 6.25mg-15mg/5mL

CONTRAINDICATIONS: Concomitant MAOIs, comatose states, treatment of lower respiratory tract symptoms (eg, asthma), pediatric patients <2 yrs.

WARNINGS/PRECAUTIONS: Caution in pediatrics ≥2 yrs. Avoid in pediatric patients whose signs and symptoms may suggest Reye's syndrome or other hepatic diseases. May impair mental/physical abilities. May lower seizure threshold; caution with seizure disorders. May lead to potentially fatal respiratory depression; avoid with compromised respiratory function (eg, COPD, sleep apnea). Caution with bone marrow depression; leukopenia and agranulocytosis reported. Neuroleptic malignant syndrome reported. Caution with narrow-angle glaucoma, prostatic hypertrophy, stenosing peptic ulcer, bladder neck or pyloroduodenal obstruction, cardiovascular disease, hepatic impairment, atopic children, sedated, elderly, or debilitated patients, and patients confined to supine position. Cholestatic jaundice reported. May alter HCG pregnancy test reading. May increase blood glucose. Avoid prolonged exposure to sunlight.

ADVERSE REACTIONS: Drowsiness, dizziness, sedation, GI disturbance, blurred vision, dry mouth, increased or decreased BP, rash, nausea, vomiting.

INTERACTIONS: See Contraindications. Hyperpyrexia, hypotension and death associated with MAOIs. May increase, prolong, or intensify sedative action of other CNS depressants, such as alcohol, sedatives/hypnotics (including barbiturates), narcotics, narcotic analgesics, general anesthetics, TCAs, and tranquilizers; avoid such agents or administer in reduced dosages. Reduce barbiturate dose by at least one-half and narcotic analgesics by one-quarter to one-half. May reverse epinephrines's vasopressor effect. May lower seizure threshold; caution with concomitant medications which may also affect seizure threshold (eg, narcotics, local anesthetics). Avoid concomitant administration with other respiratory depressants in pediatrics. Caution with concomitant use of other agents with anticholinergic properties.

PREGNANCY: Category C, caution in nursing.

MECHANISM OF ACTION: Dextromethorphan: Antitussive agent; acts centrally and elevates the threshold for coughing. Promethazine: Phenothiazine derivative, (antihistaminic); H_1 receptor blocking agent and provides clinically useful sedative and antiemetic effects.

PHARMACOKINETICS: Absorption: Dextromethorphan (rapid); Promethazine (well-absorbed). **Metabolism:** Promethazine: Liver. Dextromethorphan: Liver via O-demethylation, N-demethylation, and partial conjugation with glucuronic acid and sulfate. **Elimination:** Promethazine: Urine (sulfoxides and N-demethylpromethazine). Dextromethorphan: Urine.

P

NURSING CONSIDERATIONS

Assessment: Assess for drug hypersensitivity, sedated or comatose patients, compromised respiratory function (eg, COPD, sleep apnea), seizures, liver/renal function, bone marrow depression, atopic children, and for signs/symptoms of Reye's syndrome or encephalopathy, narrow-angle glaucoma, prostatic hypertrophy, stenosing peptic ulcer, pyloroduodenal obstruction, bladder neck obstruction, CVD, DM, pregnancy status, and potential drug/lab test interactions.

Monitoring: Monitor for CNS/respiratory depression and sleep apnea, signs/symptoms of NMS, seizures, cholestatic jaundice. Monitor children for hallucinations, convulsions, extrapyramidal symptoms, and dystonias. Monitor false positive and false negative pregnancy tests, blood glucose, and CBCs.

Patient Counseling: Advise to use caution during hazardous tasks (eg, operating machinery/driving). Instruct to report involuntary muscle movements. Avoid alcohol; limit sunlight exposure.

Administration: Oral route. **Storage:** 20-25°C (68-77°F).

PROMETHAZINE VC — RX

phenylephrine HCl - promethazine HCl (Various)

THERAPEUTIC CLASS: Phenothiazine derivative/sympathomimetic

INDICATIONS: Temporary relief of upper respiratory symptoms (eg, nasal congestion) associated with allergy or the common cold.

DOSAGE: *Adults:* 5mL q4-6h. Max: 30mL/24 hr.
Pediatrics: ≥12 yrs: 5mL q4-6h. Max: 30mL/24 hr. 6-11 yrs: 2.5-5mL q4-6h. Max: 30mL/24 hr. 2-5 yrs: 1.25-2.5mL q4-6h.

HOW SUPPLIED: Syrup: (Promethazine-Phenylephrine) 6.25mg-5mg/5mL

CONTRAINDICATIONS: Concomitant MAOIs, comatose states, treatment of lower respiratory tract symptoms (eg, asthma), HTN, peripheral vascular insufficiency, pediatric patients <2 yrs.

WARNINGS/PRECAUTIONS: Caution in pediatrics ≥2 yrs. Avoid in pediatric patients whose signs and symptoms may suggest Reye's syndrome or other hepatic diseases. May impair mental/physical abilities. May lower seizure threshold; caution with seizure disorders. May lead to potentially fatal respiratory depression; avoid with compromised respiratory function (eg, COPD, sleep apnea). Caution with bone marrow depression; leukopenia and agranulocytosis reported. Neuroleptic maliganant syndrome reported. Caution with narrow-angle glaucoma, prostatic hypertrophy, stenosing peptic ulcer, bladder neck or pyloroduodenal obstruction, cardiovascular disease, and elderly patients. Cholestatic jaundice reported. May alter HCG pregnancy test reading. May increase blood glucose. Avoid prolonged exposure to sunlight.

ADVERSE REACTIONS: Drowsiness, dizziness, anxiety, tremor, sedation, blurred vision, dry mouth, increased or decreased blood pressure, rash, nausea, vomiting.

INTERACTIONS: See Contraindications. May increase, prolong, or intensify the sedative action of other CNS depressants, such as alcohol, sedatives/hypnotics (including barbiturates), narcotics, narcotic analgesics, general anesthetics, TCAs, and tranquilizers; avoid such agents or administer in reduced dosages. Reduce barbiturate dose by at least one-half and narcotic analgesics by one-quarter to one-half. Cardiac pressor response potentiated and possible hypertensive crisis with MAOIs. Pressor response increased with TCAs. Excessive rise in BP with ergot alkaloids. Tachycardia or other arrhythmias may occur with sympathomimetics. Reflex bradycardia blocked and pressor response enhanced with atropine. Cardiostimulating effects blocked with β-blockers. Pressor response decreased with α-adrenergic blockers. Synergistic adrenergic response with amphetamines or phenylpropanolamine. Avoid concomitant administration with other respiratory depressants in pediatrics. May lower seizure threshold; caution with concomitant medications which may also affect seizure threshold (eg, narcotics, local anesthetics). Reflex bradycardia blocked; pressor response enhanced with atropine.

PREGNANCY: Category C, caution in nursing.

MECHANISM OF ACTION: Promethazine: Phenothiazine derivative; H_1-receptor blocking agent. Phenylephrine: Sympathomimetic; α-receptor agonist with little effect on β-receptors of heart; increases resistance and decreases capacitance of blood vessels; has mild central stimulant effect.

PHARMACOKINETICS: Absorption: Promethazine: Well-absorbed (GI tract). Phenylephrine: Irregularly absorbed. **Metabolism:** Promethazine: Liver, sulfoxides and N-demethylpromethazine (metabolites). Phenylephrine: Liver and intestine via monoamine oxidase. **Elimination:** Promethazine: Urine (sulfoxides and N-demethylpromethazine).

NURSING CONSIDERATIONS

Assessment: Assess for drug hypersensitivity, sedation or comatose, compromised respiratory function (eg, COPD, sleep apnea), seizures, liver/renal function, bone marrow depression, children with Reyes Syndrome or encephalopathy, narrow-angle glaucoma, prostatic hypertrophy, stenosing peptic ulcer, pyloroduodenal obstruction, bladder neck obstruction, peripheral vascular insufficiency, HTN, CVD, DM, pregnancy status, and potential drug/lab test interactions (eg, MAO inhibitors).

Monitoring: Monitor for CNS and respiratory depression, sleep apnea, signs/symptoms of NMS, seizures, cholestatic jaundice. Monitor children for hallucinations, convulsions, extrapyramidal symptoms, and dystonias. Monitor for false positive and false negative pregnancy tests, blood glucose, and CBCs.

Patient Counseling: Advise to use caution during hazardous tasks (eg, operating machinery/driving). Instruct to report involuntary muscle movements. Avoid alcohol and other respiratory depressants; limit sunlight exposure.

Administration: Oral route. **Storage:** 20-25°C (68-77°F).

PROMETHAZINE VC/CODEINE CV

phenylephrine HCl - promethazine HCl - codeine phosphate (Various)

THERAPEUTIC CLASS: Phenothiazine derivative/antitussive/sympathomimetic

INDICATIONS: Temporary relief of cough and upper respiratory symptoms (eg, nasal congestion) associated with allergy or the common cold.

DOSAGE: *Adults:* 5mL q4-6h. Max: 30mL/24hr.
Pediatrics: ≥16 yrs: 5mL q4-6h. Max: 30mL/24hr.

HOW SUPPLIED: Syrup: (Promethazine-Codeine-Phenylephrine) 6.25mg-10mg-5mg/5mL

CONTRAINDICATIONS: Concomitant MAOIs, comatose states, treatment of lower respiratory tract symptoms (eg, asthma), HTN, peripheral vascular insufficiency, pediatric patients <16 yrs.

WARNINGS/PRECAUTIONS: May cause or aggravate constipation. May lead to potentially fatal respiratory depression; avoid with compromised respiratory function (eg, COPD, sleep apnea). Caution in atopic children. May elevate CSF pressure; caution with head injury, intracranial lesions, or pre-existing increase in ICP. Avoid with asthma, acute febrile illness with chronic cough, or with chronic respiratory disease where interference with ability to clear tracheobronchial tree of secretions would have a deleterious effect on patient's respiratory function. May cause orthostatic hypotension. May impair mental/physical abilities. May lower seizure threshold; caution with seizure disorders. Caution with bone marrow depression; leukopenia and agranulocytosis reported. Neuroleptic malignant syndrome reported. Hallucinations and convulsions have occurred in pediatrics. Cholestatic jaundice reported. Caution with acute abdominal conditions, convulsive disorders, significant hepatic/renal impairment, fever, hypothyroidism, Addison's disease, ulcerative colitis, prostatic hypertrophy, recent GI or urinary tract surgery, elderly, debilitated, narrow-angle glaucoma, stenosing peptic ulcer, pyloroduodenal or bladder-neck obstruction, cardiovascular disease, thyroid disease, DM, heart disease. Urinary retention may occur with BPH. May decrease cardiac output; use extreme caution with arteriosclerosis, elderly, and patients with initially poor cerebral or coronary circulation. May alter HCG pregnancy test reading. May increase blood glucose. Avoid prolonged exposure to sunlight.

ADVERSE REACTIONS: Drowsiness, dizziness, sedation, tremor, anxiety, blurred vision, dry mouth, increased or decreased blood pressure, rash, nausea, vomiting, constipation, urinary retention.

INTERACTIONS: See Contraindications. May increase, prolong, or intensify the sedative action of other CNS depressants such as alcohol, sedatives/hypnotics (including barbiturates), narcotics, narcotic analgesics, general anesthetics, TCAs, and tranquilizers. Reduce barbiturate dose by at least one-half and narcotic analgesics by one-quarter to one-half. Cardiac pressor response potentiated and acute hypertensive crisis may occur with MAOIs; consider small test dose. May reverse epinephrine's vasopressor effect. Caution with concomitant use of other agents with anticholinergic properties. Pressor response increased with TCAs. Excessive rise in BP with ergot alkaloids. Tachycardia or other arrhythmias may occur with other sympathomimetics. Cardiostimulating effects blocked with β-blockers. Reflex bradycardia blocked and pressor response enhanced with atropine. Pressor response decreased with α-adrenergic blockers. Synergistic adrenergic response with diet preparations (eg, amphetamines or phenylpropanolamine). Avoid concomitant administration with other respiratory agents in pediatrics. May lower seizure threshold; caution with concomitant medications which may also affect seizure threshold (eg, narcotics, local anesthetics).

PREGNANCY: Category C, caution in nursing.

MECHANISM OF ACTION: Promethazine: Phenothiazine derivative. Blocks H_1-receptor. Phenylephrine; sympathomimetic. Potent postsynaptic-α-receptor agonist with little effect on β-receptors of heart; increases resistance and decreases capacitance of blood vessels. Codeine: Narcotic analgesic/antitussive. Primary effects on central CNS and GI tract.

PHARMACOKINETICS: Absorption: Codeine: Well-absorbed. Promethazine: Well-absorbed (GI tract). Phenylephrine: Irregularly-absorbed. **Distribution:** Codeine: Found in breast milk. **Metabolism:** Promethazine: Liver. Phenylephrine: Liver and intestine, via monoamine oxidase. Codeine: Liver, via O-demethylation, N-demethylation, and partial conjugation with glucuronic acid. **Elimination:** Promethazine: Urine (sulfoxides and N-demethylpromethazine). Codeine: Urine (inactive metabolite and free/conjugated morphine), feces.

P

NURSING CONSIDERATIONS

Assessment: Assess for drug hypersensitivity or idiosyncracy, acute abdominal conditions, convulsive disorders, hepatic/renal impairment, fever, thyroid diseases, Addison's disease, ulcerative colitis, prostatic hypertrophy, history of recent GI tract surgery, narrow-angle glaucoma, prostatic hypertrophy, stenosing peptic ulcer, pyloroduodenal obstruction, and bladder neck obstruction, CVD, BP, pregnancy/nursing status, and possible drug/lab test interactions.

Monitoring: Monitor for CNS and respiratory depression, bone marrow depression, cholestatic jaundice, seizures, signs/symptoms of NMS, BP, convulsions/hallucinations and dystonias in children, false positive and false negative interpretations in pregnancy tests, blood glucose, and CBC. Inform about orthostatic hypotension and overdose symptoms such as extreme sleepiness.

Patient Counseling: Advise to use caution during hazardous tasks (eg, operating machinery/driving). Counsel to report any involuntary muscle movements. Avoid alcohol; limit sunlight exposure. Inform not to be taken by nursing mothers.

Administration: Oral route. **Storage:** 20-25°C (68-77°F).

PROMETHAZINE W/CODEINE

promethazine HCl - codeine phosphate (Various)

CV

THERAPEUTIC CLASS: Phenothiazine derivative/antitussive

INDICATIONS: Temporary relief of coughs and upper respiratory symptoms associated with allergy or the common cold.

DOSAGE: *Adults:* >12 yrs: 5mL q4-6h. Max: 30mL/24 hr.
Pediatrics: 6-<12 yrs: 2.5-5mL q4-6h. Max: 30mL/24 hr.

HOW SUPPLIED: Syrup: (Promethazine-Codeine) 6.25mg-10mg/5mL

CONTRAINDICATIONS: Comatose states, treatment of lower respiratory tract symptoms (eg, asthma), pediatric patients <6 yrs.

WARNINGS/PRECAUTIONS: May cause or aggravate constipation. May lead to potentially fatal respiratory depression; avoid with compromised respiratory function (eg, COPD, sleep apnea). Caution in atopic children. May elevate CSF pressure; caution with head injury, intracranial lesions, or pre-existing increase in ICP. Avoid with asthma, acute febrile illness with chronic cough, or with chronic respiratory disease where interference with ability to clear tracheobronchial tree of secretions would have a deleterious effect on patient's respiratory function. May cause orthostatic hypotension. May impair mental/physical abilities. May lower seizure threshold; caution with seizure disorders. Caution with bone marrow depression; leukopenia and agranulocytosis reported. Neuroleptic malignant syndrome reported. Hallucinations and convulsions have occurred in pediatrics. Cholestatic jaundice reported. Caution with acute abdominal conditions, convulsive disorders, significant hepatic/renal impairment, fever, hypothyroidism, Addison's disease, ulcerative colitis, prostatic hypertrophy, recent GI or urinary tract surgery, elderly, debilitated, narrow-angle glaucoma, stenosing peptic ulcer, pyloroduodenal or bladder-neck obstruction, or cardiovascular disease. May alter HCG pregnancy test reading. May increase blood glucose. Avoid prolonged exposure to sunlight.

ADVERSE REACTIONS: Drowsiness, dizziness, sedation, blurred vision, dry mouth, increased or decreased blood pressure, rash, nausea, vomiting, constipation, urinary retention.

INTERACTIONS: May increase, prolong, or intensify the sedative action of other CNS depressants such as alcohol, sedative/hypnotics (including barbiturates), narcotics, narcotic analgesics, general anesthetics, TCAs, and tranquilizers; avoid such agents or administer in reduced dosages. Reduce barbiturate dose by at least one-half and narcotic analgesics by one-quarter to one-half. May reverse epinehrine's vasopressor effect. Caution with concomitant use of other agents with anticholinergic properties. May lower seizure threshold; caution with concomitant medications which may also affect seizure threshold (eg, narcotics, local anesthetics). Avoid concomitant administration with other respiratory depressants in pediatrics. Possible interaction with MAOIs; consider small test dose.

PREGNANCY: Category C, caution in nursing.

MECHANISM OF ACTION: Promethazine: Phenothiazine derivative; blocks H_1 receptor (antihistaminic action) and provides sedative and antiemetic effects. Codeine: Narcotic analgesic and antitussive; primary effects are on CNS and GI tract.

PHARMACOKINETICS: Absorption: Promethazine and codeine (well absorbed). **Distribution:** Codeine: Found in breast milk. **Metabolism:** Promethazine: Liver. Codeine: Liver via O-demethylation, N-demethylation, and partial conjugation with glucuronic acid. **Elimination:** Promethazine: Urine (sulfoxides and N-demethylpromethazine). Codeine: Urine (inactive metabolites and free/conjugated morphine), feces (codeine and metabolites).

NURSING CONSIDERATIONS

Assessment: Assess for respiratory, cardiac, liver, renal, thyroid functions; convulsive disorders, Addison's disease, narrow-angle glaucoma and bone marrow depression, head injury or increased intracranial pressure, asthma,

P

drug hypersensitivity or idiosyncracy reaction, and possible drug and test interactions.

Monitoring: Monitor for CNS/respiratory depression, constipation, cholestatic jaundice, seizures, bone marrow suppression, signs/symptoms of NMS, BP, interference with pregnancy test, CBC, and glucose levels.

Patient Counseling: Caution during hazardous tasks (eg, operating machinery/driving). Report any involuntary muscle movements. Avoid alcohol; limit sunlight exposure. Not to be given to nursing women. Inform about orthostatic hypotension and overdose symptoms.

Administration: Oral route. **Storage:** 20-25°C (68-77°F).

PROPECIA RX

finasteride (Merck)

THERAPEUTIC CLASS: Type II 5 alpha-reductase inhibitor

INDICATIONS: Treatment of male pattern hair loss (androgenetic alopecia). For men only.

DOSAGE: *Adults:* 1mg qd. Continue use to sustain benefit.

HOW SUPPLIED: Tab: 1mg [ProPak, 3 x 30 tabs]

CONTRAINDICATIONS: Pregnancy or women who may potentially become pregnant.

WARNINGS/PRECAUTIONS: Caution with hepatic dysfunction. Consider doubling PSA level results in men >41 yrs of age, without BPH, who are undergoing PSA test. Women who are pregnant or may become pregnant should not handle crushed or broken tablets; potential risk to a male fetus. Do not use in pediatrics or women.

ADVERSE REACTIONS: Decreased libido, erectile dysfunction, decreased volume of ejaculate, breast tenderness, hypersensitivity reactions.

PREGNANCY: Category X, not for use in nursing.

MECHANISM OF ACTION: Competitive and specific inhibitor of type II 5-α reductase; blocks peripheral conversion of testosterone to DHT, resulting in significant decreases in serum and tissue DHT concentrations.

P

PHARMACOKINETICS: Absorption: C_{max}=9.2ng/mL; T_{max}=1-2 hrs; AUC=53ng•hr/mL. **Distribution:** V_d=76L; plasma protein binding (approximately 90%); crosses blood-brain barrier. **Metabolism:** Liver (extensive); via CYP3A4. **Elimination:** Urine (39%, metabolites), feces (57%); $T_{1/2}$=4.5 hrs.

NURSING CONSIDERATIONS

Assessment: Assess for drug hypersensitivity, liver dysfunction, and pregnancy status.

Monitoring: Monitor for breast changes (eg, lumps, pain, nipple discharge, breast enlargement, tenderness, neoplasm). Interaction with interpretation of serum PSA levels in BPH.

Patient Counseling: Caution women who are pregnant/nursing or planning to become pregnant not to handle broken or crushed tabs. Inform about risks; promptly report breast changes.

Administration: Oral route. **Storage:** 15-30°C (59-86°F).

PROPYLTHIOURACIL RX

propylthiouracil (Various)

THERAPEUTIC CLASS: Thiourea-derivative antithyroid agent

INDICATIONS: Treatment of hyperthyroidism.

DOSAGE: *Adults:* Initial: 300mg/day in 3 divided doses, q8h. Severe Hyperthyroidism/Very Large Goiters: Initial: 400mg/day in 3 divided doses; may give up to 600-900mg/day if needed. Maint: 100-150mg/day.

Pediatrics: 6-10 yrs: Initial: 50-150mg/day. ≥10 yrs: Initial: 150-300mg/day. Maint: Determine by patient response.

HOW SUPPLIED: Tab: 50mg

CONTRAINDICATIONS: Nursing mothers.

WARNINGS/PRECAUTIONS: D/C with agranulocytosis, aplastic anemia, hepatitis, fever, or exfoliative dermatitis. Rare reports of severe hepatic reactions exist. D/C with significant hepatic abnormality, including transaminases >3x ULN. Caution with pregnancy, may cause fetal harm. Monitor PT and TFTs.

ADVERSE REACTIONS: Agranulocytosis, granulopenia, thrombocytopenia, aplastic anemia, drug fever, hepatitis, periarteritis, hypoprothrombinemia, skin rash, urticaria, NV, epigastric distress, arthralgia, paresthesias.

INTERACTIONS: May potentiate anticoagulant effects. Hyperthyroidism increases clearance of β-blockers; reduce β-blocker dose when patient becomes euthyroid. Increased digitalis glycoside levels when patient becomes euthyroid; reduce digitalis dose. Decreased theophylline clearance when patient becomes euthyroid; reduce theophylline dose. Caution with other drugs that cause agranulocytosis.

PREGNANCY: Category D, contraindicated in nursing.

MECHANISM OF ACTION: Antithyroid agent; inhibits synthesis of thyroid hormones.

PHARMACOKINETICS: Absorption: GI tract (readily absorbed). **Distribution:** Found in breast milk, crosses placental membranes. **Elimination:** Urine (35%); $T_{1/2}$=24 hrs.

NURSING CONSIDERATIONS

Assessment: Assess for drug hypersensitivity, pregnancy/nursing status, and possible drug interactions.

Monitoring: Monitor for fever, sore throat, interstitial pneumonitis, exfoliative dermatitis, and ANCA-positive vasculitis. Requires frequent lab tests including CBC, PT , thyroid function, LFTs, and bone marrow function.

Patient Counseling: Instruct to inform physician if pregnant/nursing or planning to become pregnant. Advise to report signs/symptoms of illness (eg, fever, sore throat, skin eruptions, headache, general malaise).

Administration: Oral route. **Storage:** 15-30°C (59-86°F).

PROQUAD RX

varicella virus vaccine live - rubella vaccine live - measles vaccine live - mumps vaccine live (Merck)

THERAPEUTIC CLASS: Vaccine

INDICATIONS: Vaccination against measles, mumps, rubella, and varicella in children 12 months to 12 yrs of age.

DOSAGE: *Pediatrics:* 12 months-12 yrs: 0.5mL SQ. At least 1 month should elapse between dose of measles-containing vaccine and dose of ProQuad. If for any reason a 2nd dose of varicella-containing vaccine is required, at least 3 months should elapse between doses.

HOW SUPPLIED: Inj: 0.5mL

CONTRAINDICATIONS: Anaphylactic reactions to neomycin; hypersensitivity to gelatin; blood dyscrasias, leukemia, lymphomas, or other malignant neoplasms affecting the bone marrow or lymphatic system; immunosuppressive therapy; primary and acquired immunodeficiency states (e.g., AIDS/HIV); congenital or hereditary immunodeficiency; active untreated tuberculosis; active febrile illness with fever >101.3°F; pregnant. Disseminated varicella vaccine virus infection has been reported in children with underlying immunodeficiency disorders who were inadvertently vaccinated with a varicella-containing vaccine.

WARNINGS/PRECAUTIONS: Caution with egg allergy. May cause thrombocytopenia. Contains albumin, remote risk of viral infection transmission.

Have epinephrine (1:1000) available. Caution with a history of cerebral injury, history of or active convulsions or any condition in which stress due to fever should be avoided.

ADVERSE REACTIONS: Injection Site: Pain/tenderness/soreness, erythema, swelling. Systemic: Fever, irritability, measles-like rash, herpes zoster and varicella infection, anaphylactic reaction, ataxia, convulsions, febrile seizure, pruritus.

INTERACTIONS: Do not give with immune globulin. Avoid use of salicylates for 6 weeks after vaccination. Avoid use of immunosuppressive doses of corticosteriods or other immunosuppressive drugs.

PREGNANCY: Category C, not for use in nursing.

MECHANISM OF ACTION: Vaccine; stimulates immune system to elicit immune response to produce antibodies that may protect against measles, mumps, rubella, and varicella disease.

NURSING CONSIDERATIONS

Assessment: Assess for history of anaphylactic reactions to neomycin, hypersensitivity to gelatin or any other component of vaccine, congenital or hereditary immunodeficiency, health status, immunization history, and varicella. Assess for blood dyscrasias, leukemia, lymphoma or other malignant neoplasms affecting bone marrow or lymphatic system, active untreated TB, active febrile illness with fever, pregnancy status, and possible drug interactions.

Monitoring: Monitor for thrombocytopenia, Reye's syndrome, and adverse reactions at injection site (eg, pain, tenderness, soreness, erythema, swelling, ecchymosis, rash).

Patient Counseling: Inform of potential benefits/risk; report adverse reactions. Vaccine may not offer 100% protection. Inform to avoid use of salicylates for 6 weeks after vaccination, and to postpone pregnancy for 3 months after vaccination.

Administration: SQ route; 1) Inspect for particulate matter and discoloration before administration. 2) Inject SQ in outer aspect of deltoid region of upper arm or in higher anterolateral area of thigh. **Storage:** Refrigerate at 2-8°C (36-46°F) or store at room temperature, 20-25°C (68-77°F). Do not freeze. Discard within 30 min if not in use.

PROQUIN XR RX

ciprofloxacin HCl (Depomed)

Fluoroquinolones are associated with an increased risk of tendinitis and tendon rupture in all ages. Risk further increased in patients >60 yrs, patients taking corticosteroid drugs, and patients with kidney, heart or lung transplants.

THERAPEUTIC CLASS: Fluoroquinolone

INDICATIONS: Treatment of uncomplicated urinary tract infections (acute cystitis) caused by *E.coli* and *K.pneumoniae*.

DOSAGE: *Adults:* 500mg qd with pm meal for 3 days. Administer at least 4 hrs before or 2 hrs after magnesium- or aluminum-containing antacids, sucralfate, Videx (didanosine) chewable/buffered tablets of pediatric powder, metal cations (eg, iron), multivitamins with zinc. Do not split, crush, or chew. Swallow tab whole.

HOW SUPPLIED: Tab, Extended-Release: 500mg

WARNINGS/PRECAUTIONS: Convulsions, increased ICP and toxic psychosis reported. D/C if dizziness, confusion, tremors, hallucinations, depression, or suicidal thoughts/acts. Caution with CNS disorders or if predisposed to seizures. May cause CNS events (eg, agitation, insomnia, anxiety, nightmares, or paranoia). Severe, fatal hypersensitivity reactions may occur. *Clostridium difficile*-associated diarrhea, colitis, achilles and other tendon ruptures reported. D/C at first sign of rash, jaundice or if pain, inflammation, or ruptured tendon occurs. Maintain hydration; avoid alkaline urine. Avoid excessive sunlight and

UV light. Not interchangeable with immediate-release or other extended-release oral formulations. D/C if symptoms of peripheral neuropathy occur. Caution in elderly taking corticosteroids.

ADVERSE REACTIONS: Fungal infection, nasopharyngitis, headache, micturition urgency.

INTERACTIONS: Increases theophylline and caffeine levels and prolongs effects. Serious/fatal reactions have occurred with theophylline. Magnesium-or-aluminum containing antacids, sucralfate, Videx (didanosine) chewable/buffered tablets or pediatric powder, and products containing calcium, iron, or zinc decrease serum and urine levels; administer at least 4 hrs before or 2 hrs after these drugs. Altered serum levels of phenytoin. Severe hypoglycemia with glyburide (rare). Potentiated by probenecid. Transient serum creatinine elevations with cyclosporine. Enhances oral anticoagulant effects. May increase risk of methotrexate toxic reactions due to inhibition of renal tubular transport. High-dose quinolones shown to provoke convulsions with NSAIDs (not ASA).

PREGNANCY: Category C, not for use in nursing.

MECHANISM OF ACTION: Broad-spectrum fluoroquinolone; inhibits topoisomerase II (DNA gyrase) and topoisomerase IV (both type II topoisomerases), which are required for bacterial DNA replication, transcription, repair, and recombination.

PHARMACOKINETICS: Absorption: (500mg) C_{max}=0.82mcg/mL; T_{max}=6.1 hrs; AUC=7.67mcg•h/mL. (250mg bid) C_{max}=0.57mcg/mL (pm), 0.93mcg/mL (am); T_{max}=2.5 hrs; AUC=7.83mcg•h/mL. **Distribution:** Plasma protein binding (9.9-36.6%). **Metabolism:** Desethyleneciprofloxacin, sulfociprofloxacin, oxociprofloxacin and formylciprofloxacin (metabolites). **Elimination:** Urine (26.9%), feces; $T_{1/2}$=4.5 hrs.

NURSING CONSIDERATIONS

Assessment: Assess for pregnancy/nursing status, CNS disorders (severe cerebral arteriosclerosis, epilepsy), and possible drug interactions.

Monitoring: Monitor for signs/symptoms of convulsions, increased ICP, toxic psychosis, *C. difficile*-associated diarrhea, neuropathy, tendinitis or rupture of tendon, phototoxicity, and hypersensitivity reactions.

Patient Counseling: Instruct to take with evening meal; swallow whole, do not split, crush, or chew; do not take with dairy products; take 4 hrs before or 2 hrs after antacids; ensure adequate hydration to prevent crystalluria. Notify healthcare provider if symptoms of pain, swelling, or inflammation of a tendon, or weakness or inability to move joints; rest and refrain from exercise; and d/c therapy. Inform therapy treats bacterial, not viral, infections. Take as directed; skipping doses or not completing full course may decrease effectiveness and increase resistance. D/C and notify healthcare provider if skin rash, other allergic reactions, or watery and bloody stools (with or without stomach cramps and fever) occur. Notify if pregnant/nursing or taking antacids or sucralfate. Use caution in activity requiring mental alertness and coordination. Avoid excessive sun exposure. Take full course as prescribed.

Administration: Oral route. **Storage:** 25°C (77°F); excursions permitted to 15-30°C (59-86°F).

PROSCAR — RX

finasteride (Merck)

THERAPEUTIC CLASS: Type II 5 alpha-reductase inhibitor

INDICATIONS: Treatment of symptomatic benign prostatic hypertrophy (BPH) to improve symptoms, reduce the risk of acute urinary retention, and reduce the risk of the need for prostate surgery. To reduce the risk of symptomatic progression of BPH in combination with doxazosin.

DOSAGE: *Adults:* 5mg qd.

HOW SUPPLIED: Tab: 5mg

P

CONTRAINDICATIONS: Pregnancy.

WARNINGS/PRECAUTIONS: Not for use in pediatrics or women. Risk to male fetus in pregnancy. Pregnant women should not handle crushed or broken tablets. Rule out infection, prostate cancer, stricture disease, hypotonic bladder prior to initiating therapy. Caution with liver dysfunction. Decreases serum PSA levels by ~50% in patients with BPH, even with prostate cancer; adjust (double) PSA results to compare with normal values. Monitor for obstructive uropathy with large residual urinary volume and/or severely diminished urinary flow.

ADVERSE REACTIONS: Impotence, decreased libido, decreased ejaculate volume, hypersensitivity reactions (pruritus, urticaria, swelling of lips and face), testicular pain.

PREGNANCY: Category X, not for use in nursing.

MECHANISM OF ACTION: Type II 5α-reductase inhibitor; inhibits type II 5α-reductase which metabolizes testosterone to 5α-dihydrotestosterone (DHT), a potent androgen needed for development and enlargement of prostate gland.

PHARMACOKINETICS: Absorption: Absolute bioavailability (63%); C_{max}=37ng/mL; T_{max}=1-2 hrs. **Distribution:** V_d=76L; plasma protein binding (90%). **Metabolism:** CYP3A4. **Elimination:** Feces (major), urine; $T_{1/2}$=6 hrs.

NURSING CONSIDERATIONS

Assessment: Assess for pregnancy status, impaired liver function, infection, prostate cancer, stricture disease, hypotonic bladder, neurogenic disorder, possible drug interactions, large residual urinary volume, or severely diminished urinary flow.

Monitoring: Monitor PSA. Monitor for signs/symptoms of hypersensitivity reaction and changes in breasts.

Patient Counseling: Instruct pregnant women not to handle crushed or broken tablets due to potential risk to fetus. Inform males volume of ejaculate may decrease. Advise to notify physician if changes in breast (lumps, pain, nipple discharge) or hypersensitivity reactions occur.

Administration: Oral route. **Storage:** Below 30°C (86°F). Protect from light and keep container tightly closed.

PROTAMINE SULFATE — RX

protamine sulfate (Various)

> **May cause severe hypotension, cardiovascular collapse, noncardiogenic pulmonary edema, catastrophic pulmonary vasoconstriction, and pulmonary HTN; risk factors include high dose/overdose, rapid/previous administration, repeated doses, and current/previous use of protamine-containing drugs. Risk to benefit of administration should be carefully considered with presence of any risk factors. Should not be given when bleeding occurs without prior heparin use.**

THERAPEUTIC CLASS: Heparin antagonist

INDICATIONS: Management of heparin overdose.

DOSAGE: *Adults:* Administer as very slow IV infusion over 10 min in doses not to exceed 50mg. Determine dose by blood coagulation studies. Each mg neutralizes not less than 100 USP heparin units.

HOW SUPPLIED: Inj: 10mg/mL [5mL, 25mL]

WARNINGS/PRECAUTIONS: May cause allergic reactions with fish hypersensitivity. Rapid administration may cause severe hypotensive and anaphylactoid-like reactions. Caution in cardiac surgeries; hyperheparinemia or bleeding reported. Previous exposure to protamine/protamine-containing insulin may induce humoral immune response; severe hypersensitivity reaction, including life-threatening anaphylaxis reported. Increased risk of antiprotamine antibodies in infertile or vasectomized men.

ADVERSE REACTIONS: Hypotension, bradycardia, transitory flushing/feeling of warmth, lassitude, dyspnea, NV, back pain, anaphylaxis that causes severe respiratory distress, circulatory collapse, noncardiogenic pulmonary edema, acute pulmonary HTN.

INTERACTIONS: Incompatible with certain antibiotics, such as cephalosporins and penicillins. Concomitant or previous use of protamine-containing drugs (eg, NPH insulin, protamine zinc insulin, certain beta-blockers) is risk factor for severe adverse events; see Black Box Warning.

PREGNANCY: Category C, caution in nursing.

MECHANISM OF ACTION: Heparin antagonist; has anticoagulant effects when administered alone, however, when given in presence of heparin, a stable salt is formed and anticoagulant activity of both drugs is lost.

NURSING CONSIDERATIONS

Assessment: Assess for fish allergy, previous vasectomy, previous exposure, severe left ventricular dysfunction, abnormal preoperative pulmonary hemodynamics, and possible drug interactions. Assess blood coagulation studies for appropriate dosage.

Monitoring: Monitor for hypersensitivity/allergic reactions, hypotension, CV collapse, pulmonary edema, and pulmonary HTN. Monitor blood coagulation studies.

Administration: Slow IV infusion. Large-size 25mL vials are designed for antiheparin treatment only when large doses of heparin have been given during surgery. **Storage:** 20-25°C (68-77°F). Do not freeze.

PROTONIX RX

pantoprazole sodium (Wyeth)

OTHER BRAND NAMES: Protonix IV (Wyeth)

THERAPEUTIC CLASS: Proton pump inhibitor

INDICATIONS: (PO) Short-term treatment (up to 8 weeks) and maintenance of healing of erosive esophagitis associated with GERD. Long-term treatment of pathological hypersecretory conditions (eg, Zollinger-Ellison syndrome). (Inj) Short-term treatment (7-10 days) of GERD with a history of erosive esophagitis. Treatment of pathological hypersecretory conditions associated with Zollinger-Ellison syndrome or other neoplastic conditions.

DOSAGE: *Adults:* (PO) Erosive Esophagitis Treatment: 40mg qd for up to 8 weeks. May repeat for 8 weeks if needed. Maint: 40mg qd. Hypersecretory Conditions: Initial: 40mg bid. Adjust to patient's needs. Max: 240mg/day. (Inj) GERD: 40mg IV qd for 7-10 days. Pathological Hypersecretory Conditions: 80mg IV q12h. May adjust up to 80mg IV q8h based on acid output. Max: 240mg/day. Duration >6 days not studied. Do not split, crush or chew tabs.

HOW SUPPLIED: Inj: 40mg; Sus, Delayed-Release: 40mg (granules/pkt); Tab, Delayed-Release: 20mg, 40mg

WARNINGS/PRECAUTIONS: Symptomatic response does not preclude the presence of gastric malignancy. Atrophic gastritis has been noted occasionally in gastric corpus biopsies from patients treated for long-term. False (+) urine screening test for THC reported. Vitamin B-12 deficiency reported with long-term use (>3 yrs). (Inj) Immediate hypersensitivity reactions reported (eg, thrombophlebitis, LFT elevation).

ADVERSE REACTIONS: (Inj) Abdominal pain, headache, constipation, dyspepsia, nausea, inj site reactions. (PO) Headache, flatulence, diarrhea, abdominal pain.

INTERACTIONS: May alter absorption of pH-dependent drugs (eg, ketoconazole, ampicillin esters, and iron salts). May substantially decrease atazanavir levels; avoid concomitant use. May increase INR and prothrombin time with concomitant warfarin therapy.

PREGNANCY: Category B, not for use in nursing.

MECHANISM OF ACTION: Proton pump inhibitor; suppresses final step in gastric acid production by covalently binding to the (H^+,K^+)-ATPase enzyme system at the secretory surface of the gastric parietal cell. Leads to inhibition of both basal and stimulated gastric acid secretion irrespective of the stimulus.

PHARMACOKINETICS: Absorption: (PO) Well absorbed; absolute bioavailability (77%); C_{max}=2.52mcg/mL; T_{max}=2.5 hr; AUC=4.8mcg•hr/mL. (IV) C_{max}=5.52mcg/mL; AUC=5.4mcg•hr/mL. **Distribution:** V_d=11.0-23.6L; plasma protein binding (98%); found in breast milk. **Metabolism:** Liver (extensive) via CYP2C19 (demethylation), sulfation; CYP3A4 (oxidation). **Elimination:** Urine (71%), feces (18%); $T_{1/2}$=1 hr.

NURSING CONSIDERATIONS

Assessment: Assess for gastric malignancy, pregnancy/nursing status, and possible drug interactions.

Monitoring: Monitor for signs/symptoms of GI tumors, vitamin B-12 deficiency, and atrophic gastritis. In patients using IV formulation, monitor for hypersensitivity reaction (eg, anaphylaxis), injection-site reactions (eg, thrombophlebitis), zinc deficiency, and hepatic effects (eg, elevations in transaminases).

Patient Counseling: If using IV formulation, switch treatment to oral formulation as soon as patient is able. Contact physician immediately if hypersensitivity or other adverse events occur. If taking oral formulation, swallow whole, with or without food in stomach; do not split, crush, or chew tablet. Concomitant administration of antacids does not effect absorption of tablets. If using suspension formulation, administer in applesauce or apple juice approximately 30 min before meal; do not place in water, other liquids, or food.

Administration: Oral and IV route. IV lines should be flushed prior to and after administration with either 5% Dextrose Inj, USP, 0.9% NaCl Inj USP, or Lactated Ringer's Inj, USP. **Storage:** 20-25°C (68-77°F); excursions permitted to 15-30°C (59-86°F). Protect injection vials from light; do not freeze.

PROTOPIC RX

tacrolimus (Astellas)

THERAPEUTIC CLASS: Macrolide immunosuppressant

INDICATIONS: Short-term and intermittent long-term therapy of moderate to severe atopic dermatitis intolerant or unresponsive to conventional therapy.

DOSAGE: *Adults:* (0.03% or 0.1%) Apply thin layer bid. Rub in gently. Stop use when signs and symptoms resolve.
Pediatrics: ≥16 yrs: (0.03% or 0.1%) Apply thin layer bid. Rub in gently. 2-15 yrs: (0.03%) Apply thin layer bid. Rub in gently. Stop use when signs and symptoms resolve.

HOW SUPPLIED: Oint: 0.03%, 0.1% [30g, 60g, 100g]

WARNINGS/PRECAUTIONS: Do not use with occlusive dressings. Increased risk of varicella zoster, herpes simplex, or eczema herpeticum. Lymphadenopathy reported; monitor closely. D/C if unknown etiology of lymphadenopathy or presence of acute infectious mononucleosis. Avoid in Netherton's syndrome. Minimize or avoid exposure to natural or artificial sunlight. Long-term safety not established. Rare cases of malignancy (eg, skin and lymphoma) reported with topical calcineurin inhibitors; therefore, continuous long-term use should be avoided and application limited to areas of involvement. Should not use in immunocompromised adults and children. Caution in patients predisposed to renal impairment. Not indicated for use in children <2 yrs. Only 0.03% oint is indicated for use in children 2-15 yrs.

ADVERSE REACTIONS: Skin burning, pruritus, flu-like symptoms, allergic reaction, skin erythema, headache, skin infection, fever, herpes simplex, rhinitis.

INTERACTIONS: Caution with CYP3A4 inhibitors (eg, erythromycin, itraconazole, ketoconazole, fluconazole, CCBs, cimetidine) in widespread and/or erythrodermic disease. Increased risk for lymphomas in transplant patients receiving other immunosuppressive therapy.

PREGNANCY: Category C, not for use in nursing.

MECHANISM OF ACTION: Macrolide immunosuppressant; not known in atopic dermatitis. Inhibits T-lymphocyte activation by first binding to an intracellular protein, FKBP-12. A complex of tacrolimus-FKBP-12, calcium, calmodulin, and calcineurin is then formed and the phosphate activity of calcineurin is inhibited. This has been shown to prevent the dephosphorylation and translocation of nuclear factor of activated T-cells.

PHARMACOKINETICS: Absorption: Absolute bioavailability (0.5%), C_{max}<2ng/mL (90% of population). **Distribution:** V_d=99%. **Metabolism:** CYP3A (extensive); demethylation and hydroxylation; 13-demethyl tacrolimus (major metabolite). **Elimination:** Feces (major).

NURSING CONSIDERATIONS

Assessment: Assess for history of hypersensitivity to tacrolimus or any other component of the ointment, premalignant and malignant skin conditions, and renal impairment. Prior to initiation, resolve cutaneous bacterial or viral infections at treatment sites.

Monitoring: Monitor for varicella zoster virus infection (chickenpox or shingles), acute mononucleosis, lymphomas, skin malignancies (eg, cutaneous T-cell lymphoma), lymphadenopathy, and acute renal failure. Monitor improvement of signs/symptoms of atopic dermatitis within 6 weeks.

Patient Counseling: Advise to be re-examined if signs/symptoms of atopic dermatitis do not improve within 6 weeks. Instruct to d/c when signs/symptoms of eczema (eg, itching, rash and redness) occur; avoid ultraviolet therapy sun lamps and tanning beds during treatment. Advise to limit sun exposure, to wear loose-fitting clothing that protects treated area from the sun, and not to cover treated skin with bandages, dressings, or wraps.

Administration: Topical. **Storage:** 25°C (77°F); excursions permitted to 15-30°C (59-86°F).

PROVENTIL HFA — RX

albuterol sulfate (Schering)

THERAPEUTIC CLASS: $Beta_2$-agonist

INDICATIONS: Prevention and treatment of bronchospasm with reversible obstructive airway disease; prevention of exercise-induced bronchospasm (EIB) in patients ≥4 yrs.

DOSAGE: *Adults:* Bronchospasm: 2 inh q4-6h or 1 inh q4h. EIB: 2 inh 15-30 min before activity.
Pediatrics: ≥4 yrs: Bronchospasm: 2 inh q4-6h or 1 inh q4h. EIB: 2 inh 15-30 min before activity.

HOW SUPPLIED: MDI: 90mcg/inh [6.7g]

WARNINGS/PRECAUTIONS: Hypersensitivity reactions reported. Monitor for worsening asthma. Fatalities reported with excessive use. Caution with cardiovascular disorders, especially coronary insufficiency, arrhythmias and HTN. May need concomitant corticosteroids. Can produce paradoxical bronschospasm. Caution with DM, hyperthyroidism, and seizures. May cause transient hypokalemia.

ADVERSE REACTIONS: Tachycardia, tremor, dizziness, nausea/vomiting, palpitations, rhinitis, upper respiratory tract infection, fever, inhalation site and taste sensation, back pain, and nervousness.

INTERACTIONS: Avoid other sympathomimetic agents. Extreme caution wtih MAOIs and TCAs. Monitor digoxin. May worsen ECG changes and/or hypokalemia with non-K^+-sparing diuretics. Antagonized by β-blockers.

PREGNANCY: Category C, not for use in nursing.

MECHANISM OF ACTION: β_2-adrenergic bronchodilator; stimulates adenyl cylase, the enzyme that catalyzes the formation of cAMP from ATP. Increased cAMP levels are associated with relaxation of bronchial smooth muscle and inhibition of release of mediators of immediate hypersensitivity.

P

NURSING CONSIDERATIONS

Assessment: Assess for convulsive disorders, hyperthyroidism, DM, CVD, and possible drug interactions.

Monitoring: Monitor pulse rate, BP, ECG changes, for paradoxical bronchospasm and hypokalemia, hypersensitivity reactions, and deterioration of asthma.

Patient Counseling: Take as directed. Report lack of response or adverse side effects.

Administration: Oral inhalation. 1) Prime inhaler before using for first time or if inhaler has not been used for 2 weeks by releasing 4 test sprays into air, away from face. 2) Clean inhaler at least once a week. Use only with actuator supplied with product. 3) Discard inhaler after 200 sprays. **Storage:** 15-25°C (59-77°F).

PROVERA RX

medroxyprogesterone acetate (Pharmacia & Upjohn)

Not for use for prevention of cardiovascular disease or dementia. Increased risk of MI, stroke, invasive breast cancer, pulmonary emboli, and DVT in postmenopausal women (50-79 yrs) reported. Increased risk of developing probable dementia in postmenopausal women (≥65 yrs) reported.

THERAPEUTIC CLASS: Progestogen

INDICATIONS: Secondary amenorrhea and for abnormal uterine bleeding due to hormonal imbalance in the absence of organic pathology, such as fibroids or uterine cancer. To reduce the incidence of endometrial hyperplasia in non-hysterectomized postmenopausal women receiving 0.625mg conjugated estrogen.

DOSAGE: *Adults:* Secondary Amenorrhea: 5-10mg qd for 5-10 days. Abnormal Uterine Bleeding: 5-10mg qd for 5-10 days beginning on day 16 or day 21 of cycle. Endometrial Hyperplasia: 5-10mg qd for 12-14 consecutive days per month beginning on day 1 or day 16 of cycle.

HOW SUPPLIED: Tab: 2.5mg*, 5mg*, 10mg* *scored

P

CONTRAINDICATIONS: Thrombophlebitis, thromboembolic disorders, cerebral apoplexy, liver dysfunction, malignancy of breast or genital organs, undiagnosed vaginal bleeding, missed abortion, pregnancy, as a diagnostic test for pregnancy.

WARNINGS/PRECAUTIONS: D/C if develop thrombotic disorders, papilledema, or retinal vascular lesions. D/C pending exam if sudden onset of proptosis, sudden partial or complete loss of vision, diplopia, or migraine. Include pap smear in pretreatment exam. Caution with depression, DM, and conditions aggravated by fluid retention (eg, epilepsy, migraine, asthma, cardiac, renal dysfunction). Increased risk of endometrial and ovarian cancer reported.

ADVERSE REACTIONS: Abnormal uterine bleeding, breast tenderness, galactorrhea, urticaria, pruritus, edema, rash, thromboembolic phenomena, menstrual changes, change in weight, cervical changes, cholestatic jaundice, depression, insomnia, nausea, somnolence.

PREGNANCY: Category X, not for use in nursing.

MECHANISM OF ACTION: Progesterone derivative; transforms proliferative into secretory endometrium.

PHARMACOKINETICS: Absorption: (10mg) Rapid; C_{max}=0.71ng/mL; T_{max}=2.83 hrs; AUC=6.01ng•h/mL. **Distribution:** V_d=40564L; plasma protein binding (90%). **Metabolism:** hydroxylation, conjugation. **Elimination:** Urine.

NURSING CONSIDERATIONS

Assessment: Assess for undiagnosed abnormal genital bleeding; known/suspected or history of breast cancer, estrogen or progesterone-dependent neoplasia, pregnancy status, missed abortion, thromboembolic disease, CAD, asthma, DM, epilepsy, SLE, migraine, porphyria, hypocalcemia, cardiac or renal/hepatic impairment.

Monitoring: Monitor BP regularly; breast exam by physician yearly and self monthly; mammogram as required. Monitor for signs/symptoms of thromboembolic disease (eg, stroke, DVT, PE, MI), HTN, hypocalcemia, abnormal vaginal bleeding, dementia, visual abnormalities, hypersensitivity reactions, hepatic dysfunction, fluid retention, exacerbation of asthma, DM, epilepsy, SLE, migraine, and porphyria.

Patient Counseling: Inform of pregnancy risks. Advise to seek medical attention if symptoms of hepatic dysfunction (jaundice), hypocalcemia, visual abnormalities (partial/complete loss of vision, diplopia, migraines), abnormal vaginal bleeding, hypersensitivity reactions, HTN, thromboembolic disease, fluid retention, exacerbation of diseases, or dementia occur.

Administration: Oral route. **Storage:** 20-25°C (68-77°F).

PROVIGIL CIV

modafinil (Cephalon)

THERAPEUTIC CLASS: Wakefulness-promoting agent

INDICATIONS: To improve wakefulness in patients with excessive daytime sleepiness associated with narcolepsy, obstructive sleep apnea/hypopnea syndrome (OSAHS), shiftwork sleep disorder (SWSD). As adjunct treatment for underlying obstruction in OSAHS.

DOSAGE: *Adults:* 200mg qd. Narcolepsy/OSAHS: Take in AM. SWSD: Take 1 hr prior to start of work shift. Hepatic Dysfunction: 100mg qd. Elderly: Consider dose reduction.

HOW SUPPLIED: Tab: 100mg, 200mg* *scored

WARNINGS/PRECAUTIONS: Avoid in history of left ventricular hypertrophy, ischemic ECG changes, chest pain, arrhythmia or other manifestations of mitral valve prolapse with CNS stimulants. Caution if recent MI, unstable angina, history of psychosis. Monitor hypertensive patients. Rare cases of severe or life-threatening rash, including Stevens-Johnson syndrome (SJS), toxic epidermal necrolysis (TEN), and drug rash with eosinophilia and systemic symptoms (DRESS) have been reported with the use of modafinil. Angioedema and anaphylactoid reactions reported.

ADVERSE REACTIONS: Headache, infection, nausea, nervousness, anxiety, insomnia, rhinitis, diarrhea, back pain, dizziness, dyspepsia, hostility.

INTERACTIONS: Methylphenidate may delay absorption. May reduce efficacy of steroidal contraceptives up to 1 month after discontinuation. Caution with MAOIs. CYP3A4 inducers (eg, carbamazepine, phenobarbital, rifampin) may decrease levels. CYP3A4 inhibitors (eg, ketoconazole, itraconazole) may increase levels. May increase levels of drugs metabolized by CYP2C19 (eg, diazepam, propranolol, phenytoin) or CYP2C9 (eg, warfarin). Monitor for toxicity with phenytoin and PT with warfarin. May increase levels of clomipramine, desipramine. May decrease levels of drugs metabolized by CYP3A4 (eg, cyclosporine, steroidal contraceptives, theophylline). Avoid alcohol.

PREGNANCY: Category C, caution in nursing.

MECHANISM OF ACTION: Wakefulness promoting agent: Psychoactive and euphoric effects, alterations in mood, perception, thinking and feelings typical of other CNS stimulants: Modafinil binds to dopamine transporter, inhibits dopamine reuptake, and results in increased extracellular dopamine levels in some brain regions.

PHARMACOKINETICS: Absorption: T_{max}=2-4 hrs. **Distribution:** V_d=0.9L/kg; plasma protein binding (60%). **Metabolism:** Liver via hydrolytic deamination, S-oxidation, aromatic ring hydroxylation, and glucuronide conjugation through CYP3A4. **Elimination:** Urine, feces.

NURSING CONSIDERATIONS

Assessment: Assess for hypersensitivity to modafinil, armodafinil or its components, hepatic impairment, history of psychosis, depression or mania, left ventricular hypertrophy, mitral valve prolapse. Use drug only in patients who have had complete evaluation of their excessive sleepiness, and in whom a diagnosis of either narcolepsy, OSAHS, and/or SWSD has been made in accordance with ICSD or DSM diagnostic criteria.

Monitoring: Monitor serious rash, Stevens-Johnson syndrome, toxic epidermal necrolysis, drug rash with eosinophilia and systemic symptoms (DRESS), angioedema, dysphagia, bronchospasm, multi-organ hypersensitivity reactions (myocarditis, hepatitis, LFT abnormalities, hematological abnormalities such as leukopenia and thrombocytopenia, pruritus, asthenia), psychiatric adverse symptoms such as anxiety, nervousness, insomnia, confusion, agitation, and depression. Also monitor BP, possible drug interactions, and adverse reactions such as headache, nausea, dizziness, chest pain.

Patient Counseling: Advise to d/c therapy and immediately report to physician any signs/symptoms suggesting angioedema or anaphylaxis (eg, swelling of face, eyes, lips, tongue or larynx; difficulty breathing or swallowing; hoarseness). Advise that level of wakefulness may not return to normal, thus caution to avoid driving or any other potentially dangerous activity. Contact physician if experience chest pain, rash, depression, anxiety, or signs of psychosis or mania; notify if breastfeeding, if intend to become pregnant, and if taking or plan to take any Rx or OTC drugs. Avoid alcohol.

Administration: Oral route. **Storage:** Store at room temperature 20-25°C (68-77°F). Keep out of reach of children.

PROZAC — RX

fluoxetine HCl (Lilly)

Antidepressants increased the risk of suicidal thinking and behavior (suicidality) in short-term studies of children, adolescents, and young adults with major depressive disorder (MDD) and other psychiatric disorders. Fluoxetine is approved for use in pediatric patients with MDD and obsessive compulsive disorder (OCD).

P

THERAPEUTIC CLASS: Selective serotonin reuptake inhibitor

INDICATIONS: Treatment of major depressive disorder (MDD), obsessive compulsive disorder (OCD), bulimia nervosa, and panic disorder with or without agoraphobia.

DOSAGE: *Adults:* MDD: Daily Dosing: Initial: 20mg qam; increase dose if no improvement after several weeks. Doses >20mg/day, give qam or bid (am and noon). Max: 80mg/day. OCD: Initial: 20mg qam; may increase dose if no significant improvement after several weeks. Maint: 20-60mg/day given qd-bid, am and noon. Max: 80mg/day. Bulimia Nervosa: 60mg qam. Max: 60mg/day. Panic Disorder: Initial: 10mg/day. May increase to 20mg/day after 1 week. May increase further after several weeks if no clinical improvement. Max: 60mg/day. Hepatic Impairment/Elderly: Use lower or less frequent dosage. *Pediatrics:* MDD: ≥8 yrs: Higher Wt Peds: Initial: 10 or 20mg/day. After 1 week at 10mg/day, may increase to 20mg/day. Lower Wt Peds: Initial: 10mg/day. Titrate: May increase to 20mg/day after several weeks if clinical improvement is not observed. OCD: ≥7 yrs: Adolescents and Higher Wt Peds: Initial: 10mg/day. Titrate: Increase to 20mg/day after 2 weeks. Consider additional dose increases after several more weeks if clinical improvement is not observed. Usual: 20-60mg/day. Lower Wt Peds: Initial: 10mg/day. Titrate: Consider additional dose increases after several weeks if clinical improvement is not observed. Usual: 20-30mg/day. Max: 60mg/day.

HOW SUPPLIED: Cap: 10mg, 20mg, 40mg; Sol: 20mg/5mL [120mL]

CONTRAINDICATIONS: During or within 14 days of MAOI therapy. Thioridazine during or within 5 weeks of discontinuation. Concomitant use of pimozide.

WARNINGS/PRECAUTIONS: D/C if unexplained allergic reaction occurs. Monitor for symptoms of mania/hypomania. Caution with diseases or conditions that could affect metabolism or hemodynamic responses, diabetes, history of seizures, suicidal tendencies. Altered platelet function, hyponatremia reported. Periodically monitor height and weight in pediatrics. Monitor for clinical worsening and/or suicidality, especially at initiation of therapy or dose changes. Avoid abrupt withdrawal. Monitor for discontinuation symptoms. Caution in third trimester of pregnancy due to risk of serious neonatal complications. May interfere with cognitive and motor performance.

ADVERSE REACTIONS: Nausea, diarrhea, insomnia, anxiety, nervousness, dizziness, somnolence, tremor, decreased libido, sweating, anorexia, asthenia, dry mouth, dyspepsia, headache.

INTERACTIONS: See Contraindications. Antidiabetic drugs may need adjustment. May shift concentrations with plasma-bound drugs (eg, coumadin, digitoxin). May alter warfarin effects. May increase benzodiazepine, phenytoin, carbamazepine levels. Increased adverse effects with tryptophan. Caution with CNS drugs. Lithium levels may increase/decrease; monitor lithium levels. May potentiate drugs metabolized by CYP2D6, antipsychotics (eg, haloperidol, clozapine), other antidepressants. Avoid alcohol. Caution with drugs that interfere with hemostasis (eg, non-selective NSAIDs, ASA, warfarin) due to increased risk of bleeding. Serotonin syndrome reported with use of an SSRI and a triptan; monitor closely. Altered appetite and weight loss reported.

PREGNANCY: Category C, not for use in nursing.

MECHANISM OF ACTION: SSRI; inhibits CNS neuronal reuptake of serotonin.

PHARMACOKINETICS: Absorption: C_{max}=15-55ng/mL, T_{max}=6-8 hrs. **Distribution:** Plasma protein binding (94.5%); excreted in breast milk. **Metabolism:** Liver (extensive) via demethylation, norfluoxetine (active metabolite). **Elimination:** Urine; $T_{1/2}$=1-3 days (fluoxetine), 4-16 days (norfluoxetine).

NURSING CONSIDERATIONS

Assessment: Assess for bipolar disorder risk, history of mania, possible drug interactions, history of seizures, narrow-angle glaucoma, disease/condition that alters metabolism or hemodynamic response, hepatic/renal impairment.

Monitoring: Monitor for signs/symptoms of clinical worsening (suicidality, unusual changes in behavior), serotonin syndrome, abnormal bleeding, activation of mania, mydriasis, akathisia, hyponatremia, seizures, cognitive/motor impairment, hepatic/renal dysfunction. If abruptly d/c, monitor for symptoms of dysphoric mood, irritability, agitation, dizziness, sensory disturbances, anxiety, confusion, headache, lethargy, emotional lability, insomnia, and hypomania.

Patient Counseling: Advise to avoid alcohol. Seek medical attention for symptoms of serotonin syndrome (mental status changes, tachycardia, hyperthermia, NV, diarrhea, incoordination), abnormal bleeding (particularly if using NSAIDs or ASA), akathisia, hyponatremia (headaches, unsteadiness), mydriasis, activation of mania, seizures, clinical worsening (suicidal ideation, unusual changes in behavior) and discontinuation symptoms (irritability, agitation, dizziness, anxiety, headache, insomnia). Caution may impair physical/mental abilities. May notice improvement in 1-4 weeks; continue therapy as directed.

Administration: Oral route. **Storage:** 15-30°C (59-86°F).

PROZAC WEEKLY — RX

fluoxetine HCl (Lilly)

Antidepressants increased the risk of suicidal thinking and behavior (suicidality) in short-term studies in children, adolescents, and young adults with major depressive disorder (MDD) and other psychiatric disorders. Fluoxetine is approved for use in pediatric patients with MDD and obsessive compulsive disorder (OCD).

THERAPEUTIC CLASS: Selective serotonin reuptake inhibitor

INDICATIONS: Treatment of major depressive disorder (MDD).

DOSAGE: *Adults:* One 90mg cap every week starting 7 days after last daily dose of fluoxetine 20mg.

HOW SUPPLIED: Cap, Extended-Release: 90mg

CONTRAINDICATIONS: During or within 14 days of MAOI therapy. Thioridazine during or within 5 weeks of discontinuation. Concomitant use of pimozide.

WARNINGS/PRECAUTIONS: Rash with systemic involvement and urticaria reported. Anxiety, nervousness, insomnia or activation of mania/hypomania reported. Weight loss and altered appetite; monitor weight changes. Caution with diseases or conditions that could affect metabolism or hemodynamic responses, diabetes, or history of seizures. May impair judgment, thinking or motor skills. Altered platelet function and hyponatremia reported. Monitor for clinical worsening and/or suicidality, especially at initiation of therapy or dose changes. Avoid abrupt withdrawal. Monitor for discontinuation symptoms. Caution in third trimester of pregnancy due to risk of neonatal complications.

ADVERSE REACTIONS: Nausea, diarrhea, insomnia, anxiety, nervousness, dizziness, somnolence, tremor, decreased libido, sweating, anorexia, asthenia, dry mouth, dyspepsia, headache.

INTERACTIONS: See Contraindications. Antidiabetic drugs may need adjustment. May shift concentrations with plasma-bound drugs (eg, coumadin, digitoxin). May alter warfarin effects. May increase benzodiazepine, phenytoin and carbamazepine levels. Increased adverse effects with tryptophan. Caution with CNS drugs. Lithium levels may increase/decrease; monitor lithium levels. May potentiate drugs metabolized by CYP2D6, antipsychotics (eg, haloperidol, clozapine) and other antidepressants. Avoid alcohol. Caution with drugs that interfere with hemostasis (eg, non-selective NSAIDs, ASA, warfarin) due to increased risk of bleeding. Serotonin syndrome reported with use of an SSRI and a triptan; monitor closely.

PREGNANCY: Category C, not for use in nursing.

MECHANISM OF ACTION: SSRI; inhibits CNS neuronal reuptake of serotonin.

PHARMACOKINETICS: Absorption: Delayed onset by 1-2 hrs. **Distribution:** Plasma protein binding (94.5%). Excreted in breast milk. **Metabolism:** Liver (extensive) via demethylation, norfluoxetine (active metabolite). **Elimination:** Kidney. $T_{1/2}$=1-3 days (fluoxetine), 4-16 days (norfluoxetine).

NURSING CONSIDERATIONS

P

Assessment: Assess for bipolar disorder risk, history of mania, possible drug interactions, history of seizures, narrow-angle glaucoma, disease/condition that alters metabolism or hemodynamic response, hepatic/renal impairment.

Monitoring: Monitor for signs/symptoms of clinical worsening (suicidality, unusual changes in behavior), serotonin syndrome, abnormal bleeding, activation of mania, mydriasis, akathisia, hyponatremia, seizures, cognitive/motor impairment, hepatic/renal dysfunction. If abruptly d/c, monitor for symptoms of dysphoric mood, irritability, agitation, dizziness, sensory disturbances, anxiety, confusion, headache, lethargy, emotional lability, insomnia, and hypomania.

Patient Counseling: Advise to avoid alcohol. Seek medical attention for symptoms of serotonin syndrome (mental status changes, tachycardia, hyperthermia, NV, diarrhea, incoordination), abnormal bleeding (particularly if using NSAIDs or ASA), akathisia, hyponatremia (headaches, unsteadiness), mydriasis, activation of mania, seizures, clinical worsening (suicidal ideation, unusual changes in behavior) and d/c symptoms (irritability, agitation, dizziness, anxiety, headache, insomnia). Caution may impair physical/mental abilities. May notice improvement in 1-4 weeks; continue therapy as directed.

Administration: Oral route. **Storage:** 15-30°C (59-86°F).

PSORCON E — RX

diflorasone diacetate (Dermik)

THERAPEUTIC CLASS: Corticosteroid

INDICATIONS: Corticosteroid-responsive dermatoses.

DOSAGE: *Adults:* Apply qd-tid depending on severity. May use occlusive dressings for psoriasis or recalcitrant conditions. D/C dressings if infection develops.

HOW SUPPLIED: Cre: 0.05% [30g, 60g]

WARNINGS/PRECAUTIONS: May produce reversible HPA axis suppression, manifestations of Cushing's syndrome, hyperglycemia, and glucosuria. Caution when applied to large surface areas or under occlusive dressings. Use appropriate antifungal or antibacterial agent with dermatological infections; d/c if infection does not clear. Pediatrics may be more susceptible to systemic toxicity. Avoid eyes. D/C if irritation occurs. Cre has an increased risk of producing adrenal suppression than Oint. Cre should not be used in treatment of rosacea or perioral dermatitis; avoid face, groin, or axillae.

ADVERSE REACTIONS: Burning, itching, irritation, dryness, folliculitis, hypertrichosis, acneiform eruptions, hypopigmentation, perioral dermatitis, allergic contact dermatitis, skin maceration, secondary infection, skin atrophy, striae, miliaria.

PREGNANCY: Category C, caution in nursing.

MECHANISM OF ACTION: Corticosteroid; posesses anti-inflammatory, anti-pruritic, and vasoconstrictive actions. Anti-inflammatory activity not established. Suspected to act by the induction of phospholipase A_2 inhibitory proteins, lipocortins. Lipocortins control the biosynthesis of potent mediators of inflammation (eg, prostaglandins, leukotrienes) by inhibiting release of their common precursor, arachidonic acid.

PHARMACOKINETICS: Absorption: Percutaneous; inflammation, other disease states, and use of occlusive dressing may increase absorption. Use of occlusive dressings for ≤24 hrs does not increase penetration, ≥96 hrs markedly enhances penetration. **Distribution:** Bound to plasma proteins in varying degrees. Systemically administered corticosteroids secreted in breast milk. **Metabolism:** Liver. **Elimination:** Kidneys (major), bile.

NURSING CONSIDERATIONS

Assessment: Assess for rosacea or perioral dermatitis. Assess use in pregnant/nursing patients.

Monitoring: Monitor for signs/symptoms of reversible HPA-axis suppression, Cushing's syndrome, hyperglycemia, glucosuria, skin irritation, allergic contact dermatitis (eg, failure to heal), and for development of concomitant skin infections (eg, bacterial, fungal). In patients using high doses or using occlusive dressings, perform periodic monitoring for HPA-axis suppression using ACTH-stimulation, A.M. plasma cortisol, and urinary free cortisol tests. Following d/c of therapy, monitor for glucocorticosteroid insufficiencies.

Patient Counseling: Counsel to use externally and exactly as directed; avoid contact with eyes. Instruct not to bandage, cover, or wrap treatment area unless directed by physician. Counsel to notify physician for signs of local adverse reactions (eg, burning, itching, irritation).

Administration: Topical administration. **Storage:** Oint: Room temperature 20-25°C (68-77°F). Cream: Store at or below 25°C (77°F).

PULMICORT — RX

budesonide (AstraZeneca)

OTHER BRAND NAMES: Pulmicort Respules (AstraZeneca) - Pulmicort Flexhaler (AstraZeneca)

THERAPEUTIC CLASS: Corticosteroid

INDICATIONS: (Respules) Treatment of asthma and as prophylactic therapy in children 12 months to 8 yrs. (Flexhaler) Maintenance treatment of asthma as prophylactic therapy in patients ≥6 yrs and to reduce or eliminate the need for oral systemic corticosteroidal therapy.

DOSAGE: *Adults:* (Flexhaler) Initial: 180-360mcg bid. Max: 720mcg bid. Individualize dose.

Pediatrics: (Flexhaler) ≥6 yrs: Initial: 180-360mcg bid. Max: 360mcg bid. Individualize dose. (Respules) 1-8 yrs: Previous Bronchodilator Only: Initial: 0.5mg qd or 0.25mg bid. Administer via jet nebulizer. Max: 0.5mg/day. Previous Inhaled Corticosteroid: 0.5mg qd or 0.25mg bid. Max: 1mg/day. Previous Oral Corticosteroid: 1mg qd or 0.5mg bid. Max: 1mg/day. Gradually reduce PO corticosteroid after 1 week of budesonide.

HOW SUPPLIED: Powder, Inhalation: (Flexhaler) 90mcg/dose, 180mcg/dose; (Turbuhaler) 200mcg; Sus, Inhalation: (Respules) 0.25mg/2mL; 0.5mg/2mL [2mL, 30^s]

CONTRAINDICATIONS: Primary treatment of status asthmaticus or other acute episodes of asthma where intensive measures are required.

WARNINGS/PRECAUTIONS: Deaths due to adrenal insufficiency have occurred with transfer from systemic corticosteroids to inhaled corticosteroids. Resume oral corticosteroids during stress or severe asthma attack. Transferring from oral to inhalation therapy may unmask allergic conditions (eg, rhinitis, conjunctivitis, arthritis, eosinophilic conditions, eczema). Observe for adrenal insufficiency, systemic corticosteroid withdrawal effects, and growth suppression (children). Increased susceptibility to infections. Not for acute bronchospasm. D/C if bronchospasm occurs after dosing. Caution with TB of respiratory tract; untreated systemic fungal, bacterial, viral or parasitic infections; or ocular herpes simplex. *Candida* infection of mouth and pharynx reported. Patients requiring oral corticosteroids should be weaned slowly from systemic corticosteroid use.

ADVERSE REACTIONS: Nasopharyngitis, pharyngitis, headache, fever, sinusitis, pain, bronchospasm, bronchitis, respiratory infection, monoliasis.

INTERACTIONS: Oral ketoconazole increases plasma levels. CYP3A4 inhibitors (eg, itraconazole, clarithromycin, erythromycin) may inhibit metabolism and increase systemic exposure. (Respules) Slight decrease in clearance and increase in oral bioavailability with cimetidine.

PREGNANCY: (Respules) Category B, caution in nursing; (Flexhaler) Category B, caution in nursing.

MECHANISM OF ACTION: Corticosteroid; not established. Shown to have inhibitory effects on multiple cell types (mast cells, eosinophils, neutrophils, macrophages and lymphocytes) and mediators (histamine, eicosanoids, leukotrienes and cytokines) involved in inflammatory and asthmatic response.

P

PHARMACOKINETICS: Absorption: Respules: (4-6 yrs) Absolute bioavailability (6%); C_{max}=2.6nmol/L, T_{max}=20 min. Turbuhaler: T_{max}=30 min. Flexhaler: (Adults) T_{max}=10 min, (180mg qd) C_{max}=0.6nmol/L. (360mg bid) C_{max}=1.6nmol/L. (Peds) T_{max}=15-30 min, (180mg qd) C_{max}=0.4nmol/L. (360mg bid) C_{max}=1.5nmol/L. **Distribution:** V_d=3L/kg; plasma protein binding (85-90%). **Metabolism:** Liver (biotransformation), via CYP3A4. **Elimination:** (Respules) $T_{1/2}$=2.3 hrs. (Turbuhaler, Flexhaler) $T_{1/2}$=2-3 hrs.

NURSING CONSIDERATIONS

Assessment: Assess for concomitant diseases such as status asthmaticus, active or quiescent pulmonary TB, ocular herpes simplex, untreated systemic fungal, bacterial, parasitic or viral infections, hepatic dysfunction, and possible drug interactions. Obtain baseline lung function and LFTs prior to therapy.

Monitoring: Monitor lung function periodically. Perform periodic eye exams. Monitor for localized oral infections with *Candida albicans*, decreased bone mass, worsening or acutely deteriorating asthma (increased use of inhaled β_2-agonist, decreased lung function), asthma instability (serial objective measures of airflow), body height in children, development of glaucoma, increased IOP, cataracts, adrenal insufficiency (eg, fatigue, weakness, NV, hypotension), paradoxical bronchospasm, and hypersensitivity reactions.

Patient Counseling: Inform to use at regular intervals; do not alter prescribed dosage unless advised by physician. Instruct not to use a spacer or bite/chew mouthpiece. Inform that improvement will occur within 24 hrs, do not increase dosage or d/c inhaler abruptly unless directed by physician. Avoid spraying in eyes; rinse mouth after inhalation. Replace mouthpiece cover after each use and clean once weekly by wiping mouthpiece with dry cloth. Should not be used for sudden symptoms of SOB or acute bronchospasm. Inform may cause reduction in growth rate (pediatrics) and may unmask allergies (eg, rhinitis, conjunctivitis, eczema). Warn to avoid exposure to chickenpox or measles. Advise to seek medical attention if exposed to chickenpox or measles, worsening of existing TB, infections or ocular herpes simplex, if symptoms worsen or do not improve, during periods of stress or severe asthmatic attack, adrenal insufficiency (eg, fatigue, weakness, NV, hypotension), paradoxical bronchospasm, or hypersensitivity reactions occur.

Administration: Oral inhalation. (Turbuhaler, Flexhaler): Prime inhaler: Turn cover and lift off. Hold upright (mouthpiece up); twist brown grip fully to right then left. Repeat. Do not have to prime again even if prolonged period of time. 1) Loading dose: Twist cover and lift off; hold in upright position (mouthpiece up), twist brown grip fully to right and back to left, will hear click. 2) Inhaling dose: Hold upright (mouthpiece up) or horizontal position; turn head away from inhaler and breathe out; do not shake inhaler after loading; place mouthpiece between lips and inhale deeply and forcefully; remove from mouth and exhale; do not blow or exhale into mouthpiece. **Storage:** (Turbuhaler, Flexhaler): 20-25°C (68-77°F). (Respules): 20-25°C (68-77°F). Protect from light. Do not refrigerate or freeze. After aluminum foil opened; stable for 2 weeks. Before use; shake amp using a circular motion.

PULMOZYME — RX

dornase alfa (Genentech)

THERAPEUTIC CLASS: Protein

INDICATIONS: Adjunct therapy in cystic fibrosis to improve pulmonary function.

DOSAGE: *Adults:* 2.5mg qd-bid via nebulizer.
Pediatrics: ≥5 yrs: 2.5mg qd-bid via nebulizer.

HOW SUPPLIED: Sol: 2.5mg/2.5mL [2.5mL: 1^s, 30^s]

CONTRAINDICATIONS: Hypersensitivity to Chinese hamster ovary cell products.

WARNINGS/PRECAUTIONS: Use with standard therapies for cystic fibrosis.

ADVERSE REACTIONS: Voice alteration, pharyngitis, rash, laryngitis, chest pain, conjunctivitis, rhinitis, fever, dyspnea.

PREGNANCY: Category B, caution in nursing.

MECHANISM OF ACTION: Protein; hydrolyzes the DNA in sputum and reduces sputum viscoelasticity.

P

NURSING CONSIDERATIONS

Assessment: Assess for hypersensitivity to Chinese hamster ovary cell products. Assess use in nursing females and in patients <5 yrs.

Monitoring: Monitor for worsening of condition and adverse events (eg, pharyngitis, chest pain, fever, rhinitis, and voice alteration).

Patient Counseling: Instruct to refrigerate medication, including during transportation; do not expose to room temperature for 24 hrs. Instruct to discard solution if cloudy or discolored. Inform that entire contents of ampule must be used once opened and to discard unused portion. Instruct to not dilute or mix with other drugs in nebulizer. Counsel to squeeze drug ampule prior to use to check for leaks.

Administration: Inhalation route. **Storage:** 2-8°C (36-46°F). Protect from strong light. Keep refrigerated during transport; do not expose to room temperature for 24 hrs. Unused ampules should be stored in their protective foil pouch under refrigeration.

PURINETHOL — RX

mercaptopurine (Gate)

THERAPEUTIC CLASS: Purine analog

INDICATIONS: Remission induction and maintenance therapy of acute lymphatic leukemia (ALL).

DOSAGE: *Adults:* Maint: 1.5-2.5mg/kg/day as single dose. Renal/Hepatic Impairment: Reduce dose. Concomitant Allopurinol: Reduce mercaptopurine dose by 1/3-1/4 of usual dose. TPMT Deficiency: Consider dose reduction. *Pediatrics:* Maint: 1.5-2.5mg/kg/day as single dose. Renal/Hepatic Impairment: Reduce dose. Concomitant Allopurinol: Reduce mercaptopurine dose by 1/3-1/4 of usual dose. TPMT Deficiency: Consider dose reduction.

HOW SUPPLIED: Tab: 50mg* *scored

CONTRAINDICATIONS: Lack of definitive diagnosis of ALL. Prior resistance to mercaptopurine or thioguanine.

WARNINGS/PRECAUTIONS: Risk of dose-related bone marrow suppression. Monitor weekly platelet counts, Hgb, Hct, total WBC with differential; increase frequency during induction phase. Monitor closely for life-threatening infection or bleeding. Risk of hepatotoxicity, anorexia, diarrhea, jaundice, and ascites (especially with >2.5mg/kg dose). Perform LFTs weekly initially, then monthly; monitor more frequently with hepatotoxic drugs or pre-existing liver disease. Increased sensitivity to myelosuppressive effects with thiopurine-S-methyltransferase (TPMT) gene deficiency; consider TPMT testing with evidence of severe toxicity.

ADVERSE REACTIONS: Bone marrow toxicity, hepatotoxicity, hyperuricemia (reduce incidence by prehydration, urine alkalinization, prophylactic allopurinol), intestinal ulceration, rash, hyperpigmentation, alopecia, transient oligospermia.

INTERACTIONS: Reduce to 1/3-1/4 of usual dose with allopurinol to avoid toxicity. Reduce dose with myelosuppressants. Bone marrow suppression reported with trimethoprim-sulfamethoxazole. Cross-resistance with thioguanine. Increased bone marrow toxicity with concomitant TPMT inhibitors (eg, olsalazine, mesalazine, sulphasalazine). Inhibition of anticoagulant effect of warfarin with concomitant administration.

PREGNANCY: Category D, not for use in nursing.

MECHANISM OF ACTION: Purine analog; competes with hypoxanthine and guanine for hypoxanthine-guanine phosphoribosyltransferase and gets converted to thiosinic acid, which then inhibits glutamine-5-phosphoribosylpyrophosphate amidotransferase of de novo pathway for purine ribonucleotide synthesis.

PHARMACOKINETICS: Absorption: Incomplete. **Distribution:** Plasma protein binding (19%). **Elimination:** $T_{1/2}$=21 min (pediatric); 47 min (adult).

NURSING CONSIDERATIONS

Assessment: Assess for drug resistance, pre-existing liver/renal disease, thiopurine-S-methyltransferase (TPMT) gene defect, pregnancy status, and possible drug interactions. Obtain baseline WBC with differential, Hgb/Hct, platelet count, LFTs, and renal function.

Monitoring: Monitor WBC with differential, Hgb/Hct, platelet count, LFTs, and renal function weekly. Bone marrow exam for evaluation of marrow status. Consider thiopurine-S-methyltransferase (TPMT) testing if evidence of severe bone marrow toxicity. Monitor for signs/symptoms of bone marrow suppression, granulocytopenia, hepatotoxicity, and hypersensitivity reactions.

Patient Counseling: Inform of pregnancy risks; avoid pregnancy. Inform of major toxicities related to therapy (myelosuppression, hepatotoxicity, GI toxicity). Instruct to take under medical supervision. Advise to seek medical attention if symptoms of fever, sore throat, jaundice, NV, signs of local infection, bleeding from any site, or symptoms suggestive of anemia occur.

Administration: Oral route. **Storage:** 15-25°C (59-77°F). Dry place.

QUESTRAN
cholestyramine (Par)

RX

OTHER BRAND NAMES: Questran Light (Par)

THERAPEUTIC CLASS: Bile acid sequestrant

INDICATIONS: Adjunct to reduce elevated cholesterol in primary hypercholesterolemia not responding to diet or to reduce LDL in hypertriglyceridemia. Relief of pruritus associated with partial biliary obstruction.

DOSAGE: *Adults:* Initial: 1 pkt or scoopful qd or bid. Maint: 2-4 pkts or scoopfuls/day, given bid. Titrate: Adjust at no less than 4 week intervals. Max: 6 pkts/day or 6 scoopfuls/day. May also give as 1-6 doses/day. Mix with fluid or highly fluid food.
Pediatrics: Usual: 240mg/kg/day of anhydrous cholestyramine resin in 2-3 divided doses. Max: 8g/day.

HOW SUPPLIED: Powder: 4g/pkt [60^{s}, 378g], (Light) 4g/scoopful [60^{s}, 268g]

CONTRAINDICATIONS: Complete biliary obstruction.

WARNINGS/PRECAUTIONS: May produce hyperchloremic acidosis with prolonged use. Caution in renal insufficiency, volume depletion, and with concomitant spironolactone. Chronic use may produce or worsen constipation. Avoid constipation with symptomatic CAD. May increase bleeding tendency due to vitamin K deficiency. Serum or red cell folate reduced with chronic use. Constipation may aggravate hemorrhoids. Light formulation contains phenylalanine. Measure cholesterol during 1st few months; periodically thereafter. Measure TG periodically.

ADVERSE REACTIONS: Constipation, heartburn, nausea, vomiting, abdominal pain, flatulence, diarrhea, anorexia, osteoporosis, rash, hyperchloremic acidosis (children), vitamin A and D deficiency, steatorrhea, hypoprothrombinemia (vitamin K deficiency).

INTERACTIONS: May interfere with absorption of fat-soluble vitamins (A, D, E, K), drugs that undergo enterohepatic circulation, and oral phosphate supplements. Take concomitant drugs 1hr before or 4-6 hrs after. Additive effects with HMG-CoA reductase inhibitors and nicotinic acid. Caution with spironolactone. May reduce or delay absorption of phenylbutazone, warfarin, thiazide diuretics, propranolol, tetracycline, penicillin G, phenobarbital, thyroid and thyroxine agents, estrogens, progestins, digitalis.

PREGNANCY: Category C, caution in nursing.

MECHANISM OF ACTION: Bile acid sequestrant; absorbs and combines with bile acids in intestine to form insoluble complex excreted in the feces, resulting in partial removal of bile acids from enterohepatic circulation by preventing their absorption. This leads to increased oxidation of cholesterol to bile acids and decreased plasma LDL and serum cholesterol levels.

PHARMACOKINETICS: Elimination: Feces.

NURSING CONSIDERATIONS

Assessment: Prior to initiation, assess secondary causes of hypercholesterolemia (eg, poorly controlled DM, hypothyroidism, nephrotic syndrome, dysproteinemias, obstructive liver disease, other drug therapy, alcoholism), presence of biliary obstruction, pregnancy/nursing status, and possible drug interactions. Obtain baseline serum, cholesterol, and TG levels.

Monitoring: Monitor for signs/symptoms of increased bleeding tendencies (vitamin K deficiency), hyperchloremic acidosis, and worsening of pre-existing constipation. Monitor serum cholesterol and TGs periodically.

Patient Counseling: Advise to drink plenty of fluids and to mix each 9g dose of Questran in at least 2-6 oz of fluid or each 6.4g dose of Questran Light in at least 4-6 oz of fluid. Instruct not to sip or hold suspension in mouth for prolonged periods; may lead to changes on surface of teeth (eg, discoloration, erosion of enamel, or decay). Advise to maintain good oral hygiene.

Administration: Oral route. **Storage:** Room temperature.

Quixin RX
levofloxacin (Vistakon)

THERAPEUTIC CLASS: Fluoroquinolone

INDICATIONS: Treatment of bacterial conjunctivitis.

DOSAGE: *Adults:* Days 1-2: 1-2 drops q2h while awake, up to 8x/day. Days 3-7: 1-2 drops q4h while awake, up to qid.
Pediatrics: ≥1 yr: Days 1-2: 1-2 drops q2h while awake, up to 8x/day. Days 3-7: 1-2 drops q4h while awake, up to qid.

HOW SUPPLIED: Sol: 0.5% [5mL]

WARNINGS/PRECAUTIONS: D/C if hypersensitivity or superinfection occurs. Avoid contact lenses with conjunctivitis.

ADVERSE REACTIONS: Transient ocular burning, decreased vision, fever, foreign body sensation, headache, ocular pain, pharyngitis, photophobia.

INTERACTIONS: Systemic quinolone therapy may increase theophylline levels, interfere with caffeine metabolism, enhance warfarin effects, and elevate serum creatinine with cyclosporine.

PREGNANCY: Category C, caution in nursing.

MECHANISM OF ACTION: Fluoroquinolone; antibacterial active against broad spectrum of gram-positive and gram-negative organisms. Responsible for inhibition of bacterial topoisomerase IV and DNA gyrase, enzymes required for DNA replication, transcription, repair, and recombination.

PHARMACOKINETICS: Absorption: C_{max}=0.94ng/mL (single dose), 2.15ng/mL (multiple doses).

NURSING CONSIDERATIONS

Assessment: Assess for proper diagnosis (eg, slit-lamp biomicroscopy, fluorescein staining), hypersensitivity to other quinolones, possible drug interactions, and use in pregnant/nursing females.

Monitoring: Monitor for signs/symptoms of hypersensitivity or anaphylactic reaction (eg, cardiovascular collapse, loss of consciousness, angioedema, airway obstruction, dyspnea, uticaria, and itching). With prolonged therapy, monitor for overgrowth of nonsusceptible organisms (eg, fungi) and for development of superinfection. Perform periodic exam of patient using magnification (eg, slit-lamp biomicroscopy, fluorescein staining).

Patient Counseling: Instruct to avoid touching applicator tip to material from eye, fingers, or other sources to prevent contamination. Advise not to wear contact lenses if there are signs/symptoms of bacterial conjunctivitis. Instruct to d/c medication and contact physician if signs of hypersensitivity reaction (eg, rash) develop.

Administration: Ocular route. Do not inject subconjunctivally or introduce directly into anterior chamber of eye. **Storage:** 15-25°C (59-77°F). Keep out of reach of children.

Qvar RX
beclomethasone dipropionate (Teva)

THERAPEUTIC CLASS: Corticosteroid

INDICATIONS: Maintenance treatment of asthma as prophylactic therapy in patients ≥5 yrs. To reduce or eliminate the need for systemic corticosteroids in asthma patients requiring systemic corticosteroids.

DOSAGE: *Adults:* Previous Bronchodilator Only: 40-80mcg bid. Max: 320mcg bid. Previous Inhaled Corticosteroid (CS) Therapy: 40-160mcg bid. Max: 320mcg bid. Maintained on Systemic CS: May attempt gradual reduction of systemic CS dose after 1 week on inhaled therapy.
Pediatrics: Adolescents: Previous Bronchodilator Only: 40-80mcg bid. Max: 320mcg bid. Previous Inhaled Corticosteroid (CS) Therapy: 40-160mcg

bid. Max: 320mcg bid. 5-11 yrs: Previous Bronchodilator Only or Inhaled CS Therapy: 40mcg bid. Max: 80mcg bid. ≥5 yrs: Maintained on Systemic CS: May attempt gradual reduction of systemic CS dose after 1 week on inhaled therapy.

HOW SUPPLIED: MDI: 40mcg/inh, 80mcg/inh [7.3g]

CONTRAINDICATIONS: Primary treatment of status asthmaticus or other acute episodes of asthma where intensive measures are required.

WARNINGS/PRECAUTIONS: Deaths due to adrenal insufficiency have occurred with transfer from systemic corticosteroids to inhaled corticosteroids. Resume oral corticosteroids during stress or severe asthma attack. Risk of adrenal insufficiency and withdrawal symptoms when replacing systemic corticosteroids. May unmask allergic conditions previously suppressed by systemic steroid therapy. Caution with TB, ocular herpes simplex, or untreated systemic bacterial, fungal, parasitic, or viral infections. May suppress growth in children. Exposure to chickenpox or measles requires prophylactic treatment. Not for rapid relief of bronchospasm.

ADVERSE REACTIONS: Headache, pharyngitis, upper respiratory tract infection, rhinitis, increased asthma symptoms, sinusitis.

PREGNANCY: Category C, not for use in nursing.

MECHANISM OF ACTION: Corticosteroid; inhibits both inflammatory cells and release of inflammatory mediators.

PHARMACOKINETICS: Absorption: C_{max}=88pg/mL; T_{max}=0.5 hr. (17-BMP) C_{max}=1419pg/mL, T_{max}=0.7hr. **Metabolism:** Biotransformation, via CYP3A. (Metabolites) beclomethasone-17-monopropionate (17-BMP), beclonethasone-21-monopropionate (21-BMP) and beclomethasone (BOH). **Elimination:** Feces (major). (17-BMP) $T_{1/2}$=2.8 hrs.

NURSING CONSIDERATIONS

Assessment: Assess for history of IOP, glaucoma, cataracts, concomitant diseases like status asthmaticus, active or quiescent pulmonary TB, ocular herpes simplex, untreated systemic fungal, bacterial, parasitic or viral infections, and possible drug interactions.

Monitoring: Monitor for localized oral infections, asthma instability (serial objective measures of airflow), body height in children, development of glaucoma, increased IOP, cataracts, adrenal insufficiency (eg, fatigue, weakness, NV, hypotension), paradoxical bronchospasm, and hypersensitivity reactions.

Patient Counseling: Advise that drug not intended for treatment of acute asthma (sudden symptoms of SOB or acute bronchospasm). Advise to rinse mouth after using inhaler. Inform that medication may cause reduction in growth rate (pediatrics) and may also unmask allergies (eg, rhinitis, conjunctivitis, eczema). Avoid exposure to chickenpox or measles. Advise to seek medical attention if exposed to chickenpox or measles, worsening of existing TB, infections, ocular herpes simplex, symptoms do not improve or worsen, during periods of stress or severe asthmatic attack, adrenal insufficiency (eg, fatigue, weakness, NV, hypotension), paradoxical bronchospasm or hypersensitivity reactions occur.

Administration: Oral inhalation. **Storage:** 25°C (77°F); excursions permitted to 15-30° (59-86°F). For optimal results, canister should be at room temperature when used. Keep out of reach of children.

R

RANEXA

RX

ranolazine (CV Therapeutics)

THERAPEUTIC CLASS: Miscellaneous antianginal

INDICATIONS: Treatment of chronic angina; may coadminister with β-blockers, nitrates, calcium channel blockers, anti-platelet therapy, lipid-lowering therapy, ACE inhibitors, and angiotensin receptor blockers.

DOSAGE: *Adults:* Initial: 500mg bid. Titrate: May increase to 1000mg bid. Max: 1000mg bid. Concurrent With Diltiazem/Verapamil/Other Moderate CYP3A

Inhibitors: 500mg bid. Concurrent With P-gp Inhibitors: Down titrate dose based on clinical response. Swallow whole; do not crush, break, or chew.

HOW SUPPLIED: Tab, Extended-Release: 500mg, 1000mg

CONTRAINDICATIONS: Strong CYP3A inhibitors (eg, ketoconazole, clarithromycin, saquinavir), CYP3A inducers (eg, rifampin, phenobarbital, carbamazepine), and hepatic dysfunction (Child-Pugh Classes A and B).

WARNINGS/PRECAUTIONS: May prolong QTc interval in a dose-related manner; avoid with known QT prolongation (including congenital long QT syndrome, uncorrected hypokalemia), known history of ventricular tachycardia, hepatic dysfunction. Monitor BP with severe renal impairment.

ADVERSE REACTIONS: Dizziness, nausea, asthenia, constipation, and headache.

INTERACTIONS: See Contraindications. Avoid with moderate CYP3A inhibitors, fluconazole, diltiazem, verapamil, macrolide antibiotics, HIV protease inhibitors, grapefruit juice or grapefruit-containing products. May increase levels of digoxin, simvastatin; consider dosage reduction of digoxin, simvastatin. Avoid with drugs that may prolong the QTc interval, such as Class Ia (eg, quinidine) and Class III (eg, dofetilide, sotalol) antiarrhythmics, and antipsychotics (eg, thioridazine, ziprasidone). May increase levels of drugs metabolized by CYP2D6 such as TCAs and some antipsychotics; consider dosage reduction of these drugs.

PREGNANCY: Category C, not for use in nursing.

MECHANISM OF ACTION: Not established; suspected to have antianginal and antiischemic effects that do not depend upon reductions of HR and BP.

PHARMACOKINETICS: Absorption: C_{max}=2569ng/mL, T_{max}=2-5hrs. **Distribution:** Plasma protein binding (62%). **Metabolism:** Gut and liver (extensive), via CYP3A and CYP2D6. **Elimination:** Urine (75%), feces (25%), and (<5% unchanged); $T_{1/2}$=7 hrs.

NURSING CONSIDERATIONS

Assessment: Assess for renal/hepatic impairment, pre-existing QT prolongation (eg, congenital long QT syndrome, uncorrected hypokalemia) or on QT-prolonging agents (eg, quinidine), ventricular tachycardia, and possible drug interactions (eg, diltiazem, potent CYP3A inhibitors, and digoxin).

Monitoring: Monitor SrCr, transient eosinophilia, ECG changes (eg, prolongation of the QTc interval), tumor formation, and progression to malignancy.

Patient Counseling: Inform about risks/benefits of drug and not to exceed recommended dose. Swallow tab whole; do not crush, break, or chew. If a dose is missed, take the prescribed dose at the next scheduled time; do not double the next dose. Do not take with grapefruit juice. Use caution while performing hazardous tasks (operating machinery/driving). Notify physician if concurrently taking any other medications.

Administration: Oral route. **Storage:** 25°C (77°F); excursions permitted to 15-30°C (59-86°F).

RAPAFLO — RX

silodosin (Watson)

THERAPEUTIC CLASS: $Alpha_1$-antagonist

INDICATIONS: Treatment for benign prostatic hyperplasia (BPH).

DOSAGE: *Adults:* 8mg qd. Moderate Renal Impairment (CrCl <30-50mL/min): 4mg qd. Take with meal.

HOW SUPPLIED: Cap: 4mg, 8mg

CONTRAINDICATIONS: Severe renal impairment (CrCl<30mL/min), severe hepatic impairment (Child-Pugh score ≥10), and concomitant administration with strong cytochrome P450 3A4 (CYP3A4) inhibitors (eg, ketoconazole, clarithromycin, itraconazole, ritonavir).

WARNINGS/PRECAUTIONS: Postural hypotension and syncope may occur. May impair mental/physical abilities. Caution in patients with moderate renal impairment. Rule out prostrate carcinoma prior to therapy. Intraoperative floppy iris syndrome reported during cataract surgery in some patients on alpha-1 blockers or previously treated with alpha-1 blockers.

ADVERSE REACTIONS: Retrograde ejaculation, dizziness, diarrhea, orthostatic hypotension, headache, nasopharyngitis, and nasal congestion.

INTERACTIONS: See Contraindications. Concomitant administration with moderate CYP3A4 (eg, diltiazem, erythromycin, verapamil) may increase plasma concentrations. Caution with antihypertensives; monitor for possible adverse events. Avoid with strong P-gp inhibitors (eg, cyclosporine) and other alpha blockers.

PREGNANCY: Category B, not for use in women.

MECHANISM OF ACTION: Selective alpha-1 adrenoreceptor antagonist; blocks alpha-1 adrenoreceptors causing smooth muscle in bladder neck and prostate to relax, resulting in improved urine flow and decreased symptoms of BPH.

PHARMACOKINETICS: Absorption: Absolute bioavailability (32%), C_{max}=61.6ng/mL, T_{max}=2.6 hrs, AUC_{ss}=373.4ng•hr/mL. **Distribution:** V_d=49.5L; plasma protein binding (97%). **Metabolism:** Via glucuronidation (CYP3A4), KMD-3213G (main metabolite), KMD-3293 (second major metabolite). **Elimination:** Urine (33.5%), feces (54.9%); $T_{1/2}$=13.3 hrs.

NURSING CONSIDERATIONS

Assessment: Assess for severe renal/hepatic impairment, prostate cancer, possible drug interactions with strong CYP2A4 inhibitors (eg, ketoconazole, clarithromycin, itraconazole, ritonavir), and pregnancy/nursing status.

Monitoring: Monitor for retrograde ejaculation, dizziness, diarrhea, orthostatic/postural hypotension, headache, nasopharyngitis, and nasal congestion.

Patient Counseling: Counsel about possible symptoms of postural hypotension; caution about driving, operating machinery, or performing hazardous tasks. Inform that orgasm with reduced or no semen does not pose a safety concern and is reversible when drug is discontinued. Notify ophthalmologist about the use of silodosin before cataract surgery or other eye procedures, even if no longer taking silodosin.

Administration: Oral route. **Storage:** Store at 25°C (77°F); excursions permitted to 15-30°C (59-86°F). Protect from light and moisture.

RAPAMUNE

sirolimus (Wyeth)

RX

Increased susceptibility to infection and development of lymphoma.

THERAPEUTIC CLASS: Macrocyclic lactone immunosuppressant

INDICATIONS: Prophylaxis of organ rejection in renal transplant patients. Recommended to be used initially with cyclosporine and corticosteroids. In low-moderate risk patients, withdraw cyclosporine 2-4 months after transplantation and increase sirolimus dose to reach recommended blood levels.

DOSAGE: *Adults:* LD: 6mg. Maint: 2mg qd. Hepatic Impairment: Reduce maintenance dose by one-third.
Pediatrics: ≥13 yrs and <40kg: LD: 3mg/m² Maint: 1mg/m²/day. Hepatic Impairment: Reduce maintenance dose by one-third. Take 4 hrs after cyclosporine.

HOW SUPPLIED: Sol: 1mg/mL [60mL]; Tab: 1mg, 2mg

WARNINGS/PRECAUTIONS: Increased cholesterol and triglycerides that may require treatment. Reduction in renal function due to long-term concomitant cyclosporine. Proteinuria observed in maintenance renal transplant patients, periodic monitoring recommended. May delay recovery of renal function in patients with delayed graft function. Increased risk of lymphocele. Provide 1 year prophylaxis for *Pneumocystis carinii* pneumonia and 3 months for cytomegalovirus after transplant. Limit exposure to sunlight and UV light. Not for use in liver or lung transplants. Interstitial lung disease reported. Increased susceptibility to infection and the possible development of lymphoma and malignancy, especially of the skin, may result from immunosuppression. Avoid in liver or lung transplant patients. Increased risk of angioedema, caution with concomitant use of angioedema-causing drugs, such as ACEI. Impaired wound healing and fat accumulation reported.

ADVERSE REACTIONS: Hypercholesterolemia, hyperlipidemia, HTN, rash, acne, anemia, leukopenia, arthralgia, diarrhea, hypokalemia, thrombocytopenia, fever, abdominal pain, headache, constipation, creatinine increase, insomnia, dyspnea, upper respiratory infection, anaphylactic/anaphylactoid reactions, angioedema, hypersensitivity vasculitis, incisional hernia, azoospermia, pericardial effusion, tuberculosis.

INTERACTIONS: Increased levels with diltiazem. CYP3A4 inhibitors (eg, CCBs, antifungals, macrolide antibiotics) may increase levels of sirolimus, while CYP3A4 inducers (eg, anticonvulsants, rifabutin, St. John's wort) may decrease levels. Avoid live vaccines, grapefruit juice, rifampin, ketoconazole. Caution with other nephrotoxic drugs (eg, aminoglycosides, amphotericin B). Hepatic artery thrombosis reported with cyclosporine or tacrolimus, and increased death rate and graft loss with tacrolimus in liver transplant patients. Bronchial anastomotic dehiscence reported with immunosuppressives in lung transplant patients. Cyclosporine is a substrate and inhibitor of CYP3A4 and P-gp. Caution with dosing. Monitor for rhabdomyolysis with cyclosporine and HMG Co-A reductase inhibitors/fibrates. Monitor renal function with cyclosporine. Grapefruit juice reduces CYP3A4 medicated drug metabolism, should not be administered with rapamune or used for dilution. Increased risk of deterioration of renal function, serum lipid abnormalities, and urinary tract infections with calcineurin inhibitors and corticosteriods.

PREGNANCY: Category C, not for use in nursing.

MECHANISM OF ACTION: Immunosuppressant; inhibits T-lymphocyte activation and proliferation that occurs in response to antigenic and cytokine (interleukin [IL]-2, IL-4, and IL-15) stimulation by a mechanism that is distinct from that of other immunosuppressants. Also inhibits antibody production. Prolongs allograft survival and suppresses immune-mediated events (animal study).

PHARMACOKINETICS: Absorption: T_{max}=1-2 hrs. **Distribution:** V_d=12L/kg; plasma protein binding (approximately 92%). **Metabolism:** CYP3A4 and P-gp, intestinal wall, liver (extensive) via O-demethylation and hydroxylation; hydroxy, demethyl and hydroxymethyl (major metabolites). **Elimination:** Feces (91%), urine (2.2%); $T_{1/2}$=62 hrs. Different pharmacokinetic data resulted from concentration-controlled trials of pediatric renal transplants.

NURSING CONSIDERATIONS

Assessment: Assess for drug hypersensitivity, low-moderate immunologic risk or high immunological risk patients, hepatic impairment, body weight/body mass index, hyperlipidemia, risk of CMV infection, and possible drug interactions.

Monitoring: Monitor for infections including opportunistic infections such as TB, CMV, and *Pneumocystis carinii* pneumonia, fatal infections and sepsis, lymphoma, skin malignancy, anaphylactic/anaphylactoid reactions, angioedema, exfoliative dermatitis and hypersensitivity vasculitis, delayed wound healing and lymphocele, interstitial lung disease (eg, pneumonitis, bronchiolitis obliterans organizing pneumonia, and pulmonary fibrosis), lab monitoring of urinary protein excretion, renal/hepatic functions, cholesterol, triglycerides, and BP.

Patient Counseling: Instruct to avoid prolonged exposure to sunlight and UV light. Instruct not to take during pregnancy/nursing. Inform can be taken with/without food, but do not crush, chew, or split.

Administration: Oral route. **Storage:** (Oral sol) 2-8°C (36-46°F), should be used within 1 month once opened. (Tab) 20-25°C (68-77°F). Use cartons to protect blister cards and strips from light.

RAZADYNE ER

RX

galantamine hydrobromide (Ortho-McNeil)

OTHER BRAND NAMES: Razadyne (Ortho-McNeil)

INDICATIONS: Treatment of mild to moderate dementia of the Alzheimer's type.

DOSAGE: *Adults:* (Sol, Tab) Initial: 4mg bid with am and pm meals. Titrate: Increase to 8mg bid after 4 weeks if tolerated, then increase to 12mg bid after 4 weeks if tolerated. Usual: 16-24mg/day. Max: 24mg/day. (Cap, ER) Initial: 8mg qd with am meal. Titrate: Increase to 16mg qd after 4 weeks, then increase to 24mg qd after 4 weeks if tolerated. Usual: 16-24mg/day. Max: 24mg/day. If therapy is interrupted, restart at lowest dose and increase to current dose. Moderate Renal/Hepatic Impairment (Child-Pugh: 7-9): Caution during dose titration. Max: 16mg/day. Avoid use with severe renal (CrCl <9mL/min) and severe hepatic impairment (Child-Pugh: 10-15).

HOW SUPPLIED: Sol: (Razadyne) 4mg/mL [100mL]; Tab: (Razadyne) 4mg, 8mg, 12mg. Cap, Extended-Release: (Razadyne ER) 8mg, 16mg, 24mg.

WARNINGS/PRECAUTIONS: Vagotonic effects; caution with supraventricular conduction disorder. May cause bradycardia and/or heart block. Caution with asthma or obstructive pulmonary disease. Monitor for active or occult GI bleeding and ulcers due to increased gastric acid secretion. Risk of generalized convulsions or bladder outflow obstruction. Ensure adequate fluid intake during treatment. Deaths reported with mild cognitive impairment.

ADVERSE REACTIONS: NV, diarrhea, anorexia, weight loss, fatigue, dizziness, headache, depression, insomnia, abdominal pain, dyspepsia, UTI.

INTERACTIONS: Potential to interfere with anticholinergics. Synergistic effect with succinylcholine, other cholinesterase inhibitors, similar neuromuscular blockers, or cholinergic agonists (eg, bethanechol). Increased levels with cimetidine, ketoconazole, and paroxetine. Caution with drugs that slow heart rate due to vagotonic effects. Monitor for GI bleeding with NSAIDs.

PREGNANCY: Category B, not for use in nursing.

MECHANISM OF ACTION: Unknown; suspected to inhibit acetylcholinesterase-enhancing cholinergic function by increasing concentration of acetylcholine through reversible inhibition of its hydrolysis.

PHARMACOKINETICS: Absorption: Bioavailability: (90% rapid and complete), T_{max}=1 hr. **Distribution:** V_d=175L; plasma protein binding (18%). **Metabolism:** Liver (glucuronidation). CYP450 enzymes: 2D6, 3A4. **Elimination:** Urine (unchanged); $T_{1/2}$=7 hrs.

NURSING CONSIDERATIONS

R

Assessment: Assess for drug hypersensitivity, cardiovascular conduction defects, GI bleeding, ulcer disease, severe asthma or COPD, renal/hepatic function, and possible drug interactions.

Monitoring: Monitor closely for symptoms of active or occult GI bleeding, and cardiac conduction defects. Monitor for common adverse events (eg, NV, anorexia, dizziness, syncope).

Patient Counseling: Take drug preferably with morning and evening meals. Ensure adequate fluid intake during treatment. If therapy has been interrupted for several days or longer, physician must restart patient at lowest dose and gradually increase to current dose. Report any adverse effects.

Administration: Oral route. **Storage:** 25°C (77°F); excursions permitted to 15-30°C (59-86°F). Do not freeze.

REBETOL RX

ribavirin (Schering)

Not for monotherapy treatment of chronic hepatitis C. Primary toxicity is hemolytic anemia. Avoid with significant or unstable cardiac disease. Contraindicated in pregnancy and male partners of pregnant women. Use 2 forms of contraception during therapy and for 6 months after discontinuation.

THERAPEUTIC CLASS: Nucleoside analogue

INDICATIONS: In combination with Intron A® for treatment of chronic hepatitis C in patients ≥3 yrs with compensated liver disease previously untreated with alpha interferon or in patients ≥18 yrs who relapsed after alpha interferon therapy. In combination with Peg-Intron™ for treatment of chronic hepatitis C in patients ≥18 yrs with compensated liver disease previously untreated with alpha interferon.

DOSAGE: *Adults:* ≥18 yrs: With Intron A: ≤75kg: 400mg qam and 600mg qpm. >75kg: 600mg qam and 600mg qpm. Treat for 24-48 weeks interferon-naive; 24 weeks in relapse. With Peg-Intron: 400mg bid, qam and qpm with food. Reduce to 600mg qd if Hgb <10g/dL with no cardiac history, or if Hgb decreases by ≥2g/dL during a 4-week period with a cardiac history. D/C if Hgb <8.5g/dL with no cardiac history or if Hgb <12g/dL after 4 weeks of dose reduction with a cardiac history. CrCl <50mL/min: Avoid use.
Pediatrics: ≥3 yrs: 15mg/kg/day in divided doses qam and qpm. Use sol if ≤25kg or cannot swallow caps. With Intron A: 25-36kg: 200mg bid, qam and qpm. 37-49kg: 200mg qam and 400mg qpm. 50-61kg: 400mg bid, qam and qpm. >61kg: Dose as adult. Genotype 1: Treat for 48 weeks. Genotype 2/3: Treat for 24 weeks. Reduce to 7.5mg/day if Hgb <10g/dL with no cardiac history, or if Hgb decreases by ≥2g/dL during a 4-week period with a cardiac history. D/C if Hgb <8.5g/dL with no cardiac history or if Hgb <12g/dL after 4 weeks of dose reduction with a cardiac history.

HOW SUPPLIED: Cap: 200mg; Sol: 40mg/mL [100mL]

CONTRAINDICATIONS: Pregnancy, male partners of pregnant women, hemoglobinopathies (eg, thalassemia major, sickle cell anemia). When used with Intron A or PEG-Intron, refer to individual monograph.

WARNINGS/PRECAUTIONS: Severe depression, suicidal ideation, bone marrow suppression, autoimmune and infectious disorders, pulmonary dysfunction, pancreatitis, and DM reported. Assess for underlying cardiac disease (obtain EKG); fatal and nonfatal MI reported with anemia. Hemolytic anemia reported; monitor Hgb or Hct initially then at Week 2 and 4 (or more if needed) of therapy. Suspend therapy if symptoms of pancreatitis arise. Avoid if CrCl <50mL/min. Obtain negative pregnancy test prior to initiation then monthly, and for 6 months post-therapy.

ADVERSE REACTIONS: Hemolytic anemia, headache, fatigue, rigors, fever, nausea, anorexia, myalgia, arthralgia, insomnia, irritability, depression, dyspnea, alopecia.

INTERACTIONS: Dental and periodontal disorders reported with interferon or peginterferon combination therapy. Coadministration not recommended with didanosine. Caution with stavudine and zidovudine.

PREGNANCY: Category X, not for use in nursing.

MECHANISM OF ACTION: Nucleoside analog; not established.

PHARMACOKINETICS: Absorption: Rapid; (Sol) C_{max}=872ng/mL, T_{max}=1 hr, AUC=14098ng•h/mL. (Cap) C_{max}=782ng/mL, T_{max}=1.7 hrs, AUC=13400ng•h/mL; absolute bioavailability (64%). **Distribution:** (Cap) V_d=2825L. **Metabolism:** Nucleated cells (phosphorylation); deribosylation and amide hydrolysis. **Elimination:** Urine (61%), feces (12%). (Cap) $T_{1/2}$=43.6 hrs.

NURSING CONSIDERATIONS

Assessment: Assess for history of hemoglobinopathy (eg, thalassemia major, sickle-cell anemia, anemia), depression, hepatic/renal dysfunction (eg, autoimmune hepatitis), DM, autoimmune disorders, infections, bone marrow suppression, pancreatitis, pregnancy status (including female partners of male patients), cardiac and lung disease. Prior to initiation; conduct pregnancy test, hematologic test (CBC with differential, Hct, Hgb), chemistries (LFTs, TSH), and ECG.

Monitoring: Monitor CBC, LFTs, TSH, and ECG periodically. Obtain Hct and Hgb (Week 2 and 4, more if needed). Perform pregnancy test monthly and 6 months after d/c of therapy (including female partners of male patients). Schedule regular dental exams. Monitor for signs/symptoms of anemia, pancreatitis, hepatic dysfunction, cardiac deterioration, pulmonary impairment, dental/periodontal disorders, and depression.

Patient Counseling: Instruct to take with food and keep well hydrated. Counsel that if dose missed, take as soon as possible during same day; do not double dose. Inform of pregnancy risks. Use 2 forms of contraception during therapy and 6 months after d/c of therapy (including female partners of male patients). Advise that to reduce damage to teeth and oral membranes from dry mouth, brush teeth bid and if experience vomiting, rinse mouth thoroughly. Seek medical attention if signs/symptoms of pancreatitis, hepatic dysfunction, depression (suicidal ideation), anemia, cardiac deterioration, or pulmonary impairment occur.

Administration: Oral route. **Storage:** Cap: 25°C (77°F); excursions permitted to 15-30°C (59-86°F). Sol: 2-8°C (36-46°F) or 25°C (77°F); excursions permitted to 15-30°C (59-86°F).

REBIF

RX

interferon beta-1a (Pfizer/Serono)

THERAPEUTIC CLASS: Biological response modifier

INDICATIONS: Treatment of patients with relapsing forms of multiple sclerosis.

DOSAGE: *Adults:* Initial: 20% of prescribed dose SQ 3x/week (TIW); 4.4mcg for prescribed dose of 22mcg, 8.8mcg for prescribed dose of 44mcg. Titrate: Increase over a 4-week period to either 22mcg or 44mcg SQ TIW. Maint: 22mcg or 44mcg SQ TIW. Leukopenia/Elevated LFTs: Reduce dose until toxicity resolves. Administer dose at the same time every day (late afternoon, evening) on the same 3 days/week at least 48 hrs apart.

HOW SUPPLIED: Inj: 22mcg/0.5mL, 44mcg/0.5mL; Titration Pack: 8.8mcg/0.2mL [6^s] and 22mcg/0.5mL [6^s]

CONTRAINDICATIONS: Hypersensitivity to human albumin.

WARNINGS/PRECAUTIONS: Caution with depression, alcohol abuse, active hepatic disease, increased serum SGPT (>2.5x ULN), history of significant hepatic disease, seizure disorder. Consider discontinuing therapy if depression, jaundice/hepatic dysfunction develops. Reduce dose if serum SGPT >5x ULN. Contains albumin; risk of viral disease transmission. Monitor blood cell counts and LFTs at 1, 3, and 6 months after initiation, then periodically. Monitor thyroid function tests every 6 months with history of thyroid dysfunction.

ADVERSE REACTIONS: Psychiatric disorders, injection site disorders, influenza-like symptoms (eg, headache, fatigue, fever, rigors, chest pain), back pain, myalgia, abdominal pain, depression, elevation of liver enzymes, hematologic abnormalities.

INTERACTIONS: Monitor with myelosuppressive agents.

PREGNANCY: Category C, caution in nursing.

MECHANISM OF ACTION: Interferon β-1a; possesses immunomodulatory, antiviral, and antiproliferative biological activities. Its effects in MS have not been fully defined.

PHARMACOKINETICS: Absorption: C_{max}=5.1 IU/mL, T_{max}=16 hrs, AUC=294 IU•h/mL. **Elimination:** $T_{1/2}$=69 hrs.

NURSING CONSIDERATIONS

Assessment: Assess for drug hypersensitivity, depression, liver disease or increased serum glutamic pyruvic transaminase, alcohol abuse, thyroid dysfunction, preexisting seizure disorder, myelosuppression, pregnancy/nursing status, and possible drug interactions.

Monitoring: Monitor for CBC, LFTs, thyroid functions, and tests used for monitoring MS, depression, suicidal ideation, suicide attempts, hepatic dysfunction, jaundice, seizures, anaphylaxis, skin rash, urticaria, and Creutzfeldt-Jakob disease (CJD).

Patient Counseling: Do not change dosage or schedule without consulting physician. Inform about risks/benefits of drug; report any adverse reactions. Notify if pregnant/nursing or planning to become pregnant.

Administration: SQ. Rotate site of injection. **Storage:** Refrigerate 2-8°C (36-46°F). Do not freeze. If refrigerator is not available, store at or below 25°C (77°F) up to 30 days away from heat and light.

RECLAST — RX

zoledronic acid (Novartis)

THERAPEUTIC CLASS: Bisphosphonate

INDICATIONS: Treatment of osteoporosis in postmenopausal women and to reduce incidence of new clinical fractures in patients at high risk of fractures. Treatment to increase bone mass in men with osteoporosis. Treatment of Paget's disease of bone in men and women.

DOSAGE: *Adults:* Osteoporosis (Postmenopausal Women/Men): 5mg IV once a year. Paget's disease: 5mg IV as single dose. Infuse for >15 mins at constant rate. Hydrate prior to administration.

HOW SUPPLIED: Sol: 5mg/100mL [100mL]

CONTRAINDICATIONS: Hypocalcemia

WARNINGS/PRECAUTIONS: Increases risk of hypocalcemia; monitor calcium and mineral levels regularly. May need calcium and vitamin D supplements. Not recommended for use in patients with severe renal impairment (CrCl <35mL/min); monitor SrCr before each dose. May cause osteonecrosis of the jaw; routine oral or dental exam needed prior to treatment. Avoid during pregnancy. Musculoskeletal pain may occur; D/C if severe symptoms develop.

ADVERSE REACTIONS: Influenza, hypocalcemia, headache, lethargy, dyspnea, HTN, A-fib, arthralgia, myalgia, pyrexia, rigors, peripheral edema, paresthesia, dyspnea, angioedema, abdominal pain, musculoskeletal pain/stiffness, fatigue, chills, influenza like illness, malaise, and C-reactive protein increased.

R

INTERACTIONS: Caution with aminoglycosides; may have an additive effect to lower serum calcium for prolonged periods. Caution when used in combination with loop diuretics; may increase risk of hypocalcemia. Caution with other nephrotoxic drugs such as NSAIDs. Avoid use in patients treated with Zometa. Caution in patients sensitive to aspirin; may cause bronchoconstriction.

PREGNANCY: Category D, not for use in nursing.

MECHANISM OF ACTION: Bisphosphonate; acts primarily on bone. Inhibits osteoclast-mediated bone resorption.

PHARMACOKINETICS: Distribution: Plasma protein binding (28-53%). **Elimination:** Urine, $T_{1/2}$=146 hrs.

NURSING CONSIDERATIONS

Assessment: Assess for hypocalcemia, renal function, asthma, parathyroid/intestinal surgery, pregnancy status, musculoskeletal pain, and possible drug interactions.

Monitoring: Monitor renal function, serum creatinine, calcium and phosphate, C-reactive protein level, CBC, BP, HR, acute phase reactions (eg, fever, myalgia, flu-like symptoms), uveitis, osteonecrosis of the jaw, routine dental and oral exams, muscle or joint pain.

Patient Counseling: Advise to take calcium tablets in divided doses for a total of 1500mg in Paget's disease and take adequate calcium and vitamin D for osteoporosis. Take at least 2 glasses of water on day of treatment. Report any adverse effects to physician or dentist.

Administration: IV route. **Storage:** Stable for 24 hrs after opening at 2-8°C (36-46°F). If refrigerated, allow to reach room temperature before administration. Store at 25°C (77°F); excursions permitted to 15-30°C (59-86°F).

RECOMBIVAX HB

hepatitis B (recombinant) (Merck) **RX**

OTHER BRAND NAMES: Recombivax HB Adult (Merck) - Recombivax HB Dialysis (Merck) - Recombivax HB Pediatric/Adolescent (Merck)

THERAPEUTIC CLASS: Vaccine

INDICATIONS: Vaccination against hepatitis B virus.

DOSAGE: *Adults:* Give IM into deltoid muscle. Give SQ if risk of hemorrhage. ≥20 yrs: 3-Dose Regimen: 10mcg at 0,1,6 months. Predialysis/Dialysis (Dialysis Formulation): 40mcg at 0,1,6, months; consider booster if anti-HBs level <10MIU/mL.

Pediatrics: Give IM into anterolateral thigh in infants/young children. Give SQ if risk of hemorrhage. 0-19 yrs: 3-Dose Regimen (Pediatric/Adolescent Formulation) 5mcg at 0,1,6 months. 11-15 yrs: 2-Dose Regimen (Adult Formulation): 10mcg 1st dose, 10mcg 4-6 months later. Infants Born to HBsAg Positive/Unknown Status Mothers: Give 3-dose regimen vaccine and 0.5mL HBIG in opposite anterolateral thigh.

HOW SUPPLIED: Inj: (Pediatric/Adolescent-Preservative Free) 5mcg/0.5mL, (Adult) 10mcg/mL, (Dialysis) 40mcg/mL

CONTRAINDICATIONS: Yeast hypersensitivity.

WARNINGS/PRECAUTIONS: Do not continue therapy if hypersensitivity occurs after injection. May not prevent hepatitis B with unrecognized infection. Caution with severely compromised cardiopulmonary status and those where febrile or systemic reaction is a significant risk. May delay use with serious active infection (eg, febrile illness). Have epinephrine available. Do not give intradermally or IV.

ADVERSE REACTIONS: Irritability, fever, diarrhea, fatigue/weakness, diminished appetite, rhinitis, injection-site reactions.

PREGNANCY: Category C, caution in nursing.

MECHANISM OF ACTION: Stimulation of immune response to produce antibodies that may protect against all subtypes of hepatitis B virus infection.

NURSING CONSIDERATIONS

Assessment: Assess current health status, medical history, previous vaccination history, possible drug interactions, and HBsAg status in pregnancy.

Monitoring: Monitor hypersensitivity reactions, injection site for pain, swelling, pruritus and erythema, fever, headache, nausea, diarrhea, fatigue/weakness, pharyngitis, and upper respiratory tract infection.

Patient Counseling: Inform of potential benefits/risks ratio; report any adverse reactions to physician.

Administration: IM. **Storage:** 2-8°C (36-46°F). Do not freeze.

REFLUDAN

lepirudin (Bayer Healthcare) **RX**

THERAPEUTIC CLASS: Thrombin inhibitor

INDICATIONS: Anticoagulant for heparin-induced thrombocytopenia (HIT) and associated thromboembolic disease.

DOSAGE: *Adults:* LD: 0.4mg/kg (max 44mg) IV over 15-20 seconds. Initial: 0.15mg/kg/hr (max 16.5mg/hr) continuous infusion for 2-10 days. Adjust dose based on aPTT. If aPTT is above target range, stop infusion for 2 hrs and restart at 50% of previous rate. Check aPTT 4 hrs later. If aPTT is below target range, increase rate in steps of 20% and check aPTT 4 hrs later. Do not exceed 0.21mg/kg/hr. Renal Impairment: LD: 0.2mg/kg. Initial: CrCl 45-60 mL/min: 0.075mg/kg/hr. CrCl 30-44mL/min: 0.045mg/kg/hr. CrCl 15-29 mL/min: 0.0225mg/kg/hr. CrCl <15mL/min/Hemodialysis: Avoid or stop infusion. Concomitant Thrombolytic Therapy: LD: 0.2mg/kg. Initial: 0.1mg/kg/hr.

HOW SUPPLIED: Inj: 50mg

WARNINGS/PRECAUTIONS: Risk of bleeding. Weigh risks/benefits with recent puncture of large vessels or organ biopsy, anomaly of vessels or organs, recent CVA, stroke, intracerebral surgery or other neuraxial procedures, severe uncontrolled HTN, bacterial endocarditis, advanced renal impairment, hemorrhagic diathesis, recent major surgery or bleeding. Avoid with baseline aPTT ≥2.5. Monitor aPTT 4 hrs after initiating infusion and at least once daily. Liver injury may enhance anticoagulant effects. Antihirudin antibodies reported; may increase anticoagulant effects.

ADVERSE REACTIONS: Hemorrhagic events (eg, bleeding, anemia, hematoma, hematuria, epistaxis, hemothorax), fever, liver dysfunction, pneumonia, sepsis, allergic skin reactions, multiorgan failure.

INTERACTIONS: Thrombolytics increase risk of life-threatening intracranial bleeding or other bleeding complications and may enhance the effect on aPTT prolongation. Increased risk of bleeding with coumarin derivatives and other drugs that affect platelet function.

PREGNANCY: Category B, not for use in nursing.

MECHANISM OF ACTION: Thrombin inhibitor; binds to thrombin and thereby blocks its thrombogenic activity.

PHARMACOKINETICS: Absorption: C_{max}=1500ng/mL. **Distribution:** V_d=12.2L. **Metabolism:** Catabolic hydrolysis. **Elimination:** Urine(48%); $T_{1/2}$=1.3 hrs.

NURSING CONSIDERATIONS

Assessment: Assess for bleeding risk (eg, recent puncture of large vessels, recent cerebrovascular accident, severe uncontrolled HTN, bacterial endocarditis, hemorrhagic diasthesis), presence of hepatic/renal dysfunction, nursing status, and drug interactions. Obtain baseline aPTT ratio.

Monitoring: Monitor for signs/symptoms of bleeding complications (eg, intracranial bleeding) and allergic reactions (eg, anaphylactic reactions). Monitor aPTT ratio 4 hours after start of infusion and perform once daily thereafter during treatment.

Patient Counseling: Instruct to notify physician immediately if develop any type of allergic reaction (eg, anaphylaxis). Advise about increased risk of bleeding during therapy. Laboratory monitoring is needed during therapy.

Administration: IV route. Do not mix with other drugs. Reconstitute: 1) Use Sterile Water for Inj, USP; or 0.9% for NaCl Inj, USP. 2) For rapid, complete reconstitution, inject 1mL of diluent into the vial and shake it gently. 3) Further dilute to final concentration of 5mg/mL. Dilute using 0.9% NaCl Inj USP, or 5% Dextrose Inj USP. 4) Warm to room temperature prior to administration. **Storage:** Unopened vials: 2-25°C (35.6-77°F). Reconstituted: Use immediately; will remain stable for 24 hrs at room temperature.

RELENZA RX

zanamivir (GlaxoSmithKline)

THERAPEUTIC CLASS: Neuraminidase inhibitor

INDICATIONS: Treatment of uncomplicated acute illness due to influenza A and B virus in patients symptomatic for ≤2 days. Prophylaxis of influenza.

DOSAGE: *Adults:* Treatment: Usual: 2 inh (10mg) q12h for 5 days. Take 2 doses at least 2 hrs apart on 1st day. Prophylaxis: Household Setting: 2 inh (10mg) qd for 10 days. Community Setting: 2 inh (10mg) qd for 28 days. Administer at same time every day.
Pediatrics: Treatment: ≥7 yrs: Usual: 2 inh (10mg) q12h for 5 days. Take 2 doses at least 2 hrs apart on 1st day. Prophylaxis: ≥5 yrs: Household Setting: 2 inh (10mg) qd for 10 days. Community Setting: ≥12 yrs: 2 inh (10mg) qd for 28 days. Administer at same time every day.

HOW SUPPLIED: Inh: 5mg/inh [20 blisters]

WARNINGS/PRECAUTIONS: Not recommended for use with underlying airways disease (eg, asthma, COPD). Serious cases of bronchospasm reported during treatment; d/c if bronchospasm or decline in respiratory function develops. D/C if allergic reaction occurs. Postmarketing neuropsychiatric events (seizures, delirium, hallucinations) reported.

ADVERSE REACTIONS: Dizziness, headaches, diarrhea, nausea, sinusitis, bronchitis, cough, ear/nose/throat infections, nasal symptoms.

INTERACTIONS: Use inhaled bronchodilator before zanamivir. Avoid administration of live attenuated influenza vaccine within 2 weeks before or 48 hours after.

PREGNANCY: Category C, caution in nursing.

MECHANISM OF ACTION: Neuraminidase inhibitor; inhibits influenza virus neuraminidase, affecting release of particles.

PHARMACOKINETICS: Absorption: Absolute bioavailability (4-17%); C_{max}=17-142ng/mL; T_{max}=1-2 hrs; AUC=111-1364ng•hr/mL. **Distribution:** Plasma protein binding (<10%). **Elimination**: Renal; $T_{1/2}$=2.5-5.1 hrs.

NURSING CONSIDERATIONS

Assessment: Assess for history of allergic reaction to lactose (milk proteins) and airway diseases (asthma or COPD).

Monitoring: Monitor for signs/symptoms of bronchospasm (worsening wheezing, SOB), allergic-like reactions (oropharyngeal edema, serious skin rashes, anaphylaxis) and neuropsychiatric events (seizures, hallucinations, abnormal behavior). Respiratory function must be monitored.

Patient Counseling: Advise to seek medical attention if symptoms of bronchospasm (worsening wheezing, SOB), allergic reaction (oropharyngeal edema, rash), or neuropsychiatric events (seizures, confusion, abnormal behavior) occur. Instruct on proper use of diskhaler and to use inhaled bronchodilator before therapy.

Administration: Oral route. **Storage**: 25°C (77°F); excursions permitted to 15-30°C (59-86°F).

RELPAX

RX

eletriptan hydrobromide (Pfizer)

THERAPEUTIC CLASS: 5-$HT_{1B/1D}$ agonist

INDICATIONS: Acute treatment of migraine with or without aura.

DOSAGE: *Adults:* ≥18 yrs: Initial: 20 or 40mg at onset of headache. If recurs after initial relief, may repeat after 2 hrs. Max: 40mg/dose or 80mg/day. Safety of treating >3 headaches/30 days not known. Severe Hepatic Impairment: Avoid use. Avoid within 72 hrs of potent CYP3A4 inhibitors.

HOW SUPPLIED: Tab: 20mg, 40mg

CONTRAINDICATIONS: Ischemic heart disease, coronary artery vasospasm (eg, Prinzmetal's angina) or other significant underlying cardiovascular disease, peripheral vascular disease, cerebrovascular syndromes, uncontrolled HTN, hemiplegic or basilar migraine, use within 24 hrs of other 5-HT_1 agonist or ergot-type agent (eg, dihydroergotamine, methysergide), severe hepatic impairment.

WARNINGS/PRECAUTIONS: Confirm diagnosis. Supervise 1st dose and monitor cardiac function in those at risk of CAD (eg, HTN, hypercholesterolemia, smoker, obesity, diabetes, CAD family history, postmenopausal women, males >40 yrs). Consider ECG during interval immediately following initial administration in patients with CAD risk factors. Monitor cardiac function in intermittent long-term users with CAD risk factors. Serious adverse cardiac events, increased BP, cerebrovascular events, vasospastic reactions reported. Serotonin syndrome symptoms (eg, mental status changes, autonomic instability, neuromuscular aberrations, and GI symptoms) reported. Caution in elderly. Possible long-term ophthalmic effects.

ADVERSE REACTIONS: Asthenia, chest tightness, dizziness, dry mouth, headache, nausea, paresthesia, somnolence, pain/pressure/heaviness in precordium/throat/jaw.

INTERACTIONS: Prolonged vasospastic reactions reported with ergot-containing drugs; avoid within 24 hours of each other. Avoid within 72 hrs of potent CYP3A4 inhibitors (eg, ketoconazole, itraconazole, nefazodone, troleandomycin, clarithromycin, ritonavir, nelfinavir). Serotonin syndrome reported with combined use of an SSRI or SNRI. Avoid within 24 hrs of other 5-HT_1 agonists. Propranolol, erythromycin, verapamil, fluconazole may increase levels.

PREGNANCY: Category C, caution in nursing.

MECHANISM OF ACTION: Selective $5HT_{1D/1B}$ agonist; binds with high affinity to $5HT_{1D/1B/1F}$ receptors. Believed to activate receptors located on intracranial blood vessels, including those on arteriovenousananstomoses, which leads to vasoconstriction and is correlated with relief of migraine headache. Activation of receptors located on sensory nerve endings in trigeminal system results in inhibition of pro-inflammatory neuropeptide release.

PHARMACOKINETICS: Absorption: Complete; absolute bioavailability (50%); T_{max}=1.5 hrs. **Distribution:** V_d=138L; plasma protein binding (85%). **Metabolism:** N-demethylated (active metabolite). **Elimination:** $T_{1/2}$= 4 hrs (parent drug), 13 hrs (metabolite).

NURSING CONSIDERATIONS

Assessment: Confirm diagnosis of migraine before therapy. Assess for IHD (eg, angina pectoris, Prinzmetal's variant angina, MI or documented silent MI), cerebrovascular syndrome (eg, stroke, TIAs), HTN, hemiplegic or basilar migraine, PVD, presence of CAD risk factors (eg, hypercholesterolemia, smoking, obesity, DM, strong family history of CAD, female with surgical or physiological menopause, or male >49 yrs), ECG changes, hepatic/renal impairment, pregnancy/nursing status, and possible drug interactions.

Monitoring: Administration of 1st dose should be in physician's office or medically staffed and equipped facility as cardiac ischemia can occur in absence of clinical symptoms; ECG should be obtained immediately during interval in those with risk factors. Monitor for signs/symptoms of cardiac events (eg, coronary vasospasm, acute MI, arrhythmia, ECG changes, follow-up coronary angiography), cerebrovascular events (eg, hemorrhage, stroke, TIAs), peripheral vascular ischemia, colonic ischemia with bloody diarrhea and abdominal pain, serotonin syndrome (eg, mental status changes, autonomic instability, neuromuscular aberrations and/or GI symptoms), ophthalmic effects, and increased BP.

Patient Counseling: Inform about potential benefits/risks (eg, symptoms of serotonin syndrome especially if taken with SSRIs or SNRIs). Advise to take exactly as prescribed. Instruct to notify physician if pregnant/nursing or planning to become pregnant.

Administration: Oral route. **Storage:** 25°C (77°F); excursions permitted to 15-30°C (59-86°F).

REMERON RX

mirtazapine (Schering)

Antidepressants increased the risk of suicidal thinking and behavior (suicidality) in short-term studies in children, adolescents, and young adults with major depressive disorder (MDD) and other psychiatric disorders. Mirtazapine is not approved for use in pediatric patients.

OTHER BRAND NAMES: Remeron SolTab (Schering)

THERAPEUTIC CLASS: Piperazino-azepine

INDICATIONS: Treatment of MDD.

DOSAGE: *Adults:* Initial: 15mg qhs. Titrate: May increase every 1-2 weeks. Max: 45mg/day. Disintegrating tabs disintegrate rapidly on tongue and can be swallowed with saliva; no water needed. Do not cut tabs in half.

HOW SUPPLIED: Tab: 15mg*, 30mg*, 45mg; Tab, Disintegrating: 15mg, 30mg, 45mg *scored

WARNINGS/PRECAUTIONS: Risk of agranulocytosis. D/C if sore throat, fever, or stomatitis, along with low WBC count, develop. May increase appetite, cholesterol, and triglycerides. Caution in history of seizures, mania/hypomania, hepatic or renal impairment, altered metabolic or hemodynamic conditions, elderly. Somnolence, dizziness reported. Close supervision with high-risk suicide patients. May impair judgment, thinking, or motor skills.

ADVERSE REACTIONS: Somnolence, appetite increase, weight gain, dizziness, dry mouth, constipation, asthenia, flu syndrome, abnormal dreams.

INTERACTIONS: Alcohol and diazepam increase cognitive and motor skill impairment. Avoid MAOIs within 14 days of use.

PREGNANCY: Category C, caution in nursing.

MECHANISM OF ACTION: Antidepressant belonging to the piperazino-azepine group; suspected to enhance central noradrenergic and serotonergic activity.

PHARMACOKINETICS: Absorption: Rapidly and completely absorbed; Absolute bioavailability (50%); T_{max}=2 hrs. **Distribution:** Plasma protein binding (85%). **Metabolism:** Demethylation and hydroxylation followed by glucuronide conjugation. **Elimination:** Urine (75%), feces (15%); $T_{1/2}$=37 hrs (female), 26 hrs (male).

NURSING CONSIDERATIONS

Assessment: Assess for seizures, major depressive disorder, bipolar disorder, cardiac arrhythmias, MI. Note other diseases/conditions and drug therapies.

Monitoring: Monitor for worsening of depression and/or emergence of suicidal ideation or unusual changes in behavior, LFTs, renal function tests, CBC with differential, and lipid profile.

Patient Counseling: Warn about risk of developing agranulocytosis. Advise families and caregivers of the need for close observation of clinical worsening and suicidal risks. Advise to avoid alcohol, sedatives, and OTC agents. Caution against operating machinery/driving. Instruct to report adverse reactions and consult physician before taking any other medications.

Administration: Oral route. **Storage:** Store at 25°C (77°F); excursions permitted to 15-30°C (59-86°F). Protect from light and moisture.

REMICADE

RX

infliximab (Centocor)

Reports of TB, invasive fungal infections, and other opportunistic infections. Evaluate for latent TB and treat if necessary prior to initiation of therapy.

THERAPEUTIC CLASS: Monoclonal antibody/TNF-alpha receptor blocker

INDICATIONS: In combination with methotrexate (MTX), for reducing signs/symptoms, inhibiting structural damage progression and improving physical function in moderately to severely active rheumatoid arthritis (RA). For reducing signs/symptoms and inducing and maintaining clinical remission of moderately to severely active Crohn's disease, when response to conventional therapy is inadequate. For reducing the number of draining enterocutaneous and rectovaginal fistulas and maintaining fistula closure in fistulizing Crohn's disease. For reducing signs/symptoms in patients with active ankylosing spondylitis (AS). For reducing signs/symptoms of active arthritis, inhibiting structural damage progression, and improving physical function in patients with psoriatic arthritis. For reducing signs/symptoms, inducing and maintaining clinical remission and mucosal healing, and eliminating corticosteroid use in patients with moderately to severely active ulcerative colitis (UC) who have inadequate response to conventional therapy. Treatment of patients with chronic, severe plaque psoriasis who are candidates for systemic therapy and when other systemic therapies are medically less appropriate.

DOSAGE: *Adults:* RA (Combo with MTX): 3mg/kg as IV infusion; repeat at 2 and 6 weeks. Maint: 3mg/kg every 8 weeks. Incomplete Response: May increase to 10mg/kg or give every 4 weeks. Crohn's Disease/Fistulizing Crohn's Disease: Induction Regimen: 5mg/kg IV at 0, 2, and 6 weeks. Maint: 5mg/kg every 8 weeks. For patients who respond then lose their response, may increase to 10mg/kg. Consider discontinuing therapy if no response to by Week 14. Ankylosing Spondylitis: 5mg/kg as IV infusion; repeat at 2 and 6 weeks. Maint: 5mg/kg every 6 weeks. Psoriatic Arthritis: 5mg/kg as IV infusion; repeat at 2 and 6 weeks. Maint: 5mg/kg every 8 weeks. May be used with or without MTX. Ulcerative Colitis: 5mg/kg at 0, 2, and 6 weeks. Maint: 5mg/kg every 8 weeks. Plaque Psoriasis: 5mg/kg IV infusion; repeat at 2 and 6 weeks. Maint: 5mg/kg every 8 weeks.
Pediatrics: ≥6 yrs: Crohn's Disease: Induction Regimen: 5mg/kg IV at 0, 2, and 6 weeks. Maint: 5mg/kg every 8 weeks.

HOW SUPPLIED: Inj: 100mg

CONTRAINDICATIONS: Hypersensitivity to murine proteins. Moderate or severe CHF (NYHA Class III/IV) with doses >5mg/kg.

WARNINGS/PRECAUTIONS: Leukopenia, neutropenia, thrombocytopenia, and pancytopenia reported. Serious infections, including sepsis and pneumonia, reported. Avoid with active infection. Monitor for signs of infection during and after therapy; d/c if serious infection develops. Caution in patients who have resided in areas where histoplasmosis or coccidioidomycosis are endemic. Hypersensitivity reactions reported. Caution with optic neuritis, chronic and recurrent infections, CNS demyelinating disease (eg, MS) and seizure disorder. May result in autoantibody formation; d/c if lupus-like syndrome develops. Monitor closely and d/c if new or worsening symptoms of heart failure appear. Lymphoma reported; caution with malignancies. Severe hepatic reactions, including acute liver failure, jaundice, hepatitis and cholestasis reported rarely. Caution in elderly.

ADVERSE REACTIONS: Nausea, infections, infusion reactions, headache, sinusitis, pharyngitis, coughing, abdominal pain, diarrhea, bronchitis, dyspepsia, fatigue, rhinitis, pain, arthralgia, hepatotoxicity.

INTERACTIONS: Do not give concurrently with live vaccines. May increase risk of serious infections and neutropenia with anakinra.

PREGNANCY: Category B, not for use in nursing.

MECHANISM OF ACTION: Monoclonal antibody; neutralizes biological activity of TNF-α by binding with high affinity to the soluble and transmembrane forms of TNF-α and inhibiting binding of TNF-α with its receptors.

PHARMACOKINETICS: Elimination: $T_{1/2}$=7.7-9.5 days.

NURSING CONSIDERATIONS

Assessment: Assess for heart failure, active or chronic infection (eg, hepatitis B virus), history of recurrent infection, previous history of TB, risk of histoplasmosis or coccidioidomycosis infection, pregnancy/nursing status, and possible drug interactions. Assess that pediatric patients with Crohn's disease are up-to-date with vaccinations. Perform test for latent TB and treat; assess need for TB therapy in patients who have risk factors for TB and a negative test for latent TB.

Monitoring: Monitor for signs/symptoms of infection (eg, sepsis, pneumonia, TB, invasive fungal infection), hepatitis B reactivation, hepatotoxicity (eg, acute liver failure, autoimmune hepatitis, jaundice, cholestasis), hematological events (eg, leukopenia, neutropenia, thrombocytopenia, pancytopenia), hypersensitivity reactions (eg, urticaria, dyspnea, hypotension, serum sickness-like reactions), neurologic events (eg, optic neuritis, seizures, CNS demyelinating disorders), malignancies (eg, lymphoma), and lupus-like syndrome. In adolescents/young adults with Crohn's disease, monitor for T-cell lymphoma.

In patients with heart failure, monitor for worsening of symptoms. Monitor overall health at each treatment visit.

Patient Counseling: Advise to immediately contact physician if signs/symptoms of infection (fever, fatigue, cough, warm/red/painful skin), hypersensitivity reaction (eg, hives, difficulty breathing, chest pain, fever), malignancies, worsening heart failure, liver injury (eg, jaundice, dark brown urine), hematological complications (eg, bruising, fever), and CNS disorders (eg, visual changes, weakness in arms or legs) develop.

Administration: IV infusion route. Reconstitute: 1) Use 10mL of Sterile Water for Injection. 2) Further dilute to 250mL with 0.9% NaCl Inj. Infusion should begin within 3 hrs of preparation. Infusion solution must be administered over a period of not less than 2 hrs. Do not store any unused portion. Prior to infusion, premedication may be administered (eg, antihistamines, acetaminophen, corticosteroids). If hypersensitivity reactions occur, may improve by slowing or suspending infusion. Upon resolution of reaction, reinitiating at a slower rate may help. **Storage:** Lyophilized powder: 2-8°C (36-46°F). Do not freeze or use beyond expiration date. Product contains no preservative.

REMODULIN RX

treprostinil sodium (United Therapeutics)

THERAPEUTIC CLASS: Pulmonary and systemic vasodilator

INDICATIONS: Treatment of pulmonary arterial hypertension (PAH) in patients with NYHA Class II-IV symptoms to diminish symptoms associated with exercise.

DOSAGE: *Adults:* Initial: 1.25ng/kg/min SQ continuous infusion. Reduce rate to 0.625ng/kg/min if not tolerated. Titrate: Increase by no more than 1.25ng/kg/min per week for first 4 weeks, then no more than 2.5ng/kg/min per week thereafter, depending on clinical response.

HOW SUPPLIED: Inj: 1mg/mL, 2.5mg/mL, 5mg/mL, 10mg/mL [20mL]

WARNINGS/PRECAUTIONS: For SQ use only. Initiate therapy in adequate setting for monitoring and emergency care. Abrupt withdrawal or sudden large dose reduction may worsen PAH symptoms. Caution with hepatic or renal impairment.

ADVERSE REACTIONS: Infusion site pain/reactions, headache, diarrhea, nausea, rash, jaw pain, vasodilatation, dizziness, edema, pruritus, hypotension.

INTERACTIONS: Drugs that alter BP (eg, diuretics, antihypertensives, vasodilators) may potentiate BP reduction. Increased risk of bleeding with anticoagulants.

PREGNANCY: Category B, caution in nursing.

MECHANISM OF ACTION: Pulmonary and systemic vasodilator; causes direct vasodilation of pulmonary and systemic arterial vascular beds; inhibits platelet aggregation.

PHARMACOKINETICS: Absorption: (SQ): Rapid, complete. Absolute bioavailability (100%). **Distribution:** V_d=14L/70kg, plasma protein binding (91%). **Metabolism:** Liver. **Elimination:** Urine (4%).

NURSING CONSIDERATIONS

Assessment: Assess for hepatic/renal impairment and possible drug interactions. Obtain baseline LFTs and renal function.

Monitoring: Monitor LFTs and renal function. Monitor for worsening of symptoms, hepatic/renal impairment, abrupt withdrawal symptoms, and hypersensitivity reactions.

Patient Counseling: Inform infusion is continuous through a SQ or surgically placed indwelling central venous catheter, via an infusion pump. Advise to seek medical attention if worsening of symptoms, hepatic/renal impairment, abrupt withdrawal symptoms, or hypersensitivity reactions occur.

Administration: SQ, IV. **Storage:** 25°C (77°F); excursions permitted to 15-30°C (59-86°F). (Undiluted): 37°C; stable for 72 hrs. (Diluted): 37°C; stable for 48 hrs.

RenaGel — RX

sevelamer HCl (Genzyme)

THERAPEUTIC CLASS: Phosphate Binder

INDICATIONS: Reduction of serum phosphorus in end-stage renal disease.

DOSAGE: *Adults:* Patients Not Taking Phosphate Binder: Usual: 800-1600mg with each meal. Initial: Serum Phosphorus: >6 and <7.5mg/dL: 800mg tid. ≥7.5 and <9mg/dL: 1200-1600mg tid. ≥9mg/dL: 1600mg tid. Titration: Serum Phosphorus >6mg/dL: Increase by 1 tab/cap per meal at 2-week intervals. 3.5-6mg/dL: Maintain dose. <3.5mg/dL: Decrease 1 tab/cap per meal at 2-week intervals. Swallow caps and tabs whole with meals. Switching from Calcium Acetate: Initial: Based on calcium acetate dose.

HOW SUPPLIED: Tab: 400mg, 800mg

CONTRAINDICATIONS: Hypophosphatemia or bowel obstruction.

WARNINGS/PRECAUTIONS: Caution with dysphagia, swallowing disorders, severe GI motility or GI surgery. Monitor serum calcium, bicarbonate and chloride.

ADVERSE REACTIONS: NV, infection, thrombosis, cough increased, respiratory effects, constipation, diarrhea, flatulence, dyspepsia, intestinal obstruction and ileus, fecal impaction, bowel perforation.

INTERACTIONS: May bind other drugs; give drugs with narrow therapeutic index 1 hr before or 3 hrs after sevelamer. Caution with antiarrhythmic or antiseizure medications. May decrease ciprofloxacin bioavailability by 50%.

PREGNANCY: Category C, unknown use in nursing.

MECHANISM OF ACTION: Phosphate binder; binds to phosphate in the dietary tract, decreasing absorption and lowering its serum concentration.

NURSING CONSIDERATIONS

Assessment: Assess for hypophosphatemia, bowel obstruction, dysphagia, swallowing disorders, severe GI motility disorders including severe constipation, major GI tract surgery, pregnancy status, peritoneal/hemodialysis patients, possible drug interactions.

Monitoring: Monitor serum chemistries (eg, bicarbonate and chloride levels), levels of vitamin D, E, and K (clotting factors) and folic acid, and for constipation.

Patient Counseling: Counsel to take with meals and adhere to prescribed diets. Dose separately from therapy if taken with concomitant medication. Report if new onset or worsening of existing constipation occurs.

Administration: Oral route. **Storage:** 25°C (77°F); excursions permitted to 15-30°C (59-86°F); avoid moisture.

Renova — RX

tretinoin (Ortho Neutrogena)

THERAPEUTIC CLASS: Retinoid

INDICATIONS: Adjunct to comprehensive skin care and sunlight avoidance programs, for mitigation of fine facial wrinkles.

DOSAGE: *Adults:* 18-71 yrs: Wash face with mild soap, pat skin dry, and wait 20-30 min before use. Apply once daily in evening. Max: 52 weeks of therapy. May apply cosmetics 1 hr later. Use moisturizer every morning to prevent dryness.

HOW SUPPLIED: Cre: 0.02% [40g]

WARNINGS/PRECAUTIONS: Avoid with sunburned skin, eczema, chronic skin conditions, and pregnancy. Larger amounts will not lead to better or faster results and may increase adverse effects. Avoid contact with eyes, mouth, paranasal creases, and mucous membranes. D/C if sensitivity, irritation, or systemic adverse reaction develops. Minimize sunlight exposure; avoid sunlamps. Wear protective clothing and use SPF ≥15. Causes photosensitivity. Extreme weather may increase skin irritation.

ADVERSE REACTIONS: Peeling, dry skin, burning, stinging, erythema, pruritus at the site of application.

INTERACTIONS: Caution with topical agents with strong drying effects, high concentration of alcohol, astringents, spices or lime, permanent wave solutions, electrolysis, hair depilatories, waxes or medicated or abrasive soaps, shampoos and cleansers. Increased phototoxicity with photosensitizers (eg, thiazides, tetracyclines, fluoroquinolones, phenothiazines, sulfonamides).

PREGNANCY: Category C, not for use in nursing.

MECHANISM OF ACTION: Endogenous retinoid metabolite of vitamin A; binds to intracellular receptors in the cytosol and nucleus. Activates three members of the retinoic acid (RAR) nuclear receptors (RARα, RARβ, RAR-gamma), which may act to modify gene expression, subsequent protein synthesis, and epithelial cell growth and differentiation.

NURSING CONSIDERATIONS

Assessment: Assess for hypersensitivity reactions, skin eczema, pregnancy/nursing status, and possible drug interactions (eg, photosensitizing drugs such as thiazides and tetracyclines).

Monitoring: Monitor for irritation, erythema, pruritus, burning, stinging, and peeling at application site and for atypical changes in melanocytes, keratinocytes, and increased dermal elastosis.

Patient Counseling: Counsel to avoid prolonged exposure to sunlight; wear protective clothing. Inform that extreme weather such as wind or cold may cause irritation. Notify if pregnant/nursing or planning to become pregnant.

Administration: Topical application. **Storage:** 25°C (77°F); excursions permitted to 15-30°C (59-86°F).

REOPRO RX

abciximab (Lilly)

THERAPEUTIC CLASS: Glycoprotein IIb/IIIa inhibitor

INDICATIONS: Adjunct to percutaneous coronary intervention (PCI) for prevention of cardiac ischemic complications in patients undergoing PCI or with unstable angina unresponsive to conventional therapy when PCI is planned within 24 hrs. Intended for use with aspirin and heparin.

DOSAGE: *Adults:* PCI: 0.25mg/kg IV bolus given 10-60 min before start PCI, followed by 0.125mcg/kg/min IV infusion (Max: 10mcg/min) for 12 hrs. Unstable Angina: 0.25mg/kg IV bolus followed by 10mcg/min infusion for 18-24 hrs, concluding 1 hr after PCI.

HOW SUPPLIED: Inj: 2mg/mL

CONTRAINDICATIONS: Active internal bleeding, recent (within 6 weeks) significant GI or GU bleeding, CVA within 2 yrs, CVA with significant residual neurological deficit, bleeding diathesis, oral anticoagulants within 7 days (unless PT ≤1.2x control), thrombocytopenia, recent (within 6 weeks) major surgery or trauma, intracranial neoplasm, arteriovenous malformation, aneurysm, severe uncontrolled HTN, history of vasculitis, IV dextran use before PCI or during an intervention. Hypersensitivity to murine proteins.

WARNINGS/PRECAUTIONS: Increased risk of bleeding. Monitor all potential bleeding sites (eg, catheter insertion sites, arterial and venous puncture sites, cutdown sites). Minimize vascular and other trauma. D/C if serious, uncontrollable bleeding, thrombocytopenia, or emergency surgery occurs. Anaphylaxis may occur. Antibody (HACA) formation may occur; risk of hypersensitivity, thrombocytopenia, decreased benefit with readministration. Monitor platelets, PT, APTT, ACT before infusion.

ADVERSE REACTIONS: Bleeding, thrombocytopenia, hypotension, bradycardia, NV, back/chest pain, headache.

INTERACTIONS: Caution with other drugs that affect hemostasis (eg, thrombolytics, heparin, oral anticoagulants, NSAIDs, dipyridamole, ticlopidine). Increased risk of bleeding with anticoagulants, thrombolytics, and antiplatelets. If have HACA titers, possible allergic reactions with monoclonal antibody agents.

PREGNANCY: Category C, caution in nursing.

MECHANISM OF ACTION: Glycoprotein IIb/IIIa inhibitor; binds to the GPIIb/IIIa receptor and inhibits platelet aggregation by preventing the binding of fibrinogen, von Willebrand factor, and other adhesive molecules to GPIIb/IIIa receptor sites on activated platelets. Also binds to vitronectin receptor, which mediates the procoagulant properties of platelets and the proliferative properties of vascular endothelial and smooth muscle cells.

PHARMACOKINETICS: Elimination: $T_{1/2}$=30 min.

NURSING CONSIDERATIONS

Assessment: Assess for active internal bleeding, recent GI or genitourinary bleeding, history of cerebrovascular accident, bleeding diathesis, thrombocytopenia, recent major surgery or trauma, intracranial neoplasm, arteriovenous malformation, aneurysm, severe uncontrolled HTN, presence or history of vasculitis, pregnancy/nursing status, and drug interactions. Obtain baseline prothrombin time, ACT, aPTT, and platelet counts.

Monitoring: Monitor for signs/symptoms of bleeding; document and monitor vascular puncture sites. If hematoma develops, monitor for enlargement. Monitor for allergic reactions (eg, anaphylaxis) and thrombocytopenia. Check aPTT or ACT prior to arterial sheath removal; should not be removed unless aPTT ≤50 seconds or ACT ≤175 seconds. Monitor platelet counts 2-4 hrs following bolus dose and 24 hrs prior to discharge.

Patient Counseling: Counsel to contact physician if develop hypersensitivity reactions (eg, anaphylaxis). Inform may take longer than usual to stop bleeding and may bruise or bleed easier while on medication. Instruct to report any unusual bleeding to physician.

Administration: IV infusion. In case of hypersensitivity reaction, epinephrine, dopamine, theophylline, antihistamines, and corticosteroids should be available for immediate use. **Storage:** Store at 2-8°C (36-46°F). Do not freeze. Do not shake. Discard any unused portion left in vial.

REQUIP **RX**

ropinirole HCl (GlaxoSmithKline)

OTHER BRAND NAMES: Requip XL (GlaxoSmithKline)

THERAPEUTIC CLASS: Non-ergoline dopamine agonist

INDICATIONS: (Tab/Tab, Extended-Release) Treatment of signs and symptoms of idiopathic Parkinson's disease. (Tab) Treatment of moderate-to-severe primary Restless Legs Syndrome (RLS).

DOSAGE: *Adults:* Parkinson's: Tab: Initial: 0.25mg tid. Titrate: May increase weekly by 0.25mg tid (0.75mg/day) for 4 weeks. After week 4, may increase weekly by 1.5mg/day up to 9mg/day, then by 3mg/day weekly to 24mg/day. Max: 24mg/day. Withdrawal: Decrease dose to bid for 4 days, then qd for 3 days. Tab, Extended-Release: Initial: 2mg qd for 1-2 weeks. Titrate: May increase by 2mg/day at ≥1 week intervals, depending on therapeutic response and tolerability. Max: 24mg/day. Swallow whole; do not chew, crush, or divide. Switching from Immediate-Release (IR) to XL: Initial dose should match total daily dose of IR formulation. See PI for more info. RLS: Tab: Initial: 0.25mg qd, 1-3 hours before bedtime. Titrate: 0.5mg qd days 3-7, 1mg qd week 2, then increase by 0.5mg weekly. Max: 4mg.

HOW SUPPLIED: Tab: 0.25mg, 0.5mg, 1mg, 2mg, 3mg, 4mg, 5mg; Tab, Extended-Release: (XL) 2mg, 4mg, 8mg

WARNINGS/PRECAUTIONS: (Tab/Tab, Extended-Release) Falling asleep during activities of daily living reported; if significant, d/c or warn patient to refrain from dangerous activities. Syncope, symptomatic hypotension, and hallucinations reported. Caution with severe renal or hepatic dysfunction. May cause or exacerbate pre-existing dyskinesia. Neuroleptic malignant syndrome, fibrotic complications, and melanoma reported. Augmentation and rebound in RLS reported. Avoid rapid dose reduction or abrupt withdrawal. Compulsive behaviors reported. (Tab, Extended-Release) May cause elevation of BP and changes in HR.

ADVERSE REACTIONS: (Tab) Neuralgia, increased BUN, hallucinations, somnolence, vomiting, headache, sweating, asthenia, edema, fatigue, syncope, orthostatic symptoms. (Tab, Extended-Release) Nausea, somnolence, dizziness, constipation, abdominal pain/discomfort.

INTERACTIONS: Adjust dose if CYP1A2 inhibitor or estrogen is stopped or started during treatment. Potentiated by ciprofloxacin. Decreased effects with dopamine antagonists (eg, phenothiazines, butyrophenones, thioxanthenes, metoclopramide). Drowsiness increased with sedatives. Caution with dopamine antagonists or alcohol.

PREGNANCY: Category C, not for use in nursing.

MECHANISM OF ACTION: Nonergoline dopamine agonist; believed to stimulate post synaptic D_2-type receptors within the caudate-putamen in the brain.

PHARMACOKINETICS: Absorption: Rapid; absolute bioavailability (55%), T_{max}=1-2 hrs. **Distribution:** V_d=7.5L/kg, plasma protein binding (40%). **Metabolism:** Liver via CYP1A2 (extensive); N-despropylation and hydroxylation. **Elimination:** Urine, $T_{1/2}$=6 hrs.

NURSING CONSIDERATIONS

Assessment: Assess LFTs, renal function tests, and CBC. Assess for glaucoma, dyskinesia, psychosis, depression, cardiovascular complications, and possible drug interactions.

Monitoring: Perform dermatological screening periodically. Monitor eye exams and for symptoms of neuroleptic malignant syndrome, impulse control symptoms (eg, compulsive behaviors such as pathological gambling and hypersexuality), fibrotic complications, melanomas, signs/symptoms of postural hypotension, hallucinations.

Patient Counseling: Caution while operating machinery/driving. Counsel on potential for drowsiness, daytime sleepiness, falling asleep during activity; d/c if occurs. Risk of symptomatic hypotension. Take as prescribed; avoid alcohol or concurrent CNS depressants. Report lack of response or severe adverse effects.

Administration: Oral route. **Storage:** (Requip) 20-25°C (68-77°F). Protect from light and moisture. (Requip XL) 25°C (77°F); excursions permitted to 15-30°C (59-86°F). Dispense in a tight, light-resistant container.

RESCRIPTOR RX

delavirdine mesylate (Pfizer)

THERAPEUTIC CLASS: Non-nucleoside reverse transcriptase inhibitor

INDICATIONS: Treatment of HIV-1 infection in combination with other antiretrovirals.

DOSAGE: *Adults:* Usual: 400mg tid. May disperse 100mg tab in ≥3 oz of water (200mg tab is not dispersible). Take with acidic beverage (eg, orange juice) if achlorhydric.

Pediatrics: ≥16yrs: Usual: 400mg tid. May disperse 100mg tab in ≥3 oz of water (200mg tab is not dispersible). Take with acidic beverage (eg, orange juice) if achlorhydric.

HOW SUPPLIED: Tab: 100mg, 200mg

CONTRAINDICATIONS: Contraindicated with drugs that are highly dependent on CYP3A for clearance (eg, astemizole, terfenadine, dihydroergotamine, egonovine, ergotamine, methylergonovine, cisapride, pimozide, alprazolam, midazolam, triazolam).

WARNINGS/PRECAUTIONS: Caution with hepatic dysfunction. D/C if severe rash develops. May cause immune reconstitution syndrome. May confer cross-resistance to other NNRTIs. May cause body fat redistribution/accumulation.

ADVERSE REACTIONS: Headache, fatigue, NV, diarrhea, increased ALT and AST, rash, maculopapular rash, pruritus, erythema, insomnia, upper respiratory infection.

INTERACTIONS: See Contraindications. Antacids decrease absorption; separate doses by 1 hr. H_2 antagonists reduce absorption; avoid chronic use. CYP3A inducers (eg, carbamazepine, phenobarbital, phenytoin, rifabutin, rifampin) may decrease plasma levels; avoid concomitant use. Increased plasma levels of drugs metabolized by CYP3A and 2C9 and amprenavir. Certain nonsedating antihistamines, sedative hypnotics, antiarrhythmics, CCBs, ergot agents, amphetamines, cisapride, and sildenafil (max of 25mg/48hrs of sildenafil) may result in potentially serious and/or life-threatening adverse events. Reduced effects of both delavirdine and didanosine; separate doses by 1 hr. Monitor LFTs with saquinavir. Increases indinavir plasma levels; reduce indinavir dose to 600mg tid.

PREGNANCY: Category C, not for use in nursing.

MECHANISM OF ACTION: HIV-1 non-nucleoside reverse transcriptase inhibitor (NNRTI). Binds directly to reverse transcriptase (RT) and blocks RNA-dependent and DNA-dependent DNA polymerase activities.

PHARMACOKINETICS: Absorption: Rapid; C_{max}=35μM, T_{max}=1 hr, AUC=180μM•hr. Bioavailability (85%). **Distribution:** Plasma protein binding (98%). **Metabolism:** Hepatic (N-desalkylation, pyridine hydroxylation) via CYP3A (major), 2D6. **Elimination:** Urine (<5%). $T_{1/2}$=5.8 hrs.

NURSING CONSIDERATIONS

Assessment: Assess for hepatic dysfunction and possible drug interactions.

Monitoring: Monitor for signs/symptoms of hypersensitivity reactions, immune reconstitution syndrome, hepatic dysfunction, and fat redistribution.

Patient Counseling: Inform to take as prescribed, not to alter dose without consulting doctor. If miss dose, do not double next dose. Patients with achlorhydria should take with acidic beverage (orange/cranberry juice). Counsel to take at least 1 hr apart if taking antacids, and to take with/without food. Advise to seek medical attention if symptoms of hypersensitivity reaction (rash, fever, blistering, oral lesions, conjunctivitis, swelling, and muscle and joint aches), immune reconstitution syndrome, hepatic dysfunction, and fat redistribution occur.

R

Administration: Oral route. **Storage:** 20-25°C (68-77°F). Keep container tightly closed. Protect from high humidity.

RESERPINE RX

reserpine (Various)

THERAPEUTIC CLASS: Rauwolfia alkaloid

INDICATIONS: Treatment of mild essential hypertension and adjunct treatment of severe hypertension. Relief of symptoms in agitated psychotic states.

DOSAGE: *Adults:* HTN: Initial: 0.5mg/day for 1-2 weeks. Maint: reduce to 0.1-0.25mg/day. Psychotic Disorders: Initial: 0.5mg/day. Range: 0.1-1mg/day.

HOW SUPPLIED: Tab: 0.1mg, 0.25mg

CONTRAINDICATIONS: Active or history of mental depression, active peptic ulcer, ulcerative colitis, current electroconvulsive therapy.

WARNINGS/PRECAUTIONS: Caution with renal insufficiency. May cause depression; d/c at 1st sign. Caution with history of peptic ulcer, ulcerative colitis, or gallstones.

ADVERSE REACTIONS: GI effects, dry mouth, hypersecretion, arrhythmia, syncope, edema, dyspnea, muscle aches, dizziness, depression, nervousness, impotence, gynecomastia, rash.

INTERACTIONS: Avoid MAOIs or use extreme caution. Prolonged effect of direct-acting sympathomimetics (eg, epinephrine, isoproterenol). May inhibit effects of indirect-acting sympathomimetics (eg, ephedrine, tyramine). Risk of arrhythmia with quinidine or digoxin. Titrate carefully with other antihypertensives. Decreased effect with TCAs.

PREGNANCY: Category C, not for use in nursing.

MECHANISM OF ACTION: Rauwolfia alkaloid; antihypertensive, depletes stores of catecholamine and 5-hydroxytryptamine in many organs including brain and adrenal medulla, resulting in decreased HR and lowering of arterial BP.

PHARMACOKINETICS: Absorption: (0.5mg) Absolute bioavailability (50%); C_{max}=1.1ng/mL; T_{max}=2.5 hrs. **Distribution:** Plasma protein binding (95%); found in breast milk. **Metabolism:** Complete. **Elimination:** Urine (1% unchanged); $T_{1/2}$=200 hrs.

NURSING CONSIDERATIONS

Assessment: Assess for hypersensivity, mental depression (suicidal tendencies), active peptic ulcer, ulcerative colitis, renal insufficiency, possible drug interactions, and pregnancy/nursing status.

Monitoring: Monitor for signs of mental depression (eg, despondency, early morning insomnia, loss of appetite, impotence, self-depreciation); d/c if any occur. Monitor BP, GI motility/secretion, and signs/symptoms of overdose (eg, flushing, pupilary constriction, hypotension, respiratory depression, impairment of consciousness, bradycardia).

Patient Counseling: Inform of possible adverse effects; immediately notify physician if any occur. Advise to take medication regularly and continuously as directed.

Administration: Oral route. **Storage:** 20-25°C (68-77°F). Protect from moisture. Preserve in tight, light-resistant container.

RESTASIS RX

cyclosporine (Allergan)

THERAPEUTIC CLASS: Topical immunomodulator

INDICATIONS: To increase tear production in patients with suppressed tear production due to ocular inflammation associated with keratoconjunctivitis sicca.

DOSAGE: *Adults:* 1 drop bid, q12h. Concomitant Artificial Tears: Space by 15 min.

Pediatrics: ≥16 yrs: 1 drop bid, q12h. Concomitant Artificial Tears: Space by 15 min.

HOW SUPPLIED: Emul: 0.05% [0.4mL, 32[s]]

CONTRAINDICATIONS: Active ocular infections.

WARNINGS/PRECAUTIONS: Not studied in patients with a history of herpes keratitis. Not to be given while wearing contact lenses; lenses may be reinserted 15 min following administration.

ADVERSE REACTIONS: Ocular burning, conjunctival hyperemia, discharge, epiphora, eye pain, foreign body sensation, pruritus, stinging, visual disturbance (eg, blurring).

PREGNANCY: Category C, caution in nursing.

MECHANISM OF ACTION: Topical immunomodulator; not established. Systemically acts as an immunosuppressive agent.

PHARMACOKINETICS: Distribution: Following systemic administration, found in breast milk.

NURSING CONSIDERATIONS

Assessment: Assess for presence of active ocular infection. Assess use in pregnant/nursing females and in patients with a history of herpes keratitis.

Monitoring: Monitor for signs/symptoms of ocular burning.

Patient Counseling: Inform to use single-use vial immediately after opening and discard remaining contents following use. Instruct not to allow tip of vial to touch eye or any surface to avoid contamination. Advise to remove contact lenses prior to use; lenses may be reinserted 15 min following administration.

Administration: Ocular route. 1) Invert unit dose vial a few times to obtain uniform, white, opaque emulsion before using. 2) Instill 1 drop bid in each eye, approximately 12 hrs apart. May be used concomitantly with artificial tears, allowing 15 min interval between products. 3) Discard vial immediately after administration. **Storage:** 15-25°C (59-77°F).

RESTORIL CIV

temazepam (Mallinckrodt)

THERAPEUTIC CLASS: Benzodiazepine

INDICATIONS: Short-term treatment of insomnia (7-10 days).

DOSAGE: *Adults:* Usual: 7.5-30mg qhs. Transient Insomnia: 7.5mg qhs. Elderly/Debilitated: Initial: 7.5mg qhs.

HOW SUPPLIED: Cap: 7.5mg, 15mg, 22.5mg, 30mg

CONTRAINDICATIONS: Pregnancy.

WARNINGS/PRECAUTIONS: Caution in elderly, debilitated, severely depressed, those with suicidal tendencies, hepatic/renal impairment, pulmonary insufficiency. Avoid abrupt discontinuation. If no improvement after 7-10 days, may indicate primary psychiatric and/or medical condition.

ADVERSE REACTIONS: Headache, dizziness, drowsiness, fatigue, nervousness, nausea, lethargy, hangover.

INTERACTIONS: Additive CNS depressant effects with alcohol and CNS depressants. May be synergistic with diphenhydramine.

PREGNANCY: Category X, caution in nursing.

MECHANISM OF ACTION: Benzodiazepine hypnotic agent.

PHARMACOKINETICS: Absorption: Well-absorbed; C_{max}=666-982ng/mL; T_{max}=approximately 1.5 hrs. **Distribution:** Plasma protein binding (96% unchanged), crosses placenta. **Metabolism:** Conjugation (major metabolites): O-conjugate . **Elimination:** Urine (80-90%); $T_{1/2}$=8.8 hrs.

R

NURSING CONSIDERATIONS

Assessment: Assess for primary physical and/or psychiatric illness, severe depression, impaired renal/hepatic function, chronic pulmonary insufficiency (COPD), hypersensitivity reactions, possible drug interactions, and alcohol use.

Monitoring: Worsening of insomnia, severe depresssion with suicidal ideation, oversedation, dizziness, drowsiness, headache, nervousness, lethargy, confusion and/or ataxia, emergence of new abnormalities of thinking or behavior, physical/psychological dependence, and withdrawal symptoms. Monitor LFTs and pulmonary functions.

Patient Counseling: Inform about the benefits/risks and possibility of physical/psychological dependence and memory problems (eg, traveler's amnesia). Caution against hazardous tasks (eg, operating machinery/driving). Never drink alcohol. Notify physician if pregnant or planning to become pregnant. Do not take any other drug, increase dose, or d/c without direction of physician.

Administration: Oral route. **Storage:** Store at 20-25°C (68-77°F).

RETAVASE — RX

reteplase (PDL)

THERAPEUTIC CLASS: Thrombolytic agent

INDICATIONS: To improve ventricular function following acute myocardial infarction (AMI), reduce the incidence of congestive heart failure (CHF) and reduce the mortality associated with AMI.

DOSAGE: *Adults:* 10 U IV over 2 min. Repeat in 30 min.

HOW SUPPLIED: Inj: 10.4 U

CONTRAINDICATIONS: Active internal bleeding, history of CVA, recent intracranial or intraspinal surgery or trauma, intracranial neoplasm, arteriovenous malformation, aneurysm, bleeding diathesis, severe uncontrolled HTN.

WARNINGS/PRECAUTIONS: Weigh benefits/risks with recent major surgery, previous puncture of noncompressible vessels, cerebrovascular disease, recent GI or GU bleeding, recent trauma, HTN, left heart thrombus, acute pericarditis, subacute bacterial endocarditis, hemostatic defects, severe hepatic or renal dysfunction, pregnancy, diabetic hemorrhagic retinopathy or other hemorrhagic ophthalmic conditions, septic thrombophlebitis or occluded AV cannula at a seriously infected site, elderly, any other bleeding condition that is difficult to manage. Cholesterol embolism and internal/superficial bleeding reported. Arrhythmias may occur with reperfusion. Avoid IM injection, noncompressible arterial puncture, and internal jugular or subclavian venous puncture. Cholesterol embolism and internal/superficial bleeding reported.

ADVERSE REACTIONS: Bleeding, allergic reactions, dyspnea, hypotension.

INTERACTIONS: Increased risk of bleeding with heparin, vitamin K antagonists, and drugs that alter platelet function (eg, ASA, NSAIDs, dipyridamole, abciximab) before or after therapy. Weigh benefits/risks with oral anticoagulants.

PREGNANCY: Category C, caution in nursing.

MECHANISM OF ACTION: Thrombolytic agent; recombinant plasminogen activator that catalyzes the cleavage of endogenous plasminogen to generate plasmin. Plasmin, in turn, degrades the fibrin matrix of the thrombus, thereby exerting its thrombolytic action.

PHARMACOKINETICS: Metabolism: Liver. **Elimination:** Renal; $T_{1/2}$=13-16 min.

NURSING CONSIDERATIONS

Assessment: Assess for active internal bleeding, history of cerebrovascular accident, recent intracranial or intraspinal surgery or trauma, intracranial neoplasm, arteriovenous malformation, aneurysm, known bleeding diathesis, severe uncontrolled HTN, renal/hepatic function, nursing/pregnancy status, and for drug interactions. Assess use in patients at risk for bleeding events (eg, recent major surgery, acute pericarditis, recent GI bleeding).

Monitoring: Monitor for signs/symptoms of bleeding (eg, intracranial, retroperitoneal, GI, genitourinary), cholesterol embolization (eg, livedo reticularis, "purple toe" syndrome, MI, cerebral infarction, HTN), and arrhythmias. Monitor all potential bleeding sites (eg, catheter insertion sites, sites of recent surgical intervention).

Patient Counseling: Counsel about increased risk of bleeding tendencies while on therapy. Instruct to contact physician if any unusual bleeding occurs. Avoid IM injections while on therapy.

Administration: IV route. Reconstitute. 1) Transfer 10mL of sterile water for injection into vial. 2) Swirl to dissolve drug, but do not shake. 2) Withdraw 10 mL of reconstituted solution into syringe. 3) Attach sterile needle; syringe is now ready for IV bolus dose. Reconstitute just prior to administration. Do not administer in the same IV line as heparin. **Storage:** Unused vial: 2-25°C (36-77°F). Box should remain sealed until use to protect the lyophilisate from exposure to light. Reconstituted: 2-30°C (36-86°F); use within 4 hrs.

RETIN-A RX

tretinoin (Ortho Neutrogena)

OTHER BRAND NAMES: Retin-A Micro (Ortho Neutrogena)

THERAPEUTIC CLASS: Retinoid

INDICATIONS: Topical treatment of acne vulgaris.

DOSAGE: *Adults:* Cleanse area thoroughly, then apply qhs. May temporarily d/c or reduce dosing frequency if irritation occurs.
Pediatrics: ≥12 yrs: (Gel: 0.04%, 0.1%) Cleanse area thoroughly, then apply qhs. May temporarily d/c or reduce dosing frequency if irritation occurs.

HOW SUPPLIED: (Retin-A) Cre: 0.025%, 0.05%, 0.1% [20g, 45g]; Gel: 0.01%, 0.025% [15g, 45g]; Sol: 0.05% [28mL]; (Retin-A Micro) Gel: 0.04%, 0.1% [20g, 45g]

WARNINGS/PRECAUTIONS: Avoid eyes, lips, paranasal creases, mucous membranes, and sunburned skin. Acne exacerbation during 1st weeks of therapy may occur. D/C if sensitivity or irritation occurs. Severe irritation with eczematous skin. Causes photosensitivity. Extreme weather (eg, cold, wind) may irritate skin.

ADVERSE REACTIONS: Local skin reactions (red, edematous, blistered, crusted), photosensitivity, temporary skin pigmentation changes.

INTERACTIONS: Caution with topical agents with strong drying effects, high concentration of alcohol, astringents, spices, or lime. Caution with sulfur, resorcinol, or salicylic acid; allow effects of these agents to subside before application of tretinoin.

PREGNANCY: Category C, caution in nursing.

MECHANISM OF ACTION: Retinoic acid derivative; not established. Responsible for decreasing cohesiveness of follicular epithelial cells with decreased microcomedo formation. Also stimulates mitotic activity and increases turnover of follicular epithelial cells, causing extrusion of comedones.

NURSING CONSIDERATIONS

Assessment: Assess for presence of sunburn and eczematous skin, pregnancy/nursing status, and possible drug interactions.

Monitoring: Monitor for signs/symptoms of a skin sensitivity reaction (eg, red, edematous, blistered, or crusted skin) or chemical irritation.

Patient Counseling: Avoid exposure to sunlight/sunlamps during therapy. Advise using effective sunscreen when outdoors and protective clothing during extended sun exposure. If sunburn occurs, instruct to d/c until skin is recovered. Avoid excessive exposure to wind or cold. Medication is flammable; avoid fire, flame, or smoking during use. Keep away from eyes, mouth, angles of the nose, and mucous membranes. Inform to notify physician if severe skin irritation occurs (eg, excessively red, swollen, blistered, or crusted skin).

Administration: Topical administration. **Storage:** Retin A Liquid, Gel: Below 86°F; Retin A Cream: Below 80°F.

RETROVIR RX

zidovudine (GlaxoSmithKline)

Associated with hematologic toxicity (eg, neutropenia, severe anemia), especially with advanced HIV disease. Prolonged use associated with symptomatic myopathy. Lactic acidosis and severe, possibly fatal hepatomegaly with steatosis reported.

THERAPEUTIC CLASS: Nucleoside analogue

INDICATIONS: Treatment of HIV infection in combination with other antiretrovirals. Prevention of maternal-fetal HIV transmission.

DOSAGE: *Adults:* (Tab) 600mg/day in divided doses. (Inj) 1mg/kg IV over 1 hr 5-6 times/day. Prevention of Maternal-Fetal HIV Transmission: >14 weeks pregnancy: 100mg PO five times/day until start of labor. During labor and

delivery: 2mg/kg IV over 1 hr followed by 1mg/kg/hr IV infusion until clamping of umbilical cord. End-Stage Renal Disease/Dialysis: 100mg PO q6-8h or 1mg/kg IV q6-8h. Significant Anemia/Neutropenia: May require dose interruption and adjunctive epoetin therapy. Less Severe Anemia/Neutropenia: Reduce daily dose.
Pediatrics: 6 weeks to <18 yrs: 480mg/m²/day PO in divided doses (240mg/m² bid or 160mg/m² tid). Max: 480mg/m²/day. 4 to <9kg: 12mg/kg bid or 8mg/kg tid. Max: 24mg/kg/day. ≥9 to <30kg: 9mg/kg bid or 6mg/kg tid. Max: 18mg/kg/day. ≥30kg: 300mg bid or 200mg tid. Max: 600mg/day. Prevention of Maternal-Fetal HIV Transmission: Neonates: 2mg/kg PO q6h (or 1.5mg/kg IV over 30 min q6h) starting within 12 hrs after birth and continue through 6 weeks of age. End-Stage Renal Disease/Dialysis: 100mg PO q6-8h or 1mg/kg IV q6-8h. Significant Anemia/Neutropenia: May require dose interruption and adjunctive epoetin therapy. Pronounced Anemia: Reduce daily dose. Mild to Moderate Hepatic Impairment: Monitor for hematologic toxicity and reduce dose if needed.

HOW SUPPLIED: Cap: 100mg; Inj: 10mg/mL; Syrup: 50mg/5mL [240mL]; Tab: 300mg

WARNINGS/PRECAUTIONS: Adverse reactions increase with disease progression. Caution with compromised bone marrow or in elderly. Monitor for hematologic toxicity; reduce dose or stop therapy. Myopathy and myositis with pathological changes associated with prolonged use. Caution with obesity and liver disease; increased risk of lactic acidosis and hepatomegaly with steatosis. Increased risk of toxicity with prolonged exposure to nucleosides, in women, obesity, advanced HIV disease, severe hepatic impairment. Possible redistribution or accumulation of body fat. Hepatic decompensation has occurred in HIV/HCV co-infected patients receiving combination antiretroviral therapy for HIV and interferon alfa with or without ribavirin; monitor for treatment-associated toxicities. Immune reconstitution syndrome has been reported with combination antiretroviral therapy.

ADVERSE REACTIONS: Headache, NV, malaise, anorexia, asthenia, constipation, anemia, neutropenia, abdominal cramps, abdominal pain, arthralgia, chills, dyspepsia, fatigue, and insomnia.

INTERACTIONS: Increased risk of hematologic toxicities with ganciclovir, interferon-alpha, bone marrow suppressives and cytotoxic drugs. Possible increased levels with phenytoin, atovaquone, fluconazole, methadone, probenecid, valproic acid. Possible decreased levels with nelfinavir, ritonavir, rifampin. Avoid with stavudine, ribavirin, doxorubicin, other combination products containing zidovudine. Prolonged exposure to antiretroviral nucleoside analogues increases risk of lactic acidosis and hepatomegaly with steatosis. May decrease phenytoin levels.

PREGNANCY: Category C, not for use in nursing.

MECHANISM OF ACTION: Pyrimidine nucleoside analogue; inhibits reverse transcriptase via DNA chain termination.

PHARMACOKINETICS: Absorption: (Tab, Cap, Syrup): Rapid. Bioavailability (64%). T_{max}=0.5-1.5 hrs. (IV) C_{max}=1.06mcg/mL. **Distribution:** V_d=1.6L/kg; plasma protein binding (<38%). **Metabolism:** Hepatic. Metabolite (3'-azido-3'-deoxy-5'-*O*-β-*D*-glucopyranuronosylthymidine (GZDV). **Elimination:** (Tab, Cap, Syrup): Zidovudine: Urine (14%). GZDV: Urine (74%); $T_{1/2}$=0.5-3 hrs. (IV): Zidovudine: Urine (18%). GZDV: Urine (60%); $T_{1/2}$=1.1 hrs.

NURSING CONSIDERATIONS

Assessment: Assess for advanced symptomatic HIV disease, anemia, myopathy, risk of liver disease, bone marrow suppression (neutropenia, pancytopenia), risk factors for lactic acidosis, renal dysfunction, and possible drug interactions.

Monitoring: Periodic monitoring of CBC, granulocyte, Hgb, renal/hepatic function test. Monitor for signs/symptoms of hypersensitivity reaction, anemia, myopathy, liver dysfunction (decompensation, failure), bone marrow suppression (neutropenia, pancytopenia), lactic acidosis, immune reconstitution syndrome, fat redistribution and renal dysfunction.

Patient Counseling: Inform that medication does not cure HIV and may continue to develop opportunistic infections and illnesses associated with HIV. Seek medical attention if symptoms of lactic acidosis (weakness, SOB), hepatic dysfunction, anemia, myopathy, bone marrow suppression (neutropenia, pancytopenia), renal dysfunction, immune reconstitution syndrome, and fat redistribution occur. Consult physician if experience muscle weakness, shortness of breath, symptoms of hepatitis or pancreatitis, or any other adverse events.

Administration: IV or oral route. **Storage:** (Vial): 15-25°C (59-77°F) and protect from light. (Diluted): Room temperature; stable for 24 hrs. Refrigerate: 2-8°C (36-46°F); stable for 48 hrs. (Tab, Syrup): 15-25°C (59-77°F). (Cap): 15-25°C (59-77°F) and protect from moisture.

REVATIO RX

sildenafil citrate (Pfizer)

THERAPEUTIC CLASS: Phosphodiesterase type 5 inhibitor

INDICATIONS: Treatment of pulmonary arterial hypertension (WHO Group I) to improve exercise ability.

DOSAGE: *Adults:* 20mg tid 4-6 hours apart.

HOW SUPPLIED: Tab: 20mg

CONTRAINDICATIONS: Organic nitrates taken regularly and/or intermittently.

WARNINGS/PRECAUTIONS: Caution with MI, stroke, or life-threatening arrhythmia within last 6 months; with resting hypotension (BP <90/50), fluid depletion, severe left ventricular outflow obstruction, autonomic dysfunction, or HTN (BP >170/110); unstable angina due to cardiac failure or CAD; anatomical penile deformation; predisposition to priapism; and retinitis pigmentosa. Avoid in patients with veno-occlusive disease. Decrease in supine BP reported. If erection persists >4 hrs, seek immediate medical assistance; penile tissue damage and permanent loss of potency could result if priapism not treated immediately.

ADVERSE REACTIONS: Epistaxis, headache, flushing, dyspepsia, insomnia, erythema, dyspnea, rhinitis, diarrhea, myalgia, pyrexia, gastritis, sinusitis, paresthesia.

INTERACTIONS: See Contraindications. Reports of bleeding (epistaxis) with vitamin K antagonists. Increased levels with CYP3A4 inhibitors (eg, cimetidine, ketoconazole, itraconazole, erythromycin, saquinavir) and protease inhibitors (eg, ritonavir). CYP2C9 inhibitors may decrease sildenafil clearance. Decreased levels with CYP3A4 inducers (eg, bosentan; more potent inducers such as barbiturates, carbamazepine, phenytoin, efavirenz, nevirapine, rifampin, rifabutin). Co-administration with bosentan resulted in a decrease in AUC of sildenafil and increase in AUC of bosentan. Additional supine BP reduction with amlodipine reported. Simultaneous administration with α-blockers may lead to symptomatic hypotension.

PREGNANCY: Category B, caution in nursing.

MECHANISM OF ACTION: It inhibits cGMP specific phosphodiesterase type-5 (PDE5) in the smooth muscle of the pulmonary vasculature, where PDE5 is responsible for degradation of cGMP. It increases cGMP within pulmonary vascular smooth muscle cells, resulting in relaxation.

PHARMACOKINETICS: Absorption: Rapid; absolute bioavailability (40%); T_{max}=30-120 min. **Distribution:** V_d=105L; plasma protein binding (96%). **Metabolism:** Liver, via CYP3A4 (major route) and CYP2C9 (minor route); through N-desmethylation. **Elimination:** Feces (80% metabolites), urine (13%); $T_{1/2}$=4 hrs.

NURSING CONSIDERATIONS

Assessment: Assess for resting hypotension, fluid depletion, left ventricular outflow obstruction or autonomic dysfunction, pulmonary veno-occlusive disease, MI, stroke, life-threatening arrhythmia, coronary artery disease, angina, HTN, retinitis pigmentosa, anatomical deformities of the penis (eg, Peyronie's disease, angulation, cavernosal), conditions predisposed to priapism (eg, sickle cell anemia, multiple myeloma, or leukemia), drug hypersensitivity, and possible drug interactions especially with organic nitrates.

Monitoring: Monitor BP, penile tissue damage, or for permanent loss of potency, epistaxis, sudden loss of vision (a sign of nonarteritic anterior ischemic optic neuropathy), signs of pulmonary edema, decrease/or loss of hearing, dizziness, and tinnitus.

Patient Counseling: Inform about risks of drug and to consult physician if any adverse events occur. Inform that drug is also marketed as Viagra for male erectile dysfunction.

Administration: Oral route. **Storage:** 25°C (77°F); excursions permitted to 15-30°C (59-86°F).

ReVia — RX

naltrexone HCl (Duramed)

THERAPEUTIC CLASS: Opioid antagonist

INDICATIONS: Treatment of alcohol dependence and to block effects of exogenously administered opioids.

DOSAGE: *Adults:* Alcoholism: 50mg qd up to 12 weeks. Opioid Dependence: Initial: 25mg qd. Maint: 50mg qd. Naloxone Challenge Test: 0.2mg IV, observe for 30 sec, then 0.6mg IV, observe for 20 min; or 0.8mg SQ, observe for 20 min.

HOW SUPPLIED: Tab: 50mg

CONTRAINDICATIONS: Acute hepatitis, hepatic failure, patients failing naloxone challenge or opioid-dependent, concomitant opioid analgesics, acute opioid withdrawal, positive urine screen for opioids, phenanthrene sensitivity.

WARNINGS/PRECAUTIONS: Hepatotoxic with excessive doses; margin of separation between safe dose and hepatotoxic dose is 5-fold or less. Only treat patients opioid-free for 7-10 days. Attempting to overcome opiate blockade is very dangerous. More sensitive to lower doses of opioids after naltrexone is discontinued. Safety in ultra-rapid opiate detoxification is not known. Increased risk of suicide in substance abuse patients. Severe opioid withdrawal syndromes reported with accidental ingestion in opioid-dependent patients. Monitor closely during blockade reversal. Caution in renal or hepatic impairment. Perform naloxone challenge test if question of opioid dependence.

ADVERSE REACTIONS: NV, headache, dizziness, nervousness, fatigue, restlessness, insomnia, anxiety, somnolence.

INTERACTIONS: Caution with other drugs. Do not use with disulfiram unless benefits outweigh risk of hepatotoxicity. Lethargy and somnolence reported with thioridazine. Antagonizes opioid-containing cough and cold, antidiarrheal, and analgesic agents.

PREGNANCY: Category C, caution in nursing.

MECHANISM OF ACTION: Opioid antagonist; markedly attenuates or completely blocks (reversibly) the subjective effects of IV-administered opioids.

PHARMACOKINETICS: Absorption: Rapid and complete. Bioavailability (5-40%); T_{max}=1 hr. **Distribution:** V_d=1350L; plasma protein binding (21%). **Metabolism:** Liver , 6β-naltrexol (major metabolite). **Elimination:** Urine (2% unchanged), (43% conjugated); (naltrexone, β-naltrexol) $T_{1/2}$=4 hrs, 13 hrs.

NURSING CONSIDERATIONS

Assessment: Start treatment only under medical jugdment of prescribing physician, assess potential of opioid use within past 7-10 days. If question of occult opioid dependence, perform naloxone challenge test. Assess for acute hepatitis or liver failure and possible drug interactions.

Monitoring: Monitor LFTs, symptoms/signs of respiratory depression, hepatotoxicity, ideopathic thrombocytopenic purpura, suicide attempts, withdrawal symptoms in opioid-dependent patients.

Patient Counseling: Instruct to take as prescribed. Drug treats alcoholism or drug dependence. Carry identification card to alert medical personnel of naltrexone use and to ensure adequate treatment in a medical emergency. Caution against taking heroin or any other opioid drug with therapy; may lead to serious injury, including coma. Notify if pregnant/nursing.

Administration: Oral route. **Storage:** 20-25°C (68-77°F).

REVLIMID — RX

lenalidomide (Celgene)

Potential for human birth defects, hematological toxicity (neutropenia and thrombocytopenia), deep venous thrombosis (DVT) and pulmonary embolism (PE). Lenalidomide is an analogue of thalidomide. Thalidomide is a known human teratogen that causes severe life-threatening human birth defects. If taken during pregnancy, may cause birth defects or death to an unborn baby. Avoid pregnancy due to potential toxicity and to avoid fetal exposure. Only available under a special restricted distribution program called Revassist℠. Associated with significant neutropenia and thrombocytopenia in patients with del 5q MDS. CBC should be monitored weekly for the first 8 weeks of therapy and at least monthly thereafter. May require dose interruption and/or reduction and the use of blood product support and/or growth factors. Increased risk of DVT and PE in patients with multiple myeloma. Observe for signs and symptoms of thromboembolism.

THERAPEUTIC CLASS: Thalidomide Analog

INDICATIONS: Transfusion-dependent anemia due to Low- or Intermediate-1-risk myelodysplastic syndromes associated with a deletion 5q cytogenetic abnormality with or without additional cytogenetic abnormalities. In combination with dexamethasone for the treatment of multiple myeloma in patients who have received at least one prior therapy.

DOSAGE: *Adults:* ≥18 yrs: Myelodysplastic Syndromes: 10mg daily with water. Multiple Myeloma: 25mg daily with water. Administer as single dose on Days 1-21 of repeated 28-day cycles. Do not break, chew, or open capsules. Adjust dose based on platelet and/or neutrophil counts.

HOW SUPPLIED: Cap: 5mg, 10mg, 15mg, 25mg

CONTRAINDICATIONS: Pregnancy.

WARNINGS/PRECAUTIONS: Risk of adverse reactions may be greater in patients with impaired renal function.

ADVERSE REACTIONS: Thrombocytopenia, neutropenia, pruritus, rash, diarrhea, constipation, nausea, nasopharyngitis, fatigue, arthralgia, cough, pyrexia, peripheral edema, insomnia, asthenia.

INTERACTIONS: Co-administration increased digoxin C_{max} by 14%; monitoring suggested.

PREGNANCY: Category X, not for use in nursing.

MECHANISM OF ACTION: Thalidomide analogue; not established, inhibits secretion of pro-inflammatory cytokines and increases secretion of anti-inflammatory cytokines from peripheral blood mononuclear cells, inhibits cell proliferation, and inhibits growth of multiple myeloma cells by inducing cell cycle arrest and apoptosis.

PHARMACOKINETICS: Absorption: T_{max}=0.625-1.5 hrs (healthy), 0.5-4.0 hrs (multiple myeloma). **Distribution**: Plasma protein binding (30%). **Elimination**: Urine; $T_{1/2}$=3 hrs.

NURSING CONSIDERATIONS

Assessment: Assess for pregnancy status, renal impairment, and possible drug interactions. Obtain pregnancy test 10-14 days before and 24 hrs before initiating therapy. Assess if been using 2 forms of effective contraception for 4 weeks prior to therapy.

Monitoring: Perform pregnancy test weekly for first 4 weeks of use, repeated every 4 weeks with regular menstrual cycles and every 2 weeks with irregular menstrual cycles. Monitor CBC, including WBC count with differential, platelet count, Hgb, Hct weekly for first 8 weeks of therapy and monthly thereafter (MDS); every 2 weeks for 1st 3 months and monthly thereafter (multiple myeloma). Monitor for signs/symptoms of hypersensitivity reactions, thromboembolic disorders, neutropenia, and thrombocytopenia.

Patient Counseling: Instruct not to break, chew, or open. Inform of pregnancy risks; avoid pregnancy during therapy; use 2 effective contraceptive methods during therapy, during therapy interruptions, and for at least 4 weeks after completing therapy. Males must always use a latex condom during any sexual contact, even if undergone successful vasectomy. Seek medical attention if symptoms of thromboembolism (SOB, chest pain, arm or leg swelling), hypersensitivity reactions, or infection occur.

Administration: Oral route. **Storage**: 25°C (77°F); excursions permitted to 15-30°C (59-86°F).

REYATAZ

RX

atazanavir sulfate (Bristol-Myers Squibb)

THERAPEUTIC CLASS: Protease inhibitor

INDICATIONS: Treatment of HIV-1 infection in combination with other antiretrovirals.

DOSAGE: *Adults:* Therapy-Naive: 400mg qd. Concomitant Efavirenz: Give atazanavir 400mg and ritonavir 100mg with efavirenz on empty stomach hs. Concomitant Buffered Didanosine: Give atazanavir 2 hrs before or 1 hr after didanosine. Concomitant Tenofovir: Give atazanavir 300mg with ritonavir 100mg. Concomitant H_2-Receptor Antagonist: Give simultaneously with, and/or at least 10 hrs after, atazanavir 300mg with ritonavir 100mg. Max: Famotidine 40mg bid. If ritonavir intolerant, give atazanavir 400mg qd at least 2 hrs before and 10 hrs after H_2-receptor antagonist. Max: Famotidine 40mg/day. Concomitant PPIs: Give PPI 12 hrs prior to atazanavir 300mg with ritonavir 100mg. Max: Omeprazole 20mg. Therapy-Experienced: 300mg with ritonavir 100mg qd. Concomitant H_2-Receptor Antagonist: Give atazanavir 300mg with ritonavir 100mg simultaneously with, and/or at least 10 hrs after, H_2-receptor antagonist. Max: Famotidine 20mg bid. Both Tenofovir and H_2-Receptor Antagonist: Atazanavir 400mg with ritonavir 100mg qd. Treatment-Naive Hemodialysis Patients: 300mg with ritonavir 100mg qd. Moderate Hepatic Insufficiency (Child-Pugh Class B): Consider 300mg qd. Take with food.

Pediatrics: Therapy-Naive: ≥13 yrs and ≥39kg/Ritonavir Intolerant: 400mg qd without ritonavir. Therapy-Naive: 6-<18 yrs: 15-<25kg: 150mg with ritonavir 80mg. 25-<32kg: 200mg with ritonavir 100mg. 32-<39kg: 250mg with ritonavir 100mg. ≥39kg: 300mg with ritonavir 100mg. Therapy-Experienced: 6-<18 yrs: 25-<32kg: 200mg with ritonavir 100mg. 32-<39kg: 250mg with ritonavir 100mg. ≥39kg: 300mg with ritonavir 100mg qd. Take with food.

HOW SUPPLIED: Cap: 100mg, 150mg, 200mg, 300mg

CONTRAINDICATIONS: Concomitant administration with midazolam, triazolam, dihydroergotamine, ergotamine, ergonovine, methylergonovine, cisapride, pimozide, rifampin, irinotecan, St. John's wort, lovastatin, simvastatin, indinavir.

WARNINGS/PRECAUTIONS: Prolongs PR-interval; caution with pre-existing conduction system disease. New-onset DM, exacerbation of pre-existing DM, hyperglycemia, hyperbilirubinemia, increased bleeding with hemophilia Types A and B, Stevens-Johnson syndrome, erythema multiforme reported. Caution with hepatic impairment; avoid with severe hepatic insufficiency. D/C with severe rash. Possible redistribution/accumulation of body fat. Immune reconstitution syndrome reported with combination therapy. Nephrolithiasis reported.

ADVERSE REACTIONS: Headache, NV, dizziness, fever, depression, abdominal pain, diarrhea, rash, myalgia, peripheral neurologic symptoms, insomnia, jaundice/scleral icterus.

INTERACTIONS: See Contraindications. Avoid nevirapine, voriconazole, other protease inhibitors with atazanavir/ritonavir therapy. May increase levels of drugs metabolized by CYP3A or UGT1A1. CYP3A inducers may decrease levels. CYP3A inhibitors, voriconazole may increase levels. Decreased levels with buffered didanosine, tenofovir, efavirenz, antacids/buffered medications (give atazanavir 2 hrs before or 1 hr after), H_2-receptor antagonists (space dosing by 10 hrs). Increase levels of saquinavir, diltiazem (reduce dose by 50%), amiodarone, lidocaine (systemic), quinidine, warfarin, TCAs, trazodone, rifabutin (reduce dose up to 75%), CCBs, oral contraceptives (use lowest possible dose), sildenafil/tadalafil/vardenafil (reduce dose), atorvastatin, rosuvastatin, cyclosporine, sirolimus, tacrolimus, clarithromycin (reduce dose by 50%; consider alternative therapy for infections other than *M.avium* complex). Increased levels with ritonavir (give atazanavir 300mg/day with ritonavir 100mg/day with food). Caution with high doses of ketoconazole, itrazonazole with atazanavir/ritonavir therapy. Atazanavir/ritonavir therapy may significantly increase plasma fluticasone propionate exposure resulting in significantly decreased serum cortisol concentrations. Avoid use of PPIs and efavirenz in treatment-experienced patients.

PREGNANCY: Category B, not for use in nursing.

MECHANISM OF ACTION: HIV-1 protease inhibitor; inhibits virus-specific processing of viral Gag-Pol polyproteins in HIV-1 infected cells, preventing formation of mature virions.

PHARMACOKINETICS: Absorption: Rapid. T_{max}=2.5 hrs. **Distribution:** Plasma protein binding (86%). **Metabolism:** Hepatic (biotransformation: mono- and dioxygenation) via CYP3A. **Elimination:** Urine (7%), feces (20%); $T_{1/2}$=7 hrs.

NURSING CONSIDERATIONS

Assessment: Assess for hepatic impairment, HBV or HCV infection, ESRD, DM, hemophilia, conduction system disease (1-3° heart block), pregnancy/nursing status, and possible drug interactions.

Monitoring: Monitor for signs/symptoms of PR interval prolongation, exacerbation of DM and hyperglycemia, hyperbilirubinemia, rash, unexplained bleeding, nephrolithiasis, changes in body fat and immune reconstitution syndrome. Monitor hematologic tests, LFTs, CK, cholesterol profile, and chemistries.

Patient Counseling: Inform that sustained decreases in plasma HIV RNA are associated with reduced risk of progression to AIDS and death. Take with food as prescribed. Do not alter dose or d/c without consulting physician. If miss dose, take as soon as possible and return to normal schedule; do not double next dose. Inform drug does not cure HIV and may continue to develop opportunistic infections and other complications associated with HIV. Report use of any other medication (St. John's wort, PDE5 inhibitor). If taking antacids or didanosine take capsule 2 hrs before or 1 hr after. Seek medical attention if symptoms of PR interval prolongation (dizziness or lightheadedness), exacerbation of DM and hyperglycemia, hyperbilirubinemia (jaundice), rash, unexplained bleeding, nephrolithiasis, redistribution of body fat, and immune reconstitution syndrome occur.

Administration: Oral route. **Storage:** Store at 25°C (77°F); excursions permitted to 15-30°C (59-86°F).

RHINOCORT AQUA — RX

budesonide (AstraZeneca)

THERAPEUTIC CLASS: Corticosteroid

INDICATIONS: Management of seasonal or perennial allergic rhinitis.

DOSAGE: *Adults*: 1 spray per nostril qd. Max: 4 sprays/nostril/day.
Pediatrics: >12 yrs: 1 spray per nostril qd. Max: 4 sprays/nostril/day. 6-12 yrs: 1 spray per nostril qd. Max: 2 sprays/nostril/day.

HOW SUPPLIED: Spray: 32mcg/spray [8.6g]

WARNINGS/PRECAUTIONS: Risk of adrenal insufficiency and withdrawal symptoms when replacing systemic corticosteroids with a topical corticosteroid. Caution with active or quiescent TB, ocular herpes simplex, or untreated bacterial, fungal, and systemic viral infections. Avoid with recent nasal trauma, surgery, or septum ulcers. Risk of more severe/fatal course of infections (eg, chickenpox, measles) and for *Candida* infections of the nose and pharynx.

Potential for reduced growth velocity in pediatrics. Should not delay or interfere with infant feeding. Immediate and/or delayed hypersensitivity reactions may occur rarely. Larger than recommended doses should be avoided; may cause hypercorticism and adrenal suppression. D/C slowly if such changes occur. Caution with hepatic dysfunction.

ADVERSE REACTIONS: Nasal irritation, pharyngitis, cough, epistaxis, bronchospasm.

INTERACTIONS: Oral ketoconazole and cimetidine increase plasma levels. CYP3A4 inhibitors (eg, itraconazole, clarithromycin, erythromycin) may decrease metabolism and increase systemic exposure. Concomitant systemic corticosteroids increase risk of hypercorticism and/or HPA axis suppression.

PREGNANCY: Category B, caution in nursing.

MECHANISM OF ACTION: Glucocorticosteroid; mechanism not established, suspected to have a wide range of inhibitory activities against multiple cell types (eg, mast cells, eosinophils, neutrophils, macrophages, lymphocytes) and mediators (eg, histamine, leukotrienes, ecosanoids, cytokines) involved in allergic-mediated inflammation.

PHARMACOKINETICS: Absorption: Well-absorbed, T_{max}=0.7 hr. **Distribution:** V_d=2-3L/Kg, plasma protein binding (85-90%). **Metabolism:** Liver (extensive), 16α-hydroxyprednisolone and 6β-hydroxybudesonide (major metabolites) via CYP3A4-catalyzed biotransformation. **Elimination:** Urine and feces; $T_{1/2}$(22R form)=2-3 hrs.

NURSING CONSIDERATIONS

Assessment: Assess for drug hypersensitivity, active or quiescent TB, untreated localized/systemic fungal or bacterial infections, systemic viral infections, ocular herpes simplex, history of glaucoma, recent nasal septal ulcers, nasal surgery/trauma, glaucoma, cataracts, concomitant use with other inhaled or systemic corticosteroids, possible drug interactions.

Monitoring: Monitor for acute adrenal insufficiency, hypercorticism, HPA-axis suppression; chickenpox, measles, nasal/pharyngeal *Candida* infections, hypoadrenalism in infants born to mothers who received corticosteroids during pregnancy, suppression of growth velocity in children, hypersensitivity reactions, contact dermatitis, wheezing, nasal septum perforation, epistaxis, vision changes, increased IOP.

Patient Counseling: Counsel to take as directed at regular intervals. Advise to avoid exposure to chickenpox or measles; immediately consult physician if exposed, if symptoms worsen, or if episodes of epistaxis or nasal discomfort occur. Instruct to avoid spraying into eyes.

Administration: Intranasal route. **Storage:** Store at 20-25°C (68-77°F). Do not freeze.

R

RIFADIN — RX

rifampin (Sanofi-Aventis)

THERAPEUTIC CLASS: Rifamycin derivative

INDICATIONS: Treatment of all forms of TB. Treatment of asymptomatic carriers of *Neisseria meningitidis* to eliminate meningococci from nasopharynx.

DOSAGE: *Adults:* TB: 10mg/kg PO/IV qd. Max: 600mg/day. Meningococcal Carriers: 600mg bid for 2 days. Take 1 hr before or 2 hrs after a meal with a full glass of water.
Pediatrics: TB: 10-20mg/kg PO/IV qd. Max: 600mg/day. Meningococcal Carriers: ≥1 month: 10mg/kg q12h for 2 days. Max: 600mg/dose. <1 month: 5mg/kg q12h for 2 days. Take 1 hr before or 2 hrs after a meal with a full glass of water.

HOW SUPPLIED: Cap: 150mg, 300mg; Inj: 600mg

WARNINGS/PRECAUTIONS: May produce liver dysfunction. May cause hyperbilirubinemia. Not for treatment of meningococcal disease. May produce reddish coloration of the urine, sweat, sputum, and tears. May permanently stain soft contact lenses.

ADVERSE REACTIONS: GI distress, thrombocytopenia, visual disturbances, menstrual disturbances, edema of face and extremities, elevated BUN and serum uric acid levels.

INTERACTIONS: May accelerate elimination of drugs metabolized by CYP450 (eg, anticonvulsants, antiarrhythmics, anticoagulants, azole antifungals, barbiturates, β-blockers, CCBs, chloramphenicol, clarithromycin, corticosteroids, cyclosporine, cardiac glycosides, clofibrate, oral or systemic contraceptives, dapsone, diazepam, doxycycline, fluoroquinolones, haloperidol, oral hypoglycemics, levothyroxine, methadone, narcotics, nortriptyline, progestins, quinine, tacrolimus, theophylline, TCAs, and zidovudine). Give antacids at least 1 hr before rifampin. Increased hepatotoxicity with halothane or isoniazid. Increased serum levels with probenecid and cotrimoxazole. Caution with other hepatotoxic agents. Concomitant ketoconazole decreases both drug serum levels. Decreased levels of enalapril, atovaquone. Increased levels with atovaquone.

PREGNANCY: Category C, not for use in nursing.

MECHANISM OF ACTION: Rifamycin derivative; has bacterial activity against intracellular and extracellular *Mycobacterium tuberculosis*. Inhibits DNA-dependent RNA polymerase activity in susceptible cells. Interacts with bacterial RNA polymerase; does not inhibit the mammalian enzyme.

PHARMACOKINETICS: Absorption: Readily absorbed from GI tract. (PO, 600mg) C_{max}=7mcg/mL. (IV, 300mg, 600mg) C_{max}=9.0mcg/mL, 17.5mcg/mL. **Distribution:** (IV, 300mg, 600mg): V_d=0.66L/kg, 0.64L/kg; distributed in body fluids and cerebrospinal fluid; plasma protein binding 80%. **Metabolism:** Via deacetylation; 25-desacetyl-rifampin (major metabolite). **Elimination:** Urine (30%), bile; (600mg, 900mg) $T_{1/2}$=3.35 hrs, 5.08hrs.

NURSING CONSIDERATIONS

Assessment: Assess for liver and renal function, DM, possible drug interactions. Document indications for therapy, culture and sensitivity.

Monitoring: Monitor LFTs (SGPT and SGOT, bilirubin or transaminase), SrCr, CBCs, and platelet count. Monitor for hematopoietic reactions (leukopenia, thrombocytopenia or acute hemolytic anemia), cutaneous reactions, hypersensitivity reactions (Stevens-Johnson syndrome, vasculitis, anaphylaxis), renal function, serum uric acid, convulsions, visual disturbances, flu-like syndrome.

Patient Counseling: Drug treats bacterial, not viral, infections. Inform that drug may produce reddish urine, sweat, sputum, and tears. Take drug 1 hr before or 2 hrs after meal with a full glass of water. Report immediately any fever, loss of appetite, malaise, NV, darkened urine, yellowish discoloration of skin/eyes, and joint pain/swelling. Take full course of therapy, not missing doses. Reliability of oral contraceptives may be affected; use alternate contraceptive measures.

Administration: Oral and IV route. **Storage:** Avoid excessive heat (40-104°C). Protect from light.

RIFAMATE RX

rifampin - isoniazid (Sanofi-Aventis)

Isoniazid associated with severe and sometimes fatal hepatitis. Monitor LFTs on a monthly basis.

THERAPEUTIC CLASS: Isonicotinic acid hydrazide/rifamycin derivative

INDICATIONS: For pulmonary TB. Not for initial therapy or prevention.

DOSAGE: *Adults:* 2 caps qd. Take 1 hr before or 2 hrs after meals. Give with pyridoxine in the malnourished, those predisposed to neuropathy (eg, alcoholics, diabetics), and adolescents.

HOW SUPPLIED: Cap: (Isoniazid-Rifampin) 150mg-300mg

CONTRAINDICATIONS: Previous isoniazid-associated hepatic injury, severe adverse reactions to isoniazid (eg, drug fever, chills, and arthritis), acute liver disease.

WARNINGS/PRECAUTIONS: Monitor LFTs before therapy, periodically thereafter. Not for intermittent therapy. Urine, feces, saliva, sputum, sweat, and tears may be colored red-orange; may stain soft contact lenses permanently. Caution with chronic liver disease or severe renal dysfunction. Perform periodic ophthalmoscopic exams.

ADVERSE REACTIONS: Headache, drowsiness, fatigue, ataxia, dizziness, confusion, visual disturbances, weakness, GI effects, peripheral neuropathy, pyridoxine deficiency, anorexia, nausea, renal or hepatic insufficiency, blood dyscrasias.

INTERACTIONS: Anticoagulants may need dose increase. May decrease activity of methadone, oral hypoglycemics, digitoxin, quinidine, disopyramide, dapsone, and corticosteroids. Higher incidence of isoniazid hepatitis with daily alcohol ingestion. Risk of phenytoin toxicity. Caution with other hepatotoxic agents and phenytoin. May decrease effects of oral contraceptives; use alternative measures.

PREGNANCY: Safety in pregnancy not known, caution in nursing.

MECHANISM OF ACTION: Isonicotinic acid hydrazide/rifamycin derivative. Isoniazid/Rifampin: Exhibits bacterial activity against intracellular and extracellular *Mycobacterium tuberculosis.* Inhibits DNA-dependent RNA polymerase activity in susceptible cells; interacts with bacterial RNA polymerase but does not inhibit the mammalian enzyme. Inhibits mycoloic acid synthesis and acts against actively growing tubercle bacilli.

PHARMACOKINETICS: Absorption: Rifampin: C_{max}=10mcg/mL, T_{max}=$1^1/_2$-3 hrs. Isoniazid: T_{max}=1-2 hrs. **Distribution:** Isoniazid: Diffuses into body fluids; crosses placental barrier and into milk. **Metabolism:** Isoniazid: Acetylation and dehydrazination. **Elimination:** Rifampin: Bile, urine; $T_{1/2}$=3 hrs.

NURSING CONSIDERATIONS

Assessment: Assess for previous isoniazid-associated hepatic injury, acute liver disease, HIV status, pregnancy status, and drug interactions. Document reasons for therapy, culture and susceptibility.

Monitoring: Prior to therapy and periodically thereafter, measure hepatic enzymes (AST, ALT). D/C at first sign of hypersensitivity reactions (fever, skin eruptions, Stevens-Johnson syndrome, vasculitis, anaphylaxis). Monitor for peripheral neuropathy, convulsions, NV, agranulocytosis, hemolytic anemia, SLE-like syndrome, metabolic and endocrine reactions (hyperglycemia, pyridoxine deficiency, pellagra), visual disturbances, serum uric acid levels.

Patient Counseling: Advise to immediately report signs/symptoms consistent with liver damage or other adverse events (eg, unexplained anorexia, NV, dark urine, icterus, rash, persistent paresthesias of the hands and feet, persistent fatigue, weakness or fever of >3 days duration and/or abdominal tenderness). Counsel not to administer with food, take as prescribed, take pyridoxine tablets if peripheral neuropathy develops. Inform that drug may produce reddish urine, sweat, sputum, and tears. Periodic eye exams are recommended when visual symptoms occur.

Administration: Oral route. **Storage:** Keep tightly closed. Store in a dry place. Avoid excessive heat.

RIFATER RX

pyrazinamide - rifampin - isoniazid (Sanofi-Aventis)

> **Isoniazid associated with severe and sometimes fatal hepatitis. Monitor LFTs on a monthly basis.**

THERAPEUTIC CLASS: Isonicotinic acid hydrazide/rifamycin derivative/nicotinamide analogue

INDICATIONS: For initial phase of pulmonary TB treatment.

DOSAGE: *Adults:* ≤44kg: 4 tabs single dose qd. 45-54kg: 5 tabs single dose. ≥55kg: 6 tabs single dose. Give pyridoxine in malnourished, if predisposed to neuropathy (eg, alcoholics, diabetics), and adolescents. Take 1 hr before or 2 hrs after meals with full glass of water. Treatment usually lasts 2 months. *Pediatrics:* ≥15 yrs: ≤44kg: 4 tabs single dose qd. 45-54kg: 5 tabs qd single dose. ≥55kg: 6 tabs qd single dose. Give pyridoxine in malnourished, if predisposed to neuropathy (eg, alcoholics, diabetics), and adolescents. Take 1 hr before or 2 hrs after meals with full glass of water. Treatment usually lasts 2 months.

HOW SUPPLIED: Tab: (Isoniazid-Pyrazinamide-Rifampin) 50mg-300mg-120mg

CONTRAINDICATIONS: Severe hepatic damage, adverse reactions to isoniazid (eg, drug fever, chills, arthritis), acute liver disease, acute gout.

WARNINGS/PRECAUTIONS: Liver dysfunction, hyperbilirubinemia, and hyperuricemia with acute gouty arthritis reported. Monitor LFTs (every 2-4 weeks), serum uric acid. Perform regular ophthalmologic exams. Caution with DM, severe renal dysfunction. May produce reddish coloration of urine, sweat, sputum, and tears. May permanently stain soft contact lenses. Caution in elderly.

ADVERSE REACTIONS: GI effects, cutaneous reactions, musculoskeletal pain, hepatitis, CNS and cardiorespiratory effects.

INTERACTIONS: Rifampin may accelerate metabolism of anticonvulsants (eg, phenytoin), antiarrhythmics (eg, disopyramide, mexiletine, quinidine, tocainide), anticoagulants, antifungals (eg, fluconazole, itraconazole, ketoconazole), barbiturates, β-blockers, CCBs (eg, diltiazem, nifedipine, verapamil), chloramphenicol, ciprofloxacin, corticosteroids, cyclosporine, cardiac glycosides, clofibrate, oral contraceptives, dapsone, diazepam, haloperidol, oral hypoglycemics (eg, sulfonylureas), methadone, narcotic analgesics, nortriptyline, progestins, theophylline. Antacids may reduce rifampin absorption. Avoid foods containing tyramine and histamine (eg, cheese, red wine, tuna). Anticoagulants may need dose increase. Higher incidence of isoniazid (INH) hepatitis with daily alcohol ingestion. Avoid halothane. INH inhibits certain CYP450 enzymes; monitor with anticonvulsants, benzodiazepines, haloperidol, ketoconazole, warfarin. Decreased levels with corticosteroids. Exaggerates CNS effects of meperidine, cycloserine, disulfiram. Excess catecholamine stimulation with L-dopa.

PREGNANCY: Category C, not for use in nursing.

MECHANISM OF ACTION: Rifampin: Inhibits DNA-dependent RNA polymerase activity in susceptible *Mycobacterium tuberculosis* organism. Interacts with bacterial RNA polymerase, but does not inhibit the mammalian enzyme. Isoniazid: Kills growing tubercle bacilli by inhibiting the biosynthesis of mycolic acids, which are major component of the cell wall of *Mycobacterium tuberculosis*. Pyrazinamide: Inhibits growth of *Mycobacterium tuberculosis*.

PHARMACOKINETICS: Absorption: Isoniazid: Bioavailability (100.6%), C_{max}=3.09mcg/mL, T_{max}=1-2 hrs. Rifampin: Bioavailability (88.8 %), C_{max}=11.04mcg/mL. Pyrazinamide: Bioavailability (96.8%), C_{max}=28.02mcg/mL. **Distribution:** Isoniazid: Passes through placental barrier and into milk. Pyrazinamide: Plasma protein binding (10%), distributed in liver, lungs, and CSF; found in breast milk. Rifampin: Protein binding (80%). **Metabolism:** Isoniazid: Acetylation and dehydrazination. Pyrazinamide: Liver, via hydroxylation; pyrazinoic acid (major active metabolite). Rifampin: Via deacetylation; 25-desacetyl-rifampin (major metabolite). **Elimination:** Rifampin: Urine (30%), bile; $T_{1/2}$=3.35 hrs. Pyrazinamide: Urine (70%), (4-14% unchanged); $T_{1/2}$=9-10 hrs. Isoniazid: Urine (50-70%); $T_{1/2}$=1-4 hrs.

NURSING CONSIDERATIONS

Assessment: Assess for previous isoniazid-associated hepatic injury, acute gout, HIV status, pregnancy status, DM, and drug interactions. Document reasons for therapy, culture and susceptibility.

Monitoring: Prior to therapy and periodically thereafter, measure hepatic enzymes (AST, ALT). D/C at first sign of hypersensitivity reactions (fever, skin eruptions, Stevens-Johnson syndrome, vasculitis, anaphylaxis). Monitor for peripheral neuropathy, convulsions, NV, agranulocytosis, hemolytic anemia, SLE like syndrome, metabolic and endocrine reactions (hyperglycemia, pyridoxine deficiency, pellagra), visual disturbances, serum uric acid levels.

Patient Counseling: Immediately report signs/symptoms consistent with liver damage or other adverse events (unexplained anorexia, NV, dark urine, icterus, rash, persistent paresthesias of hands and feet, persistent fatigue, weakness or fever of >3 days' duration and/or abdominal tenderness). Do not administer with food; take as prescribed. Take pyridoxine tablets if peripheral neuropathy develops. Drug may produce reddish urine, sweat, sputum, and tears. Periodic ophthalmoscopic examination is recommended when visual symptoms occur. Avoid tyramine- and histamine-containing foods. Effectiveness of oral contraceptives may be decreased; consider alternative contraceptive methods.

Administration: Oral route. **Storage:** 15-30°C (59-86°F). Protect from excessive humidity.

RILUTEK — RX

riluzole (Sanofi-Aventis)

THERAPEUTIC CLASS: Benzothiazole

INDICATIONS: Treatment of amyotrophic lateral sclerosis (ALS).

DOSAGE: *Adults:* 50mg q12h. Take 1 hr before or 2 hrs after meals.

HOW SUPPLIED: Tab: 50mg

WARNINGS/PRECAUTIONS: Caution in elderly, and hepatic or renal dysfunction. Perform baseline LFTs before therapy, every month during 1st 3 months, every 3 months, every 3 months for next 9 months, then periodically thereafter. Neutropenia reported; obtain WBC count with febrile illness.

ADVERSE REACTIONS: Asthenia, NV, dizziness, decreased lung function, diarrhea, abdominal pain, pneumonia, vertigo, paresthesia, anorexia, somnolence.

INTERACTIONS: Caution with potentially hepatotoxic drugs (eg, allopurinol, methyldopa, sulfinpyrazine). CYP1A2 inhibitors (eg, caffeine, phenacetin, theophylline, amitriptyline, quinolones) may decrease elimination. CYP1A2 inducers (eg, cigarette smoke, charcoal-broiled food, rifampicin, omeprazole) may increase elimination. Drugs metabolized by CYP1A2 (eg, theophylline, caffeine, tacrine) may interact with riluzole.

PREGNANCY: Category C, not for use in nursing.

MECHANISM OF ACTION: Not established; thought to inhibit the effect on glutamate release, inactivate voltage-dependent sodium channels, and interfere with intracellular events that follow transmitter binding at excitatory amino acid receptors.

PHARMACOKINETICS: Absorption: Well absorbed; absolute bioavailability (60%). **Distribution:** Plasma protein binding (96%). **Metabolism:** Liver via CYP450-dependent hydroxylation and glucuronidation. **Elimination:** Urine (85%) glucuronides, (2%, unchanged), feces (5%); $T_{1/2}$=12 hrs.

NURSING CONSIDERATIONS

Assessment: Assess for hepatic/renal impairment, pregnancy/nursing status, alcohol intake, and possible drug interaction. Perform baseline LFTs.

Monitoring: Monitor LFTs, CBC. Monitor for signs/symptoms of febrile illness and hepatic toxicity.

Patient Counseling: Counsel to immediately notify physician any signs of febrile illness. Caution against hazardous tasks (operating machinery/driving). Take therapy on regular basis; 1 hr before meal or 2 hrs after.

Administration: Oral route. **Storage:** 20-25°C (68-77°F); protect from bright light.

R

RISPERDAL
RX

risperidone (Janssen)

Elderly patients with dementia-related psychosis treated with atypical antipsychotic drugs are at an increased risk of death; most appeared to be cardiovascular (eg, heart failure, sudden death) or infectious (eg, pneumonia) in nature. Risperidone is not approved for the treatment of patients with dementia-related psychosis.

OTHER BRAND NAMES: Risperdal M-Tab (Janssen)

THERAPEUTIC CLASS: Benzisoxazole derivative

INDICATIONS: Acute and maintenance treatment of schizophrenia in adults. Treatment of schizophrenia in adolescents 13-17 yrs. Short-term treatment of acute manic or mixed episodes associated with bipolar I disorder as monotherapy (adults and adolescents 10-17 yrs) or in combination with lithium or valproate (adults). Treatment of irritability associated with autistic disorder in children and adolescents 5-16 yrs, including symptoms of aggression towards others, deliberate self-injuriousness, temper tantrums, and quickly changing moods.

DOSAGE: *Adults:* Schizophrenia: Initial: 2mg/day given once or twice daily. Titrate: Adjust dose at intervals not <24 hrs, in increments of 1-2mg/day, as tolerated, to recommended dose of 4-8mg/day. Range: 4-16mg/day. Max: 16mg/day. Bipolar Disorder: Initial: 2-3mg qd. Titrate: Adjust dose at intervals not <24 hrs and in increments/decrements of 1mg/day. Range: 1-6mg/day. Max: 6mg/day. Elderly/Debilitated/Hypotension/Severe Renal or Hepatic Impairment: Initial: 0.5mg bid. Titrate: Adjust dose in increments not >0.5mg bid. Increases to doses >1.5mg bid should occur at intervals of ≥1 week. Periodically reassess to determine maintenance treatment.
Pediatrics: Schizophrenia: 13-17 yrs: Initial: 0.5mg qd in morning or evening. Titrate: Adjust dose, if needed, in increments of 0.5 or 1mg/day and at intervals not <24 hrs, as tolerated, to recommended dose of 3mg/day. Max: 6mg/day. Bipolar Disorder: 10-17 yrs: Initial: 0.5mg qd in morning or evening. Titrate: Adjust dose, if needed, in increments of 0.5 or 1mg/day and at intervals not <24 hrs, as tolerated, to recommended dose of 2.5mg/day. Max: 6mg/day. Irritability with Autistic Disorder: 5-16 yrs: Initial: <20kg: 0.25mg/day; ≥20kg: 0.5mg/day. Titrate: After at least 4 days, may increase dose by 0.5mg/day (<20kg) or 1mg/day (≥20kg). Maint: Minimum of 14 days. Inadequate Response: Increase at ≥2-wk intervals: <20kg: Increase by 0.25mg/day; ≥20kg: Increase by 0.5mg/day. Caution in patients <15kg. Max: <20kg: 1mg/day; ≥20kg: 2.5mg/day; >45kg: 3mg/day.

HOW SUPPLIED: Sol: 1mg/mL [30mL]; Tab: 0.25mg, 0.5mg, 1mg, 2mg, 3mg, 4mg; Tab, Disintegrating: (M-Tab) 0.5mg, 1mg, 2mg, 3mg, 4mg

CONTRAINDICATIONS: Anaphylactic reactions and angioedema.

WARNINGS/PRECAUTIONS: Neuroleptic malignant syndrome and/or tardive dyskinesia may occur. Monitor for hyperglycemia; perform fasting blood glucose testing if symptoms develop or with risk factors for DM. Cerebrovascular events (eg, stroke, TIA) reported in elderly with dementia-related psychosis. Not approved for the treatment of dementia-related psychosis. May induce orthostatic hypotension, elevate prolactin levels, have an antiemetic effect. Caution in elderly, renal/hepatic impairment, history of seizures, cardio- or cerebrovascular disease, suicidal tendencies, risk of aspiration pneumonia, conditions predisposing to hypotension (eg, hypovolemia, dehydration) or affecting metabolism or hemodynamic responses. May impair judgment, thinking, or motor skills; caution when operating hazardous machinery. May disrupt body temperature regulation; caution in patients exposed to temperature extremes. Re-evaluate periodically. Patients with Parkinson's disease or dementia with Lewy bodies who receive antipsychotics are reported to have an increased sensitivity to antipsychotic medications.

ADVERSE REACTIONS: Somnolence, increased appetite, fatigue, NV, coughing, urinary incontinence, constipation, fever, parkinsonism, abdominal pain, anxiety, dizziness, tremor, dyspepsia.

INTERACTIONS: Caution with other CNS drugs or alcohol. May potentiate antihypertensives, antagonize levodopa and dopamine agonists, or increase valproate levels. Cimetidine and ranitidine may increase bioavailability. CYP3A4 inducers (eg, carbamazepine, phenytoin, rifampin, phenobarbital) may decrease levels. Clozapine, fluoxetine, and paroxetine may increase levels. Increased mortality with furosemide in elderly patients.

PREGNANCY: Category C, not for use in nursing.

MECHANISM OF ACTION: Benzisoxazole derivative; psychotropic agent; mechanism not established. Suspected to inhibit both dopamine Type 2 (D_2) and serotonin Type 2 ($5HT_2$).

PHARMACOKINETICS: Absorption: Absolute bioavailability (70%). T_{max}=1 hr; (risperidone) T_{max}=3hrs; 9-hydroxyrisperidone (extensive metabolizers). **Distribution**: V_d=1-2L/kg; plasma protein binding (risperidone: 90%) (9-hydroxyrisperidone: 77%); found in breast milk. **Metabolism**: Liver (extensive). Hydroxylation, N-dealkylation; CYP 2D6: 9-hydroxyrisperidone (major metabolite). **Elimination**: Urine (70%), feces (14%); $T_{1/2}$=20 hrs.

NURSING CONSIDERATIONS

Assessment: Assess patient for dementia-related psychosis, history of DM, liver/renal impairment, seizures, and CVD (MI, CHF, HB), and possible drug interactions.

Monitoring: Monitor for TD, NMS, EPS, cerebrovascular events (eg, stroke, transient ischemic attacks), orthostatic hypotension, body temperature, seizures, suicidal attempts, cognitive/motor impairment. Laboratory monitoring of liver enzymes, BUN, blood glucose, prolactin.

Patient Counseling: Advise of risk of orthostatic hypotension and of nonpharmacologic interventions that help reduce its occurrence. Notify physician if taking any Rx or OTC drugs or if become or intend to become pregnant during therapy. Caution while performing hazardous tasks (operating machinery/driving). Do not breastfeed while on therapy. Avoid alcohol.

Administration: Oral route, with/without meals. Oral Solution can be administered directly from the calibrated pipette, or mixed with a beverage. Do not split or chew tab. **Storage**: Store at controlled room temperature 15-25°C (59-77°F). Protect from light, moisture, and freezing. Keep out of reach of children.

RISPERDAL CONSTA — RX

risperidone (Janssen)

R

Elderly patients with dementia-related psychosis treated with atypical antipsychotic drugs are at an increased risk of death; most appeared to be cardiovascular (eg, heart failure, sudden death) or infectious (eg, pneumonia) in nature. Risperidone is not approved for the treatment of patients with dementia-related psychosis.

THERAPEUTIC CLASS: Benzisoxazole derivative

INDICATIONS: Treatment of schizophrenia.

DOSAGE: *Adults:* 25mg IM every 2 weeks. Max: 50mg every 2 weeks. Give 1st injection with oral dosage form or other oral antipsychotic. Continue for 3 weeks, then d/c oral. Titrate: Increase at intervals of no more than every 4 weeks. Hepatic or Renal Impairment/Certain Drug Interactions/Poor Tolerability to Psychotropic Meds: Premedication: Initial: 0.5mg PO bid during the 1st week of risperidone. Titrate: May increase to 1mg bid or 2mg qd during the 2nd week. Give 1st injection with oral dosage form. Continue for 3 weeks. Treatment: Initial: 12.5mg. Elderly: Start 25mg every 2 weeks. Give 1st injection with oral dosage form or other oral antipsychotic. Continue for 3 weeks.

HOW SUPPLIED: Inj: 12.5mg, 25mg, 37.5mg, 50mg

WARNINGS/PRECAUTIONS: Cerebrovascular events (eg, stroke, TIA) reported in elderly with dementia-related psychosis. Not approved for the treatment of dementia-related psychosis. Neuroleptic malignant syndrome and/or tardive dyskinesia may occur. Monitor for hyperglycemia; perform fasting blood glucose testing if symptoms develop or with risk factors for DM. May elevate prolactin levels, induce orthostatic hypotension, have an antiemetic effect. May impair physical/mental ability. Caution in elderly, renal/hepatic impairment, history of seizures, cardio- or cerebrovascular disease, suicidal tendencies, esophageal dysmotility, risk of aspiration pneumonia, conditions predisposing to hypotension (eg, hypovolemia, dehydration) or affecting metabolism or hemodynamic responses. Severe priapism and TTP reported. May disrupt body temperature regulation; caution in patients exposed to temperature extremes. Must inject into the gluteal muscle; avoid injection into blood vessel. Monitor for suicidal attempts in high risk patients. Re-evaluate periodically. Patients who receive antipsychotics are reported to have an increased sensitivity to antipsychotic medications. Osteodystrophy, renal tubular tumors, and adrenomedullary pheochromocytomas reported in animal studies.

ADVERSE REACTIONS: Headache, dizziness, constipation, dyspepsia, akathisia, parkinsonism, weight increase, dry mouth, fatigue, and pain in extremity.

INTERACTIONS: Caution with other CNS drugs or alcohol. May potentiate antihypertensives, antagonize levodopa and dopamine agonists, or increase valproate levels. Cimetidine and ranitidine may increase bioavailability. CYP3A4 inducers (eg, carbamazepine, phenytoin, rifampin, phenobarbital) may decrease levels. Clozapine, fluoxetine, and paroxetine may increase levels. Increased mortality with furosemide in elderly patients.

PREGNANCY: Category C, not for use in nursing.

MECHANISM OF ACTION: Benzisoxazole derivative; suspected to inhibit both dopamine type 2 (D_2) and serotonin type 2 ($5HT_2$).

PHARMACOKINETICS: Distribution: Breast milk, V_d=1-2L/kg. Plasma protein binding: Risperidone (approximately 90%), 9-hydroxyrisperidone (77%). **Metabolism**: Liver (extensive). Hydroxylation, N-dealkylation; CYP 2D6: 9-hydroxyrisperidone (major metabolite). **Elimination**: Urine (70%), feces (14%); $T_{1/2}$=3-6 days.

NURSING CONSIDERATIONS

Assessment: Assess patient for dementia-related psychosis, liver/renal impairment, DM, seizures, CVD (MI, CHF, HB), and possible drug interactions.

Monitoring: Monitor signs/symptoms of hypersensitivity, TD, NMS, EPS, cerebrovascular events (eg, stroke, transient ischemic attacks), orthostatic hypotension, body temperature, seizures, suicidal attempts, osteodystrophy, renal or adrenal tumors, cognitive/motor impairment. Laboratory monitoring of liver enzymes, BUN, blood glucose, prolactin.

Patient Counseling: Advise of risk of orthostatic hypotension or nonpharmacologic interventions that help reduce its occurrence. Notify physician if taking any Rx or OTC drugs or if become or intend to become pregnant during therapy. Do not breastfeed. Caution while performing hazardous tasks (operating machinery/driving). Avoid alcohol.

Administration: IM route, injected into the gluteal muscle. **Storage**: 2-8°C (36-46°F). Protect from light. If refrigeration is unavailable, store at temperatures not exceeding 25°C (77°F) for no more than 7 days prior to administration.

RITALIN

CII

methylphenidate HCl (Novartis)

OTHER BRAND NAMES: Ritalin LA (Novartis) - Ritalin SR (Novartis)

THERAPEUTIC CLASS: Sympathomimetic amine

INDICATIONS: (Cap; Extended-Release, Tab; Tab, Extended-Release) Treatment of attention deficit disorders. (Tab; Tab, Extended-Release) Treatment of narcolepsy.

DOSAGE: *Adults:* (Tab) 10-60mg/day given bid-tid 30-45 min ac. Take last dose before 6 pm if insomnia occurs. (Tab, ER) May use in place of immediate release (IR) when the 8 hr dose corresponds to the titrated 8 hr IR dose. Swallow whole; do not chew or crush. (Cap, ER) Initial: 20mg qam. Titrate:

Adjust weekly by 10mg. Max: 60mg qam.
Pediatrics: ≥6 yrs: (Tab) Initial: 5mg bid before breakfast and lunch. Titrate: Increase gradually by 5-10mg weekly. Max: 60mg/day. (Tab, ER) May use in place of immediate release (IR) when the 8 hr dose corresponds to the titrated 8 hr IR dose. Swallow whole; do not chew or crush. (Cap, ER) Initial: 20mg qam. Titrate: Adjust weekly by 10mg. Max: 60mg qam. Previous Methylphenidate Use: May use as qd in place of IR dosed bid or daily dose of methylphenidate-SR. Swallow whole or sprinkle over spoonful of applesauce. Do not crush, chew, or divide. Reduce dose or d/c if paradoxical aggravation of symptoms occurs. D/C if no improvement after appropriate dose adjustment over 1 month.

HOW SUPPLIED: Cap, Extended-Release (Ritalin LA): 10mg, 20mg, 30mg, 40mg; Tab (Ritalin): 5mg, 10mg*, 20mg*; Tab, Extended-Release (Ritalin SR): 20mg *scored

CONTRAINDICATIONS: Marked anxiety, tension, and agitation; glaucoma; motor tics or family history or diagnosis of Tourette's syndrome; during or within 14 days of MAOI use.

WARNINGS/PRECAUTIONS: Monitor growth in children. Not for severe depression or fatigue. May exacerbate symptoms of behavior disturbance and thought disorder in psychotic children. Care should be taken in using stimulants to treat patients with comorbid bipolar disorder because of concern for possible induction of mixed/manic episode in such patients. Stimulants at usual doses can cause treatment emergent psychotic or manic symptoms (hallucinations, delusional thinking, mania) in children and adolescents without prior history of psychotic illness. Aggressive behavior or hostility reported in clinical trials and the postmarketing experience of some medications indicated for the treatment of ADHD. May lower seizure threshold, especially with prior history of seizures or with prior EEG abnormalities; d/c if seizures occur. Caution with HTN and other underlying conditions that may be compromised such as heart failure, recent MI, or hyperthyroidism. Visual disturbances may occur (rare). Monitor CBC, differential, and platelets with prolonged use. Caution with emotionally-unstable patients or prior history of drug dependence or alcoholism; chronic use may lead to tolerance and psychological dependence. Monitor during withdrawal. Periodically d/c to assess condition. Avoid with known structural cardiac abnormalities or other serious cardiac problems.

ADVERSE REACTIONS: Nervousness, insomnia, hypersensitivity reactions, anorexia, nausea, dizziness, palpitations, headache, dyskinesia, drowsiness, BP and pulse changes, tachycardia, angina, arrhythmia, abdominal pain.

INTERACTIONS: See Contraindications. May decrease hypotensive effect of guanethidine. Caution with α_2-agonists (eg, clonidine) and pressor agents. Potentiates anticoagulants, anticonvulsants (eg, phenobarbital, diphenylhydantoin, primidone), phenylbutazone, TCAs (eg, imipramine, clomipramine, desipramine); monitor plasma drug levels or PT/INR. (Cap, Extended-Release) Antacids or acid suppressants may alter release characteristics of cap.

PREGNANCY: Category C, caution in nursing.

MECHANISM OF ACTION: Sympathomimetic amine; CNS stimulant, blocks reuptake of norepinephrine and dopamine into presynaptic neuron and increases release of monoamines into extraneuronal space.

PHARMACOKINETICS: Absorption: Children: (Tab, ER) T_{max}=4.7 hrs; (Tab) 1.9 hrs. **Metabolism:** α-phenyl-2-piperidine acetic acid (major metabolite). **Elimination:** Urine (78-97%), feces (1-3%); $T_{1/2}$=3.5 hrs (adults), 2.5 hrs (children).

NURSING CONSIDERATIONS

Assessment: Assess for agitation, glaucoma, tics, family history of Tourette's syndrome, cardiovascular conditions (eg, severe HTN, angina pectoris, cardiac structural abnormalities, arrhythmias, HF, recent MI), hyperthyroidism or thyrotoxicosis, bipolar disorder, psychosis, seizures, history of drug dependence or alcoholism, possible drug interactions.

Monitoring: Monitor cardiovascular status, exacerbations of behavior disturbances and thought disorders, bipolar disorder, aggression, seizures, visual disturbances, CBC with differential and platelet counts. Monitor growth in children. Periodically d/c drug to assess child's condition.

Patient Counseling: Inform about risks of treatment, appropriate use, drug abuse/dependence. Caution while operating machinery/driving. Avoid afternoon dose; may cause insomnia. Counsel to take 30 min before food; swallow tablet whole, do not crush or chew.

Administration: Oral route. **Storage:** 15-30°C (59-86°F). Protect from light and moisture.

RITUXAN RX

rituximab (Genentech/Biogen Idec)

Serious, sometimes fatal, infusion reactions reported. Acute renal failure reported in the setting of tumor lysis syndrome (TLS) following treatment of non-Hodgkin's lymphoma. Severe mucocutaneous reactions reported. JC virus infection resulting in progressive multifocal leukoencephalopathy (PML) reported.

THERAPEUTIC CLASS: Monoclonal antibody/CD20-blocker

INDICATIONS: Treatment of non-Hodgkin's lymphoma (NHL) in patients with: 1) relapsed or refractory, low-grade or follicular, CD20-positive, B-cell NHL as a single agent; 2) previously untreated follicular, CD20-positive, B-cell NHL in combination with CVP chemotherapy; 3) nonprogressing (including stable disease), low-grade, CD20-positive, B-cell NHL, as a single agent, after 1st-line CVP chemotherapy; 4) previously untreated diffuse large B-cell, CD20-positive NHL in combination with CHOP or other anthracycline-based chemotherapy regimens. In combination with methotrexate to reduce signs and symptoms and to slow the progression of structural damage in adult patients with moderately to severely active rheumatoid arthritis (RA) who have had inadequate response to one or more TNF-antagonist therapies.

DOSAGE: *Adults:* Administer only as IV infusion. Relapsed or Refractory, Low-Grade or Follicular, CD20-Positive, B-cell NHL: 375mg/m² IV once weekly for 4 or 8 doses. Retreatment for Relapsed or Refractory, Low-Grade or Follicular, CD20-Positive, B-cell NHL: 375mg/m² IV once weekly for 4 doses. Previously Untreated, Follicular, CD20-Positive, B-cell NHL: 375mg/m² IV on Day 1 of each CVP chemotherapy cycle for up to 8 doses. Nonprogressing, Low-Grade, CD20-Positive, B-cell NHL: Following completion of 6-8 cycles of CVP chemotherapy, 375mg/m² IV once weekly for 4 doses at 6-month intervals to maximum of 16 doses. Diffuse Large B-cell NHL: 375mg/m² IV given on Day 1 of each chemotherapy cycle for up to 8 infusions. RA: Give with methotrexate. Administer two 1000mg IV infusions separated by 2 weeks. Give methylprednisolone 100mg IV (or equivalent) 30 min prior to each infusion to reduce incidence and severity of infusion reactions. Do not administer as IV push or bolus. For dosing as a component of Zevalin® please refer to PI.

HOW SUPPLIED: Inj: 10mg/mL [10mL, 50mL]

WARNINGS/PRECAUTIONS: Interrupt if severe reaction develops; may resume at a 50% rate reduction when symptoms subside. Consider the diagnosis of PML in patients presenting with new-onset neurologic manifestations; d/c and consider reduction or discontinuation of concomitant chemotherapy or immunosuppressive therapy. HBV reactivation with fulminant hepatitis, hepatic failure, and death reported; d/c if viral hepatitis develops. Additional serious viral infections, either new, reactivated, or exacerbated, reported. D/C if serious arrhythmias occur. Use caution with pre-existing cardiac conditions. Use with extreme caution in combination with cisplatin; renal failure may occur. Severe renal toxicity reported; d/c if SrCr rises or oliguria occurs. Monitor CBC and platelets regularly; more frequently with cytopenias. Abdominal pain, bowel obstruction, and perforation reported. Not recommended in patients with RA who have not had prior inadequate response to one or more TNF-antagonists.

ADVERSE REACTIONS: Fever, chills, infection, asthenia, nausea, lymphopenia, leukopenia, neutropenia, headache, abdominal pain, night sweats, rash, pruritus, pain.

INTERACTIONS: Renal toxicity reported with cisplatin. Vaccination with live virus vaccines not recommended. Observe closely for signs of infection if biologic agents and/or DMARDs are used concomitantly.

PREGNANCY: Category C, safety not known in nursing.

MECHANISM OF ACTION: Human monoclonal IgG_1 kappa antibody/CD20 antigen blocker; binds to CD20 antigen on B lymphocytes and recruits immune effector functions to mediate B-cell lysis, possibly by complement-dependent cytotoxicity and antibody-dependent, cell-mediated cytotoxicity.

PHARMACOKINETICS: Absorption: NHL: C_{max}=486mcg/mL. RA: C_{max}=183mcg/mL (2x500mg), 370mcg/mL (2x1000mg). **Distribution:** RA: V_d=4.3L. **Elimination:** NHL: $T_{1/2}$=22 days. RA: $T_{1/2}$=19 days.

NURSING CONSIDERATIONS

Assessment: Assess for pre-existing cardiac or pulmonary conditions, prior cardiopulmonary adverse events, high number of circulating malignant cells (>25000/mm^3), history of arrhythmias or angina, high tumor burden, possible drug interactions, renal impairment. Screen for HBV infection prior to therapy.

Monitoring: Monitor serum electrolytes, renal function, fluid balance, CBC and platelet counts periodically; cardiac function (history of arrhythmias, angina), for signs/symptoms of HBV reactivation, infusion reaction, tumor lysis syndrome, arrhythmias, viral infections, mucocutaneous reactions, progressive multifocal leukoencephalopathy, renal failure, cytopenias, bowel obstruction/perforation, and hypersensitivity reactions.

Patient Counseling: Instruct to use effective contraception during treatment and for 12 months after therapy; vaccinations with live vaccines are not recommended. Advise to seek medical attention if symptoms of arrhythmias, infusion reaction (urticaria, hypotension, angioedema), new onset of neurological symptoms, infection, bowel obstruction (abdominal pain), mucocutaneous reactions, or hypersensitivity reactions occur.

Administration: IV route. First infusion: Initiate rate of 50mg/hr; if no toxicity, increase by 50mg/hr increments every 30 min to maximum of 400mg/hr. Subsequent infusion: Initiate rate of 100mg/hr; if no toxicity, increase by 100mg/hr increments every 30 min to maximum of 400mg/hr. **Storage:** Vials: 2-8°C (36-46°F). Protect from direct sunlight. Do not freeze or shake. Sol: 2-8°C (36-46°F); stable for 24 hrs. Room temperature; stable for 48 hrs.

ROBAXIN RX

methocarbamol (Schwarz)

OTHER BRAND NAMES: Robaxin-750 (Schwarz) - Robaxin Injection (Baxter)

THERAPEUTIC CLASS: Muscular analgesic (central-acting)

INDICATIONS: Adjunct for relief of acute, painful musculoskeletal conditions.

DOSAGE: *Adults:* (PO) Initial: (500mg tab) 1500mg qid for 2-3 days. Maint: 1000mg qid. Initial: (750mg tab) 1500mg qid for 2-3 days. Maint: 750mg q4h or 1500mg tid. Max: 6g/d for 2-3 days; 8g/d if severe. (Inj) Moderate Symptoms: 10mL IV/IM. IV Max Rate: 3mL undiluted drug/min. IM Max: 5mL into each gluteal region. Severe/Post-Op Condition: Max: 20-30mL/day up to 3 consecutive days. If feasible, continue with PO. Tetanus: 10-20mL up to 30mL. May repeat q6h until NG tube can be inserted. Continue with crushed tabs. Max: 24g/day PO.

Pediatrics: Tetanus: Initial: 15mg/kg or 500mg/m^2. Repeat q6h prn. Max: 1.8g/m^2 for 3 consecutive days. Administer by injection into tubing or IV infusion.

HOW SUPPLIED: Inj: 100mg/mL [10mL]; Tab: 500mg, 750mg

CONTRAINDICATIONS: (Inj) Renal pathology with injection due to propylene glycol content.

WARNINGS/PRECAUTIONS: May impair mental/physical abilities required for operating machinery or driving a motor vehicle. May cause color interference in certain screening tests for 5-hydroxy-indoleacetic acid (5-HIAA) and

R

vanillylmandelic acid (VMA). Caution in epilepsy with the injection. Injection rate should not exceed 3mL/min. Avoid extravasation with injection. Avoid use of injection particularly during early pregnancy.

ADVERSE REACTIONS: Lightheadedness, dizziness, drowsiness, nausea, urticaria, pruritus, rash, conjunctivitis, nasal congestion, blurred vision, headache, fever, seizures, syncope, flushing.

INTERACTIONS: Additive adverse effects with alcohol and other CNS depressants. May inhibit effect of pyridostigmine; caution in patients with myasthenia gravis receiving anticholinergics.

PREGNANCY: Category C, caution in nursing.

MECHANISM OF ACTION: Carbamate derivative of guaifenesin; not established, suspected to have CNS depressant with sedative and musculoskeletal relaxant properties.

PHARMACOKINETICS: Distribution: Plasma protein binding (46-50%). **Distribution:** Found in breast milk. **Metabolism:** Via dealkylation, hydroxylation, and conjugation pathways. **Elimination:** Urine; $T_{1/2}$=1-2 hrs.

NURSING CONSIDERATIONS

Assessment: Assess for renal/hepatic impairment, myasthenia gravis, seizures, pregnancy/nursing status, alcohol intake, and drug interactions.

Monitoring: Monitor for congenital and fetal abnormalities if taken during pregnancy, for color interference in certain screening tests for 5-HIAA using nitrosonaphthol reagent and in screening tests for urinary VMA using Gitlow method.

Patient Counseling: Caution while performing hazardous tasks (operating machinery/driving). Avoid alcohol or other CNS depressants. Notify if pregnant/nursing or if planning to become pregnant.

Administration: Oral route, IV infusion, and IM; careful supervision of dose and rate of injection. **Storage:** 20-25°C (68-77°F), in tight container; excursions permitted to 15-30°C (59-86°F).

ROCEPHIN RX

ceftriaxone sodium (Roche Labs)

THERAPEUTIC CLASS: Cephalosporin (3rd generation)

INDICATIONS: Treatment of lower respiratory tract, skin and skin structure, bone and joint, intra-abdominal and urinary tract infections, acute otitis media, uncomplicated gonorrhea, pelvic inflammatory disease, bacterial septicemia, and meningitis caused by susceptible strains of microorganisms. Surgical prophylaxis during surgical procedures classified as contaminated or potentially contaminated.

DOSAGE: *Adults:* Usual: 1-2g/day IV/IM given qd-bid. Max: 4g/day. Gonorrhea: 250mg IM single dose. Surgical Prophylaxis: 1g IV 1/2-2 hrs before surgery. Avoid diluents containing calcium.
Pediatrics: Skin Infections: 50-75mg/kg/day IV/IM given qd-bid. Max: 2g/day. Otitis Media: 50mg/kg (up to 1g) IM single dose. Serious Infections: 50-75mg/kg/day IM/IV given q12h. Max: 2g/day. Meningitis: Initial: 100mg/kg (up to 4g), then 100mg/kg/day given qd-bid for 7-14 days. Max: 4g/day. Avoid diluents containing calcium.

HOW SUPPLIED: Inj: (Rocephin) 500mg, 1g; (Generic) 250mg, 500mg, 1g, 2g, 10g, 1g/50mL, 2g/50mL

CONTRAINDICATIONS: Avoid use in hyperbilirubinemic neonates especially if premature. Avoid concurrent use with calcium-containing solutions/products in newborns.

WARNINGS/PRECAUTIONS: Cross-sensitivity to PCNs and other cephalosporins may occur. *Clostridium difficile*-associated diarrhea reported. May result in overgrowth of nonsusceptible organisms. Altered PT, transient BUN, and serum creatinine elevations may occur. Do not exceed 2g/day and monitor blood levels with both hepatic dysfunction and significant renal disease.

Caution with history of GI disease. D/C if gallbladder disease develops. May alter PT; monitor with impaired vitamin K synthesis or low vitamin K stores.

ADVERSE REACTIONS: Injection-site reactions, eosinophilia, thrombocytosis, diarrhea, SGOT and SGPT elevations.

INTERACTIONS: See Contraindications. Do not administer calcium-containing products within 48 hrs of last administration of drug.

PREGNANCY: Category B, caution in nursing.

MECHANISM OF ACTION: Broad-spectrum cephalosporin; bactericidal activity results from inhibition of cell-wall synthesis.

PHARMACOKINETICS: Absorption: (Adults) Complete; T_{max}=2-3 hrs. (Pediatrics) Bacterial meningitis: C_{max}=216mcg/mL (50mg/kg), 275mcg/mL (75mg/mL). Middle ear fluid: C_{max}=35mcg/mL; T_{max}=24 hrs. **Distribution:** (Adults) V_d=5.78-13.5L. (Pediatrics) Bacterial meningitis: V_d=338mL/kg (50mg/kg), 373mL/kg (75mg/kg). **Elimination:** Urine (33-67%), feces. (Adults) $T_{1/2}$=5.8-8.7 hrs. (Pediatrics) Bacterial meningitis: $T_{1/2}$=4.6 hrs (50mg/kg), 4.3 hrs (75mg/kg); Middle ear fluid: $T_{1/2}$=25 hrs.

NURSING CONSIDERATIONS

Assessment: Assess for impaired vitamin K synthesis or low vitamin K stores, history of colitis, and possible drug interactions.

Monitoring: Monitor drug levels periodically; PT levels (low vitamin K). Monitor for signs/symptoms of hypersensitivity reactions, *C. difficile*-associated diarrhea, superinfection, and gallbladder disease.

Patient Counseling: Inform therapy only treats bacterial, not viral, infections. Take as directed; skipping doses or not completing full course may decrease effectiveness and increase resistance. May experience diarrhea; notify physician if watery/bloody stools, hypersensitivity reactions, superinfections, or symptoms of gallbladder disease develop.

Administration: IV, IM route. Refer to PI for storage of diluents. **Storage:** 25°C (77°F) or below; protect from light.

ROMAZICON — RX

flumazenil (Roche Labs)

THERAPEUTIC CLASS: Benzodiazepine antagonist

INDICATIONS: Complete or partial reversal of sedative effects of benzodiazepines (BZDs) given with general anesthesia, or diagnostic and therapeutic procedures, and for the management of BZD overdose in adults. For reversal of BZD-induced conscious sedation in pediatrics (1-17 yrs old).

DOSAGE: *Adults:* Reversal of Conscious Sedation/General Anesthesia: Give IV over 15 seconds. Initial: 0.2mg. May repeat dose after 45 seconds and again at 60 second intervals up to a max of 4 additional times until reach desired level of consciousness. Max Total Dose: 1mg. In event of resedation, repeated doses may be given at 20-min intervals. Max: 1mg/dose (0.2mg/min) and 3mg/hr. BZD Overdose: Give IV over 30 seconds. Initial: 0.2mg. May repeat with 0.3mg after 30 seconds and then 0.5mg at 1-min intervals until reach desired level of consciousness. Max Total Dose: 3mg. In event of resedation, repeated doses may be given at 20-min intervals. Max: 1mg/dose (0.5mg/min); 3mg/hr. *Pediatrics*: >1yr: Give IV over 15 seconds. Initial: 0.01mg/kg (up to 0.2mg). May repeat dose after 45 seconds and again at 60-second intervals up to a max of 4 additional times until reach desired level of consciousness. Max Total Dose: 0.05mg/kg or 1mg, whichever is lower.

HOW SUPPLIED: Inj: 0.1mg/mL

CONTRAINDICATIONS: Patients given BZDs for life-threatening conditions (eg, control of ICP or status epilepticus), signs of serious cyclic antidepressant overdose.

WARNINGS/PRECAUTIONS: Caution in overdoses involving multiple drug combinations. Risk of seizures, especially with long-term BZD-induced sedation, cyclic antidepressant overdose, concurrent major sedative-hypnotic drug withdrawal, recent therapy with repeated doses of parenteral BZDs, myoclonic jerking or seizure prior to flumazenil administration. Monitor for resedation, respiratory depression, or other residual BZD effects (up to 2 hrs). Avoid use in the ICU; increased risk of unrecognized BZD dependence. Caution with head injury, alcoholism, and other drug dependencies. Does not reverse respiratory depression/hypoventilation or cardiac depression. May provoke panic attacks with history of panic disorder. Adjust subsequent doses in hepatic dysfunction. Not for use as treatment for BZD dependence or for management of protracted abstinence syndromes. May trigger dose-dependent withdrawal syndromes. Extravasation may occur; administer IV into a large vein.

ADVERSE REACTIONS: N/V, dizziness, injection-site pain, increased sweating, headache, abnormal or blurred vision, agitation.

INTERACTIONS: Avoid use until neuromuscular blockade effects are reversed. Toxic effects (eg, convulsions, cardiac dysrhythmias) may occur with mixed drug overdose (eg, cyclic antidepressants).

PREGNANCY: Category C, caution in nursing.

MECHANISM OF ACTION: Benzodiazepine receptor antagonist; inhibits activity at the benzodiazepine recognition site on the GABA/benzodiazepine receptor complex.

PHARMACOKINETICS: Absorption: C_{max}=24ng/mL; AUC=15ng•hr/mL. **Distribution:** V_d=1L/kg (steady state); plasma protein binding (50%). **Metabolism:** Complete (99%). **Elimination**: Urine (90-95%), feces (5-10%); $T_{1/2}$=54 min.

NURSING CONSIDERATIONS

Assessment: Assess patients using benzodiazepine for control of potentially life-threatening condition, those showing signs of serious cyclic antidepressant overdose. Assess for head injury, history of convulsions, panic disorders, lung disease, hepatic impairment, and possible drug interactions.

Monitoring: Monitor for occurrence of seizure, re-sedation, respiratory depression, or other residual benzodiazepine effects, dizziness, injection-site pain, increased sweating, headache, and abnormal or blurred vision.

Patient Counseling: Advise not to engage in activities requiring complete alertness (eg, operating machinery/driving) during first 24 hrs after discharge. Advise not to take alcohol or non-prescription drugs first 24 hrs after flumazenil administration, or if effects of the benzodiazepine persist.

Administration: IV route. **Storage:** 25°C (77°F); excursions permitted to 15-30°C (59-86°F).

ROSAC — RX

sulfacetamide sodium - sulfur (Stiefel)

THERAPEUTIC CLASS: Sulfonamide/sulfur combination

INDICATIONS: Topical control of acne vulgaris, acne rosacea, and seborrheic dermatitis.

DOSAGE: *Adults*: Apply a thin film qd-tid.
Pediatrics: ≥12 yrs: Apply a thin film qd-tid.

HOW SUPPLIED: Cre: (Sulfacetamide-Sulfur) 10%-5% [45g]

CONTRAINDICATIONS: Kidney disease.

WARNINGS/PRECAUTIONS: D/C if irritation or hypersensitivity reaction occurs. Avoid contact with eyes. Caution if denuded or abraded skin. May cause reddening and scaling of epidermis.

ADVERSE REACTIONS: Local irritation.

PREGNANCY: Category C, caution in nursing.

MECHANISM OF ACTION: Sulfonamide/sulfur combination. Sulfacetamide: Acts as a competitive antagonist to para-aminobenzoic acid (PABA), an essential component for bacterial growth. Sulfur: Not established. Inhibits the growth of *Propionibacterium acnes* and the formation of free fatty acids.

PHARMACOKINETICS: Absorption: Sulfacetamide: (PO) Readily absorbed. **Distribution:** Small amounts of orally administered sulfonamides have been found in breast milk. **Elimination:** Sulfacetamide: Urine (unchanged).

NURSING CONSIDERATIONS

Assessment: Assess for hypersensitivity to sulfonamides or sulfur and for kidney disease. Assess pregnancy/nursing status.

Monitoring: Monitor for signs/symptoms of systemic toxic reactions (eg, agranulocytosis, acute hemolytic anemia, purpura hemorrhagica, drug fever, jaundice, and contact dermatitis) and for local irritation or sensitization.

Patient Counseling: Instruct to d/c medication and notify physician if skin irritation develops. Inform medication is for external use only and to avoid contact with eyes. Advise medication may cause skin reddening and scaling.

Administration: Topical. **Storage:** 15-30°C (59-86°F). Keep out of reach of children.

ROSULA — RX

sulfacetamide sodium - sulfur (Doak)

THERAPEUTIC CLASS: Sulfonamide/sulfur combination

INDICATIONS: Topical treatment of acne vulgaris, acne rosacea, and seborrheic dermatitis.

DOSAGE: *Adults:* (Gel) Apply thin film qd-tid. (Cleanser) Wash for 10-20 seconds qd-bid.
Pediatrics: ≥12 yrs: (Gel) Apply thin film qd-tid. (Cleanser) Wash for 10-20 seconds qd-bid.

HOW SUPPLIED: (Sulfacetamide-Sulfur) Gel: 10%-5% [45mL]; Cleanser: 10%-5% [355mL]

CONTRAINDICATIONS: Kidney disease.

WARNINGS/PRECAUTIONS: D/C if irritation or hypersensitivity reaction occurs. Avoid contact with eyes, lips, and mucous membranes. Caution with denuded or abraded skin. Can cause reddening and scaling of epidermis.

ADVERSE REACTIONS: Local irritation.

PREGNANCY: Category C, caution in nursing.

MECHANISM OF ACTION: Sulfonamide/sulfur combination. Sulfacetamide: Acts as a competitive antagonist to para-aminobenzoic acid (PABA), an essential component for bacterial growth. Sulfur: Not established. Inhibits the growth of *Propionibacterium acnes* and the formation of free fatty acids.

PHARMACOKINETICS: Absorption: (PO) Readily absorbed. **Elimination:** Urine (unchanged).

NURSING CONSIDERATIONS

Assessment: Assess for hypersensitivity to sulfonamides or sulfur and kidney disease. Assess pregnancy/nursing status.

Monitoring: Monitor for signs/symptoms of systemic toxic reactions (eg, agranulocytosis, acute hemolytic anemia, purpura hemorrhagica, drug fever, jaundice, and contact dermatitis) and for development of local irritation or sensitization (eg, skin reddening and scaling).

Patient Counseling: Avoid contact with eyes, eyelids, lips, and mucous membranes. Instruct to rinse with water if accidental contact occurs. Inform to d/c and consult physician if excessive skin irritation occurs.

Administration: Topical route. **Storage:** 15-25°C (59-77°F). Protect from freezing.

ROSULA NS RX

sulfacetamide sodium - urea (Doak)

THERAPEUTIC CLASS: Sulfonamide

INDICATIONS: Topical treatment of bacterial infections of the skin including *P.acnes* and seborrheic dermatitis.

DOSAGE: *Adults:* Apply to affected area qd-bid.
Pediatrics: ≥12 yrs: Apply to affected area qd-bid.

HOW SUPPLIED: Swab: (Sulfacetamide-Urea) 10%-10% [30^s]

CONTRAINDICATIONS: Kidney disease.

WARNINGS/PRECAUTIONS: D/C if irritation or hypersensitivity reaction occurs. Avoid contact with eyes, lips, and mucous membranes. Caution with denuded or abraded skin. Cases of Stevens-Johnson syndrome and drug-induced systemic lupus erythematosus reported.

ADVERSE REACTIONS: Local hypersensitivity, instances of Stevens-Johnson syndrome.

INTERACTIONS: Incompatible with silver preparations.

PREGNANCY: Category C, caution in nursing.

MECHANISM OF ACTION: Sulfonamide; possesses bacteriostatic activity against susceptible gram-positive and gram-negative microorganisms, including *P. acnes.* Acts as a competitive antagonist to para-aminobenzoic acid (PABA), an essential component for bacterial growth.

PHARMACOKINETICS: Absorption: Sulfacetamide: (PO) Readily absorbed. **Elimination:** Urine (unchanged).

NURSING CONSIDERATIONS

Assessment: Assess for hypersensitivity to sulfonamides, presence of kidney disease, and pregnancy/nursing status. Assess for infected, abraded, denuded, or severely burned skin. Assess for drug interactions.

Monitoring: Monitor for signs/symptoms of systemic toxic reactions (eg, agranulocytosis, acute hemolytic anemia, purpura hemorrhagica, drug fever, jaundice, contact dermatitis), Stevens-Johnson syndrome, drug-induced systemic lupus erythematosus, overgrowth of nonsusceptible organisms (eg, fungi), and hypersensitivity reactions.

Patient Counseling: Avoid contact with eyes, eyelids, lips, and mucous membranes. Rinse with water if accidental contact occurs. Advise to d/c use if condition worsens or if rash develops in treatment area. Advise to notify physician and d/c use if arthritis, fever, or sores in mouth develop.

Administration: Topical route. **Storage:** 15-30°C (59-86°F). Protect from freezing. Pads may darken after prolonged storage. Slight discoloration does not impair efficacy and safety of product.

ROTATEQ RX

rotavirus vaccine, live (Merck)

THERAPEUTIC CLASS: Vaccine

INDICATIONS: Prevention of rotavirus gastroenteritis in infants and children caused by the serotypes G1, G2, G3, and G4 when administered as a 3-dose series to infants between the ages of 6-32 weeks. The first dose should be administered between 6-12 weeks of age.

DOSAGE: *Pediatrics:* Administer series of 3 doses orally starting at 6-12 weeks of age, with subsequent doses administered at 4-10 week intervals. Third dose should not be given after 32 weeks of age. Do not mix with any other vaccines or solutions. Do not reconstitute or dilute.

HOW SUPPLIED: Sus: 2mL

WARNINGS/PRECAUTIONS: Consider delaying use with febrile illness. Vaccination may not result in complete protection in all recipients. May increase risk of intussusception. Caution when administering to individuals with immunodeficient close contacts who may be at increased risk of acquiring and transmitting rotaviruses.

ADVERSE REACTIONS: Bronchiolitis, gastroenteritis, pneumonia, fever, UTI.

INTERACTIONS: Immunosuppressive therapies including irradiation, antimetabolites, alkylating agents, cytotoxic drugs, and corticosteroids (used in greater than physiologic doses) may reduce the immune response to vaccines.

PREGNANCY: Safety in pregnancy and nursing not known.

MECHANISM OF ACTION: Immunologic mechanism not established; may replicate in small intestine and induce immunity against rotavirus gastroenteritis.

NURSING CONSIDERATIONS

Assessment: Assess immunity and current health status.

Monitoring: Monitor for hypersensitivity reactions, diarrhea, vomiting, otitis media, nasopharyngitis, bronchospasm, intussusception, hematochezia, and Kawasaki syndrome.

Patient Counseling: Inform of potential benefits/risks ratio; report any adverse reactions to physician.

Administration: Oral route. **Storage:** 2-8°C (36-46°F). Protect from light.

ROWASA RX

mesalamine (Solvay)

INDICATIONS: Treatment of active mild to moderate distal ulcerative colitis, proctosigmoiditis or proctitis.

DOSAGE: *Adults:* Use 1 enema rectally qhs for 3-6 weeks. Retain for 8 hrs. Empty bowel prior to administration.

HOW SUPPLIED: Enema: 4g/60mL

WARNINGS/PRECAUTIONS: D/C if acute intolerance syndrome develops (eg, cramping, bloody diarrhea, abdominal pain, headache); consider sulfasalazine hypersensitivity. If rechallenge is considered, perform under careful observation. Caution with sulfasalazine hypersensitivity. Carefully monitor with renal dysfunction. Contains potassium metabisulfite; caution with sulfite sensitivity especially in asthmatics. Pancolitis, pericarditis (rare) reported.

ADVERSE REACTIONS: Abdominal problems, headache, flatulence, flu, fever, nausea, malaise/fatigue.

PREGNANCY: Category B, not for use in nursing.

MECHANISM OF ACTION: Unknown, possibly diminishes inflammation by blocking cyclooxygenase and inhibiting prostaglandin production in the colon.

PHARMACOKINETICS: Absorption: Colon: Poor. Extent dependent on retention time. **Metabolism:** Acetylation, N-acetyl-5-ASA (Metabolite). **Elimination:** Urine, feces, $T_{1/2}$=0.5-1.5 hrs.

NURSING CONSIDERATIONS

Assessment: Assess for history of sulfasalazine intolerance, preexisting renal disease, and history of asthma or atopic allergies. Obtain baseline BUN, urinalysis, and creatinine.

Monitoring: Monitor BUN, urinalysis, and creatinine periodically. Signs/symptoms of acute intolerance syndrome (cramping, acute abdominal pain, bloody diarrhea), hypersensitivity or allergic reaction (rash, fever).

Patient Counseling: Best results achieved if bowel emptied immediately before. Seek medical attention if symptoms of acute intolerance syndrome (cramping, acute abdominal pain, bloody diarrhea), hypersensitivity or allergic reactions occur. If signs of rash or fever occur, d/c therapy.

Administration: Rectal. 1) Shake bottle well and remove sheath from tip. 2) Lie either on left side with left leg extended and right leg flexed or "knee-chest" position. 3) Gently insert lubricated tip into rectum, slightly toward navel;

grasp firmly, tilt so nozzle aimed at back and squeeze slowly to instill drug. 4) Remain in position for 30 min to allow distribution. Retain all night if possible. **Storage:** 20-25°C (68-77°F).

ROXANOL CII

morphine sulfate (Xanodyne)

Highly concentrated, check dose carefully.

OTHER BRAND NAMES: Roxanol-T (Xanodyne)

THERAPEUTIC CLASS: Opioid analgesic

INDICATIONS: Relief of severe acute and chronic pain.

DOSAGE: *Adults:* Usual: 10-30mg q4h. During first effective pain relief, dose should be maintained for at least 3 days before any dose reduction, if respiratory activity and other vital signs are adequate. Elderly/Very Ill/Respiratory Problems/Severe Renal and Hepatic Impairment: Lower doses may be required.

HOW SUPPLIED: Sol, Concentrate: 20mg/mL (Roxanol) [30mL, 120mL, 240mL], (Roxanol-T) [30mL, 120mL]

CONTRAINDICATIONS: Respiratory insufficiency or depression, severe CNS depression, attack of bronchial asthma, heart failure secondary to chronic lung disease, cardiac arrhythmias, increased intracranial or cerebrospinal pressure, head injuries, brain tumor, acute alcoholism, delirium tremens, convulsive disorders, after biliary tract surgery, suspected surgical abdomen, surgical anastomosis, concomitantly with MAOIs or within 14 days of such treatment.

WARNINGS/PRECAUTIONS: May cause tolerance, psychological, and physical dependence; withdrawal may occur on abrupt discontinuation. Caution with head injury, increased ICP, acute asthmatic attack, COPD, cor pulmonale, decreased respiratory reserve, pre-existing respiratory depression, hypoxia, hypercapnia, elderly, debilitated, severe hepatic/renal impairment, hypothyroidism, Addison's disease, prostatic hypertrophy, or urethral stricture. May cause orthostatic hypotension in ambulatory patients, severe hypotension with depleted blood volume. May obscure diagnosis/clinical course of acute abdominal conditions. May impair mental/physical abilities.

ADVERSE REACTIONS: Respiratory depression, lightheadedness, dizziness, sedation, NV, sweating, constipation.

INTERACTIONS: See Contraindications. Potentiated by alkalizing agents and antagonized by acidifying agents. Analgesic effect potentiated by chlorpromazine, methocarbamol. Enhanced depressant effects with other CNS depressants such as anesthetics, hypnotics, barbiturates, phenothiazines, chloral hydrate, glutethimide, sedatives, MAOIs (eg, procarbazine), antihistamines, β-blockers (eg, propranolol), alcohol, furazolidone, other narcotics, tranquilizers, and TCAs. May increase anticoagulant activity of coumarin and other anticoagulants.

PREGNANCY: Category C, caution in nursing.

MECHANISM OF ACTION: Opioid analgesic; acts as agonist interacting with stereospecific and saturable binding sites or receptors in the brain and other tissues. Major effects are on CNS and bowel.

PHARMACOKINETICS: Absorption: T_{max}=60 min. **Distribution:** Crosses placenta; found in breast milk.

NURSING CONSIDERATIONS

Assessment: Assess for respiratory depression, severe CNS depression, bronchial asthma attack, chronic obstructive pulmonary disease, heart failure secondary to chronic lung disease, cardiac arrhythmias, increased intracranial or CSF pressure, head injury, brain tumor, acute alcoholism, delirium tremens, convulsive disorder, recent biliary tract surgery, presence of surgical abdomen, surgical anastomosis, presence of debilitation (eg, elderly), hepatic/renal dysfunction, hypothyroidism, Addison's disease, prostatic hypertrophy

R

or urethral stricture, pregnancy/nursing status, and possible drug interactions (eg, MAO inhibitors).

Monitoring: Monitor for signs/symptoms of respiratory depression, hypotension, elevations in CSF pressure, tolerance, and dependence.

Patient Counseling: Instruct not to take medication if MAO inhibitors used within previous 14 days. Inform that drug may impair mental/physical abilities required to perform hazardous tasks (eg, operating machinery/driving). Advise to avoid alcohol and other CNS depressants while on medication. Counsel not to abruptly d/c medication. Instruct to contact physician if adverse events (eg, respiratory depression) develop.

Administration: Oral route. **Storage:** 25°C (77°F); excursions permitted to 15-30°C (59-86°F).

ROXICET CII

oxycodone HCl - acetaminophen (Roxane)

THERAPEUTIC CLASS: Opioid analgesic

INDICATIONS: Relief of moderate to moderately severe pain.

DOSAGE: *Adults:* Usual: 5mg-325mg (1 tab or 5mL sol) q6h prn. Titrate: May need to exceed usual dose based on individual response, pain severity, and tolerance.

HOW SUPPLIED: (Oxycodone-APAP) Sol: 5mg-325mg/5mL [5mL; 500mL]; Tab: 5mg-325mg

WARNINGS/PRECAUTIONS: May cause drug dependence and tolerance; potential for abuse. Risk of respiratory depression. Capacity to elevate CSF pressure may be exaggerated with head injury, other intracranial lesions, or a pre-existing increase in ICP. May obscure the diagnosis or clinical course with head injuries or with acute abdominal conditions. Caution with severe hepatic impairment, renal dysfunction, hypothyroidism, Addison's disease, prostatic hypertrophy, urethral stricture, the elderly or debilitated.

ADVERSE REACTIONS: Lightheadedness, dizziness, sedation, NV, euphoria, dysphoria, constipation, skin rash, pruritus.

INTERACTIONS: Additive CNS depression with narcotic analgesics, general anesthetics, phenothiazines, tranquilizers, sedatives-hypnotics, alcohol, and other CNS depressants; reduce dose of one or both agents.

PREGNANCY: Category C, caution in nursing.

MECHANISM OF ACTION: Oxycodone: Opioid analgesic; pure opioid agonist. Principle therapeutic effect is analgesia. Other effects include anxiolysis, euphoria, and feelings of relaxation. Effects mediated by CNS receptors (eg, μ and kappa) for endogenous opioid-like compounds (eg, endorphins, enkephalins). APAP: Nonopiate, nonsalicylate. Site and mechanism for analgesic effect not established. Antipyretic effect occurs through inhibition of endogenous pyrogen action on the hypothalmic heat-regulating centers.

PHARMACOKINETICS: Absorption: Oxycodone: Absolute bioavailability (87%). APAP: Rapid absorption. **Distribution:** Oxycodone: Plasma protein binding (45%); (IV) V_d=211.9 L; found in breast milk. APAP: Plasma protein binding (20-50%) (variable); found in most body fluids, breast milk. **Metabolism:** Oxycodone: N-dealkylation to norcodone (metabolite); CYP2D6 (O-emethylation) to oxymorphone (metabolite). APAP: Liver via CYP450 (conjugation), NAPQI (toxic metabolite). **Excretion:** Oxycodone: Urine (parent compound and metabolites); $T_{1/2}$=3.51 hrs. APAP: Urine (90-100%).

NURSING CONSIDERATIONS

Assessment: Assess for respiratory depression, acute or severe bronchial asthma or hypercarbia, paralytic ileus, chronic obstructive pulmonary disorder, presence of debilitation (eg, elderly), presence of head injury or other intracranial lesions, elevated intracranial pressure, circulatory shock, acute abdominal conditions, hepatic/renal dysfunction, hypothyroidism, Addison's disease, prostatic hypertrophy, urethral stricture, acute alcoholism, delirium

R

tremens, kyphoscoliosis with respiratory depression, myxedema, toxic psychosis, convulsive disorders, biliary tract disease, acute pancreatitis, pregnancy/nursing status, and possible drug interactions.

Monitoring: Monitor for signs/symptoms of respiratory depression, elevations of CSF pressure, hypotension, hepatotoxicity, convulsions, anaphylactic reactions, sphincter of Oddi spasms, tolerance, and physical dependence.

Patient Counseling: Instruct to keep out of reach of children. Counsel to dispose unused drug down toilet. Advise not to adjust dosing without consulting physician. Inform that drug may impair mental/physical abilities required to perform hazardous tasks (eg, operating machinery/driving). Counsel to avoid alcohol and other CNS depressants. If on medication for more than a few weeks, avoid abrubt withdrawal; taper dosing. Inform that medication has potential for abuse; protect from theft.

Administration: Oral route. **Storage:** Tablet: 20-25°C (68-77°F); Caplet: 15-30°C (59-86°F). Dispense in a tight, light-resistant container.

Roxicodone

CII

oxycodone HCl (Xanodyne)

THERAPEUTIC CLASS: Opioid analgesic

INDICATIONS: Relief of moderate to moderately severe pain.

DOSAGE: *Adults:* Initial: Opioid-Naive: 5mg to 15mg q4-6h prn. Titrate: Based on individual response. For chronic pain or severe chronic pain, use ATC dosing schedule at lowest effective dose.

HOW SUPPLIED: Sol: 5mg/5mL [5mL, 40^{s}; 500mL], (Intensol) 20mg/mL [30mL]; Tab: 5mg*, 15mg*, 30mg* *scored

CONTRAINDICATIONS: Significant respiratory depression (in unmonitored settings or the absence of resuscitative equipment), acute or severe bronchial asthma, hypercarbia, paralytic ileus.

WARNINGS/PRECAUTIONS: Potential for physical dependence. May markedly exaggerate respiratory depressant effects in head injuries and increased ICP. May mask symptoms of acute abdominal conditions. Caution with history of drug abuse, the elderly, debilitated, hypothyroidism, Addison's disease, BPH, urethral stricture, severe hepatic and renal impairment. May cause severe hypotension. May impair mental/physical abilities.

ADVERSE REACTIONS: Respiratory depression/arrest, circulatory depression, cardiac arrest, hypotension, shock, NV, constipation, headache, pruritus, insomnia, dizziness, asthenia, somnolence.

INTERACTIONS: Additive CNS depression with narcotic analgesics, phenothiazines, tranquilizers, sedative-hypnotics, alcohol, and other CNS depressants; reduce dose. Mixed agonist/antagonist analgesics may reduce analgesic effect and/or cause withdrawal. May enhance effect of neuromuscular blockers. Avoid within 14 days of MAOIs. Severe hypotension may occur with concurrent administration of phenothiazines or other agents which compromise vasomotor tone.

PREGNANCY: Category B, not for use in nursing.

MECHANISM OF ACTION: Opioid analgesic; pure opioid agonist whose principal therapeutic effect is analgesia. Precise mechanism of analgesic effect has not been established. Specific CNS opioid receptors for endogenous compounds with opioid-like activity are found in the brain and spinal cord and play a role in analgesic effects.

PHARMACOKINETICS: Absorption: Various doses led to altered parameters. **Distribution:** Plasma protein binding (45%), (IV): V_d=2.6L/kg; found in breast milk. **Metabolism:** Hepatic (extensively); noroxycodone (major metabolite); CYP2D6 to oxymorphone (metabolite) and glucuronides. **Elimination:** Urine (parent compound and metabolites); $T_{1/2}$=3.5-4 hrs.

NURSING CONSIDERATIONS

Assessment: Assess for respiratory depression, acute or severe bronchial asthma or hypercarbia, chronic obstructive pulmonary disease or cor pulmonale, paralytic ileus, circulatory shock, head injury or other intracranial lesions, presence of increased ICP, acute alcoholism, adrenocortical insufficiency (eg, Addison's disease), convulsive disorders, CNS depression or coma, delirium tremens, presence of debilitation, kyphoscoliosis associated with respiratory depression, myxedema or hypothyroidism, prostatic hypertrophy or urethral stricture, hepatic/renal impairment, toxic psychosis, presence of acute abdominal conditions, biliary tract disease, acute pancreatitis, pregnancy/nursing status, and possible drug interactions.

Monitoring: Monitor for signs/symptoms of respiratory depression, hypotension, elevations in CSF pressure, seizures, tolerance, physical dependence, and sphincter of Oddi spasms.

Patient Counseling: Instruct to report episodes of breakthrough pain and adverse events (eg, respiratory depression). Advise to avoid adjusting dose without consulting physician. Inform that drug may impair mental/physical abilities required to perform hazardous tasks (eg, operating machinery/driving). Instruct to avoid alcohol consumption and other CNS depressants. Advise drug has potential for abuse; protect from theft. Counsel that if on medication for more than a few weeks; taper dosing to avoid abrupt withdrawal.

Administration: Oral route. **Storage:** 25°C (77°F); excursions permitted to 15-30°C (59-86°F). Dispense in a tight, light-resistant container. Protect from moisture.

ROZEREM — RX

ramelteon (Takeda)

THERAPEUTIC CLASS: Melatonin receptor agonist

INDICATIONS: Treatment of insomnia characterized by difficulty with sleep onset.

DOSAGE: *Adults:* 8mg within 30 min of bedtime. Do not take with or after high-fat meal.

HOW SUPPLIED: Tab: 8mg

CONTRAINDICATIONS: Avoid with fluvoxamine.

WARNINGS/PRECAUTIONS: Severe anaphylactic and anaphylactoid reactions reported. Sleep disturbances may manifest as a physical and/or psychiatric disorder, symptomatic treatment of insomnia should be initiated after evaluation. Abnormal thinking, behavioral changes, hallucinations, complex behaviors (eg, sleep driving), worsening depression, suicidal ideation reported. D/C therapy if complex sleep behavior occurs. May impair physical/mental abilities. May affect reproductive hormones. Avoid with severe hepatic impairment, severe sleep apnea, and severe COPD. Caution in moderate hepatic impairment.

ADVERSE REACTIONS: Headache, somnolence, fatigue, dizziness, nausea, exacerbated insomnia, upper respiratory tract infection.

INTERACTIONS: See contraindications. Fluvoxamine increases AUC for ramelteon. Decreased efficacy with strong CYP inducers (eg, rifampin). Caution with less strong CYP1A2 inhibitors, strong CYP3A4 inhibitors (eg, ketoconazole), strong CYP2C9 inhibitors (eg, fluconazole). Additive effect with alcohol and CNS depressants.

PREGNANCY: Category C, caution in nursing.

MECHANISM OF ACTION: Melatonin receptor agonist; activity at receptors believed to contribute to sleep-promoting properties.

PHARMACOKINETICS: Absorption: Rapid; absolute bioavailabilty (1.8%); T_{max}=0.75 hr. **Distribution**: Plasma protein binding (82%); V_d=73.6 L(IV). **Metabolism**: Oxidation via CYP1A2 (major), CYP3A4 (minor). M-II (active metabolite). **Elimination**: Urine, feces (<0.1%); $T_{1/2}$=1-2.6 hrs, 2-5 hrs (M-II).

NURSING CONSIDERATIONS

Assessment: Assess for manifestations of physical or psychiatric disorders, hepatic/renal impairment, sleep apnea, COPD, depression, pregnancy/nursing status, and possible drug interactions.

Monitoring: Monitor for signs/symptoms of worsening of depression, suicidal ideations, exacerbations of insomnia, hypersensitivity reactions, emergence of cognitive behavioral abnormalities, and anaphylactic/anaphylactoid reactions.

Patient Counseling: Instruct to take just prior to bedtime on empty stomach. Caution against hazardous tasks (eg, operating machinery, driving). Seek medical attention if worsening of insomnia, symptoms of cognitive or behavioral abnormalities, hypersensitivity reactions, cessation of menses, galactorrhea, decreased libido, or infertility occur.

Administration: Oral route. **Storage**: 25°C (77°F); excursions permitted to 15-30°C (59-86°F). Protect from moisture and humidity.

RYTHMOL — RX

propafenone HCl (GlaxoSmithKline)

THERAPEUTIC CLASS: Class IC antiarrhythmic

INDICATIONS: To prolong the time to recurrence of paroxysmal atrial fibrillation/flutter (PAF) and paroxysmal supraventricular tachycardia (PSVT) associated with disabling symptoms in patients without structural heart disease. Treatment of life-threatening documented ventricular arrhythmias.

DOSAGE: *Adults:* Initial: 150mg q8h. Titrate: May increase at minimum 3-4 day intervals to 225mg q8h, then to 300mg q8h if needed. Max: 900mg/day. Elderly/Marked Myocardial Damage: Increase more gradually during initial phase. Hepatic Dysfunction: Reduce dose by 20-30%.

HOW SUPPLIED: Tab: 150mg*, 225mg*, 300mg* *scored

CONTRAINDICATIONS: Uncontrolled CHF, cardiogenic shock, bradycardia, marked hypotension, bronchospastic disorders, electrolyte imbalance, and sinoatrial, atrioventricular (AV) and intraventricular disorders of impulse generation and/or conduction (eg, sick sinus node syndrome, AV block) in the absence of an artificial pacemaker.

WARNINGS/PRECAUTIONS: Avoid with non-life-threatening ventricular arrhythmias, bronchospastic disorders. May cause new or worsened arrhythmias. Caution with hepatic or renal dysfunction. Slows AV conduction and causes 1st-degree AV block. D/C if CHF worsens. Agranulocytosis, myasthenia gravis exacerbation, positive ANA titers reported. May alter pacing and sensing thresholds of artificial pacemakers.

ADVERSE REACTIONS: Taste disturbances, nausea, vomiting, dizziness, constipation, headache, fatigue, blurred vision, blood dyscrasias.

INTERACTIONS: Inhibitors of CYP2D6 (eg, desipramine, paroxetine, ritonavir, sertraline), CYP1A2 (eg, amiodarone), CYP3A4 (eg, ketoconazole, ritonavir, saquinavir, erythromycin, grapefruit juice) may increase levels; monitor closely. May increase levels of drugs metabolized by CYP2D6 (eg, desipramine, imipramine, haloperidol, venlafaxine). May increase CNS side effects of lidocaine. May increase levels of digoxin, propranolol, warfarin; monitor closely. Cimetidine may increase plasma levels. Rifampin, orlistat may decrease plasma levels.

PREGNANCY: Category C, not for use in nursing.

MECHANISM OF ACTION: Class 1C antiarrhythmic drug with local anesthetic effects and direct stablizing action on myocardium. Reduces upstroke velocity (phase 0) of the monophasic action potential in Purkinje fibers, and to a lesser extent myocardial fibers, and reduces the fast inward current carried by Na ions. Reduces spontaneous automaticity and depresses triggered activity.

PHARMACOKINETICS: Absorption: Complete, absolute bioavailability (150mg) 3.4%, (300mg) 10.6%. T_{max}=3.5 hrs. **Metabolism:** Liver (rapid, extensive) via CYP3A4, 1A2 and 2D6. 5-hydroxypropafenone and N-depropylpropafenone (active metabolites). **Elimination:** $T_{1/2}$=2-10 hrs.

NURSING CONSIDERATIONS

Assessment: Assess for CHF, cardiogenic shock, sinoatrial, atrioventricular, intraventricular disorders of impulse generation and conduction (eg, sick sinus node syndrome, AV block), implanted functioning pacemaker, bradycardia, marked hypotension, bronchospastic disorders, manifest electrolyte imbalance, renal/hepatic dysfunction, pregnancy/nursing status, and possible drug interactions.

Monitoring: Monitor LFTs, renal functions, ANA, CBC, BP, ECG. Monitor signs/symptoms of neuromuscular dysfunction and exacerbation of myasthenia gravis, impaired spermatogenesis, convulsions, atrioventricular block and acute circulatory failure.

Patient Counseling: Inform about risks/benefits. Report any adverse reactions to physician.

Administration: Oral route. **Storage:** 25°C (77°F) excursions permitted to 15-30°C (59-86°F).

RYTHMOL SR — RX

propafenone HCl (GlaxoSmithKline)

THERAPEUTIC CLASS: Class IC antiarrhythmic

INDICATIONS: To prolong the time to recurrence of symptomatic atrial fibrillation in patients without structural heart disease.

DOSAGE: *Adults:* Initial: 225mg q12h. Titrate: May increase at minimum 5-day intervals to 325mg q12h, then to 425mg q12h if needed. Hepatic Impairment/QRS Widening/2nd- or 3rd-degree AV Block: Reduce dose.

HOW SUPPLIED: Cap, Extended-Release: 225mg, 325mg, 425mg

CONTRAINDICATIONS: CHF, cardiogenic shock, bradycardia, marked hypotension, bronchospastic disorders, electrolyte imbalance, and sinoatrial, atrioventricular (AV) and intraventricular disorders of impulse generation or conduction (eg, sick sinus node syndrome, AV block) unless paced.

WARNINGS/PRECAUTIONS: Avoid with non-life-threatening ventricular arrhythmias, bronchospastic disease, AV and intraventricular conduction defects unless paced. May cause new or worsened arrhythmias, provoke overt CHF. Caution with hepatic or renal dysfunction. 1st-degree AV block, agranulocytosis, myasthenia gravis exacerbation, positive ANA titers reported. May alter pacing and sensing thresholds of artificial pacemakers.

ADVERSE REACTIONS: Dizziness, chest pain, palpitations, taste disturbance, dyspnea, NV, constipation, anxiety, fatigue, upper respiratory tract infection, influenza, 1st-degree heart block.

INTERACTIONS: Avoid with drugs that prolong QT interval (eg, some phenothiazines, cisapride, bepridil, TCAs, oral macrolides, other antiarrhythmics), Class Ia and III antiarrhythmics (eg, quinidine, amiodarone). Inhibitors of CYP2D6 (eg, desipramine, paroxetine, ritonavir, sertraline), CYP1A2 (eg, amiodarone), CYP3A4 (eg, ketoconazole, ritonavir, saquinavir, erythromycin, grapefruit juice) may increase levels; monitor closely. May increase levels of drugs metabolized by CYP2D6 (eg, desipramine, imipramine, haloperidol, venlafaxine). May increase CNS side effects of lidocaine. May increase levels of digoxin, propranolol, warfarin; monitor closely. Cimetidine may increase plasma levels. Rifampin, orlistat may decrease plasma levels.

PREGNANCY: Category C, caution in nursing.

MECHANISM OF ACTION: Class 1C antiarrhythmic drug with local anesthetic effects and direct stabilizing action on myocardium. Reduces upstroke velocity (phase 0) of the monophasic action potential in Purkinje fiber, and to a lesser extent myocardial fibers, and reduces the fast inward current carried by Na ions. Reduces spontaneous automaticity and depresses triggered activity.

PHARMACOKINETICS: Absorption: T_{max}=3-8 hrs. **Distribution:** V_d=252L; plasma protein binding (≥95%). **Metabolism:** Rapid, extensive, via CYP2D6, 3A4 and 1A2 through hydroxylation. 5-hydroxypropafenone and

R

N-depropylpropafenone (active metabolites). **Elimination:** Urine (50% metabolites); $T_{1/2}$=2-10 hrs.

NURSING CONSIDERATIONS

Assessment: Assess for CHF, cardiogenic shock, sinoatrial, AV and intraventricular disorders of impulse generation or conduction (eg, sick sinus syndrome, AV block), implanted functioning pacemaker, bradycardia, marked hypotension, bronchospastic disorders, electrolyte imbalance, MI, supraventricular arrhythmias, renal/hepatic dysfunction, pregnancy/nursing status, and possible drug interactions. Perform ECG prior to and during therapy.

Monitoring: Monitor ECG changes, proarrhythmic effects (eg, ventricular fibrillation, ventricular tachycardia, asystole, Torsade de Pointes). Monitor for conduction disturbances, QRS interval prolongation, pacemaker threshold, signs of agranulocytosis (fever, chills, weakness, and neutropenia), signs of overdosage (eg, somnolence, hypotension and bradycardia), impaired spermatogenesis, and neuromuscular dysfunction (eg, exacerbation of myasthenia gravis). Monitor ANA, CBC, LFTs, urea, and creatinine.

Patient Counseling: Inform about risks/benefits; advise to report signs of infection or electrolyte imbalance. Notify if pregnant/nursing, hospitalized, or using new Rx/OTC medication or supplement.

Administration: Oral route. Dose should be titrated to individual's drug response and tolerance. Do not crush or further divide capsule contents.
Storage: 25°C (77°F); excursions permitted to 15-30°C (59-86°F).

RYZOLT — RX

tramadol HCl (Purdue Pharma)

THERAPEUTIC CLASS: Central acting analgesic

INDICATIONS: Management of moderate to moderately severe chronic pain.

DOSAGE: *Adults:* Individualize dose: Initial: 100mg/day. Titrate: 100mg every 2-3 days to achieve adequate pain control and tolerability. For patients requiring 300mg/day, titration should take at least 4 days. Usual: 200-300mg/day. Max: 300mg/day. Patients Currently on Tramodol IR Products: Calculate 24 hr IR dose and initiate on a total daily dose rounded down to next lowest 100mg increment. Max: 300mg/day. Elderly: Start at low end of dosing range. Swallow whole with liquid; do not split, chew, dissolve or crush.

HOW SUPPLIED: Tab, Extended-Release: 100mg, 200mg, 300mg

CONTRAINDICATIONS: Significant respiratory depression in unmonitored settings, acute or severe bronchial asthma, and hypercapnia.

R

WARNINGS/PRECAUTIONS: Seizures and anaphylactoid reactions reported. Avoid in suicidal or addiction-prone patients. May increase risk of serotonin syndrome (eg, mental changes, autonomic instability, neuromuscular aberrations, and GIT symptoms). Caution if at risk for respiratory depression, or with increased ICP or head trauma. May impair mental or physical abilities. Do not d/c abruptly; withdrawal symptoms may occur. May complicate acute abdominal conditions. Avoid in severe renal or hepatic impairment.

ADVERSE REACTIONS: Dizziness, N/V, constipation, headache, somnolence, pruritus, sweating, dry mouth, fatigue, anorexia, vertigo, insomnia, arthralgia, anxiety, hot flushes.

INTERACTIONS: CYP2D6 inhibitors (eg, quinidine, fluoxetine, paroxetine, amitriptyline) and CYP3A4 inhibitors (eg, ketoconazole, erythromycin) may reduce clearance of tramadol and increase risk for serious adverse events (eg, seizures, serotonin syndrome). Serotinergic drugs (eg, SSRIs, SNRIs, MAOIs, triptans, α2-adrenergic blockers, linzeolid, lithium, St. John's wort) may increase risk of seizures and/or serotonin syndrome; monitor closely, especially during treatment initiation and dose increases. Avoid with carbamazepine. Rare reports of digoxin toxicity and altered warfarin effects. Caution and reduce dose with CNS depressants (eg, alcohol, opioids, anesthetics, phenothiazines, tranquilizers, sedative hypnotics). Additive effects with alcohol and CNS depressants may occur.

PREGNANCY: Category C, safety in nursing not known.

MECHANISM OF ACTION: Centrally-acting synthetic opioid analgesic; MoA not fully understood. Shown to inhibit reuptake of norepinephrine and serotonin.

PHARMACOKINETICS: Absorption: Bioavailability (95%); T_{max}=4 hrs (drug), 5 hrs (M1 metabolite); C_{max}=345ng/mL (drug), 71ng/mL (M1 metabolite); AUC_{0-24}=5991ng•h/mL (drug), 1361ng•h/mL (M1 metabolite). **Distribution:** V_d=2.6L/kg (male), 2.9L/kg (female); plasma protein binding (20%). **Metabolism:** Liver (extensive); through N-and O-demethylation and glucuronidation or sulfation pathways via CYP3A4, 2D6. M1 (active metabolite). **Elimination:** Urine (30% unchanged), (60% as metabolite); $T_{1/2}$=6.3 hrs (drug), 7.4 hrs (M1).

NURSING CONSIDERATIONS

Assessment: Assess for significant respiratory depression, acute or severe bronchial asthma, hypercapnia, seizure risk, epilepsy, risk for respiratory depression, increased ICT, acute abdominal conditions, renal/hepatic impairment, pregnancy/nursing status, and possible drug interactions.

Monitoring: Monitor for anaphylactoid reactions (eg, pruritus, hives, bronchospasm, angioedema, toxic epidermal necrolysis, and Stevens-Johnson syndrome), respiratory/CNS, physical dependence/abuse, seizures, serotonin syndrome, withdrawal symptoms with abrupt d/c (eg, anxiety, sweating, insomnia, rigors, upper respiratory symptoms, diarrhea, piloerection, and, rarely, hallucinations).

Patient Counseling: Advise to use caution while performing hazardous tasks (eg, operating machinery, driving). Do not take with alcohol, tranquilizers, or hypnotics. Notify physician if pregnant/nursing or planning to become pregnant. Take as prescribed.

Administration: Oral route. **Storage:** Store at 25°C (77°F); excursions permitted between 15-30°C (59-86°F).

SAIZEN — RX

somatropin (EMD Serono)

THERAPEUTIC CLASS: Human growth hormone

INDICATIONS: Long-term treatment of children with growth failure due to inadequate secretion of endogenous growth hormone. For replacement of endogenous growth hormone in adults who have growth hormone deficiency either alone, or associated with multiple hormone deficiencies, as a result of pituitary disease, hypothalamic disease, surgery, radiation therapy or trauma; or in patients who were growth hormone deficient during childhood as a result of congenital, genetic, acquired or idiopathic causes.

DOSAGE: *Adults:* Initial: ≤0.005mg/kg/day SQ. Titrate: May increase after 4 weeks to ≤0.01mg/kg/day depending on patient tolerance. Without Consideration of Body Weight: Initial: 0.2mg/day (0.15-0.3mg/day) SQ. Titrate: May increase by increments of 0.1-0.2mg/day every 1-2 months. Consider dose reduction in elderly.

Pediatrics: Individualize dose. Usual: 0.06mg/kg IM/SQ 3x/week. If epiphyses are fused, d/c therapy.

HOW SUPPLIED: Inj: 4mg, 5mg, 8.8mg

CONTRAINDICATIONS: Acute critical illness due to complications following open heart or abdominal surgery, accidental trauma or acute respiratory failure. Active proliferative or severe non-proliferative diabetic retinopathy. Active malignancy, or evidence of progression or recurrence of intracranial tumor. Prader-Willi syndrome when severely obese or have severe respiratory impairment, and in pediatric patients with closed epiphyses. Avoid reconstitution with bacteriostatic water if sensitive to benzyl alcohol.

WARNINGS/PRECAUTIONS: Benzyl alcohol associated with toxicity in newborns; if sensitivity occurs, may reconstitute with SWFI. Insulin resistance reported; use caution with DM or family history of DM. Hypothyroidism may occur; bone maturation should be carefully followed. Increased incidence of slipped capital femoral epiphysis may develop with endocrine disorders; monitor for limping or hip/knee pain. Intracranial hypertension (IH) reported; d/c treatment if papilledema observed. Patients with Turner syndrome, chronic renal insufficiency or Prader-Willi syndrome may have increased risk for IH. If idiopathic IH confirmed, may restart therapy at lower dose after signs/symptoms resolve. Alternate injection sites to reduce development of tissue atrophy. Monitor for any malignant transformation of skin lesions.

ADVERSE REACTIONS: Arthralgia, headache, influenza-like symptoms, peripheral edema, back pain, myalgia, rhinitis, dizziness, upper respiratory tract infection, paresthesia, hypoesthesia, insomnia, nausea, generalized edema, depression.

INTERACTIONS: Diminished effects with concomitant glucocorticoid; adjust dose of accordingly. May alter clearance of CYP450 substrates (eg, corticosteroids, sex steroids, anticonvulsants, cyclosporine). May increase dose if taking oral estrogen replacement concomitantly. Adjust dose of insulin/oral antidiabetics when initiating therapy.

PREGNANCY: Category B, caution in nursing.

MECHANISM OF ACTION: Human growth hormone; stimulates skeletal growth, increases number and size of skeletal muscle cells, influences size and function of internal organs and increases red cell mass, stimulates protein synthesis, modulates carbohydrate metabolism, and mobilizes lipids.

PHARMACOKINETICS: Absorption: Absolute bioavailability (70-90%). **Distribution:** V_d=12.0L. **Metabolism:** Liver, kidneys. **Elimination:** $T_{1/2}$=1.75 hrs (SC), 3.4 hrs (IM), 0.6 hrs (IV).

NURSING CONSIDERATIONS

Assessment: Assess for history of scoliosis, DM or risk factors for it, closed epiphysis, diabetic retinopathy, active malignancy, critical illness, Prader-Willi syndrome (severely obese, respiratory impairment), hypothyroidism, and possible drug interactions. Perform baseline fundoscopic exam. (Prader-Willi) Evaluate for signs of upper airway obstruction and/or sleep apnea.

Monitoring: Monitor blood glucose, thyroid function tests, and perform fundoscopic exams periodically. Monitor for signs/symptoms of progression of scoliosis, malignant transformation of skin lesions, upper airway obstruction, sleep apnea or respiratory infections (Prader-Willi), progression or recurrence of tumors, intracranial HTN, tissue atrophy, slipped capital femoral epiphysis, and hypersensitivity reactions.

Patient Counseling: Instruct on proper handling and disposal. Seek medical attention if experience symptoms of airway obstruction, sleep apnea or respiratory infections (Prader-Willi), tissue atrophy (avoid by rotating injection site), intracranial HTN (papilledema, visual changes, headache, NV), hypersensitivity reactions, onset of limp or complaints of hip/knee pain.

Administration: IM/SQ routes. **Storage:** 15-30°C (59-86°F). After reconstitution: 2-8°C (36-46°F); stable for 14 days. Cartridge reconstituted: 2-8°C (36-46°F); stable for 21 days.

SANCTURA XR — RX

trospium chloride (Espirit/Indevus)

OTHER BRAND NAMES: Sanctura (Espirit/Indevus)

THERAPEUTIC CLASS: Muscarinic antagonist

INDICATIONS: Treatment of overactive bladder with symptoms of urge urinary incontinence, urgency, and urinary frequency.

DOSAGE: *Adults:* (Tab) 20mg bid. (Cap, Extended-Release) 60mg qd in am. Take at least 1 hour before meals or on empty stomach. (Tab) CrCl <30mL/min: 20mg qhs. Elderly ≥75 yrs: May titrate to 20mg qd based upon tolerability.

HOW SUPPLIED: Cap, Extended-Release: 60mg; Tab: 20mg

CONTRAINDICATIONS: Active or risk of urinary retention, gastric retention, uncontrolled narrow-angle glaucoma.

WARNINGS/PRECAUTIONS: (Tab, Cap) Caution with significant bladder outflow obstruction, GI obstructive disorders, ulcerative colitis, intestinal atony, myasthenia gravis, moderate or severe hepatic dysfunction. Reduce dose with severe renal insufficiency. Consider risks vs benefits with controlled narrow-angle glaucoma. (Cap) Not recommended for use with severe renal impairment (CrCl <30mL/min). Consumption of alcohol within 2 hrs is not recommended.

ADVERSE REACTIONS: Dry mouth, constipation, headache, rash.

INTERACTIONS: Increased adverse effects with other anticholinergics. May alter GI absorption of other drugs due to GI motility effects. Monitor closely with other drugs eliminated by active renal tubular secretion (eg, procainamide, pancuronium, morphine, vancomycin, metformin, tenofovir).

PREGNANCY: Category C, caution in nursing.

MECHANISM OF ACTION: Antispasmodic, antimuscarinic agent; reduces tonus of smooth muscle in bladder by antagonizing effect of acetylcholine on muscarinic receptors.

PHARMACOKINETICS: Absorption: (Tab) Absolute bioavailability (9.6%), C_{max}=3.5ng/mL, T_{max}=5.3 hrs, AUC=36.4ng•hr/mL. (Cap, Extended-Release) C_{max}=2ng/mL, T_{max}=5 hrs, AUC=18ng•hr/mL. **Distribution:** V_d ≥600L; plasma protein binding (50-85%). **Metabolism:** Ester hydrolysis. **Elimination:** Feces (major), urine. (Tab) $T_{1/2}$=18.3 hrs; (Cap, Extended-Release) $T_{1/2}$=36 hrs.

NURSING CONSIDERATIONS

Assessment: Assess for bladder outflow obstruction (urinary retention), GI obstructive disorders (gastric retention), narrow-angle glaucoma, possible drug interactions, ulcerative colitis, intestinal atony, myasthenia gravis, hepatic/renal impairment.

Monitoring: Monitor for signs/symptoms of gastric retention, urinary retention, decreased gastric motility, hypersensitivity reactions, hepatic/renal dysfunction.

Patient Counseling: Inform that heat prostration may occur in hot environment and that dizziness or blurred vision may occur. Advise alcohol may enhance drowsiness effect. Instruct to take tab 1 hr prior to meals or on empty stomach. Inform that if skip dose, take next dose 1 hr prior to next meal. Instruct to take cap in AM with water on empty stomach or 1 hr prior to meal. Counsel to avoid alcohol within 2 hrs of dosing of cap.

Administration: Oral route. **Storage:** 20-25°C (68-77°F).

SANDIMMUNE — RX

cyclosporine (Novartis)

S

Give with adrenal corticosteroids but not with other immunosuppressives. Increased susceptibility to infection and development of lymphoma. Sandimmune and Neoral are not bioequivalent. Monitor blood levels to avoid toxicity.

THERAPEUTIC CLASS: Cyclic polypeptide immunosuppressant

INDICATIONS: Prophylaxis of organ rejection in kidney, liver, and heart allogeneic transplants with concomitant adrenal corticosteroids. Treatment of chronic rejection in patients previously treated with other immunosuppressives.

DOSAGE: *Adults:* Initial: PO: 15mg/kg single dose 4-12 hrs before transplant; continue same dose qd for 1-2 weeks. Usual: Taper by 5% per week until 5-10mg/kg/day. May mix oral solution with milk, chocolate milk, or orange juice. IV: 1/3 PO dose. Initial: 5-6mg/kg/day single dose; begin 4 to 12 hrs prior to transplantation. Maint: Continue single daily dose until PO forms are tolerated. Due to risk of anaphylaxis, only use injection if unable to take oral agents.

Pediatrics: Initial: PO: 15mg/kg single dose 4-12 hrs before transplant;

continue same dose qd for 1-2 weeks. Usual: Taper by 5% per week until 5-10mg/kg/day. May mix oral solution with milk, chocolate milk, or orange juice. IV: 1/3 PO dose. Initial: 5-6mg/kg/day single dose; begin 4 to 12 hrs prior to transplantation. Maint: Continue single daily dose until PO forms are tolerated. Due to risk of anaphylaxis, only use injection if unable to take oral agents.

HOW SUPPLIED: Cap: 25mg, 100mg; Inj: 50mg/mL; Sol: 100mg/mL [50mL]

CONTRAINDICATIONS: Hypersensitivity to Cremophor EL (polyoxyethylated castor oil).

WARNINGS/PRECAUTIONS: May cause hepatotoxicity and nephrotoxicity. Convulsions, elevated SrCr, and BUN levels reported. Thrombocytopenia and microangiopathic hemolytic anemia may develop. Monitor for hyperkalemia. Increases risk for development of lymphomas and other malignancies. Observe for 30 min after start of infusion and frequently thereafter. Caution with malabsorption.

ADVERSE REACTIONS: Renal dysfunction, tremor, hirsutism, HTN, gum hyperplasia, glomerular capillary thrombosis, cramps, acne, convulsions, headache, diarrhea, hepatotoxity, abdominal discomfort, paresthesia, flushing.

INTERACTIONS: Ciprofloxacin, gentamicin, tobramycin, vancomycin, SMZ/TMP, amphotericin B, ketoconazole, melphalan, diclofenac, azapropazon, sulindac, naproxen, colchicine, cimetidine, ranitidine, tacrolimus, bezafirate, fenofibrate may potentiate renal dysfunction. Diltiazem, nicardipine, colchicine, fluconazole, itraconazole, ketoconazole, verapamil, azithromycin, clarithromycin, erythromycin, quinupristin/dalfopristin, allopurinol, amiodarone, bromocriptine, danazol, imatinib, metoclopramide, oral contraceptives, HIV protease inhibitors may increase levels. St. John's wort, grapefruit juice, carbamazepine, phenobarbital, phenytoin, rifampin, sulfinpyrazone, octreotide, orlistat, terbinafine, ticlopidine, and naficillin may decrease levels. Avoid with potassium-sparing diuretics. Caution with ACEIs, angiotensin II blockers, NSAIDs. Digitalis toxicity reported. Myotoxicity with statins, frequent gingival hyperplasia with nifedipine, and convulsions with high dose methylprednisolone reported. Increased levels of sirolimus; give 4 hrs after cyclosporine. Avoid live vaccines during therapy.

PREGNANCY: Category C, not for use in nursing.

MECHANISM OF ACTION: Cyclic polypeptide immunosuppressant; not fully established. May cause specific and reversible inhibition of immunocompetent lymphocytes in the G_0- or G_1-phase of the cell cycle. T lymphocytes are preferentially inhibited with T-helper cell as main target while also possibly suppressing T-suppressor cells. Also inhibits lymphokine production and release (eg, interleukin-2, T-cell growth factor).

PHARMACOKINETICS: Absorption: Incomplete and variable. Absolute bioavailability (30%)(PO); C_{max}=1ng/mL/mg; T_{max}=3.5 hrs. **Distribution:** Plasma protein binding (90%). **Metabolism:** Extensively metabolized via hydroxylation, cyclic ether formation, and *N*-demethylation. **Elimination:** Urine (6%); $T_{1/2}$=19 hrs.

S

NURSING CONSIDERATIONS

Assessment: Prior to injection, assess that patient cannot take oral formulations and is on concomitant therapy with adrenal corticosteroids. Assess for hypersensitivity to Cremophor EL (polyoxyethylated castor oil), pregnancy/nursing status, possible drug interactions. Assess use of oral formulations in patients with malabsorption problems.

Monitoring: Monitor for signs/symptoms of hepatotoxicity, nephrotoxicity, thrombocytopenia, microangiopathic hemolytic anemia, HTN, hyperkalemia, glomerular capillary thrombosis, lymphomas and other malignancies, convulsions, encephalopathy, and development of anaphylactic reactions (eg, facial flushing, non-cardiogenic pulmonary edema with acute respiratory distress, dyspnea, changes in blood pressure, and tachycardia). Frequently monitor cyclosporine blood levels, especially when converting from Neoral to Sandimmune, renal/hepatic function (eg, BUN, SrCr, serum bilirubin, liver enzymes), and drug blood levels.

Patient Counseling: Instruct to contact physician before changing formulations of cyclosporine, which may require dose change. Inform patient will require repeated tests while on medication. Inform drug may cause increased risk of neoplasias. Advise females about risks of use during pregnancy. Instruct patients using cyclosporine oral solution with its accompanying syringe, that syringe should not be washed before or after use; will cause variation in dosage.

Administration: Oral/IV routes. Patients receiving IV formulation should be under continuous observation for anaphylactic reactions for at least first 30 min following start of infusion and at frequent intervals thereafter. IV concentrate (1mL of Sandimmune inj) should be diluted in 20-100mL of NS or D5W and administered by slow IV infusion over 2-6 hrs. **Storage:** Cap: 25°C (77°F); excursions permitted to 15-30°C (59-86°F). Oral Sol: Store in original container, below 30°C (86°F). Do not refrigerate. Protect from freezing. Once opened, use contents within 2 months. Injection: Below 30°C (86°F), protected from light. Discard diluted infusion after 24 hrs.

SANDOSTATIN — RX

octreotide acetate (Novartis)

THERAPEUTIC CLASS: Somatostatin analog

INDICATIONS: To reduce blood levels of growth hormone and IGF-I in acromegaly inadequately responding to or cannot be treated with surgical resection, pituitary irradiation, and maximum dose bromocriptine mesylate. Symptomatic treatment of metastatic carcinoid tumors, where it suppresses or inhibits severe diarrhea and flushing episodes. Treatment of profuse watery diarrhea associated with VIP (Vasoactive Intestinal Peptide)-secreting tumors.

DOSAGE: *Adults:* Give SQ/IV. Acromegaly: Initial: 50mcg tid. Titrate: Adjust dose based on IGF-I levels every 2 weeks. Usual: 100mcg tid. Max: 500mcg tid. Reduce dose if no additional benefit with dose increase. Re-evaluate IGF-I or growth hormone levels every 6 months. Withdraw yearly for 4 weeks to assess disease activity after irradiation. Carcinoid Tumors: Initial: 100-600mcg/day given bid-qid (mean dose 300mcg/day) for 2 weeks. Max: 750mcg/day. VIPomas: Initial: 200-300mcg/day (range 150-750mcg) given bid-qid for 2 weeks. Max: 450mcg/day.

HOW SUPPLIED: Inj: 50mcg/mL, 100mcg/mL, 200mcg/mL, 500mcg/mL, 1000mcg/mL

WARNINGS/PRECAUTIONS: May inhibit gallbladder contractility and decrease bile secretions; increased risk of gallstones. May alter balance between insulin, glucagon, and growth hormone and lead to hypoglycemia or hyperglycemia. Hypothyroidism may result due to TSH suppression; monitor thyroid function at baseline and periodically. Cardiac conduction and other cardiovascular abnormalities may occur. Pancreatitis reported. Depressed vitamin B_{12} levels and abnormal Schilling's test reported. May need dose adjustment in renal failure.

ADVERSE REACTIONS: Gallbladder and cardiac abnormalities, diarrhea, nausea, vomiting, abdominal distention, flatulence, constipation, headache, dizziness, hypo- and hyperglycemia, hyperthyroidism.

INTERACTIONS: May decrease cyclosporine effects. May need dose adjustments of insulin, oral hypoglycemics, β-blockers, CCBs, or agents that control fluid and electrolyte balance. Not compatible in TPN solutions. Increased availability of bromocriptine.

PREGNANCY: Category B, caution in nursing.

MECHANISM OF ACTION: Somatostatin analog; exerts similiar actions to natural hormone somatostatin, but is more potent in inhibiting growth hormone, glucagon and insulin. Like somatostatin, it also suppresses LH response to GnRH, decreases splanchnic blood flow, and inhibits release of serotonin, gastrin, vasoactive intestinal peptide, secretin, motilin and pancreatic polypeptide.

PHARMACOKINETICS: Absorption: C_{max}=5.2ng/mL; T_{max}=0.4 hrs; Acromegaly: C_{max}=2.8ng/mL, T_{max}=0.7 hr. **Distribution:** V_d=13.6L; plasma protein binding (65%); Acromegaly: V_d=21.6±8.5L, plasma protein binding (41.2%). **Elimination:** Urine (32%, unchanged); $T_{1/2}$=1.7-1.9 hrs.

NURSING CONSIDERATIONS

Assessment: Assess baseline renal function. Obtain baseline thyroid function tests (TSH, total and/or free T_4). Assess use with cardiac dysfunction, for glycemic control with DM, and for possible drug interactions.

Monitoring: Monitor for signs/symptoms of biliary tract abnormalities (eg, gallstones, biliary duct dilitation), hypo/hyperglycemia, hypothyroidism, cardiac conduction abnormalities, and pancreatitis. With acromegaly: Monitor growth hormone levels at 1-4 hr intervals for 8-12 hrs post dose. With carcinoids: Monitor 5-HIAA (urinary 5-hydroxyindole acetic acid), plasma serotonin, and plasma substance P levels. With VIPoma: Monitor VIP (plasma vasoactive intestinal peptide). Monitor total and/or free T_4 levels and vitamin B_{12} levels with chronic therapy.

Patient Counseling: Provide careful instructions about proper sterile technique and administration of injection.

Administration: IV/SQ routes. Inspect visually for particulate matter and discoloration prior to administration. **Storage:** Refrigerate; 2-8°C (36-46°F) and protect from light. At room temperature, 20-30°C (70-86°F), stable for 14 days if protected from light. Allow solution to come to room temperature prior to administration. Do not warm artificially. After initial use, multi-dose vials should be discarded within 14 days. Open amps just prior to administration and discard unused portion.

SANDOSTATIN LAR — RX

octreotide acetate (Novartis)

THERAPEUTIC CLASS: Somatostatin analog

INDICATIONS: Maintenance therapy of acromegaly. Long-term treatment of severe diarrhea and flushing associated with metastatic carcinoid tumors. Long-term treatment of profuse watery diarrhea associated with VIP (Vasoactive Intestinal Peptide)-secreting tumors. Use in patients who have responded to and tolerated Sandostatin Injection. In patients with carcinoid treatment and VIPomas, the effect of Sandostatin Injection and Sandostatin LAR Depot on tumor size, rate of growth, and development of metastases has not been determined.

DOSAGE: *Adults:* Administer intragluteally. Acromegaly: Initial: 20mg IM every 4 weeks for 3 months. Titrate: If GH ≤2.5ng/mL, IGF-1 normal, and clinical symptoms controlled then maintain dose. If GH >2.5, IGF-1 elevated, and/or clinical symptoms uncontrolled then increase to 30mg every 4 weeks. If GH ≤1, IGF-1 normal, and clinical symptoms controlled then reduce to 10mg every 4 weeks. Max: 40mg every 4 weeks. Withdraw yearly for 8 weeks to assess disease activity after pituitary irradiation. Carcinoid Tumors/VIPomas: Initial: 20mg IM every 4 weeks for 2 months. Continue with Sandostatin® injection SQ for at least 2 weeks. Titrate: If symptoms not controlled, increase to 30mg every 4 weeks. If symptoms controlled at 20mg, reduce to 10mg. Max: 30mg every 4 weeks. For exacerbation of symptoms, give Sandostatin Injection SQ for at least 2 weeks. Patients must be considered responders and tolerate the injection before switching to the depot. Renal Failure Requiring Dialysis: Reduce dose.

HOW SUPPLIED: Inj, Depot: 10mg, 20mg, 30mg

WARNINGS/PRECAUTIONS: May inhibit gallbladder contractility and decrease bile secretions; increased risk of gallstones. May alter balance between insulin, glucagon and growth hormone and lead to hypoglycemia or hyperglycemia. Hypothyroidism may result due to TSH suppression; monitor thyroid function at baseline and periodically. Cardiac conduction and other cardiovascular abnormalities may occur. Monitor zinc levels periodically with TPNs.

Pancreatitis reported. Depressed vitamin B_{12} levels and abnormal Schilling's test reported. May need dose adjustment in renal failure.

ADVERSE REACTIONS: Diarrhea, NV, abdominal discomfort, flatulence, constipation, hyperglycemia, injection site pain, upper respiratory infection, flu-like symptoms, fatigue, dizziness, headache, malaise, fever.

INTERACTIONS: May decrease cyclosporine levels. May need dose adjustments of insulin, oral hypoglycemics, β-blockers, CCBs, or agents that control fluid and electrolyte balance. May increase availability of bromocriptine. Caution with drugs that have a low therapeutic index and metabolized by CYP3A4 (eg, quinidine, terfenadine).

PREGNANCY: Category B, caution in nursing.

MECHANISM OF ACTION: Somatostatin analog; long acting. Exerts similiar actions to natural hormone somatostatin, but is more potent in inhibiting growth hormone, glucagon, and insulin. Like somatostatin, it also suppresses LH response to GnHR, decreases splanchnic blood flow and inhibits release of serotonin, gastrin, vasoactive intestinal peptide, secretin, motilin and pancreatic polypeptide.

PHARMACOKINETICS: Absorption: Rapidly and completely absorbed; C_{max}=5.2ng/mL, 2.8ng/mL (acromegaly); T_{max}=1 hrs (acromegaly). **Distribution:** V_d=13.6L, 21.6L (acromegaly); plasma protein binding (65%), (acromegaly) (41.2%). **Elimination:** Urine (32% unchanged); $T_{1/2}$=1.7 hrs.

NURSING CONSIDERATIONS

Assessment: Assess glycemic control with DM, cardiac dysfunction, baseline thyroid function (TSH, total and/or free T_4), renal function, and for possible drug interactions.

Monitoring: Monitor for signs/symptoms of hypo/hyperglycemia, hypothyroidism, cardiac conduction abnormalities, depressed vitamin B_{12}, expansion of growth hormone secreting tumors, gallbladder abnormalities (gallstones, biliary sludge). With acromegaly: Monitor growth hormone and IGF-1 levels. With carcinoids: Monitor 5-HIAA (urinary 5-hydroxyindoleacetic acid), plasma serotonin levels, and plasma Substance P levels. With VIPoma: Monitor VIP (plasma vasoactive intestinal peptide) levels. Monitor thyroid function with chronic therapy. Monitor zinc levels if receiving TPN.

Patient Counseling: Advise patients with carcinoid tumors and VIPomas to adhere closely to scheduled return visits for reinjection to minimize exacerbation of symptoms. Advise patients with acromegaly to adhere to return visit schedule to help ensure steady control of GH and IGF-1 levels.

Administration: IM route. Do not directly inject diluent without preparing sus. Never administer via IV/SQ routes. Sandostatin LAR depot drug product kit should remain at room temperature for 30-60 min prior to preparation of drug sus. Administer sus immediately after preparation. **Storage:** Refrigerate between 2-8°C (36-46°F) and protect from light until time of use.

S

SARAFEM

RX

fluoxetine HCl (Warner Chilcott/Lilly)

Antidepressants increased the risk of suicidal thinking and behavior (suicidality) in short-term studies in children and adolescents with major depressive disorder (MDD) and other psychiatric disorders. Sarafem is not approved for use in pediatric patients.

THERAPEUTIC CLASS: Selective serotonin reuptake inhibitor

INDICATIONS: Treatment of premenstrual dysphoric disorder.

DOSAGE: *Adults:* Continuous: Initial: 20mg qd. Maint: 20mg/day up to 6 months. Max: 60mg/day. Intermittent: Initial: 20mg qd; start 14 days before menses onset through 1st full day of menses. Maint: 20mg/day up to 3 months. Max: 60mg/day. Hepatic Impairment/Concurrent Disease/Concomitant Medications: Lower dose or less frequent dosing.

HOW SUPPLIED: Cap: 10mg, 20mg

CONTRAINDICATIONS: During or within 14 days of MAOI therapy. During or within 5 weeks of thioridazine use. Concurrent use with pimozide.

WARNINGS/PRECAUTIONS: Monitor for clinical worsening and/or suicidality. Vasculitis reported. D/C if rash or allergic reaction develops. May increase risk of bleeding events with concomitant use of aspirin, NSAIDs, warfarin, etc. Hyponatremia reported. Caution in patients with history of seizures. May impair thinking, judgment, or motor skills. May alter glycemic control. Changes in weight and appetite reported. Caution with cirrhosis. Serotonin syndrome may occur; caution with concomitant use of serotonergic drugs. Rash/urticaria, pulmonary and anaphylactoid events reported.

ADVERSE REACTIONS: Headache, asthenia, pain, flu syndrome, insomnia, dizziness, nervousness, rhinitis, pharyngitis, anorexia, dry mouth, diarrhea, tremor, anxiety.

INTERACTIONS: See Contraindications. May increase benzodiazepine, thioridazine, TCAs, haloperidol, clozapine, phenytoin, and carbamazepine levels. Lithium levels may increase/decrease. Do not use with or within 14 days of MAOIs. May shift concentrations with plasma-bound drugs (eg, coumadin, digitoxin). Caution with concomitant use with other SSRIs, SNRIs, triptans, or tryptophan.

PREGNANCY: Category C, not for use in nursing.

MECHANISM OF ACTION: SSRI; not established, presumed to be linked to inhibition of CNS neuronal uptake of serotonin.

PHARMACOKINETICS: Absorption: C_{max}=15-55ng/mL; T_{max}=6-8 hrs. **Distribution:** Plasma protein binding (94.5%). **Metabolism:** CYP2D6 (demethylation); norfluoxetine (active metabolite). **Elimination:** $T_{1/2}$=1-3 days (acute), 4-6 days (chronic); 4-16 days (norfluoxetine).

NURSING CONSIDERATIONS

Assessment: Assess for possible drug interactions, DM, bipolar disorder, history of seizures, hepatic impairment, and diseases or conditions that affect metabolism or hemodynamic responses.

Monitoring: Monitor for signs/symptoms of clinical worsening, suicidality and unusual changes in behavior (especially during initial few months, and dosage changes), hypersensitivity reactions, serotonin syndrome, abnormal bleeding, altered appetite and weight, hyponatremia, seizures, hypo/hyperglycemia, and abrupt withdrawal symptoms.

Patient Counseling: Caution may impair physical/mental abilities. Seek medical attention if symptoms of agitation, irritability, unusual changes in behavior, serotonin syndrome (mental status changes, autonomic instability, neuromuscular aberrations, GI symptoms), abnormal bleeding, seizures, abrupt withdrawal symptoms (dysphoric mood, irritability, agitation), hyponatremia (headache, difficulty concentrating, confusion), and hypersensitivity reactions (rash) occur.

Administration: Oral route. **Storage:** 15-30°C (59-86°F). Protect from light.

SAVELLA — RX

milnacipran HCl (Forest)

Increased risk of suicidal ideation, thinking and behavior in children, adolescents, and young adults taking antidepressants for major depressive disorder (MDD) and other psychiatric disorders. It is not approved for use in pediatric patients.

THERAPEUTIC CLASS: Serotonin and norepinephrine reuptake inhibitor

INDICATIONS: Management of fibromyalgia.

DOSAGE: *Adults:* 100mg qd (50mg bid). Titrate: Day 1: 12.5mg qd. Days 2-3: 25mg qd (12.5mg bid). Days 4-7: 50mg qd (25mg bid). After Day 7: 100mg qd (50mg bid). May increase dose to 200mg qd (100mg bid) based on individual patient's response. Max: 200mg/day. Severe Renal Impairment (CrCl = 5-29mL/min): Reduce maintenance dose to 50mg qd (25mg bid). Titrate: May increase dose up to 100mg qd (50mg bid) based on response.

HOW SUPPLIED: Tab: 12.5mg, 25mg, 50mg, 100mg

CONTRAINDICATIONS: Uncontrolled narrow-angle glaucoma and concomitant use with monoamine oxidase inhibitors (MAOIs).

WARNINGS/PRECAUTIONS: Serotonin syndrome symptoms, increased BP, HR, liver enzymes, and severe liver injury reported. Caution with HTN or cardiac disease. BP should be measured prior to therapy and periodically. If sustained increase in BP occurs; reduce dose or d/c therapy. Caution with history of seizure disorder. D/C if jaundice or liver dysfunction occurs. Avoid with substantial alcohol use or chronic liver disease. Withdrawal and physical dependence reported; avoid abrupt discontinuation. Taper after long-term use. Hyponatremia may occur. Increased risk of bleeding events. Caution with history of mania. Caution with history of dysuria, prostatic hypertrophy, prostatitis, and other lower urinary tract obstructive disorders. Mydriasis reported; caution with controlled narrow-angle glaucoma. Caution with moderate renal and severe hepatic impairment.

ADVERSE REACTIONS: NV, headache, constipation, dizziness, insomnia, hot flush, hyperhidrosis, palpitations, tachycardia, dry mouth, and HTN.

INTERACTIONS: See contraindications. Risk of Serotonin syndrome with lithium, serotonergic drugs (eg, triptans and tramadol), and MAOIs. Concurrent use with epinephrine and norepinephrine may increase risks of paroxysmal HTN and arrhythmia. Concomitant use with other serotonin reuptake inhibitors may result in HTN and coronary artery vasoconstriction. Digoxin may potentiate adverse hemodynamic effects. Risks of postural hypotension and tachycardia with IV digoxin. May inhibit clonidine effect. Switch from clomipramine may increase risk of euphoria and postural hypotension. Caution with other centrally acting drugs. Avoid with serotonin precursors (eg, tryptophan). Concurrent use of aspirin, nonsteroidal anti-inflammatory drugs, warfarin, and other anti-coagulants may increase risk of bleeding events (eg, ecchymoses, hematomas, epistaxis, petechiae or life-threatening hemorrhages).

PREGNANCY: Category C, not for use in nursing.

MECHANISM OF ACTION: Serotonin and norepinephrine reuptake inhibition; exact mechanism of central pain inhibitory action and its ability to improve symptoms of fibromyalgia in humans are not established.

PHARMACOKINETICS: Absorption: Complete; absolute bioavailability (85%-90%); T_{max}=2-4 hrs. **Distribution:** V_d=400L; plasma protein binding (13%). **Metabolism:** Via liver; *l*-milnacipran carbamoyl-O-glucuronide (major metabolite). **Elimination:** Urine (unchanged, 55%), $T_{1/2}$=6-8 hrs (milnacipran); 8-10 hrs (*d*-milnacipran); 4-6 hrs (*l*-milnacipran).

NURSING CONSIDERATIONS

Assessment: Assess for suicidality, worsening of depression, uncontrolled narrow-angle glaucoma, taking MAOIs, pre-existing tachyarrhythmias, other cardiac diseases, history of seizure disorder, pre-existing liver disease, pregnancy/nursing status, and possible drug interactions. Assess BP, HR, and LFTs (eg, AST, ALT).

Monitoring: Monitor BP, HR, LFTs, sodium levels. Monitor for emergence of agitation, irritability, unusual changes in behavior, serotonin syndrome (eg, mental status changes, autonomic instability, neuromuscular aberrations, GIT symptoms), withdrawal symptoms, physical dependence, hyponatremia, and abnormal bleeding.

Patient Counseling: Counsel patients, families, and caregivers about the risks and benefits of therapy. Instruct families and caregivers of patients to notify a healthcare provider if emergence of agitation, irritability, suicidality or unusual changes in behavior occur. Inform patients about the risk of serotonin syndrome with concomitant use of triptans, tramadol, or other serotonergic agents. Advise to monitor BP and PR periodically. Caution about the increased risk of abnormal bleeding with concomitant use of NSAIDs, aspirin, and other anticoagulation drugs. Caution against operating machinery or driving motor vehicles until effects of drug known. Avoid consumption of alcohol. Advise that withdrawal symptoms may occur with abrupt discontinuation. Notify physician if pregnant or intend to become pregnant, or if breastfeeding.

Administration: Oral route. **Storage:** Store at 25°C (77°F); excursions permitted to 15-30°C (59-86°F).

SEASONALE RX

ethinyl estradiol - levonorgestrel (Duramed)

THERAPEUTIC CLASS: Estrogen/progestogen combination

INDICATIONS: Prevention of pregnancy.

DOSAGE: *Adults:* Sunday start regimen. 1 tablet qd for 91 days, then repeat.

HOW SUPPLIED: Tab: (Ethinyl Estradiol-Levonorgestrel) 0.03mg/0.15mg

CONTRAINDICATIONS: Thrombophlebitis, DVT or thromboembolic disorders, pregnancy, cerebrovascular or CAD, valvular heart disease with complications, uncontrolled HTN, DM with vascular involvement, headaches with focal neurological symptoms, major surgery with prolonged immobilization, undiagnosed abnormal genital bleeding, cholestatic jaundice of pregnancy or jaundice with prior pill use, hepatic adenomas or carcinomas, active liver disease, breast cancer, endometrial carcinoma, or other estrogen-dependent neoplasia.

WARNINGS/PRECAUTIONS: Cigarette smoking increases risk of serious CV side effects. This risk increases with age (especially >35 yrs) and heavy smoking. Increased risk of MI, vascular disease, thromboembolism, stroke, HTN, and gallbladder disease. Retinal thrombosis, hepatic neoplasia, carcinoma of breast and reproductive organs reported. May cause glucose intolerance, fluid retention, breakthrough bleeding, and spotting. May increase BP, elevate LDL levels or cause other lipid changes. May cause or exacerbate migraine. May develop visual changes with contact lens. Increased risk of morbidity and mortality with certain inherited thrombophilias, HTN, hyperlipidemia, obesity, and diabetes. D/C if jaundice, significant depression, recurrent/persistent new headache patterns, or ophthalmic irregularities develop. Perform annual physical exam. Not for use before menarche or with uncontrolled HTN. May affect certain endocrine, LFTs, and blood components. Weigh benefit of fewer planned menses against inconvenience of increased intermenstrual bleeding or spotting.

ADVERSE REACTIONS: NV, breakthrough bleeding, spotting, amenorrhea, migraine, depression, vaginal candidiasis, edema, weight changes.

INTERACTIONS: Reduced effects, increased breakthrough bleeding with rifampin, barbiturates, phenylbutazone, phenytoin, carbamazepine, felbamate, oxcarbazepine, griseofulvin, topiramate, St. John's wort, and possibly with ampicillin and tetracyclines. Atorvastatin, ascorbic acid, acetaminophen, CYP3A4 inhibitors (eg, itraconazole, ketoconazole) may increase hormone levels. Protease inhibitors may increase or decrease levels. May increase levels of cyclosporine, prednisolone, theophylline. May decrease levels of acetaminophen. Increases clearance of temazepam, salicylic acid, morphine, clofibric acid.

PREGNANCY: Category X, not for use in nursing.

MECHANISM OF ACTION: Estrogen/progestogen combination oral contraceptive; suppresses gonadotropins and primarily inhibits ovulation. Causes changes in cervical mucus (increases difficulty of sperm entry into uterus) and endometrium (reduces likelihood of implantation).

PHARMACOKINETICS: Absorption: Levonorgestrel: Rapid and complete, absolute bioavailability (100%), C_{max}=5.6ng/mL, T_{max}=1.4 hrs, AUC=60.8ng•hr/mL. Ethinyl estradiol: Rapid, absolute bioavailability (43%), C_{max}=145ng/mL, T_{max}=1.6 hrs, AUC=1307pg•hr/mL. **Distribution:** Levonorgestrel: V_d=1.8L/kg, plasma protein binding (97.5-99%). Ethinyl estradiol: V_d=4.3L/kg, plasma protein binding (95-97%). **Metabolism:** Levonogestrel: Sulfate and glucuronide conjugates. Ethinyl estradiol: First-pass metabolism, hepatic via CYP3A4 (hydroxylation), methylation, conjugation. **Elimination:** Levonogestrel: Urine (45%), feces (32%); $T_{1/2}$=30 hrs. Ethinyl estradiol: Urine, feces; $T_{1/2}$=15 hrs.

NURSING CONSIDERATIONS

Assessment: Assess for current or history of thrombophlebitis or thromboembolic disorder, cerebrovascular disease, CAD, valvular heart disease with thrombogenic complications, uncontrolled HTN, DM with vascular involvement, headache with focal neurological symptoms, major surgery with prolonged immobilization, history of or known/suspected carcinoma of breast, endometrium, or other known/suspected estrogen-dependent neoplasia, undiagnosed abnormal genital bleeding, cholestatic jaundice of pregnancy or jaundice with prior pill use, hepatic adenomas or carcinomas, active liver disease, and known/suspected pregnancy. Assess use in patients ≥35 yrs who smoke ≥15 cigarettes/day. Assess for possible drug and lab interactions.

Monitoring: Monitor for venous or arterial thrombotic or thromboembolic events (eg, MI, thromboembolism, stroke), hepatic neoplasia, ocular lesions, bleeding irregularities, fluid retention, onset or exacerbation of headaches or migraines, gallbladder disease, HTN, and hypertriglyceridemia. Monitor glucose levels in DM and prediabetic patients, lipid levels with history of hyperlipidemia, signs of liver dysfunction (eg, jaundice), and signs of worsening depression with a history. Refer patients with contact lenses to ophthalmologist if visual changes occur. Perform annual history and physical exam.

Patient Counseling: Inform about possible serious cardiovascular and pulmonary effects. Instruct to avoid smoking while on medication. Counsel to take medication at same time daily. Instruct that if miss 1 pill, take as soon as possible; take next dose at regular time. Advise that stomach upset, spotting, or light bleeding may develop when initiating therapy; continue taking medication. Advise to notify physician if bleeding lasts longer than 7 days. If vomiting, diarrhea, or taking other medications, advise may need backup form of contraception. Inform patient will have 4 menstrual periods per yr while on medication.

Administration: Oral route. 1) Take 1 pill at same time every day until last pill in dispenser taken. 2) After taking last white pill, start 1st pink pill from new extended-cycle tab dispenser the next day regardless of when period started. This should be on a Sunday. **Storage:** Controlled temperature 20-25°C (68-77°F).

SEASONIQUE RX

ethinyl estradiol - levonorgestrel (Duramed)

THERAPEUTIC CLASS: Estrogen/progestogen combination

INDICATIONS: Prevention of pregnancy.

DOSAGE: *Adults*: 1 tablet qd for 91 days, then repeat. During first cycle of medication, start on 1st Sunday after onset of menstruation. Begin next and all subsequent 91-day courses without interruption on same day of week (Sunday) upon which first course began, following the same schedule.

HOW SUPPLIED: Tab: (Ethinyl Estradiol-Levonorgestrel) 0.03mg-0.15mg; Tab: (Ethinyl Estradiol) 0.01mg

CONTRAINDICATIONS: Thrombophlebitis, DVT or thromboembolic disorders, cerebrovascular or CAD, valvular heart disease with thrombogenic complications, uncontrolled HTN, DM with vascular involvement, headaches with focal neurological symptoms, major surgery with prolonged immobilization, breast cancer, endometrial cancer or other estrogen-dependent neoplasia, undiagnosed abnormal genital bleeding, cholestatic jaundice of pregnancy or jaundice with prior pill use, hepatic adenomas or carcinomas, active liver disease, or pregnancy.

WARNINGS/PRECAUTIONS: Cigarette smoking increases risk of serious CV side effects. This risk increases with age (especially >35 yrs) and heavy smoking. Increased risk of MI, vascular disease, thromboembolism, stroke, HTN, and gallbladder disease. Retinal thrombosis, hepatic neoplasia, carcinoma of breast and reproductive organs reported. May cause glucose intolerance, fluid retention, breakthrough bleeding, and spotting. May increase BP, elevate LDL levels or cause other lipid changes. May cause or exacerbate migraine. May

S

develop visual changes with contact lenses. Increased risk of morbidity and mortality with certain inherited thrombophilias, HTN, hyperlipidemia, obesity, and diabetes. D/C if jaundice, significant depression, recurrent/persistent new headache patterns, or ophthalmic irregularities develop. Perform annual physical exam. Not for use before menarche or with uncontrolled HTN. May affect certain endocrine, LFTs, and blood components. Weigh benefit of fewer planned menses against inconvenience of increased intermenstrual bleeding or spotting.

ADVERSE REACTIONS: NV, breakthrough bleeding, spotting, amenorrhea, migraine, depression, vaginal candidiasis, edema, weight changes.

INTERACTIONS: Reduced effects, increased breakthrough bleeding, and menstrual irregularities with rifampin, barbiturates, phenylbutazone, phenytoin, carbamazepine, felbamate, oxcarbazepine, topiramate, hypericum perforatum, griseofulvin, ampicillin, and tetracyclines. Increased levels with atorvastatin, ascorbic acid, APAP, and CYP3A4 (eg, itraconazole, ketoconazole) inhibitors. Anti-HIV protease inhibitors may increase or decrease levels. May increase plasma levels of cyclosporine, prednisolone, and theophylline. May decrease levels of APAP. Increased clearance of temazepam, salicylic acid, morphine, and clofibric acid.

PREGNANCY: Category X, not for use in nursing.

MECHANISM OF ACTION: Estrogen/progestogen combination oral contraceptive; acts by suppressing gonadotropins. Primarily inhibits ovulation. Also responsible for causing changes in cervical mucus (increases difficulty of sperm entry into uterus) and endometrium (reduces likelihood of implantation).

PHARMACOKINETICS: Absorption: Rapid; T_{max}=2 hrs; Levonorgestrel: Absolute bioavailability (100%). Ethinyl estradiol: Absolute bioavailability (43%). Oral administration of variable doses resulted in different parameters. **Distribution:** Levonorgestrel: V_d=1.8L/kg; plasma protein binding (97.5-99%). Ethinyl estradiol: V_d=4.3L/kg; plasma protein binding (95-97%). **Metabolism:** Levonogestrel: Sulfate and glucuronide conjugates. Ethinyl estradiol: 1st pass metabolism in gut wall, Hepatic, via CYP3A4 (hydroxylation), methylation, conjugation. **Elimination:** Levonorgestrel: Urine (45%), feces (32%); $T_{1/2}$=34 hrs. Ethinyl estradiol: Urine, feces; $T_{1/2}$=18 hrs.

NURSING CONSIDERATIONS

Assessment: Assess for current or history of thrombophlebitis or thromboembolic disorders, CAD, cerebrovascular disease, valvular heart disease with thrombogenic complications, uncontrolled HTN, DM with vascular involvement, headache with focal neurological symptoms, major surgery with prolonged immobilization, known/suspected or history of carcinoma of breast, endometrium or other known/suspected estrogen-dependent neoplasia, undiagnosed abnormal genital bleeding, cholestatic jaundice of pregnancy or jaundice with prior pill use, hepatic adenomas or carcinomas or active liver disease, and known or suspected pregnancy. Assess use in patients ≥35yrs who smoke ≥15 cigarettes/day. Assess use in patients with inherited thrombophilias, HTN, hyperlipidemias, obesity, or DM. Assess for possible drug or lab interactions.

Monitoring: Monitor for venous or arterial thrombotic and thromboembolic events (eg, MI, thromboembolism, stroke), vascular disease, hepatic neoplasia, ocular lesions, bleeding irregularities, fluid retention, onset or exacerbation of migraines or headaches, gallbladder disease, hypertriglyceridemia, and HTN. Monitor glucose levels in DM or prediabetic patients, lipid levels with history of hyperlipidemia, for signs/symptoms of liver dysfunction (eg, jaundice), and for signs of worsening depression with previous history. Perform annual physical exam. Refer patients who wear contact lenses to an ophthalmologist if visual changes develop.

Patient Counseling: Inform that drug does not protect against HIV infection (AIDS) and other STDs. Advise not to smoke while on medication. Inform about possible side effects of medication (eg, blood clots, HTN, liver tumors). Instruct patients will only have 4 menstrual cycles per yr while on medication. Instruct to take medication at same time daily. Counsel if dose is missed, to take as soon as possible, then take next dose at regularly scheduled time. Inform may have nausea, spotting, or light bleeding when starting therapy; continue taking medication and notify physician if bleeding persists more than 7 days. If vomiting, diarrhea, or taking concomitant medications use backup form of contraception.

Administration: Oral route. **Storage:** 20-25°C (68-77°F).

SECTRAL RX

acebutolol HCl (ESP Pharma)

THERAPEUTIC CLASS: Selective $beta_1$-blocker

INDICATIONS: Management of hypertension, ventricular arrhythmias.

DOSAGE: *Adults:* HTN: Initial: 400mg/day, given qd-bid. Usual: 200-800mg/day. Max: 1200mg/day. Ventricular Arrhythmia: Initial: 200mg bid. Maint: Increase gradually to 600-1200mg/day. Elderly: Lower daily doses. Max: 800mg/day. CrCl <50mL/min: Decrease daily dose by 50%. CrCl <25mL/min: Decrease daily dose by 75%.

HOW SUPPLIED: Cap: 200mg, 400mg

CONTRAINDICATIONS: Persistently severe bradycardia, 2nd- and 3rd-degree heart block, overt cardiac failure, cardiogenic shock.

WARNINGS/PRECAUTIONS: Withdrawal before surgery is controversial. Caution with bronchospastic disease, peripheral or mesenteric vascular disease, aortic or mitral valve disease, left ventricular dysfunction, heart failure controlled by digitalis and/or diuretics, hepatic or renal dysfunction. May mask hypoglycemia or hyperthyroidism symptoms. Avoid abrupt discontinuation. May develop antinuclear antibodies (ANA).

ADVERSE REACTIONS: Fatigue, dizziness, headache, constipation, diarrhea, dyspepsia, flatulence, nausea, dyspnea, urinary frequency, insomnia.

INTERACTIONS: Possible additive effects with catecholamine-depleting drugs. NSAIDs may reduce effects. Exaggerated hypertensive responses with alpha stimulants. May antagonize epinephrine. May potentiate insulin-induced hypoglycemia.

PREGNANCY: Category B, not for use in nursing.

MECHANISM OF ACTION: Cardioselective β-adrenoreceptor blocking agent; causes reduction in HR and systolic BP.

PHARMACOKINETICS: Absorption: Well-absorbed; absolute bioavailability (40%); T_{max}=2.5 hrs. **Distribution:** Plasma protein binding (26%); crosses placental barrier; secreted in breast milk. **Metabolism:** Diacetolol (major metabolite). **Elimination:** Renal (30-40%), nonrenal (50-60%). (Sectral, Diacetolol) $T_{1/2}$=(3-4, 8-13 hrs).

NURSING CONSIDERATIONS

S

Assessment: Assess for bradycardia, cardiogenic shock, 2nd- and 3rd-degree heart block, overt cardiac failure, impaired hepatic/renal function, bronchospastic disease, PVD, DM, thyrotoxicosis, valvular heart disease, and possible drug interactions.

Monitoring: Monitor for cardiac failure, HTN, renal dysfunction, exacerbation of ischemia following abrupt withdrawal, bronchospastic disease, PVD, ANA, anaphylactoid reactions, hypersensitivity reactions.

Patient Counseling: Instruct not to interrupt or d/c therapy without consulting physician. Advise to consult physician if signs/symptoms of impending CHF or unexplained respiratory symptoms develop. Inform about hypertensive reactions from concomitant use of α-adrenergic stimulants, such as nasal decongestants used in OTC cold preparations.

Administration: Oral route. **Storage:** 20-25°C (68-77°F). Protect from light.

SELZENTRY RX

maraviroc (Pfizer)

Hepatotoxicity reported; may be preceded by evidence of allergic reaction. Evaluate patients immediately with signs or symptoms of hepatitis or allergic reaction (eg, pruritic rash, eosinophilia, elevated IgE).

THERAPEUTIC CLASS: CCR5 co-receptor antagonist

INDICATIONS: Combination antiretroviral treatment of adults infected with only CCR5-tropic HIV-1 detectable, who have evidence of viral replication and HIV-1 strains resistant to multiple antiretroviral agents.

DOSAGE: *Adults:* >16 yrs: Give in combination with other antiretroviral medications. With Strong CYP3A Inhibitors (with or without CYP3A inducers) Including PIs (except tipranavir/ritonavir), Delavirdine: 150mg bid. With NRTIs, Tipranavir/Ritonavir, Nevirapine, Other Drugs That Are Not Strong CYP3A Inhibitors/Inducers: 300mg bid. With CYP3A Inducers (without strong CYP3A inhibitor): 600mg bid.

HOW SUPPLIED: Tab: 150mg, 300mg

WARNINGS/PRECAUTIONS: D/C if signs or symptoms of hepatitis or with increased liver transaminases combined with rash or other systemic symptoms. Caution with pre-existing liver dysfunction or co-infection with viral hepatitis B or C. Caution with increased risk for CV events especially with history of postural hypotension or on concomitant medication to lower BP. Immune reconstitution syndrome reported. May increase risk of developing infections; monitor closely for evidence of infections.

ADVERSE REACTIONS: Cough, pyrexia, upper respiratory tract infections, rash, musculoskeletal symptoms, abdominal pain, dizziness, diarrhea, edema, esophageal candidiasis, sleep disorders, rhinitis, urinary abnormalities.

INTERACTIONS: Coadministration with CYP3A inhibitors, including protease inhibitors (except tipranavir/ritonavir) and delaviridine, will increase levels. Coadministration with CYP3A inducers, including efavirenz, may decrease levels. Concomitant use with St. John's wort is not recommended.

PREGNANCY: Category B, not for use in nursing.

MECHANISM OF ACTION: CCR5 co-receptor antagonist; selectively binds to human chemokine receptor CCR5 present on cell membranes, preventing interaction of HIV-1 gp120 and CCR5 necessary for CCR5-tropic HIV-1 to enter cells.

PHARMACOKINETICS: Absorption: (1-1200mg) T_{max}=0.5-4 hrs. (100mg, 300mg) Absolute bioavailability (23%, 33%). **Distribution:** V_d=194L; plasma protein binding (76%). **Metabolism:** CYP3A; secondary amine (N-dealkylation metabolite). **Elimination:** Urine: 20% (8% unchanged), feces: 76% (25% unchanged); $T_{1/2}$=14-18 hrs.

S

NURSING CONSIDERATIONS

Assessment: Assess for known liver dysfunction or co-infection with HBV or HCV, known history of postural hypotension, pregnancy status, increased risk of CV events, and possible drug interactions.

Monitoring: Monitor for signs/symptoms of hepatotoxicity, allergic reactions, immune reconstitution syndrome, CV events, and infections.

Patient Counseling: Inform that therapy is not cure for HIV, does not reduce risk of transmission of HIV, and that opportunistic infections may develop. Advise to take as prescribed, swallow whole, do not chew. Report use of other prescription or nonprescription medication; take missed dose as soon as possible and next dose at regular time. Caution that physical/mental abilities may be impaired. Seek medical attention if signs/symptoms of infections, CV events, hepatitis (yellow eyes/skin, dark urine, vomiting, abdominal pain) or allergic reactions (rash) occur.

Administration: Oral route. **Storage:** 25°C (77°F); excursions permitted 15-30°C (59-86°F). Shelf-life is 24 months.

SENSIPAR
cinacalcet HCl (Amgen)

RX

THERAPEUTIC CLASS: Calcimimetic agent

INDICATIONS: Secondary hyperparathyroidism in patients with chronic kidney disease on dialysis. Hypercalcemia in parathyroid carcinoma.

DOSAGE: *Adults:* Take with food. Swallow whole. Secondary Hyperparathyroidism: Initial: 30mg qd. Titrate: Increase no more frequently than every 2-4 weeks through sequential doses of 60, 90, 120, and 180mg qd to target iPTH of 150-300pg/mL. Parathyroid Carcinoma: Initial: 30mg bid. Titrate: Increase every 2-4 weeks through sequential doses of 30mg bid, 60mg bid, 90mg bid, and 90mg tid-qid prn to normalize serum Ca levels. Adjust based on serum Ca levels (see PI). May be used alone or in combination with vitamin D sterols and/or phosphate binders.

HOW SUPPLIED: Tab: 30mg, 60mg, 90mg

WARNINGS/PRECAUTIONS: Monitor closely for hypocalcemia, especially with history of seizure disorder. Do not initiate with serum Ca <8.4mg/dL. Measure serum Ca and phosphorus within 1 week and iPTH 1-4 weeks after initiation or dose adjustment. After maintenance dose reached, measure serum Ca and phosphorus monthly and iPTH every 1-3 months. Adynamic bone disease may develop with iPTH levels <100pg/mL; reduce dose or d/c therapy if iPTH <150pg/mL. Caution with moderate/severe hepatic impairment. Hypotension and worsening heart failure, and/or arrhythmia with impaired cardiac function reported.

ADVERSE REACTIONS: NV, diarrhea, myalgia, dizziness, HTN, asthenia, anorexia, chest pain (non-cardiac), access infection.

INTERACTIONS: Drugs metabolized by CYP2D6 (eg, flecainide, vinblastine, thioridazine, most TCAs) may require dose adjustment. Increased amitriptyline, nortriptyline levels in CYP2D6 extensive metabolizers. Increased levels with strong CYP3A4 inhibitors (eg, ketoconazole, erythromycin, itraconazole); may require dose adjustments.

PREGNANCY: Category C, not for use in nursing.

MECHANISM OF ACTION: Calcimimetic agent; lowers PTH levels by increasing the sensitivity of the calcium-sensing receptor to extracellular calcium.

PHARMACOKINETICS: Absorption: T_{max}=2-6 hrs. **Distribution:** V_d=1000L; plasma protein binding (93-97%); found in breast milk. **Metabolism:** Rapid and extensively metabolized. Liver via CYP450 enzymes 3A4, 2D6, and 1A2. Oxidation, conjugation, and glucuronidation. **Elimination**: Urine (80%), feces (15%); $T_{1/2}$=30-40 hrs.

NURSING CONSIDERATIONS

Assessment: Assess for a history of seizure disorder, hepatic impairment, and for possible drug interactions. Assess serum calcium levels prior to administration.

Monitoring: Monitor for seizures, signs/symptoms of hypocalcemia (paresthesias, myalgias, cramping, tetany, and convulsions), and adynamic bone disease. Monitor hepatic function with a history of hepatic insufficiency. In patients with chronic kidney disease on dialysis, monitor serum calcium levels within 1 week after initiation of therapy or dose adjustment and iPTH levels within 1 to 4 weeks after initiation of therapy or dose adjustment. In patients with parathyroid carcinoma, measure serum calcium levels within 1 week after drug initiation or dose adjustment; measure serum calcium levels every 2 months after maintenance dose levels have been established. All patients on therapy require periodic monitoring of serum calcium levels.

Patient Counseling: Instruct to report any adverse reactions. Advise to take drug with food or shortly after meal; should be taken whole and not divided.

Administration: Oral route. **Storage:** 25°C (77°F); excursions permitted to 15-30°C (59-86°F).

SEPTRA RX

sulfamethoxazole - trimethoprim (King)

OTHER BRAND NAMES: Sulfatrim Pediatric (Alpharma) - Septra DS (King)

THERAPEUTIC CLASS: Sulfonamide/tetrahydrofolic acid inhibitor

INDICATIONS: Treatment of urinary tract infections (UTI), acute otitis media, acute exacerbations of chronic bronchitis (AECB), *Pneumocystis carinii* pneumonia (PCP), traveler's diarrhea, and shigellosis caused by susceptible strains of microorganisms.

DOSAGE: *Adults:* UTI/Shigellosis: 800mg-160mg PO q12h for 10-14 days (UTI) or 5 days (shigellosis). AECB: 800mg-160mg PO q12h for 14 days. Traveler's Diarrhea: 800mg-160mg PO q12h for 5 days. PCP Treatment: 15-20mg/kg TMP and 75-100mg/kg SMX per 24 hrs given PO q6h for 14-21 days. PCP Prophylaxis: 800mg-160mg PO qd. Renal Impairment: CrCl 15-30mL/min: 50% usual dose. CrCl <15mL/min: Not recommended.
Pediatrics: ≥2 months: UTI/Otitis Media/Shigellosis: 4mg/kg TMP and 20mg/kg SMX q12h for 10 days (UTI/otitis media) or 5 days (shigellosis). PCP Treatment: 15-20mg/kg TMP and 75-100mg/kg SMX per 24 hrs given q6h for 14-21 days. PCP Prophylaxis: 150mg/m²/day TMP and 750mg/m²/day SMX PO given bid, on 3 consecutive days per week. Max: 320mg TMP and 1600mg SMX per day. Renal Impairment: CrCl 15-30mL/min: 50% usual dose. CrCl <15mL/min: Not recommended.

HOW SUPPLIED: (Sulfamethoxazole [SMX]-Trimethoprim [TMP]) Sus: (Sulfatrim Pediatric, Septra) 200mg-40mg/5mL [100mL, 473mL]; Tab: (Septra) *400mg-80mg**; Tab, DS: (Septra DS) *800mg-160mg** **scored*

CONTRAINDICATIONS: Megaloblastic anemia due to folate deficiency, pregnancy at term, nursing, infants <2 months old.

WARNINGS/PRECAUTIONS: Fatal hypersensitivity reactions (eg, Stevens-Johnson syndrome, toxic epidermal necrolysis, fulminant hepatic necrosis, agranulocytosis, aplastic anemia) may occur. Cough, SOB, and pulmonary infiltrates reported. Avoid with group A β-hemolytic streptococcal infections. *Clostridium difficile*-associated diarrhea reported. Caution with hepatic/renal impairment, elderly, folate deficiency (eg, chronic alcoholics, anticonvulsants, malabsorption, malnutrition), bronchial asthma, and other allergies. In G6PD deficiency, hemolysis may occur. Increased incidence of adverse events in AIDS patients. Maintain adequate fluid intake.

ADVERSE REACTIONS: Anorexia, NV, rash, urticaria, cough, SOB, cholestatic jaundice, agranulocytosis, anemia, hyperkalemia, renal failure, interstitial nephritis, hyponatremia, convulsions.

INTERACTIONS: Increased risk of thrombocytopenia with purpura with diuretics (especially thiazides) in the elderly. Caution with warfarin; may prolong PT. Increased effects of phenytoin, methotrexate. Concomitant ACE inhibitor therapy may cause hyperkalemia.

PREGNANCY: Category C, not for use in nursing.

MECHANISM OF ACTION: Sulfamethoxazole: Inhibits bacterial synthesis of dihydrofolic acid by competing with para-aminobenzoic acid (PABA). Trimethoprim: Blocks production of tetrahydrofolic acid from dihydrofolic acid by binding to and reversibly inhibiting required enzyme, dihydrofolate reductase; thus drug blocks 2 consecutive steps in biosynthesis of nucleic acids and proteins essential to many bacteria.

PHARMACOKINETICS: Absorption: Rapid; T_{max}=1-4 hrs. **Distribution:** Trimethoprim: Plasma protein binding (44%); Sulfamethoxazole: Plasma protein binding (70%). Crosses placenta, found in breast milk. **Metabolism:** Sulfamethoxazole: N_4 acetylation. Trimethoprim: 1-and 3-oxide, 3'-and 4'-hydroxy derivative (principal metabolites). **Elimination:** Urine, trimethoprim (66.8%), sulfamethoxazole (84.5%; 30% as free and remaining as N_4 acetylated metabolite); $T_{1/2}$=10 hr (sulfamethoxazole), 8-10 hr (trimethoprim).

NURSING CONSIDERATIONS

Assessment: Assess for previous drug hypersensitivity, megaloblastic anemia, renal/hepatic impairment, folate deficiency (eg, elderly, chronic alcoholics, patients on anticonvulsants, malabsorption syndrome, malnutrition states), glucose-6-phosphate-dehydrogenase-deficient individuals, severe allergy or bronchial asthma, pregnancy/nursing status, and possible drug interactions.

Monitoring: Monitor for severe reactions (eg, Stevens-Johnson syndrome, toxic epidermal necrolysis, fulminant hepatic necrosis, agranulocytosis), *C.difficile*-associated diarrhea (may range from mild diarrhea to fatal colitis), development of drug resistance, superinfection, signs of bone marrow depression or specific decrease in platelets with or without pupura, hyperkalemia, hyponatremia, kernicterus, and clinical signs (eg, skin rash, sore throat, fever, arthralgia, pallor, jaundice) that may be early indications of serious reactions. Frequent monitoring of CBC; d/c if significant reduction is noted, perform urinalysis with careful microscopic exam and renal function tests (particularly for renal impairment).

Patient Counseling: Inform that drug only treats bacterial, not viral, infections. Take exactly as directed; skipping doses or not completing full course may decrease effectiveness and increase resistance. Instruct to maintain adequate fluid intake to prevent crystalluria and stone formation. Inform about potential benefits/risks of therapy. D/C and notify physician if skin rash, watery/bloody diarrhea (with/without muscle cramps), or fever occurs (may occur up to 2 months after therapy). Notify if pregnant/nursing.

Administration: Oral route. **Storage:** 15-25°C (59-77°F); protect from light.

SEREVENT — RX

salmeterol xinafoate (GlaxoSmithKline)

Long-acting β_2-adrenergic agonists, such as salmeterol, may increase the risk of asthma-related deaths.

THERAPEUTIC CLASS: $Beta_2$-agonist

INDICATIONS: Long-term maintenance treatment of asthma and COPD. Prevention of bronchospasm with reversible obstructive airway disease (including nocturnal asthma) when regular treatment with inhaled short-acting β_2-agonists is required. Prevention of exercise-induced bronchospasm (EIB).

DOSAGE: *Adults:* Asthma/COPD: 1 inh bid, am and pm (12 hrs apart). EIB Prevention: 1 inh 30 min before exercise (do not give preventive doses if already on bid dose).

Pediatrics: ≥4 yrs: Asthma: 1 inh bid, am and pm (12 hrs apart). EIB Prevention: 1 inh 30 min before exercise (do not give preventive doses if already on bid dose).

HOW SUPPLIED: Disk: 50mcg [28, 60 blisters]

S

WARNINGS/PRECAUTIONS: Avoid with significantly worsening or acutely deteriorating asthma. Not for acute treatment or substitute for oral/inhaled corticosteroids. Monitor for increasing use of inhaled β_2-agonists. QTc interval prolongation reported when recommended dose exceeded. D/C if paradoxical bronchospasm occurs. Immediate hypersensitivity and upper airway symptom reactions reported. Caution with cardiovascular disorder (eg, coronary insufficiency, arrhythmia, HTN), convulsive disorders, thyrotoxicosis, if usually unresponsive to sympathomimetic amines. May cause hypokalemia.

ADVERSE REACTIONS: Nasal/sinus congestion, pallor, rhinitis, headache, tracheitis/bronchitis, influenza, throat irritation.

INTERACTIONS: Caution with non-potassium-sparing diuretics. Extreme caution within 14 days of using MAOIs or TCAs. Avoid with β-blockers. Caution with >8 inhalations of short-acting β_2-agonists.

PREGNANCY: Category C, not for use in nursing.

MECHANISM OF ACTION: β_2-adrenergic agonist; increases cAMP levels causing relaxation of bronchial smooth muscles and inhibits the release of mediators of immediate hypersensitivity from mast cells.

PHARMACOKINETICS: Absorption: C_{max}=167pg/mL; T_{max}=20 min. **Distribution:** Plasma protein binding (96%). **Metabolism:** Liver (aliphatic oxidation) via CYP3A4. (Metabolite) α-hydroxysalmeterol. **Elimination:** $T_{1/2}$=5.5 hrs.

NURSING CONSIDERATIONS

Assessment: Assess for CVD (coronary insufficiency, cardiac arrhythmia, HTN), convulsive disorder, thyrotoxicosis, DM, and possible drug interactions. Obtain baseline lung function before therapy.

Monitoring: Monitor lung function periodically. Monitor for upper airway symptoms (laryngeal spasm, irritation, swelling), worsening or acutely deteriorating asthma (increased use of inhaled β_2-agonist, decreased lung function), asthma instability (serial objective measures of airflow), paradoxical bronchospasm, and hypersensitivity reactions.

Patient Counseling: Inform drug may increase risk of asthma-related death. Do not use with a spacer device. Do not stop therapy unless directed by health provider. Never exhale into Diskus, never take Diskus apart. Activate and use in a level, horizontal position. Never wash mouthpiece or any part; keep dry. Inform not to use for sudden symptoms of SOB or acute bronchospasm. Advise to rinse mouth after inhalation. Seek medical attention if symptoms worsen or do not improve, severe asthmatic attack, paradoxical bronchospasm, or hypersensitivity reaction occur.

Administration: Oral inhaled route. 1) Hold with one hand and put thumb of other hand on thumb grip. Push thumb away from self until mouthpiece appears and snaps into position 2) Hold in level, flat position with mouthpiece toward self. Slide lever away from self until it clicks 3) Exhale fully, then put mouthpiece in lips and breath in quickly and deeply. Hold breath for 10 seconds or as long as comfortable. Breath out slowly. **Storage:** 20-25°C (68-77°F). Keep in dry place, away from heat or sunlight.

SEROQUEL — RX

quetiapine fumarate (AstraZeneca)

Elderly patients with dementia-related psychosis treated with atypical antipsychotic drugs are at an increased risk of death; most appeared to be cardiovascular (eg, heart failure, sudden death) or infectious (eg, pneumonia) in nature. Quetiapine is not approved for the treatment of patients with dementia-related psychosis. Antidepressants increased the risk of suicidal thinking and behavior (suicidality) in short-term studies in children, adolescents, and young adults with major depressive disorder (MDD) and other psychiatric disorders. Quetiapine is not approved for use in pediatric patients.

THERAPEUTIC CLASS: Dibenzapine derivative

INDICATIONS: Treatment of schizophrenia. Treatment of depressive episodes associated with bipolar disorder. Treatment of acute manic episodes associated with bipolar I disorder, as monotherapy or adjunct therapy to lithium or divalproex. Maintenance treatment of bipolar I disorder as adjunct therapy to lithium or divalproex.

DOSAGE: *Adults:* Bipolar Disorder: Depressive Episodes: Give once daily hs. Day 1: 50mg/day. Day 2: 100mg/day. Day 3: 200mg/day. Day 4: 300mg/day. Bipolar Mania: Monotherapy/Adjunctive: Give bid. Initial: 100mg/day on Day 1. Titrate: Increase to 400mg/day on Day 4 in increments of up to 100mg/day in bid divided doses. Adjust doses up to 800mg/day by Day 6 in increments ≤200mg/day. Max: 800mg/day. Maintenance for Bipolar I Disorder: Give bid. 400-800mg/day. Schizophrenia: Initial: 25mg bid. Titrate: Increase by 25-50mg bid-tid on the 2nd and 3rd day to 300-400mg/day given bid-tid by the 4th day. Adjust doses by 25-50mg bid at intervals of at least 2 days. Maint: Lowest effective dose. Max: 800mg/day. Hepatic Impairment: Initial: 25mg/day. Titrate: Increase by 25-50mg/day to effective dose. Elderly/Debilitated/Predisposition to Hypotension: Consider slower rate of dose titration and lower target dose. Reinitiation of Treatment: If off >1 week: Follow initial dosing schedule. If <1 week: No dose escalation required, reinitiate the maintenance dose.

HOW SUPPLIED: Tab: 25mg, 50mg, 100mg, 200mg, 300mg, 400mg

WARNINGS/PRECAUTIONS: Hyperglycemia, in some cases extreme and associated with ketoacidosis or hyperosmolar coma or death, has been reported; monitor DM patients regularly for worsening of glucose control and all patients for symptoms of hyperglycemia. Increases in cholesterol and TG, weight gain reported in clinical trials. NMS reported. May develop tardive dyskinesia. May induce orthostatic hypotension. Caution with cardiovascular or cerebrovascular disease, conditions that predispose to hypotension (eg, dehydration, hypovolemia, treatment with antihypertensives), history of seizures. Leukopenia, neutropenia, and agranulocytosis reported. Monitor for cataracts at initiation, then every 6 months. Possible hypothyroidism. Asymptomatic, transient and reversible elevations in serum transaminase, primarily ALT, have been reported. Caution in patients at risk for aspiration pneumonia. May impair judgment, thinking, and motor skills. Priapism reported. May disrupt body's ability to reduce core temperature. Caution in patients at risk for aspiration, elderly, debilitated. May increase prolactin levels. Close supervision of high-risk patients should accompany drug therapy due to possibility of suicide attempt. Acute withdrawal symptoms (eg, N/V, insomnia) may occur after abrupt cessation.

ADVERSE REACTIONS: Headache, somnolence, dizziness, dry mouth, postural hypotension, constipation, dyspepsia, tachycardia, asthenia, agitation, abdominal pain, pharyngitis, weight gain, lethargy, nasal congestion.

INTERACTIONS: Caution with other CNS drugs. May increase cognitive and motor effects of alcohol. May antagonize effects of levodopa and dopamine agonists. May enhance effects of antihypertensives. Phenytoin or other hepatic enzyme inducers (eg, carbamazepine, barbiturates, glucocorticoids) may reduce levels. Divalproex may increase mean maximum plasma levels without affecting absorption or mean oral clearance. Caution with CYP3A inhibitors (eg, itraconazole, ketoconazole, fluconazole, erythromycin). May reduce oral clearance of lorazepam. Thioridazine may increase clearance.

PREGNANCY: Category C, not for use in nursing.

MECHANISM OF ACTION: Dibenzothiapine derivative; mechanism not established. Believed that actions are mediated through antagonism of both serotonin type 2 ($5HT_2$) and dopamine type 2 (D_2) receptors in the brain.

PHARMACOKINETICS: Absorption: Rapid, T_{max}=1.5 hrs. **Distribution:** V_d=10±4L/kg; plasma protein binding (83%). **Metabolism:** Liver (extensive) via sulfoxidation and oxidation; CYP3A4. **Elimination:** Urine (73%), feces (20%, <1% unchanged).

NURSING CONSIDERATIONS

Assessment: Assess for history of dementia-related psychosis, major depressive disorder, bipolar mania, DM, pre-existing low WBCs or drug-induced leukopenia/neutropenia, liver impairment, CVD, possible drug interactions, and mammary neoplasms (female), seizures (or conditions that may lower seizure threshold). Assess for risk of aspiration pneumonia.

Monitoring: Monitor for signs/symptoms of TD, clinical manifestation of NMS, EPS, suicidal attempts, orthostatic hypotension, body temperature, ECG changes, worsening depression, behavioral changes, agitation, irritability, priapism, esophageal dysmotility, and aspiration. Perform periodic monitoring of FBG with risk for DM. Monitor for lenticular changes; perform lens exam (eg, slit lamp exam) at initiation of treatment and at 6-month intervals during chronic treatment. Monitor for acute withdrawal symptoms (eg, N/V, insomnia) with abrupt withdrawal. Lab monitoring of liver enzymes, BUN, thyroid function, cholesterol, TG, CBC, and prolactin.

Patient Counseling: Advise of risk of orthostatic hypotension and DM. Counsel to avoid activities requiring mental alertness. Instruct to notify physician if taking other drugs, pregnant (or intend to become pregnant), or if signs of NMS, overheating, or dehydration occur. Instruct to avoid breastfeeding or alcohol intake. Advise to monitor for clinical worsening or suicide attempts; notify physician if these occur.

Administration: Oral route. **Storage:** 25°C (77°F); excursions permitted to 15-30°C (59-86°F).

SEROQUEL XR

RX

quetiapine fumarate (AstraZeneca)

Elderly patients with dementia-related psychosis treated with atypical antipsychotic drugs are at an increased risk of death; most deaths appeared to be cardiovascular (eg, heart failure, sudden death) or infectious (eg, pneumonia) in nature. Seroquel XR is not approved for the treatment of patients with dementia-related psychosis. Antidepressants increased the risk of suicidal thinking and behavior (suicidality) in short-term studies in children, adolescents, and young adults with major depressive disorder (MDD) and other psychiatric disorders. Seroquel XR is not approved for use in pediatric patients.

THERAPEUTIC CLASS: Dibenzapine derivative

INDICATIONS: Acute and maintenance treatment of schizophrenia. Treatment of acute depressive episodes associated with bipolar disorder. Treatment of acute manic or mixed episodes associated with bipolar I disorder, as monotherapy and as adjunct to lithium or divalproex. Maintenance treatment of bipolar I disorder as adjunct therapy to lithium or divalproex.

DOSAGE: *Adults:* Schizophrenia: Give once daily, preferably in evening. Initial: 300mg/day. Titrate: Within range of 400-800mg/day depending on response and tolerance. Dose increases may be made at intervals as short as 1 day and in increments up to 300mg/day. Maint: 400-800mg/day for 16 weeks. Bipolar Disorder: Depressive Episodes: Give once daily in evening. Day 1: 50mg/day. Day 2: 100mg/day. Day 3: 200mg/day. Day 4: 300mg/day. Bipolar Mania: Monotherapy/Adjunct: Give once daily in evening. Day 1: 300mg. Day 2: 600mg. Titrate: May adjust dose between 400-800mg beginning on Day 3 depending on response and tolerance. Maintenance of Bipolar I Disorder: 400-800mg/day given bid. Re-evaluate periodically. Elderly/Hepatic Impairment: Initial: 50mg/day; may increase in increments of 50mg/day depending on response and tolerance. Reinitiation of Treatment: If off >1 week: Follow initial dosing schedule. If <1 week: No dose escalation required, reinitiate the maintenance dose. Switching from Seroquel: May switch to Seroquel XR at equivalent total daily dose given once daily. Swallow tab whole; do not split, crush, or chew.

HOW SUPPLIED: Tab, Extended-Release: 50mg, 150mg, 200mg, 300mg, 400mg

WARNINGS/PRECAUTIONS: Hyperglycemia, in some cases extreme and associated with ketoacidosis or hyperosmolar coma or death, has been reported; monitor DM patients regularly for worsening of glucose control and all patients for symptoms of hyperglycemia. Increases in cholesterol and TG; weight gain reported in clinical trials. NMS reported. May develop tardive dyskinesia. May induce orthostatic hypotension. Caution with cardiovascular or cerebrovascular disease, conditions that predispose to hypotension (eg, dehydration, hypovolemia, treatment with antihypertensives), history of seizures. Leukopenia, neutropenia, and agranulocytosis reported. Monitor for cataracts at initiation, then every 6 months. Possible hypothyroidism. Asymptomatic, transient and reversible elevations in serum transaminase, primarily ALT, have been reported. May impair judgment, thinking, and motor skills. Priapism reported. May disrupt body's ability to reduce core temperature. Caution in patients at risk for aspiration, elderly, debilitated. May increase prolactin levels. Close supervision of high-risk patients should accompany drug therapy due to possibility of suicide attempt. Acute withdrawal symptoms (eg, N/V, insomnia) may occur after abrupt cessation.

ADVERSE REACTIONS: Dry mouth, constipation, dyspepsia, somnolence, dizziness, orthostatic hypotension, weight gain, increased appetite, fatigue, dysarthria, nasal congestion, insomnia, headache.

INTERACTIONS: Caution with other CNS drugs. May increase cognitive and motor effects of alcohol. May antagonize effects of levodopa and dopamine agonists. May enhance effects of antihypertensives. Phenytoin or other hepatic enzyme inducers (eg, carbamazepine, barbiturates, glucocorticoids) may reduce levels. Divalproex may increase mean maximum plasma levels without affecting absorption or mean oral clearance. Caution with CYP3A inhibitors (eg, itraconazole, ketoconazole, fluconazole, erythromycin). May reduce oral clearance of lorazepam. Thioridazine may increase clearance.

PREGNANCY: Category C, caution in nursing.

MECHANISM OF ACTION: Dibenzothiapine derivative; mechanism not established. Believed that actions are mediated through antagonism of both serotonin type 2 ($5HT_2$) and dopamine type 2 (D_2) receptors in the brain.

PHARMACOKINETICS: Absorption: T_{max}=6 hrs. **Distribution:** V_d=10±4L/kg; plasma protein bound (83%). **Metabolism:** Liver (extensive) via sulfoxidation and oxidation; CYP 450(3A4), N-desalkyl quetiapine (major metabolite). **Elimination:** Urine (73%, <1% unchanged), feces (20%).

NURSING CONSIDERATIONS

Assessment: Assess for history of dementia-related psychosis, major depressive disorder, bipolar mania, DM, pre-existing low WBCs or drug-induced leukopenia/neutropenia, liver impairment, CVD, possible drug interactions, mammary neoplasms (female), and seizures (or conditions that may lower seizure threshold). Assess for risk of aspiration pneumonia.

Monitoring: Monitor for signs/symptoms of TD, clinical manifestation of NMS, EPS, suicidal attempts, orthostatic hypotension, body temperature, ECG changes, worsening depression, behavioral changes, agitation, irritability, priapism, esophageal dysmotility, and aspiration. Perform periodic monitoring of FBG with risk for DM. Monitor for lenticular changes; perform lens exam (eg, slit lamp exam) at initiation of treatment and at 6-month intervals during chronic treatment. Monitor for acute withdrawal symptoms (eg, N/V, insomnia) with abrupt withdrawal. Lab monitoring of liver enzymes, BUN, thyroid function, cholesterol, TG, CBC, and prolactin.

Patient Counseling: Advise of risk of orthostatic hypotension and DM. Counsel to avoid activities requiring mental alertness. Instruct to notify physician if taking other drugs; pregnant (or intend to become pregnant); or if signs of NMS, overheating, or dehydration occur. Instruct to avoid breastfeeding and alcohol. Advise to monitor for clinical worsening or suicide attempts; notify physician if these occur.

Administration: Oral route. **Storage:** Store at 25°C (77°F); excursions permitted to 15-30°C (59-86°F).

SEROSTIM — RX

somatropin (EMD Serono)

THERAPEUTIC CLASS: Human growth hormone

INDICATIONS: Treatment of AIDS wasting or cachexia.

DOSAGE: *Adults:* >55kg: 6mg SQ qhs. 45-55kg: 5mg SQ qhs. 35-44kg: 4mg SQ qhs. <35kg: 0.1mg/kg SQ qhs. Dose Reductions Due to Side Effects: Reduce total daily dose or number of doses/week. Rotate injection sites. Re-evaluate for infection if weight loss continues after 2 weeks of therapy.

HOW SUPPLIED: Inj: 4mg, 5mg, 6mg, 8.8mg

CONTRAINDICATIONS: Acute critical illness due to complications after open heart or abdominal surgery, accidental trauma, acute respiratory failure.

WARNINGS/PRECAUTIONS: Monitor malnutrition, malabsorption and hypogonadism; may contribute to catabolism. Maintain nucleoside analogue therapy throughout treatment. Carpal tunnel syndrome reported. Perform periodic funduscopic exams.

ADVERSE REACTIONS: Musculoskeletal discomfort, increased tissue turgor, edema, arthralgia, extremity pain, hypoesthesia, myalgia, hyperglycemia, arthrosis, diarrhea, headache, paresthesia, insomnia, upper respiratory tract infection.

PREGNANCY: Category B, caution in nursing.

MECHANISM OF ACTION: Human growth hormone; anabolic and anticatabolic agent exerting influence by interacting with specific receptors on variety of cell types.

PHARMACOKINETICS: Absorption: Absolute bioavailabilty (70-90%). **Distribution:** V_d=12.0L. **Metabolism:** Kidneys (major), liver (minor). **Elimination:** $T_{1/2}$=4.28 hrs.

NURSING CONSIDERATIONS

Assessment: Assess for acute critical illness due to complications of surgery, multiple accidental trauma, acute respiratory failure, active malignancy, inadequate nutritional intake, malabsorption, hypogonadism, risk factors for glucose tolerance, preexisting DM, and possible drug interactions. Perform baseline fundoscopic exam.

Monitoring: Periodically perform fundoscopic exam. Monitor for signs/symptoms of carpal tunnel syndrome, increased tissue turgor, musculoskeletal discomfort, hypersensitivity/allergic reactions, and acute pancreatitis.

Patient Counseling: Instruct on proper disposal and how to rotate injection site. Seek medical attention if symptoms of carpal tunnel syndrome, swelling, musculoskeletal discomfort (pain, swelling, stiffness), hypersensitivity reactions, or pancreatitis occur.

Administration: SQ route. **Storage:** Before reconstitution: 15-30°C (59-86°F). After reconstitution: 2-8°C (36-46°F); stable for 14 days. Avoid freezing.

SILVADENE RX

silver sulfadiazine (King)

OTHER BRAND NAMES: SSD (Par)

THERAPEUTIC CLASS: Sulfonamide

INDICATIONS: Adjunct for prevention and treatment of wound sepsis in patients with 2nd- and 3rd-degree burns.

DOSAGE: *Adults:* Apply under sterile conditions qd-bid to thickness of approximately 1/16 inch. Re-apply if removed by patient activity. Continue until wound is healed.

HOW SUPPLIED: Cre: 1% [20g, 50g, 85g, 400g, 1000g]

CONTRAINDICATIONS: Late pregnancy, premature infants, newborns during first 2 months of life.

WARNINGS/PRECAUTIONS: Potential cross-sensitivity with other sulfonamides. Hemolysis may occur in G6PD deficient patients. Drug accumulation with hepatic and renal dysfunction. Monitor renal function and serum sulfa levels with extensive burns.

ADVERSE REACTIONS: Transient leukopenia, skin necrosis, erythema multiforme, skin discoloration, burning sensation, rash, interstitial nephritis, fungal superinfection, systemic sulfonamide reactions.

INTERACTIONS: May inactivate topical proteolytic enzymes. Leukopenia increased with cimetidine.

PREGNANCY: Category B, contraindicated in late pregnancy, and not for use in nursing.

MECHANISM OF ACTION: Topical antimicrobial of sulfonamide class; acts on cell membrane and cell wall of many gram-negative and gram-positive bacteria and yeast to produce bactericidal effect.

NURSING CONSIDERATIONS

Assessment: Assess pregnancy status, patient is not premature infant or a newborn infant ≤2 months old, renal/hepatic dysfunction, glucose-6-phosphate dehydrogenase deficiency, and for possible drug interactions.

Monitoring: Monitor fungal proliferation, renal/hepatic function, urine to identify sulfa crystals, serum sulfa concentrations with wounds involving extensive body surface areas, and signs/symptoms of sulfonamide reaction (eg, agranulocytosis, aplastic anemia, thrombocytopenia, leukopenia, Stevens-Johnson syndrome, exfoliative dermatitis, hepatitis and hepatocellular necrosis, CNS reactions, and toxic nephrosis).

Patient Counseling: Instruct to clean wound with soap and water and dry thoroughly prior to application; do not place tongue blades back into jar after touching wound. Inform to stop using if wounds are size of a quarter or smaller, and use a moisturizer cream or other lotion after wounds have healed.

Administration: Topical. Using a tongue blade, apply a thin layer of cream enough to cover wound. If more is needed, a new tongue blade is to be used. Place a gauze dressing over wound and keep wound clean and dry. **Storage:** At room temperature. Store only for 6 months after opening.

SIMCOR — RX

simvastatin - niacin (Abbott)

THERAPEUTIC CLASS: HMG-CoA reductase inhibitor/Nicotinic acid

INDICATIONS: Adjunct to diet for the reduction of elevated total-C, LDL-C, Apo B, non-HDL-C, TG, or to increase HDL-C with primary hypercholesterolemia, mixed dyslipidemia (Types IIa and IIb), and for reduction of elevated TG with hypertriglyceridemia when treatment with monotherapy components is inadequate.

DOSAGE: *Adults:* Patients not currently on niacin extended-release or switching from immediate-release niacin: Initial: 500mg/20mg qd hs, with a low-fat snack. Titrate: Adjust dose at ≥4 weeks. After Week 8, titrate to response and tolerance. Maint: 1000mg/20mg to 2000mg/40mg qd. Max: 2000mg/40mg qd. Do not break, crush, or chew before swallowing.

HOW SUPPLIED: Tab, Extended Release: (Niacin-Simvastatin) 500mg/20mg, 750mg/20mg, 1000mg/20mg

CONTRAINDICATIONS: Active liver disease (unexplained persistent elevations of serum transaminases), active peptic ulcer disease, arterial bleeding, pregnancy/nursing.

WARNINGS/PRECAUTIONS: Do not substitute for equivalent dose of immediate-release niacin. Myopathy and rhabdomyolysis reported; monitor serum creatine kinase (CK) periodically. D/C therapy if myopathy is suspected or diagnosed, if transaminase levels increase ≥3 ULN persist, or a few days prior to major surgery or when any major medical or surgical condition supervenes. Increased risk with higher doses, advanced age (≥65 yrs), hypothyroidism, renal impairment. Caution with heavy alcohol use, or history of liver disease; monitor LFTs prior to therapy, every 12 weeks for the first 6 months and periodically thereafter. Severe hepatic toxicity may occur in patients substituting sustained-release niacin for immediate-release niacin at equivalent doses. May increase serum glucose levels in diabetic or potentially diabetic patients, particularly in the first few months of therapy; adjust diet and/or hypoglycemic therapy or d/c if necessary. May reduce platelet count. Caution with those predisposed to gout.

ADVERSE REACTIONS: Flushing, headache, back pain, diarrhea, nausea, pruritus.

INTERACTIONS: Avoid use with concomitant CYP3A4 inhibitors including itraconazole, ketoconazole, and other antifungal azoles, erythromycin, clarithromycin, telithromycin, HIV protease inhibitors, nefazodone, grapefruit juice (>1 quart/day), cyclosporine, danazol, and fibrates; increased risk of myopathy/rhabdomyolysis. Max 20mg/day with amiodarone or verapamil. Concurrent use with propanolol decreases simvastatin levels. Potentiates effects of coumarin anticoagulants; monitor PT/INR. May increase digoxin levels; monitor appropriately. Concomitant use with aspirin decreases niacin levels. Colestipol and cholestyramine may increase niacin-binding capacity. Potentiates adverse effects with nutritional supplements containing large doses of niacin or related compounds.

PREGNANCY: Category X, not for use in nursing.

MECHANISM OF ACTION: Niacin: Nicotinic acid; not well established. May partially inhibit release of free fatty acids from adipose tissue, and increases lipoprotein lipase activity, which increases rate of chylomicron triglyceride removal from plasma. Decreases rate of hepatic synthesis of VLDL and LDL.

Simvastatin: HMG-CoA reductase inhibitor; lipid-lowering agent. Inhibits conversion of HMG-CoA to mevalonate. Also reduces VLDL, TG, and increases HDL.

PHARMACOKINETICS: Absorption: Niacin: T_{max}=4.6-4.9 hrs. Simvastatin: T_{max}=1.9-2.0 hrs. Simvastatin acid (active metabolite): C_{max} =3.29ng/mL, T_{max}= 6.56 hrs, AUC =30.81 ng•hr/mL. **Metabolism:** Rapid and extensive first-pass metabolism. **Elimination:** Niacin: Urine (54%). Simvastatin: Feces (60%), urine (13%), $T_{1/2}$ =4.2-4.9 hrs; (simvastatin acid) $T_{1/2}$ =4.6-5.0 hrs.

NURSING CONSIDERATIONS

Assessment: Prior to initiation, assess for active liver disease or unexplained elevations in serum transaminases, renal dysfunction, active peptic ulcer disease, arterial bleeding, and pregnancy/nursing status. Obtain baseline lipid profile (TC, HDL-C, LDL-C, TG) and LFTs. Assess use in patients who consume substantial quantities of alcohol and/or have a past history of liver disease, and for possible drug interactions.

Monitoring: Monitor for signs/symptoms of myopathy (eg, muscle pain, tenderness, weakness), rhabdomyolysis, decrease in platelet counts, increase in prothrombin time, and decrease in phosphorus levels. Perform periodic monitoring of lipid profile, CK, and blood glucose levels. Monitor LFTs every 12 weeks for the first 6 months and periodically every 6 months thereafter.

Patient Counseling: Counsel to take at bedtime after a low-fat snack. Inform that flushing may occur but should subside after several weeks of therapy; taking an NSAID 30 min prior may minimize. Instruct to avoid ingestion of alcohol or hot drinks with administration to prevent flushing. Advise not to break, crush, or chew, and to swallow whole. Instruct to contact physician if discontinuing drug for extended period of time, taking vitamins, other nutritional supplements, or if dizziness occurs. Notify diabetics that change in blood glucose may occur.

Administration: Oral route. **Storage:** 20-25°C (68-77°F).

SIMULECT — RX

basiliximab (Novartis)

Manage patient in facility with adequate lab and supportive resources. Prescribing physician should be experienced with immunosuppressives and transplantation. Physician should have complete information requisite for patient follow-up.

THERAPEUTIC CLASS: Monoclonal antibody/IL-2R alpha (CD25) blocker

INDICATIONS: Prophylaxis of acute organ rejection in renal transplantation.

DOSAGE: *Adults:* 20mg within 2 hrs prior to transplant, repeat 4 days after transplant. Withhold 2nd dose if graft loss or complications occur.
Pediatrics: ≥35kg: 20mg within 2 hrs prior to transplant, repeat 4 days after transplant. <35kg: 10mg within 2 hrs prior to transplant, repeat 4 days after transplant. Withhold 2nd dose if graft loss or complications occur.

HOW SUPPLIED: Inj: 10mg, 20mg

WARNINGS/PRECAUTIONS: Only administer under qualified medical supervision. Increased risk of developing lymphoproliferative disorder and opportunistic infections. Anaphylaxis and other severe hypersensitivity reactions (eg, hypotension, cardiac failure, bronchospasm, respiratory failure, etc) reported and may necessitate discontinuation. Anti-idiotype antibodies may develop.

ADVERSE REACTIONS: GI effects, peripheral edema, fever, viral infection, hyperkalemia, hypokalemia, hyperglycemia, hypercholesterolemia, hypophosphatemia, hyperuricemia, UTI, dyspnea, upper respiratory infection, acne, HTN, headache, tremor, insomnia, anemia.

PREGNANCY: Category B, not for use in nursing.

MECHANISM OF ACTION: Monoclonal antibody/IL-2Rα (CD25) blocker; acts as an IL-2 receptor antagonist by binding to the IL-2 receptor complex and inhibiting IL-2 binding. Specifically targeted against IL-2Rα, which is selectively expressed on the surface of activated T-lymphocytes. Binding to

IL-2Rα causes competitive inhibition of IL-2-mediated activation of lymphocytes, a critical pathway in the cellular immune response involved in allograft rejection.

PHARMACOKINETICS: Absorption: C_{max}=7.1ng/mL (adult). **Distribution:** V_d=8.6L (adult); 4.8L (1-11 yrs); 7.8L (12-16 yrs). **Elimination:** $T_{1/2}$=7.2 days (adult); 9.5 days (1-11 yrs); 9.1 days (12-16 yrs).

NURSING CONSIDERATIONS

Assessment: Assess use in patients who were on previous therapy with this drug, and in pregnant/nursing females. Assess for possible drug interactions.

Monitoring: Monitor for signs/symptoms of lymphoproliferative disorders, opportunistic infections, and hypersensitivity reactions (eg, hypotension, tachycardia, cardiac failure, dyspnea, pulmonary edema, respiratory failure, urticaria, and rash).

Patient Counseling: Counsel about risks/benefits. Inform to contact physician immediately if signs/symptoms of hypersensitivity reaction (eg, dyspnea, uticaria, rash) occur. Instruct females of child-bearing potential to use effective form of contraceptive before starting therapy, during therapy, and for 4 months following d/c. Advise may experience NV during administration.

Administration: Central or peripheral IV administration. Reconstituted drug should be given as a bolus injection or diluted to a volume of 25mL (10mg vial) or 50mL (20mg vial) (normal saline or dextrose 5%). Administer as IV infusion over 20-30 min. **Storage**: Lyophilized Simulect: Under refrigerated condition, 2-8°C (36-46°F). Reconstituted: Use immediately. If not used immediately, store at 2-8°C (36-46°F) for 24 hrs or at room temperature for 4 hrs. Discard reconstituted solution if not used within 24 hrs.

SINEMET CR — RX

levodopa - carbidopa (Bristol-Myers Squibb)

OTHER BRAND NAMES: Sinemet (Bristol-Myers Squibb)

THERAPEUTIC CLASS: Dopa-decarboxylase inhibitor/dopamine precursor

INDICATIONS: Treatment of symptoms of idiopathic Parkinson's disease, postencephalitic parkinsonism, and symptomatic parkinsonism.

DOSAGE: *Adults:* ≥18 yrs: Initial: (25mg-100mg tab) 1 tab tid. Titrate: Increase by 1 tab qd or every other day until 8 tabs/day. 10mg-100mg tab: Initial: 1 tab tid-qid. Titrate: Increase 1 tab qd or every other day until 2 tabs qid. 70-100mg/day carbidopa required. Max: 200mg/day carbidopa. (Tab, Extended-Release) No Prior Levodopa Use: Initial: 1 tab 50mg-200mg bid at intervals >6 hrs. Titrate: Increase or decrease dose or interval accordingly. Adjust dose every 3 days. Usual: 400-1600mg/day levodopa, given in 4-8 hr intervals while awake. Conversion to Extended-Release Tabs: See PI.

S

HOW SUPPLIED: Tab: (Carbidopa-Levodopa) 10mg-100mg*, 25mg-100mg*, 25mg-250mg*; Tab, Extended-Release: (Carbidopa-Levodopa) 25mg-100mg, 50mg-200mg* *scored

CONTRAINDICATIONS: MAOIs during or within 14 days of use, narrow-angle glaucoma, suspicious, undiagnosed skin lesions, history of melanoma.

WARNINGS/PRECAUTIONS: D/C levodopa 12 hrs before initiating therapy. Dyskinesias and mental disturbances may occur. Caution with severe cardiovascular or pulmonary disease, bronchial asthma, renal or hepatic disease, endocrine disease, chronic wide-angle glaucoma, peptic ulcer, and MI with residual arrhythmias. NMS reported during dose reduction or withdrawal. Dark color may appear in saliva, urine, or sweat. May cause false (+) ketonuria or false (-) glucosuria (glucose-oxidase method). May cause melanoma in patients with Parkinson's disease.

ADVERSE REACTIONS: Dyskinesias, nausea, cardiac irregularities, hypotension, dark saliva, GI bleeding, psychotic episodes, NMS, confusion, agitation, dizziness, somnolence, dream abnormalities.

INTERACTIONS: See Contraindications. Risk of postural hypotension with antihypertensives, selegiline. HTN and dyskinesia may occur with TCAs. Reduced effects with dopamine D_2 antagonists (eg, phenothiazines, butyrophenones, risperidone), isoniazid. Antagonized by phenytoin, papaverine, metoclopramide. Reduced bioavailability with iron salts, high-protein diets.

PREGNANCY: Category C, caution in nursing.

MECHANISM OF ACTION: Dopa-decarboxylase inhibitor/dopamine precursor. Carbidopa: Inhibits decarboxylation of peripheral levodopa. Levodopa: Rapidly decarboxylated to dopamine in extracerebral tissue so that only portion of a given dose is transported unchanged to the CNS.

PHARMACOKINETICS: Absorption: Levodopa: Absolute availability: 70-75%; C_{max}=1151ng/mL; T_{max}=2 hrs. Carbidopa: Absolute bioavailability (58%). **Elimination:** Levodopa and carbidopa: $T_{1/2}$ ≥ 1.5 hrs.

NURSING CONSIDERATIONS

Assessment: Assess LFTs, renal function, CBC, glaucoma, dyskinesia, psychosis, depression, cardiovascular complications, melanomas, and asthma.

Monitoring: Monitor LFTs, renal function, CBC, BP, biliary obstruction, depression and suicidal ideations, worsening of dyskinesia, rhabdomyolysis, diarrhea, hallucinations, fibrotic complications, hyperpyrexia, melanomas, IOP, and hypersensitivity reactions.

Patient Counseling: Instruct to take as prescribed. Caution while operating machinery/driving. Discoloration of bodily fluids may occcur. High-protein diet, excessive acidity, and iron salts reduce clinical effectiveness. Wearing-off effect may be seen at end of dosing interval. Report any adverse effects. Swallow tablet; do not chew or crush. Inform patients about the development of new or increased gambling urges, sexual urges or other urges.

Administration: Oral route. **Storage:** 30°C (86°F). Store in tightly closed container.

SINGULAIR RX

montelukast sodium (Merck)

THERAPEUTIC CLASS: Leukotriene receptor antagonist

INDICATIONS: Prophylaxis and chronic treatment of asthma (≥12 months). Relief of symptoms of seasonal allergic rhinitis (≥2 yrs) and perennial allergic rhinitis (≥6 months). Prevention of exercise-induced bronchoconstriction (EIB [≥15 yrs]).

DOSAGE: *Adults:* Asthma: 10mg qpm. Allergic Rhinitis: 10mg qd. EIB: 10mg 2 hrs before exercise. Do not take additional dose within 24 hrs of previous dose.

S

Pediatrics: Asthma: ≥15 yrs: 10mg qpm. 6-14 yrs: 5mg qpm. 2-5 yrs: 4mg qpm. 6-23 months: 4mg qpm. Seasonal/Perennial Allergic Rhinitis: ≥15 yrs: 10mg qd. 6-14 yrs: 5mg qd. 2-5 yrs: 4mg qd. Perennial Allergic Rhinitis: 6-23 months: 4mg qd. EIB: ≥15 yrs: 10mg 2 hrs before exercise. Do not take additional dose within 24 hrs of previous dose. Granules may be mixed with applesauce, carrots, rice, or ice cream; give within 15 min of opening pkt.

HOW SUPPLIED: Granules: 4mg/pkt; Tab, Chewable: 4mg, 5mg; Tab: 10mg

WARNINGS/PRECAUTIONS: Not for treatment of acute asthma attacks, including status asthmaticus. Avoid abrupt substitution for inhaled or oral corticosteroids. Continue therapy during acute exacerbations of asthma. Eosinophilic conditions reported (rare).

ADVERSE REACTIONS: Headache, abdominal pain, dyspepsia, cough, pharyngitis, flu, fever, sinusitis, nausea, diarrhea, dyspepsia, otitis, viral infection, laryngitis, epitaxis, and increase bleeding tendency.

INTERACTIONS: Monitor with potent CYP450 inducers (eg, phenobarbital, rifampin). Avoid with known ASA sensitivity.

PREGNANCY: Category B, caution in nursing.

MECHANISM OF ACTION: Leukotriene receptor antagonist; binds to cysteinyl leukotriene receptors found on airway smooth muscle cells and macrophages and other pro-inflammatory cells (eg, eosinophils); inhibits physiologic actions of leukotrienes.

PHARMACOKINETICS: Absorption: Rapid. (10mg) Bioavailability (64%) T_{max}=3-4 hrs. (5mg) T_{max}=2-2.5 hrs. Bioavailability (73%, fasted), (63%, fed). Fasted 2-5 yrs: (4mg Chewable) T_{max}=2 hrs. (4mg Granules) T_{max}=2.3 hrs (fasted), 6.4 hrs (fed). **Distribution:** V_d=8-11L; plasma protein binding (99%). **Metabolism:** Liver (extensive); CYP3A4, 2C9. **Elimination:** Biliary (major); $T_{1/2}$=2.7-5.5 hrs.

NURSING CONSIDERATIONS

Assessment: Assess for hepatic dysfunction, history of phenylketonuria, bronchospasm (status asthmaticus), and possible drug interactions. Obtain baseline LFTs.

Monitoring: Monitor for signs/symptoms of eosinophilia, vasculitic rash, worsening pulmonary symptoms, cardiac complications, neuropathy, and hypersensitivity reactions (eg, urticaria, angioedema, rash).

Patient Counseling: Inform not for treatment of acute asthma attacks and exercise-induced bronchoconstriction; appropriate rescue drug (eg, short acting β_2-agonist) should be available to prevent worsening. Take directly or mix granules with applesauce, carrots, rice, or ice cream. Advise that chewable tablets contain phenylalanine with phenylketonuria. Instruct not to decrease dose or d/c other anti-asthma medications unless instructed by physician. Seek medical attention if symptoms of eosinophilia, vasculitic rash, worsening pulmonary symptoms, cardiac complications, neuropathy, and hypersensitivity reactions occur.

Administration: Oral route. **Storage:** 25°C (77°F); excursions permitted to 15-30°C (59-86°F). Protect from light and moisture.

SKELAXIN RX

metaxalone (King)

THERAPEUTIC CLASS: Muscular analgesic (central-acting)

INDICATIONS: Adjunct for acute, painful musculoskeletal conditions.

DOSAGE: *Adults:* 800mg tid-qid.
Pediatrics: >12 yrs: 800mg tid-qid.

HOW SUPPLIED: Tab: 800mg* *scored

CONTRAINDICATIONS: Tendency for drug-induced, hemolytic, and other anemias. Significant renal or hepatic impairment.

WARNINGS/PRECAUTIONS: Caution with pre-existing liver damage. Monitor hepatic function. Serial liver function reported. False-positive Benedict's test reported. May impair mental/physical abilities.

ADVERSE REACTIONS: NV, GI upset, drowsiness, dizziness, headache, nervousness, leukopenia, hemolytic anemia, jaundice.

INTERACTIONS: May enhance the effects of alcohol, barbiturates and other CNS depressants.

PREGNANCY: Not for use in pregnancy or nursing.

MECHANISM OF ACTION: Centrally acting muscular analgesic; not established; activity may be due to general depression of CNS.

PHARMACOKINETICS: Absorption: (400mg) C_{max}=983ng/mL, T_{max}= 3.3 hrs, AUC=7479ng•hr/mL. (800mg) C_{max}=1816ng/mL, T_{max}=3.0 hrs, AUC=15044ng•hr/mL. **Distribution:** V_d=800L; extensive in tissues. **Metabolism:** Liver. **Elimination**: Urine (metabolites); $T_{1/2}$=9 hrs.

NURSING CONSIDERATIONS

Assessment: Assess for hemolytic or other anemia, renal/hepatic impairment, pregnancy/nursing status, alcohol intake, and possible drug interactions.

Monitoring: Perform frequent monitoring of LFTs. Monitor for signs/symptoms of CNS depression and lab test interactions (eg, false-positive Benedict's test).

Patient Counseling: Caution against performing hazardous tasks (operating machinery/driving). Advise to avoid alcohol or other CNS depressants. Instruct to notify if pregnant/nursing or planning to become pregnant.

Administration: Oral route; taking with food may enhance CNS depression. **Storage:** 15-30°C (59-86°F).

SKELID — RX

tiludronate disodium (Sanofi-Aventis)

THERAPEUTIC CLASS: Bisphosphonate

INDICATIONS: Treatment of Paget's disease when serum alkaline phosphatase is ≥2x ULN, or if symptomatic, or if at risk for future complications.

DOSAGE: *Adults:* 400mg qd for 3 months. After therapy, wait 3 months to assess response. Take with 6-8oz of water. Take 2 hrs after food.

HOW SUPPLIED: Tab: 200mg

WARNINGS/PRECAUTIONS: May cause GI disorders (eg, dysphagia, esophagitis, esophageal or gastric ulcers). Maintain adequate vitamin D and calcium intake. Avoid in severe renal failure. May cause osteonecrosis, primarily in jaw, and musculoskeletal pain.

ADVERSE REACTIONS: Pain, headache, dizziness, paresthesia, diarrhea, NV, dyspepsia, rhinitis, upper respiratory infection.

INTERACTIONS: Increased bioavailability with indomethacin; space dosing by 2 hrs. Decreased bioavailability with calcium supplements, ASA, and aluminum- or magnesium-containing antacids; space dosing by 2 hrs.

PREGNANCY: Category C, caution in nursing.

MECHANISM OF ACTION: Bisphosphonate; acts primarily on bone to inhibit osteoclastic activity, with a probable reduction in the enzymatic and transport processes that lead to resorption of mineralized matrix. Inhibits osteoclasts through inhibiting protein-tyrosine-phosphatase and through inhibition of the osteoclastic proton pump.

PHARMACOKINETICS: Absorption: Rapidly absorbed; C_{max}=3mg/L; T_{max}=2 hrs. **Distribution:** Plasma protein binding (90%). **Elimination:** Urine (60%); $T_{1/2}$=150 hrs.

NURSING CONSIDERATIONS

Assessment: Assess for severe renal impairment (eg, CrCl <30mL/min), risk of osteonecrosis (eg, cancer, anemia, pre-existing dental disease), pregnancy/nursing status, and possible drug interactions.

Monitoring: Monitor for signs/symptoms of upper GI disorders (eg, dysphagia, esophagitis, esophageal ulcer, gastric ulcer), osteonecrosis (eg, jaw), and musculoskeletal pain.

Patient Counseling: Instruct to take with 6-8 oz of plain water. Do not take within 2 hrs of food. Maintain vitamin D and calcium intake. Do not take calcium supplements, aspirin, and indomethacin 2 hrs before or 2 hrs after medication. If aluminum or magnesium-containing antacids are needed, take at least 2 hrs after medication. Medication should be taken for a period of 3 months, followed by another 3 months to assess response.

Administration: Oral route. **Storage:** 25°C (77°F); excursions permitted to 15-30°C (59-86°F). Do not remove tablets from foil strips until ready to be used.

SOLIRIS RX
eculizumab (Alexion)

Increases risk of meningococcal infections. Vaccinate 2 weeks prior to receiving first dose; revaccinate according to current guidelines. Monitor for early signs of meningococcal infections, evaluate, and treat if necessary.

THERAPEUTIC CLASS: Monoclonal antibody/Protein C5 blocker

INDICATIONS: Treatment of paroxysmal nocturnal hemoglobinuria (PNH) to reduce hemolysis.

DOSAGE: *Adults:* Initial: 600mg every 7 days for first 4 weeks, then 900mg as 5th dose 7 days later, then 900mg every 14 days thereafter. Administer by IV infusion over 35 min.

HOW SUPPLIED: Inj: 10mg/mL [30mL]

CONTRAINDICATIONS: Patients with unresolved serious *Neisseria meningitis* infection and patients not vaccinated against it.

WARNINGS/PRECAUTIONS: Caution in patients with any systemic infection. After discontinuation, monitor for signs and symptoms of intravascular hemolysis and serum LDH levels.

ADVERSE REACTIONS: Meningococcal infections, headache, nasopharyngitis, back pain, nausea, fatigue, cough, herpes simplex infections, sinusitis, respiratory tract infection, constipation, myalgia, pain in extremities, influenza-like illness.

PREGNANCY: Category C, caution in nursing.

MECHANISM OF ACTION: Monoclonal antibody/protein C5 blocker; binds to the complement C5 with high affinity, thereby inhibiting its cleavage to C5a and C5b and preventing the generation of the terminal complement C5b-9. Inhibits terminal complement-mediated intravascular hemolysis in PNH patient.

PHARMACOKINETICS: Absorption: C_{max}=194mcg/mL. **Distribution:** V_d=7.7L. **Elimination:** $T_{1/2}$=272 hrs.

NURSING CONSIDERATIONS

Assessment: Assess unresolved serious *Neisseria meningitis* infection and patients who are not vaccinated against *Neisseria meningitis*. Assess pregnancy status.

Monitoring: Monitor for meningococcal infections, infections caused by encapsulated bacteria, serum LDH levels, infusion reactions, hypersensitivity reactions.

Patient Counseling: Must receive a meningococcal vaccination at least 2 weeks prior to receiving the first dose if not previously vaccinated. Vaccination may not prevent meningococcal infection. Educate about signs/symptoms of meningococcal infection and need for immediate medical attention if any occur. Inform of potential for serious hemolysis when drug is discontinued; stress need for monitoring by healthcare professional for at least 8 weeks following d/c. Advise to carry Patient Safety Card at all times.

Administration: IV infusion. **Storage:** Refrigerate at 2-8°C (36-46°F) and protect from light.

SOLODYN RX
minocycline HCl (Medicis)

THERAPEUTIC CLASS: Tetracycline derivative

INDICATIONS: Treatment of inflammatory lesions of non-nodular moderate to severe acne vulgaris in patients ≥12 yrs.

DOSAGE: *Adults:* 1mg/kg qd for 12 weeks. Reduce dose with renal impairment. *Pediatrics:* ≥12 yrs: 1mg/kg qd for 12 weeks. Reduce dose with renal impairment.

HOW SUPPLIED: Tab, Extended-Release: 45mg, 90mg, 135mg.

WARNINGS/PRECAUTIONS: May cause fetal harm during pregnancy. Use during tooth development (last half of pregnancy, infancy, <8yrs) may cause permanent discoloration of the teeth or enamel hypoplasia; avoid use during this period. May decrease bone growth in premature infants. May cause pseudomembranous colitis. Renal toxicity, hepatotoxicity, photosensitivity, increased BUN, superinfection, pseudotumor cerebri may occur. Caution in renal impairment; may lead to azotemia, hyperphosphatemia, and acidosis. Long-term use has been associated with lupus-like syndrome, autoimmune hepatitis and vasculitis. May cause serum sickness. May induce hyperpigmentation.

ADVERSE REACTIONS: Headache, fatigue, dizziness, pruritus, malaise, mood alteration, Stevens-Johnson syndrome, photosensitivity.

INTERACTIONS: May require downward regulation of anticoagulant therapy. May interfere with bactericidal action of penicillin; avoid concurrent use. May decrease efficacy of oral contraceptives. Impaired absorption with antacids containing aluminum, calcium or magnesium, and iron-containing preparations. Fatal renal toxicity with methoxyflurane reported.

PREGNANCY: Category D, not for use in nursing.

MECHANISM OF ACTION: Tetracycline derivative; inhibits bacterial protein synthesis.

PHARMACOKINETICS: Absorption: C_{max}=2.63mcg/mL; T_{max}=3.5-4 hrs; AUC=33.32mcg•hr/mL.

NURSING CONSIDERATIONS

Assessment: Assess for pregnancy/nursing status, tooth development status in pediatrics/children, hepatic/renal impairment, possible drug interactions, visual disturbances prior to initiation of therapy. Routinely check for papilledema during therapy.

Monitoring: Monitor for fetal harm if given to pregnant women, permanent tooth discoloration if given during tooth development, enamel hypoplasia, photosensitivity, CNS symptoms, symptoms/signs of pseudomotor cerebri (blurred vision and headache or bulging fontanels in infants, permanent loss of vision), papilledema, decrease in fibula growth if given to premature infants, increase in BUN (azotemia, hyperphosphatemia, and acidosis). In patients with impaired renal function, monitor overgrowth of nonsusceptible organisms, pseudomembranous colitis or *C.difficile*-associated diarrhea, and development of drug resistance, hepatotoxicity, autoimmune syndromes, serious skin/hypersensitivity reactions such as Stevens-Johnson syndrome, tissue hyperpigmentation, interference with fluorescence test that can lead to false elevations of urinary catecholamines. Periodically monitor organ systems, including hematopoietic, renal and hepatic, ANC via lab tests to evaluate autoimmune syndromes.

Patient Counseling: Use caution while performing hazardous tasks (operating machinery/driving). Inform about potential benefits/risks of therapy. D/C and notify physician if erythema or symptoms of autoimmune syndromes (eg, fever, arthralgia, malaise and rash) occur. Avoid prolonged or direct exposure to sunlight and wear loose-fitting clothes. Take drug exactly as prescribed to avoid developing drug resistance and to maintain effectiveness of therapy. Notify if pregnant/nursing, planning to become pregnant, or if taking oral contaceptives. Advise men who are attempting to father a child to not take the drug.

Administration: Oral route. **Storage:** 25°C (77°F); excursions permitted to 15-30° (59-86°F); tight, light- and child-resistant containers.

SOLTAMOX RX

tamoxifen citrate (Savient)

For women with ductal carcinoma in situ (DCIS) and women at high risk for breast cancer. Fatal uterine malignancies (eg, endometrial adenocarcinoma, uterine sarcoma), stroke, and PE reported with use in risk reduction setting. Discuss benefits/risks of events with this patient population. Benefits of tamoxifen outweigh risks in women already diagnosed with breast cancer.

THERAPEUTIC CLASS: Antiestrogen

INDICATIONS: Treatment of metastatic breast cancer in women and men. Treatment of node-positive and axillary node-negative breast cancer in women following mastectomy, axillary dissection and breast irradiation. To reduce risk of invasive breast cancer in women with DCIS. Reduction of breast cancer incidence in high risk women. Use for up to 5 yrs.

DOSAGE: *Adults:* Breast Cancer Treatment: 20-40mg qd. Divide dosages >20mg into AM and PM doses. Breast Cancer Risk Reduction/DCIS: 20mg qd for 5 yrs.

HOW SUPPLIED: Sol: 10mg/5mL

CONTRAINDICATIONS: Reduction in breast cancer incidence in high risk women and women with DCIS who require coumarin-type anticoagulant therapy or have a history of DVT, PE.

WARNINGS/PRECAUTIONS: Hypercalcemia reported in patients with bone metastases. Increased incidence of uterine malignancies (eg, endometrial cancer, uterine sarcoma) and endometrial changes including hyperplasia and polyps reported. Increased incidence of thromboembolic events (eg, DVT, PE). Malignant and non-malignant effects on the liver and ocular disturbances reported. Leukopenia, anemia, thrombocytopenia, neutropenia, pancytopenia reported. Promptly evaluate abnormal vaginal bleeding if receiving or previously received tamoxifen. Patients receiving or previously received tamoxifen should have annual gynecological exam. Do not become pregnant within 2 months of therapy. May cause fetal harm during pregnancy. Does not cause infertility even with menstrual irregularity.

ADVERSE REACTIONS: (Females) Hot flashes, increased bone and tumor pain, vaginal discharge, irregular menses; (Males) loss of libido, impotence.

INTERACTIONS: Increases effects of coumarin-type anticoagulant; monitor PT. Increased risk of thromboembolic events with cytotoxic agents. Increased levels with bromocriptine. May decrease letrozole levels. Decreased levels with rifampin and aminoglutethimide. Decreased plasma levels of major metabolite, N-desmethyl tamoxifen with medroxyprogesterone.

PREGNANCY: Category D, not for use in nursing.

MECHANISM OF ACTION: Nonsteroidal antiestrogen; competes with estrogen for binding sites in target tissues.

PHARMACOKINETICS: Absorption: C_{max}=40mg/mL; T_{max}=5 hrs. N-desmethyl tamoxifen: C_{max}=15ng/mL. **Metabolism:** N-desmethyl tamoxifen (major metabolite). **Elimination:** Feces (primary); $T_{1/2}$=5-7 days.

S

NURSING CONSIDERATIONS

Assessment: Assess for pregnancy status, history of DVT or PE, hepatic impairment, and possible drug interactions. Perform baseline breast and gynecologic exam; obtain baseline mammogram.

Monitoring: Monitor CBC with platelets and LFTs periodically; perform breast exams, mammograms, and gynecologic exams routinely. Monitor for signs/symptoms of hypercalcemia, strokes, PE, uterine malignancies, and hypersensitivity reactions.

Patient Counseling: Inform of pregnancy risks; advise to use nonhormonal contraception during therapy and for 2 months after d/c. Instruct to seek medical attention for symptoms of menstrual irregularities, abnormal vaginal bleeding, changes in vaginal discharge, pelvic pain or pressure, new breast lumps, leg swelling/tenderness, SOB, changes in vision, or hypersensitivity reactions.

Administration: Oral route. **Storage:** Below 25°C (77°F). Protect from light; use within 3 months of opening; do not freeze or refrigerate.

SOLU-CORTEF — RX
hydrocortisone sodium succinate (Pharmacia & Upjohn)

THERAPEUTIC CLASS: Corticosteroid

INDICATIONS: Steroid-responsive disorders.

DOSAGE: *Adults:* Initial: 100-500mg IV/IM, depending on condition severity. May repeat dose at 2, 4, or 6 hrs based on clinical response. High-dose therapy usually not >48-72 hrs; may use antacids prophylactically.
Pediatrics: Use lower adult doses. Determine dose by severity of condition and response. Dose should not be <25mg/day.

HOW SUPPLIED: Inj: 100mg, 250mg, 500mg, 1g

CONTRAINDICATIONS: Premature infants, systemic fungal infections.

WARNINGS/PRECAUTIONS: May need to increase dose before, during, and after stressful situations. May mask signs of infection or cause new infections. Prolonged use may produce glaucoma, optic nerve damage, secondary ocular infections. Increases BP, salt/water retention, potassium and calcium excretion. More severe/fatal course of infections reported with chickenpox, measles. Enhanced effect with hypothyroidism or cirrhosis. Caution with *Strongyloides,* latent TB, ocular herpes simplex, HTN, diverticulitis, fresh intestinal anastomoses, ulcerative colitis, osteoporosis, myasthenia gravis, renal insufficiency, peptic ulcer disease. Kaposi's sarcoma reported. Monitor for psychic disturbances. Acute myopathy with high doses. Avoid abrupt withdrawal. Monitor growth and development of children on prolonged therapy. Hypernatremia may occur with high-dose therapy >48-72 hrs.

ADVERSE REACTIONS: Fluid and electrolyte disturbances, HTN, osteoporosis, muscle weakness, cushingoid state, menstrual irregularities, vertigo, headache, impaired wound healing, DM, ulcerative esophagitis, peptic ulcer, pancreatitis, increased sweating, increased ICP, carbohydrate intolerance, glaucoma, cataracts.

INTERACTIONS: Reduced efficacy and increased clearance with hepatic enzyme inducers (eg, phenobarbital, phenytoin, and rifampin). Increases clearance of chronic high dose ASA. Caution with ASA in hypoprothrombinemia. Effects on oral anticoagulants are variable; monitor PT/INR. Increased insulin and oral hypoglycemic requirements in DM. Avoid live vaccines with immunosuppressive doses. Possible decreased vaccine response with killed or inactivated vaccines with immunosuppressive doses. Decreased clearance with ketoconazole and troleandomycin.

PREGNANCY: Safety in pregnancy and nursing not known.

S

MECHANISM OF ACTION: Anti-inflammatory glucocorticoid; causes profound and varied metabolic effects and modifies the body's immune responses to diverse stimuli.

PHARMACOKINETICS: Absorption: (IM) Rapidly absorbed. T_{max}=1 hr. **Distribution:** Found in breast milk. **Elimination:** $T_{1/2}$=12 hrs.

NURSING CONSIDERATIONS

Assessment: Assess for systemic fungal infections, other current infections, active TB, vaccination history, hypersensitivity to drug components, unusual stress, IOP, ulcerative colitis, diverticulitis, HTN, recent MI, fresh intestinal anastomoses, peptic ulcer with/without impending perforation, osteoporosis, myasthenia gravis, existing psychotic tendencies, hepatic/renal impairment, and for possible drug interactions.

Monitoring: Anaphylactoid reactions (gasping syndrome, kernicterus) in premature infants, growth/development in children, glucocorticosteroid insufficiency, fluid retention, hypokalemic alkalosis, intestinal perforation with/without hemorrhage, appearance of new or exacerbation of current infections, cataracts, osteoporosis, psychic derangements, Kaposi's sarcoma, acute myopathy. Perform frequent tests of LFTs, glucose, Ca, K^+, TSH, with BP and ECG.

Patient Counseling: Inform susceptibility to infections may increase. Avoid exposure to chickenpox and measles; report immediately if exposed. Do not d/c abruptly or without medical supervision. Advise for dietary restriction of salt with K^+ supplementation.

Administration: IM and IV route. **Storage:** 20-25°C (68-77°F). Protect from light.

SOLU-MEDROL RX

methylprednisolone sodium succinate (Pharmacia & Upjohn)

THERAPEUTIC CLASS: Glucocorticoid

INDICATIONS: Steroid-responsive disorders.

DOSAGE: *Adults:* Usual: Initial: 10-40mg IV over several min. May repeat IV/IM dose at intervals based on clinical response. High-Dose Therapy: 30mg/kg IV over at least 30 min, may repeat q4-6h for 48 hrs. High-dose therapy usually not >48-72 hrs. Give antacids prophylactically. Multiple Sclerosis: (4mg methylprednisolone=5mg prednisolone): 200mg/day prednisolone for 1 week, then 80mg every other day for 1 month.
Pediatrics: Use lower adult doses. Determine dose by severity of condition and response. Dose should not be <0.5mg/kg q24h.

HOW SUPPLIED: Inj: 40mg, 125mg, 500mg, 1g, 2g

CONTRAINDICATIONS: Premature infants (due to benzyl alcohol diluent) and systemic fungal infections.

WARNINGS/PRECAUTIONS: May need to increase dose before, during, and after stressful situations. May mask signs of infection or cause new infections. Prolonged use may produce cataracts, glaucoma, secondary ocular infections. Increases BP, salt/water retention, calcium/potassium excretion. More severe/fatal course of infections reported with chickenpox, measles. Caution with latent TB, hypothyroidism, cirrhosis, ocular herpes simplex, HTN, diverticulitis, fresh intestinal anastomoses, ulcerative colitis, osteoporosis, myasthenia gravis, renal insufficiency, peptic ulcer disease. Kaposi's sarcoma reported. Growth and development of children on prolonged therapy should be monitored. Monitor for psychic disturbances. Avoid abrupt withdrawal. Reports of cardiac arrhythmias, circulatory collapse, cardiac arrest following rapid administration of large IV doses. Effectiveness not established for the treatment of sepsis syndrome and septic shock. Bradycardia reported with high doses.

ADVERSE REACTIONS: Fluid and electrolyte disturbances, HTN, osteoporosis, muscle weakness, cushingoid state, menstrual irregularities, insomnia, impaired wound healing, DM, ulcerative esophagitis, excessive sweating, increased intracranial pressure, carbohydrate intolerance, glaucoma, cataracts, nausea.

INTERACTIONS: Reduced efficacy with hepatic enzyme inducers (eg, phenobarbital, phenytoin, and rifampin). Increases clearance of chronic high dose ASA. Caution with ASA in hypoprothrombinemia. Effects on oral anticoagulants are variable; monitor PT/INR. Increased insulin and oral hypoglycemic requirements in DM. Avoid live vaccines with immunosuppressive doses. Possible decreased vaccine response with killed or inactivated vaccines with immunosuppressive doses. Mutual inhibition of metabolism with cyclosporine; convulsions reported. Decreased clearance with ketoconazole and troleandomycin.

PREGNANCY: Safety in pregnancy and nursing not known.

MECHANISM OF ACTION: Anti-inflammatory glucocorticoid; causes profound and varied metabolic effects and modifies the body's immune responses to diverse stimuli.

NURSING CONSIDERATIONS

Assessment: Assess for hypersensitivity to drug, unusual stress, infection, active TB, vaccination status, thyroid status, hepatic/renal impairment, HTN, ulcerative colitis, diverticulitis, intestinal anastomoses, hypoprothrombinemia, peptic ulcer with/without impending perforation, osteoporosis, myasthenia gravis, psychotic tendencies, glaucoma, and possible drug interactions.

Monitoring: Monitor for anaphylactic reactions. In pediatrics, monitor for gasping syndrome, hypoadrenalism, growth and development. Monitor for adrenocortical insufficiency, infection, intestinal perforation and hemorrhage, cataracts, acute myopathy, psychiatric derangements, Kaposi's sarcoma, creatinine kinase, BP, HR, serum electrolytes, IOP, TSH, LFTs, glucose, and ECG for cardiac arrhythmias and bradycardia.

Patient Counseling: Instruct to avoid exposure to chickenpox and measles; report immediately if exposed, or for fever/signs of infection. Advise regarding dietary salt restriction and K^+ supplementation.

Administration: IM/IV routes. **Storage:** 20-25°C (68-77°F) for unreconstituted product and solution. Use within 48 hrs after mixing.

SOMA — RX

carisoprodol (Meda)

THERAPEUTIC CLASS: Skeletal muscle relaxant (central-acting)

INDICATIONS: Relief of discomfort associated with acute, painful musculoskeletal conditions.

DOSAGE: *Adults:* ≤65 yrs: 250-350mg tid and hs for 2-3 weeks.
Pediatrics: ≥16 yrs: 250-350mg tid and hs for 2-3 weeks.

HOW SUPPLIED: Tab: 250mg, 350mg

CONTRAINDICATIONS: Acute intermittent porphyria and hypersensitivity to a carbamate.

WARNINGS/PRECAUTIONS: May have sedative properties. Cases of drug abuse, dependence and withdrawal reported. Caution in addiction-prone patients. First-dose idiosyncratic reactions reported (rare). Occasionally within period of 1st-4th dose, allergic reactions have occurred. Rare reports of seizures in postmarketing surveillance. Caution with liver or renal dysfunction. Seizures reported.

ADVERSE REACTIONS: Drowsiness, dizziness, headache, NV, tachycardia, postural hypotension, agitation, irritability, insomnia, seizures.

INTERACTIONS: Additive effects with alcohol, other CNS depressants, and psychotropic drugs. Concomitant use with meprobamate not recommended. Coadministration with CYP2C19 inhibitors (eg, omeprazole, fluvoxamine); may increase levels and CYP2C19 inducers (eg, St.Johns wort, rifampin); may decrease levels.

PREGNANCY: Category C, caution in nursing.

S

MECHANISM OF ACTION: Skeletal muscle relaxant; not clearly identified, suspected to relieve discomfort associated with acute painful musculoskeletal conditions.

PHARMACOKINETICS: Absorption: Carisoprodol: (250mg) C_{max}=1.2mcg/mL, T_{max}=1.5 hrs, AUC=4.5mcg•hr/mL; (350mg) C_{max}=1.8mcg/mL, T_{max}=1.7 hrs, AUC=7.0mcg•hr/mL. Meprobamate: (250mg) C_{max}=1.8mcg/mL, T_{max}= 3.6 hrs, AUC=32mcg•hr/mL; (350mg) C_{max}=2.5mcg/mL, T_{max}=4.5 hr, AUC=46mcg•hr/mL. **Distribution:** Found in breast milk. **Metabolism:** Liver via CYP2C19. Meprobamate (metabolite). **Elimination:** Urine, carisoprodol: $T_{1/2}$=1.7 hrs (250mg), 2.0 hrs (350mg). Meprobamate: $T_{1/2}$=9.7 hrs (250mg), 9.6 hrs (350mg).

NURSING CONSIDERATIONS

Assessment: Assess for acute intermittent porphyria, renal/hepatic impairment, pregnancy/nursing status, seizures, addiction-prone patients, alcohol or illegal drugs, and possible drug interactions.

Monitoring: Monitor for signs/symptoms of CNS depression, drug abuse/dependence, and seizures.

Patient Counseling: Caution against engaging in hazardous tasks (operating machinery/driving). Avoid alcohol, illegal drugs, or other CNS depressants. Notify if pregnant/nursing or planning to become pregnant. Drug is limited to acute use; notify physician if symptoms persist. Inform of drug dependence/abuse potential.

Administration: Oral route. **Storage:** 25°C (77°F); excursions permitted to 15-30°C (59-86°F).

SOMATULINE DEPOT — RX

lanreotide (Ipsen/Tercica)

THERAPEUTIC CLASS: Somatostatin analog

INDICATIONS: Long term treatment of acromegalic patients who have had inadequate response to surgery and/or radiotherapy, or for whom surgery and/or radiotherapy is not an option.

DOSAGE: Adults: Initial: 90mg deep SQ at 4 week intervals for 3 months. Titrate: Adjust dose based on IGF and GH levels. GH >1 to ≤2.5ng/mL, IGF-1 Normal and Controlled Clinical Symptoms: 90mg every 4 weeks. GH >2.5ng/mL, IGF-1 Elevated and/or Clinical Symptoms Uncontrolled: 120mg every 4 weeks. GH ≤1ng/mL, IGF-1 Normal and Clinical Symptoms Controlled: 60mg every 4 weeks. Moderate to Severe Renal/Hepatic Impairment: Initial: 60mg deep SQ at 4 week intervals for 3 months.

HOW SUPPLIED: Inj: 60mg, 90mg, 120mg

WARNINGS/PRECAUTIONS: May reduce gallbladder motility and lead to gallstone formation; monitor periodically. Hypo- and/or hyperglycemia may occur; monitor glucose levels. Decreased thyroid function reported. May decrease HR; caution with bradycardia.

ADVERSE REACTIONS: Diarrhea, abdominal pain, NV, constipation, flatulence, loose stools, cholethiasis, injection-site reactions.

INTERACTIONS: May decrease cyclosporine levels. May reduce intestinal absorption of concomitant drugs. Dose adjustments for concomitant antidiabetic treatment and drugs that induce bradycardia may be needed. Caution with drugs metabolized by CYP3A4 (eg, quinidine, terfenadine) and have low therapeutic index. Drugs metabolized by liver may need dose reduction.

PREGNANCY: Category C, caution in nursing.

MECHANISM OF ACTION: Somatostatin analog; acts mainly at the human somatostatin receptors (SSTR) 2 and 5 to inhibit growth hormone. Like somatostatin, lanreotide is an inhibitor of various endocrine, neuroendocrine, exocrine, and paracrine functions.

PHARMACOKINETICS: Absorption: SQ administration of variable doses resulted in different parameters. **Elimination:** Urine (<0.5%), feces (<5% unchanged). Biliary excretion.

NURSING CONSIDERATIONS

Assessment: Assess for cardiac disease, DM, impaired hepatic/renal function, and possible drug interactions.

Monitoring: Monitor for cholethiasis, gallbladder sludge, hyper/hypoglycemia, hypothyroidism, and cardiovascular abnormalities. Monitor blood glucose levels when dosages are adjusted. Monitor serum GH, and IGF-1 levels to assess effectiveness of treatment.

Patient Counseling: Instruct to report any adverse reactions or if condition persists or worsens. Rotate injection site between right and left side. Instruct to notify physician if dose is missed,

Administration: SQ. **Storage:** Refrigerate at 2-8°C (36-46°F). Protect from light in original package.

SOMAVERT — RX

pegvisomant (Pharmacia & Upjohn)

THERAPEUTIC CLASS: Growth hormone receptor antagonist

INDICATIONS: Treatment of acromegaly in those who have had an inadequate response to surgery and/or radiation therapy, and/or other medical therapies, or for whom these therapies are not appropriate.

DOSAGE: *Adults:* LD: 40mg SQ. Maint: 10mg SQ qd. Titrate: Adjust dose by 5mg increments/decrements, based on IGF-I levels, every 4-6 weeks. Max: 30mg/day. LFTs ≥3x/<5x ULN (without symptoms of liver dysfunction): Monitor LFTs weekly. LFTs ≥5x ULN/Transaminase Elevations ≥3x ULN: D/C immediately and evaluate. Do not initiate if baseline LFTs >3x ULN until cause is determined.

HOW SUPPLIED: Inj: 10mg, 15mg, 20mg

WARNINGS/PRECAUTIONS: May expand and cause serious complications of tumors that secrete GH; monitor with periodic imaging scans of the sella turcica. May increase glucose tolerance and risk of hypoglycemia in diabetics. May result in functional GH deficiency. AST/ALT elevations reported; obtain baseline ALT, AST, TBIL, and ALP levels prior to initiation. Monitor LFTs monthly for first 6 months, quarterly for next 6 months, then biannually; monitor more frequently if elevations occur. D/C if liver injury confirmed. Monitor IGF-I levels 4-6 weeks after initiation or dose adjustments; every 6 months after levels are normalized. Interferes with the measurement serum GH levels by commercially available GH assays; do not adjust dosage based on serum GH levels.

ADVERSE REACTIONS: Infection, abnormal LFTs, pain, injection site reactions, back pain, diarrhea, nausea, flu syndrome, chest pain, dizziness, paresthesia, HTN, sinusitis, peripheral edema.

INTERACTIONS: May need to reduce dosage of insulin and/or hypoglycemic agents. Concomitant opioids may increase dosage requirements of pegvisomant.

PREGNANCY: Category B; caution in nursing.

MECHANISM OF ACTION: Growth hormone receptor antagonist; selectively binds to growth hormone (GH) receptors on cell surfaces, where it blocks binding of endogenous GH and interferes with GH signal transduction. This decreases serum concentrations of insulin such as growth factor-I (IGF-I), as well as other GH-responsive proteins, including IGF binding protein-3 (IGFBP-3), and acid labile subunit (ALS).

PHARMACOKINETICS: Absorption: Absolute bioavailability (57%). **Distribution:** V_d=7L. **Elimination:** Urine (<1%); $T_{1/2}$=6 days.

S

NURSING CONSIDERATIONS

Assessment: Assess for latex allergy before therapy (due to stopper on vial). Assess use with tumors that secrete growth hormone. Assess proper glucose control with DM prior to therapy. Obtain baseline serum liver tests (ALT, AST, TBIL, ALP). Assess for possible drug interactions.

Monitoring: Monitor for tumor growth in patients who have growth hormone-secreting tumors. Perform periodic image scans of the sella turcica. Monitor for increased glucose tolerance while on medication (hypoglycemia). Monitor for signs/symptoms of a GH-deficient state. Serum IGF-I concentrations should be evaluated 4-6 weeks after initiation of treatment, or when dose adjustments are made, and at least every 6 months after IGF-I levels have normalized. Monitor for signs/symptoms of liver dysfunction. Evaluate periodic serum levels of ALT, AST, TBIL, and ALP.

Patient Counseling: Counsel on signs/symptoms of liver dysfunction. Instruct that if jaundice develops, immediately contact physician and d/c therapy. Inform that serial monitoring of LFTs will be required. Instruct on how to properly administer drug. Inform patients will require periodic monitoring of serial IGF-I levels in order to adjust dosing.

Administration: SQ route. Reconstitute. 1) Withdraw 1mL of SWFI and inject it into vial; 2) Roll vial; do not shake. Assess that solution is clear after reconstitution. Administer within 6 hrs after reconstitution. **Storage:** Refrigerate at 2-8°C (36-46°F). Protect from freezing.

SONATA
zaleplon (King)

CIV

THERAPEUTIC CLASS: Pyrazolopyrimidine (non-benzodiazepine)

INDICATIONS: Short-term treatment of insomnia.

DOSAGE: *Adults:* Insomnia: 10mg qhs. Low Weight Patients: Start with 5mg hs. Max: 20mg/day. Elderly/Debilitated/Concomitant Cimetidine: 5mg qhs. Max: 10mg/day. Mild to Moderate Hepatic Dysfunction: 5mg qhs. Take immediately prior to bedtime.

HOW SUPPLIED: Cap: 5mg, 10mg

WARNINGS/PRECAUTIONS: Monitor elderly/debilitated closely. Abnormal thinking and behavioral changes reported. Avoid abrupt withdrawal. Abuse potential exists. Caution in respiratory disorders, depression, conditions affecting metabolism or hemodynamic responses, and mild-to-moderate hepatic insufficiency. Not for use in severe hepatic impairment. May cause impaired coordination even the following day. Re-evaluate if no improvement of insomnia after 7-10 days of therapy. Contains tartrazine.

ADVERSE REACTIONS: Headache, asthenia, nausea, dizziness, amnesia, somnolence, eye pain, dysmenorrhea, abdominal pain.

INTERACTIONS: Potentiates CNS depression with psychotropics (eg, thioridazine, imipramine), anticonvulsants, antihistamines, alcohol and other CNS depressants. CYP3A4 inducers (eg, rifampin, phenytoin, carbamazepine and phenobarbital) decreases levels. Potentiated by cimetidine.

PREGNANCY: Category C, not for use in nursing.

MECHANISM OF ACTION: Pyrazolopyrimidine class; interacts with GABA-benzodiazepine receptor complex.

PHARMACOKINETICS: Absorption: Rapid and complete. T_{max}=1 hr. Absolute bioavailability (approximately 30%) (IV). **Distribution:** V_d=1.4L/kg; plasma protein binding (60%). **Metabolism:** Extensive, liver via aldehyde oxidase. **Elimination:** Urine (71%), feces (17%); $T_{1/2}$=1 hrs.

NURSING CONSIDERATIONS

Assessment: Assess for primary psychiatric and/or medical illness; hypersensitivity to drug, compromised respiratory function (COPD, sleep apnea), depression, suicidal tendencies, hepatic/renal impairment, drug abuse/addiction, alcohol intake, and drug interactions.

Monitoring: Monitor for anaphylactic/anaphylactoid reactions, worsening of insomnia, abnormal thinking and behavior changes, complex behaviors (eg, sleep-driving), physical/psychological dependence, withdrawal symptoms, amnesia, headache, abdominal pain, asthenia, nausea and somnolence, hepatic and pulmonary functions.

Patient Counseling: Take drug immediately prior to bedtime. Caution against hazardous tasks (eg, operating machinery/driving). Inform about the benefits/risks, possibility of physical/psychological dependence and memory disturbances. Notify if pregnant/nursing or planning to become pregnant. Do not increase dose or d/c drug before consulting physician. Avoid alcohol.

Administration: Oral route. **Storage:** 20-25°C (68-77°F).

SORIATANE RX

acitretin (Stiefel)

Avoid in pregnancy or becoming pregnant ≤3 yrs after discontinuation of therapy; use 2 reliable forms of contraception. Only use in females of reproductive potential with severe psoriasis unresponsive or contraindicated to other therapies, if receive warnings of therapy hazards and risk of contraception failure, if negative pregnancy test within 1 week before therapy, will begin therapy on the 2nd or 3rd day of next menstrual cycle, are capable of complying with contraceptive measures and are reliable. Repeat pregnancy testing and contraception counseling on a regular basis. The patient must have a negative result from a urine or serum pregnancy test. before receiving Soriatane prescription. It is not known whether residual acitretin in seminal fluid poses risk to fetus with male patients during or after therapy. Females should avoid ethanol during and 2 months after therapy. Severe birth defects reported.

THERAPEUTIC CLASS: Retinoid

INDICATIONS: Treatment of severe psoriasis, including erythrodermic and generalized pustular types.

DOSAGE: *Adults:* Initial: 25-50mg single dose qd with main meal. Individualize dose based on intersubject variation in pharmacokinetics, clinical efficacy, and incidence of side effects. Maint: 25-50mg qd. Terminate therapy when lesions resolve. May treat relapses as outlined for initial therapy.

HOW SUPPLIED: Cap: 10mg, 25mg

CONTRAINDICATIONS: See Black Box Warnings. Pregnancy.

WARNINGS/PRECAUTIONS: Risk of hepatotoxicity, hyperostosis, pancreatitis, and pseudotumor cerebri. D/C if visual difficulties occur; decreased night vision and reduced tolerance to contact lenses reported. Bone abnormalities of the vertebral column, knees, and ankles reported. Increases TG and cholesterol and decreases HDL; perform lipid tests before therapy every 1-2 weeks until establish lipid response. Caution with severe hepatic/renal impairment. Transient worsening of psoriasis may occur initially. Do not donate blood during and for 3 yrs after therapy. Avoid sun lamps and excessive sun exposure. Depression and/or psychiatric symptoms (eg, aggressive feelings, thoughts of self-harm) reported. Thinning of the skin observed.

ADVERSE REACTIONS: Ophthalmologic effects, cheilitis, rhinitis, dry mouth, epistaxis, alopecia, dry skin, rash, skin peeling, nail disorder, pruritus, paresthesia, paronychia, skin atrophy, sticky skin, xerophthalmia, arthralgia, rash, acute myocardial infarction, stroke, vulvo-vaginitis.

INTERACTIONS: Caution with oral hypoglycemics. May increase risk of hepatotoxicity with methotrexate. Interferes with microdosed progestin "minipill" oral contraceptives. Females should avoid ethanol during and 2 months after therapy. Possible additive toxic effects with vitamin A doses that exceed minimum RDAs.

PREGNANCY: Category X, not for use in nursing.

MECHANISM OF ACTION: Retinoid antipsoriatic; not established.

PHARMACOKINETICS: Absorption: C_{max}=416ng/mL; T_{max}=2-5 hrs. **Distribution:** Plasma protein binding (99.9%); found in breast milk. **Metabolism:** Extensive; via isomerization to cis-acitretin; metabolized with the parent drug into chain-shortened breakdown metaboilites and conjugates. **Elimination:** Chain-shortened breakdown metabolites and conjugates; feces (34-54%), urine (16-53%). Acitretin: $T_{1/2}$=49 hrs. Cis-acitretin: $T_{1/2}$=63 hrs.

NURSING CONSIDERATIONS

Assessment: Prior to therapy, must have had 2 negative urine or serum pregnancy tests. Assess for exclusion of pregnancy/nursing. Assess for renal/liver impairment, chronic abnormally elevated blood lipid values, DM, obesity, increased alcohol intake, or a familial history of these conditions, cardiovascular status, pre-existing abnormalities of the spine or knees or ankles, and possible drug interactions (eg, tetracyclines). Blood lipids and LFT levels should be evaluated prior to therapy and again at intervals of 1-2 weeks.

Monitoring: Monitor for hepatotoxicity, hyperostosis, hypertriglyceridemia, radiological changes of pre-exsiting abnormalities of the spine (eg, degenerative spurs, anterior bridging of spinal vertebrae, diffuse idiopathic skeletal hyperostosis, ligament calcification, and narrowing/destruction of the cervical disc space), MI or other thromboembolic events, pancreatitis, psychiatric problems, and signs/symptoms of pseudotumor cerebri (eg, headache, NV, visual disturbances, papilledema). Monitor the eye for dryness, lash loss, irritation, Bell's Palsy, blepharitis, blurred vision, cataracts, and papilledema. Careful monitoring for LFTs, lipids, and blood sugar. Pregnancy test must be repeated every month during therapy and for at least 3 yrs after d/c.

Patient Counseling: Inform about the Pregnancy Prevention Actively Required During and After Treatment (P.A.R.T) program and about the risks of therapy. Advise to use 2 effective forms of contraception at least 1 month prior to initiation of therapy. Do not donate blood during or at least 3 yrs following completion of therapy. Required by law that medication guide must be given to patient each time therapy is dispensed. Do not ingest beverages or products containing ethanol while taking therapy and for 2 months after d/c of therapy. Notify physician if nursing. Caution when driving or operating a vehicle at night. Advise against taking vitamin A supplements to avoid additive toxic effects. Avoid excessive exposure to sunlight.

Administration: Oral route. Take with food. **Storage:** 15-25°C (59-77°F). Avoid light or humidity exposure after opening bottle.

SPIRIVA — RX

tiotropium bromide (Boehringer Ingelheim/Pfizer)

THERAPEUTIC CLASS: Anticholinergic bronchodilator

INDICATIONS: Long-term, once-daily, maintenance treatment of bronchospasm associated with chronic obstructive pulmonary disease (COPD), including chronic bronchitis and emphysema.

DOSAGE: *Adults:* Inhale contents of one capsule (18mcg) qd, with HandiHaler device.

HOW SUPPLIED: Cap, Inhalation: 18mcg

CONTRAINDICATIONS: Hypersensitivity to atropine or its derivatives (eg, ipratropium).

WARNINGS/PRECAUTIONS: Not for initial treatment of acute episodes. D/C if hypersensitivity (eg, angioedema) or paradoxical bronchospasm occurs. Caution with narrow-angle glaucoma, prostatic hyperplasia, bladder-neck obstruction. Monitor with moderate to severe renal impairment (CrCl ≤50mL/min). Contents of caps are for oral inhalation only and must not be swallowed.

ADVERSE REACTIONS: Dry mouth, arthritis, cough, flu-like symptoms, sinusitis, constipation, abdominal pain, UTI, moniliasis, rash, dizziness, dysphagia, hoarseness, intestinal obstruction-ileus paralytic, increased IOP, oral candidiasis, tachycardia, throat irritation.

INTERACTIONS: Avoid with other anticholinergics (eg, ipratropium).

PREGNANCY: Category C, caution in nursing.

MECHANISM OF ACTION: Anticholinergic; inhibits M_3-receptors on smooth muscle leading to bronchodilation.

PHARMACOKINETICS: Absorption: Absolute bioavailability (19.5%); T_{max}=5 min. **Distribution:** V_d=32L/kg; plasma protein binding (72%). **Metabolism:** Liver (oxidation, conjugation) via CYP2D6, 3A4. **Elimination:** (Inhalation): Urine (14%); (IV): Urine (74%). $T_{1/2}$=5-6 days.

NURSING CONSIDERATIONS

Assessment: Assess for hypersensitivity of atropine or its derivatives, narrow-angle glaucoma, prostatic hyperplasia, bladder-neck obstruction, renal impairment, and possible drug interactions.

Monitoring: Monitor for urinary retention, mydriasis, GI distress (diarrhea, NV), paradoxical bronchospasm and allergic type-reaction (pruritus, angioedema of tongue, lips and face, urticaria, laryngospasm, anaphylaxis).

S

Patient Counseling: Inform that contents of capsule are for oral inhalation only and must not be swallowed. Do not increase dose or frequency. Not for acute periods of bronchospasm. Seek medical attention if experience symptoms of precipitation or worsening of narrow-angle glaucoma, mydriasis, increased IOP, acute eye pain/discomfort, blurring of vision, visual halos or colored images with red eyes from conjunctival and corneal congestion, and allergic/hypersensitivity reactions.

Administration: Oral inhalation. 1) Press green piercing button to open cap; pull cap up to expose mouthpiece. Open mouthpiece by pulling ridge up. 2) Remove one Cap immediately before use; insert in center chamber. 3) Close mouthpiece firmly until hear click. 4) Hold device with mouthpiece up; press green piercing button against base and release. 5) Exhale (not into mouthpiece); put mouthpiece in lips; keep head upright, device in horizontal position; breathe in slowly and deeply to hear or feel Cap vibrate; breathe in until lungs are full; hold breath as long as comfortable, and remove device from lips. 6) To ensure full dose, must breathe out again completely and inhale once again as described above. 7) After finished taking dose, open mouthpiece and tip out used Cap and discard. 8) Clean mouthpiece once a month. **Storage:** 25°C (77°F); excursions permitted to 15-30°C (59-86°F). Do not expose Cap to extreme temperatures or moisture.

SPORANOX — RX

itraconazole (Janssen/Ortho Biotech)

Contraindicated with cisapride, pimozide, quinidine, dofetilide, or levacetylmethadol. Serious cardiovascular events (eg, QT prolongation, torsades de pointes, ventricular tachycardia, cardiac arrest, and/or sudden death) reported with cisapride, pimozide, quinidine, and other CYP3A4 inhibitors. Do not use caps for onychomycosis with ventricular dysfunction.

THERAPEUTIC CLASS: Azole antifungal

INDICATIONS: (Cap) Onychomycosis of the toenail and fingernail in immunocompetent patients. Confirm diagnosis before therapy. (Cap) Treatment of blastomycosis and histoplasmosis. Treatment of aspergillosis if refractory to or intolerant to amphotericin B. (Sol) Treatment of oropharyngeal and esophageal candidiasis. (Sol) Empiric therapy of febrile, neutropenic patients with suspected fungal infections (ETFN).

DOSAGE: *Adults:* Cap: Take with full meal. If patient has achlorhydria or taking gastric acid suppressors, give with cola beverage. Onychomycosis: Toenail: 200mg qd for 12 consecutive weeks. Fingernail: 200mg bid for 1 week, skip 3 weeks, then repeat. Blastomycosis/Histoplasmosis: 200mg qd. May increase by 100mg increments if no improvement. Max: 400mg/day. Give bid if dose >200mg/day. Aspergillosis: 200-400mg/day. Life-Threatening Infections: LD: 200mg tid for 1st 3 days. Continue for at least 3 months and until infection subsides. Sol: Take on empty stomach. Swish 10mL at a time for several seconds, then swallow. Candidiasis: Oropharyngeal: 200mg/day for 1-2 weeks. If refractory to fluconazole, give 100mg bid (response in 2-4 weeks; may relapse shortly after d/c). Esophageal: 100-200mg/day for at least 3 weeks. Continue for 2 weeks after symptoms resolve.

S

HOW SUPPLIED: Cap: 100mg; Sol: 10mg/mL [150mL]

CONTRAINDICATIONS: (Cap, Sol) Concomitant cisapride, oral midazolam, pimozide, quinidine, dofetilide, triazolam, and HMG-CoA reductase inhibitors metabolized by CYP3A4 (eg, lovastatin, simvastatin). (Cap) Treatment of onychomycosis if pregnant or contemplating pregnancy, ventricular dysfunction (eg, CHF).

WARNINGS/PRECAUTIONS: Rare cases of hepatotoxicity reported. Monitor LFTs; d/c if hepatic dysfunction develops. Avoid with liver disease. D/C if neuropathy or CHF occurs. Sol and caps not interchangeable. Consider alternative therapy if unresponsive in patients with cystic fibrosis. Avoid with ventricular dysfunction. Caution with ischemic/valvular disease, pulmonary disease, renal failure, other edematous disorders. Avoid injection if CrCl <30mL/min.

ADVERSE REACTIONS: NV, diarrhea, abdominal pain, fever, cough, rash, increased sweating, headache, hypokalemia.

INTERACTIONS: See Contraindications. Increased levels with cisapride, pimozide, quinidine, dofetilide, oral midazolam, triazolam, HMG-CoA reductase inhibitors; concurrent use contraindicated. Increases levels of rifabutin, immunosuppressants, protease inhibitors, alfentanil, buspirone, methylprednisolone, trimetrexate, carbamazepine, HMG-CoA reductase inhibitors, digoxin, warfarin, busulfan, docetaxel, vinca alkaloids, astemizole, alprazolam, diazepam, oral midazolam, triazolam, dihydropyridine CCBs, verapamil, oral hypoglycemics. CYP3A4 inducers (eg, carbamazepine, phenobarbital, phenytoin, isoniazid, rifabutin, rifampin, nevirapine) decrease itraconazole levels. CYP3A4 inhibitors (eg, erythromycin, clarithromycin, indinavir, ritonavir) may increase itraconazole levels. Severe hypoglycemia with oral hypoglycemics. Additive negative inotropic effects with CCBs. Edema reported with dihydropyridine CCBs; adjust dose. Decreased absorption of caps with antacids or gastric secretion suppressors.

PREGNANCY: Category C, not for use in nursing.

MECHANISM OF ACTION: Azole antifungal agent; inhibits the CYP450-dependent synthesis of ergosterol, which is a vital component of fungal cell membranes.

PHARMACOKINETICS: Absorption: Absolute bioavailabilty (55%). Oral administration of variable doses resulted in different parameters. **Metabolism:** Liver via CYP3A4; hydroxyitraconazole (major metabolite). **Distribution:** Plasma protein binding (99.8%). **Elimination:** Urine (40%), feces (3-18%) (inactive metabolites).

NURSING CONSIDERATIONS

Assessment: Assess for proper diagnosis of fungal infection (eg, cultures, microscopic studies), cardiac function (eg, ventricular dysfunction, CHF) prior to administration. Assess pregnancy status prior to use.

Monitoring: Monitor for signs/symptoms of CHF including QT prolongation, torsade de pointes, ventricular tachycardia, cardiac arrest, and liver dysfunction, for possible drug interactions, and LFTs. Blood glucose concentrations should also be monitored when coadminstered with hypoglycemic agents. Monitor for signs of rash (Stevens-Johnson syndrome).

Patient Counseling: Instruct to take drug with a full meal. Counsel on signs/symptoms of CHF and liver dysfunction, which include unusual fatigue, anorexia, NV, jaundice, dark urine or pale stools. Counsel females to avoid pregnancy while on medication and to remain on contraceptives for 2 months following completion of therapy. Notify physician if rash develops.

Administration: Oral route. **Storage:** 15-25°C (59-77°F). Protect from light and moisture.

S

SPRYCEL — RX

dasatinib (Bristol-Myers Squibb)

THERAPEUTIC CLASS: Tyrosine kinase inhibitor

INDICATIONS: Treatment of chronic, accelerated, or myeloid or lymphoid blast phase chronic myeloid leukemia (CML) with resistance or intolerance to prior therapy including imatinib. Treatment of Philadelphia chromosome-positive acute lymphoblastic leukemia (Ph+ ALL) with resistance or intolerance to prior therapy.

DOSAGE: *Adults:* Chronic Phase CML: 100mg qd. Accelerated Phase CML/Myeloid or Lymphoid Blast Phase CML/Ph+ ALL: 70mg bid. Swallow whole; do not crush. Concomitant Strong CYP3A4 Inducers: Consider dose increase. Concomitant Strong CYP3A4 Inhibitors: Consider dose decrease to 20mg daily. Refer to PI for dose modifications for neutropenia and thrombocytopenia.

HOW SUPPLIED: Tab: 20mg, 50mg, 70mg

WARNINGS/PRECAUTIONS: Severe thrombocytopenia, neutropenia, and anemia reported; monitor CBC weekly for first 2 months, then monthly thereafter. Severe CNS hemorrhages including fatalities, GI hemorrhage, and other hemorrhage cases reported; caution in patients on medications that inhibit platelet function or anticoagulants. Pleural and pericardial effusion reported. Severe ascites, generalized edema, severe pulmonary edema reported. QT prolongation reported; caution in patients at risk (eg, hypokalemia or hypomagnesemia, congenital long QT syndrome, concomitant antiarrhythmics or other QT prolonging agents, cumulative high-dose anthracycline therapy); correct hypokalemia or hypomagnesemia prior to administration. Caution with hepatic impairment. Fetal harm may occur; avoid pregnancy.

ADVERSE REACTIONS: Fluid retention events, diarrhea, nausea, headache, abdominal pain, vomiting, bleeding events, pyrexia, pleural effusion, neutropenia, thrombocytopenia, dyspnea, anemia, skin rash, fatigue, myelosuppression, QT prolongation.

INTERACTIONS: Increased levels with CYP3A4 inhibitors (eg, ketoconazole, itraconazole, erythromycin, clarithromycin, ritonavir, atazanavir, indinavir, nefazodone, nelfinavir, saquinavir, telithromycin). Decreased levels with CYP3A4 inducers (eg, dexamethasone, phenytoin, carbamazepine, rifampicin, phenobarbital, St. John's wort). Avoid antacids; if necessary, administer 2 hrs prior to or 2 hrs after dose. Concomitant use of H_2 blockers or PPIs not recommended. Caution with CYP3A4 substrates with narrow therapeutic windows (eg, alfentanil, astemizole, terfenadine, cisapride, cyclosporine, fentanyl, pimozide, quinidine, sirolimus, tacrolimus, or ergot alkaloids such as ergotamine and dihydroergotamine).

PREGNANCY: Category D, not for use in nursing.

MECHANISM OF ACTION: Tyrosine kinase inhibitor; inhibits BCR-ABL and SRC family kinases.

PHARMACOKINETICS: Absorption: T_{max}=0.5-6 hrs. **Distribution:** V_d=2505L; plasma protein binding (96%). **Metabolism:** Extensive via CYP3A4. **Elimination:** Urine (4%), feces (85%); $T_{1/2}$=3-5 hrs.

NURSING CONSIDERATIONS

Assessment: Assess for possible drug interactions, pregnancy/nursing status, hepatic impairment, prolonged QTc, lactose intolerance, hypokalemia, and hypomagnesemia. Obtain baseline CBC, LFTs, and electrolytes.

Monitoring: Monitor CBC weekly for first 2 months and monthly afterward and LFTs periodically. Monitor for signs/symptoms of hemorrhage, myelosuppression, pleural effusion, fluid retention, QT prolongation, and hypersensitivity reactions. If symptoms of pleural effusion are present, perform CXR.

Patient Counseling: Inform of pregnancy risks and that drug contains lactose. Take whole; do not break, cut, or crush. Do not take with grapefruit juice. Advise to seek medical attention if experience symptoms of hemorrhage (unusual bleeding, easy bruising), myelosuppression (fever, infection), pleural effusion (dyspnea, dry cough), fluid retention (swelling, weight gain, SOB), QT prolongation, hypersensitivity reactions, significant NV, diarrhea, headache, musculoskeletal pain, fatigue, or rash.

Administration: Oral route. **Storage:** 25°C (77°F); excursions permitted to 15-30°C (59-86°F).

STALEVO — RX

entacapone - levodopa - carbidopa (Novartis)

THERAPEUTIC CLASS: Dopa-decarboxylase inhibitor/dopamine precursor/ COMT inhibitor

INDICATIONS: Treatment of idiopathic Parkinson's disease to substitute for equivalent doses of previously administered carbidopa/levodopa and entacapone or for those experiencing signs and symptoms of end-of-dose "wearing off" and are taking up to 600mg/day levodopa without experiencing dyskinesias.

DOSAGE: *Adults:* Currently Taking Carbidopa/Levodopa and Entacapone: May switch directly to corresponding strength of carbidopa/levodopa.

Currently Taking Carbidopa/Levodopa but not Entacapone: First titrate individually with carbidopa/levodopa product and entacapone product then transfer to corresponding dose. Max: Stalevo 50/Stalevo 75/Stalevo 100/ Stalevo 125/Stalevo 150: 8 tabs/day. Stalevo 200: 6 tabs/day.

HOW SUPPLIED: Tab: (Carbidopa/Levodopa/Entacapone): Stalevo 50: 12.5mg/50mg/200mg; Stalevo 75: 18.75mg/75mg/200mg; Stalevo 100: 25mg/100mg/200mg; Stalevo 125: 31.25mg/125mg/200mg; Stalevo 150: 37.5mg/150mg/200mg; Stalevo 200: 50mg/200mg/200mg

CONTRAINDICATIONS: MAOIs during or within 14 days of use, narrow-angle glaucoma, undiagnosed skin lesions, history of melanoma.

WARNINGS/PRECAUTIONS: Dyskinesia, mental disturbances, hypotension/ syncope, hallucinations, rhabdomyolysis, hyperpyrexia, confusion, and fibrotic complications reported. Caution with biliary obstruction, severe cardiovascular or pulmonary disease, bronchial asthma, renal, hepatic or endocrine disease, chronic wide-angle glaucoma, history of MI with residual arrhythmias, peptic ulcer. Neuroleptic malignant syndrome reported with dose reductions or withdrawal. Avoid rapid withdrawal or abrupt dose reduction. May cause dark color to appear in saliva, urine, or sweat. May cause false (+) ketonuria, false (-) glucosuria (glucose-oxidase method), elevated LFTs, abnormal BUN, positive Coombs' test. May depress prolactin secretion and increase growth hormone levels. Have higher risk of developing melanoma with Parkinson's disease.

ADVERSE REACTIONS: Dyskinesia, hyperkinesia, hypokinesia, dizziness, nausea, diarrhea, abdominal pain, constipation, vomiting, urine discoloration, back pain, fatigue, dry mouth, dyspnea.

INTERACTIONS: See Contraindications. Increased HR, arrhythmias, and BP changes with drugs metabolized by COMT (eg, isoproterenol, epinephrine, norepinephrine, dopamine, dobutamine, alpha-methyldopa, apomorphine, isoetherine, bitolterol). Probenecid, cholestyramine, and some antibiotics (eg, erythromycin, rifampicin, ampicillin, chloramphenicol) may interfere with biliary excretion. Risk of postural hypotension with antihypertensives, selegiline. HTN and dyskinesia may occur with TCAs. Reduced effect with phenytoin, papaverine, metoclopramide, isoniazid, dopamine D_2 antagonists (eg, phenothiazines, butyrophenones, risperidone). Reduced bioavailability with iron salts. Caution with highly protein-bound drugs (eg, warfarin, salicylic acid, phenylbutazone, diazepam).

PREGNANCY: Category C, caution in nursing.

MECHANISM OF ACTION: Dopa-decarboxylase inhibitor/dopamine precursor/COMT inhibitor. Carbidopa: Inhibits the decarboxylation of peripheral levodopa, making more levodopa available for brain transport. Levodopa: Crosses blood-brain barrier and presumably converted to dopamine in brain. Entacapone: Sustains plasma levels of levodopa, resulting in more constant dopaminergic stimulation in brain.

PHARMACOKINETICS: Absorption: Levodopa: Rapidly absorbed. (PO) Administration of variable doses resulted in different parameters. Entacapone: Rapidly absorbed; C_{max}=1200-1500ng/mL; T_{max}=0.8-1.2 hrs; AUC=1250-1750ng•hr/mL. Carbidopa: Slightly absorbed; C_{max}=40-225ng/mL; T_{max}=2.5-3.4 hrs; AUC=170-1200ng•hr/mL. **Distribution:** Levodopa: Plasma protein binding (10-30%). Entacapone: (98%). Carbidopa: (Approximately 36%). **Metabolism:** Levodopa: Extensive decarboxylation by dopa decarboxylase and O-methylation by catechol-O-methyltransferase. Entacapone: Completely metabolized. Carbidopa: Main metabolites: α-methyl-3-methoxy-4-hydroxyphenylpropionic acid, and α-methyl-3,4-dihydroxyphenylpropionic acid. **Elimination:** Levodopa: $T_{1/2}$=1.7 hrs. Entacapone: Feces (90%), urine (10%); $T_{1/2}$=0.8-1 hr. Carbidopa: Urine (30%, unchanged); $T_{1/2}$=1.6-2 hrs.

NURSING CONSIDERATIONS

Assessment: Assess LFTs, renal function, CBC, chronic wide-angle glaucoma, dyskinesia, psychosis, depression, cardiovascular complications, and biliary obstructions.

S

Monitoring: Monitor LFTs, renal function, CBC, BP, biliary obstruction, depression and suicidal ideations, worsening of dyskinesia, rhabdomyolysis, diarrhea, hallucinations, fibrotic complications, and hyperpyrexia.

Patient Counseling: Instruct to take as prescribed. Caution while operating machinery/driving. Discoloration of bodily fluids may occcur. High-protein diet, excessive acidity, and iron salts reduce clinical effectiveness. Wearing-off effect may be seen at end of dosing interval. Report any adverse effects. Advise to notify physicians if need to breastfeed or breastfeeding an infant. Inform that hallucinations may occur. Inform physicians if experiencing gambling, increased sexual and other urges.

Administration: Oral route. **Storage:** Store at 25°C (77°F); excursions permitted to 15-30°C (59-86°F). Dispense in tight container.

STARLIX RX

nateglinide (Novartis)

THERAPEUTIC CLASS: Meglitinide

INDICATIONS: Adjunct to diet and exercise, as monotherapy, to improve glycemic control in type 2 diabetics who have not been chronically treated with other antidiabetic agents. May be used in combination with metformin or a thiazolidinedione (TZD).

DOSAGE: *Adults:* Initial/Maint: 120mg tid before meals (with or without metformin or TZD). Take 1-30 min before meals. May use 60mg tid (with or without metformin or TZD) in patients near goal HbA_{1c}. Skip dose if meal is skipped.

HOW SUPPLIED: Tab: 60mg, 120mg

CONTRAINDICATIONS: Type 1 diabetes, diabetic ketoacidosis.

WARNINGS/PRECAUTIONS: Caution in moderate to severe hepatic impairment. Transient loss of glucose control with trauma, surgery, fever, and infection; may need insulin therapy. Secondary failure may occur in prolonged therapy. Hypoglycemia risk in elderly, debilitated, malnourished, strenuous exercise, and with adrenal or pituitary insufficiency. Autonomic neuropathy may mask hypoglycemia.

ADVERSE REACTIONS: Upper respiratory infection, flu symptoms, dizziness, arthropathy, diarrhea, hypoglycemia, back pain, jaundice, cholestatic hepatitis, elevated liver enzymes.

INTERACTIONS: Potentiated hypoglycemia with alcohol, NSAIDs, salicylates, MAOIs, and non-selective β-blockers. Risk of hyperglycemia with thiazides, corticosteroids, thyroid products and sympathomimetics. May potentiate tolbutamide. Peak plasma levels reduced with liquid meals. β-blockers may mask hypoglycemic effects. Caution with highly protein-bound drugs.

PREGNANCY: Category C, not for use in nursing.

MECHANISM OF ACTION: Meglitinide; lowers blood glucose levels by stimulating insulin secretion from the pancreas.

PHARMACOKINETICS: Absorption: Absolute bioavailability (73%); C_{max}=1 hr. **Distribution:** V_d=10L; plasma protein binding (98%). **Metabolism:** CYP2C9, 3A4; hydroxylation, glucuronide conjugation. **Elimination:** Urine (75%), feces; $T_{1/2}$=1.5 hrs.

NURSING CONSIDERATIONS

Assessment: Assess FPG, HbA_{1c}, renal function, LFTs, diabetic ketoacidosis, pregnancy status, and for possible drug interactions.

Monitoring: Monitor FPG, HbA_{1c}, renal function, LFTs, uric acid levels, diabetic ketoacidosis, upper respiratory infection, back pain, flu symptoms, dizziness, arthropathy, diarrhea, accidental trauma, bronchitis, or coughing.

Patient Counseling: Inform about importance of adherence to meal planning, regular physical activity, regular blood glucose monitoring, periodic HbA_{1c} testing, recognition and management of hypo/hyperglycemia, and periodic assessment for diabetes complications. During periods of stress (eg, trauma, infection, surgery) medication requirements may change; seek prompt medical advice. Instruct to take 30 min before meals.

Administration: Oral route. **Storage:** 25°C (77°F); excursions permitted to 15-30°C (59-86°F).

STAVZOR

RX

valproic acid (Noven)

Fatal hepatotoxicity, usually during first 6 months, reported (children <2 yrs are at higher risk); monitor closely and perform LFTs prior to therapy and periodically thereafter. Teratogenic effects (eg, neural tube defects) and life-threatening pancreatitis reported.

THERAPEUTIC CLASS: Carboxylic acid derivative

INDICATIONS: Acute treatment of manic episodes associated with bipolar disorder; monotherapy, or adjunctive therapy for complex partial seizures and simple/complex absence seizures; adjunct therapy for multiple seizure types; migraine prophylaxis.

DOSAGE: *Adults*: Mania: Initial: 750mg daily in divided doses. Titrate: Increase rapidly to produce the desired clinical effect or plasma level (50-125mcg/mL). Max: 60mg/kg/day. Complex Partial Seizures (monotherapy/adjunctive): Initial: 10-15mg/kg/day. Titrate: Increase by 5-10mg/kg/week until optimal response (50-100mcg/mL). Max: 60mg/kg/day. Conversion to Monotherapy: Reduce concomitant antiepileptic drug (AED) dosage by 25% q2 weeks; withdrawal of AED highly variable, monitor closely for seizure frequency. Simple/Complex Absence Seizures: Initial: 15mg/kg/day. Titrate: Increase by 5-10mg/kg/week until optimal response (50-100mcg/mL). Max: 60mg/kg/day. If dose >250mg/day, give in divided doses. Migraine: Initial: 250mg bid. Max: 1000mg/day. Elderly: Reduce initial dose. Swallow whole. *Pediatrics*: ≥10 yrs: Complex Partial Seizures (monotherapy/adjunctive): Initial: 10-15mg/kg/day. Titrate: Increase by 5-10mg/kg/week until optimal response (50-100mcg/mL). Max: 60mg/kg/day. Simple/Complex Absence Seizures: Initial: 15mg/kg/day. Titrate: Increase by 5-10mg/kg/week until optimal response (50-100mcg/mL). Max: 60mg/kg/day. If dose > 250mg/day, give in divided doses. Swallow whole.

HOW SUPPLIED: Cap, Delayed-Release: 125mg, 250mg, and 500mg.

CONTRAINDICATIONS: Hepatic disease, significant hepatic dysfunction, and known urea cycle disorders (UCD).

WARNINGS/PRECAUTIONS: Monitor LFTs before therapy and during first 6 months; d/c if hepatic dysfunction and hemorrhagic pancreatitis occur. Increased risk of hepatotoxicity with multiple anticonvulsants, congenital metabolic disorders, severe seizure disorders with mental retardation, organic brain disease, and children <2 yrs. Avoid abrupt withdrawal. Fatal hyperammonemic encephalopathy observed with UCD; d/c if ammonia levels increase. Prior to therapy, evaluate for UCD in high-risk patients (eg, history of unexplained encephalopathy, coma). Dose-related thrombocytopenia may occur; measure platelets and coagulation tests prior to initiation and periodically thereafter. Measure ammonia levels if unexplained lethargy, vomiting or mental status changes develop. Somnolence in elderly may occur; increase dose slowly and monitor for fluid and nutritional intake. Hyperammonemia, hypothermia, multi-organ hypersensitivity reactions reported. May interfere with urine ketone and thyroid function tests.

S

ADVERSE REACTIONS: Headache, asthenia, rash, ataxia, nausea, vomiting, abdominal pain, dyspepsia, diarrhea, anorexia, somnolence, tremor, dizziness, diplopia, and flu syndrome.

INTERACTIONS: Phenytoin, carbamazepine, phenobarbital, or primidone may increase clearance. May potentiate amitriptyline/nortriptyline, carbamazepine-10, 11-epoxide, diazepam, ethosuximide, lamotrigine, tolbutamide, warfarin, and zidovudine. Potentiated by ASA and felbamate. Antagonized by rifampin, carbamazepine, phenobarbital, phenytoin, warfarin, and tolbutamide. Additive CNS depression with other CNS depressants (eg, alcohol). Carbapenum antibiotics may reduce serum levels. Clonazepam may induce absence status in patients with absence seizures. Concomitant topiramate may induce hyperammonemia.

PREGNANCY: Category D, not for use in nursing.

MECHANISM OF ACTION: Carboxylic acid derivative; not fully established. Suggested that increased brain concentrations of GABA contribute to its activity in epilepsy.

PHARMACOKINETICS: Absorption: T_{max}=2 hrs (with food), 4.8 hrs (without food). **Distribution:** V_d=11L/1.73m^2; plasma protein binding (10% at 40mcg/mL and 18.5% at 130mcg/mL), CSF distribution (10%). **Metabolism:** Hepatic via glucuronidation and beta-oxidation. **Elimination:** Urine (30-50% glucuronide conjugate); $T_{1/2}$=9-16 hrs.

NURSING CONSIDERATIONS

Assessment: Assess LFTs prior to therapy, plasma ammonia levels, hepatic dysfunction/disease, pancreatitis, risk of hepatoxicity and encephalopathy, and pregnancy/nursing status.

Monitoring: Monitor LFTs (at frequent intervals during first 6 months), CBC with platelets, coagulation parameters, pancreatitis, ketone and thyroid function tests, plasma drug levels, hyperammonemia, and hypersensitivity reactions.

Patient Counseling: Inform to take exactly as prescribed to get the most benefit and to reduce side effects. Counsel about signs/symptoms of hepatotoxicity, pancreatitis, and hyperammonemic encephalopathy. Avoid CNS depressants (eg, alcohol). Advise to exercise caution in driving or operating machinery.

Administration: Oral route. Do not chew. **Storage:** 25°C (77°F); excursions permitted to 15°-30°C (59°-86°F).

STRATTERA — RX

atomoxetine HCl (Lilly)

> **Increased risk of suicidal ideation in short-term studies in children or adolescents with ADHD. Closely monitor for suicidality, clinical worsening, or unusual changes in behavior. Close observation/communication with prescriber by families and caregivers is advised.**

THERAPEUTIC CLASS: Selective norepinephrine reuptake inhibitor

INDICATIONS: Treatment of attention-deficit hyperactivity disorder (ADHD).

DOSAGE: *Adults:* Initial: 40mg/day given qam or evenly divided doses in the am and late afternoon/early evening. Titrate: Increase after minimum of 3 days to target dose of about 80mg/day. After 2-4 weeks, may increase to max of 100mg/day. Max: 100mg/day. Hepatic Insufficiency: Moderate (Child-Pugh Class B): Reduce initial and target doses to 50% of normal dose. Severe (Child-Pugh Class C): Reduce initial and target doses to 25% of normal dose. Concomitant CYP450 2D6 inhibitor (eg, paroxetine, fluoxetine, quinidine): Initial: 40mg/day. Titrate: Only increase to 80mg/day if symptoms fail to improve after 4 weeks.

Pediatrics: ≥6 yrs: ≤70kg: Initial: 0.5mg/kg/day given qam or evenly divided doses in the am and late afternoon or early evening. Titrate: Increase after minimum of 3 days to target dose of about 1.2mg/kg/day. Max: 1.4mg/kg/day or 100mg, whichever is less. >70kg: Initial: 40mg/day given qam or evenly divided doses in the am and late afternoon/early evening. Titrate: Increase after minimum of 3 days to target dose of about 80mg/day. After 2-4 weeks, may increase to max of 100mg/day. Max: 100mg/day. Hepatic Insufficiency: Moderate (Child-Pugh Class B): Reduce initial and target doses to 50% of the normal dose. Severe (Child-Pugh Class C): Reduce initial and target doses to 25% of normal dose. Concomitant CYP450 2D6 inhibitor (eg, paroxetine, fluoxetine, quinidine): ≥6 yrs: ≤70kg: Initial: 0.5mg/kg/day. Titrate: Only increase to 1.2mg/kg/day if symptoms fail to improve after 4 weeks. >70kg: Initial: 40mg/day. Titrate: Only increase to 80mg/day if symptoms fail to improve after 4 weeks.

HOW SUPPLIED: Cap: 10mg, 18mg, 25mg, 40mg, 60mg, 80mg, 100mg

CONTRAINDICATIONS: During or within 14 days of MAOI use; narrow angle glaucoma.

WARNINGS/PRECAUTIONS: Monitor for clinical worsening and/or suicidality. Allergic reactions, orthostatic hypotension and syncope reported. Monitor growth. May increase BP and HR; caution with HTN, tachycardia, cardiovascular or cerebrovascular disease. May increase urinary retention and urinary hesitation. Rare cases of priapism reported. May cause severe liver injury in rare cases; monitor liver enzymes and d/c with jaundice or liver injury. Reports of MI, stroke and sudden death in adults. Avoid with known structural cardiac abnormalities or other serious cardiac problems. Physical exam and evaluation of patient history is necessary. Stimulants at usual doses can cause treatment-emergent psychotic or manic symptoms (eg, hallucinations, delusional thinking, mania) in children and adolescents without prior history of psychotic illness. Monitor for appearance or worsening of aggressive behavior or hostility.

ADVERSE REACTIONS: (Adults) Dry mouth, headache, insomnia, nausea, decreased appetite, constipation, dysmenorrhea, erectile disturbance, urinary retention. (Pediatrics) Upper abdominal pain, headache, vomiting, decreased appetite, irritability, dizziness, somnolence.

INTERACTIONS: See Contraindications. May potentiate the cardiovascular effects of albuterol or other β_2 agonists. Caution with pressor agents. Increased levels in extensive metabolizers with CYP2D6 inhibitors (eg, paroxetine, fluoxetine, quinidine); atomoxetine may need dose adjustment.

PREGNANCY: Category C, caution in nursing.

MECHANISM OF ACTION: Selective norepinephrine reuptake inhibitor; inhibits the presynaptic norepinephrine transporter, as determined in *ex vivo* uptake.

PHARMACOKINETICS: Absorption: (PO) rapid; T_{max}=1-2 hrs. **Distribution:** Plasma protein binding (98%). **Metabolism:** Via CYP2D6; 4-hydroxyatomoxetine (major metabolite). **Elimination:** Urine (>80%), feces (<17%); $T_{1/2}$=5 hrs;

NURSING CONSIDERATIONS

Assessment: Assess for agitation, glaucoma, tics, family history of Tourette's syndrome, cardiovascular conditions (eg, severe HTN, angina pectoris, cardiac abnormalities, arrhythmias, heart failure, recent MI), cerebrovascular disease, hyperthyroidism or thyrotoxicosis, bipolar disorder, history of drug dependence or alcoholism, renal function, LFTs, pregnancy status, and possible drug interactions.

Monitoring: Monitor for cardiac abnormalities, exacerbations of behavior disturbances and thought disorders, bipolar disorder, aggression, seizures, and visual disturbances. Monitor height and weight in children, LFTs, hypersensitivity reactions (angioneurotic edema), urinary retention, and priapism.

Patient Counseling: Inform about risks of treatment, appropriate use, drug abuse/dependence. Drug is an occular irritant. Use caution while operating machinery/driving. Avoid late evening doses to prevent insomnia. Inform of side effects (eg, suicidal ideation, depression, liver injury, priapism) and advise to report any. Take as prescribed; swallow tablet, do not chew or crush.

Administration: Oral route. **Storage:** 25°C (77°F); excursions permitted to 15-30°C (59-86°F).

STREPTOMYCIN RX

streptomycin sulfate (Various)

Risk of severe neurotoxic reactions (eg, vestibular and cochlear disturbances) increased significantly with renal dysfunction or pre-renal azotemia. Optic nerve dysfunction, peripheral neuritis, arachnoiditis, and encephalopathy may occur. Monitor renal function; reduce dose with renal impairment and/or nitrogen retention. Do not exceed peak serum level of 20-25mcg/mL with kidney damage. Avoid other neurotoxic and/or nephrotoxic drugs (eg, neomycin, kanamycin, gentamicin, cephaloridine, paromomycin, viomycin, polymyxin B, colistin, tobramycin, cyclosporine). Respiratory paralysis can occur, especially if given soon after anesthesia or muscle relaxants. Reserve parenteral form when adequate lab and audiometric testing is available.

THERAPEUTIC CLASS: Aminoglycoside

INDICATIONS: Treatment of moderate to severe infections such as mycobacterium tuberculosis (TB) and non-TB infections (eg, plague, tularemia, chancroid, granuloma inguinale, *H.influenzae* and *K.pneumoniae* infections, UTI, gram-negative bacillary bacteremia, endocardial infections).

DOSAGE: *Adults:* IM only. TB: 15mg/kg/day (Max: 1g), or 25-30mg/kg twice weekly (Max: 1.5g), or 25-30mg/kg three times weekly (Max: 1.5g). Do not exceed a total dose of 120g over the course of therapy unless no other therapeutic options exist. Elderly (>60 yrs): Reduce dose. Treat for minimum of 1 year if possible. Tularemia: 1-2g/day in divided doses for 7-14 days until afebrile for 5-7 days. Plague: 1g bid for minimum of 10 days. Streptococcal Endocarditis: With PCN, 1g bid for week 1, then 500mg bid for week 2. Elderly (>60 yrs): 500mg bid for 2 weeks. Enterococcal Endocarditis: With PCN, 1g bid for 2 weeks, then 500mg bid for 4 weeks. Renal Impairment: Reduce dose. Moderate/Severe Infections: 1-2g/day in divided doses q6-12h. Max: 2g/day. *Pediatrics:* IM only. TB: 20-40mg/kg/day (Max: 1g), or 25-30mg/kg twice weekly (Max: 1.5g), or 25-30mg/kg three times weekly (Max: 1.5g). Do not exceed a total dose of 120g over the course of therapy unless no other therapeutic options exist. Treat for minimum of 1 year if possible. Moderate/Severe Infections: 20-40mg/kg/day (8-20mg/lb/day) in divided doses q6-12h.

HOW SUPPLIED: Inj: 1g

WARNINGS/PRECAUTIONS: Vestibular and auditory dysfunction may occur. Contains sodium metabisulfite. Can cause fetal harm in pregnancy. Caution with dose selection in renal impairment. Alkalinize urine to minimize or prevent renal irritation with prolonged therapy. CNS depression (eg, stupor, flaccidity) reported in infants with higher than recommended doses. If syphilis is suspected when treating venereal infections, perform dark field exam before initiating treatment, and monthly serologic tests for at least 4 months. Overgrowth of nonsusceptible organisms may occur. Terminate therapy when toxic symptoms appear, when impending toxicity is feared, when organisms become resistant, or when full treatment effect has been obtained. Contains sodium metabisulfite, a sulfite that may cause allergic-type reactions including anaphylaxis.

ADVERSE REACTIONS: Vestibular ototoxicity (N/V, vertigo), paresthesia of face, rash, fever, urticaria, angioneurotic edema, eosinophilia, nephrotoxicity (rare).

INTERACTIONS: See Black Box Warning. Increased ototoxicity with ethacrynic acid, furosemide, mannitol, and possibly other diuretics.

PREGNANCY: Category D, not for use in nursing.

MECHANISM OF ACTION: Aminoglycoside agent; interferes with normal protein synthesis.

PHARMACOKINETICS: Absorption: C_{max}=25-50mcg/mL; T_{max}=1 hr. **Distribution:** Passes through placenta; found in breast milk. **Elimination:** Urine (29-89%).

S

NURSING CONSIDERATIONS

Assessment: Assess for pre-existing auditory dysfunction, renal impairment, pregnancy/nursing status, and possible drug interactions. Perform baseline and periodic caloric stimulation/audiometric tests; perform dark field exam if concomitant syphilis is suspected prior to initiation of therapy and thereafter for at least 4 months.

Monitoring: Monitor for signs/symptoms of ototoxicity (vestibular/auditory dysfunction), headache, NV, and disequilibrium, CNS depression (stupor and flaccidity), overgrowth of nonsusceptible organisms, development of drug resistance, fetal harm if taken during pregnancy, skin sensitivity reactions and *C.difficile*-associated diarrhea.

Patient Counseling: Inform drug only treats bacterial, not viral, infections. Instruct to take exactly as prescribed; skipping doses or not completing full course may decrease effectiveness and increase resistance. Notify physician if pregnant/nursing or planning to become pregnant. Counsel about potential risks of therapy. Advise to d/c therapy and consult physician if any clinical signs of ototoxicity occur.

Administration: IM route. **Storage:** 15-30°C (59-86°F). Protect from light.

STROMECTOL RX
ivermectin (Merck)

THERAPEUTIC CLASS: Avermectins derivative

INDICATIONS: Treatment of strongyloidiasis of the intestinal tract due to *Strongyloides stercoralis*, and onchocerciasis due to *Onchocerca volvulus*. Has no activity against adult *Onchocerca volvulus* parasites.

DOSAGE: *Adults:* Strongyloidiasis/ ≥80kg: 200mcg/kg single dose. 15-24kg: 1 tab (3mg). 25-35kg: 2 tabs. 36-50kg: 3 tabs. 51-65kg: 4 tabs. 66-79kg: 5 tabs. Onchocerciasis/ ≥85kg: 150mcg/kg single dose. 15-25kg: 1 tab (3mg). 26-44kg; 2 tabs. 45-64kg: 3 tabs. 65-84kg: 4 tabs. For mass distribution in international treatment programs, the usual dosing interval is 12 months. Usual dosing interval for retreatment for individual patients can be as short as 3 months. Take on empty stomach with water. To verify eradication of infection perform follow-up stool exams.
Pediatrics: ≥15kg: Strongyloidiasis: 200mcg/kg single dose. Onchocerciasis: 150mcg/kg single dose. For mass distribution in international treatment programs, the usual dosing interval is 12 months. Usual dosing interval for retreatment for individual patients can be as short as 3 months. Take on empty stomach with water. To verify eradication of infection perform follow-up stool exams.

HOW SUPPLIED: Tab: 3mg

WARNINGS/PRECAUTIONS: May cause cutaneous and/or systemic reactions of varying severity (the Mazzotti reaction) and ophthalmological reactions. Patients with hyperreactive onchodermatitis (sowda) may be more likely to experience severe adverse reactions, especially edema and aggravation of onchodermatitis. Risk of serious or even fatal encephalopathy with onchocerciasis and *Loa loa* infection. Pretreatment assessment for loiasis and careful post-treatment follow-up should be performed in patients who were exposed to *Loa loa*-endemic areas of West or Central Africa.

ADVERSE REACTIONS: Diarrhea, orthostatic hypotension, nausea, dizziness, pruritis, decrease in leukocyte count, arthralgia/synovitis, axillary/cervical/inguinal lymph node enlargement, rash, fever, peripheral edema, tachycardia, seizures, elevated LFTs and bilirubin.

INTERACTIONS: Increased INR with concomitant warfarin.

PREGNANCY: Category C, not for use in pregnancy and safety not known in nursing.

MECHANISM OF ACTION: Avermectin derivative; binds selectively and with high affinity to glutamate-gated chloride ion channels, which occur in invertebrate nerve and muscle cells. This leads to increase in permeability of cell membrane to chloride ions with hyperpolarization of nerve and muscle cell, resulting in paralysis and death of parasite.

PHARMACOKINETICS: Absorption: Administration of variable doses resulted in different parameters. **Metabolism:** Liver. **Elimination:** Feces, urine (≤1%); $T_{1/2}$=18 hrs.

NURSING CONSIDERATIONS

Assessment: Document reasons for therapy. Assess HIV status, pregnancy status, and possible drug interactions.

Monitoring: Conduct stool exams following therapy to ensure eradication. Monitor for cutaneous and/or systemic reactions, ophthalmological reactions, hyperreactive onchodermatitis (edema, aggravation of onchodermatitis), encephalopathy, and other adverse reactions (eg, back pain, conjunctival hemorrhage, dyspnea, urinary and/or fecal incontinence, difficulty in standing/walking, mental status changes, confusion, lethargy, stupor, or coma),

S

hypersensitivity reactions, Stevens-Johnson syndrome, hypotension, elevated LFTs and bilirubin.

Patient Counseling: Advise to take tab on empty stomach. Counsel about need for repeated stool exams to document clearance of infection. Inform that for patients with onchocerciasis, repeated follow up and retreatment is needed; drug does not kill adult onchocerca parasite.

Administration: Oral route; take on empty stomach with water. **Storage:** Below 30°C (86°F).

SUBLIMAZE

CII

fentanyl citrate (Akorn)

THERAPEUTIC CLASS: Opioid analgesic

INDICATIONS: For analgesic action of short duration during the anesthetic periods, premedication, induction and maintenance, and in the immediate postoperative period (recovery room) as the need arises. For use as a narcotic analgesic supplement in general or regional anesthesia. For administration with a neuroleptic as an anesthetic premedication, for the induction of anesthesia and as an adjunct in the maintenance of general and regional anesthesia. For use as an anesthetic agent with oxygen in selected high risk patients, such as those undergoing open heart surgery or certain complicated neurological or orthopedic procedures.

DOSAGE: *Adults:* ≥12 yrs: Individualize dose. Premedication: 50-100mcg IM 30-60 min prior to surgery. Adjunct to General Anesthesia: Low-Dose: Total Dose: 2mcg/kg for minor surgery. Maint: 2mcg/kg. Moderate Dose: Total Dose: 2-20mcg/kg for major surgery. Maint: 2-20mcg/kg or 25-100mcg IM or IV if surgical stress or lightening of analgesia. High-Dose: Total Dose: 20-50mcg/kg for open heart surgery, complicated neurosurgery, or orthopedic surgery. Maint: 20-50mcg/kg. Adjunct to Regional Anesthesia: 50-100mcg IM or slow IV over 1-2 min. Post-op: 50-100mcg IM, repeat q 1-2 hrs as needed. General Anesthetic: 50-100mcg/kg with oxygen and a muscle relaxant, up to 150mcg/kg may be used.
Pediatrics: 2-12 yrs: Individualize dose. Induction/Maint: 2-3mcg/kg.

HOW SUPPLIED: Inj: 50mcg/mL

WARNINGS/PRECAUTIONS: Should only be administered by persons specifically trained in the use of IV anesthetics and management of the respiratory effects of potent opioids. An opioid antagonist, resuscitative and intubation equipment and oxygen should be readily available. Fluids and other countermeasures to manage hypotension should be available with tranquilizers. Initial dose reduction recommended with narcotic analgesia for recovery. May cause muscle rigidity particularly with muscles used for respiration. Adequate facilities should be available for postoperative monitoring and ventilation. Caution in respiratory depression susceptible patients (eg, comatose patients with head injury or brain tumor). Reduce dose for elderly and debilitated patients. Caution with obstructive pulmonary disease, decreased respiratory reserve, liver and kidney dysfunction, cardiac bradyarrhythmias. Monitor vital signs routinely.

S

ADVERSE REACTIONS: Respiratory depression, apnea, rigidity, bradycardia, HTN, hypotension, dizziness, blurred vision, nausea, emesis, diaphoresis, pruritus, urticaria, laryngospasms, anaphylaxis, euphoria, miosis, bradycardia, and bronchoconstriction.

INTERACTIONS: Severe and unpredictable potentiation by MAOIs has been reported. Appropriate monitoring and availability of vasodilators and β-blockers for the treatment of hypertension is indicated. Additive or potentiating effects with other CNS depressants (eg, barbiturates, tranquilizers, narcotics, general anesthetics). Reduce dose of other CNS depressants. Reports of cardiovascular depression with nitrous oxide. Alteration of respiration with certain forms of conduction anesthesia (eg, spinal anesthesia, some peridural anesthesia). Decreased pulmonary arterial pressure and hypotension with tranquilizers. Elevated BP, with and without pre-existing hypertension, slower normalcy of EEG patterns with neuroleptics. Extreme caution with neuroleptics in presence of risk factors for development of prolonged QT syndrome and torsade de pointes; ECG monitoring indicated.

PREGNANCY: Category C, caution with nursing.

MECHANISM OF ACTION: Opioid analgesic; produces analgesic and sedative effects. Alters respiratory rate and aveolar ventilation, which may last longer than analgesic effects.

PHARMACOKINETICS: Distribution: V_d=4L/kg; found in skeletal muscle and fat. **Metabolism:** Liver. **Elimination:** Urine (75%, <10% unchanged), feces (10%); $T_{1/2}$=219 min.

NURSING CONSIDERATIONS

Assessment: Assess for intolerance to other opioid agonists, risk of respiratory depression (eg, comatose patients, presence of head injury, brain tumor), impaired respiration (eg, COPD), presence of debilitation (eg, elderly), bradyarrhythmias, impaired hepatic or renal function, nursing/pregnancy status, and possible drug interactions. If combined with a neuroleptic, assess for risk of QT prolongation (eg, bradycardia, cardiac disease, electrolyte imbalance).

Monitoring: Monitor for signs/symptoms of respiratory depression, muscle rigidity, euphoria, miosis, bradycardia, bronchoconstriction, medication abuse, and drug dependence. If given with nitrous oxide, monitor for cardiovascular depression. If administered with a tranquilizer, monitor for hypotension and hypovolemia. If combined with a neuroleptic, monitor for increases in BP; perform ECG monitoring. Monitor for severe and unpredictable potentiation by MAO inhibitors if used within previous 14 days. Perform routine monitoring of vital signs.

Patient Counseling: Inform drug should be administered by persons specifically trained in use of IV anesthetics and management of respiratory effects of potent opioids. An opioid antagonist, resuscitative and intubation equipment, and oxygen should be readily available. If given with tranquilizers, fluids and other countermeasures to manage hypotension should be available.

Administration: IM/IV route. **Storage:** 20-25°C (68-77°F). Protect from light.

SUBOXONE **CIII**

buprenorphine - naloxone (Reckitt Benckiser)

OTHER BRAND NAMES: Subutex (Reckitt Benckiser)

THERAPEUTIC CLASS: Partial opioid agonist/opioid antagonist

INDICATIONS: Opioid dependence.

DOSAGE: *Adults:* Give either agent SL as a single daily dose in the range of 12-16mg/day. Hold tabs under tongue until dissolved; swallowing tabs reduces bioavailability. Induction: Subutex: Give at least 4 hrs after last short-acting opioid (eg, heroin) use or preferably when early signs of opioid withdrawal appear. Maint: Suboxone: Range: 4mg-24mg/day. Target dose: 16mg/day. Titrate: Adjust by 2mg or 4mg to a level that maintains treatment and suppresses opioid withdrawal effects. Hepatic Impairment: Adjust dose and observe for precipitated opioid withdrawal. Concomitant CNS Depressants: Consider dose reduction.

Pediatrics: ≥16 yrs: Give either agent SL as a single daily dose in the range of 12-16mg/day. Hold tabs under tongue until dissolved; swallowing tabs reduces bioavailability. Induction: Subutex: Give at least 4 hrs after last short-acting opioid (eg, heroin) use or preferably when early signs of opioid withdrawal appear. Maint: Suboxone: Range: 4mg-24mg/day. Target dose: 16mg/day. Titrate: Adjust by 2mg or 4mg to a level that maintains treatment and suppresses opioid withdrawal effects. Hepatic Impairment: Adjust dose and observe for precipitated opioid withdrawal. Concomitant CNS Depressants: Consider dose reduction.

HOW SUPPLIED: Suboxone (Buprenorphine-Naloxone) Tab, SL: 2mg-0.5mg, 8mg-2mg. Subutex (Buprenorphine) Tab, SL: 2mg, 8mg

WARNINGS/PRECAUTIONS: Significant respiratory depression reported with buprenorphine; caution with compromised respiratory function. Naloxone may not be effective in reversing any respiratory depression produced by buprenorphine. Cytolytic hepatitis and hepatitis with jaundice reported. Obtain LFTs prior to initiation and periodically thereafter. Acute and chronic hypersensitivity reactions reported. May increase CSF pressure; caution with head injury, intracranial lesions. May cause miosis, changes in level of consciousness, and orthostatic hypotension. Caution with elderly, debilitated, myxedema, hypothyroidism, acute alcoholism, Addison's disease, CNS depression or coma, toxic psychoses, prostatic hypertrophy, urethral stricture, delirium tremens, kyphoscoliosis, biliary tract dysfunction or severe hepatic/renal/pulmonary impairment. Suboxone may cause opioid withdrawal symptoms. May obscure diagnosis of acute abdominal conditions. May produce dependence.

ADVERSE REACTIONS: Headache, infection, pain (general, abdomen, back), withdrawal syndrome, constipation, nausea, insomnia, sweating, asthenia, anxiety, depression, rhinitis.

INTERACTIONS: May need dose reduction with CYP3A4 inhibitors (eg, azole antifungals, macrolides and HIV protease inhibitors). General anesthetics, other narcotic analgesics, benzodiazepines, phenothiazines, other tranquilizers, sedative/hypnotics or other CNS depressants (including alcohol) may increase risk of CNS depression; consider dose reduction of one or both agents. Monitor closely with CYP3A4 inducers (eg, phenobarbital, carbamazepine, phenytoin, rifampicin).

PREGNANCY: Category C, not for use in nursing.

MECHANISM OF ACTION: Buprenorphine: Partial agonist at the μ-opioid receptor, antagonist at the kappa-opioid receptor. Naloxone: Inhibits μ-opioid receptor activity.

PHARMACOKINETICS: Absorption: (Suboxone 16mg) C_{max}=5.95ng/mL, AUC=34.89 hr•ng/mL. (Subtex 16mg) C_{max}=5.47ng/mL, AUC=32.63 hr•ng/mL. Refer to PI for more detailed information. **Distribution:** Plasma protein binding 96% (buprenorphine), 45% (naloxone). **Metabolism:** Buprenorphine: Through N-dealkylation and glucuronidation pathways; norbuprenorphine (active metabolite). Naloxone: Through glucuronidation, N-dealkylation, and reduction. **Elimination:** Urine (30%), feces (69%); $T_{1/2}$=37 hrs (Buprenorphine), 1.1 hrs (Naloxone).

NURSING CONSIDERATIONS

Assessment: Assess for hepatic/renal and pulmonary impairment, myxedema or hypothyroidism, Addison's disease, toxic psychosis, CNS depression or coma, prostatic hypertrophy or uretheral stricture, biliary tract dysfunction, acute abdominal conditions, pregnancy/nursing status, head injury or intracranial lesions, increased CSF, alcohol intake, possible drug interactions. Perform LFTs prior to therapy and periodically thereafter.

Monitoring: Monitor LFTs. Monitor for signs/symptoms of respiratory/CNS depression, drug dependence, hepatitis, allergic reactions or anaphylactic shock, orthostatic hypotension, elevation of CSF.

S

Patient Counseling: Caution against hazardous tasks (eg, operating machinery/driving). Notify if pregnant/nursing. Concurrent administration of sedatives or alcohol may lead to serious overdose or death. Notify if taking or planning to take other medication.

Administration: Oral route. **Storage:** 25°C (77°F); excursions permitted to 15-30°C (59-86°F).

SULAR — RX

nisoldipine (Sciele)

THERAPEUTIC CLASS: Calcium channel blocker (dihydropyridine)

INDICATIONS: Treatment of hypertension.

DOSAGE: *Adults:* Initial: 20mg qd. Titrate: Increase by 10mg weekly or longer. Maint: 20-40mg qd. Max: 60mg/day. Elderly (>65 yrs)/Hepatic Dysfunction: Initial: Do not exceed 10mg/day. Do not chew, divide, or crush tabs.

HOW SUPPLIED: Tab, Extended-Release: 10mg, 20mg, 30mg, 40mg

WARNINGS/PRECAUTIONS: May increase angina or MI with severe obstructive CAD. May cause hypotension; monitor BP initially or with titration. Caution with heart failure or compromised ventricular function, especially with concomitant β-blockers. Caution with severe hepatic dysfunction or in elderly.

ADVERSE REACTIONS: Peripheral edema, headache, dizziness, pharyngitis, vasodilation, sinusitis, palpitations.

INTERACTIONS: Increased AUC and Cmax with cimetidine. Avoid phenytoin or CYP3A4 inducers. Decreased bioavailability with quinidine. High-fat meals increase peak drug levels. Avoid high-fat meals, grapefruit juice.

PREGNANCY: Category C, not for use in nursing.

MECHANISM OF ACTION: Dihydropyridine class of calcium channel antagonist (calcium ion antagonist or slow channel blocker) that inhibits transmembrane influx of calcium into vascular smooth muscle and cardiac muscle. Inhibition of Ca^+ channel results in dilation of arterioles and decreased peripheral vascular resistance.

PHARMACOKINETICS: Absorption: Well absorbed; absolute bioavailability (5%); T_{max}=6-12 hrs. **Metabolism:** CYP3A4 via hydroxylation. **Elimination:** Urine: (60-80%); $T_{1/2}$=7-12 hrs.

NURSING CONSIDERATIONS

Assessment: Assess for CAD, CHF, LFTs, BP, and possible drug interactions.

Monitoring: Monitor BP, LFTs. Monitor for peripheral edema, headache, dizziness, vasodilation, chest pain, rash, CBC with differential and platelet count, DM, thyroiditis, atrial fibrillation, hypokalemia, hematuria, sinusitis.

Patient Counseling: Instruct to swallow whole; do not chew, divide, or crush. Counsel about adverse effects; seek medical attention if any develop. Take as prescribed. Avoid concomitant intake of high-fat meal. Do not take with grapefruit juice.

Administration: Oral route. **Storage:** 20-25°C (68-77°F); excursions permitted to 15-30°C (59-86°F). Protect from moisture. Dispense in tight, light-resistant container.

SULINDAC

sulindac (Various)

RX

> **NSAIDs may cause an increased risk of serious cardiovascular thrombotic events, MI, stroke and serious GI adverse events including bleeding, ulceration, and perforation of the stomach or intestines. Contraindicated for the treatment of perioperative pain in the setting of coronary artery bypass graft (CABG) surgery.**

OTHER BRAND NAMES: Clinoril (Merck)

THERAPEUTIC CLASS: NSAID

INDICATIONS: Acute or long-term use for osteoarthritis (OA), rheumatoid arthritis (RA), ankylosing spondylitis (AS), acute painful shoulder, and acute gouty arthritis.

DOSAGE: *Adults:* OA/RA/AS: Initial: 150mg bid. Acute Painful Shoulder/Acute Gouty Arthritis: 200mg bid for 7-14 days. Max: 400mg/day. Give with food.

HOW SUPPLIED: Tab: 150mg, 200mg* *scored

CONTRAINDICATIONS: ASA or other NSAID allergy that precipitates acute asthmatic attack, urticaria, or rhinitis. Treatment of perioperative pain in the setting of CABG surgery.

WARNINGS/PRECAUTIONS: May lead to onset of new HTN or worsening of pre-existing HTN; monitor BP closely. Fluid retention and edema reported; caution with fluid retention or heart failure. Renal papillary necrosis and other renal injury reported after long-term use. Not recommended for use with advanced renal disease; if therapy must be initiated, monitor renal function. Anaphylactoid reactions may occur. May cause serious skin adverse events (eg, exfoliative dermatitis, Stevens-Johnson syndrome, and toxic epidermal necrolysis). Avoid in late pregnancy; may cause premature closure of ductus arteriosis. May cause elevations of LFTs; d/c if abnormal LFTs persist/worsen, liver disease develops, or systemic manifestations occur. Caution in elderly. Anemia may occur; monitor Hgb/Hct with long-term use. May inhibit platelet aggregation and prolong bleeding time; monitor with coagulation disorders. Caution with asthma and avoid with ASA-sensitive asthma. Keep patients well-hydrated and caution with renal lithiasis. Pancreatitis reported; if pancreatitis suspected, d/c and do not restart. Adverse eye findings reported. Monitor closely with poor liver function and consider dose reduction. Increased risk of aseptic meningitis in patients with systemic lupus erythematosus (SLE) and mixed connective tissue disease. Risk of GI ulceration, bleeding, and perforation.

ADVERSE REACTIONS: GI pain, dyspepsia, NV, diarrhea, constipation, rash, dizziness, headache, tinnitus, edema.

INTERACTIONS: Avoid DMSO, ASA, and other NSAIDs. May increase methotrexate and cyclosporine toxicities. Probenecid may increase plasma levels. Diflunisal may decrease plasma levels. May diminish antihypertensive effect of ACE inhibitors and reduce natriuretic effect of diuretics. May elevate plasma lithium levels. Increased risk of GI bleeding with warfarin.

PREGNANCY: Category C, not for use in nursing.

MECHANISM OF ACTION: NSAID; suspected to inhibit prostaglandin synthetase; exerts anti-inflammatory, analgesic, and antipyretic actions.

PHARMACOKINETICS: Absorption: PO administration of variable doses resulted in different parameters. **Distribution:** Penetrates placental and blood brain barrier. Plasma protein binding: Sulindac (93.1%), sulindac sulfone (95.4%), sulindac sulfide (97.9%). **Metabolism:** Via oxidation and reduction. **Elimination:** Urine (50%), feces 25% (metabolites); $T_{1/2}$ (sulindac, sulindac sulfide)=7.8, 16.4 hrs.

NURSING CONSIDERATIONS

Assessment: Assess LFTs, renal function, CBC, and coagulation profile. Assess for history of CABG surgery, asthma and allergic reactions to aspirin or other NSAIDs, active ulceration or chronic inflammation of GI tract, CVD (CHF, MI), asthma, pregnancy status, SLE, possible drug interactions.

Monitoring: Monitor for hypersensitivity reactions (anaphylaxis), cardiac complications, stroke, GI bleeding, asthma, skin reactions (Stevens-Johnson syndrome, toxic epidermal necrolysis). Monitor BP, LFTs, renal function, CBC with differential and platelet count, coagulation profile, ophthalmologic studies.

Patient Counseling: Counsel about potential side effects (anaphylaxis, edema, jaundice, GI discomfort, MI, stroke); seek medical attention if any develop. Avoid alcohol and smoking during treatment. Take drug as prescribed. Caution women against using drug late in pregnancy.

Administration: Oral route. **Storage:** 15-30°C (59-86°F). Store in well-closed container.

SUMYCIN — RX

tetracycline HCl (Par)

THERAPEUTIC CLASS: *Streptomyces* derived bacteriostatic agent

INDICATIONS: Treatment of respiratory tract, urinary tract, and skin and skin structure infections, lymphogranuloma, psittacosis, trachoma, uncomplicated urethral/endocervical/rectal infection caused by *Chlamydia*, nongonococcal urethritis, chancroid, plague, cholera, brucellosis, and others. When PCN is contraindicated, treatment of uncomplicated gonorrhea, syphilis, listeriosis, anthrax, *Clostridium* species, and others. Adjunct therapy for amebicides and severe acne.

DOSAGE: *Adults:* Mild-Moderate: 250mg qid or 500mg bid. Severe: 500mg qid. Continue for 24-48 hrs after symptoms subside (minimum 10 days with Group A β-hemolytic streptococci). Severe Acne: Initial: 1g/day in divided doses. Maint: After improvement, 125-500mg/day. Brucellosis: 500mg qid for 3 weeks plus streptomycin 1g IM bid for 1 week, then qd for 1 week. Syphilis:

30-40g equally divided over 10-15 days. Gonorrhea: 500mg q6h for 7 days. *Chlamydia*: 500mg qid for at least 7 days. Renal Dysfunction: Reduce dose or extend dose interval.
Pediatrics: >8 yrs: Usual: 25-50mg/kg divided bid-qid. Continue for 24-48 hrs after symptoms subside (minimum 10 days with Group A β-hemolytic streptococci). Severe Acne: Initial: 1g/day in divided doses. Maint: After improvement, 125-500mg/day. Renal Dysfunction: Reduce dose or extend dose interval.

HOW SUPPLIED: Sus: 125mg/5mL; Tab: 250mg, 500mg

WARNINGS/PRECAUTIONS: May cause fetal harm with pregnancy, permanent tooth discoloration during tooth development (last half of pregnancy and children <8 yrs). May increase BUN. Photosensitivity, enamel hypoplasia reported. Superinfection with prolonged use. Suspension contains sodium metabisulfite. Bulging fontanels in infants and benign intracranial HTN in adults reported. Monitor renal/hepatic and hematopoietic function with long-term use. Caution with history of asthma, hay fever, urticaria, and allergy.

ADVERSE REACTIONS: GI effects, photosensitivity, increased BUN, hypersensitivity reactions, blood dyscrasias, dizziness, headache.

INTERACTIONS: May decrease PT; adjust anticoagulants. May interfere with bactericidal agents (eg, penicillin). May decrease effects of oral contraceptives. Take 1 hr before or 2 hrs after dairy products. Aluminum-, calcium-, iron- and magnesium-containing products impair absorption. Fatal renal toxicity reported with concurrent methoxyflurane.

PREGNANCY: Category D, not for use in nursing.

MECHANISM OF ACTION: Tetracycline agent; inhibits bacterial protein synthesis.

PHARMACOKINETICS: Absorption: Adequate/incomplete. **Distribution:** Plasma protein binding (65%); excellent penetration into most bodily fluids and tissues; crosses placental barrier and enters fetal circulation and amniotic fluid; found in breast milk. **Elimination:** Urine, feces.

NURSING CONSIDERATIONS

Assessment: Assess pregnancy/nursing status, tooth development status in pediatrics and children, hepatic/renal impairment, asthma, hay fever, urticaria, and for possible drug interactions. Perform dark field exam in venereal diseases when coexistence of syphilis is suspected; repeat monthly thereafter for at least 4 months.

Monitoring: Monitor for allergic-type reactions, including anaphylactic symptoms and life-threatening or less severe asthmatic episodes in susceptible patients. Fetal harm if given to pregnant women, permanent tooth discoloration if given during tooth development (last half of pregnancy, infancy, childhood to 8 yrs), enamel hypoplasia, erythema, photosensitivity, symptoms/signs of pseudomotor cerebri (eg, blurred vision and headache or bulging fontanels in infants), increase in BUN (eg, azotemia, hyperphosphatemia, acidosis) in patients with impaired renal function, nephrotoxicity; Fanconi-like syndrome, overgrowth of nonsusceptible organisms, *C.difficile*-associated diarrhea and development of drug resistance. Periodically monitor hematopoietic, renal, hepatic organ function during long-term therapy. All patients with gonorrhea should have serologic test for syphilis at the time of diagnosis and follow-up test after 3 months.

Patient Counseling: Inform about potential risks/benefits of therapy. Instruct to d/c and notify physician if erythema occurs. Avoid prolonged or direct exposure to sunlight. Advise to notify physician if pregnant/nursing, planning to become pregnant, and/or if taking oral contraceptives. Inform that drug only treats bacterial, not viral, infections. Instruct to take medication exactly as prescribed to avoid developing drug resistance and to maintain effectiveness of therapy.

Administration: Oral route. **Storage:** 30°C (86°F); tightly closed container.

SUPARTZ RX
sodium hyaluronate (Smith & Nephew)

THERAPEUTIC CLASS: Hyaluronan

INDICATIONS: Treatment of pain in osteoarthritis of the knee in patients who have failed to respond adequately to conservative non-pharmacologic therapy and simple analgesics (eg, APAP).

DOSAGE: *Adults:* Administer 2.5mL by intra-articular injection once a week for a total of 5 injections. Some patients may experience benefit with 3 injections given at weekly intervals. Use strict aseptic technique.

HOW SUPPLIED: Inj: 2.5mL

CONTRAINDICATIONS: Avoid with knee infections or skin diseases in the area of the injection site.

WARNINGS/PRECAUTIONS: Avoid disinfectants containing quaternary ammonium salts for skin preparation; hyaluronic acid can precipitate in their presence. Transient pain and/or swelling of the injected joint may occur. Safety and effectiveness in joints other than the knee or concomitantly with other intra-articular injectables have not been established. Caution in patients who are allergic to avian proteins, feathers, and egg products. Avoid any strenuous activities or prolonged (eg, more than 1 hr) weight-bearing activities within 48 hours following the intra-articular injection. Remove any joint effusion before injecting. Safety and effectiveness have not been demonstrated in children.

ADVERSE REACTIONS: Arthralgia, arthropathy, arthrosis, arthritis, back pain, pain (non-specific), injection site reaction, headache, injection site pain.

PREGNANCY: Safety in pregnancy and nursing not known.

MECHANISM OF ACTION: Hyaluronan.

NURSING CONSIDERATIONS

Assessment: Assess for skin infections or disease in area of injection site, use of disinfectants containing quaternary ammonium salts, knee joint infections, and pregnancy/nursing status.

Monitoring: Monitor for knee joint swelling/effusion and local skin reaction.

Patient Counseling: Inform that drug may cause transient pain/swelling at injection site. Avoid strenuous activities or prolonged weight-bearing activities (jogging, tennis) within 48 hrs following injection.

Administration: Intra-articular. **Storage:** Below 25°C (77°F). Do not freeze. Shelf life is 42 months.

S

SUPRAX RX
cefixime (Lupin)

THERAPEUTIC CLASS: Cephalosporin (3rd generation)

INDICATIONS: Otitis media, pharyngitis, tonsillitis, acute bronchitis, acute exacerbation of chronic bronchitis, uncomplicated UTIs, and cervical/urethral gonorrhea caused by susceptible strains.

DOSAGE: *Adults:* Usual: 400mg qd. Gonorrhea: 400mg single dose. CrCl 21-60mL/min/Hemodialysis: Give 75% of standard dose. CrCl <20mL/min/CAPD: Give 50% of standard dose.
Pediatrics: >12 yrs or >50kg: (Tab/Sus) Usual: 400mg qd. ≥6 months: (Sus) 8mg/kg qd or 4mg/kg bid. Treat for at least 10 days with *S.pyogenes*. CrCl 21-60mL/min/Hemodialysis: Give 75% of standard dose. CrCl <20mL/min/CAPD: Give 50% of standard dose.

HOW SUPPLIED: Tab: 400mg; Sus: 100mg/5mL [50mL, 75mL, 100mL]

WARNINGS/PRECAUTIONS: Caution with PCN or other allergy, GI disease (eg, colitis). Anaphylactic/anaphylactoid reactions, pseudomembranous colitis reported. May cause false (+) direct Coombs test or false (+) reaction for urinary glucose using Benedict's/Fehling's solution or Clinitest.

ADVERSE REACTIONS: Diarrhea, abdominal pain, nausea, dyspepsia, flatulence, superinfection.

INTERACTIONS: May increase carbamazepine levels. Increased PT with anticoagulants (eg, warfarin).

PREGNANCY: Category B, not for use in nursing.

MECHANISM OF ACTION: 3rd-generation cephalosporin; inhibits cell-wall synthesis.

PHARMACOKINETICS: Absorption: 40-50% absorbed. C_{max}=2mcg/mL (200mg tab), 3.7mcg/mL (400mg tab), 3mcg/mL (200mg sus), 4.6mcg/mL (400mg sus); T_{max}=2-6 hrs (200mg tab, 400mg tab/sus), 2-5 hrs (200mg sus). **Distribution:** Serum protein binding (65%). **Elimination:** Urine (50% unchanged); $T_{1/2}$=3-4 up to 9 hrs.

NURSING CONSIDERATIONS

Assessment: Assess for previous hypersensitivity to cephalosporins/PCNs or other drugs, renal/hepatic impairment, GI tract disease (eg, colitis), nutritional status, those receiving protracted course of antibiotics or anticoagulants, pregnancy/nursing status, possible drug interactions.

Monitoring: Monitor for PT with vitamin K administration as indicated. Monitor for signs/symtoms of anaphylatic/anaphylactoid reactions, pseudomembranous colitis or CDAD, development of drug resistance, superinfection, pancytopenia, agranulocytosis and lab test interference (eg, false (+) reaction of urinary ketones if using nitroprusside, false (+) reaction for urinary glucose if using Clinitest, Benedict's or Fehling's solution, false (+) Coombs' test. Monitor renal function tests, LFTs, LDH, and CBC.

Patient Counseling: Inform that therapy only treats bacterial, not viral, infections. Take exactly as directed; skipping doses or not completing full course may decrease effectiveness and increase resistance. Inform about benefits/risks. D/C and notify physician if diarrhea or allergic reactions occur. Notify if pregnant/nursing.

Administration: Oral route. **Storage:** Sus/Tab, 20-25°C (68-77°F). After mixing, store sus at room temperature or under refrigeration for 14 days; keep tightly closed and shake well before use.

SURMONTIL — RX

trimipramine maleate (Odyssey)

Antidepressants increased the risk of suicidal thinking and behavior (suicidality) in short-term studies in children, adolescents, and young adults with major depressive disorder (MDD) and other psychiatric disorders. Trimipramine is not approved for use in pediatric patients.

THERAPEUTIC CLASS: Tricyclic antidepressant

INDICATIONS: Relief of symptoms of depression.

DOSAGE: *Adults:* Outpatient: Initial: 75mg/day in divided doses. Titrate: Increase to 150mg/day. Maint: 50-150mg/day. Max: 200mg/day. Hospitalized Patients: Initial: 100mg/day in divided doses. Titrate: Increase gradually to 200mg/day. If no improvement after 2-3 weeks, may increase up to 250-300mg/day. Elderly: Initial: 50mg/day. Titrate: Increase gradually to 100mg/day. Take hs for at least 3 months.
Pediatrics: Adolescents: Initial: 50mg/day. Titrate: Increase gradually to 100mg/day. Take hs for at least 3 months.

HOW SUPPLIED: Cap: 25mg, 50mg, 100mg

CONTRAINDICATIONS: Acute recovery period post-MI, within 14 days of MAOI therapy.

WARNINGS/PRECAUTIONS: Caution with cardiovascular disease, increased IOP, urinary retention, narrow-angle glaucoma, hyperthyroidism, seizure disorder, liver dysfunction. May impair ability to operate machinery. May alter

...ucose levels. May activate psychosis in schizophrenia. Manic or hypomanic episodes may occur. May increase hazards with electroshock therapy.

ADVERSE REACTIONS: Hypotension, HTN, arrhythmia, confusion, insomnia, incoordination, GI complaints, allergic reactions, gynecomastia, blood dyscrasias, dry mouth, blurred vision, urinary retention.

INTERACTIONS: Cimetidine inhibits elimination. Alcohol may exaggerate effects. May potentiate catecholamine or anticholinergic effects. Potentiated by CYP2D6 inhibitors (eg, quinidine) and substrates (eg, other antidepressants, phenothiazines, propafenone, fleccainide). Caution with SSRIs; wait 5 weeks after fluoxetine withdrawal before initiating therapy. Avoid MAOIs.

PREGNANCY: Category C, safety in nursing not known.

MECHANISM OF ACTION: Tricyclic antidepressant with anxiety-reducing sedative component to its action.

NURSING CONSIDERATIONS

Assessment: Assess renal function tests, LFTs, IOP, for seizures, major depressive disorder, cardiovascular disorders, urinary retention, thyroid disorders. Note other diseases/conditions and drug therapies.

Monitoring: Monitor for clinical worsening, suicidality, or unusual changes in behavior, seizures, increased restlessness, agitation, anxiety, insomnia, neuropsychiatric signs/symptoms (eg, delusions, hallucinations, psychosis, concentration disturbance, paranoia, and confusion), ECG, CBC with differential and platelet count, blood sugar levels.

Patient Counseling: Advise families and caregivers of the need for close observation of clinical worsening and suicidal risks. Avoid alcohol, sedatives, OTC agents. Caution against operating machinery/driving. Report adverse reactions. Consult physician before taking any other medication. Avoid excessive exposure to sunlight.

Administration: Oral route. **Storage:** 20-25°C (68-77°F). Keep bottle tightly closed. Dispense in tight container.

SUSTIVA RX

efavirenz (Bristol-Myers Squibb)

THERAPEUTIC CLASS: Non-nucleoside reverse transcriptase inhibitor

INDICATIONS: Treatment of HIV-1 infection in combination with other antiretrovirals.

DOSAGE: *Adults:* Initial: 600mg qd. Take on an empty stomach, preferably at bedtime.

Pediatrics: ≥3 yrs: 10 to <15kg: 200mg qd. 15 to <20kg: 250mg qd. 20 to <25kg: 300mg qd. 25 to <32.5kg: 350mg qd. 32.5 to <40kg: 400mg qd. ≥40kg: 600mg qd. Take on an empty stomach, preferably at bedtime.

HOW SUPPLIED: Cap: 50mg, 200mg; Tab: 600mg

CONTRAINDICATIONS: Concomitant astemizole, bepridil, cisapride, midazolam, pimozide, triazolam, ergot derivatives, or standard doses of voriconazole.

WARNINGS/PRECAUTIONS: Not for monotherapy. Severe skin rash reported. Avoid pregnancy; use barrier contraception with other contraception methods and obtain (-) pregnancy test before therapy. Monitor LFTs with known or suspected hepatitis B or C. Monitor cholesterol and triglycerides. High fat meals may increase absorption. Possible redistribution or accumulation of body fat. Serious psychiatric and CNS adverse events (eg, dizziness, insomnia, impaired concentration) reported. Caution in patients with seizure history; convulsions have been reported. May impair physical/mental abilities. Immune reconstitution syndrome reported.

ADVERSE REACTIONS: CNS symptoms (eg, dizziness, insomnia, impaired concentration, somnolence, abnormal dreams), psychiatric symptoms (eg, severe depression), rash, GI effects.

INTERACTIONS: Avoid astemizole, cisapride, midazolam, triazolam, voriconazole, St. John's wort, or ergot derivatives. St. John's wort decreases efavirenz to suboptimal levels; increases risk of resistance. Significantly decreased levels of voriconazole. CYP3A4 inducers (eg, phenobarbital, rifampin, rifabutin) may decrease plasma levels. Increased levels of ethinyl estradiol. Decreased levels of clarithromycin; consider alternative. Decreased levels of indinavir and rifabutin; adjust doses. Increased levels of ritonavir and efavirenz with concomitant use; monitor LFTs. Decreased levels of saquinavir, sertraline. May decrease methadone levels; monitor for signs of withdrawal. May affect warfarin levels. May decrease itraconazole, ketoconazole, amprenavir, atazanavir, indinavir, and lopinavir levels. Decreased levels of anticonvulsants (eg, phenytoin, phenobarbital, carbamazepine) and efavirenz; monitor anticonvulsant levels.

PREGNANCY: Category D, not for use in nursing.

MECHANISM OF ACTION: Non-nucleoside reverse transcriptase inhibitor.

PHARMACOKINETICS: Absorption: C_{max}=12.9μM, T_{max}=3-5 hrs; AUC=184μM•h. **Distribution:** Plasma protein binding (99.5-99.75%). **Metabolism:** CYP3A4, 2B6 (hydroxylation, glucuronidation). **Elimination:** Urine, feces; $T_{1/2}$=40-55 hrs.

NURSING CONSIDERATIONS

Assessment: Assess for possible drug interactions, history of HBV, HCV, injection drug use, seizures, psychiatric illness, pregnancy status, and hepatic impairment. Perform pregnancy test prior to therapy.

Monitoring: Monitor LFTs periodically. Monitor for signs and symptoms of seizures, plasma anticonvulsant drug levels, serious psychiatric events, severe rashes, fat redistribution or accumulation, immune reconstitution syndrome, nervous system symptoms, and hypersensitivity reactions.

Patient Counseling: Inform patient may continue to develop opportunistic infections; no data on therapy reducing risk of transmitting HIV. Instruct to take every day as prescribed; take on empty stomach at bedtime to reduce CNS symptoms (eg, dizziness, insomnia, impaired concentration, abnormal dreams) that may occur during 1st weeks of therapy. Instruct to avoid potentially hazardous tasks such as driving or operating machinery. Inform of pregnancy risks; use reliable barrier and oral contraception during therapy. Advise to seek medical attention if symptoms of seizures, rash, serious psychiatric events (severe depression, suicidal ideation, aggressive behavior), fat redistribution or accumulation, immune reconstitution syndrome, or hypersensitivity reactions occur. Notify physician of any history of mental illness or substance abuse.

Administration: Oral route. **Storage:** 25°C (77°F); excursions permitted to 15-30°C (59-86°F).

SUTENT — RX

sunitinib malate (Pfizer)

S

THERAPEUTIC CLASS: Multikinase inhibitor

INDICATIONS: Treatment of gastrointestinal stromal tumor (GIST) after disease progression on or intolerance to imatinib mesylate. Treatment of advanced renal cell carcinoma (RCC).

DOSAGE: *Adults:* 50mg once daily; 4 weeks on, 2 weeks off. Dose increase/reduction in 12.5mg increments is recommended. Concomitant Strong CYP3A4 Inhibitors: Consider dose reduction to minimum of 37.5mg daily. Concomitant CYP3A4 Inducer: Consider dose increase to maximum of 87.5mg daily.

HOW SUPPLIED: Cap: 12.5mg, 25mg, 50mg

WARNINGS/PRECAUTIONS: Cases of decreased left ventricular ejection fraction (LVEF) reported. Patients with cardiac risk factors should be carefully monitored for signs and symptoms of CHF; baseline and periodic evaluation of LVEF should be considered. D/C if clinical manifestations of CHF occur. Prolongation of QT interval and torsade de pointes observed; consider monitoring ECG and electrolytes (magnesium, potassium). Cases of hemorrhagic events reported. Serious, sometimes fatal GI complications including GI perforation have occurred with intra-abdominal malignancies. Cases of HTN reported; monitor for HTN and treat as needed with standard antihypertensive therapy. Temporary suspension recommended if severe HTN occurs. Adrenal toxicity reported; monitor for adrenal insufficiency with stress, trauma, or severe infection. Myelosuppression, hypothyroidism, increases in serum lipase/amylase, and pancreatitis reported. Monitor CBCs, platelet count, thyroid function, and serum chemistries beginning each treatment cycle. May cause fetal harm; avoid pregnancy. Closely observed signs and/or symptoms of thyroid dysfunction; laboratory monitoring performed and treated as per standard medical practice.

ADVERSE REACTIONS: Fatigue, asthenia, diarrhea, NV, mucositis/stomatitis, dyspepsia, abdominal pain, HTN, rash, hand-foot syndrome, skin discoloration, altered taste, anorexia, bleeding.

INTERACTIONS: Concomitant CYP3A4 inhibitors (eg, ketoconazole) may increase plasma concentrations; consider dose reduction. CYP3A4 inducers (eg, rifampin) may decrease plasma concentrations; consider dose increase. Avoid concurrent St. John's wort; may decrease plasma concentrations unpredictably.

PREGNANCY: Category D, not for use in nursing.

MECHANISM OF ACTION: Multikinase inhibitor; inhibits multiple receptor tyrosine kinase, implicated in tumor growth, pathologic angiogenesis, and metastatic cancer progression.

PHARMACOKINETICS: Absorption: T_{max}=6-12 hrs. **Distribution:** V_d=2230L; plasma protein binding (95%). **Metabolism:** CYP3A4. **Elimination:** Feces (61%), renal (16%); $T_{1/2}$=40-60 hrs, 80-110 hrs (metabolite).

NURSING CONSIDERATIONS

Assessment: Assess for risk factors or history of CVD (QT prolongation, bradycardia, HTN, MI, CABG), seizures, liver dysfunction, pregnancy status, hypothyroidism and possible drug interactions. Obtain baseline left ventricular ejection fraction (LVEF) (no risk factors: EF), thyroid function, LFTs, BP, CBC with platelet count, chemistries with phosphate, and renal function.

Monitoring: Monitor LVEF, ECG, CBC with platelets, chemistries (Mg^{2+}, K^+, phosphate), thyroid function, and LFTs periodically. Monitor for signs/symptoms of CVD, electrolyte imbalance, hemorrhagic events, hypothyroidism, adrenal insufficiency, reversible posterior leukoencephalopathy syndrome (RPLS), pancreatitis, muscle toxicity, hypersensitivity reactions, renal/hepatic dysfunction.

Patient Counseling: Inform of pregnancy risks. Instruct not to take with grapefruit juice or grapefruit. Advise to seek medical attention if symptoms of CVD (eg, QT prolongation, HTN), electrolyte imbalance, hemorrhagic events (eg, GI perforation; black, tarry stools), hypothyroidism, adrenal insufficiency (during stress), RPLS (eg, HTN, headache, AMS, visual loss), pancreatitis, muscle toxicity, hypersensitivity reactions, renal/hepatic dysfunction occur.

S

Administration: Oral route. **Storage:** 25°C (77°F); excursions permitted to 15-30°C (59-86°F).

SYMBICORT RX

formoterol fumarate dihydrate - budesonide (AstraZeneca)

Long-acting β_2-adrenergic agonists (formoterol) may increase the risk of asthma-related death. Symbicort should only be used for patients not adequately controlled on other asthma-controller medications or whose disease severity clearly needs initiation of treatment with two maintenance therapies.

THERAPEUTIC CLASS: Corticosteroid/beta$_2$ agonist

INDICATIONS: (80/4.5mcg, 160/4.5mcg) Long-term maintenance treatment of asthma in patients ≥12 yrs. (160/4.5mcg) Maintenance treatment of airflow obstruction in patients with chronic obstructive pulmonary disease (COPD) including chronic bronchitis and emphysema.

DOSAGE: *Adults:* Asthma: Initial: Individualize dose based on asthma severity. 2 inh bid of 80/4.5 or 160/4.5. Maint: 2 inh bid of 80/4.5 or 160/4.5. No Current Inhaled Corticosteroid (CS): 2 inh bid of 80/4.5 or 160/4.5 depending on asthma severity. Max: 160/4.5mcg bid. Patients not responding to the starting dose after 1-2 weeks of therapy with 80/4.5, replace with 160/4.5 for better asthma control. COPD: 2 inh bid of 160/4.5. If asthma or shortness of breath occurs in the period between doses, inhale short-acting $beta_2$-agonist immediately. Rinse mouth after use.
Pediatrics: ≥12 yrs: Asthma: Initial: Individualize dose based on asthma severity. 2 inh bid of 80/4.5 or 160/4.5. Maint: 2 inh bid of 80/4.5 or 160/4.5. No Current Inhaled Corticosteroid (CS): 2 inh bid of 80/4.5 or 160/4.5 depending on asthma severity. Max: 160/4.5mcg bid. Patients not responding to the starting dose after 1-2 weeks of therapy with 80/4.5, replace with 160/4.5 for better asthma control. If asthma occurs in the period between doses, inhale short-acting $beta_2$-agonist immediately. Rinse mouth after use.

HOW SUPPLIED: MDI: (Budesonide-Formoterol) 80mcg-4.5mcg/inh, 160mcg-4.5mcg/inh [10.2g]

CONTRAINDICATIONS: Primary treatment of status asthmaticus or other acute asthma attacks or COPD requiring intensive measures.

WARNINGS/PRECAUTIONS: Not for asthma managed by inhaled CS with occasional use of short-acting $beta_2$-agonists. Do not use in patients with significantly worsening or acutely deteriorating asthma or COPD. Not for acute treatment of symptoms. Monitor for increasing use of inhaled, short-acting β_2-agonists. Deaths due to adrenal insufficiency have occurred with transfer from systemic corticosteroids to inhaled corticosteroids. Resume oral corticosteroids during stress or severe asthma attack. Transferring from oral to inhalation therapy may unmask allergic conditions (eg, rhinitis, conjunctivitis, eczema). Observe for adrenal insufficiency, systemic corticosteroid withdrawal effects, and growth suppression (pediatrics). Increased susceptibility to infections. Not for acute bronchospasm. Do not use any additional inhaled long-acting β_2-agonist for prevention of exercise-induced bronchospasm or the maintenance treatment of asthma. D/C if paradoxical bronchospasm occurs. Immediate hypersensitivity and upper airway symptom reactions reported. Caution with cardiovascular disorder (eg, coronary insufficiency, arrhythmia, HTN), seizures, thyroid and hepatic problems, diabetes, osteoporosis. QTc interval prolongation reported. Glaucoma, increased IOP, and cataracts reported. Caution in patients with active or quiescent TB infection, untreated systemic fungal, bacterial, viral, or parasitic infections, or ocular herpes simplex. Localized infections with *Candida albicans* may occur in mouth and pharynx. Lower respiratory tract infections, including pneumonia, reported in patients with COPD. Reduction in bone mineral density reported; monitor periodically. Eosinophilic conditions and Churg-Strauss syndrome reported. Hypokalemia and hyperglycemia may occur.

ADVERSE REACTIONS: Nasopharyngitis, headache, upper respiratory tract infections, sinusitis, back pain, nasal/sinus congestion, oral candidiasis, influenza, rhinitis, pharyngolaryngeal pain, vomiting, and bronchitis.

S

INTERACTIONS: Oral ketoconazole increases plasma levels. CYP3A4 inhibitors (eg, itraconazole, clarithromycin, erythromycin) may inhibit metabolism and increase systemic exposure. Caution with non-K^+-sparing diuretics. Extreme caution within 14 days of using MAOIs or TCAs. Avoid with β-blockers.

PREGNANCY: Category C, not for use in nursing.

MECHANISM OF ACTION: Budesonide: Corticosteroid; shown to have inhibitory effects on multiple cell types (mast cells, eosinophils, neutrophils, macrophages and lymphocytes) and mediators (histamine, eicosanoids, leukotrienes and cytokines) involved in inflammatory and asthmatic response. Formoterol: β_2-adrenergic agonist; stimulates intracellular adenyl cyclase, which catalyzes conversion of ATP to cAMP, to produce relaxation of bronchial smooth muscle and inhibition of release of mediators of immediate hypersensitivity from cells (mast cells).

PHARMACOKINETICS: Absorption: (Asthma) Budesonide: Rapid (lungs). C_{max}=4.5nmol/L; T_{max}=20 min. Formoterol: Rapid (GI). C_{max}=136pmol;

T_{max}=5-10 min. (COPD) Budesonide: Rapid (lungs). C_{max}=3.3nmol/L; T_{max}=30 min. Formoterol: Rapid (GI). C_{max}=167pmol/L; T_{max}=15 min. **Distribution:** Budesonide: V_d=3L/kg; plasma protein binding (85-90%). Formoterol: Plasma protein binding (RR enantiomer, 46%), (SS enantiomer, 58%). **Metabolism:** Budesonide: Liver (biotransformation) via CYP3A4. Formoterol: Liver (direct glucuronidation and O-demethylation) via CYP2D6, 2C. **Elimination:** Budesonide: $T_{1/2}$=2-3 hrs. Formoterol: Urine (8%).

NURSING CONSIDERATIONS

Assessment: Assess if asthma controlled by inhaled corticosteroids and occasional use of short-acting β_2-agonists. Assess for risk factors for decreased bone mineral content (eg, tobacco use, advanced age, sedentary lifestyle, family history of osteoporosis, drugs that decrease bone mass), CVD (eg, coronary insufficiency, cardiac arrhythmia, HTN), convulsive disorder, thyrotoxicosis, DM, concomitant diseases like status asthmaticus, active or quiescent pulmonary TB, ocular herpes simplex, untreated systemic fungal, bacterial, parasitic, or viral infections, and possible drug interactions. Obtain baseline bone mineral density and lung function prior to therapy.

Monitoring: Monitor bone mineral density and lung function periodically. Perform periodic eye exams. Monitor for localized oral infections with *Candida albicans*, decreased bone mass, upper airway symptoms (eg, laryngeal spasm, irritation, swelling), worsening or acutely deteriorating asthma (increased use of inhaled β_2-agonist, decreased lung function), asthma instability (serial objective measures of airflow), body height in children, development of glaucoma, increased IOP, posterior subcapsular cataracts, adrenal insufficiency (eg, fatigue, weakness, NV and hypotension), paradoxical bronchospasm, eosinophilic conditions, pneumonia, and hypersensitivity reactions.

Patient Counseling: Avoid spraying in eyes. Advise to rinse mouth after inhalation. Replace mouthpiece cover after each use and clean inhaler every 7 days by wiping mouthpiece with dry cloth. Do not d/c therapy unless directed by physician. Should not be used for sudden symptoms of SOB or acute bronchospasm. Inform may cause reduction in growth rate (pediatric). May unmask allergies (eg, rhinitis, conjunctivitis, eczema). Avoid exposure to chickenpox or measles; seek medical attention if exposed to chickenpox or measles, or if experience worsening of existing TB, infections or ocular herpes simplex, symptoms do not improve or worsen, during periods of stress or severe asthmatic attack, adrenal insufficiency (fatigue, weakness, NV and hypotension), paradoxical bronchospasm or hypersensitivity reactions.

Administration: Oral inhalation. **Storage:** 20-25°C (68-77°F). Store with mouthpiece down. Shake well.

SYMBYAX RX

fluoxetine HCl - olanzapine (Lilly)

Antidepressants increased the risk of suicidal thinking and behavior (suicidality) in short-term studies in children, adolescents, and young adults with major depressive disorder (MDD) and other psychiatric disorders. Symbyax is not approved for use in pediatric patients. Elderly patients with dementia-related psychosis treated with atypical antipsychotic drugs are at an increased risk of death; most appeared to be cardiovascular (eg, heart failure, sudden death) or infectious (eg, pneumonia) in nature. Symbyax is not approved for the treatment of patients with dementia-related psychosis.

THERAPEUTIC CLASS: Thienobenzodiazepine/selective serotonin reuptake inhibitor

INDICATIONS: Acute treatment of depressive episodes associated with bipolar disorder I, and treatment-resistant depression (Major Depressive Disorder [MDD] who do not respond to 2 separate trials of different antidepressants of adequate dose and duration in the current episode) in adults.

DOSAGE: *Adults:* ≥18 yrs: Depressive Episodes Associated with Bipolar I Disorder/Treatment Resistant Depression: Initial: 6mg-25mg qd in evening. Titrate: Adjust dose based on efficacy and tolerability. Max: 18mg-75mg/day. Hypotension Risk/Hepatic Impairment/Slow Metabolizers: Initial: 3mg-

25mg to 6mg-25mg qd in evening. Titrate: Increase cautiously. Re-evaluate periodically.

HOW SUPPLIED: Cap: (Olanzapine-Fluoxetine): 3mg-25mg, 6mg-25mg, 6mg-50mg, 12mg-25mg, 12mg-50mg

CONTRAINDICATIONS: During or within 14 days of MAOI use; during or within 5 weeks of discontinuation of thioridazine use; concomitant pimozide use.

WARNINGS/PRECAUTIONS: Monitor for clinical worsening and/or suicidality. Monitor for hyperglycemia, worsening of glucose control with DM, FBG levels with diabetes risk, hyperlipidemia, weight gain, serotonin syndrome or neuroleptic malignant syndrome (NMS) like signs/symptoms. Ketoacidosis, hyperosmolar coma, or fatality reported. Risk of orthostatic hypotension, NMS, tardive dyskinesia, hyperprolactinemia, hyponatremia, seizures and elevated transaminases reported. Caution with cardio- or cerebrovascular disease, hypotension risk (eg, dehydration, hypovolemia), history of seizures or conditions that lower seizure threshold, elderly (especially with dementia), hepatic impairment, risk of aspiration pneumonia, conditions that affect metabolism or hemodynamic responses, prostatic hypertrophy, narrow-angle glaucoma, history of paralytic ileus, suicidal tendencies. D/C if unexplained allergic reaction, tardive dyskinesia occur. Monitor for symptoms of mania/hypomania. May cause disruption of body temperature regulation and may increase risk of bleeding events. Serotonin syndrome or NMS-like reactions reported; caution with MAOIs and other serotonergic drugs. Caution when prescribing olanzapine and fluoxetine products concomitantly. May impair judgment, thinking, or motor skills. Gradual dose reduction rather than abrupt cessation is recommended upon discontinuation.

ADVERSE REACTIONS: Asthenia, somnolence, weight gain, increased appetite, peripheral edema, tremor, diarrhea, dry mouth, amblyopia, twitching, arthralgia, abnormal ejaculation.

INTERACTIONS: See Contraindications. Risk of orthostatic hypotension with antihypertensives, benzodiazepines, alcohol. May antagonize levodopa, dopamine agonists. Increased clearance with carbamazepine, omeprazole, rifampin, other inducers of CYP1A2 or glucuronyl transferase. Increase in clozapine, haloperidol, phenytoin levels. Caution with other CNS-active drugs, other highly protein-bound drugs (eg, warfarin, digitoxin), hepatotoxic drugs, other olanzapine- or fluoxetine-containing products. Decreased clearance with fluvoxamine. Monitor lithium levels. May increase TCA levels; may require reduction in TCA dose. Increased risk of bleeding with NSAIDs, ASA, warfarin. Inhibits drugs metabolized by CYP2D6 (eg, flecainide, vinblastine, TCAs); initiate at lower end of dosage range.

PREGNANCY: Category C, not for use in nursing.

MECHANISM OF ACTION: Not established; proposed to activate serotonin, norepinephrine, and dopamine, enhancing antidepressant effect. Olanzepine: Thienobenzodiazepine; psychotropic agent with high affinity binding to $5HT_{2a/2c}$, $5HT_6$, D_{1-4}, H_1, and adrenergic $(\alpha)_1$-receptors. Fluoxetine: SSRI; inhibits serotonin transport; weak inhibitor of norepinephrine and dopamine transporters.

PHARMACOKINETICS: Absorption: Olanzepine: Well absorbed; T_{max}=approximately 6 hrs. Fluoxetine: C_{max}=15-55ng/mL, T_{max}=6-8 hrs. **Distribution:** Olanzepine: V_d=1000L; plasma protein binding (93%). Fluoxetine: Plasma protein binding (94.5%). **Metabolism:** Olanzapine: Extensively metabolized, via glucuronidation and CYP450 mediated oxidation, 10-N-glucuronide and 4'-N-desmethyl olanzapine (major metabolites). Fluoxetine: Liver (extensive); CYP 2D6 pathway, norfluoxetine (active metabolite). **Elimination:** Olanzapine: Urine (57%), feces (30%); $T_{1/2}$=21-54 hrs. Fluoxetine: Kidneys; (acute administration) $T_{1/2}$=1-3 days; (chronic administration) $T_{1/2}$=4-6 days.

NURSING CONSIDERATIONS

Assessment: Assess for dementia-related psychosis, major depressive disorder, bipolar mania, DM, bleeding disorders, seizures, cardio/cerebrovascular disorders, renal/hepatic impairment, drug interactions (eg, MAOIs).

Monitoring: Monitor for clinical worsening, suicidality, and unusual changes in behavior, signs/symptoms of TD, extrapyramidal symptoms, clinical

S

manifestations of NMS, serotonin syndrome, orthostatic hypotension, bleeding tendency. Monitor body temperature, weight, CBC, glucose, liver enzymes, BUN, cholesterol, TG, Na^+, and prolactin.

Patient Counseling: Advise of risk of orthostatic hypotension. Counsel to avoid hazardous tasks (eg, operating machinery/driving), alcohol use, overheating, dehydration. Instruct to notify physician before taking any other drugs, if pregnant, or intend to become pregnant. Notify physician if rash or hives develop. Take exactly as prescribed; continue even if symptoms improve.

Administration: Oral route. **Storage:** 25° (77°F); excursions permitted to 15-30°C (59-86°F). Keep tightly closed; protect from moisture.

SYMLIN — RX

pramlintide acetate (Amylin)

Use with insulin. Risk of insulin-induced severe hypoglycemia, particularly with type 1 DM. Severe hypoglycemia usually occurs within 3 hrs of injection. Serious injuries may occur if severe hypoglycemia occurs while operating a motor vehicle, heavy machinery, or other high-risk activities. Appropriate patient selection, careful patient instruction, and insulin dose adjustments are necessary to reduce this risk.

OTHER BRAND NAMES: SymlinPen (Amylin)

THERAPEUTIC CLASS: Synthetic amylin analog

INDICATIONS: Adjunct treatment in patients with type 1 or type 2 DM who use mealtime insulin therapy and who have failed to achieve desired glucose control despite optimal insulin therapy. May be used with or without sulfonylurea and/or metformin in type 2 DM.

DOSAGE: *Adults:* Before initiating therapy, reduce insulin dose by 50%. Monitor blood glucose frequently. Adjust insulin dose once target dose of pramlintide is maintained. Type 2 DM: Initial: 60mcg SQ immediately prior to meals. Titrate: 120mcg as tolerated. Type 1 DM: Initial: 15mcg SQ immediately prior to meals. Titrate: Increase by 15mcg increments to 30mcg or 60mcg as tolerated.

HOW SUPPLIED: Inj: 600mcg/mL [5mL]; Pen injector: 1000mcg/mL [1.5mL, 2.7mL]

CONTRAINDICATIONS: Confirmed diagnosis of gastroparesis; hypoglycemia unawareness.

WARNINGS/PRECAUTIONS: Do not mix with insulin; administer as separate injections.

ADVERSE REACTIONS: NV, headache, anorexia, abdominal pain, fatigue, dizziness, coughing, pharyngitis.

S

INTERACTIONS: Do not administer with agents that alter gastrointestinal motility (eg, anticholinergic agents such as atropine), and agents that slow intestinal absorption of nutrients (eg, α-glucosidase inhibitors). Administer analgesics and other oral agents that require rapid onset 1 hr before or 2 hrs after injection.

PREGNANCY: Category C, caution in nursing.

MECHANISM OF ACTION: Amylinomimetic agent that modulates gastric emptying, prevents postprandial rise in plasma glucagon, and produces satiety, which leads to a decreased caloric intake.

PHARMACOKINETICS: Absorption: Absolute bioavailability (30-40%); SQ administration of variable doses resulted in different parameters. **Distribution:** Not extensively bound to blood cells or albumin (40% unbound). **Metabolism:** Kidneys (primarily). Des-lys pramlintide (primary active metabolite). **Elimination:** $T_{1/2}$=48 min.

NURSING CONSIDERATIONS

Assessment: Assess patient does not have confirmed diagnosis of gastroparesis or hypoglycemia unawareness. Evaluate patient's HbA_{1c}, recent blood glucose monitoring data, history of insulin-induced hypoglycemia, current insulin regimen, and body weight. Assess if patient has failed to achieve proper glycemic control despite individualized insulin management. Assess use in patients with visual or dexterity impairment. Assess for possible drug interactions and pregnancy/nursing status.

Monitoring: Monitor for signs/symptoms of hypoglycemia (eg, hunger, headache, sweating, tremor) when using in combination with insulin. Monitor proper glucose control through serum blood glucose levels and HbA_{1c} test.

Patient Counseling: Instruct to never mix with insulin and not to transfer from pen-injector to syringe. If dose missed, wait until next scheduled dose and administer usual amount. Instruct to administer immediately prior to each major meal (≥250 calories or ≥30g of carbohydrates). Instruct that insulin dose adjustments should be made only by healthcare professional. Patients should have fast-acting sugar (eg, hard candy, glucose tablet, juice) at all times. Self-glucose monitoring should be done on a daily basis. Counsel about signs/symptoms of hypoglycemia (eg, hunger, headache, sweating, tremor, irritability). Instruct regarding the critical importance of maintaining proper glucose control, especially when operating heavy machinery (eg, motor vehicles).

Administration: SQ injection to abdomen or thigh; administration to the arm is not recommended because of variable absorption. Rotate injection sites and do not use any site for any concomitant insulin injection. Allow to come to room temperature before injecting. **Storage:** Pen injectors and vials not in use: 2-8°C (36-40°F). Do not freeze. Do not use if frozen. Unused drug (opened or unopened) should not be used after expiration date. Pen-injectors and vials in use: After 1st use, refrigerate or keep at a temperature <30°C (86°F). Use within 30 days.

SYMMETREL RX
amantadine HCl (Endo)

THERAPEUTIC CLASS: Dopamine agonist

INDICATIONS: Prophylaxis and treatment of uncomplicated influenza A infections. Treatment of parkinsonism and drug-induced extrapyramidal reactions.

DOSAGE: *Adults:* Influenza A Virus Prophylaxis/Treatment: 200mg qd given as a single dose of two 100-mg tabs (or 4 tsps of syrup). May give 100mg (or 2 tsps) bid if CNS effects develop. Elderly: ≥65 yrs: 100mg qd. Parkinsonism: Initial: 100mg bid. Serious Associated Illness/Concomitant High Dose Antiparkinson Agent: Initial: 100mg qd. Titrate: May increase to 100mg bid after 1 to several weeks. Max: 400mg/day. Drug-Induced Extrapyramidal Reactions: 100mg bid. Titrate: May increase to 300mg/day in divided doses. CrCl 30-50mL/min: 200mg on Day 1, then 100mg qd. CrCl 15-29mL/min: 200mg on Day 1, then 100mg every other day. CrCl <15mL/min/Hemodialysis: 200mg every 7 days.
Pediatrics: Influenza A Virus Prophylaxis/Treatment: 9-12 yrs: 100mg (or 2 tsps of syrup) bid. 1-9 yrs: 4.4-8.8mg/kg/day. Max: 150mg/day.

S

HOW SUPPLIED: Syrup: 50mg/5mL; Tab: 100mg

WARNINGS/PRECAUTIONS: Deaths reported from overdose. Suicide attempts, neuroleptic malignant syndrome (NMS) reported. Caution with CHF, peripheral edema, orthostatic hypotension, renal or hepatic dysfunction, recurrent eczematoid rash, uncontrolled psychosis or severe psychoneurosis. Avoid in untreated angle closure glaucoma. Do not d/c abruptly in Parkinson's disease. May increase seizure activity. Melanoma reported; monitor frequently. May impair mental/physical abilities.

ADVERSE REACTIONS: Nausea, dizziness, insomnia, depression, anxiety, hallucinations, confusion, anorexia, dry mouth, constipation, ataxia, livedo reticularis, peripheral edema, orthostatic hypotension, irritability, and headache.

INTERACTIONS: Caution with CNS stimulants. Anticholinergic agents may potentiate the anticholinergic side effects. Increased tremor in elderly Parkinson's patients with thioridazine. Reduced renal clearance by about 30% with quinine or quinidine. Avoid use of Attenuated Influenza Vaccine within 2 weeks before or 48 hours after.

PREGNANCY: Category C, not for use in nursing.

MECHANISM OF ACTION: Antiviral; appears to prevent release of infectious viral nucleic acid into host cell by interfering with function of transmembrane domain of viral M2 protein, preventing virus assembly during replication. Parkinson's disease; may have direct/indirect effect on dopamine neurons and is a weak, non-competitive NMDA receptor antagonist.

PHARMACOKINETICS: Absorption: (Tab) C_{max}=0.51mcg/mL, T_{max}=2-4 hrs. (Syrup) C_{max}=0.24mcg/mL, T_{max}=2-4 hrs. **Distribution:** (IV) V_d=3-8L/Kg; plasma protein binding (67%). **Metabolism:** N-acetylation; acetylamantadine (metabolite). **Elimination:** Urine; excreted unchanged; $T_{1/2}$=16 hrs.

NURSING CONSIDERATIONS

Assessment: Assess for history of CHF, peripheral edema, epilepsy or other "seizures," recurrent eczematoid rash, psychiatric illness, untreated angle-closure glaucoma, pregnancy/nursing status, possible drug interactions, renal/hepatic impairment.

Monitoring: Monitor for signs/symptoms of CHF, peripheral edema, epilepsy or other "seizures", recurrent eczematoid rash, psychiatric illness, untreated angle-closure glaucoma, NMS (eg, fever, muscle rigidity, altered mental status), renal/hepatic impairment, and melanoma. Monitor lab tests such as CPK, WBC, serum myoglobin, BUN, SrCr, alkaline phosphatase, LDH, bilirubin, GGT, SGOT and SGPT.

Patient Counseling: Advise blurry vision and impaired mental acuity may occur. Avoid excessive alcohol use, getting up suddenly from sitting or lying position, and abrupt d/c. Notify physician if no improvement in a few days or appears less effective after a few weeks. Seek medical attention if experience symptoms of CHF (eg, lightheadedness, SOB), peripheral edema, epilepsy or other "seizures," recurrent eczematoid rash, psychiatric illness (suicidal ideation, mood changes), untreated angle-closure glaucoma, hypersensitivity reaction, NMS (eg, fever, muscle rigidity, altered mental status), renal/hepatic impairment. Consult a physician before discontinuing medication. Caution against driving/working where alertness and adequate motor coordination are important. Notify physician if new or increased gambling urges, increased sexual urges or other intense urges occur.

Administration: Oral route. Influenza A: Treatment: should be started within 24-48 hrs after onset and after disappearance of signs and symptoms; continue for at least 10 days after known exposure. Prophylaxis: Administer for 2-4 weeks after vaccine is given. If vaccine unavailable, continue for entire duration of exposure in community. **Storage:** 25°C (77°F); excursions permitted to 15-30°C (59-86°F).

SYNAGIS — RX

palivizumab (MedImmune)

THERAPEUTIC CLASS: Monoclonal antibody/RSV F-protein blocker

INDICATIONS: Prevention of serious lower respiratory tract disease caused by respiratory syncytial virus (RSV) in pediatrics at high risk of RSV. Safety and efficacy established in infants with bronchopulmonary dysplasia (BPD) and infants with history of prematurity (≤35 weeks gestational age).

DOSAGE: *Pediatrics:* 15mg/kg IM; give 1st dose before start of RSV season (November-April), then monthly throughout season. Give monthly also if develop RSV infection.

HOW SUPPLIED: Inj: 50mg [0.5mL], 100mg [1mL]

WARNINGS/PRECAUTIONS: Anaphylactoid reactions (cyanosis, dyspnea, respiratory failure) reported. Administer appropriate medications (eg, epinephrine) in the event of anaphylaxis. Caution with thrombocytopenia or any coagulation disorder due to IM injection. Safety and efficacy not demonstrated for treatment of established RSV disease.

ADVERSE REACTIONS: Upper respiratory infection, otitis media, rash, cough, diarrhea, vomiting, liver function abnormality, fever, rhinitis, hernia, gastroenteritis, wheezing, anaphylaxis, thrombocytopenia.

PREGNANCY: Category C, safety in nursing not known.

MECHANISM OF ACTION: Monoclonal antibody; exhibits neutralizing and fusion-inhibitory activity against RSV.

PHARMACOKINETICS: Elimination: $T_{1/2}$=20 days.

NURSING CONSIDERATIONS

Assessment: Assess for thrombocytopenia and coagulation disorders.

Monitoring: Monitor for anaphylaxis or acute hypersensitivity reactions and platelet count.

Patient Counseling: Advise to seek medical attention if hypersensitivity reactions occur.

Administration: IM (anterolateral aspect of thigh). Administer immediately after withdrawal from vial; do not re-enter vial; gluteal muscle should not be used because of risk of damage to sciatic nerve. Do not dilute, shake, or vigorously agitate vial. **Storage:** 2-8°C (35.5-46.4°F). Do not freeze; or use beyond expiration date.

SYNALAR RX

fluocinolone acetonide (Medicis)

THERAPEUTIC CLASS: Corticosteroid

INDICATIONS: Corticosteroid-responsive dermatoses.

DOSAGE: *Adults:* Apply bid-qid. May use occlusive dressings for psoriasis or recalcitrant conditions; d/c dressings if infection develops.
Pediatrics: Apply bid-qid. May use occlusive dressings for psoriasis or recalcitrant conditions; d/c dressings if infection develops.

HOW SUPPLIED: Cre, Oint: 0.025% [15g, 60g]; Sol: 0.01% [20mL, 60mL]

WARNINGS/PRECAUTIONS: May produce reversible HPA axis suppression, manifestations of Cushing's syndrome, hyperglycemia, and glucosuria. Caution when applied to large surface areas or under occlusive dressings. Use appropriate antifungal or antibacterial agent with dermatological infections; d/c if infection does not clear. Peds may be more susceptible to systemic toxicity. Avoid eyes. D/C if irritation occurs.

ADVERSE REACTIONS: Burning, itching, irritation, dryness, folliculitis, hypertrichosis, acneiform eruptions, premolar dermatitis, hypopigmentation, allergic dermatitis, skin maceration, secondary infection, skin atrophy.

PREGNANCY: Category C, caution with nursing.

MECHANISM OF ACTION: Corticosteroid; possesses anti-inflammatory, antipruritic, and vasoconstrictive actions. Anti-inflammatory activity not established.

PHARMACOKINETICS: Absorption: Percutaneous; occlusion, inflammation, and other disease states may increase absorption. **Distribution:** Systemically administered corticosteroids are found in breast milk. **Metabolism:** Liver. **Excretion:** Kidneys, bile.

NURSING CONSIDERATIONS

Assessment: Assess pregnancy/nursing status.

Monitoring: Monitor for signs/symptoms of HPA-axis suppression, Cushing's syndrome, hyperglycemia, glucosuria, treatment-site irritation, and for development of dermatological infections (eg, bacterial, fungal). If on prolonged therapy, monitor for atrophy of skin and subcutaneous tissues. If on high doses or applying to large surface area, perform periodic monitoring for HPA-axis suppression using urinary free cortisol and ACTH stimulation tests. In pediatric patients, monitor for signs/symptoms of systemic toxicity, HPA-

S

axis suppression (eg, linear growth retardation, delayed weight gain); and intracranial HTN.

Patient Counseling: Instruct to use externally and exactly as directed; avoid contact with eyes. Counsel not to bandage or wrap treatment area as to be occlusive unless directed by physician. Advise to report any local adverse reactions (eg, irritation). Instruct caregivers of pediatrics to avoid using tight-fitting diapers or plastic pants on treatment area.

Administration: Topical route. **Storage:** Room temperature; avoid freezing and excessive heat, above 40°C (104°F).

SYNERA RX

tetracaine - lidocaine (Endo)

THERAPEUTIC CLASS: Acetamide local anesthetic

INDICATIONS: For use on intact skin to provide local dermal analgesia for superficial venous access and superficial dermatological procedures such as excision, electrodessication, and shave biopsy of skin lesions.

DOSAGE: *Adults:* Venipuncture or IV Cannulation: Apply to intact skin for 20-30 min prior to procedure. Superficial Dermatological Procedures: Apply to intact skin for 30 min prior to procedure.
Pediatrics: ≥3 yrs: Venipuncture or IV Cannulation: Apply to intact skin for 20-30 min prior to procedure. Superficial Dermatological Procedure: Apply to intact skin for 30 min prior to procedure.

HOW SUPPLIED: Patch: (Lidocaine-Tetracaine) 70mg-70mg

CONTRAINDICATIONS: PABA hypersensitivity.

WARNINGS/PRECAUTIONS: Serious adverse events may occur in children or pets if ingested. Caution in acutely ill or debilitated. Risk of allergic/anaphylactoid reactions (urticaria, angioedema, bronchospasm, shock). Increased risk of toxicity in severe hepatic disease. Avoid broken or inflamed skin, eye contact, larger area or longer duration than recommended.

ADVERSE REACTIONS: Erythema, blanching, edema, urticaria, angioedema, bronchospasm, shock.

INTERACTIONS: Additive toxic effect with concomitant Class I antiarrhythmics (eg, tocainide, mexiletine). Consider total amount absorbed from all formulations with other local anesthetics.

PREGNANCY: Category B, caution in nursing.

MECHANISM OF ACTION: Lidocaine: Amide-type local anesthetic; blocks Na^+ channels required for initiation and conduction of neuronal impulses. Tetracaine: Ester-type local anesthetic; blocks Na^+ channels required for initiation and conduction of neuronal impulses.

S

PHARMACOKINETICS: Absorption: C_{max}=1.7ng/mL (lidocaine), <0.9ng/mL (tetracaine); T_{max}=1.7 hrs. (lidocaine). **Distribution:** Lidocaine: V_d=0.8-1.3 L/kg; plasma protein binding (75%); crosses placenta. **Metabolism:** Lidocaine: CYP1A2, CYP3A4 (N-deethylation). Monoethylglycinexylidide, glycinexylidide (active metabolites). Tetracaine: Plasma esterases (hydrolysis). **Elimination:** Lidocaine: Urine; $T_{1/2}$=1.8 hrs.

NURSING CONSIDERATIONS

Assessment: Assess for pseudocholinesterase deficiency, possible drug interactions, cardiac and hepatic impairment.

Monitoring: Monitor for allergic or anaphylactoid reactions (eg, erythema, blanching, edema), cardiac and hepatic dysfunction.

Patient Counseling: Inform that use may lead to diminished or blocked sensation in treated skin. Instruct to wash hands after application; avoid contact with eyes; remove patch before MRI.

Administration: Transdermal. **Storage:** 25°C (77°F) excursions permitted to 15-30°C (59-86°F).

SYNERCID

RX

dalfopristin - quinupristin (King)

THERAPEUTIC CLASS: Streptogramin

INDICATIONS: Treatment of serious or life-threatening infections associated with vancomycin-resistant *Enterococcus faecium* (VREF) bacteremia and complicated skin and skin structure infections (cSSSI) caused by *Staphylococcus aureus* (methicillin-susceptible) or *Streptococcus pyogenes*.

DOSAGE: *Adults:* ≥16 yrs: VREF: 7.5mg/kg IV q8h. Duration depends on site and severity of infection. cSSSI: 7.5mg/kg IV q12h for at least 7 days. Hepatic Cirrhosis (Child Pugh A or B): May need dose reduction.
Pediatrics: ≥16 yrs: VREF: 7.5mg/kg IV q8h. Duration depends on site and severity of infection. cSSSI: 7.5mg/kg IV q12h for at least 7 days. Hepatic Cirrhosis (Child Pugh A or B): May need dose reduction.

HOW SUPPLIED: Inj: (Dalfopristin-Quinupristin) 350mg-150mg per 500mg vial

WARNINGS/PRECAUTIONS: Pseudomembranous colitis reported. Flush vein with 5% dextrose after infusion to minimize venous irritation. Arthralgia, myalgia, and bilirubin elevation reported.

ADVERSE REACTIONS: Infusion-site reactions (inflammation, pain, edema), nausea, diarrhea, rash.

INTERACTIONS: Significant inhibiton of CYP3A4; caution with drugs metabolized by this enzyme system (eg, cyclosporine A, tacrolimus, midazolam, nifedipine, verapamil, diltiazem, astemizole, terfenadine, delaviridine, nevirapine, indinavir, ritonavir, vinca alkaloids, docetaxel, paclitaxel, diazepam, HMG-CoA reductase inhibitors, methylprednisolone, carbamazepine, quinidine, lidocaine, disopyramide). Monitor cyclosporine levels. Avoid drugs metabolized by CYP3A4 that prolong QTc interval. May inhibit gut metabolism of digoxin.

PREGNANCY: Category B, caution in nursing.

MECHANISM OF ACTION: Bacteriostatic agent; acts on bacterial ribosome. Dalfopristin: Inhibits the early phase of protein synthesis. Quinipristin: Inhibits the late phase of protein synthesis.

PHARMACOKINETICS: Absorption: Quinipristin: C_{max}=3.2mcg/mL, AUC=7.2mcg•hr/mL; Dalfopristin: C_{max}=7.96mcg/mL, AUC=10.57mcg•hr/mL. **Distribution:** Quinipristin: V_d=0.45L/kg, plasma protein binding (moderate); Dalfopristin: V_d=0.24L/kg, plasma protein binding (moderate). **Metabolism:** Quinipristin: 2 conjugated metabolites (1 with glutathione; 1 with cysteine); Dalfopristin: 1 nonconjugated metabolite; active metabolites. **Elimination:** Urine: 15% (quinipristin), 19% (dalfopristin), feces (75-77%); $T_{1/2}$=0.85 hrs. (quinipristin), 0.7 hrs. (dalfopristin).

NURSING CONSIDERATIONS

Assessment: Assess for hepatic/renal impairment, pregnancy/nursing status, and for possible drug interactions (eg, concurrent administration with cyclosporine).

Monitoring: Monitor for pseudomembranous colitis or C.*difficile*-associated diarrhea (may range from mild diarrhea to fatal colitis), venous irritation, arthralgia/myalgia, development of superinfection or drug resistance, isolated hyperbilirubinemia, and therapeutic monitoring of cyclosporine levels if used concurrently. Lab monitoring of LFTs, renal function, glucose, CBC, and blood chemistry.

Patient Counseling: Inform about risks/benefits of therapy. D/C and notify physician if any adverse reactions occur. Notify if pregnant/nursing.

Administration: IV route. Infuse over 60 min; inspect for particulate matter or discoloration; flush only with D5W to minimize venous irritation. Do not dilute with saline solution. **Storage:** Before reconstitution, at 2-8°C (36-46°F); diluted solution stable for 5 hrs at room temperature or for 54 hrs if refrigerated at 2-8°C (36-46°F). Do not freeze.

SYNTHROID RX

levothyroxine sodium (Abbott)

THERAPEUTIC CLASS: Thyroid replacement hormone

INDICATIONS: Replacement or supplemental therapy in congenital or acquired hypothyroidism. As a pituitary TSH suppressant in the treatment and prevention of euthyroid goiters, including thyroid nodules, lymphocytic thyroiditis, and multinodular goiter. Adjunct to surgery and radioiodine therapy for thyrotropin-dependent well-differentiated thyroid cancer.

DOSAGE: *Adults:* Hypothyroidism: Usual: 1.7mcg/kg/day PO. >200mcg/day (seldom). Patients ≥50 Years/<50 Years With Cardiac Disease: May start with 25-50mcg/day and gradually increase every 6-8 weeks until euthyroid. Elderly With Cardiac Disease: Initial: 12.5-25mcg qd PO. Titrate: Increase by 12.5-25mcg every 4-6 weeks until euthyroid. Severe Hypothyroidism: Initial: 12.5-25mcg/day. Titrate: Increase by 25mcg/day every 2-4 weeks. Secondary (Pituitary) or Tertiary (Hypothalamic) Hypothyroidism: Titrate: Increase until clincally euthyroid. Give 1/2 of oral dose for IV/IM. Pregnancy: May require increased doses. Subclinical Hypothyroidism: Lower doses required.
Pediatrics: Hypothyroidism: 0-3 months: 10-15mcg/kg/day.
3-6 months: 8-10mcg/kg/day. 6-12 months: 6-8mcg/kg/day. 1-5 yrs: 5-6mcg/kg/day. 6-12 yrs: 4-5mcg/kg/day. >12 yrs (growth/puberty incomplete): 2-3mcg/kg/day. Growth/Puberty Complete: 1.7mcg/kg/day. Cardiac Risk: Lower starting dose. Infants with Serum T_4 <5mcg/dL: Initial: 50mcg/day. Chronic/Severe Hypothyroidism: Children: Initial: 25mcg/day. Titrate: Increase by 25mcg for 2 weeks then every 2-4 weeks until euthyroid. May crush tab and sprinkle over food (applesauce) or mix with 5-10mL water, formula (non-soy), or breast milk.

HOW SUPPLIED: Tab: 25mcg*, 50mcg*, 75mcg*, 88mcg*, 100mcg*, 112mcg*, 125mcg*, 137mcg*, 150mcg*, 175mcg*, 200mcg*, 300mcg* *scored

CONTRAINDICATIONS: Untreated thyrotoxicosis, acute MI, uncorrected adrenal insufficiency.

WARNINGS/PRECAUTIONS: Do not use in the treatment of obesity or for weight loss; larger doses in euthyroid patients can cause serious or even life threatening toxicity. Not for the treatment of infertility unless associated with hypothyroidism. Caution with cardiovascular disorders, angina, CAD, HTN and the elderly. May aggravate DM, diabetes insipidus, or adrenal cortical insufficiency. Myxedema coma may not be treated with oral thyroid hormone products; administer IV products. May lower seizure threshold.

ADVERSE REACTIONS: Fatigue, weight loss, headache, hyperactivity, anxiety, tremors, muscle weakness, palpitations, arrhythmias, diarrhea, hair loss, flushing, decreased bone mineral density, craniosynostosis in infants, pseudotumor cerebri in pediatrics (rare), hypersensitivity reactions, seizures (rare).

INTERACTIONS: Increased risk of coronary insufficiency with sympathomimetics and CAD. May potentiate oral anticoagulant effects; adjust dose and monitor PT/INR. Lithium blocks release of T_4 and T_3. Antidiabetic agents may need adjustment. Decreased absorption with cholestyramine resin, colestipol, ferrous sulfate, aluminum hydroxide, sodium polystyrene sulfonate, soybean flour (infant formula), sucralfate. Altered protein binding with clofibrate, estrogens, androgens/anabolic hormones, asparaginase, 5-FU, furosemide, glucocorticoids, meclofenamic acid, mefenamic acid, methadone, perphenazine, phenytoin, phenylbutazone, tamoxifen, salicylates. Altered thyroid hormone or TSH levels with aminoglutethimide, p-aminosalicyclic acid, amiodarone, androgens/anabolic hormones, complex anions (eg, thiocyanate, perchlorate, pertechnetate), antithyroid drugs, β-adrenergic blockers, carbamazepine, chloral hydrate, diazepam, dopamine/dopamine agonists, ethionamide, glucocorticoids, heparin, hepatic enzyme inducers, insulin, iodinated cholestographic agents, iodine-containing compounds, levodopa, lovastatin, lithium, 6-mercaptopurine, metoclopramide, mitotane, nitroprusside, phenobarbital, phenytoin, resorcinol, rifampin, somatostatin analogs, sulfonamides, sulfonylureas, thiazide diuretics. Adrenocorticoid clearance is decreased with hypothyroidism and increased with hyperthyroidism. Cytokines, amiodarone may induce hypo- or hyperthyroidism. Increased risk of arrhythmias with maprotiline. HTN and tachycardia reported with ketamine. Sympathomimetics may increase risk of coronary insufficiency with CAD. Adverse effects of both drugs with TCAs. Decreased clearance of theophylline with hypothyroidism. Impaired β-blocker effects. Decreased digitalis effects. Decreased uptake of iodine-containing radiolabeled ions. Altered levels of theophylline may occur. Use with somatrem/somatropin may accelerate epiphyseal closure. Additive effects of both agents with TCAs. Avoid mixing crushed tabs with foods/formula with large amounts of iron, soybean or fiber.

PREGNANCY: Category A, caution in nursing.

MECHANISM OF ACTION: Thyroid hormone; not understood, suspected to control DNA transcription and protein synthesis.

PHARMACOKINETICS: Distribution: Plasma protein binding (99%); found in breast milk. **Metabolism:** Deiodination and conjugation in the liver (mainly), kidneys, and other tissues. **Elimination:** Urine, feces; (approximately 20% unchanged). (T_4) $T_{1/2}$=6-7 days, and (T_3) $T_{1/2}$≤2 days.

NURSING CONSIDERATIONS

Assessment: Assess for suppressed TSH level with normal T_3 and T_4 or overt thyrotoxicosis, hypersensitivity history, cardiovascular disease (angina or acute MI), uncorrected adrenal insufficiency, thyroid diseases (nontoxic diffuse or nodular goiter), endocrine disorders (hypothalamic/pituitary hormone deficiencies and/or autoimmune polyglandular disorders), DM, clotting status, upcoming surgery and possible drug and test interactions. Assess infants for associated congenital anomalies.

Monitoring: Perform frequent lab tests and clinical evaluation of thyroid functions (TSH and free T_4 levels), glucose/lipid metabolism, blood and/or urinary glucose in diabetics, and clotting parameters. Monitor for cardiovascular signs (eg, arrhythmia, coronary insufficiency), growth development, bone metabolism, cognitive function, emotional status, GI functions, reproductive functions, partial hair loss in infants, and signs/symptoms of thyrotoxicosis.

Patient Counseling: Inform that drug is to be taken for life and not to be taken for treatment of obesity or weight reduction. Take 1 hr before breakfast on empty stomach with full glass of water. Notify if pregnant/nursing or planning to become pregnant. Notify if taking any other drugs. Do not d/c or change dose without consulting physician. Report any signs/symptoms of thyroid toxicity.

Administration: Oral route. **Storage:** Store at 25°C (77°F); excursions permitted to 15-30°C (59-86°F). Protect from light and moisture.

SYNVISC

RX

hylan G-F 20 (Wyeth)

S

THERAPEUTIC CLASS: Hylan polymer

INDICATIONS: Treatment of osteoarthritis (OA) knee pain inadequately responsive to conservative nonpharmacologic therapy and simple analgesics.

DOSAGE: *Adults:* Usual: Intra-articular injection once weekly (one week apart) for total of three injections.

HOW SUPPLIED: Inj: 8mg/mL

CONTRAINDICATIONS: Knee joint infections, hyaluronan hypersensitivity, skin diseases or infections in injection site area.

WARNINGS/PRECAUTIONS: Avoid with skin disinfectants containing quaternary ammonium salts; hyaluronan can precipitate in their presence. Do not inject extra-articularly or into synovial tissue and capsule. Intravascular injections may cause systemic adverse events. Caution with allergies to avian proteins, feathers, and egg products. Avoid with severely inflamed knee joints. Remove synovial fluid or effusion, if present, before injecting. Follow strict aseptic administration. Caution with lymphatic or venous stasis. Avoid strenuous activity or prolonged weight-bearing activities after injection. Packaging contains dry natural rubber latex.

ADVERSE REACTIONS: Injection site pain, knee swelling/effusion, rash, calf cramps, ankle edema, muscle pain.

INTERACTIONS: Do not inject anesthetics or other drugs into knee joint during therapy.

PREGNANCY: Safety in pregnancy and nursing not known.

MECHANISM OF ACTION: Hylan polymer.

NURSING CONSIDERATIONS

Assessment: Assess for knee joint infection, skin disease, or infection in area of injection site, pregnancy status, lymphatic or venous stasis.

Monitoring: Monitor for signs/symptoms of allergic reaction (eg, rash, hives, itching, fever), knee joint effusion/swelling, and local skin reactions.

Patient Counseling: Inform that use may cause transient pain/swelling of injected joint. Instruct to avoid any strenuous or prolonged weight-bearing activity (eg, jogging, tennis) within 48 hrs of injection. Seek medical attention if symptoms of allergic reaction occur.

Administration: Intra-articular. **Storage:** 30°C (86°F). Do not freeze. Protect from light.

TALACEN

pentazocine HCl - acetaminophen (Sanofi-Aventis) **CIV**

THERAPEUTIC CLASS: Opioid agonist-antagonist analgesic

INDICATIONS: Relief of mild to moderate pain.

DOSAGE: *Adults:* 1 tab q4h prn. Max: 6 tabs/day.

HOW SUPPLIED: Tab: (Pentazocine-APAP) 25mg-650mg* *scored

WARNINGS/PRECAUTIONS: Contains sodium metabisulfite. Caution with head injury, increased ICP, acute CNS manifestations, MI, certain respiratory conditions, renal/hepatic dysfunction, biliary surgery, seizure disorders, and alcohol use. Potential for physical and psychological dependence.

ADVERSE REACTIONS: NV, constipation, abdominal distress, anorexia, diarrhea, dizziness, lightheadedness, hallucinations, sedation, euphoria, headache, confusion, disorientation, sweating, tachycardia.

INTERACTIONS: Increased CNS depressant effects with alcohol. Withdrawal symptoms with narcotics.

PREGNANCY: Category C, caution in nursing.

MECHANISM OF ACTION: Pentazocine: Acts as analgesic and sedative. APAP: Acts as analgesic and antipyretic.

PHARMACOKINETICS: Absorption: Pentazocine: Well-absorbed; T_{max}=1.7 hrs. APAP: Rapid and complete; T_{max}=0.5-2.5 hrs. **Distribution:** Pentazocine: Crosses placental barrier. APAP: Plasma protein binding (8-43%). **Metabolism:** Pentazocine: Liver. APAP: Liver via conjugation. **Elimination:** Pentazocine: Renal excretion, $T_{1/2}$=3.6 hrs. APAP: Urine (80% conjugated drug, 3% unchanged); $T_{1/2}$=2.8 hrs.

NURSING CONSIDERATIONS

Assessment: Assess for head injury, MI, respiratory depression, impaired renal/hepatic function, biliary surgery, seizures, pregnancy status, and possible drug interactions.

Monitoring: Monitor vital signs, sedation, seizures, respiratory depression, NV, BP, HR, allergic reactions, leukopenia, drug abuse or dependence.

Patient Counseling: Inform that drug may cause sedation, dizziness, and occasional euphoria. Counsel about drug abuse and dependence. Avoid alcohol and do not abruptly d/c drug as there could be withdrawal symptoms. Exercise caution while driving or operating machinery.

Administration: Oral route. **Storage:** 25°C (77°F); excursions permitted to 15-30°C (59-86°F).

TALWIN NX

CIV

pentazocine HCl - naloxone HCl (Sanofi-Aventis)

For oral use only. Severe, potentially lethal reactions may result from misuse by injection alone, or in combination with other agents.

THERAPEUTIC CLASS: Opioid agonist-antagonist analgesic

INDICATIONS: Relief of moderate to severe pain.

DOSAGE: *Adults:* Usual: 1 tab q3-4h. May increase to 2 tabs q3-4h. Max: 12 tabs/day.
Pediatrics: ≥12 yrs: Usual: 1 tab q3-4h. May increase to 2 tabs q3-4h. Max: 12 tabs/day.

HOW SUPPLIED: Tab: (Pentazocine-Naloxone) 50mg-0.5mg* *scored

WARNINGS/PRECAUTIONS: Caution with elderly, drug dependence, head injury, increased ICP, certain respiratory conditions, acute CNS manifestations, renal or hepatic dysfunction, biliary surgery, and MI.

ADVERSE REACTIONS: Hypotension, tachycardia, hallucinations, dizziness, sedation, euphoria, sweating, NV, constipation, diarrhea, anorexia, facial edema, dermatitis, visual problems, chills, insomnia, urinary retention, paresthesia.

INTERACTIONS: Increased CNS depressant effects with alcohol. Withdrawal symptoms with narcotics.

PREGNANCY: Category C, caution in nursing.

MECHANISM OF ACTION: Pentazocine: Acts as analgesic and sedative. Naloxone: Acts as antagonist to pentazocine and pure antagonist to narcotic analgesics.

PHARMACOKINETICS: Absorption: Pentazocine: GI tract (well absorbed), T_{max}=1-3 hrs. **Distribution:** Pentazocine: Crosses placenta. **Metabolism:** Pentazocine: Liver. **Elimination:** Pentazocine: Urine; $T_{1/2}$=2-3 hrs.

NURSING CONSIDERATIONS

Assessment: Assess for head injury, MI, respiratory depression, impaired renal/hepatic function, biliary surgery, seizures, pregnancy status, and possible drug interactions.

Monitoring: Monitor vital signs, sedation, seizures, respiratory depression, NV, BP, HR, allergic reactions, leukopenia, drug abuse or dependence.

Patient Counseling: Inform that drug may cause sedation, dizziness, and occasional euphoria. Counsel about drug abuse and dependence. Avoid alcohol and do not abruptly d/c drug as there could be withdrawal symptoms. Exercise caution while driving or operating machinery.

Administration: Oral route. **Storage:** 25°C (77°F); excursions permitted to 15-30°C (59-86°F).

T

TAMBOCOR

RX

flecainide acetate (Graceway)

THERAPEUTIC CLASS: Class IC antiarrhythmic

INDICATIONS: Prevention of paroxysmal supraventricular tachycardias (PSVT), paroxysmal atrial fibrillation/flutter (PAF) associated with disabling symptoms in patients without structural heart disease. Prevention of life-threatening ventricular arrhythmias such as sustained ventricular tachycardia (VT).

DOSAGE: *Adults:* PSVT/PAF: Initial: 50mg q12h. Titrate: May increase by 50mg bid every 4 days. Max: 300mg/day. Sustained VT: Initial: 100mg q12h. Titrate: May increase by 50mg bid every 4 days. Max: 400mg/day. CrCl ≤35mL/min: Initial: 100mg qd or 50mg bid. Reduce dose by 50% with amiodarone.
Pediatrics: <6 months: Initial: 50mg/m²/day given bid-tid. ≥6 months: Initial:

100mg/m²/day given bid-tid. Max: 200mg/m²/day. Reduce dose by 50% with amiodarone.

HOW SUPPLIED: Tab: 50mg, 100mg*, 150mg* *scored

CONTRAINDICATIONS: Right bundle branch block associated with left hemiblock (without a pacemaker), pre-existing 2nd- or 3rd-degree AV block, cardiogenic shock.

WARNINGS/PRECAUTIONS: Avoid with non-life-threatening ventricular arrhythmias. Increased mortality and non-cardiac arrests reported. Ventricular proarrhythmic effects may occur with atrial fibrillation/flutter. May cause or worsen CHF, arrhythmias. Slows cardiac conduction; dose related increases in PR, QRS, and QT intervals reported. Conduction changes may cause sinus pause, sinus arrest, bradycardia, 2nd- or 3rd-degree AV block. Extreme caution with sick sinus syndrome. May increase endocardial pacing thresholds and suppress ventricular escape with pacemakers. Correct hypokalemia or hyperkalemia before therapy. Monitor with significant hepatic impairment. Initiate treatment of sustained VT in the hospital.

ADVERSE REACTIONS: Arrhythmias, hepatic dysfunction, cardiac arrest, CHF, flushing, anxiety, vomiting, diarrhea, tinnitus.

INTERACTIONS: Additive negative inotropic effects with β-blockers (eg, propranolol). Potentiated by cimetidine, amiodarone, CYP2D6 inhibitors (eg, quinidine). Increases digoxin levels. Increased elimination with phenytoin, phenobarbital, carbamazepine. Diltiazem, nifedipine, verapamil, disopyramide not recommended.

PREGNANCY: Category C, safety in nursing unknown.

MECHANISM OF ACTION: Class 1C antiarrhythmic agent with local anesthetic activity; decreases intracardiac conduction in all parts of the heart with greatest effect on His-Purkinje system (H-V conduction).

PHARMACOKINETICS: Absorption: Complete. T_{max}=3 hrs. **Metabolism:** Extensive, via CYP2D6. Meta-O-dealkylated flecainide (active metabolite). **Elimination:** Urine (30% unchanged), feces (5%); $T_{1/2}$=20 hrs, 29 hrs (at birth), 11-12 hrs (3 months), 6 hrs (1 yr), 8 hrs (1-12 yrs), and 11-12 hrs (12-15 yrs).

NURSING CONSIDERATIONS

Assessment: Assess for pre-existing 2nd- or 3rd-degree AV block, right bundle branch block associated with a left hemiblock, implanted pacemaker, cardiogenic shock, MI, asymptomatic non-life threatening ventricular arrhythmia, atrial fibrillation/flutter, cardiomyopathy, pre-existing severe HF or low ejection fraction, sick sinus syndrome, supraventricular tachycardia, pregnancy/nursing status, and possible drug interactions. Correct hypokalemia or hyperkalemia prior to therapy.

Monitoring: Determine pacing threshold in patients with pacemaker prior to therapy, after 1 week, and at regular intervals thereafter. Periodically monitor plasma levels with renal/hepatic impairment, CHF, and/or those on concurrent amiodarone therapy. Monitor for HR, ECG changes, paradoxical increase in ventricular rate, proarrhythmic effects (new or worsened supraventricular or ventricular arrhythmia), worsening of CHF, effects on cardiac conduction, and bradycardia.

Patient Counseling: Advise about importance of initiating therapy in hospital with continuous rhythmic monitoring. Inform about risks/benefits and report any adverse reactions to physician.

Administration: Oral route. **Storage:** 15-30°C (59-86°F).

TAMIFLU RX

oseltamivir phosphate (Roche Labs)

THERAPEUTIC CLASS: Neuraminidase inhibitor

INDICATIONS: Treatment of uncomplicated acute illness due to influenza in adults and children ≥1 yr who have been symptomatic for no more than 2 days. Prophylaxis of influenza in adults and children ≥1 yr.

DOSAGE: *Adults:* Prophylaxis: Begin within 2 days of exposure to infection. 75mg qd for at least 10 days, up to 6 weeks with community outbreak. CrCl 10-30mL/min: 75mg every other day or 30mg qd. Treatment: Begin therapy within 2 days of symptom onset. 75mg bid for 5 days. CrCl 10-30mL/min: 75mg qd for 5 days.
Pediatrics: Prophylaxis: ≥13 yr: Begin within 2 days of exposure to infection. 75mg qd for at least 10 days, up to 6 weeks with community outbreak. ≥1 yr: (Sus) ≤15kg: 30mg qd. >15-23kg: 45mg qd. >23-40kg: 60mg qd. >40kg: 75mg qd. Duration: 10 days. Treatment: ≥13 yrs: Begin therapy within 2 days of symptom onset. 75mg bid for 5 days. ≥1 yr: (Sus) ≤15kg: 30mg bid. >15-23kg: 45mg bid. >23-40kg: 60mg bid. >40kg: 75mg bid. Duration: 5 days.

HOW SUPPLIED: Cap: 30mg, 45mg, 75mg; Sus: 12mg/mL [25mL]

WARNINGS/PRECAUTIONS: Efficacy not known with chronic cardiac disease, respiratory disease, and immunocompromised. Not a substitute for influenza vaccine. Adjust dose with renal dysfunction. Postmarketing neuropsychiatric events (self-injury and delirium) reported. Caution with kidney disease, heart disease, respiratory disease, or any serious health condition. Sorbitol in Tamiflu may cause upset stomach and diarrhea in patients with history of fructose intolerance.

ADVERSE REACTIONS: NV, diarrhea, cough, headache, fatigue, abdominal pain, bronchitis, dizziness.

INTERACTIONS: Avoid administration of attenuated influenza vaccine within 2 weeks before or 48 hours after; may inhibit replication of live vaccine virus.

PREGNANCY: Category C, caution in nursing.

MECHANISM OF ACTION: Neuraminidase inhibitor; inhibits influenza virus neuraminidase, affecting release of viral particles.

PHARMACOKINETICS: Absorption: (GI tract). Oseltamivir: C_{max}=65.2ng/mL; AUC_{0-12h}=112ng•hr/mL Oseltamivir carboxylate (metabolite). C_{max}=348ng/mL; AUC_{0-12h}=2719ng•hr/mL. **Distribution:** Oseltamivir carboxylate: (IV): V_d=23-26L; plasma protein binding (3%). Oseltamivir: Plasma protein binding (42%). **Metabolism:** Oseltamivir: Hepatic (esterases). Metabolite: (Oseltamivir carboxylate). **Elimination:** Oseltamivir carboxylate: Renal (>99%); feces (<20%).

NURSING CONSIDERATIONS

Assessment: Assess for renal impairment, neuropsychiatric events, hereditary fructose intolerance, and possible drug interactions.

Monitoring: Monitor for signs/symptoms of neuropsychiatric events (eg, hallucinations, delirium, abnormal behavior), anaphylaxis/serious skin reactions, renal impairment, and fructose intolerance (eg, dyspepsia, diarrhea).

Patient Counseling: Instruct to begin treatment as soon as 1st appearance of flu symptoms. Advise to take missed doses as soon as possible, except if near next scheduled dose (within 2 hrs). Drug may be taken with/without food. Seek medical attention if symptoms of neuropsychiatric events (eg, hallucinations, delirium, abnormal behavior), anaphylaxis/serious skin reactions, renal impairment, and fructose intolerance (eg, dyspepsia, diarrhea) occur.

Administration: Oral route. **Storage:** Refrigerate 2-8°C (36-46°F); stable for 5 weeks. Room temperature: 25°C (77°F); stable for 5 days. Do not freeze.

TAMOXIFEN RX

tamoxifen citrate (Various)

For women with ductal carcinoma in situ (DCIS) and women at high risk for breast cancer; fatal uterine malignancies (eg, endometrial adenocarcinoma, uterine sarcoma), stroke, and PE reported with use in risk reduction setting. Discuss benefits/risks of events with this patient population. Benefits of tamoxifen outweigh risks in women already diagnosed with breast cancer.

THERAPEUTIC CLASS: Antiestrogen

INDICATIONS: Treatment of metastatic breast cancer in women and men. Treatment of node-positive and axillary node-negative breast cancer in women following mastectomy, axillary dissection and breast irradiation. To reduce risk of invasive breast cancer in women with DCIS. Reduction of breast cancer incidence in high risk women. Use for up to 5 yrs.

DOSAGE: *Adults:* Breast Cancer Treatment: 20-40mg qd. Divide dosages >20mg into AM and PM doses. Breast Cancer Risk Reduction/DCIS: 20mg qd for 5 yrs.

HOW SUPPLIED: Tab: 10mg, 20mg

CONTRAINDICATIONS: Reduction in breast cancer incidence in high risk women and women wtih DCIS who require coumarin-type anticoagulant therapy or have a history of DVT, PE.

WARNINGS/PRECAUTIONS: Hypercalcemia reported in patients with bone metastases. Increased incidence of uterine malignancies (eg, endometrial cancer, uterine sarcoma) and endometrial changes including hyperplasia and polyps reported. Increased incidence of thromboembolic events (eg, DVT, PE). Malignant and non-malignant effects on the liver and ocular disturbances reported. Leukopenia, anemia, thrombocytopenia, neutropenia, pancytopenia reported. Promptly evaluate abnormal vaginal bleeding if receiving or previously received tamoxifen. Patients receiving or who previously received tamoxifen should have annual gynecological exam. Do not become pregnant within 2 months of therapy. May cause fetal harm during pregnancy. Does not cause infertility even with menstrual irregularity.

ADVERSE REACTIONS: Hot flashes, increased bone and tumor pain, vaginal discharge, fatigue/asthenia, mood disturbances, nausea/vomiting, irregular menses; (men) loss of libido, impotence.

INTERACTIONS: Increases effects of coumarin-type anticoagulant; monitor PT. Increased risk of thromboembolic events with cytotoxic agents. Increased levels with bromocriptine. May decrease letrozole levels. Decreased levels with rifampin and aminoglutethimide. Decreased plasma levels of major metabolite, N-desmethyl tamoxifen with medroxyprogesterone. Avoid administering with anastrozole.

PREGNANCY: Category D, not for use in nursing.

MECHANISM OF ACTION: Non-steroidal antiestrogen; competes with estrogen for binding sites in target tissues.

PHARMACOKINETICS: Absorption: C_{max}=40ng/mL; T_{max}=5 hrs. N-desmethyl tamoxifen: C_{max}=15ng/mL. **Metabolism:** N-desmethyl tamoxifen (major metabolite). **Elimination:** Feces (primary); $T_{1/2}$=5-7 days.

NURSING CONSIDERATIONS

Assessment: Assess for pregnancy status, history of DVT and PE, hepatic impairment, and possible drug interactions. Perform baseline breast exam, gynecologic exam; obtain baseline mammogram.

Monitoring: Monitor CBC with platelets and LFTs periodically; perform breast exam, mammogram, and gynecologic exam routinely. Monitor for signs/symptoms of hypercalcemia, stroke, PEs, uterine malignancies, and hypersensitivity reactions.

Patient Counseling: Inform of pregnancy risks; advise to use nonhormonal contraception during therapy and for 2 months after d/c. Instruct to seek medical attention if symptoms of menstrual irregularities, abnormal vaginal bleeding, changes in vaginal discharge, pelvic pain/pressure, new breast lumps, leg swelling/tenderness, SOB, changes in vision, or hypersensitivity reactions occur.

Administration: Oral route. **Storage:** 20-25°C (68-77°F); avoid excessive heat; protect from light.

TAPAZOLE RX

methimazole (King)

THERAPEUTIC CLASS: Thyroid hormone synthesis inhibitor

INDICATIONS: Treatment of hyperthyroidism. To ameliorate hyperthyroidism prior to subtotal thyroidectomy or radioactive iodine therapy. Also indicated when thyroidectomy is contraindicated or not advisable.

DOSAGE: *Adults:* Initial: Mild Hyperthyroidism: 5mg q8h. Moderately Severe Hyperthyroidism: 30-40mg/day, in divided doses q8h. Severe Hyperthyroidism: 20mg q8h. Maint: 5-15mg/day.
Pediatrics: Initial: 0.4mg/kg/day, in divided doses q8h. Maint: 1/2 of initial dose.

HOW SUPPLIED: Tab: 5mg*, 10mg* *scored

CONTRAINDICATIONS: Nursing mothers.

WARNINGS/PRECAUTIONS: Can cause fetal harm. Agranulocytosis, leukopenia, thrombocytopenia, aplastic anemia may occur; monitor bone marrow function. D/C with agranulocytosis, aplastic anemia, or exfoliative dermatitis. D/C with liver abnormality (eg, hepatitis) including transaminases >3x ULN. Monitor thyroid function periodically. May cause hypoprothrombinemia and bleeding; monitor PT.

ADVERSE REACTIONS: Rash, urticaria, NV, arthralgia, paresthesia, myalgia, neuritis, vertigo, edema, altered taste, hair loss, lymphadenopathy, lupus-like syndrome, insulin autoimmune syndrome.

INTERACTIONS: May potentiate anticoagulants. β-blockers, digitalis, theophylline may need dose reduction when patient becomes euthyroid. Caution with other drugs that cause agranulocytosis.

PREGNANCY: Category D, contraindicated in nursing.

MECHANISM OF ACTION: Inhibits synthesis of thyroid hormones.

PHARMACOKINETICS: Absorption: Readily absorbed (GI tract). **Distribution:** Crosses placenta and found in breast milk. **Elimination:** Urine.

NURSING CONSIDERATIONS

Assessment: Assess for drug hypersensitivity, pregnancy/nursing status, and possible drug interactions.

Monitoring: Monitor for signs of illness (eg, fever, sore throat, malaise, skin eruptions, headache), and hepatic dysfunction (eg, anorexia, upper quadrant pain), with frequent lab testing of CBC, TSH, LFTs, PT, and bone marrow function.

Patient Counseling: Instruct to inform physician if pregnant/nursing or planning to become pregnant. Report signs/symptoms of illness (eg, fever, general malaise, sore throat) to physician.

Administration: Oral route. **Storage:** 15-30°C (59-86°F).

TARCEVA — RX

erlotinib (Genentech/OSI)

THERAPEUTIC CLASS: Epidermal growth factor receptor tyrosine kinase inhibitor

INDICATIONS: Treatment of patients with locally advanced or metastatic non-small cell lung cancer (NSCLC) after failure of at least one prior chemotherapy regimen. 1st-line treatment of patients with locally advanced, unresectable, or metastatic pancreatic cancer in combination with gemcitabine.

DOSAGE: *Adults:* NSCLC: 150mg at least 1 hr before or 2 hrs after ingestion of food. Pancreatic Cancer: 100mg at least 1 hr before or 2 hrs after ingestion of food, in combination with gemcitabine. Continue until disease progression or unacceptable toxicity. Acute Onset of New or Progressive Pulmonary Symptoms: D/C therapy. Severe Diarrhea/Severe Skin Reactions: May require dose reduction or temporary interruption of therapy. Strong CYP3A4 Inhibitors: Consider dose reduction. When dose reduction is necessary, reduce dose in 50-mg decrements.

HOW SUPPLIED: Tab: 25mg, 100mg, 150mg

WARNINGS/PRECAUTIONS: Serious interstitial lung disease (ILD), including fatalities, reported; d/c if ILD diagnosed. Caution in patients with total bilirubin >3x ULN; monitor closely with hepatic impairment (total bilirubin >ULN or Child-Pugh A,B,C). Consider dose reduction or interruption if changes in liver function are severe. Hepatic failure, hepatorenal syndrome, acute renal failure, and renal insufficiency reported. Caution in patients at risk of dehydration; monitor renal function and serum electrolytes periodically. May increase risk of MI and cerebrovascular accident. Elevations in INR and infrequent reports of bleeding reported. Monitor closely with concomitant anticoagulants. May cause fetal harm; avoid pregnancy. May cause MI/ischemia.

ADVERSE REACTIONS: Rash, diarrhea, anorexia, fatigue, dyspnea, cough, NV, infection, stomatitis, pruritus, dry skin, conjunctivitis, keratoconjunctivitis sicca, abdominal pain, and myalgia.

INTERACTIONS: Co-treatment with ketoconazole increases erlotinib AUC by 2/3. Caution with ketoconazole, atazanavir, clarithromycin, indinavir, itraconazole, nefazodone, nelfinavir, ritonavir, saquinavir, telithromycin, troleandomycin, voriconazole, and grapefruit or grapefruit juice. Rifampicin decreases erlotinib AUC by 2/3 to 4/5. Cigarette smoking may reduce erlotinib AUC. Drugs that alter pH of upper GI tract may alter solubility and bioavailability; concomitant use of PPIs or H_2 blockers should be avoided.

PREGNANCY: Category D, not for use in nursing.

MECHANISM OF ACTION: Human epidermal growth factor receptor tyrosine kinase inhibitor; inhibits intracellular phosphorylation of tyrosine kinase associated with epidermal growth factor receptor, which is expressed on cell surface of normal and cancer cells.

PHARMACOKINETICS: Absorption: Absolute bioavailability (60%); T_{max}=4 hrs. **Distribution:** V_d=232L; plasma protein binding (93%). **Metabolism:** CYP3A4 (major); CYP1A2, 1A1 (minor). **Elimination:** Feces (1%), urine (0.3%); $T_{1/2}$=36 hrs.

NURSING CONSIDERATIONS

Assessment: Assess for lung disease, hepatic/renal impairment, pregnancy/nursing status, and possible drug interactions. Obtain baseline LFTs and renal function. If on anticoagulants, obtain baseline PT/INR.

Monitoring: Periodically monitor LFTs, renal function, and serum electrolytes. Monitor for acute onset of new or progressive pulmonary symptoms, hepatotoxicity, and hypersensitivity reactions.

Patient Counseling: Instruct to seek medical attention if symptoms of severe or persistent diarrhea, NV, onset or worsening of SOB, cough, or eye irritation occur. Advise to stop smoking. Inform of pregnancy risks; avoid pregnancy. If an antacid is necessary, the antacid dose should be seperated by several hours.

Administration: Oral route. **Storage**: 25°C (77°F); excursions permitted to 15-30° (59-86°F).

TARKA RX

verapamil HCl - trandolapril (Abbott)

ACE inhibitors can cause death/injury to developing fetus during 2nd and 3rd trimesters. Stop therapy if pregnancy detected.

THERAPEUTIC CLASS: ACE inhibitor/calcium channel blocker (nondihydropyridine)

INDICATIONS: Treatment of hypertension. Not for initial therapy.

DOSAGE: *Adults:* Replacement Therapy: 1 tab qd with food. Severe Hepatic Dysfunction: Give 30% of normal dose.

HOW SUPPLIED: Tab: (Trandolapril-Verapamil) 2mg-180mg, 1mg-240mg, 2mg-240mg, 4mg-240mg

CONTRAINDICATIONS: Severe ventricular dysfunction, hypotension, cardiogenic shock, sick sinus syndrome or 2nd- or 3rd-degree AV block (except with functioning ventricular pacemaker), A-Fib/Flutter with an accessory bypass tract, history of ACE inhibitor-associated angioedema.

WARNINGS/PRECAUTIONS: Monitor for hypotension with surgery or anesthesia. Risk of hyperkalemia with renal insufficiency, DM. D/C if jaundice develops. Avoid with moderate to severe cardiac failure and ventricular dysfunction if taking a β-blocker. May cause angioedema, cough, fetal/neonatal morbidity, hypotension, AV block, anaphylactoid reactions, transient bradycardia, PR-interval prolongation. Monitor LFTs periodically. Give 30% of normal dose with severe hepatic dysfunction. Caution with CHF, hypertrophic cardiomyopathy, renal or hepatic dysfunction. Decrease dose in those with decreased neuromuscular transmission. Monitor WBC with collagen-vascular disease and/or renal disease.

ADVERSE REACTIONS: AV block, constipation, cough, dizziness, fatigue, headache, increased hepatic enzymes, chest pain, upper respiratory tract infection/congestion.

INTERACTIONS: May increase alcohol blood levels and prolong effects. Additive effects on HR, AV conduction, and contractility with β-blockers. Potentiates other antihypertensives. May increase digoxin, carbamazepine, theophylline, and cyclosporine levels. Avoid disopyramide within 48 hrs before or 24 hrs after verapamil. Additive negative inotropic effects and AV conduction prolongation with flecainide. Avoid quinidine with hypertrophic cardiomyopathy. Monitor lithium. Increased clearance with phenobarbital. Rifampin may reduce oral bioavailability. May potentiate neuromuscular blockers; both agents may need dose reduction. Risk of hyperkalemia with K^+-sparing diuretics, K^+ supplements. Caution with inhalation anesthetics.

PREGNANCY: Category C (1st trimester) and D (2nd and 3rd trimesters), not for use in nursing.

MECHANISM OF ACTION: ACE inhibitor; inhibition results in decreased plasma angiotensin II, which leads to decreased vasopressor activity and decreased aldosterone secretion. Calcium channel blocker; inhibits calcium ion influx into cardiac muscle and smooth muscle.

PHARMACOKINETICS: Absorption: Verapamil: Absolute bioavailability (20-35%), T_{max}=4-15 hrs. Trandolopril: Absolute bioavailability (~10%), T_{max}=0.5-2 hrs. **Distribution:** Verapamil: Plasma protein binding (90%). Trandolapril: Plasma protein binding (80%). **Metabolism:** Verapamil: Liver. **Elimination:** Verapamil: Urine 70% (metabolite), 3-4% (unchanged), feces 16% (metabolite). Trandolapril: Urine 33% (metabolite), 1% (unchanged), feces 66% (metabolite).

NURSING CONSIDERATIONS

Assessment: Assess for severe left ventricular dysfunction, hypotension, cardiogenic shock, sick sinus syndrome, 2nd- or 3rd-degree AV block, atrial flutter or atrial fibrillation, history of angioedema, heart failure, hypotension, LFTs, renal function, CHF, accessory bypass tract, hypertrophic cardiomyopathy, CBC with platelets and differential, pregnancy status, neuromuscular disorders (Duchenne's), and possible drug interactions.

Monitoring: Monitor for angioedema, cough, anaphylactoid reactions, LFTs, renal function, headaches, URI, heart block, CP, CBC with platelets and differential count, serum electrolytes.

Patient Counseling: Counsel regarding adverse effects (eg, angioedema, neutropenia, jaundice) and instruct to report any signs/symptoms. Inform of risks when taken during pregnancy. Instruct to take as prescribed with food. Educate about need for periodic follow-ups and blood tests to rule out adverse effects and monitor therapeutic effects.

Administration: Oral route. **Storage:** 15-25°C (59-77°F).

TASMAR RX

tolcapone (Valeant)

Risk of fatal, acute fulminant liver failure. Withdraw if patients fail to show benefit within 3 weeks of initiation. D/C if hepatotoxicity develops, and do not consider retreatment. Perform LFTs before therapy, then every 2 weeks for 1st year, every 4 weeks for next 6 months, then every 8 weeks thereafter. Perform LFTs before increase dose to 200mg tid. Avoid with liver disease or if LFTs ≥2x ULN. Caution with severe dyskinesia or dystonia.

THERAPEUTIC CLASS: COMT inhibitor

INDICATIONS: Adjunct to levodopa/carbidopa for the treatment of symptoms of idiopathic Parkinson's disease.

DOSAGE: *Adults:* Initial: 100mg tid. Use 200mg tid only if clinical benefit is justified. May need to decrease levodopa dose.

HOW SUPPLIED: Tab: 100mg, 200mg

CONTRAINDICATIONS: Liver disease, patients withdrawn from therapy due to drug-induced hepatocellular injury. History of non-traumatic rhabdomyolysis, hyperpyrexia or confusion related to medication.

WARNINGS/PRECAUTIONS: Hypotension/syncope, rhabdomyolysis, hallucinations, confusion, diarrhea, hematuria reported. Fibrotic complications can occur. Avoid with liver dysfunction. Caution with severe renal dysfunction. Closely monitor when discontinuing therapy.

ADVERSE REACTIONS: Dyskinesia, nausea, dystonia, excessive dreaming, anorexia, muscle cramps, orthostatic complaints, diarrhea, confusion, hallucination, vomiting, constipation, fatigue, increased sweating, xerostomia, urine discoloration, hepatotoxicity.

INTERACTIONS: Dobutamine, apomorphine and isoproterenol may need a dose reduction. Avoid non-selective MAOIs (eg, phenelzine, tranylcypromine). May increase risk of orthostatic hypotension and dyskinesia with levodopa. Caution with tolbutamide, desipramine, warfarin.

PREGNANCY: Category C, caution in nursing.

MECHANISM OF ACTION: Cathecol-*O*-methyltransferase inhibitor; suspected to alter the plasma pharmacokinetics of levodopa, leading to more sustained plasma levels of drug.

PHARMACOKINETICS: Absorption: (PO) Rapidly absorbed; absolute bioavailability (65%); T_{max}=2 hrs; C_{max}=3mcg/mL (100mg, 200mg); C_{max}=6mcg/mL (100mg, 200mg). **Distribution:** V_d=9L; plasma protein binding (>99.9%). **Metabolism:** Liver (glucuronidation) via CYP450 enzymes 3A4, 2A6. **Elimination:** Urine (60%, 0.5% unchanged), feces (40%); $T_{1/2}$=2-3 hrs.

NURSING CONSIDERATIONS

Assessment: Assess LFTs, renal function test, dyskinesia, psychosis, depression, and cardiovascular complications.

Monitoring: LFTs (SGPT/ALT, SGOT/AST), renal function test, hypotension/syncope, diarrhea, dyskinesia, rhabdomyolysis, hematuria, hyperpyrexia, confusion, fibrotic complications, and depression.

Patient Counseling: Instruct to take as prescribed. Caution while operating machinery/driving. Regular follow-up needed. Avoid alcohol, OTC agents, and CNS depressants. Report adverse effects.

Administration: Oral route. **Storage:** 20-25°C (68-77°F). Keep in tight container.

TAXOL RX

paclitaxel (Bristol-Myers Squibb)

Anaphylaxis, severe hypersensitivity reactions reported. Pretreat with corticosteroids, diphenhydramine, and H_2 antagonists. Do not rechallenge if severe hypersensitivity reaction occurs. Monitor CBC frequently.

THERAPEUTIC CLASS: Antimicrotubule agent

INDICATIONS: First-line (with cisplatin) treatment of advanced ovarian carcinoma and non-small cell lung cancer. Subsequent treatment in advanced ovarian carcinoma. Treatment of breast cancer after failure with combination chemotherapy for metastatic disease or relapse within 6 months of adjuvant chemotherapy. Adjuvant treatment of node-positive breast cancer administered sequentially to doxorubicin-containing chemotherapy. Second-line treatment of AIDS-related Kaposi's sarcoma.

DOSAGE: *Adults:* IV: Ovarian Carcinoma: Previously Untreated: 175mg/m² over 3 hrs or 135mg/m² over 24 hrs every 3 weeks followed by cisplatin. Previous Treatment: 135mg/m² or 175mg/m² over 3 hrs every 3 weeks. Breast Cancer: 175mg/m² over 3 hrs every 3 weeks for 4 courses. Non-Small Cell Lung Cancer: 135mg/m² over 24 hrs every 3 weeks followed by cisplatin. Kaposi's Sarcoma: 135mg/m² over 3 hrs every 3 weeks or 100mg/m² over 3 hrs every 2 weeks. Reduce dose of subsequent courses by 20% if neutrophils <500 cells/mm³ for ≥1 week or severe peripheral neuropathy occurs. Premedicate prior to administration to prevent severe hypersensitivity reactions; dexamethasone 20mg PO 12 and 6 hrs before, diphenhydramine 50mg IV 30-60 min prior, and cimetidine 300mg or ranitidine 50mg IV 30-60 min before.

HOW SUPPLIED: Inj: 6mg/mL

CONTRAINDICATIONS: Hypersensitivity to drugs formulated in Cremophor® EL (eg, cyclosporine for injection concentrate, teniposide for injection concentrate), solid tumor patients with baseline neutrophils <1500 cells/mm³, AIDS-related Kaposi's sarcoma patients with baseline neutrophils <1000 cells/mm³.

WARNINGS/PRECAUTIONS: Severe conduction abnormalities, injection site reactions, peripheral neuropathy (more common in elderly) reported. Bone marrow suppression is dose dependent, dose limiting, and more common in elderly. Can cause fetal harm. Hypotension, bradycardia, and HTN may occur during administration. Toxicity enhanced with elevated liver enzymes. Contains dehydrated alcohol.

ADVERSE REACTIONS: Neutropenia, leukopenia, thrombocytopenia, anemia, infections, bleeding, bradycardia, hypotension, peripheral neuropathy, myalgia/arthralgia, nausea, vomiting, diarrhea, mucositis, alopecia.

INTERACTIONS: Increases doxorubicin levels. Caution with CYP450 2C8 and 3A4 substrates or inhibitors (eg, ritonavir, saquinavir, indinavir, nelfinavir). Myelosuppression more profound with cisplatin.

PREGNANCY: Category D, not for use in nursing.

MECHANISM OF ACTION: Antimicrotubule; promotes assembly of microtubules from tubulin dimers and stabilizes microtubules by preventing depolymerization inhibiting microtubule network essential for vital interphase and mitotic cellular functions.

PHARMACOKINETICS: Absorption: IV administration of multiple doses resulted in different parameters. **Distribution:** V_d=227-688L/m²; plasma protein binding (89-98%). **Metabolism:** CYP2C8 (major), CYP3A4 (minor). 6α-hydroxy paclitaxel (metabolite). **Elimination:** Urine (1.3-12.6%), feces.

NURSING CONSIDERATIONS

Assessment: Assess for pregnancy status, possible drug interactions, neutrophil count (>1500 cells/mm³ for solid tumors; >1000 cells/mm³ for Kaposi's sarcoma), hypersensitivity to Cremophor EL, and hepatic impairment.

Monitoring: Monitor blood count frequently; vital signs frequently during 1st hr of infusion. Monitor for signs/symptoms of anaphylaxis/hypersensitivity reactions, injection-site reaction, conduction abnormalities, bone marrow suppression, infections, neutropenia, and hepatic dysfunction.

Patient Counseling: Inform of pregnancy risks. Advise to seek medical attention if symptoms of infection, anaphylaxis/hypersensitivity reactions (eg, dyspnea, hypotension, angioedema, urticaria), conduction abnormalities, or injection site reactions (eg, erythema, tenderness, swelling, discoloration) occur.

Administration: IV route. **Storage:** 20-25°C (68-77°F). Protect from light.

TAXOTERE RX

docetaxel (Sanofi-Aventis)

Increased treatment-related mortality reported with hepatic dysfunction, high-dose therapy, and in non-small cell lung carcinoma previously treated with platinum-based chemotherapy with docetaxel 100mg/m². Avoid if neutrophils <1500 cells/mm³, bilirubin >ULN, or SGOT/SGPT >1.5x ULN with alkaline phosphatase >2.5x ULN. Severe hypersensitivity reactions reported. Severe fluid retention may occur despite dexamethasone.

THERAPEUTIC CLASS: Antimicrotubule agent

INDICATIONS: Treatment of locally advanced or metastatic breast cancer and non-small cell lung cancer (NSCLC) after failure of prior chemotherapy. In combination with doxorubicin and cyclophosphamide for the adjuvant treatment of operable, node-positive breast cancer. In combination with cisplatin for treatment of unresectable, locally advanced or metastatic NSCLC in those previously untreated with chemotherapy. In combination with prednisone for treatment of androgen independent (hormone refractory) metastatic prostate cancer. In combination with cisplatin and fluorouracil for the treatment of advanced gastric adenocarcinoma, including adenocarcinoma of the gastroesophageal junction, in patients who have not received prior chemotherapy for advanced disease. In combination with cisplatin and fluorouracil for the induction treatment of patients with locally advanced squamous cell carcinoma of the head and neck (SCCHN).

DOSAGE: *Adults:* Premedicate with oral corticosteroids. Adjust dose based on febrile neutropenia, neutrophil count, cutaneous reactions, peripheral neuropathy, neurosensory signs/symptoms, or GI toxicities (see PI). Breast Cancer: 60-100mg/m² IV over 1 hr every 3 weeks. Adjuvant Treatment Operable Node-Positive Breast CA: 75mg/m² 1 hr after doxorubicin 50mg/m² and cyclophosphamide 500mg/m² every 3 weeks for 6 courses. NSCLC: 75mg/m² IV over 1 hr every 3 weeks. Prostate Cancer: 75mg/m² every 3 weeks over 1 hr with prednisone 5mg bid. Gastric Adenocarcinoma: Premedicate with antiemetics and appropriate hydration. 75mg/m² IV over 1 hr, followed by cisplatin 75mg/m² IV over 1-3 hrs (both on Day 1 only), followed by fluorouracil 750mg/m²/day IV over 24 hrs for 5 days, starting at end of cisplatin infusion. Repeat treatment every 3 weeks. SCCHN: Induction followed by Radiotherapy: 75mg/m² IV over 1 hr, followed by cisplatin 75mg/m² IV over 1 hr, on Day 1, followed by fluorouracil as a continuous IV infusion at 750mg/m²/day for 5 days. Administer every 3 weeks for 4 cycles. Induction followed by Chemoradiotherapy: 75mg/m² IV over 1 hr on Day 1, followed by cisplatin 100mg/m² IV over 30 min to 3 hrs, followed by fluorouracil 1000mg/m²/day as a continuous IV infusion from Day 1 to Day 4. Administer every 3 weeks for 3 cycles.

HOW SUPPLIED: Inj: 20mg/0.5mL, 80mg/2mL

CONTRAINDICATIONS: Neutrophils <1500 cells/mm³, hypersensitivity to polysorbate 80.

T

WARNINGS/PRECAUTIONS: Toxic deaths, febrile neutropenia, neutropenia, localized erythema of extremities with edema and desquamation, severe neurosensory symptoms, severe asthenia reported. Monitor for hypersensitivity reactions. Can cause fetal harm. Caution in elderly. Monitor CBC frequently; avoid subsequent cycles until neutrophils recover to >1500 cells/mm³ and platelets recover to >100,000 cells/mm³.

ADVERSE REACTIONS: Arthralgia, myalgia, alopecia, stomatitis, nausea, vomiting, diarrhea, nail changes, cutaneous and neurosensory reactions, fluid retention, hypersensitivity reaction, leukopenia, thrombocytopenia, anemia, neutropenia, fever.

INTERACTIONS: Caution with agents that induce, inhibit, or are metabolized by CYP450 3A4 (eg, ketoconazole, erythromycin, terfenadine, astemizole, cyclosporine).

PREGNANCY: Category D, not for use in nursing.

MECHANISM OF ACTION: Antimicrotubule agent; disrupts microtubular network in cells that is essential for mitotic and interphase cellular functions.

Binds to free tubulin and promotes assembly of tubulin into stable microtubules while simultaneously inhibiting their disassembly.

PHARMACOKINETICS: Distribution: V_d=113L; plasma protein binding (94%). **Metabolism:** CYP3A4. **Elimination:** Urine, feces (80%); $T_{1/2}$=11.1 hrs.

NURSING CONSIDERATIONS

Assessment: Assess CBC with platelet count and differential, LFTs, bilirubin levels, non-small cell lung carcinoma, pregnancy status, and possible drug interactions.

Monitoring: Monitor LFTs, bilirubin, CBC with platelets and differential count. Monitor for fluid retention, neurosensory symptoms, skin toxicity, and hypersensitivity reactions.

Patient Counseling: Counsel about side effects of drug; report signs/symptoms of side effects. Advise about need for routine blood tests and follow ups. Inform physician before taking any other medications. Advise women of childbearing age not to become pregnant when taking this drug.

Administration: IV route; infuse over 1 hr. **Storage:** 2-25°C (36-77°F). Protect from bright light.

TAZICEF — RX

ceftazidime (Hospira)

THERAPEUTIC CLASS: Cephalosporin (3rd generation)

INDICATIONS: Treatment of lower respiratory tract (eg, pneumonia), skin and skin structure (SSSI), bone and joint, gynecologic, intra-abdominal, CNS (eg, meningitis), and urinary tract infections (UTI), bacterial septicemia, and sepsis caused by susceptible strains of microorganisms.

DOSAGE: *Adults:* Usual: 1g IV q8-12h. Uncomplicated UTI: 250mg IM/IV q12h. Complicated UTI: 500mg IM/IV q8-12h. Bone and Joint Infections: 2g IV q12h. Uncomplicated Pneumonia/SSSI: 500mg-1g IM/IV q8h. Gynecological/Intra-Abdominal/Meningitis/Severe Life-Threatening Infection: 2g IV q8h. Lung Infection caused by *Pseudomonas* in Cystic Fibrosis (normal renal function): 30-50mg/kg IV q8h. Max: 6g/day. Renal Impairment: CrCl 31-50mL/min: 1g q12h. CrCl 16-30mL/min: 1g q24h. CrCl 6-15mL/min: 500mg q24h. CrCl <5mL/min: 500mg q48h. For severe infections (6g/day), increase renal impairment dose by 50% or increase dosing interval. Apply reduced dosage recommendations after initial 1g LD is given. Hemodialysis: Give 1g LD before and 1g after each hemodialysis period. Intra-Peritoneal Dialysis/Continuous Ambulatory Peritoneal Dialysis: Give 1g LD followed by 500mg q24h, or add to fluid at 250mg/2L.

Pediatrics: Neonates (0-4 weeks): 30mg/kg IV q12h. 1 month-12 yrs: 30-50mg/kg IV q8h. Max: 6g/day. Higher doses for patients with cystic fibrosis or when treating meningitis. Renal Impairment: CrCl 31-50mL/min: 1g q12h. CrCl 16-30mL/min: 1g q24h. CrCl 6-15mL/min: 500mg q24h. CrCl <5mL/min: 500mg q48h. Hemodialysis: Give 1g before and 1g after each hemodialysis. For severe infections (6g/day), increase renal impairment dose by 50% or increase dosing interval. Apply reduced dosage recommendations after initial 1g LD is given. Hemodialysis: Give 1g LD before and 1g after each hemodialysis period. Intra-Peritoneal Dialysis/Continuous Ambulatory Peritoneal Dialysis: Give 1g followed by 500mg q24h, or add to fluid at 250mg/2L.

HOW SUPPLIED: Inj: 1g, 2g, 6g

WARNINGS/PRECAUTIONS: Monitor renal function; potential for nephrotoxicity. May result in overgrowth of nonsusceptible organisms. Possible cross-sensitivity between PCNs, cephalosporins, and other β-lactams. Pseudomembranous colitis reported. Elevated levels with renal insufficiency can lead to seizures, encephalopathy, asterixis, and neuromuscular excitability. Possible decrease in PT; caution with renal or hepatic impairment, poor nutritional state; monitor PT and give vitamin K if needed. Caution with colitis and other GI diseases. Distal necrosis may occur after inadvertent intra-arterial administration. Continue for 2 days after signs/symptoms of infection

T

resolve; may require longer therapy with complicated infections. Caution in elderly.

ADVERSE REACTIONS: Phlebitis and inflammation at injection site, pruritus, rash, fever, diarrhea, NV.

INTERACTIONS: Nephrotoxicity reported with aminoglycosides or potent diuretics (eg, furosemide). Avoid with chloramphenicol; may decrease effect of β-lactam antibiotics.

PREGNANCY: Category B, caution in nursing.

MECHANISM OF ACTION: 3rd-generation cephalosporin; inhibits enzymes responsible for cell-wall synthesis.

PHARMACOKINETICS: Absorption: C_{max}=90mcg/mL (1g IV), 39mcg/mL (1g IM); see PI for detailed info. **Distribution:** Plasma protein binding (<10%); found in breast milk. **Elimination:** Urine (80-90% unchanged); $T_{1/2}$=1.9 hrs (IV).

NURSING CONSIDERATIONS

Assessment: Assess for previous hypersensitivity reaction to cephalosporins/PCNs or other drugs, renal/hepatic impairment, poor nutritional status, patients receiving protracted course of antibiotics, GI disease (particularly colitis), pregnancy/nursing status, and possible drug interactions.

Monitoring: Monitor PT; vitamin K administration as indicated. Monitor for signs/symptoms of allergic reactions (eg, Stevens-Johnson syndrome, toxic epidermal necrolysis), pseudomembranous colitis or *C.difficile*-associated diarrhea (may range in severity from mild diarrhea to fatal colitis), development of drug resistance, overgrowth of nonsusceptible organisms, seizures, encephalopathy, asterixis, neuromuscular excitability, distal necrosis in inadvertent intra-atrial injection, and lab test interactions (eg, false (+) urinary glucose test when using Clinitest, Benedict's solution, or Fehling's solution), (+) Coombs' test without hemolysis, LFTs, renal function tests, and CBC).

Patient Counseling: Only treats bacterial, not viral, infections. Take exactly as directed; skipping doses or not completing full course may decrease effectiveness and increase resistance. Inform about risks/benefits. D/C and notify physician if experience allergic reaction or diarrhea. Notify if pregnant/nursing.

Administration: IV and IM route. Do not use flexible container in series connections. **Storage**: Dry state 20-25°C (68-77°F), reconstituted solution for 24 hrs at room temperature, or for 7 days at 5°C; stable for 3 months if frozen at -20°C; thawed solution, store for up to 8 hrs at room temperature or for 4 days at 5°C; do not refreeze thawed solution.

TAZORAC RX

tazarotene (Allergan)

T

THERAPEUTIC CLASS: Retinoid

INDICATIONS: (Gel 0.05%, 0.1%) Stable plaque psoriasis of up to 20% body surface area involvement. (Gel 0.1%) Acne vulgaris of mild to moderate severity.

DOSAGE: *Adults:* Psoriasis: Start with 0.05% Gel, increase to 0.1% if tolerated. Apply thin film to psoriatic lesions qpm. Acne: Cleanse and dry skin. Apply thin film of 0.1% Gel to acne lesions qpm.
Pediatrics: ≥12 yrs: Psoriasis: Start with 0.05% Gel, increase to 0.1% if tolerated. Apply thin film to psoriatic lesions qpm. Acne: Cleanse and dry skin. Apply thin film of 0.1% Gel to acne lesions qpm.

HOW SUPPLIED: Gel: 0.05%, 0.1% [30g, 100g]

CONTRAINDICATIONS: Women who are or may become pregnant.

WARNINGS/PRECAUTIONS: Use adequate birth control measures. Avoid mouth, eyes, eyelids, exposure to sunlight or sunlamps, or eczematous skin. D/C if pruritus, burning, skin redness, or peeling. Weather extremes (eg, wind, cold) may be irritating.

ADVERSE REACTIONS: Pruritus, burning/stinging, erythema, worsening of psoriasis, irritation, skin pain, desquamation, dry skin, rash, fissuring, localized edema, skin discoloration.

INTERACTIONS: Avoid topical agents that have a strong drying effect. Caution with photosensitizers (eg, thiazides, tetracyclines, fluoroquinolones, phenothiazines, sulfonamides).

PREGNANCY: Category X, caution in nursing.

MECHANISM OF ACTION: Retinoic acid derivative; binds to all 3 members of the retinoic acid receptor RAR (RARα, RARβ, and RAR_{gamma}). Treatment of psoriasis not established. Suppresses expression of MRP8, a marker of inflammation; induces expression of a gene which may be a growth suppressor in keratinocytes, and may inhibit epidermal hyperproliferation in treated plaques. Treatment of acne not established; may be due to anti-hyperproliferative, normalizing-of-differentiation, and anti-inflammatory actions.

PHARMACOKINETICS: Absorption: Percutaneous; C_{max}=18.9ng/mL; AUC_{0-24hr}=172ng•hr/mL. **Distribution:** Plasma protein binding (>99%). **Metabolism:** Esterase hydrolysis to form tazarotenic acid (active metabolite). **Excretion:** Urine, feces; $T_{1/2}$=18 hrs.

NURSING CONSIDERATIONS

Assessment: Assess that treatment is not for more than 20% of BSA, and not on eczematous skin. Two weeks prior to treatment, assess pregnancy status in females of childbearing potential. Assess that sexually active females are using effective form of contraception during therapy. Initiate therapy in childbearing females during a normal menstrual period. Assess use in pediatric and nursing patients. Assess for possible drug interactions.

Monitoring: Monitor for excessive pruritus, burning, skin redness, or peeling.

Patient Counseling: Instruct to avoid contact with eyes, eyelids, and mouth; do not cover treated areas with dressings or bandages. Wash hands following administration. Do not take if pregnant, planning to become or suspected to be pregnant. Instruct females to use effective form of contraception while on medication; advise to begin therapy during menstrual period. Avoid exposure to sunlight/sunlamps while on therapy; wear protective clothing and use sunscreen (minimum SPF15) when exposed to sunlight. Avoid using medication on sunburned skin. Exposure to weather extremes (eg, wind, cold) may cause skin irritation. Contact physician if excessive skin irritation develops. If dose is missed, do not make it up; instead, continue with normal dosing schedule.

Administration: Topical route. **Storage:** 25°C (77°F). Excursions permitted to 15-30°C (59-86°F). Keep tube tightly closed when not in use.

TEGRETOL — RX

carbamazepine (Novartis)

Serious and fatal dermatologic reactions, including toxic epidermal necrolysis (TEN), Stevens-Johnson syndrome (SJS), and presence of HLA-B*1502 allele reported. Aplastic anemia and agranulocytosis reported. Obtain complete pretreatment hematological testing as a baseline. D/C if evidence of bone marrow depression develops.

OTHER BRAND NAMES: Tegretol-XR (Novartis)

THERAPEUTIC CLASS: Carboxamide

INDICATIONS: Treatment of partial seizures with complex symptomatology, general tonic-clonic seizures, and mixed seizure patterns of these or other partial or generalized seizures. Treatment of trigeminal or glossopharyngeal neuralgia pain.

DOSAGE: *Adults:* Epilepsy: Initial: (Immediate- or Extended-Release Tabs) 200mg bid or (Sus) 100mg qid. Titrate: (Immediate-Release Tabs/Sus) Increase weekly by 200mg/day given tid-qid. (Extended-Release Tabs) Increase weekly by 200mg/day given bid. Maint: 800-1200mg/day. Max: 1200mg/day. Trigeminal Neuralgia: Initial (Day 1): (Immediate- or Extended-Release Tabs) 100mg bid or (Sus) 50mg qid. Titrate: May increase by 100mg

q12h (Tabs) or 50mg qid (Sus). Maint: 400-800mg/day. Max: 1200mg/day. Re-evaluate every 3 months. Extended-Release tabs should be swallowed whole and not crushed or chewed.
Pediatrics: Epilepsy: >12 yrs: Initial: (Immediate- or Extended-Release Tabs) 200mg bid or (Sus) 100mg qid. Titrate: (Immediate-Release Tabs/Sus) Increase weekly by 200mg/day given tid-qid. (Extended-Release Tabs) Increase weekly by 200mg/day given bid. Max: 12-15 yrs: 1000mg/day. >15 yrs: 1200mg/day. 6-12 yrs: Initial: (Immediate- or Extended-Release Tabs) 100mg bid or (Sus) 50mg qid. Titrate: (Immediate-Release Tabs/Sus) Increase weekly by 100mg/day given tid-qid. (Extended-Release Tabs) Increase weekly by 100mg/day given bid. Maint: 400-800mg/day. Max: 1000mg/day. 6 months-6 yrs: Initial: (Immediate-Release Tabs) 10-20mg/kg/day given bid-tid or (Sus) 10-20mg/kg/day given qid. Titrate: (Immediate-Release Tabs/Sus) Increase weekly tid-qid. Max: 35mg/kg/day. Extended-Release tabs should be swallowed whole and not crushed or chewed.

HOW SUPPLIED: Sus: 100mg/5mL [450mL]; Tab: (Tegretol) 200mg*; Tab, Chewable: 100mg*; Tab, Extended-Release: (Tegretol-XR) 100mg, 200mg, 400mg *scored

CONTRAINDICATIONS: History of bone marrow depression, MAOI use within 14 days, hypersensitivity to TCAs. Co-administration with nefazodone.

WARNINGS/PRECAUTIONS: Lyell's syndrome, Stevens-Johnson syndrome, multi-organ hypersensitivity reactions, and presence of HLA-B*1502 reported. Caution with history of adverse hematologic reaction to any drug, increased IOP, the elderly, mixed seizure disorder with atypical absence seizure. Fetal harm with pregnancy. May activate latent psychosis. Caution with cardiac (eg, conduction disturbance including 2nd and 3rd degree AV block), hepatic, or renal damage. Perform eye exam and monitor LFTs and renal function at baseline and periodically. Suspension produces higher peak levels than the tablet. Avoid in hepatic porphyria (eg, acute intermittent porphyria, variegate porphyria, porphyria cutanea tarda). Withdraw gradually to minimize the potential of increased seizure frequency.

ADVERSE REACTIONS: Dizziness, drowsiness, unsteadiness, nausea, vomiting, bone marrow depression, rash, urticaria, photosensitivity reactions, CHF, edema, HTN, hypotension, Stevens-Johnson syndrome, toxic epidermal necrolysis.

INTERACTIONS: Do not give suspension with other medicinal liquids or diluents. Metabolism is inhibited by CYP3A4 inhibitors (eg, cimetidine, macrolides) and induced by CYP3A4 inducers (eg, rifampin, phenytoin). Decreases oral contraceptive effectiveness. Increases plasma levels of clomipramine, phenytoin, and primidone. Decreases levels of APAP, alprazolam, clonazepam, clozapine, dicumarol, doxycycline, ethosuximide, haloperidol, lamotrigine, methsuximide, oral contraceptives, phensuximide, phenytoin, theophylline, tiagabine, topiramate, valproate, and warfarin. Increased risk of neurotoxic side effects with lithium. Avoid MAOIs.

PREGNANCY: Category D, not for use in nursing.

T

MECHANISM OF ACTION: Anticonvulsant; reduces polysynaptic response and blocks post-tetanic potentiation.

PHARMACOKINETICS: Absorption: T_{max}=1.5 hrs (oral); T_{max}=4-5 hrs (conventional tab); T_{max}=3-12 hrs (XR tab). **Distribution:** Plasma protein binding (76%). Found in placenta and breast milk. **Metabolism:** Liver via cytochrome P450 3A4. Carbamazepine-10,11-epoxide (metabolite). **Elimination:** Urine (3% unchanged); $T_{1/2}$=25-65 hrs (single dose); $T_{1/2}$=12-17 hrs (multiple doses).

NURSING CONSIDERATIONS

Assessment: Assess use with history of bone marrow depression, hepatic porphyria, hypersensitivity to any tricyclic compound, previous adverse hematological and dermatological reactions with other medications, history of mixed seizure disorders, cardiac damage or cardiac conduction disturbances, renal/hepatic damage. Assess renal function (complete urinalysis, BUN), CBC (platelets, reticulocytes), serum iron, LFTs; perform eye exam (slit lamp, fundoscopy, tonometry) prior to therapy. Assess pregnancy status prior to medication.

Monitoring: Monitor for hepatic failure, multiorgan hypersensitivity reactions, bone marrow depression, aplastic anemia, agranulocytosis, dermatological reactions (Stevens-Johnson syndrome), latent psychosis, and confusion or agitation in elderly patients. Monitor LFTs, SrCr, BUN, IOP.

Patient Counseling: Counsel about signs/symptoms of hematological, dermatological, and hepatic complications (eg, fever, sore throat, easy bruising, jaundice). May cause drowsiness or dizziness; caution against using heavy machinery/driving. Avoid alcohol or abrupt d/c.

Administration: Oral route. Oral sus should not be administered with other liquid medications or diluents. Conversion of patients from tabs to sus should be done by administering same number of mg/day in smaller, more frequent doses. XR tabs must be swallowed whole; do not chew or crush. **Storage:** 15-30°C (59-86°F). Protect from moisture. Dispense in tightly sealed container.

TEKTURNA — RX

aliskiren (Novartis)

When used in pregnancy, drugs that act directly on the renin-angiotensin system can cause injury and even death to the developing fetus. D/C therapy when pregnancy is detected.

THERAPEUTIC CLASS: Renin inhibitor

INDICATIONS: Treatment of hypertension. May be used alone or with other antihypertensives.

DOSAGE: *Adults:* Usual: 150mg qd. Titrate: May increase to 300mg/day if needed. High-fat meals decrease absorption.

HOW SUPPLIED: Tab: 150mg, 300mg

WARNINGS/PRECAUTIONS: Caution with greater than moderate renal dysfunction (SCr >1.7mg/dL [women] or >2mg/dL [men] and/or GFR <30mL/min), history of dialysis, nephrotic syndrome, or renovascular hypertension. May increase serum K^+, especially when used in combination with ACE inhibitors in diabetics. Angioedema of face, extremities, lips, tongue, glottis, and/or larynx reported; d/c and monitor until complete resolution of signs and symptoms. Hypotension rarely seen.

ADVERSE REACTIONS: Diarrhea, headache, nasopharyngitis, dizziness, fatigue, upper respiratory tract infection, back pain, cough.

INTERACTIONS: Coadministration with atorvastatin may increase C_{max} up to 50% after multiple dosing. Coadministration of irbesartan may reduce C_{max} up to 50% after multiple dosing. Coadministration of ketoconazole 200mg bid may result in an approximate 80% increase in plasma level. Coadministration with furosemide may reduce AUC and C_{max} by 30% and 50%, respectively. Concomitant use with cyclosporine is not recommended. Concomitant use with K^+-sparing diuretics, K^+ supplements, salt substitutes containing K^+, or other drugs that increase K^+ levels may lead to increases in serum K^+; caution with concomitant use.

PREGNANCY: Category C (1st trimester) and D (2nd and 3rd trimesters); not for use in nursing.

MECHANISM OF ACTION: Potent renin inhibitor; lowers BP by directly inhibiting renin, decreasing plasma renin activity, and inhibiting conversion of angiotensinogen to angiotensin I.

PHARMACOKINETICS: Absorption: Poor, T_{max}=1-3 hrs, bioavailability (2.5%), accumulation $T_{1/2}$=24 hrs. **Metabolism:** via CYP3A4 enzyme. **Elimination:** Urine (25% of absorbed dose as parent drug).

NURSING CONSIDERATIONS

Assessment: Assess BP, renal functions, renal artery stenosis, pregnancy status, and for possible drug interactions.

Monitoring: Monitor BP, renal functions, serum K^+ levels. Monitor for angioedema of head/neck and NV.

Patient Counseling: Counsel about fetal risks during pregnancy and signs/symptoms of angioedema (eg, laryngeal or tongue edema); advise to seek prompt medical attention if any develop. Inform about adverse effects (eg, hypotension, hyperkalemia). Infants with histories of in-utero exposure should be closely observed for hypotension, oliguria, hyperkalemia. Inform about need for periodic monitoring of electrolytes.

Administration: Oral route. **Storage:** 25°C (77°F). Excursions permitted to 15-30°C (59-86°F). Protect from moisture. Dispense in tight container.

TEKTURNA HCT RX

aliskiren - hydrochlorothiazide (Novartis)

Drugs that act directly on the renin-angiotensin system can cause injury and even death to the developing fetus. D/C therapy when pregnancy is detected.

THERAPEUTIC CLASS: Renin inhibitor/thiazide diuretic

INDICATIONS: Treatment of hypertension as add-on therapy or replacement therapy. Not for initial therapy.

DOSAGE: Adults: Initial: Not Controlled on Monotherapy: 150mg-12.5mg qd. Titrate: May increase to 150mg-25mg, 300mg-12.5mg qd if uncontrolled after 2-4 weeks. Max: 300mg-25mg. Avoid with CrCl ≤30mL/min.

HOW SUPPLIED: Tab: (Aliskiren-HCTZ) 150mg-12.5mg, 150mg-25mg, 300mg-12.5mg, 300mg-25mg

CONTRAINDICATIONS: Anuria, sulfonamide hypersensitivity.

WARNINGS/PRECAUTIONS: Angioedema of head and neck may occur; d/c therapy and monitor until signs and symptoms resolve. May cause symptomatic hypotension in volume- and/or salt-depleted patients; correct condition prior to therapy. Avoid with CrCl <30mL/min. Caution with hepatic impairment, or history of allergy or bronchial asthma. May exacerbate or activate SLE. Monitor serum electrolytes periodically to detect possible electrolyte imbalance.

ADVERSE REACTIONS: Dizziness, influenza, diarrhea, cough, vertigo, asthenia, arthralgia.

INTERACTIONS: (Aliskiren) Ketoconazole and atorvastatin may increase plasma levels. Irbesartan may reduce levels. Co-administration may diminish furosemide levels. (HCTZ) Potentiation of orthostatic hypotension may occur with alcohol, barbiturates, and narcotics. Dosage adjustment of insulin or oral hypoglycemic agents may be required. Potentiates effects of other antihypertensives. Cholestyramine and colestipol resins may impair absorption. Corticosteroids and ACTH deplete electrolytes. May decrease response to pressor amines (eg, norepinephrine). May increase responsiveness to skeletal muscle relaxants (eg, tubocurarine). Increased risk of lithium toxicity; avoid concurrent use. NSAIDs may reduce diuretic effects; monitor closely.

T

PREGNANCY: Category D, not for use in nursing.

MECHANISM OF ACTION: Aliskiren: Direct renin inhibitor. HCTZ: Thiazide diuretic, affects renal tubular mechanisms of electrolyte reabsorption, directly increasing excretion of Na^+ and Cl^- in approximately equivalent amounts.

PHARMACOKINETICS: Absorption: Aliskiren: T_{max}=1 hr. HCTZ: T_{max}=2.5 hrs. **Metabolism**: Aliskiren: CYP3A4 enzyme. HCTZ: Not metabolized. **Elimination**: Aliskiren: Urine (25% of absorbed dose as parent drug). HCTZ: Urine, $T_{1/2}$=5.8-18.9 hrs.

NURSING CONSIDERATIONS

Assessment: Assess for signs/symptoms of dizziness, flu-like symptoms, diarrhea, cough, and tiredness.

Monitoring: Monitor for hypersensitivity and anaphylaxis reactions, anuria, urticaria, head/neck angioedema. Lab tests such as BUN, creatinine, Hg, Hct, LFTs, serum uric acid, and electrolytes should be monitored.

Patient Counseling: Instruct to notify physician or pharmacist if any unusual symptoms develop or if any known symptoms persist or worsen. Caution that lightheadedness may occur, especially during 1st days of therapy. If syncope occurs, d/c until physician consulted. Caution that inadequate fluid intake, excessive perspiration, diarrhea, or vomiting can lead to an excessive fall in BP, with same consequences as lightheadedness and possible syncope. Establish routine pattern for taking medication with regard to meals.

Administration: Oral route. **Storage**: 15-30°C (59-86°F).

TEMODAR — RX
temozolomide (Schering)

THERAPEUTIC CLASS: Alkylating agent (imidazotetrazine derivative)

INDICATIONS: Treatment of newly diagnosed glioblastoma multiforme (GBM) concomitantly with radiotherapy and as maintenance treatment. Treatment of refractory anaplastic astrocytoma in patients experiencing disease progression with nitrosourea and procarbazine regimen.

DOSAGE: *Adults:* Adjust according to nadir neutrophil and platelet counts of previous cycle and at time of initiating next cycle. Newly Diagnosed GBM: (IV/PO) 75mg/m^2 qd for 42 days with focal radiotherapy; dose may continue up to 49 days if absolute neutrophil count ≥1.5 x 10^9/L, platelet count ≥100 x 10^9/L, common toxicity criteria (CTC) non-hematological toxicity ≤Grade 1 (except alopecia, NV) are met. Maint: Cycle 1 (28 days): 150mg/m^2 qd for 1st 5 days of each 28-day cycle. Cycle 2-6 (28 days): If Cycle 1 toxicity Grade ≤2, ANC ≥1.5 x 10^9/L and platelets ≥100 x 10^9/L, increase to 200mg/m^2/day for 5 consecutive days per 28-day cycle. Do not increase dose in subsequent cycles if dose not escalated at Cycle 2. If Cycle 1 toxicity Grade 3, ANC <1.0 x 10^9/L and platelets <50 x 10^9/L, reduce to 100mg/m^2/day for 5 consecutive days per 28-day cycle. D/C if Cycle 1 toxicity Grade 4, dose reduction to <100mg/m^2/day is required or if same Grade 3 toxicity recurs after dose reduction. Refractory Anaplastic Astrocytoma: Initial: (IV/PO) 150mg/m^2 qd for 5 consecutive days per 28-day cycle. If ANC ≥1.5 x 10^9/L and platelets ≥100 x 10^9/L for both the nadir and Day 29 (Day 1 of next cycle), may increase to 200mg/m^2/day for 5 consecutive days per 28-day cycle. Start next cycle when ANC >1.5 x 10^9/L and platelets >100 x 10^9/L . If ANC <1 x 10^9/L or platelets <50 x 10^9/L during any cycle, reduce next cycle by 50mg/m^2. If ANC 1.0-1.5 x 10^9/L or platelets 50-100 x 10^9/L during any cycle, maintain initial dose. If ANC >1.5 x 10^9/L or platelets >100 x 10^9/L during any cycle, increase to or maintain at 200mg/m^2/day for 5 days. CBC on Day 22, and weekly until ANC is >1.5 x 10^9/L and platelets >100 x 10^9/L. Swallow whole with water. IV infusion over 90 minutes.

HOW SUPPLIED: Cap: 5mg, 20mg, 100mg, 140mg, 180mg, 250mg. Inj: 100mg

CONTRAINDICATIONS: Hypersensitivity to DTIC (dacarbazine).

WARNINGS/PRECAUTIONS: Before therapy, must have ANC ≥1.5 x 10^9/L and platelets ≥100 x 10^9/L. Myelosuppression may occur; obtain CBC on Day 22 (21 days after 1st dose) or within 48 hrs of that day, repeat weekly until ANC >1.5 x 10^9/L and platelets >100 x 10^9/L. Greater risk of myelosuppression in women and elderly. May cause fetal harm during pregnancy. Very rare cases of myelodysplastic syndrome and secondary malignancies, including myeloid leukemia, have been observed. Do not open capsules. Caution in elderly, or severe renal/hepatic impairment. *Pneumocytis carinii* pneumonia (PCP) prophylaxis required in all patients with newly diagnosed GBM receiving concomitant radiotherapy for 42 days regimen. Monitor for lymphopenia and PCP. Increased risk of infusion-related adverse reactions, and suboptimal dosing with shorter or longer infusion time.

ADVERSE REACTIONS: Anorexia, alopecia, headache, fatigue, myelosuppression (thrombocytopenia, neutropenia), NV, convulsions, hemiparesis, asthenia, fever, peripheral edema, constipation, dizziness, diarrhea, abnormal coordination, viral infection, amnesia, insomnia, lymphopenia, leukopenia, and allergic reactions.

INTERACTIONS: Valproic acid may decrease clearance.

PREGNANCY: Category D, not for use in nursing.

MECHANISM OF ACTION: Alkylating agent (imidazotetrazine derivative); exerts action by alkylation of DNA.

PHARMACOKINETICS: Absorption: Rapid and complete, T_{max}=1 hr. **Distribution:** V_d=0.4L/kg; plasma protein binding (15%). **Metabolism:** Via hydroxylation; 3-methyl-(triazen-1-yl)imidazole-4-carboxamide (major metabolite) **Elimination:** Urine, feces; $T_{1/2}$=1.8 hrs.

NURSING CONSIDERATIONS

Assessment: Assess for CBC with differential and platelet counts, hepatic/renal functions, pregnancy status. Note other diseases/conditions and possible drug interactions.

Monitoring: Monitor for CBC with differential and platelet counts, lymphopenia, PCP, secondary malignancies, hypersensitivity reactions, convulsions, hemiparesis.

Patient Counseling: Counsel about adverse effects (eg, NV); seek medical attention if any develop. Take as prescribed. Swallow whole; never chew. Instruct not to open capsule. Avoid inhalation or contact with skin or mucous membranes. Regular follow-ups needed. Keep away from children and pets.

Administration: Oral and IV route. See PI for reconstitution. **Storage:** (Cap) 25°C (77°F); excursions permitted to 15-30°C (59-96°F). (IV) Refrigerate at 2-8°C (36-46°F). After reconstitution, store at room temperature (25°C [77°F]). Reconstituted product must be used within 14 hrs.

TEMOVATE RX

clobetasol propionate (GlaxoSmithKline)

OTHER BRAND NAMES: Temovate Scalp (GlaxoSmithKline) - Temovate-E (GlaxoSmithKline)

THERAPEUTIC CLASS: Corticosteroid

INDICATIONS: Corticosteroid-responsive dermatoses. Temovate-E is also used to treat moderate to severe plaque-type psoriasis.

DOSAGE: *Adults:* Apply bid. Max: 50g/week or 50mL/week. Moderate-Severe Psoriasis: (Temovate-E) Apply bid for up to 4 weeks. May use on 5-10% of BSA. Max: 50g/week. Limit treatment to 2 consecutive weeks. Avoid with occlusive dressings.
Pediatrics: ≥12 yrs: Apply bid. Max: 50g/week or 50mL/week. Moderate-Severe Psoriasis: ≥16 yrs: (Temovate-E) Apply bid for up to 4 weeks. May use on 5-10% of BSA. Max: 50g/week. Limit treatment to 2 consecutive weeks. Avoid with occlusive dressings.

HOW SUPPLIED: (Temovate) Cre, Oint: 0.05% [15g, 30g, 45g, 60g]; Gel: 0.05% [15g, 30g, 60g]; Sol: 0.05% [25mL]; (Temovate-E) Cre: 0.05% [15g, 30g, 60g]; (Temovate Scalp) Sol: 0.05% [25mL, 50mL]

CONTRAINDICATIONS: (Scalp Sol) Primary scalp infections.

WARNINGS/PRECAUTIONS: Not for use on face, groin, or axillae, or for treatment of rosacea or perioral dermatitis. May produce reversible HPA axis suppression, manifestations of Cushing's syndrome, hyperglycemia, and glucosuria. Use appropriate antifungal or antibacterial agent with dermatological infections; d/c if infection does not clear. Peds may be more susceptible to systemic toxicity. Avoid eyes. D/C if irritation occurs.

ADVERSE REACTIONS: Burning, stinging, pruritus, skin atrophy, cracking/fissuring of the skin, erythema, folliculitis, numbness of fingers, telangiectasia, tingling (Sol), folliculitis (Sol).

PREGNANCY: Category C, caution in nursing.

MECHANISM OF ACTION: Corticosteroid; possesses anti-inflammatory, antipruritic, and vasoconstrictive properties. Anti-inflammatory effects not established. Suspected to act by induction of phospholipase A_2 inhibitory proteins, lipocortins. Lipocortins control biosynthesis of potent inflammation mediators (eg, prostaglandins, leukotrienes) by inhibiting release of their common precursor, arachidonic acid.

PHARMACOKINETICS: Absorption: Occlusion, inflammation, other disease states may increase absorption. Use of occlusive dressings ≤24 hrs does not increase penetration, use for 96 hrs markedly enhances penetration.

NURSING CONSIDERATIONS

Assessment: Assess medication not for treatment of perioral dermatitis or rosacea. Assess pregnancy/nursing status.

Monitoring: Monitor for signs/symptoms of reversible HPA-axis suppression, Cushing's syndrome, hyperglycemia, glucosuria, skin irritation, allergic contact dermatitis (eg, failure to heal), and concomitant skin infections (eg, fungal, bacterial). With large doses or use of occlusive dressings, perform periodic monitoring for HPA-axis suppression using ACTH stimulation, A.M. plasma cortisol, and urinary free cortisol tests. Following d/c, monitor for glucocorticosteroid insufficiencies. In pediatric patients, monitor for systemic toxicity, HPA-axis suppression (linear growth retardation, delayed weight gain), Cushing's syndrome, and intracranial HTN.

Patient Counseling: Counsel to use externally and exactly as directed; avoid contact with eyes, face, groin, or axillae. Advise not to bandage, cover, or wrap treated skin area. Contact physician if adverse reactions occur or improvement not seen after 2 weeks of therapy.

Administration: Topical route. **Storage:** 15-30°C (59-86°F). Do not refrigerate.

TENORETIC — RX
chlorthalidone - atenolol (AstraZeneca)

THERAPEUTIC CLASS: Selective $beta_1$-blocker/monosulfamyl diuretic

INDICATIONS: Treatment of hypertension. Not for initial therapy.

DOSAGE: *Adults:* Initial: 50mg-25mg tab qd. May increase to 100mg-25mg tab qd. CrCl 15-35mL/min: Max: 50mg atenolol/day. CrCl <15mL/min: Max: 50mg atenolol qod.

HOW SUPPLIED: Tab: (Atenolol-Chlorthalidone) 50mg-25mg*, 100mg-25mg *scored

CONTRAINDICATIONS: Sinus bradycardia, >1st-degree heart block, cardiogenic shock, overt cardiac failure, anuria, sulfonamide hypersensitivity.

WARNINGS/PRECAUTIONS: Withdrawal before surgery is not recommended. Caution with bronchospastic disease, conduction abnormalities, left ventricular dysfunction. Caution in patients with impaired renal and hepatic function. Can cause heart failure with prolonged use. May mask hypoglycemia or hyperthyroidism symptoms. Avoid abrupt discontinuation. Avoid with untreated pheochromocytoma. Possible fetal harm in pregnancy. May aggravate peripheral arterial circulatory disorders. Enhanced effects in postsympathectomy patient. Neonates born to mothers receiving atenolol may be at risk of hypoglycemia and bradycardia.

ADVERSE REACTIONS: Bradycardia, dizziness, fatigue, and nausea.

INTERACTIONS: Additive effects with catecholamine-depleting drugs (eg, reserpine), CCBs, and digitalis. Bradycardia, heart block, and LVEDP can rise with verapamil or diltiazem. Coadministration with disopyramide has been associated with severe bradycardia, asystole, and heart failure. Additive negative chronotropic effects with amiodarone. Exacerbates rebound HTN with clonidine withdrawal. Prostaglandin synthase inhibitors (eg, indomethacin) may decrease hypotensive effects. Caution with anesthetic agents. May block epinephrine effects. May decrease arterial response to norepinephrine. May increase risk of lithium toxicity. Possible hypokalemia with corticosteroids or ACTH. May alter insulin requirements.

PREGNANCY: Category D, caution in nursing.

MECHANISM OF ACTION: Atenolol: Cardioselective β-adrenoreceptor blocking agent; causes reduction in HR and systolic BP. Chlorthalidone: Monosulfamyl diuretic; acts on distal convoluted tubule and produces diuresis with increased excretion of Na^+ and Cl^-.

PHARMACOKINETICS: Absorption: Atenolol: Rapid, incomplete (50%). T_{max}=2-4 hrs. Chlorthalidone: Onset of action within 2 hrs. **Distribution**: Atenolol: Plasma protein binding (6-16%). **Elimination:** Atenolol: Renal excretion; $T_{1/2}$=approximately 6-7 hrs. **Distribution:** Plasma protein binding (75%). **Elimination:** Urine (unchanged), $T_{1/2}$=40-60 hrs.

NURSING CONSIDERATIONS

Assessment: Assess for bradycardia, cardiogenic shock, 2nd- and 3rd-degree heart block, overt cardiac failure, impaired renal/hepatic function, bronchospastic disease, PVD, DM, thyrotoxicosis, pheochromocytoma, anuria, hypersensitivity to sulfonamide-derived drugs, serum electrolytes, parathyroid disease, pregnancy status, SLE, and possible drug interactions.

Monitoring: Monitor for cardiac failure, HTN, renal function, exacerbation of ischemia following abrupt withdrawal, bronchospastic disease, arrhythmias, CBC with platelets and differential count, hypersensitivity reactions, mesenteric arterial thrombosis, reversible mental depression, hyperuricemia or acute gout, signs/symptoms of electrolyte imbalance, serum glucose, lipid profile, toxic epidermal necrolysis, impotence, HR, orthostatic hypotension, pancreatitis, LFTs.

Patient Counseling: Instruct not to interrupt or d/c therapy without consulting physician. Notify physician if signs/symptoms of impending CHF or unexplained respiratory symptoms develop. Counsel about signs/symptoms of electrolyte imbalance (eg, dry mouth, thirst, weakness, lethargy, drowsiness, restlessness, muscle pains/cramps, muscular fatigue, hypotension, oliguria, tachycardia, GI disturbances such as NV), and advise to seek prompt medical attention. Advise to take as prescribed.

Administration: Oral route. **Storage:** Store at controlled room temperature, 20-25°C (68-77°F).

TENORMIN — RX

atenolol (AstraZeneca)

Avoid abrupt discontinuation of therapy in coronary artery disease. Severe exacerbation of angina and occurrence of MI and ventricular arrhythmias reported in angina patients following abrupt discontinuation of therapy with β-blockers.

THERAPEUTIC CLASS: Selective $beta_1$-blocker

INDICATIONS: Management of hypertension. Long-term management of angina pectoris. To reduce cardiovascular mortality in hemodynamically stable patients with definite or suspected AMI.

DOSAGE: *Adults:* HTN: Initial: 50mg qd. Titrate: May increase after 1-2 weeks. Max: 100mg qd. Angina: Initial: 50mg qd. Titrate: May increase to 100mg after 1 week. Max: 200mg qd. AMI: Initial: 5mg IV over 5 min, repeat 10 min later. If tolerated, give 50mg PO 10 min after the last IV dose, followed by another 50mg PO 12 hrs later. Maint: 100mg qd or 50mg bid for 6-9 days. Renal Impairment/Elderly: HTN: Initial: 25mg qd. HTN/Angina/AMI: Max: CrCl 15-35mL/min: 50mg/day. CrCl <15mL/min: 25mg/day. Hemodialysis: 25-50mg after each dialysis.

HOW SUPPLIED: Tab: 25mg, 50mg*, 100mg *scored

CONTRAINDICATIONS: Sinus bradycardia, >1st-degree heart block, cardiogenic shock, overt cardiac failure.

WARNINGS/PRECAUTIONS: Withdrawal before surgery is not recommended. Caution with bronchospastic disease, conduction abnormalities, left ventricular dysfunction, heart failure controlled by digitalis and/or diuretics, renal or hepatic dysfunction. Can cause heart failure with prolonged use, hyperuricemia, hypercalcemia, hypokalemia, hypophosphatemia. May mask hypoglycemia or hyperthyroidism symptoms. Avoid abrupt discontinuation. Avoid with untreated pheochromocytoma. Possible fetal harm in pregnancy. May aggravate peripheral arterial circulatory disorders. May manifest latent DM. Monitor for fluid or electrolyte imbalance. May develop antinuclear antibodies (ANA).

Neonates born to mothers receiving atenolol may be at risk of hypoglycemia and bradycardia.

ADVERSE REACTIONS: Bradycardia, hypotension, dizziness, fatigue, nausea, depression, dyspnea.

INTERACTIONS: Additive effects with catecholamine-depleting drugs (eg, reserpine), CCBs, amiodarone, and digitalis. Use with disopyramide may be associated with severe bradycardia, asystole, and heart failure. Bradycardia, heart block, and LVEDP can rise with verapamil or diltiazem. Exacerbates rebound HTN with clonidine withdrawal. Prostaglandin synthase inhibitors (eg, indomethacin) may decrease hypotensive effects. Caution with drugs that depress myocardium (eg, anesthesia). May block epinephrine effects. Concomitant use with digitalis glycosides may increase risk of bradycardia.

PREGNANCY: Category D, caution in nursing.

MECHANISM OF ACTION: Cardioselective β-adrenoreceptor blocking agent; causes reduction in HR and systolic BP.

PHARMACOKINETICS: Absorption: Rapid, incomplete (50%); T_{max} = 2-4 hrs. **Distribution**: Plasma protein binding (6-16%). **Elimination:** Kidneys; $T_{1/2}$=6-7 hrs.

NURSING CONSIDERATIONS

Assessment: Assess for bradycardia, cardiogenic shock, 2nd- and 3rd-degree heart block, overt cardiac failure, impaired renal/hepatic function, bronchospastic disease, PVD, DM, thyrotoxicosis, pregnancy status, pheochromocytoma, and possible drug interactions.

Monitoring: Monitor for cardiac failure, HTN, renal function, exacerbation of ischemia following abrupt withdrawal, bronchospastic disease, arrhythmias, CBC with platelets and differential count, hypersensitivity reactions, mesenteric arterial thrombosis, reversible mental depression.

Patient Counseling: Instruct not to interrupt or d/c therapy without consulting physician. Notify physician if signs/symptoms of impending CHF or unexplained respiratory symptoms develop. Educate about signs/symptoms of adverse effects.

Administration: Oral route. **Storage:** 20-25°C (68-77°F). Dispense in well-closed, light-resistant containers.

TERAZOL 3 — RX

terconazole (Ortho-McNeil)

THERAPEUTIC CLASS: Azole antifungal

INDICATIONS: Treatment of vulvovaginal candidiasis.

DOSAGE: *Adults:* 1 applicatorful or sup vaginally qhs for 3 nights.

HOW SUPPLIED: Cre: 0.8% [20g]; Sup: 80mg [3^{s}]

WARNINGS/PRECAUTIONS: D/C if sensitization, irritation, fever, chills, or flu-like symptoms occur. Confirm diagnosis by KOH smears and/or cultures; reconfirm if no response. Do not use diaphragm with suppository.

ADVERSE REACTIONS: Sup: Localized burning, pruritus, genital pain, headache. Cre: Dysmenorrhea, headache, pruritus, burning, abdominal pain.

PREGNANCY: Category C, not for use in nursing.

MECHANISM OF ACTION: Terconazole (antifungal agent); uncertain, suspected to exert activity by disruption of normal fungal cell membrane permeability.

PHARMACOKINETICS: Absorption: C_{max}=5.9ng/mL, T_{max}=6.6 hrs. **Distribution:** Plasma protein binding (94.9%).

NURSING CONSIDERATIONS

Assessment: Assess for hypersensitivity and possible drug interactions.

Monitoring: Monitor for sensitization, irritation, fever, chills, and flu-like symptoms. If lack of response to drug, standard KOH smear and cultures should be repeated to confirm diagnosis.

Patient Counseling: Do not concurrently use with rubber or latex products (eg, condoms, diaphragms).

Administration: (Intravaginal) 1) Lie on back, knees drawn up toward chest. 2) Cre: Insert filled applicator into vagina and press plunger to release cre into vagina. Sup: Insert sup into vagina with finger at hs as directed by physician. **Storage:** 15-30°C (59-86°F).

Terazol 7 — RX

terconazole (Ortho-McNeil)

THERAPEUTIC CLASS: Azole antifungal

INDICATIONS: Treatment of vulvovaginal candidiasis.

DOSAGE: *Adults:* 1 applicatorful vaginally qhs for 7 nights.

HOW SUPPLIED: Cre: 0.4% [45g]

WARNINGS/PRECAUTIONS: D/C if sensitization, irritation, fever, chills, or flu-like symptoms occur. Confirm diagnosis by KOH smears and/or cultures; reconfirm if no response.

ADVERSE REACTIONS: Headache, body pain, burning, itching, irritation.

PREGNANCY: Category C, not for use in nursing.

MECHANISM OF ACTION: Terconazole (antifungal agent); uncertain; suspected to exert activity by disruption of normal fungal cell membrane permeability.

PHARMACOKINETICS: Absorption: C_{max}=5.9ng/mL, T_{max}=6.6 hrs. **Distribution:** Plasma protein binding (94.9%).

NURSING CONSIDERATIONS

Assessment: Assess for hypersensitivity and possible drug interactions.

Monitoring: Monitor for sensitization, irritation, fever, chills, flu-like symptoms. If lack of response to drug, standard KOH smear and cultures should be repeated to confirm diagnosis.

Patient Counseling: Do not concurrently use rubber or latex products (eg, condoms, vaginal diaphragms).

Administration: 1) Lie on back with knees drawn up towards chest. 2) Insert filled applicator into vagina as far as it will comfortably go. 3) Press plunger to release cre into vagina. 4) Apply at bedtime as directed by doctor. **Storage:** 15-30°C (59-86°F).

Terbutaline — RX

terbutaline sulfate (Various)

THERAPEUTIC CLASS: $Beta_2$-agonist

INDICATIONS: Prevention and reversal of bronchospasm in asthma, and reversible bronchospasm in bronchitis and emphysema.

DOSAGE: *Adults:* (PO) Usual: 5mg tid. May reduce to 2.5mg tid. Max: 15mg/24hrs. (Inj) Usual: 0.25mg SQ into lateral deltoid area. May repeat within 15-30 min if no improvement. Max: 0.5mg/4hrs.
Pediatrics: (PO) 12-15 yrs: Usual: 2.5mg tid. Max: 7.5mg/24hrs. (Inj) ≥12 yrs: Usual: 0.25mg SQ into lateral deltoid area. May repeat within 15-30 min if no improvement. Max: 0.5mg/4hrs.

HOW SUPPLIED: Inj: 1mg/mL [1mL]; Tab: 2.5mg*, 5mg* *scored

CONTRAINDICATIONS: Hypersensitivity to sympathomimetic amines.

WARNINGS/PRECAUTIONS: Caution with ischemic heart disease, HTN, arrhythmias, hyperthyroidism, DM, seizures. Not approved for tocolysis.

Hypersensitivity and exacerbation of bronchospasm reported. Monitor for transient hypokalemia.

ADVERSE REACTIONS: Nervousness, tremor, headache, somnolence, palpitations, dizziness, tachycardia, nausea.

INTERACTIONS: Avoid other sympathomimetic agents (except aerosol bronchodilators). Extreme caution with MAOIs and TCAs during or within 14 days of treatment. Decreased effects with β-blockers. Possible ECG changes and hypokalemia with loop or thiazide diuretics.

PREGNANCY: Category B, caution in nursing.

MECHANISM OF ACTION: β_2-adrenergic agonist; stimulates intracellular adenyl cyclase, which catalyzes conversion of ATP to cAMP, to produce relaxation of bronchial smooth muscle and inhibition of release of mediators of immediate hypersensitivity from cells (mast cells).

PHARMACOKINETICS: Absorption: (SC) C_{max}=9.6ng/mL; T_{max}=0.5 hrs; AUC=29.4h•ng/mL. (Tab) C_{max}=8.3ng/mL; T_{max}=2 hrs; AUC=54.6h•ng/mL. (Sol) C_{max}=8.6ng/mL; T_{max}=1.5 hrs; AUC=53.1h•ng/mL. **Metabolism:** Sulfate conjugate (metabolite). **Elimination:** SC: Urine (60%); $T_{1/2}$=5.7 hrs. (PO) Urine (30-50%), feces; $T_{1/2}$=3.4 hrs (asthmatics).

NURSING CONSIDERATIONS

Assessment: Assess for ischemic heart disease, CVD (eg, coronary insufficiency, cardiac arrhythmia, HTN), convulsive disorders, hyperthyroidism, DM, and possible drug interactions.

Monitoring: Monitor for signs/symptoms of CV effects (eg, increased BP, palpitations), worsening of symptoms, paradoxical bronchospasm, and hypersensitivity reactions (eg, anaphylactic, urticaria, angioedema, rash, bronchospasm).

Patient Counseling: Advise to seek medical attention if symptoms worsen, therapy becomes less effective, need more inhalation from short-acting β_2-agonist than usual, paradoxical bronchospasm, or hypersensitivity reactions (eg, anaphylaxis, urticaria, angioedema, rash, bronchospasm) occur.

Administration: SC, oral route. **Storage:** 20-25°C (68-77°F). Protect from light.

TESSALON — RX

benzonatate (Forest)

THERAPEUTIC CLASS: Non-narcotic antitussive

INDICATIONS: Symptomatic relief of cough.

DOSAGE: *Adults:* Usual: 100-200mg tid as needed. Max: 600mg/day. *Pediatrics:* >10 yrs: Usual: 100-200mg tid as needed. Max: 600mg/day.

HOW SUPPLIED: Cap: 100mg, 200mg

WARNINGS/PRECAUTIONS: Severe hypersensitivity reactions; confusion and hallucinations reported in combination with other prescribed drugs. Swallow capsules without sucking/chewing to avoid local anesthesia adverse effects.

ADVERSE REACTIONS: Sedation, headache, dizziness, confusion, hallucinations, constipation, nausea, GI upset, pruritus.

PREGNANCY: Category C, caution in nursing.

MECHANISM OF ACTION: Non-narcotic/antitussive agent; acts peripherally by anesthetizing stretch receptors located in respiratory passages, lungs, and pleura by dampening their activity, thereby reducing cough reflex at its source.

NURSING CONSIDERATIONS

Assessment: Assess for drug hypersensitivity.

Monitoring: Monitor for hypersensitivity (eg, bronchospasm, laryngospasm, cardiovascular collapse), mental confusion, visual hallucinations, overdose signs/symptoms (eg, restlessness, tremors, clonic convulsions followed by profound CNS depression).

Patient Counseling: Caution to swallow caps whole; do not chew or dissolve cap in mouth; may lead to temporary anasthesia of the oral mucosa, hypersensitivity reactions, or choking.

Administration: Oral route. **Storage:** 25°C (77°F); excursions permitted to 15-30°C (59-86°F).

Testim

testosterone (Auxilium)

CIII

THERAPEUTIC CLASS: Androgen

INDICATIONS: Testosterone replacement in males with primary or hypogonadotropic hypogonadism.

DOSAGE: *Adults:* ≥18 yrs: Apply 5g qd, preferably in the am, to clean, dry, intact skin of shoulders and/or upper arms. Allow to dry prior to dressing. Titrate: May increase to 10g qd if response not achieved or serum concentration is below normal range. Do not apply to genitals or abdomen. To maintain serum testosterone levels, do not wash site of application for at least 2 hrs.

HOW SUPPLIED: Gel: 1% [5g (50mg)/tube, 30^s]

CONTRAINDICATIONS: Breast or prostate carcinoma in men. Not for use by women. Pregnant and nursing women should avoid skin contact with application sites on men. Hypersensitivity to soy products.

WARNINGS/PRECAUTIONS: Caution in elderly; increased risk of prostatic hypertrophy/carcinoma. Risk of edema with pre-existing cardiac, renal, or hepatic disease; d/c if edema occurs, diuretic therapy may be required. Risk of gynecomastia. May potentiate sleep apnea especially with obesity or chronic lung diseases. Transfer of testosterone can occur with skin to skin contact. Risk of virilization of female partner. Advise patients to report persistent penis erections, changes in skin color, ankle swelling, unexplained nausea and vomiting, or breathing disturbances. Monitor serum testosterone, LFTs, Hgb, Hct, PSA, cholesterol, lipids. Prolonged use associated with serious hepatic effects (peliosis hepatitis, hepatic neoplasms, cholestatic hepatitis, jaundice).

ADVERSE REACTIONS: Application site reactions, benign prostatic hyperplasia, decreased DBP, increased BP, gynecomastia, headache, Hct/Hgb increases, hot flushes, insomnia, increased lacrimation, mood swings, smell disorder.

INTERACTIONS: May elevate oxyphenbutazone levels. May decrease blood glucose and insulin requirements. May increase clearance of propranolol. Corticosteroids may enhance edema; caution with cardiac or hepatic disease.

PREGNANCY: Category X, not for use in nursing.

MECHANISM OF ACTION: Endogenous androgen; responsible for normal growth and development of male sex organs and for maintenance of secondary sex characteristics.

PHARMACOKINETICS: Metabolism: Skin, liver, male urogenital tract via 5α-reductase; estradiol and dihydrotestosterone (metabolites). **Elimination:** Urine, feces; $T_{1/2}$=10-100 min.

NURSING CONSIDERATIONS

Assessment: Assess for hypersensitivity to soy, breast or prostate carcinoma, cardiac or renal/hepatic disease, obesity; chronic lung disease, pregnancy/nursing status of female partner, and possible drug interactions.

Monitoring: Periodically monitor Hgb, Hct, LFTs, PSA, cholesterol, and HDL. Obtain serum testosterone levels 14 days after initiation of therapy. Monitor for signs/symptoms of hypersensitivity reactions, edema with/without CHF, gynecomastia, prostatic hyperplasia/carcinoma in geriatrics, and potentiation of sleep apnea.

Patient Counseling: Inform of pregnancy risks; avoid contact with application sites if pregnant/nursing. If contact occurs, wash area immediately with soap and water. Instruct not to apply to the scrotum, penis, or abdomen. Cover application site after gel dries with clothing; wash application site with soap and water prior to direct skin-to-skin contact. Advise to wash or swim ≥2 hrs after application. Inform to contact physician if changes in body hair distribution, increase in acne, virilization of female partner, too frequent or persistent erections, changes in skin color, ankle swelling, unexplained NV, breathing disturbances, or hypersensitivity reactions occur.

Administration: Transdermal. Apply every day at same time to clean, dry skin of shoulder or upper arms. **Storage:** 25°C (77°F); excursions permitted to 15-30°C (59-86°F).

TESTRED
methyltestosterone (Valeant)

CIII

THERAPEUTIC CLASS: Androgen

INDICATIONS: Testosterone replacement therapy in males with primary hypogonadism or hypogonadotrophic hypogonadism. To stimulate puberty in males with delayed puberty. Secondary treatment of advancing inoperable metastatic (skeletal) breast cancer in females 1-5 yrs postmenopausal.

DOSAGE: *Adults:* Dose based on age, sex and diagnosis. Adjust dose according to clinical response and adverse events. Male Replacement Therapy: 10-50mg/day. Breast Carcinoma: 50-200mg/day.
Pediatrics: Dose based on age, sex and diagnosis. Adjust dose according to clinical response and adverse events. Delayed Puberty: Use lower range of 10-50mg/day for 4-6 months. Caution in children.

HOW SUPPLIED: Cap: 10mg

CONTRAINDICATIONS: Pregnancy. Males with breast or prostate carcinoma.

WARNINGS/PRECAUTIONS: D/C if hypercalcemia occurs in breast cancer; monitor calcium levels. Monitor for virilization in females. Risk of compromised stature in children; monitor bone growth every 6 months. Risk of hepatic damage with long-term use. D/C if jaundice, cholestatic hepatitis occur. Risk of edema; caution with pre-existing cardiac, renal or hepatic disease. Caution in the elderly; increased risk of prostatic hypertrophy and prostatic carcinoma. Should not be used for enhancement of athletic performance. Monitor LFTs, Hct, and Hgb periodically.

ADVERSE REACTIONS: Amenorrhea, virilization, menstrual irregularities, gynecomastia, excessive frequency/duration of penile erections, male pattern baldness, increased/decreased libido, oligospermia, hirsutism, acne, fluid and electrolyte disturbances, nausea, hypercholesterolemia, clotting factor suppression, polycythemia, altered LFTs, priapism, anxiety, depression.

INTERACTIONS: Potentiates oral anticoagulants and oxyphenbutazone. May decrease blood glucose and insulin requirements in diabetics.

PREGNANCY: Category X, not for use in nursing.

MECHANISM OF ACTION: Endogenous androgen (derivative of testosterone); responsible for normal growth and development of male sex organs and maintenance of secondary sex characteristics.

PHARMACOKINETICS: Metabolism: Gut, liver. **Elimination:** Urine, feces; $T_{1/2}$=10-100 min.

NURSING CONSIDERATIONS

Assessment: Assess for known or suspected carcinoma of prostate or male breast, pregnancy status, pre-existing cardiac or renal/hepatic disease, and possible drug interactions.

Monitoring: Periodically monitor urine and serum calcium levels (female breast cancer), LFTs, Hgb and Hct, and bone age of left wrist and hand every 6 months (bone maturation in pediatrics). Monitor for signs/symptoms of hypersensitivity reactions, peliosis hepatitis, hepatic dysfunction, prostatic hyperplasia/carcinoma in geriatrics, edema (with or without CHF), hypercalcemia, and virilization of females.

Patient Counseling: Inform of pregnancy risks. Instruct to contact physician if any hypersensitivity reactions, NV, ankle swelling, changes in skin color, symptoms of hepatotoxicity, frequent or persistent erections (males), hoarseness (females), acne, changes in menstrual periods (females), or more facial hair occur.

Administration: Oral route. **Storage:** 25°C (77°F); excursions permitted to 15-30°C (59-86°F).

TETANUS & DIPHTHERIA TOXOIDS ADSORBED RX

diphtheria toxoid - tetanus toxoid (Sanofi Pasteur)

THERAPEUTIC CLASS: Toxoid combination

INDICATIONS: Active immunization against tetanus and diphtheria (Td).

DOSAGE: *Adults:* 0.5mL IM in the vastus lateralis or deltoid. Repeat 4-8 weeks later. Give 3rd dose 6-12 months after 2nd dose. Booster: 0.5mL IM every 10 yrs.

Pediatrics: >7 yrs: 0.5mL IM in the vastus lateralis or deltoid. Repeat 4-8 weeks later. Give 3rd dose 6-12 months after 2nd dose. Booster: 0.5mL IM every 10 yrs.

HOW SUPPLIED: Inj: 5LFU-2LFU/0.5mL

CONTRAINDICATIONS: Neurological or systemic allergic reaction to previous dose. Defer during febrile illness, acute infection, or an outbreak of poliomyelitis. Thimerosal hypersensitivity.

WARNINGS/PRECAUTIONS: Suboptimal response may occur in immunocompromised patients. Avoid booster more frequently than every 10 yrs especially with Arthus-type hypersensitivity reactions or temperature >39.4°C after a previous dose of tetanus toxoid. Caution with IM injection in thrombocytopenia or any coagulation disorder. Increased risk of local/systemic reactions to boosters doses. Have epinephrine available.

ADVERSE REACTIONS: Injection-site reactions, fever, malaise, hypotension, nausea, arthralgia.

INTERACTIONS: Immunosuppressive therapy may reduce response to active immunization. Caution with anticoagulants.

PREGNANCY: Category C, safety in nursing not known.

MECHANISM OF ACTION: Toxoid combination; activates neutralizing antibodies to diphtheria and tetanus toxins for protection against diphtheria and tetanus.

PHARMACOKINETICS: Absorption: Complete.

NURSING CONSIDERATIONS

Assessment: Assess for history of hypersensitivity including thimerosal (mercury derivative), systemic or neurologic reactions following previous dose of vaccine, acute illness, bleeding disorders (eg, hemophilia, thrombocytopenia), anticoagulant therapy, immunosuppressive therapy, and outbreak of poliomyelitis.

Monitoring: Monitor for acute anaphylactic reactions, Arthus-type hypersensitivity reactions, injection-site redness, warmth, edema, induration with/without tenderness, urticaria and rash, malaise, transient fever, pain, hypotension, nausea, arthralgia, and neurological complications (eg, cochlear lesion, brachial plexus neuropathies, paralysis of radical nerve, EEG disturbances, encephalopathy).

Patient Counseling: Inform of the benefits and risks of immunization and of importance of completing the primary immunization series or receiving recommended booster doses. Does not treat diphtheria or tetanus infections. Instruct to report any severe or unusual adverse reactions (eg, hives, swelling of mouth, difficulty breathing, hypotension, shock).

Administration: IM. Inspect for particulate matter and/or discoloration prior to administration. Shake well before withdrawing each dose. Inject IM only in anterolateral aspect of thigh or deltoid muscle of upper arm. **Storage:** 2-8°C (35-46°F). Do not freeze.

TETANUS TOXOID ADSORBED
RX

tetanus toxoid (Sanofi Pasteur)

THERAPEUTIC CLASS: Toxoid

INDICATIONS: Active immunization against tetanus.

DOSAGE: *Adults:* Primary Immunization: 0.5mL IM. Repeat 4-8 weeks later. Give 3rd dose 6-12 months after 2nd dose. Booster: 0.5mL IM every 10 yrs. *Pediatrics:* <1 yr: 3 doses of 0.5mL IM 4 to 8 weeks apart, then 4th dose (0.5mL) 6 to 12 months after the 3rd dose. Last dose before 4 yrs. Give booster of 0.5mL at 4-6 yrs. No booster needed if last primary dose was given after 4 yrs. ≥1 yrs: Primary Immunization: 0.5mL IM. Repeat 4-8 weeks later. Give 3rd dose 6-12 months after 2nd dose. Booster: 0.5mL IM every 10 yrs.

HOW SUPPLIED: Inj: 5 LFU/0.5mL

CONTRAINDICATIONS: Neurological or systemic allergic reaction to previous dose. Defer during febrile illness, acute infection, or an outbreak of poliomyelitis. Thimerosal hypersensitivity.

WARNINGS/PRECAUTIONS: Suboptimal response may occur in immunocompromised patients. Avoid booster more frequently than every 10 yrs especially with Arthus-type hypersensitivity reactions or temperature >103°F after a previous dose of tetanus toxoid. Caution with IM injections in thrombocytopenia or any coagulation disorders. Have epinephrine injection available. Increased incidence of local/systemic reaction to booster doses.

ADVERSE REACTIONS: Local erythema, malaise, transient fever, pain, hypotension, nausea, arthralgia.

INTERACTIONS: Caution with anticoagulants. Immunosuppressive therapy (eg, radiation, corticosteroids, chemotherapy) may reduce antibody response to vaccine; defer routine vaccination. Separate syringes and sites should be used when Tetanus Immune Globulin (human) and vaccine are given concurrently.

PREGNANCY: Category C, safety in nursing not known.

MECHANISM OF ACTION: Development of neutralizing antibodies against tetanus toxin.

NURSING CONSIDERATIONS

Assessment: Review current health status, previous sensitivity/immunization events (eg, Guillain-Barre syndrome, convulsions), and possible drug interactions.

Monitoring: Monitor adverse events such as severe Arthus-type hypersensitivity reactions; anaphylactic reactions; injection site for hematoma, redness, warmth, edema, induration, and tenderness; urticaria; rash; malaise; fever; pain; hypotension; nausea; arthralgia; Guillain-Barre syndrome; brachial neuritis; EEG disturbances.

Patient Counseling: Inform patient and caregiver of potential benefits/risk ratio; report any adverse reactions to physician. Stress importance of completing vaccination series.

Administration: IM in the area of the vastus lateralis or deltoid. **Storage**: 2-8°C (36-46°F). Do not freeze.

TEVETEN
RX

eprosartan mesylate (Abbott/Kos)

Can cause death/injury to developing fetus during 2nd and 3rd trimesters. Stop therapy if pregnancy detected.

THERAPEUTIC CLASS: Angiotensin II receptor antagonist

INDICATIONS: Treatment of hypertension, alone or with other antihypertensives.

DOSAGE: *Adults:* Initial: 600mg qd. Usual: 400-800mg/day, given qd-bid. Moderate to Severe Renal Impairment: Max: 600mg/day.

HOW SUPPLIED: Tab: 400mg, 600mg

WARNINGS/PRECAUTIONS: Can cause fetal injury/death. Correct volume or salt depletion before therapy. Changes in renal function may occur; caution with renal artery stenosis, severe CHF.

ADVERSE REACTIONS: Upper respiratory infection, rhinitis, pharyngitis, cough.

INTERACTIONS: Risk of hypotension with diuretics.

PREGNANCY: Category C (1st trimester) and D (2nd and 3rd trimesters), not for use in nursing.

MECHANISM OF ACTION: Angiotensin II receptor antagonist; blocks vasoconstrictor and aldosterone-secreting effects of angiotensin II by selectively blocking binding of angiotensin II to AT_1 receptor found in many tissues.

PHARMACOKINETICS: Absorption: Absolute bioavailability (approximately 13%); T_{max}=1-2 hrs. **Distribution:** V_{ss}=308L; plasma protein binding (approximately 98%). **Elimination:** Feces (90%), urine (7%), (600mg); $T_{1/2}$=20 hrs.

NURSING CONSIDERATIONS

Assessment: Assess LFTs, renal function, BP, pregnancy status, and possible drug interactions.

Monitoring: Monitor BP, LFTs, renal function, CBC with platelet count and differential, serum K^+ levels. Monitor for angina, bradycardia, angioneurotic edema, hypersensitivity reactions, upper respiratory tract infection, constipation, rhinitis, eczema. Hypotension, oliguria, and hyperkalemia should be closely observed in infants with histories of angiotensin II receptor antagonist exposure.

Patient Counseling: Counsel about signs/symptoms of adverse effects; advise to seek prompt medical attention. Inform about fetal risks if taken during pregnancy.

Administration: Oral route. **Storage:** Store at controlled room temperature of 20-25°C (68-77°F).

TEVETEN HCT RX

eprosartan mesylate - hydrochlorothiazide (Abbott/Kos)

Can cause death/injury to developing fetus during 2nd and 3rd trimesters. Stop therapy if pregnancy detected.

THERAPEUTIC CLASS: Angiotensin II receptor antagonist/thiazide diuretic

INDICATIONS: Treatment of hypertension. Not for initial therapy.

T

DOSAGE: *Adults:* Usual (Not Volume Depleted): 600mg-12.5mg qd. Titrate: May increase to 600mg-25mg qd if needed. Renal Impairment: Max: 600mg/day (eprosartan).

HOW SUPPLIED: Tab: (Eprosartan-HCTZ) 600mg-12.5mg, 600mg-25mg

CONTRAINDICATIONS: Anuria, sulfonamide hypersensitivity.

WARNINGS/PRECAUTIONS: Hypersensitivity reactions reported. Fetal/neonatal morbidity and death reported. Monitor for hypotension in volume/salt depletion. Caution with CHF, renal or hepatic dysfunction. May exacerbate or activate SLE. Monitor electrolytes periodically. Hypercalcemia, hypomagnesemia, hyperuricemia, hyperglycemia may occur. Enhanced effects in post-sympathectomy patient.

ADVERSE REACTIONS: Dizziness, headache, back pain, fatigue, myalgia, upper respiratory tract infection, sinusitis, viral infection.

INTERACTIONS: Increased risk of hyperkalemia with K^+-sparing diuretics, K^+ supplements, or K^+-containing salt substitutes. Potentiated orthostatic hypotension with alcohol, barbiturates, and narcotics. May need to adjust insulin and antidiabetic drugs. Impaired absorption with cholestyramine, colestipol. Corticosteroids and ACTH deplete electrolytes. May decrease response to pressor amines (eg, norepinephrine). Potentiated effect with other antihypertensives. May increase responsiveness to nondepolarizing skeletal muscle relaxants (eg, tubocurarine). Risk of lithium toxicity; avoid use. NSAIDs may decrease diuretic/antihypertensive effects.

PREGNANCY: Category C (1st trimester) and D (2nd and 3rd trimesters), not for use in nursing.

MECHANISM OF ACTION: Eprosartan: Angiotensin II receptor antagonist; blocks vasoconstrictor and aldosterone-secreting effects of angiotensin II by selectively blocking binding of angiotensin II to AT_1 receptor in vascular smooth muscle and adrenal gland. HCTZ: Thiazide diuretic; affects renal tubular mechanism of electrolyte reabsorption, directly increasing excretion of Na^+ and Cl^-.

PHARMACOKINETICS: Absorption: Eprosartan: Absolute bioavailability (13%); T_{max}=1-2 hrs. **Distribution:** Eprosartan: V_{ss}=308L; plasma protein binding (approximately 98%). HCTZ: Crosses placenta; excreted in breast milk. **Elimination:** Eprosartan: Feces (90%), urine (7%); (600mg) $T_{1/2}$=20 hrs. HCTZ: Urine (61% unchanged); $T_{1/2}$=5.6-14.8 hrs.

NURSING CONSIDERATIONS

Assessment: Assess for anuria, hypersensitivity to other sulfonamide-derived drugs, renal/hepatic insufficiency, hypotension, hyperuricemia, electrolyte imbalance, and possible drug interactions.

Monitoring: Monitor BP, LFTs, renal function, CBC with platelet count and differential, serum electrolytes, hyperuricemia, lipid profile. Monitor for MI, CHF, angioneurotic edema, hypersensitivity reactions, upper respiratory tract infection, diarrhea, sinusitis, pancreatitis, Stevens-Johnson syndrome, xanthopsia. Infants with history of angiotensin II receptor antagonist exposure should be closely observed for hypotension, oliguria, and hyperkalemia.

Patient Counseling: Inform of risks if taken during pregnancy. Advise that inadequate fluid intake, excessive perspiration, diarrhea, or vomiting can lead to excessive fall in BP, leading to lightheadedness or possible syncope. Advise not to use K^+ supplements or salt substitutes containing K^+ without consulting physician. Inform about signs/symptoms of adverse effects and advise to seek prompt medical attention.

Administration: Oral route. **Storage:** Controlled room temperature, 20-25°C (68-77°F).

TEV-TROPIN — RX

somatropin (Gate)

THERAPEUTIC CLASS: Human growth hormone

INDICATIONS: Long-term treatment of children who have growth failure due to an inadequate secretion of normal endogenous growth hormone.

DOSAGE: *Pediatrics:* 0.1mg/kg (0.3 IU/kg) SQ 3x week.

HOW SUPPLIED: Inj: 5mg

CONTRAINDICATIONS: Prader-Willi syndrome (PWS) with severe obesity or severe respiratory impairment. Growth failure due to PWS. Acute critical illness due to complications following open heart or abdominal surgery, multiple accidental traumas, acute respiratory failure; closed epiphyses; progression of an underlying intracranial lesion; active neoplasia, benzyl alcohol sensitivity.

WARNINGS/PRECAUTIONS: Reports of fatalities in pediatric patients with PWS. In PWS, evaluate for upper airway obstruction prior to initiation; monitor weight, for sleep apnea, signs of upper airway obstruction (eg, suspend therapy with onset of or increased snoring), respiratory infections (treat early and aggressively if occur). Monitor GHD secondary to intracranial lesion for progression/recurrence; glucose intolerance; hypothyroidism; intracranial hypertension (perform fundoscopic exam at start and periodically). Slipped capital femoral epiphysis may occur. Monitor for malignant transformation of any skin lesion. When injected SQ in same site over long period of time, may cause tissue atrophy; rotate injection site.

ADVERSE REACTIONS: Headaches, injection site reactions (pain, bruise), leukemia.

INTERACTIONS: Decreased effects with glucocorticoids.

PREGNANCY: Category C, caution with nursing.

MECHANISM OF ACTION: Human growth hormone; stimulates linear growth synthesis, metabolizes lipids, reduces body fat stores by increasing cellular protein, and increases plasma fatty acids.

PHARMACOKINETICS: Absorption: C_{max}=80ng/mL; T_{max}=7 hrs. **Elimination:** (IV) $T_{1/2}$=0.42 hrs. (SQ) $T_{1/2}$=2.7 hrs.

NURSING CONSIDERATIONS

Assessment: Assess for hypersensitivity to benzyl alcohol, closed epiphyses (pediatric), proliferative diabetic retinopathy, active malignancy, acute critical illness (complications of surgery, multiple accidental trauma, or acute respiratory failure), pre-existing type 1 or type 2 DM or impaired glucose tolerance, history of scoliosis, pre-existing papilledema, hypothyroidism, diagnostic imaging (rule out pituitary or intracranial tumor), hypopituitarism, and possible drug interactions. Obtain baseline fundoscopic exam. Prader-Willi syndrome: Evaluate for signs of upper airway obstruction or sleep apnea before initiation. Turner syndrome: Evaluate for otitis media or other ear disorders, and for cardiovascular disorders before initiation.

Monitoring: Monitor fasting blood glucose and thyroid function tests periodically, periodic fundoscopic exam, weight control (Prader-Willi syndrome), signs/symptoms of malignant transformation of skin lesions, intracranial HTN, slipped capital femoral epiphysis (eg, onset of limp, hip or knee pain), hypersensitivity/allergic reactions, respiratory infections (Prader-Willi syndrome), otitis media or ear disorders (Turner syndrome), CV disorders (Turner syndrome), and progression of scoliosis.

Patient Counseling: Instruct thoroughly as to proper usage, proper disposal; caution against any reuse of needles and syringes. Seek medical attention if symptoms of slipped capital femoral epiphysis (eg, onset of limp, hip or knee pain), hypersensitivity/allergic reactions, respiratory infections (Prader-Willi syndrome), otitis media or ear disorders (Turner syndrome), CV disorders (Turner syndrome), and progression of scoliosis occur.

Administration: SQ. **Storage:** Refrigerate at 2-8°C (36-46°F). Do not freeze. (After reconstitution): Refrigerate; stable for up to 14 days.

THALOMID RX

thalidomide (Celgene)

T

Severe, life-threatening human birth defects if taken during pregnancy. Women of childbearing potential should have a pregnancy test before starting therapy, then weekly for 1st month, and monthly thereafter. Males must use latex condoms during sexual contact with females of childbearing potential. Effective contraception must be used 4 weeks before, during, and 4 weeks after therapy. Only prescribers and pharmacists registered with the *S.T.E.P.S.®* distribution program can prescribe and dispense. The use of thalidomide in multiple myeloma results in an increased risk of venous thromboembolic events (eg, DVT, PE).

THERAPEUTIC CLASS: Immunomodulatory agent

INDICATIONS: Acute treatment of the cutaneous manifestations of moderate to severe erythema nodosum leprosum (ENL). Maintenance therapy for prevention and suppression of the cutaneous manifestations of ENL recurrence. In combination with dexamethasone for the treatment of newly diagnosed multiple myeloma.

DOSAGE: *Adults:* Acute ENL: Initial: 100-300mg qhs with water at least 1 hr after evening meal. <50kg: Start therapy at lower end of dosing range. Severe Cutaneous ENL: Initial: 400mg qhs with water at least 1 hr after evening meal.

Use with corticosteroids in moderate to severe neuritis with severe ENL. Taper steroid where neuritis is ameliorated. Duration of therapy is usually 2 weeks. Taper Dose: Decrease by 50mg every 2-4 weeks. Maintenance Therapy for Prevention/Suppression of ENL Recurrence: Use minimum dose to control reaction. Taper Dose: Every 3-6 months, attempt to decrease dose by 50mg every 2-4 weeks. Multiple Myeloma: 200mg qhs at least 1 hr after evening meal. Give with dexamethasone in 28-day treatment cycles.
Pediatrics: ≥12 yrs: Acute ENL: Initial: 100-300mg qhs with water at least 1 hr after evening meal. <50kg: Start therapy at lower end of dosing range. Severe Cutaneous ENL: Initial: 400mg qhs with water at least 1 hour after evening meal. Use with corticosteroids in moderate to severe neuritis with severe ENL. Taper steroid where neuritis is ameliorated. Duration of therapy is usually 2 weeks. Taper Dose: Decrease by 50mg every 2-4 weeks. Maintenance Therapy for Prevention/Suppression of ENL Recurrence: Use minimum dose to control reaction. Taper Dose: Every 3-6 months, attempt to decrease dose by 50mg every 2-4 weeks. Multiple Myeloma: 200mg qhs at least 1 hr after evening meal. Give with dexamethasone in 28-day treatment cycles.

HOW SUPPLIED: Cap: 50mg, 100mg, 200mg

CONTRAINDICATIONS: Women of childbearing potential unless alternative therapies are considered inappropriate and if precautions are taken to avoid pregnancy. Sexually mature males unless they comply with the *S.T.E.P.S.*® program and mandatory contraceptive measures.

WARNINGS/PRECAUTIONS: See Black Box Warning. If hypersensitivity reaction occurs such as rash, fever, or tachycardia, d/c drug. Stevens-Johnson syndrome and toxic epidermal necrolysis reported. May cause severe birth defects. Drowsiness and somnolence reported, caution when operating machinery. May cause neuropathy, monitor for symptoms. If symptoms of neuropathy arise, d/c immediately. Do not initiate if ANC <750/mm^3. Measure viral load of HIV patients after 1st and 3rd month of therapy and every 3 months thereafter.

ADVERSE REACTIONS: Drowsiness, somnolence, peripheral neuropathy, dizziness, orthostatic hypotension, neutropenia, increased HIV viral load, rash, constipation, hypocalcemia, thrombosis/embolism, dyspnea.

INTERACTIONS: Enhanced sedation with barbiturates, alcohol, chlorpromazine, and reserpine. Caution with drugs associated with peripheral neuropathy.

PREGNANCY: Category X, not for use in nursing.

MECHANISM OF ACTION: Immunomodulatory agent; not fully established. Possesses immunomodulatory, anti-inflammatory, and anti-angiogenic properties. Immunologic effects may be caused by suppression of excessive TNF-α production and down-modulation of selected cell surface adhesion molecules involved in leukocyte migration. Also causes suppression of macrophage involvement in prostaglandin synthesis and modulation of interleukin-10 and 12 production by peripheral blood mononuclear cells. In multiple myeloma, increased circulating natural killer cells and plasma levels of interleukin-2 and INF-gamma are also seen.

PHARMACOKINETICS: Absorption: Slow; T_{max}=2.9-5.7 hrs. **Distribution:** Plasma protein binding (55-66%); found in semen. **Metabolism:** Non-enzymatic hydrolysis. **Elimination:** Urine (<0.7% unchanged); $T_{1/2}$=5-7 hrs.

NURSING CONSIDERATIONS

Assessment: Assess use in those capable of reproduction. Assess that females are committed to either abstaining from heterosexual contact or willing to use 2 forms of reliable contraception including 1 highly effective method (eg, IUD, hormonal contraception, tubal ligation, or partner's vasectomy) and 1 additional effective method (eg, latex condom, diaphragm, or cervical cap) beginning 4 weeks prior to treatment, during treatment, and continuing 4 weeks after treatment. Prior to therapy, assess that males will wear latex condom during any sexual contact with women of childbearing potential, even if they have undergone a vasectomy. Assess pregnancy status 24 hours prior to therapy. Prior to therapy, assess nursing status, absolute neutrophil count (ANC), and drug interactions.

Monitoring: Monitor for signs/symptoms of VTE events (eg, SOB, chest pain, arm or leg swelling), drowsiness, somnolence, peripheral neuropathy, dizziness, orthostatic hypotension, neutropenia, hypersensitivity reactions (eg, erythematous macular rash), bradycardia, seizures, Stevens-Johnson syndrome, toxic epidermal necrolysis. Perform periodic monitoring of WBC count with differential. Perform pregnancy test weekly during first 4 weeks of therapy, then at 4-week intervals (regular menstrual cycle) or every 2 weeks (irregular menstrual cycle). Monitor for missed periods or abnormal menstrual bleeding.

Patient Counseling: Instruct females they must use 2 forms of contraception beginning 4 weeks prior to treatment, during treatment, and 4 weeks following end of therapy. Instruct males to use latex condom during any heterosexual contact. Counsel to not extensively handle thalidomide caps and maintain medication in blister packs until ingestion. May cause drowsiness and somnolence, impair mental/physical abilities. Avoid hazardous tasks (eg, operating machinery/driving) and avoid alcohol or medications which may cause CNS depression. May cause dizziness; sit upright for a few min prior to standing up from recumbent position. Instruct about signs/symptoms of peripheral neuropathies (eg, numbness, tingling) and thromboembolism (eg, SOB, chest pain, leg or arm swelling). Inform that not allowed to donate blood and males not allowed to donate sperm while on medication.

Administration: Oral route. **Storage:** 25°C (77°F); excursions permitted to 15-30°C (59-86°F). Protect from light.

THEO-24 — RX

theophylline (UCB)

THERAPEUTIC CLASS: Xanthine bronchodilator

INDICATIONS: Treatment of symptoms and reversible airflow obstruction associated with chronic asthma and other chronic lung diseases.

DOSAGE: *Adults:* Initial: 300-400mg/day. Titrate: After 3 days increase to 400-600mg/day if tolerated. May increase to >600mg/day if needed and tolerated after 3 more days. Renal/Liver Dysfunction/Elderly/CHF: Max: 400mg/day. May give in divided doses q12h in fast metabolizers. Swallow tab whole with full glass of water, do not crush. Dose should be titrated based on serum levels.

Pediatrics: 12-15 yrs: <45kg: Initial: 12-14mg/kg/day. Max: 300mg/day. Titrate: After 3 days increase to 16mg/kg/day. Max: 400mg/day. May increase to 20mg/kg/day if tolerated and needed after 3 more days. Max: 600mg/day. 12-15 yrs (>45kg): Follow adult dose schedule. Renal/Liver Dysfunction/CHF: Max: 16mg/kg/day or 400mg/day. May give in divided doses q12h in fast metabolizers. Swallow tab whole with full glass of water, do not crush. Dose should be titrated based on serum levels.

HOW SUPPLIED: Cap, Extended-Release: 100mg, 200mg, 300mg, 400mg

WARNINGS/PRECAUTIONS: Extreme caution in PUD, seizure disorders, and/or cardiac arrhythmias (except bradycardia). Caution in neonates, children <1 yr, and the elderly. Caution in pulmonary edema, CHF, fever ≥102°F for 24 hrs, cor pulmonale, hypothyroidism, liver disease, reduced renal function, sepsis, shock, and HTN. If toxicity develops (eg, repetitive vomiting) monitor serum levels and adjust dosage.

ADVERSE REACTIONS: Diarrhea, NV, abdominal pain, nervousness, headache, insomnia, seizures, dizziness, tachycardia, arrhythmias, restlessness, tremor, transient diuresis.

INTERACTIONS: Potentiated by propranolol, allopurinol, erythromycin, cimetidine, interferon, ciprofloxacin, clarithromycin, disulfiram, enoxacin, methotrexate, β-adrenergic blockers, oral contraceptives, fluvoxamine, CCBs, corticosteroid, thyroid hormones, thiabendazole, ticlopidine, troleandomycin, carbamazepine, pentoxifylline, diuretics, tacrine, and isoniazid. Diminishes the effects of adenosine, diazepam, lithium, lorazepam, midazolam, and pancuronium. Synergistic CNS effects with ephedrine. Diminished effects with aminoglutethemide, phenytoin, phenobarbital, carbamazepine, rifampin, barbiturates, hydantoins, ketoconazole, diuretics, sympathomimetics, and isoproterenol.

PREGNANCY: Category C, caution in nursing.

MECHANISM OF ACTION: Methylxanthine; not established, suspected to act by relaxation of smooth muscle and suppression of response of airways to stimuli.

PHARMACOKINETICS: Absorption: Rapid, complete; C_{max}=18.1mcg/mL. **Distribution:** V_d=0.45L/kg; plasma protein binding (40%); crosses placenta; excreted in breast milk. **Metabolism:** Liver (N-demethylation); metabolite: Caffeine. Liver (demethylation) via CYP1A2; metabolite: 3-methylxanthine. Liver (hydroxylation) via CYP2E1 and 3A3. **Elimination:** (Neonates) Urine (50%). (>3mo) Urine (10%).

NURSING CONSIDERATIONS

Assessment: Assess physiologic conditions that may alter theophylline clearance. Assess for acute pulmonary edema, CHF, hypo/hyperthyroidism, renal/hepatic dysfunction, CF, peptic ulcer, seizure disorders, cardiac arrhythmias, recent cessation of smoking, cor pulmonale, shock, decreased protein binding, sepsis with multi-organ failure, pregnancy status, and possible drug interactions. Obtain baseline serum theophylline concentration and unbound theophylline concentrations (conditions with decreased protein binding; cirrhosis, pregnancy in 3rd trimester).

Monitoring: Monitor serum theophylline concentrations frequently in acutely ill patients, periodically during long-term therapy, before increasing dose, signs/symptoms of toxicity present, new illness, worsening of chronic illness, or change in treatment regimen. Signs/symptoms of toxicity (persistent NV), persistent fever, worsening of chronic illness; if start or d/c smoking cigarettes or marijuana, or if start or d/c other medication.

Patient Counseling: Instruct not to alter dose, timing of dose, or frequency of administration without informing physician. If dose missed, take next dose at scheduled time; do not make up missed dose. Seek medical attention if symptoms of toxicity (persistent NV), persistent fever, worsening of chronic illness; if start or stop smoking cigarettes or marijuana, or if start or d/c other medication.

Administration: Oral route. **Storage:** Below 25°C (77°F).

THIORIDAZINE RX

thioridazine HCl (Various)

Prolongation of QTc interval reported in a dose-related manner. Associated with torsade de pointes and sudden death; reserve for patients who fail to respond to or cannot tolerate other antipsychotics.

THERAPEUTIC CLASS: Piperidine phenothiazine

INDICATIONS: Management of schizophrenia in patients not responsive to or intolerant to other antipsychotics.

DOSAGE: *Adults:* Initial: 50-100mg tid. Titrate: Increase gradually. Usual: 200-800mg/day given bid-qid. Max: 800mg/day.
Pediatrics: Initial: 0.6mg/kg/day given in divided doses. Titrate: Increase gradually. Max: 3mg/kg/day.

HOW SUPPLIED: Tab: 10mg, 15mg, 25mg, 50mg, 100mg, 150mg, 200mg

CONTRAINDICATIONS: Severe CNS depression, comatose states, severe hypo- or hypertensive heart disease. Drugs that prolong QTc interval, congenital long QT syndrome, cardiac arrhythmias, drugs that inhibit CYP450 2D6 (eg, fluoxetine, paroxetine), patients with reduced activity of CYP450 2D6.

WARNINGS/PRECAUTIONS: Perform baseline ECG and measure baseline potassium level; monitor periodically thereafter. May develop tardive dyskinesia. NMS, seizures, leukopenia, agranulocytosis reported. Caution with activities requiring alertness. May elevate prolactin levels.

ADVERSE REACTIONS: Tardive dyskinesia, ECG changes, drowsiness, dry mouth, blurred vision, peripheral edema, galactorrhea, NV, gynecomastia, impotence, constipation, diarrhea.

INTERACTIONS: See Contraindications. May potentiate CNS depressants, alcohol, atropine, and phosphorus insecticides. Propranolol, fluvoxamine, and pindolol increase thioridazine plasma levels; avoid concomitant use. Avoid CYP2D6 inhibitors (eg, fluoxetine, paroxetine); increased risk of arrhythmias.

PREGNANCY: Safety in pregnancy and nursing not known.

MECHANISM OF ACTION: Phenothiazine; associated with minimal extrapyramidal stimulation.

NURSING CONSIDERATIONS

Assessment: Before treatment, strongly recommend at least 2 trials, each with a different antipsychotic, at adequate dose at adequate duration. Assess for history of cardiac arrhythmias, congenital long QT syndrome, severe CNS depression, comatose states, hypotensive heart disease, HTN, possible drug interactions. Normalize serum K^+ and perform ECG before initiating treatment. Those with QTc interval ≥450 msec should not receive drug.

Monitoring: Periodically monitor ECGs for proarrhythmic effect, Holter monitoring if symptoms associated with occurrence of torsade de pointes (eg, dizziness, palpitations, syncope). Signs/symptoms of TD, NMS, CNS depression, convulsions, pigmentary retinopathy, drowsiness, EPS, pseudoparkinsonism, dry mouth, constipation, NV, galactorrhea, breast engorgement, amenorrhea. Monitor CBC and prolactin levels.

Patient Counseling: Advise about risk for potentially fatal heart rhythm disturbance; inform physician if receiving thioridazine treatment before taking any new medication. Avoid hazardous tasks.

Administration: Oral route. **Storage:** Controlled room temperature 15-30°C (59-86°F). Protect from light.

THYROLAR RX

liotrix (Forest)

THERAPEUTIC CLASS: Thyroid replacement hormone

INDICATIONS: Hypothyroidism. As a pituitary TSH suppressant in the treatment or prevention of euthyroid goiters. Diagnostic agent in suppression tests to differentiate suspected hyperthyroidism or thyroid gland autonomy. Management of thyroid cancer.

DOSAGE: *Adults:* Hypothyroidism: Usual: 12.5mcg-50mcg to 25mcg-100mcg qd. Elderly/Coronary Artery Disease: Initial: 6.25mcg-25mcg qd. Chronic Myxedema: 3.1mcg-12.5mcg qd. Titrate: Increase by 3.1mcg-12.5mcg/d q 2-3 weeks. Reduce dose if angina occurs. Myxedema Coma: 400mcg IV levothyroxine sodium (100mcg/mL rapidly) followed by 100-200mcg/day IV. Switch to PO when stable. Thyroid Suppression: 1.56mg/kg/d levothyroxine (T_4) for 7-10 days.

Pediatrics: Hypothyroidism: >12 yrs: 18.75mcg-75mcg qd. 6-12 yrs: 12.5mcg-50mcg to 18.75mcg-75mcg qd. 1-5 yrs: 9.35mcg-37.5mcg to 12.5mcg-50mcg qd. 6-12 months: 6.25mcg-25mcg to 9.35mcg-37.5mcg qd. 0-6 months: 3.1mcg-12.5mcg to 6.25mcg-25mcg qd.

HOW SUPPLIED: (T3-T4) Tab: (1/4) 3.1mcg-12.5mcg, (1/2) 6.25mcg-25mcg, (1) 12.5mcg-50mcg, (2) 25mcg-100mcg, (3) 37.5mcg-150mcg

CONTRAINDICATIONS: Untreated thyrotoxicosis, uncorrected adrenal cortical insufficiency.

WARNINGS/PRECAUTIONS: Do not use in the treatment of obesity; larger doses in euthyroid patients can cause serious or even life-threatening toxicity. Caution with angina pectoris and elderly; use lower doses. May aggravate diabetes mellitus or insipidus and adrenal cortical insufficiency. Excessive doses may cause craniosynostosis. Extreme caution with long-standing myxedema especially with cardiovascular impairment.

INTERACTIONS: May increase insulin or oral hypoglycemic requirements. Decreased absorption with cholestyramine and colestipol; space dosing by 4-5 hrs. Altered effect of oral anticoagulants; monitor PT/INR. Estrogens increase thyroxine-binding globulin; increase in thyroid dose may be needed.

Serious or life-threatening side effects can occur with sympathomimetic amines. Androgens, corticosteroids, estrogens, iodine-containing preparations, and salicylates may interfere with thyroid lab tests.

PREGNANCY: Category A, caution in nursing.

MECHANISM OF ACTION: Thyroid hormone; not understood, suspected to enhance oxygen consumption by most body tissues, increase basal metabolic rate and metabolism of carbohydrates, lipids, and proteins.

PHARMACOKINETICS: Distribution: Plasma protein binding (99%), found in breast milk. **Metabolism:** Deiodination and conjugation in liver, kidneys, and other tissues.

NURSING CONSIDERATIONS

Assessment: Assess for adrenal corticoid insufficiency, untreated thyrotoxicosis, and appropriate lab tests in addition to full clinical evaluation and possible drug interactions.

Monitoring: Frequent lab tests and clinical evaluation of thyroid function, including TSH and free T_4 levels, blood and/or urinary glucose, clotting parameters, reproductive function, and signs/symptoms of thyrotoxicity.

Patient Counseling: Inform that drug is to be taken for life; not for treatment of obesity or weight loss. Take on empty stomach. Notify physician if pregnant/nursing, planning to become pregnant, or taking any other drugs. Do not d/c or change dose unless directed by physician. Report any signs/symptoms of toxicity (eg, increased pulse rate, palpitations, excessive sweating, heat intolerance, nervousness).

Administration: Oral route. **Storage:** 2-8°C (36-46°F) in tight, light-resistant container.

TIAZAC — RX

diltiazem HCl (Forest)

OTHER BRAND NAMES: Taztia XT (Andrx)

THERAPEUTIC CLASS: Calcium channel blocker (nondihydropyridine)

INDICATIONS: Hypertension. Chronic stable angina.

DOSAGE: *Adults:* HTN: Initial: 120-240mg qd. Titrate: Adjust at 2-week intervals. Usual: 120-540mg qd. Max: 540mg qd. Angina: Initial: 120-180mg qd. Titrate: Increase over 7-14 days. Max: 540mg qd.

HOW SUPPLIED: Cap, Extended-Release: (Taztia XT, Tiazac) 120mg, 180mg, 240mg, 300mg, 360mg; (Tiazac) 420mg

CONTRAINDICATIONS: Sick sinus syndrome and 2nd- or 3rd-degree AV block (except with functioning pacemaker), severe hypotension (<90mmHg systolic), acute MI, pulmonary congestion.

WARNINGS/PRECAUTIONS: Caution in renal, hepatic, or ventricular dysfunction. Monitor LFTs and renal function with prolonged use. D/C if persistent rash occurs. Symptomatic hypotension may occur. Acute hepatic injury reported.

ADVERSE REACTIONS: Headache, peripheral edema, vasodilation, dizziness, rash, dyspepsia.

INTERACTIONS: Increased levels of buspirone, quinidine, carbamazepine, midazolam, triazolam, lovastatin, and propranolol. Increased levels of diltiazem with cimetidine. Monitor digoxin, cyclosporine. Potentiates cardiac contractility, conductivity, and automaticity; and vascular dilation with anesthetics. Additive cardiac conduction effects with digitalis or β-blockers. Avoid rifampin and other CYP3A4 inducers. Potential additive effects with agents known to affect cardiac contractility and/or conduction.

PREGNANCY: Category C, not for use in nursing.

MECHANISM OF ACTION: Calcium channel blocker; inhibits cellular influx of calcium ions during membrane depolarization of cardiac and vascular smooth muscle.

PHARMACOKINETICS: Absorption: Well-absorbed. Absolute bioavailability (~40%). **Distribution:** Plasma protein binding (70-80%). **Metabolism:** Hepatic; desacetyldiltiazem, desmethyldiltiazem (major metabolites). **Elimination:** Urine, bile; $T_{1/2}$=3.0-4.5 hrs.

NURSING CONSIDERATIONS

Assessment: Assess for sick sinus syndrome and 2nd- or 3rd-degree AV block without functional ventricular pacemaker, severe hypotension, AMI, pulmonary congestion (documented by x-ray), CHF, renal/hepatic function, drug hypersensitivity, and possible drug interactions.

Monitoring: Monitor LFTs, renal function, BP, HR. Monitor for angina, heart block, photosensitivity, ECG abnormalities, headache, edema, pain.

Patient Counseling: Counsel about signs/symptoms of adverse effects. Instruct to take as prescribed. Educate on need for routine checkup and lab exams.

Administration: Oral route. **Storage:** Controlled room temperature, 20-25°C (68-77°F). Avoid excessive humidity.

TICLID — RX

ticlopidine HCl (Roche Labs)

Can cause life-threatening hematological adverse reactions, including neutropenia/agranulocytosis, thrombotic thrombocytopenic purpura (TTP), and aplastic anemia. Monitor for evidence of neutropenia or TTP during first 3 months; d/c if any seen.

THERAPEUTIC CLASS: Platelet aggregation inhibitor

INDICATIONS: To reduce risk of thrombotic stroke in stroke patients or those with stroke precursors who are ASA intolerant, allergic, or failed ASA therapy. Adjunct to ASA to reduce incidence of subacute stent thrombosis in patients undergoing successful coronary artery stent implantation.

DOSAGE: *Adults:* Take with food. Stroke: 250mg bid. Coronary Artery Stenting: 250mg bid with ASA up to 30 days after stent implant.

HOW SUPPLIED: Tab: 250mg

CONTRAINDICATIONS: Hematopoietic disorders (eg, neutropenia, thrombocytopenia), history of TTP or aplastic anemia, hemostatic disorders, active pathological bleeding, severe liver impairment.

WARNINGS/PRECAUTIONS: Monitor for hematologic toxicity before treatment, then every 2 weeks for 1st 3 months, and 2 weeks after discontinuation. Monitor more frequently if signs of hematological adverse reactions; d/c if neutrophils <1200/mm^3, aplastic anemia or TTP occurs. D/C 10-14 days before surgery. Caution in trauma, surgery, bleeding disorders. May need dose adjustment with renal or hepatic impairment. May elevate LFTs, TG, and cholesterol.

ADVERSE REACTIONS: Diarrhea, rash, nausea, GI pain, dyspepsia, neutropenia.

INTERACTIONS: Adjust dose with drugs metabolized by CYP450 with low therapeutic ratios or with hepatic impairment. Potentiates ASA and NSAIDs effect on platelet aggregation. Antacids reduce plasma levels. Cimetidine reduces clearance. Decreases digoxin plasma levels. Significant decrease of theophylline plasma clearance. Caution with phenytoin, propranolol. D/C anticoagulants or fibrinolytics. Increased bioavailability with food.

PREGNANCY: Category B, not for use in nursing.

MECHANISM OF ACTION: Platelet aggregation inhibitor; interferes with platelet membrane function by inhibiting ADP-induced platelet fibrinogen binding and subsequent platelet-platelet interactions. Effect on platelet function is irreversible. Responsible for prolonging bleeding time.

PHARMACOKINETICS: Absorption: Rapid; T_{max}=2 hrs. **Distribution:** Plasma protein binding (98%). **Metabolism:** Liver (extensive). **Elimination:** Urine (60%), feces (23%); $T_{1/2}$=12.6 hrs (single dose), 4-5 days (multiple dose).

NURSING CONSIDERATIONS

Assessment: Assess for presence of hematopoietic disorders (eg, neutropenia, thrombocytopenia), history of TTP, aplastic anemia, presence of hemostatic disorder or active bleeding (eg, bleeding peptic ulcer, intracranial bleeding), severe liver impairment, renal impairment, nursing status, and drug interactions. Obtain baseline CBC including ANC, platelet count, and peripheral smear.

Monitoring: Monitor for signs/symptoms of thrombocytopenia, TTP (eg, weakness, petechiae, purpura, dark urine, neurological changes), aplastic anemia, agranulocytosis, pancytopenia, leukemia, liver dysfunction, and serum cholesterol elevations. During first 3 months of therapy, monitor CBC including ANC, platelet count, and peripheral smear every 2 weeks. If therapy discontinued before 3 months, monitor for 2 weeks following discontinuation. If liver dysfunction suspected, perform liver function testing (eg, ALT, AST, GGT).

Patient Counseling: Counsel about possible adverse effects (eg, thrombocytopenia, neutropenia). Contact physician immediately if any signs/symptoms of infection or TTP syndrome (eg, fever, weakness, difficulty speaking, seizures, yellowing of skin or eyes, bloody urine, petechiae) develop. Inform that lab testing is required during therapy. Advise it may take longer than usual to stop bleeding while on medication. Instruct to contact physician if any unusual bleeding occurs. Advise to notify all other physicians of medication. Take with food.

Administration: Oral route. **Storage:** 15-30°C (59-86°F).

TIGAN — RX

trimethobenzamide HCl (King)

THERAPEUTIC CLASS: Emetic response modifier

INDICATIONS: Treatment of postoperative nausea and vomiting and for nausea associated with gastroenteritis.

DOSAGE: *Adults:* (Cap) 300mg tid-qid. (Inj) 200mg IM tid-qid.

HOW SUPPLIED: Cap: 300mg; Inj: 100mg/mL

CONTRAINDICATIONS: Injection in children.

WARNINGS/PRECAUTIONS: Caution in children; may cause EPS, which may be confused with CNS signs of undiagnosed primary disease (eg, Reye's syndrome) and may unfavorably alter the course of Reye's syndrome due to hepatotoxic potential. Caution with acute febrile illness, encephalitides, gastroenteritis, dehydration, electrolyte imbalance, and in elderly; CNS reactions reported. May produce drowsiness.

ADVERSE REACTIONS: Hypersensitivity reactions, Parkinson-like symptoms, hypotension (inj), blood dyscrasias, blurred vision, coma, convulsions, mood depression, diarrhea, disorientation, dizziness, drowsiness, headache, jaundice, muscle cramps, opisthotonos.

INTERACTIONS: Caution with CNS agents (eg, phenothiazines, barbiturates, belladonna derivatives) in acute febrile illness, encephalitides, gastroenteritis, dehydration, and electrolyte imbalance. Adverse drug interactions reported with alcohol.

PREGNANCY: Safety in pregnancy and nursing not known.

MECHANISM OF ACTION: Mechanism not established; thought to involve chemoreceptor trigger zone, an area in medulla oblongata through which emetic impulses are conveyed to vomiting center (direct impulses to vomiting center apparently not similarly inhibited).

PHARMACOKINETICS: Absorption: T_{max}=30 min (IM 200mg). **Elimination:** $T_{1/2}$=7-9 hrs.

NURSING CONSIDERATIONS

Assessment: Assess for hepatic impairment, Reye's syndrome in children, pregnancy/nursing status, alcohol intake, acute febrile illness, encephalitides,

T

gastroenteritis, dehydration, electrolyte imbalance, appendicitis, toxicity, possible drug interactions.

Monitoring: Monitor for signs of hepatotoxicity, CNS reactions such as opisthotonos, convulsions, coma, EPS, and cerebral edema.

Patient Counseling: Caution against performing hazardous tasks (operating machinery/driving). Notify if pregnant/nursing.

Administration: Oral route and IM. **Storage:** 25°C (77°F); excursions permitted to 15-30°C (59-86°F).

TIKOSYN RX
dofetilide (Pfizer)

To minimize risk of arrhythmia, place patients initiated or reinitiated on therapy for minimum of 3 days in a facility that can provide CrCl, ECG monitoring, and cardiac resuscitation. Dofetilide is available only to hospitals and prescribers who have received appropriate dofetilide dosing and treatment initiation education.

THERAPEUTIC CLASS: Class III antiarrhythmic

INDICATIONS: Conversion to and maintenance of normal sinus rhythm in atrial fibrillation/flutter.

DOSAGE: *Adults:* CrCl: >60mL/min: 500mcg bid. CrCl 40-60mL/min: 250mcg bid. CrCl 20 to <40mL/min: 125mcg bid. Determine QTc interval 2-3 hrs after 1st dose and adjust dose if QTc >500msec or if >15% increase from baseline. QTc/Renal Dose Adjustment: Reduce 500mcg bid to 250mcg bid. Reduce 250mcg bid to 125mcg bid. Reduce 125mcg bid to 125mcg qd. D/C any time after 2nd dose if QTc >500msec (550msec with ventricular conduction abnormalities).

HOW SUPPLIED: Cap: 125mcg, 250mcg, 500mcg

CONTRAINDICATIONS: Long QT syndromes, baseline QT interval or QTc >440msec (500msec with ventricular conduction abnormalities), severe renal impairment (CrCl <20mL/min). Concomitant verapamil, cimetidine, trimethoprim, ketoconazole, and inhibitors of renal cation transport system (eg, megesterol, prochlorperazine).

WARNINGS/PRECAUTIONS: Can cause serious ventricular arrhythmia. Calculate CrCl before 1st dose; adjust dose based on CrCl. Caution in severe hepatic impairment. Maintain normal K^+ levels.

ADVERSE REACTIONS: Headache, chest pain, dizziness, arrhythmia, conduction disturbances, dyspnea, nausea, insomnia.

INTERACTIONS: See Contraindications. Hypokalemia or hypomagnesemia may occur with K^+-depleting diuretics. CYP3A4 inhibitors (eg, macrolides, protease inhibitors, grapefruit juice, etc) may potentiate dofetilide. Avoid verapamil, cimetidine, trimethoprim, ketoconazole, and inhibitors of renal cationic secretion. Caution with drugs actively secreted by cationic secretion (eg, amiloride, triamterene, metformin). Not recommended with drugs that prolong the QT interval. Hold Class I and III antiarrhythmics for at least 3 half-lives before initiating dofetilide. Reduce amiodarone to <0.3mcg/mL or withdraw at least 3 months before initiating dofetilide.

PREGNANCY: Category C, not for use in nursing.

MECHANISM OF ACTION: Class III antiarrhythmic; blocks cardiac ion channel carrying rapid component of delayed rectifier K^+ current, I_{Kr}.

PHARMACOKINETICS: Absorption: Bioavailability (>90%); T_{max}=2-3 hrs. **Distribution:** V_d=3L/kg; plasma protein binding (60-70%). **Metabolism:** Liver via CYP3A4 though N-dealkylation and N-oxidation pathways. **Elimination:** Urine (80% unchanged), (20% metabolites); T_{max}=10 hrs.

NURSING CONSIDERATIONS

Assessment: Assess for congenital or acquired long QT syndrome, ventricular arrhythmia, CHF, recent MI, structural heart disease, atrial flutter/fibrillation, baseline QT interval or QTc ≥440 msec (500 msec), sick sinus syndrome, HB,

T

implanted pacemaker, renal/hepatic impairment, pregnancy/nursing status, and possible drug interactions. Correct K^+ levels prior to therapy.

Monitoring: Patient should be in a facility for minimum of 3 days where CrCl, continuous ECG monitoring, and cardiac resuscitation are available. Monitor for ventricular arrhythmias (eg, torsade de pointes and polymorphic ventricular tachycardia associated with QT interval prolongation).

Patient Counseling: Inform about risks/benefits and need for compliance with prescribed dosing. Periodic monitoring of QTc and renal function required. Notify physician if pregnant/nursing or if taking concurrent administration of any OTC medication. Advise to not double next dose if dose is missed.

Administration: Oral route. **Storage:** 15-30°C (59-86°F). Protect from humidity and moisture.

TIMENTIN

RX

ticarcillin disodium - clavulanate potassium (GlaxoSmithKline)

THERAPEUTIC CLASS: Broad-spectrum penicillin/beta-lactamase inhibitor

INDICATIONS: Treatment of lower respiratory tract, bone and joint, skin and skin structure, urinary tract (UTI), gynecologic, and intra-abdominal infections, and septicemia caused by susceptible strains of microorganisms.

DOSAGE: *Adults:* ≥60kg: UTI/Systemic Infection: 3g-100mg (3.1g vial) IV q4-6h. Gynecologic Infections: Moderate: 200mg/kg/day ticarcillin IV given q6h. Severe: 300mg/kg/day ticarcillin IV given q4h. <60kg: Usual: 200-300mg/kg/day ticarcillin IV given q4-6h. Renal Impairment (based on ticarcillin): LD: 3.1g. Maint: CrCl >60mL/min: 3.1g q4h. CrCl 30-60mL/min: 2g IV q4h. CrCl 10-30mL/min: 2g IV q8h. CrCl <10mL/min: 2g IV q12h (2g IV q24h with hepatic dysfunction). Peritoneal Dialysis: 3.1g IV q12h. Hemodialysis: 2g IV q12h, and 3.1g after each dialysis.
Pediatrics: ≥3 months: ≥60kg: Mild to Moderate: 3g-100mg (3.1g vial) IV q6h. Severe: 3g-100mg (3.1g vial) IV q4h. <60 kg: Mild to Moderate: 50mg/kg ticarcillin IV q6h. Severe: 50mg/kg ticarcillin IV q4h. Renal Impairment (based on ticarcillin): LD: 3.1g vial. Maint: CrCl >60mL/min: 3.1g q4h. CrCl 30-60mL/min: 2g IV q4h. CrCl 10-30mL/min: 2g IV q8h. CrCl <10mL/min: 2g IV q12h (2g IV q24h with hepatic dysfunction). Peritoneal Dialysis: 3.1g IV q12h. Hemodialysis: 2g IV q12h, and 3.1g after each dialysis.

HOW SUPPLIED: Inj: (Ticarcillin-Clavulanate) 3g-100mg, 3g-100mg/100mL, 30g-1g

WARNINGS/PRECAUTIONS: Serious, sometimes fatal, hypersensitivity reactions reported with PCN therapy. *Clostridium difficile*-associated diarrhea reported. Prolonged use may result in overgrowth of nonsusceptible organisms. Risk of convulsions with high doses, especially with renal impairment. Monitor renal, hepatic, hematopoietic functions, and serum K^+ with prolonged therapy. Caution with fluid and electrolyte imbalance; hypokalemia reported. Clotting time, platelet aggregation, and PT abnormalities may occur especially with renal impairment; d/c therapy. Continue therapy for at least 2 days after signs/symptoms disappear. Caution in elderly patients with impaired renal function.

ADVERSE REACTIONS: Hypersensitivity reactions, headache, giddiness, taste/smell disturbances, stomatitis, flatulence, N/V, diarrhea, hematologic disturbances, hepatic/renal function tests abnormalities, local reactions.

INTERACTIONS: May inactivate aminoglycoside if mixed together in parenteral solution. Increased serum levels and prolonged half-life with probenecid. May reduce efficacy of combined oral estrogen/progesterone contraceptives.

PREGNANCY: Category B, caution in nursing.

MECHANISM OF ACTION: Ticarcillin: Broad-spectrum antibiotic with bactericidal activity against many gram-positive and gram-negative aerobic and anerobic bacteria. Clavulanic acid: β-lactam, which possesses ability to inactivate wide range of β-lactamase enzymes.

PHARMACOKINETICS: Absorption: Ticarcillin: C_{max}=330mcg/mL, AUC=485mcg•hr/mL. Clavulanic acid: C_{max}=8mcg/mL, AUC=8.2mcg•hr/mL. **Distribution:** Ticarcillin: Plasma protein binding (45%). Clavulanic acid: Plasma

T

protein binding (25%). **Elimination:** Ticarcillin: Urine (unchanged 60-70%); $T_{1/2}$=1.1 hrs, 4.4 hrs (neonates), 1 hr (infants/ children). Clavulanic acid: Urine (35-45% unchanged); $T_{1/2}$=1.1 hrs, 1.9 hrs (neonates), 0.9 hr (infants/children).

NURSING CONSIDERATIONS

Assessment: Assess for previous hypersensitivity reactions to cephalosporins, PCNs, or other allergens, renal/hepatic impairment, presence of fluid/electrolyte imbalance, pregnancy/nursing status, and possible drug interactions.

Monitoring: Periodically monitor renal, hepatic, hematopoietic function and serum K^+ levels. Monitor for signs/symptoms of anaphylactic/anaphylactoid reactions, CDAD, drug resistance or superinfection, bleeding manifestations, electrolyte abnormalities, lab test interactions (eg, false (+) Coombs' test).

Patient Counseling: Inform drug only treats bacterial, not viral, infections. Take as directed; skipping doses or not completing full course may decrease effectiveness and increase resistance. Inform about risks/benefits. D/C and notify physician if allergic reactions or watery/bloody diarrhea (with/without muscle cramps) occur. Notify if pregnant/nursing.

Administration: IV infusion (30 min). Do not use flexible container in series connections. **Storage:** 24°C (75°F). Avoid freezing or excessive heat.

TIMOLOL GFS — RX

timolol maleate (Falcon)

THERAPEUTIC CLASS: Nonselective beta-blocker

INDICATIONS: Treatment of elevated IOP in patients with open-angle glaucoma or ocular hypertension.

DOSAGE: *Adults:* Initial: 1 drop 0.25-0.5% qd. Evaluate IOP 4 weeks after starting treatment. Max: 1 drop 0.5% qd. Dose other ophthalmic drugs 10 min prior to gel-forming drops.

HOW SUPPLIED: Sol, Gel Forming: 0.25%, 0.5% [2.5mL, 5mL]

CONTRAINDICATIONS: Bronchial asthma, history of bronchial asthma, severe COPD, sinus bradycardia, 2nd- or 3rd-degree AV block, overt cardiac failure, cardiogenic shock.

WARNINGS/PRECAUTIONS: May be absorbed systemically. Caution with cardiac failure, DM, and cerebrovascular insufficiency. May mask symptoms of hypoglycemia and hyperthyroidism. Avoid with COPD, bronchospastic disease. Not for use alone in angle-closure glaucoma. May potentiate muscle weakness. D/C if cardiac failure develops. Withdrawal before surgery is controversial.

ADVERSE REACTIONS: Ocular burning, ocular stinging, transient blurred vision.

INTERACTIONS: May potentiate systemic/ophthalmic β-blockers and catecholamine-depleting drugs (eg, reserpine). Oral/IV calcium antagonists can cause AV conduction disturbances, left ventricular failure, or hypotension. Digitalis can cause additive effects in prolonging AV conduction time. Quinidine may potentiate β-blockade. May antagonize epinephrine. Give other ophthalmic drugs 10 min before use.

PREGNANCY: Category C, not for use in nursing.

MECHANISM OF ACTION: Nonselective β-adrenergic receptor blocker; reduces IOP. Actions may also be related to reduced aqueous formation.

PHARMACOKINETICS: Absorption: C_{max}≤5ng/mL. **Distribution:** Found in breast milk.

NURSING CONSIDERATIONS

Assessment: Assess for presence or history of bronchial asthma, severe COPD, sinus bradycardia, 2nd- or 3rd-degree AV block, overt cardiac failure, or cardiogenic shock. Assess use with cardiac failure, cerebrovascular insufficiencies, mild to moderate COPD (eg, chronic bronchitis, emphysema), elective surgery, risk for spontaneous hypoglycemia, DM, angle-closure glaucoma, or hyperthyroidism. Assess for possible drug interactions.

Monitoring: Monitor for signs/symptoms of cardiac failure, reduced cerebral blood flow, severe respiratory reactions, choroidal detachment, muscle weakness, bacterial keratitis, and anaphylaxis. With suspected thyrotoxicosis, avoid abrupt withdrawal from medication which may precipitate thyroid storm.

Patient Counseling: Inform that transient blurring may occur; caution when performing hazardous tasks (eg, driving). Counsel those who have ocular surgery or develop intercurrent ocular condition (eg, trauma, infection) to contact physician prior to continuing use of present multidose container. Instruct to invert closed medication container and shake once prior to use. Administer concomitant topical ophthalmic medications at least 10 min apart. Counsel those with DM that signs/symptoms of hypoglycemia may be masked.

Administration: Ocular route. **Storage:** 2-25°C (36-77°F). Protect from light.

TIMOLOL MALEATE — RX

timolol maleate (Various)

THERAPEUTIC CLASS: Nonselective beta-blocker

INDICATIONS: Treatment of hypertension. To reduce cardiovascular mortality and risk of reinfarction with previous MI. Migraine prophylaxis.

DOSAGE: *Adults:* HTN: Initial: 10mg bid. Maint: 20-40mg/day. Wait at least 7 days between dose increases. Max: 60mg/day given bid. MI: 10mg bid. Migraine: Initial: 10mg bid. Maint: 20mg qd. Max: 30mg/day in divided doses. May decrease to 10mg qd. D/C if inadequate response after 6-8 weeks with max dose.

HOW SUPPLIED: Tab: 5mg, 10mg*, 20mg* *scored

CONTRAINDICATIONS: Active or history of bronchial asthma, severe COPD, sinus bradycardia, 2nd- and 3rd-degree AV block, overt cardiac failure, cardiogenic shock.

WARNINGS/PRECAUTIONS: Caution with well-compensated cardiac failure, DM, mild to moderate COPD, bronchospastic disease, dialysis, hepatic/renal impairment, or cerebrovascular insufficiency. Exacerbation of ischemic heart disease with abrupt cessation. May mask hyperthyroidism or hypoglycemia symptoms. Withdrawal before surgery is controversial. May potentiate weakness with myasthenia gravis. Can cause cardiac failure. Caution and consider monitoring renal function in elderly.

ADVERSE REACTIONS: Fatigue, headache, nausea, arrhythmia, pruritus, dizziness, dyspnea, asthenia, bradycardia.

INTERACTIONS: Possible additive effects and hypotension and/or marked bradycardia with catecholamine-depleting drugs. NSAIDs may reduce antihypertensive effects. Quinidine may potentiate β-blockade. AV conduction time prolonged with digitalis and either diltiazem or verapamil. Hypotension, AV conduction disturbances, left ventricular failure reported with oral calcium antagonists. Caution with IV calcium antagonists, insulin, oral hypoglycemics. Avoid calcium antagonists with cardiac dysfunction. May exacerbate rebound HTN following clonidine withdrawal. May block effects of epinephrine.

PREGNANCY: Category C, not for use in nursing.

MECHANISM OF ACTION: β_1 and β_2 adrenergic receptor blocking agent; reduces cardiac output and plasma renin activity.

PHARMACOKINETICS: Absorption: (PO) Completely absorbed (90%); T_{max}=2 hrs. **Metabolism:** Partially, by liver. **Excretion:** Kidneys; $T_{1/2}$= 4 hrs.

NURSING CONSIDERATIONS

Assessment: Assess for bradycardia, cardiogenic shock, 2nd- and 3rd-degree heart block, overt cardiac failure, impaired hepatic/renal function, bronchospastic disease, PVD, DM, thyrotoxicosis, valvular heart disease, and possible drug interactions.

T

Monitoring: Monitor for cardiac failure, HTN, renal function, exacerbation of ischemia following abrupt withdrawal, bronchospastic disease, PVD, anaphylactoid reactions, hypersensitivity reactions.

Patient Counseling: Counsel if signs suggest reduced cerebral blood flow; may need to d/c therapy. Instruct not to interrupt or d/c therapy without consulting physician. Counsel about signs/symptoms of CHF; notify physician if signs/symptoms of impending CHF or unexplained respiratory symptoms occur.

Administration: Oral route. **Storage:** 20-25°C (68-77°F); tight, light-resistant container.

TIMOPTIC

timolol maleate (Merck)

RX

OTHER BRAND NAMES: Timoptic-XE (Merck) - Timoptic Ocudose (Merck)

THERAPEUTIC CLASS: Nonselective beta-blocker

INDICATIONS: Treatment of elevated IOP in patients with open-angle glaucoma or ocular hypertension.

DOSAGE: *Adults:* (Sol) Initial: 1 drop 0.25% bid. May increase to a max of 1 drop 0.5% bid. Maint: If adequate control, may attempt 1 drop 0.25-0.5% qd. (Sol, Gel Forming) Initial: 1 drop 0.25-0.5% qd. Max: 1 drop 0.5% qd. Dose other ophthalmic drugs 10 min prior to gel-forming drops.

HOW SUPPLIED: Sol: (Timoptic) 0.25%, 0.5% [5mL, 10mL]; Sol: (Timoptic Ocudose) 0.25%, 0.5% [0.2mL 60ˢ]; Sol, Gel Forming: (Timoptic-XE) 0.25%, 0.5% [5mL]

CONTRAINDICATIONS: Bronchial asthma, history of bronchial asthma, severe COPD, sinus bradycardia, 2nd- or 3rd-degree AV block, overt cardiac failure, cardiogenic shock.

WARNINGS/PRECAUTIONS: Severe cardiac and respiratory reactions reported. Caution with cardiac failure and cerebrovascular insufficiency; d/c if cardiac failure develops. May mask symptoms of hypoglycemia or hyperthyroidism; caution with DM or thyrotoxicosis. Avoid with COPD, bronchospastic disease. Not for use alone in angle-closure glaucoma. May potentiate muscle weakness. Withdrawal before surgery is controversial.

ADVERSE REACTIONS: Ocular: burning, stinging, blurred vision, pain, conjunctivitis, discharge, foreign body sensation, itching, tearing. Systemic: headache, dizziness, upper respiratory infections.

INTERACTIONS: May potentiate systemic/ophthalmic β-blockers and catecholamine-depleting drugs (eg, reserpine). Oral/IV calcium antagonists may cause AV conduction disturbances, left ventricular failure, or hypotension. Digitalis may cause additive effects in prolonging AV conduction time. Potentiated systemic β-blockade reported with concomitant CYP2D6 inhibitors. Quinidine may potentiate systemic β-blockade. May antagonize epinephrine. May exacerbate rebound hypertension following clonidine withdrawal. Give other ophthalmic drugs 10 min before use.

PREGNANCY: Category C, not for use in nursing.

MECHANISM OF ACTION: Nonselective β-blocker; reduces elevated and normal IOP.

PHARMACOKINETICS: Absorption: C_{max}=0.46ng/mL (morning dosing), 0.35ng/mL (afternoon dosing). **Distribution:** Found in breast milk.

NURSING CONSIDERATIONS

Assessment: Assess for history of asthma or COPD, sinus bradycardia, heart block, cardiac failure, DM, pregnancy/nursing status, undergoing major surgery, hyperthyroidism or thyrotoxicosis, cerebrovascular insufficiency, angle-closure glaucoma, myasthenia gravis or myasthenic syndrome, and possible drug interactions.

Monitoring: Monitor BP, HR, IOP, for signs/symptoms of anaphylaxis, increasing muscle weakness in susceptible patients, bronchospasm with severe

T

respiratory and cardiac reactions, thyroid storm, masked symptoms of acute hypoglycemia, psychiatric disturbances, and bacterial keratitis.

Patient Counseling: Instruct to avoid touching tip of container to eye or surrounding structures. Remove contact lenses prior to administration and reinsert 15 min following administration.

Administration: Ocular route. **Storage:** 15-30°C (59-86°F); avoid freezing/light. Keep out of reach of children.

TINDAMAX RX

tinidazole (Mission)

Avoid unnecessary use. Reserve only for indicated conditions. Although none reported, potential risk of carcinogenicity exists and has been observed in rats and mice treated chronically with metronidazole, a structurally related drug with similar biologic effects.

THERAPEUTIC CLASS: Antiprotozoal agent

INDICATIONS: Treatment of trichomoniasis caused by *Trichomonas vaginalis*, giardiasis caused by *Giardia duodenalis*, intestinal amebiasis and amebic liver abscess caused by *Entamoeba histolytica*, and bacterial vaginosis in non-pregnant women.

DOSAGE: *Adults:* Take with food. Trichomoniasis/Giardiasis: 2g single dose. Amebiasis: Intestinal: 2g qd for 3 days. Amebic Liver Abscess: 2g qd for 3-5 days. Hemodialysis: Give additional dose equivalent to one-half of recommended dose at the end of dialysis. For trichomoniasis, treat sexual partner with the same dose. Bacterial Vaginosis: 2g qd for 2 days or 1g qd for 5 days. *Pediatrics:* >3 yrs: Take with food. Giardiasis: 50mg/kg single dose. Amebiasis: Intestinal: 50mg/kg qd for 3 days. Amebic Liver Abscess: 50mg/kg qd for 3-5 days. Max (for all): 2g/day. May crush tabs in cherry syrup.

HOW SUPPLIED: Tab: 250mg*, 500mg* *scored

CONTRAINDICATIONS: Treatment during 1st trimester of pregnancy, nursing mothers during therapy and 3 days following last dose.

WARNINGS/PRECAUTIONS: Seizures, peripheral neuropathy reported. D/C if abnormal neurological signs occur. Caution with hepatic impairment, blood dyscrasias, or CNS diseases. May develop vaginal candidiasis. May develop drug resistance if prescribed in absence of proven or strongly suspected bacterial infection.

ADVERSE REACTIONS: Metallic/bitter taste, nausea, anorexia, flatulence, urinary tract infection, pelvic pain, vulvo-vaginal discomfort, vaginal odor, menorrhagia, upper respiratory infection, convulsions, peripheral neuropathy.

INTERACTIONS: Avoid alcohol during and for 3 days after use and within 2 weeks of disulfiram. May potentiate oral anticoagulants. May reduce clearance of phenytoin (IV), fluorouracil. May increase levels of lithium, cyclosporine, tacrolimus, fluorouracil. Separate dosing with cholestyramine. Phenobarbital, rifampin, phenytoin, other hepatic enzyme inducers may decrease levels. Cimetidine, ketoconazole, other hepatic enzyme inhibitors may increase levels. Antagonized by oxytetracycline.

PREGNANCY: Category C, not for use in nursing.

MECHANISM OF ACTION: Antiprotozoal; antibacterial agent; nitro group of tinidazole is reduced by cell extracts of *Trichomonas*. Free nitro radical generated as a result of this reduction may be responsible for antiprotozoal activity.

PHARMACOKINETICS: Absorption: Rapid, complete. (Fasted) C_{max}=47.7mcg/mL, T_{max}=1.6 hrs, AUC=901.6mcg/hr/mL. **Distribution:** V_d= 50L; plasma protein binding (12%); crosses blood-brain and placental barrier; found in breast milk. **Metabolism:** Mainly via oxidation, hydroxylation, conjugation; CYP3A4 mainly involved. **Elimination:** Urine (20-25% unchanged), feces (12%); $T_{1/2}$=12-14 hrs.

NURSING CONSIDERATIONS

Assessment: Assess for blood dyscrasias, seizures, pregnancy status, possible drug interactions. Document indications for therapy.

T

Monitoring: Monitor for convulsive seizures, peripheral neuropathy, vaginal candidiasis, drug resistance, hypersensitivity reactions (urticaria, erythema multiforme, Stevens-Johnson syndrome).

Patient Counseling: Advise to take with food to minimize epigastric discomfort and other GI side effects. Avoid alcohol and preps containing ethanol and propylene during therapy and for 3 days afterward to prevent abdominal cramps, NV, headache, and flushing. Counsel that therapy only treats bacterial, not viral, infections. Instruct to take as directed; skipping doses or not completing full course may decrease effectiveness and increase resistance.

Administration: Oral route. **Storage:** 20-25°C (68-77°F); excursions permitted to 15-30°C (59-86°F). Protect contents from light.

TNKase — RX

tenecteplase (Genentech)

THERAPEUTIC CLASS: Thrombolytic agent

INDICATIONS: To reduce mortality with AMI.

DOSAGE: *Adults:* Administer as single IV bolus over 5 seconds. <60kg: 30mg. ≥60 to <70kg: 35mg. ≥70 to <80kg: 40mg. ≥80 to <90kg: 45mg. ≥90kg: 50mg. Max: 50mg/dose.

HOW SUPPLIED: Inj: 50mg

CONTRAINDICATIONS: Active internal bleeding, history of CVA, intracranial or intraspinal surgery or trauma within 2 months, intracranial neoplasm, arteriovenous malformation, aneurysm, bleeding diathesis, severe uncontrolled HTN .

WARNINGS/PRECAUTIONS: Weigh benefits/risks with recent major surgery, cerebrovascular disease, recent GI or GU bleeding, recent trauma, HTN, left heart thrombus, acute pericarditis, subacute bacterial endocarditis, hemostatic defects, severe hepatic dysfunction, pregnancy, diabetic hemorrhagic retinopathy or other hemorrhagic ophthalmic conditions, septic thrombophlebitis or occluded AV cannula at a seriously infected site, elderly, any other bleeding condition that is difficult to manage. Cholesterol embolism and internal/superficial bleeding reported. Arrhythmias may occur with reperfusion. Avoid IM injection, noncompressible arterial puncture, and internal jugular or subclavian venous puncture. Caution with readministration.

ADVERSE REACTIONS: Bleeding.

INTERACTIONS: Increased risk of bleeding with heparin, vitamin K antagonists, and drugs that alter platelet function (eg, ASA, NSAIDs, dipyridamole, GP IIb/IIIa inhibitors) before or after therapy. Weigh benefits/risks with oral anticoagulants, GP IIb/IIIa inhibitors.

PREGNANCY: Category C, caution in nursing.

MECHANISM OF ACTION: Thrombolytic agent; modified form of human tissue plasminogen activator (tPA) that binds to fibrin and converts plasminogen to plasmin.

PHARMACOKINETICS: Metabolism: Liver. **Elimination:** $T_{1/2}$=90-130 min.

NURSING CONSIDERATIONS

Assessment: Assess for active internal bleeding, history of CVA, intracranial or intraspinal surgery or trauma within previous 2 months, intracranial neoplasm, arteriovenous malformation, aneurysm, known bleeding diathesis, acute pericarditis, subacute bacterial endocarditis, hemorrhagic ophthalmic conditions (eg, diabetic hemorrhagic retinopathy), severe uncontrolled HTN, hepatic function, pregnancy/nursing status, advanced age, and drug interactions.

Monitoring: Monitor for signs/symptoms of bleeding (internal or superficial), cholesterol embolization (eg, livedo reticularis, "purple toe syndrome," acute renal failure), arrhythmia, and hypersensitivity reactions (eg, anaphylaxis).

Patient Counseling: Counsel about increased risk of bleeding while on therapy. Contact physician if any type of unusual bleeding or hypersensitivity reactions develop. Inform that arterial and venous punctures should be minimized while on therapy. Avoid noncompressible arterial punctures and subclavian venous punctures. Instruct that if arterial puncture is necessary following the 1st few hours of therapy, it is preferable to use upper extremity vessel that is accessible to manual compression. Following arterial puncture, instruct to apply pressure for at least 30 min and check puncture site for evidence of bleeding. Instruct that if any serious bleeding occurs, concomitant heparin or antiplatelet agents should be discontinued immediately.

Administration: IV route. Reconstitute just prior to use. 1) Inject 10mL of SWFI into vial. 2) Do not shake; gently swirl until contents completely dissolved. 3) May be administered as reconstituted solution (5mg/mL). **Storage:** Lyophilized vial: Store at controlled room temperature not exceeding 30°C (86°F), or under refrigeration 2-8°C (36-46°F). Reconstituted: 2-8°C (36-46°F); use within 8 hrs.

TOBI

tobramycin (Chiron) **RX**

THERAPEUTIC CLASS: Aminoglycoside

INDICATIONS: Management of cystic fibrosis patients with *P.aeruginosa*.

DOSAGE: *Adults:* Inhale via nebulizer 300mg q12h for 28 days, then stop for 28 days. Resume therapy for next 28-day on/28-day off cycle.
Pediatrics: ≥6 yrs: Inhale via nebulizer 300mg q12h for 28 days, then stop for 28 days. Resume therapy for next 28-day on/28-day off cycle.

HOW SUPPLIED: Sol: 60mg/mL (300mg/amp)

WARNINGS/PRECAUTIONS: Caution with muscular disorders (eg, myasthenia gravis, Parkinson's disease), and renal, auditory, vestibular, or neuromuscular dysfunction. May cause hearing loss, bronchospasm. Can cause fetal harm in pregnancy. D/C if nephrotoxicity occurs until serum level <2mcg/mL.

ADVERSE REACTIONS: Voice alteration, taste perversion, tinnitus.

INTERACTIONS: Avoid neurotoxic or ototoxic drugs. Hearing loss reported with previous or concomitant systemic aminoglycosides. Avoid ethacrynic acid, furosemide, urea, and mannitol.

PREGNANCY: Category D, not for use in nursing.

MECHANISM OF ACTION: Aminoglycoside antibiotic; inhibits protein synthesis in bacterial cell.

PHARMACOKINETICS: Absorption: C_{max}=1237mcg/g (sputum), 0.95mcg/mL (serum). **Distribution**: Crosses placenta. **Elimination**: Glomerular filtration, sputum expectoration (unchanged); $T_{1/2}$=approximately 2 hrs (IV).

NURSING CONSIDERATIONS

Assessment: Assess and document bacterial infection using culture and susceptibility techniques. Assess renal function, CF, neuromuscular disorders, pregnancy status, and possible drug interactions.

Monitoring: Monitor for ototoxicity, neurotoxicity, nephrotoxicity, bronchospasm, hypersensitivity reactions.

Patient Counseling: Counsel pregnant patients of potential hazard to fetus. Advise to immediately report signs of hearing loss, dizziness, or any hearing changes. Instruct to thoroughly clean and disinfect nebulizer after each treatment to reduce risk of infection, illness, or injury from contamination.

Administration: Administered by inhalation. Refer to PI for administration and disinfecting techniques. **Storage**: Do not use beyond expiration date when refrigerated 2-8°C (36-46°F) or beyond 28 days when stored at room temperature 25°C (77°F). Do not expose to intense light.

TOBRADEX RX

tobramycin - dexamethasone (Alcon)

THERAPEUTIC CLASS: Aminoglycoside/corticosteroid

INDICATIONS: Ocular inflammation associated with infection or risk of infection.

DOSAGE: *Adults:* (Sus) 1-2 drops q4-6h. May increase to 1-2 drops q2h for first 24-48 hrs. (Oint) Apply 1/2 inch in conjunctival sac up to tid-qid. Max: 20mL or 8g for initial RX.
Pediatrics: ≥2 yrs: (Sus) 1-2 drops q4-6h. May increase to 1-2 drops q2h for first 24-48 hrs. (Oint) Apply 1/2 inch in conjunctival sac up to tid-qid. Max: 20mL or 8g for initial RX.

HOW SUPPLIED: Oint: (Tobramycin-Dexamethasone) 0.3-0.1% [3.5g]; Sus: 0.3-0.1% [2.5mL, 5mL, 10mL]

CONTRAINDICATIONS: Viral diseases of the cornea and conjunctiva including epithelial herpes simplex keratitis, vaccinia, and varicella. Mycobacterial infection and fungal diseases of the eye.

WARNINGS/PRECAUTIONS: Not for injection into the eye. Prolonged use may result in glaucoma, optic nerve damage, visual acuity and fields of vision defects, cataracts, secondary ocular infections (eg, fungal infections).

ADVERSE REACTIONS: Conjunctival erythema, hypersensitivity, lid itching and swelling, secondary infection.

PREGNANCY: Category C, caution in nursing.

MECHANISM OF ACTION: Tobramycin: Aminoglycoside antibiotic; inhibits synthesis of proteins in bacterial cells. Dexamethasone: Corticoid; suppresses inflammatory response and probably delays or slows healing.

NURSING CONSIDERATIONS

Assessment: Assess for dendritic keratitis, vaccinia, varicella, other viral diseases of cornea or conjunctiva, mycobacterial infection, fungal diseases of eye, and possible drug interactions.

Monitoring: Routinely monitor IOP. Monitor for signs/symptoms of hypersensitivity reactions, glaucoma, defects in visual acuity and fields of vision, posterior subcapsular cataracts, perforations, and superinfections.

Patient Counseling: Instruct not to touch dropper or tube tip to any surface to avoid contaminating contents and not to wear contact lenses during therapy. Advise to seek medical attention if symptoms of glaucoma, defects in vision, perforations, or superinfections occur.

Administration: Ocular route. Shake well before use. **Storage:** 8-27°C (46-80°F). Store upright.

T

TOBRAMYCIN RX

tobramycin sulfate (Various)

Potential ototoxicity, nephrotoxicity, and neurotoxicity. Monitor peak and trough serum levels to avoid toxicity. Avoid prolonged serum levels >12mcg/mL. Rising trough levels (>2mcg/mL) may indicate tissue accumulation. Tissue accumulation, excessive peak levels, advanced age, and cumulative dose may contribute to ototoxicity and nephrotoxicity. Monitor urine, BUN, SrCr, and CrCl periodically. Obtain serial audiograms. D/C or adjust dose with renal, vestibular, or auditory dysfunction. Caution in premature and neonatal infants, advanced age, and dehydration. Avoid other neurotoxic or nephrotoxic agents, particularly other aminoglycosides, cephaloridine, viomycin, polymyxin B, colistin, cisplatin, and vancomycin. Avoid potent diuretics (eg, ethacrynic acid, furosemide). Risk of fetal harm during pregnancy.

THERAPEUTIC CLASS: Aminoglycoside

INDICATIONS: Treatment of serious lower respiratory tract, CNS (eg, meningitis), intra-abdominal, bone, skin and skin structure, and complicated/recurrent urinary tract infections, and septicemia.

DOSAGE: *Adults:* IM/IV: Serious Infections: 3mg/kg/day given q8h. Life-Threatening Infections: Up to 5mg/kg/day given tid-qid. Reduce to 3mg/kg/day as soon as clinically indicated. Max: 5mg/kg/day unless serum levels monitored. Treat for 7-10 days; may need longer course in difficult and complicated infections. Severe Cystic Fibrosis: Initial: 10mg/kg/day given qid. Measure levels to determine subsequent doses. Renal Impairment: LD: 1mg/kg, followed by reduced doses given q8h or normal doses given at prolonged intervals based on either CrCl or SrCr. Do not use either method during dialysis. Obese Patients: Calculate dose based on estimated LBW plus 40% of excess as basic wt on which to figure mg/kg. ADD-Vantage vials not for IM use.
Pediatrics: >1 week: IM/IV: 6-7.5mg/kg/day given tid-qid (eg, 2-2.5mg/kg q8h or 1.5-1.89mg/kg q6h). ≤1 week: Up to 2mg/kg q12h. Treat for 7-10 days; may need longer course in difficult and complicated infections. Severe Cystic Fibrosis: Initial: 10mg/kg/day given qid. Measure levels to determine subsequent doses. Renal Impairment: LD: 1mg/kg, followed by reduced doses given q8h or normal doses given at prolonged intervals based on either CrCl or SrCr. Do not use either method during dialysis. Obese Patients: Calculate dose based on estimated LBW plus 40% of excess as basic wt on which to figure mg/kg. ADD-Vantage vials not for IM use.

HOW SUPPLIED: Inj: 10mg/mL, 40mg/mL, 1.2g

CONTRAINDICATIONS: History of serious toxic reactions to aminoglycosides.

WARNINGS/PRECAUTIONS: Increased risk of ototoxicity, nephrotoxicity, and neurotoxicity if treatment >10 days. Contains sodium bisulfite. D/C if allergic reaction occurs. Monitor serum calcium, magnesium, and sodium. For peak levels, measure about 30 min after IV infusion or 1 hr after IM injection. For trough levels, measure at 8 hrs or just before next dose. Prolonged or secondary apnea may occur with massive transfusions of citrated blood. Caution with muscular disorders (eg, myasthenia gravis, parkinsonism). Increased risk of neurotoxicity and nephrotoxicity after absorption from body surfaces with local irrigation or application. Not for intraocular and/or subconjunctival use. Overgrowth of nonsusceptible organisms may occur.

ADVERSE REACTIONS: Neurotoxicity (eg, dizziness, tinnitus, hearing loss, numbness, skin tingling, muscle twitching, convulsions), nephrotoxicity (eg, rising BUN/nonprotein nitrogen/serum creatinine, oliguria, cylindruria, increased proteinuria), blood dyscrasias, fever, rash, exfoliative dermatitis, urticaria, NV, diarrhea, headache, lethargy, injection-site pain, confusion, disorientation, increased serum transaminases.

INTERACTIONS: See Black Box Warning. Increased nephrotoxicity with cephalosporins. Do not premix with other drugs; administer separately. Possibility of prolonged or secondary apnea in anesthetized patients receiving neuromuscular blockers (eg, succinylcholine, tubocurarine, decamethonium).

PREGNANCY: Category D, safety not known in nursing.

MECHANISM OF ACTION: Aminoglycoside antibiotic; inhibits synthesis of proteins in bacterial cells.

PHARMACOKINETICS: Absorption: (IM) Rapidly absorbed; C_{max}=4mcg/mL; T_{max}=30-90 min. **Distribution:** Crosses placenta, distributed in body fluids. **Elimination**: Renal, biliary; $T_{1/2}$=2 hrs.

NURSING CONSIDERATIONS

Assessment: Assess and document bacterial infection using culture and susceptibility techniques. Assess renal function, CF, neuromuscular disorders, extensive burns, possible drug interactions, pregnancy status. Periodically evaluate serum calcium, magnesium, sodium, peak and trough serum levels of tobramycin.

Monitoring: Monitor for ototoxicity, neurotoxicity, nephrotoxicity, blood dyscraias, injection-site pain, hypersensitivity reactions, LFTs, superinfections.

Patient Counseling: Inform drug only treats bacterial, not viral, infections. Instruct to take as directed; skipping doses or not completing full course may decrease effectiveness and increase resistance. Inform may experience adverse effects (eg, tinnitus, vertigo, hearing loss, nephrotoxicity); advise to seek prompt medical attention.

Administration: IM/IV route. Dilute vials with 30mL SWFI. **Storage:** 15-30°C (59-86°F). After reconstitution, store in refrigerator and use within 96 hrs. Stored at room temperature, solution must be used within 24 hrs.

TOBREX RX
tobramycin (Alcon)

THERAPEUTIC CLASS: Aminoglycoside

INDICATIONS: External infections of the eye and its adnexa.

DOSAGE: *Adults:* Mild to Moderate Infection: Apply half-inch oint bid-tid or 1-2 drops q4h. Severe Infection: Apply half-inch oint q3-4h or 2 drops hourly until improvement, reduce frequency prior to discontinuation.

HOW SUPPLIED: Oint: 0.3% [3.5g]; Sol: 0.3% [5mL]

WARNINGS/PRECAUTIONS: Oint may retard corneal wound healing.

ADVERSE REACTIONS: Hypersensitivity, lid itching, swelling, conjunctival erythema, superinfection.

INTERACTIONS: Cross-sensitivity to other aminoglycoside antibiotics may occur.

PREGNANCY: Category B, not for use in nursing.

MECHANISM OF ACTION: Aminoglycoside antibiotic; inhibits synthesis of proteins in bacterial cells.

NURSING CONSIDERATIONS

Assessment: Assess for proper diagnosis of causative organisms. Assess use in pregnancy/nursing.

Monitoring: Monitor for sensitivity reactions while on therapy. With prolonged therapy, monitor for overgrowth of nonsusceptible organisms (eg, fungi) and for development of superinfection. Monitor total serum drug concentrations with concomitant systemic aminoglycoside antibiotics.

Patient Counseling: Advise not to wear contact lenses if signs/symptoms of ocular infections develop. Instruct to notify physician if any sensitivity reactions occur. To avoid contamination, avoid touching tube or dropper tip to any surface.

Administration: Ocular route. Do not inject into eye. **Storage:** 8-27°C (46-80°F).

TOFRANIL RX
imipramine HCl (Mallinckrodt)

T

Antidepressants increased the risk of suicidal thinking and behavior (suicidality) in short-term studies in children, adolescents, and young adults with major depressive disorder (MDD) and other psychiatric disorders. Imipramine HCl is not approved for use in pediatric patients except for patients with nocturnal enuresis.

THERAPEUTIC CLASS: Tricyclic antidepressant

INDICATIONS: Treatment of depression. Temporary adjunct in childhood enuresis in ≥6 yrs.

DOSAGE: *Adults:* Depression: Initial: (Inpatient) 100mg/day in divided doses. Titrate: Increase to 200mg/day; up to 250-300mg/day after 2 weeks if needed. (Outpatient) 75mg/day. Titrate: Increase to 150mg/day. Maint: 50-150mg/day. Max: 200mg/day. Elderly/Adolescents: Initial: 30-40mg/day. Max: 100mg/day.
Pediatrics: Depression: Adolescents: Initial: 30-40mg/day. Max: 100mg/day. Enuresis: ≥6 yrs: Initial: 25mg/day 1 hour before bedtime. Titrate: 6-12 yrs: If inadequate response in 1 week, increase to 50mg before bedtime. ≥12 yrs: Increase to 75mg before bedtime after 1 week if needed. Max: 2.5mg/kg/day.

HOW SUPPLIED: Tab: 10mg, 25mg, 50mg

CONTRAINDICATIONS: Within 14 days of MAOI therapy, or during acute recovery period following MI.

WARNINGS/PRECAUTIONS: Caution with elderly, serious depression, cardiovascular disease, hyperthyroidism, urinary retention, narrow-angle glaucoma, increased IOP, seizure disorders, renal and hepatic impairment. May activate psychosis in schizophrenia; reduce dose. Limit electroshock therapy. May alter blood glucose levels. Photosensitivity reported. D/C prior to elective surgery, or with hypomanic or manic episodes. D/C with pathological neutrophil depression.

ADVERSE REACTIONS: Orthostatic hypotension, HTN, confusion, hallucinations, numbness, tremors, dry mouth, urticaria, NV, diarrhea, gynecomastia (male), breast enlargement (female), galactorrhea.

INTERACTIONS: See Contraindications. Increased levels with methylphenidate, CYP2D6 inhibitors (eg, quinidine, cimetidine, SSRIs) and enzyme substrates (eg, phenothiazines, other antidepressants, propafenone, flecainide). Wait 5 weeks after discontinuing SSRIs before initiating TCAs. Decreased levels with enzyme inducers (eg, barbiturates, phenytoin). May block effects of clonidine, guanethidine. Additive effects with anticholinergics, CNS depressants, alcohol. Caution with drugs that lower BP and thyroid drugs. Paralytic ileus with anticholinergics. Avoid preparations that contain a sympathomimetic amine (eg, epinephrine, norepinephrine); may potentiate catecholamine effect.

PREGNANCY: Safety in pregnancy not known; not for use in nursing.

MECHANISM OF ACTION: Tricyclic antidepressant; mechanism unknown. Suspected to potentiate adrenergic synapses by blocking uptake of norepinephrine at nerve endings.

NURSING CONSIDERATIONS

Assessment: Assess renal/hepatic function, LFTs, ECG, IOP, major depressive disorder, and for seizures. Note other diseases/conditions and drug therapies.

Monitoring: Monitor for clinical worsening, suicidality, or unusual changes in behavior, seizures, increased restlessness, agitation, anxiety, insomnia, neuropsychiatric signs/symptoms (eg, delusions, hallucinations, psychosis, concentration disturbances, paranoia, confusion), ECG, CBC with differential and platelets, blood sugar levels.

Patient Counseling: Advise families and caregivers of need for close observation of clinical worsening and suicidal risks. Avoid alcohol, sedatives, OTC agents. Caution against operating machinery/driving. Report adverse reactions. Consult physician before taking any other medications. Avoid excessive exposure to sunlight.

Administration: Oral route. **Storage:** 20-25°C (68-77°F).

TOFRANIL-PM — RX

imipramine pamoate (Mallinckrodt)

T

Antidepressants increased the risk of suicidal thinking and behavior (suicidality) in short-term studies in children, adolescents, and young adults with major depressive disorder (MDD) and other psychiatric disorders. Imipramine pamoate is not approved for use in pediatric patients.

THERAPEUTIC CLASS: Tricyclic antidepressant

INDICATIONS: Treatment of depression.

DOSAGE: *Adults:* (Inpatient) Initial: 100-150mg/day. Titrate: May increase to 200mg/day. After 2 weeks may increase up to 250-300mg/day if needed. (Outpatient) Initial: 75mg/day. Titrate: May increase to 150mg/day. Max: 200mg/day. (Inpatient/Outpatient) Maint: Following remission, maintain at lowest possible dose. Usual: 75-150mg/day. Elderly/Adolescents: Initiate with Tofranil 25-50mg/day. Switch to Tofranil-PM with doses ≥75mg. Max: 100mg/day.

Pediatrics: Adolescents: Initiate with Tofranil 25-50mg/day. Switch to Tofranil-PM with doses ≥75mg. Max: 100mg/day.

HOW SUPPLIED: Cap: 75mg, 100mg, 125mg, 150mg

CONTRAINDICATIONS: Within 14 days of MAOI therapy or during acute recovery period following MI.

WARNINGS/PRECAUTIONS: Caution with elderly, serious depression, cardiovascular disease, hyperthyroidism, urinary retention, narrow-angle glaucoma, increased IOP, seizure disorders, renal and hepatic impairment. May activate psychosis in schizophrenia; reduce dose. Limit electroshock therapy. May alter blood glucose levels. Photosensitivity reported. D/C prior to elective surgery, or with hypomanic or manic episodes. D/C with pathological neutrophil depression.

ADVERSE REACTIONS: Orthostatic hypotension, HTN, confusion, hallucinations, numbness, tremors, dry mouth, urticaria, nausea, vomiting, diarrhea, gynecomastia (male), breast enlargement (female), galactorrhea.

INTERACTIONS: See Contraindications. Increased levels with methylphenidate, CYP2D6 inhibitors (eg, quinidine, cimetidine, SSRIs) and enzyme substrates (eg, phenothiazines, other antidepressants, propafenone, flecainide). Wait 5 weeks after discontinuing SSRIs before initiating TCAs. Decreased levels with enzyme inducers (eg, barbiturates, phenytoin). Blocks effects of clonidine, guanethidine. Additive effects with anticholinergics, CNS depressants, alcohol. Caution with drugs that lower BP and thyroid drugs. Paralytic ileus with anticholinergics. Avoid preparations that contain a sympathomimetic amine (eg, epinephrine, norepinephrine); may potentiate catecholamine effect.

PREGNANCY: Safety in pregnancy not known; not for use in nursing.

MECHANISM OF ACTION: Tricyclic antidepressant; mechanism unknown. Suspected to potentiate adrenergic synapses by blocking uptake of norepinephrine at nerve endings.

NURSING CONSIDERATIONS

Assessment: Assess renal function test, LFTs, ECG, IOP, seizures, major depressive disorder. Note other diseases/conditions and drug therapies.

Monitoring: Monitor for clinical worsening, suicidality, unusual changes in behavior, seizures, increased restlessness, agitation, anxiety, insomnia, neuropsychiatric signs/symptoms (delusions, hallucinations, psychosis, concentration disturbance, paranoia, confusion), ECG, CBC with differential and platelets, blood sugar levels.

Patient Counseling: Advise families and caregivers of need for close observation of clinical worsening and suicidal risks. Avoid alcohol, sedatives, OTC agents. Caution against operating machinery/driving. Report adverse reactions. Consult physician before taking any other medications. Avoid excessive exposure to sunlight.

Administration: Oral route. **Storage**: 20-25°C (68-77°F). Dispense in a tight container.

T

TOLMETIN — RX

tolmetin sodium (Various)

NSAIDs may cause an increased risk of serious cardiovascular thrombotic events, MI, stroke, and serious GI adverse events including bleeding, ulceration and perforation of the stomach or intestines. Contraindicated for the treatment of perioperative pain in the setting of coronary artery bypass graft (CABG) surgery.

THERAPEUTIC CLASS: NSAID

INDICATIONS: Treatment of acute flares and the long-term management of rheumatoid arthritis (RA) and osteoarthritis (OA). Treatment of juvenile rheumatoid arthritis (JRA).

DOSAGE: *Adults:* OA/RA: Initial: 400mg tid. Usual: 200-600mg tid. Max: 1800mg/day. Take with antacids other than sodium bicarbonate if GI upset occurs.

Pediatrics: JRA: ≥2 yrs: Initial: 20mg/kg/day given tid-qid. Usual: 15-

30mg/kg/day. Max: 30mg/kg/day. Take with antacids other than sodium bicarbonate if GI upset occurs.

HOW SUPPLIED: Cap: (DS) 400mg; Tab: 200mg*, 600mg *scored

CONTRAINDICATIONS: ASA or other NSAID allergy that precipitates asthma, rhinitis, urticaria, or allergic-type reactions. Treatment of perioperative pain in the setting of CABG surgery.

WARNINGS/PRECAUTIONS: May cause adverse ocular events. Prolongs bleeding time. Risk of renal toxicity with heart failure, liver dysfunction, and elderly. Caution with compromised cardiac function, HTN, or other conditions predisposing to fluid retention. Borderline LFT elevations may occur. Decreased bioavailability with milk or food. Can cause serious skin adverse reactions such as exfoliative dermatitis, SJS, and TEN, which can be fatal. Avoid with ASA-sensitive asthma and caution with preexisting asthma. Cannot be expected to substitute for corticosteroids or to treat corticosteroid insufficiency. Notable elevations of ALT or AST reported. Rare cases of severe hepatic reactions, including jaundice and fatal fulminant hepatitis, liver necrosis, and hepatic failure. Patients on long-term treatment should have Hgb or Hct checked if exhibit signs or symptoms of anemia.

ADVERSE REACTIONS: Dyspepsia, GI distress, diarrhea, flatulence, vomiting, headache, asthenia, elevated blood pressure, dizziness, edema, weight gain/loss.

INTERACTIONS: Increased PT and bleeding with warfarin. May enhance methotrexate toxicity. May diminish the antihypertensive effect of ACEIs. Concomitant administration with ASA not recommended; potential for increased adverse effects. Can reduce the natriuretic effect of furosemide and thiazides. Can produce elevation of plasma lithium levels and reduction in renal lithium clearance.

PREGNANCY: Category C, not for use in nursing.

MECHANISM OF ACTION: NSAID; not established, suspected to inhibit prostaglandin synthetase, lowers plasma level of PGE.

PHARMACOKINETICS: Absorption: Rapid; C_{max}=40mcg/mL (400 mg); T_{max}=30-60 min. **Elimination:** Urine; $T_{1/2}$=5 hrs.

NURSING CONSIDERATIONS

Assessment: Assess for NSAID or ASA allergy (ASA triad), HTN, risk factors for CV disease, history of ulcer disease or GI bleeding, fluid retention, CHF, possible drug interactions, pregnancy status, renal/hepatic impairment. Obtain baseline BP.

Monitoring: Monitor BP and renal function periodically. Monitor for signs/symptoms of CV events (eg, thrombosis, MI, stroke), HTN, fluid retention, edema, GI events (eg, ulceration, perforation, bleeding), skin reactions, visual disturbances, anemia, hypersensitivity reactions, renal/hepatic dysfunction.

Patient Counseling: Instruct to seek medical attention if experience symptoms of CV events (eg, chest pain, SOB, weakness, slurred speech), ulceration or bleeding (eg, epigastric pain, dyspepsia, melena, hematemesis), skin reactions (eg, rash, blisters, fever, itching), anaphylactoid reactions (eg, swelling, difficulty breathing), hepatotoxicity (eg, nausea, fatigue, pruritus, RUQ pain), weight gain, or edema. Inform of pregnancy risks.

Administration: Oral route. **Storage**: 15-30°C (59-86°F). Protect from light.

TOPAMAX — RX

topiramate (Ortho-McNeil)

OTHER BRAND NAMES: Topamax Sprinkle Capsules (Ortho-McNeil)

THERAPEUTIC CLASS: Sulfamate-substituted monosaccharide antiepileptic

INDICATIONS: Monotherapy in patients 10 yrs of age and older with partial onset or primary generalized tonic-clonic seizures. Adjunct therapy in patients 2-16 yrs of age and older with partial onset seizures, primary generalized tonic-clonic seizures, and seizures associated with Lennox-Gastaut syndrome. Migraine prophylaxis in adults.

DOSAGE: *Adults:* Seizures: Monotherapy: Initial: 25mg qam and qpm for 1 week. Titrate: Increase am and pm dose by 25mg every week until 200mg/day, then increase by 50mg every week until 400mg/day. Adjunct Therapy: ≥17 yrs: Initial: 25-50mg/day. Titrate: Increase by 25-50mg/week. Usual: Partial: 100-200mg bid. Tonic-Clonic: 200mg bid. Max: 1600mg/day. Migraine Prophylaxis: Titrate: Week 1: 25mg qpm. Week 2: 25mg bid. Week 3: 25mg qam and 50mg qpm. Week 4: 50mg bid. Usual: 50mg bid. Renal Dysfunction: 50% of usual dose. Swallow caps whole or sprinkle over food. *Pediatrics:* Seizures: Monotherapy: ≥10 yrs: Initial: 25mg qam and qpm for 1 week. Titrate: Increase am and pm dose by 25mg every week until 200mg/day, then increase by 50mg every week until 400mg/day. Adjunct Therapy: 2-16 yrs: Initial: 1-3mg/kg nightly for 1 week. Titrate: Increase by 1-3mg/kg/day every 1-2 weeks. Usual: 2.5-4.5mg/kg bid. Swallow caps whole or sprinkle over food.

HOW SUPPLIED: Cap, Sprinkle: 15mg, 25mg; Tab: 25mg, 50mg, 100mg, 200mg

WARNINGS/PRECAUTIONS: Hyperchloremic, nonanion gap, metabolic acidosis reported; obtain baseline and periodic serum bicarbonate levels. Withdraw gradually. Psychomotor slowing, difficulty with concentration, speech/language problems, paresthesia, acute myopia with secondary angle-closure glaucoma, oligohidrosis, hyperthermia, and dose-related depression or mood problems reported. May cause hyperammonemia and encephalopathy if used concomitantly with valproic acid. Risk of kidney stones; maintain adequate fluid intake. Caution with renal or hepatic dysfunction.

ADVERSE REACTIONS: Somnolence, fatigue, dizziness, ataxia, speech disorders, psychomotor slowing, abnormal vision, memory difficulty, paresthesia, diplopia, depression, anorexia, anxiety, mood problems, pancreatitis, hepatic failure.

INTERACTIONS: Phenytoin, carbamazepine, valproic acid decrease levels. Increases phenytoin, decreases valproic acid levels. May decrease AUC of digoxin. May potentiate CNS depression with alcohol, other CNS depressants. Increased risk of kidney stones with carbonic anhydrase inhibitors. May increase metformin levels; monitor diabetics regularly.

PREGNANCY: Category C, caution in nursing.

MECHANISM OF ACTION: Sulfamate-substituted monosaccharide; unknown mechanism. Suspected to block voltage-dependent Na^+ channels, augment activity of the neurotransmitter gamma-aminobutyrate at some subtypes of the GABA-A receptor, antagonizes the AMPA/kainate subtype of the glutamate receptor, and inhibits the carbonic anhydrase enzyme, particularly isoenzymes II and IV.

PHARMACOKINETICS: Absorption: Rapid; T_{max}=2 hrs. **Distribution:** Plasma protein binding (15-41%); found in breast milk. **Metabolism:** Metabolized via hydroxylation, hydrolysis, and glucuronidation. **Elimination:** Urine: (70% unchanged); $T_{1/2}$=21 hrs. For pediatric parameters refer to PI.

NURSING CONSIDERATIONS

Assessment: Assess for renal/hepatic impairment, glaucoma, diarrhea, depression/mood disorders, metabolic acidosis, osteoporosis, lung problems, pregnancy status, high-fat diet, growth problems, and possible drug interactions.

Monitoring: Monitor for signs/symptoms of acute myopia, secondary angle glaucoma (decreased visual acuity, ocular pain), oligohidrosis, hyperthermia (eg, decreased sweating, increased body temperature), cognitive or neuropsychiatric impairment (eg, psychomotor slowing, speech difficulty, somnolence), kidney stones, renal dysfunction, LFTs, parasthesias.

Patient Counseling: Inform to take with/without food. Instruct caregivers of pediatric/adolescent patients that medication may cause decreased sweating and increased body temperature. Advise to take proper precautions and maintain adequate hydration to prevent development of kidney stones. Avoid alcohol use, abrupt d/c, and operating machinery/driving when initiating therapy. Instruct to seek immediate medical attention if blurred vison, visual disturbances, or periorbital pain occur. Instruct to increase food intake if weight loss occurs. Inform females medication may decrease efficacy of oral contraceptives.

Administration: Oral route. Sprinkle caps may be swallowed whole or administered by carefully opening cap and sprinkling entire contents on small amount (teaspoonful) of food. The drug/food mixture should be swallowed, not chewed. **Storage:** Tab: 15-30°C (59-86°F). Protect form moisture. Cap, Sprinkle: Below 25°C (77°F). Protect from moisture.

TOPICORT — RX

desoximetasone (Taro)

OTHER BRAND NAMES: Topicort LP (Taro)

THERAPEUTIC CLASS: Corticosteroid

INDICATIONS: Corticosteroid-responsive dermatoses.

DOSAGE: *Adults:* Apply bid.
Pediatrics: (Cre, Gel) Apply bid. ≥10 yrs: (Oint) Apply bid.

HOW SUPPLIED: Cre: (LP) 0.05% [15g, 60g], 0.25% [15g, 60g, 100g]; Gel: 0.05% [15g, 60g]; Oint: 0.25% [15g, 60g]

WARNINGS/PRECAUTIONS: May produce reversible HPA axis suppression, manifestations of Cushing's syndrome, hyperglycemia, and glucosuria. Caution when applied to large surface areas or under occlusive dressings. Use appropriate antifungal or antibacterial agent with dermatological infections; d/c if infection does not clear or if irritation occurs. Peds may be more susceptible to systemic toxicity. Avoid eyes.

ADVERSE REACTIONS: Burning, itching, irritation, dryness, folliculitis, hypertrichosis, acneiform eruptions, hypopigmentation, perioral dermatitis, allergic contact dermatitis, skin maceration, secondary infection, skin atrophy, striae, miliaria.

PREGNANCY: Category C, caution in nursing.

MECHANISM OF ACTION: Corticosteroid; possesses anti-inflammatory, anti-pruritic, and vasoconstrictive properties. Anti-inflammatory activity not established.

PHARMACOKINETICS: Absorption: Percutaneous; occlusion, inflammation, and other disease states may increase absorption. **Metabolism:** Liver. **Excretion:** Urine (major), bile.

NURSING CONSIDERATIONS

Assessment: Assess pregnancy/nursing status.

Monitoring: Monitor for signs/symptoms of reversible HPA-axis suppression, Cushing's syndrome, hyperglycemia, glucosuria, skin irritation, and for dermatological infections (eg, bacterial, fungal). In patients on large doses or using occlusive dressings, monitor for HPA-axis suppression by using urinary free cortisol and ACTH stimulation tests. Following d/c, monitor for signs of steroid withdrawal. In pediatrics, monitor for signs/symptoms of systemic toxicity, HPA-axis suppression (eg, linear growth retardation, delayed weight gain), Cushing's syndrome, and intracranial HTN.

Patient Counseling: Instruct to use externally and exactly as directed; avoid contact with eyes. Report adverse reactions (eg, burning, itching, irritation). Do not bandage, cover, or wrap treated skin unless directed by physician. Advise caregivers of pediatric patients not to use tight-fitting diapers or plastic pants on treatment area.

Administration: Topical route. **Storage:** 15-30°C (59-86°F).

TOPROL-XL

RX

metoprolol succinate (AstraZeneca)

THERAPEUTIC CLASS: Selective $beta_1$-blocker

INDICATIONS: Treatment of hypertension, angina pectoris, and stable symptomatic (NYHA Class II or III) heart failure of ischemic, hypertensive, or cardiomyopathic origin.

DOSAGE: *Adults:* HTN: Initial: 25-100mg qd. Titrate: May increase weekly or at longer intervals. Max: 400mg/day. Angina: Initial: 100mg qd. Titrate: May increase weekly. Max: 400mg/day. Heart Failure: Initial: (NYHA Class II) 25mg qd for 2 weeks. Severe Heart Failure: 12.5mg qd for 2 weeks. Titrate: Double dose every 2 weeks as tolerated. Max: 200mg/day.
Pediatrics: ≥6 yrs: HTN: 1mg/kg qd. Max: 50mg/day. Dose adjust according to BP response. Doses above 2mg/kg have not been studied.

HOW SUPPLIED: Tab, Extended-Release: 25mg*, 50mg*, 100mg*, 200mg*
*scored

CONTRAINDICATIONS: Severe bradycardia, >1st-degree heart block, cardiogenic shock, sick sinus syndrome (unless a pacemaker is present), decompensated cardiac failure.

WARNINGS/PRECAUTIONS: Exacerbation of angina pectoris and MI reported following abrupt withdrawal; taper over 1-2 weeks. Caution with heart failure, bronchospastic disease, DM, hepatic dysfunction, hyperthyroidism, or peripheral vascular disease. May mask symptoms of hyperthyroidism and hypoglycemia. Withdrawal prior to surgery is controversial. Worsening cardiac failure may occur during up titration; lower dose or temporarily d/c.

ADVERSE REACTIONS: Bradycardia, SOB, fatigue, dizziness, depression, diarrhea, pruritus, rash, hepatitis, arthralgia.

INTERACTIONS: Additive effects with catecholamine-depleting drugs (eg, reserpine, MAOIs). CYP2D6 inhibitors (eg, quinidine, fluoxetine, paroxetine, propafenone) may increase levels. May exacerbate rebound hypertension following clonidine withdrawal. Caution when used with CCBs of the verapamil and diltiazem type. Concomitant use of digitalis glycosides and β-blockers can increase the risk of bradycardia.

PREGNANCY: Category C, caution with nursing.

MECHANISM OF ACTION: β_1-selective (cardioselective) adrenergic receptor blocking agent; slows sinus rate and decreases AV nodal conduction.

PHARMACOKINETICS: Absorption: Rapid and complete. **Distribution:** Plasma protein binding (12%); crosses blood-brain barrier. **Metabolism:** Metabolized via CYP2D6. **Elimination:** Liver; urine; $T_{1/2}$=3-7 hrs.

NURSING CONSIDERATIONS

Assessment: Assess for bradycardia, heart block, cardiogenic shock, cardiac failure, sick sinus syndrome (without pacemaker), ischemic heart disease, bronchospastic disease, DM, hyperthyroidism, PVD, arterial insufficiency, impaired hepatic function, pheochromocytoma, anaphylactic reactions, and possible drug interactions.

Monitoring: Monitor BP, ejection fraction, hepatic function, serum transaminase, alkaline phosphatase, LDH. Monitor for signs/symptoms of hypotension, MI, hypoglycemia, tachycardia, bronchospastic disease, DM, PVD.

Patient Counseling: Instruct not to interrupt or d/c therapy without consulting physician. Advise to take drug regularly and continuously, as directed, preferably with or immediately following meals. If dose is missed, take only next scheduled dose (without doubling). Avoid engaging in tasks requiring mental alertness (eg, operating machinery/driving). Contact physician if any difficulty in breathing occurs. Inform physician or dentist of any medication use before any type of surgery. Advise HF patients to consult physician if they experience signs/symptoms of worsening HF (eg, weight gain, increasing SOB). Exercise caution when administering to nursing women.

Administration: Oral route. Tabs are scored and may be divided. Whole or half-tab should be swallowed whole, not chewed or crushed. **Storage:** 25°C (77°F); excursions permitted to 15-30°C (59-86°F).

TORISEL
temsirolimus (Wyeth)

RX

THERAPEUTIC CLASS: Kinase inhibitor

INDICATIONS: Treatment of advanced renal cell carcinoma.

DOSAGE: *Adults:* 25mg infused over 30-60 min once a week. Hold if ANC <1,000/mm³, platelet count <75,000/mm³, or NCI CTCAE grade 3 or greater adverse reactions. Once toxicities resolve to grade 2 or less, restart with dose reduced by 5mg/week to a dose no lower than 15mg/week. Concomitant Strong CYP3A4 Inhibitors: Consider dose reduction to 12.5mg/week. If strong inhibitor is discontinued, allow wash out period of about 1 week before dose adjustment. Concomitant Strong CYP3A4 Inducers: Consider dose increase to 50mg/week. If strong inducer is discontinued, return to dose used prior to initiation of strong inducer.

HOW SUPPLIED: Inj: 25mg/mL

WARNINGS/PRECAUTIONS: Hypersensitivity reactions such as anaphylaxis, dyspnea, flushing, and chest pain have been observed. Give H_1 antihistamine before starting infusion. Hyperglycemia, glucose intolerance, and hyperlipemia may occur; monitor glucose and lipid profiles. Infections may result from immunosuppression. Monitor for interstitial lung disease (ILD); if ILD is suspected, d/c and consider use of corticosteroids and/or antibiotics. Bowel perforation may occur; monitor closely. Renal failure, sometimes fatal, reported; monitor renal function. May cause abnormal wound healing; caution during perioperative period. Caution with CNS tumors and/or anticoagulant therapy. Avoid live vaccines and close contact with those who have received live vaccines. Monitor CBC weekly and chemistry panel every 2 weeks. May cause fetal harm; avoid pregnancy during, and for 3 months after, therapy.

ADVERSE REACTIONS: Rash, asthenia, mucositis, nausea, edema, anorexia, anemia, hyperlipidemia, hyperglycemia, hypertriglyceridemia, lymphopenia, elevated alkaline phosphatase, AST, serum creatinine , leukopenia, hypophosphatemia, thrombocytopenia.

INTERACTIONS: Strong inducers of CYP3A4/5 (eg, dexamethasone, carbamazepine, phenytoin, phenobarbital, rifampacin) may decrease levels. Strong CYP3A4 inhibitors (eg, atazanavir, clarithromycin, indinavir, itraconazole, ketoconazole) may increase levels. If alternative treatment cannot be administered, dose adjustment should be considered. Concomitant use with sunitinib may result in dose-limiting toxicity.

PREGNANCY: Category D, not for use in nursing.

MECHANISM OF ACTION: Kinase inhibitor; binds to intracellular protein and protein-drug complex, inhibits mTOR activity that controls cell division, reduces levels of hypoxia-inducible factors HIF-1 and HIF-2 α, and vascular endothelial growth factor.

PHARMACOKINETICS: Absorption: C_{max}=585ng/mL, AUC=1627ng•h/mL. **Distribution:** V_d=172L. **Metabolism:** Liver CYP3A4; sirolimus (active metabolite). **Elimination:** Urine (4.6%), feces (78%); $T_{1/2}$(temsirolimus, sirolimus)=17.3, 54.6 hrs.

NURSING CONSIDERATIONS

Assessment: Assess renal function, serum glucose, serum cholesterol, CBC, pregnancy status. Note other diseases/conditions and drug therapies.

Monitoring: Monitor for hypersensitivity reactions, blood glucose levels, infections, interstitial lung disease, increased cholesterol levels, bowel perforation, renal failure, intracerebral bleeding, wound healing complications.

Patient Counseling: Counsel about adverse effects; report if any develop. Advise to use reliable contraception throughout treatment and continue

T

for 3 months after last dose. Inform to avoid use of live vaccines and close contact with those who receive live vaccines while on this drug.

Administration: IV route. Infuse over 30-60 min. **Storage:** 2-8°C (36-46°F). Protect from light.

Toviaz RX

fesoterodine fumarate (Pfizer)

THERAPEUTIC CLASS: Muscarinic antagonist

INDICATIONS: Treatment of overactive bladder with symptoms of urge urinary incontinence, urgency, and frequency.

DOSAGE: *Adults:* Usual: 4mg qd. Titrate: May increase to 8mg based on individual response and tolerability. Severe Renal Insufficiency (CrCl<30mL/min)/ Potent CYP3A4 Inhibitors: Should not exceed 4mg. Swallow whole; do not chew, divide, or crush.

HOW SUPPLIED: Tab, Extended Release: 4mg, 8mg

CONTRAINDICATIONS: Urinary retention, gastric retention, or uncontrolled narrow-angle glaucoma.

WARNINGS/PRECAUTIONS: Caution with bladder outlet obstruction, decreased GI motility, patients treated for narrow-angle glaucoma, and myasthenia gravis. Avoid in severe hepatic dysfunction.

ADVERSE REACTIONS: Dry mouth, constipation, urinary tract infection, and dry eyes.

INTERACTIONS: Combining with other antimuscarinic agents may increase the frequency and/or severity of dry mouth, constipation, urinary retention, and other anticholinergic pharmacologic effects (including gastrointestinal motility). Doses >4mg are not recommended with concomitant administration of potent CYP3A4 inhibitors (eg, ketoconazole, itraconazole, clarithromycin). Caution with dose titration when taking concomitant weak or moderate CYP3A4 inhibitors (eg, erythromycin).

PREGNANCY: Category C, not for use in nursing.

MECHANISM OF ACTION: Muscarinic antagonist; plays a role in contraction of urinary bladder smooth muscle and stimulation of salivary secretion.

PHARMACOKINETICS: Absorption: Absolute bioavailability (52%), T_{max}=5 hrs. **Distribution:** Plasma protein binding (50%). **Metabolism:** Liver (hydrolysis) via CYP2D6 and CYP3A4; carboxy-N-desisopropyl and N-desisopropyl metabolites. **Excretion:** Urine (70%), feces (7%); $T_{1/2}$=7 hrs. Refer to PI for pharmacokinetics parameters for extensive and poor CYP2D6 metabolizers.

NURSING CONSIDERATIONS

Assessment: Assess for history of urinary retention, gastric retention, uncontrolled narrow-angle glaucoma, myasthenia gravis, hepatic/renal impairment, pregnancy/nursing status, HR and possible drug interactions.

Monitoring: Monitor for dry mouth, constipation, urinary tract infection, blurred vision, and dry eyes and HR.

Patient Counseling: Instruct to swallow whole; do not chew, divide, or crush. Counsel about clinically significant adverse effects (eg, constipation and urinary retention). Heat prostration may occur when used in a hot environment. Avoid alcohol. Advise to read the patient leaflet before starting treatment.

Administration: Oral route. **Storage:** Store at 20-25°C (68-77°F); excursions permitted between 15-30°C (59-86°F). Protect from moisture.

TRACLEER RX

bosentan (Actelion)

Potential liver injury; monitor LFTs before therapy, then monthly. Contraindicated in pregnancy; obtain monthly pregnancy tests. May cause fetal harm. Prescribe through Tracleer Access Program.

THERAPEUTIC CLASS: Endothelin receptor antagonist

INDICATIONS: Treatment of pulmonary arterial hypertension in patients with WHO Class III or IV symptoms, to improve exercise ability and decrease rate of clinical worsening.

DOSAGE: *Adults:* Initial: 62.5mg bid. Titrate/Maint: Increase to 125mg bid after 4 weeks. Low Weight (<40kg): Initial/Maint: 62.5mg bid. Adjust if Develop LFT abnormality: >3 to ≤5x ULN: Reconfirm LFTs. Reduce dose or interrupt therapy. Monitor LFTs every 2 weeks. If LFTs return to pre-treatment levels, reintroduce or continue therapy. >5 to ≤8x ULN: Reconfirm LFTs. Stop treatment and monitor LFTs every 2 weeks. If LFTs return to pre-treatment values, may reintroduce therapy. >8x ULN: Stop treatment, do not reintroduce. *Pediatrics:* >12 yrs: <40kg: Initial/Maint: 62.5mg bid.

HOW SUPPLIED: Tab: 62.5mg, 125mg

CONTRAINDICATIONS: Concomitant use of cyclosporine A, glyburide, lopinavir/ritonavir or other ritonavir-containing HIV regimens, and pregnancy.

WARNINGS/PRECAUTIONS: May decrease Hgb and Hct; monitor 1 and 3 months after initiation, then every 3 months. Caution in elderly or mild hepatic impairment. Avoid with moderate to severe hepatic impairment, or LFTs >3x ULN. D/C gradually. Patients with severe chronic heart failure had an increased incidence of hospitalization for CHF associated with weight gain and increased leg edema during the first 4-8 weeks of treatment. Consider intervention with diuretic, fluid management, or hospitalization for decompensating heart failure. If signs of pulmonary edema occur, possibility of associated Pulmonary Veno-Occlusive Disease should be considered; d/c therapy. May decrease sperm count after 3 or 6 months of therapy.

ADVERSE REACTIONS: Headache, nasopharyngitis, flushing, hepatic dysfunction, lower limb edema, hypotension, palpitations, dyspepsia, edema, fatigue, pruritus, thrombocytopenia.

INTERACTIONS: See Contraindications. Concomitant use of hormonal contraceptives may decrease norethindrone and ethinyl estradiol levels. May reduce statin efficacy; monitor cholesterol levels. May decrease levels of drugs metabolized by CYP450 3A4 (eg, statins) and 2C9. CYP450 3A4 inhibitors (eg, ketoconazole) increase levels. Sildenafil may increase levels; and decrease sildenafil levels. Caution with tacrolimus. Rifampicin may increase through levels after the first concomitant dose, but 60% decrease at steady state.

PREGNANCY: Category X, not for use in nursing.

MECHANISM OF ACTION: Endothelin receptor antagonist; a neurohormone; binds to ET_A and ET_B receptors in the endothelium and vascular smooth muscle. Specific and competitive antagonist at endothelin receptor types with slightly higher affinity for ET_A receptors than ET_B receptors.

PHARMACOKINETICS: Absorption: Absolute bioavailabilty (50%); T_{max}=3-5 hrs. **Distribution:** V_d=18L; plasma protein binding (>98%). **Metabolism:** Liver via (CYP2C9, CYP3A4, and CYP2C19). **Elimination:** Biliary, urine (<3%); $T_{1/2}$=5 hrs.

NURSING CONSIDERATIONS

Assessment: Prior to therapy, perform serum aminotransferase levels/bilirubin and pregnancy test. Assess for chronic heart failure, hepatic impairment, drug hypersensitivity, pregnancy/nursing status, and possible drug interactions.

Monitoring: Monitor Hgb and Hct levels after 1 and 3 months of treatment, then every 3 months. Monitor for signs of fluid retention, CHF (eg, weight gain, increased leg edema), pulmonary edema, and pulmonary veno-occlusive disease. Perform monthly pregnancy tests for women of childbearing potential. Monitor liver enzymes and bilirubin monthly; alter treatment if elevated or d/c treatment if associated with liver injury symptoms (eg, NV, fever, jaundice, fever, abdominal pain, unusual fatigue).

Patient Counseling: Counsel that this medication is only prescribed through TRACLEER Access Program. Counsel about benefits/risks of therapy with importance of monthly lab monitoring and reporting any adverse reactions. Do not use during pregnancy; notify physician if pregnant/nursing or planning to become pregnant. Advise women to practice additional methods of contraception and not rely on hormonal contraception alone.

Administration: Oral route. **Storage:** 20-25°C (68-77°F); excursions permitted to 15-30°C (59-86°F).

TRANDATE — RX

labetalol HCl (Prometheus)

THERAPEUTIC CLASS: Nonselective beta-blocker/alpha$_1$ blocker

INDICATIONS: Management of hypertension.

DOSAGE: *Adults:* PO: Initial: 100mg bid. Titrate: May increase by 100mg bid every 2-3 days. Maint: 200-400mg bid. Severe HTN: 1200-2400mg/day given bid-tid. Titrate: Do not increase by more than 200mg bid. Elderly: Initial: 100mg bid. Titrate: May increase by 100mg bid. Maint: 100-200mg bid.

HOW SUPPLIED: Tab: 100mg*, 200mg*, 300mg* *scored

CONTRAINDICATIONS: Bronchial asthma, overt cardiac failure, greater than first degree heart block, cardiogenic shock, severe bradycardia, other conditions associated with hypotension, history of obstructive airway disease.

WARNINGS/PRECAUTIONS: Caution with hepatic dysfunction. Avoid abrupt withdrawal; may exacerbate ischemic heart disease. Caution with latent cardiac insufficiency, may exacerbate cardiac failure, reduce sinus HR, and slow AV conduction. Avoid in overt CHF. Avoid with bronchospastic disease. Paradoxical HTN in pheochromocytoma reported. D/C prior to surgery. Caution with DM; may mask symptoms of hypoglycemia.

ADVERSE REACTIONS: Dizziness, fatigue, NV, dyspepsia, paresthesia, nasal stuffiness, ejaculation failure, impotence, edema, dyspnea, headache, vertigo, postural hypotension, increased sweating.

INTERACTIONS: Increased tremor with TCAs. Antagonizes effects of β-agonists (bronchodilators). Potentiated by cimetidine; may need to reduce dose. Synergistic effects with halothane. Synergistic antihypertensive effects blunts the reflex tachycardia with nitroglycerin. Caution with calcium antagonists. May need to adjust dose of antidiabetic drugs.

PREGNANCY: Category C, caution in nursing.

MECHANISM OF ACTION: Selective α_1-adrenergic and nonselective β-adrenergic receptor blocking agent.

T

PHARMACOKINETICS: Absorption: Complete; T_{max}=1-2 hrs. **Distribution:** Plasma protein binding (50%); crosses placenta. **Metabolism:** Liver (conjugation, glucuronidation). **Elimination:** Feces, urine (55-60%); $T_{1/2}$=6-8 hrs.

NURSING CONSIDERATIONS

Assessment: Assess for bradycardia, heart block, cardiogenic shock, cardiac failure, ischemic heart disease, severe hypotension, bronchospastic disease, DM, pheochromocytoma, anaphylactic reactions, and possible drug interactions.

Monitoring: Monitor for cardiac failure, HTN, renal function, exacerbation of ischemia following abrupt withdrawal, bronchospastic disease, arrhythmias, hypersensitivity reactions, CBC with platelets and differential, anaphylactic reactions.

Patient Counseling: Instruct not to interrupt or d/c without consulting physician. Instruct to report signs/symptoms of cardiac failure or hepatic dysfunction (eg, pruritus, dark urine, persistent anorexia, jaundice, RUQ tenderness, or unexplained flu-like symptoms). Transient scalp itching may occur, usually when treatment initiated.

Administration: Oral route. **Storage:** 2-30°C (36-86°F); protect from moisture.

Transderm Scop — RX

scopolamine (Novartis Consumer)

THERAPEUTIC CLASS: Anticholinergic

INDICATIONS: Prevention of nausea and vomiting associated with motion sickness or recovery from anesthesia and surgery.

DOSAGE: *Adults:* Motion Sickness: Apply 1 patch 4 hrs before travel. Replace after 3 days. Post-OP N/V: Apply 1 patch the evening before surgery or 1 hr prior to cesarean section. Keep in place for 24 hrs. Apply patch to a hairless area behind the ear. Do not cut patch in half.

HOW SUPPLIED: Patch: 0.33mg/24 hrs [4[s]]

CONTRAINDICATIONS: Angle-closure (narrow angle) glaucoma, hypersensitivity to belladonna alkaloids.

WARNINGS/PRECAUTIONS: Monitor IOP with open-angle glaucoma. Not for use in children. Caution with pyloric obstruction, urinary bladder neck or intestinal obstruction, and in elderly. Increased CNS effects with liver or kidney dysfunction. May aggravate seizures or psychosis. Idiosyncratic reactions reported (rare). Remove patch before MRI.

ADVERSE REACTIONS: Dry mouth, drowsiness, blurred vision, dilation of pupils, dizziness, disorientation, confusion.

INTERACTIONS: Caution with anticholinergic drugs (eg, other belladonna alkaloids, antihistamines, TCAs, and muscle relaxants). Increased CNS effects with sedatives, tranquilizers, and alcohol. May decrease absorption of oral medications due to delayed gastric emptying or decreased gastric motility.

PREGNANCY: Category C, caution in nursing.

MECHANISM OF ACTION: Anticholinergic agent; acts as competitive inhibitor at postganglionic muscarinic receptor sites of parasympathetic nervous system and on smooth muscle that responds to acetylcholine but lacks cholinergic innervation. Acts in the CNS by blocking cholinergic transmission from vestibular nuclei to higher centers in the CNS and from reticular formation to the vomiting center.

PHARMACOKINETICS: Absorption: Well-absorbed; C_{max}=87pg/mL (free), 354pg/mL (total); T_{max}=24 hrs. **Distribution:** Crosses placenta and blood brain barrier; plasma protein binding (reversibly bound); found in breast milk. **Metabolism:** Extensively metabolized. **Elimination:** Urine (10%) parent and metabolite, (5%, unchanged); $T_{1/2}$=9.5 hrs.

NURSING CONSIDERATIONS

Assessment: Assess for angle-closure/chronic open-angle glaucoma, pyloric obstruction or urinary bladder neck obstruction, intestinal obstruction, hepatic/renal impairment, pregnancy/nursing status, seizures, psychosis, alcohol intake, and possible drug interactions.

Monitoring: Monitor for interference with gastric secretion test, IOP and glaucoma therapy in chronic open-angle glaucoma during patch use, acute toxic psychosis (eg, confusion, agitation, rambling speech, hallucinations, paranoid behaviors, delusions), drowsiness, and disorientation.

Patient Counseling: Caution against performing hazardous tasks (eg, operating machinery/driving). Wash hands thoroughly with soap and water immediately after handling patch; remove patch and consult physician if symptoms of acute-angle glaucoma or difficulty in urinating occur. Dispose properly and keep away from children or pets.

Administration: Transdermal route; apply on hairless area behind ear. Do not cut patch. **Storage:** 20-25°C (68-77°F).

TRANXENE-SD

CIV

clorazepate dipotassium (Ovation)

OTHER BRAND NAMES: Tranxene T-Tab (Ovation) - Tranxene-SD Half Strength (Ovation)

THERAPEUTIC CLASS: Benzodiazepine

INDICATIONS: Management of anxiety disorders. Adjunct therapy for partial seizures. Symptomatic relief of acute alcohol withdrawal.

DOSAGE: *Adults:* Anxiety: Initial: (Tab) 15mg qhs. Usual: 30mg/day in divided doses. Max: 60mg/day. Elderly/Debilitated: Initial: 7.5-15mg/day. (Tab, Extended-Release) 22.5mg q24h, (may substitute for 7.5mg tid) or 11.25mg q24h (may substitute for 3.75mg tid). Do not use Extended-Release for initial therapy. Alcohol Withdrawal: Day 1: (Tab) 30mg, then 30-60mg/day. Day 2: 45-90mg/day. Day 3: 22.5-45mg/day. Day 4: 15-30mg. Give in divided doses. Reduce dose and continue with 7.5-15mg/day; discontinue when stable. Max: 90mg/day. Antiepileptic Adjunct: Initial: (Tab) 7.5mg tid. Titrate: Increase by no more than 7.5mg/week. Max: 90mg/day.
Pediatrics: >9 yrs: Anxiety: Initial: (Tab) 15mg qhs. Usual: 30mg/day in divided doses. Max: 60mg/day. (Tab, Extended-Release) 22.5mg q24h, (may substitute for 7.5mg tid) or 11.25mg q24h (may substitute for 3.75mg tid). Do not use Extended-Release for initial therapy. >12 yrs: Antiepileptic Adjunct: Initial: (Tab) 7.5mg tid. Titrate: Increase by no more than 7.5mg/week. Max: 90mg/day. 9-12 yrs: Initial: 7.5mg bid. Titrate: Increase by no more than 7.5mg/week. Max: 60mg/day.

HOW SUPPLIED: Tab: (Tranxene T-Tab) 3.75mg*, 7.5mg*, 15mg*; Tab, Extended-Release: (Tranxene-SD) 22.5mg, (Tranxene-SD Half Strength) 11.25mg *scored

CONTRAINDICATIONS: Acute narrow-angle glaucoma.

WARNINGS/PRECAUTIONS: Avoid with depressive neuroses or psychotic reactions. Withdrawal symptoms with abrupt withdrawal; taper gradually. Caution with known drug dependency, renal/hepatic impairment. Suicidal tendencies reported; give lowest effective dose. Monitor LFTs and blood counts periodically with long-term therapy. Use lowest effective dose in elderly.

ADVERSE REACTIONS: Drowsiness, dizziness, GI complaints, nervousness, blurred vision, dry mouth, headache, mental confusion.

INTERACTIONS: Additive CNS depression with CNS depressants, alcohol. Potentiated by barbiturates, narcotics, phenothiazines, MAOIs, other antidepressants. Increased sedation with hypnotics.

PREGNANCY: Safety in pregnancy not known, not for use in nursing.

MECHANISM OF ACTION: Benzodiazepine; antianxiety/hypnotic agent which has CNS depressant effect.

PHARMACOKINETICS: Absorption: Orally absorbed; completely decarboxylated to nordiazepam. **Distribution:** Plasma protein binding (97-98%). **Metabolism:** Hydroxylation. **Elimination:** Urine (62-67%), feces (15-19%); $T_{1/2}$=40-50 hrs.

T

NURSING CONSIDERATIONS

Assessment: Assess for acute narrow-angle glaucoma, renal function tests, LFTs, depressive neurosis, psychotic reactions, pregnancy status. Note other diseases/conditions and drug therapies.

Monitoring: Monitor hypersensitivity reactions, renal function, LFTs, CBC, psychological dependence, suicidal ideations.

Patient Counseling: Avoid alcohol, sedatives. Caution against operating machinery/driving. Counsel about drug abuse/dependence. Report side effects.

Administration: Oral route. **Storage:** 25°C (77°F). Protect from moisture; keep bottle tightly closed. Dispense in light-resistant container.

TRASYLOL RX

aprotinin (Bayer Healthcare)

May cause fatal anaphylactic or anaphylactoid reactions; increased risk if re-exposed to aprotinin-containing products. Weigh benefit against risks in primary CABG surgery if second exposure to aprotinin is required. Administer only in operative settings where cardiopulmonary bypass can be rapidly initiated.

THERAPEUTIC CLASS: Broad-spectrum protease inhibitor

INDICATIONS: Prophylactic use to reduce perioperative blood loss and the need for blood transfusion in patients undergoing cardiopulmonary bypass in the course of coronary artery bypass graft (CABG) surgery who are at an increased risk for blood loss and blood transfusion.

DOSAGE: *Adults:* IV: Administer through central line. Do not administer other drugs in same line. Test Dose: 1mL 10 min before LD. Regimen A: LD: 200mL IV over 20-30 min. Pump Prime Dose: Add 200mL to recirculating priming fluid. Constant Infusion Dose: 50mL/hr. Regimen B: Give 1/2 doses of Regimen A.

HOW SUPPLIED: Inj: 10,000 KIU/mL

CONTRAINDICATIONS: Exposure to aprotinin within previous 12 months. Obtain full patient medical history as aprotinin may be a component in fibrant sealant products.

WARNINGS/PRECAUTIONS: D/C if hypersensitivity reactions occur. Take precautions with re-exposure to aprotinin: have emergency anaphylactic treatment available; give test dose and LD only when conditions for rapid cannulation present; delay aprotinin addition into pump prime solution until after LD safely given. Consider giving H_1 and H_2 blockers 15 minutes before test dose. Greater risk of hypersensitivity to aprotinin if history of allergic reactions to other agents. Administer test dose 10 minutes before LD. Administer LD in supine position over 20-30 minutes. Rapid IV administration may cause hypotension. May increase risk of renal dysfunction and possibly cause an increased need for dialysis in the perioperative period.

ADVERSE REACTIONS: Fever, infection, arrhythmia, hypotension, MI, CHF, pericarditis, peripheral edema, GI effects, confusion, insomnia, lung disorder, pleural effusion, atelectasis, dyspnea, pneumothorax, nausea, abnormal LFTs and renal function, urinary retention.

INTERACTIONS: May inhibit effects of fibrinolytic agents. May block acute hypotensive effect of captopril. Concomitant heparin may prolong activated clotting time. Caution with drugs that affect renal function (eg, aminoglycosides).

PREGNANCY: Category B, safety in nursing not known.

MECHANISM OF ACTION: Broad-spectrum protease inhibitor; modulates systemic inflammatory response (SIR) associated with cardiopulmonary bypass surgery, resulting in decreased need for blood transfusion, reduced bleeding, and decreased mediastinal re-exploration for bleeding. Inhibits multiple mediators (kallikrein, plasmin), pro-inflammatory cytokine release, and maintains glycoprotein homeostasis.

PHARMACOKINETICS: Elimination: Urine (25-40%, 2% unchanged).

NURSING CONSIDERATIONS

Assessment: Assess for possible allergic reaction, history of previous (past year) exposure to drug, potential benefits/risks in those who have experienced allergic reaction after previous administration, history of renal impairment and/or drugs that may alter renal function, and possible drug interactions (eg, heparin). Perform heparin titration-protamine titration prior to administration to determine heparin LD.

Monitoring: Monitor for signs of fatal hypersensitivity reactions (eg, hypotension, anaphylactic shock with circulatory failure). During surgery, monitor for deep hypothermic circulatory arrest, anticoagulation test. Regular monitoring of SrCr, glucose, LDH, alkaline phosphatase, AST, PTT, celite ACT, and CPK-MB.

Patient Counseling: Inform about the benefits/risks of therapy and the need to report adverse reactions.

Administration: IV route. **Storage:** 2-25°C (36-77°F). Avoid freezing.

TRAVATAN RX
travoprost (Alcon)

OTHER BRAND NAMES: Travatan Z (Alcon)

THERAPEUTIC CLASS: Prostaglandin analog

INDICATIONS: Reduction of elevated IOP in open-angle glaucoma and ocular hypertension if intolerant to or unresponsive to other IOP therapies.

DOSAGE: *Adults:* 1 drop in affected eye(s) qd in pm. Max: Once daily dosing.

HOW SUPPLIED: Sol: (Travatan) 0.004% [2.5mL]; (Travatan Z) 0.004% [2.5mL, 5mL]

WARNINGS/PRECAUTIONS: Contains benzalkonium chloride; remove contact lenses prior to administration, may reinsert after 15 min (Travatan). Avoid with active intraocular inflammation. Caution with history of intraocular inflammation (eg, iritis/uveitis), aphakia, pseudophakia with torn posterior lens capsule, risk of macular edema. Increased ocular pigmentation (iris, eyelid, eyelashes) reported; may be permanent. Other eyelash changes reported. Not for the treatment of angle-closure, inflammatory, or neovascular glaucoma.

ADVERSE REACTIONS: Ocular hyperemia/pruritus/discomfort, foreign body sensation, decreased visual acuity, blepharitis, blurred vision, cataract, dry eye, photophobia, tearing.

INTERACTIONS: Space dosing of other ophthalmics by 5 min.

PREGNANCY: Category C, caution in nursing.

MECHANISM OF ACTION: Selective FP prostanoid receptor agonist; believed to reduce IOP by increasing outflow of aqueous humor.

PHARMACOKINETICS: Absorption: C_{max}=0.018ng/mL; T_{max}=30 min. **Metabolism:** Cornea, via esterases to active free acid and systemically to inactive metabolites via β-oxidation and reduction. **Elimination:** Urine (2%); $T_{1/2}$=45 min.

NURSING CONSIDERATIONS

Assessment: Assess for intraocular inflammation (iritis/uveitis), active macular edema, aphakic/pseudophakic patient with torn posterior lens capsules, angle-closure, inflammatory, or neovascular glaucoma, pregnancy/nursing status, and possible drug interactions.

Monitoring: Monitor for increased brown pigmentation of the iris, periorbital tissue, and eyelid tissue; changes in eyelashes (eg, increased length, thickness, or growth; brown pigmentation; change in number of lashes; or misdirected growth of lashes); macular edema (cystoid macular edema); and bacterial keratitis.

T

Patient Counseling: Inform about risk of brown pigmentation of iris, which may be permanent, and about darkening of eyelid skin. Instruct to avoid touching tip of applicator to eye or surrounding areas. Advise to remove contact lenses prior to administration; reinsert 15 min after administration. Administer at least 5 min apart if using >1 topical ophthalmic drug. Consult physician if having ocular surgery, if intercurrent ocular condition (eg, trauma or infection) develops, or if ocular reaction occurs.

Administration: Ocular route. **Storage:** 2-25°C (36-77°F).

TRAZODONE RX

trazodone HCl (Various)

Antidepressants increased the risk of suicidal thinking and behavior (suicidality) in short-term studies in children and adolescents with major depressive disorder (MDD) and other psychiatric disorders. Trazodone is not approved for use in pediatric patients.

THERAPEUTIC CLASS: Triazolopyridine derivative

INDICATIONS: Treatment of depression.

DOSAGE: *Adults:* Initial: 150mg/day in divided doses pc. Titrate: May increase by 50mg/day every 3-4 days. Max: (Outpatient) 400mg/day, (Inpatient) 600mg/day.

HOW SUPPLIED: Tab: 50mg*, 100mg*, 150mg*, 300mg* *scored

WARNINGS/PRECAUTIONS: Avoid during initial recovery phase of MI. Caution in cardiac disease. D/C prior to elective surgery.

ADVERSE REACTIONS: Dry mouth, edema, constipation, blurred vision, fatigue, nervousness, drowsiness, dizziness, headache, insomnia, NV, musculoskeletal pain, hypotension, confusion, priapism.

INTERACTIONS: Potent CYP3A4 inhibitors (eg, ritonavir, ketoconazole, indinavir, itraconazole, nefazodone) may increase levels. Carbamazepine decreases levels. Increases digoxin and phenytoin serum levels. Caution with antihypertensives and MAOIs. May enhance response to alcohol, barbiturates and other CNS depressants. May affect PT in patients on warfarin.

PREGNANCY: Category C, caution in nursing.

MECHANISM OF ACTION: Triazolopyridine derivative; suspected to inhibit serotonin uptake by brain synaptosomes and potentiate behavioral changes.

PHARMACOKINETICS: Absorption: Well absorbed; T_{max}=1 hr. **Metabolism:** Metabolized to m-chlorophenylpiperazine (active metabolite) by CYP3A4 enzyme.

NURSING CONSIDERATIONS

Assessment: Assess for seizures, MDD, bipolar disorder, cardiac arrhythmias, MI. Note other diseases/conditions and drug therapies.

Monitoring: Monitor for worsening of depression and/or emergence of suicidal ideation or unusual changes in behavior. Monitor for priapism, erectile dysfunction, cardiac arrhythmias, BP.

Patient Counseling: Advise families and caregivers of need for close observation of clinical worsening and suicidal risks. Avoid alcohol, sedatives, OTC agents. Caution against operating machinery/driving. Report adverse reactions. Consult physician before taking any other medications. Males with prolonged or inappropriate erections should d/c drug and contact physician.

Administration: Oral route. **Storage:** Store at 20-25°C (68-77°F).

TRECATOR RX

ethionamide (Wyeth)

THERAPEUTIC CLASS: Peptide synthesis inhibitor

INDICATIONS: Treatment of active TB in patients with *M.tuberculosis* resistant to isoniazid or rifampin, or where there is intolerance to other drugs.

DOSAGE: *Adults:* 15-20mg/kg qd with food. May give in divided doses with poor GI tolerance. Max: 1g/day. Alternate Regimen: Initial: 250mg qd then titrate gradually to optimal doses as tolerated, or 250mg qd for 1-2 days, then 250mg bid for 1-2 days, then 1g/day in 3-4 divided doses. Continue therapy until bacteriological conversion has become permanent and maximal clinical improvement occurs.

Pediatrics: ≥12 yrs: 10-20 mg/kg/day in divided doses given bid or tid with food, or 15mg/kg/day as single dose. Continue therapy until bacteriological conversion has become permanent and maximal clinical improvement occurs.

HOW SUPPLIED: Tab: 250mg

CONTRAINDICATIONS: Severe hepatic impairment.

WARNINGS/PRECAUTIONS: Rapid development of resistance if used alone; should be used with at least 1 or 2 other drugs. Perform ophthalmologic exams before and periodically during therapy. Measure serum transaminases prior to initiation and monthly thereafter. Risk of hypoglycemia in diabetics; monitor blood glucose prior to initiation then periodically. Hypothyroidism reported; monitor TFTs.

ADVERSE REACTIONS: NV, diarrhea, abdominal pain, excessive salivation, metallic taste, stomatitis, anorexia, psychotic disturbances, drowsiness, dizziness, hypersensitivity reactions, increase in serum bilirubin, SGOT or SGPT.

INTERACTIONS: Discontinue all antituberculous medication with elevated serum transaminases until resolved; reintroduce sequentially to determine which drug is responsible. May raise isoniazid levels. May potentiate adverse effects of other antituberculous drugs. Convulsions reported with cycloserine. Risk of psychotic reactions with excessive ethanol ingestion. Give with pyridoxine.

PREGNANCY: Category C, not for use in nursing.

MECHANISM OF ACTION: Peptide synthesis inhibitor; may be bacteriostatic or bactericidal in action.

PHARMACOKINETICS: Absorption: Completely absorbed; C_{max}=2.16mcg/mL, T_{max}=1.02 hrs, AUC=7.67mcg•hr/mL. **Distribution:** V_d=93.5L; plasma protein binding (30%); widely distributed into body tissues. **Metabolism:** Liver (extensive). **Elimination:** Urine ≤1%; $T_{1/2}$=1.92 hrs.

NURSING CONSIDERATIONS

Assessment: Assess for severe hepatic impairment, DM, susceptibility test, and possible drug interactions.

Monitoring: Monitor for hypersensitivity reactions (eg, rash, photosensitivity), GI (eg, N/V, diarrhea) and psychotic disturbances (eg, mental depression). Determination of serum transaminases (SGOT, SGPT), blood glucose, thyroid function, and eye exams should be done periodically.

Patient Counseling: Advise to report vision loss or blurriness, with/without eye pain. Instruct to avoid excessive ethanol ingestion to avoid psychotic reaction. Take as directed; skipping doses or not completing full course may decrease effectiveness and increase resistance.

Administration: Oral route. **Storage:** 20-25°C (68-77°F). Dispense in tight container.

TRELSTAR RX

triptorelin pamoate (Watson)

OTHER BRAND NAMES: Trelstar LA (Watson) - Trelstar Depot (Watson)

THERAPEUTIC CLASS: Luteinizing hormone-releasing hormone agonist

INDICATIONS: Palliative treatment of advanced prostate cancer.

DOSAGE: *Adults:* (Depot) 3.75mg IM every month or (LA) 11.25mg IM every 84 days.

HOW SUPPLIED: Inj: (Depot) 3.75mg, (LA) 11.25mg

CONTRAINDICATIONS: Pregnancy.

WARNINGS/PRECAUTIONS: Anaphylactic shock, angioedema, urethral obstruction, spinal cord compression, renal impairment reported. May worsen symptoms during 1st few weeks of treatment. Closely monitor patients with metastatic vertebral lesions and/or urinary tract obstruction during 1st few weeks of therapy. Monitor serum testosterone levels, PSA.

ADVERSE REACTIONS: Hot flushes, HTN, headache, skeletal pain, dysuria, leg edema, pain, impotence.

INTERACTIONS: Avoid hyperprolactinemic drugs.

PREGNANCY: Category X, not for use in nursing.

MECHANISM OF ACTION: Luteinizing hormone-releasing hormone agonist; potent inhibitor of gonadotropin secretion.

PHARMACOKINETICS: Absorption: (IM) C_{max}=28.43, T_{max}=1 hr. **Distribution**: V_d=30-33L. **Elimination**: Liver and kidneys; $T_{1/2}$=3 hrs.

NURSING CONSIDERATIONS

Assessment: Assess serum testosterone levels, PSA levels, metastatic vertebral lesions, urinary tract obstruction, pregnancy status.

Monitoring: Monitor serum levels of testosterone and PSA. Monitor for new onset of symptoms, bone pain, neuropathy, hematuria, spinal cord compression, pituitary apoplexy, hypersensitivity reactions.

Patient Counseling: Counsel about side effects; report if any occur. Counsel about potential hazards to fetus if drug used during pregnancy or if pregnancy occurs during therapy.

Administration: IM route. Reconstitute with SWFI. Discard if not used immediately after reconstitution. **Storage**: 20-25°C (68-77°F); excursions permitted to 15-30°C (59-86°F).

TRENTAL RX

pentoxifylline (Sanofi-Aventis)

THERAPEUTIC CLASS: Blood viscosity reducer

INDICATIONS: Treatment of intermittent claudication due to chronic occlusive arterial disease of the limbs.

DOSAGE: *Adults:* 400mg tid with meals for at least 8 weeks. Reduce to 400mg bid if digestive and CNS side effects occur; discontinue if side effects persist.

HOW SUPPLIED: Tab, Extended-Release: 400mg

CONTRAINDICATIONS: Recent cerebral and/or retinal hemorrhage, intolerance to methylxanthines (eg, caffeine, theophylline, theobromine).

WARNINGS/PRECAUTIONS: Monitor Hgb and Hct with risk factors complicated by hemorrhage (eg, recent surgery, peptic ulceration, cerebral/retinal bleeding). Occasional reports of angina, hypotension, and arrhythmia in patients with concurrent coronary artery and cerebrovascular diseases.

ADVERSE REACTIONS: Bloating, dyspepsia, NV, dizziness, headache.

INTERACTIONS: Increase risk of bleeding with warfarin; monitor PT/INR more frequently. May increase in theophylline levels; risk of theophylline toxicity. May increase effect of antihypertensives.

PREGNANCY: Category C, not for use in nursing.

MECHANISM OF ACTION: Blood viscosity reducer; not established. Increases blood flow to affected microcirculation and enhances tissue oxygenation. Improves erythrocyte flexibility, increases leukocyte deformability, and inhibits neutrophil adhesion and activation.

PHARMACOKINETICS: Absorption: T_{max}=1 hr. **Distribution:** Found in breast milk. **Metabolism:** 1st pass; metabolites (major): Metabolite 1(1-[5-hydroxyhexyl]-3,7-dimethylxanthine); metabolite V (1-[3-carboxypropyl]-3,7-dimethylxanthine). **Elimination:** Urine (major), feces (<4%); $T_{1/2}$=0.4-0.8 hrs; $T_{1/2}$=0.4-0.8 hrs (metabolites).

NURSING CONSIDERATIONS

Assessment: Assess for recent cerebral and/or retinal hemorrhage, hypersensitivity to methylxanthines (eg, caffeine, theophylline, theobromine), nursing/pregnancy status, renal function, and drug interactions.

Monitoring: In presence of concurrent coronary artery disease and cerebrovascular disease, monitor for signs/symptoms of angina, arrhythmia, and hypotension. If on concomitant warfarin therapy, perform more frequent monitoring of prothrombin time. If risk for bleeding (eg, recent surgery, peptic ulceration, recent cerebral and/or retinal bleeding), periodically monitor Hgb and/or Hct. Perform periodic monitoring of renal function elderly (≥65 yrs).

Patient Counseling: Inform to take with meals. Instruct to report if any digestive (eg, dyspepsia, nausea) or CNS (eg, headaches) side effects develop; dose adjustment may be needed. Instruct to report any signs/symptoms of angina or hypotension.

Administration: Oral administration. **Storage**: 15-30°C (59-86°F). Dispense in well-closed, light-resistant container. Protect blisters from light.

TRIAZ — RX

benzoyl peroxide (Medicis)

THERAPEUTIC CLASS: Antibacterial/keratolytic

INDICATIONS: Topical treatment of acne vulgaris.

DOSAGE: *Adults:* (Cleanser) Wash for 10-20 seconds qd-bid. (Gel) Apply qd-bid after washing with cleanser.

HOW SUPPLIED: Gel: 3%, 6%, 9% [42.5g]; Cleanser: 3%, 6%, 9% [170.3g, 340.2g]; Pads: 3%, 6%, 9% [30^s]

WARNINGS/PRECAUTIONS: External use only. Avoid contact with eyes, lips, and mucous membranes. Avoid sun exposure and use sunscreen. D/C if severe irritation develops.

ADVERSE REACTIONS: Dryness, contact dermatitis.

PREGNANCY: Category C, caution in nursing.

MECHANISM OF ACTION: Antibacterial/keratolytic; not established. Produces antibacterial activity against *Propionibacterium acnes*. Also found to reduce lipids and free fatty acids, and produce mild desquamation (drying and peeling activity) with simultaneous reduction in comedones and acne lesions.

PHARMACOKINETICS: Absorption: Percutaneous. **Metabolism:** Metabolized to benzoic acid. **Elimination:** Urine (benzoate).

NURSING CONSIDERATIONS

Assessment: Assess use in pregnancy/nursing.

Monitoring: Monitor for signs/symptoms of severe skin irritation and for allergic contact dermatitis.

Patient Counseling: Instruct to avoid contact with eyes, eyelids, lips, and mucous membranes. If accidental contact occurs, rinse area with water. Contact with hair or fabric may result in bleaching and discoloration. If excessive irritation develops, d/c and consult physician. Avoid unnecessary sun exposure; use sunscreen.

Administration: Topical route. For external use only. **Storage:** 15-25°C (59-77°F).

TRICOR — RX

fenofibrate (Abbott)

THERAPEUTIC CLASS: Fibric acid derivative

INDICATIONS: Adjunct to diet, for treatment of hypertriglyceridemia (Types IV and V) and to reduce elevated Total-C, LDL-C, Apo B, TG, and to increase HDL-C in primary hypercholesterolemia or mixed dyslipidemia (Types IIa and IIb).

DOSAGE: *Adults:* Hypercholesterolemia/Mixed Dyslipidemia: Initial: 145mg qd. Hypertriglyceridemia: Initial: 48-145mg/day. Titrate: Adjust if needed after repeat lipid levels at 4-8 week intervals. Max: 145mg/day. Renal Dysfunction/Elderly: Initial: 48mg/day. Take without regard to meals.

HOW SUPPLIED: Tab: 48mg, 145mg

CONTRAINDICATIONS: Pre-existing gallbladder disease, unexplained persistent hepatic function abnormality, hepatic or severe renal dysfunction (including primary biliary cirrhosis).

WARNINGS/PRECAUTIONS: Monitor LFTs regularly; d/c if >3x ULN. May cause cholelithiasis; d/c if gallstones found. D/C if myopathy or marked CPK elevation occurs. Decreased Hgb, Hct, WBCs, thrombocytopenia, and agranulocytosis reported; monitor CBC during first 12 months of therapy. Acute hypersensitivity reactions (rare) and pancreatitis reported. Monitor lipids periodically initially, d/c if inadequate response after 2 months on 145mg/day. Minimize dose in severe renal impairment. Caution in elderly.

ADVERSE REACTIONS: Abdominal pain, back pain, headache, abnormal LFTs, respiratory disorder, increased creatinine phosphokinase.

INTERACTIONS: Potentiates coumarin anticoagulants; reduce anticoagulant dose and monitor PT/INR. Avoid HMG-CoA reductase inhibitors unless benefits outweigh risks. Bile acid sequestrants may impede absorption; take at least 1 hr before or 4-6 hrs after the resin. Evaluate benefits/risks with immunosuppressants (eg, cyclosporine) and other nephrotoxic agents.

PREGNANCY: Category C, not for use in nursing.

MECHANISM OF ACTION: Fibric acid derivative; activates peroxisome proliferator-activated receptor α (PPARα), increasing lipolysis and elimination of triglyceride-rich particles from plasma by activating lipoprotein lipase and reducing production of apoprotein C-III (lipoprotein lipase inhibitor). The resulting fall in triglycerides produces an alteration in size and composition of LDL particles, from small dense particles to large buoyant particles, which have greater affinity for cholesterol receptors and are catabolized rapidly. Activation of PPARα also induces an increase in synthesis of apoproteins A-I, A-II, and HDL-cholesterol.

PHARMACOKINETICS: Absorption: Well absorbed; T_{max}=6-8 hrs. **Distribution:** Plasma protein binding (99%). **Metabolism:** Hydrolysis, conjugation; fenofibric acid (active metabolite). **Elimination:** Urine (60%), feces (25%); $T_{1/2}$=20 hrs.

NURSING CONSIDERATIONS

Assessment: Assess for hepatic/renal dysfunction, pre-existing gallbladder disease, pregnancy/nursing status, and drug interactions. Obtain baseline lipid levels.

Monitoring: Monitor for signs/symptoms of liver dysfunction, cholelithiasis, pancreatitis, hypersensitivity reactions (eg, Stevens-Johnson syndrome, toxic epidermal necrosis), hematological changes (eg, thrombocytopenia, agranulocytosis), myopathies, rhabdomyolysis, PE, DVT, and elevations in SrCr. Periodically monitor liver function (eg, ALT, AST), cholesterol levels, and blood counts. Evaluate CPK levels in patients suspected of having myopathies. Monitor for clinical response; if adequate response not seen after 2 months with maximum dose, d/c therapy.

Patient Counseling: Advise to immediately contact physician if unexplained muscle pain, tenderness, or weakness develop, particularly when accompanied by malaise or fever. Recommend appropriate lipid-lowering diet. Instruct to take with/without meals.

Administration: Oral route. **Storage:** 25°C (77°F); excursions permitted to 15-30°C (59-86°F). Keep out of reach of children. Protect from moisture.

TRIGLIDE — RX

fenofibrate (Sciele)

THERAPEUTIC CLASS: Fibric acid derivative

INDICATIONS: Adjunct to diet for treatment of hypertriglyceridemia (Types IV and V) and for the reduction of LDL-C, Total-C, TG, and Apo B in primary hypercholesterolemia or mixed dyslipidemia (Types IIa and IIb).

DOSAGE: *Adults:* Hypercholesterolemia/Mixed Hyperlipidemia: 160mg qd. Hypertriglyceridemia: Initial: 50-160mg/day. Titrate: Adjust if needed after repeat lipid levels at 4-8 week intervals. Max: 160mg/day. Renal Dysfunction/Elderly: Initial: 50mg/day. Take without regard to meals.

HOW SUPPLIED: Tab: 50mg, 160mg

CONTRAINDICATIONS: Severe renal dysfunction, hepatic dysfunction (including primary biliary cirrhosis and unexplained persistent liver function abnormality), pre-existing gallbladder disease.

WARNINGS/PRECAUTIONS: Monitor LFTs regularly; d/c if >3x ULN. May cause cholelithiasis; d/c if gallstones found. D/C if myopathy or marked CPK elevation occurs. Decreased Hgb, Hct, WBCs, thrombocytopenia, and agranulocytosis reported; monitor CBCs during first 12 months of therapy. Acute hypersensitivity reactions (rare) and pancreatitis reported. Monitor lipids periodically initially; d/c if inadequate response after 2 months on 160mg/day. Minimize dose in severe renal impairment. Caution in elderly.

ADVERSE REACTIONS: Abdominal pain, back pain, headache, abnormal LFTs, respiratory disorder, increased creatinine phosphokinase/SGPT/SGOT.

INTERACTIONS: May potentiate coumarin anticoagulants; reduce anticoagulant dose and monitor PT/INR. Avoid HMG-CoA reductase inhibitors unless benefits outweigh risks. Bile acid sequestrants may impede absorption; take at least 1 hr before or 4-6 hrs after the resin. Evaluate benefits/risks with immunosuppressants (eg, cyclosporine) and other nephrotoxic agents; use lowest effective dose.

PREGNANCY: Category C, not for use in nursing.

MECHANISM OF ACTION: Fibric acid derivative; activates peroxisome proliferator-activated receptor α (PPARα). Causes increase in lipolysis and elimination of triglyceride-rich particles from plasma by activating lipoprotein lipase and reducing production of apoprotein C-III. Decreases in triglycerides then produce an alteration in size and composition of LDL particles, from small and dense to large, buoyant particles. Larger particles have a greater affinity for cholesterol receptors and are catabolized rapidly. Activation of PPARα also induces an increase in the synthesis of apoproteins A-1, A-II, and HDL cholesterol.

PHARMACOKINETICS: Absorption: Well absorbed; T_{max}=3 hrs. **Distribution:** Plasma protein binding (99%). **Metabolism:** Hydrolysis to fenofibric acid (active metabolite); conjugation. **Elimination:** Urine (60%), feces (25%); $T_{1/2}$=16 hrs (metabolite).

NURSING CONSIDERATIONS

Assessment: Assess for severe renal dysfunction, hepatic dysfunction (primary biliary cirrhosis, unexplained persistent liver function abnormality), pre-existing gallbladder disease, and pregnancy/nursing status. Obtain baseline liver function (including ALT) and lipid levels. Assess for drug interactions.

Monitoring: Monitor for signs/symptoms of liver dysfunction (chronic active and cholestatic hepatitis), cholelithiasis, pancreatitis, hypersensitivity reactions (Stevens-Johnson syndrome, toxic epidermal necrolysis), hematological changes (agranulocytosis, thrombocytopenia), myopathies, rhabdomyolysis. Perform periodic monitoring of liver function (including ALT) and blood counts. If cholelithiasis suspected, gallbladder studies are indicated; d/c therapy if gallstones are found. Perform periodic monitoring of serum lipid levels; if adequate response not seen following 2 months of therapy with maximum dose, d/c therapy. If myopathy suspected, obtain CPK levels.

Patient Counseling: Advise to immediately contact physician if unexplained muscle pain, tenderness, or weakness develop, particularly if accompanied by malaise or fever. Recommend appropriate lipid-lowering diet. Instruct drug may be taken with/without food.

Administration: Oral route. **Storage:** 20-25°C (68-77°F); excursions permitted between 15-30°C (59-86°F). Protect from light and moisture.

TRILEPTAL

RX

oxcarbazepine (Novartis)

THERAPEUTIC CLASS: Dibenzazepine

INDICATIONS: Monotherapy or adjunct therapy in adults and children 4-16 yrs with partial seizures.

DOSAGE: *Adults:* Monotherapy: Initial: 300mg bid. Titrate: Increase by 300mg/day every 3rd day. Maint: 1200mg/day. Adjunct Therapy: Initial: 300mg bid. Titrate: Increase weekly by a maximum of 600mg/day. Maint: 600mg bid. Conversion to Monotherapy: Initial: 300mg bid while reducing other AEDs. Titrate: Increase weekly by 600mg/day. Withdraw other AEDs over 3-6 weeks. Maint: 2400mg/day. Renal Impairment: CrCl <30mL/min: Initial: 300mg qd. Titrate: Increase gradually.
Pediatrics: 4-16yrs: Monotherapy: Initial: 4-5mg/kg bid. Titrate: Increase by 5mg/kg/day every 3rd day. Maint (mg/day): 20kg: Initial: 600mg. Max: 900mg. 25-30kg: Initial: 900mg. Max: 1200mg. 35-40kg: Initial: 900mg. Max: 1500mg. 45kg: Initial: 1200mg. Max: 1500mg. 50-55kg: Initial: 1200mg. Max: 1800mg. 60-65kg: Initial: 1200mg. Max: 2100mg. 70kg: Initial: 1500mg. Max: 2100mg. Adjunct Therapy: Initial: 4-5mg/kg bid. Max: 600mg/day. Titrate: Increase over 2 weeks. Maint (mg/day): 20-29kg: 900mg. 29.1-39kg: 1200mg. >39kg: 1800mg. Conversion to Monotherapy: Initial: 4-5mg/kg bid while reducing other AEDs. Titrate: Increase weekly by max of 10mg/kg/day to target dose. Withdraw other AEDs over 3-6 weeks. Renal Impairment: CrCl <30mL/min: Initial: 300mg qd. Titrate: Increase gradually.

HOW SUPPLIED: Sus: 300mg/5mL [250mL]; Tab: 150mg*, 300mg*, 600mg*
*scored

WARNINGS/PRECAUTIONS: Risk of hyponatremia. Cross-sensitivity with carbamazepine. Avoid abrupt withdrawal. Adjust dose in renal impairment. Reports of serious dermatologic reactions (eg, Stevens-Johnson syndrome, toxic epidermal necrolysis). CNS effects reported (eg, psychomotor slowing, concentration difficulty, speech or language problems, somnolence or fatigue, coordination abnormalities). Reports of multi-organ hypersensitivity reactions in close temporal association to initiation of therapy. Rare cases of anaphylaxis and angioedema involving the larynx, glottis, lips and eyelids reported.

ADVERSE REACTIONS: Dizziness, somnolence, diplopia, NV, asthenia, nystagmus, ataxia, abnormal vision, tremor, abnormal gait, headache.

INTERACTIONS: Additive sedative effect with alcohol. Verapamil, carbamazepine, phenytoin, phenobarbital, valproic acid may decrease levels. Decreased plasma levels of felodipine and oral contraceptives. Increased plasma levels of phenytoin, phenobarbital.

PREGNANCY: Category C, not for use in nursing.

MECHANISM OF ACTION: Dibenzazepine; mechanism unknown. Oxcarbazepine and 10-monohydroxy metabolite (MHD) suspected to exert antiseizure effects through blockade of voltage-sensitive Na^+ channels, resulting in stabilization of hyperexcited neural membranes, inhibition of repetitive neuronal firing, and diminution of propagation of synaptic impulses. Also, increased K^+ conductance and modulation of high-voltage activated calcium channels may contribute to anticonvulsant activity.

PHARMACOKINETICS: Absorption: Completely absorbed. T_{max}=4.5 hrs (Tab), 6 hrs (Sus). **Distribution:** V_d=49L (MHD); plasma protein binding (40%) (metabolite); found in breast milk. **Metabolism:** Liver; reduced to MHD (active metabolite), then conjugated. **Elimination:** Urine (>95%), feces (<4%); $T_{1/2}$=2 hrs (parent drug), 9 hrs (MHD). In pediatrics, MHD clearance decreases as age/weight increase, approaching that of adults.

NURSING CONSIDERATIONS

Assessment: Assess renal function, possible drug interactions, and drug allergy to carbamazepine.

Monitoring: Monitor serum Na^+ levels with maintenance treatment, particularly with other medications also known to reduce levels. Monitor for signs/

T

symptoms of hyponatremia, anaphylaxis and angioedema, severe dermatological reactions, cognitive or neuropsychiatric events, multiorgan hypersensitivity, and hematological effects (eg, agranulocytosis, aplastic anemia).

Patient Counseling: Advise to immediately report signs/symptoms suggesting angioedema. Instruct to notify physician if fever with other organ system involvement or serious skin reaction develop. Counsel females that efficacy of oral contraceptives may decrease; use another form of contraception. Avoid operating heavy machinery until gauging effects of drug. Instruct to avoid alcohol. Inform medication can be taken with/without food.

Administration: Oral route. **Storage:** 25°C (77°F); excursions permitted to 15-30°C (59-86°F). Dispense in tight container. Use sus within 7 weeks after opening.

TRI-LEVLEN RX

ethinyl estradiol - levonorgestrel (Bayer Healthcare)

THERAPEUTIC CLASS: Estrogen/progestogen combination

INDICATIONS: Prevention of pregnancy.

DOSAGE: *Adults:* Start 1st Sunday after menses begin or 1st day of menses. 21-day: 1 tab qd for 21 days, stop 7 days, then repeat. 28-day: 1 tab qd for 28 days, then repeat.

HOW SUPPLIED: Tab: (Ethinyl Estradiol-Levonorgestrel) 0.03mg-0.05mg, 0.04mg-0.075mg, 0.03mg-0.125mg

CONTRAINDICATIONS: Thrombophlebitis, DVT or thromboembolic disorders, pregnancy, cerebrovascular or coronary artery disease, undiagnosed abnormal genital bleeding, cholestatic jaundice of pregnancy or jaundice with prior pill use, hepatic adenomas or carcinomas, breast cancer or other estrogen-dependent neoplasia.

WARNINGS/PRECAUTIONS: Cigarette smoking increases risk of serious cardiovascular side effects. This risk increases with age (especially >35 yrs) and heavy smoking. Increased risk of MI, vascular disease, thromboembolism, stroke and gallbladder disease. Retinal thrombosis, hepatic neoplasia, carcinoma of breast and reproductive organs reported. May cause glucose intolerance. May increase BP, elevate LDL levels or cause other lipid changes, fluid retention, breakthrough bleeding, and spotting. May cause or exacerbate migraine. May develop visual changes with contact lens. Increased risk of MI with HTN, hyperlipidemia, obesity, and diabetes. D/C if develop jaundice, significant depression or ophthalmic irregularities. Perform annual physical exam. Use before menarche is not indicated. May affect certain endocrine, LFTs and blood components.

ADVERSE REACTIONS: NV, breakthrough bleeding, spotting, amenorrhea, migraine, depression, vaginal candidiasis, edema, weight changes.

INTERACTIONS: Reduced effects, increased breakthrough bleeding, and menstrual irregularities with rifampin, barbiturates, phenylbutazone, phenytoin, and possibly with griseofulvin, ampicillin, and tetracyclines. Increases or decreases levels of cyclosporine and theophylline.

PREGNANCY: Category X, not for use in nursing.

MECHANISM OF ACTION: Oral contraceptive combination; suppresses gonadotropins, inhibits ovulation. Causes changes in cervical mucus (increases difficulty of sperm entry into uterus) and endometrium (reduces likelihood of implantation).

PHARMACOKINETICS: Distribution: Found in breast milk.

NURSING CONSIDERATIONS

Assessment: Assess for history of DVT, thromboembolic disorders, thrombophlebitis, cerebrovascular disease, CAD, carcinoma of breast, endometrium or other estrogen-dependent neoplasia, abnormal genital bleeding, cholestatic jaundice of pregnancy or jaundice with prior pill use, hepatic adenoma/carcinoma, and pregnancy status. Obtain complete medical history and physical exam with special reference to BP, breasts, abdomen, and pelvic organs, including cervical cytology and relevant lab tests.

Monitoring: Monitor for thromboembolic disorders and other vascular problems, malignant neoplasms, MI, stroke, hepatic neoplasia, ocular lesions, bleeding irregularities, migraine headaches, gallbladder disease, elevated BP, jaundice, emotional disorders, carbohydrate and lipid metabolic effects, lipid profile (HDL, LDL, TG), LFTs, PT, TBG, T3/T4, blood glucose, and serum folate levels.

Patient Counseling: Counsel not to smoke; smoking increases risk of cardiovascular side effects. Instruct to take at same time daily. Inform that drug does not protect against HIV infection/AIDS, and other STDs. Educate that light bleeding is possible. Caution that some medications decrease efficacy; consult physician to determine appropriate back-up contraceptive method. Instruct to immediately report any sharp CP, coughing of blood, sudden SOB, pain in calf, severe headache and vomiting, dizziness or fainting, disturbances of vision or speech, severe pain or tenderness in stomach area, difficulty sleeping, weakness, changes in mood, or jaundice.

Administration: Oral route. **Storage:** 20-25°C (68-77°F).

TRILIPIX

fenofibric acid (Abbott)

RX

THERAPEUTIC CLASS: Fibric acid derivative

INDICATIONS: Adjunctive therapy to diet to reduce TG in patients with severe hypertriglyceridemia. Adjunctive therapy to diet to reduce elevated LDL-C, Total-C, TG, and Apo B, and to increase HDL-C in patients with primary hyperlipidemia or mixed dyslipidemia. Adjunct to diet in combination with a statin to reduce TG and increase HDL-C in patients with mixed dyslipidemia and coronary heart disease (CHD) or a CHD risk equivalent who are on optimal statin therapy to achieve LDL-C goal.

DOSAGE: *Adults:* Severe Hypertriglyceridemia: Individualize dose. Initial (Usual): 45-135mg qd. Titrate: May adjust dose if necessary following repeat lipid determinations at 4- to 8- week intervals. Max: 135mg/day. Primary Hyperlipidemia or Mixed Dyslipidemia: 135mg qd. Co-administered with Statins in Mixed Dyslipidemia: 135mg qd. Mild-to-Moderate Renal Impairment: Initial: 45mg qd. Titrate: May increase dose after evaluation of effects on renal function and lipid levels. Elderly: Base dose selection on renal function. May take with/without meals. May be taken at same time as statin.

HOW SUPPLIED: Tab, Delayed-Release: 45mg, 135mg

CONTRAINDICATIONS: Severe renal impairment (including dialysis), active liver disease (including primary biliary cirrhosis and unexplained persistent liver function abnormalities), nursing mothers, and pre-existing gallbladder disease.

WARNINGS/PRECAUTIONS: Increases risk of myositis/myopathy in elderly, DM, renal failure, or hypothyroidism; d/c therapy if myopathy or marked CPK elevation occurs. Reversible elevations of serum creatinine reported; monitor renal function. Increase in serum transaminases (eg, ALT, AST) reported; monitor liver function, and d/c therapy if enzyme levels >3x ULN. Myalgia reported. May increase cholesterol excretion into bile; d/c if cholelithiasis occurs. Acute hypersensitivity reactions (rare) and pancreatitis reported. Decreased Hgb, Hct, WBCs, rare thrombocytopenia and agranulocytosis reported. Avoid in severe renal impairment and caution in elderly.

ADVERSE REACTIONS: Headache, back pain, nasopharyngitis, nausea, myalgia, diarrhea, upper respiratory tract infection.

INTERACTIONS: May potentiate anticoagulant effects; caution with oral coumarin anticoagulant and monitor PT/INR. Bile acid resins may impede absorption; take at least 1 hr before or 4-6 hrs after the resin. Evaluate benefits/risks with immunosuppressants (eg, cyclosporine) and other potentially nephrotoxic agents; use lowest effective dose.

PREGNANCY: Category C, not for use in nursing.

MECHANISM OF ACTION: Fibric acid derivative; activates peroxisome proliferator-activated receptor α (PPARα). Causes increase in lipolysis and elimination of triglyceride-rich particles from plasma by activating lipoprotein lipase and reducing production of APO C-III (an inhibitor of lipoprotein lipase activity).

PHARMACOKINETICS: Absorption: Well-absorbed, absolute bioavailability (81%); T_{max}=4-5 hrs. **Distribution:** Plasma protein binding (99%). **Metabolism:** Conjugation. **Elimination:** $T_{1/2}$=20 hrs.

NURSING CONSIDERATIONS

Assessment: Assess for severe renal impairment, active liver disease (eg, primary biliary cirrhosis, unexplained liver function abnormality), pre-existing gallbladder disease, pregnancy/nursing status, and possible drug interactions. Obtain baseline LFTs (including ALT/AST), renal function, and lipid levels.

Monitoring: Monitor for signs/symptoms of active liver disease, cholelithiasis, pancreatitis, hypersentivity reactions (eg, Stevens-Johnson syndrome, toxic epidermal necrolysis), hematological changes (eg, agranulocytosis, thrombocytopenia), myopathies, rhabdomyolysis. Perform periodic monitoring of liver function (including ALT/AST) and blood counts. If cholelithiasis suspected, gallbladder studies are indicated; d/c therapy if gallstones present. Perform periodic monitoring of serum lipid levels. If myopathy suspected, obtain CPK levels.

Patient Counseling: Instruct to notify physician if unexplained muscle pain, tenderness, or weakness develop, particularly if accompanied by malaise or fever. Recommend appropriate lipid-lowering diet. Inform that drug may be taken with/without food and may be taken at same time as statin.

Administration: Oral route. **Storage:** 25°C (77°F); excursions permitted to 15-30°C (59-86°F). Protect from moisture.

TRI-LUMA RX

fluocinolone acetonide - hydroquinone - tretinoin (Galderma)

THERAPEUTIC CLASS: Corticosteroid/depigmenting agent/keratolytic

INDICATIONS: Short-term treatment of moderate to severe melasma of the face.

DOSAGE: *Adults:* Gently wash face and neck with mild cleanser. Apply thin film to hyperpigmented areas of melasma including 1/2 inch of normal skin surrounding lesion, at least 30 min before bedtime.

HOW SUPPLIED: Cre: (Fluocinolone-Hydroquinone-Tretinoin) 0.01%-4%-0.05% [30g]

WARNINGS/PRECAUTIONS: Contains sodium metabisulfite. D/C if ochronosis, sensitivity, or irritation occurs. Cutaneous hypersensitivity reported. May produce reversible HPA axis suppression, manifestations of Cushing's syndrome, hyperglycemia, and glucosuria. Avoid eyes, nose, angles of mouth, occlusive dressings, or sunlight/UV exposure. Extreme weather (eg, cold, wind) may irritate skin.

ADVERSE REACTIONS: Erythema, desquamation, burning, dryness, pruritus, acne, paresthesia, telangiectasia.

INTERACTIONS: Avoid medicated/abrasive soaps or cleansers, soaps/cosmetics with drying effects, products with high concentration of alcohol/astringent, and other irritants or keratolytic agents. Caution with other photosensitizers. Use non-hormonal birth control.

PREGNANCY: Category C, caution in nursing.

MECHANISM OF ACTION: Fluocinolone: Corticosteroid; acts as anti-inflammatory agent. Hydroquinone: Depigmenting agent; interrupts 1 or more steps in tyrosine-tyrosinase pathway in melanin systhesis. Tretinoin: Keratolytic.

PHARMACOKINETICS: Absorption: Hydroquinone: C_{max}=25.55-86.52ng/mL. Tretinoin: (gp I) C_{max}=2,01-5.34ng/mL, (gp II) C_{max}=2-4.99ng/mL. **Distribution:** Corticosteroid; (found in breast milk).

NURSING CONSIDERATIONS

Assessment: Assess for drug or sulfite hypersensitivity, pregnancy/nursing status, and for possible drug interactions with photosensitizer drugs.

Monitoring: Monitor for allergic-type reactions (eg, anaphylactic symptoms, life-threatening asthmatic attacks), local irritation (eg, reddening, peeling, burning sensation, dryness, pruritus), ochronosis (gradual blue-black darkening of skin), HPA-axis suppression with potential for glucocorticoid insufficiency after withdrawal, manifestations of Cushing's syndrome, hyperglycemia, and glucosuria. Lab monitoring of HPA-axis supression by ACTH or cosyntropin stimulation test, morning plasma cortisol test, urinary free cortisol test.

Patient Counseling: Instruct to avoid sunlight, sunlamp, and UV light exposure. Wearing protective clothing and using sunscreen essential during therapy. Avoid contact with eyes, nose, or angles of mouth. Notify physician if pregnant/nursing or planning to become pregnant.

Administration: Topical route. **Storage:** 20-25°C (68-77°F). Avoid freezing.

TRI-NORINYL RX

ethinyl estradiol - norethindrone (Watson)

THERAPEUTIC CLASS: Estrogen/progestogen combination

INDICATIONS: Prevention of pregnancy.

DOSAGE: *Adults:* 1 tab qd for 28 days, then repeat. Start 1st Sunday after menses begin or 1st day of menses.

HOW SUPPLIED: Tab: (Ethinyl Estradiol-Norethindrone) 0.035mg-0.5mg, 0.035mg-1mg

CONTRAINDICATIONS: Thrombophlebitis, DVT or thromboembolic disorders, pregnancy, cerebrovascular or coronary artery disease, undiagnosed abnormal genital bleeding, cholestatic jaundice of pregnancy or jaundice with prior pill use, hepatic adenomas or carcinomas, breast cancer or other estrogen-dependent neoplasia.

WARNINGS/PRECAUTIONS: Cigarette smoking increases risk of serious cardiovascular side effects. This risk increases with age (especially >35 yrs) and heavy smoking. Increased risk of MI, vascular disease, thromboembolism, stroke and gallbladder disease. Retinal thrombosis, hepatic neoplasia, carcinoma of breast and reproductive organs reported. May cause glucose intolerance. May increase BP, elevate LDL levels or cause other lipid changes, fluid retention, breakthrough bleeding, and spotting. May cause or exacerbate migraine. May develop visual changes with contact lens. Increased risk of MI with HTN, hyperlipidemia, obesity, and diabetes. D/C if jaundice, significant depression or ophthalmic irregularities develop. Perform annual physical exam. Use before menarche is not indicated. May affect certain endocrine, LFTs and blood components.

ADVERSE REACTIONS: NV, breakthrough bleeding, spotting, amenorrhea, migraine, depression, vaginal candidiasis, edema, weight changes.

INTERACTIONS: Reduced effects, increased breakthrough bleeding, and menstrual irregularities with rifampin, barbiturates, phenylbutazone, phenytoin, and possibly with griseofulvin, ampicillin, and tetracyclines.

PREGNANCY: Category X, not for use in nursing.

MECHANISM OF ACTION: Combination oral contraceptive; acts by suppressing gonadotropins. Primarily inhibits ovulation. Also causes changes in cervical mucus (increases difficulty of sperm entry into uterus) and endometrium (reduces likelihood of implantation).

NURSING CONSIDERATIONS

Assessment: Assess family history of breast cancer, presence of certain inherited or acquired thrombophilias, HTN, hyperlipidemia, obesity, DM, renal disease, depression, heavy smoking, and potential drug interactions. Conduct personal and family history and complete physical exam.

T

Monitoring: Monitor for MI, thromboembolism, cerebrovascular disease, benign hepatic adenomas, retinal thrombosis, HTN, headache, bleeding irregularities, jaundice, fluid retention, and emotional disorders. Conduct periodic complete physical exam with emphasis on BP, breasts, abdomen, and pelvic organs including cervical cytology and relevant lab tests (eg, TG, prothrombin clotting factors such as VII, VIII, IX, and X, renal/hepatic functions, TBG, sex steroid binding globulins).

Patient Counseling: Inform drug does not protect against HIV infection (AIDS) and other STDs. Inform of potential risks/benefits of oral contraceptives. Do not smoke while on treatment. Take 1 pill at same time daily.

Administration: Oral route. **Storage:** 15-25°C (59-77°F).

TRIPEDIA RX

pertussis vaccine, acellular - diphtheria toxoid - tetanus toxoid (Sanofi Pasteur)

THERAPEUTIC CLASS: Vaccine/toxoid combination

INDICATIONS: Active immunization against diphtheria, tetanus, and pertussis in pediatrics 6 weeks to 7 yrs of age (prior to 7th birthday). Combined with ActHIB for active immunization in pediatrics 15-18 months previously immunized against diphtheria, tetanus, and pertussis with 3 doses of whole-cell pertussis DTP or acellular pertussis vaccine and 3 or fewer doses of ActHIB® within 1st year of life for prevention of *H. influenzae* type b, diphtheria, tetanus, and pertussis.

DOSAGE: *Pediatrics:* ≥6 weeks up to 7 yrs: Primary Series: 3 doses of 0.5mL IM at 4-8 week intervals. 1st dose usually at 2 months, but can give at 6 weeks up to 7th birthday. Booster: 4th dose (0.5mL IM) at 15-20 months, at least 6 months after 3rd dose, 5th dose at 4-6 yrs; prior to school entry. May give to complete 4th or 5th dose of primary series of 3 doses of whole-cell pertussis DTP (4th dose at 15-20 months and 5th dose before school if 4th dose not given on or before 4th birthday). May combine with ActHIB® for 4th dose at 15-18 months.

HOW SUPPLIED: Inj: 0.5mL

CONTRAINDICATIONS: Hypersensitivity to thimersal and gelatin, immediate anaphylactic reaction associated with previous dose, encephalopathy not due to an identifiable cause within 7 days of prior pertussis immunization. Defer during poliomyelitis outbreak or acute febrile illness.

WARNINGS/PRECAUTIONS: Caution if within 48 hrs of previous whole-cell DTP or acellular DTP vaccine, fever ≥105°F not due to another identifiable cause, collapse or shock-like state, or inconsolable crying lasting ≥3 hrs occurs, or if convulsions occur within 3 days. For high seizure risk, give APAP at time of vaccination and q4-6h for 24 hrs. Caution with neurologic or CNS disorders. Avoid with coagulation disorders. Have epinephrine available. Suboptimal response may occur in immunocompromised patients.

T

ADVERSE REACTIONS: Local erythema and swelling, irritability, drowsiness, anorexia, fever.

INTERACTIONS: Avoid with anticoagulants. Immunosuppressive therapy (eg, irradiation, antimetabolites, alkylating agents, cytotoxic drugs, corticosteroids) may decrease response. Do not combine through reconstitution with any vaccine for infants <15 months.

PREGNANCY: Category C, safety in nursing not known.

MECHANISM OF ACTION: Active immunization against diphtheria, tetanus, and pertussis (whooping cough).

NURSING CONSIDERATIONS

Assessment: Review current health status, previous sensitivity/immunization events (eg, fever, shock, persistent crying, convulsions, Guillain-Barre syndrome), and possible drug interactions.

Monitoring: Monitor for Arthus-type hypersensitivity reactions, injection site for erythema, swelling, and tenderness, fever, irritability, drowsiness, anorexia, NV, high-pitched/persistent crying, and neurological complications.

Patient Counseling: Inform of potential benefits/risks; report any adverse reactions to physician. May not offer 100% protection.

Administration: IM route. Inject into anterolateral aspect of thigh or deltoid region. **Storage:** 2-8°C (36-46°F). Do not freeze.

TRIPHASIL RX

ethinyl estradiol - levonorgestrel (Wyeth)

OTHER BRAND NAMES: Enpresse (Barr)

THERAPEUTIC CLASS: Estrogen/progestogen combination

INDICATIONS: Prevention of pregnancy.

DOSAGE: *Adults:* 1 tab qd for 28 days, then repeat. Start 1st Sunday after menses begin or 1st day of menses.

HOW SUPPLIED: Tab: (Ethinyl Estradiol-Levonorgestrel) 0.03mg-0.05mg, 0.04mg-0.075mg, 0.03mg-0.125mg

CONTRAINDICATIONS: Thrombophlebitis, DVT or thromboembolic disorders, pregnancy, cerebrovascular or coronary artery disease, undiagnosed abnormal genital bleeding, cholestatic jaundice of pregnancy or jaundice with prior pill use, hepatic adenomas or carcinomas, breast cancer or other estrogen-dependent neoplasia, thrombogenic valvulopathies, thrombogenic rhythm disorders, diabetes with vascular involvement, uncontrolled HTN, endometrium carcinoma, active liver disease if liver function has not returned to normal.

WARNINGS/PRECAUTIONS: Cigarette smoking increases risk of serious cardiovascular side effects; risk increases with age (especially >35 yrs) and heavy smoking. Increased risk of MI, vascular disease, thromboembolism, stroke and gallbladder disease. Retinal thrombosis, hepatic neoplasia, carcinoma of breast and reproductive organs reported. May cause glucose intolerance. May increase BP, elevate LDL levels or cause other lipid changes, fluid retention, breakthrough bleeding, and spotting. May cause or exacerbate migraine. May develop visual changes with contact lens. Diarrhea and vomiting may decrease hormone absorption. Increased risk of MI with HTN, hyperlipidemia, obesity, and diabetes. D/C if jaundice, significant depression or ophthalmic irregularities develop. Perform annual physical exam. Use before menarche is not indicated. May affect certain endocrine, LFTs and blood components.

ADVERSE REACTIONS: NV, breakthrough bleeding, spotting, amenorrhea, migraine, depression, vaginal candidiasis, edema, weight changes.

INTERACTIONS: Reduced effects, increased breakthrough bleeding, and menstrual irregularities with rifampin, rifabutin, barbiturates, phenylbutazone, phenytoin, griseofulvin, topiramate, some protease inhibitors, modafinil, ampicillin, other penicillins, tetracyclines and possibly with St. John's wort. Troleadomycin may increase risk of intrahepatic cholestasis. Increased levels with ascorbic acid, APAP, CYP3A4 inhibitors (eg, indinavir, fluconazole, troleandomycin), and atorvastatin. May alter levels of cyclosporine, theophylline, and corticosteroids.

PREGNANCY: Category X, not for use in nursing.

MECHANISM OF ACTION: Combination oral contraceptive; acts by suppressing gonadotropins. Inhibits ovulation and produces changes in cervical mucus (increasing difficulty of sperm entry into uterus) and endometrium (reducing likelihood of implantation).

PHARMACOKINETICS: Absorption: (LNG): Rapid and complete. (50/30mcg LNG/EE single dose): C_{max}=1.7ng/mL, T_{max}=1.3 hr, AUC=17ng•hr/mL; (EE) Rapid and complete, (50/30mcg LNG/EE single dose): C_{max}=141pg/mL, T_{max}=1.5 hr, AUC=1126pg•hr/mL. **Distribution**: Found in breast milk, (EE) plasma protein binding (97%). **Metabolism**: (LNG) reduction, hydroxylation, conjugation; (EE) in liver via CYP3A4 through hydroxylation (major), methylation, glucuronidation. **Elimination**: (LNG) Urine (40%-68%), feces (16-48%); $T_{1/2}$=approximately 36 hrs. (EE) Urine, feces; $T_{1/2}$=18 hrs.

NURSING CONSIDERATIONS

Assessment: Assess family history of breast cancer, presence of certain inherited or acquired thrombophilias, HTN, hyperlipidemia, obesity, DM, renal disease, depression, heavy smoking, and potential drug interactions. Conduct personal/family history and complete physical exam.

Monitoring: Monitor for MI, thromboembolism, cerebrovascular disease, benign hepatic adenomas, retinal thrombosis, HTN, headache, bleeding irregularites, jaundice, fluid retention, and emotional disorders. Conduct periodic complete physical exam with emphasis on BP, breasts, abdomen, and pelvic organs including cervical cytology and relevant lab tests (eg, TG, prothrombin and clotting factors as VII, VIII, IX, and X, renal/hepatic functions, TBG, sex steroid binding globulins).

Patient Counseling: Inform drug does not protect against HIV infection (AIDS) and other STDs. Inform of potential risks/benefits of oral contraceptives. Do not smoke while on treatment. Take 1 pill at same time daily.

Administration: Oral route. **Storage**: 20-25°C (68-77°F).

TRIVORA — RX

ethinyl estradiol - levonorgestrel (Watson)

OTHER BRAND NAMES: Enpresse (Barr)

THERAPEUTIC CLASS: Estrogen/progestogen combination

INDICATIONS: Prevention of pregnancy.

DOSAGE: *Adults:* 1 tab qd for 28 days, then repeat. Start 1st Sunday after menses begin or 1st day of menses.

HOW SUPPLIED: Tab: (Ethinyl Estradiol-Levonorgestrel) 0.03mg-0.05mg, 0.04mg-0.075mg, 0.03mg-0.125mg

CONTRAINDICATIONS: Thrombophlebitis, deep vein thrombophlebitis, thromboembolic disorders, pregnancy, cerebrovascular or coronary artery disease, undiagnosed abnormal genital bleeding, cholestatic jaundice of pregnancy or jaundice with prior pill use, hepatic carcinoma, benign liver tumor, breast cancer, endometrial cancer, or other estrogen-dependent neoplasia.

WARNINGS/PRECAUTIONS: Cigarette smoking increases risk of serious cardiovascular side effects. This risk increases with age (especially >35 yrs) and heavy smoking. Increased risk of MI, vascular disease, thromboembolism, stroke, and gallbladder disease. Retinal thrombosis, hepatic neoplasia reported. May cause glucose intolerance. May increase BP, elevate LDL levels or cause other lipid changes, fluid retention, breakthrough bleeding, and spotting. May cause or exacerbate migraine. May develop visual changes with contact lens. Morbidity and mortality risk increased with HTN, hyperlipidemia, obesity, and diabetes. D/C if jaundice, significant depression or ophthalmic irregularities develop. Perform annual physical exam. Use before menarche is not indicated. May affect certain endocrine, LFTs, and blood components.

ADVERSE REACTIONS: NV, breakthrough bleeding, spotting, amenorrhea, migraine, depression, vaginal candidiasis, edema, weight changes.

INTERACTIONS: Reduced effects, increased breakthrough bleeding, and menstrual irregularities with rifampin, barbiturates, phenylbutazone, phenytoin, and possibly with griseofulvin, ampicillin, and tetracyclines.

PREGNANCY: Category X, not for use in nursing.

MECHANISM OF ACTION: Combination oral contraceptive; acts by suppressing gonadotropins, primarily inhibits ovulation. Also causes changes in cervical mucus (increasing difficulty of sperm entry into uterus) and endometrium (reducing likelihood of implantation).

PHARMACOKINETICS: Absorption: Triphasic pharmacokinetic parameters varied according to variable dosing. Levonorgestrel: Rapidly and completely absorbed. Absolute bioavailability (100%). Ethinyl: Rapid and almost completely absorbed. Absolute bioavailabilty (38-48%). **Distribution:** Found in breast milk. Levonorgestrel: SHBG binding (60%). Ethinyl: Albumin binding (97%). **Metabolism:** Levonorgestrel: Via hydroxylation and conjugation. Ethinyl: Liver via CYP3A4 enzyme through hydroxylation, methylation and glucuronidation. **Elimination:** Levonorgestrel: Urine (40-68%), feces (16-48%); $T_{1/2}$=36 hrs. Ethinyl: Urine, feces; $T_{1/2}$=18 hrs.

NURSING CONSIDERATIONS

Assessment: Assess family history of breast cancer, presence of inherited or acquired thrombophilias, HTN, hyperlipidemia, obesity, DM, renal disease, depression, heavy smoking, and potential drug interactions. Conduct personal/family history and complete physical exam.

Monitoring: Monitor for MI, thromboembolism, cerebrovascular disease, benign hepatic adenomas, retinal thrombosis, HTN, headache, bleeding irregularites, jaundice, fluid retention, and emotional disorders. Conduct periodic complete physical exam with emphasis on BP, breasts, abdomen, and pelvic organs, including cervical cytology and relevant lab tests.

Patient Counseling: Inform that drug does not protect against HIV infection and other STDs. Counsel on benefits/risks of drug. Advise to avoid smoking while taking medication. Instruct to take 1 pill at same time daily.

Administration: Oral route. **Storage:** 20-25°C (68-77°F).

TRIZIVIR

RX

abacavir sulfate - zidovudine - lamivudine (GlaxoSmithKline)

Fatal hypersensitivity reactions reported; discontinue if hypersensitivy reaction suspected and do not restart. Hematologic toxicities, lactic acidosis, and severe hepatomegaly with steatosis (including fatal cases) reported. Severe exacerbations of hepatitis B in patients co-infected with HIV upon discontinuation; monitor hepatic function.

THERAPEUTIC CLASS: Nucleoside analog combination

INDICATIONS: Treatment of HIV-1 infection alone or in combination with other antiretrovirals.

DOSAGE: *Adults:* >40kg and CrCl >50mL/min: 1 tab bid.
Pediatrics: Adolescents: >40kg and CrCl >50mL/min: 1 tab bid.

HOW SUPPLIED: Tab: (Abacavir-Lamivudine-Zidovudine) 300mg-150mg-300mg

WARNINGS/PRECAUTIONS: Hypersensitivity; d/c if suspected and register patients by calling 1-800-270-0425. Caution with bone marrow compromise. Prolonged use associated with myopathy and myositis with pathological changes. Avoid with mild to moderate hepatic impairment or liver cirrhosis. Recurrent hepatitis upon discontinuation of lamivudine reported in hepatitis B patients. Lamivudine-resistant hepatitis B virus reported.

ADVERSE REACTIONS: NV, diarrhea, loss of appetite, insomnia, fever, chills, fatigue.

INTERACTIONS: Ethanol decreases elimination. Ganciclovir, interferon-alpha, and other bone marrow suppressants or cytotoxic agents may increase hematologic toxicity. Antagonistic effects with stavudine. Increased lamivudine exposure with trimethoprim 160mg/sulfamethoxazole 800mg. Avoid zalcitabine. Hepatic decompensation reported in patients on combination antiretroviral therapy for HIV and interferon alfa with or without ribavarin; monitor closely for treatment-associated toxicities.

PREGNANCY: Category C, not for use in nursing.

MECHANISM OF ACTION: Abacavir: Carbocyclic nucleoside analogue; inhibits HIV-1 reverse transcriptase (RT) by competing with natural substrate dGTP and incorporating into viral DNA. Lamivudine/Zidovudine: Nucleoside analogue; inhibits RT via DNA chain termination.

PHARMACOKINETICS: Absorption: Abacavir: Rapid; bioavailability (86%). Lamivudine: Rapid; bioavailability (86%). Zidovudine: Rapid; bioavailability (64%). **Distribution:** Abacavir: V_d=0.86L/kg; plasma protein binding (50%).

T

Lamivudine: V_d=1.3L/kg; plasma protein binding (low). Zidovudine: V_d=1.6L/kg; plasma protein binding (low). **Metabolism:** Abacavir: Hepatic, via alcohol dehydrogenase and glucuronyl transferase. Lamivudine: Metabolite (trans-sulfoxide). Zidovudine: Hepatic, via glucuronyl transferase. Major metabolite: (3'-azido-3'-deoxy-5'-*O*-β-*D*-glucopyranuronosylthymidine (GZDV). **Elimination:** Abacavir: $T_{1/2}$=1.45 hrs. Lamivudine: (IV): Urine (70%); $T_{1/2}$=5-7 hrs. Zidovudine: Urine (14%); (GZDV): Urine (74%); $T_{1/2}$=0.5-3 hrs.

NURSING CONSIDERATIONS

Assessment: Assess for impaired hepatic/renal function, bone marrow suppression, risk factors for lactic acidosis, myopathy, and drug interactions.

Monitoring: Signs/symptoms of hypersensitivity reactions (eg, fever, rash, NV, diarrhea, generalized malaise, fatigue, dyspnea, cough), lactic acidosis, myopathy, exacerbations of hepatitis, immune reconstitution syndrome, hepatic dysfunction (eg, decompensation, failure), and fat redistribution.

Patient Counseling: If treatment interrupted, advise not to restart therapy to avoid more severe symptoms (eg, life-threatening hypotension, death). Seek medical attention if symptoms of hypersensitivity reactions (eg, fever, rash, NV, diarrhea, generalized malaise, fatigue, dyspnea, cough), lactic acidosis, myopathy, exacerbations of hepatitis, immune reconstitution syndrome, hepatic dysfunction (eg, decompensation, failure), and fat redistribution occur.

Administration: Oral route. **Storage:** 25°C (77°F); excursions permitted to 15-30°C (59-86°F).

TRUSOPT

RX

dorzolamide HCl (Merck)

THERAPEUTIC CLASS: Carbonic anhydrase inhibitor

INDICATIONS: Treatment of open-angle glaucoma and ocular hypertension.

DOSAGE: *Adults:* 1 drop tid. Space dosing of other ophthalmic drugs by 10 min.
Pediatrics: 1 drop tid. Space dosing of other ophthalmic drugs by 10 min.

HOW SUPPLIED: Sol: 2% [5mL, 10mL]

WARNINGS/PRECAUTIONS: Systemically absorbed. Avoid with sulfonamide allergy or severe renal impairment. Caution with hepatic impairment. Not studied in acute angle-closure glaucoma. Local ocular adverse effects (eg, conjunctivitis, lid reactions) reported with chronic use. Bacterial keratitis reported with contaminated containers.

ADVERSE REACTIONS: Ocular burning, stinging, discomfort, superficial punctate keratitis, bitter taste, blurred vision, eye redness, tearing, dryness, photophobia, ocular allergic reactions, lid reactions, conjunctivitis.

INTERACTIONS: Caution with high-dose salicylates. Acid-base disturbances with oral carbonic anhydrase inhibitors. Avoid oral carbonic anhydrase inhibitors due to additive effects. Wait 10 min before using another ophthalmic drug.

PREGNANCY: Category C, not for use in nursing.

MECHANISM OF ACTION: Carbonic anhydrase inhibitor; catalyzes reversible reaction involving hydration of carbon dioxide and dehydration of carbonic acid; also decreases aqueous humor secretion in ciliary processes of the eye by slowing the formation of bicarbonate ions with subsequent reduction in Na^+ and fluid transport, which results in reduction in IOP.

PHARMACOKINETICS: Distribution: Plasma protein binding (33%). **Metabolism:** Metabolites: N-desethyl. **Elimination:** Urine (unchanged, metabolite).

NURSING CONSIDERATIONS

Assessment: Assess for sulfonamide hypersensitivity reaction, acute angle-closure glaucoma, renal/hepatic dysfunction, pregnancy/nursing status, and possible drug interactions.

Monitoring: Monitor for hypersensitivity reactions (eg, Stevens-Johnson syndrome, toxic epidermal necrosis), agranulocytosis, aplastic anemia, and other blood dyscrasias. Monitor for ocular reactions such as conjunctivitis, lid reactions, bacterial keratitis, and choroidal detachment with administration of aqueous suppressant therapy after filtration procedures.

Patient Counseling: Advise to d/c and notify physician if allergic/ocular reactions or concurrent ocular conditions (eg, surgery, trauma, infection) occur. Avoid touching container tip to eye or surrounding surfaces. Instruct to remove contact lenses and reinsert 15 min after administration. Separate use by 10 min if using >1 topical ophthalmic drug.

Administration: Ocular route. **Storage:** 15-30°C (59-86°F); avoid light.

TRUVADA RX

tenofovir disoproxil fumarate - emtricitabine (Gilead)

Lactic acidosis and severe hepatomegaly with steatosis, including fatal cases, reported with nucleoside analogs alone or with concomitant antiretrovirals. Severe acute exacerbations of hepatitis B reported in patients coinfected with HBV and HIV upon discontinuation of emtricitabine or tenofovir disoproxil fumarate (DF).

THERAPEUTIC CLASS: Nucleoside analog combination

INDICATIONS: Treatment of HIV-1 infection in combination with other antiretrovirals.

DOSAGE: *Adults:* ≥18 years: CrCl ≥50mL/min: 1 tab qd. CrCl 30-49mL/min: 1 tab q48h.

HOW SUPPLIED: Tab: (Emtricitabine-Tenofovir Disoproxil Fumarate) 200mg-300mg

WARNINGS/PRECAUTIONS: Obesity and prolonged nucleosides exposure may be risk factors for lactic acidosis and severe hepatomegaly with steatosis. Avoid in patients with CrCl <30mL/min or patients requiring hemodialysis. Tenofovir DF may cause renal impairment. Monitor CrCl and phosphorous in patients at risk or with a history of renal dysfunction and those receiving concomitant nephrotoxic agents. May decrease in bone mineral density; monitor bone density in patients with history of pathologic bone fracture or at risk for osteopenia. Possible redistribution/accumulation of body fat. Hepatic function should be monitored closely for at least several months in patients who are coinfected with HIV and HBV and d/c Viread.

ADVERSE REACTIONS: Dizziness, diarrhea, NV, anxiety, fever, headache, asthenia, abdominal pain, depression, flatulence, rash, paresthesia, dyspepsia, insomnia, neuropathy, increased cough, rhinitis.

INTERACTIONS: May increase levels of didanosine; use caution when coadministering, monitor for didanosine-associated adverse effects, and d/c if these adverse effects develop. Atazanavir and lopinavir/ritonavir may increase tenofovir DF-concentrations; monitor for emtricitabine/tenofovir DF associated adverse effects. Atazanavir without ritonavir should not be coadministered with emtricitabine/tenofovir DF. Drugs that reduce renal function or compete for active tubular secretion may increase serum levels of emtricitabine, tenofovir DF, and/or other renally eliminated drugs (eg, adefovir, dipivoxil, cidofovir, acyclovir, valacyclovir, ganciclovir, valganciclovir). Avoid coadministration with other drugs containing lamivudine. Avoid with concurrent or recent use of nephrotoxic agents. Do not coadminister with Atripla, Emtriva or Viread.

PREGNANCY: Category B, not for use in nursing.

MECHANISM OF ACTION: Emtricitabine: Nucleoside analog of cytidine. Inhibits activity of HIV-1 reverse transcriptase (RT) by competing with natural substrate deoxycytidine 5'-triphosphate and incorporating into nascent viral DNA, resulting in chain termination. Tenofovir disoproxil: Acyclic nucleoside phosphonate diester analog of adenosine monophosphate. Inhibits activity of HIV-1 RT by competing with natural substrate deoxydenosine 5'-triphosphate and incorporating into DNA, by DNA chain termination.

PHARMACOKINETICS: Absorption: Emtricitabine: Bioavailability (92%); C_{max}=1.8mcg/mL, T_{max}=1-2 hrs, AUC=10mcg•h/mL. Tenofovir disoproxil: Bioavailability (25%), C_{max}=0.3mcg/mL, T_{max}=1 hr, AUC=2.29mcg•h/mL. **Distribution:** Emtricitabine: Plasma protein binding (<4%). Tenofovir disoproxil: Plasma protein binding (<0.7%). **Elimination:** Emtricitabine: Urine (86%); $T_{1/2}$=10 hrs. Tenofovir disoproxil: (IV) Urine (70-80%); $T_{1/2}$=17 hrs.

NURSING CONSIDERATIONS

Assessment: Assess for risk factors for lactic acidosis, liver disease/dysfunction (eg, decompensation, failure), severe acute exacerbation of HBV, renal disease/dysfunction, history of pathologic bone fracture or osteopenia, inflammatory response, HIV status, and possible drug interactions.

Monitoring: Perform routine monitoring of CrCl and serum phosphorus if risk for renal impairment. Monitor hepatic/renal function and bone density. Monitor LFTs for several months after d/c therapy, signs/symptoms of pancreatitis, neuropathy, fat redistribution/accumulation, immune reconstitution syndrome, exacerbation of HBV, lactic acidosis, liver/renal dysfunction.

Patient Counseling: Inform should not be coadministered with drugs containing lamivudine. Seek medical attention if symptoms of pancreatitis, neuropathy, fat redistribution/accumulation, immune reconstitution syndrome, exacerbation of HBV, lactic acidosis, hepatic/renal dysfunction occur.

Administration: Oral route. **Storage:** 25°C (77°F), excursions permitted to 15-30°C (59-86°F).

TUSSIONEX PENNKINETIC

CIII

hydrocodone polistirex - chlorpheniramine polistirex (UCB)

THERAPEUTIC CLASS: Opioid antitussive/antihistamine

INDICATIONS: Relief of cough and upper respiratory symptoms associated with allergy and cold.

DOSAGE: *Adults:* ≥12 yrs: 5mL q12h. Max: 10mL/24 hrs.
Pediatrics: 6-11 yrs: 2.5mL q12h. Max: 5mL/24 hrs.

HOW SUPPLIED: Sus, Extended-Release: (Chlorpheniramine-Hydrocodone) 8mg-10mg/5mL

CONTRAINDICATIONS: Should not be used in children less than 6 years of age due to risk of fatal respiratory depression.

WARNINGS/PRECAUTIONS: May produce dose-related respiratory depression. Caution with pulmonary disease, post-surgery, head injury, intracranial lesions or pre-existing increase in ICP, narrow-angle glaucoma, asthma, BPH, elderly, debilitated, impaired hepatic/renal functions, hypothyroidosis, Addison's disease or urethral stricture. May mask acute abdominal conditions and the clinical course of head injuries. May cause obstructive bowel disease. Consider risk/benefit ratio in pediatrics, especially with croup. Impairment of mental and physical performance.

ADVERSE REACTIONS: Sedation, drowsiness, lethargy, anxiety, dysphoria, euphoria, dizziness, psychotic dependence, rash, pruritus, NV, ureteral spasm, urinary retention, respiratory depression, dryness of the pharynx, tightness of the chest.

INTERACTIONS: Additive CNS depression with narcotics, antipsychotics, antianxiety agents, and alcohol. Increased effect of antidepressant or hydrocodone with MAOIs or TCAs. Concurrent anticholinergics may cause paralytic ileus.

PREGNANCY: Category C, not for use in nursing.

MECHANISM OF ACTION: Hydrocodone: Opioid antitussive/antihistamine; not established. Suspected to act directly on cough center. Chlorpheniramine: H_1-receptor antagonist; possesses anticholinergic and sedative activity. Prevents released histamine from dilating capillaries and causing edema of the respiratory mucosa.

PHARMACOKINETICS: Absorption: Hydrocodone: C_{max}=22.8ng/mL, T_{max}=3.4 hrs. Chlorpheniramine: C_{max}=58.4ng/mL, T_{max}=6.3 hrs. **Elimination:** Hydrocodone: $T_{1/2}$=4 hrs. Chlorpheniramine: $T_{1/2}$=16 hrs.

NURSING CONSIDERATIONS

Assessment: Assess that patient is ≥6 yrs and females are not nursing. Assess use with pulmonary disease, depressed ventilatory functions, post-op patients, presence of head injury, intracranial lesions, increased intracranial pressure, acute abdominal conditions, elderly/debilitated, severe hepatic/renal impairment, hypothyroidism, Addison's disease, prostatic hypertrophy, urethral stricture, and during pregnancy. Assess for drug interactions.

Monitoring: Monitor for signs/symptoms of respiratory depression and development of obstructive bowel disease.

Patient Counseling: Inform medication may produce drowsiness and impair mental/physical abilities; use caution when performing hazardous tasks (eg, operating machinery/driving). Instruct not to dilute with fluids or mix with other drugs.

Administration: Oral route. Shake well before use. **Storage:** 20-25°C (68-77°F); excursions permitted to 15-30°C (59-86°F). Dispense in a well-closed container.

TWINJECT — RX

epinephrine (Verus)

THERAPEUTIC CLASS: Sympathomimetic catecholamine

INDICATIONS: Emergency treatment of severe allergic reactions (type 1) including anaphylaxis to insect stings or bites, allergens, foods, drugs, diagnostic testing substances, as well as idiopathic or exercise-induced anaphylaxis.

DOSAGE: *Adults:* Administer SQ or IM into thigh. 15-30kg: (Twinject 0.15mg) 0.15mg. May repeat if needed. ≥30kg: (Twinject 0.3mg) 0.3mg. May repeat if needed.
Pediatrics: Administer SQ or IM into thigh. 15-30kg: (Twinject 0.15mg) 0.15mg. May repeat if needed. ≥30kg: (Twinject 0.3mg) 0.3mg. May repeat if needed.

HOW SUPPLIED: Inj: (Twinject 0.15mg, Twinject 0.3mg) 1mg/mL

WARNINGS/PRECAUTIONS: Inject into anterolateral aspect of thigh; avoid injecting into hands, feet, or buttock. Avoid IV use. Contains sodium bisulfite. Caution with cardiac arrhythmias, coronary artery or organic heart disease, or HTN. May precipitate/aggravate angina pectoris or produce ventricular arrhythmias with coronary insufficiency or ischemic heart disease. Light-sensitive; store in tube provided.

ADVERSE REACTIONS: Anxiety, apprehensiveness, restlessness, tremor, weakness, dizziness, sweating, palpitations, pallor, nausea, vomiting, headache, respiratory difficulties, HTN.

INTERACTIONS: Monitor for cardiac arrhythmias with cardiac glycosides or diuretics. Effects may be potentiated by TCAs, MAOIs, levothyroxine, and certain antihistamines (notably chlorpheniramine, tripelennamine, diphenhydramine). Cardiostimulating and bronchodilating effects antagonized by β-adrenergic blockers (eg, propranolol). Vasoconstricting and hypertensive effects antagonized by α-adrenergic blockers (eg, phentolamine). Ergot alkaloids and phenothiazines may reverse pressor effects.

PREGNANCY: Category C, safety in nursing not known.

MECHANISM OF ACTION: Acts on α- and β-adrenergic receptors.

NURSING CONSIDERATIONS

Assessment: Assess for arrhythmias, ischemic/organic heart disease, HTN, DM, hyperthyroidism, pregnancy status, Parkinson's disease, and drug interactions (eg, medications that may sensitize heart to arrhythmia such as digitalis).

Monitoring: Monitor BP, HR, blood glucose, signs of cerebral hemorrhage, ventricular arrhythmia, HTN, and anginal pain.

Patient Counseling: Inform about side effects of therapy (eg, increased pulse rate, sense of forceful heartbeat, palpitations, throbbing headache, pallor, anxiety, shakiness). Side effects may subside rapidly, especially with rest, quiet, and recumbency but may be severe or persistent with HTN or hyperthyroidism. Never inject into buttocks or by IV route.

Administration: IM or SQ route. Inject into anterolateral administration. **Storage:** 20-25°C (68-77°F); excursions permitted to 15-30°C (59-86°F). Protect from light. Avoid freezing or refrigeration. Discard if discolored.

TWINRIX — RX

hepatitis A vaccine (inactivated) - hepatitis B (recombinant) (GlaxoSmithKline)

THERAPEUTIC CLASS: Vaccine

INDICATIONS: Active immunization against hepatitis A virus and hepatitis B virus in patients ≥18 yrs of age.

DOSAGE: *Adults:* ≥18 yrs: 3-Dose Schedule: 1mL IM in deltoid region at 0, 1, and 6 months. Alternative 4-Dose Schedule: 1 mL IM in deltoid region on Days 0, 7, and 21-30, followed by booster dose at 12 months.

HOW SUPPLIED: Inj: (Hepatitis A-Hepatitis B) 720 ELISA U-20mcg/mL

CONTRAINDICATIONS: Hypersensitivity to monovalent hepatitis A or B vaccines or any component, including yeast and neomycin.

WARNINGS/PRECAUTIONS: Anaphylaxis reported (rare). Hepatitis A and B have long incubation periods, so vaccine may be ineffective with unrecognized hepatitis. May not prevent disease if protective antibody titers are not achieved. Delay vaccine with moderate to severe acute illness. Caution with thrombocytopenia or bleeding disorders. Suboptimal response may occur in immunocompromised patients. Have epinephrine (1:1000) available.

ADVERSE REACTIONS: Injection-site reactions (soreness, redness, swelling, induration), respiratory infection, headache, fatigue, diarrhea, nausea, fever.

INTERACTIONS: Caution with anticoagulants. Immunosuppressive therapy may reduce response.

PREGNANCY: Category C, caution in nursing.

MECHANISM OF ACTION: Produces immune response against hepatitis A and all subtypes of hepatitis B virus.

NURSING CONSIDERATIONS

Assessment: Assess for hypersensitivity to any component of vaccine, including yeast and neomycin, adverse reactions related to previous vaccination history, potential benefits/risks, bleeding disorders (eg, hemophilia, thrombocytopenia), and possible drug interactions.

Monitoring: Monitor for possible anaphylactoid reactions, injection-site reactions, respiratory infection.

Patient Counseling: Inform about potential benefits/risks; report severe or unusual adverse reactions. Counsel on importance of completing vaccination series.

Administration: IM route. **Storage:** 2-8°C (36-46°F).

TYGACIL — RX

tigecycline (Wyeth)

THERAPEUTIC CLASS: Glycylcycline

INDICATIONS: Treatment of complicated skin and skin structure infections (cSSSI), complicated intra-abdominal infections (cIAI), and community-acquired bacterial pneumonia (CABP) caused by susceptible strains of indicated pathogens in patients ≥18 yrs.

DOSAGE: *Adults:* Initial:100mg IV over 30-60 min then 50mg q12h over 30-60 min for 5-14 days (cSSSI/cIAI) and for 7-14days (CABP). Severe Hepatic Impairment (Child-Pugh C): 100mg IV over 30-60 min then 25mg q12h.

HOW SUPPLIED: Inj: 50mg/5mL

WARNINGS/PRECAUTIONS: Anaphylaxis/anaphylactoid reactions reported. Structurally similar to tetracyclines and may have similar adverse effects: photosensitivity, pseudotumor cerebri, pancreatitis, and anti-anabolic action (may lead to increased BUN, azotemia, acidosis, and hyperphosphatemia). Caution with known hypersensitivity to tetracyclines. May cause fetal harm and permanent tooth discoloration (yellow-gray-brown) when administered during tooth development (last half of pregnancy to 8 yrs). *Clostridium difficile*-associated diarrhea reported. Caution when used for cIAI secondary to clinical apparent intestinal perforations. May result in overgrowth of non-susceptible organisms, including fungi; monitor during therapy.

ADVERSE REACTIONS: NV, diarrhea, abdominal pain, infection, fever, headache, HTN, thrombocythemia, anemia, hypoproteinemia, increased lactic dehydrogenase, increased SGOT, increased SGPT.

INTERACTIONS: Decreased effectiveness of oral contraceptives. Monitor PT with warfarin.

PREGNANCY: Category D, caution in nursing.

MECHANISM OF ACTION: Glycylcycline; inhibits protein translation in bacteria by binding to the 30S ribosomal subunit and blocking entry of amino-acyl tRNA molecules into A site of ribosome.

PHARMACOKINETICS: Absorption: IV infusion of variable doses resulted in different parameters. **Distribution:** V_{ss}=7-9L/kg; plasma protein binding (71-89%). **Metabolism:** Liver. **Elimination:** Bile (primary), urine; $T_{1/2}$(100mg)=27.1 hrs.

NURSING CONSIDERATIONS

Assessment: Assess with known hypersensitivity to tetracycline class of antibiotics, complicated intra-abdominal infections secondary to clinically apparent intestinal perforation. Document indications for therapy, culture and susceptibility testing.

Monitoring: Monitor for signs/symptoms of hypersensitivity reactions (eg, anaphylaxis), PT, pancreatitis, photosensitivity, superinfection, *C. difficile*-associated diarrhea, vaginal candidiasis, benign intracranial HTN, LFTs, renal function, HTN, CBC with platelets and differential, hyperglycemia.

Patient Counseling: Inform of pregnancy risks (eg, fetal harm, discoloration of teeth) and photosensitivity reactions. Inform that therapy treats bacterial, not viral, infections. Take as directed; skipping doses or not completing full course of therapy may decrease effectiveness and increase resistance. May experience diarrhea; notify physician if watery/bloody stools, hypersensitivity reactions, superinfection, or photosensitivity develops.

Administration: IV route. Reconstituted solution should be yellow to orange in color; if not, discard solution. **Storage:** Room temperature for up to 24 hrs (reconstituted). Store refrigerated 2-8°C (36-46°F) up to 45 hrs following immediate transfer of reconstituted solution into IV bag.

TYKERB RX

lapatinib (GlaxoSmithKline)

Severe hepatotoxicity and deaths have been reported.

THERAPEUTIC CLASS: Kinase inhibitor

INDICATIONS: Treatment of patients with advanced or metastatic breast cancer, in combination with capecitabine, whose tumors overexpress HER2 and who received prior therapy including an anthracycline, a taxane, and trastuzumab.

DOSAGE: *Adults:* Usual: 1250mg qd on Days 1-21 continuously with capecitabine 2000mg/m²/day (administered orally in 2 doses 12 hrs apart) on Days 1-14 in a repeating 21-day cycle. Give at least 1 hr before or after a meal (however, give capecitabine with food). ≥Grade 2 LVEF: D/C dose. If LVEF recovers and asymptomatic after 2 weeks, restart at 1000mg/day. Hepatic Impairment (Child-Pugh Class C): Consider dose reduction to 750mg/day. Concomitant Strong CYP3A4 Inhibitors: Avoid use. Concomitant Strong CYP3A4 Inducers: Avoid use and if must coadminister titrate gradually from 1250mg/day up to 4500mg/day based on tolerability. ≥Grade 2 NCI CTC Toxicity: D/C or interrupt dose and restart with 1250mg/day when toxicity <Grade 1. Restart at 1000mg/day if toxicity recurs.

HOW SUPPLIED: Tab: 250mg

WARNINGS/PRECAUTIONS: Decreased left ventricular ejection fraction reported; confirm normal LVEF prior to therapy and evaluate during treatment. Reduce dose in patients with severe hepatic impairment. Severe diarrhea reported; manage with antidiarrheals, replace electrolytes. Prolongs the QT interval in some patients; consider ECG and electrolyte monitoring. Fetal harm may occur if administered to pregnant women; women should not become pregnant during therapy. Has been associated with interstitial lung disease and pneumonitis in monotherapy or in combination with other chemotherapies.

ADVERSE REACTIONS: Diarrhea, NV, stomatitis, dyspepsia, palmar-plantar erythrodysesthesia, rash, dry skin, mucosal inflammation, pain in extremity, back pain, dyspnea, insomnia.

INTERACTIONS: May increase exposure to concomitant drugs metabolized by CYP3A4 or CYP2C8. Avoid coadministration with strong CYP3A4 inhibitors and inducers; if unavoidable, consider dose reduction with concomitant CYP3A4 inhibitors, and gradual dose increase with concomitant CYP3A4 inducers. Levels may increase if given with a P-glycoprotein inhibitor.

PREGNANCY: Category D, not for use in nursing.

MECHANISM OF ACTION: Kinase inhibitor; acts by inhibiting intracellular tyrosine kinase domains of both Epidermal Growth Factor Receptor (EGFR) and Human Epidermal Receptor Type 2 (HER2) receptors.

PHARMACOKINETICS: Absorption: Incomplete and variable. C_{max}=2.43mcg/mL, T_{max}=4 hrs, AUC=36.2mcg•hr/mL. **Distribution**: Plasma protein binding (>99%). **Metabolism**: CYP3A4, CYP3A5. **Elimination**: Feces (27%), urine (<2%); $T_{1/2}$ (single dose, repeated dose)=14.2 hrs, 24 hrs.

NURSING CONSIDERATIONS

Assessment: Assess for severe hepatic impairment, hypokalemia or hypomagnesemia (correct prior to therapy), baseline left ventricular ejection fraction (LVEF), interstitial lung disease, and possible drug interactions.

Monitoring: Continue evaluation of LVEF and electrolyte monitoring during treatment. Monitor for toxicities such as severe diarrhea, palmar-plantar erythrodysesthesia, pulmonary symptoms, and QT prolongation.

T

Patient Counseling: Advise females of childbearing age not to become pregnant during therapy. Notify physician if SOB, palpitations, fatigue, persistent cough, or diarrhea occurs. Report use of any Rx/OTC drugs or herbal products. Instruct to take at least 1 hr before or 1 hr after a meal; take capecitabine with food or within 30 min after food.

Administration: Oral route. **Storage**: 25°C (77°F); excursions permitted to 15-30°C (59-86°F). Keep container tightly closed and out of reach of children.

TYLENOL WITH CODEINE — CIII

codeine phosphate - acetaminophen (Ortho-McNeil)

OTHER BRAND NAMES: Acetaminophen w/Codeine Elixir (Various)

THERAPEUTIC CLASS: Opioid analgesic

INDICATIONS: Relief of mild to moderately severe pain.

DOSAGE: *Adults:* (Tab) Usual: 15-60mg codeine/dose and 300-1000mg APAP/dose up to q4h prn. Max: 60mg codeine/dose, 360mg codeine/day,

and 4g APAP/day. (Elixir): 15mL q4h prn.
Pediatrics: (Elixir): Usual: 7-12 yrs: 10mL tid-qid. 3-6 yrs: 5mL tid-qid.

HOW SUPPLIED: (Codeine-APAP) Elixir: (CV) 12-120mg/5mL; Tab: (#3, CIII) 30-300mg, (#4, CIII) 60-300mg

WARNINGS/PRECAUTIONS: Respiratory depressant effects may be exacerbated with head injury or increased ICP. May obscure head injuries, acute abdominal conditions. Caution in the elderly, debilitated, severe hepatic or renal dysfunction, hypothyroidism, Addison's disease, prostatic hypertrophy, or urethral stricture. Potential for physical dependence, tolerance. Tabs contain sulfites.

ADVERSE REACTIONS: Lightheadedness, dizziness, sedation, SOB, NV, allergic reactions, euphoria, dysphoria, constipation, abdominal pain, pruritus.

INTERACTIONS: Additive CNS depression with narcotic analgesics, antipsychotics, antianxiety agents, alcohol, other CNS depressants. Anticholinergics may produce paralytic ileus.

PREGNANCY: Category C, caution in nursing.

MECHANISM OF ACTION: Codeine: Narcotic analgesic and antitussive; produces centrally-acting analgesic effects. APAP: Nonopiate, nonsalicyclate analgesic and antipyretic.

PHARMACOKINETICS: Absorption: Codeine: Rapidly absorbed. APAP: Rapidly absorbed. **Distribution:** Codeine: Found in liver, spleen, kidneys; crosses blood brain barrier; found in fetal tissue and breast milk. APAP: Found in breast milk. **Metabolism:** APAP: Liver (conjugation). **Elimination:** Codeine: Urine (90%) (parent compound and metabolites); $T_{1/2}$=2.9 hrs. APAP: Urine (85%); $T_{1/2}$=1.25-3 hrs.

NURSING CONSIDERATIONS

Assessment: Assess for head injury or other intracranial lesions, presence of increased ICP, acute abdominal conditions, sulfite hypersensitivity, presence of debilitation (eg, elderly), renal/hepatic impairment, hypothyroidism, urethral stricture, Addison's disease, prostatic hypertrophy, pregnancy/nursing status, and possible drug interactions.

Monitoring: Monitor for signs/symptoms of respiratory depression, elevations in CSF pressure, drowsiness, allergic type reactions (eg, anaphylaxis), elevations in serum amylase levels, medication abuse, and medication dependence. Monitor hepatic/renal function with severe hepatic/renal disease.

Patient Counseling: Inform that drug may be habit forming; take only for as long as prescribed, in amounts prescribed, and no more frequently than prescribed. Advise drug may impair mental/physical abilities required to perform hazardous tasks (eg, operating machinery/driving). Counsel to avoid alcohol and other CNS depressants during therapy. Counsel about possible adverse events if used during pregnancy/nursing.

Administration: Oral route **Storage:** Controlled room temperature 15-30°C (59-86°F). Dispense in tight, light-resistant container.

TYLOX

CII

oxycodone HCl - acetaminophen (Ortho-McNeil)

OTHER BRAND NAMES: Roxilox (Roxane)

THERAPEUTIC CLASS: Opioid analgesic

INDICATIONS: Moderate to moderately severe pain.

DOSAGE: *Adults:* Usual: 1 cap q6h prn.

HOW SUPPLIED: Cap: (Oxycodone-APAP) 5mg-500mg

WARNINGS/PRECAUTIONS: Contains sulfites. Monitor with head injury; may increase respiratory depressant effects and CSF pressure. Caution in elderly, debilitated, severe hepatic or renal dysfunction, hypothyroidism, Addison's disease, prostatic hypertrophy, or urethral stricture. Potential for physical dependence, tolerance. Inappropriate for intractable/severe pain.

ADVERSE REACTIONS: Dizziness, sedation, NV, euphoria, dysphoria, constipation, abdominal pain, pruritus.

INTERACTIONS: Additive CNS depression with alcohol, tranquilizers, sedative-hypnotics, narcotic analgesics, general anesthetics, phenothiazines, antipsychotics, antianxiety agents, other CNS depressants. May produce paralytic ileus with anticholinergics.

PREGNANCY: Category C, caution in nursing.

MECHANISM OF ACTION: Oxycodone: Narcotic analgesic. Produces similiar action to morphine, prominently in CNS and smooth muscle organs. Produces analgesia and sedative effects. APAP: Nonopiate, nonsalicylate analgesic and antipyretic.

NURSING CONSIDERATIONS

Assessment: Assess for sulfite sensitivity, presence of head injury or other intracranial lesions, elevations in ICP, acute abdominal conditions, presence of debilitation, hepatic/renal impairment, hypothyroidism, Addison's disease, prostatic hypertrophy or urethral stricture, pregnancy/nursing status, and possible drug interactions.

Monitoring: Monitor for signs/symptoms of hypersensitivity reactions (eg, anaphylaxis), elevations in CSF pressure, respiratory depression, drug dependence, and drug abuse. Monitor for paralytic ileus if used in combination with anticholinergics.

Patient Counseling: Instruct to report any adverse reactions (eg, allergic reactions, respiratory depression). May impair mental/physical abilities required for the performance of potentially hazardous tasks (eg, operating machinery/driving). May produce dependence and has potential for abuse.

Administration: Oral route. **Storage:** 15-30°C (59-86°F). Protect from moisture. Dispense in tight, light-resistant container.

TYSABRI RX

natalizumab (Biogen Idec/Elan)

Increases risk of progressive multifocal leukoencephalopathy (PML). Because of risk of PML, natalizumab is available only through a special restricted distribution program called the TOUCH™ Prescribing Program. Administer only to patients who are enrolled in and meet all conditions of the TOUCH™ Prescribing Program. Monitor patients for any new signs or symptoms that may be suggestive of PML. Dosing should be withheld immediately at the first sign or symptom suggestive of PML.

THERAPEUTIC CLASS: Monoclonal antibody/VCAM-1 blocker

INDICATIONS: Treatment of patients with relapsing forms of multiple sclerosis (MS) to delay the accumulation of physical disability and reduce the frequency of clinical exacerbations. Treatment for inducing and maintaining clinical response and remission in adult patients with moderately to severely active Crohn's disease (CD) with evidence of inflammation who have had an inadequate response to, or are unable to tolerate, conventional CD therapies and TNF-α inhibitors.

T

DOSAGE: *Adults:* MS/CD: 300mg IV infusion over 1 hr every 4 weeks. (CD) D/C therapy if no therapeutic benefit by 12 weeks, if patient cannot be tapered off corticosteroids within 6 months, or in patients who require additional steroid use that exceeds 3 months within a calendar year to control their CD.

HOW SUPPLIED: Inj: 300mg/15mL

CONTRAINDICATIONS: Progressive multifocal leukoencephalopathy (PML).

WARNINGS/PRECAUTIONS: Possible hypersensitivity reactions, including anaphylaxis. Concurrent use with antineoplastic, immunosuppressive, or immunomodulating agents may further increase the risk of infections. Liver injury reported. Induces increases in circulating lymphocytes, monocytes, eosinophils, basophils, and nucleated RBCs.

ADVERSE REACTIONS: Headache, fatigue, UTI, depression, lower respiratory tract infection, arthralgia, abdominal discomfort, rash, gastroenteritis, vaginitis, allergic reaction, urinary urgency/frequency, irregular menstruation/ dysmenorrhea, dermatitis, abnormal LFTs.

INTERACTIONS: Avoid with concomitant immunosuppresants (eg, 6-mercaptopurine, azathioprine, cyclosporine, or methotrexate) or inhibitors of TNF-α. Taper corticosteroids in CD patients before starting therapy.

PREGNANCY: Category C, caution in nursing.

MECHANISM OF ACTION: Monoclonal antibody; not defined. Binds to α4-subunit of α4β1 and α4β7 integrins expressed on surface of all leukocytes except neutrophils. Inhibits α4-mediated adhesion of leukocytes to their counter-receptor(s).

PHARMACOKINETICS: Absorption: (MS) C_{max}=110mcg/mL; (CD) C_{max}=101mcg/mL. **Distribution:** (MS) V_d=5.7L; (CD) V_d=5.2L. **Elimination:** (MS) $T_{1/2}$=11 days; (CD) $T_{1/2}$=10 days.

NURSING CONSIDERATIONS

Assessment: Assess for risk of progressive multifocal leukoencephalopathy, history of chronic immunosuppressant or immunomodulatory therapy and immunocompromised status, drug hypersensitivity, and drug interactions. MRI should be done prior to initiating therapy in MS.

Monitoring: Monitor for progressive multifocal leukoencephalopathy (eg, progressive weakness on 1 side of body, clumsiness, vision problems, changes in thinking, memory, and orientation leading to confusion and personality changes); a gadolinium-enhanced MRI scan of brain and CSF analysis for JC viral DNA recommended for diagnosis. Monitor for anaphylactic reactions, infections (eg, pneumonia, UTI), opportunistic infections, hepatotoxicity. Antibody testing recommended if presence of persistent antibodies suspected. Monitor CBC, LFTs, and bilirubin.

Patient Counseling: Inform about TOUCH™ Prescribing Program. Educate on risks/benefits. Instruct to report signs of infections, progressive multifocal leukoencephalopathy, hypersensitivity reactions, liver toxicity. Counsel on importance of follow-up schedule (3 and 6 months after 1st infusion, then every 6 months). Inform if pregnant/nursing or planning to become pregnant.

Administration: IV infusion. **Storage:** 2-8°C (36-46°F). Do not shake or freeze.

TYZEKA — RX

telbivudine (Idenix)

Lactic acidosis and severe hepatomegaly with steatosis reported. Discontinuation may result in severe acute exacerbations of hepatitis; monitor hepatic function closely for at least several months following discontinuation of therapy.

THERAPEUTIC CLASS: Nucleoside analogue

INDICATIONS: Treatment of chronic hepatitis B.

DOSAGE: *Adults:* CrCl ≥50mL/min: 600mg qd. CrCl 30-49mL/min: 600mg every 48 hrs. CrCl <30mL/min (not requiring dialysis): 600mg every 72 hrs. ESRD: 600mg every 96 hrs.
Pediatrics: ≥16 yrs: CrCl ≥50mL/min: 600mg qd. CrCl 30-49mL/min: 600mg every 48 hrs. CrCl <30mL/min (not requiring dialysis): 600mg every 72 hrs. ESRD: 600mg every 96 hrs.

HOW SUPPLIED: Tab: 600mg

WARNINGS/PRECAUTIONS: Myopathy reported; interrupt therapy if myopathy suspected and d/c if myopathy diagnosed. Monitor renal function.

ADVERSE REACTIONS: Upper respiratory tract infection, fatigue, malaise, abdominal pain, nasopharyngitis, headache, elevated blood CPK, cough, nausea, vomiting, influenza, flu-like symptoms, diarrhea, loose stools, pharyngolaryngeal pain.

INTERACTIONS: Drugs that alter renal function may alter plasma concentrations of telbivudine.

PREGNANCY: Category B, not for use in nursing.

MECHANISM OF ACTION: Thymidine nucleoside analogue; inhibits HBV DNA polymerase by competing with thymidine 5'-triphosphate and inhibits viral replication by incorporating into viral DNA causing DNA chain termination.

PHARMACOKINETICS: Absorption: C_{max}=3.69mcg/mL, T_{max}=2 hrs, AUC=26.1mcg•h/mL. **Distribution:** Plasma protein binding (3.3%). **Elimination:** Urine; $T_{1/2}$=40-49 hrs.

NURSING CONSIDERATIONS

Assessment: Assess for possible drug interactions and renal impairment.

Monitoring: Monitor LFTs periodically and for several months after d/c. Monitor for signs/symptoms of exacerbation of HBV after d/c, hepatotoxicity, hypersensitivity reactions, and myopathy.

Patient Counseling: Inform of possibility of liver disease deterioration; not shown to reduce risk of HBV transmission to others through sexual contact or blood contamination. Advise not to change dose or d/c without consultation. If dose missed, instruct to take as soon as remembered and next dose at regular time. If almost time for next dose, skip missed dose (do not take 2 doses at same time). Advise to seek medical attention if symptoms of exacerbation, hepatotoxicity, hypersensitivity reactions, or myopathy (eg, myalgia, muscle tenderness, weakness) occur.

Administration: Oral route. **Storage:** 25°C (77°F); excursions permitted to 15-30°C (59-86°F).

ULORIC RX

febuxostat (Takeda)

THERAPEUTIC CLASS: Xanthine oxidase inhibitor

INDICATIONS: Chronic management of hyperuricemia in patients with gout.

DOSAGE: *Adults:* Hyperuricemia with Gout: Initial: 40mg qd. Range: 40-80mg qd. Serum Uric Acid (sUA) >6mg/dL After 2 Weeks at 40mg: 80mg qd.

HOW SUPPLIED: Tab: 40mg, 80mg

CONTRAINDICATIONS: Patients treated with azathioprine, mercaptopurine, or theophylline.

WARNINGS/PRECAUTIONS: May increase risk of gout flares; prophylactic treatment with NSAIDs or colchicine is recommended. Higher rate of CV thromboembolic events (eg, cardiovascular deaths, non-fatal MI, non-fatal strokes) vs. allopurinol reported; monitor for signs and symptoms of MI and stroke. Elevated serum transaminase levels observed; monitor LFTs periodically. Caution with severe hepatic impairment. Avoid with asymptomatic or secondary hyperuricemia (eg, malignant disease, Lesch-Nyhan syndrome).

ADVERSE REACTIONS: Liver function abnormalities, nausea, arthralgia, rash.

INTERACTIONS: See Contraindications. Concomitant use with xanthine oxidase substrates may increase plasma concentrations of these drugs, resulting in severe toxicity.

PREGNANCY: Category C, caution in nursing.

U

MECHANISM OF ACTION: Xanthine oxidase inhibitor; achieves therapeutic effect by decreasing serum uric acid.

PHARMACOKINETICS: Absorption: (40mg) C_{max}= 1.6mcg/mL. (80mg) C_{max}= 2.6mcg/mL. T_{max}=1-1.5 hrs. **Distribution:** V_d=50L; plasma protein binding (99.2%). **Metabolism:** Conjugation via uridine diphosphate glucuronosyltransferase (UGT), and oxidation via CYP450 enzymes. **Elimination:** Hepatic and renal pathways; Urine (49%), feces (45%); $T_{1/2}$=5-8 hrs.

NURSING CONSIDERATIONS

Assessment: Assess for treatment with azathioprine, mercaptopurine, or theophylline, secondary/asymptomatic hyperuricemia, hepatic/renal impairment, possible drug interactions, and pregnancy/nursing status. Assess for sUA, LFTs, and ECG.

Monitoring: Monitor for sUA levels, LFTs, QTc interval, MI, and stroke.

Patient Counseling: May take without regard to food or antacid use. Counsel about potential benefits and risks. Inform that gout flares, elevated liver enzymes, and adverse cardiovascular events may occur. Counsel about concomitant prophylaxis with NSAIDs or colchicine for gout flares. Instruct to notify physician if rash, chest pain, SOB, or neurologic symptoms occur. Advise to inform physician of any other medications currently taking, including OTC drugs.

Administration: Oral route. **Storage:** Store at 25°C (77°F); excursions permitted to 15°-30°C (59°-86°F). Protect from light.

ULTIVA
remifentanil HCl (Abbott)

CII

THERAPEUTIC CLASS: Opioid analgesic

INDICATIONS: As an analgesic agent for use during the induction and maintenance of general anesthesia. For continuation as an analgesic into the immediate postoperative period in adults under the direct supervision of an anesthesia practitioner in a postoperative anesthesia care unit or intensive care setting. As an analgesic component of monitored anesthesia care in adults.

DOSAGE: *Adults:* Continuous IV Infusion: Induction: 0.5-1mcg/kg/min. Maint: 0.4mcg/kg with nitrous oxide 66%; 0.25mcg/kg with isoflurane (0.4-1.25 MAC); 0.25 with propofol (100-200mcg/kg/min). Post-Op Continuation: 0.1mcg/kg/min. CABG: Induction/Maint/Continuation: 1mcg/kg/min. Elderly (>65 yrs): Use 50% of adult dose. Titrate carefully.
Pediatrics: Anesthesia Maint: Continuous IV Infusion: 1-12 yrs: 0.25mcg/kg/min with halothane (0.3-1.5 MAC), sevoflurane (0.3-1.5 MAC, or isoflurane (0.4-1.5 MAC). Range: 0.05-1.3mcg/kg/min. Birth-2 months: 0.4mcg/kg/min. Range: 0.4-1mcg/kg/min.

HOW SUPPLIED: Inj: 1mg, 2mg, 5mg

CONTRAINDICATIONS: Epidural or intrathecal administration, hypersensitivity to fentanyl analogs.

WARNINGS/PRECAUTIONS: Administer only with infusion device. IV bolus administration should be used only during the maintenance of general anesthesia. Interruption of infusion will result in rapid offset of effect. Use associated with apnea and respiratory depression. Not for use in diagnostic or therapeutic procedures outside the monitored anesthesia care setting. Resuscitative and intubation equipment, oxygen, and opioid antagonist must be readily available. May cause skeletal muscle rigidity and is related to the dose and speed of administration. Do not administer into the same IV tubing with blood due to potential inactivation by nonspecific esterases in blood products. Continuously monitor vital signs and oxygenation. Bradycardia, hypotension, intraoperative awareness reported. Not recommended as sole agent for induction of anesthesia.

ADVERSE REACTIONS: NV, hypotension, muscle rigidity, bradycardia, shivering, fever, dizziness, visual disturbances, respiratory depression, apnea.

INTERACTIONS: Synergism with thiopental, propofol, isoflurane, midazolam; reduce doses of these drugs by up to 75%.

PREGNANCY: Category C, caution in nursing.

MECHANISM OF ACTION: Opioid analgesic.

PHARMACOKINETICS: Distribution: V_d=100mL/kg, 350mL/kg (initial, steady-state), plasma protein binding (70%). **Metabolism**: Hydrolysis via nonspecific blood and tissue esterases to carboxylic acid metabolite. **Elimination**: $T_{1/2}$=10-20 min.

NURSING CONSIDERATIONS

Assessment: Assess for pulmonary disease, decreased respiratory reserve, and possible drug interactions.

Monitoring: Monitor for cardiovascular depression (eg, bradycardia, hypotension), respiratory depression, muscle rigidity of neck and extremities, NV, chills, arrhythmias, chest wall rigidity. Monitor vital signs routinely. Appropriate post-op monitoring should ensure adequate spontaneous breathing established and maintained prior to discharge.

Patient Counseling: Advise to use caution while performing potentially hazardous tasks (eg, operating machinery/driving). Counsel about side effects of drug and abuse potential.

Administration: IV infusion. Continuous infusions should only be administered using an infusion device. **Storage**: 2-25°C (36-77°F).

ULTRACET — RX

tramadol HCl - acetaminophen (Ortho-McNeil)

THERAPEUTIC CLASS: Central acting analgesic

INDICATIONS: Short-term management of acute pain.

DOSAGE: *Adults:* 2 tabs q4-6h prn for 5 days or less. Max: 8 tabs/24 hrs. CrCl <30mL/min: Max: 2 tabs q12h.

HOW SUPPLIED: Tab: (Tramadol-APAP) 37.5mg-325mg

CONTRAINDICATIONS: Acute intoxication with any of the following: alcohol, hypnotics, narcotics, centrally-acting analgesics, opioids or psychotropic drugs.

WARNINGS/PRECAUTIONS: Seizures and anaphylactic reactions reported. May complicate acute abdominal conditions. Caution with risk of respiratory depression, increased ICP, or head injury. Avoid abrupt withdrawal. Caution in elderly. Avoid use in opioid-dependent patients and with hepatic impairment.

ADVERSE REACTIONS: Constipation, diarrhea, nausea, somnolence, anorexia, increased sweating, dizziness.

INTERACTIONS: See Contraindications. Caution and reduce dose with CNS depressants (eg, alcohol, opioids, anesthetics, phenothiazines, tranquilizers, sedatives, hypnotics). May need dose adjustment with carbamazepine. Possible digoxin toxicity and altered warfarin effects. Caution with quinidine. CYP2D6 inhibitors (eg, fluoxetine, paroxetine, amitriptyline) may potentiate tramadol. May potentiate seizure risk with MAOIs, SSRIs, naloxone (with overdose), TCAs, tricyclics (eg, cyclobenzaprine, promethazine), neuroleptics, opioids and drugs that lower seizure threshold. Avoid other APAP-containing products and alcohol.

PREGNANCY: Category C, not for use in nursing.

MECHANISM OF ACTION: Tramadol: Centrally acting synthetic opioid analgesic; mechanism not fully understood. Binds to μ-opioid receptors and inhibits reuptake of norepinephrine and serotonin. APAP: Non-opiate, non-salicylate analgesic.

PHARMACOKINETICS: Absorption: Tramadol: Bioavailability (75%), T_{max}=2 hrs, 3 hrs (M1). APAP: Small intestines; T_{max}=1 hr. **Distribution:** (IV) Tramadol: V_d=2.4L/kg (male), 2.9L/kg (female); Plasma protein binding (20%). APAP: V_d=0.9L/kg; Plasma protein binding (20%). **Metabolism:** Tramadol: CYP2D6, 3A4 (N-and O-demethylation, glucuronidation or sulfation); M1 (active metabolite). APAP: CYP2E1, 1A2, 3A4 (conjugation, sulfation, oxidation). **Elimination:** Tramadol: $T_{1/2}$=5-6 hrs, 7 hrs (M1); urine (30%). APAP: $T_{1/2}$=2-3 hrs; urine (<9%).

U

NURSING CONSIDERATIONS

Assessment: Assess for acute intoxication, CNS/respiratory depression, seizures, head trauma, metabolic disorders, CNS infection, acute abdominal conditions, increased ICP, drug abuse, opioid dependence, possible drug interactions, renal/hepatic impairment.

Monitoring: Monitor for signs/symptoms of seizures, respiratory depression, withdrawal symptoms, hepatotoxicity, and hypersensitivity reactions.

Patient Counseling: Caution that drug may impair physical/mental abilities. Instruct to avoid alcohol. Advise to seek medical attention if symptoms of seizures, respiratory depression, hypersensitivity reactions, hepatotoxicity, or withdrawal symptoms (eg, anxiety, sweating, insomnia, rigors) occur.

Administration: Oral route. **Storage:** 25°C (77°F); excursions permitted to 15-30°C (59-86°F).

ULTRAM — RX

tramadol HCl (Ortho-McNeil)

OTHER BRAND NAMES: Ultram ER (PRICARA)

THERAPEUTIC CLASS: Central acting analgesic

INDICATIONS: Management of moderate to moderately severe pain.

DOSAGE: *Adults:* ≥17 yrs: (Tab) Initial: 25mg qam. Titrate: May increase by 25mg every 3 days to 25mg qid, then may increase by 50mg every 3 days to 50mg qid. Usual: 50-100mg q4-6h as needed. Max: 400mg/day. Elderly: Start at low end of dosing range. >75 yrs: Max: 300mg/day. CrCl <30mL/min: Dose q12h. Max: 200mg/day. Cirrhosis: 50mg q12h. ≥18 yrs: (Tab, ER) Initial: 100mg qd. Titrate: May increase by 100mg every 5 days. Max: 300mg/day. Elderly: Start at low end of dosing range. Avoid in CrCl <30mL/min and severe hepatic impairment (Child-Pugh Class C).

HOW SUPPLIED: Tab: 50mg*; Tab, Extended-Release: 100mg, 200mg, 300mg *scored

CONTRAINDICATIONS: Acute intoxication with any of the following: alcohol, hypnotics, narcotics, centrally acting analgesics, opioids or psychotropic drugs.

WARNINGS/PRECAUTIONS: Seizures and anaphylactoid reactions reported. Do not use in opioid-dependent patients. Caution if at risk for respiratory depression, or with increased ICP or head trauma. May complicate acute abdominal conditions. Do not d/c abruptly. Adjust dose with renal or hepatic impairment.

ADVERSE REACTIONS: Dizziness, NV, constipation, headache, somnolence, nervousness, sweating, asthenia, dyspepsia, dry mouth, diarrhea, CNS stimulation, pruritus.

INTERACTIONS: See Contraindications. Caution and reduce dose with CNS depressants (eg, alcohol, opioids, anesthetics, phenothiazines, tranquilizers, sedatives, hypnotics). Avoid with carbamazepine. Possible digoxin toxicity and altered warfarin effects. Caution with quinidine. CYP2D6 inhibitors (eg, fluoxetine, paroxetine, amitriptyline) may potentiate tramadol. May potentiate seizure risk with MAOIs, SSRIs, naloxone (with overdose), TCAs, tricyclics (eg, cyclobenzaprine, promethazine), neuroleptics, opioids and drugs that lower seizure threshold.

PREGNANCY: Category C, not for use in nursing.

MECHANISM OF ACTION: Centrally acting synthetic opioid analgesic; mechanism not fully understood. Shown to inhibit reuptake of norepinephrine and serotonin.

PHARMACOKINETICS: Absorption: Rapid, complete. Bioavailability (75%); T_{max}=2 hrs (drug), 3 hrs (M1). **Distribution:** V_d=2.6L/kg (male), 2.9L/kg (female); plasma protein binding (20%). **Metabolism:** Liver (extensive); through N-and O-demethylation and glucuronidation or sulfation pathways via CYP3A4, 2D6. M1 (active metabolite). **Elimination:** Urine: (30% unchanged), (60% as metabolite); $T_{1/2}$=6.3 hrs (drug), 7.4 hrs (M1).

NURSING CONSIDERATIONS

Assessment: Assess for acute intoxication with alcohol, hypnotics, centrally acting analgesics, opioids, or psychotropic drugs. Assess for epilepsy, risk for seizure (eg, head trauma, metabolic disorders, alcohol and drug withdrawal, CNS infections), risk for respiratory depression, increased ICT, acute abdominal conditions, renal/hepatic impairment, pregnancy/nursing status, and possible drug interactions (eg, MAOIs, SSRIs).

Monitoring: Monitor for anaphylactoid reactions (eg, pruritus, hives, bronchospasm, angioedema, toxic epidermal necrolysis and Stevens-Jonhson syndrome), repiratory/CNS, physical dependence/abuse, seizures, serotonin syndrome, withdrawal symptoms with abrupt d/c (eg, anxiety, sweating, insomnia, rigors, upper respiratory symptoms, diarrhea, piloerection and rarely, hallucinations).

Patient Counseling: Advise to use caution while performing hazardous tasks (operating machinery/driving). Do not take with alcohol, tranquilizers, or hypnotics. Notify physician if pregnant/nursing or planning to become pregnant. Take as prescribed.

Administration: Oral route. **Storage:** 25°C (77°F); excursions permitted to 15-30°C (59-86°F); in tight container.

ULTRAVATE RX

halobetasol propionate (Ranbaxy)

THERAPEUTIC CLASS: Corticosteroid

INDICATIONS: Corticosteroid-responsive dermatoses.

DOSAGE: *Adults:* Apply qd-bid. Rub in gently. Limit treatment to 2 weeks. Max: 50g/week.
Pediatrics: ≥12 yrs: Apply qd-bid. Rub in gently. Limit treatment to 2 weeks. Max: 50g/week.

HOW SUPPLIED: Cre, Oint: 0.05% [15g, 50g]

WARNINGS/PRECAUTIONS: Avoid face, groin, or axillae. Not for treatment of rosacea or perioral dermatitis. May produce reversible HPA axis suppression, manifestations of Cushing's syndrome, hyperglycemia, and glucosuria. Caution when applied to large surface areas or under occlusive dressings. Use appropriate antifungal or antibacterial agent with dermatological infections; d/c if infection does not clear. Pediatrics may be more susceptible to systemic toxicity. Avoid eyes. D/C if irritation occurs. Re-assess if no improvement after 2 weeks.

ADVERSE REACTIONS: Stinging, burning, itching, irritation, dryness, folliculitis, hypertrichosis, acneiform eruptions, hypopigmentation, perioral dermatitis, allergic contact dermatitis, skin maceration, secondary infection, skin atrophy, striae, miliaria.

PREGNANCY: Category C, caution in nursing.

MECHANISM OF ACTION: Corticosteroid; possesses anti-inflammatory, antipruritic, and vasoconstrictive properties. Anti-inflammatory activity not established; suspected to act by induction of phospholipase A_2 inhibitory proteins called lipocortins. Lipocortins control biosynthesis of potent inflammation mediators (eg, prostaglandins, leukotrienes) by inhibiting release of their common precursor, arachidonic acid.

PHARMACOKINETICS: Absorption: Percutaneous; occlusion, inflammation, and other disease states may increase absorption. **Distribution:** Systemically administered corticosteroids appear in breast milk.

NURSING CONSIDERATIONS

Assessment: Assess for pregnancy/nursing status and for presence of concomitant skin infections. Assess that treatment is not for rosacea or perioral dermatitis.

Monitoring: Monitor for signs/symptoms of reversible HPA-axis suppression, Cushing's syndrome, hyperglycemia, glucosuria, treatment-site irritation, allergic contact dermatitis (eg, failure to heal), and for dermatological infections (eg, bacterial, fungal). Monitor for glucocorticosteroid insufficiencies and treat appropriately. If applying to large area or to areas under occlusion, perform periodic monitoring for HPA-axis suppression using ACTH stimulation, AM plasma cortisol, and urinary free cortisol tests. In pediatric patients, monitor for signs/symptoms of systemic toxicity, HPA-axis suppression (linear growth retardation, delayed weight gain), Cushing's syndrome, and intracranial HTN. Monitor for signs of clinical improvement; if no improvement within 2 weeks, reassess diagnosis.

Patient Counseling: Instruct to use externally and as directed; avoid contact with eyes, use on face, groin, or axillae. Counsel not to bandage or wrap treatment area so as to be occlusive unless directed by physician. Instruct to report signs of local adverse reactions (eg, irritation).

Administration: Topical route. **Storage**: 15-30°C (59-86°F).

Unasyn — RX

ampicillin sodium - sulbactam sodium (Pfizer)

THERAPEUTIC CLASS: Semisynthetic penicillin/beta-lactamase inhibitor

INDICATIONS: Treatment of skin and skin structure (SSSI), intra-abdominal, and gynecological infections caused by susceptible microorganisms.

DOSAGE: *Adults:* 1.5-3g (ampicillin+sulbactam) IM/IV q6h. Max: 4g sulbactam/day. Renal Impairment: CrCl ≥30mL/min: 1.5-3g q6-8h. CrCl 15-29mL/min: 1.5-3g q12h. CrCl 5-14mL/min: 1.5-3g q24h.
Pediatrics: ≥1 yr: 300mg/kg/day (ampicillin+sulbactam) IV in equally divided doses q6h. Max: 4g sulbactam/day. ≥40kg: Dose according to adult recommendations.

HOW SUPPLIED: Inj: (Ampicillin-Sulbactam) 1g-0.5g, 2g-1g, 10g-5g

WARNINGS/PRECAUTIONS: Serious, sometimes fatal, hypersensitivity reactions reported with PCN therapy. *Clostridium difficile*-associated diarrhea reported. Increased risk of skin rash with mononucleosis; use alternate agent.

ADVERSE REACTIONS: Injection site pain, thrombophlebitis, diarrhea.

INTERACTIONS: Probenecid increases and prolongs blood levels. Increased incidence of rash with allopurinol. Do not reconstitute with aminoglycosides; may inactivate aminoglycosides.

PREGNANCY: Category B, caution in nursing.

MECHANISM OF ACTION: Ampicillin: Broad-spectrum antibacterial agent; inhibits cell-wall mucopeptide biosynthesis. Sulbactam: Broad-spectrum antibacterial agent; good inhibitory activity against clinically important plasmid mediated β-lactamases most frequently responsible for transferred drug resistance.

PHARMACOKINETICS: Absorption: IV/IM administration of variable doses resulted in different parameters. **Distribution**: Plasma protein binding (28% ampicillin), (38% sulbactam). **Elimination:** Urine (75-80% unchanged); $T_{1/2}$=1 hr.

NURSING CONSIDERATIONS

Assessment: Assess for history of hypersensitivity to cephalosporins/PCNs, pregnancy status, possible drug interactions, hepatic/renal function, hematopoietic function, mononucleosis. Document indications for therapy, culture, and susceptibility testing.

Monitoring: Monitor for signs/symptoms of hypersensitivity reactions (eg, anaphylaxis, urticaria), *C. difficile*-associated diarrhea, agranulocytosis, renal function, serum albumin, LDH, superinfections, and convulsions.

Patient Counseling: Inform that drug only treats bacterial, not viral, infections. Take as directed; skipping doses or not completing full course may decrease effectiveness and increase resistance. May experience diarrhea; contact physician if watery/bloody stools, superinfection, or hypersensitivity reactions occur. Report any adverse reactions.

Administration: IV/IM route. IM: Reconstitute with SWFI or lidocaine 0.5% or 2%. For 1.5g vial, add 3.2mL diluent; withdrawal volume is 4mL. For 3g vial, add 6.4mL diluent; withdrawal volume is 8mL. **Storage:** IM: Use only freshly prepared solutions and administer within 1 hr after preparation. IV: See PI.

UNIPHYL RX

theophylline (Purdue Pharmaceutical)

THERAPEUTIC CLASS: Xanthine bronchodilator

INDICATIONS: Treatment of the symptoms and reversible airflow obstruction associated with chronic asthma and other chronic lung disease (eg, emphysema, chronic bronchitis).

DOSAGE: *Adults:* Initial: 300-400mg qd for 3 days with meals. Titrate: Increase to 400-600mg qd. After 3 days and if needed/tolerated, increase dose according to blood levels. Tab may be split in half; do not chew or crush. Renal Dysfunction/Elderly (>60 yrs): Max: 400mg/day. Conversion from Immediate-Release Theophylline: Give same daily dose as once daily. *Pediatrics:* 12-15 yrs: (<45kg): Initial: 12-14mg/kg/day up to 300mg qd for 3 days with meals. Titrate: Increase to 16mg/kg/day up to 400mg qd. After 3 days if needed/tolerated increase to 20mg/kg/day up to 600mg qd. (>45kg): Follow adult dose schedule. Tab may be split in half; do not chew or crush. Conversion from Immediate-Release Theophylline: ≥12 yrs: Give same daily dose as once daily. Renal Dysfunction: Max: 400mg qd.

HOW SUPPLIED: Tab, Extended-Release: 400mg*, 600mg* *scored

WARNINGS/PRECAUTIONS: Extreme caution in peptic ulcer disease, seizure disorders and/or cardiac arrhythmias (except bradycardia). Caution in neonates, children <1 yr, and the elderly. Caution in pulmonary edema, CHF, fever ≥102°F for 24 hrs, cor pulmonale, hypothyroidism, liver disease, reduced renal function, sepsis, shock, and HTN. If toxicity develops (eg, repetitive vomiting) monitor serum levels and adjust dosage.

ADVERSE REACTIONS: Vomiting, headache, insomnia, diarrhea, restlessness, tremors, hematemesis, hypokalemia, hyperglycemia, tachycardia, hypotension/shock, nervousness, disorientation, arrhythmias, seizures.

INTERACTIONS: Diminished effects with charcoal broiled food, phenytoin, carbamazepine, phenobarbital, hydantoins, rifampin, ritonavir, aminoglutethimide, barbiturates, ketoconazole, sulfinpyrazone, INH, loop diuretics, sympathomimetics, high protein/low carbohydrate diet, St. John's wort. Potentiated by propranolol, allopurinol, erythromycin, troleandomycin, ciprofloxacin, quinolone antibiotics, oral contraceptives, CCBs, corticosteroids, disulfiram, ephedrine, influenza virus vaccine, interferon, macrolides, mexiletine, thiabendazole, thyroid hormones, carbamazepine, loop diuretics.

PREGNANCY: Category C, caution in nursing.

MECHANISM OF ACTION: Methylxanthine; acts via smooth muscle relaxation and suppression of airway response to stimuli. Bronchodilatation suggested to be mediated by inhibiting isozymes of phosphodiesterase. Also increases the force of contraction of diaphragmatic muscles due to enhancement of calcium uptake through adenosine-mediated channel.

PHARMACOKINETICS: Absorption: Rapid, complete; (800 qam, fed) C_{max}=12.1mcg/mL, C_{min}=4.5mcg/mL, T_{max}=8.8 hrs, AUC=203mcg•hr/mL. (600 qd, fed) C_{max}=12.91mcg/mL, C_{min}=5.52mcg/mL, T_{max}=8.62 hrs, AUC=209mcg•hr/mL. Bioavailability Ratio 600/400: 98.8%. **Distribution:** V_d= 0.45L/kg; plasma protein binding (40%). **Metabolism:** Extensive; CYP1A2, 2E1, 3A3; Caffeine and 3-methylxanthine (active metabolites). **Elimination:** Urine (10% unchanged), $T_{1/2}$=8 hrs.

U

NURSING CONSIDERATIONS

Assessment: Assess risk of exacerbation of concurrent conditions (eg, active PUD, seizure disorder, cardiac arrhythmias). Assess use with neonates, children <1 yr, elderly, pulmonary edema, CHF, fever ≥102°F for 24 hrs, cor pulmonale, hypothyroidism, liver disease (eg, cirrhosis, acute hepatitis), reduced renal function, sepsis, shock, and HTN. Assess known hypersensitivity, renal/hepatic functions, and possible drug interactions.

Monitoring: Carefully monitor serum drug levels (target unbound concentration: 6-12mcg/mL) for dose adjustments, drug toxicity, worsening of chronic illness, hepatic dysfunction. Monitor plasma glucose, uric acid, free fatty acids, cholesterol, HDL, LDL, LFTs and urine free cortisol excretion. If toxicity develops (eg, repetitive vomiting), adjust dosage based on serum levels.

Patient Counseling: Instruct to seek medical attention if NV, persistent headache, insomnia, or rapid heartbeat occur. Counsel not to take St. John's wort concurrently; may result in decreased drug levels. Inform to take once daily in morning or evening. Advise to consistently take with/without food, do not chew or crush, and inform physician if new illness (especially if accompanied with persistent fever) or worsening of chronic illness occurs. Advise to inform all physicians of theophylline use especially if medication is being added or removed from treatment.

Administration: Oral route. **Storage:** 25°C (77°F); excursions permitted to 15-30°C (59-86°F).

UNIRETIC RX

moexipril HCl - hydrochlorothiazide (Schwarz)

ACE inhibitors can cause death/injury to developing fetus during 2nd and 3rd trimesters. Stop therapy if pregnancy detected.

THERAPEUTIC CLASS: ACE inhibitor/thiazide diuretic

INDICATIONS: Treatment of hypertension. Not for initial therapy.

DOSAGE: *Adults:* Initial (if not controlled on moexipril/HCTZ monotherapy): Switch to 7.5mg-12.5mg tab, 15mg-12.5mg tab, or 15mg-25mg tab qd. Titrate: May increase after 2-3 weeks. Initial (if controlled on 25mg HCTZ/day with hypokalemia): 3.75mg-6.25mg (1/2 of 7.5mg-12.5mg tab). If excessive reduction with 7.5mg-12.5mg tab, may switch to 3.75mg-6.25mg. Replacement Therapy: Substitute combination for titrated components. Take 1 hr before meals.

HOW SUPPLIED: Tab: (Moexipril-HCTZ) 7.5mg-12.5mg*, 15mg-12.5mg*, 15mg-25mg* *scored

CONTRAINDICATIONS: History of ACE inhibitor-associated angioedema, anuria, sulfonamide hypersensitivity.

WARNINGS/PRECAUTIONS: D/C if angioedema, jaundice, or if marked LFT elevation occurs. Intestinal angioedema reported. Risk of hyperkalemia with DM, renal dysfunction. Persistent nonproductive cough reported. Monitor WBCs in renal and collagen vascular disease. Anaphylactoid reactions reported. Fetal/neonatal morbidity and death reported. Monitor for hypotension in high-risk patients (eg, surgery/anesthesia, volume/salt depletion). Caution in elderly, CHF, renal or hepatic dysfunction. More reports of angioedema in blacks than nonblacks. May exacerbate or activate SLE. Monitor electrolytes. Avoid if CrCl ≤40mL/min/1.73m^2. May increase cholesterol, TG. Hypercalcemia, hypomagnesemia, hyperuricemia may occur.

ADVERSE REACTIONS: Cough, dizziness, fatigue.

INTERACTIONS: Increase risk of hyperkalemia with K^+-sparing diuretics, K^+ supplements, or K^+-containing salt substitutes. Potentiates orthostatic hypotension with alcohol, barbiturates, and narcotics. Adjust antidiabetic drugs. Reduced absorption with cholestyramine, colestipol. Corticosteroids, ACTH deplete electrolytes. May decrease response to pressor amines. Potentiates other antihypertensives. May increase responsiveness to skeletal muscle relaxants. Risk of lithium toxicity. NSAIDs reduce effects. Increased absorption of HCTZ with guanabenz and propantheline.

PREGNANCY: Category C (1st trimester) and D (2nd and 3rd trimesters), not for use in nursing.

MECHANISM OF ACTION: Moexipril: ACE inhibitor; inhibition results in decreased plasma angiotensin II, leading to decreased vasopressor activity and decreased aldosterone secretion. HCTZ: Thiazide diuretic; affects renal tubular mechanism of electrolyte reabsorption, directly increasing excretion of Na^+ and Cl^-.

PHARMACOKINETICS: Absorption: Moexipril: Incomplete, T_{max}=0.8 hrs. **Distribution:** Moexiprilat: V_d=2.8L/kg; plasma protein binding (50%). HCTZ: V_d=1.5-4.2L/kg; plasma protein binding (21-24%). **Metabolism:** Moexiprilat (active metabolite). **Elimination**: Moexipril: Urine (24%), feces (20%); $T_{1/2}$=2-9 hrs (Moexiprilat). HCTZ: Renal excretion; $T_{1/2}$=5.6-14.8 hrs.

NURSING CONSIDERATIONS

Assessment: Assess BP, LFTs, renal function, CHF, renal artery stenosis, SLE, serum electrolytes, pregnancy status, history of allergy to sulfonamides, bronchial asthma, parathyroid disorders, and possible drug interactions.

Monitoring: Monitor BP, LFTs, renal function, CBC with platelet count and differential, serum electrolytes. Monitor for MI, CHF, angioedema of head, neck, or intestines, anaphylactoid reactions, hepatic failure, hyperuricemia, hyperglycemia, hypersensitivity reactions, cough, N/V, dizziness, Stevens-Johnson syndrome.

Patient Counseling: Inform about fetal risks if taken during pregnancy. Caution that inadequate fluid intake, excessive perspiration, diarrhea, or vomiting can lead to excessive fall in BP, with same consequences of lightheadedness and possible syncope. Advise not to use K^+ supplements or salt substitutes containing K^+ without consulting physician. Counsel about signs/symptoms of neutropenia (eg, infections, sore throat, fever), angioedema, electrolyte imbalance (eg, thirst, weakness, lethargy), and other adverse effects; advise to seek prompt medical attention if any occur. Instruct to take medication 1 hr before meals.

Administration: Oral route. **Storage:** 20-25°C (68-77°F). Protect from excessive moisture.

UNITHROID RX

levothyroxine sodium (Lannett)

THERAPEUTIC CLASS: Thyroid replacement hormone

INDICATIONS: Hypothyroidism. As a pituitary TSH suppressant in the treatment and prevention of euthyroid goiters, including thyroid nodules, lymphocytic thyroiditis, and multinodular goiter. Adjunct to surgery and radioiodine therapy for thyrotropin-dependent well-differentiated thyroid cancer.

DOSAGE: *Adults:* Take in AM at least 1/2-1 hr before food. Hypothyroid: Usual: 1.7mcg/kg/day. >200mcg/day (seldom). >50 yrs/<50 yrs with Cardiac Disease: Initial: 25-50mcg/day. Titrate: Increase by 12.5-25mcg/day every 6-8 weeks until euthyroid. Elderly with Cardiac Disease: Initial: 12.5-25mcg/day. Titrate: Increase by 12.5-25mcg/day every 4-6 weeks until euthyroid. Severe Hypothyroidism: Initial: 12.5-25mcg/day. Titrate: Increase by 25mcg/day every 2-4 weeks until euthyroid. Pregnancy: May increase dose requirements. Subclinical Hypothyroidism: Lower doses required.
Pediatrics: Take in AM at least 1/2-1 hr before food. Hypothyroidism: 0-3 months: 10-15mcg/kg/day. 3-6 months: 8-10mcg/kg/day. 6-12 months: 6-8mcg/kg/day. 1-5 yrs: 5-6mcg/kg/day. 6-12 yrs: 4-5mcg/kg/day. >12 yrs: 2-3mcg/kg/day. Growth/Puberty Complete: 1.7mcg/kg/day. Cardiac Risk: Initial: Use lower dose. Titrate: Increase dose every 4-6 weeks until euthyroid. Infants with Serum T_4 <5mcg/dL: Initial: 50mcg/day. Chronic/Severe Hypothyroidism: Children: Initial: 25mcg/day. Titrate: Increase by 25mcg/day every 2-4 weeks until desired effect. Minimize Hyperactivity in Older Children: Initial: Give 1/4 of full replacement dose. Titrate: Increase by same amount weekly until full dose achieved. May crush tab and mix with 5-10mL water.

HOW SUPPLIED: Tab: 25mcg*, 50mcg*, 75mcg*, 88mcg*, 100mcg*, 112mcg*, 125mcg*, 150mcg*, 175mcg*, 200mcg*, 300mcg* *scored

CONTRAINDICATIONS: Untreated thyrotoxicosis, acute MI, uncorrected adrenal insufficiency.

WARNINGS/PRECAUTIONS: Do not use in the treatment of obesity; larger doses in euthyroid patients can cause serious or even life threatening toxicity. Caution with cardiovascular disease, CAD, adrenal insufficiency, autonomous thyroid tissue, hypothalamic/pituitary hormone deficiencies, and the elderly with risk of occult cardiac disease. Carefully titrate dose to avoid over or under treatment. Decreased bone mineral density with long term use. With adrenal insufficiency supplement with glucocorticoids before therapy.

INTERACTIONS: Sympathomimetics may increase risk of coronary insufficiency with CAD. Upward dose adjustments needed for insulin and oral hypoglycemic agents. Decreased absorption with soybean flour (infant formula), cotton seed meal, walnuts, and fiber. May potentiate oral anticoagulant effects; adjust dose and monitor PT/INR. May decrease levels and effects of digitalis glycosides. Cholestyramine, colestipol, ferrous sulfate, aluminum hydroxide, sodium polystyrene, soybean flour, sucralfate may decrease absorption. Reduced TSH secretion with dopamine/dopamine agonists, glucocorticoids, octreotide. Decreased thyroid hormone secretion with aminoglutethimide, amiodarone, iodine (including iodine-containing radiographic contrast agents), lithium, methimazole, PTU, sulfonamides, tolbutamide. Increased thyroid hormone secretion with amiodarone, iodide (including iodine-containing radiographic contrast agents). Decreased T_4 absorption with antacids (aluminum & magnesium hydroxides), simethicone, bile acid sequestrants (cholestyramine, colestipol), calcium carbonate, cation exchange resins (eg, Kayexalate), ferrous sulfate, sucralfate. Increased serum TBG concentration with clofibrate, estrogens, heroin/methadone, 5-FU, mitotane, tamoxifen. Decreased serum TBG concentration with androgens/anabolic steroids, asparaginase, glucocorticoids, nicotinic acid (slow-release). Protein-binding site displacement with furosemide, heparin, hydantoins, NSAIDs, salicylates. Increased hepatic metabolism with carbamazepine, hydantoins, phenobarbital, rifampin. Decreased conversion of T_4 to T_3 levels with amiodarone, β-adrenergic antagonists (propranolol >160mg/day), glucocorticoids (dexamethasone >4mg/day), PTU. Additive effects of both agents with antidepressants. Interferon-(alpha) may cause development of antithyroid microsomal antibodies causing transient hypothyroidism, hyperthyroidism, or both. Interleukin-2 has been associated with transient painless thyroiditis. Excessive use with growth hormones may accelerate epiphyseal closure. Ketamine use may produce marked HTN and tachycardia. May reduce uptake of iodine-containing radiographic contrast agents. Altered levels of thyroid hormone and/or TSH level with choral hydrate, diazepam, ethionamide, lovastatin, metoclopramide, 6-mercaptopurine, nitroprusside, para-aminosalicylate sodium, perphenazine, resorcinol (excessive topical use), thiazide diuretics.

PREGNANCY: Category A, caution in nursing.

MECHANISM OF ACTION: Thyroid hormone; not understood, suspected to control DNA transcription and protein synthesis.

PHARMACOKINETICS: Distribution: Plasma protein binding (99%), found in breast milk. **Metabolism:** Liver via sequential deiodination (major pathway), conjugation in liver (mainly), kidneys, other tissues. **Elimination:** Urine, feces (20% unchanged); (T_4) $T_{1/2}$=6-7 days, (T_3) $T_{1/2}$≤2days.

NURSING CONSIDERATIONS

Assessment: Assess for suppressed serum TSH with normal T_3 and T_4 levels, overt thyrotoxicosis, thyroid diseases (eg, nontoxic diffuse or nodular goiter), endocrine disorders (eg, hypothalmic/pituitary hormone deficiencies, autoimmune polyglandular disorders), infants for congenital anomalies, cardiovascular diseases (eg, angina pectoris, acute MI), DM, hypersensitivity history, clotting status, upcoming surgery, and for possible drug and test interactions.

U

Monitoring: Perform frequent lab tests and clinical evaluations of thyroid functions (TSH and free T_4 levels, lipid metabolism, blood/urinary glucose in DM, clotting parameters). Monitor cardiovascular signs (eg, arrhythmias, coronary insufficiency), growth/development, bone metabolism, cognitive function, emotional status, GI functions, reproductive functions, partial hair loss in infants, and signs/symptoms of thyroid toxicity.

Patient Counseling: Inform that drug is to be taken for life and not for treatment of obesity or weight loss. Take on empty stomach, 1 hr before breakfast with full glass of water. Notify physician if pregnant/nursing or planning to become pregnant. Notify if taking any other drugs. Do not d/c or change dosage unless directed by physician. Report any signs/symptoms of thyroid toxicity to physician.

Administration: Oral route. **Storage**: 20-25°C (68-77°F); excursions permitted to 15-30°C (59-86°F).

UNIVASC RX
moexipril HCl (Schwarz)

ACE inhibitors can cause death/injury to developing fetus during 2nd and 3rd trimesters. Stop therapy if pregnancy detected.

THERAPEUTIC CLASS: ACE inhibitor

INDICATIONS: Treatment of hypertension.

DOSAGE: *Adults:* If possible, d/c diuretic 2-3 days prior to therapy. Take 1 hr before meals. Initial: 7.5mg qd, 3.75mg with concomitant diuretic therapy. Maint: 7.5-30mg/day given qd-bid. Resume diuretic if BP not controlled. Max: 60mg/day. CrCl ≤40mL/min: Initial: 3.75mg qd. Max: 15mg/day.

HOW SUPPLIED: Tab: 7.5mg*, 15mg* *scored

CONTRAINDICATIONS: History of ACE inhibitor-associated angioedema.

WARNINGS/PRECAUTIONS: D/C if angioedema, jaundice, or if marked LFT elevation occurs. Intestinal angioedema reported. Risk of hyperkalemia with DM, renal dysfunction. Persistent nonproductive cough reported. Monitor WBCs in renal and collagen vascular disease. Anaphylactoid reactions reported. Fetal/neonatal morbidity and death reported. Monitor for hypotension in high-risk patients (heart failure, surgery/anesthesia, prolonged diuretic therapy, volume and/or salt depletion, etc.). Caution with CHF, renal dysfunction, and renal artery stenosis. Less effective on BP in blacks and more reports of angioedema than nonblacks.

ADVERSE REACTIONS: Cough, dizziness, diarrhea, flu syndrome, fatigue, pharyngitis, flushing, rash, myalgia.

INTERACTIONS: May increase lithium levels. Hypotension risk with diuretics. Increased risk of hyperkalemia with K^+-sparing diuretics, K^+-containing salt substitutes, or K^+ supplements.

PREGNANCY: Category C (1st trimester) and D (2nd and 3rd trimesters), not for use in nursing.

MECHANISM OF ACTION: ACE inhibitor; inhibition results in decreased plasma angiotensin II, which leads to decreased vasopressor activity and decreased aldosterone secretion.

PHARMACOKINETICS: Absorption: Incomplete; T_{max}=90 min (moexiprilat). **Distribution:** Moexiprilat: V_d=183L; plasma protein binding (80%). **Metabolism:** Moexiprilat (active metabolite). **Elimination:** Moexiprilat: Urine (7%), feces (52%); $T_{1/2}$=2-9 hrs.

NURSING CONSIDERATIONS

Assessment: Assess BP, LFTs, renal function, CHF, renal artery stenosis, pregnancy status, and possible drug interactions.

Monitoring: Monitor BP, LFTs, renal function, CBC with platelet count and differential, serum K^+ levels. Monitor for MI, CHF, head/neck and intestinal angioedema, anaphylactoid reactions, hepatic failure, hypersensitivity reactions, cough, NV, dizziness.

Patient Counseling: Counsel about fetal risks during pregnancy and signs/symptoms of angioedema (eg, laryngeal/tongue edema, abdominal pain); advise to seek prompt medical attention if symptoms develop. Inform about adverse effects (eg, anaphylaxis, cough, hypotension, hyperkalemia). Infants with histories of in utero exposure should be closely observed for hypotension, oliguria, hyperkalemia. Inform about need for periodic monitoring of electrolytes and blood counts. Caution that inadequate fluid intake, excessive perspiration, diarrhea, vomiting may lead to excessive fall in BP, resulting in lightheadedness and possible syncope. Advise not to use K^+ supplements or salt substitutes. Instruct to take 1 hr before meals.

Administration: Oral route. **Storage:** Room temperature; protect from excessive moisture.

UROXATRAL
alfuzosin HCl (Sanofi-Aventis) **RX**

THERAPEUTIC CLASS: $Alpha_1$-antagonist

INDICATIONS: Treatment of signs and symptoms of benign prostatic hyperplasia.

DOSAGE: *Adults:* 10mg qd, taken immediately after same meal each day.

HOW SUPPLIED: Tab, Extended-Release: 10mg

CONTRAINDICATIONS: Moderate or severe hepatic insufficiency. Concomitant potent CYP3A4 inhibitors (eg, ketoconazole, itraconazole, ritonavir).

WARNINGS/PRECAUTIONS: Increase risk of hypotension/postural hypotension and syncope; monitor for any occurrences. Rule out prostate cancer and BPH. D/C with new or worsening angina. Caution with severe renal insufficiency. Caution in patients with congenital or aquired QT prolongation.

ADVERSE REACTIONS: Dizziness, upper respiratory tract infection, headache, fatigue, urticaria, angioedema, pruritus, rhinitis, tachycardia, chest pain, priapism, diarrhea, flushing, edema, angina pectoris.

INTERACTIONS: Increased levels with potent CYP3A4 inhibitors (eg, ketoconazole, itraconazole, ritonavir); concomitant use is contraindicated. Avoid use with other α-blockers. Increased levels with cimetidine, diltiazem, atenolol. Possibility of significant hypotension with other antihypertensives. Caution with medications which prolong the QT interval.

PREGNANCY: Category B, not for use in nursing.

MECHANISM OF ACTION: Post-synaptic α_1-adrenoreceptor antagonist; inhibits adrenoreceptors in lower urinary tract causing smooth muscle in bladder neck and prostate to relax resulting in improved urine flow and decreased symptoms of BPH.

PHARMACOKINETICS: Absorption: Absolute bioavailability (49%); C_{max}=13.6ng/mL; T_{max}=8 hrs; AUC=194ng•hr/mL. **Distribution:** V_d=3.2L/kg; plasma protein binding (82-90%). **Metabolism:** CYP3A4 (Oxidation, O-demethylation, N-dealkylation). **Elimination:** Urine (11%); $T_{1/2}$=10 hrs.

NURSING CONSIDERATIONS

Assessment: Assess for symptomatic hypotension, prostate cancer, BPH, history of QT prolongation, hepatic/renal impairment, possible drug interactions, and pregnancy/nursing status.

Monitoring: Monitor for postural hypotension (syncope), hypersensitivity reactions, QT prolongation, hepatic/renal dysfunction.

Patient Counseling: Advise to take after same meal each day; do not chew or crush. Caution while driving, operating machinery, or performing hazardous tasks. Notify physician if symptoms of postural hypotension, CV effects, hypersensitivity reactions, or hepatic/renal dysfunction occur.

Administration: Oral route. **Storage:** 25°C (77°F); excursions permitted to 15-30°C (59-86°F). Protect from light and moisture.

VAGIFEM
estradiol (Novo Nordisk) **RX**

Estrogens increase the risk of endometrial cancer.

THERAPEUTIC CLASS: Estrogen

INDICATIONS: Treatment of atrophic vaginitis.

DOSAGE: *Adults:* Initial: Insert 1 tab vaginally qd for 2 weeks. Maint: Insert 1 tab twice weekly. Attempt to d/c or taper at 3-6 month intervals.

HOW SUPPLIED: Tab, Vaginal: 25mcg

CONTRAINDICATIONS: Breast carcinoma or other estrogen dependent neoplasia, abnormal genital bleeding, pregnancy, porphyria, thrombophlebitis, thromboembolic disorders. History of thrombophlebitis, thrombosis, or thromboembolic disorders associated with estrogen use.

WARNINGS/PRECAUTIONS: Risk of gallbladder disease, thromboembolism, thrombotic disease. Elevated BP and hepatic adenomas reported. Monitor for hypercalcemia in breast cancer and bone metastases. Caution in asthma, epilepsy, migraine, cardiac or renal dysfunction due to fluid retention. Excessive uterine bleeding and mastodynia reported. Caution in liver dysfunction, metabolic bone disease associated with hypercalcemia, diabetes. May cause hypercoagulability and hyperlipoproteinemia. Caution in young patients.

ADVERSE REACTIONS: Vaginal spotting, vaginal discharge, allergic reactions, headache, abdominal pain, respiratory infection, genital moniliasis, back pain, rash.

PREGNANCY: Category X, caution in nursing.

MECHANISM OF ACTION: Estrogen (estradiol); binds and activates estrogen receptors, regulating growth, differentiation and functioning of different tissues within and outside reproductive system.

PHARMACOKINETICS: Absorption: C_{max}=50pg/mL. **Metabolism:** Liver; estrone, estriol (metabolites). **Elimination:** Urine.

NURSING CONSIDERATIONS

Assessment: Assess for abnormal genital bleeding, strong family history of breast cancer, abnormal mammograms, breast nodules, known/suspected breast or estrogen-dependent neoplasia, cerebral vascular disease, thromboembolic disorders, CAD, DM, atrophic vaginal mucosa, porphyria, asthma, epilepsy, migraine, vaginal infections, fibrocystic disease, cardiac, hepatic/renal impairment, pregnancy status, and possible drug interactions. Perform exam of breast, abdomen, and pelvic organs; obtain baseline Pap smear and BP.

Monitoring: Monitor BP periodically; perform exams routinely. Monitor for abnormal vaginal bleeding, gallbladder disease, hepatic adenoma, HTN, hyperglycemia, fluid retention, trauma from applicator, hypercalcemia, hepatic dysfunction, and hypersensitivity reactions.

Patient Counseling: Advise to seek medical attention for symptoms of abnormal vaginal bleeding, gallbladder disease, hepatic adenoma (abdominal pain/tenderness, abdominal mass), HTN, hyperglycemia, fluid retention, trauma from applicator, hypercalcemia, hepatic dysfunction (eg, jaundice), or hypersensitivity reactions. Instruct to insert applicator carefully if atrophic vaginal mucosa present.

Administration: Intravaginal route. **Storage:** 25°C (77°F); excursions permitted to 15-30°C (59-86°F).

VALCYTE — RX

valganciclovir HCl (Roche Labs)

V

Granulocytopenia, anemia, and thrombocytopenia reported. Carcinogenic, teratogenic, and may cause aspermatogenesis based on animal studies.

THERAPEUTIC CLASS: Synthetic guanine derivative nucleoside analogue

INDICATIONS: Treatment of cytomegalovirus (CMV) retinitis in AIDS patients. Prevention of CMV disease in kidney, heart, and kidney-pancreas transplant patients at high risk (Donor CMV seropositive/recipient CMV seronegative).

DOSAGE: *Adults:* Treatment of CMV retinitis: Initial: 900mg bid for 21 days. Maint: 900mg qd. Prevention of CMV disease: 900mg qd starting within 10 days of transplantation until 100 days post-transplantation. CrCl 40-59mL/min: Initial: 450mg bid. Maint: 450mg qd. CrCl 25-39mL/min: Initial: 450mg qd. Maint: 450mg every 2 days. CrCl 10-24mL/min: Initial: 450mg every 2 days. Maint: 450mg twice weekly. CrCl <10mL/min: Not recommended. Take with food.

HOW SUPPLIED: Tab: 450mg

CONTRAINDICATIONS: Hypersensitivity to ganciclovir.

WARNINGS/PRECAUTIONS: Avoid if the neutrophils <500cells/mcL, platelet count <25,000/mcL or hemoglobin >8g/dL. Severe leukopenia, neutropenia, anemia, thrombocytopenia, pancytopenia, bone marrow depression, and aplastic anemia observed. Adjust dose in renal impairment. Do not substitute with ganciclovir caps. May cause temporary or permanent inhibition of spermatogenesis.

ADVERSE REACTIONS: Diarrhea, NV, graft rejection, abdominal pain, pyrexia, headache, neutropenia, leukopenia, anemia, insomnia, peripheral neuropathy, HTN.

INTERACTIONS: Greater risk for neutropenia and anemia with zidovudine. Monitor for toxicity with probenecid. Increased levels of metabolites of both drugs with mycophenolate mofetil. Increased risk of didanosine toxicity. Caution with myelosuppressive drugs or irradiation.

PREGNANCY: Category C, not for use in nursing.

MECHANISM OF ACTION: Guanine derivative; inhibits viral DNA synthesis, resulting in inhibition of human CMV replication.

PHARMACOKINETICS: Absorption: Absolute bioavailability (59.4%); C_{max}=5.61mcg/mL; T_{max}=1-3 hrs; AUC=29.1mcg•h/mL. **Distribution:** (Ganciclovir) V_d=0.703L/kg; plasma protein binding (1-2%). **Metabolism:** Intestinal wall, liver (hydrolysis). **Elimination:** Renal; $T_{1/2}$=4.08 hrs.

NURSING CONSIDERATIONS

Assessment: Assess for renal impairment, pre-existing cytopenia, pregnancy/nursing status, prior/current irradiation, or use of myelosuppressive drugs. Obtain baseline neutrophil (≥500cells/µL), platelet (≥25000/µL), and Hgb (≥8g/dL) count.

Monitoring: Monitor CBC and renal function (SrCr) frequently. Perform ophthalmologic exams every 4-6 weeks during therapy. Monitor for signs/symptoms of drug toxicity (eg, granulocytopenia, anemia, thrombocytopenia), infertility, renal dysfunction, and hypersensitivity reactions.

Patient Counseling: Instruct to take with food; do not break or crush. Avoid direct contact of broken or crushed tab with skin or mucous membranes; if contact occurs, wash thoroughly with soap and water. Advise to use effective contraception and practice barrier contraception during and for ≥90 days following therapy due to pregnancy risks. Strict adherence to dosage recommendations is essential to avoid OD; cannot be substituted for ganciclovir caps on 1:1 basis. Inform of major toxicities (eg, anemia, granulocytopenia, thrombocytopenia). Caution may impair physical/mental abilities.

Administration: Oral route. **Storage:** 25°C (77°F); excursions permitted to 15-30°C (59-86°F).

VALIUM

CIV

diazepam (Roche Labs)

V

THERAPEUTIC CLASS: Benzodiazepine

INDICATIONS: Management of anxiety disorders and short-term relief of anxiety symptoms. Symptomatic relief of acute alcohol withdrawal. Adjunct therapy in skeletal muscle spasm and convulsive disorders.

DOSAGE: *Adults:* Anxiety: 2-10mg bid-qid. Alcohol Withdrawal: 10mg tid-qid for 24 hours. Maint: 5mg tid-qid prn. Skeletal Muscle Spasm: 2-10mg tid-qid: Seizure Disorders: 2-10mg bid-qid. Elderly/Debilitated: 2-2.5mg qd-bid initially; may increase gradually as needed and tolerated.
Pediatrics: ≥6 months: 1-2.5mg tid-qid initially; may increase gradually as needed and tolerated.

HOW SUPPLIED: Tab: 2mg*, 5mg*, 10mg* *scored

CONTRAINDICATIONS: Acute narrow-angle glaucoma, untreated open-angle glaucoma, patients <6 months.

WARNINGS/PRECAUTIONS: Monitor blood counts and LFTs in long-term use. Neutropenia and jaundice reported. Increase in grand mal seizures reported. Avoid abrupt withdrawal. Caution with kidney or hepatic dysfunction.

ADVERSE REACTIONS: Drowsiness, fatigue, ataxia, paradoxical reactions, minor EEG changes.

INTERACTIONS: Phenothiazines, narcotics, barbiturates, MAOIs, and other antidepressants may potentiate effects. Delayed clearance with cimetidine. Avoid alcohol and other CNS-depressants. Risk of seizure with flumazenil.

PREGNANCY: Not for use during pregnancy, safety in nursing not known.

MECHANISM OF ACTION: Benzodiazepine; exerts anxiolytic, sedative, muscle-relaxant, anticonvulsant and amnestic effect. Facilitates GABA, an inhibitory neurotransmitter in CNS.

PHARMACOKINETICS: Absorption: T_{max}=0.25-2.5 hrs. **Distribution:** V_d=0.8-1.0 L/kg, plasma protein binding (98%), crosses blood-brain and placental barrier, appears in breast milk. **Metabolism:** Via N-desmethylation, hydroxylation, glucuronidation to N-desmethyldiazepam, temazepam, oxazepam by CYP3A4, CYP2C19 enzymes. **Elimination:** Urine; $T_{1/2}$=48 hrs, $T_{1/2}$(N-desmethyldiazepam)=100 hrs.

NURSING CONSIDERATIONS

Assessment: Assess for acute narrow-angle glaucoma; renal, hepatic, and pulmonary function; pregnancy status. Note other diseases/conditions and drug therapies.

Monitoring: Monitor hypersensitivity reactions, rebound or withdrawal symptoms, seizures, renal function tests, LFTs, pulmonary function tests, HR, insomnia.

Patient Counseling: Avoid alcohol, sedatives. Caution while operating machinery/driving. Counsel about drug abuse/dependence and side effects, report if any occur.

Administration: Oral route. **Storage:** 15-30°C (59-86°F). Dispense in tight, light-resistant containers.

VALTREX — RX

valacyclovir HCl (GlaxoSmithKline)

THERAPEUTIC CLASS: Nucleoside analogue

INDICATIONS: Treatment of herpes zoster (shingles) and herpes labialis (cold sores). Treatment of initial and recurrent episodes of genital herpes in immunocompetent adults, chronic suppressive therapy of recurrent episodes of genital herpes in immunocompetent and in HIV-infected adults, and reduction of transmission of genital herpes in immunocompetent adults. Treatment of chickenpox in immunocompetent patients ≥2 yrs.

DOSAGE: *Adults:* Herpes Zoster: 1g q8h for 7 days. Start within 48 hrs after onset of rash. CrCl 30-49mL/min: 1g q12h. CrCl 10-29mL/min: 1g q24h. CrCl <10mL/min: 500mg q24h. Genital Herpes: Initial: 1g q12h for 10 days. Start within 48 hrs after onset of symptoms. CrCl ≤10-29mL/min: 1g q24h. CrCl <10mL/min: 500mg q24h. Recurrent Episodes: Treatment: 500mg q12h for 3 days. Start at the 1st sign or symptom of episode. CrCl ≤10-29mL/min: 500mg q24h. Suppressive Therapy with Normal Immune Function: 1g q24h. CrCl ≤10-29mL/min: 500mg q24h. Alternative: (≤9 episodes/yr) 500mg q24h. CrCl ≤10-29mL/min: 500mg q48h. Suppressive Therapy with HIV and CD4 ≥100cells/mm³: 500mg q12h. CrCl ≤10-29mL/min: 500mg q24h. Reduction of Transmission of Genital Herpes (≤9 episodes/yr): 500mg qd for the source partner. Herpes Labialis: 2g q12h for 1 day. Start at earliest symptom of cold sore. CrCl 30-49mL/min: 1g q12h. CrCl 10-29mL/min: 500mg q12h. <10mL/min: 500mg single dose. Administer therapy for 1 day. Initiate at earliest

symptom of cold sore.
Pediatrics: Herpes Labialis: ≥12 yrs: 2g q12h for 1 day. Start at earliest symptom of cold sore. Chickenpox: 2 to <18 yrs: 20mg/kg q8h for 5 days. Max 1g q8h. Initiate at the earliest sign or symptom of chickenpox.

HOW SUPPLIED: Tab: 500mg, 1g

CONTRAINDICATIONS: Acyclovir hypersensitivity.

WARNINGS/PRECAUTIONS: Thrombotic thrombocytopenic purpura/hemolytic uremic syndrome reported with advanced HIV disease, allogenic bone marrow or renal transplants. Reduce dose with renal dysfunction. Possible renal and CNS toxicity in elderly.

ADVERSE REACTIONS: Headache, nausea, and abdominal pain.

INTERACTIONS: Caution with other potentially nephrotoxic drugs.

PREGNANCY: Category B, caution in nursing.

MECHANISM OF ACTION: Nucleoside analogue; inhibits replication of herpes viral DNA by inhibiting viral DNA polymerase, incorporating and terminating growing viral DNA chain, and inactivating viral DNA polymerase.

PHARMACOKINETICS: Absorption: Rapid (GI tract). Oral administration of variable doses resulted in different parameters. **Distribution:** Plasma protein binding (13.5-17.9%). **Metabolism:** Hepatic/Intestinal (1st pass). **Elimination:** Urine (45.6%), feces (47.12%); $T_{1/2}$=2.5-3.3 hrs.

NURSING CONSIDERATIONS

Assessment: Assess for renal/hepatic impairment, immunocompromised (transplant, advanced HIV, AIDS), and possible drug interactions.

Monitoring: Monitor for thrombotic thrombocytopenic purpura/hemolytic uremic syndrome (TTP/HUS).

Patient Counseling: Advise to maintain adequate hydration. Avoid contact when lesions or symptoms are present to avoid infecting partner(s); use safe sex practice in combination with suppressive therapy. Instruct to initiate treatment at earliest symptom of cold sores (eg, tingling, itching, burning).

Administration: Oral route. **Storage:** 15-25°C (59-77°F). Dispense in tightly closed container.

VALTROPIN — RX

somatropin (LG Life)

THERAPEUTIC CLASS: Human growth hormone

INDICATIONS: Treatment of pediatric patients who have growth failure due to inadequate secretion of endogenous growth hormone. Treatment of growth failure associated with Turner syndrome in pediatric patients who have open epiphyses. Long-term replacement therapy in adults with growth hormone deficiency (GHD) of either adult or childhood onset etiology.

DOSAGE: *Adults:* Individualize dose. Initial: 0.33mg/day SQ 6 days a week. Dosage may be increased to individual patient requirement to maximum of 0.66mg/day after 4 weeks. Alternative Dosing: 0.2mg/day (Range: 0.15-0.3mg/day). May increase gradually every 1-2 months by 0.1-0.2mg/day based on individual patient requirements.
Pediatrics: Individualize dose. Divide weekly dose into equal amounts given either daily or 6 days a week by SQ injection. GHD: 0.17-0.3mg/kg of body weight/week. Turner Syndrome: Up to 0.375mg/kg of body weight/week.

HOW SUPPLIED: Inj: 5mg

CONTRAINDICATIONS: Pediatrics with closed epiphyses. Active proliferative and severe non-proliferative diabetic retinopathy. Presence of active malignancy. Acute critical illness due to complications following open heart surgery, abdominal surgery, or multiple accidental trauma, or those with acute respiratory failure. Patients with Prader-Willi syndrome who are severely obese or have severe respiratory impairment.

WARNINGS/PRECAUTIONS: Known sensitivity to supplied diluent (meta-cresol). Caution in pediatric pateints with Prader-Willi syndrome with 1 or more risk factors (severe obesity, history of upper airway destruction or sleep apnea, or unidentified respiratory infection). May decrease insulin sensitivity. Patients with GHD secondary to intracranial lesion should be monitered closely for progression or recurrence of underlying disease process. Intracranial HTN reported. Monitor closely with DM, glucose intolerance, hypopituitarism. Funduscopic exam recommended at initiation and periodically during course of therapy. Monitor carefully for any malignant transformation of skin lesions.

ADVERSE REACTIONS: Headache, pyrexia, cough, respiratory tract infection, diarrhea, vomiting, pharyngitis.

INTERACTIONS: Growth-promoting effects may be inhibited by glucocorticoids. May alter clearance of compounds metabolized by CP450 liver enzymes (eg, corticosteroids, sex steroids, anticonvulsants, cyclosporine); monitor closely. May need insulin adjustment.

PREGNANCY: Category B, caution in nursing.

MECHANISM OF ACTION: Human growth hormone; stimulates linear growth synthesis, metabolizes lipids, reduces body fat stores by increasing cellular protein, and increases plasma fatty acids.

PHARMACOKINETICS: Absorption: C_{max}=43.97ng/mL, T_{max}=4 hrs, AUC=369.9ng•hr/mL. **Metabolism:** Liver, kidneys (protein catabolism). **Elimination:** $T_{1/2}$=3.03 hrs.

NURSING CONSIDERATIONS

Assessment: Assess for hypersensitivity to benzyl alcohol, closed epiphyses (pediatric), proliferative diabetic retinopathy, active malignancy, acute critical illness (complications of surgery, multiple accidental trauma, or acute respiratory failure), pre-existing type 1 or type 2 DM or impaired glucose tolerance, history of scoliosis, pre-existing papilledema, hypothyroidism, diagnostic imaging (pituitary or intracranial tumor), hypopituitarism, and possible drug interactions. Obtain baseline funduscopic exam. Prader-Willi syndrome: Evaluate for signs of upper airway obstruction or sleep apnea before initiation. Turner syndrome: Evaluate for otitis media or other ear disorders, and cardiovascular disorders before initiation.

Monitoring: Monitor fasting blood glucose and thyroid function tests periodically, periodic fundoscopic exam, weight control (Prader-Willi syndrome), signs/symptoms of malignant transformation of skin lesions, intracranial HTN, slipped capital femoral epiphysis (eg, onset of limp, hip or knee pain), hypersensitivity/allergic reactions, respiratory infections (Prader-Willi syndrome), otitis media or ear disorders (Turner syndrome), CV disorders (Turner syndrome), and progression of scoliosis.

Patient Counseling: Instruct thoroughly as to proper usage, proper disposal, caution against any reuse of needles and syringes. Seek medical attention if signs/symptoms of slipped capital femoral epiphysis (eg, onset of limp, hip or knee pain), hypersensitivity/allergic reactions, respiratory infections (Prader-Willi syndrome), otitis media or ear disorders (Turner syndrome), CV disorders (Turner syndrome), or progression of scoliosis occur.

Administration: SQ route (thighs). **Storage:** Before reconstitution: 2-8°C (36-46°F). Do not freeze. After reconstitution: 2-8°C (36-46°F) for up to 21 days. Do not freeze.

VANCOCIN ORAL — RX

vancomycin HCl (Viro Pharma)

THERAPEUTIC CLASS: Tricyclic glycopeptide antibiotic

INDICATIONS: Treatment of enterocolitis caused by *Staphylococcus aureus* and antibiotic-associated pseudomembranous colitis caused by *C.difficile.*

DOSAGE: *Adults:* 500mg-2g/day given tid-qid for 7-10 days.
Pediatrics: 40mg/kg/day given tid-qid for 7-10 days. Max: 2g/day.

HOW SUPPLIED: Cap: 125mg, 250mg

WARNINGS/PRECAUTIONS: Not effective for other types of infection. Caution with inflammatory disorders of intestinal mucosa, renal impairment; increased risk of systemic absorption. Ototoxicity reported. Monitor auditory function.

ADVERSE REACTIONS: Nephrotoxicity, ototoxicity, reversible neutropenia, anaphylactoid reactions (hypotension, wheezing, "Red Man Syndrome," pruritus), superinfection.

INTERACTIONS: Monitor renal function with aminoglycosides.

PREGNANCY: Category B, not for use in nursing.

MECHANISM OF ACTION: Tricyclic glycopeptide antibiotic; inhibits cell-wall biosynthesis, altering bacterial cell membrane permeabilty and RNA synthesis.

PHARMACOKINETICS: Absorption: Poor. **Elimination:** Urine, feces.

NURSING CONSIDERATIONS

Assessment: Assess for inflammatory intestinal disorders, renal function, ototoxicity, and possible drug interactions. Document indications for therapy, culture, and susceptibility testing.

Monitoring: Monitor for hypersensitivity reactions (Stevens-Johnson syndrome, vasculitis, "Red Man Syndrome"), ototoxicity, renal function, CBC with platelets and differential, superinfection.

Patient Counseling: Inform that therapy treats bacterial, not viral, infections. Take as directed; skipping doses or not completing full course may decrease effectiveness and increase resistance. May experience diarrhea; notify physician if watery/bloody stools, hypersensitivity reactions, or superinfection occur.

Administration: Oral route. **Storage:** 15-30°C (59-86°F).

VANCOMYCIN INJECTION — RX

vancomycin HCl (Various)

THERAPEUTIC CLASS: Tricyclic glycopeptide antibiotic

INDICATIONS: Treatment of serious or severe infections caused by susceptible strains of methicillin-resistant (β-lactam resistant) staphylococci. Indicated for PCN-allergic patients, for patients who cannot receive or have failed to respond to other drugs, and for infections caused by vancomycin-susceptible organisms that are resistant to other antimicrobials. Indicated for initial therapy when methicillin-resistant staphylococci are suspected, but after susceptibility data are available, therapy should be adjusted accordingly. Effective in the treatment of staphylococcal endocarditis; effectiveness has been documented in other infections due to staphylococci, including septicemia, bone infections, lower respiratory tract infections, and skin and skin-structure infections. Reported to be effective alone or incombination with an aminoglycoside for endocarditis caused by *S.viridans* or *S.bovis*. Reported to be effective only in combination with an aminoglycoside for endocarditis caused by enterococci (eg, *E.faecalis*). Reported to be effective for treatment of diphtheroid endocarditis. Successfully used in combination with either rifampin, an aminoglycoside, or both in early-onset prosthetic valve endocarditis caused by *S.epidermidis* or diphtheroids. Parenteral form may be administered orally for treatment of antibiotic-associated pseudomembranous colitis produced by *C.difficile* and for staphylococcal enterocolitis.

DOSAGE: *Adults*: Inj: Usual: 500mg IV q6h or 1g IV q12h. Administer at not >10mg/min or over at least 60 min, whichever is longer. Max Conc: 5mg/mL. Max Rate: 10mg/min. Renal Impairment: Initial: Not <15mg/kg. Dosage per day in mg is about 15x the GFR in mL/min (refer to table in PI). Elderly: Require greater dose reductions than expected. Functionally Anephric: Initial: 15mg/kg, then 1.9mg/kg/24 hrs. Marked Renal Impairment: 250-1000mg every several days. Anuria: 1000mg every 7-10 days. PO: 500-2000mg/day in 3-4 divided doses for 7-10 days. Max: 2000mg/day. May dilute in 1oz of water. *Pediatrics*: Inj: Usual: 10mg/kg IV q6h. Infants/Neonates: Initial: 15mg/kg, then 10mg/kg q12h for neonates in 1st week of life and q8h thereafter until 1 month of age. Administer over at least 60 min. Renal Impairment: Initial: Not <15mg/kg. Dosage per day in mg is about 15x the GFR in mL/min (refer to table in PI). Premature Infants: Require greater dose reduction. ADD-Vantage vials should not be used in neonates, infants, and pediatrics who require doses <500mg. PO: 40mg/kg/day in 3-4 divided doses for 7-10 days. Max: 2000mg/day. May dilute in 1oz of water.

HOW SUPPLIED: Inj: 500mg, 1g, 5g, 500mg/100mL, 1g/200mL

WARNINGS/PRECAUTIONS: Rapid bolus administration may cause hypotension and cardiac arrest (rare); administer in diluted solution over ≥60 min. Frequency of infusion-related events may increase with concomitant use of anesthetic agents. Ototoxicity reported; monitor auditory function. Caution with renal insufficiency and adjust dose with renal dysfunction. Pseudomembranous colitis reported. Alters the normal flora of the colon and may permit overgrowth of clostridia. Prolonged use may result in overgrowth of nonsusceptible organisms. Reversible neutropenia reported; monitor leukocyte count. Administer via IV route; pain, avoid IM route. Thrombophlebitis may occur; rotate injection sites. Safety and efficacy of administration via the intraperitoneal and intrathecal (intralumbar and intraventricular) routes has not been established. Administration via intraperitoneal route during CAPD has resulted in a syndrome of chemical peritonitis. Adjust dosing schedules in elderly.

ADVERSE REACTIONS: Infusion-related events, hypotension, wheezing, pruritus, pain, chest and head muscle spasm, dyspnea, urticaria, "Red Man Syndrome," nephrotoxicity, pseudomembranous colitis, ototoxicity, neutropenia, phlebitis.

INTERACTIONS: Concomitant use of anesthetic agents has been associated with erythema, histamine-like flushing, and anaphylactoid reactions. Concurrent and/or sequential systemic or topical use of other potentially neurotoxic and/or nephrotoxic drugs (eg, amphotericin B, aminoglycosides, bacitracin, polymyxin B, colistin, viomycin, cisplatin) requires careful monitoring.

PREGNANCY: Category C, not for use in nursing.

MECHANISM OF ACTION: Tricyclic glycopeptide antibiotic; inhibits cell-wall biosynthesis, alters bacterial cell membrane permeability and RNA synthesis.

PHARMACOKINETICS: Absorption: (1g at 2 hrs) C_{max} =23mcg/mL; (500mg at 2 hrs) C_{max} = 19mcg/mL. **Distribution:** Serum protein binding (55%). **Elimination:** Urine (75% in 24 hrs); $T_{1/2}$=4-6 hrs.

NURSING CONSIDERATIONS

Assessment: Assess for renal function, ototoxicity, and possible drug interactions. Document indications for therapy, culture, and susceptibility testing.

Monitoring: Monitor for hypersensitivity reactions (eg, Stevens-Johnson syndrome, vasculitis), infusion reactions (eg, hypotension, arrhythmias, "Red Man Syndrome"), ototoxicity, renal function, *C. difficile*-associated diarrhea, pseudomembranous colitis, CBC with platelets and differential, superinfection, and chemical peritonitis (intraperitoneal route).

Patient Counseling: Inform that drug treats bacterial, not viral, infections. Take as directed; skipping doses or not completing full course may decrease effectiveness and increase resistance. Inform that may experience diarrhea; notify physician if watery/bloody stools, hypersensitivity reactions, or superinfection develops.

Administration: IV route; infuse over at least 60 min. **Storage:** Store at or below -4°C (20°F).

VANOS — RX

fluocinonide (Medicis)

THERAPEUTIC CLASS: Corticosteroid

INDICATIONS: Corticosteroid-responsive dermatoses.

DOSAGE: *Adults:* Apply thin layer to affected area qd-bid. Max: 60g/week. Do not exceed 2 weeks.
Pediatrics: ≥12 yrs: Appy thin layer to affected area qd-bid. Max: 60g/week. Do not exceed 2 weeks.

HOW SUPPLIED: Cre: 0.1% [30g, 60g]

WARNINGS/PRECAUTIONS: May produce reversible HPA axis suppression, manifestations of Cushing's syndrome, hyperglycemia, and glucosuria. Caution when applied to large surface areas or under occlusive dressings. Use appropriate antifungal or antibacterial agent with dermatological infections. D/C if infection does not clear or irritation develops. Do not use for more than 2 weeks at a time.

ADVERSE REACTIONS: Headache, application site burning, nasopharyngitis, nasal congestion, unspecified application site reaction.

PREGNANCY: Category C, not for use in nursing.

MECHANISM OF ACTION: Corticosteroid; possesses anti-inflammatory, antipruritic, and vasoconstrictive properties. Anti-inflammatory activity not established; suspected to act by induction of phospholipase A_2 inhibitory proteins, lipocortins. Lipocortins control biosynthesis of potent inflammation mediators (eg, prostaglandins, leukotrienes) by inhibiting release of their common precursor, arachidonic acid.

PHARMACOKINETICS: Absorption: Percutaneous; inflammation and/or other disease states may increase absorption. **Distribution:** Systemically administered corticosteroids appear in breast milk.

NURSING CONSIDERATIONS

Assessment: Assess for rosacea or perioral dermatitis. Assess use in pregnancy/nursing.

Monitoring: Monitor for signs/symptoms of reversible HPA-axis suppression, Cushing's syndrome, hyperglycemia, glucosuria, skin irritation, allergic contact dermatitis (eg, failure to heal), and for development of concomitant skin infections (eg, bacterial, fungal). With large doses or use of occlusive dressings, monitor for HPA-axis suppression using cosyntropin ($ACTH_{1-24}$) stimulation test. Following withdrawal of therapy, monitor for glucocorticosteroid insufficiency. In pediatric patients, monitor for systemic toxicity, HPA-axis suppression (linear growth retardation, delayed weight gain), Cushing's syndrome, and intracranial HTN.

Patient Counseling: Counsel to use externally and exactly as directed; avoid contact with eyes, face, groin, and underarms. Instruct not to cover, wrap, or bandage treatment areas unless directed by physician. Wash hands following application. Contact physician if adverse reactions (eg, burning, itching, irritation) occur or no clinical improvement after 2 weeks. Contact physician before using other corticosteroid-containing products. Notify physician if planning surgery during therapy.

Administration: Topical route. **Storage:** 15-30°C (59-86°F).

VANTAS

RX

histrelin acetate (Indevus)

THERAPEUTIC CLASS: Luteinizing hormone-releasing hormone agonist

V

INDICATIONS: Palliative treatment of advanced prostate cancer.

DOSAGE: *Adults:* 50mg every 12 months. Inject SQ into inner aspect of the upper arm. Refrain from wetting the inserted arm for 24 hours. Refrain from heavy lifting or strenuous exercise of the inserted arm for 7 days after implant insertion. Must remove after 12 months of therapy.

HOW SUPPLIED: Implant: 50mg

CONTRAINDICATIONS: Women and pediatric patients.

WARNINGS/PRECAUTIONS: Transient increase in serum testosterone and worsening of symptoms of prostate cancer with initial therapy. Urethral obstruction and spinal cord compression reported. Anaphylactic reactions may occur.

ADVERSE REACTIONS: Hot flashes, fatigue, implant site reaction, testicular atrophy, renal impairment, gynecomastia, constipation, erectile dysfunction.

PREGNANCY: Category X, not for use in nursing.

MECHANISM OF ACTION: LH-RH agonist; acts as potent inhibitor of gonadotropin secretion, desensitizes responsiveness of pituitary gonadotropin, causing reduction in testicular steroidogenesis.

PHARMACOKINETICS: Absorption: C_{max}=1.1ng/mL; T_{max}=12 hrs. **Distribution:** V_d=58.4L. **Elimination:** $T_{1/2}$=3.92 hrs.

NURSING CONSIDERATIONS

Assessment: Assess pregnancy status, for metastatic vertebral lesions, urinary tract obstruction, and possible drug interactions. Obtain baseline serum testosterone and PSA levels.

Monitoring: Periodically monitor serum testosterone and PSA levels. Monitor for signs/symptoms of anaphylactoid reactions, transient worsening of symptoms, and implant-site reaction.

Patient Counseling: Instruct to refrain from wetting arm for 24 hrs and from heavy lifting or strenuous exertion for 7 days after implant insertion. Monitor for signs/symptoms of anaphylactoid reactions, transient worsening of symptoms, and implant-site reaction.

Administration: Dermal implant. Inserting implant: 1) Clean and anesthesize area; make 2-3mm incision SQ and perpendicular to shoulder. 2) Grasp tool by handle; insert tip into incision with bevel up and advance along track to inscribed line on cannula. 3) Hold tool in place; move thumb to green retraction button; press down to release lock; draw button back to back stop. Withdraw tool from incision. Check implant by palpation. **Storage:** Refrigerate; 2-8°C (36-46°F). Protect from light. Do not freeze.

VANTIN RX

cefpodoxime proxetil (Pharmacia & Upjohn)

THERAPEUTIC CLASS: Cephalosporin (3rd generation)

INDICATIONS: Treatment of acute otitis media, pharyngitis/tonsillitis, community-acquired pneumonia (CAP), acute bacterial exacerbation of chronic bronchitis (ABECB), acute uncomplicated urethral and cervical gonorrhea, acute uncomplicated anorectal infections in women, uncomplicated skin and skin structure infections (SSSI), acute maxillary sinusitis, and uncomplicated urinary tract infections (UTI) caused by susceptible strains of microorganisms.

DOSAGE: *Adults:* Take tabs with food. Pharyngitis/Tonsillitis: 100mg q12h for 5-10 days. CAP: 200mg q12h for 14 days. ABECB: 200mg q12h for 10 days. Uncomplicated Gonorrhea (Men/Women)/Rectal Gonococcal Infections (Women): 200mg single dose. SSSI: 400mg q12h for 7-14 days. Sinusitis: 200mg q12h for 10 days. UTI: 100mg q12h for 7 days. CrCl <30mL/min: Increase interval to q24h. Hemodialysis: Dose 3 times weekly after dialysis. *Pediatrics:* ≥12 yrs: Take tabs with food. Pharyngitis/Tonsillitis: 100mg q12h for 5-10 days. CAP: 200mg q12h for 14 days. ABECB: 200mg q12h for 10 days. Uncomplicated Gonorrhea (Men/Women)/Rectal Gonococcal Infections (Women): 200mg single dose. SSSI: 400mg q12h for 7-14 days. Sinusitis: 200mg q12h for 10 days. UTI: 100mg q12h for 7 days. 2 months-12 yrs: Otitis Media: 5mg/kg q12h for 5 days. Max: 200mg/dose. Pharyngitis/Tonsillitis: 5mg/kg q12h for 5-10 days. Max: 100mg/dose. Sinusitis: 5mg/kg q12h for 10 days. Max: 200mg/dose. CrCl <30mL/min: Increase interval to q24h. Hemodialysis: Dose 3 times weekly after dialysis.

HOW SUPPLIED: Sus: 50mg/5mL [50mL, 75mL, 100mL], 100mg/5mL [50mL, 75mL, 100mL]; Tab: 100mg, 200mg

WARNINGS/PRECAUTIONS: Cross-sensitivity to PCNs and other cephalosporins may occur. *Clostridium difficile*-associated diarrhea reported. Positive direct Coombs' tests reported. Caution with renal impairment;

dose reduction may be needed. May result in overgrowth of nonsusceptible organisms.

ADVERSE REACTIONS: Diarrhea, nausea.

INTERACTIONS: Decreased plasma levels and absorption with antacids and H_2-blockers. Delayed peak plasma levels with anticholinergics. Probenecid inhibits renal excretion. Closely monitor renal function with nephrotoxic agents. Caution with potent diuretics.

PREGNANCY: Category B, not for use in nursing.

MECHANISM OF ACTION: Cephalosporin; inhibits cell-wall synthesis.

PHARMACOKINETICS: Absorption: C_{max}(100mg)=1.4mcg/mL, T_{max}=2-3 hrs. **Distribution:** Plasma protein binding (22-31%). **Metabolism:** Via desterification. **Elimination**: Urine; $T_{1/2}$= 2.09-2.84 hrs.

NURSING CONSIDERATIONS

Assessment: Assess for history of hypersensitivity to cephalosporins/PCNs, pregnancy status, possible drug interactions, renal impairment. Document indications for therapy, culture, and susceptibility testing.

Monitoring: Monitor for signs/symptoms of hypersensitivity reactions (anaphylaxis, Stevens-Johnsons syndrome), *C.difficile*-associated diarrhea, seizures, LFTs, CBC with platelets and differential, renal function, PT, LDH, superinfections.

Patient Counseling: Inform that drug only treats bacterial, not viral, infections. Instruct to take as directed; skipping doses or not completing full course may decrease effectiveness and increase resistance. Inform may experience diarrhea; contact physician if watery/bloody stools, superinfections, or hypersensitivity reactions occur.

VAQTA RX

hepatitis B immune globulin (Merck)

THERAPEUTIC CLASS: Vaccine

INDICATIONS: Active immunization against hepatitis A virus. Give primary immunization at least 2 weeks before expected exposure.

DOSAGE: *Adults:* ≥19 yrs: 1mL (50 U) IM followed by a booster of 1mL (50 U) 6-18 months later.
Pediatrics: 1-18 yrs: 0.5mL (25 U) IM followed by a booster of 0.5mL (25 U) 6-18 months later.

HOW SUPPLIED: Inj: 25 U/0.5mL, 50 U/mL

WARNINGS/PRECAUTIONS: Have epinephrine (1:1000) available. May not prevent hepatitis A with unrecognized infection. Caution with bleeding disorders (eg, hemophilia or thrombocytopenia or patients on anticoagulant therapy). Defer use with acute infection or febrile illness. Suboptimal response may occur in immunocompromised patients.

ADVERSE REACTIONS: Injection-site pain, tenderness, erythema, swelling, warmth, fever.

INTERACTIONS: Immunosuppressive therapy may reduce response to active immunization.

PREGNANCY: Category C, caution in nursing.

MECHANISM OF ACTION: Vaccine; produces an antibody response against hepatitis A virus.

NURSING CONSIDERATIONS

Assessment: Assess for immune status, vaccination history, bleeding disorders (eg, hemophilia, thrombocytopenia), acute infection or febrile illness, pregnancy/nursing status, and possible drug interactions (eg, anticoagulants).

Monitoring: Monitor for signs/symptoms of hypersensitivity reactions (eg, anaphylaxis), injection-site reactions, or hematoma, immune response, fever, elevated LFTs, eosinophilia, and increased urine protein.

Patient Counseling: Inform of potential risks/benefits; report any adverse reactions to physician. Primary immunization should be given 2 weeks prior to expected exposure to hepatitis A virus.

Administration: IM route; inject preferably into deltoid muscle. Do not inject intravascularly, intradermally, or SQ. **Storage:** 2-8°C (36-46°F). Do not freeze.

VARIVAX RX

varicella virus vaccine live (Merck)

THERAPEUTIC CLASS: Vaccine

INDICATIONS: Vaccination against varicella.

DOSAGE: *Adults:* 0.5mL SQ at elected date, repeat 4-8 weeks later. *Pediatrics:* 12 months-12 yrs: 0.5mL SQ. If a second dose is given; administer a minimum of 3 months later. ≥13 yrs: 0.5mL SQ at elected date, repeat 4-8 weeks later.

HOW SUPPLIED: Inj: 1350PFU/0.5mL

CONTRAINDICATIONS: Pregnancy (avoid pregnancy for 3 months after vaccine); gelatin hypersensitivity; anaphylactoid reactions to neomycin, blood dyscrasias, leukemia, lymphomas, malignant neoplasms affecting bone marrow or lymphatic system, febrile respiratory illness or other active febrile infection, active untreated TB, immunosuppressive therapy, immunosuppressant doses of corticosteroids, immunodeficiency states and family history of congenital or hereditary immunodeficiency.

WARNINGS/PRECAUTIONS: Children and adolescents with ALL in remission can receive the vaccine under an investigational protocol. Defer vaccine for at least 5 months after blood or plasma transfusions, or administration of immune globulin or varicella zoster immune globulin. Defer vaccine with family history of congenital, hereditary immunodeficiency until immune system evaluated. Rarely, vaccine virus transmission through varicella-like rash can occur; avoid close association with susceptible high-risk individuals for up to six weeks (eg, immunocompromised patients, pregnant women without history of chickenpox, newborns of mothers without documented history of chickenpox). Have epinephrine available. Do not inject into a blood vessel.

ADVERSE REACTIONS: Fever, local reactions, pain, varicella-like rashes.

INTERACTIONS: Avoid immune globulins for 2 months after vaccination. Avoid salicylates for 6 weeks after vaccination. Contraindicated with immunosuppressive therapy or immunosuppressant doses of corticosteroids.

PREGNANCY: Category C, caution in nursing.

MECHANISM OF ACTION: Vaccine; cell-mediated immune response stimulation against varicella zoster virus (VZV) infection.

NURSING CONSIDERATIONS

Assessment: Assess for immunity, health status, blood dyscrasias, immunization/family history, and possible drug interactions.

Monitoring: Monitor for signs/symptoms of allergic reactions, injection-site reactions (eg, pain, swelling, rash, hematoma, pruritus), fever, URI, irritability, diarrhea, anorexia, NV, headache, and thrombocytopenia.

Patient Counseling: Inform of potential benefits/risks; report adverse reactions to physician. May not offer 100% protection.

Administration: SQ route; inject into outer aspect of deltoid region. **Storage:** Frozen at -15°C (+5°F) or colder; diluent stored at room temperature or refrigerated.

VASERETIC RX

enalapril maleate - hydrochlorothiazide (Merck)

ACE inhibitors can cause death/injury to developing fetus during 2nd and 3rd trimesters. Stop therapy if pregnancy detected.

THERAPEUTIC CLASS: ACE inhibitor/thiazide diuretic

INDICATIONS: Treatment of hypertension.

DOSAGE: *Adults:* Initial (if not controlled with enalapril/HCTZ monotherapy): 10mg-25mg tab qd. Titrate: May increase after 2-3 weeks. Max: 20mg enalapril/50mg HCTZ per day. Replacement Therapy: Substitute combination for titrated components.

HOW SUPPLIED: Tab: (Enalapril-HCTZ) 10mg-25mg

CONTRAINDICATIONS: History of ACE inhibitor-associated angioedema and hereditary or idiopathic angioedema. Anuria, sulfonamide hypersensitivity.

WARNINGS/PRECAUTIONS: D/C if angioedema, jaundice, or if marked LFT elevation occurs. Risk of hyperkalemia with DM, renal dysfunction. Persistent nonproductive cough reported. Monitor WBCs in renal and collagen vascular disease. Anaphylactoid reactions reported. Fetal/neonatal morbidity and death reported. Monitor for hypotension in high-risk patients (heart failure, surgery/anesthesia, hyponatremia, severe volume/salt depletion, etc). Caution with CHF, renal or hepatic dysfunction, obstruction to left ventricle outflow tract, elderly, renal artery stenosis. More reports of angioedema in blacks than nonblacks. May exacerbate or activate SLE. Monitor serum electrolytes. Avoid if CrCl ≤30mL/min/1.73m^2. May increase cholesterol, TG, uric acid levels, and blood glucose. Intestinal angioedema reported. Oliguria, progressive azotemia, acute renal failure, and death (rare) may occur in patients with CHF. Not for initial therapy. Caution with severe renal disease, impaired hepatic function, progressive liver disease.

ADVERSE REACTIONS: Dizziness, cough, fatigue, and headache.

INTERACTIONS: Increase risk of hyperkalemia with K^+-sparing diuretics, K^+ supplements, or K^+-containing salt substitutes. Potentiates orthostatic hypotension with alcohol, barbiturates, and narcotics. Adjust insulin and antidiabetic drugs. Impaired absorption with cholestyramine, colestipol. Corticosteroids and ACTH deplete electrolytes. May decrease response to pressor amines. Potentiates other antihypertensives. May increase responsiveness to skeletal muscle relaxants, nondepolarizing (eg, tubocurarine). Risk of lithium toxicity. NSAIDs may reduce antihypertensive effect and worsen renal dysfunction. Nitritoid reactions (eg, facial flushing, NV, hypotension) reported rarely with injectable gold. Concomitant use of diuretic may increase blood urea and serum creatinine with HTN or CHF.

PREGNANCY: Category C (1st trimester) and D (2nd and 3rd trimesters), not for use in nursing.

MECHANISM OF ACTION: Enalapril: ACE inhibitor; inhibition results in decreased plasma angiotensin II, which leads to decreased vasopressor activity and decreased aldosterone secretion. HCTZ: Thiazide diuretic; affects renal tubular mechanism of electrolyte reabsorption, directly increasing excretion of Na^+ and chloride.

PHARMACOKINETICS: Absorption: T_{max} (enalapril, enalaprilat)=1, 3-4 hrs. **Distribution:** HCTZ: Crosses placental barrier. **Metabolism:** Via hydrolysis; Enalaprilat (metabolite). **Elimination:** Urine, feces; $T_{1/2}$ (enalaprilat)=11 hrs. HCTZ: Kidneys; $T_{1/2}$=5.6-14.8 hrs.

V

NURSING CONSIDERATIONS

Assessment: Assess BP, LFTs, renal function, CVD (eg, cardiomyopathy, aortic stenosis), renal artery stenosis, SLE, serum electrolytes, pregnancy status, history of allergy to sulfonamides, bronchial asthma, parathyroid disorders, and for possible drug interactions.

Monitoring: Monitor BP, LFTs, renal function, CBC with platelet count and differential, serum electrolytes. Monitor for MI, CHF, angioedema (head, neck, intestinal), anaphylactoid reactions, hepatic failure, hyperuricemia, hyperglycemia, hypersensitivity reactions, cough, NV, dizziness.

Patient Counseling: Inform about fetal risks if taken during pregnancy. Caution that inadequate fluid intake, excessive perspiration, diarrhea, or vomiting may lead to excessive fall in BP, resulting in lightheadedness and possible syncope. Advise not to use K^+ supplements or salt substitutes containing K^+ without consulting physician. Counsel about signs/symptoms of neutropenia (eg, fever sore throat, infection), angioedema, electrolyte imbalance (eg, thirst, weakness, lethargy) and other adverse effects; advise to seek prompt medical attention if any occur.

Administration: Oral route. **Storage:** 25°C (77°F). Keep container tightly closed. Protect from moisture.

VASOTEC **RX**

enalapril maleate (Merck)

ACE inhibitors can cause death/injury to developing fetus during 2nd and 3rd trimesters. Stop therapy if pregnancy detected.

THERAPEUTIC CLASS: ACE inhibitor

INDICATIONS: Treatment of hypertension. Treatment of symptomatic chronic heart failure (CHF) usually in combination with diuretics and digitalis. To decrease overt heart failure development and hospitalization in stable asymptomatic left ventricular dysfunction.

DOSAGE: *Adults:* HTN: If possible, d/c diuretic 2-3 days prior to therapy. Initial: 5mg qd, 2.5mg qd with concomitant diuretic. Usual: 10-40mg/day given qd or bid. Resume diuretic if BP not controlled. CrCl>80mL/min: Initial: 5mg/day. CrCl≤80>30mL/min: Initial: 5mg. CrCl ≤30mL/min: Initial: 2.5mg/day. Dialysis: Initial: 2.5mg/day on dialysis days. Max: 40mg/day. Heart Failure: Initial: 2.5mg/day. Usual: 2.5-20mg given bid. Max: 40mg/day. Asymptomatic Left Ventricular Dysfunction: Initial: 2.5mg bid. Titrate: Increase to 20mg/day. Hyponatremia or SrCr 1.6mg/dL with Heart Failure: Initial: 2.5mg/day. Titrate: Increase to 2.5mg bid, then 5mg bid. Max: 40mg/day.
Pediatrics: HTN: Initial: 0.08mg/kg (up to 5mg) qd. Titrate: Adjust according to response. Max: 0.58mg/kg/dose (or 40mg/dose).

HOW SUPPLIED: Tab: 2.5mg*, 5mg*, 10mg,* 20mg* *scored

CONTRAINDICATIONS: History of ACE inhibitor associated angioedema and hereditary or idiopathic angioedema.

WARNINGS/PRECAUTIONS: D/C if angioedema, jaundice, or if marked LFT elevation occurs. Risk of hyperkalemia with DM, renal dysfunction. Persistent nonproductive cough reported. Monitor WBCs in renal or collagen vascular disease. Anaphylactoid reactions reported. Fetal/neonatal morbidity and death reported. Monitor for hypotension in high-risk patients (heart failure, surgery/anesthesia, hyponatremia, high-dose diuretic therapy, severe volume and/or salt depletion, etc). Caution with CHF, obstruction to left ventricle outflow tract, renal dysfunction, and renal artery stenosis. Less effective on BP in blacks and more reports of angioedema than nonblacks. Intestinal angioedema reported. Oliguria, progressive azotemia, acute renal failure, and death (rare) may occur in patients with CHF. Avoid if GFR <30mL/min/1.73m² in pediatric patients.

ADVERSE REACTIONS: Fatigue, orthostatic effects, asthenia, diarrhea, NV, headache, dizziness, cough, rash, hypotension.

INTERACTIONS: May increase lithium levels. Hypotension risk with diuretics. May further decrease renal dysfunction with NSAIDs. Increase risk of hyperkalemia with K^+-sparing diuretics, K^+-containing salt substitutes, or K^+ supplements. Augmented effect by antihypertensives that cause renin release (eg, thiazides). NSAIDs may diminish antihypertensive effect. Nitritoid reactions (eg, facial flushing, NV, hypotension) reported rarely with injectable gold. Concomitant use of diuretic may increase blood urea and serum creatinine with HTN or CHF.

PREGNANCY: Category C (1st trimester) and D (2nd and 3rd trimesters), not for use in nursing.

MECHANISM OF ACTION: ACE inhibitor; inhibition results in decreased plasma angiotensin II, which leads to decreased vasopressor activity and decreased aldosterone secretion.

PHARMACOKINETICS: Absorption: T_{max}=1, 3-4 hrs (enalapril, enalaprilat). **Metabolism:** Via hydrolysis, enalaprilat (metabolite). **Elimination:** Urine, feces; $T_{1/2}$=11 hrs (enalaprilat).

NURSING CONSIDERATIONS

Assessment: Assess BP, LFTs, renal function, CHF, renal artery stenosis, pregnancy status, and possible drug interactions.

Monitoring: Monitor BP, LFTs, renal function, CBC with platelet count and differential, serum K^+ levels. Monitor for MI, CHF, angioedema (head, neck, intestinal), anaphylactoid reactions, hepatic failure, hypersensitivity reactions, cough, NV, dizziness.

Patient Counseling: Counsel about fetal risks during pregnancy and signs/symptoms of angioedema (eg, laryngeal/tongue edema, abdominal pain); advise to seek prompt medical attention if symptoms develop. Inform about adverse effects (eg, anaphylaxis, cough, hypotension, hyperkalemia). Infants with histories of *in utero* exposure should be closely observed for hypotension, oliguria, hyperkalemia. Inform about need for periodic monitoring of electrolytes and blood counts. Caution that inadequate fluid intake, excessive perspiration, diarrhea, vomiting may lead to excessive fall in BP, which can result in lightheadedness or possible syncope. Advise not to use K^+ supplements or salt substitutes containing K^+ without consulting physician.

Administration: Oral route. See PI for preparation of suspension. **Storage:** (Cap)25°C (77°F); excursions permitted to 15-30°C (59-86°F). Protect from moisture. Dispense in tight container. (Sus) Refrigerate at 2-8°C (36-46°F) and can be stored for up to 30 days. Shake the suspension before each use.

VASOTEC I.V. RX

enalaprilat (Merck)

ACE inhibitors can cause death/injury to developing fetus during 2nd and 3rd trimesters. Stop therapy if pregnancy detected.

THERAPEUTIC CLASS: ACE inhibitor

INDICATIONS: Treatment of hypertension when oral therapy is not practical.

DOSAGE: *Adults:* Administer IV over 5 min. Usual: 1.25mg q6h for no longer than 48 hrs. Max: 20mg/day. Concomitant Diuretic/CrCl ≤30mL/min: Initial: 0.625mg, may repeat after 1 hr. Maint: 1.25mg q6h. Risk of Excessive Hypotension: Initial: 0.625mg over 5 min to 1 hr. PO/IV Conversion: Give 5mg/day PO for 1.25mg IV q6h and 2.5mg/day PO for 0.625mg q6h IV.

HOW SUPPLIED: Inj: 1.25mg/mL

CONTRAINDICATIONS: History of ACE inhibitor associated angioedema and hereditary or idiopathic angioedema.

WARNINGS/PRECAUTIONS: D/C if angioedema, jaundice, or if marked LFT elevation occurs. Risk of hyperkalemia with DM, renal dysfunction. Persistent nonproductive cough reported. Monitor WBCs in renal or collagen vascular disease. Anaphylactoid reactions reported. Fetal/neonatal morbidity and death reported. Monitor for hypotension in high risk patients (heart failure, surgery/anesthesia, hyponatremia, high dose diuretic therapy, severe volume and/or salt depletion, etc). Caution with CHF, obstruction to left ventricle outflow tract, renal dysfunction, and renal artery stenosis. Less effective on BP in blacks and more reports of angioedema than nonblacks.

ADVERSE REACTIONS: Hypotension, headache, angioedema, myocardial infarction, fatigue, dizziness, fever, rash, constipation, cough.

INTERACTIONS: May increase lithium levels. Hypotension risk with diuretics. May further decrease renal dysfunction with NSAIDs. Increase risk of hyperkalemia with K^+-sparing diuretics, K^+-containing salt substitutes or K^+ supplements. Augmented effect by antihypertensives that cause renin release (eg, thiazides). NSAIDs may diminish antihypertensive effect.

PREGNANCY: Category C (1st trimester) and D (2nd and 3rd trimesters), not for use in nursing.

MECHANISM OF ACTION: ACE inhibitor; inhibition results in decreased plasma angiotensin II, which leads to decreased vasopressor activity and decreased aldosterone secretion.

PHARMACOKINETICS: Absorption: (PO) Poorly absorbed. **Elimination:** Urine (90% unchanged); $T_{1/2}$=11 hrs.

NURSING CONSIDERATIONS

Assessment: Assess BP, LFTs, renal function, CVD (eg, aortic stenosis, cardiomyopathy), renal artery stenosis, pregnancy status, and possible drug interactions.

Monitoring: Monitor BP, LFTs, renal function, CBC with platelet count and differential, serum K^+ levels. Monitor for MI, CHF, angioedema (head, neck, intestinal), anaphylactoid reactions, hepatic failure, hypersensitivity reactions, cough, NV, dizziness.

Patient Counseling: Counsel about fetal risks during pregnancy and signs/symptoms of angioedema (eg, laryngeal/tongue edema, abdominal pain); seek prompt medical attention if any develop. Inform about adverse effects (eg, anaphylaxis, cough, hypotension, hyperkalemia, neutropenia). Infants with histories of *in utero* exposure should be closely observed for hypotension, oliguria, hyperkalemia. Inform about need for periodic monitoring of electrolytes and blood counts. Advise not to use K^+ supplements or salt substitutes containing K^+ without consulting physician.

Administration: IV route; inject over 5 min. **Storage:** Store below 30°C (86°F).

VECTIBIX — RX

panitumumab (Amgen)

> **Dermatologic toxicities and severe infusion reactions reported; d/c if severe dermatologic or infusion reaction occurs.**

THERAPEUTIC CLASS: Monoclonal antibody/EGFR-blocker

INDICATIONS: Treatment of EGFR-expressing, metastatic colorectal carcinoma with disease progression on or following fluoropyrimidine-, oxaliplatin-, and irinotecan-containing chemotherapy regimens.

DOSAGE: *Adults:* 6mg/kg IV infusion over 60 min every 14 days. Infuse doses >1000mg over 90 min. Reduce infusion rate by 50% with mild or moderate (Grade 1 or 2) infusion reaction for duration of that infusion. Immediately and permanently d/c infusion with severe (Grade 3 or 4) infusion reactions. Withhold for dermatologic toxicities that are ≥Grade 3 or considered intolerable. If toxicity does not improve to ≤Grade 2 within 1 month, permanently d/c. If dermatologic toxicity improves to ≤Grade 2 and symptoms improve after withholding no more than 2 doses, treatment may be resumed at 50% of original dose. If toxicities recur, permanently d/c. If toxicities do not recur, subsequent doses may be increased by increments of 25% of original dose until recommended dose of 6mg/kg is reached.

HOW SUPPLIED: Inj: 20mg/mL

WARNINGS/PRECAUTIONS: See Black Box Warning. Toxicity involving GI mucosa, eye, and nail reported. Pulmonary fibrosis reported; d/c with interstitial lung disease, pneumonitis, or lung infiltrates. Diarrhea may occur; incidence and severity may increase when used in combination with irinotecan. Use with leucovorin not recommended. Hypomagnesemia and hypocalcemia reported; monitor electrolytes during and for 8 weeks following therapy. Sunlight may exacerbate any skin reactions that may occur; use sunscreen and/or hats and limit sun exposure during therapy. Detection of EGFR protein expression is necessary for selection of appropriate patients. Avoid in combination with chemotherapy with or without bevacizumab.

ADVERSE REACTIONS: Rash, hypomagnesemia, paronychia, fatigue, abdominal pain, NV, diarrhea, constipation, erythema, acneiform dermatitis, pruritus, skin exfoliation, skin fissures, cough.

PREGNANCY: Category C, not for use in nursing.

MECHANISM OF ACTION: IgG2 kappa monoclonal antibody; binds specifically to epidermal growth factor receptor (EGFR) on both normal and tumor cells, and competitively inhibits binding of ligands for EGFR.

PHARMACOKINETICS: Absorption: C_{max}=213mcg/mL, AUC=1306mcg•day/mL. **Elimination:** $T_{1/2}$=7.5 days.

NURSING CONSIDERATIONS

Assessment: Assess for EGFR protein expression, underlying pulmonary disease, pregnancy/nursing status, and possible drug interactions. Obtain baseline electrolyte levels.

Monitoring: Monitor electrolytes periodically during, and for 8 weeks after, therapy. Monitor for signs/symptoms of dermatologic toxicities (eg, dermatitis acneiform, pruritus, erythema, rash, skin exfoliation, paronychia, dry skin, skin fissures), severe infusion reactions (eg, anaphylactic reactions, bronchospasm, fever, chills, hypotension), and pulmonary fibrosis.

Patient Counseling: Advise to report skin/ocular changes and dyspnea. Sunlight can exacerbate any skin reactions, instruct to wear sunscreen and hats and to limit sun exposure while on therapy. Instruct to d/c nursing during, and 2 months after, therapy.

Administration: IV infusion; do not administer as bolus or push. Administer through IV pump using low-protein binding 0.2µm or 0.22µm in-line filter.
Storage: 2-8°C (36-46°F). Protect from sunlight. (Diluted): Room temperature; stable for 6 hrs, or at 2-8°C (36-46°F); stable for 24 hrs. Do not freeze.

VELCADE — RX

bortezomib (Millennium)

THERAPEUTIC CLASS: Proteasome inhibitor

INDICATIONS: Treatment of multiple myeloma and mantle cell lymphoma in patients who have received at least 1 prior therapy.

DOSAGE: *Adults:* Initial 1.3mg/m²/dose IV bolus twice weekly for 2 weeks (Days 1, 4, 8, and 11) followed by a 10-day rest period (Days 12-21). At least 72 hrs should elapse between consecutive doses. Grade 3 Non-Hematological/ Grade 4 Hematological Toxicities (excluding neuropathy): Withhold therapy until symptoms of toxcitiy resolve. Reinitiate at 25% reduced dose. Peripheral Neuropathy: Grade 1 with pain or Grade 2 (interfering with function but not activities of daily living): Reduce dose to 1mg/m². Grade 2 with pain or Grade 3 (interfering with activities of daily living): Withhold dose until toxicity resolves. Reinitiate at 0.7mg/m² once weekly. Grade 4 (permanent sensory loss interfering with funtion): D/C therapy.

HOW SUPPLIED: Inj: 3.5mg

CONTRAINDICATIONS: Hypersensitivity to boron or mannitol.

WARNINGS/PRECAUTIONS: Avoid pregnancy. May cause or worsen peripheral neuropathy along with reports of severe sensory and motor peripheral neuropathy. Thrombocytopenia and neutropenia reported; monitor CBC and platelets frequently. May cause orthostatic/postural hypotension; caution with history of syncope or dehydration. May cause acute development or exacerbation of CHF and/or new onset of decreased left ventricular ejection fraction. Rare reports of acute diffuse infiltrative pulmonary disease of unknown etiology such as pneumonitis, interstitial pneumonia, lung infiltration and ARDS. May cause nausea, diarrhea, constipation, and vomiting; use of antiemetic and antidiarrheal medications may be necessary. Rare reports of Reversible Posterior Leukoencephalopathy syndrome. May cause tumor lysis syndrome. Hepatic impairment may decrease clearance. Closely monitor if CrCl <13mL/min or on hemodialysis. Patients on oral antidiabetic agents may require close monitoring of blood glucose levels. Monitor CBC frequently. Dosing adjustments not necessary for patients with renal impairment. Should be administered after dialysis procedure.

ADVERSE REACTIONS: Asthenic disorders, diarrhea, nausea, constipation, peripheral neuropathy, vomiting, pyrexia, thrombocytopenia, psychiatric disorders, anorexia/decreased appetite, paresthesia/dysesthesia, anemia, headache, cough, dyspnea.

INTERACTIONS: Caution with concomitant use of medications associated with peripheral neuropathy (eg, amiodarone, antivirals, isoniazid, nitrofurantoin, statins) or hypotension. Oral antidiabetic agents may require dosage adjustment. Caution with CYP3A4 inducers and inhibitors; may alter levels.

PREGNANCY: Category D, not for use in nursing.

MECHANISM OF ACTION: Proteasome inhibitor; inhibits chymotrypsin-like activity of 26S proteosome cell.

PHARMACOKINETICS: Absorption: (Twice weekly: 1mg/m^2; 1.3mg/m^2) C_{max}=67-106ng/mL; 89-120ng/mL. **Distribution:** V_d=498-1884L/m^2; plasma protein binding (83%). **Metabolism:** Oxidation via CYP3A4, 2C19, 1A2; 2D6, 2C9 (minor). Deboronation (major). **Elimination:** (1mg/m^2; 1.3mg/m^2) $T_{1/2}$=40-193 hrs; 76-108 hrs.

NURSING CONSIDERATIONS

Assessment: Assess for peripheral neuropathy, hypersensitivity to boron or mannitol, syncope, dehydration, risk factors for or existing heart disease (eg, CHF, hypotension, HTN), DM, hepatic dysfunction, pregnancy status, and possible drug interactions.

Monitoring: Monitor CBC, blood glucose, and LFTs periodically. Monitor for signs/symptoms of dehydration, hypoglycemia, hyperglycemia, new/worsening neuropathy, cardiopulmonary symptoms, reversible posterior leukoencephalopathy syndrome (RPLS), tumor lysis syndrome, and hypersensitivity reactions.

Patient Counseling: Caution may impair mental/physical abilities. Inform of pregnancy risks and to use contraceptives. Advise to avoid dehydration. Seek medical attention if symptoms of new/worsening neuropathy (eg, burning, paresthesia, weakness), cardiopulmonary symptoms (eg, SOB, cough, swelling of feet), RPLS (eg, seizure, HTN, headache, blindness), hypersensitivity reactions, or hypotension (eg, dizziness, fainting spells) occur.

Administration: IV route. **Storage:** 25°C (77°F); excursions permitted to 15-30°C (59-86°F). Protect from light. Reconstituted: 25°C (77°F); stable for 8 hrs.

VENTAVIS — RX

iloprost (Actelion)

THERAPEUTIC CLASS: Systemic and pulmonary arterial vascular bed dilator

INDICATIONS: Treatment of pulmonary arterial hypertension (WHO Group I) in patients with NYHA Class III or IV symptoms.

V

DOSAGE: *Adults:* Initial: 2.5mcg via Prodose AAD System. Maint: 5mcg. Max: 45mcg/day. Should be taken 6 to 9 times per day. Elderly: Start at lower end of dosing range.

HOW SUPPLIED: Sol, Inhalation: 20mcg/2mL

WARNINGS/PRECAUTIONS: Risk of syncope and hypotension. If signs of pulmonary edema occur; d/c therapy. Avoid oral ingestion and contact with skin or eyes. I-neb AAD or Prodose AAD System administration only. May induce acute bronchospasm in patients with hyperreactive airways. Monitor those with COPD, asthma, acute pulmonary infections. Caution in elderly.

ADVERSE REACTIONS: Vasodilation, increased cough, headache, trismus, insomnia, NV, hypotension, flu syndrome, back pain, syncope, palpitations, muscle cramps, increased GGT, increased alk phos.

INTERACTIONS: Iloprost has the potential to increase the hypotensive effect of vasodilators and antihypertensive agents. Increased risk of bleeding with anticoagulants.

PREGNANCY: Category C, not for use in nursing.

MECHANISM OF ACTION: Synthetic prostacyclin PGI_2 analogue; dilates systemic and pulmonary arterial vascular beds. Affects platelet aggregation.

PHARMACOKINETICS: Absorption: C_{max}=150pg/mL. **Distribution:** V_d=0.7-0.08L/kg; plasma protein binding (60%). **Metabolism:** β-oxidation. Tetranor-iloprost (main metabolite). **Elimination:** Urine (68%), feces (12%).

NURSING CONSIDERATIONS

Assessment: Assess for renal/hepatic impairment, hypotension; not to be taken if systolic BP <85 mmHg. Assess risk of syncope, pregnancy status, and possible drug interactions (eg, anticoagulants).

Monitoring: Monitor vital signs. While initiating treatment, monitor for signs of pulmonary edema (may be a sign of pulmonary venous HTN). Monitor for further hypotension and increased risk of syncope.

Patient Counseling: Counsel to use drug as prescribed, including dosing frequency, amp dispensing, and equipment cleaning. Caution about fall in BP and possible dizziness or fainting; consult physician if fainting gets worse and use caution in standing up or getting out of bed or chair.

Administration: Inhalation route. **Storage:** 20-25°C (68-77°F); excursions permitted to 15-30°C (59-86°F).

VENTOLIN HFA — RX

albuterol sulfate (GlaxoSmithKline)

THERAPEUTIC CLASS: $Beta_2$-agonist

INDICATIONS: Prevention and treatment of bronchospasm with reversible obstructive airway disease. Prevention of Exercise-Induced Bronchospasm (EIB).

DOSAGE: *Adults:* Bronchospasm: 2 inh q4-6h or 1 inh q4h. EIB: 2 inh 15-30 min before activity.

Pediatrics: ≥4 yrs: Bronchospasm: 2 inh q4-6h or 1 inh q4h. EIB: 2 inh 15-30 min before activity.

HOW SUPPLIED: MDI: 90mcg/inh [18g]

WARNINGS/PRECAUTIONS: D/C if paradoxical bronchospasm or cardiovascular events occur. Avoid excessive use. Caution with coronary insufficiency, arrhythmias, HTN, DM, hyperthyroidism, seizures, sensitivity to sympathomimetics. Hypersensitivity reactions may occur. May cause transient hypokalemia.

ADVERSE REACTIONS: Throat irritation, viral respiratory infections, upper respiratory inflammation, cough, musculoskeletal pain.

INTERACTIONS: Avoid other short-acting sympathomimetic bronchodilators; caution with oral sympathomimetics. Extreme caution with MAOIs, TCAs during or within 2 weeks of discontinuation. May cause severe bronchospasm with β-blockers. Decreases digoxin levels. ECG changes and/or hypokalemia with non-K^+-sparing diuretics.

PREGNANCY: Category C, not for use in nursing.

MECHANISM OF ACTION: β_2-adrenergic bronchodilator; stimulates adenyl cyclase, the enzyme that catalyzes formation of cAMP from ATP. Increased cAMP levels associated with relaxation of bronchial smooth muscle and inhibition of release of mediators of immediate hypersensitivity.

PHARMACOKINETICS: Absorption: C_{max}=3ng/mL; T_{max}=0.42 hrs.

NURSING CONSIDERATIONS

Assessment: Assess for renal/hepatic function, history of hypersensitivity to drug, CVD (eg, coronary insufficiency, HTN, cardiac arrhythmias), convulsive disorders, hyperthyroidism, DM and ketoacidosis, and possible drug interactions.

Monitoring: Monitor for possible paradoxical bronchospasm, deterioration of asthma, cardiovascular effects, and immediate hypersensitivity reactions.

Patient Counseling: Instruct to shake inhaler well before using. Prime inhaler before using for 1st time, when not used >2 weeks, or when dropped. To prime, release 4 test sprays into air away from face. Keep plastic actuator clean to prevent build-up and blockage. Wash actuator by running warm water through top and bottom for 30 seconds at least once a week; shake after to remove excess water and air-dry thoroughly. Avoid spraying in eyes.

Administration: Oral inhalation. 1) Remove cap from mouthpiece of actuator. 2) Breathe out through mouth. 3) Breathe in through mouth and at same time spray product into mouth. 4) Hold breath for 10 seconds and remove mouthpiece. 5) Wait 1 min before next spray. 6) Replace cap and keep mouthpiece clean. 7) Discard after 200 sprays. **Storage:** 15-20°C (59-77°F). Do not puncture. Do not use or store near heat or open flame. Exposure to temp above 120°F may cause bursting. Store inhaler with mouthpiece down, away from children.

VERAMYST RX

fluticasone furoate (GlaxoSmithKline)

THERAPEUTIC CLASS: Corticosteroid

INDICATIONS: Treatment of the symptoms of seasonal and perennial allergic rhinitis in patients ≥2 yrs.

DOSAGE: *Adults:* Initial: 2 sprays per nostril qd. Maint: 1 spray per nostril qd. *Pediatrics:* ≥12 yrs: Initial: 2 sprays per nostril qd. Maint: 1 spray per nostril qd. 2-11 yrs: Initial: 1 spray per nostril qd. Titrate: If inadequate response, may increase to 2 sprays per nostril.

HOW SUPPLIED: Spray: 27.5mcg/spray [10g]

WARNINGS/PRECAUTIONS: Excessive use may cause hypercorticism and adrenal suppression. Risk of adrenal insufficiency and withdrawal symptoms when replacing systemic corticosteroids with topical corticosteroids. Caution with active or quiescent TB, ocular herpes simplex, or untreated bacterial, fungal, and systemic viral infections. Risk for more severe/fatal course of infections (eg, chickenpox, measles); avoid exposure in patients who have not had disease or have not been properly immunized. Epistaxis and nasal ulcerations may occur. *Candida* infection of nose reported. Avoid with recent nasal trauma, ulcers, or surgery. May result in glaucoma and cataracts. Potential for reduced growth velocity in pediatrics.

ADVERSE REACTIONS: Headache, epistaxis, nasopharyngitis, pyrexia, pharynolaryngeal pain, cough, nasal ulceration, back pain.

INTERACTIONS: Ketoconazole or other potent CYP3A4 inhibitors may increase serum fluticasone levels; co-administer with caution. Increased levels with ritonavir; avoid use.

PREGNANCY: Category C, caution in nursing.

MECHANISM OF ACTION: Corticosteroid; unknown. Anti-inflammatory agent with wide range of effects on multiple cell types (eg, mast cells, eosinophils, neutrophils, macrophages, lymphocytes) and mediators (eg, histamine, eicosanoids, cytokines, leukotrienes) involved in inflammation.

PHARMACOKINETICS: Absorption: Incomplete absorption, absolute bioavailability (0.5%). **Distribution:** Plasma protein binding (99%). **Metabolism:** Hepatic (extensive) via CYP3A4. **Elimination:** Feces.

NURSING CONSIDERATIONS

Assessment: Assess for active or quiescent TB, untreated localized or systemic fungal/bacterial infection, systemic viral infection, ocular herpes simplex, history of glaucoma or cataracts, history of nasal polyps, recent nasal septal ulcers, nasal surgery/trauma, glaucoma, concomitant use with other inhaled or systemic corticosteroids, hepatic function, possible drug interactions.

Monitoring: Monitor for acute adrenal insufficiency, hypercorticism, HPA-axis suppression, chickenpox, measles, nasal or pharyngeal *Candida* infections, epistaxis, nasal ulceration, nasal septal perforation, hypoadrenalism (in infant born to mother who received corticosteroids during pregnancy), suppression of growth velocity in children, vision changes, increased IOP.

Patient Counseling: Counsel to take as directed. Avoid exposure to chickenpox and measles; consult physician immediately if exposed, if symptoms worsen, or if adverse reactions (eg, epistaxis, nasal ulceration, nasal/pharyngeal candida infection, vision changes) occur. Avoid spraying into eyes.

Administration: Intranasal route. **Storage:** Store device in upright position, cap in place, between 15-30°C (59-86°F). Do not freeze or refrigerate.

VERELAN RX

verapamil HCl (UCB)

THERAPEUTIC CLASS: Calcium channel blocker (nondihydropyridine)

INDICATIONS: Management of hypertension.

DOSAGE: *Adults:* Usual: 240mg qam. Titrate: May increase by 120mg qam. Max: 480mg qam. Elderly/Small People: Initial: 120mg qam. Titrate: May increase to 180mg qam, then 240mg qam, then 360mg qam, then 480mg qam. May sprinkle on applesauce; do not crush or chew.

HOW SUPPLIED: Cap, Extended-Release: 120mg, 180mg, 240mg, 360mg

CONTRAINDICATIONS: Severe ventricular dysfunction, hypotension, cardiogenic shock, sick sinus syndrome or 2nd- or 3rd-degree AV block (except with functioning ventricular pacemaker), A-Fib/Flutter with an accessory bypass tract.

WARNINGS/PRECAUTIONS: Avoid with moderate to severe cardiac failure, and ventricular dysfunction if taking a β-blocker. May cause hypotension, AV block, transient bradycardia, PR interval prolongation. Monitor LFTs periodically; hepatocellular injury reported. Give 30% of normal dose with severe hepatic dysfunction. Caution with hypertrophic cardiomyopathy, renal or hepatic dysfunction. Decrease dose in those with decreased neuromuscular transmission.

ADVERSE REACTIONS: Constipation, dizziness, nausea, hypotension, headache, peripheral edema, infection, flu syndrome, fatigue, bradycardia, AV block.

INTERACTIONS: Additive negative effects on HR, AV conduction, and contractility with β-blockers. Potentiates other antihypertensives. May increase digoxin, carbamazepine, theophylline, cyclosporine, and alcohol levels. Avoid disopyramide within 48 hrs before or 24 hrs after verapamil. Additive negative inotropic effects and AV conduction prolongation with flecainide. Avoid quinidine with hypertrophic cardiomyopathy. Monitor lithium levels. Increased clearance with phenobarbital. Rifampin may reduce oral bioavailability. May potentiate neuromuscular blockers; both agents may need dose reduction. Caution with inhalation anesthetics. Increased bleeding time with ASA. Increased efficacy of doxorubicin. Reduced absorption with COPP and VAC cytotoxic drug regimens. May decrease clearance of paclitaxel. CYP3A4 inhibitors (eg, erythromycin, ritonavir) or grapefruit juice may increase levels. CYP3A4 inducers (eg, rifampin) may lower levels.

PREGNANCY: Category C, not for use in nursing.

NURSING CONSIDERATIONS

Assessment: Assess for left ventricular dysfunction, hypotension, sick sinus syndrome, 2nd- or 3rd-degree AV block, atrial flutter, accessory bypass tract, CHF, LFTs, cardiomyopathy, attenuated neuromuscular transmission, renal impairment, and possible drug interactions.

Monitoring: Monitor for hypotension, CHF, arrhythmias, heart block, LFTs, constipation, headache, dizziness.

Patient Counseling: Counsel about adverse effects. Instruct to take as prescribed. Advise to swallow cap whole; do not crush or chew. May administer by opening and sprinkling pellets on spoonful of applesauce (should not be hot), and swallow immediately without chewing with a glass of cool water. Subdividing contents of capsule not recommended.

VERELAN PM — RX

verapamil HCl (UCB)

THERAPEUTIC CLASS: Calcium channel blocker (nondihydropyridine)

INDICATIONS: Management of hypertension.

DOSAGE: *Adults:* Usual: 200mg qhs. Titrate: May increase to 300mg qhs, then 400mg qhs. Renal or Hepatic Dysfunction/Elderly/Small People: Initial: 100mg qhs. Max: 400mg qhs. May sprinkle on applesauce; do not crush or chew.

HOW SUPPLIED: Cap, Extended-Release: 100mg, 200mg, 300mg

CONTRAINDICATIONS: Severe ventricular dysfunction, hypotension, cardiogenic shock, sick sinus syndrome or 2nd- or 3rd-degree AV block (except with functioning ventricular pacemaker), A-Fib/Flutter with an accessory bypass tract.

WARNINGS/PRECAUTIONS: Avoid with moderate to severe cardiac failure, and ventricular dysfunction if taking a β-blocker. May cause hypotension, AV block, transient bradycardia, PR interval prolongation. Monitor LFTs periodically; hepatocellular injury reported. Give 30% of normal dose with severe hepatic dysfunction. Caution with hypertrophic cardiomyopathy, renal or hepatic dysfunction. Decrease dose in those with decreased neuromuscular transmission.

ADVERSE REACTIONS: Constipation, dizziness, nausea, hypotension, headache, peripheral edema, infection, flu syndrome, fatigue, bradycardia, AV block.

INTERACTIONS: Additive negative effects on HR, AV conduction, and contractility with β-blockers. Potentiates other antihypertensives. May increase digoxin, carbamazepine, theophylline, cyclosporine, and alcohol levels. Avoid disopyramide within 48 hrs before or 24 hrs after verapamil. Additive negative inotropic effects and AV conduction prolongation with flecainide. Avoid quinidine with hypertrophic cardiomyopathy. Monitor lithium levels. Increased clearance with phenobarbital. Rifampin may reduce oral bioavailability. May potentiate neuromuscular blockers; both agents may need dose reduction. Caution with inhalation anesthetics. Increased bleeding time with ASA. Increased efficacy of doxorubicin. Reduced absorption with COPP and VAC cytotoxic drug regimens. May decrease clearance of paclitaxel. CYP3A4 inhibitors (eg, erythromycin, ritonavir) or grapefruit juice may increase levels. CYP3A4 inducers (eg, rifampin) may decrease levels.

PREGNANCY: Category C, not for use in nursing.

MECHANISM OF ACTION: Calcium channel blocker (non-dihydropyridine); inhibits transmembrane influx of ionic calcium into arterial smooth muscle and contractile myocardial cells without altering serum calcium concentrations.

PHARMACOKINETICS: Absorption: Absolute bioavailability (33-65% R), (13-34% S); C_{max}=77.8ng/mL (R), 16.8ng/mL (S); AUC=1037ng•h/mL (R-enantiomer), 195ng•h/mL (S-enantiomer). **Distribution:** Plasma protein binding (94% R), (88% S); α-1-acid glycoprotein binding (92% R), (86% S); found in breast milk. **Metabolism:** Liver via CYP450; demethylation, and dealkylation; norverapamil (active metabolite). **Elimination:** Urine (70%), feces (16%); $T_{1/2}$=14-16 hrs.

NURSING CONSIDERATIONS

Assessment: Assess for left ventricular dysfunction, hypotension, cardiogenic shock, sick sinus syndrome, 2nd- or 3rd-degree AV block, atrial flutter/fibrillation, accessory bypass tract, CHF, LFTs, hypertrophic cardiomyopathy, attenuated neuromuscular transmission, impaired renal function, and possible drug interactions.

Monitoring: Monitor for hypotension, CHF, arrhythmias, AV block, angina pectoris, MI, ECG, LFTs, constipation, headache, dizziness, and infections.

Patient Counseling: Advise to immediately seek medical help if a drop in BP, chest pain, headache, dizziness, NV, or edema develops. Instruct to take as prescribed. Swallow capsule whole; do not crush or chew. May administer by opening and sprinkling pellets on spoonful of applesauce (should not be hot), and swallow immediately, without chewing, with a glass of cool water.

Administration: Oral route. **Storage:** 25°C (77°F); excursions permitted to 15-30°C (59-86°F). Protect from moisture. Dispense in tight, light-resistant container.

VESANOID RX

tretinoin (Roche Labs)

Administer under strict supervision of experienced physician and institution. Risk of retinoic acid-APL syndrome and leukocytosis. High risk of teratogenic effects.

THERAPEUTIC CLASS: Retinoid

INDICATIONS: Induction of remission in acute promyelocytic leukemia (APL) in those resistant to anthracycline therapy or those where anthracycline-based therapy is contraindicated.

DOSAGE: *Adults:* 45mg/m²/day in 2 divided doses. D/C 30 days after achieving complete remission or after 90 days of therapy, whichever occurs 1st. *Pediatrics:* ≥1 yrs: 45mg/m²/day in 2 divided doses. D/C 30 days after achieving complete remission or after 90 days of therapy, whichever occurs 1st.

HOW SUPPLIED: Cap: 10mg

CONTRAINDICATIONS: Sensitivity to parabens.

WARNINGS/PRECAUTIONS: May cause abortion or fetal abnormalities. Females should use contraception during and 1 month after therapy. Confirm APL diagnosis. Pseudotumor cerebri reported, especially in pediatrics. Reversible hypercholesterolemia, hypertriglyceridemia reported. Elevated LFTs reported; d/c if >5x ULN. Monitor for signs of respiratory compromise or leukocytosis. Check hematologic profile, coagulation profile, LFTs, and cholesterol frequently.

ADVERSE REACTIONS: Malaise, shivering, hemorrhage, infections, peripheral edema, pain, chest discomfort, edema, disseminated intravascular coagulation, weight change, injection site reactions, dyspnea, pleural effusion, respiratory insufficiency, pneumonia.

INTERACTIONS: Possible interactions with drugs that affect CYP450 system. Aggravated symptoms of hypervitaminosis A with vitamin A. Cases of fatal thrombotic complications with antifibrinolytic agents (eg, tranexamic acid, aminocaproic acid). Increased risk of pseudotumor cerebri/intracranial HTN with tetracyclines.

PREGNANCY: Category D, not for use in nursing.

MECHANISM OF ACTION: Retinoid; not known. Induces cytodifferentiation and decreases proliferation of APL cells.

PHARMACOKINETICS: Absorption: C_{max}=394ng/mL; T_{max}=1-2 hrs; AUC=537ng•h/mL. **Distribution:** Plasma protein binding (>95%). **Metabolism:** Oxidation via CYP450. **Elimination:** $T_{1/2}$=0.5-2 hrs.

NURSING CONSIDERATIONS

Assessment: Assess for hypersensitivity to parabens (preservatives), detection of t(15;17) genetic marker, elevated WBC levels, pregnancy status, and possible drug interactions. Obtain baseline WBC, hematologic profile, coagulation profile, LFTs, triglyceride and cholesterol levels.

Monitoring: Frequently monitor WBC, hematologic profile, coagulation profile, LFTs, triglyceride and cholesterol levels. Monitor for signs/symptoms of pseudotumor cerebri, leukocytosis, retinoic acid-APL syndrome (RA-APL), thrombosis, respiratory compromise, and hypersensitivity reactions.

Patient Counseling: Caution may impair mental/physical abilities. Inform of pregnancy risks; advise to use 2 forms of contraception during, and for 1 month after d/c, even if history of infertility or menopause (unless prior hysterectomy). Inform "mini-pill" is inadequate. Advise to seek medical attention if symptoms of pseudotumor cerebri (eg, papilledema, headache, NV), leukocytosis (eg, bleeding), RA-APL (eg, fever, dyspnea, ARD, weight gain), thrombosis, respiratory compromise, or hypersensitivity reactions occur.

Administration: Oral route. **Storage:** 15-30°C (59-86°F). Protect from light.

VESICARE RX

solifenacin succinate (Astellas/GlaxoSmithKline)

THERAPEUTIC CLASS: Muscarinic antagonist

INDICATIONS: Treatment of overactive bladder with symptoms of urge urinary incontinence, urgency, and urinary frequency.

DOSAGE: *Adults:* Usual: 5mg qd. Max: 10mg qd. Renal Impairment (CrCl <30mL/min)/Moderate Hepatic Impairment (Child-Pugh B)/Potent CYP3A4 Inhibitors: Max: 5mg qd. Do not use in severe hepatic impairment (Child-Pugh C).

HOW SUPPLIED: Tab: 5mg, 10mg

CONTRAINDICATIONS: Urinary retention, gastric retention, uncontrolled narrow-angle glaucoma.

WARNINGS/PRECAUTIONS: Caution with bladder outflow obstruction, GI obstructive disorders, decreased gastrointestinal motility, and narrow-angle glaucoma. Caution with renal and hepatic impairment.

ADVERSE REACTIONS: Dry mouth, constipation, nausea, dyspepsia, UTI, blurred vision.

INTERACTIONS: Do not exceed 5mg daily dose when administered with therapeutic doses of ketoconazole or other potent CYP3A4 inhibitors.

PREGNANCY: Category C, not for use in nursing.

MECHANISM OF ACTION: Muscarinic receptor antagonist; inhibits muscarinic receptors, resulting in decreased urinary smooth muscle contraction and salivary secretion.

PHARMACOKINETICS: Absorption: Absolute bioavailabilty (90%); T_{max}=3-8 hrs. **Distribution:** V_d=600L; plasma protein binding (98%). **Metabolism:** CYP3A4 (N-oxidation; 4R-hydroxylation), 4R-hydroxy solifenacin (active metabolite). **Elimination:** Urine (<15%), feces; $T_{1/2}$=45-68 hrs.

NURSING CONSIDERATIONS

Assessment: Assess for bladder outflow obstruction (eg, urinary retention), gastric retention, narrow-angle glaucoma, decreased GI motility, possible drug interactions, renal/hepatic impairment.

Monitoring: Monitor for signs/symptoms of urinary retention, gastric retention, blurred vision, hypersensitivity reaction, renal/hepatic dysfunction.

Patient Counseling: Inform that therapy associated with constipation and blurred vision. Inform may impair mental/physical abilities. Advise to seek medical attention if symptoms of severe abdominal pain, constipation (>3 days), blurred vision, heat prostration (eg, decreased sweating), or hypersensitivity reactions occur.

Administration: Oral route. **Storage:** 25°C (77°F); excursions permitted to 15-30°C (59-86°F).

VFEND

voriconazole (Pfizer)

RX

THERAPEUTIC CLASS: Azole antifungal

INDICATIONS: Treatment of invasive aspergillosis, esophageal candidiasis. Treatment of candidemia in nonneutropenic patients and the following *Candida* infections: disseminated infections in skin and infections in abdomen, kidney, bladder wall, and wounds. Treatment of serious fungal infections caused by *Scedosporium apiospermum* and *Fusarium* spp. including *Fusarium solani* in patients intolerant of, or refractory to, other therapy.

DOSAGE: *Adults:* (Inj) LD: 6mg/kg IV q12h x 2 doses. Maint: 4mg/kg IV q12h. Switch to PO when appropriate. (PO) Maint: ≥40kg: 200mg q12h; 300mg q12h if inadequate response. <40kg: 100mg q12h; 150 mg q12h if inadequate response. Esophageal Candidiasis: (PO) ≥40kg: 200mg q12h. <40kg: 100mg q12h. Treat for minimum of 14 days and at least 7 days following resolution of symptoms. Intolerant: (Inj/PO) Maint: IV: 3mg/kg q12h. PO: Reduce by 50mg steps to minimum of 200mg q12h for >40kg or 100mg q12h for <40kg. Concomitant Phenytoin: Maint: IV: 5mg/kg q12h. PO: ≥40kg: 400mg q12h. <40kg: 200mg q12h. Concomitant Efavirenz: Maint: 400mg q12h and efavirenz should be decreased to 300mg q24h. Mild to Moderate Hepatic Cirrhosis: Maint: 1/2 of maint dose. CrCl <50mL/min: Use PO. Give PO 1 hr before or 1 hr after a meal. Base duration on severity of underlying disease, recovery from immunosuppression, and clinical response.

HOW SUPPLIED: Inj: 200mg; Sus: 40mg/mL; Tab: 50mg, 200mg

CONTRAINDICATIONS: Concomitant CYP3A4 substrates (terfenadine, astemizole, cisapride, pimozide, quinidine), sirolimus, rifampin, carbamazepine, long-acting barbiturates, high-dose ritonavir (400mg q12h), low-dose ritonavir (100mg q12h; assess benefit/risk), rifabutin, ergot alkaloids, St. John's wort.

WARNINGS/PRECAUTIONS: Monitor visual function with treatment >28 days. Hepatic reactions (clinical hepatitis, cholestasis, fulminant hepatic failure) reported; monitor LFTs at initiation and during therapy. D/C if liver dysfunction occurs. Tabs contain lactose; avoid with galactose intolerance, Lapp lactase deficiency, or glucose-galactose malabsorption. Anaphylactoid-type reactions reported with infusion. Avoid strong, direct sunlight. Monitor renal function. May prolong QT interval; caution with proarrhythmic conditions. Correct electrolyte disturbances before starting therapy. If rash develops, monitor closely and consider discontinuation of voriconazole.

ADVERSE REACTIONS: Visual disturbances, fever, chills, rash, headache, NV, sepsis, peripheral edema, abdominal pain, respiratory disorder, increased LFTs and alkaline phosphatase.

INTERACTIONS: See Contraindications. Avoid with low-dose ritonavir (100mg q12h). Efavirenz reduces levels. May increase levels of CYP3A4 inhibitors; monitor for adverse events and toxicity with HIV protease inhibitors, NNRTIs, benzodiazepines, HMG-CoA reductase inhibitors, dihydropyridine CCBs, and vinca alkaloids. May increase levels of CYP2C9 inhibitors; monitor phenytoin, warfarin, hypoglycemics, tacrolimus (reduce tacrolimus to 1/3 of initial dose), and cyclosporine (reduce cyclosporine to 1/2 of initial dose). Omeprazole is CYP2C19/3A4 inhibitor; reduce omeprazole by 1/2 if voriconazole ≥40mg. Proton pump inhibitors that are CYP2C19 substrates may increase levels. Phenytoin may decrease levels. Oral contraceptives containing ethinyl estradiol and norethindrone may increase levels. May increase levels of oral contraceptives containing ethinyl estradiol and norethindrone. May increase levels of methadone; may prolong QT interval; dose reduction may be needed. Do not infuse into same line or cannula with other drug infusions or parenteral nutrition. Do not infuse simultaneously with blood products or electrolyte supplements.

PREGNANCY: Category D, not for use in nursing.

MECHANISM OF ACTION: Triazole antifungal agent; inhibits fungal CYP450 mediated 14α-lanosterol demethylation, an essential step in fungal ergosterol biosynthesis. Accumulation of 14-α methyl-sterols correlates with subsequent loss of ergosterol in fungal cell wall and may be responsible for antifungal activity of vorconizole.

PHARMACOKINETICS: Absorption: Administration of different doses led to varying parameters. T_{max}=1-2 hrs. **Distribution:** V_d=4.6L/kg; plasma protein binding (58%). **Metabolism:** Hepatic, via CYP2C19, CYP2C9, CYP3A4; N-oxide (major metabolite). **Elimination:** <2% excreted unchanged in urine.

NURSING CONSIDERATIONS

Assessment: Obtain fungal cultures prior to therapy to properly identify causative organisms. Assess for possible drug interactions. Assess pregnancy status, renal (SrCr) and hepatic function (LFTs, bilirubin), serum electrolytes (K^+, Mg, Ca), and correct deficiencies. Assess use with proarrhythmic conditions. Give oral formulation to patients with CrCl<50mL/min unless benefits of IV use outweigh risks. Assess with known hypersensitivity to drug or excipient, history of cardiotoxic chemotherapy, cardiomyopathy, hypokalemia, concomitant medications, arrhythmias, hepatic insufficiency (CrCl 50mL/min), and renal insufficiency.

Monitoring: Monitor visual acuity, visual field, and color perception with therapy for longer than 28 days. Monitor for infusion-related reactions, hepatotoxicity, arrhythmias, QT prolongation, acute renal failure, and dermatological reactions (eg, Stevens-Johnson syndrome). Monitor for drug toxicity with hepatic insufficiencies. Monitor renal function (SrCr) and hepatic function (LFTs, bilirubin) during therapy.

Patient Counseling: Counsel to take tabs or oral sus at least 1 hr before or after a meal. Avoid driving at night; drug may affect vision. Counsel to avoid hazardous tasks if visual changes occur and avoid direct sunlight. Oral sus contains sucrose and is not recommended with rare problems of fructose intolerance, sucrase-isomalate deficiency, or glucose-galactose malabsorption. Counsel females to use proper contraception during therapy.

Administration: Oral and IV route. IV: Do not infuse concomitantly into same line or cannula with other drug infusions, including parenteral nutrition. Reconstitute. 1) Add 19mL of SWFI to vial for a concentration of 10mg/mL. 2) Further dilute so final concentration is ≤5mg/mL. Infusion should be administered at maximum rate of 3/mg/kg/hr over 1 hr. Refer to prescribing guidelines. Oral Sus: Reconstitute: 1) Add 46mL of water to bottle and shake. **Storage:** IV: (unreconstituted) 15-30°C (59-86°F). Tab: 15-30°C (59-86°F). Oral Sus: (reconstituted) 15-30°C (59-86°F) for 14 days; (refrigerate before reconstitution) 2-8°C (36-46°F).

VIADUR — RX

leuprolide acetate (Bayer Healthcare)

THERAPEUTIC CLASS: Synthetic gonadotropin releasing hormone analog

INDICATIONS: Palliative treatment of advanced prostate cancer.

DOSAGE: *Adults:* Insert 1 implant SQ in upper arm every 12 months.

HOW SUPPLIED: Implant: 65mg

CONTRAINDICATIONS: Women, pregnancy, pediatrics.

WARNINGS/PRECAUTIONS: Transient worsening of symptoms may occur during 1st few weeks of therapy. Closely monitor patients with metastatic vertebral lesions and/or urinary tract obstruction during 1st few weeks of therapy. Monitor serum testosterone, PSA. Ureteral obstruction and spinal cord decompression reported.

ADVERSE REACTIONS: Headache, asthenia, hot flashes, ecchymosis, peripheral edema, depression, sweating, gynecomastia, nocturia, testis atrophy, breast pain, urinary retention/frequency, local bruising/burning.

PREGNANCY: Category X, safety in nursing not known.

MECHANISM OF ACTION: LH-RH agonist; acts as a potent inhibitor of gonadotropin secretion resulting in suppression of testicular and ovarian steroidogenesis.

PHARMACOKINETICS: Absorption: C_{max}=16.9ng/mL; T_{max}=4 hrs. **Distribution:** V_d=27L; plasma protein binding (43-49%). **Metabolism:** (Major metabolite): M-I. **Elimination:** $T_{1/2}$=3 hrs.

NURSING CONSIDERATIONS

Assessment: Assess pregnancy status, metastatic vertebral lesions, urinary tract obstruction, and possible drug interactions. Obtain baseline serum testosterone and PSA levels.

Monitoring: Periodically monitor serum testosterone and PSA levels and for signs/symptoms of anaphylactoid reactions, transient worsening of symptoms, and insertion-site reaction.

Patient Counseling: Inform to keep site clean and dry for 24 hrs; do not bathe or swim for 24 hrs. Avoid heavy lifting and physical activity for 48 hrs. Avoid bumping site for few days. After healed, should be able to go back to normal activities. Inform of pregnancy risks. Advise to seek medical attention if symptoms of hot flushes, transient worsening of symptoms (eg, bone pain, increased difficulty in urinating, onset or aggravation of nerve symptoms), insertion-site reaction (eg, unusual bleeding, redness, pain, weakness, numbness), or anaphylactoid reaction occurs.

Administration: Dermal implant. Inserting implant: 1) After cleansing and anesthetizing area, make 5mm incision just through dermis in groove between biceps and triceps. 2) Grasp handle and extend index finger to rest on back of actuator. Insert cannula tip into incision with level up and advance into intended track. Advance to depth indicator on cannula. 3) Hold handle in place; using index finger slide actuator back until stops. Do not pull back on handle. Withdraw implanter from incision. Check implant by palpation. **Storage:** 25°C (77°F); excursions permitted to 15-30°C (59-86°F).

VIAGRA — RX

sildenafil citrate (Pfizer)

THERAPEUTIC CLASS: Phosphodiesterase type 5 inhibitor

INDICATIONS: Treatment of erectile dysfunction (ED).

DOSAGE: *Adults:* Usual: 50mg 1 hr (range 0.5-4 hrs) prior to sexual activity at frequency of up to once daily. Titrate: May decrease to 25mg qd or increase to 100mg qd. Max: 100mg qd. Elderly/Hepatic Impairment/CrCl <30mL/min/Concomitant CYP450 3A4 Inhibitors (eg, ketoconazole, itraconazole, erythromycin, saquinavir): Initial: 25mg qd. Concomitant Ritonavir: Max: 25mg q48h. Concomitant α-blocker: Avoid doses >25mg sildenafil within 4 hours of an α-blocker.

HOW SUPPLIED: Tab: 25mg, 50mg, 100mg

CONTRAINDICATIONS: Organic nitrates taken regularly and/or intermittently.

WARNINGS/PRECAUTIONS: Caution with MI, stroke or life-threatening arrhythmia within last 6 months; with resting hypotension (BP<90/50) or HTN (BP>170/110); unstable angina due to cardiac failure or CAD; anatomical penile deformation; predisposition to priapism; and retinitis pigmentosa. Avoid in men where sexual activity is inadvisable due to underlying CV status. Decrease in supine BP reported. Rare reports of non-arteritic anterior ischemic optic neuropathy (NAION) with PDE5 inhibitors. Caution when PDE5 inhibitors are given concomitantly with α-blockers. PDE5 inhibitors and α-adrenergic blocking agents are both vasodilators with BP-lowering effects; additive effect on BP may be anticipated. Patients should be stable on α-blocker therapy prior to initiating a PDE5 inhibitor. Cases of sudden decrease or loss of hearing reported. D/C if experienced these symptoms.

ADVERSE REACTIONS: Headache, flushing, dyspepsia, nasal congestion, UTI, abnormal vision (eg, color tinge, increased light sensitivity, blurred vision), diarrhea, cardiovascular events, sudden decrease or loss of hearing.

INTERACTIONS: See Contraindications. Increased levels with CYP3A4 inhibitors (eg, cimetidine, ketoconazole, itraconazole, erythromycin, saquinavir) and protease inhibitors (eg, ritonavir). CYP2C9 inhibitors may decrease sildenafil clearance. CYP3A4 inducers (eg, rifampin) may decrease levels. Potentiates hypotensive effects of nitrates. Additional supine BP reduction with amlodipine reported. Simultaneous administration with α-blockers may lead to symptomatic hypotension; sildenafil dose should not exceed 25mg and should not be taken within 4 hrs of taking an α-blocker. Avoid with other ED treatments.

PREGNANCY: Category B, not for use in nursing.

MECHANISM OF ACTION: Phosphodiesterase type 5 inhibitor; enhances effect of nitric oxide by inhibiting phosphodiesterase type 5, which is responsible for the degradation of cGMP in corpus cavernosum.

PHARMACOKINETICS: Absorption: Rapid; absolute bioavailability (40%). **Distribution:** V_d=105L; plasma protein binding (96%). **Metabolism:** Liver, via CYP450 3A4 (major), 2C9 (minor); N-desmethyl. **Elimination:** Feces (80% metabolites), urine (13%); $T_{1/2}$=4 hrs.

NURSING CONSIDERATIONS

Assessment: Assess for CVD, retinitis pigmentosa, bleeding disorders, active peptic ulceration, anatomical deformation of penis, renal/hepatic impairment, potential underlying causes of ED, possible drug interactions, and pregnancy/nursing status.

Monitoring: Monitor potential for cardiac risk due to sexual activity, postural hypotension, color vision changes, hypersensitivity reactions, stomach ulcers. Monitor therapeutic effect when used in combination with other drugs.

Patient Counseling: Instruct to seek medical assistance if erection persists >4 hrs. Advise of potential BP-lowering effect of α-blockers and antihypertensive drugs, and cardiac risk of sexual activity. Counsel about protective measures necessary to guard against STDs, including HIV. D/C and inform physician if sudden loss of vision, color vision, or hearing occur. Counsel to take tab 1 hr before intercourse.

Administration: Oral route. **Storage:** 25°C (77°F); excursions permitted to 15-30°C (59-86°F). Keep out of reach of children.

VIBRAMYCIN RX

doxycycline hyclate (Pfizer)

OTHER BRAND NAMES: Vibra-Tabs (Pfizer)

THERAPEUTIC CLASS: Tetracycline derivative

INDICATIONS: Treatment of the following infections caused by susceptible microorganisms: Rocky Mountain spotted fever; typhus fever and the typhus group; Q fever; rickettsialpox; tick fevers; respiratory tract infections; lymphogranuloma venereum; psittacosis (ornithosis); trachoma; inclusion conjunctivitis; uncomplicated urethral, endocervical, or rectal infections; nongonococcal urethritis; relapsing fever; chancroid; plague; tularemia; cholera; *Campylobacter fetus* infections; brucellosis; bartonellosis; granuloma inguinale; respiratory tract and urinary tract infections; anthrax. Treatment of infections caused by *Escherichia coli*, *Enterobacter aerogenes*, *Shigella* species, *Acinetobacter* species. When penicillin is contraindicated, treatment of the following infections caused by susceptible microorganisms: uncomplicated gonorrhea, syphilis, yaws, listeriosis, Vincent's infection, actinomycosis, infections caused by *Clostridium* species. Adjunct in acute intestinal amebiasis and severe acne. Prophylaxis of malaria.

DOSAGE: *Adults:* Usual: 100mg q12h on Day 1, then 100mg qd or 50mg q12h. Severe Infection: 100mg q12h. Treat for 10 days with strep infection. Uncomplicated Gonococcal Infection (Except Anorectal in Men): 100mg bid for 7 days or 300mg followed by 300mg in 1 hr. Uncomplicated Urethral/Endocervical/Rectal Infection and Nongonococcal Urethritis: 100mg bid for 7 days. Syphilis: 100mg bid for 2 weeks. Syphilis for >1 yr: 100mg bid for

4 weeks. Acute Epididymo-orchitis: 100mg bid for at least 10 days. Inhalation Anthrax (Post-Exposure): 100mg bid for 60 days. Malaria Prophylaxis: 100mg qd. Begin 1-2 days before travel and continue for 4 weeks after leaving malarious area.
Pediatrics: >8 yrs: ≤100 lbs: 1mg/lb bid on Day 1, then 1mg/lb qd or 0.5mg/lb bid. Severe Infections: Maint: 2mg/lb. >100 lbs: Usual: 100mg q12h on Day 1, then 100mg qd or 50mg q12h. Severe Infection: 100mg q12h. Treat for 10 days with strep infection. Inhalation Anthrax (Post-Exposure): <100 lbs: 1mg/lb bid for 60 days. ≥100 lbs: 100mg bid for 60 days. Malaria Prophylaxis: >8 yrs: 2mg/kg qd. Max: 100mg/day. Begin 1-2 days before travel and continue for 4 weeks after leaving malarious area.

HOW SUPPLIED: Cap: (Doxycycline Hyclate) 50mg, 100mg; Syrup: (Doxycycline Calcium) 50mg/5mL; Sus: (Doxycycline Monohydrate) 25mg/5mL [60mL]; Tab: (Vibra-Tabs) 100mg

WARNINGS/PRECAUTIONS: May cause fetal harm with pregnancy. Permanent tooth discoloration during tooth development (last half of pregnancy, infancy, and children <8 yrs) reported. *Clostridium difficile*-associated diarrhea reported. May increase BUN. Photosensitivity, enamel hypoplasia reported. Superinfection with prolonged use. Syrup contains sodium metabisulfite. Bulging fontanels in infants and benign intracranial HTN in adults reported. Monitor renal/hepatic and hematopoietic function with long-term use. Take adequate fluids with caps or tabs to reduce esophageal irritation. Take with food or milk if GI irritation occurs.

ADVERSE REACTIONS: GI effects (eg, anorexia, nausea, vomiting, diarrhea), photosensitivity, increased BUN, hypersensitivity reactions, hemolytic anemia, thrombocytopenia, neutropenia, eosinophilia.

INTERACTIONS: May decrease PT, adjust anticoagulants. May interfere with bactericidal agents (eg, penicillin). May decrease effects of oral contraceptives. Aluminum-, calcium-, iron-, and magnesium-containing products and bismuth subsalicylate impair absorption. Decreased half-life with barbiturates, carbamazepine, and phenytoin. Fatal renal toxicity with methoxyflurane.

PREGNANCY: Category D, not for use in nursing.

MECHANISM OF ACTION: Tetracycline derivative; thought to inhibit protein synthesis.

PHARMACOKINETICS: Absorption: (PO) completely absorbed, C_{max}=2.6 mcg/mL, T_{max}=2 hrs. **Distribution:** Crosses placenta. **Elimination:** Urine, feces.

NURSING CONSIDERATIONS

Assessment: Assess for pregnancy status, possible drug interactions, and renal impairment. Document indications for therapy, culture, and susceptibility testing. Perform incision and drainage in conjunction with antibiotic therapy when indicated.

Monitoring: Monitor for signs/symptoms of hypersensitivity reactions, photosensitivity, superinfection, *C. difficile*-associated diarrhea, vaginal candidiasis, benign intracranial HTN, LFTs, renal function. In venereal disease with coexistent syphilis, conduct dark field exam before treatment and monthly for 4 months.

Patient Counseling: Inform of pregnancy risks and photosensitivity reactions (d/c at 1st sign of skin erythema). Advise to avoid excessive sunlight and UV light and wear sunscreen/sunblock. Instruct to drink fluids liberally to reduce risk of esophageal irritation or ulceration. Inform that therapy only treats bacterial, not viral, infections. Take as directed; skipping doses or not completing full course may decrease effectiveness and increase resistance. Inform may experience diarrhea; notify physician if watery/bloody stools, hypersensitivity reactions, superinfections, photosensitivity, or benign intracranial HTN occur. Advise to avoid foods with calcium. Advise patients on malaria prophylaxis to begin therapy 2 days before travel, continue while in malarious area, and continue for 4 weeks after returning from area. Therapy should not exceed 4 months.

Administration: Oral route. **Storage:** Below 30°C (86°F); dispense in tight, light-resistant container.

VICODIN CIII

hydrocodone bitartrate - acetaminophen (Abbott)

OTHER BRAND NAMES: Vicodin HP (Abbott) - Vicodin ES (Abbott)

THERAPEUTIC CLASS: Opioid analgesic

INDICATIONS: Relief of moderate to moderately severe pain.

DOSAGE: *Adults:* Usual: Vicodin: 1-2 tabs q4-6h prn. Max: 8 tabs/day. Vicodin HP: 1 tab q4-6h prn. Max: 6 tabs/day. Vicodin ES: 1 tab q4-6h prn. Max: 5 tabs/day.

HOW SUPPLIED: (Hydrocodone-APAP) Tab: Vicodin: 5mg-500mg*; Vicodin HP: 10mg-660mg*; Vicodin ES: 7.5mg-750mg* *scored

WARNINGS/PRECAUTIONS: Caution in elderly, debilitated, severe hepatic or renal dysfunction, hypothyroidism, Addison's disease, prostatic hypertrophy, urethral stricture, pulmonary disease and postoperative use. May obscure acute abdominal conditions or head injuries. May produce dose-related respiratory depression. Monitor for tolerance. Suppresses cough reflex.

ADVERSE REACTIONS: Lightheadedness, dizziness, sedation, NV, constipation, rash, respiratory depression.

INTERACTIONS: Additive CNS depression with other narcotic analgesics, antihistamines, antipsychotics, antianxiety agents, alcohol and other CNS depressants. Increased effect of antidepressant or hydrocodone with MAOIs or TCAs.

PREGNANCY: Category C, not for use in nursing.

MECHANISM OF ACTION: Hydrocodone: Opioid analgesic; precise mechanism not known. Suspected to relate to existence of opiate receptors in CNS. APAP: Nonopiate, nonsalicylate analgesic and antipyretic. Analgesic action involves peripheral influences; specific mechanism not established. Antipyretic activity mediated through hypothalmic heat-regulating centers. Inhibits prostaglandin synthetase.

PHARMACOKINETICS: Absorption: Hydrocodone: C_{max}=23.6ng/mL; T_{max}=1.3 hrs. APAP: Rapidly absorbed. **Distribution:** APAP: Found in breast milk. **Metabolism:** Hydrocodone: O-demethylation, N-demethylation and 6-keto reduction. APAP: Liver (conjugation). **Elimination:** Hydrocodone: $T_{1/2}$=3.8 hrs. APAP: Urine (85%) (parent compound and metabolites); $T_{1/2}$=1.25-3 hrs.

NURSING CONSIDERATIONS

Assessment: Assess for hypersensitivity to other opioids, head injury or other intracranial lesions, elevated ICP, acute abdominal conditions, pulmonary disease, presence of debilitation (eg, elderly), hepatic/renal impairment, hypothyroidism, Addison's disease, prostatic hypertrophy or urethral stricture, nursing/pregnancy status, potential for misuse or abuse, and possible drug interactions.

Monitoring: Monitor for signs/symptoms of respiratory depression, elevations in CSF pressure, drug abuse, and drug dependence. In presence of severe hepatic/renal disease, monitor serial liver and/or renal function tests.

Patient Counseling: Caution that may impair mental/physical abilities required for performance of potentially hazardous tasks (eg, operating machinery). Avoid alcohol and other CNS depressants. Advise that drug may be habit forming; should only take for as long as prescribed, in amounts prescribed, and no more frequently than prescribed.

Administration: Oral route. **Storage:** 25°C (77°F); excursions permitted to 15-30°C (59-86°F). Dispense in tight, light-resistant container.

VICOPROFEN CIII

hydrocodone bitartrate - ibuprofen (Abbott)

OTHER BRAND NAMES: Reprexain (Centrix)

THERAPEUTIC CLASS: Opioid analgesic

INDICATIONS: Short-term (generally <10 days) management of acute pain.

DOSAGE: *Adults:* Usual: 1 tab q4-6h prn. Max: 5 tabs/day. Elderly: Use lowest dose or longest interval.
Pediatrics: ≥16 yrs: Usual: 1 tab q4-6h prn. Max: 5 tabs/day.

HOW SUPPLIED: (Hydrocodone-Ibuprofen) Tab: (Vicoprofen) 7.5mg-200mg; (Reprexain) 5mg-200mg, 7.5mg-200mg *scored

CONTRAINDICATIONS: ASA or other NSAID allergy that precipitates asthma, urticaria, or other allergic reaction.

WARNINGS/PRECAUTIONS: May produce dose-related respiratory depression. May obscure acute abdominal conditions or head injuries. Avoid with ASA triad, late pregnancy, advanced renal disease, ASA-sensitive asthma. Caution in elderly, debilitated, dehydration, renal disease, intrinsic coagulation defects, severe hepatic dysfunction, asthma, hypothyroidism, Addison's disease, prostatic hypertrophy, urethral stricture, heart failure, HTN, ulcer disease, pulmonary disease, postoperative use. May be habit-forming. Suppresses cough reflex. Risk of GI ulceration, bleeding, perforation. Anemia, fluid retention, edema, severe hepatic reactions reported. Possible risk of aseptic meningitis, especially in SLE patients. Increased risk of serious cardiovascular thrombotic events, MI and stroke. Fluid retention and edema observed. Skin reactions (eg, exfoliative dermatitis, TEN, SJS) can occur.

ADVERSE REACTIONS: Headache, somnolence, dizziness, constipation, dyspepsia, NV, infection, edema, nervousness, anxiety, pruritus, diarrhea, asthenia, abdominal pain, insomnia, dry mouth, sweating.

INTERACTIONS: Additive CNS depression with other narcotics, antihistamines, antipsychotics, antianxiety agents, alcohol, CNS depressants. Increased effect of antidepressant or hydrocodone with MAOIs or TCAs. May produce paralytic ileus with anticholinergics. May decrease effects of furosemide and thiazide diuretics, ACE-inhibitors. Avoid ASA. Risk of serious GI bleeding with warfarin. May enhance methotrexate toxicity. Monitor for lithium toxicity.

PREGNANCY: Category C, not for use in nursing.

MECHANISM OF ACTION: Hydrocodone: Opioid analgesic and antitussive. Not known; suspected to be related to existence of opiate receptors in CNS. Produces actions similiar to codeine; most occur in CNS and smooth muscle. Ibuprofen: Non-steroidal anti-inflammatory agent. Not established; suspected to inhibit cyclooxygenase activity and prostaglandin synthesis. Peripherally acting analgesic; has no known effects on opiate receptors. Possesses antipyretic activity.

PHARMACOKINETICS: Absorption: Hydrocodone: C_{max}=27ng/mL; T_{max}=1.7 hrs. Ibuprofen: C_{max}=30mcg/mL; T_{max}=1.8 hrs. **Distribution:** Ibuprofen: Plasma protein binding (99%). **Metabolism:** Hydrocodone: CYP2D6, via O-demethylation to hydromorphone (active metabolite); CYP3A4 via N-demethylation; 6-keto reduction. Ibuprofen: Interconversion from R-isomer to S-isomer; (+)-2-4'-(2-hydroxy-2-methyl-propyl) phenyl propionic acid and (+)-2-4-(2-carboxypropyl) phenyl propionic acid (primary metabolites). **Elimination:** Hydrocodone: Urine (primary); $T_{1/2}$=4.5 hrs. Ibuprofen: Urine (50-60% metabolites, 15% unchanged, conjugate), $T_{1/2}$=2.2 hrs.

NURSING CONSIDERATIONS

V

Assessment: Assess for hypersenstivity to other opioids, previous reaction to ASA or NSAIDs (eg, asthma, urticaria), type of pain (eg, CABG surgery), cardiovascular disease, HTN, heart failure, fluid retention, drug abuse potential, head injury, intracranial lesions, presence of increased ICP, acute abdominal conditions, history of peptic ulcers and/or GI bleeding, impaired renal/hepatic function, presence of debilitation (eg, elderly), hypothyroidism, Addison's disease, prostatic hypertrophy or urethral stricture, pulmonary disease (eg, asthma), SLE, pregnancy/nursing status, and possible drug interactions. Obtain baseline BP.

Monitoring: Monitor for signs/symptoms of cardiovascular thrombotic events, MI, stroke, HTN, fluid retention and edema, drug abuse and dependence, respiratory depression, elevations in CSF pressure, GI effects (eg, inflammation, bleeding, ulceration, perforation of stomach, small intestine, or large intestine), renal effects (eg, renal papillary necrosis), anaphylactoid reactions, skin reactions (eg, exfoliative dermatitis, Stevens-Johnson syndrome, toxic epidermal necrolysis), hepatic effects (eg, elevations in hepatic enzymes, jaundice, liver necrosis), hematological effects (eg, anemia), bronchospasm, and aseptic meningitis. If signs/symptoms of anemia develop, evaluate Hgb or Hct. Monitor BP while on therapy. If on long-term therapy, perform periodic monitoring of CBC and chemistry profile.

Patient Counseling: Inform drug cannot be substitute for corticosteroids or treat corticosteroid insufficiency. Caution that may impair mental and/or physical abilities required to perform potentially hazardous tasks (eg, operating machinery/driving). Avoid alcohol and other CNS depressants while on therapy. Advise drug may be habit forming; only take for as long as prescribed, and no more frequently than prescribed. Inform to contact physician if cardiovascular events (eg, CP, SOB, slurring of speech), GI effects (eg, ulcers, bleeding), edema, or weight gain occur. Immediately stop therapy and contact physician if signs/symptoms of skin reactions or hepatotoxicity (eg, nausea, fatigue, jaundice) develop. Seek immediate medical attention if any anaphylactoid reactions (eg, difficulty breathing, facial swelling) develop. Report any signs of blurred vision or other eye symptoms.

Administration: Oral route. **Storage:** 25°C (77°F); excursions permitted to 15-30°C (59-86°F). Dispense in a tight, light-resistant container.

VIDAZA — RX

azacitidine (Pharmion)

THERAPEUTIC CLASS: Pyrimidine nucleoside analog

INDICATIONS: Treatment of myelodysplastic syndrome subtypes: refractory anemia or refractory anemia with ringed sideroblasts (if accompanied by neutropenia or thrombocytopenia or requiring transfusions), refractory anemia with excess blasts, refractory anemia with excess blasts in transformation, and chronic myelomonocytic leukemia.

DOSAGE: *Adults:* Initial: 75mg/m² SQ or IV (administer over 10-40 min) daily for 7 days. Repeat cycle every 4 weeks. May increase to 100mg/m² after 2 cycles if no beneficial effect and no toxicity. Treat ≥4 cycles. Adjust dose based on hematology lab values, renal function, and serum electrolytes.

HOW SUPPLIED: Inj: 100mg

CONTRAINDICATIONS: Advanced malignant hepatic tumors.

WARNINGS/PRECAUTIONS: May cause fetal harm. Avoid pregnancy in women of childbearing potential. Neutropenia and thrombocytopenia may occur; monitor CBC periodically (at minimum, before each cycle). May cause hepatotoxicity; caution with liver disease. Renal abnormalities reported; reduce dose or hold for unexplained reductions in serum bicarbonate <20mEq/L or elevations of BUN or SrCr occur. Monitor for toxicity with renal impairment.

ADVERSE REACTIONS: (SQ) N/V, anemia, thrombocytopenia, pyrexia, leukopenia, diarrhea, fatigue, inj site erythema, constipation, neutropenia, ecchymosis, cough, dyspnea, weakness. (IV) Petechiae, rigors, weakness, hypokalemia.

PREGNANCY: Category D, not for use in nursing.

MECHANISM OF ACTION: Pyrimidine analogue; believed to cause hypomethylation of DNA and direct cytotoxicity on abnormal hematopoietic cells in bone marrow.

PHARMACOKINETICS: Absorption: (SQ) Rapid; Bioavailability (89%). C_{max}=750ng/mL; T_{max}=0.5 hr. **Distribution:** (IV) V_d=76L. **Elimination:** (SQ) $T_{1/2}$=41 min.

NURSING CONSIDERATIONS

Assessment: Assess for hypersensitivity to mannitol, advanced malignant hepatic tumors, renal/hepatic impairment, pregnancy status, and possible drug interactions. Obtain baseline CBC, LFTs, and SrCr.

Monitoring: Monitor CBC, platelet count, renal/hepatic function periodically. Monitor for signs/symptoms of renal/hepatic dysfunction.

Patient Counseling: Inform of pregnancy risks; advise women to avoid pregnancy and men not to father children while on therapy.

Administration: IV/SQ route. **Storage:** 25°C (77°F); excursions permitted to 15-30°C (59-86°F). Reconstituted: Vials: Stable for 1 hr at 25°C (77°F); stable for 8 hrs at 2-8°C (36-46°F).

VIDEX

didanosine (Bristol-Myers Squibb)

RX

Fatal/nonfatal pancreatitis, lactic acidosis, and severe hepatomegaly with steatosis reported. Suspend therapy if suspect pancreatitis and discontinue if pancreatitis confirmed. Fatal lactic acidosis reported in pregnant women receiving concomitant stavudine.

OTHER BRAND NAMES: Videx EC (Bristol-Myers Squibb)

THERAPEUTIC CLASS: Nucleoside analogue

INDICATIONS: Treatment of HIV-1 infection in combination with other antiretrovirals.

DOSAGE: *Adults:* ≥60kg: (Cap) 400mg qd; (Sol) 200mg bid or 400mg qd. 25-<60kg: (Cap) 250mg qd; (Sol) 125mg bid or 250mg qd. 20-<25kg: (Cap) 200mg qd. CrCl 30-59mL/min: ≥60kg: (Cap) 200mg qd; (Sol) 200mg qd or 100mg bid. <60kg: (Cap) 125mg qd; (Sol) 150mg qd or 75mg bid. CrCl 10-29mL/min: ≥60kg: (Cap) 125mg qd; (Sol) 150mg qd. <60kg: (Cap) 125mg qd; (Sol) 100mg qd. CrCl <10mL/min: ≥60kg: (Cap) 125mg qd; (Sol) 100mg qd. <60kg: (Sol) 75mg qd. Continous Ambulatory Peritoneal Dialysis/ Hemodialysis: ≥60kg: (Cap) 125mg qd. Concomitant Tenofovir Disoproxil Fumarate: CrCl 60mL/min : ≥60kg: 250mg qd; <60kg: 200mg qd. (Cap) Take on empty stomach; swallow caps whole. (Sol) Take on empty stomach, at least 30 minutes before or 2 hours after eating.
Pediatrics: 2 weeks-8 months: (Sol) 100mg/m² bid. >8 months: 120mg/m² bid. 6-18 yrs: 20-<25kg: (Cap) 200mg qd. 25-<60kg: 250mg qd. ≥60kg: 400mg qd. Renal Impairment: (Cap) dose reduction recommended. (Cap) Take on empty stomach; swallow caps whole. (Sol) Take on empty stomach, at least 30 min before or 2 hrs after meals.

HOW SUPPLIED: Sol: 2g, 4g; Cap, Delayed-Release: (Videx EC) 125mg, 200mg, 250mg, 400mg

WARNINGS/PRECAUTIONS: Risk of toxicity with CrCl <60mL/min; reduce dose. Retinal changes and optic neuritis reported; perform periodic retinal exams. Peripheral neuropathy reported. Caution with hepatic dysfunction. May cause asymptomatic hyperuricemia. Twice daily dosing is preferred over once daily dosing. Monitor for lactic acidosis in pregnancy if used with stavudine. Possible redistribution or accumulation of fat. Immune reconstitution syndrome has been reported in patients treated with combination antiretroviral therapy. Fatal and non-fatal pancreatitis reported; increased risk in combination with stavudine, with or without hydroxyurea. Fatal hepatic events (eg, hepatic toxicity) reported; increased risk with hydroxyurea and stavudine.

ADVERSE REACTIONS: Pancreatitis, lactic acidosis, hepatomegaly, visual changes, diarrhea, neuropathy, abdominal pain, headache, NV, rash, elevated LFTs.

INTERACTIONS: Extreme caution with drugs that may cause pancreatitis. Increase risk of peripheral neuropathy with neurotoxic agents (eg, stavudine). Aluminum- and magnesium-containing antacids may potentiate adverse events. Space dose by 2 hrs of drugs whose absorption can be affected by stomach acidity (eg, ketoconazole, itraconazole). Increased serum levels with oral ganciclovir. Space dose by 2 hrs after or 6 hrs before ciprofloxacin. Avoid allopurinol. Decreased serum levels with methadone. Caution with tenofovir or ribavirin; monitor closely for didanosine-related toxicities and suspend therapy if signs of pancreatitis, symptomatic hyperlactatemia, or lactic acidosis develop.

PREGNANCY: Category B, not for use in nursing.

MECHANISM OF ACTION: Antiviral agent; inhibits activity of HIV-1 reverse transcriptase both by competing with natural substrate deoxyadenosine 5-triphosphate and by incorporation into viral DNA, causing termination of viral DNA chain elongation.

PHARMACOKINETICS: Absorption: Rapid. T_{max}=0.25-1.5 hrs. Oral bioavailability: Adults (42%); 8 months-19 yrs (25%). **Distribution:** (Sol) V_d= (Adults) 43.70L/m²; (8 months-19 yrs) 28L/m², plasma protein bound (<5%). (Cap) V_d= (Adults) 308.26L; (20-<25kg) 98.1L; (25-<60kg) 154.69L; (≥60kg) 363L. (Cap) AUC= (Adults) 2.65mg•h/L; (20-<25kg) 2.38mg•h/L; (25-<60kg) 2.36mg•h/L; (≥60kg) 2.25mg•h/L. **Elimination:** (Sol) $T_{1/2}$= (Adults) 1.5 hrs; (8 months-19 yrs) 0.8 hrs. (Cap) $T_{1/2}$= (Adults) 1.19 hrs; (20-<25kg) 0.75 hrs; (25-<60kg) 0.92 hrs; (≥60kg) 1.26 hrs.

NURSING CONSIDERATIONS

Assessment: Assess renal/hepatic function and possible drug interactions.

Monitoring: Monitor for possible pancreatitis, lactic acidosis, severe hepatomegaly, steatosis, retinal changes, optic neuritis, peripheral neuropathy, fat redistribution, immune reconstitution syndrome, hyperuricemia. Closely monitor renal/hepatic function. Perform periodic retinal exams.

Patient Counseling: Preferred dosing frequency is twice daily, but some adults may require once-daily dosing. Instruct to take 2 appropriate strength tabs at each dose but not to take more than 4 tabs at each administration. Inform about possible serious toxicity of pancreatitis and about signs/symptoms of lactic acidosis, liver failure, peripheral neuropathy. Caution about use of medications or other substances, including alcohol. Inform that medication does not cure HIV and may continue to develop opportunistic infections and other complications of HIV. Notify physician if changes in visual acuity occur. Inform about fat redistribution effect. HIV-infected females should avoid nursing to reduce risk of transmission. Advise to take on empty stomach, at least 30 min before or 2 hrs after eating.

Administration: Oral Chewable/Dispersible Buffered Tabs: 1) Tabs must be chewed or thoroughly dispersed in at least 1oz water or clear apple juice. Buffered Powder for Oral Sol: 1) Add contents to 4oz water and disperse. Do not mix with fruit juice or other acid-containing liquid. Pediatric Powder for Oral Sol: 1) Constitute dry powder with purified water, USP, to initial concentration of 20mg/mL. 2) Immediately mix resulting sol with antacids to final concentration of 10mg/mL. **Storage:** Tabs: 59-86°F (15-30C°) Store in tightly closed container. If dispersed in water, dose may be stored at ambient room temperature for up to 1 hr. Buffered Powder: 59-86°F (15-30°C). After dispersed in water, dose may be stored at ambient room temperature for up to 4 hrs. Pediatric Powder: 15-30°C (59-86°F). Admixture may be stored up to 30 days in refrigerator at 2-8°C (36-46°F). Discard unused medication after 30 days.

V

VIGAMOX
RX

moxifloxacin HCl (Alcon)

THERAPEUTIC CLASS: Fluoroquinolone

INDICATIONS: Treatment of bacterial conjunctivitis.

DOSAGE: *Adults:* 1 drop tid for 7 days.
Pediatrics: ≥1 yr: 1 drop tid for 7 days.

HOW SUPPLIED: Sol: 0.5% [3mL]

WARNINGS/PRECAUTIONS: Not for injection. Do not inject subconjunctivally or into the anterior chamber of the eye. Superinfection may result with prolonged use. Fatal hypersensitivity reactions reported after first dose of systemic quinolone therapy. Avoid contact lenses when symptoms are present.

ADVERSE REACTIONS: Conjunctivitis, decreased visual acuity, dry eye, keratitis, ocular discomfort/hyperemia, ocular pain/pruritus, subconjunctival hemorrhage, tearing.

PREGNANCY: Category C, caution in nursing.

MECHANISM OF ACTION: Fluoroquinolone antibiotic; inhibits topoisomerase II (DNA gyrase) and topoisomerase IV. DNA gyrase is essential enzyme involved in replication, transcription, and repair of bacterial DNA. Topoisomerase IV is enzyme known to play key role in partitioning of chromosomal DNA during bacterial cell division.

PHARMACOKINETICS: Absorption: C_{max}=2.7ng/mL; AUC=45ng•hr/mL. **Distribution:** Presumed to be excreted in breast milk.

NURSING CONSIDERATIONS

Assessment: Assess for proper diagnosis of causative organisms (eg, slit lamp biomicroscopy, fluorescein staining). Assess for allergies to other quinolones. Assess use in pregnant/nursing females.

Monitoring: Monitor for signs/symptoms of hypersensitivity or anaphylactic reactions (eg, cardiovascular collapse, angioedema, airway obstruction, dyspnea, urticaria). With prolonged therapy, monitor for overgrowth of nonsusceptible organisms (eg, fungi) and for development of superinfection.

Patient Counseling: Instruct to avoid contaminating applicator tip with material from eye, fingers, or other sources. Instruct to d/c medication and contact physician if rash or allergic reaction occurs. Advise with bacterial conjunctivitis not to wear contact lenses.

Administration: Ocular route. Do not inject into eye. **Storage:** Store at 2-25°C (36-77°F).

VIMPAT — RX

lacosamide (UCB)

THERAPEUTIC CLASS: Sodium channel inactivator

INDICATIONS: (Tab/Inj) Adjunctive therapy for the treatment of partial-onset seizures in patients ≥17 yrs with epilepsy.

DOSAGE: *Adults:* Partial-Onset Seizures: (PO/Inj) Initial: 50mg bid (100mg/day). Titrate: May increase at weekly intervals by 100mg/day given as two divided doses. Maint: 200-400mg/day based on response and tolerability. CrCl ≤30mL/min or Mild/Moderate Hepatic Impairment: Max: 300mg/day. Switching from Oral to IV Dosing: Initial total daily IV dosage should be equivalent to total daily dosage and frequency of PO dosing and infused over 30-60 min. Switching from IV to Oral Dosing: Oral administration may be given at equivalent daily dosage and frequency of IV treatment.

HOW SUPPLIED: Tab, Delayed Release: 50mg, 100mg, 150mg, 200mg. Inj: 200mg/20mL

WARNINGS/PRECAUTIONS: May increase risk of suicidal behavior and ideation. Monitor emergence or worsening of depression, suicidal thoughts/behavior, and changes in mood/behavior. May cause dizziness, ataxia, and syncope. May impair physical/mental abilities. Caution with known conduction abnormalities (eg, AV block, sick sinus syndrome), or severe cardiac disease (eg, myocardial ischemia, heart failure). May predispose to atrial arrythmias especially in patients with diabetic neuropathy and/or CV disease. Withdraw gradually over minimum of 1 week to minimize potential of increased seizure frequency in patients with seizure disorders. Multiorgan hypersensitivity reactions (Drug Reaction with Eosinophilia and Systemic Symptoms [DRESS]) reported. Caution in elderly. Avoid use with severe hepatic impairment. Monitor closely during dose titration with co-existing hepatic or renal impairment.

ADVERSE REACTIONS: Dizziness, headache, N/V, fatigue, diplopia, vertigo, somnolence, ataxia, tremor, diarrhea, contusion, and pruritus.

INTERACTIONS: Caution with drugs known to induce PR interval prolongation.

PREGNANCY: Category C, not for use in nursing.

MECHANISM OF ACTION: Not established; selectively enhances slow inactivation of voltage-gated sodium channels, resulting in stabilization of hyperexcitable neuronal membranes and inhibition of repetitive neuronal firing (in vitro studies).

PHARMACOKINETICS: Absorption: Complete; absolute bioavailability (100%); (Tab) T_{max}=1-4 hrs. **Distribution:** V_d=0.6L/kg; plasma protein binding (15%). **Metabolism:** CYP2C19; O-desmethyl-lacosamide (major metabolite). **Elimination:** Urine (95%), feces (0.5%); $T_{1/2}$=13 hrs.

NURSING CONSIDERATIONS

Assessment: Assess renal function, LFTs, PR interval prolongation, diabetic neuropathy, AV block, atrial fibrillation and atrial flutter, hepatitis and nephritis, and pregnancy/nursing status. Obtain baseline AST/ALT, bilirubin.

Monitoring: Monitor renal function, LFTs, ECG abnormalities, emergence or worsening of depression, suicidal thoughts or behavior, and/or any unusual changes in mood or behavior.

Patient Counseling: Instruct to take only as prescribed with or without food. Counsel about high risk of suicidal thoughts and behavior. Carefully monitor emergence or worsening symptoms of depression, unusual changes in behavior or mood, suicidal thoughts, behavior, or self-harm. Counsel about dizziness, blurred vision, somnolence. Advise not to drive, operate complex machinery, or engage in other hazardous activities until effects of drug are known. Counsel that electrocardiographic changes may predispose to irregular HR and syncope. Inform about DRESS and to d/c therapy immediately if it occurs. Instruct to seek consultation if symptoms of live toxicity (eg, fatigue, jaundice, dark urine) occur. Notify physician if pregnant or intend to get pregnant.

Administration: Oral/IV route. **Storage:** Store at 20-25°C (68-77°F); excursions permitted between 15-30°C (59-86°F).

VINBLASTINE RX

vinblastine sulfate (Various)

For IV use only; fatal if given intrathecally. Considerable irritation if leakage occurs into surrounding tissue. If this occurs, d/c and restart in another vein. Heat and hyaluronidase minimize discomfort and cellulitis.

THERAPEUTIC CLASS: Vinca alkaloid

INDICATIONS: Palliative treatment of generalized Hodgkin's disease (Stages III and IV), lymphocytic lymphoma, histiocytic lymphoma, advanced mycosis fungoides, advanced testis carcinoma, Kaposi's sarcoma, Letterer-Siwe disease, and resistant choriocarcinoma and unresponsive breast carcinoma.

DOSAGE: *Adults:* Dose at intervals of ≤7 days. 1st Dose: 3.7mg/m². 2nd Dose: 5.5mg/m². 3rd Dose: 7.4mg/m². 4th Dose: 9.25mg/m². 5th Dose: 11.1mg/m². Max: 18.5mg/m². Do not increase dose after that dose which reduces WBC to 3000 cells/mm³. Maint: Use dose of 1 increment smaller than this dose at weekly intervals. Reduce to 50% dose if direct serum bilirubin >3mg/100mL. Only dose if WBC ≥4000 cells/mm³.
Pediatrics: Letterer-Swine Disease as Single Agent: Initial: 6.5mg/m². Hodgkin's Disease in Combination Therapy: Initial: 6mg/m². Testicular Germ Cell Carcinoma in Combination Therapy: Initial: 3mg/m².

HOW SUPPLIED: Inj: 1mg/mL [10mL]

CONTRAINDICATIONS: Significant granulocytopenia (unless result of disease being treated), bacterial infections.

WARNINGS/PRECAUTIONS: Avoid pregnancy. Acute shortness of breath, severe bronchospasm, aspermia, stomatitis, neurologic toxicity reported. Increased toxicity with hepatic insufficiency. Monitor for infection with WBC

<2000 cells/mm³. Avoid with malignant-cell infiltration of bone marrow, or in older persons with cachexia or ulcerated skin. Small daily amounts for long periods is not advised. Avoid eye contamination. Monitor WBCs. May cause fetal harm during pregnancy. Caution with ischemic cardiac disease.

ADVERSE REACTIONS: Leukopenia (granulocytopenia), anemia, thrombocytopenia, alopecia, constipation, anorexia, NV, abdominal pain, diarrhea, HTN, paresthesis.

INTERACTIONS: May increase phenytoin metabolism/elimination, or decrease phenytoin absorption. Caution with CYP3A inhibitors (eg, erythromycin, doxorubicin, etoposide), or with hepatic dysfunction; may cause earlier onset and/or an increased severity of side effects. Increased risk of acute shortness of breath and severe bronchospasm with mitomycin-C.

PREGNANCY: Category D, not for use in nursing.

MECHANISM OF ACTION: Vinca alkaloid; inhibits microtubule formation in mitotic spindle, resulting in cell division arrest.

PHARMACOKINETICS: Metabolism: CYP3A. **Elimination:** $T_{1/2}$=24.8 hrs.

NURSING CONSIDERATIONS

Assessment: Assess for hepatic dysfunction, granulocytopenia, bacterial infection, ischemic heart disease, pulmonary dysfunction, malignant-cell infiltration of bone marrow, elderly with cachexia or ulcerated area of skin, pregnancy status, and possible drug interactions.

Monitoring: Monitor CBC and LFTs periodically and for signs/symptoms of leukopenia (infection), extravasation, hepatic dysfunction, and hypersensitivity reactions.

Patient Counseling: Instruct to avoid pregnancy during therapy. Inform that alopecia, jaw pain, and pain in organs containing tumor tissue may occur during treatment. Avoid contact with eyes; if contamination occurs, wash immediately and thoroughly. Advise to seek medical attention if symptoms of sore throat, fever, chills, or sore mouth occur.

Administration: IV route. **Storage:** 2-8°C (36-46°F).

VINCRISTINE — RX

vincristine sulfate (Various)

Properly position IV needle or catheter before injection; considerable irritation with extravasation. Use hyaluronidase and heat to minimize discomfort and cellulitis with extravasation. Fatal with intrathecal use. For IV use only.

THERAPEUTIC CLASS: Vinca alkaloid

INDICATIONS: For treatment of acute leukemia. As an adjunct in the treatment of Hodgkin's disease, non-Hodgkin's malignant lymphomas, rhabdomyosarcoma, neuroblastoma, and Wilms' tumor.

DOSAGE: *Adults:* Usual: 1.4mg/m² IV at weekly intervals. Bilirubin >3mg/dL: 50% dose reduction. If given together with L-asparaginase, give 12-24 hrs before the enzyme.
Pediatrics: Usual: 2mg/m2 IV at weekly intervals. ≤10kg: Initial: 0.05mg/kg IV once weekly. Bilirubin >3mg/dL: 50% dose reduction. If given together with L-asparaginase, give 12-24 hrs before the enzyme.

HOW SUPPLIED: Inj: 1mg/mL

CONTRAINDICATIONS: Demyelinating form of Charcot-Marie-Tooth syndrome.

WARNINGS/PRECAUTIONS: Acute uric acid nephropathy may occur. May require additional agents with CNS leukemia. Neurotoxicity is dose-limiting toxicity. Perform CBC before each dose. Determine serum uric acid levels frequently during 1st 3-4 weeks. Acute shortness of breath, severe bronchospasm reported. Monitor with pre-existing neuromuscular disease. Avoid eye contamination. May cause fetal harm during pregnancy.

ADVERSE REACTIONS: Alopecia, abdominal cramps, weight loss, nausea, vomiting, diarrhea, constipation, paralytic ileus, HTN, hypotension, polyuria, dysuria, urinary retention, sensory impairment, paresthesia, neuritic pain, motor difficulties, rash, fever.

INTERACTIONS: Reduced levels of phenytoin and increased seizures reported. Increased risk of acute shortness of breath and severe bronchospasm with mitomycin-C. Monitor with other neurotoxic agents. Discontinue drugs known to cause urinary retention for 1st few days after administration. Give 12-24 hrs before L-asparaginase therapy to minimize toxicity. Do not give with radiation therapy through ports that include the liver. Do not dilute in solutions that raise or lower the pH outside the range of 3.5-5.5.

PREGNANCY: Category D, not for use in nursing.

MECHANISM OF ACTION: Antineoplastic agent; inhibits microtubule formation in mitotic spindle, resulting in cell division arrest at metaphase stage.

PHARMACOKINETICS: Distribution: Crosses blood-brain barrier. **Metabolism:** Liver, via CYP450 isoenzyme 3A **Elimination:** Feces (80%), urine (10-20%); $T_{1/2}$=85 hrs.

NURSING CONSIDERATIONS

Assessment: Assess for hepatic dysfunction, presence of leukopenia or complicating infection, demyelinating form of Charcot-Marie-Tooth syndrome and possible drug interactions.

Monitoring: Monitor for acute uric acid nephropathy, acute SOB, and severe bronchospasm. Monitor bone marrow function and CBC (WBC, platelet). Acute elevation of serum uric acid may occur, thus such levels should be determined frequently during first 3-4 weeks of treatment.

Patient Counseling: Avoid contamination of eye with concentrated drug. If accidental contamination occurs, severe irritation (or if drug was delivered under pressure, even corneal ulceration) may result. Wash eye immediately and thoroughly.

Administration: IV route. **Storage:** Refrigerate between 2-8°C (36-46°F).

VIRACEPT RX

nelfinavir mesylate (Pfizer)

THERAPEUTIC CLASS: Protease inhibitor

INDICATIONS: Treatment of HIV infection in combination with other antiretrovirals.

DOSAGE: *Adults:* 1250mg bid or 750mg tid. Concomitant rifabutin: Reduce rifabutin dose by one-half and nelfinavir 1250mg bid is preferred dose. Take with a meal or light snack. May crush or dissolve whole tab in water or mix in food and consume immediately. May store mixture under refrigeration up to 6 hrs.

Pediatrics: 2-13 yrs: 45-55mg/kg bid or 25-35mg/kg tid. Take with a meal or light snack. May mix powder with non-acidic liquid (eg, water, milk, formula, etc.); consume immediately. May store up to 6 hrs under refrigeration.

HOW SUPPLIED: Sus: (powder) 50mg/g [144g]; Tab: 250mg, 625mg

CONTRAINDICATIONS: Concomitant pimozide, triazolam, midazolam, ergot derivatives, amiodarone or quinidine.

WARNINGS/PRECAUTIONS: Powder contains phenylalanine. New-onset DM, exacerbation of DM and hyperglycemia reported. Register pregnant patients (800-258-4263). Caution with hepatic dysfunction. Increased bleeding reported. Possible redistribution or accumulation of fat.

ADVERSE REACTIONS: Diarrhea, nausea, flatulence, rash, redistribution of body fat, jaundice, hypersensitivity reactions, bilirubinemia, hyperglycemia, metabolic acidosis.

INTERACTIONS: See Contraindications. Avoid pimozide, triazolam, midazolam, ergot derivatives, amiodarone or quinidine; potential for life-threatening adverse events. Avoid rifampin. Avoid lovastatin or simvastatin; caution with other HMG-CoA reductase inhibitors. May increase sildenafil or other PDE5 inhibitor levels and adverse effects. Avoid St. John's wort; may decrease levels of nelfinavir. May increase levels of drugs metabolized by CYP450 3A (eg, dihydropyridine CCBs, immunosuppressants, etc). Use alternative or additional contraception with oral contraceptives. May increase levels of cyclosporine, tacrolimus, sirolimus, atorvastatin, cerivastatin, fluticasone, azithromycin. Carbamazepine, phenobarbital may decrease levels of nelfinavir. May decrease levels of phenytoin, methadone. Give didanosine 1 hr before or 2 hrs after nelfinavir. Omeprazole decreases levels of nelfinavir; concomitant use with proton pump inhibitors may lead to loss of virologic response and development of resistance.

PREGNANCY: Category B, not for use in nursing.

MECHANISM OF ACTION: HIV-1 protease inhibitor; prevents cleavage of *gag* and *gag-pol* polyprotein resulting in production of immature, non-infectious virus.

PHARMACOKINETICS: Absorption: (1250mg bid) C_{max}=4mg/L; AUC=52.8mg•h/L. (750mg tid) C_{max}=3mg/L; AUC=43.6mg•h/L. **Distribution:** V_d=2-7L/kg; plasma protein binding (>98%). **Metabolism:** CYP3A, 2C19 (oxidation). **Elimination:** Feces (22%), urine (1-2%); $T_{1/2}$=3.5-5 hrs.

NURSING CONSIDERATIONS

Assessment: Assess for possible drug interactions, hepatic impairment, PKU, DM, and hemophilia.

Monitoring: Monitor for signs/symptoms of hypersensitivity reactions, new onset or exacerbation of DM and hyperglycemia, immune reconstitution syndrome, bleeding, fat redistribution/accumulation, and hepatic dysfunction.

Patient Counseling: Inform that therapy does not cure HIV; may continue to develop opportunistic infections. Inform that therapy does not reduce risk of transmitting HIV. Instruct to take every day with food; do not alter dose or d/c without consulting physician. Advise if dose is missed, take as soon as possible; do not double dose. Report use of Rx and OTC medications and seek medical attention if symptoms of hypersensitivity reactions, infections, fat redistribution/accumulation occur.

Administration: Oral route. **Storage:** Tab/Oral Powder: 15-30°C (59-86°F).

VIRAMUNE — RX

nevirapine (Boehringer Ingelheim)

Severe, life-threatening, in some cases fatal, hepatotoxicity and skin reactions (eg, Stevens-Johnson syndrome, toxic epidermal necrolysis, hypersensitivity) reported. Women, including pregnant women, and/or patients with higher CD4 counts are at higher risk of hepatotoxicity. Permanently d/c following severe hepatitis, skin or hypersensitivity reactions. Monitoring during the first 18 weeks of therapy is essential; extra vigilance is warranted during the first 6 weeks of therapy.

THERAPEUTIC CLASS: Non-nucleoside reverse transcriptase inhibitor

INDICATIONS: Treatment of HIV-1 infection in combination with other antiretrovirals.

DOSAGE: *Adults:* 200mg qd for 14 days (lead-in period), then 200mg bid. If severe rash occurs, d/c therapy. If mild-to-moderate rash occurs during 14-day lead-in period, do not increase dose until rash resolves. If dosing interrupted for >7 days, restart 14-day lead-in dosing.
Pediatrics: ≥15 days:150mg/m² qd for 14 days, followed by 150mg/m² bid. Max: 400mg/day. If severe rash occurs, d/c therapy. If mild-to-moderate rash occurs during 14-day lead-in period, do not increase dose until rash resolves. If dosing interrupted for >7 days, restart lead-in dosing.

HOW SUPPLIED: Sus: 50mg/5mL [240mL]; Tab: 200mg* *scored

CONTRAINDICATIONS: Moderate or severe (Child Pugh Class B or C) hepatic impairment.

WARNINGS/PRECAUTIONS: Avoid with severe hepatic impairment. Caution with moderate impairment and dialysis. Perform laboratory tests (eg, LFTs) at baseline and during first 18 weeks of therapy. Possible redistribution or accumulation of body fat.

ADVERSE REACTIONS: Headache, fever, severe rash, GI effects, fatigue, thrombocytopenia, fatigue, hepatotoxicity, granulocytopenia (pediatrics), rhabdomyolysis.

INTERACTIONS: Avoid use of prednisone for prevention of therapy-associated rash. Decreased levels of clarithromycin; consider alternative. Decreased levels of efavirenz, indinavir, nelfinavir, saquinavir. May decrease effectiveness of oral contraceptives and other hormonal contraceptives; use alternate or additional method of contraception. Increased levels with fluconazole. Avoid with ketoconazole, St. John's wort, rifampin. Decreased levels of lopinavir; adjust lopinavir/ritonavir doses. May decrease levels of methadone; monitor for signs of withdrawal. Increased levels of rifabutin. Possible decreased levels with antiarrhythmics (eg, amiodarone, disopyramide, lidocaine), anticonvulsants (eg, carbamazepine, clonazepam, ethosuximide), itraconazole, CCBs (eg, diltiazem, nifedipine, verapamil), cyclophosphamide, ergotamine, immunosuppressants (eg, cyclosporine, tacrolimus, sirolimus), cisapride, fentanyl. Monitor with warfarin.

PREGNANCY: Category B, not for use in nursing.

MECHANISM OF ACTION: Non-nucleoside reverse transcriptase inhibitor; binds directly to reverse transcriptase and blocks RNA-dependent DNA polymerase activities by causing disruption of the enzyme's catalytic site.

PHARMACOKINETICS: Absorption: Absolute bioavailability: 93+/- 9% (tab), 91+/-8% (sol); C_{max}=2+/-0.4 Mcg/mL; T_{max}=4 hrs. **Distribution:** V_d=1.21±0.09L/Kg; plasma protein binding (60%); readily crosses placenta; found in breast milk. **Metabolism:** Liver; oxidative metabolism, via CYP3A4 and CYP2B6 (extensively); glucuronide metabolites. **Elimination:** Urine (<3% excreted as parent drug); $T_{1/2}$=45 hrs.

NURSING CONSIDERATIONS

Assessment: Assess for possible drug interactions prior to therapy (St. John's wort, methadone). Assess baseline LFTs and CD4 count.

Monitoring: Monitor for hepatotoxicity and skin reactions (eg, Steven-Johnson syndrome, toxic epidermal necrolysis) during therapy. Perform LFTs prior to dose escalation and 2 weeks following dose escalation. Monitor patients on methadone for evidence of narcotic withdrawal.

Patient Counseling: Counsel about signs/symptoms of hepatoxicity. Notify physician immediately if any rash or skin reactions develop. Inform may experience redistribution or accumulation of fat tissue during medication. Counsel that drug does not cure HIV and may continue to develop opportunistic infections and other complications of HIV. Instruct females to avoid nursing to reduce risk transmission. Inform females that oral contraceptives and other hormonal methods of birth control should not be used as sole method of birth control since drug may lower plasma levels of those medications.

Administration: Oral route. **Storage:** 25°C (77°F); excursions permitted to 15-30°C (59-86°F).

VIRAZOLE

RX

ribavirin (Valeant)

Sudden deterioration of respiratory function associated with initiation in infants. Monitor respiratory function carefully. Not for use in adults. Use with mechanical ventilator assistance with staff familiar with mode of administration and specific type of ventilator.

THERAPEUTIC CLASS: Nucleoside analogue

INDICATIONS: Treatment of hospitalized infants and young children with severe lower respiratory tract infections due to respiratory syncytial virus.

DOSAGE: *Pediatrics:* Continuous aerosol administration of 20mg/mL in the drug reservoir of the SPAG-2 unit for 12-18 hrs/day for 3-7 days.

HOW SUPPLIED: Sol, Inhalation: 6g

CONTRAINDICATIONS: Women who are or may become pregnant during exposure to drug.

WARNINGS/PRECAUTIONS: Monitor respiratory function and fluid status according to SPAG-2 manual. Accumulation of drug precipitate can result in mechanical ventilator dysfunction and associated increased pulmonary pressures.

ADVERSE REACTIONS: Worsening of respiratory status, bronchospasm, pulmonary edema, hypoventilation, cyanosis, dyspnea, bacterial pneumonia, pneumothorax, apnea, atelectasis, ventilator dependence, cardiac arrest, hypotension, bradycardia.

INTERACTIONS: Digoxin toxicity reported.

PREGNANCY: Category X, safety in nursing not known.

MECHANISM OF ACTION: Nucleoside analogue; mechanism unknown. Suspected to be analogue of guanosine or xanthosine.

PHARMACOKINETICS: Elimination: $T_{1/2}$=9.5 hrs.

NURSING CONSIDERATIONS

Assessment: Assess for pregnancy status and possible drug interactions.

Monitoring: Monitor respiratory function and fluid status periodically.

Administration: Inhalation route. **Storage:** 25°C (77°F); excursions permitted to 15-30°C (59-86°F). Reconstituted: 20-30°C (68-86°F); stable for 24 hrs.

VIREAD — RX

tenofovir disoproxil fumarate (Gilead)

> **Lactic acidosis and severe hepatomegaly with steatosis, including fatal cases, reported with nucleoside analogs alone or with concomitant antiretrovirals. Severe acute exacerbations of hepatitis B have been reported in patients coinfected with HBV and HIV and have discontinued Viread. Monitor hepatic function closely for at least several months in patients who d/c anti-hepatitis B therapy, including Viread. If appropriate, resumption of anti-hepatitis B therapy may be warranted.**

THERAPEUTIC CLASS: Nucleotide analog reverse transcriptase inhibitor

INDICATIONS: Treatment of HIV-1 infection in combination with other antiretrovirals and for chronic hepatitis B in adults.

DOSAGE: *Adults:* 300mg qd without regard to food. Renal Impairment: CrCl 30-49mL/min: 300mg q48 hrs. CrCl 10-29mL/min: 300mg q72-96 hrs. Hemodialysis: 300mg every 7 days after total of approximately 12 hrs of dialysis.

HOW SUPPLIED: Tab: 300mg

WARNINGS/PRECAUTIONS: Obesity and prolonged nucleoside exposure may be risk factors for lactic acidosis and severe hepatomegaly with steatosis. Caution if risk factors for hepatic disease present or with hepatic insufficiency. Monitor hepatic function with both clinical and lab follow-up for at least several months in patients who are coinfected with HIV and HBV and d/c Viread. All patients should have CrCl calculated prior to and during therapy. Dose adjust and monitor renal function when CrCl <50mL/min. May cause renal impairment. Monitor SrCr and phosphorous in patients at risk for, or with history of, renal dysfunction and those receiving concomitant nephrotoxic agents. Bone monitoring should be considered for HIV patients at risk for osteopenia. Cases of osteomalacia reported. Possible fat redistribution and accumulation of body fat. Immune reconstitution syndrome observed in HIV infected patients.

ADVERSE REACTIONS: N/V, diarrhea, flatulence, asthenia, headache, abdominal pain, anorexia.

INTERACTIONS: Increases levels of didanosine; use caution when coadministering, monitor for didanosine-associated adverse effects (suppression of

CD4 cell counts), and discontinue if these adverse events develop. Renally eliminated drugs (eg, cidofovir, acyclovir, valacyclovir, ganciclovir, valganciclovir) may increase levels of itself or tenofovir. Indinavir, lopinavir/ritonavir, and drugs that decrease renal function may increase tenofovir plasma levels. May decrease lamivudine, indinavir, lopinavir, and ritonavir plasma levels. Avoid with concurrent or recent use of nephrotoxic agents. Avoid use with Truvada or Atripla.

PREGNANCY: Category B, not for use in nursing.

MECHANISM OF ACTION: Nucleotide analog reverse transcriptase inhibitor; inhibits activity of HIV-1 reverse transcriptase by competing with natural substrate deoxyadenosine 5'-triphosphate and, after incorporation into DNA, by DNA termination.

PHARMACOKINETICS: Absorption: C_{max}=296±90ng/mL; T_{max}=1.0±0.4 hrs; AUC=2287±685ng•hr/mL. **Distribution:** Serum protein bound (<7.2%); V_d=1.3±0.6L/kg (after 1mg/kg dose); V_d=1.2±0.4L/kg (after 3mg/kg dose). **Elimination:** Urine (70-80% unchanged); $T_{1/2}$=17 hrs.

NURSING CONSIDERATIONS

Assessment: Assess HBV status, renal function (SrCr, serum phosphorus), and for possible drug interactions.

Monitoring: Monitor for signs/symptoms of lactic acidosis, severe hepatomegaly with steatosis, and immune reconstitution syndrome. Perform routine monitoring of CrCl and serum phosphorus if at risk for renal impairment. Monitor hepatic function closely with clinical and lab follow-up for several months if coinfected with HIV and HBV and d/c drug. Monitor cholesterol levels, creatine kinase levels, and serum amylase levels. Monitor bone mineral density if previous history of fractures or osteopenia.

Patient Counseling: Inform that drug not approved for treatment of HBV infection. Advise that redistribution or accumulation of fat tissue may occur. Supplementation with calcium with vitamin D may be beneficial with previous history of bone fractures/osteopenia. Counsel about importance of adherence to antiretroviral regimen. Inform that therapy does not cure HIV and may continue to acquire opportunistic infections. Intruct HIV-infected mothers to avoid nursing to reduce risk of transmission.

Administration: Oral route. **Storage:** 25°C (77°F); excursions permitted to 15-30°C (59-86°F).

VIROPTIC RX

trifluridine (King)

THERAPEUTIC CLASS: Fluorinated pyrimidine nucleoside antiviral

INDICATIONS: Treatment of primary keratoconjunctivitis and recurrent epithelial keratitis due to herpes simplex virus, types 1 and 2.

DOSAGE: *Adults:* 1 drop q2h while awake until re-epithelialization. Max: 9 drops/day. Following Re-epithelialization: 1 drop q4h while awake for 7 days; minimum of 5 drops/day. If no improvement after 7 days or if complete re-epithelialization has not occurred after 14 days, consider other therapy. Avoid using >21 days.

Pediatrics: ≥6 yrs: 1 drop q2h while awake until re-epithelialization. Max: 9 drops/day. Following Re-epithelialization: 1 drop q4h while awake for 7 days; minimum of 5 drops/day. If no improvement after 7 days or if complete re-epithelialization has not occurred after 14 days, consider other therapy. Avoid using >21 days.

HOW SUPPLIED: Sol: 1% [7.5mL]

WARNINGS/PRECAUTIONS: Only use with a clinical diagnosis of herpetic keratitis. May cause transient, mild local irritation of the conjunctiva and cornea when instilled.

ADVERSE REACTIONS: Burning, stinging, palpebral edema, superficial punctate keratopathy, epithelial keratopathy, hypersensitivity reaction, stromal edema, irritation, keratitis sicca, hyperemia, increased IOP.

PREGNANCY: Category C, caution in nursing.

MECHANISM OF ACTION: Fluorinated pyrimidine nucleoside antiviral; unknown, suspected to interfere with DNA synthesis.

PHARMACOKINETICS: Absorption: Penetrates intact cornea. **Metabolism:** 5-carboxy-2'-deoxyuridine (major metabolite).

NURSING CONSIDERATIONS

Assessment: Prior to therapy, assess for clinical diagnosis of herpetic keratitis. Assess use in pregnancy/nursing.

Monitoring: Monitor for clinical signs of improvement after 7 days of therapy. Monitor for complete re-epithelialization after 14 days of therapy. Monitor for signs/symptoms of mild local irritation of conjunctiva and cornea. Monitor for signs of viral resistance.

Patient Counseling: Advise that recommended dosage and frequency of administration should not be exceeded. Inform that continuous administration for periods exceeding 21 days should be avoided because of potential for ocular toxicity.

Administration: Ocular route. **Storage:** Store under refrigeration 2-8°C (36-46°F).

VISICOL RX

sodium phosphate (Salix)

Serious acute phosphate nephropathy (rare) reported. Some cases resulted in permanent renal impairment requiring long-term dialysis. Increased risk of acute phosphate nephropathy may occur with increased age, hypovolemia, increased bowel transit time (eg, bowel obstruction), active colitis, or baseline kidney disease, and using medicines that affect renal perfusion or function (eg, diuretics, ACE inhibitors, ARBs, and possibly NSAIDs). Use the recommended dose and dosing regimen (pm/am split dose).

THERAPEUTIC CLASS: Bowel cleanser

INDICATIONS: For cleansing the colon in preparation for colonoscopy in adults ≥18 yrs.

DOSAGE: *Adults:* ≥18 yrs: Adequately hydrate before, during, and after use. Evening Before Colonoscopy Procedure: 3 tabs with 8 oz clear liquids every 15 min for total of 20 tabs (last dose is 2 tabs). Day of Colonoscopy Procedure: Repeat dosing on day of exam 3-5 hrs before procedure. May retreat after 7 days.

HOW SUPPLIED: Tab: (Sodium Phosphate Monobasic Monohydrate-Sodium Phosphate Dibasic Anhydrous) 1.102g-0.398g* *scored

CONTRAINDICATIONS: Patients with biopsy-proven acute phosphate nephropathy.

WARNINGS/PRECAUTIONS: Fatalities reported due to significant fluid shift, severe electrolyte imbalances and arrhythmias with administration of sodium phosphate products. Caution with severe renal insufficiency (CrCl <30 mL/minute), CHF, ascites, unstable angina, acute bowel obstruction, bowel perforation, toxic megacolon, gastric retention, ileus, pseudo-obstruction of the bowel, severe chronic constipation, acute colitis, gastric bypass, stapling surgery, or hypomotility syndrome. Caution with impaired renal function, history of acute phosphate nephropathy, known or suspected electrolyte disturbances (eg, dehydration) or concomitant medications that may affect electrolyte levels (eg, diuretics). Correct electrolyte disturbance before use. Reports of generalized tonic-clonic seizures and/or loss of consciousness in patients with no prior history of seizures. Caution in patients with history of seizures and in patients at high risk of seizure (eg, withdrawing from alcohol or benzodiazepines, known or suspected hyponatremia). Caution in patients with higher risk of arrhythmias (eg, history of cardiomyopathy, prolonged QT interval, uncontrolled arrhythmias, recent MI). Pre-dose and post-colonoscopy ECGs should be done in patients with high risk of serious, cardiac arrhythmias. May induce colonic mucosal aphthous ulcerations and exacerbate IBS. Do not use additional enema or laxative. Difficulty of swallowing may occur in patients with a history of difficulties or anatomic narrowing of the esophagus (eg, stricture). Caution with recent cardiac surgery (eg, coronary artery bypass graft surgery). Caution in elderly.

ADVERSE REACTIONS: NV, abdominal bloating, dizziness, headache, abdominal pain.

INTERACTIONS: May reduce absorption of other drugs. Caution with sodium phosphate-containing products, agents that prolong QT interval or affect electrolyte levels. Caution with concomitant use of medications lowering seizure threshold (eg, tricyclic antidepressants).

PREGNANCY: Category C, safety not known in nursing.

MECHANISM OF ACTION: Osmotic laxative; causes large amounts of water to be drawn into colon, promoting colon evacuation.

NURSING CONSIDERATIONS

Assessment: Assess for acute phosphate nephropathy, known hypersensitivity to sodium phosphates, cardiac arrhythmias, severe electrolyte abnormalities, severe renal insufficiency, CHF, unstable angina, bowel obstruction, bowel perforation, gastric retention, severe chronic constipation, acute colitis, history of seizures, and possible drug interactions.

Monitoring: Monitor CrCl, phosphate, calcium, K^+, Na^+ and BUN levels, vomiting, arrhythmias, and seizures.

Patient Counseling: Drink 8 oz clear liquid with each 3-tab dose. Ingest total of 3.6 quarts clear liquid. Do not use within 7 days of previous administration. Do not take additional laxatives or purgatives.

Administration: Oral route. **Storage:** 25°C (77°F); excursions permitted to 15-30°C (59-86°F). Discard any unused portion.

VISTIDE — RX

cidofovir (Gilead)

Renal impairment is a major toxicity; prehydrate with IV normal saline (NS) and administer probenecid with each dose. Monitor serum creatinine (SCr) and urine protein within 48 hrs prior to each dose. Modify dose with renal function changes. Contraindicated with nephrotoxic agents. Neutropenia reported; monitor neutrophils. Carcinogenic, teratogenic, and hypospermatic in animal studies.

THERAPEUTIC CLASS: Viral DNA synthesis inhibitor

INDICATIONS: Treatment of cytomegalovirus (CMV) retinitis in AIDS patients.

DOSAGE: *Adults:* IV: Induction: 5mg/kg once weekly for 2 weeks. Maint: 5mg/kg once every 2 weeks. Reduce maint from 5mg/kg to 3mg/kg for an increase in SCr of 0.3-0.4mg/dL above baseline. D/C with increase in SCr ≥0.5mg/dL above baseline or ≥3+ proteinuria. Administer probenecid 2g PO 3 hrs before cidofovir, then 1g at 2 hrs and 8 hrs after completion of cidofovir infusion. Administer at least 1L 0.9% NS immediately before infusion. If tolerated, give 2nd liter at start of or immediately after infusion.

HOW SUPPLIED: Inj: 75mg/mL

CONTRAINDICATIONS: SCr >1.5mg/dL, CrCl ≤55mL/min, or urine protein ≥100mg/dL (≥2+ proteinuria) with therapy initiation. Nephrotoxic agents (discontinue at least 7 days before therapy), severe hypersensitivity to probenecid or other sulfa-containing agents, direct intraocular use.

WARNINGS/PRECAUTIONS: Dose-dependent nephrotoxicity. Monitor IOP, visual acuity, ocular symptoms, uveitis/iritis, and renal function periodically. Monitor WBC with differential before each dose. Avoid during pregnancy. Adequate contraception for both sexes during and following treatment is advised. May cause male infertility. Potentially carcinogenic.

ADVERSE REACTIONS: NV, neutropenia, proteinuria, decreased IOP/ocular hypotony, anterior uveitis/iritis, metabolic acidosis, nephrotoxicity, pneumonia, dyspnea, infection, fever, creatinine ≥2mg/dL, decreased sodium bicarbonate.

INTERACTIONS: Avoid nephrotoxic agents (aminoglyosides, amphotericin B, foscarnet, IV pentamidine, vancomycin, and NSAIDs); discontinue nephrotoxic agents at least 7 days before therapy. Temporarily discontinue zidovudine or decrease zidovudine by 50% with probenecid.

PREGNANCY: Category C, not for use in nursing.

MECHANISM OF ACTION: Viral DNA synthesis inhibitor; suppresses CMV replication by selective inhibition of viral DNA synthesis.

PHARMACOKINETICS: Administration: Variable doses resulted in altered parameters. **Absorption:** 5mg/kg: AUC=28.3 mcg•mL/hr (without probenecid), AUC=40.8+/-+9.0 mcg•mL/hr (with probenecid); C_{max}=11.5mcg/mL (without probenecid), C_{max}=19.6+/-7.2 mcg/mL (with probenecid); 3mg/kg: AUC=20.0+/-2.3mcg•mL/hr (without probenecid), AUC=25.7+/-8.5mcg•mL/hr (with probenecid); C_{max}=7.3+/-1.4 mcg/mL (without probenecid), C_{max}=9.8+/-3.7mcg/mL (with probenecid). **Distribution:** V_d=537±126mL/kg (without probenecid), V_d= 410+/-102mL/kg (with probenecid); Plasma protein binding (≤6%). **Elimination:** 80-100% excreted unchanged in urine.

NURSING CONSIDERATIONS

Assessment: Assess renal function prior to therapy.

Monitoring: Monitor renal function, SrCr, urine protein, WBC, neutrophils, serum bicarbonate, IOP, and visual acuity. Monitor for signs/symptoms of nephrotoxicity, metabolic acidosis, uveitis, or iritis. Monitor for allergic reactions when using in combination with probenecid.

Patient Counseling: Counsel to take full course of probenecid with drug. If nausea develops, take with food. Inform drug does not cure CMV retinitis; may continue to experience progression of retinitis during, and following, treatment. Advise for regular follow-up ophthalmologic exams. Advise females to use proper contraception while on medication and to continue using contraception for at least 1 month following therapy. Counsel males to use proper contraception while on medication and for 3 months following therapy. Advise drug is not for direct intraocular injection.

Administration: IV route. 1) Inspect for particulate matter and discoloration. 2) Add appropriate volume to 100mL 0.9% NS. 3) Infuse over 1 hr at constant rate. 4) Probenecid and IV saline prehydration must be administered with each infusion. **Storage:** Vial: 20-25°C (68-77°F). Admixture: Under refrigeration, 2-8°C, for no more than 24 hrs. If refrigerated, allow admixture to reach room temperature prior to use.

VISUDYNE — RX

verteporfin (Novartis Ophthalmics)

THERAPEUTIC CLASS: Photosensitizing agent

INDICATIONS: Treatment of age-related macular degeneration with subfoveal choroidal neovascularization.

DOSAGE: *Adults:* 6mg/m^2 IV over 10 min at 3mL/min. Photoactivation with laser light therapy with nonthermal diode laser 15 min after start IV infusion. Re-evaluate every 3 months and repeat if choroidal neovascular leakage detected on fluorescein angiography.

HOW SUPPLIED: Inj: 15mg

CONTRAINDICATIONS: Porphyria.

WARNINGS/PRECAUTIONS: Avoid direct sunlight or bright indoor light for 5 days. Avoid extravasation. If extravasation occurs, protect area from direct light until swelling and discoloration fade. Protect from intense light if surgery within 48 hrs after therapy. Do not retreat if severe vision decrease of 4 lines or more occurs within 1 week after therapy. Only use compatible lasers. Caution with moderate to severe hepatic dysfunction. Reduced effects with increasing age.

ADVERSE REACTIONS: Headache, injection site reactions, visual disturbances, asthenia, HTN, eczema, constipation, nausea, anemia, arthralgia, vertigo, pharyngitis.

INTERACTIONS: CCBs, polymyxin B, and radiation therapy may enhance rate of uptake by vascular endothelium. Increased photosensitivity with tetracyclines, sulfonamides, phenothiazines, sulfonylureas, thiazide diuretics, and griseofulvin. Decreased effects with dimethyl sulfoxide, β-carotene, ethanol, formate, mannitol, and drugs that decrease clotting, vasoconstriction, or platelet aggregation (eg, thromboxane A_2 inhibitors).

PREGNANCY: Pregnancy C, not for use in nursing.

MECHANISM OF ACTION: Photosensitizing agent; transported into plasma by lipoproteins. Activated by light in presence of oxygen; light activation causes local damage to neovascular endothelium, subsequently leading to vessel occlusion. Damaged endothelium releases procoagulant and vasoactive factors through lipo-oxygenase and cyclo-oxygenase pathways, resulting in platelet aggregation, fibrin clot formation, and vasoconstriction.

PHARMACOKINETICS: Absorption: Dose proportional. **Distribution:** Found in breast milk. **Metabolism:** Liver and plasma esterases; diacid metabolite. **Elimination:** Feces (major), urine (≤0.01%); $T_{1/2}$=5-6 hrs.

NURSING CONSIDERATIONS

Assessment: Assess patient does not have porphyria and that females are not nursing. Assess use in pregnancy, with severe hepatic impairment, or biliary obstruction. Assess for drug interactions.

Monitoring: Monitor for signs/symptoms of extravasation or injection site reactions, severe decreases in vision, severe CP, vasovagal and hypersensitivity reactions (eg, syncope, rash, dyspnea, flushing, changes in BP and HR). Monitor that IV line is free-flowing.

Patient Counseling: Instruct to avoid exposure of unprotected skin, eyes, or other body organs to direct sunlight, bright light (eg, tanning salon, bright halogen lighting, high powered lighting), or light-emitting medical devices (eg, pulse oximeters) for 5 days following therapy. Instruct to protect eyes and skin if going outdoors during first 5 days following treatment. Instruct to avoid staying in dark when indoors; skin should be exposed to ambient indoor lighting. Darkness inactivates drug in skin through process called photobleaching. Inform that visual changes may occur; avoid using machinery/driving until symptoms have subsided.

Administration: IV route. Reconstitute. 1) Use 7mL SWFI to provide 7.5mL containing 2mg/mL; do not use NS or other parenteral solutions. Do not mix in same sol with other drugs. 2) Dilute using D5W to total infusion volume of 30mL. **Storage:** 20-25°C (68-77°F). Following dilution, protect from light and use within maximum of 4 hrs.

VITRASERT — RX

ganciclovir (Bausch & Lomb)

THERAPEUTIC CLASS: Nucleoside analogue

INDICATIONS: Treatment of cytomegalovirus (CMV) retinitis in AIDS patients.

DOSAGE: *Adults:* Each implant releases 4.5mg over 5-8 months. Remove and replace when there is evidence of progression of retinitis.
Pediatrics: ≥9 yrs: Each implant releases 4.5mg over 5-8 months. Remove and replace when there is evidence of progression of retinitis.

HOW SUPPLIED: Implant: 4.5mg

CONTRAINDICATIONS: Hypersensitivity to acyclovir, patients with contraindication for intraocular surgery (eg, external infection, severe thrombocytopenia).

WARNINGS/PRECAUTIONS: For intravitreal implantation only. Monitor for extraocular CMV disease. Implant does not treat systemic CMV. Complications from surgery include vitreous loss or hemorrhage, cataract formation, retinal detachment, uveitis, endophthalmitis, decrease in visual acuity. Immediate decrease in visual acuity will last 2-4 weeks postop. Maintain sterility of the surgical field, implant. Handle implant by suture tab to avoid damage to polymer coating. Handling and disposal of the implant should follow guidelines for antineoplastics.

ADVERSE REACTIONS: Visual acuity loss, vitreous hemorrhage, retinal detachments, cataract formation/lens opacities, macular abnormalities, IOP spikes, optic disk/nerve changes, uveitis, hyphemas.

PREGNANCY: Category C, not for use in nursing.

MECHANISM OF ACTION: Nucleoside analogue antiviral; inhibits replication of herpes viruses.

NURSING CONSIDERATIONS

Assessment: Assess for proper diagnosis of CMV retinitis (eg, indirect opthalmoscopy). Assess patient does not have contraindications for intraocular surgery (eg, external infection, severe thrombocytopenia) and does not have allergy to acyclovir. Assess use in pregnancy/nursing.

Monitoring: Monitor for extraocular CMV disease and infections (eg, pneumonitis, colitis), vitreous loss or hemorrhage, cataract formation, retinal detachment, uvelitis, intraocular infection, and decrease in visual acuity.

Patient Counseling: Advise that implant is not a cure for CMV retinitis; some patients may continue to experience progression of retinitis. Counsel about potential complications following intraocular surgery (eg, intraocular infection, retina detachment, formation of cataracts). Inform patient will experience immediate and temporary decrease in visual acuity for 2-4 weeks after surgery and will require follow-up ophthalmological exams at regular intervals following surgery. Inform medication may cause infertility and may be carcinogenic.

Administration: Ocular implant. **Storage:** 15-30°C (59-86°F). Protect from freezing, excessive heat, and light.

VIVELLE — RX

estradiol (Novartis)

Estrogens increase risk of endometrial cancer in postmenopausal women. Estrogens, with or without progestins, should not be used for the prevention of cardiovascular disease. Increased risks of MI, stroke, invasive breast cancer, PE, and DVT in postmenopausal women (50-79 yrs of age) reported. Increased risk of developing probable dementia in postmenopausal women ≥65 yrs of age reported.

OTHER BRAND NAMES: Vivelle-Dot (Novartis)

THERAPEUTIC CLASS: Estrogen

INDICATIONS: Treatment of moderate to severe vasomotor symptoms and/or vulvar/vaginal atrophy associated with menopause. Treatment of hypoestrogenism due to hypogonadism, castration, or primary ovarian failure. Prevention of postmenopausal osteoporosis.

DOSAGE: *Adults:* Vasomotor Symptoms/Vulvar/Vaginal Atrophy: Initial: 0.0375mg/day twice weekly. Titrate: Adjust after at least 1 month. D/C or taper at 3-6 month intervals. Wait 1 week after withdrawal of oral therapy before initiating therapy. Osteoporosis Prevention: Minimum Effective Dose: 0.025mg/day twice weekly. Apply to clean, dry area of the trunk; avoid breasts and waistline. Rotate sites; allow 1 week between same site. Without intact uterus, may give continuously; with intact uterus, may give cyclically (3 weeks on, 1 week off) with a progestin.

HOW SUPPLIED: Patch: (Vivelle) 0.05mg/day, 0.1mg/day [8^{s}, 48^{s}]; (Vivelle-Dot) 0.025mg/day, 0.0375mg/day, 0.05mg/day, 0.075mg/day, 0.1mg/day [8^{s}, 24^{s}]

CONTRAINDICATIONS: Pregnancy, undiagnosed abnormal genital bleeding, breast cancer, estrogen dependent neoplasia, DVT/PE, active or recent (eg, within past year) arterial thromboembolic disease (eg, stroke, MI), liver dysfunction or disease.

WARNINGS/PRECAUTIONS: May increase risk of cardiovascular events (eg, MI, stroke), venous thrombosis, and PE; d/c immediately if any of these events occur or are suspected. May increase risk of breast/endometrial cancer and gallbladder disease. May lead to severe hypercalcemia with breast cancer and bone metastases; monitor and d/c if hypercalcemia occurs. Retinal vascular thrombosis reported; monitor and d/c if papilledema or retinal vascular lesions occur. Consider addition of a progestin if no hysterectomy. May elevate BP; monitor at regular intervals. May cause elevations of plasma triglycerides with pre-existing hypertriglyceridemia. Caution with history of cholestatic jaundice associated with past estrogen use or with pregnancy; d/c with recurrence. May lead to increased thyroid-binding globulin levels; monitor thyroid function. May cause fluid retention; caution with cardiac/renal dysfunction. Caution with severe hypocalcemia. May increase risk of ovarian cancer. May exacerbate endometriosis, asthma, DM, epilepsy, migraine, porphyria, SLE, and hepatic hemangiomas; use with caution.

ADVERSE REACTIONS: Altered vaginal bleeding, vaginal candidiasis, breast tenderness/enlargement, NV, melasma, headache, weight changes, edema, altered libido.

INTERACTIONS: CYP3A4 inducers (eg, St. John's wort, phenobarbital, carbamazepine, rifampin) may decrease levels which may decrease therapeutic effects and/or change uterine bleeding profile. CYP3A4 inhibitors (eg, erythromycin, clarithromycin, ketoconazole, itraconazole, ritonavir, grapefruit juice) may increase levels which may result in side effects.

PREGNANCY: Contraindicated in pregnancy, caution in nursing.

MECHANISM OF ACTION: Estrogen; responsible for development and maintenance of female reproductive system, and secondary sexual characteristics by modulating pituitary secretion of gonadotropins, LH and FSH.

PHARMACOKINETICS: Absorption: Transdermal administration of variable doses resulted in different parameters. **Metabolism**: Liver, estrone (metabolite), estriol (major urinary metabolite). **Elimination**: Urine; $T_{1/2}$=4.4 hrs, 5.9-7.7 hrs (Dot).

NURSING CONSIDERATIONS

Assessment: Assess for abnormal bleeding, breast or estrogen-dependent neoplasia, CAD, asthma, endometriosis, DM, epilepsy, migraine, porphyrias, SLE, hypothyroidism, pregnancy status, thromboembolic disease, hypocalcemia, and hepatic impairment.

Monitoring: Monitor BP regularly; TFTs periodically. Breast exam by physician yearly and self-exam monthly; mammogram as required. Monitor for signs/symptoms of dementia, gallbladder disease, hypercalcemia, CV events (eg, MI, stroke), abnormal vaginal bleeding, thromboembolic disorders, fluid retention, visual abnormalities, hypersensitivity reactions, hepatic dysfunction, exacerbation of asthma, DM, epilepsy, SLE, migraines, and porphyria.

Patient Counseling: Inform of pregnancy risks. Advise to seek medical attention if symptoms of hepatic dysfunction (eg, jaundice), hypercalcemia, visual abnormalities (eg, partial/complete loss of vision, diplopia), migraines, abnormal vaginal bleeding, hypersensitivity reactions, HTN, thromboembolic disorders, fluid retention, exacerbation of diseases, CV events, or dementia occur.

Administration: Transdermal route. Apply immediately after removed from pouch. **Storage**: Below 30°C (86°F). Dot: 25°C (77°F).

VIVITROL — RX

naltrexone (Cephalon)

THERAPEUTIC CLASS: Opioid antagonist

INDICATIONS: Treatment of alcohol dependence.

DOSAGE: *Adults:* Administer 380mg IM gluteal inj every 4 weeks or once a month using alternating buttocks.

HOW SUPPLIED: Inj, Extended-Release: 380mg

CONTRAINDICATIONS: Concomitant opioid analgesics, physiologic opioid dependence, acute opiate withdrawal, positive urine screen for opioids.

WARNINGS/PRECAUTIONS: Hepatotoxic with excessive doses; margin of separation between safe dose and hepatotoxic dose is 5-fold or less. May cause eosinophilic pneumonia. Only treat patients opioid-free for 7-10 days. Perform naloxone challenge test if risk of precipitating withdrawal. Attempting to overcome the opiate blockade using opioids is very dangerous. More sensitive to lower doses of opioids after naltrexone is discontinued. In emergency situation, suggested plan for pain management is regional analgesia, conscious sedation with a benzodiazepine, or use of non-opioid analgesics or general anesthesia. Monitor for development of depression or suicidal thinking. Caution in renal or hepatic impairment. Administration will not eliminate or diminish alcohol withdrawal symptoms.

ADVERSE REACTIONS: NV, diarrhea, abdominal pain, upper respiratory tract infection, pharyngitis, insomnia, anxiety, depression, injection site reactions, arthralgia, muscle cramps, dizziness, syncope, appetite disorder, retinal artery occlusion.

INTERACTIONS: See Contraindications.

PREGNANCY: Category C, not for use in nursing.

MECHANISM OF ACTION: Opioid antagonist; high affinity for μ-opioid receptor.

PHARMACOKINETICS: Absorption: T_{max}=2 hrs. **Distribution:** Plasma protein binding (21%). **Metabolism:** Extensive, via dihydrodiol dehydrogenase, 6β-naltrexol (primary metabolite). **Elimination:** Urine; $T_{1/2}$=5-10 days.

NURSING CONSIDERATIONS

Assessment: Assess opioid use or dependence, acute opiate withdrawal, hepatic failure or hepatitis, renal impairment, pre-existing subclinical abstinence syndrome, pregnancy/nursing status, alcohol intake, and for possible drug interactions.

Monitoring: Monitor for injection-site reactions, signs/symptoms of hepatotoxicity, respiratory arrest, eosinophilic pneumonia, suicidal ideation attempt, and acute abstinence syndrome. Monitor CBC, LFTs, and CPK.

Patient Counseling: Alert families and caregivers to monitor for emergence of symptoms of depression or suicidality. Advise to carry documentation to alert medical personnel on therapy. Advise that concomitant large doses of heroin, or other opioids, may lead to serious injury, coma, or death; reduced sensitivity to lower doses of opioids. Notify if pregnant/nursing or planning to become pregnant. Inform about risks of therapy and to d/c and immediately consult physician if symptoms/signs of hepatotoxicity, pneumonia, or worsening skin reactions occur. Counsel that therapy treats alcohol dependence only when used as part of treatment program.

Administration: IM route; gluteal region. Must be administrated by health care professional. Not for IV use. **Storage:** 2-8°C (36-46°F). Do not freeze.

VOLTAREN GEL — RX

diclofenac sodium (Novartis Consumer)

V

NSAIDs may cause an increased risk of serious cardiovascular thrombotic events, MI, stroke and serious GI adverse events including bleeding, ulceration, and perforation of the stomach or intestines. Contraindicated for the treatment of perioperative pain in the setting of coronary artery bypass graft (CABG) surgery.

THERAPEUTIC CLASS: NSAID

INDICATIONS: Relief of the pain of osteoarthritis of joints amenable to topical treatment, such as knees and hands. Not evaluated for use on spine, hip, or shoulder.

DOSAGE: *Adults:* Measure onto enclosed dosing card to appropriate 2g or 4g line. Lower Extremities: Apply 4g to affected foot, knee, or ankle qid. Max: 16g/day to any single joint. Upper Extremities: Apply 2g to affected hand, elbow, or wrist qid. Max: 8g/day to any single joint. Total dose should not exceed 32g/day over all affected joints. Avoid showering or bathing for at least 1 hour after application. Avoid open wounds, eyes, mucous membranes, external heat, and/or occlusive dressings. Avoid wearing clothing or gloves for at least 10 min after application.

HOW SUPPLIED: Gel: 1%

CONTRAINDICATIONS: ASA or other NSAID allergy that precipitates asthma, urticaria, or allergic-type reactions. Treatment of perioperative pain in the setting of CABG surgery.

WARNINGS/PRECAUTIONS: May lead to onset of new HTN or worsening of pre-existing HTN; monitor BP closely. Fluid retention and edema reported; caution with fluid retention or heart failure. Renal papillary necrosis and other renal injury reported after long-term use. Not recommended for use with advanced renal disease; if therapy must be initiated, monitor renal function. Anaphylactoid reactions may occur. May cause serious skin adverse events (eg, exfoliative dermatitis, Stevens-Johnson syndrome, and toxic epidermal necrolysis). Avoid in late pregnancy; may cause premature closure of ductus arteriosus. May cause elevations of LFTs; d/c if liver disease develops or systemic manifestations occur. Caution in elderly. Anemia may occur; with long-term use, monitor Hgb/Hct if signs or symptoms of anemia develop. May inhibit platelet aggregation and prolong bleeding time; monitor with coagulation disorders. Caution with asthma and avoid with ASA-sensitive asthma. Patients should minimize or avoid exposure to natural or artificial sunlight on treated areas. Monitor for signs or symptoms of GI bleeding.

ADVERSE REACTIONS: Application-site reactions, including dermatitis.

INTERACTIONS: Avoid with other diclofenac products. Increased adverse effects with ASA; avoid use. May enhance methotrexate toxicity; caution when coadministering. May increase nephrotoxicity of cyclosporine; caution when coadministering. May diminish antihypertensive effect of ACE-inhibitors. May reduce natriuretic effect of furosemide and thiazides; monitor for renal failure. May increase lithium levels; monitor for toxicity. Synergistic effects on GI bleeding with warfarin. Avoid concomitant use with other topical products, including topical medications, sunscreens, lotions, moisturizers, and cosmetics, on the same skin site.

PREGNANCY: Category C, not for use in nursing.

MECHANISM OF ACTION: NSAID; inhibits cyclooxygenase, resulting in reduced formation of prostaglandins, thromboxanes, and prostacylin.

PHARMACOKINETICS: Absorption: (4g) C_{max}=15ng/mL; T_{max}=14 hrs; AUC=233ng•h/mL. (12g)C_{max}=53.8ng/mL; T_{max}=10 hrs; AUC=807ng•h/mL.

NURSING CONSIDERATIONS

Assessment: Assess for hypersensitivity to ASA or NSAIDs, history of ulcer or GI bleeding, HTN, fluid retention, CHF, asthma, cardiovascular disease (or risk factors), pregnancy status, possible drug interactions, renal/hepatic impairment. Obtain baseline BP.

Monitoring: Monitor BP, LFTs, and renal function periodically. Monitor for signs/symptoms of cardiovascular events, GI events (eg, ulcerations, bleeding), hepatotoxicity, renal dysfunction, HTN, skin reactions, anemia, blood loss, and hypersensitivity reactions.

Patient Counseling: Instruct to avoid contact with eyes; if contact occurs, wash with water or saline and if irritation persists for >1 hr call physician. Advise to minimize sun exposure. Seek medical attention for symptoms of cardiovascular events (eg, chest pain, SOB, weakness, slurring of speech), GI events (eg, epigastric pain, dyspepsia, melena, hematemesis), hepatotoxicity (eg, RUQ pain, pruritus, fatigue), skin reactions (eg, rash, blisters, fever), unexplained weight gain or edema, or hypersensitivity reactions (eg, difficulty breathing, swelling of face/throat).

Administration: Topical route. **Storage:** 25°C (77°F), excursions permitted to 15-30°C (59-86°F). Avoid freezing.

VOLTAREN OPHTHALMIC RX

diclofenac sodium (Novartis Ophthalmics)

THERAPEUTIC CLASS: NSAID

INDICATIONS: Treatment of postoperative inflammation following cataract surgery. Temporary relief of pain and photophobia in corneal refractive surgery.

DOSAGE: *Adults:* Cataract Surgery: 1 drop qid, start 24 hrs after surgery and continue for 2 weeks. Corneal Refractive Surgery: 1-2 drops within 1 hr prior to, and within 15 min after surgery. Continue qid for up to 3 days.

HOW SUPPLIED: Sol: 0.1% [2.5mL, 5mL]

WARNINGS/PRECAUTIONS: May delay wound healing. Caution with bleeding tendencies. Monitor for 1 yr after use in corneal refractive procedures. May increase bleeding of ocular tissues. No significant increase in tumor incidence. No differences in safety and effectiveness observed between elderly and younger adult patients.

ADVERSE REACTIONS: Transient burning/stinging, keratitis, elevated IOP, lacrimation, abnormal vision, conjunctivitis, eyelid swelling, discharge, iritis, itching.

INTERACTIONS: Caution with agents that prolong bleeding time (eg, NSAIDs). Potential for cross-sensitivity to acetylsalicylic acid, phenylacetic acid derivatives, and other NSAIDs.

PREGNANCY: Category C, safety in nursing not known.

MECHANISM OF ACTION: NSAID; anti-inflammatory and analgesic that inhibits the enzyme cyclo-oxygenase, which is essential for biosynthesis of prostaglandins.

PHARMACOKINETICS: Absorption: C_{max}<10ng/mL; T_{max}=4 hrs.

NURSING CONSIDERATIONS

Assessment: Assess for hypersensitivity or cross-sensitivity with some drugs (eg, ASA), history of complicated or repeated ocular surgeries, corneal denervation, corneal epithelial defects, DM, ocular surface diseases (eg, dry eye syndrome), RA, bleeding tendencies, and history of concomitant use of medications that may prolong bleeding time or delay wound healing.

Monitoring: Monitor for corneal thinning, erosion, ulceration, or perforation and for hypersensitivity reactions, wound healing problems, keratitis, increased bleeding time, bleeding of ocular tissues (hyphemas) in conjunction with ocular surgery, and increased IOP after cataract surgery.

Patient Counseling: Instruct not to administer while wearing contact lenses.

Administration: Ocular route. **Storage:** 15-25°C (59-77°F).

VOLTAREN-XR RX

diclofenac sodium (Novartis)

V

NSAIDs may cause an increased risk of serious cardiovascular thrombotic events, MI, stroke and serious GI adverse events including bleeding, ulceration, and perforation of the stomach or intestines. Contraindicated for the treatment of perioperative pain in the setting of coronary artery bypass graft (CABG) surgery.

OTHER BRAND NAMES: Voltaren (Novartis)

THERAPEUTIC CLASS: NSAID

INDICATIONS: (Voltaren) Relief of signs and symptoms of osteoarthritis (OA), rheumatoid arthritis (RA), and ankylosing spondylitis (AS). (Voltaren-XR) Relief of signs and symptoms of OA and RA.

DOSAGE: *Adults:* (Voltaren) OA: 50mg bid-tid or 75mg bid. Max: 150mg/day. RA: 50mg tid-qid or 75mg bid. Max: 200mg/day. AS: 25mg qid and 25mg qhs prn. Max: 125mg/day. (Voltaren-XR) OA: 100mg qd. RA: 100mg qd-bid.

HOW SUPPLIED: Tab, Delayed-Release: (Voltaren) 75mg; (Generic) 25mg, 50mg, 75mg; Tab, Extended-Release: (Voltaren-XR)100mg

CONTRAINDICATIONS: ASA or other NSAID allergy that precipitates asthma, urticaria, or allergic-type reactions. Treatment of perioperative pain in the setting of CABG surgery.

WARNINGS/PRECAUTIONS: Cannot replace corticosteroid or to treat corticosteroid insufficiency. May lead to onset of new HTN or worsening of pre-existing HTN; monitor BP closely. Fluid retention and edema reported; caution with fluid retention or heart failure. Caution with considerable dehydration. Renal papillary necrosis and other renal injury reported after long-term use. Not recommended for use with advanced renal disease; if therapy must be initiated, monitor renal function. Anaphylactoid reactions may occur. May cause serious skin adverse events (eg, exfoliative dermatitis, Stevens-Johnson syndrome, and toxic epidermal necrolysis). Avoid in late pregnancy; may cause premature closure of ductus arteriosus. May cause elevations of LFTs; d/c if liver disease develops or systemic manifestations occur. Caution in elderly. Anemia may occur; with long-term use, monitor Hgb/Hct if signs or symptoms of anemia develop. May inhibit platelet aggregation and prolong bleeding time; monitor with coagulation disorders. Caution with asthma and avoid with ASA-sensitive asthma. Risk of GI ulceration, bleeding, and perforation.

ADVERSE REACTIONS: Abdominal pain, constipation, diarrhea, dyspepsia, flatulence, gross bleeding/perforation, heartburn, N/V, GI ulcers (gastric/duodenal), renal function abnormalities, anemia, dizziness, edema, elevated liver enzymes, headaches, increased bleeding time, pruritus, rashes, and tinnitus.

INTERACTIONS: Avoid with other diclofenac products. Increased adverse effects with ASA; avoid use. May enhance methotrexate toxicity; caution when co-administering. May increase nephrotoxicity of cyclosporine; caution when co-administering. May diminish antihypertensive effect of ACE-inhibitors. May reduce natriuretic effect of furosemide and thiazides; monitor for renal failure. May increase lithium levels; monitor for toxicity. Synergistic effects on GI bleeding with warfarin.

PREGNANCY: Category C, not for use in nursing.

MECHANISM OF ACTION: NSAID; not known, suspected to inhibit prostaglandin synthetase.

PHARMACOKINETICS: Absorption: Absolute bioavailability (55%); T_{max}=5.3 hrs. **Distribution:** V_d=1.4L/kg; plasma protein binding (99%). **Metabolism:** Liver (glucuronidation and sulfation). **Elimination:** Urine (65%), bile (35%); $T_{1/2}$=2.3 hrs.

NURSING CONSIDERATIONS

Assessment: Assess for history of asthma, cardiovascular thrombotic events, CABG surgery, stroke, MI, CVD (eg, pre-existing HTN, CHF) or risk factors, fluid retention, edema, pregnancy status, GI events (eg, bleeding, ulceration, perforation) or risk factors, possible drug interactions, renal/hepatic impairment.

Monitoring: Monitor BP, CBC, LFTs, renal function, and chemistries periodically. Monitor for signs/symptoms of GI events (eg, bleeding, ulceration, perforation), cardiovascular thrombotic events, CHF, HTN, salt depletion, allergic reactions (eg, rash, eosinophilia), renal/liver dysfunction.

Patient Counseling: Advise to seek medical attention if symptoms of hepatotoxicity (eg, nausea, fatigue, pruritus), anaphylactic reactions (eg, difficulty breathing, swelling of face/throat), hypersensitivity reactions (eg, rash), cardiovascular events (eg, chest pain, SOB, weakness, slurring of speech), GI ulceration or bleeding (eg, epigastric pain, dyspepsia, melena, hematemesis), weight gain, or edema occur. Inform of pregnancy risks.

Administration: Oral route. **Storage:** Below 30°C (86°F). Protect from moisture.

VOSPIRE ER

RX

albuterol sulfate (Dava)

THERAPEUTIC CLASS: Beta$_2$-agonist

INDICATIONS: Treatment of bronchospasm in reversible obstructive airway disease.

DOSAGE: *Adults:* Usual: 4-8mg q12h. Low Body Weight: Initial: 4mg q12h. Titrate: May increase to 8mg q12h. Max: 32mg/day in divided doses. Swallow whole with liquids; do not chew or crush.

Pediatrics: >12 yrs: Usual: 4-8mg q12h. Low Body Weight: Initial: 4mg q12h. Titrate: May increase to 8mg q12h. Max: 32mg/day in divided doses. 6-12 yrs: Usual: 4mg q12h. Max: 24mg/day in divided doses. Swallow whole with liquids; do not chew or crush.

HOW SUPPLIED: Tab, Extended-Release: 4mg, 8mg

WARNINGS/PRECAUTIONS: Hypersensitivity reactions reported. Caution with cardiovascular disorders, especially coronary insufficiency, arrhythmias and HTN. Increased doses may signify need for concomitant corticosteroids. Can produce paradoxical bronchospasm. Caution with DM, hyperthyroidism, seizures. May produce transient hypokalemia. Erythema multiforme and Stevens-Johnson (rare) reported in children.

ADVERSE REACTIONS: Tremor, headache, nervousness, tachycardia, palpitations, N/V, muscle cramps.

INTERACTIONS: Avoid oral sympathomimetic agents. Extreme caution within 14 days of MAOI or TCA therapy. Monitor digoxin. May worsen ECG changes and/or hypokalemia with non-K^+-sparing diuretics. Antagonized by β-blockers.

PREGNANCY: Category C, not for use in nursing.

MECHANISM OF ACTION: β_2-adrenergic bronchodilator; stimulates adenyl cylase, enzyme that catalyzes formation of cAMP from ATP. Increased cAMP levels associated with relaxation of bronchial smooth muscle and inhibition of release of mediators of immediate hypersensitivity.

PHARMACOKINETICS: Absorption: C_{max}=13.7ng/mL; T_{max}=6 hrs; AUC=134ng•hr/mL. **Elimination:** $T_{1/2}$=9.3 hrs.

NURSING CONSIDERATIONS

Assessment: Assess for renal/hepatic functions, history of hypersensitivity to drug, cardiovascular disorder (coronary insufficiency, HTN, cardiac arrhythmias), convulsive disorders, hyperthyroidism, DM and ketoacidosis, and possible drug interactions.

Monitoring: Monitor for possible paradoxical bronchospasm, asthma deterioration, cardiovascular effects, immediate hypersensitivity reactions, CBC with differential count, ketoacidosis, hypokalemia, serum glucose concentrations, tremors.

Patient Counseling: Instruct to swallow tablet; do not chew or crush. Report lack of response or adverse effects.

Administration: Oral route. **Storage:** Store at 20-25°C (68-77°F). Dispense in well-closed, light-resistant container.

VYTORIN

RX

simvastatin - ezetimibe (Merck/Schering-Plough)

THERAPEUTIC CLASS: Cholesterol absorption inhibitor/HMG-CoA reductase inhibitor

INDICATIONS: When treatment with both components is appropriate, used as an adjunct to diet for the reduction of elevated total-C, LDL-C, Apo B, TG, non-HDL-C, and to increase HDL-C in primary hypercholesterolemia (heterozygous familial and non-familial) or mixed hyperlipidemia. For the reduction of elevated total-C, LDL-C in homozygous familial hypercholesterolemia as an adjunct to other lipid-lowering treatments or if such treatments are unavailable.

DOSAGE: *Adults:* Take once daily in the evening. Initial: 10mg-20mg qd. Less Aggressive LDL-C Reductions: Initial: 10mg-10mg qd. LDL-C Reduction >55%: Initial: 10mg-40mg qd. Titrate: Adjust at ≥2 weeks. Homozygous Familial Hypercholesterolemia: 10mg-40mg or 10mg-80mg qd. Severe Renal Insufficiency: Avoid unless tolerant of ≥5mg of simvastatin; monitor closely. Concomitant Bile Acid Sequestrant: Take either ≥2 hrs before or ≥4 hrs after bile acid sequestrant. Concomitant Cyclosporine: Avoid unless tolerant of ≥5mg of simvastatin. Max: 10mg-10mg/day. Concomitant Amiodarone/ Verapamil: Max: 10mg-20mg/day.

HOW SUPPLIED: Tab: (ezetimibe-simvastatin) 10mg-10mg, 10mg-20mg, 10mg-40mg, 10mg-80mg

CONTRAINDICATIONS: Active liver disease, unexplained persistent elevations in serum transaminases, pregnancy, lactation.

WARNINGS/PRECAUTIONS: Rhabdomyolysis (rare), myopathy reported. D/C therapy if myopathy is suspected or diagnosed, if AST or ALT ≥3x ULN persists, a few days prior to major surgery or when any major medical or surgical condition supervenes. Monitor LFTs prior to therapy and thereafter when clinically indicated. With 10mg-80mg dose, monitor LFTs prior to titration, 3 months after titration and periodically thereafter for 1st yr. Caution with heavy alcohol use, severe renal insufficiency, or history of hepatic disease. Avoid use in moderate or severe hepatic insufficiency.

ADVERSE REACTIONS: Headache, upper respiratory tract infection, myalgia, CK and transaminase elevations, urticaria, arthralgia.

INTERACTIONS: Avoid use with concomitant itraconazole, ketoconazole, erythromycin, clarithromycin, telithromycin, HIV protease inhibitors, nefazodone, grapefruit juice (>1 quart/day); increased risk of myopathy/rhabdomyolysis. Max 10mg-10mg daily with gemfibrozil, cyclosporine, danazol. Max 10mg-20mg daily with amiodarone, verapamil. Caution with other fibrates, ≥1g/day of niacin. Incremental LDL-C reductions with concomitant cholestyramine. Monitor digoxin, warfarin.

PREGNANCY: Category X, not for use in nursing.

MECHANISM OF ACTION: Ezetimibe: Cholesterol absorption inhibitor. Reduces blood cholesterol by inhibiting absorption of cholesterol by small intestine. Molecular target is sterol transporter, Niemann-Pick C1-Like 1 (NPC1L1), which is involved in intestinal uptake of cholesterol and phytosterols. Simvastatin: HMG-CoA reductase inhibitor. Inhibits conversion of HMG-CoA to mevalonate. Also reduces VLDL, TG, and increases HDL-C.

PHARMACOKINETICS: Distribution: Ezetimibe: Plasma protein binding (>90%). Simvastatin: Plasma protein binding (95%); crosses blood-brain barrier. **Metabolism:** Ezetimibe: Small intestine, liver via glucuronide conjugation, ezetimibe-glucuronide (active metabolite). Simvastatin: Hydrolysis; β-hydroxyacid; 6'-hydroxy; 6'hydroxymethyl, and 6'-exomethylene (major active metabolites). **Elimination:** Ezetimibe: Feces (78%), urine (11%). Simvastatin: Feces (60%), urine (13%).

NURSING CONSIDERATIONS

Assessment: Assess for secondary causes of dyslipidemia (eg, DM, hypothyroidism, obstructive liver disease, chronic renal failure, drugs that increase LDL-C and decrease HDL-C), active liver disease or unexplained persistent elevations of serum transaminases, pregnancy/nursing status. Obtain baseline lipid profile (total-C, LDL-C, HDL-C, TG) and liver function (eg, AST, ALT). Assess use in patients who consume excessive amounts of alcohol or have history of liver disease. Assess for drug interactions.

Monitoring: Monitor for signs/symptoms of myopathy (unexplained muscle pain, tenderness, weakness), rhabodomyolysis, liver dysfunction, and CNS toxicity (eg, optic nerve degeneration). Perform periodic monitoring of CK levels, LFTs, and lipid profile.

Patient Counseling: Recommend cholesterol-lowering diet while taking drug. Instruct to take in evening, with/without food. Advise to contact physician immediately if unexplained muscle pain, tenderness, or weakness develops. Advise about possible drug interactions and interaction with grapefruit juice.

Administration: Oral route. **Storage:** 20-25°C (68-77°F). Keep container tightly closed.

VYVANSE

CII

lisdexamfetamine dimesylate (Shire)

High abuse potential; prolonged periods of administration may lead to dependence. Misuse of amphetamine may cause sudden death and serious cardiovascular events.

THERAPEUTIC CLASS: Sympathomimetic amine

INDICATIONS: Treatment of ADHD.

DOSAGE: *Adults:* Individualize dose. Usual: 30mg qam. Titrate: If needed, may increase in increments of 10mg or 20mg at weekly intervals. Max: 70mg/day. Swallow caps or dissolve contents in glass of water; do not store once dissolved. Re-evaluate periodically.

Pediatrics: 6-12 yrs: Individualize dose. Usual: 30mg qam. Titrate: If needed, may increase in increments of 10mg or 20mg at weekly intervals. Max: 70mg/day. Swallow caps or dissolve contents in glass of water; do not store once dissolved. Re-evaluate periodically.

HOW SUPPLIED: Cap: 20mg, 30mg, 40mg, 50mg, 60mg, 70mg

CONTRAINDICATIONS: Advanced arteriosclerosis, symptomatic CVD, moderate to severe HTN, hyperthyroidism, glaucoma, agitated states, history of drug abuse, during or within 14 days of MAOI use.

WARNINGS/PRECAUTIONS: Avoid use with structural cardiac abnormalities, cardiomyopathy, serious heart rhythm abnormalities, or other serious cardiac problems; sudden death reported. Assess presence of cardiac disease through cardiac evaluation. Caution with HTN, heart failure, recent MI, or ventricular arrhythmia; monitor BP and HR. May exacerbate symptoms of behavior disturbance and thought disorder in psychotic patients. Caution with comorbid bipolar disorder; concern for possible induction of mixed/manic episode. Treatment emergent psychotic or manic symptoms (eg, hallucinations, delusional thinking, or mania, without prior history of psychotic illness) may occur; d/c treatment if needed. Aggressive behavior or hostility reported; monitor condition as it worsens. Monitor growth in children. Stimulants may lower the convulsive threshold; d/c in the presence of seizures. Difficulties with accommodation and blurring of vision reported. May exacerbate motor or phonic tics and Tourette's syndrome.

ADVERSE REACTIONS: Ventricular hypertrophy, tic, NV, psychomotor hyperactivity, insomnia, rash, upper abdominal pain, decreased appetite, dizziness, dry mouth, irritability, weight loss, headache, affect lability.

INTERACTIONS: Urinary acidifying agents (eg, ammonium chloride, sodium acid phosphate) and methenamine decrease efficacy. Inhibits adrenergic blockers, antihistamines, and antihypertensives (veratrum alkaloids). Potentiated effects of both agents with TCAs. MAOIs and furazolidone metabolite may cause hypertensive crisis. Antagonized by chlorpromazine, haloperidol, and lithium carbonate. May delay absorption of ethosuximide, phenobarbital, and phenytoin. Potentiates meperidine, norepinephrine, phenobarbital, and phenytoin. Potentiated by propoxyphene overdose; fatal convulsions may occur.

PREGNANCY: Category C, not for use in nursing.

MECHANISM OF ACTION: Dextroamphetamine; blocks reuptake of norepinephrine and dopamine into presynaptic neuron and increases release of these monoamines into extraneuronal space.

PHARMACOKINETICS: Absorption: Rapidly absorbed; T_{max}=1 hr. **Metabolism:** 1st-pass intestinal and/or hepatic metabolism to dextroamphetamine and L-lysine. **Elimination:** Urine, feces; $T_{1/2}$≤1 hr.

NURSING CONSIDERATIONS

Assessment: Assess for agitation, glaucoma, tics, family history of Tourette's syndrome, cardiovascular conditions (eg, severe HTN, angina pectoris, cardiac structural abnormalities, arrhythmias, HF, recent MI), hyperthyroidism or thyrotoxicosis, bipolar disorder, psychosis, history of drug dependence or alcoholism, possible drug interactions.

Monitoring: Monitor HR, BP, cardiovascular abnormalities, exacerbation of behavioral disturbances and thought disorders, bipolar disorder, aggression, seizures, visual disturbances, impotence, and changes in libido. Monitor growth in children.

Patient Counseling: Inform about risks of treatment, appropriate use, and drug abuse/dependence. Use caution while operating machinery/driving. Avoid afternoon dose to reduce potential insomnia. May be taken with/without food.

Administration: Oral route. **Storage:** Store at 25°C (77°F); excursions permitted to 15-30°C (59-86°F).

WelChol RX

coleseveIam HCl (Daiichi Sankyo)

THERAPEUTIC CLASS: Bile acid sequestrant

INDICATIONS: Adjunct to diet and exercise to reduce elevated LDL-cholesterol in primary hyperlipidemia as monotherapy or with an HMG-CoA reductase inhibitor and to improve glycemic control in adults with type 2 diabetes mellitus (DM).

DOSAGE: *Adults:* Hyperlipidemia/Type 2 DM: 3 tabs bid or 6 tabs qd. Take with liquids and a meal.

HOW SUPPLIED: Tab: 625mg

CONTRAINDICATIONS: Bowel obstruction, hypertriglyceridemia-induced pancreatitis, serum TG concentrations >500mg/dL.

WARNINGS/PRECAUTIONS: Monitor lipids, including TG and non-HDL-cholesterol levels prior to initiation of treatment and periodically thereafter. Caution in TG levels >300mg/dL, dysphagia or swallowing disorders, gastroparesis, GI motility disorders, major GI tract surgery, bowel obstruction, and those susceptible to vitamin K or fat-soluble vitamin deficiencies. Coadministered drugs should be given at least 4 hrs prior to treatment; monitor drug levels. Not for use in treatment of type 1 DM or for diabetic ketoacidosis.

ADVERSE REACTIONS: Asthenia, constipation, dyspepsia, pharyngitis, myalgia, nausea, hypoglycemia, bowel obstruction, dysphagia, esophageal obstruction, fecal impaction, hypertriglyceridemia, pancreatitis, increased transaminases.

INTERACTIONS: May increase TG levels when used with insulin or sulfonylureas. May decrease level of glyburide, levothyroxine, and oral contraceptives containing ethinyl estradiol and norethindrone. Concomitant use with warfarin decreases INR; monitor INR. May elevate TSH in patients receiving thyroid hormone replacement therapy. May decrease phenytoin levels.

PREGNANCY: Category B, caution in nursing.

MECHANISM OF ACTION: Bile acid sequestrant; non-absorbed, lipid-lowering polymer that binds bile acids in intestine, impeding their reabsorption. Consequently, compensatory effects lead to increased LDL-C clearance from blood, resulting in decreased serum LDL-C levels.

PHARMACOKINETICS: Absorption: Not hydrolyzed by digestive enzymes and not absorbed. **Distribution:** Limited to GI tract. **Metabolism:** Not metabolized systemically. **Excretion:** Urine.

NURSING CONSIDERATIONS

Assessment: Prior to initiation, assess history of bowel obstruction, gastroparesis, other GI motility disorder, or hypertriglyceridemia-induced pancreatitis;

serum TG concentrations >500mg/dL; possible drug interactions. Obtain baseline lipid parameters (eg, TG, non-HDL-C).

Monitoring: Monitor signs/symptoms of increased TG levels (eg, hypertriglyceridemia-induced pancreatitis), hypoglycemia, vitamin K or fat-soluble vitamin deficiencies, dysphagia, or esophageal obstruction. Periodically monitor lipid profile (eg, TG, non-HDL-C), HbA_{1c}, and coadministered drug levels.

Patient Counseling: Instruct to take with meal/liquid and consume diet that promotes bowel regularity; take drugs that may interact (eg, glyburide, levothyroxine, oral contraceptives) ≥4 hrs prior. Instruct to promptly d/c and seek medical attention if severe abdominal pain or constipation occurs. Inform that dysphagia or esophageal obstruction may occur because of tab size; caution with swallowing disorders.

Administration: Oral route. **Storage:** 25°C (77°F); excursions permitted to 15-30°C (59-86°F). Protect from moisture.

WELLBUTRIN SR — RX

bupropion HCl (GlaxoSmithKline)

Antidepressants increased the risk of suicidal thinking and behavior (suicidality) in short-term studies in children, adolescents, and young adults with major depressive disorder (MDD) and other psychiatric disorders. Bupropion is not approved for use in pediatric patients.

OTHER BRAND NAMES: Wellbutrin (GlaxoSmithKline)

THERAPEUTIC CLASS: Aminoketone

INDICATIONS: Treatment of MDD.

DOSAGE: *Adults:* ≥18 yrs: (Tab, Extended-Release) Initial: 150mg qd, may increase to 150mg bid after 3 days. Usual: 150mg bid. Max: 200mg bid. Separate doses by at least 8 hrs. Severe Hepatic Cirrhosis: 100mg/day or 150mg every other day. Mild-Moderate Hepatic Cirrhosis/Renal Impairment: Reduce frequency and/or dose. (Tab) Initial: 100mg bid, may increase to 100mg tid after 3 days. Usual: 100mg tid. Max: 450mg/day, given in divided doses of not more than 150mg each. Severe Hepatic Cirrhosis: Max: 75mg qd.

HOW SUPPLIED: Tab: 75mg, 100mg; Tab, Extended-Release: 100mg, 150mg, 200mg

CONTRAINDICATIONS: Seizure disorder, bulimia or anorexia nervosa, within 14 days of MAOIs, other forms of bupropion, abrupt discontinuation of alcohol or sedatives.

WARNINGS/PRECAUTIONS: Dose-related risk of seizures. D/C and do not restart if seizure occurs. Extreme caution with history of seizure, cranial trauma, severe hepatic cirrhosis. Agitation, insomnia, psychosis, confusion and other neuropsychiatric signs reported. Caution with bipolar disorder, recent MI, unstable heart disease, renal impairment. Altered appetite/weight, allergic reactions, HTN reported. Monitor for clinical worsening and/or suicidality, especially at initiation of therapy or dose changes.

ADVERSE REACTIONS: Headache, dry mouth, nausea, insomnia, dizziness, pharyngitis, infection, abdominal pain, constipation, diarrhea, tinnitus, agitation, anxiety, rash, anorexia.

INTERACTIONS: See Contraindications. Extreme caution with drugs that lower seizure threshold (eg, antidepressants, antipsychotics, theophylline, systemic steroids). Increased seizure risk with opioid, cocaine, or stimulant addiction, OTC stimulants or anorectics, oral hypoglycemics, insulin, excessive use or abrupt discontinuation of alcohol or sedatives. Caution with levodopa, amantadine, and drugs that are metabolized by CYP2D6 (eg, SSRIs, TCAs, antipsychotics, β-blockers, type 1C antiarrhythmics); use low initial dose and gradually titrate. Avoid other bupropion-containing drugs. Monitor HTN with transdermal nicotine. Caution with CYP2B6 substrates or inhibitors (eg, orphenadrine, cyclophosphamide, thiotepa). Carbamazepine, phenytoin, cimetidine, and phenobarbital may induce metabolism of bupropion. Minimize or avoid alcohol.

PREGNANCY: Category C, not for use in nursing.

MECHANISM OF ACTION: Aminoketone antidepressant; suspected to inhibit neuronal uptake of norepinephrine and dopamine.

PHARMACOKINETICS: Absorption: T_{max}=3 hrs (bupropion, hydroxybupropion). **Distribution**: Plasma protein binding (84%). **Metabolism**: Hydroxylation, hydroxybupropion (CYP2B6); Reduction of carbonyl group, threohydrobupropion, eythrohydrobupropion. **Elimination**: Urine (87%), feces (10%), (0.5% unchanged); $T_{1/2}$=21 hrs, 20 hrs, 33 hrs, 37 hrs (bupropion, hydroxybupropion, erythrohydrobupropion, threohydrobupropion, respectively).

NURSING CONSIDERATIONS

Assessment: Assess for history of seizures, bulimia/anorexia nervosa, LFTs, renal function tests, DM, head trauma, use of alcohol, opiate sedatives. Note other diseases/conditions and drug therapies.

Monitoring: Monitor for clinical worsening, suicidality, or unusual changes in behavior, seizures, increased restlessness, agitation, anxiety, insomnia, neuropsychiatric signs/symptoms (eg, delusions, hallucinations, psychosis, concentration disturbance, paranoia, confusion), weight loss, loss of appetite, arthralgia, myalgia, HTN, and fever with rash.

Patient Counseling: Advise families and caregivers of need for close observation of clinical worsening and/or suicidal risks. Avoid alcohol, sedatives, OTC drugs. Exercise caution while operating machinery/driving. Report adverse reactions. Consult physician before taking any other medications.

Administration: Oral route. **Storage:** Store SR tab at controlled room temperature, 20-25°C (68-77°F). Dispense in a tight, light-resistant container.

WELLBUTRIN XL — RX

bupropion HCl (GlaxoSmithKline)

Antidepressants increased the risk of suicidal thinking and behavior (suicidality) in short-term studies in children, adolescents, and young adults with major depressive disorder (MDD) and other psychiatric disorders. Bupropion is not approved for use in pediatric patients.

THERAPEUTIC CLASS: Aminoketone

INDICATIONS: Treatment of MDD and prevention of seasonal major depressive episodes in patients diagnosed with seasonal affective disorder (SAD).

DOSAGE: *Adults:* ≥18 yrs: Give in AM. Swallow whole. MDD: Initial: 150mg qd. May increase to 300mg qd on Day 4. Usual: 300mg qd. Max: 450mg qd. SAD: Start in autumn; stop in early spring. Initial: 150mg qd. May increase to 300mg after 1 week. Usual/Max: 300mg qd. Taper dose for 2 weeks prior to discontinuation. Mild-Moderate Hepatic Cirrhosis/Renal Impairment: Reduce frequency and/or dose. Severe Hepatic Cirrhosis: Max: 150mg every other day.

HOW SUPPLIED: Tab, Extended-Release: 150mg, 300mg

CONTRAINDICATIONS: Seizure disorder, bulimia or anorexia nervosa, within 14 days of MAOIs, other forms of bupropion, abrupt discontinuation of alcohol or sedatives.

WARNINGS/PRECAUTIONS: Dose-related risk of seizures. D/C and do not restart if seizure occurs. Extreme caution with history of seizure, cranial trauma, severe hepatic cirrhosis. Agitation, insomnia, psychosis, confusion and other neuropsychiatric signs reported. Caution with bipolar disorder, recent MI, unstable heart disease, renal impairment. Altered appetite/weight, allergic reactions, HTN reported. Monitor for clinical worsening and/or suicidality, especially at initiation of therapy or dose changes.

ADVERSE REACTIONS: Headache, dry mouth, nausea, insomnia, dizziness, pharyngitis, abdominal pain, agitation, diarrhea, palpitations, myalgia, anxiety, tinnitus, constipation, sweating, rash.

INTERACTIONS: See Contraindications. Extreme caution with drugs that lower seizure threshold (eg, antidepressants, antipsychotics, theophylline, systemic steroids). Increased seizure risk with opioid, cocaine, or stimulant addiction, OTC stimulants or anorectics, oral hypoglycemics, insulin, excessive use or abrupt discontinuation of alcohol or sedatives. Caution with levodopa, amantadine, and drugs that are metabolized by CYP2D6 (eg, SSRIs, TCAs, antipsychotics, β-blockers, type 1C antiarrhythmics); use low initial dose and gradually titrate. Monitor HTN with transdermal nicotine. Caution with CYP2B6 substrates or inhibitors (eg, orphenadrine, cyclophosphamide, thiotepa). Carbamazepine, phenytoin, cimetidine, and phenobarbital may induce metabolism of bupropion. Minimize or avoid alcohol.

PREGNANCY: Category C, not for use in nursing.

MECHANISM OF ACTION: Aminoketone antidepressant; suspected to inhibit neuronal uptake of norepinephrine and dopamine.

PHARMACOKINETICS: Absorption: T_{max}=2 hrs. **Distribution**: Plasma protein binding (84%). **Metabolism**: Extensive to hydroxybupropion (CYP2B6) via hydroxylation; threohydrobupropion, eythrohydrobupropion via reduction of carbonyl group. **Elimination**: Urine (87%), feces (10%), (0.5% unchanged); $T_{1/2}$=21 hrs, 20 hrs, 33 hrs, 37 hrs (bupropion, hydroxybupropion, erythrohydrobupropion, threohydrobupropion respectively).

NURSING CONSIDERATIONS

Assessment: Assess for history of seizures, bulimia/anorexia nervosa, LFTs, renal function tests, DM, head trauma, use of alcohol, opiate sedatives, history of MI or unstable heart disease, psychosis, mixed/manic eposodes. Note other diseases/conditions and drug therapies, especially other bupropion products.

Monitoring: Monitor for clinical worsening, suicidality, unusual changes in behavior, seizures, increased restlessness, agitation, anxiety, insomnia, neuropsychiatric signs/symptoms (eg, delusions, hallucinations, psychosis, concentration disturbances, paranoia, confusion), weight loss, loss of appetite, arthralgia, myalgia, HTN, and fever with rash.

Patient Counseling: Advise families and caregivers of need for close observation of clinical worsening and suicidal risks. Avoid alcohol, sedatives, OTC drugs. Exercise caution while operating machinery/driving. Report adverse reactions and consult physician before taking any other medications or plan to become pregnant. Advise to swallow tablets whole; do not chew, divide, or crush. D/C and do not restart if experience seizure while on treatment.

Administration: Oral route. **Storage**: 15-30°C (59-77°F). Protect from light and moisture.

WESTCORT — RX

hydrocortisone valerate (Ranbaxy)

THERAPEUTIC CLASS: Corticosteroid

INDICATIONS: Corticosteroid-responsive dermatoses.

DOSAGE: *Adults:* Apply bid-tid. May use occlusive dressings for psoriasis or recalcitrant conditions; d/c dressings if infection develops.
Pediatrics: Apply bid-tid. May use occlusive dressings for psoriasis or recalcitrant conditions; d/c dressings if infection develops.

HOW SUPPLIED: Cre, Oint: 0.2% [15g, 45g, 60g]

WARNINGS/PRECAUTIONS: May produce reversible HPA axis suppression, manifestations of Cushing's syndrome, hyperglycemia, and glucosuria. Caution when applied to large surface areas or under occlusive dressings. Use appropriate antifungal or antibacterial agent with dermatological infections; d/c if infection does not clear. Pediatrics may be more susceptible to systemic toxicity. Avoid eyes. D/C if irritation occurs.

ADVERSE REACTIONS: Burning, itching, dryness, irritation, folliculitis, hypertrichosis, acneiform eruptions, hypopigmentation, allergic contact dermatitis, skin maceration, secondary infection, skin atrophy, striae, miliaria.

PREGNANCY: Category C, caution in nursing.

MECHANISM OF ACTION: Corticosteroid; possesses anti-inflammatory, antipruritic, and vasoconstrictive properties. Anti-inflammatory effects not established; suspected to act by induction of phospholipase A_2 inhibitory proteins, lipocortins. Lipocortins control biosynthesis of potent inflammation mediators (eg, prostaglandins, leukotrienes) by inhibiting release of their common precursor, arachidonic acid.

PHARMACOKINETICS: Absorption: Percutaneous; inflammation and other disease states may increase absorption. Use of occlusive dressings for ≤24 hrs not shown to increase penetration; use for ≥96 hrs markedly enhances penetration. **Distribution:** Systemically administered corticosteroids found in breast milk.

NURSING CONSIDERATIONS

Assessment: Assess use in pregnant/nursing patients.

Monitoring: Monitor for signs/symptoms of reversible HPA-axis suppression, Cushing's syndrome, hyperglycemia, glucosuria, skin irritation, allergic contact dermatitis (eg, failure to heal), and concomitant skin infections (eg, bacterial, fungal). If large doses or using occlusive dressings, monitor for HPA-axis suppression using ACTH stimulation test, AM plasma cortisol test, and urinary free cortisol test. Monitor for glucocorticosteroid insufficiencies following d/c of therapy. In pediatric patients, monitor for signs/symptoms of systemic toxicity, HPA-axis suppression (linear growth retardation, delayed weight gain), Cushing's syndrome, and intracranial HTN.

Patient Counseling: Instruct to use externally and exactly as directed; avoid contact with eyes or using on face, underarms, or groin areas. Instruct not to bandage or wrap treatment areas unless directed by physician. Contact physician if adverse reactions or if no clinical improvement within 2 weeks. Instruct parents of pediatric patients not to apply medication to diaper areas.

Administration: Topical route. **Storage:** 20-25°C (68-77°F); excursions permitted to 15-30°C.

XALATAN RX

latanoprost (Pharmacia & Upjohn)

THERAPEUTIC CLASS: Prostaglandin analog

INDICATIONS: Reduction of elevated IOP in open-angle glaucoma or ocular hypertension.

DOSAGE: *Adults:* Usual: 1 drop in affected eye(s) qd in the evening. Max: Once daily dosing. Space dosing with other ophthalmic drugs by at least 5 min.

HOW SUPPLIED: Sol: 0.005% [2.5mL, 2.5mL x 3]

CONTRAINDICATIONS: Hypersensitivity to benzalkonium chloride.

WARNINGS/PRECAUTIONS: Changes to pigmented tissues, growth of eyelashes, and macular edema reported. May change eye color. Caution with history of intraocular inflammation, aphakic patients, pseudophakic patients with a torn posterior lens capsule, patients at risk of macular edema. Avoid with active intraocular inflammation. Remove contact lenses prior to use and reinsert 15 min after administration.

ADVERSE REACTIONS: Eyelash changes (increased length, thickness, pigmentation, number of lashes), eyelid skin darkening, intraocular inflammation, iris pigmentation changes, macular edema.

INTERACTIONS: Administer at least 5 min apart from other topical ophthalmic agents.

PREGNANCY: Category C, caution in nursing.

MECHANISM OF ACTION: Selective FP prostanoid receptor agonist; believed to reduce IOP by increasing outflow of aqueous humor.

PHARMACOKINETICS: Absorption: C_{max}=2 hrs. **Distribution:** V_d=0.16L/kg. **Metabolism:** Cornea, via esterases to active free acid; Liver, via fatty acid β-oxidation to 1,2-dinor and 1,2,3,4-tetranor (metabolites). **Elimination:** Urine (88-98%).

NURSING CONSIDERATIONS

Assessment: Assess for intraocular inflammation (iritis/uveitis), active macular edema, aphakic/pseudophakic patient with torn posterior lens capsules, angle-closure inflammatory or neovascular glaucoma, pregnancy/nursing status, and possible drug interactions.

Monitoring: Monitor for increased brown pigmentation of iris, periorbital tissue, and eyelid tissue; changes in eyelashes (eg, increased length, thickness, or growth; brown pigmentation; change in number of lashes; misdirected growth of lashes); macular edema (cystoid macular edema); bacterial keratitis.

Patient Counseling: Inform about risk of brown pigmentation of iris, which may be permanent, and about darkening of eyelid skin. Instruct to avoid touching tip of applicator to eye or surrounding areas. Advise to remove contact lenses prior to administration; reinsert 15 min after administration. Administer at least 5 min apart if using >1 topical ophthalmic drug. Consult physician if having ocular surgery, if intercurrent ocular condition (eg, trauma or infection) develops, or if ocular reaction occurs.

Administration: Ocular route. **Storage:** 2-8°C (36-46°F); may store for 6 weeks at room temperature.

XANAX

alprazolam (Pharmacia & Upjohn) **CIV**

THERAPEUTIC CLASS: Benzodiazepine

INDICATIONS: Anxiety disorders and short-term relief of anxiety symptoms. Panic disorder with or without agoraphobia.

DOSAGE: *Adults:* Anxiety: Initial: 0.25-0.5mg tid. Titrate: May increase every 3-4 days. Max: 4mg/day. Elderly/Advanced Liver Disease/Debilitated: Initial: 0.25mg bid-tid. Titrate: Increase gradually as tolerated. Panic Disorder: Initial: 0.5mg tid. Titrate: Increase by no more than 1mg/day every 3-4 days; slower titration if ≥4mg/day. Usual: 1-10mg/day. Decrease dose slowly (no more than 0.5mg every 3 days).

HOW SUPPLIED: Tab: 0.25mg*, 0.5mg*, 1mg*, 2mg* *scored

CONTRAINDICATIONS: Acute narrow-angle glaucoma, untreated open-angle glaucoma, concomitant ketoconazole or itraconazole.

WARNINGS/PRECAUTIONS: Risk of dependence. Withdrawal symptoms, including seizures, reported with dose reduction or abrupt discontinuation; avoid abrupt withdrawal. Caution with impaired renal, hepatic, or pulmonary function, severe depression, obesity, elderly, and debilitated. May cause fetal harm. Hypomania/mania reported with depression. Weak uricosuric effect. Periodically reassess usefulness.

ADVERSE REACTIONS: Drowsiness, lightheadedness, depression, headache, confusion, insomnia, dry mouth, constipation, diarrhea, nausea/vomiting, tachycardia/palpitations, blurred vision, nasal congestion.

INTERACTIONS: See Contraindications. Increases plasma levels of imipramine, desipramine. Additive CNS depressant effects with psychotropics, anticonvulsants, antihistamines, ethanol. Potentiated by fluoxetine, fluvoxamine, nefazodone, cimetidine, oral contraceptives. Propoxyphene decreases plasma levels. Caution with diltiazem, isoniazid, macrolides, grapefruit juice, sertraline, paroxetine, ergotamine, cyclosporine, amiodarone, nicardipine, nifedipine and other CYP3A inhibitors. Avoid azole antifungals.

PREGNANCY: Category D, not for use in nursing.

MECHANISM OF ACTION: Benzodiazepine; mechanism unknown, suspected to bind at stereo specific receptors at several sites within the CNS.

PHARMACOKINETICS: Absorption: (PO) Readily absorbed; T_{max}=1-2 hrs; C_{max}(0.5-3mg)=8-37ng/mL. **Distribution:** Plasma protein binding (80%). **Metabolism:** Liver via CYP3A4; 4-hydroxyalprazolam and α-hydroxyalprazolam (metabolites). **Elimination:** Urine; $T_{1/2}$=11.2 hrs.

NURSING CONSIDERATIONS

Assessment: Assess for acute narrow-angle glaucoma, renal/hepatic/pulmonary function, pregnancy status. Note other diseases/conditions and drug therapies.

Monitoring: Monitor hypersensitivity reactions, rebound/withdrawal symptoms (eg, seizures), renal function, LFTs, pulmonary function tests, HR, insomnia.

Patient Counseling: Avoid alcohol, sedatives, smoking. Caution while operating machinery/driving. Take as directed. Counsel about drug abuse/dependence, potential side effects, advise to report if any occur.

Administration: Oral route. **Storage:** 20-25°C (68-77°F).

XANAX XR CIV

alprazolam (Pharmacia & Upjohn)

THERAPEUTIC CLASS: Benzodiazepine

INDICATIONS: Panic disorder with or without agoraphobia.

DOSAGE: *Adults:* ≥18 yrs: Initial: 0.5-1mg qd, preferably in the am. Titrate: Increase by no more than 1mg/day every 3-4 days. Maint: 1-10mg/day. Usual: 3-6mg/day. Decrease dose slowly (no more than 0.5mg every 3 days). Elderly/Advanced Liver Disease/Debilitated: Initial: 0.5mg qd.

HOW SUPPLIED: Tab, Extended-Release: 0.5mg, 1mg, 2mg, 3mg

CONTRAINDICATIONS: Acute narrow-angle glaucoma, untreated open-angle glaucoma, concomitant ketoconazole or itraconazole.

WARNINGS/PRECAUTIONS: Risk of dependence. Withdrawal symptoms, including seizures, reported with dose reduction or abrupt discontinuation; avoid abrupt withdrawal. Caution with impaired renal, hepatic, or pulmonary function, severe depression, obesity, elderly, and debilitated. May cause fetal harm. Hypomania/mania reported with depression. Weak uricosuric effect. Periodically reassess usefulness.

ADVERSE REACTIONS: Sedation, somnolence, memory impairment, dysarthria, abnormal coordination, fatigue, depression, constipation, mental impairment, ataxia, dry mouth, decreased libido, increased/decreased appetite.

INTERACTIONS: See Contraindications. Increases plasma levels of imipramine, desipramine. Additive CNS depressant effects with psychotropics, anticonvulsants, antihistamines, ethanol. Potentiated by fluoxetine, fluvoxamine, nefazodone, cimetidine, oral contraceptives. Decreased levels with CYP3A inducers (eg, carbamazepine) or propoxyphene. Caution with diltiazem, isoniazid, macrolides, grapefruit juice, sertraline, paroxetine, ergotamine, cyclosporine, amiodarone, nicardipine, nifedipine and other CYP3A inhibitors. Avoid azole antifungals.

PREGNANCY: Category D, not for use in nursing.

MECHANISM OF ACTION: Benzodiazepine; mechanism unknown, suspected to bind at stereo specific receptors at several sites within the CNS.

PHARMACOKINETICS: Absorption: Readily absorbed; absolute bioavailability (90%); C_{max}(0.5-3mg)=8-37ng/mL; T_{max}=1-2 hrs. **Distribution:** Plasma protein binding (80%). **Metabolism:** Liver, via CYP3A4; 4-hydroxyalprazolam and α-hydroxyalprazolam (metabolites). **Elimination:** Urine (unchanged and metabolites); $T_{1/2}$=10.7-15.58 hrs.

NURSING CONSIDERATIONS

Assessment: Assess for acute narrow-angle glaucoma, seizures, renal/hepatic/pulmonary function, and pregnancy status. Note other diseases/conditions and drug therapies.

Monitoring: Monitor for hypersensitivity reactions, rebound or withdrawal symptoms, seizures, LFTs, renal/pulmonary function tests, HR, insomnia.

Patient Counseling: Instruct to avoid alcohol, sedatives, smoking. Caution while operating machinery/driving. Take as directed. Counsel about drug abuse/dependence, side effects, and advise to report if any signs/symptoms occur. Advise to take in the AM; do not crush or chew tabs.

Administration: Oral route. **Storage:** 25°C (77°F); excursions permitted to 15-30°C (59-86°F).

XELODA RX

capecitabine (Roche Labs)

Altered coagulation parameters and/or bleeding, including death, reported with coumarin-derivative anticoagulants (eg, warfarin). Monitor PT/INR frequently to adjust anticoagulant dose.

THERAPEUTIC CLASS: Fluoropyrimidine carbamate

INDICATIONS: First-line treatment of metastatic colorectal carcinoma when fluoropyrimidine therapy alone is preferred. Adjuvant treatment in patients with Dukes' C colon cancer who have undergone complete resection of the primary tumor when treatment with fluoropyrimidine therapy alone is preferred. Treatment of metastatic breast cancer in combination with docetaxel after failure of prior anthracycline-containing chemotherapy. Treatment of metastatic breast cancer in patients resistant to paclitaxel and anthracycline-containing chemotherapy or resistant to paclitaxel and for whom further anthracycline therapy is not indicated.

DOSAGE: *Adults:* Take with water within 30 min after meals. Usual/Concomitantly w/ docetoxel: 1250mg/m^2 bid for 2 weeks, then 1 week off. Give as 3-week cycles. For adjuvant treatment of Dukes' C colon cancer give as 3-week cycles for a total of 8 cycles (24 weeks). CrCl 30-50mL/min: Reduce to 75% of starting dose. Interrupt and/or reduce dose if toxicity occurs. Readjust according to adverse effects (see PI for details).

HOW SUPPLIED: Tab: 150mg, 500mg

CONTRAINDICATIONS: Hypersensitivity to 5-FU, dihydropyrimidine dehydrogenase (DPD) deficiency, severe renal impairment (CrCl <30mL/min).

WARNINGS/PRECAUTIONS: Reduce dose with moderate renal dysfunction. Carefully monitor for adverse events with mild to moderate renal dysfunction. Carefully monitor with severe diarrhea fluid/electrolyte balance; may need dose adjustment. Patients ≥80 yrs may experience increased Grade 3 and 4 adverse events (see full prescribing info). Possible fetal harm with pregnancy. Monitor for hand-and-foot syndrome. Cardiotoxicity reported; more common with history of CAD. Carefully monitor with mild to moderate hepatic dysfunction due to hepatic metastases. Hyperbilirubinemia, neutropenia, thrombocytopenia, and decrease in hemoglobin reported.

ADVERSE REACTIONS: Diarrhea, hand and foot syndrome, pyrexia, anemia, nausea, fatigue, vomiting, dermatitis, neutropenia, thrombocytopenia, stomatitis, anorexia, hyperbilirubinemia, abdominal pain, paresthesia.

INTERACTIONS: May increase phenytoin levels; reduce phenytoin dose. Leucovorin may increase levels and toxicity of 5-FU. Altered coagulation parameters and/or bleeding reported with anticoagulants (eg, coumarin, phenprocoumon); monitor PT/INR frequently. Caution with CYP2C9 substrates. Aluminum and/or magnesium antacids may increase levels.

PREGNANCY: Category D, not for use in nursing.

MECHANISM OF ACTION: Fluoropyrimidine carbamate (prodrug of 5-FU) antineoplastic; binds to thymidylate synthetase, forming covalently bound ternary complex that inhibits formation of thymidylate from 2-deoxyuridylate, inhibits DNA synthesis, and interferes with RNA processing and protein synthesis.

PHARMACOKINETICS: Absorption: T_{max}=1.5 hrs. **Distribution:** Plasma protein binding (<60%). **Metabolism:** Extensive enzymatic conversion to 5-FU; hydrogenated to less toxic metabolite via dihydropyrimidine dehydrogenase. 5-FU (metabolite). **Elimination:** Urine (3%).

NURSING CONSIDERATIONS

Assessment: Assess for hypersensitivity to 5-FU, dihydropyrimidine dehydrogenase deficiency, renal/hepatic impairment, history of CAD, pregnancy status, and possible drug interactions.

Monitoring: Monitor LFTs, CBC, and renal functions periodically. Monitor for signs/symptoms of renal/hepatic impairment, fever (≥100.5°F), infections, hand-and-foot syndrome, and hypersensitivity reactions.

Patient Counseling: Inform of pregnancy risks; avoid pregnancy during therapy. Advise to seek medical attention if symptoms of NV, diarrhea, hand-and-foot syndrome, fever (≥100.5°F), infections, or hypersensitivity reactions occur.

Administration: Oral route. **Storage:** 25°C (77°F); excursions permitted to 15-30°C (59-86°F).

XENICAL RX

orlistat (Roche Labs)

THERAPEUTIC CLASS: Lipase inhibitor

INDICATIONS: For weight loss and weight maintenance and to reduce risk of weight regain after weight loss in obese patients with initial BMI ≥30kg/m² or ≥27kg/m² in presence of other risk factors.

DOSAGE: *Adults:* 120mg tid with each main meal containing fat. Take during or up to 1 hr after meals. Use with reduced-calorie diet with about 30% of calories from fat. Omit dose if meal is missed or contains no fat. Separate multivitamin (containing fat-soluble vitamins) by at least 2 hrs, separate by 4 hrs if taking levothyroxine concomitantly.
Pediatrics: ≥12 yrs: 120mg tid with each main meal containing fat. Take during or up to 1 hr after meals. Use with reduced-calorie diet with about 30% of calories from fat. Omit dose if meal is missed or contains no fat. Separate multivitamin (containing fat-soluble vitamins) by at least 2 hrs, separate by 4 hrs if taking levothyroxine concomitantly.

HOW SUPPLIED: Cap: 120mg

CONTRAINDICATIONS: Chronic malabsorption syndrome, cholestasis.

WARNINGS/PRECAUTIONS: Exclude organic causes of obesity. Caution with history of hyperoxaluria or calcium oxalate nephrolithiasis. GI effects may increase with a high-fat diet (>30%). Weight loss may improve metabolic control; monitor dosage of antidiabetic agents. Increased risk of cholelithiasis due to substantial weight loss.

ADVERSE REACTIONS: Oily spotting, flatus with discharge, fecal urgency, fatty/oily stool, oily evacuation, increased defecation, fecal incontinence.

INTERACTIONS: Monitor warfarin and cyclosporine (separate cyclosporine dose by 2 hrs). May decrease absorption of fat-soluble vitamins and β-carotene; supplement with fat-soluble multivitamin.

PREGNANCY: Category B, not for use in nursing.

MECHANISM OF ACTION: Lipase inhibitor; inhibits absorption of dietary fats. Acts in lumen of stomach and small intestine by forming covalent bond with active serine residue site of gastric and pancreatic lipases, inactivating enzymes making them unavailable to hydrolyze dietary fats.

PHARMACOKINETICS: Distribution: Plasma protein binding (>99%). **Metabolism:** GI wall. **Elimination:** Feces (83%); $T_{1/2}$=1-2 hrs.

NURSING CONSIDERATIONS

Assessment: Assess for chronic malabsorption syndrome, cholestasis, hypothyroidism, calcium oxalate nephrolithiasis, hyperoxaluria, anorexia nervosa, bulimia, and possible drug interactions.

Monitoring: Monitor urinary oxalate levels and for signs/symptoms of hypersensitivity reactions.

Patient Counseling: Inform may increase GI events when taken with high-fat diet. Advise that daily intake of fat should be distributed for 3 main meals. Encourage to take multivitamin supplement containing fat-soluble vitamins.

Administration: Oral route. **Storage:** 25°C (77°F); excursions permitted to 15-30°C (59-86°F).

XIBROM RX
bromfenac (Ista)

THERAPEUTIC CLASS: NSAID

INDICATIONS: Treatment of postoperative inflammation after cataract extraction.

DOSAGE: *Adults:* 1 drop bid in affected eye(s), start 24 hours post-op and continue for 2 weeks.

HOW SUPPLIED: Sol: 0.09% [5mL]

WARNINGS/PRECAUTIONS: Contains sodium sulfite; may cause allergic-type reactions including anaphylactic symptoms and life-threatening or less severe asthmatic episodes. Potential cross-sensitivity to acetylsalicylic acid, phenylacetic acid derivatives, and other NSAIDs. May cause increased bleeding of ocular tissues; slow or delay healing; keratitis. Continued use may lead to sight-threatening epithelial breakdown, corneal thinning, corneal erosion, corneal ulceration, corneal perforation; d/c if this occurs. Caution in complicated ocular surgeries, corneal denervation, corneal epithelial defects, DM, ocular surface diseases (eg, dry eye syndrome), RA, repeat ocular surgeries within a short period of time, bleeding tendencies, or receiving other medication which may prolong bleeding time.

ADVERSE REACTIONS: Abnormal sensation in eye, conjunctival hyperemia, eye irritation (burning/stinging), eye pain, eye pruritus, eye redness, headache, iritis.

INTERACTIONS: Concomitant use of topical NSAIDs and topical steroids may increase potential for healing problems. Caution with other medications which may prolong bleeding time.

PREGNANCY: Category C, caution in nursing.

MECHANISM OF ACTION: NSAID; thought to block prostaglandin synthesis by inhibiting cyclooxygenase 1 and 2.

NURSING CONSIDERATIONS

Assessment: Assess for hypersensitivity reactions (eg, sulfite) or cross-sensitivity (eg, ASA), history of complicated or repeated ocular surgeries, corneal denervation, corneal epithelial defects, DM, ocular surface diseases (eg, dry eye syndrome), RA, bleeding tendencies, and concomitant medications that may prolong bleeding time or delay wound-healing.

Monitoring: Monitor for anaphylactic symptoms, severe asthma attacks, wound-healing problems, keratitis, corneal thinning, corneal erosion/ulceration/perforation, increased bleeding time, and bleeding of ocular tissues (hyphemas) in conjunction with ocular surgery.

Patient Counseling: Advise not to wear contact lenses during therapy.

Administration: Ocular route. **Storage:** Store at 15-25°C (59-77°F).

XIFAXAN RX
rifaximin (Salix)

THERAPEUTIC CLASS: Semisynthetic rifampin analog

INDICATIONS: Traveler's diarrhea caused by noninvasive strains of *E.coli*

DOSAGE: *Adults:* 1 tab tid for 3 days.
Pediatrics: ≥12 yrs: 1 tab tid for 3 days.

HOW SUPPLIED: Tab: 200mg

WARNINGS/PRECAUTIONS: Avoid in diarrhea complicated by fever or blood in the stool or diarrhea due to pathogens other than *E.coli*. D/C if diarrhea symptoms worsen or persist >24-48 hrs; consider alternative antibiotic therapy. Pseudomembranous colitis reported.

ADVERSE REACTIONS: Flatulence, headache, abdominal pain, rectal tenesmus, defecation urgency, nausea, constipation, pyrexia.

PREGNANCY: Category C; not for use in nursing.

MECHANISM OF ACTION: Antibacterial agent; binds to β-subunit of bacterial DNA-dependent RNA polymerase, resulting in inhibition of bacterial RNA synthesis.

PHARMACOKINETICS: Absorption: C_{max}=4.3ng/mL; T_{max}=1.25 hrs. **Metabolism:** CYP3A4. **Elimination:** Feces (97%), urine (0.32%).

NURSING CONSIDERATIONS

Assessment: Assess for pregnancy status, diarrhea complicated by fever or blood in stool, diarrhea by pathogens other than *Escherichia coli* (eg, *Campylobacter jejuni*, *Shigella* spp. *Salmonella* spp).

Monitoring: Monitor for pseudomembranous colitis, antibiotic-associated colitis, worsening of symptoms, superinfection, pyrexia. Monitor CBC.

Patient Counseling: Inform to take with/without food. D/C and seek medical attention for persistent diarrhea (>24-48 hrs), blood in stools.

Administration: Oral route. **Storage:** 20-25°C (68-77°F); excursions permitted to 15-30°C (59-86°F).

XIGRIS RX

drotrecogin alfa (Lilly)

THERAPEUTIC CLASS: Activated protein C

INDICATIONS: For reduction of mortality in severe sepsis (associated with acute organ dysfunction) in patients at a high risk of death.

DOSAGE: *Adults:* 24mcg/kg/hr IV for 96 hrs.

HOW SUPPLIED: Inj: 5mg, 20mg

CONTRAINDICATIONS: Active internal bleeding, hemorrhagic stroke within 3 months, intracranial or intraspinal surgery or severe head trauma within 2 months, trauma with an increased risk of life-threatening bleeding, epidural catheter, intracranial neoplasm or mass lesion, evidence of cerebral herniation.

WARNINGS/PRECAUTIONS: Increased risk of bleed with platelets <30,000 x 10^6/L (even if platelets increased by transfusions), PT/INR >3, GI bleed within 6 weeks, ischemic stroke within 3 months, intracranial arteriovenous malformation or aneurysm, known bleeding diathesis, chronic severe hepatic disease, or condition where bleeding is a significant hazard or difficult to manage due to location. If bleeding occurs, stop infusion. D/C 2 hrs before invasive surgical procedures or procedures with risk of bleeding. Avoid noncompressible puncture sites.

ADVERSE REACTIONS: Bleeding.

INTERACTIONS: Caution with drugs that affect hemostasis; increased risk of bleed with therapeutic heparin, thrombolytic therapy within 3 days, and oral anticoagulants, ASA >650mg, platelet inhibitors or glycoprotein IIb/IIIa inhibitors within 7 days.

PREGNANCY: Category C, not for use in nursing.

MECHANISM OF ACTION: Activated protein C; exerts antithrombotic effect by inhibiting Factors Va and VIIIa.

NURSING CONSIDERATIONS

Assessment: Assess for internal bleeding, recent (within 3 months) hemorrhagic stroke, recent (within 2 months) intracranial or intraspinal surgery, severe head trauma, trauma with increased risk of life-threatening bleeding, presence of epidural catheter, intracranial neoplasm or mass lesion or evidence of cerebral herniation, platelet count, bleeding diathesis, LFTs, GI bleeding, recent administration of heparin, ASA, thrombolytic therapy, oral anticoagulants. Assess for possible drug interactions.

Monitoring: Monitor for hypersensitivity reactions and active bleeding. Monitor thromboplastin time (APTT) and PTT .

Patient Counseling: Advise to report any side effects

Administration: IV route; infuse at rate of 24mcg/kg/hr over 96 hrs. Refer to PI. **Storage:** 2-8°C (36-46°F). Do not freeze. Protect reconstituted vials from light.

XOLAIR RX

omalizumab (Genentech/Novartis)

Anaphylaxis, presenting as bronchospasm, hypotension, syncope, urticaria, and/or angioedema of the throat or tongue has been reported. Monitor patients closely for an appropriate time period after administration.

THERAPEUTIC CLASS: Monoclonal antibody/IgE-blocker

INDICATIONS: Moderate-severe persistent asthma in those who have a positive skin test or *in vitro* reactivity to a perennial aeroallergen and whose symptoms are inadequately controlled with inhaled corticosteroids.

DOSAGE: *Adults:* 150-375mg SQ every 2 or 4 weeks based on body weight and pretreatment serum total IgE level. Max: 150mg/site. 30-90kg & IgE ≥30-100 IU/mL: 150mg every 4 weeks. >90-150kg & IgE ≥30-100 IU/mL OR 30-90kg & IgE >100-200 IU/mL OR 30-60kg & IgE >200-300 IU/mL: 300mg every 4 weeks. >90-150kg & IgE >100-200 IU/mL OR >60-90kg & IgE >200-300 IU/mL OR 30-70kg & IgE >300-400 IU/mL: 225mg every 2 weeks. >90-150kg & IgE >200-300 IU/mL OR >70-90kg & IgE >300-400 IU/mL OR 30-70kg & IgE >400-500 IU/mL OR 30-60kg & IgE >500-600 IU/mL: 300mg every 2 weeks. >70-90kg & IgE >400-500 IU/mL OR >60-70kg & IgE >500-600 IU/mL OR 30-60kg & IgE >600-700 IU/mL: 375mg every 2 weeks.
Pediatrics: ≥12 yrs: 150-375mg SQ every 2 or 4 weeks based on body weight and pretreatment serum total IgE level. Max: 150mg/site. 30-90kg & IgE ≥30-100 IU/mL: 150mg every 4 weeks. >90-150kg & IgE ≥30-100 IU/mL OR 30-90kg & IgE >100-200 IU/mL OR 30-60kg & IgE >200-300 IU/mL: 300mg every 4 weeks. >90-150kg & IgE >100-200 IU/mL OR >60-90kg & IgE >200-300 IU/mL OR 30-70kg & IgE >300-400 IU/mL: 225mg every 2 weeks. >90-150kg and IgE >200-300 IU/mL OR >70-90kg & IgE >300-400 IU/mL OR 30-70kg & IgE >400-500 IU/mL OR 30-60kg & IgE >500-600 IU/mL: 300mg every 2 weeks. >70-90kg & IgE >400-500 IU/mL OR >60-70kg & IgE >500-600 IU/mL OR 30-60kg & IgE >600-700 IU/mL: 375mg q2 weeks.

HOW SUPPLIED: Inj: 150mg [5mL]

WARNINGS/PRECAUTIONS: Malignant neoplasms reported. Not for use in treatment of acute bronchospasm or status asthmaticus. Systemic or inhaled corticosteroids should not be abruptly discontinued when initiating therapy.

ADVERSE REACTIONS: Anaphylaxis, malignancies, injection-site reactions, viral infections, upper respiratory infection, sinusitis, headache, pharyngitis, pain, arthralgia.

PREGNANCY: Category B, caution in nursing.

MECHANISM OF ACTION: Monoclonal antibody/IgE blocker; inhibits binding of IgE to high-affinity IgE receptor on surface of mast cells and basophils and limits degree of release of mediators of allergic response.

PHARMACOKINETICS: Absorption: (SQ) Absolute bioavailability (62%); T_{max}=7-8 days. **Distribution:** V_d=78mL/kg; crosses placental barrier. **Elimination:** $T_{1/2}$=26 days.

NURSING CONSIDERATIONS

Assessment: Assess for acute asthma, malignancies, IgE levels, pregnancy status.

Monitoring: Monitor IgE levels, hypersensitivity reactions, injection-site reactions, viral infections, sinusitis, pharyngitis, headaches, malignancies, upper respiratory tract infections.

Patient Counseling: Instruct to report any adverse reactions. Take as directed. Decreases in corticosteroid therapy should be gradual and under medical supervision.

Administration: SQ route. **Storage:** 2-8°C (36-46°F), or within 4 hrs of reconstitution when stored at room temperature.

XOPENEX RX
levalbuterol HCl (Sepracor)

THERAPEUTIC CLASS: $Beta_2$-agonist

INDICATIONS: Prevention and treatment of bronchospasm with reversible obstructive airway disease.

DOSAGE: *Adults:* Initial: 0.63mg tid, q6-8h. Severe Asthma: 1.25mg tid, q6-8h. Administer by nebulizer.
Pediatrics: ≥12 yrs: Initial: 0.63mg tid, q6-8h. Severe Asthma: 1.25mg tid, q6-8h. 6-11 yrs: 0.31mg tid. Max: 0.63mg tid. Administer by nebulizer.

HOW SUPPLIED: Sol, Inhalation: 0.31mg/3mL, 0.63mg/3mL, 1.25mg/3mL [3mL, 24^s]

WARNINGS/PRECAUTIONS: Hypersensitivity reactions reported. D/C immediately if paradoxical bronchospasm occurs. May produce ECG changes; caution with cardiovascular disorders, coronary insufficiency, arrhythmias, and HTN. Caution with convulsive disorders, hyperthyroidism, and diabetes. May produce transient hypokalemia.

ADVERSE REACTIONS: Tachycardia, migraine, dyspepsia, leg cramps, nervousness, dizziness, tremor, rhinitis, increased cough, chest pain, HTN, hypotension, diarrhea, dry mouth, anxiety, insomnia, paresthesia, wheezing.

INTERACTIONS: Avoid other sympathomimetic agents. Extreme caution with MAOIs and TCAs. Monitor digoxin. ECG changes and/or hypokalemia with non-K^+-sparing diuretics. Antagonized by β-blockers.

PREGNANCY: Category C, not for use in nursing.

MECHANISM OF ACTION: β_2-adrenergic bronchodilator; stimulates adenyl cyclase, the enzyme that catalyzes formation of cAMP from ATP. Increased cAMP levels associated with relaxation of bronchial smooth muscle and inhibition of release of mediators of immediate hypersensitivity.

PHARMACOKINETICS: Absorption: C_{max}(1.25, 5mg)=1.1, 4.5ng/ml; T_{max}(1.25, 5mg)=0.2, 0.2 hrs. **Metabolism:** GI tract by SULT1A3. **Elimination:** Renal (80-100%), urine (25-46% unchanged), feces (≤20%); $T_{1/2}$(1.25, 5mg)=3.3, 4 hrs.

NURSING CONSIDERATIONS

Assessment: Assess for convulsive disorders, hyperthyroidism, DM, CVD, renal/hepatic impairment, and possible drug interactions.

Monitoring: Monitor cardiovascular effects (eg, HR, BP, arrhythmias), paradoxical bronchospasm, hypersensitivity reactions, deterioration of asthma, tremors.

Patient Counseling: Take as directed. Report lack of response or any adverse side effects.

Administration: Inhalation route. 1) Open unit dose vial and squeeze contents into nebulizer reservoir. 2) Connect nebulizer to compressor and nebulizer reservoir to mouthpiece or face mask. 3) Breathe as calmly and deeply as possible until no more mist is formed. 4) Clean nebulizer. **Storage:** 20-25°C (68-77°F). Protect from light and excessive heat.

XOPENEX HFA RX
levalbuterol tartrate (Sepracor)

THERAPEUTIC CLASS: $Beta_2$-agonist

INDICATIONS: Prevention and treatment of bronchospasm with reversible obstructive airway disease.

DOSAGE: *Adults:* 2 inh (90mcg) q4-6h or 1 inh (45mcg) q4h may be sufficient. *Pediatrics:* ≥4 yrs: 2 inh (90mcg) q4-6h or 1 inh (45mcg) q4h may be sufficient.

HOW SUPPLIED: MDI: 45mcg/inh [15g]

WARNINGS/PRECAUTIONS: D/C immediately if paradoxical bronchospasm occurs. May produce ECG changes; caution with cardiovascular disorders, coronary insufficiency, arrhythmias, and HTN. Caution with convulsive disorders, hyperthyroidism, and diabetes. May produce transient hypokalemia.

ADVERSE REACTIONS: Asthma, pharyngitis, rhinitis, pain, vomiting.

INTERACTIONS: Avoid other sympathomimetic agents. Extreme caution with MAOIs and TCAs. Monitor digoxin. ECG changes and/or hypokalemia with non-K^+-sparing diuretics. Antagonized by β-blockers.

PREGNANCY: Category C, not for use in nursing.

MECHANISM OF ACTION: β_2-adrenergic bronchodilator; stimulates adenyl cylase, the enzyme that catalyzes formation of cAMP from ATP. Increased cAMP levels associated with relaxation of bronchial smooth muscle and inhibition of release of mediators of immediate hypersensitivity.

PHARMACOKINETICS: Absorption: C_{max}=0.199ng/mL (≥12 yrs), 0.163ng/mL (4-11 yrs); T_{max}=0.54 hrs (≥12 yrs), 0.76 hrs (4-11 yrs); AUC=0.695ng•hr/mL (≥12 yrs), 0.579ng•hr/mL (4-11 yrs). **Metabolism:** GI tract by SULT1A3. **Elimination:** Renal (80-100%), urine (25-46% unchanged), feces (≤20%).

NURSING CONSIDERATIONS

Assessment: Assess for convulsive disorders, hyperthyroidism, DM and ketoacidosis, CVD (eg, coronary insufficiency, HTN, cardiac arrhythmias), renal/hepatic impairment, history of hypersensitivity to drug, and possible drug interactions.

Monitoring: Monitor cardiovascular effects (eg, BP, HR, arrhythmias), for possible paradoxical bronchospasm, asthma deterioration, tremors, and immediate hypersensitivity reactions.

Patient Counseling: Instruct to shake inhaler well before using. If first time or inhaler not used >3 days, release 4 test sprays into air, away from face. Keep plastic actuator clean to prevent build-up and blockage. Wash actuator by running warm water through top and bottom for 30 seconds at least once a week. Shake to remove excess water and air-dry thoroughly. Avoid spraying in eyes.

Administration: Oral inhalation. 1) Shake and test spray into air 4 times. 2) Shake inhaler well. 3) Breathe out through mouth. 4) Breathe in through mouth and at same time spray product into mouth. 5) Hold breath for 10 seconds and remove mouthpiece. 6) Wait for 1 min before next spray. 7) Replace cap and keep mouthpiece clean. 8) Discard after 200 sprays. **Storage:** 20-25°C (68-77°F). Protect from freezing and direct sunlight.

XYLOCAINE INJECTION — RX

lidocaine HCl (Abraxis)

OTHER BRAND NAMES: Xylocaine-MPF (Abraxis)

THERAPEUTIC CLASS: Local anesthetic

INDICATIONS: For production of local or regional anesthesia by infiltration techniques such as percutaneous injection and IV regional anesthesia by peripheral nerve block techniques such as brachial plexus and intercostal and by central neural techniques such as lumbar and caudal epidural blocks.

DOSAGE: *Adults:* Dosage varies depending on procedure, depth, and duration of anesthesia, degree of muscular relaxation, and patient physical condition. Max: 4.5mg/kg or total dose of 300mg. Epidural/Caudal Anesthesia: Max: Intervals not less than 90 min. Paracervical Block: Max: 200mg/90 min. Regional Anesthesia: IV: Max: 4mg/kg. Children/Elderly/Debilitated/Cardiac or Liver Disease: Reduce dose.
Pediatrics: >3 yrs: Max: 1.5-2mg/lb. Regional Anesthesia: IV: Max: 3mg/kg.

HOW SUPPLIED: Inj: 0.5%, 1%, 2%; (MPF) 0.5%, 1%, 1.5%, 2%

WARNINGS/PRECAUTIONS: Acidosis, cardiac arrest, death reported from delay in toxicity management. Local anesthetic solutions containing antimicrobial preservatives should not be used for epidural or spinal anesthesia. Use lowest effective dose. During epidural anesthesia, administer initial test dose and monitor for CNS and cardiovascular toxicity as well as for signs of unintended intrathecal administration. Reduce dose with debilitated, elderly, acutely ill, and children. Extreme caution when using lumbar and caudal epidural anesthesia with existing neurological disease, spinal deformities, septicemia, and severe HTN. Monitor cardiovascular and respiratory vital signs and state of consciousness after each injection. Caution with hepatic disease, cardiovascular disorders. Monitor circulation and respiration with injections into head and neck area.

ADVERSE REACTIONS: Lightheadedness, nervousness, euphoria, confusion, dizziness, drowsiness, tinnitus, blurred vision, vomiting, heat/cold sensations, twitching, tremors, convulsions, respiratory depression, bradycardia, hypotension, urticaria, edema, anaphylactoid reactions.

PREGNANCY: Category B, caution in nursing.

MECHANISM OF ACTION: Anesthetic; stabilizes neuronal membrane by inhibiting ionic fluxes required for initiation and conduction of impulses, thereby effecting local anesthetic action.

PHARMACOKINETICS: Absorption: Complete. **Distribution:** Crosses blood-brain and placental barriers. **Metabolism:** Liver (rapid), oxidative N-alkylation (major pathway), yields monoethylglycinexylidide and glycinexylidide (metabolites). **Elimination:** Urine, (90% metabolites), (≤10% unchanged); $T_{1/2}$=1.5-2.0 hrs.

NURSING CONSIDERATIONS

Assessment: Assess for drug hypersensitivity, hepatic functions, pregnancy/nursing status, shock, heart block, and possible drug/test interactions.

Monitoring: Monitor for allergic-type reactions, cardiac/respiratory vital signs (eg, adequacy of ventilation, tachypnia, tachycardia, labile BP), state of consciousness, signs of CNS toxicity (restlessness, anxiety, tinnitus, dizziness, blurred vision, tremors, depression, drowsiness), confusion, convulsions, and increased creatine phosphokinase levels after IM injection, which interacts with diagnosis of MI.

Patient Counseling: Counsel about possibilty of temporary loss of sensation and muscle function following injection; avoid inadvertent trauma until normal functions return. Consult physician/dentist if anesthesia persists or rash occurs.

Administration: IM/IV routes. **Storage:** 25°C (77°F).

Xylocaine Jelly — RX

lidocaine HCl (AstraZeneca)

THERAPEUTIC CLASS: Acetamide local anesthetic

INDICATIONS: Prevention and control of pain in procedures involving the male and female urethra. Topical treatment of painful urethritis. Anesthetic lubricant for endotracheal intubation.

DOSAGE: *Adults:* Max: 600mg/12 hrs. Surface Anesthesia of Male Urethra: Instill about 15mL (300mg). Instill an additional dose of not more than 15mL if needed. Prior to Sounding or Cystoscopy: A total dose of 30mL (600mg) is usually required. Prior to Catheterization: 5-10mL usually adequate. Surface Anesthesia of Female Urethra: Instill 3-5mL. Elderly/Debilitated: Reduce dose. *Pediatrics:* Determine dose by age and weight. Max: 4.5mg/kg.

HOW SUPPLIED: Jelly: 2% [Tube: 5mL, 30mL; Syringe: 10mL, 20mL]

WARNINGS/PRECAUTIONS: Avoid excessive dosage or frequent administration; may result in serious adverse effects requiring resuscitative measures. Caution with heart block and severe shock. Extreme caution if mucosa traumatized or sepsis is present in the area of application; risk of rapid systemic absorption.

ADVERSE REACTIONS: Lightheadedness, nervousness, confusion, euphoria, dizziness, drowsiness, blurred vision, tremors, convulsions, respiratory depression, bradycardia, hypotension, urticaria, edema, anaphylactoid reactions.

PREGNANCY: Category B, caution in nursing.

MECHANISM OF ACTION: Local anesthetic; stabilizes neuronal membrane by initiating ionic fluxes required for initiation and conduction of impulses.

PHARMACOKINETICS: Absorption: Rapid. **Metabolism:** Biotransformation. **Distribution:** Plasma protein binding (60-80%); crosses placenta. **Elimination:** Urine; $T_{1/2}$=1.5-2 hrs.

NURSING CONSIDERATIONS

Assessment: Assess for acidosis, severe shock, heart block, possible drug interactions, renal/hepatic impairment.

Monitoring: Monitor for signs/symptoms of hypersensitivity reactions, malignant hyperthermia, renal/hepatic dysfunction.

Patient Counseling: Instruct not to ingest food or drink within 60 min of using local anesthetics in mouth or throat area. Numbness of tongue or buccal mucosa may enhance danger of unintentional biting trauma. Inform to strictly adhere to dosing instructions and keep out of reach of children. Instruct to notify physician if pregnant/nursing or planning to become pregnant.

Administration: Topical route. **Storage:** 20-25°C (68-77°F).

XYLOCAINE VISCOUS RX

lidocaine HCl (AstraZeneca)

THERAPEUTIC CLASS: Acetamide local anesthetic

INDICATIONS: Topical anesthesia of irritated or inflamed mucous membranes of the mouth and pharynx. To reduce gagging during X-ray or dental procedures.

DOSAGE: *Adults:* Irritated/Inflamed Mucous Membranes: Usual: 15mL undiluted. (Mouth) Swish and spit out. (Pharynx) Gargle and may swallow. Do not administer in <3 hr intervals. Max: 8 doses/24hr; (Single Dose) 4.5mg/kg or total of 300mg.

Pediatrics: >3 yrs: Max: Determine by age and weight. Infants <3 yrs: Apply 1.25mL with cotton-tipped applicator to immediate area. Do not administer in <3 hour intervals. Max: 8 doses/24hr.

HOW SUPPLIED: Sol: 2% [100mL, 450mL]

WARNINGS/PRECAUTIONS: Reduce dose in elderly, debilitated, acutely ill and children. Caution with heart block, severe shock, and known drug sensitivities. Excessive dosage or too frequent administration may result in high plasma levels and serious adverse effects requiring resuscitative measures. Extreme caution if mucosa traumatized; risk of rapid systemic absorption. Overdose reported in pediatrics due to inappropriate dosing.

ADVERSE REACTIONS: Lightheadedness, nervousness, confusion, euphoria, dizziness, drowsiness, blurred vision, tremors, convulsions, respiratory depression, bradycardia, hypotension, urticaria, edema, anaphylactoid reactions.

PREGNANCY: Category B, caution in nursing.

MECHANISM OF ACTION: Local anesthetic; stabilizes neuronal membrane by inhibiting ionic fluxes required for initiation and conduction of nerve impulses.

PHARMACOKINETICS: Absorption: Well-absorbed. **Distribution:** Crosses blood-brain and placental barriers; plasma protein binding (60-80%). **Metabolism:** Liver (rapid), oxidative N-alkylation, ring hydoxylation, cleavage of amide linkage, conjugation; monoethylglycinexylidide and glyciexylidide (metabolites). **Elimination:** Urine (90% metabolites, <10% unchanged); $T_{1/2}$=1.5-2 hrs.

NURSING CONSIDERATIONS

Assessment: Assess for renal/hepatic function, shock, heart block, acutely ill/debilitated/elderly, and pregnancy/nursing status.

Monitoring: Monitor for anaphylactoid reactions.

Patient Counseling: Instruct not to ingest food or drink within 60 min of using local anesthetics in mouth or throat area. Numbness of tongue or buccal mucosa may enhance danger of unintentional biting trauma. Inform to strictly adhere to dosing instructions and keep out of reach of children. Instruct to notify physician if pregnant/nursing or planning to become pregnant.

Administration: Topical route. Shake well. **Storage**: 15-30°C (59-86°F); tight container.

XYZAL RX

levocetirizine dihydrochloride (Sanofi-Aventis/UCB)

THERAPEUTIC CLASS: H_1-antagonist

INDICATIONS: Relief of symptoms associated with seasonal and perennial allergic rhinitis. Treatment of uncomplicated skin manifestations of chronic idiopathic urticaria.

DOSAGE: *Adults:* 5mg qd in evening. Adjust dose with decreased renal function.

Pediatrics: ≥12 yrs: 5mg qd in evening. Adjust dose with decreased renal function. 6-11 yrs: 2.5mg (1/2 tab) qd in evening.

HOW SUPPLIED: Sol: 2.5mg/5mL; Tab: 5mg* *scored

CONTRAINDICATIONS: End stage renal disease (CrCl <10mL/min) or hemodialysis. Pediatrics 6-11 yrs with renal impairment.

WARNINGS/PRECAUTIONS: May impair mental/physical abilities.

ADVERSE REACTIONS: Somnolence, fatigue, dry mouth, headache, nasopharyngitis, abdominal pain, cough, epistaxis, asthenia, pharyngitis.

INTERACTIONS: Avoid alcohol and CNS depressants. Possible decreased clearance with large doses of theophylline.

PREGNANCY: Category B, not for use in nursing.

MECHANISM OF ACTION: Antihistamine; inhibits H_1-receptor.

PHARMACOKINETICS: Absorption: Rapid, extensive; C_{max}=270ng/mL (single dose), 308ng/mL (multiple doses); T_{max}=0.9 hrs. **Distribution:** V_d=0.4L/kg; plasma protein binding (91-92%). Found in breast milk. **Metabolism**: Through aromatic oxidation, N and O- dealkylation and taurine conjugation pathways, via CYP3A4. **Elimination:** Urine (58.4%), feces (12.9%); $T_{1/2}$=8 hrs.

NURSING CONSIDERATIONS

Assessment: Assess for renal impairment, ESRD or hemodialysis, nursing status, alcohol consumption, and possible drug interactions (eg, CNS depressants).

Monitoring: Monitor for allergic reactions and LFTs.

Patient Counseling: Caution against performing hazardous tasks requiring mental alertness and motor coordination (eg, operating machinery, driving). Advise against concurrent use of alcohol or other CNS depressants since additional reduction in mental alertness may occur. Notify physician if nursing.

Administration: Oral route. **Storage:** 20-25°C (68-77°F), excursions permitted to 15-30°C (59-86°F).

YASMIN RX

drospirenone - ethinyl estradiol (Bayer Healthcare)

THERAPEUTIC CLASS: Estrogen/progestogen combination

INDICATIONS: Prevention of pregnancy.

DOSAGE: *Adults:* 1 tab qd for 28 days, then repeat. Start 1st Sunday after menses begin or 1st day of menses.

HOW SUPPLIED: Tab: (Ethinyl Estradiol-Drospirenone) 0.03mg-3mg

CONTRAINDICATIONS: Renal or adrenal insufficiency, hepatic dysfunction, thrombophlebitis, thromboembolic disorders, history of deep vein thrombophlebitis, cerebrovascular or CAD, breast carcinoma, endometrial carcinoma, estrogen-dependent neoplasia, undiagnosed abnormal genital bleeding, cholestatic jaundice of pregnancy or jaundice with prior pill use, liver tumor, active liver disease, pregnancy, heavy smoking (≥15 cigarettes daily) and >35 yrs.

WARNINGS/PRECAUTIONS: Cigarette smoking increases risk of serious CV side effects; risk increases with age (especially >35 yrs) and heavy smoking. Increased risk of MI, thromboembolism, thrombotic disease, cerebrovascular events, and gallbladder disease. Monitor K^+ levels during first cycle with conditions predisposing to hyperkalemia. Retinal thrombosis, hepatic neoplasia, carcinoma of breast and reproductive organs reported. May cause glucose intolerance. May increase BP, elevate LDL levels or cause other lipid changes, fluid retention, breakthrough bleeding and spotting. May cause or exacerbate migraine. May develop visual changes with contact lens. Increased risk of MI with HTN, hyperlipidemia, obesity and DM. D/C if jaundice, significant depression or ophthalmic irregularities develop. Use before menarche is not indicated.

ADVERSE REACTIONS: NV, breakthrough bleeding, spotting, amenorrhea, migraine, depression, vaginal candidiasis, edema, weight changes.

INTERACTIONS: Reduced effects, increased breakthrough bleeding, and menstrual irregularities with rifampin, phenobarbital, phenytoin, carbamazepine, possibly with griseofulvin, ampicillin, tetracycline, St. John's wort, and phenylbutazone. Increased levels with atorvastatin, ascorbic acid and APAP. Risk of hyperkalemia with ACE inhibitors, angiotensin-II receptor antagonists, K^+-sparing diuretics, heparin, aldosterone antagonists, and NSAIDs; monitor K^+ levels during 1st cycle. May increase levels of cyclosporine, prednisolone, and theophylline. May decrease APAP levels and increase clearance of temazepam, salicylic acid, morphine, and clofibric acid.

PREGNANCY: Category X, not for use in nursing.

MECHANISM OF ACTION: Combination oral contraceptive; acts by suppressing gonadotropins. Inhibits ovulation and produces changes in cervical mucus (increasing difficulty of sperm entry into uterus) and endometrium (reducing likelihood of implantation).

PHARMACOKINETICS: Absorption: Drospirenone (DRSP): Absolute bioavailability (76%); (Cycle 13/Day 21) C_{max}=78.7ng/mL; T_{max}=1.6 hrs; AUC=968ng•h/mL. Ethinyl estradiol (EE): Absolute bioavailability (40%); (Cycle 13/Day 21) C_{max}=90.5pg/mL; T_{max}=1.6 hrs; AUC=469.5pg•h/mL. **Distribution:** DRSP: V_d=4L/kg; serum protein binding (97%). EE: V_d=4-5L/kg; serum albumin binding (98.5%). **Metabolism:** DRSP: Liver, via CYP3A4 (minor). EE: Hydroxylation (via CYP3A4), conjugation (glucuronidation and sulfation). **Elimination:** DRSP: Urine, feces; $T_{1/2}$=30 hrs. EE: Urine, feces; $T_{1/2}$=24 hrs.

NURSING CONSIDERATIONS

Assessment: Assess family history of breast cancer, presence of inherited or acquired thrombophilias, HTN, hyperlipidemias, obesity, DM, renal disease, depression, heavy smoking, and potential drug interactions. Assess personal/family history, complete physical exam.

Monitoring: Monitor for MI, thromboembolism, cerebrovascular disease, benign hepatic adenomas, retinal thrombosis, HTN, headache, bleeding irregularites, jaundice, fluid retention, and emotional disorders. Conduct periodic complete physical exam with emphasis on BP, breasts, abdomen, and pelvic organs including cervical cytology and relevant lab tests (eg, K^+ levels, prothrombin time and clotting factors VII, VIII, IX, X, cholesterol, TG, serum folate, TBG, glucose tolerance).

Patient Counseling: Inform that drug does not protect against HIV infection (AIDS) and other STDs. Inform of potential risks/benefits of oral contraceptives. Counsel not to smoke while on treatment. Take 1 pill at same time daily. Notify physician if nursing or need more info about therapy.

Administration: Oral route. **Storage:** 25°C (77°F); excursions permitted to 15-30° (59-86°F).

YAZ RX

drospirenone - ethinyl estradiol (Bayer Healthcare)

THERAPEUTIC CLASS: Estrogen/progestogen combination

INDICATIONS: Prevention of pregnancy. Treatment of symptoms of premenstrual dysphoric disorder (PMDD). Treatment of moderate acne vulgaris in women ≥14 yrs.

DOSAGE: *Adults:* 1 tab qd for 28 days (24 active plus 4 inert pills), then repeat. Start 1st Sunday after menses begin or 1st day of menses.
Pediatrics: ≥14 yrs: Acne: 1 tab qd for 28 days (24 active plus 4 inert pills), then repeat. Start 1st Sunday after menses begin or 1st day of menses.

HOW SUPPLIED: Tab: (Ethinyl Estradiol-Drospirenone) 0.02mg-3mg

CONTRAINDICATIONS: Renal or adrenal insufficiency, hepatic dysfunction, thrombophlebitis, thromboembolic disorders, history of deep vein thrombophlebitis, valvular heart disease with thrombogenic complications, severe HTN, DM with vascular involvement, HA with focal neurological symptoms, major surgery with prolonged immobilization, cerebrovascular or CAD, breast carcinoma, endometrial carcinoma, estrogen-dependent neoplasia, undiagnosed abnormal genital bleeding, cholestatic jaundice of pregnancy or jaundice with prior pill use, liver tumor, active liver disease, pregnancy, heavy smoking (>15 cigarettes daily) and >35 yrs.

WARNINGS/PRECAUTIONS: Cigarette smoking increases risk of serious CV side effects. Risk increases with age (especially >35 yrs) and with heavy smoking. Increased risk of MI, thromboembolism, thrombotic disease, cerebrovascular events, and gallbladder disease. Monitor K^+ levels during first cycle with conditions predisposing to hyperkalemia. Retinal thrombosis, hepatic neoplasia, carcinoma of breast and reproductive organs reported. May cause glucose intolerance. May increase BP, elevate LDL levels or cause other lipid changes, fluid retention, breakthrough bleeding and spotting. May cause or exacerbate migraine. May develop visual changes with contact lens. Increased risk of MI with HTN, hyperlipidemia, obesity and DM. D/C if jaundice, significant depression or ophthalmic irregularities develop. Use before menarche is not indicated.

ADVERSE REACTIONS: NV, breakthrough bleeding, spotting, amenorrhea, migraine, mental depression, vaginal candidiasis, edema, weight changes, depression decrease in serum folate levels, aggravation of varicose veins, uritcaria, angioedema, severe reactions with respiratory and circulatory symptoms, dysmenorrhea.

INTERACTIONS: Reduced effects, increased breakthrough bleeding, and menstrual irregularities with rifampin, phenobarbital, phenytoin, carbamazepine, possibly with griseofulvin, ampicillin, tetracycline, St. John's wort, and phenylbutazone. Increased levels with atorvastatin, ascorbic acid and APAP. Risk of hyperkalemia with ACE inhibitors, angiotensin-II receptor antagonists, potassium-sparing diuretics, heparin, aldosterone antagonists, and NSAIDs; monitor K^+ levels during 1st cycle. Increased levels of cyclosporine, prednisolone, and theophylline. May decrease APAP levels and increase clearance of temazepam, salicylic acid, morphine, and clofibric acid.

PREGNANCY: Category X, not for use in nursing.

MECHANISM OF ACTION: Estrogen/progestogen oral contraceptive; acts by suppressing gonadotropins, inhibiting ovulation. Also causes changes in cervical mucus (increases difficulty of sperm entry into uterus) and endometrium (reduces likelihood of implantation).

PHARMACOKINETICS: Absorption: Drospirenone (DRSP): Absolute bioavailability (76%); (Cycle 1/Day 21) C_{max}=70.3ng/mL; T_{max}=1.5 hrs; AUC=763ng•h/mL. Ethinyl estradiol (EE): Absolute bioavailability (40%); (Cycle 1/Day 21)

C_{max}=45.1pg/mL; T_{max}=1.5 hrs; AUC=220pg•h/mL. **Distribution:** DRSP: V_d=4L/kg; serum protein binding (97%). EE: V_d=4-5L/kg; serum albumin binding (98.5%). **Metabolism:** DRSP: Liver, via CYP3A4 (minor). EE: Hydroxylation (via CYP3A4), conjugation (glucuronidation and sulfation). **Elimination:** DRSP: Urine, feces; $T_{1/2}$=30 hrs. EE: Urine, feces; $T_{1/2}$=24 hrs.

NURSING CONSIDERATIONS

Assessment: Assess family history of breast cancer, presence of inherited or acquired thrombophilias, HTN, hyperlipidemias, obesity, DM, renal disease, depression, heavy smoking, and potential drug interactions. Assess personal/family history; complete physical exam.

Monitoring: Monitor for MI, thromboembolism, cerebrovascular disease, benign hepatic adenomas, retinal thrombosis, HTN, headache, bleeding irregularites, jaundice, fluid retention, and emotional disorders. Conduct periodic complete physical exam with emphasis on BP, breasts, abdomen, and pelvic organs including cervical cytology and relevant lab tests (eg, K^+ levels, prothrombin time, clotting factors VII, VIII, IX, X, cholesterol, TG, serum folate, TBG, glucose tolerance).

Patient Counseling: Inform that drug does not protect against HIV infection (AIDS) and other STDs. Inform of potential risks/benefits of oral contraceptives. Counsel not to smoke while on treatment. Take 1 pill at same time daily. Notify physician if nursing or need more information about therapy.

Administration: Oral route. **Storage:** 25°C (77°F); excursions permitted to 15-30°C (59-86°F).

ZANAFLEX — RX

tizanidine HCl (Acorda)

THERAPEUTIC CLASS: Centrally acting $alpha_2$-adrenergic agonist

INDICATIONS: Short-term treatment of spasticity.

DOSAGE: *Adults:* Initial: 4mg single dose q6-8h. Titrate: Increase by 2-4mg. Usual: 8mg single dose q6-8h. Max: 3 doses/24h or 36mg/day.

HOW SUPPLIED: Cap: 2mg, 4mg, 6mg; Tab: 2mg*, 4mg* *scored

CONTRAINDICATIONS: Concomitant use with fluvoxamine, ciprofloxacin or potent inhibitors of CYP1A2.

WARNINGS/PRECAUTIONS: May prolong QT interval. May cause liver damage; monitor baseline LFTs and at 1, 3, and 6 months. Retinal degeneration and corneal opacities reported. Caution with renal impairment or elderly. May cause hypotension, caution with antihypertensives; avoid ciprofloxacin and fluvoxamine. Use with extreme caution in patients with hepatic impairment. May cause sedation and hallucinations. Avoid concomitant use with oral contraceptives. When discontinuing, taper dose to avoid withdrawal and rebound HTN, tachycardia, and hypertonia.

ADVERSE REACTIONS: Dry mouth, somnolence, asthenia, dizziness, UTI, urinary frequency, flu-like syndrome, rhinitis.

INTERACTIONS: See Contraindications. Potentiated depressant effect with alcohol. Potentiated by oral contraceptives. Avoid α-adrenergic agonists. Avoid with CYP1A2 inhibitors.

PREGNANCY: Category C, caution in nursing.

MECHANISM OF ACTION: Centrally acting α_2-adrenergic agonist; reduces spasticity by increasing presynaptic inhibition of motor neurons.

PHARMACOKINETICS: Absorption: Complete; (Fasting) T_{max}=1 hr. (Fed) Absolute bioavailability (40%); C_{max} increased by 30%; T_{max}=1.25 hrs. **Distribution:** V_d=2.4L/kg; plasma protein binding (30%); excreted in breast milk. **Metabolism:** CYP1A2. **Elimination:** Urine (60%), feces (20%); $T_{1/2}$=2.5 hrs.

NURSING CONSIDERATIONS

Assessment: Assess for hypersensitivity, hypotension, hepatic/renal dysfunction, corneal opacities, retinal degeneration, CVD, QT prolongation, pregnancy/nursing status, and possible drug interactions. Obtain baseline LFTs.

Monitoring: Monitor for hypotension, bradycardia, lightheadedness/dizziness, syncope, hepatic impairment, sedation, hallucinosis/psychotic-like symptoms, corneal opacities, retinal degeneration, dry mouth, somnolonce, asthenia, and withdrawal symptoms (eg, rebound HTN, tachycardia, hypertonia). Evaluate LFTs at 1, 3, and 6 months, BP, HR, ECG.

Patient Counseling: Counsel to take exactly as directed, not to increase dose unless directed by physician, and about possibility of orthostatic hypotension. Caution against performing hazardous tasks (eg, operating machinery/driving). To avoid withdrawal symptoms, do not suddenly d/c therapy. Avoid alcohol and CNS depressants. Advise that food changes absorption; may lead to potentiation in efficacy and adverse effects. Instruct to inform physician if taking oral contraceptives, fluvoxamine, ciprofloxacin, or if pregnant/nursing.

Administration: Oral route. **Storage:** 25°C (77°F); excursions permitted to 15-30°C (59-86°F). Dispense in tight, child-resistant container.

ZANTAC RX

ranitidine HCl (GlaxoSmithKline)

THERAPEUTIC CLASS: H_2-blocker

INDICATIONS: (PO) Short-term treatment of active duodenal (DU) and benign gastric ulcers (GU). Maintenance therapy for duodenal and gastric ulcers. Treatment of pathological hypersecretory conditions (eg, Zollinger-Ellison) and GERD. Treatment and maintenance of erosive esophagitis. (Inj) Hospitalized patients with pathological hypersecretory conditions or intractable duodenal ulcer. Short-term alternate to oral therapy.

DOSAGE: *Adults:* (PO) DU/GU: 150mg bid or (DU) 300mg after evening meal or qhs. Maint: 150mg qhs. GERD: 150mg bid. Erosive Esophagitis: 150mg qid. Maint: 150mg bid. Hypersecretory Conditions: 150mg bid. May give up to 6g/day with severe disease. (Inj) Usual: 50mg IV/IM q6-8 hrs or 6.25mg/hr continuous IV. Max: 400mg/day. Zollinger-Ellison: Initial: 1mg/kg/hr. Titrate: May increase after 4 hrs by 0.5mg/kg/hr increments. Max: 2.5mg/kg/hr or 220mg/hr. CrCl <50mL/min: 50mg IV q18-24 hrs or 150mg PO q24h. Give more frequent (q12h) if necessary. Hemodialysis: Give dose at end of treatment. Dissolve each 150mg effervescent tab in 6-8oz of water before administration.

Pediatrics: 1 month-16 yrs: (PO) DU/GU: 2-4mg/kg bid. Max: 300mg/day. Maint: 2-4mg/kg qd. Max: 150mg/day. GERD/Erosive Esophagitis: 2.5-5mg/kg bid. (Inj) DU: 2-4mg/kg/day IV given q6-8 hrs. Max: 50mg q6-8 hrs. CrCl <50mL/min: 50mg IV q18-24 hrs or 150mg PO q24h. Give more frequent (q12h) if necessary. Hemodialysis: Give dose at end of treatment. Dissolve each 25mg effervescent tab in 5mL of water before administration.

HOW SUPPLIED: Inj: 1mg/mL, 25mg/mL; Syrup: 15mg/mL; Tab: 150mg, 300mg; Tab, Effervescent: 25mg

WARNINGS/PRECAUTIONS: Do not exceed recommended infusion rates; bradycardia reported with rapid infusion. Caution with liver and renal dysfunction. Monitor SGPT if on IV therapy for ≥5 days at dose >100mg qid. Avoid use with history of acute porphyria. Symptomatic response does not preclude the presence of gastric malignancy. May cause false (+) urine protein test. Granules and effervescent tablets contain phenylalanine.

ADVERSE REACTIONS: Headache, constipation, diarrhea, nausea, abdominal discomfort, vomiting, hepatitis, blood dyscrasias, rash, injection site reactions (IV/IM).

INTERACTIONS: Increases plasma levels of triazolam. Monitor anticoagulants.

PREGNANCY: Category B, caution with nursing.

MECHANISM OF ACTION: H_2-blocker; competitive, reversible inhibitor of histamine at histamine H_2-receptors, including those found on gastric cells.

PHARMACOKINETICS: Absorption: (PO, 150mg) C_{max}=440-545ng/mL, T_{max}=2-3 hrs; (IM) Rapid; C_{max}=576ng/mL, T_{max}=15 min. **Distribution**: V_d=1.4L/kg;

plasma protein binding (15%); found in breast milk. **Metabolism**: Liver, N-oxide (principal metabolite). **Elimination**: Urine: (PO 30% unchanged); (IV 70% unchanged); (PO) $T_{1/2}$=2.5-3 hrs, (IV) $T_{1/2}$=2-2.5 hrs. Refer to PI for pediatric parameters.

NURSING CONSIDERATIONS

Assessment: Assess for renal/hepatic dysfunction, gastric malignancy, history of acute porphyria, pregnancy/nursing status, and possible drug interactions.

Monitoring: Monitor for signs/symptoms of hepatic effects (eg, elevations in SGPT values), CV effects, headache, and GI effects (eg, constipation, diarrhea). In patients receiving IV formulation at dosages ≥100mg qid for ≥5 days, monitor SGPT daily from Day 5 to the conclusion of IV therapy.

Patient Counseling: Antacids may be given as pain relief for GI symptoms. If taking efferdose tab formulation, do not chew tab; swallow whole, or dissolve on tongue; should be completely dissolved in ≥5mL of water before administration; may be given by medicine dropper or oral syringe. Notify physician if any adverse events develop.

Administration: Oral/IM/IV routes. **Storage:** Tab: 15-30°C (59-86°F) in dry place; protect from light. Replace cap securely after each use. Efferdose Tab: 2-30°C (36-86°F); Syrup: 4-25°C (39-77°F), dispense in tight, light resistant container. Injection: 4-25°C (39-77°F); excursions permitted to 30°C (86°F); protect from light. Premixed Injection: 2-25°C (36-77°F); protect from light.

ZARONTIN RX

ethosuximide (Parke-Davis)

THERAPEUTIC CLASS: Succinimide

INDICATIONS: Control of absence (petit mal) epilepsy.

DOSAGE: *Adults:* 500mg qd. Titrate: May increase daily dose by 250mg every 4-7 days. Max: 1.5g/day.
Pediatrics: Initial: 3-6 yrs: 250mg qd. ≥6 yrs: 500mg qd. Titrate: May increase daily dose by 250mg every 4-7 days. Usual: 20mg/kg/day. Max: 1.5g/day.

HOW SUPPLIED: Cap: 250mg; Syrup: 250mg/5mL

WARNINGS/PRECAUTIONS: Extreme caution in liver and renal dysfunction. Monitor blood counts, liver and renal function periodically. SLE, blood dyscrasias reported. Adjust dose slowly and avoid abrupt withdrawal. May increase grand mal seizures in mixed types of epilepsy when used alone. Caution with mental/physical activities.

ADVERSE REACTIONS: Anorexia, NV, abdominal pain, blood dyscrasias, drowsiness, headache, urticaria, SLE, myopia.

INTERACTIONS: May increase phenytoin levels. Valproic acid may alter levels.

PREGNANCY: Safety in pregnancy and nursing not known.

MECHANISM OF ACTION: Succinimide anticonvulsant; suppresses paroxysmal 3 cycles/second spike and wave activity associated with lapses of consciousness, which is common in absence (petit mal) seizures. Frequency of attacks is reduced through depression of motor cortex and elevation of the CNS threshold to convulsive stimuli.

PHARMACOKINETICS: Distribution: Crosses placenta, found in breast milk.

NURSING CONSIDERATIONS

Assessment: Assess renal/hepatic function prior to therapy. Assess for drug interactions. Obtain baseline CBC.

Monitoring: Monitor for blood dyscrasias and signs/symptoms of SLE. Monitor for occurrence of grand mal seizures in patients with mixed types of epilepsy who are on monotherapy. Monitor CBC, LFTs, urinalysis, and signs/symptoms of infection (eg, sore throat, fever).

Patient Counseling: Advise to contact physician if any signs/symptoms of infection develop. Counsel not to abruptly d/c therapy. Inform that therapy may impair mental/physical abilities; avoid activities requiring alertness (eg, operating vehicles).

Administration: Oral. **Storage:** (Oral Sol) Below 30°C (86°F). Preserve in tight containers. Protect from freezing and light. (Caps) 25°C (77°F); excursions permitted to 15-30°C (59-86°F).

ZAROXOLYN **RX**

metolazone (Celltech)

Do not interchange rapid and complete bioavailability metolazone formulations for other slow and incomplete bioavailability metolazone formulations; they are not therapeutically equivalent.

THERAPEUTIC CLASS: Quinazoline diuretic

INDICATIONS: Treatment of hypertension and of salt and water retention in edema accompanying CHF or renal disease.

DOSAGE: *Adults:* Edema: 5-20mg qd. HTN: 2.5-5mg qd. Elderly: Start at low end of dosing range.

HOW SUPPLIED: Tab: 2.5mg, 5mg, 10mg

CONTRAINDICATIONS: Anuria, hepatic coma or precoma.

WARNINGS/PRECAUTIONS: Risk of hypokalemia, orthostatic hypotension, hypercalcemia, hyperuricemia, azotemia, and rapid-onset hyponatremia. Cross-allergy with sulfonamide-derived drugs, thiazides, or quinethazone. Sensitivity reactions may occur with 1st dose. Monitor electrolytes. May cause hyperglycemia and glycosuria in diabetics. Caution in elderly or severe renal impairment. May exacerbate or activate SLE.

ADVERSE REACTIONS: Chest pain/discomfort, orthostatic hypotension, syncope, neuropathy, necrotizing angiitis, hepatitis, jaundice, pancreatitis, blood dyscrasias, joint pain.

INTERACTIONS: Furosemide and other loop diuretics prolong fluid and electrolyte loss. Adjust dose of other antihypertensives. Potentiates hypotensive effects of alcohol, barbiturates, and narcotics. Lithium, digitalis toxicity. Corticosteroids and ACTH increase hypokalemia and salt and water retention. Enhanced neuromuscular blocking effects of curariform drugs. Salicylates and NSAIDs decrease effects. Decreased arterial response to norepinephrine. Decrease in methenamine efficacy. Adjust anticoagulants, antidiabetics.

PREGNANCY: Category B, not for use in nursing.

MECHANISM OF ACTION: Quinazoline diuretic; acts primarily to inhibit Na^+ reabsorption at cortical diluting site and, to a lesser extent, in proximal convoluted tubule.

PHARMACOKINETICS: Absorption: T_{max}=8 hrs. **Elimination:** Urine (unchanged).

NURSING CONSIDERATIONS

Assessment: Assess for anuria, SLE, DM, sulfonamide hypersensitivity, history of allergy or bronchial asthma, hepatic/renal impairment, possible drug interactions.

Monitoring: Monitor serum electrolytes periodically. Monitor for signs/symptoms of electrolyte imbalance, exacerbation or activation of SLE, hyperglycemia, hyperuricemia or precipitation of gout, hypersensitivity reactions (eg, angioedema, bronchospasm, toxic epidermal necrolysis, Stevens-Johnson syndrome), orthostatic hypotension, renal/hepatic dysfunction.

Patient Counseling: Counsel to take medication as directed and promptly report adverse reactions. Advise not to interchange formulations. Instruct to seek medical attention if symptoms of electrolyte imbalance (eg, dry mouth, thirst, weakness) or hypersensitivity reactions occur.

Administration: Oral route. **Storage:** 25°C (77°F); excursions permitted to 15-30°C (59-86°F). Protect from light.

ZEBETA — RX
bisoprolol fumarate (Duramed)

THERAPEUTIC CLASS: Selective $beta_1$-blocker

INDICATIONS: Management of hypertension.

DOSAGE: *Adults:* Initial: 2.5-5mg qd. Max: 20mg/day. Hepatic Dysfunction or CrCl <40mL/min: Initial: 2.5mg qd; caution with dose titration.

HOW SUPPLIED: Tab: 5mg*, 10mg *scored

CONTRAINDICATIONS: Cardiogenic shock, overt cardiac failure, 2nd- or 3rd-degree AV block, marked sinus bradycardia.

WARNINGS/PRECAUTIONS: Avoid abrupt withdrawal. May mask hypoglycemia or hyperthyroidism symptoms. Caution with compensated cardiac failure, DM, bronchospastic disease, hepatic/renal impairment, or peripheral vascular disease. May precipitate cardiac failure. Both digitalis glycosides and β-blockers slow atrioventricular conduction and decrease HR. Concomitant use can increase risk of bradycardia.

ADVERSE REACTIONS: Diarrhea, URI, fatigue.

INTERACTIONS: May block epinephrine effects. Caution with clonidine withdrawal. Excessive reduction of sympathetic activity with catecholamine-depleting drugs. Avoid other β-blockers. Caution with CCBs (eg, verapamil, diltiazem), antiarrhythmics (eg, disopyramide), and anesthetics that depress myocardial function. Rifampin increases clearance. Antidiabetic agents may need adjustment.

PREGNANCY: Category C, caution in nursing.

MECHANISM OF ACTION: Synthetic β_1-selective (cardioselective) adrenoreceptor blocking agent; inhibits β_2-adrenoreceptors, chiefly in bronchial and vascular musculature.

PHARMACOKINETICS: Absorption: Absolute bioavailability 80%; T_{max}=2-4 hrs. **Distribution:** Plasma protein binding (30%). **Elimination:** Urine, feces (≤2%); $T_{1/2}$=9-12 hrs.

NURSING CONSIDERATIONS

Assessment: Assess for bradycardia, cardiogenic shock, 2nd- and 3rd-degree heart block, overt cardiac failure, impaired renal/hepatic function, bronchospastic disease, PVD, DM, thyrotoxicosis, pregnancy status, and possible drug interactions.

Monitoring: Monitor for cardiac failure, HTN, renal function, exacerbation of ischemia following abrupt withdrawal, bronchospastic disease, arrhythmias, CBC with platelet count and differential, hypersensitivity reactions, mesenteric arterial thrombosis, reversible mental depression.

Patient Counseling: Instruct not to interrupt or d/c therapy without consulting physician. Notify physician if signs/symptoms of impending CHF or unexplained respiratory symptoms develop. Educate about signs/symptoms of drug's potential adverse effects. Advise to exercise caution while driving or operating machinery.

Administration: Oral route. **Storage**: 20-25°C (68-77°F). Protect from moisture. Dispense in tight container.

ZEGERID — RX
sodium bicarbonate - omeprazole (Santarus)

THERAPEUTIC CLASS: Proton pump inhibitor

INDICATIONS: (Cap, Powder) Short-term treatment of erosive esophagitis diagnosed by endoscopy, active duodenal ulcer, and active benign gastric ulcer. Treatment of heartburn and other symptoms associated with GERD. Maintain healing of erosive esophagitis. (Powder, 40mg-1680mg) Reduction of risk of upper GI bleeding in critically ill patients.

DOSAGE: *Adults:* Cap/Powder: Duodenal Ulcer: 20mg qd for 4-8 weeks. Gastric Ulcer: 40mg qd for 4-8 weeks. GERD: 20mg qd for up to 4 weeks without esophageal lesions and for 4-8 weeks with erosive esophagitis. Maintenance of Healing Erosive Esophagitis: 20mg qd. Powder (40mg-1680mg): Risk Reduction of Upper GI Bleeding in Critically Ill Patients: Initial: 40mg, followed by 40mg after 6-8 hrs. Maint: 40mg qd for 14 days. Take 1 hr before a meal. Add pkt contents to 2 tablespoons of water; do not use other liquids or foods. Stir powder well and drink immediately. Swallow caps whole with water.

HOW SUPPLIED: (Omeprazole-Sodium Bicarbonate) Cap: 20mg-1100mg, 40mg-1100mg; Powder: 20mg-1680mg/pkt [30^s], 40mg-1680mg/pkt [30^s].

WARNINGS/PRECAUTIONS: Atrophic gastritis reported with long-term use. Symptomatic response does not preclude the presence of gastric malignancy. Due to sodium bicarbonate content, avoid with metabolic alkalosis, hypocalcemia and use caution with a sodium-restricted diet, Bartter's syndrome, hypokalemia, respiratory alkalosis. Long-term use of bicarbonate with calcium or milk may cause milk-alkali syndrome.

ADVERSE REACTIONS: Abdominal pain, headache, nausea, vomiting.

INTERACTIONS: May prolong elimination of diazepam, warfarin, phenytoin, and drugs metabolized by oxidation. May increase PT and INR if given concomitantly with warfarin. May alter absorption of pH-dependent drugs (eg, ketoconazole, ampicillin esters, and iron salts). Monitor when given with drugs metabolized by CYP450 (eg, cyclosporine, disulfiram, benzodiazepines). Clarithromycin may increase levels. May increase levels of tacrolimus, clarithromycin. May reduce levels of atazanavir.

PREGNANCY: Category C, not for use in nursing.

MECHANISM OF ACTION: Omeprazole: Proton-pump inhibitor; suppresses gastric acid secretion by specific inhibition of the (H^+/K^+)-ATPase enzyme at secretory surface of gastric parietal cell. Sodium Bicarbonate: Acts as antacid.

PHARMACOKINETICS: Absorption: Omeprazole: Rapid absorption; T_{max}=30 min; (Sus) Absolute bioavailability (30-40%); C_{max}=1954ng/mL. (Cap) C_{max}=1526ng/mL. **Distribution:** Omeprazole: Plasma protein binding (95%); found in breast milk. **Metabolism:** Omeprazole: Hydroxyomeprazole and corresponding carboxylic acid (metabolites). **Elimination:** Omeprazole: Urine (77% as metabolites), feces; $T_{1/2}$=1 hr.

NURSING CONSIDERATIONS

Assessment: Assess for hepatic impairment, gastric malignancy, Na^+-restricted diet, metabolic alkalosis, respiratory alkalosis, problems with acid-base balance, hypocalcemia, Bartter's syndrome, hypokalemia, pregnancy/nursing status, and possible drug interactions. Assess dosing in Asian patients.

Monitoring: Monitor for signs/symptoms of atrophic gastritis. Monitor for milk-alkali syndrome in presence of long-term use of bicarbonate with calcium or milk.

Patient Counseling: Counsel to take on empty stomach at least 1 hr before meals. If taking cap, swallow whole, do not open cap and sprinkle contents on food. For sus, empty packet contents into small cup containing 1-2 tbl of water; do not use other liquids or foods; stir well and drink immediately; refill cup with water and drink. Notify physician of adverse events (eg, GI effects).

Administration: Oral route. **Storage:** 25°C (77°F); excursions permitted to 15-30°C (59-86°F).

ZELAPAR — RX

selegiline HCl (Valeant)

THERAPEUTIC CLASS: Monoamine oxidase inhibitor (Type B)

INDICATIONS: Adjunct in the management of Parkinson's disease in patients exhibiting a deteriorated response to levodopa/carbidopa therapy.

DOSAGE: *Adults:* 1.25mg qd for 6 weeks. Titrate: After 6 weeks, may increase to 2.5mg if desired benefit not achieved. Max: 2.5mg/day.

HOW SUPPLIED: Tab, Orally Disintegrating: 1.25mg

CONTRAINDICATIONS: Concomitant meperidine, tramadol, methadone, propoxyphene dextromethorphan, and other MAOIs.

WARNINGS/PRECAUTIONS: Do not exceed 2.5mg/day; risk of non-selective MAO inhibition. Greater risk of orthostatic hypotension and dizziness in geriatric patients. Decrease levodopa/carbidopa to prevent exacerbation of levodopa side effects (eg, preexisting dyskinesias). Melanoma reported; perform periodic dermatologic screening. May increase frequency of mild oropharyngeal abnormality. Caution with renal or hepatic impairment. Neuroleptic malignant syndrome reported in association with rapid dose reduction, withdrawal of, or changes in antiparkinsonian therapy.

ADVERSE REACTIONS: Nausea, dizziness, pain, headache, insomnia, rhinitis, skin disorders, dyskinesia, backache, dyspepsia, stomatitis, constipation, hallucinations, pharyngitis, rash.

INTERACTIONS: See Contraindications. Serious, sometimes fatal, reactions have been precipitated with meperidine, tramadol, methadone, and propoxyphene; avoid concomitant use. Episodes of psychosis or bizarre behavior reported with dextromethorphan; avoid concomitant use. Severe toxicity reported with SSRIs or TCAs; avoid concurrent use and allow 2 weeks between discontinuation of selegiline and initiation of TCAs or SSRIs. Allow 5 weeks for fluoxetine due to a longer half-life. Caution with sympathomimetics and CYP3A4 inducers (eg, phenytoin, carbamazepine, nafcillin, phenobarbital, and rifampin).

PREGNANCY: Category C, not for use in nursing.

MECHANISM OF ACTION: Irreversible MAO inhibitor; blocks catabolism of dopamine and increases net amount of dopamine available.

PHARMACOKINETICS: Absorption: C_{max}(1.25mg, 2.5mg, 5mg)=3.34, 4.47, 1.12ng/mL. T_{max}(1.25mg, 2.5mg, 5mg)=10-15 min, 10-15 min, 40-90 min. **Distribution:** Plasma protein binding (85%). **Metabolism:** Liver (1st-pass metabolism). **Elimination:** Urine; $T_{1/2}$=10 hrs (steady state).

NURSING CONSIDERATIONS

Assessment: Assess renal function, LFTs, dyskinesia, phenylalanine levels, BP, melanomas, pregnancy/nursing status, and possible drug interactions.

Monitoring: Monitor LFTs, renal function, BP, exacerbation of pre-existing dyskinesia, melanomas, hyperpyrexia, hallucinations.

Patient Counseling: Should be taken every morning before breakfast without liquid. Do not remove blister from outer pouch until just prior to dosing. Report any side effects. Notify physician if new or increased gambling urges, sexual urges, or other urges occur.

Administration: Oral route; dissolve on tongue. **Storage:** 25°C (77°F); excursions permitted to 15-30°C (59-86°F). Use within 3 months after opening.

ZEMPLAR IV — RX

paricalcitol (Abbott)

THERAPEUTIC CLASS: Vitamin D analog

INDICATIONS: Prevention and treatment of secondary hyperparathyroidism associated with chronic kidney disease Stage 5.

DOSAGE: *Adults:* Initial: 0.04-0.1mcg/kg bolus no more frequently than every other day during dialysis. Max: 0.24mcg/kg (16.8mcg). Titrate: May increase by 2-4mcg at 2-4 week intervals. Monitor serum Ca and phosphorus more frequently during dose adjustments. Reduce or interrupt dose if elevated Ca level or Ca x P product >75, may reinitiate at lower dose once normalized. May need dose decrease as PTH levels decrease (see PI).
Pediatrics: ≥5 yrs: (Inj) Initial: 0.04-0.1mcg/kg bolus no more frequently than every other day during dialysis. Max: 0.24mcg/kg (16.8mcg). Titrate: May

increase by 2-4mcg at 2-4 week intervals. Monitor serum Ca and phosphorus more frequently during dose adjustments. Reduce or interrupt dose if elevated Ca level or Ca x P product >75, may reinitiate at lower dose once normalized. May need dose decrease as PTH levels decrease (see PI).

HOW SUPPLIED: Inj: 2mcg/mL, 5mcg/mL

CONTRAINDICATIONS: Vitamin D toxicity, hypercalcemia.

WARNINGS/PRECAUTIONS: Overdose may cause progressive hypercalcemia. Should supplement with calcium and restrict phosphorus. May need phosphate-binding compounds to control serum phosphorus levels. Avoid concomitant phosphate or vitamin D-related compounds.

ADVERSE REACTIONS: NV, edema, chills, flu, GI bleeding, lightheadedness, pneumonia, pain, allergic reaction, headache, HTN, diarrhea, arthritis, rash.

INTERACTIONS: Digitalis toxicity potentiated by hypercalcemia. Avoid excessive use of aluminum containing compounds.

PREGNANCY: Category C, caution in nursing.

MECHANISM OF ACTION: Synthetic vitamin D analog; binds to vitamin D receptor, which results in selective activation of vitamin D pathways. Shown to reduce parathyroid hormone levels by inhibiting PTH synthesis and secretion.

PHARMACOKINETICS: Absorption: C_{max}=1.680ng/mL (hemodialysis), 1.832ng/mL (peritoneal dialysis); AUC=14.51ng•h/mL (hemodialysis), 16.01ng•h/mL (peritoneal dialysis). **Distribution:** V_d=23.8L (healthy), 31L (hemodialysis), and 35L (peritoneal dialysis); plasma protein binding (≥99.8%). **Metabolism:** Hepatic, via hydroxylation and glucuronidation; CYP24, CYP3A4, UGT1A4. **Elimination:** Hepatobiliary excretion (primary), urine (19%), feces (63%); $T_{1/2}$=13.9 hrs (hemodialysis), 15.4 hrs (peritoneal dialysis).

NURSING CONSIDERATIONS

Assessment: Assess for vitamin D toxicity and hypercalcemia prior to therapy. Assess for possible drug interactions.

Monitoring: Monitor for signs/symptoms of hypercalcemia, hyperphosphatemia, and metastatic calcification. If hypercalcemia develops, monitor for fluid and electrolyte imbalances, ECG abnormalities, and serum calcium levels; monitor serum calcium levels frequently until levels normalized. Monitor for adynamic bone lesions with suppressed PTH levels. Monitor calcium and phosphorus levels twice weekly when initiating therapy. Once dosage established, monitor serum calcium and phosphorus monthly. Monitor serum/plasma PTH levels every 3 months.

Patient Counseling: Inform about compliance with dosing instructions, diet and phosphorus restrictions, and avoidance of unapproved OTC drugs. Counsel about signs/symptoms of hypercalcemia. Advise to avoid taking phosphate- or vitamin D-containing compounds. Avoid excessive aluminum-containing compounds.

Administration: IV route. **Storage:** 25°C (77°F); excursions permitted to 15-30°C (59-86°F).

ZEMPLAR ORAL — RX

paricalcitol (Abbott)

THERAPEUTIC CLASS: Vitamin D analog

INDICATIONS: Prevention and treatment of secondary hyperparathyroidism associated with Stage 3 and 4 chronic kidney disease.

DOSAGE: *Adults:* Initial: Baseline iPTH Level ≤500pg/mL: 1mcg qd or 2mcg tiw. Baseline iPTH Level >500pg/mL: 2mcg qd or 4mcg tiw. May need dose adjustment based on iPTH level relative to baseline (see PI).

HOW SUPPLIED: Cap: 1mcg, 2mcg, 4mcg

CONTRAINDICATIONS: Vitamin D toxicity, hypercalcemia.

WARNINGS/PRECAUTIONS: May cause over suppression of PTH, hypercalcemia, hypercalciuria, hyperphosphatemia, and adynamic bone disease. Overdose may cause progressive hypercalcemia.

ADVERSE REACTIONS: Pain, allergic reactions, headache, infection, hypotension, HTN, diarrhea, NV, constipation, edema, arthritis, dizziness, vertigo, rhinitis, rash.

INTERACTIONS: Digitalis toxicity potentiated by hypercalcemia. Caution with strong CYP3A inhibitors (ketoconazole, atazanavir, clarithromycin, indinavir, itraconazole, nefazodone, nelfinavir, ritonavir, saquinavir, telithromycin, voriconazole). Drugs that may impair intestinal absorption of fat-soluble vitamins (cholestyramine) may intefere with absorption.

PREGNANCY: Category C, not for use in nursing.

MECHANISM OF ACTION: Synthetic vitamin D analog; binds to vitamin D receptor (VDR), which results in selective activation of vitamin D pathways. Shown to reduce parathyroid hormone levels by inhibiting PTH synthesis and secretion.

PHARMACOKINETICS: Absorption: Well absorbed; absolute bioavailability (72%); C_{max}=0.630ng/mL; T_{max}=3 hrs; AUC=5.25ng•h/mL. **Distribution:** V_d=34L (healthy); 44-46L (CKD stage 3 and 4); plasma protein binding (≥99.8%). **Metabolism:** Hepatic, via hydroxylation and glucuronidation; extensively metabolized by CYP24, as well as CYP3A4, UGT1A4. 24(R)-hydroxy paracalcitol (minor metabolite). **Elimination:** Hepatobiliary excretion (primary); urine (18%), feces (70%); $T_{1/2}$=17 hrs (CKD Stage 3), 20 hrs (CKD Stage 4).

NURSING CONSIDERATIONS

Assessment: Assess for vitamin D toxicity or hypercalcemia prior to therapy. Assess for possible drug interactions (digitalis compounds).

Monitoring: Monitor for signs/symptoms of hypercalcemia (eg, cardiac arrhythmias, seizures, vascular calcification, soft tissue calcification). Monitor for PTH suppression, hypercalciuria, hyperphosphatemia and adynamic bone disease. Monitor serum calcium, serum phosphorus, and serum/plasma PTH every 2 weeks for 3 months after initiation of therapy or following dosage adjustment. Levels should then be assessed monthly for 3 months, and then every 3 months thereafter.

Patient Counseling: Inform about compliance with dosage instructions, proper diet, phosphorus restrictions, and avoidance of unapproved OTC drugs. Advise about signs/symptoms of hypercalcemia. Instruct to avoid use of aluminum-containing compounds and pharmacological doses of vitamin D and its derivatives while on therapy. Inform medication may be taken without regard to food.

Administration: Oral route. **Storage:** 25°C (77°F); excursions permitted to 15-30°C (59-86°F).

ZERIT RX

stavudine (Bristol-Myers Squibb)

Lactic acidosis and severe, fatal hepatomegaly reported. Fatal and non-fatal pancreatitis reported with didanosine.

THERAPEUTIC CLASS: Synthetic thymidine nucleoside analogue

INDICATIONS: Treatment of HIV-1 infection in combination with other antiretrovirals.

DOSAGE: *Adults:* ≥60kg: 40mg q12h. <60kg: 30mg q12h. Interrupt therapy if develop peripheral neuropathy, resume at 1/2 dose when neuropathy resolves. D/C permanently if neuropathy recurs after resumption. Suspend therapy if lactic acidosis or hepatotoxicity occurs. CrCl 26-50mL/min: ≥60kg: 20mg q12h. <60kg: 15mg q12h. CrCl 10-25mL/min: ≥60kg: 20mg q24h. <60kg: 15mg q24h.

Pediatrics: ≥60kg: 40mg q12h. 30-59 kg: 30mg q12h. ≥14 days and <30kg: 1mg/kg q12h. Birth-13 days: 0.5mg/kg q12h. Interrupt therapy if develop peripheral neuropathy, resume with 1/2 dose when neuropathy resolves. D/C permanently if neuropathy recurs after resumption. Suspend therapy if lactic acidosis or hepatotoxicity occurs. Renal Impairment: Reduce dose and/or increase interval.

HOW SUPPLIED: Cap: 15mg, 20mg, 30mg, 40mg; Sus: 1mg/mL [200mL]

WARNINGS/PRECAUTIONS: Obesity and prolonged nucleoside exposure may increase risk to lactic acidosis and hepatomegaly. Caution with risk factors for hepatic disease. Peripheral neuropathy reported. Monitor for lactic acidosis in pregnancy if used with didanosine. D/C if motor weakness develops.

ADVERSE REACTIONS: Peripheral neuropathy, rash, elevated LFTs and amylase, headache, diarrhea, NV.

INTERACTIONS: Avoid zidovudine. Increased risk of neuropathy with neurotoxic drugs (eg, didanosine). Increased risk of hepatotoxicity with didanosine and hydroxyurea. Motor weakness reported with other antiretrovirals.

PREGNANCY: Category C, not for use in nursing.

MECHANISM OF ACTION: Thymidine nucleoside analogue; inhibits activity of HIV-1 reverse transcriptase by competing with natural substrate thymidine triphosphate and by DNA chain termination following incorporation into viral DNA. Inhibits cellular DNA polymerases β and gamma and markedly reduces synthesis of mitochondrial DNA.

PHARMACOKINETICS: Absorption: Rapidly absorbed; C_{max}=536±146ng/mL; T_{max}=1 hr; AUC=2568±454ng.h/mL. **Distribution**: V_d=46±21L (adults); V_d=0.73+/-0.32L/kg (age 5 weeks to 15 yrs). **Elimination**: Renal (40%); $T_{1/2}$=1.15±0.35 hrs (IV, adult), 1.6±0.23 hrs (PO, adult); $T_{1/2}$=1.11+/-0.28 hrs (IV, age 5 weeks to 15 yrs); $T_{1/2}$= 0.96+/-0.26 hrs (PO, age 5 weeks to 15 yrs).

NURSING CONSIDERATIONS

Assessment: Assess for liver dysfunction, chronic active hepatitis, and possible drug interactions.

Monitoring: Monitor for signs of lactic acidosis, severe hepatomegaly with steatosis, pancreatitis, and immune reconstitution syndrome. Monitor for neurologic symptoms (eg, motor weakness, peripheral neuropathy). Monitor LFTs, renal function, and evidence of worsening liver disease.

Patient Counseling: Inform to seek medical attention if early recognition of symptoms of hyperlactatemia or lactic acidosis syndrome (eg, unexplained weight loss, abdominal discomfort, NV, fatigue, dyspnea, motor weakness, peripheral neuropathy). Counsel that redistribution or accumulation of fat tissue may occur. Advise patients and caregivers to importance of adherence to any antiretroviral regimen. Inform that therapy does not cure HIV; may continue to develop opportunistic infections and other complications of HIV. Inform HIV-infected mothers not to nurse to reduce risk of transmission.

Administration: Oral route. May be taken with/without food. Preparation of Oral Sol: 1) Add 202mL purified water to container. Shake well. Final concentration is 1mg/mL. 2) Dispense in original container. Shake prior to use.
Storage: Caps: Store in tightly closed containers at 25°C (77°F); excursions permitted to 15-30°C (59-86°F). Oral Sol: Protect from excessive moisture and store in tightly closed container at 25°C (77°F); excursions permitted to 15-30°C (59-86°F). After reconstitution, refrigerate at 2-8°C (36-46°F). Discard any unused portion after 30 days.

ZESTORETIC — RX

lisinopril - hydrochlorothiazide (AstraZeneca)

ACE inhibitors can cause death/injury to developing fetus during 2nd and 3rd trimesters. Stop therapy if pregnancy detected.

THERAPEUTIC CLASS: ACE inhibitor/thiazide diuretic

INDICATIONS: Treatment of hypertension. Not for initial therapy.

DOSAGE: *Adults:* Initial (If Not Controlled with Lisinopril/HCTZ Monotherapy): 10mg-12.5mg tab or 20mg-12.5mg tab daily. Titrate: May increase after

2-3 weeks. Initial (If Controlled on 25mg HCTZ/Day with Hypokalemia): 10mg-12.5mg tab. Replacement Therapy: Substitute combination for titrated components.

HOW SUPPLIED: Tab: (Lisinopril-HCTZ) 10mg-12.5mg, 20mg-12.5mg, 20mg-25mg

CONTRAINDICATIONS: History of ACE inhibitor-associated angioedema, hereditary or idiopathic angioedema, anuria, sulfonamide hypersensitivity.

WARNINGS/PRECAUTIONS: D/C if angioedema, jaundice, or marked LFT elevation occur. Risk of hyperkalemia with DM, renal dysfunction. Persistent nonproductive cough reported. Monitor WBCs in renal and collagen vascular disease. Anaphylactoid reactions during membrane exposure reported. Fetal/neonatal morbidity and death reported. Monitor for hypotension in high-risk patients (eg, surgery/anesthesia, volume/salt depletion). Caution with CHF, renal or hepatic dysfunction. More reports of angioedema in blacks than nonblacks. May exacerbate or activate SLE. Monitor electrolytes. Avoid if CrCl ≤30mL/min/1.7m². May increase cholesterol, TG. Hypercalcemia, hypomagnesemia, hyperuricemia may occur. Caution with left ventricle outflow obstruction.

ADVERSE REACTIONS: Dizziness, headache, cough, fatigue, orthostatic effects, diarrhea, nausea, muscle cramps, angioedema, cutaneous pseudolymphoma.

INTERACTIONS: Increases risk of hyperkalemia with K^+-sparing diuretics, K^+ supplements, or K^+-containing salt substitutes. Potentiates orthostatic hypotension with alcohol, barbiturates, and narcotics. Adjust antidiabetic drugs. Reduced absorption with cholestyramine, colestipol. Corticosteroids, ACTH deplete electrolytes. May decrease response to pressor amines. Potentiates other antihypertensives. May increase responsiveness to skeletal muscle relaxants. Risk of lithium toxicity. NSAIDs reduce effects and worsen renal dysfunction. Nitritoid reactions with gold.

PREGNANCY: Category C (1st trimester) and D (2nd and 3rd trimesters), not for use in nursing.

MECHANISM OF ACTION: Lisinopril: ACE inhibitor; inhibition results in decreased plasma angiotensin II, which leads to decreased vasopressor activity and decreased aldosterone secretion. HCTZ: Thiazide diuretic; affects renal tubular mechanism of electrolyte reabsorption, directly increasing excretion of Na^+ and Cl^-.

PHARMACOKINETICS: Absorption: Lisinopril: T_{max}=7 hrs. **Distribution:** HCTZ: Crosses placenta. **Elimination:** Lisinopril: Urine (unchanged); $T_{1/2}$=12 hrs. HCTZ: Kidneys; $T_{1/2}$=5.6-14.8 hrs.

NURSING CONSIDERATIONS

Assessment: Assess BP, LFTs, renal function, CVD (eg, cardiomyopathy, aortic stenosis), renal artery stenosis, SLE, serum electrolytes, pregnancy status, history of allergy to sulfonamides, bronchial asthma, parathyroid disorders, and for possible drug interactions.

Monitoring: Monitor BP, LFTs, renal function, CBC with platelet count and differential, serum electrolytes. Monitor for MI, CHF, angioedema (head/neck, intestinal), anaphylactoid reactions, hepatic failure, hyperuricemia, hyperglycemia, hypersensitivity reactions, cough, NV, dizziness.

Patient Counseling: Inform about fetal risks if taken during pregnancy. Caution that inadequate fluid intake, excessive perspiration, diarrhea, and vomiting may lead to excessive fall in BP, resulting in lightheadedness or possible syncope. Advise not to use K^+ supplements or salt substitutes containing K^+ without consulting physician. Counsel about signs/symptoms of neutropenia (eg, infection, sore throat, fever), angioedema, electrolyte imbalance (eg, thirst, weakness, lethargy), and other potential adverse effects; seek prompt medical attention if any occur.

Administration: Oral route. **Storage:** 20-25°C (68-77°F).

ZESTRIL **RX**

lisinopril (AstraZeneca)

ACE inhibitors can cause injury/death to developing fetus during 2nd and 3rd trimesters. D/C if pregnancy is detected.

THERAPEUTIC CLASS: ACE inhibitor

INDICATIONS: Treatment of HTN. Adjunct therapy in heart failure if inadequately controlled by diuretics and digitalis. Adjunct therapy in stable patients within 24 hrs of AMI to improve survival.

DOSAGE: *Adults:* HTN: If possible, d/c diuretic 2-3 days prior to therapy. Initial: 10mg qd, 5mg qd with diuretic. Usual: 20-40mg qd. Resume diuretic if BP not controlled. Max: 80mg/day. CrCl 10-30mL/min: Initial: 5mg/day. Max: 40mg/day. CrCl <10mL/min: Initial: 2.5mg/day. Max: 40mg/day. Heart Failure: Initial: 5mg qd. Usual: 5-40mg qd. May increase by 10mg every 2 weeks. Max: 40mg/day. Hyponatremia or CrCl ≤30mL/min or SrCr >3mg/dL: Initial: 2.5mg qd. AMI: Initial: 5mg within 24 hrs, then 5mg after 24 hrs, then 10mg after 48 hrs, then 10mg qd. Use 2.5mg during first 3 days with low SBP. Maint: 10mg qd for 6 weeks, 2.5-5mg with hypotension. D/C with prolonged hypotension. Elderly: Caution with dose adjustment.
Pediatrics: ≥6 yrs: HTN: Initial: 0.07mg/kg qd up to 5mg total. Dose adjust according to response. Max: 0.61mg/kg or 40mg.

HOW SUPPLIED: Tab: 2.5mg, 5mg, 10mg, 20mg, 30mg, 40mg

CONTRAINDICATIONS: History of ACE inhibitor-associated angioedema, hereditary or idiopathic angioedema.

WARNINGS/PRECAUTIONS: D/C if angioedema, jaundice, or marked LFT elevation occur. Risk of hyperkalemia, hypoglycemia with DM, renal dysfunction. Persistent nonproductive cough reported. Monitor WBCs in renal and collagen vascular disease. Anaphylactoid reactions during membrane exposure reported. Fetal/neonatal morbidity and death reported. Monitor for hypotension in high-risk patients (heart failure with SBP <100mmHg, surgery/anesthesia, hyponatremia, high-dose diuretic therapy, severe volume and/or salt depletion, etc). Caution with CHF, aortic stenosis/hypertrophic cardiomyopathy, renal dysfunction, and renal artery stenosis. Less effective on BP in blacks and more reports of angioedema than nonblacks.

ADVERSE REACTIONS: Hypotension, diarrhea, headache, dizziness, hyperkalemia, chest pain, cough, cutaneous pseudolymphoma.

INTERACTIONS: May increase lithium levels. Hypotension risk with diuretics. Concomitant use with antidiabetic medications may increase risk of hypoglycemia. Coadministration with NSAIDs in patients with compromised renal function may further deteriorate renal function. Increase risk of hyperkalemia with K^+-sparing diuretics, K^+-containing salt substitutes, or K^+ supplements. Indomethacin may reduce effects. Nitritoid reactions with gold.

PREGNANCY: Category C (1st trimester) and D (2nd and 3rd trimesters), not for use in nursing.

MECHANISM OF ACTION: ACE inhibitor; inhibition results in decreased plasma angiotensin II, which leads to decreased vasopressor activity and aldosterone secretion.

PHARMACOKINETICS: Absorption: T_{max}=7 hrs. **Elimination:** Urine (unchanged); $T_{1/2}$=12 hrs.

NURSING CONSIDERATIONS

Assessment: Assess BP, LFTs, renal function, CVD (eg, aortic stenosis, cardiomyopathy), renal artery stenosis, pregnancy status, and for possible drug interactions.

Monitoring: Monitor BP, LFTs, renal function, CBC with platelet count and differential, serum K^+ levels. Monitor for MI, CHF, angioedema (head, neck, intestinal), anaphylactoid reactions, hepatic failure, hypersensitivity reactions, cough, NV, dizziness.

Patient Counseling: Counsel about fetal risks during pregnancy and signs/symptoms of angioedema (laryngeal/tongue edema, abdominal pain); advise to seek prompt medical attention if symptoms develop. Inform about potential adverse effects (eg, anaphylaxis, cough, hypotension, hyperkalemia). Infants with history of *in utero* exposure should be closely observed for hypotension, oliguria, hyperkalemia. Inform about need for periodic monitoring of electrolytes and blood counts. Caution that inadequate fluid intake, excessive perspiration, diarrhea, vomiting may lead to excessive fall in BP, which can result in lightheadedness or possible syncope. Advise not to use K^+ supplements or salt substitutes containing K^+ without consulting physician.

Administration: Oral route. **Storage:** Store at controlled room temperature, 20-25°C (68-77°F). Protect from moisture, freezing, and excessive heat.

ZETIA — RX

ezetimibe (Merck/Schering-Plough)

THERAPEUTIC CLASS: Cholesterol absorption inhibitor

INDICATIONS: Adjunct to diet, as monotherapy or with concomitant HMG-CoA reductase inhibitors, to reduce total-C, LDL-C, and Apo B levels in primary (heterozygous familial and nonfamilial) hypercholesterolemia. Adjunct to diet, with concomitant fenofibrate, to reduce elevated total-C, LDL-C, Apo B, and non-HDL-C in mixed hyperlipidemia. Adjunct to other lipid-lowering treatments or if such treatments are unavailable, with concomitant atorvastatin or simvastatin, to reduce total-C and LDL-C in homozygous familial hypercholesterolemia. Adjunct to diet, to reduce sitosterol and campesterol levels in homozygous familial sitosterolemia.

DOSAGE: *Adults:* 10mg qd. May give with HMG-CoA reductase inhibitor (with primary hypercholesterolemia) or fenofibrate (with mixed hyperlipidemia) for incremental effect. Concomitant Bile Sequestrant: Give either ≥2 hrs before or ≥4 hrs after bile acid sequestrant.

HOW SUPPLIED: Tab: 10mg

CONTRAINDICATIONS: When used with a statin, refer to the HMG-CoA reductase inhibitor monographs.

WARNINGS/PRECAUTIONS: Monitor LFTs with concurrent statin therapy. Not recommended with moderate or severe hepatic insufficiency.

ADVERSE REACTIONS: Back pain, arthralgia, diarrhea, sinusitis, abdominal pain, myalgia.

INTERACTIONS: Incremental LDL-C reduction may be reduced with concomitant cholestyramine. Fibrates may increase cholesterol excretion into the bile; concurrent use is not recommended. Increased levels with fenofibrate and gemfibrozil. Monitor cyclosporine levels with concomitant use of cyclosporine. Monitor INR when administered with warfarin.

PREGNANCY: Category C, contraindicated in nursing.

MECHANISM OF ACTION: Cholesterol absorption inhibitor; inhibits absorption of cholesterol by small intestine. Targets the sterol transporter, Neimann-Pick C1-like 1 (NPC1L1), which is involved in intestinal uptake of cholesterol and phytosterol; inhibited uptake leads to decrease of intestinal cholesterol to the liver, causing reduction of hepatic cholesterol stores and increase in clearance of cholesterol from the blood.

PHARMACOKINETICS: Absorption: Ezetimibe: C_{max}=3.4-5.5ng/mL; T_{max}=4-12 hrs. Ezetimibe-glucuronide (active metabolite) C_{max}=45-71ng/mL; T_{max}=1-2 hrs. **Distribution:** Plasma protein binding (>90%). **Metabolism:** Small intestine, liver via glucuronide conjugation; Ezetimibe-glucuronide (major active metabolite). **Elimination:** Feces (78%), urine (11%); $T_{1/2}$=22 hrs.

NURSING CONSIDERATIONS

Assessment: Assess for secondary causes of dyslipidemia (eg, DM, hypothyroidism, obstructive liver disease, chronic renal failure, drugs that increase LDL-C and decrease HDL-C), presence of active liver disease or unexplained elevations in serum transaminases, and pregnancy/nursing status. Obtain baseline lipid profile (total-C, LDL-C, HDL-C, TG). Obtain baseline LFTs if co-administered with HMG-CoA reductase inhibitor. Assess for possible drug interactions.

Monitoring: Monitor for signs/symptoms of elevated liver enzymes, myopathy, and rhabdomyolysis. Periodically monitor LFTs if on concomitant therapy with HMG-CoA reductase inhibitor. Monitor lipid profile while on therapy.

Patient Counseling: Recommend standard cholesterol-lowering diet before and during treatment. Advise drug may be taken with/without food. Counsel about risk of myopathy and instruct to contact physician promptly if any unexplained muscle pain, tenderness, or weakness occur. Inform patients who become pregnant while taking drug of potential risk to fetus. Instruct that if on concomitant therapy with bile acid sequestrant, dosing of drug should occur either ≥2 hrs before or ≥4 hrs after administration of the bile acid sequestrant.

Administration: Oral route. **Storage:** 25°C; excursions permitted to 15-30°C (59-86°F). Protect from moisture.

ZEVALIN RX

ibritumomab tiuxetan (Biogen Idec)

Discontinue if severe infusion reactions occur. Severe and prolonged cytopenias reported; avoid if ≥25% lymphoma marrow involvement and/or impaired bone marrow reserve. Severe, some fatal, cutaneous and mucocutaneous reactions reported. Do not exceed the maximum dose. Avoid patients with altered biodistribution.

THERAPEUTIC CLASS: Monoclonal antibody

INDICATIONS: Treatment of relapsed or refractory low grade, follicular, or transformed B-cell non-Hodgkin's lymphoma, including rituximab refractory follicular non-Hodgkin's lymphoma.

DOSAGE: *Adults:* Day 1: Rituximab 250mg/m^2 IV single infusion. Within 4 hrs, give 5mCi of In-111 ibritumomab IV. Assess biodistribution by conducting 1st image at 2-24 hrs, 2nd image at 48-72 hrs, and optional 3rd image at 90-120 hrs. If biodistribution acceptable, Day 7-9: Rituximab 250mg/m^2 IV. Within 4 hrs, give Y-90 Ibritumomab 0.4mCi/kg (or 0.3mCi/kg if platelets 100,000-149,000 cells/mm^3). Max: Y-90 ibritumomab 32mCi.

HOW SUPPLIED: Inj: 3.2mg/2mL

CONTRAINDICATIONS: Type I hypersensitivity or anaphylactic reactions to murine proteins or to any component of this product including rituximab, yttrium chloride, and indium chloride.

WARNINGS/PRECAUTIONS: Use with rituximab, contains albumin; remote risk of transmission of viral disease and CJD. Single course treatment only. Minimize radiation exposure during and after radiolabeling. Monitor CBC and platelets weekly until levels recover. Increased risk of hypersensitivity reactions with HAMA from prior murine protein use. Caution with transfusion. Secondary leukemia and mylodysplastic syndrome reported. Monitor closely for evidence of extravasation. Immediately terminate infusion if signs or symptoms of extravasation occurred.

ADVERSE REACTIONS: Neutropenia, thrombocytopenia, anemia, NV, abdominal pain, diarrhea, increased cough, dyspnea, dizziness, arthralgia, anorexia, anxiety, ecchymosis, infusion site erythema, ulceration following extravasation, radiation injury, tissue complications.

INTERACTIONS: Increased risk of bleeding and hemorrhage with drugs that interfere with platelet function or coagulation; monitor for thrombocytopenia more frequently. Safety of immunization with live viral vaccines not studied.

PREGNANCY: Category D, not for use in nursing.

MECHANISM OF ACTION: Monoclonal antibody; binds specifically to CD20 antigen, which is expressed on pre-B and mature B lymphocytes, and on B-cell non-Hodgkin's lymphomas.

PHARMACOKINETICS: Elimination: Urine (7.5%); $T_{1/2}$=30 hrs.

NURSING CONSIDERATIONS

Assessment: Assess for hypersensitivity, infusion reactions, cytopenia, hemorrhage, severe infections, erythema multiforme, Stevens-Johnson syndrome, lymphoma marrow involvement and/or impaired bone marrow reserves, history of failed stem cell collection, altered biodistribution, and pregnancy status.

Monitoring: Monitor for infusion reactions (eg, urticaria, hypotension, angioedema, hypoxia, bronchospasm, pulmonary infiltrates, acute respiratory distress, MI, ventricular filtration, cardiogenic shock), thrombocytopenia, neutropenia, hemorrhage, cerebral hemorrhage, severe infections, Stevens-Johnson syndrome, exfoliative dermatitis, toxic epidermal necrolysis, leukemia, myelodysplastic syndrome, pregnancy, extravasation during drug infusion, radiation exposure, viral diseases (Creutzfeldt-Jakob disease), and lab tests (eg, CBC, platelets).

Patient Counseling: Counsel about risk of allergic or serious hypersensitivity, to avoid pregnancy/nursing, and use of effective contraceptives in females of childbearing potential. Advise to immediately seek medical intervention if bleeding, easy bruising, painful sores, ulcers, blisters or peeling skin, hives, swelling, dizziness, blurred vision, drowsiness, headache, cough, wheezing, difficulty breathing, weakness, fatigue, or infection occur. Caution against immunization with live vaccines.

Administration: IV route. Refer to PI for specific instructions. **Storage:** 2-8°C (36-46°F). Do not freeze.

ZIAC RX

bisoprolol fumarate - hydrochlorothiazide (Duramed)

THERAPEUTIC CLASS: Selective $beta_1$-blocker/thiazide diuretic

INDICATIONS: Management of hypertension.

DOSAGE: *Adults:* Initial: 2.5mg-6.25mg tab qd. Maint: May increase every 14 days. Max: 20mg bisoprolol-12.5mg HCTZ/day. Renal/Hepatic Dysfunction: Caution in dosing/titrating.

HOW SUPPLIED: Tab: (Bisoprolol-HCTZ) 2.5mg-6.25mg, 5mg-6.25mg, 10mg-6.25mg

CONTRAINDICATIONS: Cardiogenic shock, overt cardiac failure, 2nd- or 3rd-degree AV block, marked sinus bradycardia, anuria, sulfonamide hypersensitivity.

WARNINGS/PRECAUTIONS: Caution with compensated cardiac failure, DM, bronchospastic disease, hepatic/renal impairment, or peripheral vascular disease. Avoid abrupt withdrawal. Photosensitivity reactions, hypokalemia, hypercalcemia, hypophosphatemia reported. May activate/exacerbate SLE. Enhanced effects in post-sympathectomy patients. May mask hyperthyroidism or hypoglycemia symptoms. Monitor for fluid/electrolyte imbalance. May precipitate hyperuricemia, acute gout, cardiac failure.

ADVERSE REACTIONS: Cough, diarrhea, myalgia, headache, dizziness, fatigue, upper respiratory infection.

INTERACTIONS: Alcohol, barbiturates, or narcotics may potentiate orthostatic hypotension. Adjust dose of antidiabetic drugs. Potentiates other antihypertensives. Avoid other β-blockers. Impaired absorption with cholestyramine, colestipol. Corticosteroids, ACTH intensify electrolyte depletion. May decrease response to pressor amines. May increase response to nondepolarizing muscle relaxants. Risk of lithium toxicity. NSAIDs may reduce effects. May block epinephrine effects. Excessive reduction of sympathetic activity with catecholamine-depleting drugs. Caution with clonidine withdrawal. Increased clearance with rifampin. Caution with CCBs, myocardial depressants, anesthesia, and antiarrhythmics. Digitalis glycosides and β-blockers slow atrioventricular conduction and decrease HR; concomitant use can increase the risk of bradycardia.

PREGNANCY: Category C, not for use in nursing.

MECHANISM OF ACTION: Bisoprolol: β_1-selective, cardioselective, adrenoreceptor-blocking agent; decreases HR, increases sinus node recovery time, prolongs AV-node refractory periods, and prolongs AV-nodal conduction with rapid atrial stimulation. HCTZ: Thiazide diuretic; affects renal tubular mechanisms of electrolyte reabsorption and increases excretion of Na^+ and Cl^-.

PHARMACOKINETICS: Absorption: Bisoprolol: Absolute bioavailability (80%); (2.5mg) C_{max}=9ng/mL, T_{max}=3 hrs. HCTZ: Well-absorbed; C_{max}=30ng/mL, T_{max}=2.5 hrs. **Distribution**: Bisoprolol: Plasma protein binding (30%). HCTZ: Plasma protein binding (40-68%). **Elimination:** Bisoprolol: $T_{1/2}$=7-15 hrs; urine (55% unchanged). HCTZ: $T_{1/2}$=4-10 hrs; urine (60% unchanged).

NURSING CONSIDERATIONS

Assessment: Assess for bradycardia, cardiogenic shock, 2nd- or 3rd-degree heart block, overt cardiac failure, impaired renal/hepatic function, bronchospastic disease, PVD, DM, thyrotoxicosis, anuria, sulfonamide hypersensitivity, history of allergy or bronchial asthma, parathyroid disease, possible drug interactions.

Monitoring: Monitor for cardiac failure, HTN, exacerbation of ischemia following abrupt withdrawal, bronchospastic disease, arrhythmias, CBC with platelet count and differential, hypersensitivity reactions, reversible mental depression, serum electrolytes periodically. Monitor for signs/symptoms of electrolyte imbalance, hyperglycemia, hyperuricemia or precipitation of gout, hypersensitivity reactions, and renal/hepatic dysfunction.

Patient Counseling: Instruct not to interrupt or d/c therapy without consulting physician. Notify physician if signs/symptoms of impending CHF or unexplained respiratory symptoms develop. Educate about signs/symptoms of adverse effects. Advise to exercise caution while operating machinery/driving. Advise to seek medical attention if symptoms of electrolyte imbalance (eg, dry mouth, thirst, weakness) or hypersensitivity/photosensitivity reactions occur. Inform diabetics that drug may mask symptoms of hypoglycemia; caution during treatment.

Administration: Oral route. **Storage**: 20-25°C (68-77°F). Dispense in tight container.

ZIAGEN RX

abacavir sulfate (GlaxoSmithKline)

Fatal hypersensitivity reactions, lactic acidosis, severe hepatomegaly with steatosis, including fatal cases reported. D/C if hypersensitivity reaction is suspected and do not restart. Patients who carry the HLA-B*5701 allele are at high risk for experiencing a hypersensitivity reaction.

THERAPEUTIC CLASS: Synthetic carbocyclic nucleoside analogue

INDICATIONS: Treatment of HIV-1 infection in combination with other antiretrovirals.

DOSAGE: *Adults:* 300mg bid or 600mg qd. Mild Hepatic Impairment: 200mg bid.
Pediatrics: >3 months: 8mg/kg bid. Max: 300mg bid. 14-21 kg: 150mg (1/2 tablet) bid. Max: 300mg/day. >21-<30 kg: 150mg (1/2 tablet) in AM, 300mg (1 tablet) in PM. Max: 450mg/day. ≥30 kg: 300mg bid. Max: 600mg/day.

HOW SUPPLIED: Sol: 20mg/mL [240mL]; Tab: 300mg* *scored

CONTRAINDICATIONS: Moderate or severe hepatic impairment.

WARNINGS/PRECAUTIONS: Register abacavir hypersensitive patients at 800-270-0425. Immune reconstitution syndrome and redistribution/accumulation of fat reported. Increased risk of myocardial infarction; caution in patients with underlying risk of coronary heart disease.

ADVERSE REACTIONS: Nausea, headache, malaise and fatigue, NV, dreams/sleep disorders, drug hypersensitivity, diarrhea, rashes, abdominal pain/gastritis/gastrointestinal signs and symptoms, depressive disorders, dizziness, musculoskeletal pain, bronchitis, fever and/or chills, ear/nose/throat infections, and viral respiratory infections.

INTERACTIONS: Decreased elimination with ethanol. Increase methadone dose with abacavir.

PREGNANCY: Category C, not for use in nursing.

MECHANISM OF ACTION: Carbocyclic nucleoside analogue; inhibits HIV-1 reverse transcriptase (RT) by competing with natural substrate dGTP and incorporating into viral DNA.

PHARMACOKINETICS: Absorption: Rapid; absolute bioavailabilty (83%). (BID dosing) C_{max} = 3mcg/mL, AUC_{0-12h}=6.02mcg•hr/mL. (QD dosing) C_{max}= 4.26mcg/mL, AUC=11.95mcg•hr/mL. **Distribution:** (IV) V_d=0.86L/kg; plasma protein binding (50%). **Metabolism:** Hepatic, via alcohol dehydrogenase and glucuronyl transferase. **Elimination:** Urine (1.2%); (QD dosing) $T_{1/2}$=1.54 hrs.

NURSING CONSIDERATIONS

Assessment: Assess for HLA-B* allele, moderate or severe hepatic impairment, risk factors for coronary heart disease (eg, hypertension, hyperlipidemia, diabetes mellitus, smoking) and possible drug interaction.

Monitoring: Monitor for signs/symptoms of hypersensitivity (eg, fever, rash, NV, diarrhea, generalized malaise, fatigue, dyspnea, cough), lactic acidosis, immune reconstitution syndrome, fat redistribution/accumulation, and hepatic dysfunction (eg, decompensation, failure).

Patient Counseling: Inform that treatment does not reduce risk of HIV transmission to others through sexual contact or blood contamination. Inform if treatment is interrupted, do not restart or replace with any drug containing abacavir to avoid more serious symptoms (eg, life-threatening hypotension, death). Seek medical attention if symptoms of hypersensitivity (eg, fever, rash, NV, diarrhea, generalized malaise, fatigue, dyspnea, cough), lactic acidosis, immune reconstitution syndrome, fat redistribution, and hepatic dysfunction (eg, decompensation, failure) occur.

Administration: Oral route. **Storage**: 20-25°C (68-77°F). Do not freeze. May be refrigerated.

ZIANA RX

clindamycin phosphate - tretinoin (Medicis)

THERAPEUTIC CLASS: Lincosamide derivative/retinoid

INDICATIONS: Topical treatment of acne vulgaris.

DOSAGE: *Adults:* Apply pea-sized amount to entire face qd at bedtime. Avoid eyes, mouth, angles of nose, or mucous membranes. Not for oral, ophthalmic, or intravaginal use.
Pediatrics: ≥12 yrs: Apply pea-sized amount to entire face qd at bedtime. Avoid eyes, mouth, angles of nose, or mucous membranes. Not for oral, ophthalmic, or intravaginal use.

HOW SUPPLIED: Gel: (Clindamycin-Tretinoin) 1.2%-0.025% [2g, 30g, 60g]

CONTRAINDICATIONS: Regional enteritis, ulcerative colitis, or history of antibiotic-associated colitis.

WARNINGS/PRECAUTIONS: May cause severe colitis; d/c if significant diarrhea occurs. Avoid exposure to sunlight and sunlamps; wear sunscreen daily.

ADVERSE REACTIONS: Nasopharyngitis, erythema, scaling, itching, burning.

INTERACTIONS: Caution with concomitant topical medications, medicated/abrasive soaps and cleansers, soaps/cosmetics with strong drying effect, products with high concentrations of alcohol, astringents, spices, or lime. Avoid with erythromycin-containing products. Caution with neuromuscular blocking agents.

PREGNANCY: Category C, not for use in nursing.

MECHANISM OF ACTION: Clindamycin: Lincosamide antibiotic; binds to 50S ribosomal subunits of susceptible bacteria and prevents elongation of peptide chains by interfering with peptidyl transfer, thereby suppressing bacterial protein synthesis. Found to have activity against *P.acnes*. Tretinoin: Retinoid; not established. Suspected to decrease cohesiveness of follicular epithelial cells with decreased microcomedo formation. Also responsible for stimulating miotic activity and increasing turnover of follicular epithelial cells, causing extrusion of comedones.

PHARMACOKINETICS: Absorption: Tretinoin: Percutaneous (minimal). **Distribution:** Orally and parenterally administered clindamycin found in breast milk. **Metabolism:** Tretinoin: 13-cis-retinoic acid and 4-oxo-13-cis-retinoic acid (metabolites).

NURSING CONSIDERATIONS

Assessment: Assess for regional enteritis, ulcerative colitis, or history of antibiotic-associated colitis. Assess use in pregnancy/nursing and for possible drug interactions.

Monitoring: Monitor for signs/symptoms of diarrhea, bloody diarrhea, and colitis (including pseudomembranous colitis). Perform stool cultures to identify *Clostridium difficile* and stool assay to identify *C.difficile* toxin. Monitor for signs/symptoms of skin irritation (eg, erythema, scaling, burning, stinging).

Patient Counseling: Instruct to wash face gently with mild soap and warm water at bedtime before applying. Advise not to use excessive amount; may cause skin irritation. Avoid washing face more than 2-3 times a day; may worsen acne. Advise to avoid exposure to sunlight/sunlamps; use sunscreen and protective clothing outdoors. Inform that weather extremes, such as wind or cold, may irritate skin during therapy.

Administration: Topical route. **Storage:** Store at room temperature, 15-30°C (59-86°F). Do not freeze. Keep away from heat and light.

ZINACEF RX

cefuroxime (GlaxoSmithKline)

THERAPEUTIC CLASS: Cephalosporin (2nd generation)

INDICATIONS: Treatment of septicemia; meningitis; gonorrhea; lower respiratory tract, urinary tract, skin and skin structure (SSSI), and bone and joint infections caused by susceptible strains of microorganisms. For preoperative and perioperative surgical prophylaxis.

DOSAGE: *Adults:* Usual: 750mg-1.5g q8h for 5-10 days. Uncomplicated Pneumonia and UTI/SSSI/Disseminated Gonococcal Infections: 750mg q8h. Severe/Complicated Infections: 1.5g q8h. Bone and Joint Infections: 1.5g q8h. Life-Threatening Infections/Infections With Susceptible Organisms: 1.5g q6h. Meningitis: Max: 3g q8h. Uncomplicated Gonococcal Infection: 1.5g IM single dose at 2 different sites with 1g PO probenecid. Surgical Prophylaxis: 1.5g IV 0.5-1 hr before incision, then 750mg IM/IV q8h with prolonged procedure. Open Heart Surgery (Perioperative): 1.5g IV at induction of anesthesia and q12h thereafter, for total of 6g. Renal Impairment: CrCl 10-20mL/min: 750mg q12h. CrCl <10mL/min: 750mg q24h. Hemodialysis: Give further dose at end of dialysis.
Pediatrics: >3 months: Usual: 50-100mg/kg/day in divided doses q6-8h. Severe Infections: 100mg/kg/day (not to exceed max adult dose). Bone and Joint Infections: 150mg/kg/day in divided doses q8h (not to exceed max adult dose). Meningitis: 200-240mg/kg/day IV in divided doses q6-8h. Renal Dysfunction: Modify dosing frequency consistent with adult recommendations.

HOW SUPPLIED: Inj: 750mg, 1.5g, 7.5g, 750mg/50mL, 1.5g/50mL

WARNINGS/PRECAUTIONS: Cross-sensitivity to PCNs and other cephalosporins may occur. *Clostridium difficile*-associated diarrhea reported, ranging in severity from mild diarrhea to fatal colitis. Monitor renal function. May result in overgrowth of nonsusceptible organisms. Caution with history of GI disease, particularly colitis. Hearing loss in peds being treated for meningitis. Risk of decreased prothrombin activity with renal or hepatic impairment, poor nutritional state, or protracted course of therapy. False (+) urine glucose with copper reduction tests and false (-) with ferricyanide test.

ADVERSE REACTIONS: Thrombophlebitis, GI symptoms, decreased Hgb and Hct, eosinophilia. Transient rise in SGOT, SGPT, alkaline phosphatase, bilirubin, and LDH.

INTERACTIONS: Possible nephrotoxicity with concomitant aminoglycosides. Caution with potent diuretics; may adversely affect renal function. May decrease prothrombin activity; caution with anticoagulants. May reduce efficacy of combined estrogen/progesterone oral contraceptives.

PREGNANCY: Category B, caution in nursing.

MECHANISM OF ACTION: 2nd-generation cephalosporin; inhibits cell-wall synthesis.

PHARMACOKINETICS: Absorption: C_{max}(750mg IM, IV)=27mcg/mL, 50mcg/mL; T_{max}(750mg IM, IV)=45 min, 15 min. **Distribution:** Plasma protein binding (50%). **Elimination**: Urine; $T_{1/2}$=80 min.

NURSING CONSIDERATIONS

Assessment: Assess for history of hypersensitivity to cephalosporins/PCNs, pregnancy status, possible drug interactions, renal impairment, colitis. Document indications for therapy, culture, and susceptibility testing.

Monitoring: Monitor for signs/symptoms of hypersensitivity reactions (eg, anaphylaxis, Stevens-Johnson syndrome), *C.difficile*-associated diarrhea, seizures, LFTs, CBC with platelet count and differential, renal function, PT, LDH, superinfections, hearing loss.

Patient Counseling: Inform therapy only treats bacterial, not viral, infections. Take as directed; skipping doses or not completing full course may decrease effectiveness and increase resistance. May experience diarrhea; notify physician if watery/bloody stools, superinfections, or hypersensitivity reactions occur.

Administration: IV/IM routes. Refer to PI for administration procedures.
Storage: 15-30°C (59-86°F). Protect from light (dry state).

ZINECARD — RX

dexrazoxane (Pharmacia & Upjohn)

THERAPEUTIC CLASS: EDTA derivative

INDICATIONS: To reduce the incidence and severity of cardiomyopathy associated with doxorubicin in women with metastatic breast cancer who received a cumulative doxorubicin dose of 300mg/m^2 and who will continue doxorubicin therapy.

DOSAGE: *Adults:* IV: 10:1 ratio of dexrazoxane:doxorubicin (eg, 500mg/m^2 dexrazoxane:50mg/m^2 doxorubicin). Hepatic Impairment: Reduce dose proportionally. Give by slow IV push or rapid IV infusion. Give doxorubicin within 30 min after start of infusion.

HOW SUPPLIED: Inj: 250mg, 500mg

CONTRAINDICATIONS: Chemotherapy regimens not containing an anthracycline.

WARNINGS/PRECAUTIONS: Not for use with initiation of doxorubicin therapy. Monitor cardiac function. May cause secondary malignancies. Obtain frequent CBCs. Caution with moderate or severe renal insufficiency; reduce dose by 50% if CrCl <40mL/min.

ADVERSE REACTIONS: Alopecia, nausea, vomiting, fatigue, malaise, anorexia, stomatitis, fever, infection, diarrhea, pain on injection, sepsis, neurotoxicity, streaking/erythema.

INTERACTIONS: Avoid use during the initiation of FAC (fluorouracil, doxorubicin, cyclophosphamide) therapy. Additive myelosuppression with other chemotherapies.

PREGNANCY: Category C, not for use in nursing.

MECHANISM OF ACTION: EDTA derivative; suspected to interfere with iron-mediated free radical generation.

PHARMACOKINETICS: Absorption: C_{max}(500mg/m²)=36.5mcg/ml. **Distribution**: V_d=25L/m². **Elimination:** Urine (42%).

NURSING CONSIDERATIONS

Assessment: Assess renal/hepatic function, CBC with differential and platelet count, LVEF, pregnancy status, and for possible drug interactions. Should not be used with chemotherapy regimens that do not contain an anthracycline.

Monitoring: Monitor for myelosuppression, abnormalities in hepatic/renal function, neurotoxicity, infections, stomatitis, diarrhea, LVEF.

Patient Counseling: Instruct to avoid nursing during therapy. Discuss signs/symptoms of adverse side effects and advise to report any if they develop.

Administration: IV route. Refer to PI for details. **Storage:** 25°C (77°F); excursions permitted to 15-30°C (59-86°F). Reconstituted solutions stable for 6 hrs at room temperature or 2-8°C (36-46°F). Discard unused solutions.

ZITHROMAX RX

azithromycin (Pfizer)

THERAPEUTIC CLASS: Macrolide

INDICATIONS: Treatment of the following infections caused by susceptible microorganisms: (PO) Acute bacterial exacerbations of COPD, acute bacterial sinusitis (ABS), community-acquired pneumonia (CAP), pharyngitis/tonsillitis, uncomplicated skin and skin structure, urethritis/cervicitis, genital ulcer disease (men), acute otitis media. Prevention (alone) or treatment (with ethambutol) of disseminated *Mycobacterium avium* complex (MAC) disease in advanced HIV infection. (IV) CAP and pelvic inflammatory disease (PID).

DOSAGE: *Adults:* PO: CAP/Pharyngitis/Tonsillitis (2nd-line therapy)/SSSI: 500mg on Day 1, then 250mg qd on Days 2-5. COPD: 500mg qd for 3 days or 500 mg on Day 1, then 250ng qd on Days 2-5. ABS: 500mg qd for 3 days. Genital Ulcer Disease and Nongonococcal Urethritis/Cervicitis: 1g single dose. Gonococcal Urethritis/Cervicitis: 2g single dose. MAC Prophylaxis: 1200mg once weekly. MAC Treatment: 600mg qd with ethambutol 15mg/kg/day. IV: CAP: 500mg qd for at least 2 days, then 500mg PO qd to complete 7-10 day course. PID: 500mg qd for 1-2 days, then 250mg PO qd to complete 7 day course.

Pediatrics: Sus: Otitis Media: ≥6 months: 30mg/kg single dose; 10mg/kg qd for 3 days; or 10mg/kg qd on Day 1, then 5mg/kg qd on Days 2-5. ABS: ≥6 months: 10mg/kg qd for 3 days. CAP: ≥6 months: 10mg/kg qd on Day 1, then 5mg/kg qd on Days 2-5. Sus/Tab: Pharyngitis/Tonsillitis: ≥2 yrs: 12mg/kg qd for 5 days. 1g sus not for pediatric use.

HOW SUPPLIED: Inj: 500mg; Sus: 100mg/5mL [15mL], 200mg/5mL [15mL, 22.5mL, 30mL], 1g/pkt [3[s], 10[s]]; Tab: 250mg [Z-PAK, 6 tabs], 500mg [TRI-PAK, 3 tabs], 600mg

WARNINGS/PRECAUTIONS: D/C if allergic reaction occurs. Oral therapy only for CAP of mild severity. Hypersensitivity reactions may recur after initial successful symptomatic treatment. *Clostridium difficile*-associated diarrhea reported. Caution with renal/hepatic dysfunction. 1g sus not for pediatric use.

ADVERSE REACTIONS: Diarrhea/loose stools, nausea, abdominal pain, taste/smell perversion.

INTERACTIONS: Monitor theophylline, terfenadine, cyclosporine, hexobarbital, phenytoin, warfarin. May increase digoxin, carbamazepine levels. Potentiates triazolam. Aluminum- and magnesium-containing antacids may reduce PO levels. Acute ergot toxicity may occur with ergotamine or dihydroergotamine. Monitor for side effects (eg, liver enzyme abnormalities, hearing impairment) with nelfinavir.

PREGNANCY: Category B, caution in nursing.

MECHANISM OF ACTION: Macrolide; inhibits protein synthesis by binding 50S ribosomal subunits of susceptible organisms.

PHARMACOKINETICS: Absorption: Administration of variable doses resulted in different parameters. **Distribution:** Plasma protein binding (7-51%). **Elimination:** Biliary (major), urine; $T_{1/2}$=68 hrs.

NURSING CONSIDERATIONS

Assessment: Assess for nosocomial infections, CF, immunodeficiency states, functional asplenia, LFTs, prolonged QT interval, and possible drug interactions. Document indications for therapy, culture and susceptibility testing.

Monitoring: Monitor for signs/symptoms of hypersensitivity reactions (eg, angioedema, Stevens-Johnson syndrome), *C. difficile*-associated diarrhea, anemia, arrhythmias, jaundice, fungal dermatitis, LFTs, hearing loss, seizures.

Patient Counseling: Caution not to take aluminum- or magnesium-containing antacids. Inform that therapy treats bacterial, not viral, infections. Take as directed; skipping doses or not completing full course may decrease effectiveness and increase resistance. Inform may experience diarrhea; notify physician if watery/bloody stools, superinfection, or hypersensitivity reactions occur.

Administration: Oral/IV routes. **Storage:** Store tabs between 15-30°C (59-86°F). Store dry powder below 30°C (86°F); reconstituted sus between 5-30°C (41-86°F).

ZMAX — RX

azithromycin (Pfizer)

THERAPEUTIC CLASS: Macrolide

INDICATIONS: Treatment of community-acquired pneumonia in adults and children >6 months and mild-to-moderate acute bacterial sinusitis in adults caused by susceptible bacteria.

DOSAGE: *Adults:* 2g single dose. Take on empty stomach (1 hr before or 2 hrs after a meal).
Pediatrics: >6 months: 60mg/kg single dose. Take on empty stomach (1 hr before or 2 hrs after a meal). Max: 2g single dose. Patients weighing >34kg should receive the adult dose. See PI for specific information of pediatric dosage.

HOW SUPPLIED: Sus, Extended-Release: 2g, 27mg/mL

CONTRAINDICATIONS: Hypersensitivity to macrolide or ketolide antibiotics.

WARNINGS/PRECAUTIONS: Rare reports of angioedema, anaphylaxis, and dermatologic reactions including Stevens-Johnson syndrome and toxic epidermal necrolysis. D/C if allergic reaction occurs. Hypersensitivity reactions may recur after initial successful symptomatic treatment. *Clostridium difficile*-associated diarrhea reported. Caution with renal/hepatic dysfunction and patients with increased risk for prolonged cardiac repolarization. Exacerbation and new onset of symptoms of myasthenia gravis reported.

ADVERSE REACTIONS: Diarrhea/loose stools, NV, abdominal pain, headache, and taste/smell perversion.

INTERACTIONS: Monitor for azithromycin side effects (eg, liver enzyme abnormalities, hearing impairment) with nelfinavir. Monitor cyclosporine, hexobarbital, phenytoin, warfarin concentrations. May increase digoxin levels. Acute ergot toxicity may occur with ergotamine or dihydroergotamine.

PREGNANCY: Category B, caution in nursing.

MECHANISM OF ACTION: Macrolide antibiotic; inhibits protein synthesis by binding 50S ribosomal subunits of susceptible organisms.

PHARMACOKINETICS: Absorption: Oral administration of variable doses resulted in different parameters. **Distribution:** V_d=31.1L/kg; plasma protein binding (7-51%). **Elimination:** Bile (major route), urine; $T_{1/2}$=59 hrs.

NURSING CONSIDERATIONS

Assessment: Assess LFTs, prolonged QT interval, and possible drug interactions. Document indications for therapy, culture and susceptibility testing.

Monitoring: Monitor for signs/symptoms of hypersensitivity reactions (eg, angioedema, Stevens-Johnson syndrome), *C.difficile*-associated diarrhea, neutropenia, arrhythmia, jaundice, LFTs, hearing loss, seizures, and myasthenia gravis.

Patient Counseling: Inform to take on empty stomach. Instruct to immediately report any signs of allergic reaction. Contact physician if vomiting occurs within 1st hr. Advise to keep bottle tightly closed, use within 12 hrs of reconstitution, shake well before use, and to consume entire contents of bottle. Instruct that drug may be taken without regard to magnesium- or aluminum-containing antacids. Inform that therapy treats bacterial, not viral, infections. Take as directed; skipping doses or not completing full course may decrease effectiveness and increase resistance. Inform may experience diarrhea; notify physician if watery/bloody stools, superinfection, or hypersensitivity reactions occur.

Administration: Oral route. Reconstitute with 60mL water. Shake well.
Storage: Store dry powder at or below 30°C (86°F). Reconstituted sus should be consumed within 12 hrs and stored at 25°C (77°F); excursions permitted to 15-30°C (59-86°F). Do not refrigerate or freeze.

Zocor RX

simvastatin (Merck)

THERAPEUTIC CLASS: HMG-CoA reductase inhibitor

INDICATIONS: May initiate with diet in patients with, or at high-risk for, coronary heart disease (CHD). In high risk patients with CHD, diabetes, peripheral vessel disease, history of stroke or other cerebrovascular disease, to reduce risk of total mortality by reducing CHD deaths, risk of non-fatal MI and stroke, need for revascularization procedures. To reduce elevated total-C, LDL-C, Apo B, TG, and increase HDL-C in primary hypercholesterolemia (heterozygous familial and nonfamilial) and mixed dyslipidemia (Types IIa and IIb). To treat hypertriglyceridemia (Type IV) and primary dysbetalipoproteinemia (Type III). To reduce total-C, LDL-C in homozygous familial hypercholesterolemia as adjunct to other lipid-lowering agents or if such treatments are unavailable. To reduce total-C, LDL-C, Apo B in adolescents 10-17 yrs old, at least 1 yr postmenarche, with heterozygous familial hypercholesterolemia. To reduce elevated LDL-C, TG in Type IIb hyperlipidemia.

DOSAGE: *Adults:* Initial: 20-40mg qpm. Usual: 5-80mg/day. Titrate: Adjust at ≥4-week intervals. High Risk for CHD Events: Initial: 40mg/day. Homozygous Familial Hypercholesterolemia: 40mg qpm or 80mg/day given as 20mg bid plus 40mg qpm. Concomitant Cyclosporine: Initial: 5mg/day. Max: 10mg/day. Concomitant Gemfibrozil (try to avoid): Max: 10mg/day. Concomitant Amiodarone/Verapamil: Max: 20mg/day. Severe Renal Insufficiency: 5mg/day; monitor closely.
Pediatrics: Heterozygous Familial Hypercholesterolemia: 10-17 yrs (at least 1 yr postmenarchal): Initial: 10mg qpm. Usual: 10-40mg/day. Titrate: Adjust at ≥4-week intervals. Max: 40mg/day.

HOW SUPPLIED: Tab: 5mg, 10mg, 20mg, 40mg, 80mg

CONTRAINDICATIONS: Active liver disease, unexplained persistent elevations of serum transaminases, pregnancy, nursing mothers.

WARNINGS/PRECAUTIONS: Caution with heavy alcohol use, severe renal insufficiency or history of hepatic disease. Monitor LFTs prior to therapy, periodically thereafter for 1st yr, or until 1 yr after last dose elevation (additional test at 3 months for 80mg dose). D/C if AST or ALT ≥3x ULN persists, if myopathy is suspected or diagnosed, a few days prior to major surgery. Rhabdomyolysis (rare), myopathy reported.

ADVERSE REACTIONS: Abdominal pain, headache, CK and transaminase elevations, constipation, upper respiratory infection, hepatic failure.

INTERACTIONS: Avoid use with concomitant itraconazole, ketoconazole, erythromycin, clarithromycin, telithromycin, HIV protease inhibitors, nefazodone, grapefruit juice (>1 quart/day); increased risk of myopathy/rhabdomyolysis. Max 10mg/day with gemfibrozil, cyclosporine, danazol. Max

20mg/day with amiodarone, verapamil. Caution with other fibrates, ≥1g/day of niacin. Monitor digoxin, warfarin.

PREGNANCY: Category X, not for use in nursing.

MECHANISM OF ACTION: HMG-CoA reductase inhibitor; lipid-lowering agent.

PHARMACOKINETICS: Absorption: T_{max}=1.3-2.4 hrs. **Distribution:** Plasma protein binding (95%); crosses blood-brain barrier. **Metabolism:** Liver (1st pass); β-hydroxyacid; 6'hydroxy. 6'-hydroxymethyl, 6'-exomethylene (active metabolites). **Elimination:** Feces (60%), urine (13%).

NURSING CONSIDERATIONS

Assessment: Assess for secondary causes of hypercholesterolemia (eg, hypothyroidism, nephrotic syndrome, dysproteinemias, obstructive liver disease, other drug therapy, alcoholism), active liver disease or unexplained elevations in serum transaminases, renal insufficiencies, pregnancy/nursing status. Obtain baseline lipid profile (total-C, HDL-C, TG) and LFTs. Assess for drug interactions.

Monitoring: Monitor for signs/symptoms of myopathy (eg, muscle pain, tenderness, weakness), rhabdomyolysis, liver dysfunction, and CNS toxicity (eg, optic nerve degeneration, CNS vascular lesions). Periodically monitor lipid levels (LDL-C), creatine kinase levels (CK), and LFTs. Patients titrated to 80mg dose should have LFTs evaluated prior to titration, 3 months after titration, and periodically thereafter.

Patient Counseling: Recommend standard cholesterol-lowering diet. Counsel to contact physician immediately if unexplained muscle pain, tenderness, or weakness occurs. Advise about possible drug interactions and interaction with grapefruit juice. Notify all physicians of all concurrently taken medications. Counsel about risks during pregnancy/nursing.

Administration: Oral route. **Storage:** 5-30°C (41-86°F).

ZOFRAN RX

ondansetron (GlaxoSmithKline)

THERAPEUTIC CLASS: 5-HT_3 receptor antagonist

INDICATIONS: (Inj) Prevention of nausea and vomiting associated with initial and repeat courses of emetogenic cancer chemotherapy, including high-dose cisplatin. Prevention of postoperative nausea and/or vomiting. (Sol/Tab) Prevention of nausea and vomiting associated with: highly emetogenic cancer chemotherapy, including cisplatin ≥50mg/m²; initial and repeat courses of moderately emetogenic cancer chemotherapy; and radiotherapy in patients receiving either total body irradiation, single high-dose fraction to the abdomen, or daily fractions to the abdomen. Prevention of postoperative nausea and/or vomiting.

DOSAGE: *Adults:* Prevention of Chemotherapy-Induced Nausea/Vomiting: (Inj) 32mg single dose or three 0.15mg/kg doses, 1st dose 30 min before chemotherapy, then 4 and 8 hrs after 1st dose. Prevention of Nausea/Vomiting Associated With Highly Emetogenic Cancer Chemotherapy: (Tab) 24mg single dose tab 30 min before chemotherapy. Prevention of Nausea/Vomiting Associated With Moderately Emetogenic Cancer Chemotherapy: (Sol/Tab) 8mg bid, 1st dose 30 min before chemotherapy, then 8 hrs later, then bid for 1-2 days after chemotherapy. Prevention of Post-Op Nausea/Vomiting: (Inj) 4mg IM/IV immediately before anesthesia or post-op after surgery if nausea or vomiting occurs. (Sol/Tab) 16mg 1 hr before anesthesia. Prevention of Nausea/Vomiting Associated with Radiation Therapy: (Sol/Tab) Usual: 8mg tid. Total Body Irradiation: 8mg 1-2 hrs before therapy daily. Single High-Dose Therapy To Abdomen: 8mg 1-2 hrs before therapy then q8h after 1st dose for 1-2 days after completion of therapy. Daily Fractionated Therapy To Abdomen: 8mg 1-2 hrs before therapy then q8h after 1st dose. Severe Hepatic Dysfunction (Child-Pugh ≥10): Max: 8mg/day IV single dose infused over 15 min, start 30 min before chemotherapy or 8mg/day PO.
Pediatrics: Prevention of Chemotherapy-Induced Nausea/Vomiting: (Inj)

6 months-18 yrs: Three 0.15mg/kg doses, 1st dose 30 min before chemotherapy, then 4 and 8 hrs after the 1st dose. (Sol/Tab) Prevention of Nausea/Vomiting Associated With Moderately Emetogenic Cancer Chemotherapy: ≥12 yrs: 8mg bid, 1st dose 30 min before chemotherapy, then 8mg 8 hrs later, then bid for 1-2 days. 4-11 yrs: 4mg tid, 1st dose 30 min before chemotherapy, then 4 and 8 hrs after 1st dose, then tid for 1-2 days. Prevention of Post-Op Nausea/Vomiting: (Inj) >12 yrs: 4mg IM/IV immediately before anesthesia or post-op after surgery if nausea or vomiting occurs. 1 month-12 yrs: ≤40kg: 0.1mg/kg single dose. >40kg: 4mg single dose. Severe Hepatic Dysfunction: Max: 8mg/day IV single dose infused over 15 min, start 30 min before chemotherapy or 8mg/day PO.

HOW SUPPLIED: Inj: 2mg/mL, 32mg/50mL; Sol: 4mg/5mL [50mL]; Tab: 4mg, 8mg, 24mg; Tab, Disintegrating: 4mg, 8mg

WARNINGS/PRECAUTIONS: Hypersensitivity reactions reported in those hypersensitive to other 5-HT_3 receptor antagonists. Transient ECG changes including QT interval prolongation reported with IV administration. May mask progressive ileus or gastric distension. Orally disintegrating tabs contain phenylalanine; caution in phenylketonurics.

ADVERSE REACTIONS: Headache, diarrhea, dizziness, drowsiness, malaise/fatigue, constipation, LFT abnormalities.

INTERACTIONS: Ondansetron is metabolized by CYP450 enzymes; inducers or inhibitors of these enzymes may change the clearance and half-life of ondansetron.

PREGNANCY: Category B, caution in nursing.

MECHANISM OF ACTION: Serotonin 5-HT_3 receptor blocker; not established. Blocks 5-HT_3 receptors from serotonin which may stimulate vagal afferents through 5-HT_3 receptors which initiate vomiting reflex.

PHARMACOKINETICS: Absorption: IV and oral administration of variable ages resulted in different parameters. **Distribution:** Plasma protein binding (70-76%). **Metabolism:** Hydroxylation, conjugation. **Elimination:** Urine.

NURSING CONSIDERATIONS

Assessment: Assess for possible drug interactions, PKU, and hepatic impairment.

Monitoring: Monitor for signs/symptoms of hypersensitivity reactions, progressive ileus, and gastric distention.

Patient Counseling: Instruct not to remove tab from blister until just prior to dosing; do not push through foil. Remove gently and immediately place on tongue to dissolve and swallow. Inform that tab contains phenylalanine. Advise to seek medical attention if symptoms of hypersensitivity reactions, progressive ileus, or gastric distention occur.

Administration: IM/IV/Oral routes. **Storage:** Inj/Tab: 2-30°C (36-86°F). Protect from light. Avoid excessive heat. Protect from freezing. Sol: 15-30°C (59-86°F). Protect from light; store upright.

ZOLADEX 1-MONTH RX

goserelin acetate (AstraZeneca)

THERAPEUTIC CLASS: Synthetic gonadotropin releasing hormone analog

INDICATIONS: Palliative treatment of advanced prostate cancer and advanced breast cancer in pre-and perimenopausal women. Adjunct to and during radiotherapy and in combination with flutamide for management of locally confined Stage T2b-T4 (Stage B2-C) prostate cancer. Management of endometriosis, including pain relief and reduction of endometriotic lesions. Use as an endometrial thinning agent prior to ablation for dysfunctional uterine bleeding.

DOSAGE: *Adults:* Inject SQ into anterior abdominal wall below navel line. Advanced Prostate/Breast Cancers: 3.6mg every 28 days. Stage B2-C Prostate Cancer: 3.6mg starting 8 weeks before radiotherapy then 10.8mg formulation 28 days after 1st injection or 3.6mg at 28-day intervals for 4 doses (2 before and 2 during radiotherapy). Endometriosis: 3.6mg every 28 days for up to 6 months. Endometrial Thinning: 3.6mg then surgery 4 weeks later, or 3.6mg for 2 doses (4 weeks apart) followed by surgery 2-4 weeks after 2nd dose.

HOW SUPPLIED: Implant: 3.6mg

CONTRAINDICATIONS: Pregnancy, nursing.

WARNINGS/PRECAUTIONS: Exclude pregnancy before initiating therapy. Premenopausal women should use nonhormonal contraception during and 12 weeks post-therapy. Worsening of symptoms of prostate and breast cancer with initial therapy. Ureteral obstruction and spinal cord compression reported with prostate cancer. Temporary increases in bone pain may occur. Ovarian cysts reported. Hypercalcemia reported in prostate and breast cancer patients with bone metastases. May increase cervical resistance. Hypersensitivity, antibody formation, and acute anaphylactic reactions may occur.

ADVERSE REACTIONS: (Males) Hot flashes, sexual dysfunction, decreased erections, lower urinary tract symptoms, lethargy, pain (worsened in the first 30 days), edema, URI, rash, sweating, diarrhea, nausea. (Females, Endometriosis Treatment) Hot flashes, vaginitis, emotional lability, decreased libido, sweating, depression, headache, acne, breast atrophy. (Breast Cancer Treatment) Hot flashes, tumor flare, nausea, edema, malaise/fatigue/lethargy, vomiting.

INTERACTIONS: Ovarian hyperstimulation syndrome reported when used concomitantly with other gonadotropins.

PREGNANCY: Category X (endometriosis and endometrial thinning), Category D (breast cancer), not for use in nursing.

MECHANISM OF ACTION: Synthetic analog of luteinizing hormone-releasing hormone (LHRH); acts as potent inhibitor of pituitary gonadotropin secretion. In males, causes initial increase in serum LH and FSH levels, causing increase in testosterone. In females, causes decrease in serum estradiol levels consistent with postmenopausal state, reduction of ovarian size and function, reduction in size of uterus and mammary gland, and regression of sex hormone-responsive tumors.

PHARMACOKINETICS: Absorption: C_{max}=2.84ng/mL (male), 1.46ng/mL (female); T_{max}=12-15 days (male), 8-22 days (female); AUC=27.8ng•hr/mL (male), 18.5ng•hr/mL (female). **Distribution:** V_d=44.1L (male), 20.3L (female); plasma protein binding (27.3%). **Metabolism:** Liver. **Elimination:** Urine: 90% (20% unchanged); $T_{1/2}$=4.2 hrs (male), 2.3 hrs (female).

NURSING CONSIDERATIONS

Assessment: Assess for endometriosis, serum testosterone levels, PSA, pregnancy status. Note other diseases/conditions and drug therapies.

Monitoring: Monitor for ureteral obstruction, spinal cord compression, renal impairment, BMD, hypersensitivity reactions, pituitary apoplexy, sexual dysfunction, serum cholesterol levels.

Patient Counseling: Counsel about potential side effects; seek medical attention if any occur.

Administration: SQ route. Inject into anterior abdominal wall below navel line. **Storage:** Room temperature; do not exceed 25°C (77°F).

ZOLADEX 3-MONTH — RX

goserelin acetate (AstraZeneca)

THERAPEUTIC CLASS: Synthetic gonadotropin releasing hormone analog

INDICATIONS: Palliative treatment of advanced prostate cancer. Adjunct to radiotherapy and flutamide for management of locally confined Stage T2b-T4 (Stage B2-C) prostate cancer.

DOSAGE: *Adults:* Inject SQ into anterior abdominal wall below navel line. Advanced Prostate Cancer: 10.8mg every 12 weeks. Stage B2-C Prostate Cancer: 3.6mg depot formulation 8 weeks before radiotherapy then 10.8mg 28 days after 1st injection.

HOW SUPPLIED: Implant: 10.8mg

CONTRAINDICATIONS: Pregnancy, 10.8mg implant is not indicated in women.

WARNINGS/PRECAUTIONS: Worsening of symptoms of prostate cancer with initial therapy. Ureteral obstruction and spinal cord compression reported. Temporary increase in bone pain may occur. Hypersensitivity, antibody formation, and acute anaphylactic reactions may occur.

ADVERSE REACTIONS: Hot flashes, sexual dysfunction, decreased erections, osteoporosis, pain, asthenia, gynecomastia.

PREGNANCY: Category X, not for use in nursing.

MECHANISM OF ACTION: Synthetic analog of luteinizing hormone-releasing hormone (LHRH); acts as potent inhibitor of pituitary gonadotropin secretion. In males, causes initial increase in serum LH and FSH levels, causing increase in testosterone. In females, causes decrease in serum estradiol levels consistent with postmenopausal state, reduction of ovarian size and function, reduction in size of uterus and mammary gland, and regression of sex hormone-responsive tumors.

PHARMACOKINETICS: Absorption: C_{max}=8.85ng/mL; T_{max}=1.8 hrs. **Distribution:** V_d=44.1 L; plasma protein binding (27%). **Metabolism:** Hydrolysis of C-terminal amino acids. **Elimination:** Urine (90%, 20% unchanged); $T_{1/2}$=4.16 hrs.

NURSING CONSIDERATIONS

Assessment: Assess serum testosterone levels, PSA, DM, CVD. Note other diseases/conditions and drug therapies.

Monitoring: Monitor for ureteral obstruction, spinal cord compression, renal impairment, BMD, hypersensitivity reactions, pituitary apoplexy, sexual dysfunction, serum cholesterol levels, CVD, CBC.

Patient Counseling: Counsel about potential side effects; seek medical attention if any occur.

Administration: SQ route. Inject into anterior abdominal wall below navel line. **Storage:** Room temperature; do not exceed 25°C (77°F).

ZOLINZA RX

vorinostat (Merck)

THERAPEUTIC CLASS: Histone deacetylase inhibitor

INDICATIONS: Treatment of cutaneous manifestations in patients with cutaneous T-cell lymphoma who have progressive, persistent, or recurrent disease on or following two systemic therapies.

DOSAGE: *Adults:* 400mg PO qd with food. Intolerant to Therapy: May reduce dose to 300mg PO qd with food. If necessary, may further reduce dose to 300mg PO qd with food for 5 consecutive days each week.

HOW SUPPLIED: Cap: 100mg

WARNINGS/PRECAUTIONS: Pulmonary embolism and DVT reported; monitor for signs and symptoms. Dose-related thrombocytopenia and anemia may occur; consider dose modification or discontinuation. GI disturbances reported. Hyperglycemia observed; monitor glucose levels. QTc prolongation reported; monitor electrolytes and ECGs at baseline and periodically during treatment. Monitor CBC and chemistry tests every 2 weeks during first 2 months of therapy and monthly thereafter.

ADVERSE REACTIONS: Diarrhea, fatigue, nausea, thrombocytopenia, anorexia, dysgeusia, decreased weight, muscle spasms, alopecia, dry mouth, increased SrCr, chills, vomiting, constipation, dizziness.

INTERACTIONS: Prolongation of PT and INR observed with coumarin-derivative anticoagulants; monitor closely. Severe thrombocytopenia and GI bleeding reported with concomitant use of other histone deacetylase inhibitors (eg, valproic acid); monitor platelet count every 2 weeks for the first two months of therapy.

PREGNANCY: Category D, not for use in nursing.

MECHANISM OF ACTION: Histone deacetylase inhibitor; inhibits activity of histone deacetylases (HDAC) allowing for accumulation of acetyl groups on the histone lysine residues, resulting in open chromatin structure and transcriptional activation.

PHARMACOKINETICS: Absorption: Fasted: C_{max}=1.2μM, T_{max}=1.5 hrs, AUC=4.2μM•hr. Fed: C_{max}=1.2μM, T_{max}=4 hrs, AUC=6.0μM•hr. **Distribution:** Plasma protein binding (71%). **Metabolism:** Liver, via glucuronidation and β-oxidation. **Elimination:** Urine (unchanged); $T_{1/2}$=2 hrs.

NURSING CONSIDERATIONS

Assessment: Assess for congenital long QT syndrome, intake of anti-arrhythmics (or other medicinal products that may lead to QT prolongation), pre-existing renal impairment, hypokalemia, hypomagnesemia, fluid imbalance, and cardiac symptoms.

Monitoring: Monitor for PE, DVT, thrombocytopenia, anemia, NV, diarrhea, anorexia, weight decrease, hyperglycemia, GI bleeding. Monitor serum glucose, CBC, platelet count, electrolytes, glucose, and SrCr every 2 weeks for first 2 months. Obtain baseline and periodic ECGs.

Patient Counseling: Counsel to take with food, not to open or crush, and to drink at least 2L of fluid per day to prevent dehydration. Instruct to promptly report any adverse effects (eg, NV, diarrhea, weight loss, fatigue, chills, dry mouth, dysgeusia, unusual bleeding), or if signs of DVT develop.

Administration: Oral route. **Storage:** 20-25°C (68-77°F); excursions permitted to 15-30°C (59-86°F).

ZOLOFT — RX

sertraline HCl (Pfizer)

Antidepressants increased the risk of suicidal thinking and behavior (suicidality) in short-term studies in children, adolescents, and young adults with major depressive disorder (MDD) and other psychiatric disorders. Sertraline HCl is not approved for use in pediatric patients except for patients with obsessive compulsive disorder (OCD).

THERAPEUTIC CLASS: Selective serotonin reuptake inhibitor

INDICATIONS: Treatment of major depressive disorder (MDD), social anxiety disorder (SAD), obsessive compulsive disorder (OCD), panic disorder with or without agoraphobia, premenstrual dysphoric disorder (PMDD) and post-traumatic stress disorder (PTSD).

DOSAGE: *Adults:* MDD/OCD: 50mg qd. Titrate: Adjust dose at 1 week intervals. Max: 200mg/day. Panic Disorder/PTSD/SAD: Initial: 25mg qd. Titrate: Increase to 50mg qd after 1 week. Adjust dose at 1 week intervals. Max: 200mg/day. PMDD: Initial: 50mg qd continuous or limited to luteal phase of cycle. Titrate: Increase 50mg/cycle if needed up to 150mg/day for continuous or 100mg/day for luteal phase dosing. If 100mg/day is established for luteal phase dosing, a 50mg/day titration step for 3 days should take place at the beginning of each luteal phase dosing period. Hepatic Impairment: Use lower or less frequent doses. Dilute sol with 4oz water, ginger ale, lemon/lime soda, lemonade or orange juice. Take immediately after mixing.
Pediatrics: OCD: Initial: 6-12 yrs: 25mg qd. 13-17 yrs: 50mg qd. Titrate: Adjust dose at 1 week intervals. Max: 200mg/day. Hepatic Impairment: Use lower or less frequent doses. Dilute sol with 4oz water, ginger ale, lemon/lime soda, lemonade or orange juice. Take immediately after mixing.

HOW SUPPLIED: Sol: 20mg/mL [60mL]; Tab: 25mg*, 50mg*, 100mg* *scored

CONTRAINDICATIONS: Concomitant use of MAOIs or pimozide. Concomitant disulfiram with solution.

WARNINGS/PRECAUTIONS: Avoid abrupt withdrawal. May increase risk of bleeding events. Activation of mania/hypomania, SIADH, hyponatremia, altered platelet function reported. Caution with diseases or conditions that could affect hemodynamic responses or metabolism, seizure disorder, suicidal tendensies. Decrease appetite and weight loss reported. Caution in third trimester of pregnancy due to risk of serious neonatal complications. Serotonin syndrome may occur. Monitor for clinical worsening and/or suicidality, especially at initiation of therapy or dose changes.

ADVERSE REACTIONS: Ejaculation failure, dry mouth, increased sweating, somnolence, tremor, anorexia, dizziness, headache, vomiting, diarrhea, dyspepsia, nausea, agitation, insomnia, nervousness, abnormal vision.

INTERACTIONS: See Contraindications. Avoid alcohol, tryptophan, other SNRIs, and SSRIs. Caution with other centrally acting drugs, TCAs. May shift concentrations with plasma-bound drugs (eg, warfarin, digitoxin). May alter warfarin effects. Increased levels with cimetidine. Decreases clearance of tolbutamide. Rare reports of weakness, hyperreflexia, incoordination with an SSRI and sumatriptan. May potentiate drugs metabolized by CYP2D6 (eg, TCAs, Type 1C antiarrhythmics). Monitor lithium. Caution with OTC products. May induce metabolism of cisapride. Increase risk of bleeding with NSAIDs, ASA, warfarin. Concomitant use of serotonergic drugs and with drugs that impair metabolism of serotonin may cause serotonin syndrome. Caution with other agents that may affect serotonergic neurotransmitter systems (eg, triptans, linezolid, tramadol, or ST. John's Wort).

PREGNANCY: Category C, caution in nursing.

MECHANISM OF ACTION: SSRI; inhibits CNS neuronal uptake of serotonin.

PHARMACOKINETICS: Absorption: T_{max}=4.5-8.4 hrs. **Distribution:** Plasma protein binding (98%). **Metabolism:** Liver (extensive). **Elimination:** Feces (12-14% unchanged), urine (minor); $T_{1/2}$=26 hrs.

NURSING CONSIDERATIONS

Assessment: Assess for risk of bipolar disorder, history of seizures, disease/condition that alters metabolism or hemodynamic response, hepatic/renal impairment, MAOI, thioridazine, or pimozide therapy, renal/hepatic impairment, pregnancy/nursing status, and possible drug interactions.

Monitoring: Monitor for worsening of depression, emergence of suicidal ideation and behavior (suicidality), or unusual changes in behavior. Monitor for possible serotonin syndrome and hyponatremia (eg, headache, difficulty concentrating, memory impairment, confusion, weakness, and unsteadiness, which may lead to falls), and NMS-like reactions. Monitor platelets, body weight, Na^+, and uric acid.

Patient Counseling: Advise to avoid alcohol. Seek medical attention for symptoms of serotonin syndrome (mental status changes, tachycardia, hyperthermia, NV, diarrhea, incoordination), abnormal bleeding (eg, NSAIDs or ASA), hyponatremia, activation of mania, seizures, clinical worsening (suicidal ideation, unusual changes in behavior) and discontinuation symptoms (irritability, agitation, dizziness, anxiety, headache, insomnia). May cause motor/mental skills impairment; use caution when operating machinery/driving. May notice improvement in 1-4 weeks; continue therapy as directed. Notify physician if pregnant/intend to become pregnant, or breastfeeding. Counsel about benefits and risks of therapy. Inform physician if taking, or plan to take any over-the-counter prescriptions.

Administration: Oral route. Mix sol with 4oz water, ginger ale, lemon/lime soda, lemonade, or orange juice. Do not mix with anything other than liquids listed. Dose should be taken immediately after mixing. **Storage:** 25°C (77°F); excursions permitted to 15-30°C (59-86°F).

Zolpimist RX

zolpidem tartrate (NovaDel Pharma)

THERAPEUTIC CLASS: Imidazopyridine hypnotic

INDICATIONS: Short-term treatment of insomnia characterized by difficulties with sleep initiation.

DOSAGE: *Adults:* Individualize dose. 10mg qhs. Max: 10mg/day. Elderly/Debilitated/Hepatic Insufficiency: 5mg qhs.

HOW SUPPLIED: Spray: 5mg/spray [8.2g]

WARNINGS/PRECAUTIONS: Evaluate for primary psychiatric and/or medical illness if insomnia fails to remit after 7-10 days of treatment. Severe anaphylactic and anaphylactoid reactions reported. Visual/auditory hallucinations, complex behavior (eg, sleep-driving), abnormal thinking and behavior changes reported. Worsening of depression, including suicidal thoughts and actions have been reported in depressed patients. Caution with conditions that could affect metabolism or hemodynamic responses, sleep apnea syndrome, myasthenia gravis, and worsening depression. Signs and symptoms of withdrawal reported with abrupt discontinuation of sedative/hypnotics. Monitor elderly and debilitated patients for impaired motor and/or cognitive performance.

ADVERSE REACTIONS: Drowsiness, dizziness, headache, N/V, diarrhea.

INTERACTIONS: CNS-active drugs may potentially enhance effects. Additive effects seen with alcohol use. Decreased alertness observed with combination use of imipramine/chlorpromazine. Ketoconazole may enhance sedative effects; consider lowering zolpidem dose when given with ketoconazole.

PREGNANCY: Category C, safety not known in nursing.

MECHANISM OF ACTION: Imidazopyridine, non-benzodiazepine hypnotic; interacts with a GABA-BZ receptor complex and preferentially binds to the BZ_1 receptor subtype at the α_1/α_5 subunits.

PHARMACOKINETICS: Absorption: Rapid; (5mg) C_{max}=114ng/mL, (10mg) C_{max}=210ng/mL; T_{max}=0.9 hrs. **Distribution:** Plasma protein binding (92.5%). **Elimination:** Renal; (5mg) $T_{1/2}$=2.7 hrs, (10mg) $T_{1/2}$= 3.

NURSING CONSIDERATIONS

Assessment: Assess for primary psychiatric and/or medical illness, pre-existing respiratory impairment (eg, sleep apnea syndrome), myasthenia gravis, hypersensitivity reactions, hepatic impairment, possible drug interactions, history of alcohol abuse, and pregnancy/nursing status.

Monitoring: Monitor for anaphylactic/anaphylactoid reactions, abnormal thinking, behavioral changes, complex behavior (eg, sleep-driving, hallucinations). Monitor patients with hepatic impairment, and those on long-term treatment for drug abuse/dependence.

Patient Counseling: Instruct not to take with or immediately after meals. Counsel to take just before bedtime (prior to a full 7-8 hrs of sleep) without food and do not take with alcohol. Caution against hazardous tasks (eg, driving/operating machines). Inform about risks/benefits of use.

Administration: Oral route. **Storage:** Store upright at 25°C (77°F); with excursions permitted to 15-30°C (59-86°F). Do not freeze. Avoid prolonged exposure to heat.

Zometa RX

zoledronic acid (Novartis)

THERAPEUTIC CLASS: Bisphosphonate

INDICATIONS: Treatment of hypercalcemia of malignancy. Treatment of multiple myeloma and bone metastases from solid tumors, in conjunction with antineoplastic therapy.

DOSAGE: *Adults:* Hypercalcemia of Malignancy: Max: 4mg IV over no less than 15 min. Retreatment (if necessary): Wait at least 7 days from initial dose. Multiple Myeloma/Bone Metastases: 4mg IV over 15 min every 3-4 weeks. CrCl 50-60mL/min: 3.5mg; CrCl 40-49mL/min: 3.3mg; CrCl 30-39mL/min: 3mg. Measure SrCr prior to each dose. Withhold dose with renal deterioration; resume when SrCr returns to within 10% of baseline. Take with oral calcium 500mg/day and vitamin D 400 IU/day.

HOW SUPPLIED: Inj: 4mg/5mL

CONTRAINDICATIONS: Urticaria, angioedema, anaphylactic shock.

WARNINGS/PRECAUTIONS: Caution with hepatic insufficiency, ASA-sensitive asthma, and the elderly. Risk of renal toxicity/failure. In severe renal impairment, avoid with bone metastases and use caution with hypercalcemia of malignancy. Rehydrate before use with hypercalcemia of malignancy. Monitor SrCr before each dose, and serum calcium, electrolytes, phosphate, magnesium, and Hct/Hgb regularly. May cause fetal harm during pregnancy. Osteonecrosis of the jaw reported in cancer patients treated with bisphosphonates; avoid invasive dental procedures during therapy. Severe and occasionally incapacitating bone, joint, and/or muscle pain reported.

ADVERSE REACTIONS: Fever, chills, bone pain, arthralgia, myalgia, NV, diarrhea, constipation, injection site reactions, conjunctivitis, hypomagnesemia, abnormal serum creatinine, hypophosphatemia, hypokalemia, anorexia, anemia, insomnia, anxiety, dyspnea.

INTERACTIONS: Additive effect/risk of hypocalcemia with aminoglycosides and loop diuretics. Caution with other nephrotoxic drugs. Increased risk of renal dysfunction with thalidomide in multiple myeloma patients.

PREGNANCY: Category D, not for use in nursing.

MECHANISM OF ACTION: Bisphosphonate; inhibits bone resorption through osteoclastic activity and induces osteoclast apoptosis. Also blocks osteoclastic resorption of mineralized bone and cartilage through binding to bone.

PHARMACOKINETICS: Absorption: IV administration of different doses resulted in different parameters. **Distribution:** Plasma protein binding: 28-53%. **Elimination:** Urine; $T_{1/2}$=146 hrs.

NURSING CONSIDERATIONS

Assessment: Assess hydration status, serum levels of calcium, phosphate, magnesium, SrCr, renal function, LFTs, asthma, pregnancy status, and for possible drug interactions.

Monitoring: Monitor serum levels of calcium, phosphate, magnesium, SrCr, renal function, LFTs. Monitor adverse events (eg, osteonecrosis of jaw, musculoskeletal pain, bronchoconstriction, fever, nausea, constipation, anemia, and dyspnea).

Patient Counseling: Advise to take oral calcium supplement of 500mg and multiple vitamin containing 400IU vitamin D daily. Cancer patients should maintain good oral hygiene, have dental exam with preventive dentistry prior to therapy with bisphosphonates, and avoid invasive dental procedures. Inform about importance of blood tests. Advise to avoid pregnancy during course of therapy.

Administration: IV route. Single doses should not exceed 4mg and duration of infusion should not be less than 15 min. **Storage:** 25°C (77°F); excursions permitted to 15-30°C (59-86°F).

ZOMIG RX

zolmitriptan (AstraZeneca)

OTHER BRAND NAMES: Zomig Nasal Spray (AstraZeneca) - Zomig-ZMT (AstraZeneca)

THERAPEUTIC CLASS: 5-$HT_{1B/1D}$ agonist

INDICATIONS: Acute treatment of migraine attacks with or without aura.

DOSAGE: *Adults:* ≥18 yrs: (Spray) 5mg single dose; may repeat once after 2 hrs. Max: 10mg/24 hrs. Safety of treating >4 headaches/30 days unknown. (Tab) Initial: 2.5mg or lower (2.5mg tab may be broken in 1/2); may repeat after 2 hrs. Max: 10mg/24 hrs. Safety of treating >3 headaches/30 days unknown. (ZMT) 2.5mg single dose; may repeat after 2 hrs. Max: 10mg/24 hrs. Dissolve on tongue without water. Safety of treating >3 headaches/30 days unknown. Hepatic Impairment: Use low dose and monitor blood pressure.

HOW SUPPLIED: Nasal Spray: 5mg [0.1mL, 6[s]]; Tab: 2.5mg*, 5mg; Tab, Disintegrating: (ZMT) 2.5mg, 5mg *scored

CONTRAINDICATIONS: Ischemic heart disease, coronary artery vasospasm (eg, Prinzmetal's angina), uncontrolled HTN, cerebrovascular syndromes, other significant cardiovascular disease, hemiplegic or basilar migraine, MAOI use during or within 14 days, other 5-HT_1 agonist or ergot-type agent (eg, dihydroergotamine, methysergide) use within 24 hrs.

WARNINGS/PRECAUTIONS: Confirm migraine diagnosis. Supervise 1st dose and monitor cardiac function in those at risk of CAD (eg, HTN, hypercholesterolemia, smoker, obesity, diabetes, CAD family history, postmenopausal women, males >40 yrs). Serious adverse cardiac events, cerebrovascular events, vasospastic reactions reported with 5-HT_1 agonists. Disintegrating tabs contain phenylalanine. Caution with hepatic dysfunction. Reconsider diagnosis before 2nd dose, if no response seen after 1st dose. Serotonin syndrome symptoms (eg, mental status changes, autonomic instability, neuromuscular aberrations, and GI symptoms) reported. Avoid in patients with symptomatic Wolff-Parkinson-White syndrome or arrhythmias associated with other cardiac accessory conduction pathway disorders.

ADVERSE REACTIONS: Paresthesia, hyperesthesia, paresthesia, asthenia, warm/cold sensation, neck/throat/jaw pain, dry mouth, nausea, dizziness, somnolence, unusual taste (nasal spray).

INTERACTIONS: Ergot-containing agents may prolong vasospastic reactions. Avoid MAOIs during or within 14 days of therapy. Serotonin syndrome reported with combined use of an SSRI or SNRI. Half-life and AUC doubled with cimetidine. Avoid 5-$HT_{1D/1B}$ agonists within 24 hrs.

PREGNANCY: Category C, caution in nursing.

MECHANISM OF ACTION: 5-$HT_{1D/1B}$ agonist; binds with high affinity to 5-$HT_{1D/1B}$ receptors on intracranial vessels (including arteriovenous anastomoses) and sensory nerves of trigeminal system, which results in cranial vessel constriction and inhibition of pro-inflammatory neuropeptide release.

PHARMACOKINETICS: Absorption: Well-absorbed; absolute bioavailability (40%); T_{max}=3 hrs (ODT/Nasal Spray), 1.5 hrs (Tab). **Distribution:** (Oral) V_d=7L/kg, (Nasal Spray) V_d=8.4L/kg. Plasma protein binding (25%). **Metabolism:** N-desmethyl (active metabolite). **Elimination:** Urine (65%, 8% unchanged), feces (30% Oral); $T_{1/2}$=3 hrs (Nasal Spray).

NURSING CONSIDERATIONS

Assessment: Confirm diagnosis of migraine before therapy. Assess for ischemic heart disease (eg, angina pectoris, Prinzmetal's variant angina, MI or documented silent MI), HTN, hemiplegic or basilar migraine, presence of risk factors (eg, hypercholesterolemia, smoking, obesity, DM, strong family history of CAD, female with surgical or physiological menopause, or male >40 yrs), ECG changes, hepatic/renal impairment, pregnancy/nursing status, and possible drug interactions.

Monitoring: Administration of 1st dose should be in physician's office or medically staffed and equipped facility as cardiac ischemia may occur in absence of clinical symptoms. ECG should be obtained immediately after administration in those with risk factors. Monitor for signs/symptoms of cardiac events (eg, coronary vasospasm, acute MI, arrhythmia, ECG changes, follow-up coronary angiography), cerebrovascular events (eg, hemorrhage, stroke, TIAs), peripheral vascular ischemia, colonic ischemia with bloody diarrhea and abdominal pain, serotonin syndrome (eg, mental status changes, autonomic instability, neuromuscular aberrations and/or GI symptoms), ophthalmic effects, and increased BP.

Patient Counseling: Inform about risk of serotonin syndrome, especially if taken with SSRIs or SNRIs. Advise to notify physician if pregnant/nursing or planning to become pregnant. Counsel on proper administration technique for nasal spray.

Administration: Oral/Nasal routes. ODT: Immediately prior to dosing, remove blister from outer pouch with dry hands. Dissolve on tongue and swallow. **Storage:** 20-25°C (68-77°F).

ZONEGRAN RX
zonisamide (Eisai)

THERAPEUTIC CLASS: Sulfonamide anticonvulsant

INDICATIONS: Adjunctive therapy in the treatment of partial seizures.

DOSAGE: *Adults:* Initial: 100mg qd for 2 weeks. Titrate: May increase to 200mg/day for at least 2 weeks. May then increase to 300mg/day, then to 400mg/day for at least 2-week intervals. Max: 400mg/day.
Pediatrics: ≥16 yrs: Initial: 100mg qd for 2 weeks. Titrate: May increase to 200mg/day for at least 2 weeks. May then increase to 300mg/day, then to 400mg/day for at least 2-week intervals. Max: 400mg/day.

HOW SUPPLIED: Cap: 25mg, 100mg

CONTRAINDICATIONS: Sulfonamide hypersensitivity.

WARNINGS/PRECAUTIONS: Sulfonamide hypersensitivity reactions (eg, Stevens-Johnson syndrome, toxic epidermal necrolysis, fulminant hepatic necrosis, blood dyscrasias), cognitive/neuropsychiatric effects, kidney stones, sudden death reported. D/C with unexplained rash. Increased risk of oligohidrosis and hyperthermia in pediatrics; monitor for decreased sweating and increased body temperature. Advise females to use contraceptives to prevent pregnancy. Caution with renal/hepatic impairment. Avoid abrupt withdrawal. May cause cognitive/neuropsychiatric adverse events. Caution while driving, operating machinery, or performing hazardous tasks. Taper and d/c if CPK levels elevated or if patient manifests clinical signs and symptoms of pancreatitis.

ADVERSE REACTIONS: Headache, abdominal pain, anorexia, nausea, dizziness, ataxia, confusion, difficulty concentrating, memory difficulties, agitation/irritability, depression, insomnia, somnolence, fatigue, tiredness.

INTERACTIONS: Liver enzyme inducers increase metabolism and clearance and decrease half-life. Caution with drugs that predispose patients to heat-related disorders (eg, carbonic anhydrase inhibitors, anticholinergic drugs).

PREGNANCY: Category C, not for use in nursing.

MECHANISM OF ACTION: Sulfonamide; mechanism unknown. Found to block Na^+ channels and reduce voltage-dependent, transient inward currents (T-type Ca^{2+} currents), which then stabilize neuronal membranes and suppress neuronal hypersynchronization. Facilitates both dopaminergic and serotonergic neurotransmission.

PHARMACOKINETICS: Absorption: C_{max}=2-5mcg/mL; T_{max}=2 to 6 hrs. **Distribution:** V_d=1.45L/kg; plasma protein binding (40%). **Metabolism:** Liver, via acetylation and reduction by CYP3A4; N-acetyl zonisamide, 2-sulfamoylacetyl phenol (metabolites). **Elimination**: Urine (62%), feces (3%); $T_{1/2}$=63 hrs.

NURSING CONSIDERATIONS

Assessment: Assess renal/hepatic function, drug allergy to sulfonamides, and possible drug interactions prior to therapy.

Monitoring: Monitor for signs/symptoms of Stevens-Johnson syndrome, toxic epidermal necrolysis, fulminant hepatic necrosis, agranulocytosis, aplastic anemia, cognitive and neuropsychiatric disorders (eg, depression, psychosis, psychomotor slowing), kidney stones, status epilepticus, and pancreatitis. Monitor renal function (SrCr, BUN) while on therapy, pancreatic lipase and serum amylase levels if signs/symptoms of pancreatitis develop, serum CPK levels and aldolase levels if muscle pain or weakness develops.

Patient Counseling: Advise to avoid alcohol while on medication and operating machinery/driving until accustomed to effects. Counsel caretakers of adolescents/pediatric patients that medication may decrease sweating and increase body temperature; hydrate properly when exposed to these conditions to help avoid development of kidney stones. Advise females of need to use proper contraception while on therapy. Notify physican if seizures worsen, signs/symptoms of kidney stones develop, infection, muscle pain, or easy bruising develops.

Administration: Oral route. **Storage:** 25°C (77°F), excursions permitted to 15-30°C (59-86°F). Store in dry area; protect from light.

ZORBTIVE — RX

somatropin (EMD Serono)

THERAPEUTIC CLASS: Human growth hormone

INDICATIONS: Treatment of Short Bowel Syndrome in patients receiving specialized nutritional support.

DOSAGE: *Adults:* 0.1mg/kg qd SC for 4 weeks. Max: 8mg qd. Rotate injection site.

HOW SUPPLIED: Inj: 8.8mg

CONTRAINDICATIONS: Acute critical illness due to complications following open heart or abdominal surgery, multiple accidental trauma, or acute respiratory failure; active neoplasia (either newly diagnosed or recurrent); benzyl alcohol sensitivity.

WARNINGS/PRECAUTIONS: Associated with acute pancreatitis. New onset impaired glucose intolerance, new onset type 2 DM, exacerbation of pre-existing DM, ketoacidosis, diabetic coma reported; closely monitor with risk factors for glucose intolerance. Perform funduscopic evaluations periodically. Increased tissue turgor, musculoskeletal discomfort, and carpal tunnel syndrome may occur.

ADVERSE REACTIONS: Peripheral/facial edema, chest/back pain, fever, flu-like disorder, malaise, flatulence, abdominal pain, nausea, vomiting, viral infection, dizziness, headache, rash.

PREGNANCY: Category B, caution in nursing.

MECHANISM OF ACTION: Human growth hormone; anabolic and anticatabolic agent, exerts influence by interacting with specific receptors. On gut, actions may be direct or mediated via local or systemic production of IGF-1; also enhances transmucosal transport of water, electrolytes, and nutrients.

PHARMACOKINETICS: Absorption: (SQ) Absolute bioavailability (70-90%). **Distribution:** V_d=12.0L. **Metabolism:** Liver, kidneys. **Elimination:** Urine; (SQ) $T_{1/2}$=3.94 hrs. (IV) $T_{1/2}$=0.58 hrs.

NURSING CONSIDERATIONS

Assessment: Assess for acute critical illness (eg, complications after open heart or abdominal surgery, multiple accidental trauma, acute respiratory failure), active malignancy, hypersensitivity to benzyl alcohol, and possible drug interactions. Perform baseline fundoscopic exam.

Monitoring: Perform fundoscopic exam periodically. Monitor for signs/symptoms of impaired glucose intolerance, new onset type 2 DM, exacerbation of pre-existing DM, diabetic ketoacidosis, diabetic coma, carpal tunnel syndrome, acute pancreatitis, tissue atrophy at injection site, increased tissue turgor (swelling), musculoskeletal discomfort (eg, pain, swelling, stiffness), and hypersensitivity/allergic reactions.

Patient Counseling: Instruct thoroughly as to proper usage and disposal; caution against any reuse of needles or syringes. Advise to seek medical attention if symptoms of impaired glucose intolerance, new onset type 2 DM, exacerbation of pre-existing DM, diabetic ketoacidosis, diabetic coma, carpal tunnel syndrome, acute pancreatitis, tissue atrophy at injection site, increased tissue turgor (swelling), musculoskeletal discomfort (pain, swelling, stiffness), or hypersensitivity/allergic reactions occur.

Administration: SQ route. **Storage:** (Before reconstitution): 15-30°C (59-86°F). (After reconstitution): Refrigerate; 2-8°C (36-46°F) for up to 14 days. Avoid freezing.

ZOSTAVAX RX

zoster vaccine live (Merck)

THERAPEUTIC CLASS: Vaccine

INDICATIONS: Prevention of herpes zoster in individuals ≥60.

DOSAGE: *Adults:* ≥60 yrs: Inject SQ immediately after reconstitution with supplied diluent.

HOW SUPPLIED: Inj: 19,400 PFU/0.65mL

CONTRAINDICATIONS: Anaphylactic/anaphylactoid reactions to gelatin or neomycin. Primary or acquired immunodeficiency states (eg, leukemia); lymphomas or other malignant neoplasms affecting the bone marrow or lymphatic system; AIDS or other clinical manifestations HIV infections. Immunosuppressive therapy, including high-dose corticosteroids. Active untreated tuberculosis. Pregnancy.

WARNINGS/PRECAUTIONS: More extensive vaccine-associated rash or disseminated disease with immunosuppression. Anaphylactic/anaphylactoid reaction may occur. Deferral of vaccination should be considered in acute illness. Not indicated for prevention of primary varicella infection. Have epinephrine (1:1000) available.

ADVERSE REACTIONS: Erythema, pain, tenderness, swelling, pruritus.

INTERACTIONS: See Contraindications.

PREGNANCY: Category C, caution in nursing.

MECHANISM OF ACTION: Vaccine; stimulates immune system to produce antibodies that may protect against herpes zoster infection (shingles).

NURSING CONSIDERATIONS

Assessment: Assess current health status and previous vaccination history.

Monitoring: Monitor for hypersensitivity reactions, injection-site reactions (eg, hematoma, pain, swelling, erythema, pruritus), and headache.

Patient Counseling: Inform of potential benefits/risks; report any adverse reactions to physician. Inform may not provide protection in all vaccine recipients.

Administration: SQ route. Inject into deltoid region of upper arm. **Storage:** Frozen at average temperature of 15°C (+5°F) or colder; diluent stored at room temperature 20-25°C (68-77°F) or refrigerated 2-8°C (36-46°F).

ZOSYN RX

piperacillin sodium - tazobactam (Wyeth)

THERAPEUTIC CLASS: Broad-spectrum penicillin/beta-lactamase inhibitor

INDICATIONS: Treatment of appendicitis, peritonitis, uncomplicated/complicated skin and skin structure infections, postpartum endometritis, pelvic inflammatory disease, moderate severity of community-acquired pneumonia (CAP), and moderate to severe nosocomial pneumonia caused by susceptible strains of microorganisms.

DOSAGE: *Adults:* Usual: 3.375g q6h for 7-10 days. CrCl 20-40mL: 2.25g q6h. CrCl <20mL/min: 2.25g q8h. Hemodialysis/CAPD: 2.25g q12h. Give 1 additional 0.75g dose after each dialysis period. Nosocomial Pneumonia: 4.5g q6h for 7-14 days plus aminoglycoside. CrCl 20-40mL/min: 3.375g q6h. CrCl <20mL/min: 2.25g q6h. Hemodialysis/CAPD: Max: 2.25g q8h. Give 1 additional 0.75g dose after each dialysis period.

Pediatrics: Appendicitis/Peritonitis: ≤40kg: ≥9 months: 100mg piperacillin-12.5mg tazobactam/kg q8h. 2-9 months: 80mg piperacillin-10mg tazobactam/kg q8h. ≥40kg: Use adult dose.

HOW SUPPLIED: Inj: (Piperacillin-Tazobactam) 40mg-5mg/mL, 60mg-7.5mg/mL, 2g-0.25g, 3g-0.375g, 4g-0.5g, 2g-0.25g/50mL, 3g-0.375g/50mL, 4g-0.5g/100mL, 36g-4.5g

CONTRAINDICATIONS: History of allergic reactions to cephalosporins.

WARNINGS/PRECAUTIONS: Serious, fatal hypersensitivity reactions may occur with PCN allergy. *Clostridium difficile*-associated diarrhea reported. D/C if bleeding manifestations occur. May experience neuromuscular excitability or convulsions with higher doses. Contains 2.79mEq/g Na; caution with restricted salt intake. Increased incidence of rash and fever in cystic fibrosis. Monitor electrolyte periodically with low K^+ reserves. Therapy may lead to emergence of resistant organisms that can cause superinfections. Caution with renal impairment (CrCl <40mL/min).

ADVERSE REACTIONS: Diarrhea, headache, constipation, NV, insomnia, rash, dyspepsia, pruritus.

INTERACTIONS: May inactivate aminoglycosides. Probenecid prolongs half-life. Monitor coagulation parameters with heparin, oral anticoagulants, or drugs that affect blood coagulation system or thrombocyte function. May prolong neuromuscular blockade of vecuronium.

PREGNANCY: Category B, caution in nursing.

MECHANISM OF ACTION: Piperacillin: Broad-spectrum penicillin; exerts bactericidal activity by inhibiting septum formation and cell-wall synthesis of susceptible bacteria. Tazobactam: β-lactamase enzyme inhibitor.

PHARMACOKINETICS: Absorption: (2.25g, 3.375g, 4.5g of piperacillin): C_{max}=134mcg/mL, 242mcg/mL, 298mcg/mL. (2.25g, 3.375g, 4.5g of tazobactam): C_{max}= 15mcg/mL, 24mcg/mL, 34mcg/mL. **Distribution:** V_d=0.243L/kg; plasma protein binding (30%); wide distribution into tissues and bodily fluids; crosses placental barrier; found in breast milk. **Elimination:** Kidneys; Piperacilin: Urine (68% unchanged); Tazobactam: Urine (80% unchanged, 20% as single metabolite); $T_{1/2}$=0.7-1.2 hrs.

NURSING CONSIDERATIONS

Assessment: Assess for previous hypersensitivity reaction to cephalosporins, PCNs or other allergens, renal/hepatic impairment, pregnancy/nursing status, hypokalemia, cytotoxic therapy, diuretic therapy, and possible drug interactions.

Monitoring: Periodically monitor renal/hepatic function, hematopoietic function, and serum K^+ levels. Monitor for signs/symptoms of anaphylactic/anaphylactoid reactions, CDAD, drug resistance or superinfection, bleeding manifestations, and electrolyte abnormalities.

Patient Counseling: Inform drug only treats bacterial, not viral, infections. Instruct to take as directed; skipping doses or not completing full course may decrease effectiveness and increase resistance. Inform about risks/benefits. Advise to d/c and notify physician if allergic reaction or watery/bloody diarrhea (with or without muscle cramps) occur. Notify if pregnant/nursing.

Administration: IV route. Administer as infusion over 30 min. **Storage:** 20-25°C (68-77°F); discard any unused portion of reconstituted solution after 24 hrs if at room temperature or 48 hrs if refrigerated at 2-8°C (36-46°).

ZOVIRAX CREAM — RX

acyclovir (Biovail)

THERAPEUTIC CLASS: Nucleoside analogue

INDICATIONS: Treatment of recurrent herpes labialis (cold sores).

DOSAGE: *Adults:* Apply 5x/day for 4 days. Initiate with 1st sign/symptom. *Pediatrics:* ≥12 yrs: Apply 5x/day for 4 days. Initiate with 1st sign/symptom.

HOW SUPPLIED: Cre: 5% [2g, 5g]

WARNINGS/PRECAUTIONS: Cutaneous use only; not for use in the eye, mouth or nose.

ADVERSE REACTIONS: Dry lips, desquamation, dryness of skin, cracked lips, burning skin, pruritus, flakiness of skin, stinging on skin.

PREGNANCY: Category B, caution in nursing.

MECHANISM OF ACTION: Synthetic purine nucleoside analogue; possesses inhibitory activity against herpes simplex virus types 1 and 2, and varicella-zoster virus. Stops replication of herpes viral DNA by competitive inhibition of viral DNA polymerase, incorporation into and termination of growing viral DNA chain, and inactivation of viral DNA polymerase.

PHARMACOKINETICS: Absorption: Minimal systemic absorption.

NURSING CONSIDERATIONS

Assessment: Assess nursing and immunocompromised status.

Monitoring: Monitor for signs/symptoms of irritation and contact sensitization.

Patient Counseling: Inform that medication is for treatment of cold sores. Instruct that medication for external use only; avoid application to eyes, inside mouth or nose, or unaffected skin areas. Inform that drug not for treatment of genital herpes and not a cure for cold sores. Instruct to use at first sign of cold sore (eg, tingling, redness, bump, or itch). Counsel to wash hands prior to and following administration, apply to clean/dry skin, and do not cover cold sores with bandages or dressings unless directed by physician. Advise to avoid applying another type of skin product (eg, cosmetics, sunscreen, lip balms) or medication to cold sore area during therapy, unless directed by physician. Instruct not to bathe, shower, or swim immediately after application.

Administration: Topical route. **Storage:** 25°C (77°F); excursions permitted to 15-30°C (59-86°F).

ZOVIRAX INJECTION RX

acyclovir sodium (GlaxoSmithKline)

THERAPEUTIC CLASS: Nucleoside analogue

INDICATIONS: Treatment of neonatal herpes simplex infections and herpes simplex encephalitis. Treatment of varicella-zoster (shingles), initial and recurrent mucosal and cutaneous herpes simplex in immunocompromised patients. Treatment of severe initial clinical episodes of herpes genitalis in immunocompetent patients.

DOSAGE: *Adults:* Initiate with 1st sign/symptom. Max: 20mg/kg q8h for any patient. Mucosal/Cutaneous Herpes Simplex Infections: 5mg/kg q8h for 7 days. Herpes Genitalis: 5mg/kg q8h for 5 days. Herpes Simplex Encephalitis: 10mg/kg q8h for 10 days. Varicella Zoster: 10mg/kg q8h for 7 days. Obese Patients: Dose according to IBW. CrCl 25-50mL/min: Give 100% of recommended dose q12h. CrCl 10-25: Give 100% of recommended dose q24h. CrCl 0-10mL/min: Give 50% of recommended dose q24h. Elderly: Reduce dose and monitor renal function.

Pediatrics: Initiate with 1st sign/symptom. Max: 20mg/kg q8h for any patient. Mucosal/Cutaneous Herpes Simplex: ≥12 yrs: 5mg/kg q8h for 7 days. <12 yrs: 10mg/kg q8h for 7 days. Herpes Genitalis: ≥12 yrs: 5mg/kg q8h for 5 days. Herpes Simplex Encephalitis: ≥12 yrs: 10mg/kg q8h for 10 days. 3 months-12 yrs: 20mg/kg q8h for 10 days. Neonatal Herpes Simplex: Birth-3 months: 10mg/kg q8h for 10 days. Varicella Zoster: ≥12 yrs: 10mg/kg q8h for 7 days. <12 yrs: 20mg/kg q8h for 7 days. Obese Patients: Dose according to IBW. CrCl 25-50mL/min: Give 100% of recommended dose q12h. CrCl 10-25: Give 100% of recommended dose q24h. CrCl 0-10mL/min: Give 50% of recommended dose q24h.

HOW SUPPLIED: Inj: 500mg, 1000mg

CONTRAINDICATIONS: Hypersensitivity to valacyclovir.

WARNINGS/PRECAUTIONS: Do not administer topically, IM, PO, SQ, or in the eye. Adjust dose in renal impairment and the elderly. Renal failure and death reported. Thrombotic thrombocytopenic purpura/hemolytic uremic syndrome in immunocompromised patients reported. Patient must be adequately hydrated. Caution with underlying neurologic abnormalities, electrolyte abnormalities, significant hypoxia, and serious renal or hepatic abnormalities. Infusion must not be given over <1 hr.

ADVERSE REACTIONS: Injection site inflammation, phlebitis, transient serum creatinine and BUN elevations, NV.

INTERACTIONS: Increased serum levels with probenecid. Avoid with nephrotoxic drugs.

PREGNANCY: Category B, caution in nursing.

MECHANISM OF ACTION: Synthetic purine nucleoside analogue; possesses inhibitory activity against herpes simplex virus types 1 and 2, and varicella-zoster virus. Stops replication of herpes viral DNA by competitive inhibition of viral DNA polymerase, incorporation into and termination of growing viral DNA chain, and inactivation of viral DNA polymerase.

PHARMACOKINETICS: Absorption: C_{max}=9.8mcg/mL (5mg/kg), 22.9mcg/mL (10mg/kg). **Distribution:** Plasma protein binding (9-33%); found in breast milk. **Metabolism:** 9-carboxymethoxymethylguanine (major metabolite). **Elimination:** Urine (62-91% unchanged) (14.1% metabolite). Refer to PI for detailed info regarding renal function and pediatrics.

NURSING CONSIDERATIONS

Assessment: Assess for immunosuppression, renal/hepatic disease, electrolyte abnormalities, significant hypoxia, pregnancy/nursing status, hydration status, possible drug interactions.

Monitoring: Monitor signs/symptoms of renal failure, thrombocytopenic purpura/hemolytic uremic syndrome, encephalopathic changes (eg, lethargy, obtundation, tremors, confusion, hallucinations, agitation, seizures, or coma). Monitor renal function (CrCl), LFTs, and CBC.

Patient Counseling: Notify physician if pregnant/nursing. Inform about potential risks of therapy and advise to report any adverse reactions.

Administration: IV route. Infuse over period of ≥ 1 hr to reduce risk of renal tubular damage, with adequate hydration. Not for topical, IM, oral, ocular, or SQ use. **Storage:** 15-25°C (59-77°F).

ZOVIRAX OINTMENT — RX

acyclovir (Biovail)

THERAPEUTIC CLASS: Nucleoside analogue

INDICATIONS: Management of initial genital herpes and in limited non-life-threatening mucocutaneous herpes simplex infections in immunocompromised patients.

DOSAGE: *Adults:* Apply to all lesions q3h, 6x/day for 7 days. Apply with finger cot or rubber glove to prevent autoinoculation and transmission. Initiate with 1st sign/symptom.

HOW SUPPLIED: Oint: 5% [15g]

WARNINGS/PRECAUTIONS: Not for use for the prevention of recurrent HSV infections. Cutaneous use only; avoid eyes.

ADVERSE REACTIONS: Pain with application, transient burning and stinging, pruritus.

PREGNANCY: Category B, not for use in nursing.

MECHANISM OF ACTION: Synthetic purine nucleoside analogue; possesses inhibitory activity against herpes simplex virus types 1 and 2, and varicella-zoster virus. Stops replication of herpes viral DNA by competitive inhibition of viral DNA polymerase, incorporation into and termination of growing viral DNA chain, and inactivation of viral DNA polymerase.

PHARMACOKINETICS: Absorption: Minimal systemic absorption.

NURSING CONSIDERATIONS

Assessment: Assess for active signs/symptoms of herpes simplex virus. Assess nursing status.

Monitoring: Monitor for signs/symptoms of mild pain (eg, transient burning, stinging) and for pruritus at treatment site.

Patient Counseling: Counsel that ointment is for cutaneous administration only; should not be used in eyes. Advise to initiate as soon as possible following onset of signs/symptoms; not to use in absence of signs/symptoms. Counsel to use finger cot or rubber glove when applying to prevent autoinoculation of other body sites and transmission of infection to others.

Administration: Topical route. **Storage:** 15-25°C (59-77°F); store in dry place.

ZOVIRAX ORAL — RX

acyclovir (GlaxoSmithKline)

THERAPEUTIC CLASS: Nucleoside analogue

INDICATIONS: Acute treatment of herpes zoster (shingles). Treatment of initial and recurrent episodes of genital herpes. Treatment of chickenpox (varicella).

DOSAGE: *Adults:* Herpes Zoster: 800mg q4h, 5x/day for 7-10 days. Start within 72 hrs after onset of rash. Genital Herpes: Initial: 200mg q4h, 5x/day for 10 days. Chronic Therapy: 400mg bid or 200mg 3-5x/day up to 12 months, then re-evaluate. Intermittent Therapy: 200mg q4h, 5x/day for 5 days. Start with 1st sign/symptom of recurrence. Chickenpox: 800mg qid for 5 days. CrCl 10-25mL/min: For a dose of 800mg q4h, give 800mg q8h. CrCl 0-10mL/min: For a dose of 200mg q4h, give 200mg q12h. For a dose of 400mg q12h, give 200mg q12h. For a dose of 800mg q4h, give 800mg q12h. Elderly: Reduce dose.

Pediatrics: ≥2 yrs: ≤40kg: Chickenpox: 20mg/kg qid for 5 days. >40kg: 800mg qid for 5 days.

HOW SUPPLIED: Cap: 200mg; Sus: 200mg/5mL; Tab: 400mg, 800mg

CONTRAINDICATIONS: Hypersensitivity to valacyclovir.

WARNINGS/PRECAUTIONS: Adjust dose in renal impairment, elderly. Renal failure and death reported. Thrombotic thrombocytopenic purpura/hemolytic uremic syndrome in immunocompromised patients reported.

ADVERSE REACTIONS: Nausea, diarrhea, headache, malaise, and renal dysfunction, seizures, tremors, anemia, leukopenia, elevated LFTs.

INTERACTIONS: Probenecid increased levels of IV formulation. Caution with potentially nephrotoxic agents.

PREGNANCY: Category B, caution in nursing.

MECHANISM OF ACTION: Synthetic purine nucleoside analogue; possesses inhibitory activity against herpes simplex virus types 1 and 2, and varicella-zoster virus. Stops replication of herpes viral DNA by competitive inhibition of viral DNA polymerase, incorporation into and termination of growing viral DNA chain, and inactivation of viral DNA polymerase.

PHARMACOKINETICS: Absorption: Absolute bioavailability (10-20%). Oral administration of variable doses resulted in different parameters. **Distribution:** Plasma protein binding (9-33%). **Elimination:** $T_{1/2}$=2.5-3.3 hrs.

NURSING CONSIDERATIONS

Assessment: Assess if immunocompromised (eg, transplant, advanced HIV, AIDS), renal impairment, and possible drug interactions.

Monitoring: Monitor for signs/symptoms of thrombotic thrombocytopenic purpura/hemolytic syndrome. Check renal function, LFTs, BUN, and SrCr.

Patient Counseling: Inform may be taken with/without food and to maintain adequate hydration. Advise to avoid contact when lesions or symptoms are present to avoid infecting partners. Advise to use safe sex practice in combination with suppressive therapy. Instruct to initiate treatment at earliest symptom of cold sores (eg, tingling, itching, burning).

Administration: Oral route. **Storage:** 15-25°C (59-77°F); protect from moisture.

ZYBAN

bupropion HCl (GlaxoSmithKline)

RX

> **Antidepressants increased the risk of suicidal thinking and behavior (suicidality) in short-term studies in children, adolescents, and young adults with major depressive disorder (MDD) and other psychiatric disorders. Bupropion is not approved for use in pediatric patients.**

THERAPEUTIC CLASS: Aminoketone

INDICATIONS: Aid to smoking cessation treatment.

DOSAGE: *Adults:* ≥18 yrs: Initial: 150mg qd for 3 days. Usual: 150mg bid; separate dose intervals by at least 8 hrs. Max: 300mg/day. Initiate treatment while patient is still smoking. Patients should set a "target quit date" within the first 2 weeks. Treat for 7 to 12 weeks; d/c at 7 weeks if no progress seen. Renal/Hepatic Dysfunction: Reduce dose. Severe Hepatic Cirrhosis: 150mg every other day.

HOW SUPPLIED: Tab, Extended-Release: 150mg

CONTRAINDICATIONS: Seizure disorder, bulimia or anorexia nervosa, within 14 days of MAOIs, other forms of bupropion, abrupt discontinuation of alcohol or sedatives.

WARNINGS/PRECAUTIONS: Dose-related risk of seizures. D/C and do not restart if seizure occurs. Extreme caution with history of seizure, cranial trauma, severe hepatic cirrhosis. Caution with recent MI, unstable heart disease, renal impairment. Agitation, insomnia, psychosis, confusion and other neuropsychiatric phenomena reported. Allergic reactions, HTN reported. May precipitate manic episodes in bipolar disorder.

ADVERSE REACTIONS: Anxiety, dizziness, anorexia, myalgia, pruritus, dry mouth, insomnia, nausea, constipation, tremor, dream abnormality, rash, confusion.

INTERACTIONS: Extreme caution with drugs that lower seizure threshold (eg, antidepressants, antipsychotics, theophylline, systemic steroids). Increased seizure risk with opioid, cocaine, or stimulant addiction, OTC stimulants or anorectics, oral hypoglycemics or insulin, excessive use or abrupt discontinuation of alcohol or sedatives. Caution with levodopa, amantadine, and drugs that are metabolized by CYP2D6 (eg, SSRIs, TCAs, antipsychotics, β-blockers, type 1C antiarrhythmics); use low initial dose and gradually titrate. Avoid other bupropion-containing drugs and MAOIs. Monitor HTN with transdermal nicotine. Caution with CYP2B6 substrates or inhibitors (eg, orphenadrine, cyclophosphamide). Carbamazepine, phenytoin, cimetidine, and phenobarbital may induce metabolism of bupropion. Minimize or avoid alcohol.

PREGNANCY: Pregnancy B, not for use in nursing.

MECHANISM OF ACTION: Mechanism unknown; suspected to inhibit neuronal uptake of norepinephrine and dopamine.

PHARMACOKINETICS: Absorption: C_{max}=136ng/mL; T_{max}=3 hrs. **Distribution:** V_d=1,950L; plasma protein binding (84%); found in breast milk. **Metabolism:** Extensive, through hydroxylation and reduction pathways. Hydroxybupropion, threohydrobupropion, and erythrohydrobupropion (active metabolites). **Elimination:** Urine; $T_{1/2}$=21 hrs.

NURSING CONSIDERATIONS

Assessment: Assess for hepatic/renal dysfunction, seizure disorder, cranial trauma, presence or history of bulimia or anorexia nervosa, major depressive disorder, bipolar disorders. Detailed psychiatric history (eg, family history of suicide, bipolar disorder, depression) should be taken. Assess HTN, pregnancy/nursing status, if undergoing discontinuation of alcohol/sedatives, and for drug interactions (eg, MAOIs). 14 days should elapse between d/c of MAOIs and initiation of therapy.

Monitoring: Monitor for anaphylactoid/anaphylactic reactions, worsening of depression, emergence of suicidal ideation and unusual behavior, insomnia, signs/symptoms of hepatotoxicity, psychosis, confusion, activation of psychosis and/or mania, HTN, and seizures.

Patient Counseling: Instruct to read patient guide and discuss with physician. Advise to be alert to emergence of anxiety, clinical worsening, suicidal risk, and to report any to physician. Instruct to notify physician if pregnant/nursing.

Administration: Oral route. **Storage:** 20-25°C (68-77°F); tightly closed, light-resistant containers.

ZYDONE CIII

hydrocodone bitartrate - acetaminophen (Endo)

THERAPEUTIC CLASS: Opioid analgesic

INDICATIONS: Relief of moderate to moderately severe pain.

DOSAGE: *Adults:* (5/400): 1-2 tabs q4-6h prn. Max: 8 tabs/day. (7.5/400, 10/400): 1 tab q4-6h prn. Max: 6 tabs/day.

HOW SUPPLIED: Tab: (Hydrocodone-APAP) 5mg-400mg, 7.5mg-400mg, 10mg-400mg

WARNINGS/PRECAUTIONS: May produce dose-related respiratory depression. May obscure diagnosis of acute abdominal conditions or head injuries. Caution in elderly, debilitated, severe hepatic or renal dysfunction, hypothyroidism, Addison's disease, prostatic hypertrophy, urethral stricture, pulmonary disease, and postoperative use. May be habit-forming. May impair mental/physical abilities. Suppresses cough reflex.

ADVERSE REACTIONS: Lightheadedness, dizziness, sedation, NV.

INTERACTIONS: Additive CNS depression with opioids, antihistamines, antipsychotics, antianxiety agents, or other CNS depressants (including alcohol). Increased effect of antidepressant or hydrocodone with MAOIs or TCAs.

PREGNANCY: Category C, not for use in nursing.

MECHANISM OF ACTION: Hydrocodone: Opioid analgesic and antitussive; not established. Possibly related to existence of opiate receptors in CNS. Most actions involve CNS and smooth muscle. APAP: Nonopiate, nonsalicylate analgesic and antipyretic. Mechanism of analgesic effect not established; involves peripheral influences. Antipyretic activity mediated through hypothalamic heat-regulating centers. Inhibits prostaglandin synthetase.

PHARMACOKINETICS: Absorption: Hydrocodone: C_{max}=23.6ng/mL; T_{max}=1.3 hrs. APAP: Rapidly absorbed. **Distribution:** APAP: Found in breast milk. **Metabolism:** Hydrocodone: O-demethylation, N-demethylation and 6-keto reduction. APAP: Liver (conjugation). **Elimination:** Hydrocodone: $T_{1/2}$=3.8 hrs. APAP: Urine (85%); $T_{1/2}$=1.25-3 hrs.

NURSING CONSIDERATIONS

Assessment: Assess for hypersensitivity to other opioids, head injury or other intracranial lesions, presence of increased ICP, acute abdominal conditions, presence of debilitation (eg, elderly), hepatic/renal impairment, hypothyroidism, Addison's disease, prostatic hypertrophy or urethral stricture, pulmonary disease, pregnancy/nursing status, and possible drug interactions.

Monitoring: Monitor for signs/symptoms of respiratory depression, elevations in CSF pressure, hepatic/renal dysfunction, drug abuse and dependence.

Patient Counseling: Inform that drug may impair mental/physical abilities required for performing potentially hazardous tasks (eg, operating machinery/driving). Advise to avoid alcohol and other CNS depressants. Counsel drug may be habit forming; take only as long as prescribed, in amounts prescribed, and no more frequently than prescribed.

Administration: Oral route. **Storage:** 25°C (77°F); excursions permitted to 15-30°C (59-86°F). Dispense in a tight, light-resistant container with child-resistant closure.

ZYFLO CR — RX

zileuton (Critical Therapeutics)

THERAPEUTIC CLASS: Leukotriene inhibitor

INDICATIONS: Prophylaxis and chronic treatment of asthma.

DOSAGE: *Adults:* 1200mg bid within 1 hr after am and pm meals. Max: 2400mg/day.
Pediatrics: ≥12 yrs: 1200mg bid within 1 hr after am and pm meals. Max: 2400mg/day.

HOW SUPPLIED: Tab: Extended-Release: 600mg *scored

CONTRAINDICATIONS: Active liver disease or transaminase elevations (≥3x ULN).

WARNINGS/PRECAUTIONS: Not for treatment of acute attacks. Evaluate liver function prior to therapy and periodically thereafter. D/C if signs of liver disease occur.

ADVERSE REACTIONS: Headache, ALT elevation, dyspepsia, pain, nausea, asthenia, myalgia, sinusitis, pharyngolaryngeal pain.

INTERACTIONS: Monitor drugs metabolized by CYP450 3A4. Increases theophylline levels; reduce theophylline by 50% and monitor levels. Potentiates warfarin, propranolol.

PREGNANCY: Category C, not for use in nursing.

MECHANISM OF ACTION: Leukotriene inhibitor; anti-asthmatic agent, inhibits leukotriene (LTB_4, LTC_4, LTD_4, and LTE_4) formation by inhibiting the enzyme 5-lipoxygenase.

PHARMACOKINETICS: Absorption: T_{max}=4.3 hrs. **Distribution:** V_d=1.2L/kg; plasma protein binding (93%). **Metabolism:** Liver, via oxidation by CYP1A2, CYP2C9, CYP3A4; glucuronidation. **Elimination:** Urine, feces; $T_{1/2}$=3.2 hrs.

NURSING CONSIDERATIONS

Assessment: Assess for hepatic impairment, acute asthma, status asthmaticus, pregnancy status, alcoholism.

Monitoring: Monitor hepatic function (eg, hepatic enzymes, bilirubin), hypersensitivity reactions, sinusitis, pharyngolaryngeal pain.

Patient Counseling: Inform that drug is indicated for chronic treatment of asthma; take regularly as prescribed after meals. Advise to swallow tab whole; do not crush or chew. Advise to report adverse side effects. Counsel about possibilities of liver damage and need for liver enzyme monitoring on regular basis. Avoid alcohol.

Administration: Oral route. **Storage:** 20-25°C (68-77°F); excursions permitted to 15-30°C (59-86°F). Protect from light.

ZYLET — RX

loteprednol etabonate - tobramycin (Bausch & Lomb)

THERAPEUTIC CLASS: Aminoglycoside/corticosteroid

INDICATIONS: Treatment of steroid-responsive inflammatory ocular conditions for which a corticosteroid is indicated and where superficial bacterial ocular infection or a risk of bacterial ocular infection exists.

DOSAGE: *Adults:* Initial: 1-2 drops q4-6h. May increase to 1-2 drops q1-2h for first 24-48 hrs. Max: 20mL for initial Rx.

HOW SUPPLIED: Sus: 2.5mL, 5mL, 10mL

CONTRAINDICATIONS: Viral diseases of the cornea and conjunctiva including epithelial herpes simplex keratitis (dendritic keratitis), vaccinia, and varicella, and also in mycobacterial infection of the eye and fungal diseases of ocular structures.

WARNINGS/PRECAUTIONS: Not for injection into the eye. Prolonged use may result in glaucoma, optic nerve damage, visual acuity and fields of vision defects, cataracts, secondary ocular infections. May exacerbate the severity of many viral infections of the eye (including herpes simplex). May delay healing and increase incidence of bleb formation after cataract surgery.

ADVERSE REACTIONS: Injection and superficial punctate keratitis, increased IOP, burning, stinging, headache, secondary infection, vision disorders, discharge, itching, lacrimation disorder, photophobia, corneal deposits, ocular discomfort, eyelid disorder.

PREGNANCY: Category C, caution in nursing.

MECHANISM OF ACTION: Loteprednol: Corticosteroid; not understood. Thought to act by induction of phospholipase A_2 inhibitory proteins, lipocortins. Tobramycin: Aminoglycoside antibiotic; inhibits synthesis of proteins in bacterial cells.

NURSING CONSIDERATIONS

Assessment: Assess for viral disease of cornea and conjunctiva (eg, dendritic keratitis, vaccinia, varicella), mycobacterial infection of eye, fungal disease of eye, glaucoma, and possible drug interactions.

Monitoring: Routinely monitor IOP (use >10 days). Monitor for signs/symptoms of hypersensitivity reactions, glaucoma, defects in visual acuity and fields of vision, posterior subcapsular cataracts, perforations, and superinfections.

Patient Counseling: Instruct not to touch dropper tip to any surface to avoid contamination and not to wear contact lenses during therapy. Advise to seek medical attention if pain develops, if itching/inflammation becomes aggravated, or if hypersensitivity reactions, defects in vision, glaucoma, perforations, or superinfections occur.

Administration: Ocular route. **Storage:** 15-25°C (59-77°F). Protect from freezing; store upright.

ZYLOPRIM RX

allopurinol (Prometheus)

THERAPEUTIC CLASS: Xanthine oxidase inhibitor

INDICATIONS: Management of symptoms of primary and secondary gout. Management of hyperuricosuria and hyperuricemia due to chemotherapy. Management of recurrent calcium oxalate calculi in those with hyperuricosuria (uric acid excretion >800mg/day in males and >750mg/day in females).

DOSAGE: *Adults:* Gout: Initial: 100mg/day. Titrate: Increase by 100mg/week until serum uric acid level is ≤6mg/dL. Mild Gout: Usual: 200-300mg/day. Moderately Severe Gout: Usual: 400-600mg/day. Max: 800mg/day. Recurrent Calcium Oxalate Stones: Usual: 200-300mg/day. Prevention of Uric Acid Nephropathy with Chemotherapy: Usual: 600-800mg/day for 2-3 days with high fluid intake. CrCl 10-20mL/min: 200mg/day. CrCl <10mL/min: Max: 100mg/day. CrCl <3mL/min: Also increase dosing intervals. Take after meals. Divide dose if >300mg.
Pediatrics: Hyperuricemia with Malignancies: 6-10 yrs: 300mg/day. <6 yrs: 150mg/day. Evaluate response after 48 hrs. Take after meals.

HOW SUPPLIED: Tab: 100mg*, 300mg* *scored

WARNINGS/PRECAUTIONS: D/C if skin rash occurs. Severe hypersensitivity reactions, hepatotoxicity, and bone marrow depression reported. Monitor LFTs during early stages of therapy with liver disease. Caution with activities that require alertness. Caution with renal impairment. Renal failure reported with hyperuricemia secondary to neoplastic diseases. Fluid intake should yield ≥2L of urinary output/day. Maintain neutral or slightly alkaline urine. Acute gout attacks increase during early stages of therapy; give colchicine.

ADVERSE REACTIONS: Acute gout attacks, rash, diarrhea, SGOT/SGPT increase, alkaline phosphatase increase, nausea.

INTERACTIONS: Increased toxicity with thiazide diuretics or renal impairment; monitor renal function. Reduce mercaptopurine or azathioprine to 1/3 or 1/4 of usual dose. Potentiates dicumarol, chlorpropamide and cyclosporine. Decreased effects with uricosurics. Increased skin rash with ampicillin, amoxicillin. Enhanced bone marrow suppression with cytotoxic agents (eg, cyclophosphamide). Caution with sulfinpyrazone.

PREGNANCY: Category C, caution in nursing.

MECHANISM OF ACTION: Xanthine oxidase inhibitor; acts on purine catabolism; reduces production of uric acid by inhibiting biochemical reactions immediately preceding its formation.

PHARMACOKINETICS: Absorption: C_{max}=3mcg/mL, T_{max}=1.5 hrs. Oxipurinol: C_{max}=6.5mcg/mL, T_{max}=4.5 hrs. **Metabolism:** Oxidation, oxipurinol (metabolite). **Elimination:** Kidneys, feces (20%); $T_{1/2}$=1-2 hrs. Oxipurinol: $T_{1/2}$=15 hrs.

NURSING CONSIDERATIONS

Assessment: Assess for HTN, DM, multiple myeloma, congestive myocardial diseases, possible drug interactions, pre-existing hepatic/renal disease.

Monitoring: Monitor LFTs, serum uric acid, and renal function periodically. Monitor for signs/symptoms of hepatotoxicity, hypersensitivity/allergic reaction, bone marrow depression, and renal dysfunction.

Patient Counseling: Inform that full benefit will not be seen until after 2-6 weeks of therapy. Increase fluid intake during therapy to prevent renal stones. Caution that drowsiness may occur and physical/mental abilities may be impaired. Instruct to take after meals to minimize gastric irritation. Advise to seek medical attention immediately at 1st sign of allergic reaction (skin rash), painful urination, blood in urine, irritation of eyes, swelling of lips/mouth, or hepatotoxicity (anorexia, weight loss, pruritus).

Administration: Oral route. **Storage:** 15-25°C (59-77°F); store in dry place and protect from light.

ZYMAR — RX

gatifloxacin (Allergan)

THERAPEUTIC CLASS: Fluoroquinolone

INDICATIONS: Treatment of bacterial conjunctivitis.

DOSAGE: *Adults:* 1 drop q2h while awake, up to 8x/day for 2 days; then 1 drop up to qid while awake for 5 days.
Pediatrics: ≥1 yr: 1 drop q2h while awake, up to 8x/day for 2 days; then 1 drop up to qid while awake for 5 days.

HOW SUPPLIED: Sol: 0.3% [5mL]

WARNINGS/PRECAUTIONS: Not for injection. Do not inject subconjunctivally or into the anterior chamber of the eye. Superinfection may result with prolonged use. Fatal hypersensitivity reactions reported after 1st dose of systemic quinolone therapy. Avoid contact lenses when symptoms are present.

ADVERSE REACTIONS: Conjunctival irritation, increased lacrimation, keratitis, papillary conjunctivitis, chemosis, conjunctival hemorrhage, dry eye, eye discharge/irritation/pain, red eye, eyelid edema, headache, reduced visual acuity, taste disturbance.

INTERACTIONS: Systemic quinolone therapy may increase theophylline levels, interfere with caffeine metabolism, enhance warfarin effects, and elevate serum creatinine with cyclosporine.

PREGNANCY: Category C, caution in nursing.

MECHANISM OF ACTION: Fluoroquinolone antibiotic; inhibits topoisomerase II (DNA gyrase) and topoisomerase IV. DNA gyrase is essential enzyme involved in replication, transcription, and repair of bacterial DNA. Topoisomerase IV is enzyme known to play key role in partitioning of chromosomal DNA during bacterial cell division.

NURSING CONSIDERATIONS

Assessment: Assess for proper diagnosis of causative organisms (eg, slit lamp biomicroscopy, fluorescein staining). Assess for hypersensitivity to other quinolones, possible drug interactions, and use in pregnancy/nursing.

Monitoring: Monitor for signs/symptoms of hypersensitivity or anaphylactic reactions (eg, cardiovascular collapse, loss of consciousness, angioedema). Monitor for overgrowth of nonsusceptible organisms (eg, fungi) with prolonged therapy.

Patient Counseling: Advise to avoid contaminating applicator tip with material from eye, fingers, or other sources. Instruct to d/c therapy and contact physician at first sign of rash or allergic reaction. Advise not to wear contact lenses if there are signs/symptoms of bacterial conjunctivitis.

Administration: Ocular route. Do not inject into eye. **Storage:** Store at 15-25°C (59-77°F). Protect from freezing.

ZYPREXA RX

olanzapine (Lilly)

Elderly patients with dementia-related psychosis treated with atypical antipsychotic drugs are at an increased risk of death; most appeared to be cardiovascular (eg, heart failure, sudden death) or infectious (eg, pneumonia) in nature. Olanzapine is not approved for the treatment of patients with dementia-related psychosis.

OTHER BRAND NAMES: Zyprexa IntraMuscular (Lilly) - Zyprexa Zydis (Lilly)

THERAPEUTIC CLASS: Thienobenzodiazepine

INDICATIONS: (PO) Treatment of schizophrenia. Treatment of acute mixed or manic episodes in bipolar I disorder. Short-term treatment of acute manic episodes associated with bipolar I disorder in combination with lithium or valproate. (Inj) Agitation associated with schizophrenia, bipolar I mania.

DOSAGE: *Adults:* (PO) Schizophrenia: Initial/Usual: 5-10mg qd. Titrate: Adjust by 5mg daily at weekly intervals. Max: 20mg/day. Bipolar Disorder: Initial: 10-15mg qd. Titrate: May increase/decrease dose by 5mg daily. Max: 20mg/day. With Lithium or Valproate: Initial/Usual: 10mg qd. Max: 20mg/day. Debilitated/Hypotension Risk/Slow Metabolizers/Sensitivity to Olanzapine Effects: Initial: 5mg qd. Titrate: Increase cautiously. (IM) Agitation: Initial: 10mg IM. Usual: 2.5-10mg IM. Max: 3 doses of 10mg q 2-4h. Elderly: 5mg IM. Debilitated/Hypotension Risk/Sensitivity to Olanzapine Effects: 2.5mg IM. May initiate PO therapy when clinically appropriate.

HOW SUPPLIED: Inj: 10mg; Tab: 2.5mg, 5mg, 7.5mg, 10mg, 15mg, 20mg; Tab, Disintegrating: (Zydis) 5mg, 10mg, 15mg, 20mg

WARNINGS/PRECAUTIONS: Monitor for hyperglycemia, worsening of glucose control with DM, FBG levels with diabetes risk. Risk of NMS, tardive dyskinesia, orthostatic hypotension, seizures. Caution in hepatic impairment, prostatic hypertrophy, narrow-angle glaucoma, history of paralytic ileus, elderly patients with dementia, cardio- or cerebrovascular disease, hypotension risk (eg, hypovolemia, dehydration), risk for aspiration pneumonia, suicidal tendencies. May cause alterations in lipid levels and weight gain; monitor regularly. May cause cognitive and motor impairment. Elevated transaminases, hyperprolactinemia reported. May cause disruption of body temperature regulation. Re-evaluate periodically.

ADVERSE REACTIONS: Postural hypotension, constipation, dry mouth, weight gain, somnolence, dizziness, personality disorder, akathisia, asthenia, dyspepsia, tremor, increased appetite, ecchymosis, rhinitis, joint pain.

INTERACTIONS: May potentiate antihypertensives. Decreased levels with activated charcoal. Increased clearance with carbamazepine. Increased levels with fluvoxamine; lower olanzapine dose. Caution with other CNS drugs, alcohol. May antagonize levodopa, dopamine agonists. Inducers of CYP1A2 or glucuronyl transferase (eg, omeprazole, rifampin) may increase clearance. Inhibitors of CYP1A2 may decrease clearance.

PREGNANCY: Category C, not for use in nursing.

MECHANISM OF ACTION: Thienobenzodiazepine; psychotropic agent; mechanism unknown. Selective monoaminergic antagonist with high affinity binding to selective serotonin, dopamine, histamine, muscarinic, and α-adrenergic receptors.

PHARMACOKINETICS: Absorption: Well-absorbed. (PO) T_{max}=6 hrs; (IM) T_{max}=15-45 min. **Distribution:** V_d=1000L; plasma protein binding (93%). **Metabolism**: Via CYP450 mediated oxidation and direct glucuronidation; 10-N-glucuronide, 4'-N-desmethyl (major metabolites). **Elimination:** Urine (57%, 7% unchanged), feces (30%); $T_{1/2}$=21-54 hrs.

NURSING CONSIDERATIONS

Assessment: Assess for dementia-related psychosis in elderly, DM, baseline lipid panel, CVD, seizures, hepatic/renal impairment, and possible drug interactions.

Monitoring: Monitor for clinical manifestations of NMS, TD, hyperglycemia, hyperlipidemia, seizures, orthostatic hypotension, periodic assessment of transaminases, serum prolactin levels. Regular monitoring of weight and close supervision of high-risk patients for suicide attempt.

Patient Counseling: Inform of benefits/risks of therapy, potential risk of hypoglycemia-related adverse events and orthostatic hypotension; report any adverse events. Counsel to avoid alcohol, overheating, and dehydration. Advise that weight gain may occur. Instruct to use caution while operating machinery/driving. Advise to notify physician if taking, or planning to take, any Rx drugs or OTC products.

Administration: Oral/IM routes. **Storage:** 20-25°C (68-77°F). Protect from light. Do not freeze (vial).

Zyvox — RX

linezolid (Pharmacia & Upjohn)

THERAPEUTIC CLASS: Oxazolidinone class antibacterial

INDICATIONS: Treatment of vancomycin-resistant *Enterococcus faecium* (VRE) infections, nosocomial pneumonia caused by *Staphylococcus aureus* (methicillin-susceptible and -resistant strains) or *Streptococcus pneumoniae* (including multi drug-resistant strains [MDRSP]), complicated skin and skin structure infections (SSSI) including diabetic foot infections without concomitant osteomyelitis caused by *Staphylococcus aureus* (methicillin-susceptible and -resistant strains), *Streptococcus pyogenes*, or *Streptococcus agalactiae*, uncomplicated SSSI caused by *Staphylococcus aureus* (methicillin-susceptible only) or *Streptococcus pyogenes*, community-acquired pneumonia (CAP) caused by *Streptococcus pneumoniae* (MDRSP), including concurrent bacteremia, or *Staphylococcus aureus* (methicillin-susceptible strains only).

DOSAGE: *Adults:* Complicated SSSI/CAP/Nosocomial Pneumonia: 600mg IV/PO q12h for 10-14 days. VRE: 600mg IV/PO q12h for 14-28 days. Uncomplicated SSSI: 400mg PO q12h for 10-14 days.
Pediatrics: Complicated SSSI/CAP/Nosocomial Pneumonia: Treat for 10-14 days. ≥12 yrs: 600mg IV/PO q12h. Birth-11 yrs: 10mg/kg IV/PO q8h. VRE: Treat for 14-28 days: ≥12 yrs: 600mg IV/PO q12h; Birth-11 yrs: 10mg/kg IV/PO q8h. Uncomplicated SSSI: Treat for 10-14 days: ≥12 yrs: 600mg PO q12h; 5-11 yrs: 10mg/kg PO q12h; <5 yrs: 10mg/kg PO q8h. Neonates <7 days: Initiate with dosing regimen of 10mg/kg q12h; may increase to 10mg/kg q8h if suboptimal response. All neonatal patients should receive 10mg/kg q8h by 7 days of life.

HOW SUPPLIED: Inj: 2mg/mL [100mL, 200mL, 300mL]; Sus: 100mg/5mL [150mL]; Tab: 400mg, 600mg

WARNINGS/PRECAUTIONS: Myelosuppression, including anemia, thrombocytopenia, pancytopenia, and leukopenia reported; monitor CBC weekly. *Clostridium difficile*-associated diarrhea reported. Oral sus contains phenylalanine. Peripheral and optic neuropathy reported; monitor visual function if on for extended periods (≥3 months). Lactic acidosis and convulsions reported. May promote overgrowth of nonsusceptible organisms.

ADVERSE REACTIONS: Diarrhea, headache, N/V.

INTERACTIONS: Potential interaction with adrenergic and serotonergic agents. May enhance pressor response to sympathomimetics, vasopressors, and dopaminergic agents; caution with dopamine, epinephrine, pseudoephedrine, and phenylpropanolamine. Serotonin syndrome may occur with concomitant serotonergic agents, including antidepressants such as SSRIs. Avoid large quantities of tyramine-containing foods or beverages.

PREGNANCY: Category C, caution in nursing.

MECHANISM OF ACTION: Oxazolidinone antibacterial; inhibits bacterial protein synthesis; binds to a site on the bacterial 23S ribosomal RNA of the 50S subunit and prevents formation of functional 70S initiation complex, which is an essential component of the bacterial translation process.

PHARMACOKINETICS: Absorption: Rapid/extensive; absolute bioavailability (100%); T_{max}=1-2 hrs. **Distribution:** V_d=40-50L; plasma protein binding (31%); distributes to well-perfused tissues. **Metabolism:** Via oxidation; aminoethoxyacetic acid (A), hydroxyethyl glycine (B) (inactive metabolites). **Elimination:** Urine (30% as parent drug, 40% as B, 10% as A), feces (6% as B, 3% as A).

NURSING CONSIDERATIONS

Assessment: Assess for pre-existing myelosuppression (including anemia, leukopenia, pancytopenia, thrombocytopenia), concomitant drugs that produce myelosuppression, presence of chronic infections, previous or concomitant antibiotic therapy, catheter-related bloodstream infections or catheter-site infections, pregnancy/nursing status, uncontolled HTN, carcinoid syndrome, pheochromocytoma, untreated hyperthyroidism, phenylketonuria, renal/hepatic impairment, and possible drug interactions (eg, SSRIs).

Monitoring: Perform weekly monitoring of CBC. Monitor for signs/symptoms of myelosuppresion (eg, anemia, leukopenia, pancytopenia, thrombocytopenia), pseudomembranous colitis or *C.difficile*-associated diarrhea (may range from mild diarrhea to fatal colitis), lactic acidosis with repeated NV, convulsions, development of drug resistance or superinfection, serotonin syndrome (eg, cognitive dysfunction, hyperrexia, hyperreflexia, incoordination), blurred vision, optic/peripheral neuropathy. Monitor visual function with long-term therapy or if new visual symptoms occur.

Patient Counseling: Instruct to notify if pregnant/nursing, have HTN or history of seizures, or if taking cold remedies, decongestants or SSRIs. Inform about risks/benefits of therapy. D/C and notify physician if visual changes or other side effects occur. Inform that drug treats bacterial, not viral, infections. Instruct to take drug exactly as directed to prevent drug resistance and maintain effectiveness. Caution to avoid large quantities of food or beverages with high tyramine content.

Administration: IV/Oral routes. **Storage:** 25°C (77°F); excursions permitted to 15-30°C (59-86°F); store in tightly closed bottles.

Appendix: Reference Tables

ABBREVIATIONS, MEASUREMENTS, AND CALCULATIONS

Abbreviations, Acronyms, and Symbols A1
Calculations and Formulas A7
Tables for Pharmacy Calculations A15

PROFESSIONAL ORGANIZATIONS, BOARDS, AND OTHER INFORMATION CENTERS

Drug Information Centers A17
Poison Control Centers A23
Certification Programs for Nurses A29
Professional Associations for Nurses A31
Nurse Practitioner Programs by State A33
Professional Associations for NPs A37

OTC DRUG COMPARISON CHARTS

Central Nervous System
Antipyretic Products A39
Headache/Migraine Products A43
Insomnia Products A49
Smoking Cessation Products A51
Weight Management Products A53

Dermatology
Acne Products A59
Antifungal Products A63
Contact Dermatitis Products A65
Dandruff Products A67
Diaper Rash Products A69
Dry Skin Products A71
Psoriasis Products A83
Wound Care Products A85

Gastrointestinal
Antacid and Heartburn Products A87
Antidiarrheal Products A91
Antiflatulant Products A93
Hemorrhoidal Products A95
Laxative Products A97

Ophthalmic
Artificial Tear Products A101
Ophthalmic Decongestant/ Antihistamine Products A103

Respiratory
Allergic Rhinitis Products A105
Is it a Cold, the Flu, or an Allergy? A109
Cough-Cold-Flu Products A110
Nasal Decongestant/ Moisturizing Products A125

Miscellaneous
Analgesic Products A129
Canker and Cold Sore Products A135

RX DRUG COMPARISON CHARTS

Cardiology
ACE Inhibitors A137
Antiarrhythmic Agents A138
Angiotensin II Receptor Blockers (ARBs) and Combinations A145
Beta-Blockers A147
Calcium Channel Blockers A151
Cholesterol-Lowering Agents A153
Coagulation Modifiers A155
Diuretics A161
Lipid Management A163

Dermatology
Acne Management: Systemic Therapies A165
Acne Management: Topical Therapies A167
Psoriasis Management: Systemic Therapies A169
Psoriasis Management: Topical Therapies A171
Topical Corticosteroids A173

Endocrinology
Insulin Formulations A175
Oral Antidiabetic Agents A177

Gastroenterology
Antiemetics A179
H_2 Antagonists and Proton Pump Inhibitors (PPIs) Comparison A185

Infectious Disease
Antibiotic Sensitivity Chart
Aminoglycosides A186
Carbapenems/Monobactams A190
Cephalosporins A194
Fluoroquinolones A199
Macrolides and Clindamycin A203
Penicillins A207
Sulfonamides A211
Tetracyclines A211
Miscellaneous A215
Drug Treatments for Common STDs A219
Flu Vaccines A223
HIV/AIDS Pharmacotherapy A225
HIV/AIDS Complications Therapy A229
Management of Hepatitis B and Hepatitis C A231
Oral Antibiotics A235
Systemic Antibiotics A237
Systemic Antifungals A269

Musculoskeletal
Ankylosing Spondylitis Agents A273
Bone Mineral Density Classification/Tests A275
Dietary Calcium Intake A277
Gout Agents A279
Osteoarthritis Agents A281
Osteoporosis Agents A283
Rheumatoid Arthritis Agents A287

Obstetrics and Gynecology
Gynecological Anti-Infectives A289
Hormone Therapy A291
Oral Contraceptives A293

Oncology
Breast Cancer Treatment Options A295
Breast Cancer Risk Factors A301
Chemotherapy Regimens A303
Colorectal Cancer Treatment Options A307

Ophthalmology
Administration Guidelines for Eye Drops & Ointment A309
Glaucoma Agents A311

Neurology and Pain Management
ADHD Agents A313
Alzheimer's Disease Agents A317
Antiparkinson's Agents A318
Opioid Products A322
Oral Anticonvulsants A327
Oral Narcotic Analgesics A329
Triptans for Acute Migraine A331

Psychiatry
Antidepressants A333
Antipsychotic Agents A335
Bipolar Disorder Pharmacotherapy A337

Pulmonology
Administration Guidelines for Dry Powder Inhalers A341
Administration Guidelines for Metered-Dose Inhalers A343
Asthma Management A345
Asthma Treatment Plan A347

Urology
Urological Therapies A349

IMMUNIZATION CHARTS
Recommended Immunization Schedule for Persons Aged 0-6 Years A351
Recommended Immunization Schedule for Persons Aged 7-18 Years A353
Catch-up Immunization Schedule for Persons Aged 4 Months–18 Years Who Start Late or Who Are More Than 1 Month Behind A355
Recommended Adult Immunization Schedule, by Vaccine and Age Group A357
Vaccines That Might Be Indicated for Adults Based on Medical and Other Indications A361

MISCELLANEOUS
Alcohol-Free Products A365
Common Laboratory Test Values A369
Cytochrome P450 Enzymes: Substrates, Inducers, and Inhibitors A373
Drugs Excreted in Breast Milk A383
Drugs That May Cause Photosensitivity A385
Drugs That May Cause QT Prolongation A389
Drugs That May Cause Stevens-Johnson Syndrome and Toxic Epidermal Necrolysis (TEN) A391
Drugs That Should Not Be Crushed A393
Generic Availability Guide A399
Lactose- and Galactose-Free Drugs A405
Poison Antidote Chart A407
Sugar-Free Products A413
Sulfite-Containing Products A419
Use-in-Pregnancy Ratings A421
Vitamin Comparison Table A428

ABBREVIATIONS, ACRONYMS, AND SYMBOLS

ABBREVIATIONS	DESCRIPTIONS
- (eg, 6-8)	to (eg, 6 to 8)
/	per
<	less than
>	greater than
≤	less than or equal to
≥	greater than or equal to
α	alpha
β	beta
5-FU	5-fluorouracil
5-HT	5-hydroxytryptamine (serotonin)
ABECB	acute bacterial exacerbation of chronic bronchitis
aa	of each
ACTH	adrenocorticotrophic hormone
ad	right ear
ADHD	attention-deficit/hyperactivity disorder
A-fib	atrial fibrillation
A-flutter	atrial flutter
AIDS	acquired immunodeficiency syndrome
ALT	alanine transaminase (SGPT)
am	morning
AMI	acute myocardial infarction
ANA	antinuclear antibodies
ANC	absolute neutrophil count
APAP	acetaminophen
as	left ear
ASA	aspirin
AST	aspartate transaminase (SGOT)
au	each ear
AUC	area under the curve
AV	atrioventricular
bid	twice daily
BMI	body mass index
BP	blood pressure
BPH	benign prostatic hypertrophy
BSA	body surface area
BUN	blood urea nitrogen
CABG	coronary artery bypass graft
CAD	coronary artery disease
Cap	capsule or gelcap
CAP	community-acquired pneumonia
CBC	complete blood count
CF	cystic fibrosis
CHF	congestive heart failure
cm	centimeter
CMV	cytomegalovirus
C_{max}	peak plasma concentration
CNS	central nervous system
COPD	chronic obstructive pulmonary disease
CrCl	creatinine clearance
Cre	cream
CRF	chronic renal failure

(Continued)

ABBREVIATIONS	DESCRIPTIONS
CSF	cerebrospinal fluid
CVA	cerebrovascular accident
CVD	cardiovascular disease
CYP450	cytochrome P450
d/c	discontinue
DHEA	dehydroepiandrosterone
DM	diabetes mellitus
DVT	deep vein thrombosis
ECG	electrocardiogram
EEG	electroencephalogram
eg	for example
EPS	extrapyramidal symptom
ESRD	end-stage renal disease
FSH	follicle-stimulating hormone
g	gram
GABA	gamma-aminobutyric acid
GAD	general anxiety disorder
GERD	gastroesophageal reflux disease
GFR	glomerular filtration rate
GI	gastrointestinal
GnRH	gonadotropin-releasing hormone
GVHD	graft versus host disease
HCG	human chorionic gonadotropin
Hct	hematocrit
HCTZ	hydrochlorothiazide
HDL	high-density lipoprotein
Hgb	hemoglobin
HIV	human immunodeficiency virus
HMG-CoA	3-hydroxy-3-methylglutaryl-coenzyme A
HR	heart rate
hr or hrs	hour or hours
hs	bedtime
HSV	herpes simplex virus
HTN	hypertension
IBD	inflammatory bowel disease
IBS	irritable bowel syndrome
ICH	intracranial hemorrhage
ICP	intracranial pressure
IM	intramuscular
INH	isoniazid
Inj	injection
INR	international normalized ratio
IOP	intraocular pressure
IU	international units
IV	intravenous/intravenously
K^+	potassium
kg	kilogram
KIU	kallikrein inhibitor unit
L	liter
lbs	pounds
LD	loading dose
LDL	low-density lipoprotein
LFT	liver function test
LH	luteinizing hormone

(Continued)

ABBREVIATIONS	DESCRIPTIONS
LHRH	luteinizing-hormone releasing hormone
Lot	lotion
Loz	lozenge
LVH	left ventricular hypertrophy
M	molar
MAC	mycobacterium avium complex
Maint	maintenance
MAOI	monoamine oxidase inhibitor
Max	maximum
mcg	microgram
mEq	milli-equivalent
mg	milligram
MI	myocardial infarction
min	minute (usually as mL/min)
mL	milliliter
mm	millimeter
mM	millimolar
MRI	magnetic resonance imaging
MS	multiple sclerosis
msec	millisecond
MTX	methotrexate
Na	sodium
NaCl	sodium chloride
NG	nasogastric
NKA	no known allergies
NMS	neuroleptic malignant syndrome
NPO	nothing by mouth
NSAID	nonsteroidal anti-inflammatory drug
NV	nausea and vomiting
OA	osteoarthritis
OCD	obsessive-compulsive disorder
od	right eye
Oint	ointment
os	left eye
ou	each eye
PAT	paroxysmal atrial tachycardia
pc	after meals
PCN	penicillin
PCP	*Pneumocystis carinii* pneumonia
PD	Parkinson's disease
PID	pelvic inflammatory disease
pkt, pkts	packet, packets
pm	evening
po	orally
PONV	postoperative nausea and vomiting
pr	rectally
prn	as needed
PSA	prostate-specific antigen
PSVT	paroxysmal supraventricular tachycardia
PT	prothrombin time
PTSD	post-traumatic stress disorder
PTT	partial thromboplastin time
PTU	propylthiouracil
PUD	peptic ulcer disease

(Continued)

ABBREVIATIONS	DESCRIPTIONS
PVD	peripheral vascular disease
q4h, q6h, q8h, etc.	every four hours, every six hours, every eight hours, etc.
qd	once daily
qh	every hour
qid	four times daily
qod	every other day
qs	a sufficient quantity
qs ad	a sufficient quantity up to
RA	rheumatoid arthritis
RBC	red blood cells
RDIs	reference daily intakes
RDS	respiratory distress syndrome
REM	rapid eye movement
SAH	subarachnoid hemorrhage
SBP	systolic blood pressure
sec	second(s)
SGOT	serum glutamic-oxaloacetic transaminase (AST)
SGPT	serum glutamic-pyruvic transaminase (ALT)
SIADH	syndrome of inappropriate antidiuretic hormone secretion
SLE	systemic lupus erythematosus
SOB	shortness of breath
Sol	solution
SQ, SC	subcutaneous
SrCr	serum creatinine
SSRI	selective serotonin reuptake inhibitor
SSSI	skin and skin structure infection
STD	sexually transmitted disease
Sup	suppository
Sus	suspension
SVT	supraventricular tachycardia
$T_{1/2}$	half-life
Tab	tablet or caplet
Tab, SL	sublingual tablet
TB	tuberculosis
TBG	thyroxine binding globulin
tbl	tablespoon
TCA	tricyclic antidepressant
TD	tardive dyskinesia
TFT	thyroid function test
TG	triglyceride
tid	three times daily
T_{max}	time to maximum concentration
TNF	tumor necrosis factor
TPN	total parenteral nutrition
TSH	thyroid stimulating hormone
tsp	teaspoonful
TTP	thrombotic thrombocytopenic purpura

(Continued)

ABBREVIATIONS	DESCRIPTIONS
U	unit
ud	as directed
ULN	upper limit of normal
URTI/URI	upper respiratory tract infection
UTI	urinary tract infection
UV	ultraviolet
WBC	white blood cell count
Vd	volume of distribution
VTE	venous thromboembolism
X	times (eg, >2X ULN)
yr or yrs	year or years

CALCULATIONS AND FORMULAS

WEIGHTS AND MEASURES

METRIC MEASURES	
1 kilogram (kg)	1000 g
1 gram (g)	1000 mg
1 milligram (mg)	0.001 g
1 microgram (mcg or μg)	0.001 mg; 1 x 10^{-6} g
1 liter (L)	1000 mL
1 milliliter (mL)	0.001 L; 1 cc (cubic centimeter)
APOTHECARY MEASURES (AP)	
1 scruple	20 grains (gr)
1 drachm	3 scruples; 60 gr
1 ounce (oz)	8 drachms; 24 scruples; 480 gr
1 pound (lb)	12 oz; 96 drachms; 288 scruples; 5760 gr
U.S. FLUID MEASURES	
1 fluidrachm	60 minim
1 fluidounce	8 fluidrachm; 480 minim
1 pint (pt)	16 fl oz; 7680 minim
1 quart (qt)	2 pt; 32 fl oz
1 gallon (gal)	4 qt; 128 fl oz
AVOIRDUPOIS WEIGHT (AV)	
1 ounce	437.5 gr
1 pound	16 oz
CONVERSION FACTORS	
1 gram	15.4 gr
1 grain	64.8 mg
1 ounce (Av)	28.35 g; 437.5 gr
1 ounce (Ap)	31.1 g; 480 gr
1 pound (Av)	453.6 g; 2.68 lb (Ap); 2.20 lb (Av)
1 fluidounce	29.57 mL
1 fluidrachm	3.697 mL
1 minim	0.06 mL
COMMON MEASURES	
1 teaspoonful	5 mL; 1/6 fl oz
1 tablespoonful	15 mL; 1/2 fl oz
1 wineglassful	60 mL; 2 fl oz
1 teacupful	120 mL; 4 fl oz
1 gallon	3800 mL; 128 fl oz
1 quart	960 mL; 32 fl oz
1 pint	480 mL; 16 fl oz (exactly 473.2 mL)
8 fluid ounces	240 mL
4 fluid ounces	120 mL
2.2 lb	1 kg

DOSE EQUIVALENTS

WEIGHT (METRIC)	WEIGHT (APOTHECARY)
30 g	1 ounce
15 g	4 drams
10 g	2 1/2 drams
7.5 g	2 drams
6 g	90 grains
5 g	75 grains
4 g	60 grains; 1 dram
3 g	45 grains
2 g	30 grains; 1/2 dram
1.5 g	22 grains
1 g	15 grains
750 mg	12 grains
600 mg	10 grains
500 mg	7 1/2 grains
400 mg	6 grains
300 mg	5 grains
250 mg	4 grains

(Continued)

DOSE EQUIVALENTS *(Continued)*

WEIGHT (METRIC)	WEIGHT (APOTHECARY)
200 mg	3 grains
150 mg	2 1/2 grains
125 mg	2 grains
100 mg	1 1/2 grains
75 mg	1 1/4 grains
60 mg	1 grain
50 mg	3/4 grain
40 mg	2/3 grain
30 mg	3/8 grain
25 mg	3/8 grain
20 mg	1/3 grain
15 mg	1/5 grain
12 mg	1/5 grain
10 mg	1/6 grain
8 mg	1/8 grain
6 mg	1/10 grain
5 mg	1/12 grain
4 mg	1/15 grain
3 mg	1/20 grain
2 mg	1/30 grain
1.5 mg	1/40 grain
1.2 mg	1/50 grain
1 mg	1/60 grain

LIQUID MEASURES (METRIC)	LIQUID MEASURES (APOTHECARY)
1000 mL	1 quart
750 mL	1 1/2 pints
500 mL	1 pint
230 mL	8 fluid ounces
200 mL	7 fluid ounces
100 mL	3 1/2 fluid ounces
50 mL	1 3/4 fluid ounces
30 mL	1 fluid ounces
15 mL	4 fluid drams
10 mL	2 1/2 fluid drams
8 mL	2 fluid drams
5 mL	1 1/4 fluid drams
4 mL	1 fluid dram
3 mL	45 minims
2 mL	30 minims
1 mL	15 minims
0.75 mL	12 minims
0.6 mL	10 minims
0.5 mL	8 minims
0.3 mL	5 minims
0.25 mL	4 minims
0.2 mL	3 minims
0.1 mL	1 1/2 minims
0.06 mL	1 minim
0.05 mL	3/4 minim
0.03 mL	1/2 minim

MILLIEQUIVALENT (mEq) AND MILLIMOLE (mmol)

CALCULATIONS

$$\text{moles} = \frac{\text{weight of a substance (grams)}}{\text{molecular weight of that substance (grams)}} \quad \textbf{OR} \quad = \frac{\text{equivalent}}{\text{valence of ion}}$$

$$\text{millimoles} = \frac{\text{weight of a substance (milligrams)}}{\text{molecular weight of that substance (milligrams)}} \quad \textbf{OR} \quad = \frac{\text{milliequivalents}}{\text{valence of ion}} \quad \textbf{OR} \quad = \text{moles} \times 1000$$

equivalents = moles x valence of ion

milliequivalents = millimoles x valence of ion **OR** = equivalents x 1000

(Continued)

CONVERSIONS

mg/100mL to mEq/L	$\text{mEq/L} = \frac{(\text{mg/100mL}) \times 10 \times \text{valence}}{\text{atomic weight}}$
mEq/L to mg/100mL	$\text{mg/100mL} = \frac{(\text{mEq/L}) \times \text{atomic weight}}{10 \times \text{valence}}$
mEq/L to volume percent of a gas	$\text{volume \%} = \frac{(\text{mEq/L}) \times 22.4}{10}$

ACID-BASE ASSESSMENT

DEFINITIONS

PIO_2	Oxygen partial pressure of inspired gas (mmHg); 150 mmHg in room air at sea level
FiO_2	Fractional pressure of oxygen in inspired gas (0.21 in room air)
PAO_2	Alveolar oxygen partial pressure
$PACO_2$	Alveolar carbon dioxide partial pressure
PaO_2	Arterial oxygen partial pressure
$PaCO_2$	Arterial carbon dioxide partial pressure
R	Respiratory exchange quotient (typically 0.8, increases with high carbohydrate diet, decreases with high fat diet)

HENDERSON-HASSELBALCH EQUATION

$pH = 6.1 + \log [HCO_3^- / (0.03)(pCO_2)]$

ALVEOLAR GAS EQUATION

$PIO_2 = FiO_2 \times (\text{total atmospheric pressure - vapor pressure of } H_2O \text{ at } 37°C)$
$= FiO_2 \times (760 \text{ mmHg} - 47 \text{ mmHg})$

$PaO_2 = PIO_2 - PaCO_2/R$

ALVEOLAR/ARTERIAL OXYGEN GRADIENT

$PAO_2 - PaO_2$

ACID-BASE DISORDERS

Disorder	pH	HCO_3^-	PCO_2	Compensation
Metabolic acidosis	< 7.35	Primary decrease	Compensatory decrease	1.2-mmHg decrease in PCO_2 for every 1-mmol/L decrease in HCO_3^- **or** $PCO_2 = (1.5 \times HCO_3^-) + 8\ (\pm 2)$ **or** $PCO_2 = HCO_3^- + 15$ **or** PCO_2 = last 2 digits of pH x 100
Metabolic alkalosis	> 7.45	Primary increase	Compensatory increase	0.6-0.75 mmHg increase in PCO_2 for every 1-mmol/L increase in HCO_3^-. PCO_2 should not rise above 60 mm Hg in compensation.
Respiratory acidosis	< 7.35	Compensatory increase	Primary increase	***Acute:*** 1-2 mmol decrease in HCO_3^-. for every 10-mmHg decrease in PCO_2. ***Chronic:*** 3-4 mmol increase in HCO_3^-. for every 10-mmHg increase in PCO_2.
Respiratory alkalosis	> 7.45	Compensatory decrease	Primary decrease	***Acute:*** 1-2 mmol increase in HCO_3^-. for every 10-mmHg increase in PCO_2. ***Chronic:*** 4-5 mmol decrease in HCO_3^-. for every 10-mmHg decrease in PCO_2.

ACID-BASE EQUATION

H^+ (in mEq/L) = $(24 \times PaCO_2)$ divided by HCO_3^-

(Continued)

OTHER CALCULATIONS

ANION GAP

Anion gap = $Na^+ - (Cl^- + HCO_3^-$ measured)

AA GRADIENT

Aa gradient [(713) (FiO_2 - ($PaCO_2$ divided by 0.8))] - PaO_2

OSMOLALITY

Definition:
Osmolality is a measure of the total number of particles in a solution.

U.S. units (sodium as mEq/L, BUN (blood urea nitrogen) and glucose as (mg/dL)
Plasma osmolality (mOsm/kg) = 2([Na^+] + [K^+]) + ([BUN]/2.8) + ([glucose]/18)

SI units (all variables in mmol/L):
Plasma osmolality (mOsm/kg) = 2[Na^+] + [urea] + [glucose]
Normal range plasma osmolality: 280 - 303 mOsm/kg

Corrected Sodium
Corrected Na+ = measured Na^+ + [1.5 x (glucose - 150 divided by 100)]*
*Do not correct for glucose <150.

Total Serum Calcium Corrected for Albumin Level
[(Normal albumin - patient's albumin) x 0.8] + patient's measured total calcium

Water Deficit
Water deficit = 0.6 x body weight [1 - (140 divided by Na^+)]*
*Body weight is estimated weight in kg; Na^+ is serum or plasma sodium.

Bicarbonate Deficit
HCO_3^- deficit = [0.4 x weight (kg)] x (HCO_3^- desired - HCO_3^- measured)

CHILD-PUGH SCORE

The Child-Pugh classification used to assess the prognosis of chronic liver disease, mainly cirrhosis. Child-Pugh is also used to determine the required strength of treatment and the necessity of liver transplantation.

Score:
The score employs five clinical measures of liver disease. Each measure is scored 1-3, with 3 indicating most severe derangement.

Measure	1 point	2 points	3 points	Units
Bilirubin (total)*	<34 (<2)	34-50 (2-3)	>50 (>3)	mol/L (mg/dL)
Serum albumin	>35	28-35	<28	mg/L
INR**	<1.7	1.71-2.20	> 2.20	no unit
Ascites	None	Suppressed with medication	Refractory	no unit
Hepatic encephalopathy	None	Grade I-II (or suppressed with medication)	Grade III-IV (or refractory)	no unit

* In primary sclerosing cholangitis and primary biliary cirrhosis, the bilirubin references are changed to reflect the fact that these diseases feature high conjugated bilirubin levels. The upper limit for 1 point is 68 mol/L (4 mg/dL) and the upper limit for 2 points is 170 mol/L (10 mg/dL).

** Some older reference works substitute PT prolongation for INR.

Interpretation:
Chronic liver disease is classified into Child-Pugh class A to C, employing the added score from above.

Points	Class	One year survival	Two year survival
5-6	A	100%	85%
7-9	B	81%	57%
10-15	C	45%	35%

CREATININE CLEARANCE

Clinically, creatinine clearance is a useful measure for estimating the glomerular filtration rate (GFR) of the kidneys.

Factors	Abbreviations
Creatinine clearance	Cl_{Cr}
Plasma creatinine concentration	P_{Cr}
Serum creatinine concentration	S_{Cr}
Urine creatinine concentration	U_{Cr}
Urine flow rate	V
Plasma creatinine concentration	P_{Cr}

(Continued)

CREATININE CLEARANCE *(Continued)*

Calculations:

$$Cl_{Cr} = \frac{U_{Cr} \times V}{P_{Cr}}$$

Example:

Patient with P_{Cr} 1 mg/dL, U_{Cr} 60 mg/dL, and V of 0.5 dL/hr.

$$Cl_{Cr} = \frac{60 \text{ mg/dL} \times 0.5 \text{ dL/hr} = 30 \text{ dL/hr}}{1 \text{ mg/dL}}$$

Cockcroft-Gault formula: Estimates creatinine clearance (mL/min).

Male:

$$Cl_{Cr} = \frac{(140 - \text{age}) \times \text{mass (kg)}}{72 \times S_{Cr} \text{ (mg/dL)}}$$

Example:

Male patient, 67 years of age, weight 75 kg, and S_{Cr} 1 mg/dL.

$$Cl_{Cr} = \frac{(140 - 67) \times 75}{72 \times 1} = 76 \text{ mL/min}$$

Female:

$$Cl_{Cr} = \frac{(140 - \text{age}) \times \text{mass (kg)} \times 0.85}{72 \times S_{Cr} \text{ (mg/dL)}}$$

Example:

Female patient, 67 years of age, weight 75 kg, and S_{Cr} 1 mg/dL.

$$Cl_{Cr} = \frac{(140 - 67) \times 75}{72 \times 1} \times 0.85 = 64.6 \text{ mL/min}$$

Note: Using actual body weight (ABW) in obese patients can significantly overestimate creatinine clearance. Adjusted ideal body weight (IBW) can provide more approximate estimate. Adjusted IBW = IBW + 0.4 (ABW - IBW).

BASAL ENERGY EXPENDITURE (BEE)

Basal energy expenditure: the amount of energy required to maintain the body's normal metabolic activity (ie, respiration, maintenance of body temperature, etc).

H = height (cm), W = weight (kg), A = age (years)

Male:

BEE = 66.67 + 13.75W + 5H - 6.76A

Female:

BEE = 665.1 + 9.56W +1.85H -4.68A

BODY MASS INDEX (BMI)

$$BMI = \frac{\text{weight (kg)}}{[\text{height (m)}]^2}$$

BODY SURFACE AREA (BSA)

$$BSA\ (m^2) = \sqrt{\frac{\text{height (in)} \times \text{weight (lb)}}{3131}}$$

OR

$$BSA\ (m^2) = \sqrt{\frac{\text{height (cm)} \times \text{weight (kg)}}{3600}}$$

IDEAL BODY WEIGHT (IBW)

Adults (18 years and older; IBW is in kg):

- IBW (male) = 50 + (2.3 x height [inches] over 5 feet)
- IBW (female) = 45.5 + (2.3 x height [inches] over 5 feet)

Children (IBW is in kg; height is in cm):

1-18 years of age:

$$IBW = \frac{(\text{height}^2 \times 1.65)}{100}$$

5 feet and taller:

- IBW (male) = 39 + (2.27 x height [inches] over 5 feet)
- IBW (female) = 42.2 + (2.27 x height [inches] over 5 feet)

(Continued)

POUNDS/KILOGRAM CONVERSION

1 pound = 0.45359 kilogram				1 kilogram = 2.2 pounds			
lb	kg	lb	kg	lb	kg	lb	kg
1	0.45	105	47.63	210	95.25	315	142.88
5	2.27	110	49.89	215	97.52	320	145.15
10	4.54	115	52.16	220	99.79	325	147.42
15	6.80	120	54.43	225	102.06	330	149.68
20	9.07	125	56.70	230	104.33	335	151.95
25	11.34	130	58.97	235	106.59	340	154.22
30	13.61	135	61.23	240	108.86	345	156.49
35	15.88	140	63.50	245	111.13	350	158.76
40	18.14	145	65.77	250	113.40	355	161.02
45	20.41	150	68.04	255	115.67	360	163.29
50	22.68	155	70.31	260	117.93	365	165.56
55	24.95	160	72.57	265	120.20	370	167.83
60	27.22	165	74.84	270	122.47	375	170.10
65	29.48	170	77.11	275	124.74	380	172.36
70	31.75	175	79.38	280	127.01	385	174.63
75	34.02	180	81.65	285	129.27	390	176.90
80	36.29	185	83.91	290	131.54	395	179.17
85	38.56	190	86.18	295	133.81	400	181.44
90	40.82	195	88.45	300	136.08	405	183.70
95	43.09	200	90.72	305	138.34	410	185.97
100	45.36	205	92.99	310	140.61	415	188.24

TEMPERATURE CONVERSION

Fahrenheit to Celsius = (°F - 32) x 5/9 = °C				Celsius to Fahrenheit = (°C x 9/5) + 32 = °F			
°F	°C	°F	°C	°C	°F	°C	°F
0.0	-17.8	92.0	33.3	0.0	32.0	49.0	120.2
5.0	-15.0	93.0	33.9	5.0	41.0	50.0	122.0
10.0	-12.2	94.0	34.4	10.0	50.0	51.0	123.8
15.0	-9.4	95.0	35.0	15.0	59.0	52.0	125.6
20.0	-6.7	96.0	35.6	20.0	68.0	53.0	127.4
25.0	-3.9	97.0	36.1	25.0	77.0	54.0	129.2
30.0	-1.1	98.0	36.7	30.0	86.0	55.0	131.0
35.0	1.7	98.6	37.0	35.0	95.0	56.0	132.8
40.0	4.4	99.0	37.2	36.0	96.8	57.0	134.6
45.0	7.2	100.0	37.8	37.0	98.6	58.0	136.4
50.0	10.0	101.0	38.3	38.0	100.4	59.0	138.2
55.0	12.8	102.0	38.9	39.0	102.2	60.0	140.0
60.0	15.6	103.0	39.4	40.0	104.0	65.0	149.0
65.0	18.3	104.0	40.0	41.0	105.8	70.0	158.0
70.0	21.1	105.0	40.6	42.0	107.6	75.0	167.0
75.0	23.9	106.0	41.1	43.0	109.4	80.0	176.0
80.0	26.7	107.0	41.7	44.0	111.2	85.0	185.0
85.0	29.4	108.0	42.2	45.0	113.0	90.0	194.0
90.0	32.2	109.0	42.8	46.0	114.8	95.0	203.0
91.0	32.8	110.0	43.3	47.0	116.6	100.0	212.0
				48.0	118.4	105.0	221.0

(Continued)

PEDIATRIC DOSAGE ESTIMATION FORMULAS

The following formulas can be used to estimate the approximate pediatric dosage of a medication. These formulas are based on the adult dose and either the child's age or weight. These formulas should be used with caution as the response to any drug is not always directly proportional to the age or weight of the child relative to the usual adult dose. Dosage will also vary based on the formula used. Care should be taken when using any of these methods to calculate the child's dosage. Some products have FDA approved pediatric indications and dosages, always refer to full prescribing information first before calculating a pediatric dosage.

BASED ON WEIGHT

Augsberger's Rule:

$$\frac{[(1.5 \times \text{weight [kg]}) + 10]}{100} \times \text{adult dose} = \text{approximate child's dose}$$

Example: If the child's weight is 15 kg (33 lb) and the adult dose is 50 mg then the child's dose is 16.25 mg.

$$\frac{[(1.5 \times 15 \text{ kg}) + 10]}{100} \times 50 \text{ mg} = 0.325 \times 50 \text{ mg} = 16.25 \text{ mg}$$

Clark's Rule:

(weight [lb]/150) x adult dose = approximate child's dose

Example: If the child's weight is 15 kg (33 lb) and the adult dose is 50 mg then the child's dose is 11 mg.

(33/150) x 50 mg = 0.22 x 50 mg = 11 mg

Based on Age

Augsberger's Rule:

$$\frac{[(4 \times \text{age [years]}) + 20]}{100} \times \text{adult dose} = \text{approximate child's dose}$$

Example: If the child's age is 8 years and the adult dose is 50 mg then the child's dose is 26 mg.
[(4 x 8) + 20)/100] x 50 mg = 0.52 X 50 mg = 26 mg

Dilling's Rule:

(age [years]/20) x adult dose = approximate child's dose

Example: If the child's age is 8 years and the adult dose is 50 mg then the child's dose is 20 mg.
(8/20) x 50 mg = 0.40 x 50 mg = 20 mg

Cowling's Rule:

$$\frac{[\text{age at next birthday (years)}]}{24} \times \text{adult dose} = \text{approximate child's dose}$$

Example: If the child is going to turn 8 years old in few months and the adult dose is 50 mg then the child's dose is 16.7 mg. (8/24) x 50 mg = 0.33 x 50 mg = 16.7 mg

Younge's Rule:

$$\frac{[\text{age (years)}]}{\text{age} + 12} \times \text{adult dose} = \text{approximate child's dose}$$

Example: If the child's age is 8 years and the adult dose is 50 mg then the child's dose is 20 mg.
[8/(8+12)] x 50 mg = 0.4 x 50 mg = 20 mg

Fried's Rule (younger than 1 year):

$$\frac{[\text{age (months)}]}{150} \times \text{adult dose} = \text{approximate infant's dose}$$

Example: If the child's age is 10 months and the adult dose is 50 mg then the child's dose is 3.33 mg.
(10/150) x 50 mg = 0.067 x 50 mg = 3.33 mg

TABLES FOR PHARMACY CALCULATIONS

WEIGHTS AND MEASURES

Metric Measure

Weight

1 kilogram (kg)	=	1,000 g
1 gram (g)	=	1,000 mg
1 milligram (mg)	=	0.001 g
1 microgram (mcg)	=	0.001 mg
1 gamma	=	1 mcg

Liquid

1 liter (L)	=	1,000 mL
1 milliliter (mL)	=	1 cc (cubic centimeter)

Apothecary (Ap)

Weight

1 scruple	=	20 grains (gr)
1 drachm	=	3 scruples
	=	60 gr
1 ounce (oz)	=	8 drachms
	=	24 scruples
	=	480 gr
1 pound (lb)	=	12 oz
	=	96 drachms
	=	288 scruples
	=	5,760 gr

U.S. Fluid Measure

1 fluidrachm	=	60 minim (min)
1 fluidounce	=	8 fld drachm
	=	480 min
1 pint (pt)	=	16 fl oz
	=	7,680 min
1 quart (qt)	=	2 pt
	=	32 fl oz
1 gallon (gal)	=	4 qts
	=	128 fl oz

Avoirdupois (Av)

Weight

1 ounce	=	437.5 gr
1 pound	=	16 oz

Conversion Factors

1 gram	=	15.4 gr
1 grain	=	64.8 mg
1 ounce (Av)	=	28.35 g
	=	437.5 gr
1 ounce (Ap)	=	31.1 g
	=	480 gr
1 pound (Av)	=	453.6 g
1 kilogram	=	2.68 pounds Ap
	=	2.20 lbs Av
1 fluidounce	=	29.57 mL
1 fluidrachm	=	3.697 mL
1 minim	=	0.06 mL

Converting °F to °C

For °F to °C, the formula is:

5/9 (°F minus 32) = °C

For °C to °F, the formula is:

9/5 (°C plus 32) = °F

Common Measures

1 teaspoonful	=	5 mL
	=	1/6 fl oz
1 tablespoonful	=	15 mL
	=	1/2 fl oz
1 wineglassful	=	60 mL
	=	2 fl oz
1 teacupful	=	120 mL
	=	4 fl oz

TABLE OF SATURATED SOLUTIONS

This table shows the quantity of the substance and milliliters (mL) of water for 100 mL of a saturated solution at about 25° C.

Substance	Gram	mL Water
Alum	13.00	92.0
Ammonium Carbonate	22.00	88.0
Ammonium Chloride	28.30	79.3
Ammonium Nitrate	90.20	41.8
Ammonium Sulfate	53.10	71.7
Borax	5.90	98.0
Boric Acid	5.10	97.0
Calcium Lactate	5.00	96.0
Chloral Hydrate	120.00	31.0
Citric Acid	88.60	42.7
Copper Sulfate	22.30	98.7
Dextrose	59.00	60.0
Ferric Chloride	125.00	29.0
Ferrous Sulfate	52.80	72.7
Lactose	17.00	90.0
Lead Acetate	55.00	79.0
Lithium Chloride	59.50	70.2
Lithium Sulfate	33.00	88.5
Magnesium Sulfate	72.00	58.5
Manganese Chloride	90.00	54.0
Mercuric Chloride	6.96	98.5
Methylene Blue	4.30	97.0
Oxalic Acid	10.30	94.2
Potassium Bromide	56.00	82.0
Potassium Carbonate	82.20	73.5
Potassium Chloride	8.41	96.6
Potassium Citrate	92.00	56.5
Potassium Iodide	103.20	69.1
Potassium Nitrate	33.40	86.0
Potassium Permanganate	7.43	97.3
Resorcinol	67.20	47.2
Rochelle Salt	51.90	78.8
Silver Nitrate	164.00	65.5
Sodium Acetate	65.00	53.0
Sodium Benzoate	41.50	73.9
Sodium Bicarbonate	8.80	97.6
Sodium Bromide	73.00	78.0
Sodium Carbonate	27.50	96.0
Sodium Chloride	31.50	88.1
Sodium Citrate	55.50	72.5
Sodium Iodide	124.30	67.7
Sodium Nitrate	62.30	73.8
Sodium Salicylate	67.00	58.0
Sodium Sulfate	33.30	87.0
Sodium Thiocyanate	87.00	51.0
Sodium Thiosulfate	93.00	46.0
Tartaric Acid	76.90	54.7
Urea	62.00	53.5
Zinc Sulfate	93.00	56.0

DOSE EQUIVALENTS

These approximate dose equivalents have been adopted by U.S.P. XXII, N.F. XVII. They are approved by the Food and Drug Administration.

When converting specific quantities or a prescription that requires compounding, or when converting a pharmaceutical formula from one system of weights or measures to the other, the following must be used.

Weight

Metric	Apothecary
30 g	1 ounce
15 g	4 drachms
10 g	2½ drachms
7.5 g	2 drachms
6 g	90 grains
5 g	75 grains
4 g	60 grains (1 drachm)
3 g	45 grains
2 g	30 grains (½ drachm)
1.5 g	22 grains
1 g	15 grains
750 mg	12 grains
600 mg	10 grains
500 mg	7½ grains
400 mg	6 grains
300 mg	5 grains
250 mg	4 grains
200 mg	3 grains
150 mg	2½ grains
125 mg	2 grains
100 mg	1½ grains
75 mg	1¼ grains
60 mg	1 grain
50 mg	¾ grain
40 mg	⅔ grain
30 mg	½ grain
25 mg	⅜ grain
20 mg	⅓ grain
15 mg	¼ grain
12 mg	⅕ grain
10 mg	⅙ grain
8 mg	⅛ grain
6 mg	1/10 grain
5 mg	1/12 grain
4 mg	1/15 grain
3 mg	1/20 grain
2 mg	1/30 grain
1.5 mg	1/40 grain
1.2 mg	1/50 grain
1 mg	1/60 grain

(Continued)

Liquid Measure

Metric	Apothecary
1000 mL	1 quart
750 mL	1½ pints
500 mL	1 pint
250 mL	8 fluidounces
200 mL	7 fluidounces
100 mL	3½ fluidounces
50 mL	1¾ fluidounces
30 mL	1 fluidounce
15 mL	4 fluidrachms
10 mL	2½ fluidrachms
8 mL	2 fluidrachms
5 mL	1¼ fluidrachms
4 mL	1 fluidrachm
3 mL	45 minims
2 mL	30 minims
1 mL	15 minims
0.75 mL	12 minims
0.6 mL	10 minims
0.5 mL	8 minims
0.3 mL	5 minims
0.25 mL	4 minims
0.2 mL	3 minims
0.1 mL	1½ minims
0.06 mL	1 minim
0.05 mL	¾ minim
0.03 mL	½ minim

DRUG INFORMATION CENTERS

ALABAMA

BIRMINGHAM

Drug Information Service
University of Alabama
UAB Hospital Pharmacy

Drug Information-JT1720
619 S. 19th St.
Birmingham, AL 35249-6860
Mon.-Fri. 7 AM-4 PM
205-934-2162
www.health.uab.edu/pharmacy

Global Drug
Information Service
Samford University
McWhorter School
of Pharmacy

800 Lakeshore Dr.
Birmingham, AL 35229-7027
Mon. 8 AM-9 PM
Tues.-Fri. 8 AM-4:30 PM
205-726-2519 or 2891
www.samford.edu/schools/
pharmacy/dic/index.html

HUNTSVILLE

Huntsville Hospital Drug
Information Center

101 Sivley Rd.
Huntsville, AL 35801
Mon.-Fri. 8 AM-4:30 PM
256-265-8284

ARIZONA

TUCSON

Arizona Poison and Drug
Information Center

1259 N. Martin Ave.
Drachman Hall B308
Tucson, AZ 85724
7 days/week, 24 hours
520-626-6016
800-222-1222 (Emergency)
www.pharmacy.arizona.edu

ARKANSAS

LITTLE ROCK

Arkansas Drug Information Center

4301 W. Markham St.
Slot 522-2
Little Rock, AR 72205
Mon.-Fri. 8:30 AM-5 PM
501-686-6161
(Little Rock area only -
for healthcare
professionals only)
888-228-1233
(AR only - for healthcare
professionals only)

CALIFORNIA

LOS ANGELES

Los Angeles Regional
Drug Information Center
LAC & USC Medical Center

1200 N. State St.
Trailer 25
Los Angeles, CA 90033
Mon.-Fri. 8 AM-4 PM
Closed 12 PM to 1 PM
323-226-7741

SAN DIEGO

Drug Information Service
University of California
San Diego Medical Center

200 West Arbor Dr.
MC 8925
San Diego, CA 92103-8925
Mon.-Fri. 9 AM-5 PM
619-543-6971
(for healthcare
professionals only)

STANFORD

Drug Information Center
University of California
Stanford Hospital and Clinics

300 Pasteur Dr.
Room H-0301
Stanford, CA 94305
Mon.-Fri. 8 AM-4 PM
650-723-6422

COLORADO

DENVER

Rocky Mountain Poison
and Drug Center

990 Bannock St.
(Physical address)
777 Bannock St.
(Mailing address)
Denver, CO 80264
303-739-1100
800-222-1222 (Emergency)
www.rmpdc.org

CONNECTICUT

HARTFORD

Drug Information Center Hartford
Hospital

P.O. Box 5037
80 Seymour St.
Hartford, CT 06102
Mon.-Fri. 8:30 AM-5 PM
860-545-2221
860-545-2961(After 5 PM)
www.hartfordhospital.org

NEW HAVEN

Drug Information Center
Yale-New Haven Hospital

20 York St.
New Haven, CT 06540-3202
Mon.-Fri. 9 AM-5 PM
203-688-2248
www.ynhh.org/patients/pharmacy.html

DISTRICT OF COLUMBIA

Drug Information Service
Howard University Hospital

Room BB06
2041 Georgia Ave. NW
Washington, DC 20060
Mon.-Fri. 8:30 AM-4 PM
202-865-7413

FLORIDA

FT. LAUDERDALE

Nova Southeastern University
College of Pharmacy
Drug Information Center

3200 S. University Dr.
Ft. Lauderdale, FL 33328
Mon.-Fri. 9 AM-5 PM
954-262-3103
http://pharmacy.nova.edu

GAINESVILLE

Drug Information &
Pharmacy Resource Center
Shands Hospital at
University of Florida

1600 SW Archer Rd.
Gainesville, FL 32610-0316
Mon.-Fri. 9 AM-5 PM
352-265-0408
(for healthcare
professionals only)
http://shands.org/professional/
druginfo

JACKSONVILLE

Drug Information Service
Shands Jacksonville

655 W. 8th St.
Jacksonville, FL 32209
Mon.-Fri. 8:30 AM-5 PM
904-244-4185
(for healthcare
professionals only)
904-244-4700
(for consumers,
Mon.-Fri. 9:30 AM-4 PM)

http://jax.shands.org/
education/pharmacy/contact.asp

ORLANDO

Orlando Regional Drug Information Service
Orlando Regional Healthcare System

1414 Kuhl Ave., MP 192
Orlando, FL 32806
Mon.-Fri. 8 AM-4 PM
321-841-8715

TALLAHASSEE

Drug Information Education Center
Florida Agricultural and Mechanical University
College of Pharmacy and Pharmaceutical Sciences

Tallahassee, FL 32307
Mon.-Fri. 9 AM-5 PM
850-599-3064

WEST PALM BEACH

Drug Information Center
Nova Southeastern University, West Palm Beach

3970 RCA Blvd., Suite 7006A
Palm Beach Gardens, FL 33410
Mon.-Fri. 9 AM-5 PM
561-622-8682, ext 5655
(for healthcare professionals only)

GEORGIA

ATLANTA

Emory University Hospital
Dept. of Pharmaceutical Services-Drug Information

1364 Clifton Rd. NE
Atlanta, GA 30322
Mon.-Fri. 9 AM-4 PM
404-712-4644
(for healthcare professionals only)

Drug Information Service Northside Hospital

1000 Johnson Ferry Rd. NE
Atlanta, GA 30342
Mon.-Fri. 9 AM-4 PM
404-851-8676 (GA only)

COLUMBUS

Columbus Regional Drug Information Center

710 Center St.
Columbus, GA 31902
Mon.-Fri. 8 AM-4:30 PM
706-571-1934
(for healthcare professionals only)

IDAHO

POCATELLO

Idaho Drug Information Service
Idaho State University
College of Pharmacy

970 S. 5th Ave.
Campus Box 8092
Pocatello, ID 83209
Mon.-Thur. 8:30 AM-5 PM
Fri. 8:30 AM-3 PM
208-282-4689
800-334-7139 (ID only)
http://pharmacy.isu.edu

ILLINOIS

CHICAGO

Drug Information Center
Northwestern Memorial Hospital

Feinberg Pavilion, LC 700
251 E. Huron St.
Chicago, IL 60611
Mon.-Fri. 8:30 AM-5 PM
312-926-7573

Drug Information Center
University of Illinois at Chicago

833 S. Wood St.
MC 886
Chicago, IL 60612-7231
Mon.-Fri. 8 AM-4 PM
312-996-3681
(for healthcare professionals only)
312-996-5332
(for consumers,
Mon.-Fri. 9 AM-12 PM)
www.uic.edu/pharmacy

HARVEY

Drug Information Center
Ingalls Memorial Hospital

1 Ingalls Dr.
Harvey, IL 60426
Mon.-Fri. 8 AM-7 PM
Sat. 9 AM-3:30 PM
708-915-4300

HINES

Drug Information Service
Hines Veterans Administration Hospital

Pharmacy Services
MC119
P.O. Box 5000
Hines, IL 60141-5000
Mon.-Fri. 8 AM-4:30 PM
708-202-2573

PARK RIDGE

Drug Information Center
Advocate Lutheran General Hospital

1775 Dempster St.
Park Ridge, IL 60068
Mon.-Fri. 7:30 AM-4 PM
847-723-8128
(for healthcare professionals only)

INDIANA

INDIANAPOLIS

Drug Information Center
St. Vincent Hospital and Health Services

2001 W. 86th St.
Indianapolis, IN 46260
Mon.-Fri. 8 AM-4 PM
317-338-3200
(for healthcare professionals only)

Drug Information Service
Clarian Health Partners

Pharmacy Department I-65
at 21st St.
Room CG04
Indianapolis, IN 46202
Mon.-Fri. 8 AM-4:30 PM
317-962-1750

MUNCIE

Drug Information Center
Ball Memorial Hospital

2401 University Ave.
Muncie, IN 47303
Mon.-Fri. 8 AM-4:30 PM
765-747-3033

IOWA

DES MOINES

Regional Drug Information Center
Mercy Medical Center-Des Moines

1111 Sixth Ave.
Des Moines, IA 50314
Mon.-Fri. 8 AM-4:30 PM
(regional service; in-house service answered 7 days/ week, 24 hours)
515-247-3286

IOWA CITY

Drug Information Center
University of Iowa Hospitals and Clinics

200 Hawkins Dr.
Iowa City, IA 52242
Mon.-Fri. 8 AM-4:30 PM
319-356-2600

KANSAS

KANSAS CITY

Drug Information Center
University of Kansas
Medical Center

3901 Rainbow Blvd.
Kansas City, KS 66160
Mon.-Fri. 8:30 AM-4:30 PM
913-588-2328

KENTUCKY

LEXINGTON

University of Kentucky
Central Pharmacy
Chandler Medical Center

800 Rose St., C-114
Lexington, KY 40536-0293
7 days/week, 24 hours
859-323-5642
859-323-6289

LOUISIANA

MONROE

Louisiana Drug and Poison
Information Center
University of Louisiana at Monroe
College of Pharmacy

Sugar Hall
Monroe, LA 71209-6430
Mon.-Thur. 8 AM-4:30 PM
Fri. 8 AM-11:30 AM
318-342-1710

NEW ORLEANS

Xavier University Drug Information
Center
Tulane University
Hospital and Clinic

1440 Canal St.
Suite 808
New Orleans, LA 70112
Mon.-Fri. 9 AM-5 PM
504-588-5670

MARYLAND

ANDREWS AFB

Drug Information Services

79 MDSS/SGQP
1050 W. Perimeter Rd.
Suite D1-119
Andrews AFB, MD 20762-6660
Mon.-Fri. 7:30 AM-5 PM
240-857-4565

BALTIMORE

Drug Information Service
Johns Hopkins Hospital

600 N. Wolfe St.
Carnegie 180
Baltimore, MD 21287-6180
Mon.-Fri. 8:30 AM-5 PM
410-955-6348
www.hopkinsmedicine.org/pharmacy

Drug Information Service
University of Maryland

School of Pharmacy
Pharmacy Hall Room 760
20 North Pine St.
Baltimore, MD 21201
Mon.-Fri. 8:30 AM-5 PM
410-706-7568
(consumers only)
410-706-0898
(for healthcare professionals only)
www.pharmacy.umaryland.edu/umdi

EASTON

Drug Information
Pharmacy Dept.
Memorial Hospital

219 S. Washington St.
Easton, MD 21601
7 days/week, 7 AM-5:30 PM
410-822-1000, ext. 5645

MASSACHUSETTS

WORCESTER

Drug Information Pharmacy
UMass Memorial Medical Center
Healthcare Hospital

55 Lake Ave. North
Worcester, MA 01655
Mon.-Fri. 8:30 AM-5 PM
508-856-3456
508-856-2775 (24-hour)

MICHIGAN

ANN ARBOR

Drug Information Service Dept. of
Pharmacy Services
University of Michigan Health System

1500 East Medical
Center Dr.
UH B2D301
Box 0008
Ann Arbor, MI 48109-0008
Mon.-Fri. 8 AM-5 PM
734-936-8200

DETROIT

Drug Information Center
Department of Pharmacy Services
Detroit Receiving Hospital and
University Health Center

4201 St. Antoine Blvd.
Detroit, MI 48201
Mon.-Fri. 9 AM-5 PM
313-745-4556
www.dmcpharmacy.org

LANSING

Drug Information Services
Sparrow Hospital

1215 East Michigan Ave.
Lansing, MI 48912
7 days/week, 24 hours
517-364-2444
www.sparrow.org

ROYAL OAK

Drug Information Services
William Beaumont Hospital

3601 West 13 Mile Rd.
Royal Oak, MI 48073-6769
Mon.-Fri. 8 AM-4:30 PM
248-898-4077

SOUTHFIELD

Drug Information Service
Providence Hospital

16001 West 9 Mile Rd.
Southfield, MI 48075
Mon.-Fri. 8 AM-4 PM
248-849-3125

MISSISSIPPI

JACKSON

Drug Information Center
University of Mississippi
Medical Center

2500 N. State St.
Jackson, MS 39216
Mon.-Fri. 8 AM-4:30 PM
601-984-2060

MISSOURI

KANSAS CITY

University of Missouri-Kansas City Drug Information Center

2464 Charlotte St., Suite 1220
Kansas City, MO 64108
Mon.-Fri. 9 AM-4 PM
816-235-5490

SPRINGFIELD

Drug Information Center
St. John's Hospital
1235 E. Cherokee St.
Springfield, MO 65804
Mon.-Fri. 8 AM-4:30 PM
417-820-3488

ST. JOSEPH

Regional Medical Center Pharmacy

5325 Faraon St.
St. Joseph, MO 64506
7 days/week, 24 hours
816-271-6141

MONTANA

MISSOULA

Drug Information Service University of Montana School of Pharmacy and Allied Health Sciences

32 Campus Dr.
1522 Skaggs Bldg.
Missoula, MT 59812-1522
Mon.-Fri. 8 AM-5 PM
406-243-5254
800-501-5491
www.health.umt.edu/dis

NEBRASKA

OMAHA

Drug Informatics Service School of Pharmacy Creighton University

2500 California Plaza
Health Science Library
Room 204
Omaha, NE 68178
Mon.-Fri. 8:30 AM-4:30 PM
402-280-5101
http://druginfo.creighton.edu

NEW JERSEY

NEWARK

New Jersey Poison Information and Education System

140 Bergen St.
Newark, NJ 07107
Mon.-Fri. 8 AM- 5 PM
973-972-9280
800-222-1222 (Emergency)
www.njpies.org

NEW BRUNSWICK

Drug Information Service Robert Wood Johnson University Hospital

Pharmacy Department
1 Robert Wood Johnson Pl.
New Brunswick, NJ 08901
Mon.-Fri. 8:30 AM-4:30 PM
732-937-8842

NEW MEXICO

ALBUQUERQUE

New Mexico Poison Center University of New Mexico Health Sciences Center

MSC09 5080
1 University of New Mexico
Albuquerque, NM 87131
7 days/week, 24 hours
505-272-4261
800-222-1222 **(Emergency)**
http://hsc.unm.edu/pharmacy/poison

NEW YORK

BROOKLYN

International Drug Information Center Long Island University Arnold & Marie Schwartz College of Pharmacy & Health Sciences

75 DeKalb Ave.
RM-HS509
Brooklyn, NY 11201
Mon.-Fri. 9 AM-5 PM
718-488-1064
www.liu.edu

NEW HYDE PARK

Drug Information Center St. John's University at Long Island Jewish Medical Center

270-05 76th Ave.
New Hyde Park, NY 11040
Mon.-Fri. 8 AM-3 PM
718-470-DRUG (3784)

NEW YORK CITY

Drug Information Center Memorial Sloan-Kettering Cancer Center

1275 York Ave.
RM S-702
New York, NY 10021
Mon.-Fri. 9 AM-5 PM
212-639-7552

Drug Information Center Mount Sinai Medical Center

1 Gustave Levy Pl.
New York, NY 10029
Mon.-Fri. 9 AM-5 PM
212-241-6619
(for in-house healthcare professionals only)

ROCHESTER

Finger Lakes
Poison and Drug
Information Center
University of Rochester

601 Elmwood Ave.
Rochester, NY 14642
Mon.-Fri. 8 AM-5 PM
585-275-3718
www.fingerlakespoison.org

NORTH CAROLINA

BUIES CREEK

Drug Information Center School of Pharmacy Campbell University

P.O. Box 1090
Buies Creek, NC 27506
Mon.-Fri. 8:30 AM-5:00 PM
910-893-1200, ext. 2701
800-760-9697, ext. 2701
800-327-5467 (NC only)
www.campbellpharmacy.net/resources/drug_info_center.html

CHAPEL HILL

University of North Carolina Hospitals Drug Information Center Dept. of Pharmacy

101 Manning Dr.
Chapel Hill, NC 27514
Mon.-Fri. 8 AM-4:30 PM
919-966-2373

DURHAM

Drug Information Center Duke University Health Systems

DUMC Box 3089
Durham, NC 27710
Mon.-Fri. 8 AM-5 PM
919-684-5125

GREENVILLE

Eastern Carolina Drug Information Center
Pitt County Memorial Hospital
Dept. of Pharmacy Service

P.O. Box 6028
2100 Stantonsburg Rd.
Greenville, NC 27835
Mon.-Fri. 8 AM-5 PM
252-847-4257

WINSTON-SALEM

Drug Information Service Center
Wake-Forest University Baptist Medical Center

Medical Center Blvd.
Winston-Salem, NC 27157
Mon.-Fri. 8 AM-5 PM
336-716-2037
(for healthcare professionals only)

OHIO

ADA

Drug Information Center
Raabe College of Pharmacy
Ohio Northern University

Ada, OH 45810
Mon.-Thurs. 8:30 AM-5 PM
Fri. 8:30 AM-4 PM
419-772-2307
www.onu.edu/pharmacy/druginfo

CINCINNATI

Drug and Poison Information Center

Children's Hospital Medical Center

3333 Burnet Ave.
Cincinnati, OH 45229
Mon.-Fri. 9 AM-5 PM
513-636-5063
(Administration)
513-636-5111
(7 days/week, 24 hours)

CLEVELAND

Drug Information Service
Cleveland Clinic Foundation

9500 Euclid Ave.
Cleveland, OH 44195
Mon.-Fri. 8:30 AM-4:30 PM
216-444-6456
(for healthcare professionals only)

COLUMBUS

Drug Information Center
Ohio State University Hospital
Dept. of Pharmacy

Doan Hall 368
410 W. 10th Ave.
Columbus, OH 43210-1228
Mon.-Fri. 8 AM-4:30 PM
614-293-8679
(for in-house healthcare professionals only)

Drug Information Center
Riverside Methodist Hospital

3535 Olentangy River Road
Columbus, OH 43214
7 days/week, 24 hours
614-566-5425

TOLEDO

Drug Information Services
St. Vincent Mercy Medical Center

2213 Cherry St.
Toledo, Ohio 43608-2691
Mon.-Fri. 7 AM-5 PM
419-251-4227
www.rx.medctr.ohio-state.edu

OKLAHOMA

OKLAHOMA CITY

Drug Information Service
Integris Health

3300 Northwest Expressway
Oklahoma City, OK 73112
Mon.-Fri. 8 AM-4:00 PM
405-949-3660
(for healthcare professionals of Integris Health only)

Drug Information Center
OU Medical Center

1200 Everett Dr.
Oklahoma City, OK 73104
Mon.-Fri. 8 AM-4:30 PM
405-271-6226
Fax: 405-271-6281

TULSA

Drug Information Center
Saint Francis Hospital

6161 S. Yale Ave.
Tulsa, OK 74136
Mon.-Fri. 8 AM-4:30 PM
918-494-6339
(for healthcare professionals only)

PENNSYLVANIA

PHILADELPHIA

Drug Information Center
Temple University Hospital
Dept. of Pharmacy

3401 N. Broad St.
Philadelphia, PA 19140
Mon.-Fri. 8 AM-4:30 PM
215-707-4644

Drug Information Service
Dept. of Pharmacy
Thomas Jefferson University Hospital

111 S. 11th St.
Philadelphia, PA 19107-5089
Mon.-Fri. 8 AM-5 PM
215-955-8877

University of Pennsylvania Health System Drug Information Service
Hospital of the University of Pennsylvania
Department of Pharmacy

3400 Spruce St.
Philadelphia, PA 19104
Mon.-Fri. 8:30 AM-4 PM
215-662-2903

PITTSBURGH

Pharmaceutical Information Center
Mylan School of Pharmacy
Duquesne University

431 Mellon Hall
Pittsburgh, PA 15282
Mon.-Fri. 8 AM-4 PM
412-396-4600

UPLAND

Drug Information Center
Crozer-Chester Medical Center
Dept. of Pharmacy

1 Medical Center Blvd.
Upland, PA 19013
Mon.-Fri. 8 AM-4:30 PM
610-447-2851
(for in-house healthcare professionals only)

PUERTO RICO

SAN JUAN

Centro de Informacion de Medicamentos-CIM
Escuela de Farmacia-RCM

P.O. Box 365067
San Juan, PR 00936-5067
Mon.-Fri. 8 AM-4:30 PM
787-758-2525, ext. 1516

SOUTH CAROLINA

CHARLESTON

Drug Information Service
Medical University of South Carolina

150 Ashley Ave.
Rutledge Tower Annex
Room 604
P.O. Box 250584
Charleston, SC 29425-0810
Mon.-Fri. 9 AM-5:30 PM
843-792-3896
800-922-5250

SPARTANBURG

Drug Information Center
Spartanburg Regional Healthcare System

101 E. Wood St.
Spartanburg, SC 29303
Mon.-Fri. 8 AM-4:30 PM
864-560-6910

TENNESSEE

KNOXVILLE

Drug Information Center
University of Tennessee
Medical Center at Knoxville

1924 Alcoa Highway
Knoxville, TN 37920-6999
Mon.-Fri. 8 AM-4:30 PM
865-544-9124

MEMPHIS

South East Regional Drug Information Center
VA Medical Center

1030 Jefferson Ave.
Memphis, TN 38104
Mon.-Fri. 6:30 AM-4 PM
901-523-8990, ext. 6720

Drug Information Center
University of Tennessee

875 Monroe Ave.
Suite 109
Memphis, TN 38163
Mon.-Fri. 8 AM-5 PM
901-448-5556

TEXAS

AMARILLO

Drug Information Center
Texas Tech Health Sciences Center

School of Pharmacy
1300 Coulter Rd.
Amarillo, TX 79106
Mon.-Fri. 8 AM-5 PM
806-356-4008

GALVESTON

Drug Information Center
University of Texas
Medical Branch

301 University Blvd.
Galveston, TX 77555-0701
Mon.-Fri. 8 AM-5 PM
409-772-2734

HOUSTON

Drug Information Center
Ben Taub General Hospital
Texas Southern University/HCHD

1504 Taub Loop
Houston, TX 77030
Mon.-Fri. 8:30 AM-5 PM
713-873-3710

LACKLAND A.F.B.

Drug Information Center
Dept. of Pharmacy
Wilford Hall Medical Center

2200 Bergquist Dr.
Suite 1
Lackland A.F.B., TX 78236
7 days/week, 24 hours
210-292-5414

LUBBOCK

Drug Information and Consultation Service
Covenant Medical Center

3615 19th St.
Lubbock, TX 79410
7 days/week, 24 hours
806-725-0408

SAN ANTONIO

Drug Information Service
University of Texas
Health Science Center at San Antonio
Department of Pharmacology

7703 Floyd Curl Drive
San Antonio, TX 78229-3900
Mon.-Fri. 8 AM-4 PM
210-567-4280

TEMPLE

Drug Information Center
Scott and White Memorial Hospital

2401 S. 31st St.
Temple, TX 76508
Mon.-Fri. 8 AM-5 PM
254-724-4636

UTAH

SALT LAKE CITY

Drug Information Service
University of Utah Hospital

421 Wakara Way
Suite 204
Salt Lake City, UT 84108
Mon.-Fri. 7:30 AM-5 PM
801-581-2073

VIRGINIA

HAMPTON

Drug Information Center
Hampton University School of Pharmacy

Hampton Harbors Annex
Hampton, VA 23668
Mon.-Fri. 9 AM-4 PM
757-728-6693

WEST VIRGINIA

MORGANTOWN

West Virginia Center for Drug and Health Information
West Virginia University
Robert C. Byrd Health Sciences Center

1124 HSN, P.O. Box 9520
Morgantown, WV 26506
Mon.-Fri. 8:30 AM-5 PM
304-293-6640
800-352-2501 (WV)
www.hsc.wvu.edu/SOP

WYOMING

LARAMIE

Drug Information Center
University of Wyoming

1000 East University Ave.
Dept 3375
Laramie, WY 82071
Mon.-Fri. 8:30 AM-4:30 PM
307-766-6988

POISON CONTROL CENTERS

The American Association of Poison Control Centers (AAPCC) uses a single, nationwide emergency number to automatically link callers with their regional poison center. This toll-free number, **800-222-1222**, also works for **teletype lines (TTY)** for the hearing-impaired and **telecommunication devices (TTD)** for individuals who are deaf. However, a few local poison centers and the ASPCA/Animal Poison Control Center are not part of this nationwide system and continue to use separate numbers.

Most of the centers listed below are certified by the AAPCC. **Certified centers are marked by an asterisk after the name.** Each has to meet certain criteria. It must, for example, serve a large geographic area; it must be open 24 hours a day and provide direct-dial or toll-free access; it must be supervised by a medical director; and it must have registered pharmacists or nurses available to answer questions from the public.

Within each state, centers are listed alphabetically by city. Some state poison centers also list their original emergency numbers (including TTY/TDD), which only work within that state. For these listings, callers may use either the state number or the nationwide 800 number.

ALABAMA

BIRMINGHAM

Regional Poison Control Center, The Children's Hospital of Alabama (*)

1600 7th Ave. South
Birmingham, AL 35233-1711
Business: 205-939-9201
Emergency: 800-222-1222
www.chsys.org

TUSCALOOSA

Alabama Poison Center (*)

2503 Phoenix Dr.
Tuscaloosa, AL 35405
Business: 205-345-0600
Emergency: 800-222-1222
800-462-0800 (AL)
www.alapoisoncenter.org

ALASKA

JUNEAU

Alaska Poison Control System

Section of Injury Prevention and EMS
410 Willoughby Ave., Room 103
Box 110616
Juneau, AK 99811-0616
Business: 907-465-3027
Emergency: 800-222-1222
www.chems.alaska.gov

(PORTLAND, OR)

**Oregon Poison Center (*)
Oregon Health and Science University**

3181 SW Sam Jackson Park Rd.
Portland, OR 97239
Business: 503-494-8600
Emergency: 800-222-1222
www.oregonpoison.com

ARIZONA

PHOENIX

**Banner Poison Control Center (*)
Banner Good Samaritan Medical Center**

901 E. Willetta St.
Suite 207-A
Phoenix, AZ 85006
Business: 602-253-3334
Emergency: 800-222-1222
www.bannerpoisoncontrol.com

TUCSON

Arizona Poison and Drug Information Center

1295 N. Martin Ave.
Tucson, AZ 85724
Business: 520-626-7899
Emergency: 800-222-1222
www.pharmacy.arizona.edu/outreach/poison/

ARKANSAS

LITTLE ROCK

**Arkansas Poison and Drug Information Center
College of Pharmacy - UAMS**

4301 West Markham St.
Mail Slot 522-2
Little Rock, AR 72205-7122
Business: 501-686-6161
Emergency: 800-222-1222
800-376-4766 (AR)
TDD/TTY: 800-641-3805

ASPCA/Animal Poison Control Center

1717 South Philo Rd.
Suite 36
Urbana, IL 61802
Business: 217-337-5030
Emergency: 888-426-4435
800-548-2423
www.aspca.org/apcc

CALIFORNIA

FRESNO/MADERA

**California Poison Control System-Fresno/Madera Div.(*)
Valley Children's Hospital**

9300 Valley Children's Place
MB15
Madera, CA 93638-8762
Business: 559-622-2300
Emergency: 800-222-1222
800-876-4766 (CA)
TDD/TTY: 800-972-3323
www.calpoison.org

SACRAMENTO

**California Poison Control System-Sacramento Div.(*)
UC Davis Medical Center**

2315 Stockton Blvd.
Sacramento, CA 95817
Business: 916-227-1400
Emergency: 800-222-1222
800-876-4766 (CA)
TDD/TTY: 800-972-3323
www.calpoison.org

SAN DIEGO

**California Poison Control System-San Diego Div. (*)
UC San Diego Medical Center**

200 West Arbor Dr.
San Diego, CA 92103-8925
Business: 858-715-6300
Emergency: 800-222-1222
800-876-4766 (CA)
TDD/TTY: 800-972-3323
www.calpoison.org

SAN FRANCISCO

**California Poison Control System-San Francisco Div.(*)
San Francisco General Hospital
University of California San Francisco**

Box 1369
San Francisco, CA 94143-1369
Business: 415-502-6000
Emergency: 800-222-1222
800-876-4766 (CA)
TDD/TTY: 800-972-3323
www.calpoison.org

COLORADO

DENVER

Rocky Mountain Poison and Drug Center (*)

777 Bannock St.
Mail Code 0180
Denver CO 80204-4028
Business: 303-739-1100
Emergency: 800-222-1222
TDD/TTY: 303-739-1127 (CO)
www.RMPDC.org

CONNECTICUT

FARMINGTON

Connecticut Regional Poison Control Center (*)
University of Connecticut Health Center

263 Farmington Ave.
Farmington, CT 06030-5365
Business: 860-679-4540
Emergency: 800-222-1222
TDD/TTY: 866-218-5372
http://poisoncontrol.uchc.edu

DELAWARE

(PHILADELPHIA, PA)

The Poison Control Center (*)
Children's Hospital of Philadelphia

34th St. & Civic Center Blvd.
Philadelphia, PA 19104-4399
Business: 215-590-2100
Emergency: 800-222-1222
TDD/TTY: 215-590-8789
www.poisoncontrol.chop.edu

DISTRICT OF COLUMBIA

WASHINGTON, DC

National Capital Poison Center (*)

3201 New Mexico Ave.
Suite 310
Washington, DC 20016
Business: 202-362-3867
Emergency: 800-222-1222
www.poison.org

FLORIDA

Jacksonville

Florida Poison Information Center-Jacksonville (*)
Shands Jacksonville Medical Center

655 West 8th St.
Box C23
Jacksonville, FL 32209
Business: 904-244-4465
Emergency: 800-222-1222
http://fpicjax.org

MIAMI

Florida Poison Information Center-Miami (*)
University of Miami–Department of Pediatrics

P.O. Box 016960
Miami, FL 33101
Business: 305-585-5250
Emergency: 800-222-1222
www.miami.edu/poison-center

TAMPA

Florida Poison Information Center-Tampa (*)
Tampa General Hospital

P.O. Box 1289
Tampa, FL 33601-1289
Business: 813-844-7044
Emergency: 800-222-1222
www.poisoncentertampa.org

GEORGIA

ATLANTA

Georgia Poison Center (*)
Hughes Spalding Children's Hospital, Grady Health System

80 Jesse Hill Jr. Dr., SE
P.O. Box 26066
Atlanta, GA 30303-3050
Business: 404-616-9237
Emergency: 800-222-1222
404-616-9000 (Atlanta)
TDD: 404-616-9287
www.georgiapoisoncenter.org

HAWAII

(DENVER, CO)

Rocky Mountain Poison and Drug Center (*)

777 Bannock St.
Mail Code 0180
Denver CO 80204-4028
Business: 303-739-1100
Emergency: 800-222-1222
www.RMPDC.org

IDAHO

(Denver, CO)

Rocky Mountain Poison and Drug Center (*)

777 Bannock St.
Mail Code 0180
Denver CO 80204-4028
Business: 303-739-1100
Emergency: 800-222-1222
www.RMPDC.org

ILLINOIS

CHICAGO

Illinois Poison Center (*)

222 South Riverside Plaza
Suite 1900
Chicago, IL 60606
Business: 312-906-6136
Emergency: 800-222-1222
TDD/TTY: 312-906-6185
www.illinoispoisoncenter.org

INDIANA

INDIANAPOLIS

Indiana Poison Control Center (*)
Clarian Health Partners Methodist Hospital

I-65 at 21st St.
Indianapolis, IN 46206-1367
Business: 317-962-2335
Emergency: 800-222-1222
800-382-9097
317-962-2323 (Indianapolis)
TTY: 317-962-2336
www.clarian.org/poisoncontrol

IOWA

Sioux City

Iowa Statewide Poison Control Center
Iowa Health System and the University of Iowa Hospitals and Clinics

401 Douglas St., Suite 402
Sioux City, IA 51101
Business: 712-279-3710
Emergency: 800-222-1222
712-277-2222 (IA)
www.iowapoison.org

KANSAS

KANSAS CITY

University of Kansas Poison Control Hospital Center

3901 Rainbow Blvd.
Room B400
Kansas City, KS 66160-7231
Business 913-588-6638
Emergency: 800-222-1222
800-332-6633 (KS)
TDD: 866-238-0677
www.kumed.com/poison

KENTUCKY

LOUISVILLE

Kentucky Regional Poison Center (*)
Kosair Children's Hospital

PO Box 35070
Louisville, KY 40232-5070
Business: 502-629-7264
Emergency: 800-222-1222
www.krpc.com

LOUISIANA

MONROE

Louisiana Drug and Poison Information Center (*)
University of Louisiana at Monroe

700 University Ave.
Monroe, LA 71209-6430
Emergency: 800-222-1222

MAINE

PORTLAND

Northern New England Poison Center

Maine Medical Center
22 Bramhall St.
Portland, ME 04102
Business: 207-662-0111
Emergency: 800-222-1222
207-871-2879 (ME)
TDD/TTY: 207-662-4900 (ME)
www.nnepc.org

MARYLAND

BALTIMORE

Maryland Poison Center (*)
University of Maryland at Baltimore School of Pharmacy

220 Arch St.
Office Level 1
Baltimore, MD 21201
Business: 410-706-7604
Emergency: 800-222-1222
TDD: 410-706-1858
www.mdpoison.com

(WASHINGTON, DC)

National Capital Poison Center (*)

3201 New Mexico Ave.
Suite 310
Washington DC 20016
Business: 202-362-3867
Emergency: 800-222-1222
TDD/TTY: 202-362-8563 (MD)
www.poison.org

MASSACHUSETTS

BOSTON

Regional Center for Poison Control and Prevention (*)
(Serving Massachusetts and Rhode Island)
Children's Hospital Boston

300 Longwood Ave.
Boston, MA 02115
Business: 617-355-6609
Emergency: 800-222-1222
TDD/TTY: 888-244-5313
www.maripoisoncenter.com

MICHIGAN

DETROIT

Regional Poison Control Center (*)
Children's Hospital of Michigan

4160 John R. Harper
Professional Office Bldg.
Suite 616
Detroit, MI 48201
Business: 313-745-5335
Emergency: 800-222-1222
TDD/TTY: 800-356-3232
www.mitoxic.org/pcc

GRAND RAPIDS

DeVos Children's Hospital Regional Poison Center (*)

100 Michigan St., NE
Grand Rapids, MI 49503
Business: 616-391-3690
Emergency: 800-222-1222
http://poisoncenter.devoschildrens.org

MINNESOTA

MINNEAPOLIS

Minnesota Poison Control System (*) Hennepin County Medical Center

701 Park Ave.
Mail Code RL
Minneapolis, MN 55415
Business: 612-873-3144
Emergency: 800-222-1222
www.mnpoison.org

MISSISSIPPI

JACKSON

Mississippi Regional Poison Control Center, University of Mississippi Medical Center

2500 North State St.
Jackson, MS 39216
Business: 601-984-1680
Emergency: 800-222-1222
http://poisoncontrol.umc.edu

MISSOURI

ST. LOUIS

Missouri Regional Poison Center (*)
Cardinal Glennon Children's Hospital

7980 Clayton Rd.
Suite 200
St. Louis, MO 63117
Business: 314-772-5200
Emergency: 800-222-1222
TDD/TTY: 314-612-5705
www.cardinalglennon.com

MONTANA

(DENVER, CO)

Rocky Mountain Poison and Drug Center (*)

777 Bannock St.
Mail Code 0180
Denver CO 80204-4028
Business: 303-739-1100
Emergency: 800-222-1222
TDD/TTY: 303-739-1127
www.RMPDC.org

NEBRASKA

OMAHA

The Poison Center (*)
Children's Hospital

8401 W. Dodge St., Suite 115
Omaha, NE 68114
Business: 402-955-5555
Emergency: 800-222-1222
www.nebraskapoison.com

NEVADA

(DENVER, CO)

Rocky Mountain Poison and Drug Center (*)

777 Bannock St.
Mail Code 0180
Denver CO 80204-4028
Business: 303-739-1100
Emergency: 800-222-1222
www.RMPDC.org

(PORTLAND, OR)

Oregon Poison Center (*)
Oregon Health and Science University

3181 SW Sam Jackson Park Rd.
Portland, OR 97239
Business: 503-494-8600
Emergency: 800-222-1222
www.oregonpoison.com

NEW HAMPSHIRE

(PORTLAND, ME)

Northern New England Poison Center

Maine Medical Center
22 Bramhall St.
Portland, ME 04102
Business: 207-662-0111
Emergency: 800-222-1222
www.nnepc.org

NEW JERSEY

NEWARK

New Jersey Poison Information and Education System (*)
UMDNJ

140 Bergen St. Suite G1600
Newark, NJ 07101
Business: 973-972-9280
Emergency: 800-222-1222
TDD/TTY: 973-926-8008
www.njpies.org

NEW MEXICO

ALBUQUERQUE

New Mexico Poison and Drug Information Center (*)

MSC09/5080
1 University of New Mexico
Albuquerque, NM 87131-0001
Business: 505-272-4261
Emergency: 800-222-1222
http://HSC.UNM.edu/pharmacy/poison

NEW YORK

BUFFALO

Western New York Regional Poison Control Center (*) Women and Children's Hospital of Buffalo

219 Bryant St.
Buffalo, NY 14222
Business: 716-878-7654
Emergency: 800-222-1222
www.wnypoison.org

MINEOLA

Long Island Regional Poison and Drug Information Center (*)
Winthrop University Hospital

259 First St.
Mineola, NY 11501
Business: 516-663-2650
Emergency: 800-222-1222
TDD: 516-747-3323 (Nassau)
631-924-8811 (Suffolk)
www.lirpdic.org

NEW YORK CITY

New York City Poison Control Center (*)
NYC Dept. of Health

455 First Ave., Room 123
New York, NY 10016
Business: 212-447-8152
Emergency: 800-222-1222
(English) 212-340-4494
212-POISONS
(212-764-7667)
Emergency: 212-VENENOS
(Spanish) (212-836-3667)
TDD: 212-689-9014
www.nyc.gov/html/doh/html/poison/poison.shtml

ROCHESTER

Finger Lakes Regional Poison and Drug Information Center (*)
University of Rochester Medical Center

601 Elmwood Ave.
Box 321
Rochester, NY 14642
Business: 585-273-4155
Emergency: 800-222-1222
TTY: 585-273-3854
www.fingerlakespoison.org

SYRACUSE

Upstate New York Poison Center (*)
SUNY Upstate Medical University

750 East Adams St.
Syracuse, NY 13210
Business: 315-464-7078
Emergency: 800-222-1222
TTY: 315-464-5424
www.upstatepoison.org

NORTH CAROLINA

CHARLOTTE

Carolinas Poison Center (*)
Carolinas Medical Center

PO Box 32861
Charlotte, NC 28232-2861
Business: 704-512-3795
Emergency: 800-222-1222
www.ncpoisoncenter.org

NORTH DAKOTA

BISMARK

ND Department of Health Injury Prevention Program
North Dakota Poison Center

600 E. Boulevard Ave.
Bismark, ND 58505
Business: 612-873-3144
Emergency: 800-222-1222
www.ndpoison.org

OHIO

CINCINNATI

Cincinnati Drug and Poison Information Center (*)
Cincinatti Children's Hospital

3333 Burnet Ave.
Cincinnati, OH 45229
Business: 513-636-5063
Emergency: 800-222-1222
TDD/TTY: 800-253-7955
www.cincinnatichildrens.org/dpic

CLEVELAND

Greater Cleveland Poison Control Center
Rainbow Babies and Children's Hospital

11100 Euclid Ave.
MP 6007
Cleveland, OH 44106-6007
Business: 216-844-1573
Emergency: 800-222-1222
www.uhhospitals.org/rainbowchildren/tabid/195/Default.aspx

COLUMBUS

Central Ohio Poison Center (*)
Nationwide Children's Hospital

700 Children's Dr.
Columbus, OH 43205-2696
Business: 614-355-0435
Emergency: 800-222-1222
TTY: 614-228-2272
www.bepoisonsmart.com

OKLAHOMA

OKLAHOMA CITY

Oklahoma Poison Control Center (*)
College of Pharmacy at OU Medical Center

940 Northeast 13th St.
Room 3N3510
Oklahoma City, OK 73104
Business: 405-271-5062
Emergency: 800-222-1222
www.oklahomapoison.org

OREGON

PORTLAND

Oregon Poison Center (*)
Oregon Health and Science University

3181 S.W. Sam Jackson Park Rd.
Portland, OR 97239
Business: 503-494-8600
Emergency: 800-222-1222
www.ohsu.edu/poison

PENNSYLVANIA

PHILADELPHIA

The Poison Control Center (*)
Children's Hospital of Philadelphia

34th Street & Civic Center Blvd.
Philadelphia, PA 19104-4399
Business: 215-590-2100
Emergency: 800-222-1222
215-386-2100 (PA)
TDD/TTY: 215-590-8789
www.poisoncontrol.chop.edu

PITTSBURGH

Pittsburgh Poison Center (*)
Children's Hospital of Pittsburgh

3705 Fifth Ave.
Pittsburgh, PA 15213
Business: 412-390-3300
Emergency: 800-222-1222
412-681-6669
www.chp.edu/clinical/03a_poison.php

RHODE ISLAND

(BOSTON, MA)

Regional Center for Poison Control and Prevention (*)
Children's Hospital Boston
(Serving Massachusetts and Rhode Island)

300 Longwood Ave., IC Smith Bldg
Boston, MA 02115
Business: 617-355-6609
Emergency: 800-222-1222
TDD/TTY: 888-244-5313
www.maripoisoncenter.com

SOUTH DAKOTA

(MINNEAPOLIS, MN)

Hennepin Regional Poison Center (*) Hennepin County Medical Center

701 Park Ave., Mail Code RL
Minneapolis, MN 55415
Business: 612-873-3144
Emergency: 800-222-1222
www.mnpoison.org

SIOUX FALLS

Sanford Poison Center (*)
USD Medical Center

1305 W. 18th St.
Box 5039
Sioux Falls, SD 57117-5039
Business: 605-328-6670
Emergency: 800-222-1222
www.sdpoison.org

TENNESSEE

NASHVILLE

Tennessee
Poison Center (*)

1161 21st Ave. South
501 Oxford House
Nashville, TN 37232-4632
Business: 615-936-0760
Emergency: 800-222-1222
www.poisonlifeline.org

TEXAS

AMARILLO

Texas Panhandle
Poison Center (*)
Texas Tech University Health Sciences Center

1501 S. Coulter Dr.
Amarillo, TX 79106
Business: 806-354-1630
Emergency: 800-222-1222
www.poisoncontrol.org

DALLAS

North Texas Poison Center (*)
Texas Poison Center Network
Parkland Health and Hospital System

5201 Harry Hines Blvd.
Dallas, TX 75235
Business: 214-589-0911
Emergency: 800-222-1222
www.poisoncontrol.org

EL PASO

West Texas Regional
Poison Center (*)
Thomason Hospital

4815 Alameda Ave.
El Paso, TX 79905
Business 915-534-3800
Emergency: 800-222-1222
www.poisoncontrol.org

GALVESTON

Southeast Texas
Poison Center (*)
The University of Texas Medical Branch

301 University Blvd.
Galveston, TX 77555-1175
Business: 409-772-9142
Emergency: 800-222-1222
www.poisoncontrol.org

SAN ANTONIO

South Texas
Poison Center (*)
The University of Texas Health Science Center–San Antonio

7703 Floyd Curl Dr., MSC 7849
San Antonio, TX 78229-3900
Business: 210-567-5762
Emergency: 800-222-1222
www.poisoncontrol.org

TEMPLE

Central Texas Poison Center (*)
Scott & White Memorial Hospital

2401 South 31st St.
Temple, TX 76508
Business: 254-724-7401
Emergency: 800-222-1222
www.poisoncontrol.org

UTAH

SALT LAKE CITY

Utah Poison Control Center (*)
University of Utah

585 Komas Dr.
Salt Lake City, UT 84108
Business: 801-587-0600
Emergency: 800-222-1222
http://uuhsc.utah.edu/poison

VERMONT

(PORTLAND, ME)

Northern New England
Poison Center

Maine Medical Center
22 Bramhall St.
Portland, ME 04102
Business: 207-662-0111
Emergency: 800-222-1222
www.nnepc.org

VIRGINIA

CHARLOTTESVILLE

Blue Ridge Poison Center (*)
University of Virginia Health System

PO Box 800774
Charlottesville, VA 22908-0774
Business: 434-924-0347
Emergency: 800-222-1222
www.healthsystem.virginia.edu/brpc

RICHMOND

Virginia Poison Center (*)
Virginia Commonwealth University Medical Center

600 E. Broad St. Suite 640
P.O. Box 980522
Richmond, VA 23298-0522
Business: 804-828-4780
Emergency: 800-222-1222
804-828-9123
www.poison.vcu.edu

WASHINGTON

SEATTLE

Washington Poison Center (*)

155 NE 100th St.
Seattle, WA 98125-8007
Business: 206-517-2359
Emergency: 800-222-1222
www.wapc.org

WEST VIRGINIA

CHARLESTON

West Virginia Poison Center (*)
WVU Charleston Division

3110 MacCorkle Ave. SE
Charleston, WV 25304
Business: 304-347-1212
Emergency: 800-222-1222
www.wvpoisoncenter.org

WISCONSIN

MILWAUKEE

Wisconsin Poison Center

Suite CC 660
P.O. Box 1997
Milwaukee, WI 53201
Business: 414-266-2952
Emergency: 800-222-1222
TDD/TTY: 414-266-2542
www.wisconsinpoison.org

Wyoming

(Omaha, NE)

The Poison Center (*)
Children's Hospital

8401 W. Dodge St., Suite 115
Omaha, NE 68114
Business: 402-955-5555
Emergency: 800-222-1222
www.nebraskapoison.com

CERTIFICATION PROGRAMS FOR NURSES

Organization	Website
American Nurses Credentialing Center (ANCC) • Acute Care Nurse Practitioner • Adult Health Clinical Nurse Specialist (formerly Med-Surg) • Adult Nurse Practitioner • Adult Psychiatric & Mental Health Clinical Nurse Specialist • Adult Psychiatric & Mental Health Nurse Practitioner • Ambulatory Care Nurse • Cardiac Vascular Nurse • Case Management Nurse • Child/Adolescent Psychiatric & Mental Health Clinical Nurse Specialist • Diabetes Management, Advanced • Family Nurse Practitioner • Family Psychiatric & Mental Health Nurse Practitioner • Gerontological Nurse • Gerontological Clinical Nurse Specialist • Gerontological Nurse Practitioner • Informatics Nurse • Medical-Surgical Nurse • Nurse Executive (*formerly Nursing Administration*) • Nurse Executive, Advanced (*formerly Nursing Administration, Advanced*) • Nursing Professional Development • Pain Management • Pediatric Nurse • Pediatric Clinical Nurse Specialist • Pediatric Nurse Practitioner • Psychiatric and Mental Health Nurse • Public/Community Health Clinical Nurse Specialist	**nursecredentialing.org**
Association of Medical Esthetic Nurses (AMEN) • Medical Esthetics-Certified (ME-C)	**www.amen-usa.org**
Association for the Advancement of Medical Instrumentation (AAMI) • Biomedical Equipment Technicians (CBET) • Radiology Equipment Specialists (CRES) • Clinical Laboratory Equipment Specialists (CLES)	**www.aami.org**
American Society of Ophthalmic Registered Nurses (ASORN) • Ophthalmic Registered Nurses (CORN)	**webeye.ophth.uiowa.edu/asorn**
American Board of Certification for Gastroenterology (ABCGN) • Certified Gastroenterology Registered Nurses (CGRN)	**www.abcgn.org**
National Council of State Boards of Nursing (NCSBN) • Nurse Practitioner Certification • Nurse Licensure Compact (NLC)	**www.ncsbn.org**
National Certification Board for Diabetes Educators (NCBDE) • Certified Diabetes Educator	**www.ncbde.org**
Board of Certification for Emergency Nursing (BCEN) • Certified Emergency Nursing (CEN) • Certified Flight Registered Nurse (CFRN)	**www.ena.org/bcen**
HIV/AIDS Nursing Certification Board (HANCB) • HIV/AIDS Nursing	**www.hancb.org**
Certification Board of Infection Control & Epidemiology (CBIC) • Infectious Disease Nursing	**www.cbic.org**
Infusion Nurses Certification Corporation (INS) • Infusion Nursing	**www.ins1.org**
National Certification Corporation (NCC) • Inpatient OB/GYN (INPT) • Maternal Newborn (MN) • Low Risk Neonatal (LRN) • Neonatal Intensive Care (NIC)	**www.nccwebsite.org**
Oncology Nursing Certification Corporation • Oncology Certified Nurse (OCN®) • Certified Pediatric Oncology Nurse (CPON®) • Advanced Oncology Certified Nurse Practitioner (AOCNP®) • Advanced Oncology Certified Clinical Nurse Specialists (AOCNS®)	**www.oncc.org**

CERTIFICATION PROGRAMS FOR NURSES

Organization	Website
American Academy of Pain Management (AAPM) • Credentialed Pain Practitioner (CPP)	**www.aapainmanage.org**
Competency & Credentialing Institute (CCI) • Perioperative Nursing (CNOR & CRNFA)	**www.cc-institute.org**
American Society of Plastic Surgical Nurses (ASPSN) • Certified Plastic Surgical Nurse (CPSN)	**www.aspsn.org**
American Board of Perianesthesia Nursing Certificate (ABPANC) • Certified Post Anesthesia Nurse (CPAN®) • Certified Ambulatory Perianesthesia Nurse (CAPA®)	**www.cpancapa.org**
National Board for Certification of School Nurses (NCSN) • School Nursing (NBCSN)	**www.nbcsn.com**
Genetic Nursing Credentialing Commission (GNCC) • Advanced Practice Nurse in Genetics (APNG) • Genetics Clinical Nurse (GCN)	**www.geneticnurse.org**
Center for Nursing Education and Testing (C-NET®) • American Legal Nurse Certification Testing (ALNCCB) • Certified Board for Urology Nurses & Associates (CBUNA) • Dermatology Nursing Certification Board (DNCB) • Certified Sexual Assault Nurse Examiner (SANE-A) • Certified Sexual Assault Nurse Examiner (SANE-P) • Certified Medical-Surgical Nurse (CMSRN) • Certified Nephrology Nurse (CNN) • Certified Dialysis Nurse (CDN) • Certified Clinical Hemodialysis Technician (CCHT) • Certified Nephrology Nurse – Nurse Practitioner (CNN-NP) • Plastic Surgical Nursing Certification Board (PSNCB) • Radiological Nurse (RNC)	**www.cnetnurse.com**
Prepared Childbirth Educators, Inc. • Certified Breastfeeding Counselor (CBC) • Certified Childbirth Educator (CCE) • Certified Labor Support Specialist (CLSS) • Certified Prenatal/Postnatal Fitness Instructor • Certified Infant Massage Instructor/Educator	**www.childbirtheducation.org**
Education of Nurse Anesthetists in the U.S. • Certified Registered Nurse Anesthetist (CRNA)	**www.aana/com**

PROFESSIONAL ASSOCIATIONS FOR NURSES

COMMUNITY HEALTH

American Academy of Ambulatory Care Nursing
East Holly Ave.
Box 56
Pitman, NJ 08071-0056
800-262-6877
www.aaacn.org

American Public Health Association
800 I St., NW
Washington, DC 20001-3710
202-777-2742
www.apha.org

CRITICAL CARE

American Association of Critical-Care Nurses
101 Columbia
Aliso Viejo, CA 92656-4109
800-899-2226
www.aacn.org

Northeast Pediatric Cardiology Nurses Association
PO Box 261
Brookline, MA 02446
www.npcna.org

Society of Critical Care Medicine
500 Midway Dr.
Mount Prospect, IL 60056
847-827-6869
www.sccm.org

EMERGENCY NURSING

Air & Surface Transport Nurses Association
7995 East Prentice Ave., Suite 100
Greenwood Village, CO 80111
800-897-6362
www.astna.org

Emergency Nurses Association
915 Lee St.
Des Plaines, IL 60016-6569
800-900-9659
www.ena.org

GERIATRICS

American Geriatrics Society
The Empire State Building
350 Fifth Ave., Suite 801
New York, NY 10118
212-308-1414
www.americangeriatrics.org

Gerontological Society of America
1220 L St. NW, Suite 901
Washington, DC 20005
202-842-1275
www.geron.org

National Conference of Gerontological Nurse Practitioners
7794 Grow Dr.
Pensacola, FL 32514
866-355-1392
www.ncgnp.org

MIDWIFERY

American College of Nurse-Midwives
8403 Colesville Rd., Suite 1550
Silver Spring, MD 20910
240-485-1800
www.acnm.org

NEONATAL

Association of Women's Health, Obstetric & Neonatal Nurses
2000 L St., NW, Suite 740
Washington, DC 20036
800-673-8499
www.awhonn.org

National Association of Neonatal Nurses
4700 W. Lake Ave.
Glenview, IL 60025-1468
800-451-3795
www.nann.org

NEPHROLOGY

American Nephrology Nurses' Association
East Holly Ave.
Box 56
Pitman, NJ 08071-0056
888-600-2662
www.annanurse.org

National Kidney Foundation
30 East 33rd St.
New York, NY 10016
800-622-9010
www.kidney.org

NEUROSCIENCE

American Association of Neuroscience Nurses
4700 West Lake Ave.
Glenview, IL 60025
888-557-2266
www.aann.org

American Association of Spinal Cord Injury Nurses
801 18th St., NW
Washington, DC 20006
202-416-7704
www.aascin.org

NURSE PRACTITIONERS

National Association of Nurse Practitioners in Women's Health
505 C St., NE
Washington, DC 20002
202-543-9693
www.npwh.org

National Association of Pediatric Nurses Associates & Practitioners
20 Brace Rd., Suite 200
Cherry Hill, NJ 08034-2634
856-857-9700
www.napnap.org

National Conference of Gerontological Nurse Practitioners
7794 Grow Dr.
Pensacola, FL 32514
866-355-1392
www.ncgnp.org

Nurse Practitioner Association of New York State
12 Corporate Dr.
Clifton Park, NY 12065
518-348-0719
www.thenpa.org

ONCOLOGY

Association of Pediatric Hematology/Oncology Nurses
4700 West Lake Ave.
Glenview, IL 60025-1485
847-375-4724
www.apon.org

Oncology Nursing Society
125 Enterprise Dr.
Pittsburgh, PA 15275
412-859-6100
www.ons.org

PALLIATIVE CARE

Hospice and Palliative Nurses Association
One Penn Center West, Suite 229
Pittsburgh, PA 15276-0100
412-787-9301
www.hpna.org

PEDIATRICS

Pediatric Nursing Certification Board
800 South Frederick Ave.
Suite 204
Gaithersburg, MD 20877-4152
888-641-2767
www.pncb.org

PREOPERATIVE & PERIOPERATIVE

American Association of Nurse Anesthetists
222 South Prospect Ave.
Park Ridge, IL 60068
Phone: 847-692-7050
Fax: 847-692-6968
www.aana.com

American Society of Perianesthesia Nurses
10 Melrose Ave., Suite 110
Cherry Hill, NJ 08003-3696
877-737-9696
www.aspan.org

American Society of Plastic Surgical Nurses
7794 Grow Dr.
Pensacola, FL 32514
800-272-0136
www.aspsn.org

Association of Perioperative Registered Nurses (AORN)
2170 South Parker Rd., Suite 300
Denver, CO 80231
800-755-2676
www.aorn.org

PSYCHIATRIC

American Psychiatric Nurses Association
1555 Wilson Blvd., Suite 530
Arlington, VA 22209
866-243-2443
www.apna.org

REHABILITATION

Association of Rehabilitation Nurses
4700 West Lake Ave.
Glenview, IL 60025
800-229-7530
www.rehabnurse.org

SCHOOL NURSING

American School Health Association
7263 State Route 43
PO Box 708
Kent, OH 44240
330-678-1601
www.ashaweb.org

National Association of School Nurses
8484 Georgia Ave., Suite 420
Silver Spring, MD 20910
866-627-6767
www.nasn.org

STATE ASSOCIATIONS/ ANESTHETISTS

California Association of Nurse Anesthetists
PO Box 1426
Boyes Hot Springs, CA 95416
206-984-1624
www.canainc.org

Connecticut Association of Nurse Anesthetists
377 Research Parkway
Suite 2D
Meriden, CT 06450
203-238-1207
www.ctana.com

New York State Association of Nurse Anesthetists
PO Box 8867
Albany, NY 12208-0867
518-861-8876
www.nysana.com

Pennsylvania Association of Nurse Anesthetists
234 North Third St.
Harrisburg, PA 17101
800-495-7262
www.pana.org

Texas Association of Nurse Anesthetists
701 Brazos St., Suite 670
Austin, TX 78701
512-495-9004
www.txana.org

STUDENT NURSING

National Student Nurses' Association
45 Main St., Suite 606
Brooklyn, NY 11201
718-210-0705
www.nsna.org

WOUND CARE

Wound, Ostomy and Continence Nurses Society
15000 Commerce Parkway, Suite C
Mt. Laurel, NJ 08054
888-224-9626
www.wocn.org

NURSE PRACTITIONER PROGRAMS BY STATE

ALABAMA

University of Alabama–Huntsville
College of Nursing
Nursing Building, Room 207
301 Sparkman Dr.
Huntsville, AL 35899
256-824-6345
onlinenurse.nb.uah.edu

ARIZONA

Arizona State University
College of Nursing & Healthcare Innovation
500 N. 3rd St.
Phoenix, AZ 85004
602-496-2200
nursing.asu.edu

University of Arizona
College of Nursing
1305 N. Martin St.
PO Box 210203
Tucson, AZ 85721
520-626-6205
www.nursing.arizona.edu

CALIFORNIA

Azusa Pacific University
School of Nursing
901 E. Alosta Ave.
Azusa, CA 91702-7000
626-969-3434
www.apu.edu/nursing

California State University–Bakersfield
Dept. of Nursing, 29 RNC
9001 Stockdale Hwy.
Bakersfield, CA 93311
661-654-3110
www.csub.edu/nursing

California State University–Fresno
Dept. of Nursing
College of Health & Human Services
2345 E. San Ramon
M/S MH26
Fresno, CA 93740
559-278-4004
www.csufresno.edu/chhs

California State University–Long Beach
Dept. of Nursing
College of Health & Human Services
1250 Bellflower Blvd.
Long Beach, CA 90840
562-985-4194
www.csulb.edu/colleges/chhs

Loma Linda University
School of Nursing, West Hall
Loma Linda, CA 92350
909-558-4923
www.llu.edu/llu/nursing

UCLA School of Nursing
Factor Building
700 Tiverton Ave.
Los Angeles, CA 90095
310-825-7181
www.nursing.ucla.edu

University of California–San Francisco
School of Nursing
2 Koret Way, #N-319X
San Francisco, CA 94143-0602
415-476-9710
www.nurseweb.ucsf.edu

University of San Diego
Hahn School of Nursing & Health Science
5998 Alcala Park
San Diego, CA 92110
619-260-4600
www.sandiego.edu

University of San Francisco
School of Nursing
2130 Fulton St.
San Francisco, CA 94117-1080
415-422-6681
www.usfca.edu/nursing

COLORADO

Regis University
Rueckert-Hartman College for Health Professions
3333 Regis Blvd.
Mail Code G-9
Denver, CO 80221-1099
303-458-4126
www.regis.edu

University of Colorado–Denver
College of Nursing
Campus Box C288
Education 2 North
13120 E. 19th Ave.
Aurora, CO 80045
303-724-1812
www.nursing.ucdenver.edu

CONNECTICUT

Quinnipiac University
Dept. of Nursing
275 Mount Carmel Ave.
Hamden, CT 06518-1908
203-582-5397
www.quinnipiac.edu

Saint Joseph College
Div. of Nursing
1678 Asylum Ave.
West Hartford, CT 06117
860-231-5211
www.sjc.edu

Yale University
School of Nursing
100 Church St. South
PO Box 9740
New Haven, CT 06536-0740
203-785-2389
www.nursing.yale.edu

DELAWARE

University of Delaware
College of Health Sciences
School of Nursing
McDowell Hall
25 N. College
Newark, DE 19716
302-831-1253
www.udel.edu/nursing

DISTRICT OF COLUMBIA

Catholic University of America
School of Nursing
125 Gowan Hall
620 Michigan Ave., NE
Washington, DC 20064
202-319-5400
nursing.cua.edu

Georgetown University
School of Nursing & Health Studies
3700 Reservoir Rd., NW
PO Box 571107
Washington, DC 20057-1107
202-687-4647
snhs.georgetown.edu

FLORIDA

Barry University
School of Nursing
11300 NE Second Ave.
Miami Shores, FL 33161-6695
305-899-3800
www.barry.edu

Florida State University
College of Nursing
98 Varsity Way
PO Box 3064310
Tallahassee, FL 32306
850-644-3299
www.nursing.fsu.edu

University of Florida
College of Nursing
PO Box 100197
Gainesville, FL 32610-0197
352-273-6001
www.con.ufl.edu

University of Miami
School of Nursing & Health Studies
PO Box 248153
Coral Gables, FL 33124
305-284-3666
www.miami.edu/sonhs

GEORGIA

Emory University
School of Nursing
1520 Clifton Rd., NE
Atlanta, GA 30322-4207
404-727-7976
www.nursing.emory.edu

Georgia State University
School of Nursing
PO Box 4019
Atlanta, GA 30302-4019
404-413-1201
www.chhs.gsu.edu/nursing

HAWAII

Hawaii Pacific University
School of Nursing
45-045 Kamehameha Hwy.
Kaneohe, HI 96744-5297
808-236-3552
www.hpu.edu

IDAHO

Boise State University
Dept. of Nursing
1910 University Dr.
Boise, ID 83725-1840
208-426-4143
www.nursing.boisestate.edu

Idaho State University
School of Nursing
650 Memorial Dr.
Building 66, Room 329
Pocatello, ID 83201
208-282-2185
www.isu.edu/nursing

ILLINOIS

DePaul University
Dept. of Nursing
990 West Fullerton Pkwy.
Chicago, IL 60614
773-325-7280
www.depaul.edu

North Park University
School of Nursing
3225 West Foster Ave.
Chicago, IL 60625-4895
773-244-5736
www.northpark.edu

Southern Illinois University–Edwardsville
School of Nursing, Alumni Hall
Room 2117
PO Box 1066
Edwardsville, IL 62026
618-650-3956
www.siue.edu/nursing

University of Illinois–Chicago
College of Nursing
845 South Damen Ave., MC 802
Chicago, IL 60612
312-996-7800
www.uic.edu/nursing

INDIANA

Indiana Wesleyan University–Marion
College of Adult & Professional Studies
4201 S. Washington St.
Marion, IN 46953
765-677-2148
www.indwes.edu

Purdue University
School of Nursing
502 N. University St.
West Lafayette, IN 47907-2069
765-494-4004
www.nursing.purdue.edu

KENTUCKY

University of Kentucky
College of Nursing
315 College of Nursing Building
Lexington, KY 40536-0232
859-323-5108
www.mcuky.edu/nursing

LOUISIANA

Louisiana State University
School of Nursing
1900 Gravier St., 4th Floor
New Orleans, LA 70112
504-568-4106
www.nursing.lsuhsc.edu

MARYLAND

Johns Hopkins University
School of Nursing
525 N. Wolfe St.
Baltimore, MD 21205
410-955-7548
www.son.jhmi.edu

MASSACHUSETTS

Northeastern University
College of Health Sciences
School of Nursing
102 Robinson Hall
Boston, MA 02115
617-373-3649
www.neu.edu

University of Massachusetts–Dartmouth
College of Nursing
285 Old Westport Rd.
North Dartmouth, MA 02747
508-999-8586
www.umassd.edu/nursing

University of Massachusetts–Worcester
Graduate School of Nursing
55 Lake Ave. North
Worcester, MA 01655
508-856-3488
www.umassmed.edu

MICHIGAN

Michigan State University
College of Nursing
A117 Life Sciences Building
East Lansing, MI 48824-1317
517-355-6527
www.nursing.msu.edu

University of Michigan
School of Nursing Building
400 North Ingalls
Ann Arbor, MI 48109-5482
734-763-5985
www.nursing.umich.edu

University of Michigan–Flint
School of Health Professions & Studies
2180 William S. White Building
303 East Kearsley St.
Flint, MI 48502
810-762-3420
www.umflint.edu

MINNESOTA

University of Minnesota
School of Nursing
5-140 Weaver-Densford Hall
308 Harvard St., SE
Minneapolis, MN 55455
612-624-9600
www.nursing.umn.edu

MISSOURI

Missouri State University
Dept. of Nursing
Professional Building, Suite 300
901 S. National Ave.
Springfield, MO 65897
417-836-5310
www.missouristate.edu

Saint Louis University
School of Nursing
3525 Caroline St.
St. Louis, MO 63104
314-977-8995
www.slu.edu

University of Missouri–Kansas City
School of Nursing
Health Sciences Building
2464 Charlotte
Kansas City, MO 64108
816-235-1700
www.nursing.umkc.edu

NEBRASKA

Creighton University
School of Nursing
2500 California Plaza
Omaha, NE 68178
402-280-2000
www.creighton.edu

NEW JERSEY

The College of New Jersey
Dept. of Nursing
Paul Loser Hall 206
PO Box 7718
Ewing, NJ 08628-0718
609-771-2591
www.tcnj.edu

Felician College
Div. of Health Sciences
262 South Main St.
Lodi, NJ 07644
201-559-6000
www.felician.edu

Monmouth University
School of Nursing & Health Studies
400 Cedar Ave.
West Long Branch, NJ 07764-1898
732-571-3443
www.monmouth.edu

Ramapo College of New Jersey
Nursing Programs at Ramapo
School of Theoretical & Applied Science
505 Ramapo Valley Rd.
Mahwah, NJ 07430
201-684-7737
www.ramapo.edu

Rutgers College of Nursing
Ackerson Hall, Rm. 102
108 University Ave.
Newark, NJ 07102
973-353-5293
www.nursingrutgers.edu

NEW MEXICO

New Mexico State University
School of Nursing
MSC 3185
PO Box 30001
Las Cruces, NM 88003-8001
575-646-3812
www.nmsu.edu

University of New Mexico
College of Nursing
MSC09 5350
Albuquerque, NM 87131-0001
505-272-4221
hsc.unm.edu/consg

NEW YORK

Adelphi University
School of Nursing
One South Ave.
Garden City, NY 11530-0701
516-877-4540
www.nursing.adelphi.edu

Binghamton University–SUNY
Decker School of Nursing
PO Box 6000
Binghamton, NY 13902-6000
607-777-2311
www.binghamton.edu

College of Mount Saint Vincent
Dept. of Nursing
6301 Riverdale Ave.
Riverdale, NY 10471
718-405-3365
www.mountsaintvincent.edu

Columbia University
School of Nursing
630 West 168th St.
PO Box 6
New York, NY 10032
212-305-5756
www.columbia.edu

D'Youville College
Nursing Department
320 Porter Ave.
Buffalo, NY 14201-9985
716-829-7613
www.dyc.edu

Long Island University–Brooklyn
School of Nursing
1 University Plaza
Brooklyn, NY 11201-8423
(718) 488-1508
www.liu.edu

Long Island University–Brookville
C.W. Post Campus
Dept. of Nursing
720 Northern Blvd.
Brookville, NY 11548
516-299-2320
www.liu.edu

New York University
College of Nursing at the College of Dentistry
246 Greene St.
New York, NY 10003
212-998-5300
www.nyu.edu/nursing

Pace University
Lienhard School of Nursing
41 Park Row, Room 300
New York, NY 10038
914-773-3552
www.pace.edu

SUNY Institute of Technology
School of Nursing & Health Systems
PO Box 3050
Utica, NY 13504
315-792-7295
www.sunyit.edu

University at Buffalo
School of Nursing
1040 Kimball Tower
SUNY at Buffalo
Buffalo, NY 14214
716-829-2533
www.nursing.buffalo.edu

University of Rochester
School of Nursing
601 Elmwood Ave.
Rochester, NY 14642
585-273-5764
www.son.rochester.edu

NORTH CAROLINA

University of North Carolina–Chapel Hill
School of Nursing
301 Carrington Hall, CB# 7460
Chapel Hill, NC 27599-7460
919-966-3734
www.nursing.ce.unc.edu

University of North Carolina–Charlotte
School of Nursing
9201 University City Blvd.
Charlotte, NC 28223-0001
704-687-7952
www.nursing.uncc.edu

OHIO

Case Western Reserve University
School of Nursing
10900 Euclid Ave.
Cleveland, OH 44106
216-368-2545
www.fpb.case.edu

Kent State University
College of Nursing
113 H Henderson Hall
Kent, OH 44242
330-672-7930
www.kent.edu/nursing

Ohio State University
College of Nursing
Newton Hall
1585 Neil Ave.
Columbus, OH 43210
614-292-4699
www.con.ohio-state.edu

University of Akron
College of Nursing
Mary Gladwin Hall
209 Carroll St.
Akron, OH 44325-3701
330-972-7551
www.uakron.edu/nursing

University of Toledo
College of Nursing
2801 W. Bancroft
Toledo, OH 43606-3390
800-586-5336
www.utoledo.edu

OKLAHOMA

University of Oklahoma
College of Nursing
PO Box 26901
1100 N. Stonewall Ave.
Oklahoma City, OK 73117
405-271-2420
www.nursing.ouhsc.edu

OREGON

Oregon Health & Science University
School of Nursing
3455 SW US Veterans Hospital Rd.
Portland, OR 97239
503-494-1043
www.ohsu.edu/nursing

University of Portland
School of Nursing
5000 North Willamette Blvd.
Portland, OR 97203-5798
503-943-7211
www.nursing.up.edu

PENNSYLVANIA

Bloomsburg University
Dept. of Nursing
3109 McCormick Center for Human Services
400 E. Second St.
Bloomsburg, PA 17815
570-389-4316
www.bloomu.edu

Drexel University
College of Nursing & Health Professions
Bellet Building
1505 Race St., Ms 501
Philadelphia, PA 19102
215-762-7822
www.drexel.edu

Millersville University
Dept. of Nursing
127 Caputo Hall
PO Box 1002
1 South George St.
Millersville, PA 17551
717-872-3410
www.millersville.edu

Pennsylvania State University
School of Nursing Graduate Programs
210 Health & Human Development East
University Park, PA 16802
814-863-2211
www.psu.edu

Temple University
College of Health Professions–Nursing Dept.
3307 N. Broad St.
Jones Hall #517
Philadelphia, PA 19140
215-707-3789
www.temple.edu

University of Pennsylvania
School of Nursing
Claire M. Fagin Hall
418 Curie Blvd.
Philadelphia, PA 19104-4217
215-898-8281
www.nursing.upenn.edu

University of Pittsburgh
School of Nursing
3500 Victoria St.
Victoria Building
Pittsburgh, PA 15261
412-624-4586
www.nursing.pitt.edu

Villanova University
College of Nursing
800 E. Lancaster Ave.
Villanova, PA 19085-1690
610-519-4933
www.villanova.edu/nursing

TENNESSEE

Belmont University
School of Nursing
1900 Belmont Blvd
Nashville, TN 37212-3757
615-460-6139
www.belmont.edu

East Tennessee State University
College of Nursing
310 Roy S. Nicks Hall
PO Box 70617
Johnson City, TN 37614-0617
423-439-7199
www.etsu.edu/nursing

Union University
School of Nursing
Nursing Admissions Coordinator
1050 Union University Dr.
Jackson, TN 38305
731-661-5029
www.uu.edu

University of Tennessee–Memphis
College of Nursing
877 Madison Ave.
Memphis, TN 38163
901-448-6135
www.utmem.edu

Vanderbilt University
School of Nursing
Godchaux Hall 207
461 21st Ave. South
Nashville, TN 37240
615-343-8876
www.vanderbilt.edu

TEXAS

Texas A&M University–Corpus Christi
College of Nursing & Health Sciences
6300 Ocean Dr.
Corpus Christi, TX 78412
361-825-2649
www.tamucc.edu

University of Texas–Austin
School of Nursing, D0100
1700 Red River St.
Austin, TX 78701
512-471-4100
www.utexas.edu/nursing

VIRGINIA

Marymount University
School of Health Professions
Dept. of Nursing
2807 North Glebe Rd.
Arlington, VA 22207
703-284-1580
www.marymount.edu

Shenandoah University
Div. of Nursing
1775 N. Sector Ct.
Winchester, VA 22601
540-665-5506
www.su.edu/nursing

University of Virginia
School of Nursing
McLeod Hall
PO Box 800782
Charlottesville, VA 22908-3388
434-924-0063
www.nursing.virginia.edu

Virginia Commonwealth University
School of Nursing
PO Box 980567
1100 E. Leigh St.
Richmond, VA 23219
www.nursing.vcu.edu

WASHINGTON

Gonzaga University
Dept. of Nursing
502 E. Boone Ave.
Spokane, WA 99258-0102
509-323-3569
www.gonzaga.edu

Pacific Lutheran University
School of Nursing
Ramstad Building #214
Tacoma, WA 98447
253-535-7674
www.plu.edu

Seattle University
College of Nursing
901 12th Ave.
PO Box 222000
Seattle, WA 98122
206-296-5676
www.seattleu.edu

University of Washington
School of Nursing
PO Box 357262
Seattle, WA 98195
206-543-8732
www.son.washington.edu

Washington State University
Intercollegiate College of Nursing
PO Box 1495
Spokane, WA 99210-1495
509-324-7292
www.nursing.wsu.edu

WISCONSIN

University of Wisconsin–Milwaukee
College of Nursing
1921 E. Hartford Ave.
PO Box 413
Milwaukee, WI 53201
414-229-4189
www.uwm.edu

WYOMING

University of Wyoming
School of Nursing
Dept. 3065
1000 E. University Ave.
Laramie, WY 82071
307-766-3903
www.uwyo.edu

PROFESSIONAL ASSOCIATIONS FOR NPs

NATIONAL ASSOCIATIONS

American Academy of Nurse Practitioners
PO Box 12846
Austin, TX 78711
512-442-4262
www.aanp.org

National Association of Nurse Practitioners in Women's Health
505 C St., NE
Washington, DC 20002
202-543-9693
www.npwh.org

National Association of Pediatric Nurse Practitioners
20 Brace Rd., Suite 200,
Cherry Hill, NJ 08034-2634
856-857-9700
www.napnap.org

National Conference of Gerontological Nurse Practitioners
7794 Grow Dr.
Pensacola, FL 32514
866-355-1392
www.ncgnp.org

Nurse Practitioner Wellness Alliance
2813 East Main Ave.
Puyallup, WA 98372
253-445-8943
www.npwellnessalliance.com

STATE ASSOCIATIONS

ALABAMA
North Alabama Nurse Practitioners Association
PO Box 14055
Huntsville, AL 35815
www.nanpainfo.com

ALASKA
Alaska Nurse Practitioner Association
3701 E. Tudor Rd., Suite #208
Anchorage, AK 99507
907-222-6847
www.alaskanp.org

ARIZONA
Arizona Nurse Practitioners Council
1850 E. Southern Ave., Suite 1
Tempe, AZ 85282
480-831-0404
www.arizonanp.com

ARKANSAS
Advanced Practice Council of the Arkansas Nurses Association
1123 South University, Suite 1015
Little Rock, AR 72204
501-244-2363
www.arna.org

CALIFORNIA
California Association for Nurse Practitioners
One Capitol Mall, Suite 320
Sacramento, CA 95814
916-441-1361
www.canpweb.org

COLORADO
Colorado Society of Advanced Practice Nurses
PO Box 100158
Denver, CO 80250-0158
303-757-7483
www.csapn.org

CONNECTICUT
Connecticut Advanced Practice Registered Nurse Society
2842 Main St., #323
Glastonbury, CT 06033
www.ctaprns.org

DELAWARE
Advanced Practice Nurse Council of Delaware
5586 Kirkwood Hwy.
Wilmington, DE 19808
800-381-0939
www.denurses.org

DISTRICT OF COLUMBIA
Nurse Practitioner Association of DC
PO Box 77424
Washington, DC 20013-7424
202-686-5514
www.npadc.org

FLORIDA
Florida Nurse Association Advanced Practice Council
1235 E. Concord St.
Orlando, FL 32803
407-896-3261
www.floridanurse.org

Florida Nurse Practitioner Network
PO Box 25422
Tampa, FL 33622
866-535-3676
www.fnpn.org

GEORGIA
Nurse Practitioner Council of Coastal Georgia
PO Box 14046
Savannah, GA 31416
912-351-7800
www.npcouncilofcoastalga.org

IDAHO
Nurse Practitioners of Idaho
2845 E. Overland Rd.
Ste 150 PMB 110
Meridian, ID 83642
208-362-3468
www.npidaho.org

ILLINOIS
Illinois Nurses Association Council of Advanced Practice Nurses
105 W. Adams St., Suite 2101
Chicago, IL 60603
312-419-2900
www.illinoisnurses.com

INDIANA
Coalition of Advanced Practice Nurses of Indiana
PO Box 10239
Fort Wayne, IN 46851
www.capni.org

IOWA
Iowa Nurse Practitioner Society
Hoskins Geriatrics, PC
53 Norwood Cir.
Iowa City, IA 52245
319-338-8189
www.iowanpsociety.org

KENTUCKY
Kentucky Coalition of Nurse Practitioners and Nurse Midwives
1017 Ash St.
Louisville, KY 40217
502-333-0076
www.kcnpnm.org

LOUISIANA
Louisiana Association of Nurse Practitioners
5713 Superior Dr., Suite A5,
Baton Rouge, LA 70816
225-293-7950
www.lanp.org

MAINE
Maine Nurse Practitioner Association
11 Columbia St.
Augusta, ME 04330
207-621-0313
www.mnpa.us

MARYLAND
Nurse Practitioner Association of Maryland
PO Box 540
Ellicott City, MD 21041-0540
410-884-3992
www.npamonline.org

MASSACHUSETTS
Massachusetts Coalition of Nurse Practitioners
PO Box 1153
Littleton, MA 01460
781-575-1565
www.mcnpweb.org

MICHIGAN
Michigan Council of Nurse Practitioners
PO Box 87934
Canton, MI 48187
734-432-9881
www.micnp.org

MINNESOTA
Association of Southeast Minnesota Nurse Practitioners
PO Box 7371
Rochester, MN 55903
www.asmnp.org

MISSISSIPPI
Mississippi Nurses Association, NP Special Interest Group
31 Woodgreen Pl.
Madison, MS 39110
601-898-0670
www.msnurses.org

MISSOURI
Missouri Coalition for Advanced Practice
PO Box 105228
1904 Bubba Lane
Jefferson City, MO 65110
573-636-4623
www.missourinurses.org

MONTANA
Montana Nurses Association/Advanced Practice
20 Old Montana State Highway
Clancy, MT 59634
406-442-6710
www.mtnurses.org

NEVADA
Nevada Nurses Association Advanced Practice Nurse Group
PO Box 34660
Reno, NV 89533
775-747-2333
www.nvnurses.org

NEW HAMPSHIRE
New Hampshire Nurse Practitioners Association
180 Mutton Rd.
Webster, NH 03303
603-648-2233
www.npweb.org

NEW JERSEY
Forum for Nurses in Advanced Practice
1479 Pennington Rd.
Trenton, NJ 08618
www.njsna.org

NEW MEXICO
New Mexico Nurse Practitioner Council
PO Box 40682
Albuquerque, NM 87196-0682
505-855-9845
www.nmnpc.org

NEW YORK
Nurse Practitioner Association New York State
12 Corporate Dr.
Clifton Park, NY 12065
518-348-0719
www.thenpa.org

NORTH CAROLINA
North Carolina Nurses Association Council of NPs
PO Box 12025
Raleigh, NC 27605
800-626-2153
www.ncnurses.org.

OHIO
Ohio Association of Advanced Practice Nurses
5818 Wilmington Pike #300
Dayton, OH 45459
866-668-3839
www.oaapn.org

OKLAHOMA
Oklahoma Nurse Practitioners Association
337 NE 4th
Oklahoma City, OK 73104
405-949-5738
www.npofoklahoma.com

OREGON
Nurse Practitioners of Oregon
18765 SW Boones Ferry Rd., Suite 200
Tualatin, OR 97062
800-634-3552
www.nursepractitionersoforegon.org

PENNSYLVANIA
Pennsylvania Coalition of Nurse Practitioners
PO Box 545
Mechanicsburg, PA 17055
717-766-4458
www.pacnp.org

SOUTH DAKOTA
Nurse Practitioner Association of South Dakota
PO Box 2822
Rapid City, SD 57709
www.npasd.org

TENNESSEE
Tennessee Nurses Association Council of Advanced Practice Nurses
545 Mainstream Dr., Suite 405
Nashville, TN 37228-1296
615-254-0350
www.tnaonline.org

TEXAS
Texas Nurse Practitioner
500 N. Capital of Texas Highway
Building 5, Suite 210
Austin, TX 78746
512-275-7153
www.texasnp.org

UTAH
Utah Nurse Practitioners
PO Box 581084
Salt Lake City, UT 84108
www.utahnp.org

VERMONT
Vermont Nurse Practitioners Association
PO Box 64773
Burlington, VT 05406
www.vtnpa.org

VIRGINIA
Virginia Council of Nurse Practitioners
2209 Dickens Rd.
Richmond, VA 23230-2005
804-565-6360
www.vcnp.net

WEST VIRGINIA
Nurses Association
405 Capitol St.,
Suite 600
Charleston, WV 25301
304-342-1169
www.wvnurses.org

WASHINGTON
ARNPs United of Washington State
10024 SE 240th St., Suite 102
Kent, WA 98031
253-480-1035
www.auws.org

WISCONSIN
Wisconsin Nurses Association
6117 Monona Dr.
Madison, WI 53716
608-221-0383
www.wisconsinnurses.org

ANTIPYRETIC PRODUCTS

BRAND	INGREDIENT/STRENGTH	DOSE
ACETAMINOPHEN		
Anacin Aspirin Free Extra Strength Tablets	Acetaminophen 500mg	**Adults & Peds ≥12 yrs:** 2 tabs q6h. **Max:** 8 tabs q24h.
Feverall Childrens' Suppositories	Acetaminophen 120mg	**Peds 3-6 yrs:** 1-2 supp. q4-6h. **Max:** 6 supp q24h.
Feverall Infants' Suppositories	Acetaminophen 80mg	**Peds 3-11 months:** 1 supp q6h. **12-36 months:** 1 supp q4h. **Max:** 6 supp q24h.
Feverall Jr. Strength Suppositories	Acetaminophen 325mg	**Peds 6-12 yrs:** 1 supp q4-6h. **Max:** 6 supp q24h.
Tylenol 8 Hour Caplets	Acetaminophen 650mg	**Adults & Peds ≥12 yrs:** 2 tabs q8h prn. **Max:** 6 tabs q24h.
Tylenol Arthritis Caplets	Acetaminophen 650mg	**Adults:** 2 tabs q8h prn. **Max:** 6 tabs q24h.
Tylenol Arthritis Geltabs	Acetaminophen 650mg	**Adults:** 2 tabs q8h prn. **Max:** 6 tabs q24h.
Tylenol Children's Suspension	Acetaminophen 160mg/5mL	**Peds 2-3 yrs (24-35 lbs):** 1 tsp (5mL). **4-5 yrs (36-47 lbs):** 1.5 tsp (7.5mL). **6-8 yrs (48-59 lbs):** 2 tsp (10mL). **9-10 yrs (60-71 lbs):** 2.5 tsp (12.5mL). **11 yrs (72-95 lbs):** 3 tsp (15mL). May repeat q4h. **Max:** 5 doses q24h.
Tylenol Extra Strength Caplets	Acetaminophen 500mg	**Adults & Peds ≥12 yrs:** 2 tabs q4-6h prn. **Max:** 8 tabs q24h.
Tylenol Extra Strength Cool Caplets	Acetaminophen 500mg	**Adults & Peds ≥12 yrs:** 2 tabs q4-6h prn. **Max:** 8 tabs q24h.
Tylenol Extra Strength Rapid Release Gelcaps	Acetaminophen 500mg	**Adults & Peds ≥12 yrs:** 2 caps q4-6h prn. **Max:** 8 caps q24h.
Tylenol Extra Strength Rapid Blast Liquid	Acetaminophen 1000mg/30mL	**Adults & Peds ≥12 yrs:** 2 tbl (30mL) q4-6h prn. **Max:** 8 tbl (120mL) q24h.
Tylenol Extra Strength EZ Tablets	Acetaminophen 500mg	**Adults & Peds ≥12 yrs:** 2 tabs q4-6h prn. **Max:** 8 tabs q24h.
Tylenol Extra Strength Go Tabs	Acetaminophen 500mg	**Adults & Peds ≥12 yrs:** 2 tabs q4-6h prn. **Max:** 8 tabs q24h.
Tylenol Infants' Suspension	Acetaminophen 80mg/0.8mL	**Peds 2-3 yrs (24-35 lbs):** 1.6 mL q4h prn. **Max:** 5 doses (8mL) q24h.
Tylenol Junior Meltaways Tablets	Acetaminophen 160mg	**Peds 6-8 yrs (48-59 lbs):** 2 tabs. **9-10 yrs (60-71 lbs):** 2.5 tabs. **11 yrs (72-95 lbs):** 3 tabs. **12 yrs (≥96 lbs):** 4 tabs. May repeat q4h. **Max:** 5 doses q24h.
Tylenol Regular Strength Tablets	Acetaminophen 325mg	**Adults & Peds ≥12 yrs:** 2 tabs q4-6h prn. **Max:** 12 tabs q24h. **Peds 6-11 yrs:** 1 tab q4-6h. **Max:** 5 tabs q24h.
NONSTEROIDAL ANTI-INFLAMMATORY DRUGS (NSAIDs)		
Advil Caplets	Ibuprofen 200mg	**Adults & Peds ≥12 yrs:** 1-2 caps q4-6h. **Max:** 6 caps q24h.
Advil Children's Chewable Tablets	Ibuprofen 50mg	**Peds 2-3 yrs (24-35 lbs):** 2 tabs q6-8h. **4-5 yrs (36-47 lbs):** 3 tabs q6-8h. **6-8 yrs (48-59 lbs):** 4 tabs q6-8h. **9-10 yrs (60-71 lbs):** 5 tabs q6-8h. **11 yrs (72-95 lbs):** 6 tabs q6-8h. **Max:** 4 doses q24h

(Continued)

BRAND	INGREDIENT/STRENGTH	DOSE
NONSTEROIDAL ANTI-INFLAMMATORY DRUGS (NSAIDs) *(Continued)*		
Advil Children's Suspension	Ibuprofen 100mg/5mL	**Peds 2-3 yrs (24-35 lbs):** 1 tsp (5mL). **4-5 yrs (36-47 lbs):** 1.5 tsp (7.5mL). **6-8 yrs (48-59 lbs):** 2 tsp (10mL). **9-10 yrs (60-71 lbs):** 2.5 tsp (12.5mL). **11 yrs (72-95 lbs):** 3 tsp (15mL). May repeat q6-8h. **Max:** 4 doses q24h.
Advil Gel Caplets	Ibuprofen 200mg	**Adults & Peds ≥12 yrs:** 1-2 caps q4-6h. **Max:** 6 caps q24h.
Advil Infants' Concentrated Drops	Ibuprofen 50mg/1.25mL	**Peds 6-11 months (12-17 lbs):** 1.25mL. **12-23 months (18-23 lbs):** 1.875mL. May repeat q6-8h. **Max:** 4 doses q24h.
Advil Junior Strength Chewable Tablets	Ibuprofen 100mg	**Peds 6-8 yrs (48-59 lbs):** 2 tabs. **9-10 yrs (60-71 lbs):** 2.5 tabs. **11 yrs (72-95 lbs):** 3 tabs. May repeat q6-8h. **Max:** 4 doses q24h.
Advil Liqui-Gels	Ibuprofen 200mg	**Adults & Peds ≥12 yrs:** 1-2 caps q4-6h. **Max:** 6 caps q24h.
Advil Tablets	Ibuprofen 200mg	**Adults & Peds ≥12 yrs:** 1-2 tabs q4-6h. **Max:** 6 tabs q24h.
Aleve Caplets	Naproxen 220mg	**Adults & Peds ≥12 yrs:** 1 tab q8-12h. May take 1 additional tab within 1 hour of first dose. **Max:** 2 caps q8-12h. 3 caps q24h.
Aleve Liquid Gels	Naproxen 220mg	**Adults & Peds ≥12 yrs:** 1 cap q8-12h. May take 1 additional tab within 1 hour of first dose. **Max:** 2 caps q8-12h. 3 caps q24h.
Aleve Smooth Gels	Naproxen 220mg	**Adults & Peds ≥12 yrs:** 1 cap q8-12h. May take 1 additional tab within 1 hour of first dose. **Max:** 2 caps q8-12h. 3 caps q24h.
Aleve Tablets	Naproxen 220mg	**Adults & Peds ≥12 yrs:** 1 tab q8-12h. May take 1 additional tab within 1 hour of first dose. **Max:** 2 caps q8-12h. 3 caps q24h.
Motrin Children's Suspension	Ibuprofen 100mg/5mL	**Peds 2-3 yrs (24-35 lbs):** 1 tsp (5mL). **4-5 yrs (36-47 lbs):** 1.5 tsp (7.5mL). **6-8 yrs (48-59 lbs):** 2 tsp (10mL). **9-10 yrs (60-71 lbs):** 2.5 tsp (12.5mL). **11 yrs (72-95 lbs):** 3 tsp (15mL). May repeat q6-8h. **Max:** 4 doses q24h.
Motrin IB Caplets	Ibuprofen 200mg	**Adults & Peds ≥12 yrs:** 1-2 tabs q4-6h. **Max:** 6 tabs q24h.
Motrin IB Tablets	Ibuprofen 200mg	**Adults & Peds ≥12 yrs:** 1-2 tabs q4-6h. **Max:** 6 tabs q24h.
Motrin Infants' drops	Ibuprofen 50mg/1.25mL	**Peds 6-11 months (12-17 lbs):** 1.25mL. **12-23 months (18-23 lbs):** 1.875mL. May repeat q6-8h. **Max:** 4 doses q24h.
Motrin Junior Strength Caplets	Ibuprofen 100mg	**Peds 6-8 yrs (48-59 lbs):** 2 tabs. **9-10 yrs (60-71 lbs):** 2.5 tabs. **11 yrs (72-95 lbs):** 3 tabs. May repeat q6-8h. **Max:** 4 doses q24h.
Motrin Junior Strength Chewable Tablets	Ibuprofen 100mg	**Peds 6-8 yrs (48-59 lbs):** 2 tabs. **9-10 yrs (60-71 lbs):** 2.5 tabs. **11 yrs (72-95 lbs):** 3 tabs. May repeat q6-8h. **Max:** 4 doses q24h.

(Continued)

BRAND	INGREDIENT/STRENGTH	DOSE
SALICYLATES		
Anacin 81 Tablets	Aspirin 81mg	**Adults & Peds ≥12 yrs:** 2 tabs q6h. **Max:** 8 tabs q24h.
Bayer Aspirin Extra Strength Caplets	Aspirin 500mg	**Adults & Peds ≥12 yrs:** 1-2 tabs q4-6h. **Max:** 8 tabs q24h.
Bayer Genuine Aspirin Caplets	Aspirin 325mg	**Adults & Peds ≥12 yrs:** 1-2 tabs q4h. **Max:** 12 tabs q24h.
Bayer Aspirin Safety Coated Caplets	Aspirin 325mg	**Adults & Peds ≥12 yrs:** 1-2 tabs q4h. **Max:** 12 tabs q24h.
Bayer Children's Aspirin Chewable Tablets	Aspirin 81mg	**Adults & Peds ≥12 yrs:** 4-8 tabs q4h. **Max:** 48 tabs q24h.
Bayer Low Dose Aspirin Tablets	Aspirin 81mg	**Adults & Peds ≥12 yrs:** 4-8 tabs q4h. **Max:** 48 tabs q24h.
Ecotrin Low Strength Tablets	Aspirin 81mg	**Adults:** 4-8 tabs q4h. **Max:** 48 tabs q24h.
Ecotrin Enteric Regular Strength Tablets	Aspirin 325mg	**Adults & Peds ≥12 yrs:** 1-2 tabs q4h. **Max:** 12 tabs q24h.
Ecotrin Maximum Strength Tablets	Aspirin 500mg	**Adults & Peds ≥12 yrs:** 2 tabs q6h. **Max:** 8 tabs q24h.
Halfprin 162mg Tablets	Aspirin 162mg	**Adults & Peds ≥12 yrs:** 2-4 tabs q4h. **Max:** 24 tabs q24h.
Halfprin 81mg Tablets	Aspirin 81mg	**Adults & Peds ≥12 yrs:** 4-8 tabs q4h. **Max:** 48 tabs q24h.
St. Joseph Aspirin Chewable Tablets	Aspirin 81mg	**Adults & Peds ≥12 yrs:** 4-8 tabs q4h. **Max:** 48 tabs q24h.
St. Joseph Enteric Safety-Coated Tablets	Aspirin 81mg	**Adults & Peds ≥12 yrs:** 4-8 tabs q4h. **Max:** 48 tabs q24h.
SALICYLATES, BUFFERED		
Bayer Extra Strength Plus Caplets	Aspirin Buffered with Calcium Carbonate 500mg	**Adults & Peds ≥12 yrs:** 1-2 tabs q4-6h. **Max:** 8 tabs q24h.
Bufferin Extra Strength Tablets	Aspirin Buffered with Calcium Carbonate/ Magnesium Oxide/Magnesium Carbonate 500mg	**Adults & Peds ≥12 yrs:** 2 tabs q6h. **Max:** 8 tabs q24h.
Bufferin Tablets	Aspirin Buffered with Benzoic Acid/Citric Acid 325mg	**Adults & Peds ≥12 yrs:** 2 tabs q4h. **Max:** 12 tabs q24h.

HEADACHE/MIGRAINE PRODUCTS

BRAND	INGREDIENT/STRENGTH	DOSE
ACETAMINOPHEN		
Anacin Extra Strength Aspirin Free Tablets	Acetaminophen 500mg	**Adults & Peds ≥12 yrs:** 2 tabs q6h. **Max:** 8 tabs q24h.
Tylenol 8 Hour Caplets	Acetaminophen 650mg	**Adults & Peds ≥12 yrs:** 2 tabs q8h prn. **Max:** 6 tabs q24h.
Tylenol Arthritis Caplets	Acetaminophen 650mg	**Adults:** 2 tabs q8h prn. **Max:** 6 tabs q24h.
Tylenol Arthritis Geltabs	Acetaminophen 650mg	**Adults:** 2 tabs q8h prn. **Max:** 6 tabs q24h.
Tylenol Children's Suspension	Acetaminophen 160mg/5mL	**Peds 2-3 yrs (24-35 lbs):** 1 tsp (5mL). **4-5 yrs (36-47 lbs):** 1.5 tsp (7.5mL). **6-8 yrs (48-59 lbs):** 2 tsp (10mL). **9-10 yrs (60-71 lbs):** 2.5 tsp (12.5mL). **11 yrs (72-95 lbs):** 3 tsp (15mL). May repeat q4h. **Max:** 5 doses q24h.
Tylenol Extra Strength Caplets	Acetaminophen 500mg	**Adults & Peds ≥12 yrs:** 2 tabs q4-6h prn. **Max:** 8 tabs q24h.
Tylenol Extra Strength Cool Caplets	Acetaminophen 500mg	**Adults & Peds ≥12 yrs:** 2 tabs q4-6h prn. **Max:** 8 tabs q24h.
Tylenol Extra Strength Rapid Release Gelcaps	Acetaminophen 500mg	**Adults & Peds ≥12 yrs:** 2 caps q4-6h prn. **Max:** 8 caps q24h.
Tylenol Extra Strength Rapid Blast Liquid	Acetaminophen 1000mg/30mL	**Adults & Peds ≥12 yrs:** 2 tbl (30mL) q4-6h prn. **Max:** 8 tbl (120mL) q24h.
Tylenol Extra Strength EZ Tabs	Acetaminophen 500mg	**Adults & Peds ≥12 yrs:** 2 tabs q4-6h prn. **Max:** 8 tabs q24h.
Tylenol Extra Strength Go Tabs	Acetaminophen 500mg	**Adults & Peds ≥12 yrs:** 2 tabs q4-6h prn. **Max:** 8 tabs q24h.
Tylenol Infants' Suspension	Acetaminophen 80mg/0.8mL	**Peds 2-3 yrs (24-35 lbs):** 1.6 mL q4h prn. **Max:** 5 doses (8mL) q24h.
Tylenol Junior Meltaways Tablets	Acetaminophen 160mg	**Peds 6-8 yrs (48-59 lbs):** 2 tabs. **9-10 yrs (60-71 lbs):** 2.5 tabs. **11 yrs (72-95 lbs):** 3 tabs. **12 yrs (≥96 lbs):** 4 tabs. May repeat q4h. **Max:** 5 doses q24h.
Tylenol Regular Strength Tablets	Acetaminophen 325mg	**Adults & Peds ≥12 yrs:** 2 tabs q4-6h prn. **Max:** 12 tabs q24h. **Peds 6-11 yrs:** 1 tab q4-6h. **Max:** 5 tabs q24h.
ACETAMINOPHEN COMBINATIONS		
Anacin Advanced Headache Formula	Acetaminophen/Aspirin/Caffeine 250mg-250mg-65mg	**Adults & Peds ≥12 yrs:** 2 tabs q6h. **Max:** 8 tabs q24h.
Excedrin Extra Strength Caplets	Acetaminophen/Aspirin/Caffeine 250mg-250mg-65mg	**Adults & Peds ≥12 yrs:** 2 tabs q6h. **Max:** 8 tabs q24h.
Excedrin Extra Strength Express Gels	Acetaminophen/Aspirin/Caffeine 250mg-250mg-65mg	**Adults & Peds ≥12 yrs:** 2 tabs q6h. **Max:** 8 tabs q24h.
Excedrin Extra Strength Geltabs	Acetaminophen/Aspirin/Caffeine 250mg-250mg-65mg	**Adults & Peds ≥12 yrs:** 2 tabs q6h. **Max:** 8 tabs q24h.
Excedrin Extra Strength Tablets	Acetaminophen/Aspirin/Caffeine 250mg-250mg-65mg	**Adults & Peds ≥12 yrs:** 2 tabs q6h. **Max:** 8 tabs q24h.
Excedrin Migraine Caplets	Acetaminophen/Aspirin/Caffeine 250mg-250mg-65mg	**Adults:** 2 tabs. **Max:** 2 tabs q24h.
Excedrin Migraine Geltabs	Acetaminophen/Aspirin/Caffeine 250mg-250mg-65mg	**Adults:** 2 tabs. **Max:** 2 tabs q24h.

(Continued)

BRAND	INGREDIENT/STRENGTH	DOSE
ACETAMINOPHEN COMBINATIONS *(Continued)*		
Excedrin Migraine Tablets	Acetaminophen/Aspirin/Caffeine 250mg-250mg-65mg	**Adults:** 2 tabs. **Max:** 2 tabs q24h.
Excedrin Sinus Headache Caplets	Acetaminophen/Phenylephrine HCl 325mg-5mg	**Adults & Peds ≥12 yrs:** 2 tabs q4h. **Max:** 12 tabs q24h.
Excedrin Sinus Headache Tablets	Acetaminophen/Phenylephrine HCl 325mg-5mg	**Adults & Peds ≥12 yrs:** 2 tabs q4h. **Max:** 12 tabs q24h.
Excedrin Tension Headache Caplets	Acetaminophen/Caffeine 500mg-65mg	**Adults & Peds ≥12 yrs:** 2 tabs q6h. **Max:** 8 tabs q24h.
Excedrin Tension Headache Express Gels	Acetaminophen/Caffeine 500mg-65mg	**Adults & Peds ≥12 yrs:** 2 tabs q6h. **Max:** 8 tabs q24h.
Excedrin Tension Headache Geltabs	Acetaminophen/Caffeine 500mg-65mg	**Adults & Peds ≥12 yrs:** 2 tabs q6h. **Max:** 8 tabs q24h.
Excedrin Tension Headache Tablets	Acetaminophen/Caffeine 500mg-65mg	**Adults & Peds ≥12 yrs:** 2 tabs q6h. **Max:** 8 tabs q24h.
Goody's Cool Orange	Acetaminophen/Aspirin/Caffeine 325mg-500mg-65mg	**Adults & Peds ≥12 yrs:** 1 powder q6h. **Max:** 4 powders q24h.
Goody's Extra Strength Headache Powders	Acetaminophen/Aspirin/Caffeine 260mg-520mg-32.5mg	**Adults & Peds ≥12 yrs:** 1 powder q4-6h. **Max:** 4 powders q24h.
Sudafed PE Sinus Headache	Acetaminophen/Phenylephrine HCl 325mg-5mg	**Adults & Peds ≥12 yrs:** 2 tabs q4h. **Max:** 12 tabs q24h.
Tylenol Sinus Congestion and Pain Daytime Cool Burst Caplet	Acetaminophen/Phenylephrine HCl 325mg-5mg	**Adults & Peds ≥12 yrs:** 2 tabs q4h. **Max:** 12 tabs q24h.
Tylenol Sinus Congestion & Pain Daytime Gelcaps	Acetaminophen/Phenylephrine HCl 325mg-5mg	**Adults & Peds ≥12 yrs:** 2 caps q4h. **Max:** 12 caps q24h.
Tylenol Sinus Congestion & Pain Daytime Rapid Release Gelcaps	Acetaminophen/Phenylephrine HCl 325mg-5mg	**Adults & Peds ≥12 yrs:** 2 caps q4h. **Max:** 12 caps q24h.
Vanquish Caplets	Acetaminophen/Aspirin/Caffeine 194mg-227mg-33mg	**Adults & Peds ≥12 yrs:** 2 tabs q6h. **Max:** 8 tabs q24h.
ACETAMINOPHEN/SLEEP AIDS		
Excedrin PM Caplets	Acetaminophen/Diphenhydramine 500mg-38mg	**Adults & Peds ≥12 yrs:** 2 tabs qhs.
Excedrin PM Geltabs	Acetaminophen/Diphenhydramine citrate 500mg-38 mg	**Adults & Peds ≥12 yrs:** 2 tabs qhs.
Excedrin PM Tablets	Acetaminophen/Diphenhydramine citrate 500mg-38 mg	**Adults & Peds ≥12 yrs:** 2 tabs qhs.
Goody's PM Powder	Acetaminophen/Diphenhydramine 1000mg-76mg/dose	**Adults & Peds ≥12 yrs:** 1 packet (2 powders) qhs.
Tylenol PM Caplets	Acetaminophen/Diphenhydramine 500mg-25mg	**Adults & Peds ≥12 yrs:** 2 tabs qhs.
Tylenol PM Vanilla Liquid	Acetaminophen/Diphenhydramine 1000mg/30mL-50mg/30mL	**Adults & Peds ≥12 yrs:** 2 tbl (30mL) qhs. **Max:** 8 tbl q24h.
Tylenol PM Rapid Release Gels	Acetaminophen/Diphenhydramine 500mg-25mg	**Adults & Peds ≥12 yrs:** 2 caps qhs.
Tylenol PM Geltabs	Acetaminophen/Diphenhydramine 500mg-25mg	**Adults & Peds ≥12 yrs:** 2 tabs qhs.
Tylenol Sinus Congestion and Pain Nighttime	Acetaminophen/Chlorpheniramine/Phenylephrine HCl 325mg-2mg-5mg	**Adults & Peds ≥12 yrs:** 2 caps q4h. **Max:** 12 caps q24h.
NONSTEROIDAL ANTI-INFLAMMATORY DRUGS (NSAIDs)		
Advil Caplets	Ibuprofen 200mg	**Adults & Peds ≥12 yrs:** 1-2 tabs q4-6h. **Max:** 6 tabs q24h.
Advil Children's Chewable Tablets	Ibuprofen 50mg	**Peds: 2-3 yr (24-35 lbs):** 2 tabs q6-8h. **4-5 yr (36-47 lbs):** 3 tabs q6-8h. **6-8 yr (48-59 lbs):** 4 tabs q6-8h. **9-10 yr (60-71 lbs):** 5 tabs q6-8h. **11 yr (72-95 lbs):** 6 tabs q6-8h. **Max:** 4 doses q24h
Advil Children's Suspension	Ibuprofen 100mg/5mL	**Peds 2-3 yrs (24-35 lbs):** 1 tsp (5mL). **4-5 yrs (36-47 lbs):** 1.5 tsp (7.5mL). **6-8 yrs (48-59 lbs):** 2 tsp (10mL). **9-10 yrs (60-71 lbs):** 2.5 tsp (12.5mL). **11 yrs (72-95 lbs):** 3 tsp (15mL). May repeat q6-8h. **Max:** 4 doses q24h.

(Continued)

BRAND	INGREDIENT/STRENGTH	DOSE
NONSTEROIDAL ANTI-INFLAMMATORY DRUGS (NSAIDs) *(Continued)*		
Advil Gel Caplets	Ibuprofen 200mg	**Adults & Peds ≥12 yrs:** 1-2 tabs q4-6h. **Max:** 6 tabs q24h.
Advil Infants' Concentrated Drops	Ibuprofen 50mg/1.25mL	**Peds 6-11 months (12-17 lbs):** 1.25mL. **12-23 months (18-23 lbs):** 1.875mL. May repeat q6-8h. **Max:** 4 doses q24h.
Advil Junior Strength Chewable Tablets	Ibuprofen 100mg	**Peds 6-8 yrs (48-59 lbs):** 2 tabs q6-8h. **9-10 yrs (60-71 lbs):** 2.5 tabs q6-8h. **11-12 yrs (72-95 lbs):** 3 tabs q6-8h. **Max:** 4 doses q24h.
Advil Liqui-Gels	Ibuprofen 200mg	**Adults & Peds ≥12 yrs:** 1-2 caps q4-6h. **Max:** 6 caps q24h.
Advil Migraine Capsules	Ibuprofen 200mg	**Adults:** 2 caps prn. **Max:** 2 caps q24h.
Advil Tablets	Ibuprofen 200mg	**Adults & Peds ≥12 yrs:** 1-2 tabs q4-6h. **Max:** 6 tabs q24h.
Aleve Caplets	Naproxen 220mg	**Adults & Peds ≥12 yrs:** 1 tab q8-12h. May take 1 additional tab within 1 hour of first dose. **Max:** 2 tabs q8-12h, 3 tabs q24h.
Aleve Liquid Gels	Naproxen 220mg	**Adults & Peds ≥12 yrs:** 1 cap q8-12h. May take 1 additional cap within 1 hr of first dose. **Max:** 3 caps q8-12hr, 3 caps q24h.
Aleve Smooth Gels	Naproxen 220mg	**Adults & Peds ≥12 yrs:** 1 cap q8-12h. May take 1 additional tab within 1 hour of first dose. **Max:** 2 tabs q8-12h, 3 tabs q24h.
Aleve Tablets	Naproxen 220mg	**Adults & Peds ≥12 yrs:** 1 tab q8-12h. May take 1 additional tab within 1 hour of first dose. **Max:** 2 tabs q8-12h, 3 tabs q24h.
Motrin Children's Suspension	Ibuprofen 100mg/5mL	**Peds 2-3 yrs (24-35 lbs):** 1 tsp (5mL). **4-5 yrs (36-47 lbs):** 1.5 tsp (7.5mL). **6-8 yrs (48-59 lbs):** 2 tsp (10mL). **9-10 yrs (60-71 lbs):** 2.5 tsp (12.5mL). **11 yrs (72-95 lbs):** 3 tsp (15mL). May repeat q6-8h. **Max:** 4 doses q24h.
Motrin IB Caplets	Ibuprofen 200mg	**Adults & Peds ≥12 yrs:** 1-2 tabs q4-6h. **Max:** 6 tabs q24h.
Motrin IB Tablets	Ibuprofen 200mg	**Adults & Peds ≥12 yrs:** 1-2 tabs q4-6h. **Max:** 6 tabs q24h.
Motrin Infants' Drops	Ibuprofen 50mg/1.25mL	**Peds 6-11 months (12-17 lbs):** 1.25mL. **12-23 months (18-23 lbs):** 1.875mL. May repeat q6-8h. **Max:** 4 doses q24h.
Motrin Junior Strength Caplets	Ibuprofen 100mg	**Peds 6-8 yrs (48-59 lbs):** 2 tabs. **9-10 yrs (60-71 lbs):** 2.5 tabs. **11 yrs (72-95 lbs):** 3 tabs. May take 6-8hrs. **Max:** 4 doses q24h.
Motrin Junior Strength Chewable Tablets	Ibuprofen 100mg	**Peds 6-8 yrs (48-59 lbs):** 2 tabs. **9-10 yrs (60-71 lbs):** 2.5 tabs. **11 yrs (72-95 lbs):** 3 tabs. May repeat q6-8h. **Max:** 4 doses q24h.
NSAID COMBINATIONS		
Advil Allergy Sinus Caplets	Ibuprofen/Chlorpheniramine/ Pseudoephedrine HCl 200mg-2mg-30mg	**Adults & Peds ≥12 yrs:** 1 tab q4-6h. **Max:** 6 tabs q24h.
Advil Cold & Sinus Caplets	Ibuprofen/Pseudoephedrine HCl 200mg-30mg	**Adults & Peds ≥12 yrs:** 1-2 tabs q4-6h. **Max:** 6 tabs q24h.
Advil Cold & Sinus Liqui-Gels	Ibuprofen/Pseudoephedrine HCl 200mg-30mg	**Adults & Peds ≥12 yrs:** 1-2 caps q4-6h. **Max:** 6 caps q24h.
Aleve-D Sinus & Cold	Naproxen Sodium/Pseudoephedrine HCl 220 mg-120 mg	**Adults & Peds ≥12 yrs:** 1 tab q12h. **Max:** 2 tabs q24h.

(Continued)

BRAND	INGREDIENT/STRENGTH	DOSE
NSAID SLEEP AIDS		
Advil PM Caplets	Ibuprofen/Diphenhydramine Citrate 200mg-38mg	**Adults & Peds ≥12 yrs:** 2 caps qhs. **Max:** 2 caps q24hrs.
Advil PM Liqui-Gels	Ibuprofen/Diphenhydramine HCl 200mg-25mg	**Adults & Peds ≥12 yrs:** 2 caps qhs. **Max:** 2 caps q24hrs.
SALICYLATES		
Anacin 81 Tablets	Aspirin 81mg	**Adults & Peds ≥12 yrs:** 2 tabs q6h. **Max:** 8 tabs q24h.
Bayer Aspirin Extra Strength Caplets	Aspirin 500mg	**Adults & Peds ≥12 yrs:** 1-2 tabs q4-6h. **Max:** 8 tabs q24h.
Bayer Aspirin Regular Strength Safety Coated	Aspirin 325mg	**Adults & Peds ≥12 yrs:** 1-2 caps q4h. **Max:** 12 caps q24h.
Bayer Genuine Aspirin Caplets	Aspirin 325mg	**Adults & Peds ≥12 yrs:** 1-2 tabs q4h or 3 tabs q6h. **Max:** 12 tabs q24h.
Bayer Aspirin Chewable Tablets	Aspirin 81mg	**Adults & Peds ≥12 yrs:** 4-8 tabs q4h. **Max:** 48 tabs q24h.
Bayer Low Dose Aspirin Tablets	Aspirin 81mg	**Adults & Peds ≥12 yrs:** 4-8 tabs q4h. **Max:** 48 tabs q24h.
Doan's Extra Strength Caplets	Magnesium Salicylate Tetrahydrate 580mg	**Adults & Peds ≥12 yrs:** 2 tabs q6h. **Max:** 8 tabs q24h.
Ecotrin Low Strength Tablets	Aspirin 81mg	**Adults:** 4-8 tabs q4h. **Max:** 48 tabs q24h.
Ecotrin Regular Strength Tablets	Aspirin 325mg	**Adults & Peds ≥12 yrs:** 1-2 tabs q4h. **Max:** 12 tabs q24h.
Ecotrin Maximum Strength Tablets	Aspirin 500mg	**Adults & Peds ≥12 yrs:** 2 tabs q6h. **Max:** 8 tabs q24h.
Halfprin 162mg Tablets	Aspirin 162mg	**Adults & Peds ≥12 yrs:** 2-4 tabs q4h. **Max:** 24 tabs q24h.
Halfprin 81mg Tablets	Aspirin 81mg	**Adults & Peds ≥12 yrs:** 4-8 tabs q4h. **Max:** 48 tabs q24h.
St. Joseph Chewable	Aspirin 81mg	**Adults & Peds ≥12 yrs:** 4-8 tabs q4h. **Max:** 48 tabs q24h.
St. Joseph Enteric	Aspirin 81mg	**Adults & Peds ≥12 yrs:** 4-8 tabs q4h. **Max:** 48 tabs q24h.
SALICYLATES, BUFFERED		
Alka-Seltzer Original Effervescent Tablets	Aspirin/Citric Acid/Sodium Bicarbonate 325mg-1000mg-1916mg	**Adults & Peds ≥12 yrs:** 2 tabs q4h. **Max:** 8 tabs q24h. **≥60 yrs: Max:** 4 tabs q24h.
Alka-Seltzer Extra Strength Effervescent Tablets	Aspirin/Citric Acid/Sodium Bicarbonate 500mg-1000mg-1985mg	**Adults & Peds ≥12 yrs:** 2 tabs q6h. **Max:** 7 tabs q24h. **≥60 yrs: Max:** 3 tabs q24h.
Ascriptin Maximum Strength Tablets	Aspirin Buffered with Maalox/Calcium Carbonate 500mg	**Adults & Peds ≥12 yrs:** 2 tabs q4h. **Max:** 8 tabs q24h.
Ascriptin Regular Strength Tablets	Aspirin Buffered with Maalox/Calcium Carbonate 325mg	**Adults & Peds ≥12 yrs:** 2 tabs q4h. **Max:** 12 tabs q24h.
Bayer Extra Strength Plus Caplets	Aspirin Buffered with Calcium Carbonate 500mg	**Adults & Peds ≥12 yrs:** 1-2 tabs q4-6h. **Max:** 8 tabs q24h.
Bayer Women's Low Dose Aspirin	Aspirin 81mg Buffered with Calcium Carbonate 777mg	**Adults & Peds ≥12 yrs:** 4-8 tabs q4h. **Max:** 10 tabs q24h.
Bufferin Extra Strength Tablets	Aspirin Buffered with Calcium Carbonate/Magnesium Oxide/Magnesium Carbonate 500mg	**Adults & Peds ≥12 yrs:** 2 tabs q6h. **Max:** 8 tabs q24h.
Bufferin Tablets	Aspirin Buffered with Benzoic Acid/Citric Acid 325mg	**Adults & Peds ≥12 yrs:** 2 tabs q4h. **Max:** 12 tabs q24h.
SALICYLATE COMBINATIONS		
Alka-Seltzer Wake-Up Call!	Aspirin/Caffeine 500mg-65mg	**Adults & Peds ≥12 yrs:** 2 tabs q6h. **Max:** 8 tabs q24h. **≥60 yrs: Max:** 4 tabs q24h.

(Continued)

BRAND	INGREDIENT/STRENGTH	DOSE
SALICYLATE COMBINATIONS *(Continued)*		
Anacin Max Strength Tablets	Aspirin/Caffeine 500mg-32mg	**Adults & Peds ≥12 yrs:** 2 tabs q6h. **Max:** 8 tabs q24h.
Anacin Tablets	Aspirin/Caffeine 400mg-32mg	**Adults & Peds ≥12 yrs:** 2 tabs q6h. **Max:** 8 tabs q24h.
Bayer Back & Body Pain Caplets	Aspirin/Caffeine 500mg-32.5mg	**Adults & Peds ≥12 yrs:** 2 tabs q6h. **Max:** 8 tabs q24h.
BC Arthritis Strength Powders	Aspirin/Caffeine/Salicylamide 742mg-38mg-222mg	**Adults & Peds ≥12 yrs:** 1 powder q3-4h. **Max:** 4 powders q24h.
BC Original Formula Powders	Aspirin/Caffeine/Salicylamide 650mg-33.3mg-195mg	**Adults & Peds ≥12 yrs:** 1 powder q3-4h. **Max:** 4 powders q24h.
SALICYLATES/SLEEP AIDS		
Alka-Seltzer PM Pain Reliever & Sleep Aid effervescent Tablets	Aspirin/Diphenhydramine Citrate 325mg-38mg	**Adults & Peds ≥12 yrs:** 2 tabs qpm.
Bayer PM Relief Caplets	Aspirin/Diphenhydramine 500mg-38.3mg	**Adults & Peds ≥12 yrs:** 2 tabs qhs.
Doan's Extra Strength PM Caplets	Magnesium Salicylate Tetrahydrate/Diphenhydramine 580mg-25mg	**Adults & Peds ≥12 yrs:** 2 tabs qhs.

INSOMNIA PRODUCTS

BRAND	INGREDIENT/STRENGTH	DOSE
DIPHENHYDRAMINE		
Nytol Quick Caps Caplets	Diphenhydramine 25mg	**Adults & Peds: ≥12 yrs:** 2 tabs qpm.
Nytol Quick Gels Capsules	Diphenhydramine 50mg	**Adults & Peds: ≥12 yrs:** 1 tab qpm.
Simply Sleep Nighttime Sleep Aid Caplets	Diphenhydramine 25mg	**Adults & Peds: ≥12 yrs:** 2 tabs qpm.
Sominex Original Formula	Diphenhydramine 25mg	**Adults & Peds: ≥12 yrs:** 2 tabs qpm.
Sominex Maximum Strength Formula	Diphenhydramine 50mg	**Adults & Peds: ≥12 yrs:** 1 tab qpm.
Unisom Nighttime Sleep-Aid Sleep Gels	Diphenhydramine 50mg	**Adults & Peds: ≥12 yrs:** 1 tab qpm.
DIPHENHYDRAMINE COMBINATION		
Alka-Seltzer PM	Aspirin/Diphenhydramine Citrate 325mg-38mg	**Adults & Peds: ≥12 yrs:** 2 tabs qpm.
Bayer PM Relief Caplets	Aspirin/Diphenhydramine Citrate 500mg-38.3mg	**Adults & Peds: ≥12 yrs:** 2 tabs qhs.
Doan's Extra Strength PM Caplets	Magnesium Salicylate Tetrahydrate/ Diphenhydramine 580mg-25mg	**Adults & Peds: ≥12 yrs:** 2 tabs qhs.
Excedrin PM Caplets	Acetaminophen/Diphenhydramine Citrate 500mg-38mg	**Adults & Peds: ≥12 yrs:** 2 tabs qhs.
Excedrin PM Geltabs	Acetaminophen/Diphenhydramine Citrate 500mg-38mg	**Adults & Peds: ≥12 yrs:** 2 tabs qhs.
Excedrin PM Tablets	Acetaminophen/Diphenhydramine Citrate 500mg-38mg	**Adults & Peds: ≥12 yrs:** 2 tabs qhs.
Goody's PM Powders	Acetaminophen/Diphenhydramine Citrate 1000mg-76mg/dose	**Adults & Peds: ≥12 yrs:** 1 packet (2 powders) qhs.
Tylenol PM Caplets	Acetaminophen/Diphenhydramine HCl 500mg-25mg	**Adults & Peds: ≥12 yrs:** 2 tabs qhs.
Tylenol PM Rapid Release Gelcaps	Acetaminophen/Diphenhydramine HCl 500mg-25mg	**Adults & Peds: ≥12 yrs:** 2 caps qhs.
Tylenol PM Geltabs	Acetaminophen/Diphenhydramine HCl 500mg-25mg	**Adults & Peds: ≥12 yrs:** 2 tabs qhs.
Tylenol PM Liquid	Acetaminophen/Diphenhydramine HCl 1000g-50mg/30mL	**Adults & Peds: ≥12 yrs:** 2 tbl (30mL) qhs. **Max:** 8 tbl (120mL) q24h.
DOXYLAMINE		
Unisom Nighttime Sleep-Aid Sleep Tabs	Doxylamine Succinate 25mg	**Adults & Peds: ≥12 yrs:** 1 tab 30 min before hs.

SMOKING CESSATION PRODUCTS

BRAND	INGREDIENT/STRENGTH	DOSE
Commit Stop Smoking 2mg Lozenges	Nicotine Polacrilex 2mg	**Adults:** If smoking first cigarettte >30 minutes after waking up use 2mg lozenge. **Weeks 1 to 6:** 1 lozenge q1-2h. **Weeks 7 to 9:** 1 lozenge q2-4h. **Weeks 10 to 12:** 1 lozenge q4-8h. **Max:** 5 lozenges/6 hours; 20 lozenges/day. Stop using at the end of 12 weeks.
Commit Stop Smoking 4mg Lozenges	Nicotine Polacrilex 4mg	**Adults:** If smoking first cigarette within 30 minutes after waking up use 4mg lozenge. **Weeks 1 to 6:** 1 lozenge q1-2h. **Weeks 7 to 9:** 1 lozenge q2-4h. **Weeks 10 to 12:** 1 lozenge q4-8h. **Max:** 5 lozenges/6 hours; 20 lozenges/day. Stop using at the end of 12 weeks.
NicoDerm CQ Step 1 Clear Patch	Nicotine 21mg	**Adults:** If smoking >10 cigarettes/day. **Weeks 1 to 6:** Apply one 21mg patch/day. **Weeks 7 to 8:** Apply one 14mg patch/day. **Weeks 9 to 10:** Apply one 7mg patch/day.
NicoDerm CQ Step 2 Clear Patch	Nicotine 14mg	**Adults:** If smoking <10 cigarettes/day. **Weeks 1 to 6:** Apply one 14mg patch/day. **Weeks 7 to 8:** Apply one 7mg patch/day.
NicoDerm CQ Step 3 Clear Patch	Nicotine 7mg	**Adults:** Apply 1 patch qd Weeks 9 to 10 if smoking >10 cigarettes/day or Weeks 7 to 8 if smoking ≤10 cigarettes/day.
Nicorette 2mg	Nicotine Polacrilex 2mg	**Adults:** If smoking <25 cigarettes/day use 2mg gum. **Weeks 1 to 6:** 1 piece q1-2h. **Weeks 7 to 9:** 1 piece q2-4h. **Weeks 10 to 12:** 1 piece q4-8h. **Max:** 24 pieces/day.
Nicorette 4mg	Nicotine Polacrilex 4mg	**Adults:** If smoking ≥25 cigarettes/day use 4mg gum. **Weeks 1 to 6:** 1 piece q1-2h. **Weeks 7 to 9:** 1 piece q2-4h. **Weeks 10 to 12:** 1 piece q4-8h. **Max:** 24 pieces/day.
Habitrol Nicotine Transdermal System Patch Step 1	Nicotine 21mg/24hr	**Adults:** If smoking >10 cigarettes/day. **Weeks 1 to 4:** Apply one 21mg patch/day. **Weeks 5 to 6:** Apply one 14mg patch/day. **Weeks 7 to 8:** Apply one 7mg patch/day.
Habitrol Nicotine Transdermal System Patch Step 2	Nicotine 14mg/24hr	**Adults:** If smoking >10 cigarettes/day. **Weeks 1 to 4:** Apply one 21mg patch/day. **Weeks 5 to 6:** Apply one 14mg patch/day. **Weeks 7 to 8:** Apply one 7mg patch/day. If smoking <10 cigarettes/day. **Weeks 1 to 6:** Apply one 14 mg patch/day. **Weeks 7 to 8:** Apply one 7mg patch/day.
Habitrol Nicotine Transdermal System Patch Step 3	Nicotine 7mg/24hr	**Adults:** If smoking >10 cigarettes/day. **Weeks 1 to 4:** Apply one 21mg patch/day. **Weeks 5 to 6:** Apply one 14mg patch/day. **Weeks 7 to 8:** Apply one 7mg patch/day. If smoking <10 cigarettes/day. **Weeks 1 to 6:** Apply one 14mg patch/day. **Weeks 7 to 8:** Apply one 7mg patch/day.

WEIGHT MANAGEMENT PRODUCTS

BRAND	INGREDIENT/STRENGTH	DOSE
Alli Weight-Loss Aid	Orlistat 60 mg	**Adults:** 1 cap with each fat-containing meal. **Max:** 3 caps per day.
Applied Nutrition Carb Blocker	Common Bean Extract, IsoPhase 3400, Soy Bean Oil, Bioperine Black Pepper Extract (95% Piperine) (Fruit), Conjugated Linoleic Acid (CLA), White Tea Extract (30% Polyphenols, 10% Caffeine) (Leaf)	**Adults:** Take 2 caps with meals bid.
Applied Nutrition Green Tea Fat Burner	Chromium (From Chromium Picolinate), Green Tea Extract (Leaf, 50% EGCG, 2% Caffeine), Natural Caffeine, Xenedrol Blend [(Bitter Orange Extract) (Fruit, 6% Synephrine), Betaine HCl, Bladderwrack Powder, Cayenne Powder (Fruit), Eleuthero Powder (Root), Ginger Powder (Root), Gotu Kola Powder (Aerial), Licorice *(Glycyrrhiza glabra)* Powder (Root, rhizome), Maté (Yerba Maté) Powder (Leaf)]	**Adults:** Take 2 caps with meals bid.
Applied Nutrition Green Tea Triple Fat Burner	Vitamin C (as Ascorbic Acid), Vitamin E (as d-Alpha Tocopheryl Acetate), Niacin (as Niacinamide), Vitamin B6 (as Pyridoxine Hydrochloride), Folic Acid, Vitamin B12 (as Cyanocobalamin), Green Tea Extract (50% EGCG) (Leaf), White Tea Extract (50% EGCG) (Leaf), Orange Pekoe (Black) Tea Extract (50% EGCG) (Leaf), Natural Caffeine, Citrus (*Citrus spp.*) Bioflavonoids (10% Bioflavonoids)	**Adults:** Take 2 caps with meals bid.
Applied Nutrition Hoodia Diet Capsules	Green Tea Extract (Leaf, 20% Caffeine), *Hoodia gordonii* (Aerial, 20:1), Natural Caffeine, Garcinia Extract (Fruit, 50% Hydroxycitric Acid), Choline (as Choline Bitartrate), Inositol, L-Methionine	**Adults:** Take 2 caps with meals bid.
Applied Nutrition Natural Fat Burner Capsules	Vitamin C (as Ascorbic Acid), Vitamin E (as d-Alpha Tocopheryl Acetate), Niacin (as Niacinamide), Vitamin B6 (as Pyridoxine Hydrochloride), Folic Acid, Vitamin B12 (as Cyanocobalamin), Green Tea Extract (leaf, 50% EGCG), Natural Caffeine, Red Leaf Lettuce-powder, Cassia Extract (6:1 bark), Cranberry *(Vaccinium macrocarpon)* Extract (fruit), Grapefruit Extract, Noni Extract, Blueberry *(Vaccinium angustifolium)* Extract (fruit), Pomegranate Extract, Apple Cider Vinegar powder, Citrus *(Citrus spp.)* Bioflavonoids (fruit)	**Adults:** Take 2 caps with meals bid.
Aqua-Ban Maximum Strength Diuretic Tablets	Pamabrom 50mg	**Adults:** Take 1 tab qid. **Max:** 4 tabs q24h.
Atkins Essential Oils Softgels	Vitamin E (from Mixed Tocopherols), Alpha Linolenic Acid (from Flaxseed Oil), Gamma Linolenic Acid (from Borage Seed Oil), Eicosapentaenoic Acid (from Fish Oil), Oleic Acid (from Flaxseed, Borage Seed and Fish Oils), Docosahexaenoic Acid (from Fish Oil), Linoleic Acid (from Flaxseed, Borage Seed and Fish Oils)	**Adults:** Take 2 caps qd.
BioMD Nutraceuticals Metabolism T3 Capsules	Calcium Phosphate, Gum Guggul Extract, L-Tyrosine, *Garcinia cambogia*, Dipotassium Phosphate, Sodium Phosphate, Disodium Phosphate, Phosphatidyl Choline	**Adults:** Take 2 caps with meal bid-tid. **Max:** 6 caps q24h.
Biotest Hot-Rox Capsules	A7-E Super-Thermogenic Gel XXX500 [Lauroyl Macrogol-32 Glycerides, P-Methylcarbonyl-ethylphenol, 3,17-Dihydroxy-Delta-5-Etiocholane-7-One Diethylcarbonate, Carbolin 19 (Forskolin 1,9-Carbonate), Piperine, Yohimbine HCl], Caffeine	**Adults:** Take 1-2 caps bid. **Max:** 4 caps q24h.

(Continued)

BRAND	INGREDIENT/STRENGTH	DOSE
Carb Cutter Original Formula Tablets	Vitamin C (as Ascorbic Acid), Chromium (as Chromium Dinicotinate Glycinate), Absorptive Vegetable Fiber, Banaba Leaf Extract *(Lagerstroemia speciosa)*, Gymnema Sylvestre Leaf and Gymnema Sylvestre Leaf Extract (25% Gymnemic Acids), Fenugreek Seed Extract, Super Hydroxycitric Extract of *Garcinia cambogia* Fruit], Vanadium (as BMOV), Guarana Seed Extract (Supplying 60mg Caffeine), Korean Ginseng Root Extract (5% Ginsenosides), Eleuthero Root Extract (0.8% Eleutherosides), Green Tea Leaf Extract (36% Total Polyphenols)	**Adults:** Take 1-2 tabs with meals bid.
Carb Cutter Phase 2 Starch Neutralizer Tablets	Phase 2 Starch Neutralizer (*Phaseolus vulgaris* from White Kidney Bean Extract), *Gymnema sylvestre* Leaf, Fenugreek Seed, *Garcina cambogia* Fruit Extract 50.0%, Hydroxycitric Acid, Vanadium (as Vanadyl Sulfate)	**Adults:** Take 1-2 tabs with meals bid.
Chroma Slim Apple Cider Vinegar Caplets	Buchu Extract (Leaf), Parsley (Leaf and Stem), Juniper (Berry), Uva-Usi (Leaf), Dandelion (Root)	**Adults:** Take 2 caps with meals qd or bid.
Dexatrim Max Caplets Evening Appetite Control	Proprietary Herbal Blend 450 mg (L-Theanine (From Green Tea Leaf); 5-HTP (Natural 5-Hydroxytryptophan From Griffonia Simplicifolia Seed); Chamomile Flower; English Lavender Flower; Lemon Balm Leaf and Orange Blossom]	**Adults:** Take 2 caps 30 minutes before evening meal. **Max:** 6 caps qd.
Dexatrim Max_2O	Thiamin (B1), Riboflavin (B2), Niacin (B3), Vitamin B6, Vitamin B12, Pantothenic Acid, Chromium, Potassium	**Adults:** Dissolve 2 tablets in 16 ounces of water.
Dexatrim Natural Extra Energy Formula Caplets	Calcium, Chromium, Green Tea Leaf Standardized Extract with Epigallocatechin Gallate (EGCG) and Caffeine, Asian (Panax), Ginseng Root	**Adults:** Take 1 cap with meals tid.
Dexatrim Natural Green Tea Formula Caplets	Calcium, Chromium, Green Tea Leaf Standardized Extract, Asian (Panax), Ginseng Root	**Adults:** Take 1 cap with meal tid.
Dexatrim Max Complex 7	Thiamine (B1), Riboflavin (B2), Niacin (B3), Vitamin B6, Vitamin B12, Pantothenic Acid, Chromium, Complex 7 Proprietary Herbal Blend (Green Tea and Oolong Tea Standardized Leaf Extracts (*Camellia sinensis*), Epigallocatechin Gallate (EGCG), Caffeine, Asian (*Panax*) Ginseng Root (4% Ginsenosides), 7-Keto [3-acetyl-7Oxo Dehydroepiandrosterone]	**Adults:** Take 2 caps qam. Second serving mid-afternoon. **Max:** 4 caps q24h.
EAS CLA Capsules	CLA (Conjugated Linoleic Acid 1.5g)	**Adults:** Take 2 caps with meals tid.
Estrin-D Capsules	Vitamin B6, Magnesium, Estrin-D Proprietary Blend (Yerbe Mate Leaf, Caffeine, Guarana Seed, Damiana Leaf and Stem, Green Tea, Ginger Root, Kola Nut, DHEA, Schisandra Fruit, Scutellaria Root, Coca Nut, Jujube Fruit, Thea Sinensis Complex Leaf)	**Adults:** Take 2 caps 30 minutes before meals. **Max:** 6 caps q24h.
Hydroxycut	Hydroxycitrate, Polynictinate, *Garcinia cambogia, Gymnema sylvestre* leaf extract, Soy Phospholipids, *Rhodiola rosea* extract, *Withania somnifera* extract, Hydroxytea, Green Tea Extract, White Tea Extract, Caffeine Anhydrous	**Adults:** Take 2 caps tid. **Max:** 6 caps q24h.
Hydroxycut Caffeine-Free Weight Loss Formula	Calcium, Chromium, Potassium, Hydroxagen Plus (Contains *Garcinia cambogia* extract, *Gymnema sylvestra* leaf extract, soy phospholipids, *Rhodiola rosea* extract, with *Ania somnifera* extract); HydroxyTea CF (Contains Caffeine-Free Green Tea Leaf Extract, Caffeine Free White Tea Extract, Caffeine Free Oolong Tea Extract	**Adults:** Take 2 caps with meals tid. **Max:** 6 caps q24h.

(Continued)

BRAND	INGREDIENT/STRENGTH	DOSE
Isatori Lean System 7 Advanced Metabolic Support Formula	Yerba Mate, Guarana Extract, Green Tea Leaf Extract, Dandelion Leaf, Advantra, 7-Keto, Bioperine	**Adults:** Take 3 caps with meals bid. **Max:** 6 caps q24h.
Metab-O-Fx Extreme	Guarana Seed, Yerba Maté Leaf, Kola Nut Seed, Bitter Orange Extract, Green Tea Extract, Cocoa Nut, Black Tea Extract, Korean Ginseng Root, *Rhodiola rodsea* Extract	**Adults:** Take 1 tab with meal bid-tid. **Max:** 3 tabs q24h.
Metabolife Break Through	Proprietary Blend of Green Tea (Leaf) Extract, L-Tyrosine, Cayenne (Fruit), Caffeine	**Adults:** Take 2 tabs 30 minutes before meals bid-tid. **Max:** 6 tabs q24h.
Metabolife Extreme Energy	Niacin, Pantothenic Acid (as D-Calcium Pantothenate), Magnesium (as Oxide/Amino Acid Chelate), Guarana Extract (Seed), Asian Ginseng Extract (Root), Green Tea Extract (Leaf), Yerba Mate Extract (Leaf), Eleuthero Extract (root), *Rhodiola* Extract (root), Theaine	**Adults:** Take 1-3 caps tid at least 3-4 hrs apart. **Max:** 4 tabs q8h.
Metabolife Ultra Caplets	Calcium (as Hydroxycitrate), Chromium (as Chromium Picolinate), Sodium, Potassium, SuperCitriMax Garcinia Extract (Fruit) (Standardized for Hydroxycitric Acid), Caffeine, Co-Enzyme Q10	**Adults:** Take 2 caps 1 hour before main meals with full glass of water. **Max:** 6 caps q24h.
Metabolife Ultra Caffeine Free Caplets	Thiamin (B1), Riboflavin (B2), Niacin (B3), Vitamin B6, Pantothenic acid, Calcium, Chromium, Potassium, Garcinia Extract (Fruit)	**Adults:** Take 2 tabs 30 minutes before meals bid-tid. **Max:** 6 tabs q24h.
MHP TakeOff, Hi-Energy Fat Burner Capsules	*Citrus aurantium* Extract, Guarana Seed Extract and Green Tea Leaf Extract, L-Tyrosine, Adrenal Support Blend, *Ginkgo biloba* Leaf Extract, Triple-Ginseng Concentrate (Contains: Panax Ginseng Root Extract, American Ginseng Root Extract and Siberian Ginseng Root Extract. Adrenal Support Blend: Licorice Root Extract, Astragalus Root Extract and Schizandra Berry Extract.)	**Adults:** Take 2 caps qd or bid.
Natrol Carb Intercept with Phase 2 Starch Neutralizer Capsules	White Kidney Bean Extract	**Adults:** Take 2 caps before carbohydrate-containing meals.
Natrol CitriMax Plus	Calcium (from (-) Hydoxycitric Acid), Chromium (as Chromium Polynicotinate), (10(-) HydroxyCitric Acid (HCA) (from Garcinia Cambogia (Fruit), Uva Ursi (Leaf), Cascara Sagrada (bark)	**Adults:** Take 1 cap ½ hr before meals tid.
Natrol Green Tea 500mg Capsules	Green Tea Extract, Polyphenols, Catechins, Caffeine	**Adults:** Take 1 cap with meals qd.
Natural Balance Fat Magnet Capsules	Chitosan, Psyllium Husk, Malic Acid, Vegetarian Lipase, Aloe Vera	**Adults:** Take 2 caps with meals bid.
Nature Made Chromium Picolinate, Extra Strength	Chromium 350mg	**Adults:** Take 1 tab qd.
Nature's Bounty Super Green Tea Diet Capsules	Green Tea *(Camellia sinensis)* (Leaf); Caffeine; Guarana *(Paullinia cupana)* (Seed); Ginger *(Zingiber officinale)* (Root); Bladderwrack Extract *(Fucus vesiculosus)* (Whole Plant); Uva Ursi *(Arctistaohylos uva-ursi)* (Leaf); Vitamin B-6 (as Pyridoxine Hydrochloride); Chromium (as Chromium Polynicotinate)	**Adults:** Take 1 cap bid.
Nature's Bounty Xtreme Lean Zn-3 Ephedra Free Capsules	Methylxanthines (Caffeine), Green Tea Extract (*Camellia Sinensis*) (Leaf) (Standardized for Epigallocatechin gallate, Caffeine, Polyphenols), Metabromine Cocoa Extract (Standardized for Theobromine, Caffeine), Bitter Orange Extract (*Citrus Aurantium*) (Fruit) (Standardized for Synepherine, N-Methyltyramine, Hordenine, Octopamine and Tyramine), Tyrosine Complex (L-Tyrosine and Acetyl L-Tyrosine), L-Methionine, Ginger Extract (*Zingiber Officinale*) (Root), Grape Seed Extract (seed), Flavone Complex (Proprietary Blend of 3, 3', 4', 5-7-Tetrahydroxyflavone), DMAE (Dimethylaminoethanol). Vitamin C as Ascorbic Acid; Vitamin B6 as Pyridoxine Hydrochloride, Pantothenic acid as d-Calcium Pantothenate, Magnesium as Magnesium Oxide	**Adults:** Take 2 caps bid.

(Continued)

BRAND	INGREDIENT/STRENGTH	DOSE
Nunaturals LevelRight for Blood Sugar Management Capsules	*Gymenema sylvestre* Extract, Fenugreek Extract, Bitter Melon Extract, Siberian Ginseng Extract, Alpha Lipoic Acid, Cinnamon Bark Extract, Banaba Leaf Extract, Biotin, Chromium Polynicotinate, Chromium Picolinate, Vanadium	**Adults:** Take 1 cap with meals tid.
One-A-Day Weight Smart Dietary Supplement Tablets	Vitamin A (30% as Beta-Carotene), Vitamin C, Vitamin D, Vitamin E, Vitamin K, Thiamin (B1), Riboflavin (B2), Niacin, Vitamin B6, Folic Acid, Vitamin B12, Pantothenic Acid, Calcium (Elemental), Iron, Magnesium, Zinc, Selenium, Copper, Manganese, Chromium, Guarana Seed (Powder & Extract), Caffeine, Green Tea Powder (Leaf) Cayenne Pepper Powder (Fruit)	**Adults:** Take 1 tab with meals qd.
PatentLean Effective and Trusted Fat and Weight Loss Supplement	3-Acetyl-7-Oxo-Dehydroepiandrosterone	**Adults:** Take 1 cap with meals bid. **Max:** 2 caps q24h.
Prolab Enhanced CLA	CLA (Conjugated Linoleic Acid), Flax Seed Oil, Alpha Linoleic Acid, Linoleic Acid, Sunflower or Safflower Oil	**Adults:** Take 3 caps with meals qd.
Stacker 2 Ephedra Free Capsules	Kola Nut (Seeds), Yerba Mate (Leaves), Casia Mimosoides Extract (Leaves/Stems/Pids), White Willow Bark, Caffeine (Anhydrous), Green Tea (Leaves), Guggulsterone (Whole Plant), Gymnema (Leaves)	**Adults:** Take 1 cap after meals. **Max:** 3 caps q24h.
Tetrazene ES-50 Ultra High-Energy Weight Loss Catalyst Capsules	Vitamin B6 (as Pyridoxine HCl); Biotin; Tetrazene Proprietary Blend: KGM-90 (Super-Class) Pharmaceutical Grade Glucomannan), Glutamine, Olive Leaf Extract. ES-50 Thermogenic Complex: L-Tyrosine, *Camellia Sinensis* (Green Tea Leaf Extract, Standardized for EGCG and Caffeine), Pharmaceutical Grade Caffeine, Vinpocetine.	**Adults:** Take 2 caps with meals tid. **Max:** 6 caps q24h.
Tetrazene KGM-90 Rapid Weight Loss Catalyst Capsules	Vitamin B6; Biotin; Propietary Blend as Follows: KGM-90 (SuperClass Pharmaceutical Grade Glucomannan)	**Adults:** Take 2 caps with meals tid. **Max:** 6 caps q24h.
ThyroStart with Thydrazine, Thyroid Support Capsules	Vitamin A 6000IU, Vit C 20mg, Vit B2 10mg Vit B1 1.65mg, Vit B6 2mg, Vit B12 10mg, Biotin: 50mcg, Pantothenic Acid 10mg, Magnesium 20mg, Zinc 10mcg, Selenium: 10mcg, Copper 20mcg, Manganese 1mg, Molybdenum 10mcg, Proprietary Blend (Contains Kelp Meal, Niacinamide, L-Tyrosine, Horsetail Root, Nettles, Radish, Parathyroid Substance, Thymus Substance, Adrenal Substance, Pancrease Substance	**Adults:** Take 2 caps with meals tid.
Twinlab GTF Chromium	Calicum from Dicalcium Phosphate Dehydrate; 200mcg tablets Chromium from Chromium Yeast; Brewers Yeast	**Adults:** Take 1 tab qd.
Twinlab Mega L-Carnitine	L-Carnitine 500mg	**Adults:** Take 1 tablet daily on an empty stomach.
Twinlab Metabolift, Ephedra Free Formula Capsules	Guarana Seed Extract, Citrus Aurantium Fruit Extract, Proprietary Thermogenic and Metabolic Blend, St. John's Wort Extract, L-Phenylalanine, Green Tea Leaf Extract, Quercetin Dihydrate, Citrus Bioflavonoid Complex, Ginger Root, Cayenne Fruit	**Adults:** Take 2 caps before each meal. **Max:** 6 caps q24h.
Ultra Diet Pep Tablets	Vitamin B12 (Cyanocobalamin), Vitamin B6 (as Pyridoxine HCl), Pantothenic Acid (as d-Calcium Pantothenate), DynaChrome Chromium (as Arginate/Chelidamate), Potassium (as Potassium Chloride), Green Tea Leaf Extract, Dandelion (Leaf); Ginger (Root), Passion Flower (Aerial Portion Extract)	**Adults:** Take 1 tab with meals bid.

(Continued)

BRAND	INGREDIENT/STRENGTH	DOSE
Xenadrine EFX Capsules	Tyroplex (Proprietary Blend of L-Tyrosine and Acetyl-L-Tyrosine), Green Tea Extract (standardized for Epigallocatechin Gallate, Caffeine and Polyphenols), Seropo (Proprietary Cocoa Extract standardized for Tyramine and Theobromine), Yerba Maté (standardized for Caffeine and Methylxanthines), dl-Methionine, Guara (Standardized for Theophylline), L-Theamine, Norabrolide Fermented Saliva Scalera Leaf Extract, Ginger Root (standardized for Gingerols), Isotherm (proprietary blend of 3, 3', 4', 5-7 Pentahydroxyflavone and 3, 3', 4', 7-Tetrahydroxyflavone), DMAE (2-Dimethylaminoethanol), Grape Seed Extract (standardized for Catechins), Long Pepper, Black Pepper, Red Cayenne Pepper (Standardized for 1% Capsaicin)	**Adults:** Take 2 caps bid, before breakfast and in mid-afternoon. **Max:** 4 caps q24h.
Xenadrine NRG 8 Hour Power Capsules	Proprietary Thermoxanthin Blend: Yerba Maté Leaf *(Ilex Paraguariensis)*, Guarana Seed *(Paullinia cupana)*, Cocoa Seed *(Theobroma cacao)*, Green Tea Leaf *(Camellia sinensis)*, Green Coffee Bean Extract *(Coffee arabica)*, Naturally Infused Caffeine	**Adults:** Take 2 caps qd.
XtremeLean Advanced Formula, Ephedra Free Capsules	Vitamin C (as Ascorbic Acid), Vitamin B-6 (as Pyridoxine Hydrochloride), Pantothenic Acid (as d-Calcium Pantothenate), Magnesium (as Magnesium Oxide), Proprietary XtremeLean, Thermo Complex (Yerba Maté Extract [Leaf])-(standardized for Methylxanthines [Caffeine])), Green Tea Extract *(Camellia sinensis)* (Leaf) (standardized for Epigallocatechin Gallate, Caffeine, Polyphenols), Metabromine Cocoa Extract (standardized for Theobromine, Caffeine), Bitter Orange Extract *(Citrus aurantium)* (Fruit) (standardized for Synepherine, N-Methyltyramine, Hordenine, Octopamine, Tyramine), Tyrosine Complex (L-Tyrosine, Acetyl L-Tyrosine), L-Methionine, Ginger Extract *(Zingiber officinale)* (Root), Grape Seed Extract (Seed); Flavone Complex (Proprietary Blend of: 3, 3', 4', 5-7- Pentahydroxyflavone, 3, 3', 4', 7 Tetrahydroxyflavone), DMAE (Dimethylaminoethanol)	**Adults:** Take 2 caps before meals bid.
Zantrex 3, Ephedrine Free	Rice Flour, Zantrex-3 Proprietary Blend Containing: Yerba Maté (Leaf), Caffeine, Guarana (Seed), Damiana (Leaf, Stem), Green Tea (Leaf), Kola Nut, *Schizonepeta* (Spica), *Piper nigrum* (Fruit), Tibetan Ginseng (Root), Panax Ginseng (Root), Maca Root, Cocoa Nut, Thea Sinensis Complex (Leaf)	**Adults:** Take 2 caps with meals qd. **Max:** 6 cap q24h.

ACNE PRODUCTS

BRAND	INGREDIENT/STRENGTH	DOSE
BENZOYL PEROXIDE		
Clean & Clear Continuous Control Acne Cleanser	Benzoyl Peroxide 10%	**Adults & Peds:** Use bid.
Clean & Clear Persa-Gel 10, Maximum Strength	Benzoyl Peroxide 10%	**Adults & Peds:** Use qd-tid.
Clearasil Daily Acne Stay Clear Cream	Benzoyl Peroxide 10%	**Adults & Peds:** Use qd-tid.
Clearasil Total Acne Control	Benzoyl Peroxide 10%	**Adults & Peds:** Use qd-tid.
Clearasil Acne Treatment Tinted Cream	Benzoyl Peroxide 10%	**Adults & Peds:** Use up to tid.
Clearasil Ultra Acne Treatment Vanishing Cream	Benzoyl Peroxide 10%	**Adults & Peds:** Use up to tid.
Neutrogena Clear Pore Cleanser Mask	Benzoyl Peroxide 3.5%	**Adults & Peds:** Use biw-tiw.
Neutrogena On-the-Spot Acne Treatment Vanishing Formula	Benzoyl Peroxide 2.5%	**Adults & Peds:** Apply qd initially, then bid-tid.
Oxy Chill Factor Daily Wash	Benzoyl Peroxide 10%	**Adults & Peds:** Use qd-tid.
Oxy Maximum Daily Wash	Benzoyl Peroxide 10%	**Adults & Peds:** Use qd.
Oxy Spot Treatment	Benzoyl Peroxide 10%	**Adults & Peds:** Use qd-tid.
PanOxyl Aqua Gel Maximum Strength gel	Benzoyl Peroxide 10%	**Adults & Peds:** Apply qd initially, then bid-tid.
PanOxyl Bar 10% Maximum Strength	Benzoyl Peroxide 10%	**Adults & Peds:** Apply qd initially, then bid-tid.
PanOxyl Bar 5%	Benzoyl Peroxide 5%	**Adults & Peds:** Use qd initially, then bid-tid.
ZAPZYT Maximum Strength Acne Treatment gel	Benzoyl Peroxide 10%	**Adults & Peds:** Use up to tid. If dryness occurs, use qd or qod.
ZAPZYT Treatment Bar	Benzoyl Peroxide 10%	**Adults & Peds:** Use qd initially, then bid-tid. If dryness occurs, use qd or qod.
SALICYLIC ACID		
Aveeno Clear Complexion Cleansing Bar	Salicylic Acid 0.5%	**Adults & Peds:** Use daily.
Aveeno Clear Complexion Foaming Cleanser	Salicylic Acid 0.5%	**Adults & Peds:** Use daily.
Aveeno Correcting Treatment, Clear Complexion	Salicylic Acid 1%	**Adults & Peds:** Use qd-tid.
Biore Blemish Fighting Cleansing Cloths	Salicylic Acid 0.5%	**Adults & Peds:** Use qd-tid.
Biore Blemish Fighting Ice Cleanser	Salicylic Acid 2%	**Adults & Peds:** Use qd.
Bye Bye Blemish Anti-Acne Serum	Salicylic Acid (strength not available)	**Adults & Peds:** Use qd-tid.
Bye Bye Blemish Drying Lotion	Salicylic Acid 2%	**Adults & Peds:** Use pm.
Bye Bye Blemish Purifying Acne Mask	Salicylic Acid 0.5%	**Adults & Peds:** Use qd.
Clean & Clear Advantage Acne Cleanser	Salicylic Acid 2%	**Adults & Peds:** Use qd.
Clean & Clear Advantage Acne Spot Treatment	Salicylic Acid 2%	**Adults & Peds:** Use qd.
Clean & Clear Advantage Cleansing Pads	Salicylic Acid 2%	**Adults & Peds:** Use qd.
Clean & Clear Blackhead Clearing Astringent	Salicylic Acid 1%	**Adults & Peds:** Use qd.
Clean & Clear Blackhead Clearing Daily Cleansing Pads	Salicylic Acid 1%	**Adults & Peds:** Use qd.

(Continued)

BRAND	INGREDIENT/STRENGTH	DOSE
SALICYLIC ACID *(Continued)*		
Clean & Clear Blackhead Clearing Scrub	Salicylic Acid 2%	**Adults & Peds:** Use qd.
Clean & Clear Advantage Oil-Free Acne Moisturizer	Salicylic Acid 0.5%	**Adults & Peds:** Use qd.
Clean & Clear Continuous Control Acne Wash, Oil Free	Salicylic Acid 2%	**Adults & Peds:** Use qd-tid.
Clearasil Stay Clear Deep Cleanse Acne Fighting Cleansing Wipes	Salicylic Acid 2%	**Adults & Peds:** Use qd-tid.
Clearasil Stay Clear Skin Perfecting Wash	Salicylic Acid 2%	**Adults & Peds:** Use bid.
Clearasil Stay Clear Oil Free Gel Wash	Salicylic Acid 2%	**Adults & Peds:** Use bid.
Clearasil Stay Clear Daily Pore Cleansing Pads	Salicylic Acid 2%	**Adults & Peds:** Use qd-tid.
Clearasil Stay Clear Daily Facial Scrub	Salicylic Acid 2%	**Adults & Peds:** Use qd.
Clearasil Ultra Acne Clearing Gel Wash	Salicylic Acid 2%	**Adults & Peds:** Use qd.
Clearasil Ultra Daily Face Wash	Salicylic Acid 2%	**Adults & Peds:** Use qd.
Clearasil Ultra Acne Clearing Scrub	Salicylic Acid 2%	**Adults & Peds:** Use qd.
Clearasil Ultra Deep Pore Cleansing Pads	Salicylic Acid 2%	**Adults & Peds:** Use qd-tid.
L'Oreal Pure Zone Skin Clearing Foaming Cleanser	Salicylic Acid 2%	**Adults & Peds:** Use tid.
Neutrogena Advanced Solutions Acne Mark Fading Peel with CelluZyme	Salicylic Acid 2%	**Adults & Peds:** Use qw-tiw.
Neutrogena Blackhead Eliminating Astringent	Salicylic Acid 0.5%	**Adults & Peds:** Use qd-tid.
Neutrogena Blackhead Eliminating Daily Scrub	Salicylic Acid 2%	**Adults & Peds:** Use bid.
Neutrogena Blackhead Eliminating Foaming Pads	Salicylic Acid 0.5%	**Adults & Peds:** Use qd.
Neutrogena Body Clear Body Scrub	Salicylic Acid 2%	**Adults & Peds:** Use qd.
Neutrogena Oil Free Acne Wash Foam Cleanser	Salicylic Acid 2%	**Adults & Peds:** Use qd.
Neutrogena Clear Pore Oil-Eliminating Astringent	Salicylic Acid 2%	**Adults & Peds:** Use qd-tid.
Neutrogena Oil Free Acne Stress Control Power Clear Scrub	Salicylic Acid 2%	**Adults & Peds:** Use qd.
Neutrogena Oil Free Acne Stress Control Power Foam Wash	Salicylic Acid 0.5%	**Adults & Peds:** Use qd-tid.
Neutrogena Acne Stress Control 3-in-1 Hydrating Acne Treatment	Salicylic Acid 2%	**Adults & Peds:** Use qd-tid.
Neutrogena Oil Free Acne Wash Cleansing Cloths	Salicylic Acid 2%	**Adults & Peds:** Use qd.
Neutrogena Oil Free Acne Wash Cream Cleanser	Salicylic Acid 2%	**Adults & Peds:** Use qd-bid.
Neutrogena Rapid Clear Acne Defense Face Lotion	Salicylic Acid 2%	**Adults & Peds:** Use qd-tid.
Neutrogena Rapid Clear Acne Eliminating Spot Gel	Salicylic Acid 2%	**Adults & Peds:** Use qd-tid.
Neutrogena Skin Polishing Acne Cleanser	Salicylic Acid 0.5%	**Adults & Peds:** Use bid.

(Continued)

BRAND	INGREDIENT/STRENGTH	DOSE
SALICYLIC ACID *(Continued)*		
Neutrogena Oil-Free Anti-Acne Moisturizer	Salicylic Acid 0.5%	**Adults & Peds:** Use qd initially, then bid-tid. If dryness occurs, use qd or qod.
Noxzema Triple Clean Anti-Blemish Astringent	Salicylic Acid 2%	**Adults & Peds:** Use qd-tid. If dryness occurs, use qd or qod.
Noxzema Triple Clean Anti-Blemish Pads	Salicylic Acid 2%	**Adults & Peds:** Use qd-tid.
Olay Daily Facials Lathering Cleansing Cloths-Clarifying for Combination/Oily Skin	Salicylic Acid (strength NA)	**Adults & Peds:** Apply qd.
Olay Regenerist Daily Regenerating Cleanser	Salicylic Acid	**Adults & Peds:** Use qd.
Olay Total Effects Plus Blemish Control Moisturizer	Salicylic Acid 1.5%	**Adults & Peds:** Apply qd-tid.
Oxy Chill Factor Cleansing Pads	Salicylic Acid 0.2%	**Adults & Peds:** Use qd-tid.
Oxy Chill Factor Face Scrub	Salicylic Acid 2%	**Adults & Peds:** Use qd-tid.
Oxy Maximum Bar Soap	Salicylic Acid 0.5%	**Adults & Peds:** Use qd-tid.
Oxy Maximum Face Scrub	Salicylic Acid 2%	**Adults & Peds:** Use qd-tid.
Oxy Maximum Daily Cleansing Pads	Salicylic Acid 2%	**Adults & Peds:** Use qd-tid.
Oxy Body Wash	Salicylic Acid 2%	**Adults & Peds:** Use qd.
Phisoderm Anti-Blemish Body Wash	Salicylic Acid 2%	**Adults & Peds:** Use qd.
St. Ives Medicated Apricot Scrub	Salicylic Acid 2%	**Adults & Peds:** Use qd.
Stridex Facewipes to Go with Acne Medication	Salicylic Acid 0.5%	**Adults & Peds:** Use qd-tid.
Stridex Triple Action Acne Pads Maximum Strength, Alcohol Free	Salicylic Acid 2%	**Adults & Peds:** Use qd-tid.
Stridex Essential Care Pads with Salicylic Acid	Salicylic Acid 1%	**Adults & Peds:** Use qd-tid.
Stridex Triple Action Medicated Acne Pads, Sensitive Skin	Salicylic Acid 0.5%	**Adults & Peds:** Use qd-tid.
ZAPZYT Acne Wash Treatment For Face & Body	Salicylic Acid 2%	**Adults & Peds:** Use bid.
ZAPZYT Pore Treatment Gel	Salicylic Acid 2%	**Adults & Peds:** Use qd-tid.
TRICLOSAN		
Noxzema Triple Clean Anti-Bacterial Cleanser	Triclosan 0.3%	**Adults & Peds ≥6 months:** Use qd each time skin is cleansed.

ANTIFUNGAL PRODUCTS

BRAND	INGREDIENT/STRENGTH	DOSE
BUTENAFINE		
Lotrimin Ultra Antifungal Cream	Butenafine HCl 1%	**Adults & Peds ≥12 yrs:** Use qd or bid.
CLOTRIMAZOLE		
FungiCure Maximum Strength Anti-Fungal Liquid Spray	Clotrimazole 1%	**Adults & Peds:** Use bid.
FungiCure Intensive Spray	Clotrimazole 1%	**Adults & Peds ≥2 yrs:** Use bid.
FungiCure Manicure/Pedicure Formula Liquid	Clotrimazole 1%	**Adults & Peds ≥2 yrs:** Use bid.
Lotrimin AF Antifungal Athlete's Foot Cream	Clotrimazole 1%	**Adults & Peds ≥2 yrs:** Use bid.
Lotrimin AF Antifungal Athlete's Foot Topical Solution	Clotrimazole 1%	**Adults & Peds ≥2 yrs:** Use bid.
Lotrimin AF For Her Antifungal Cream	Clotrimazole 1%	**Adults & Peds ≥2 yrs:** Use bid.
MICONAZOLE		
Clearly Confident Triple Action Fungus Treatment	Miconazole Nitrate 2%	**Adults:** Apply to affected area bid.
Desenex Antifungal Liquid Spray	Miconazole Nitrate 2%	**Adults:** Use bid.
Desenex Antifungal Powder	Miconazole Nitrate 2%	**Adults:** Use bid.
Desenex Antifungal Spray	Miconazole Nitrate 2%	**Adults:** Use bid.
DiabetAid Antifungal Foot Bath Tablets	Miconazole Nitrate 2%	**Adults & Peds ≥2 yrs:** Use prn.
Diabet-X Antifungal Skin Treatment Cream	Miconazole Nitrate 2%	**Adults & Peds ≥2 yrs:** Use prn.
Lotrimin AF Antifungal Aerosol Liquid Spray	Miconazole Nitrate 2%	**Adults & Peds ≥2 yrs:** Use bid.
Lotrimin AF Antifungal Jock Itch Aerosol Powder Spray	Miconazole Nitrate 2%	**Adults & Peds ≥2 yrs:** Use bid.
Lotrimin AF Antifungal Powder	Miconazole Nitrate 2%	**Adults & Peds ≥2 yrs:** Use bid.
Micatin Athlete's Foot Cream	Miconazole Nitrate 2%	**Adults:** Use bid.
Micatin Athlete's Foot Spray Liquid	Miconazole Nitrate 2%	**Adults:** Use bid.
Micatin Jock Itch Spray Powder	Miconazole Nitrate 2%	**Adults:** Use bid.
Micatin Jock Itch Antifungal Cream	Miconazole Nitrate 2%	**Adults:** Use bid.
Neosporin AF Antifungal Cream	Miconazole Nitrate 2%	**Adults & Peds ≥12 yrs:** Use bid.
Neosporin AF Athlete's Foot Antifungal Spray Liquid	Miconazole Nitrate 2%	**Adults & Peds ≥12 yrs:** Use bid.
Neosporin AF Athlete's Foot Antifungal Spray Powder	Miconazole Nitrate 2%	**Adults & Peds ≥12 yrs:** Use bid.
Neosporin AF Jock Itch Antifungal Cream	Miconazole Nitrate 2%	**Adults & Peds ≥12 yrs:** Use bid.
Zeasorb Super Absorbent Antifungal Powder	Miconazole Nitrate 2%	**Adults & Peds:** Use bid.
TERBINAFINE		
Lamisil AT Antifungal Cream	Terbinafine HCl 1%	**Adults & Peds ≥12 yrs:** Use bid.
Lamisil AT Antifungal Spray Pump	Terbinafine HCl 1%	**Adults & Peds ≥12 yrs:** Use qd or bid.
Lamisil AT Athlete's Foot Cream	Terbinafine HCl 1%	**Adults & Peds ≥12 yrs:** Use bid.
Lamisil AT Athlete's Foot Gel	Terbinafine HCl 1%	**Adults & Peds ≥12 yrs:** Use qd.

(Continued)

BRAND	INGREDIENT/STRENGTH	DOSE
TERBINAFINE *(Continued)*		
Lamisil AT Athlete's Foot Spray Pump	Terbinafine HCl 1%	**Adults & Peds ≥12 yrs:** Use bid.
Lamisil AT for Women Cream	Terbinafine HCl 1%	**Adults & Peds ≥12 yrs:** Use bid.
Lamisil AT Jock Itch Cream	Terbinafine HCl 1%	**Adults & Peds ≥12 yrs:** Use qd.
Lamisil AT Jock Itch Spray Pump	Terbinafine HCl 1%	**Adults & Peds ≥12 yrs:** Use qd.
TOLNAFTATE		
FungiCure Anti-Fungal Gel	Tolnaftate 1%	**Adults & Peds:** Use bid.
Gold Bond Antifungal Foot Swabs	Tolnaftate 1%	**Adults & Peds:** Use bid.
Miracle of Aloe Miracure Anti-Fungal	Tolnaftate 1%	**Adults & Peds ≥12 yrs:** Use bid.
Swabplus Foot Care Fungus Relief Swabs	Tolnaftate 1%	**Adults & Peds:** Use qd or bid.
Tinactin Antifungal Deodorant Powder Spray	Tolnaftate 1%	**Adults & Peds:** Use qd or bid.
Tinactin Antifungal Liquid Spray	Tolnaftate 1%	**Adults & Peds:** Use qd or bid.
Tinactin Antifungal Powder Spray	Tolnaftate 1%	**Adults & Peds:** Use qd or bid.
Tinactin Antifungal Cream	Tolnaftate 1%	**Adults & Peds:** Use qd or bid.
Tinactin Antifungal Absorbent Powder	Tolnaftate 1%	**Adults & Peds:** Use qd or bid.
Tinactin Antifungal Jock Itch Powder Spray	Tolnaftate 1%	**Adults & Peds:** Use qd or bid.
UNDECYLENIC ACID		
Fungi Nail Anti-fungal Solution	Undecylenic Acid 25%	**Adults & Peds:** Use bid.
FungiCure Anti-fungal Liquid	Undecylenic Acid 10%	**Adults & Peds ≥2 yrs:** Use bid.
FungiCure Maximum Strength Liquid	Undecylenic Acid 25%	**Adults & Peds ≥2 yrs:** Use bid.
FungiCure Professional Formula Liquid	Undecylenic Acid 15%	**Adults & Peds:** Use bid.
Tineacide Antifungal Cream	Undecylenic Acid 10%	**Adults & Peds ≥12 yrs:** Use bid.

CONTACT DERMATITIS PRODUCTS

BRAND	INGREDIENT/STRENGTH	DOSE
ANTIHISTAMINE		
Benadryl Itch Stopping Extra Strength Gel	Diphenhydramine HCl 2%	**Adults & Peds ≥2 yrs:** Apply to affected area tid-qid.
ANTIHISTAMINE COMBINATION		
Benadryl Extra Strength Itch-Stopping Cream	Diphenhydramine HCl/Zinc Acetate 2%-0.1%	**Adults & Peds ≥2 yrs:** Apply to affected area tid-qid.
Benadryl Extra Strength Spray	Diphenhydramine HCl/Zinc Acetate 2%-0.1%	**Adults & Peds ≥2 yrs:** Apply to affected area tid-qid.
Benadryl Extra Strength Itch Relief Stick	Diphenhydramine HCl/Zinc Acetate 2%-0.1%	**Adults & Peds ≥2 yrs:** Apply to affected area tid-qid.
Benadryl Original Strength Itch Stopping Cream	Diphenhydramine HCl/Zinc Acetate 1%-0.1%	**Adults & Peds ≥2 yrs:** Apply to affected area tid-qid.
CalaGel Anti-Itch Gel	Diphenhydramine HCl/Zinc Acetate/Benzenthonium Chloride 2%-0.215%-0.15%	**Adults & Peds ≥2 yrs:** Apply to affected area no more than tid.
Ivarest Double Relief Formula	Diphenhydramine HCl/Benzyl Alcohol/ Calamine 2%-10.5%-14%	**Adults & Peds ≥2 yrs:** Apply to affected area tid-qid.
ASTRINGENT		
Domeboro Powder Packets	Aluminum Acetate (combination of Calcium Acetate 893mg and Aluminum Sulfate 1191mg)	**Adults & Peds:** Dissolve 1-3 pkts and apply to affected area for 15-30 min tid.
Ivy-Dry with Zytrel Super Liquid	Zinc Acetate/Benzyl Alcohol/Camphor/ Menthol 2%-10%-0.5%-0.25%	**Adults & Peds ≥6 yrs:** Apply to affected area qd-tid.
Ivy Dry Anti-Itch Cream	Zinc Acetate/Benzyl Alcohol 2%-10%	**Adults & Peds ≥2 yrs:** Apply to affected area tid.
Ivy Dry Cream	Zinc Acetate/Benzyl Alcohol 2%-10%	**Adults & Peds ≥6 yrs:** Apply to affected area tid.
Ivy Dry Kids	Zinc Acetate 2%	**Adults & Peds ≥2 yrs:** Apply to affected area tid.
ASTRINGENT COMBINATION		
Aveeno Calamine and Pramoxine HCl Anti-Itch Cream	Calamine/Pramoxine HCl 3%-1%	**Adults & Peds ≥2 yrs:** Apply to affected area tid-qid.
Aveeno Anti-Itch Concentrated Lotion	Calamine/Pramoxine HCl/ Camphor 3%-1%-0.47%	**Adults & Peds ≥2 yrs:** Apply to affected area qid.
Caladryl Clear Anti-Itch Lotion	Zinc Acetate/Pramoxine HCl 0.1%-1%	**Adults & Peds ≥2 yrs:** Apply to affected area tid-qid.
Caladryl Anti-Itch Lotion	Calamine/Pramoxine HCl 8%-1%	**Adults & Peds ≥2 yrs:** Apply to affected area tid-qid.
Calamine Lotion (generic)	Calamine/Zinc Oxide	**Adults & Peds:** Apply to affected area prn.
Cortaid Poison Ivy Care Treatment Kit	Zinc Acetate/Pramoxine HCl 0.12%-1%	**Adults & Peds ≥2 yrs:** Apply to affected area tid-qid.
CLEANSER		
Ivy-Dry Scrub	Polyethylene, sodium lauryl sulfoacetate, cetearyl alcohol, nonoxynol-9, camellia sinensis oil, phenoxyethanol, methylparaben, propylparaben, triethanolamine, carbomer, erythorbic acid, aloe barbadensis extract, tocopheryl acetate extract, tetrasodium EDTA	**Adults & Peds:** Wash affected area prn.
Cortaid Poison Ivy Care Toxin Removal Cloths	Water, lauroyl sarcosinate, glycerin, DMDM, hydantoin, methylparaben, tetrasodium EDTA, Aloe barnadenis leaf extract, citric acid	**Adults & Peds:** Wipe affected area at least 15 seconds.
CORTICOSTEROID		
Aveeno 1% Hydrocortisone Anti-Itch Cream	Hydrocortisone 1%	**Adults & Peds ≥2 yrs:** Apply to affected area tid-qid.
Cortaid Advanced 12-Hour Anti-Itch Cream	Hydrocortisone 1%	**Adults & Peds ≥2 yrs:** Apply to affected area tid-qid.
Cortaid Intensive Therapy Cooling Spray	Hydrocortisone 1%	**Adults & Peds ≥2 yrs:** Apply to affected area tid-qid.
Cortaid Intensive Therapy Moisturizing Cream	Hydrocortisone 1%	**Adults & Peds ≥2 yrs:** Apply to affected area tid-qid.
Cortaid Maximum Strength Cream	Hydrocortisone 1%	**Adults & Peds ≥2 yrs:** Apply to affected area tid-qid.

(Continued)

BRAND	INGREDIENT/STRENGTH	DOSE
CORTICOSTEROID *(Continued)*		
Cortaid Maximum Strength Ointment	Hydrocortisone 1%	**Adults & Peds ≥2 yrs:** Apply to affected area tid-qid.
Cortizone-10 Easy Relief Applicator	Hydrocortisone 1%	**Adults & Peds ≥2 yrs:** Apply to affected area tid-qid.
Cortizone-10 Cooling Relief Gel	Hydrocortisone 1%	**Adults & Peds ≥2 yrs:** Apply to affected area tid-qid.
Cortizone-10 Cream	Hydrocortisone 1%	**Adults & Peds ≥2 yrs:** Apply to affected area tid-qid.
Cortizone-10 Ointment	Hydrocortisone 1%	**Adults & Peds ≥2 yrs:** Apply to affected area tid-qid.
Cortizone-10 Plus	Hydrocortisone 1%	**Adults & Peds ≥2 yrs:** Apply to affected area tid-qid.
Cortizone-10 Intensive Healing Formula	Hydrocortisone 1%	**Adults & Peds ≥2 yrs:** Apply to affected area tid-qid.
Corticool	Hydrocortisone 1%	**Adults & Peds ≥2 yrs:** Apply to affected area tid-qid.
Dermarest Eczema Medicated Lotion	Hydrocortisone 1%	**Adults & Peds ≥2 yrs:** Apply to affected area tid-qid.
COUNTERIRRITANT		
Gold Bond First Aid Quick Spray	Menthol/Benzethonium Chloride 1%-0.13%	**Adults & Peds ≥2 yrs:** Apply to affected area tid-qid.
Gold Bond Medicated Maximum Strength Anti-Itch Cream	Menthol/Pramoxine HCl 1%-1%	**Adults & Peds ≥2 yrs:** Apply to affected area tid-qid.
Ivy Block Lotion	Bentoquatam 5%	**Adults & Peds ≥6 yrs:** Apply q4h for continued protection.
LOCAL ANESTHETIC		
Solarcaine Aloe Extra Burn Relief Gel	Lidocaine HCl 0.5%	**Adults & Peds ≥2 yrs:** Apply to affected area tid-qid.
Solarcaine Aloe Extra Burn Relief Spray	Lidocaine HCl 0.5%	**Adults & Peds ≥2 yrs:** Apply to affected area tid-qid.
Solarcaine First Aid Medicated Spray	Benzocaine/Triclosan 20%-0.13%	**Adults & Peds ≥2 yrs:** Apply to affected area qd-tid.
LOCAL ANESTHETIC COMBINATION		
Bactine Cleansing Spray	Lidocaine/Benzalkonium Chloride 2.5%-0.13%	**Adults & Peds ≥2 yrs:** Apply to affected area qd-tid.
Bactine First Aid Liquid	Lidocaine HCl/Benzalkonium Chloride 2.5%-0.13%	**Adults & Peds ≥2 yrs:** Apply to affected area qd-tid.
Lanacane Maximum Strength Cream	Benzocaine/Benzethonium Chloride 20%-0.2%	**Adults & Peds ≥2 yrs:** Apply to affected area qd-tid.
Lanacane Maximum Strength Spray	Benzocaine/Benzethonium Chloride 20%-0.2%	**Adults & Peds ≥2 yrs:** Apply to affected area qd-tid.
Lanacane Original Formula Cream	Benzocaine/Benzethonium Chloride 6%-0.2%	**Adults & Peds ≥2 yrs:** Apply to affected area qd-tid.
SKIN PROTECTANT		
Aveeno Skin Relief Moisturizing Cream	Dimethicone 2.5%	**Adults & Peds ≥2 yrs:** Apply to affected area tid-qid.
Lanacane Medicated Body Lotion	Dimethicone 1%	**Adults & Peds ≥2 yrs:** Apply to affected area qd-tid.
SKIN PROTECTANT COMBINATION		
Gold Bond Extra Strength Medicated Body Lotion Triple Action Relief	Dimethicone/Menthol 5%-0.5%	**Adults & Peds:** Apply to dry, itchy skin as often as needed.
Gold Bond Medicated Body Lotion Triple Action Relief	Dimethicone/Menthol 5%-0.15%	**Adults & Peds:** Apply to affected area prn.
Gold Bond Medicated Powder	Zinc Oxide/Menthol 1%-0.15%	**Adults & Peds ≥2 yrs:** Apply to affected area tid-qid.
Gold Bond Medicated Extra Strength Powder	Zinc Oxide/Menthol 5%-0.8%	**Adults & Peds ≥2 yrs:** Apply to affected area tid-qid.
Vaseline Intensive Rescue Clinical Therapy	Dimethicone 1%	**Adults & Peds:** Apply to affected area prn.

DANDRUFF PRODUCTS

BRAND	INGREDIENT/STRENGTH	DOSE
COAL TAR		
Denorex Therapeutic Protection 2-in-1 Shampoo	Coal Tar 0.5%	**Adults & Peds:** Use biw.
DHS Tar Shampoo	Coal Tar 0.5%	**Adults & Peds:** Use biw.
DHS Tar Gel Shampoo	Coal Tar 0.5%	**Adults & Peds:** Use biw.
Ionil T Shampoo	Coal Tar 1%	**Adults & Peds:** Use biw.
Ionil T Plus Shampoo	Coal Tar 2%	**Adults & Peds:** Use biw.
Neutrogena T-Gel Shampoo Original Formula	Coal Tar 0.5%	**Adults & Peds:** Use biw.
Neutrogena T-Gel Shampoo, Extra Strength	Coal Tar 1%	**Adults & Peds:** Use biw.
Neutrogena T-Gel Stubborn Itch Shampoo	Coal Tar 0.5%	**Adults & Peds:** Use biw.
Reme-T Gel	Coal Tar 5%	**Adults & Peds:** Use biw.
CORTICOSTEROID		
Maximum Strength Scalpicin Liquid	Hydrocortisone 1%	**Adults & Peds ≥2 yrs:** Apply to affected area qd-qid.
KETOCONAZOLE		
Nizoral Anti-Dandruff Shampoo	Ketoconazole 1%	**Adults & Peds ≥12:** Use q3-4d up to 8 wks.
PYRITHIONE ZINC		
Denorex Dandruff Shampoo, Daily Protection	Pyrithione Zinc 2%	**Adults & Peds:** Use biw.
DHS Zinc Shampoo	Pyrithione Zinc 2%	**Adults & Peds:** Use biw.
Garnier Fructis Fortifying Shampoo, Anti-Dandruff	Pyrithione Zinc 1%	**Adults & Peds:** Use biw.
Head & Shoulders Dry Scalp Care Dandruff Shampoo Plus Conditioner; Shampoo; Conditioner	Pyrithione Zinc 0.5%	**Adults & Peds:** Use biw.
Head & Shoulders Smooth & Silky Dandruff Shampoo Plus Conditioner; Shampoo; Conditioner	Pyrithione Zinc 1%	**Adults & Peds:** Use biw.
Head & Shoulders Citrus Breeze Dandruff Shampoo Plus Conditioner; Shampoo	Pyrithione Zinc 1%	**Adults & Peds:** Use biw.
Head & Shoulders Classic Clean Dandruff Shampoo Plus Conditioner; Shampoo; Conditioner	Pyrithione Zinc 1%	**Adults & Peds:** Use biw.
Head & Shoulders Extra Volume Dandruff Shampoo	Pyrithione Zinc 1%	**Adults & Peds:** Use biw.
Head & Shoulders Ocean Lift Dandruff Shampoo Plus Conditioner; Shampoo	Pyrithione Zinc 1%	**Adults & Peds:** Use biw.
Head & Shoulders Dandruff Refresh Shampoo Plus Conditioner; Shampoo	Pyrithione Zinc 1%	**Adults & Peds:** Use biw.
Head & Shoulders Restoring Shine Dandruff Shampoo Plus Conditioner; Shampoo	Pyrithione Zinc 1%	**Adults & Peds:** Use biw.
Head & Shoulders Sensitive Care Dandruff Shampoo Plus Conditioner; Shampoo	Pyrithione Zinc 1%	**Adults & Peds:** Use biw.
L'Oreal VIVE Pro Anti-Dandruff for Men Shampoo	Pyrithione Zinc 1%	**Adults & Peds:** Use biw.
Neutrogena T-Gel Daily Control Dandruff Shampoo	Pyrithione Zinc 1%	**Adults & Peds:** Use biw.

(Continued)

BRAND	INGREDIENT/STRENGTH	DOSE
PYRITHIONE ZINC *(Continued)*		
Neutrogena T-Gel Daily Control 2-in-1 Dandruff Shampoo Plus Conditioner	Pyrithione Zinc 1%	**Adults & Peds:** Use biw.
Pantene Pro-V Shampoo + Conditioner, Anti-Dandruff	Pyrithione Zinc 1%	**Adults & Peds:** Use biw.
Pert Plus Shampoo Plus Conditioner, Dandruff Control	Pyrithione Zinc 1%	**Adults & Peds:** Use biw.
Pert Plus 2-in-1 Dandruff Dismissed Shampoo	Pyrithione Zinc 0.45%	**Adults & Peds:** Use biw.
Selsun Salon 2-in-1 Pyrithione Zinc Shampoo	Pyrithione Zinc 1%	**Adults & Peds:** Use biw.
Suave for Men 2 in 1 Shampoo/ Conditioner, Dandruff	Pyrithione Zinc 0.5%	**Adults & Peds:** Use biw.
SALICYLIC ACID		
Denorex Dandruff Shampoo, Extra Strength	Salicylic Acid 3%	**Adults & Peds:** Use biw.
DHS SAL Shampoo	Salicylic Acid 3%	**Adults & Peds:** Use biw.
Ionil, Ionil Plus Shampoo	Salicylic Acid 2%	**Adults & Peds:** Use biw.
Neutrogena T/Gel Therapeutic Conditioner	Salicylic Acid 2%	**Adults & Peds:** Use biw.
Neutrogena T/Sal Shampoo	Salicylic Acid 3%	**Adults & Peds:** Use biw.
Scalpicin Anti-Itch Liquid Scalp Treatment	Salicylic Acid 3%	**Adults & Peds:** Apply to affected area qd-qid.
Selsun Blue Naturals Dandruff Shampoo	Salicylic Acid 3%	**Adults & Peds:** Use biw.
SELENIUM SULFIDE		
Head & Shoulders Dandruff Shampoo, Intensive Treatment	Selenium Sulfide 1%	**Adults & Peds:** Use biw.
Selsun Blue Dandruff Shampoo, Medicated Formula	Selenium Sulfide 1%	**Adults & Peds:** Use biw.
Selsun Blue 2-in-1	Selenium Sulfide 1%	**Adults & Peds:** Use biw.
Selsun Blue Normal to Oily Formula	Selenium Sulfide 1%	**Adults & Peds:** Use biw.
Selsun Blue Dandruff Shampoo, Moisturizing Formula	Selenium Sulfide 1%	**Adults & Peds:** Use biw.
SULFUR/SALICYLIC ACID		
Sebulex Medicated Dandruff Shampoo	Sulfur/Salicylic Acid 2%-2%	**Adults & Peds ≥12yrs:** Use qod-qd.

DIAPER RASH PRODUCTS

BRAND	INGREDIENT/STRENGTH	DOSE
WHITE PETROLATUM		
Balmex Extra Protective Clear Ointment	White Petrolatum 51%	**Peds:** Apply prn.
Vaseline Baby, Baby Fresh Scent	White Petrolatum 100%	**Peds:** Apply prn.
Vaseline Petroleum Jelly	White Petrolatum 100%	**Peds:** Apply prn.
ZINC OXIDE		
Aveeno Baby Soothing Relief Diaper Rash Cream	Zinc Oxide 13%	**Peds:** Apply prn.
Balmex Diaper Rash Cream with ActivGuard	Zinc Oxide 11.3%	**Peds:** Apply prn.
Balmex Diaper Rash Ointment with Aloe & Vitamin E	Zinc Oxide 11.3%	**Peds:** Apply prn.
Boudreaux's Butt Paste, Diaper Rash Ointment	Zinc Oxide 16%	**Peds:** Apply prn.
California Baby Diaper Rash Cream	Zinc Oxide 12%	**Peds:** Apply prn.
Canus Li'l Goat's Milk Ointment	Zinc Oxide 40%	**Peds:** Apply prn.
Desitin Diaper Rash Ointment, Creamy	Zinc Oxide 10%	**Peds:** Apply prn.
Desitin Original Diaper Rash Ointment	Zinc Oxide 40%	**Peds:** Apply prn.
Huggies Diaper Rash Cream	Zinc Oxide 10%	**Peds:** Apply prn.
Huggies Gentle Care Creamy Diaper Rash Ointment	Zinc Oxide 10%	**Peds:** Apply prn.
Johnson's Baby Diaper Rash Cream with Zinc Oxide	Zinc Oxide 13%	**Peds:** Apply prn.
Mustela Bebe Vitamin Barrier Cream	Zinc Oxide 10%	**Peds:** Apply prn.
COMBINATION PRODUCTS		
A+D Original Ointment, Diaper Rash and All-Purpose Skincare Formula	Petrolatum/Lanolin 53.4%-15.5%	**Peds:** Apply prn.
A+D Zinc Oxide Diaper Rash Cream with Aloe	Dimethicone/Zinc Oxide 1%-10%	**Peds:** Apply prn.
Lansinoh Diaper Rash Ointment	Dimethicone/USP Modified Lanolin/ Zinc Oxide 5.5%-15.5%-5.5%	**Peds:** Apply prn.
Triple Paste Medicated Ointment	Beeswax/Lanolin/Zinc Oxide (strength not available)	**Peds:** Apply prn.

DRY SKIN PRODUCTS

BRAND	INGREDIENTS	DOSE
AmLactin Moisturizing Cream	Water, Lactic Acid, Ammonium Hydroxide, Light Mineral Oil, Glyceryl Stearate, PEG-100 Stearate, Glycerin, Propylene Glycol, Magnesium Aluminum Silicate, Laureth 4, Polyoxyl 40 Stearate, Cetyl Alcohol, Methylcellulose, Methyl Paraben, Propylparaben	**Adults & Peds:** Apply bid.
AmLactin Moisturizing Lotion	Water, Lactic Acid, Ammonium Hydroxide, Light Mineral Oil, Glyceryl Stearate, PEG-100 Stearate, Glycerin, Propylene Glycol, Magnesium Aluminum Silicate, Laureth 4, Polyoxyl 40 Stearate, Cetyl Alcohol, Methylcellulose, Methylparaben, Propylparaben	**Adults & Peds:** Apply bid.
AmLactin XL Moisturizing Lotion	Water, Ammonium Lactate, Potassium Lactate, Sodium Lactate, Emulsifying Wax, Light Mineral Oil, White Petrolatum, Glycerin, Propylene Glycol, Stearic Acid, Xanthum Gum, Methyl and Propylparabens	**Adults & Peds:** Apply bid.
Aquaphor Baby Healing Ointment	Petrolatum, Mineral Oil, Ceresin, Lanolin Alcohol, Panthenol, Glycerin, Bisabolol	**Adults & Peds:** Apply prn.
Aquaphor Original Ointment	Petrolatum, Mineral Oil, Ceresin, Lanolin Alcohol	**Adults & Peds:** Apply to affected area prn.
Aquaphor Healing Ointment	Petrolatum, Mineral Oil, Ceresin, Lanolin Alcohol, Panthenol, Glycerin, Bisabolol	**Adults & Peds:** Apply to affected area prn.
Aveeno Baby Calming Comfort Lotion	Dimethicone, Avena Sativa (Oat) Kernel Flour (Oat), Benzyl Alcohol, Cetyl Alcohol, Distearyldimonium Chloride, Fragrance, Glycerin, Isopropyl Palmitate, Petrolatum, Sodium Chloride, Water	**Adults & Peds:** Apply prn.
Aveeno Baby Continuous Protection Lotion SPF 55	Avobenzone, Homosalate, Octisalate, Octocrylene, Oxybenzone, Avena Sativa (Oat) Kernel Flour, Behenyl Alcohol, BHT, Butyloctyl Salicylate, Caprylyl Methicone, Diethylhexyl 2,6-Naphthalate, Dimethicone, Disodium EDTA, Ethylhexyl Stearate, Ethylhexyl Glycerin, Ethylparaben, Glyceryl Stearate, Methylparaben, PEG 100 Stearate, Phenoxyethanol, Propylparaben, Silica, Sodium Polyacrylate, Styrene Acrylate Copolymer, Trideceth 6, Trimethylsiloxysilicate, VP/Hexadecene Copolymer, Water, Xanthan Gum	**Adults & Peds ≥6 mo:** Apply before sun exposure prn.
Aveeno Baby Moisture Soothing Relief Moisture Cream	Water, Glycerin, Petrolatum, Mineral Oil, Cetyl Alcohol, Dimethicone, Avena Sativa (Oat) Kernel Flour, Carbomer, Sodium Hydroxide, Ceteareth-6, Hydrolyzed Milk Protein, Hydrolyzed Oats, Hydrolyzed Soy Protein, PEG-25 Soya Sterol, Tetrasodium EDTA, Methylparaben, Citric Acid, Sodium Citrate, Benzalkonium Chloride, Benzaldehyde, Butylene Glycol, Butylparaben, Ethylparaben, Ethyl Alcohol, Isobutylparaben, Phenoxyethanol, Propylparaben, Stearyl Alcohol	**Adults & Peds:** Apply prn.
Aveeno Baby Soothing Bath Treatment Packets	Colloidal Oatmeal 43%, Calcium Silicilate, Laureth-4 Mineral Oil	**Adults & Peds:** Bathe in 1 packet for 15-20 min qd-bid.
Aveeno Baby Daily Moisture Lotion	Dimethicone 1.2%, Water, Glycerin, Distearyldimonium Chloride, Petrolatum, Isopropyl Palmitate, Cetyl Alcohol, Oat Flour Avena Sativa, Allontoin, Benzyl Alcohol, Sodium Chloride	**Peds:** Apply prn.
Aveeno Daily Moisturizer, Ultra-Calming SPF 15	Avobenzone/Octinoxate/Octisalate (3%-7.5%-2%), Arachidyl Alcohol, Arachidyl Glucoside, Behenyl Alcohol, Benzyl Alcohol, Butylparaben, C12 15 Alkyl Benzoate, C12 16 Alkyl Hydroxyethyl Ethylcellulose, C13 14 Isoparaffin, Cetearyl Alcohol, Cetearyl Glucoside, Chrysanthemum Parthenium Extract (Feverfew), Cyclohexasiloxane, Cyclopentasiloxane, Dimethicone, Disodium EDTA, Ethylene Acrylic Acid Copolymer, Ethylparaben, Fragrance, Glycerin, Iodopropynyl Butylcarbamate, Isobutylparaben, Laureth 7, Magnesium Aspartate, Methylparaben, Panthenol, Phenoxyethanol, Phenyl Trimethicone, Polyacrylamide, Potassium Aspartate, Propylparaben, Sarcosine, Sodium Cocoyl Amino Acids, Steareth 2, Steareth 12, Tetradibutyl Pentaerithrityl Hydroxyhydrocinnamate, Water	**Adults:** Apply qd.

(Continued)

BRAND	INGREDIENTS	DOSE
Aveeno Daily Moisturizing Lotion	Dimethicone 1.25%, Avena Sativa (Oat) Kernal, Benzyl Alcohol, Cetyl Alcohol, Distearyldimonium Chloride, Glycerin, Isopropyl Palmitate, Petrolatum, Sodium Chloride, Water	**Adults:** Apply prn.
Aveeno Intense Relief Hand Cream	Water, Glycerin, Distearyldimonium Chloride, Petrolatum, Isopropyl Palmitate, Cetyl Alcohol, Aluminum Starch Octenyl Succinate, Dimethicone, Avena Sativa (Oat) Kernel Flour, Benzyl Alcohol, Sodium Chloride	**Adults & Peds:** Apply prn.
Aveeno Moisturizing Bar for Dry Skin	Avena Stativa (Oat) Flour, Water, Cetearyl Alcohol, Stearic Acid, Sodium Cocoyl Isethionate, Water, Disodium Lauryl Sulfosuccinate, Glycerin, Hydrogenated Vegetable Oil, Titanium Dioxide, Citric Acid, Sodium Trideceth Sulfate, Hydrogenated Castor Oil	**Adults & Peds:** Use qd.
Aveeno Moisturizing Lotion, Skin Relief	Dimethicone 1.25%, Allantoin, Avena Sativa Kernel Flour (Oat), Benzyl Alcohol, Cetyl Alcohol, Distearyldimonium Chloride, Glycerin, Isopropyl Palmitate, Menthol, Petrolatum, Sodium Chloride, Triticum Vulgare Germ Protein (Wheat), Water	**Adult & Peds ≥2 yrs:** Apply qd.
Aveeno Positively Radiant Moisturizing Lotion	Water, Glycerin, Emulsifying Wax, Ethylhexyl Isononanoate, Glycine Soja (Soybean) Seed Extract, Propylene Glycol Isoceteth-3 Acetate, Dimethicone, Polyacrylamide, Cyclomethicone, Stearic Acid, Phenoxyethanol, c13-14 Isoparaffin, Dimethicone Copolyol, Benzyl Alcohol, TItanium Dioxide, Fragrance, Iodopropynyl Butylcarbamate, Tocopherol Acetate, Panthenol, Panthenyl Ethylether, Glyceryl Laurate, Laureth-7, Methylparaben, Silica, Mica, Polymethyl Methacrylate, Cetearyl Alcohol, Tetrasodium EDTA, Butylparaben, Ethylparaben, Isobutylparaben, Propylparaben, DMDM Hydantoin, Panthenol, BHT, Citric Acid	**Adults:** Apply qd.
Aveeno Positively Radiant Daily Moisturizer SPF 15	Avobenzone/Octinoxate/Octisalate (3%-7.5%-2%), Arachidyl Alcohol, Arachidyl Glucoside, Behenyl Alcohol, Benzalkonium Chloride, Benzyl Alcohol, BHT, Bisphenylpropyl Dimethicone, Butylparaben, c12-15 Alkyl Benzoate, c13-14 Isoparaffin, Cetearyl Alcohol, Cetearyl Glucoside, Dimethicone, Disodium EDTA, Ethylene/Acrylic Acid Copolymer, Ethylparaben, Fragrance, Glycerin, Glycine Soja (Soybean) Seed Extract, Iodopropyl Butylcarbamate, Isobutylparaben, Laureth-7, Methylparaben, Mica, Panthenol, Phenoxyethanol, Polyacrylamide, Polymethyl Methacrylate, Propylparaben, Silica, Steareth-2, Steareth-21, Titanium Dioxide, Water, Sodium Hydroxide, Citric Acid	**Adults:** Use daily.
Aveeno Positively Smooth Facial Moisturizer	Water, C12-15 Alkyl Benzoate, Cetearyl Alcohol, Bisphenylpropyl Dimethicone, Glycine, Soja Seed Extract, Butylene Glycol, Arachidyl Alcohol, Glycine Soja Protein, Dimethicone, Glycerin, Panthenol, Polyacrylamide, Phenoxyethanol, Cetearyl Glucoside, Behenyl Alcohol, Benzyl Alcohol, C13-14 Isoparaffin, DMDM Hydantoin, Arachidyl Glucoside, Disodium EDTA, Methylparaben, Laureth 7, BHT, Ethylparaben, Butylparaben, Propylparaben, Isobutylparaben, Fragrance, Iodopropynyl Butylcarbamate	**Adults:** Apply prn.
Aveeno Positively Smooth Moisturizing Lotion	Water, Glycerin, Emulsifying Wax, Ethylhexyl Isononanoate, Glycine Soja Seed Extracts (Soybean), Propylene Glycol Isoceteth 3 Acetate, Dimethicone, Cyclomethicone, Polyacrylamide, Stearic Acid, Phenoxyethanol, C13 14 Isoparaffin, Dimethicone Copolyol, Benzyl Alcohol, Fragrance, DMDM Hydantoin, Glyceryl Laurate, Laureth 7, Methylparaben, Cetearyl Alcohol, Tetrasodium EDTA, Butylparaben, Ethylparaben, BHT, Propylparaben, Isobutylparaben, Iodopropynyl Butylcarbamate, Panthenyl Ethyl Ether, Tocopheryl Acetate, Panthenol	**Adults:** Apply prn.

(Continued)

BRAND	INGREDIENTS	DOSE
Aveeno Radiant Skin Daily Moisturizer with SPF 15	Octinoxate (Octyl Methoxycinnamate)/Avobenzone / Octisalate (Octyl Salicylate) 7.5%-3%-2%; Arachidyl Alcohol, Arachidyl Glucoside, Behenyl Alcohol, Benzalkonium Chloride, Benzyl Alcohol, BHT, Bis-phenylpropyl Dimethicone, Butylparaben, C12-15 Alkyl-Benzoate, C13-14 Isoparaffin, Cetearyl Alcohol, Cetearyl Glucoside, Dimethicone, Disodium EDTA, Ethylene/Acrylic Acid Copolymer, Ethylparaben, Fragrance, Glycerin, Glycine Soja (Soybean) Seed Extract, Iodopropynyl Butylcarbamate, Isobutylparaben, Laureth-7, Methylparaben, Mica, Panthenol, Phenoxyethanol, Polyacrylamide, Polymethylmethacrylate, Propylparaben, Silica, Steareth-2, Steareth-21, Titanium Dioxide, Water, Sodium Hydroxide, Citric Acid	**Adults:** Apply prn.
Aveeno Creamy Moisturizing Oil	Water, Sesamum Indicum Seed Oil (Sesame), Di PPG 3 Myristyl Ether Adipate, Glycerin, Hydrogenated Polydecene, Dimethicone, Cetyl Alcohol, Avena Sativa Kernel Oil (Oat), Prunus Amygdalus Dulcis Oil (Sweet Almond), Avena Sativa Kernel Flour (Oat), Glyceryl Stearate, PEG 100 Stearate, Magnesium Aluminum Silicate, Xanthan Gum, Diazolidinyl Urea, Acrylates/C10 30 Alkyl Acrylate Crosspolymer, Lauroyl Lysine, Methylparaben, Ethylparaben, Propylparaben, Sodium Hydroxide, BHT, Tetrasodium EDTA, Fragrance	**Adults:** Apply after shower/bath prn.
Aveeno Intense Relief Overnight Cream	Dimethicone (1.3%), Avena Sativa (Oat) Kernel Extract, Avena Sativa (Oat) Kernel Flour, Avena Sativa (Oat) Kernel Oil, Benzyl Alcohol, Butyrospermum Parkii (Shea Butter), Cetyl Alcohol, Chamomilla Recutita (Matricaria) Flower Extract, Distearyldimonium Chloride, Glycerin, Isopropyl Palmitate, Petrolatum, Propylene Glycol, Sodium Chloride, Steareth 20, Water	**Adults:** Apply prn.
Aveeno Skin Relief Moisturizing Cream	Dimethicone (2.5%), Water, Glycerin, Distearyldimonium Chloride, Petrolatum, Cetyl Alcohol, Theobroma Cacao (Cocoa) Seed Butter, Cetearyl Alcohol, Avena Sativa (Oat) Kernel Flour, Di PPG 3 Myristyl Ether Adipate, Benzyl Alcohol, Ceteareth 20, Avena Sativa (Oat) Kernel Oil, Hydroxyethyl Cellulose, Menthol, Sodium Chloride, Butyrospermum Parkii (Shea Butter) Extract	**Adults & Peds ≥2 yrs:** Apply tid-qid.
Aveeno Ultra-Calming Night Cream	Water, Glycerin, C12 15 Alkyl Benzoate, Cetearyl Alcohol, Dimethicone, Arachidyl Alcohol, Cetyl Alcohol, Chrysanthemum Parthenium (Feverfew) Extract, Phenoxyethanol, Phenyl Trimethicone, Behenyl Alcohol, Cetearyl Glucoside, Ethylene Acrylic Acid Copolymer, Panthenol, Polyacrylamide, Arachidyl Glucoside, Sodium Cocoyl Amino Acids, Fragrance, C13 14 Isoparaffin, Cetyl Hydroxyethylcellulose, Methylparaben, Disodium EDTA, Sodium Polyacrylate, Pentaerythrityl Tetra Di T Butyl Hydroxyhydrocinnamate, Sarcosine, Laureth 7, Propylparaben, Ethylparaben, Magnesium Aspartate, Potassium Aspartate	**Adults:** Apply prn.
Aveeno Skin Relief Body Wash, Fragrance Free	Water, Glycerin, Cocamidopropyl Betaine, Sodium Laureth Sulfate, Decyl Glucoside, Avena Sativa (Oat) Kernel Flour, Glycol Stearate, Sodium Lauroampho PG Acetate Phosphate, Guar Hydroxypropyltrimonium Chloride, Hydroxypropyltrimonium Hydrolyzed Wheat protein, PEG 20 Glycerides, Hydroxypropyltrimonium Hydrolyzed Wheat Starch, PEG 150 Pentaerythrityl Tetrastearate, PEG 120 Methyl Glucose Trioleate, Propylene Glycol, Tetrasodium EDTA, PEG 6 Caprylic/Capric Glycerides, Quaternium 15, Coriandrum Sativum Extract, Elettaria Cardamomum Seed Extract, Conmiphora Myhrrha Extract, SD Alcohol 39C, May Contain:, Sodium Hydroxide, Citric Acid	**Adults:** Apply prn.
Carmol-10 Lotion	Urea 10%, Carbomer 940, Cetyl Alcohol, Isopropyl Palmitate, PEG 8 Doleate, PEG 8 Distearate, Propylene Glycol, Propylene Glycol Dipelargonate, Sodium Laureth Sulfate, Stearic Acid, Trolamine, Xanthan Gum	**Adults & Peds:** Apply qd-bid.
Carmol-20 Cream	Urea 20%, Water, Isopropyl Myristate, Isopropyl Palmitate, Stearic Acid, Propylene Glycol, Trolamine, Sodium Laureth, Carbomer, Xanthan Gum, Fragrance	**Adults & Peds:** Apply qd-bid.

(Continued)

BRAND	INGREDIENTS	DOSE
Cetaphil Daily Facial Moisturizer SPF 15 with Parsol 1789	Avobenzone 3%, Octocrylene 10%, Water, Diisopropyl Adipate, Cyclomethicone, Glyceryl Stearate, PEG-100 Stearate, Glycerin, Polymethyl Methacrylate, Phenoxyethanol, Benzyl Alcohol, Acrylates/C10-30 Alkyl Acrylate Crosspolymer, Tocopheryl Acetate, Carbomer 940, Disodium EDTA, Triethanolamine	**Adults & Peds:** Apply prn.
Cetaphil Daily Advance Ultra Hydrating Lotion	Water, Glycerin, Hydrogenated Polyisobutene, Cetearyl Alcohol, Macadamia Integrifolia Seed Oil (Macadamia Nut Oil), Butyrospermum Parkii (Shea Butter), Acrylates/C10-30 Alkyl acrylate Crosspolymer, Sodium Polyacrylate, Phenoxyethanol, Tocopheryl Acetate, Ceteareth-20, Stearoxytrimethylsilane, Stearyl Alcohol, Benzyl Alcohol, Farnesol, Sodium PCA, Panthenol, Cyclopentasiloxane, Dimethiconol, Citric Acid, Sodium Hydroxide	**Adults & Peds:** Apply prn.
Cetaphil UVA/UVB Defense SPF 50	Octinoxate/Octocrylene/Oxybenzone/Titanium Dioxide (7.5%-5%-7%-6%-5.7%), Water, Propylene Glycol, Glycerin, Dimethicone, VP/Eicosene Copolymer, Cyclohexasiloxane, Stearic Acid, Potassium Cetyl Phosphate, Glyceryl Stearate, PEG-100 Stearate, Aluminum Hydroxide, Dimethiconol, Disodium EDTA, Tocopherol, Cyclopentasiloxane, Triethanolamine, Phenoxyethanol, Ethylparaben, Chlorphenesin, Cetyl Alcohol, Acrylates/C10-30 Alkyl Acrylate Crosspolymer, Methylparaben, Xanthan Gum	**Adults & Peds:** Apply prn.
Cetaphil Moisturizing Cream	Water, Petrolatum, Glyceryl Polymethacrylate, Dicaprylyl Ether, Glycerin, Dimethicone, Glyceryl Stearate, Cetyl Alcohol, Prunus Amygdalus Dulcis (Sweet Almond) Oil, PEG-30 Glyceryl Stearate, Tocopheryl Acetate, Benzyl Alcohol, Phenoxyethanol, Sodium Hydroxide, Acrylates/C10-30 Alkyl Acrylate Crosspolymer, Dimethiconol, Disodium EDTA, Propylene Glycol	**Adults & Peds:** Apply prn.
Cetaphil Moisturizing Lotion	Water, Glycerin, Hydrogenated Polyisobutene, Cetearyl Alcohol, Ceteareth-20, Macadamia Nut Oil, Dimethicone, Tocopheryl Acetate, Stearoxytrimethylsilane, Stearyl Alcohol, Panthenol, Farnesol, Benzyl Alcohol, Phenoxyethanol, Acrylates/C10-30Alkyl Acrylate Crosspolymer, Sodium Hydroxide, Citric Acid	**Adults & Peds:** Apply prn.
Cetaphil Therapeutic Hand Cream	Water, Glycerin, Cetearyl Alcohol, Oleth-2, PEG-2 Stearate, ButyrospermumParkii, Ethylhexyl Methoxycinnamate, Dimethicone, Stearyl Alcohol, Glyceryl Stearate, PEG-100 Stearate, Methylparaben,Tocopherol, Arginine PCA, Chlorhexidine Digluconate	**Adults & Peds:** Apply prn.
Corn Huskers Lotion	Water, Glycerin, SD Alcohol 40, Sodium Calcium Alginate, Oleyl Sarcosin, Methylparaben, Guar Gum, Triethanolamine, Calcium Sulfate, Calcium Chloride, Fumaric Acid, Boric Acid, Fragrance	**Adults & Peds:** Apply prn.
Curel Continuous Comfort Original Formula	Water, Glycerin, Distearyldimonium Chloride, Petrolatum, Isopropyl Palmitate, Cetyl Alcohol, Butyrospermum Park II (Shea Butter), Acacia Senegal Gum, Dimethicone, Fragrance, Sodium Chloride, Gelatin, Methylparaben, Propylparaben	**Adults:** Apply to skin prn.
Curel Continuous Comfort Fragrance Free	Water, Glycerin, Distearyldimonium Chloride, Petrolatum, Isopropyl Palmitate, Cetyl Alcohol, Acacia Senegal Gum, Dimethicone, Sodium Chloride, Gelatin, Methylparaben, Propylparaben	**Adults:** Apply to skin prn.
Curel Natural Healing Soothing Lotion	Water, Glycerin, Distearyldimonium Chloride, Petrolatum, Isoproptyl Palmitate, Cetyl Alcohol, Lavandula Angustifolia (Lavender) Flower Extract, Anthemis Nobilis (Chamomile) Flower Extract, Avena Sativa (Oat) Meal Extract, Propylene Glycol, Pentylene Glycol, Dimethicone, Fragrance, Sodium Chloride, Methylparaben, Propylparaben, Caramel	**Adults:** Apply to skin prn.
Curel Natural Healing Nourishing Lotion	Water, Glycerin, Distearyldimonium Chloride, Petrolatum, Isoproptyl Palmitate, Cetyl Alcohol, Butyrospermum Parkii (Shea Butter), Vanilla Planifolia Fruit Extract, Honey (Mel), Propylene Glycol, Butylene Glycol, Dipropylene Glycol, Dimethicone, Fragrance, Sodium Chloride, Methylparaben, Propylparaben, Caramel	**Adults:** Apply to skin prn.

(Continued)

BRAND	INGREDIENTS	DOSE
Curel Natural Healing Revitalizing Lotion	Water, Glycerin, Distearyldimonium Chloride, Petrolatum, Isopropryl Palmitate, Cetyl Alcohol, Camellia Sinensis (Green Tea) Leaf Extract, Aloe Barbadensis Leaf Extract, Cucumis Sativus (Cucumber) Fruit Extract, Propylene Glycol, Dimethicone, Fragrance, Sodium Chloride, Methylparaben, Propylparaben, Caramel	**Adults:** Apply to skin prn.
Curel Ultra Healing Intensive Moisture Lotion	Water, Glycerin, Petrolatum, Cetearyl Alcohol, Benhentrimonium Chloride, Cetyl-PG Hydroxyethyl Palmitamide, Isopropyl Palmitate, Butyrospermum Park II (Shea Butter), Avena Sativa (Oat) Meal Extract, Eucalyptus Globulus Leaf Extract, Citrus Aurantium Dulcis (orange) Peel Oil, Cyclopentasiloxane, Dimethicone, Acacia Senegal Gum, Gelatin, DMDM Hydantoin	**Adults:** Apply to skin prn.
Eucerin Creme Original	Water, Petrolatum, Mineral Oil, Ceresin, Lanolin Alcohol Methylchloroisothiazolinone, Methylisothiazolinone	**Adults & Peds:** Apply prn.
Eucerin Dry Skin Therapy Calming Cream	Water, Glycerin, Cetyl Palmitate, Mineral Oil, Caprylic/Capric Triglyceride, Octyldodecanol, Cetyl Alcohol, Glycerly Stearate,Colloidal Oatmeal, Dimethicone, PEG-40 Stearate, Phenoxyethanol, DMDM Hydantoin, Iodopropynyl Butylcarbamate	**Adults & Peds >2 yrs:** Apply prn.
Eucerin Plus Intensive Repair Lotion	Water, Mineral Oil, PEG-7 Hydrogenated Castor Oil, Isohexadecane, Sodium Lactate, Urea, Glycerin, Isopropyl Palmitate, Panthenol, Microcrystalline Wax, Magnesium Sulfate, Lanolin Alcohol, Bisabolol, Methylchloroisothiazolinone, Methylisothiazolinone	**Adults:** Apply prn.
Eucerin Sensitive Facial Skin Gentle Hydrating Cleanser	Water, Sodium Laureth Sulfate, Cocamidopropyl Betaine, Disodium Cocamphodiacetate, Glycol Distearate, PEG 7 Glyceryl Cocoate, PEG 5 Lanolate, Cocamide MEA, Laureth 10, Citric Acid, PEG 120 Methyl Glucose Dioleate, Lanolin Alcohol, Imidazolidinyl Urea	**Adults:** Use qd.
Eucerin Plus Intensive Repair Hand Creme	Water, Glycerin, Urea, Glyceryl Stearate, Stearyl Alcohol, Dicaprylyl Ether, Sodium Lactate, Dimethicone, PEG-40 Stearate, Cyclopentasiloxane, Cyclohexasiloxane, Auminum Starch Octenylsuccinate, Lactic Acid, Xanthan Gum, Phenoxyethanol, Methylparaben, Propylparaben	**Adults & Peds:** Apply qd.
Eucerin Lotion Daily Replenishing	Water, Sunflower Seed Oil, Petrolatum, Glycerin, Glyceryl Stearate SE, Octyldodecanol, Caprylic/Capric Triglyceride, Stearic Acid, Dimethicone, Cetearyl Alcohol, Lanolin Alcohol, Panthenol, Tocopheryl Acetate, Cholesterol, Carbomer, Disodium EDTA, Sodium Hydroxide, Phenoxyethanol, Methylparaben, Ethylparaben, Propylparaben, Butylparaben, Isobutylparaben, BHT	**Adults & Peds:** Apply qd.
Eucerin Lotion Original	Water, Mineral Oil, Isopropyl Myristate, PEG-40 Sorbitan Peroleate, Glyceryl Lanolate, Sorbitol, Propylene Glycol, Cetyl Palmitate, Magnesium Sulfate, Aluminum Stearate, Lanolin Alcohol, BHT, Methylchloroisothiazolinone, Methylisothiazolinone	**Adults & Peds:** Apply prn.
Eucerin Plus Smoothing Essentials	Water, Glycerin, Caprylic/Capric Triglyceride, Cetearyl Alcohol, Urea, Hydrogenated Coco Glycerides, Isopropyl Stearate, Octyldodecanol, Sodium Lactate, Dimethicone, Arginine HCl, Glyceryl Stearate SE, Myristyl Myristate, Carnitine, Chondrus Crispus (Carrageenan), Sodium Cetearyl Sulfate, Lactic Acid, Sodium Citrate, Citric Acid, Acrylates/C10 30 Alkyl Acrylate Crosspolymer, Phenoxyethanol, Methylparaben, Benzyl Alcohol, Propylparaben, Potassium Sorbate	**Adults:** Apply qd.
Eucerin Redness Relief Daily Perfecting Lotion SPF 15	Octinoxate, Octisalate, Titanium Dioxide, Water, Glycerine, Dimethicone, Polyglyceryl-3 Methylglucose Distearate, Butyrospermum Parkii (Shea Butter), Lauroyl Lysine, Squalane, Alcohol Denat., Sorbitan Stearate, Phenoxyethanol, Butylene Glycol, Magnesium Aluminum Silicate, Glycyrrhiza Inflata Root Extract, Xanthan Gum, Methylparaben, Propylparaben, Ethylparaben, Iodopropynyl Butylcarbamate, Trimethoxycaprylylsilane, Chromium Oxide Greens, Chromium Hydroxide Green, Ultramarines	**Adults & Peds:** Apply prn.

(Continued)

BRAND	INGREDIENTS	DOSE
Eucerin Redness Relief Soothing Cleanser	Water, Glycerin, Sodium Laureth Sulfate, Carbomer, Phenoxyethanol, PEG-40 Hydrogenated Castor Oil, Sodium Methyl Cocoyl Taurate, PEG-7 Glyceryl Cocoate, Decyl Glucoside, Glycyrrhiza Inflata Root Extract, Xanthan Gum, Sodium Hydroxide, Methylparaben, Butylparaben, Ethylparaben, Isobutylparaben, Propylparaben, Benzophenone-4	**Adults & Peds:** Use qam and qpm.
Eucerin Redness Relief Soothing Moisture Lotion SPF 15	Water, Glycerin, Dimethicone, Polyglyceryl 3 Methylglucose Distearate, Butyrospermum Parkii (Shea Butter), Squalane, Alcohol Denat., Dicaprylyl Carbonate, Sorbitan Stearate, Lauroyl Lysine, Glycyrrhiza Inflata Root Extract, Phenoxyethanol, 1, 2 Hexanediol, Magnesium Aluminum Silicate, Xanthan Gum, Trimethoxycaprylylsilane, Methylparaben, Propylparaben, Ethylparaben	**Adults & Peds:** Apply qm and qpm.
Eucerin Redness Relief Soothing Night Crème	Water, Glycerin, Panthenol, Caprylic/Capric Triglyceride, Dicaprylyl Carbonate, Octyldodecanol, C12-15 Alkyl Benzoate, Dimethicone, Squalane, Tapioca Starch, Cetearyl Alcohol, Glyceryl Stearate Citrate, Myristyl Myristate, Butylene Glycol, Benzyl Alcohol, Glycyrrhiza Inflata Root Extract, Carbomer, Phenoxyethanol, Ammonium Acryloydimethyltaurate/VP Copolymer, Sodium Hydroxide, Methylparaben, Propylparaben, Iodopropynyl Butylcarbamate	**Adults & Peds:** Apply qpm.
Gold Bond Ultimate Healing Lotion	Water, Glycerin, Dimethicone, Petrolatum, Jojoba Esters, Cetyl Alcohol, Aloe Barbadensis Leaf Juice, Stearyl Alcohol, Distearyldimonium Chloride, Cetearyl Alcohol, Steareth 21, Steareth 2, Propylene Glycol, Chamomilla Recutita Flower Extract (Matricaria), Polysorbate 60, Stearamidopropyl PG Dimonium Chloride Phosphate, Methyl Gluceth 20, Tocopheryl Acetate, Magnesium Ascorbyl Phosphate, Hydrolyzed Collagen, Hydrolyzed Elastin, Retinyl Palmitate, Hydrolyzed Jojoba Esters, Glyceryl Stearate, Dipotassium EDTA, Fragrance, Potassium Hydroxide, Diazolidinyl Urea, Methylparaben, Propylparaben	**Adults & Peds:** Apply prn.
Gold Bond Ultimate Healing Skin Therapy Powder	Corn Starch, Sodium Bicarbonate, Silica, Fragrance, Ascrobyl Palmitate, Aloe Barbadensis Leaf Extract, Lavandula Angustifolia Extract, Chamomilla Recutita Flower Extract, Rosmarinus Officinalis Leaf Extract, Acacia Farnesiana Extract, Tocopheryl Acetate, Retinyl Palmitate, Polyoxymethylene Urea, Isopropyl Myristate, Benzethonium Chloride	**Adults & Peds:** Apply prn.
Keri Moisture Therapy Advance Extra Dry Skin Lotion	Water; Glycerin, Stearic Acid, Hydrogenated Polyisobutene, Petrolatum, Cetyl Alcohol, Aloe Barbadensis Leaf Juice, Tocopheryl Acetate, Cyclopentasiloxane, Dimethicone Copolyol, Glyceryl Stearate, PEG-100 Stearate, Dimethicone, Carbomer, Methylparaben, PEG-5 Soya Sterol, Magnesium Aluminum Silicate, Propylparaben, Phenoxyethanol, Disodium EDTA, Diazolidinyl Urea, Sodium Hydroxide, Fragrance	**Adults & Peds:** Apply prn.
Keri Lotion, Sensitive Skin	Water, Glycerin, Stearic Acid, Hydrogenated Polyisobutene, Petrolatum, Cetyl Alcohol, Aloe Barbadensis Leaf Juice, Tocopheryl Acetate (Vitamin E Acetate), Cyclopenta Siloxane, Dimethicone Copolyol, Glyceryl Stearate, PEG 100 Stearate, Dimethicone, Carbomer, Methylparaben, PEG 5 Soy Sterol, Magnesium Aluminum Silicate, Propylparaben, Phenoxyethanol, Disodium EDTA, Diazolidinyl Urea, Sodium Hydroxide	**Adults:** Apply prn.
Keri Original Formula Lotion	Water, Mineral Oil, Glycerin, Glycerol Stearate, PEG-40 Stearate, PEG-4 Dilaurate, Laureth-4, Carbomer, Methylpapaben, Propylparaben, Fragrance, DMDM Hydantoin, Iodopropynyl Butylcarbamate, Aloe Barbadensis Leaf Juice, Helianthus Annuus (Sunflower) Seed Oil, Sodium Hydroxide, Disodium EDTA, Tocopheryl Acetate (Vitamin E Acetate)	**Adults & Peds:** Apply prn.
Keri Nourishing Shea Butter Lotion	Water, Mineral Oil, Glycerin, Butyrospermum Parkii, PEG-40 Stearate, Glyceryl Stearate, PEG-4 Dilaurate, Laureth 4, Aloe Barbadensis Leaf Juice, Helianthus Annuus Seed Oil, Tocopheryl Acetate, Carbomer, Methylparaben, Propylparaben, DMDM Hydantoin, Iodopropynyl Butylcarbamate, Sodium Hydroxide, Disodium EDTA, Fragrance	**Adults & Peds:** Apply prn.

(Continued)

BRAND	INGREDIENTS	DOSE
Keri Age Defy & Protect Lotion	Octinoxate/Oxybenzone (7.5%-2%), Water, Ammonium Lactate, Cetearyl Alcohol, Glycerin, Ceteth-20, Galactoarabinan, Propylene Glycol Myristyl Ether Acetate, C12-15 Alkyl Benzoate, Sodium Hydroxypropyl Starch Phosphate, Octyldodecyl Neopentanoate, Dimethicone, Neopentyl Glycol Diethylhexanoate, Neopentyl Glycol Diisostearate, Xanthan Gum, Disodium EDTA, DMDM Hydantoin, Iodopropynyl Butylcarbamate, Tocopheryl Acetate (Vitamin E Acetate), Fragrance	**Adults & Peds:** Apply prn.
Keri Long Lasting Hand Cream	Water, Cetearyl Alcohol and Polysorbate 60, Mineral Oil, Cetyl Alcohol, Caprylic/Capric Triglycerides, Propylene Glycol, Dimethicone, Methylparaben, Tocopheryl Acetate (Vitamin E Acetate), Propylparaben, Disodium EDTA	**Adults & Peds:** Apply prn.
Keri Overnight Deep Conditioning	Water, Butyrospermum Parkii (Shea Butter), Glycerin, Cetearyl Alcohol, Steareth-30, Ceteareth-10, Phenoxyethanol, Methylparaben, Ethylparaben, Butylparaben, Propylparaben, Dipentaerythrityl Tetrahydroxystearate/Tetraisostearate, Hydrogenated Polyisobutene, Cetyl Alcohol, Glycyrrhiza Glabra (Licorice) Root Extract, Butylene Glycol, Pyrus Malus (Apple) Fruit Extract, Dimethicone, Cyclopentasiloxane, Cyclohexasiloxane, Triethanolamine, Hydrogenated Castor Oil, Acrylates/C10-30 Alkyl Acrylate Crosspolymer, Disodium EDTA, Carbomer, Fragrance, Tocopheryl Acetate*, Caprylic/Capric Triglyceride, Hydrogenated Lecithin, Hydroxylated Lecithin, BHT, Lecithin, Ascorbyl Palmitate, Retinyl Palmitate, Helianthus Annuus (Sunflower) Seed Oil, Glyceryl Polymethacrylate, Propylene Glycol, Palmitoyl Oligopeptide, Panthenol, Niacinamide, Phytonadione	**Adults & Peds:** Apply prn.
Keri Renewal Milk Body Lotion	Water, Caprylic/Capric Triglyceride, Helianthus Annuus (Sunflower) Seed Oil, Glycerin, PEG-20 Methyl Glucose Sesquistearate, Methyl Glucose Sesquistearate, Sodium Pyruvate, Dimethicone, Beeswax, Phenoxythanol, Polyacrylamide, Tocopheryl Acetate, Borago Officinalis Extract, Lactic acid, Bifida Ferment Lysate, Methylparaben, C13-14 Isoparaffin, Carbomer, Sodium Hydroxide, Propylparaben, Propylene Glycol, Allantoin, Acrylates/ C10-30 Alkyl Acrylate Crosspolymer, Disodium EDTA, Laureth-7, Ethylparaben, Butylparaben, BHT, Asorbyl Palmitate, Glyceryl Stearate, Glyceryl Oleate, Citric Acid, Hydrolyzed Fibronectin, Glycosphingolipids, Phospholipids, Cholesterol, Whey Protein	**Adults & Peds:** Apply prn.
Keri Renewal Serum for Dry Skin	Water, Urea, Propylene Glycol, Cyclopentasiloxane, Cyclomethicone, Lactobionic Acid, Gluconolactone, PEG/PPG-18/18 Dimethicone, Arginine, Butylene Glycol, Glycerin, Ammonium Hydroxide, Dimethiconol, Chlorphenesin, Methylparaben	**Adults & Peds:** Apply prn.
Lac-Hydrin Five Lotion	Water, Lactic Acid, Ammonium Hydroxide, Glycerin, Petrolatum, Squalane, Steareth-2, POE-21-Stearyl Ether, Propylene Glycol Dioctanoate, Cetyl Alcohol, Dimethicone, Methylchloroisothiazoline, Methylisothiazolinone	**Adults & Peds:** Apply bid.
Lubriderm Advanced Therapy Hand Cream	Water, Glycerin, Distearyldimonium Chloride, Petrolatum, Isopropyl Palmitate, Cetyl Alcohol, Aluminum Starch Octenylsuccinate, Dimethicone, Avena Sativa (Oat) Kernel Flour, Benzyl Alcohol, Methylparaben, Sodium Chloride, Tocopheryl Acetate, Lecithin, and Retinyl Palmitate	**Adults & Peds:** Apply prn.
Lubriderm Advanced Therapy Moisturizing Lotion	Water, Mineral Oil, Glycerin, Cetyl Alcohol, Sorbitol, Caprylic/Capric Triglyceride, Cetearyl Alcohol, Stearic Acid, Dimethicone, Polysorbate 60, Tocopheryl Acetate, Panthenol, Phenoxyethanol, Lecithin, Carbomer, Sodium Hydroxide, Ceteareth-20, Diazolidinyl Urea, Sodium Citrate, Methylparaben, Titanium Dioxide, BHT, Sodium Pyruvate, Retinyl Palmitate, Propylparaben, Fragrance, Citric Acid, Ethylparaben, Tocopherol	**Adults & Peds:** Apply prn.

(Continued)

BRAND	INGREDIENTS	DOSE
Lubriderm Advanced Therapy Triple Smoothing Lotion	Water, Glycerin, Glycolic Acid, Cetyl Alcohol, Dimethicone, Stearyl Alcohol, Isopropyl Palmitate, Caprylic/Capric Triglyceride, Potassium Hydroxide, Ethylhexyl Palmitate, Glyceryl Stearate, PEG-100 Stearate, Cetearyl Alcohol, Petrolatum, Cyclopentasiloxane, Ceteareth-20, Urea, Cyclohexasiloxane, DMDM Hydantoin, Methylparaben, Disodium EDTA, Xantham Gum, Fragrance, Panthenol, Tocopheryl Acetate, Retinyl Palmitate	**Adults & Peds:** Apply prn.
Lubriderm Daily Moisture Fragrance Free Lotion	Water, Mineral Oil, Glycerin, Caprylic/Capric Triglyceride, Cetyl Alcohol, Phenoxyethanol, Panthenol, Cetearyl Alcohol, Stearic Acid, Dimethicone, Carbomer, Ceteareth-20, Sodium Hydroxide, Sodium Citrate, Methylparaben, Propylparaben, Citric Acid, Ethylparaben	**Adults & Peds:** Apply prn.
Lubriderm Daily Moisture Lotion	Water, Mineral Oil, Glycerin, Caprylic/Capric Triglyceride, Stearic Acid, Cetyl Alcohol, Phenoxyethanol, Panthenol, Cetearyl Alcohol, Dimethicone, Carbomer, Ceteareth-20, Sodium Hydroxide, Sodium Citrate, Methylparaben, Propylparaben, Fragrance, Citric Acid, Ethylparaben	**Adults & Peds:** Apply prn.
Lubriderm Sensitive Skin Therapy Moisturizing Lotion	Water, Butylene Glycol, Mineral Oil, Petrolatum, Glycerin, Cetyl Alcohol, Propylene Glycol Dicaprylate/Dicaprate, PEG-40 Stearate, C11-13 Isoparaffin, Glyceryl Stearate, Tri-PPG-3 Myristyl Ether Citrate, Emulsifying Wax, Dimethicone, DMDM Hydantoin, Methylparaben, Carbomer, Ethylparaben, Propylparaben, Titanium Dioxide, Disodium EDTA, Sodium Hydroxide, Butylparaben, Xanthan Gum	**Adults & Peds:** Apply prn.
Lubriderm Daily Moisturizer Lotion, SPF 15	Octyl Methoxycinnamate/Octyl Salicylate/Oxybenzone (7.5%-4%-3%), Purified Water, C 12-15 Alkyl Benzoate, Cetearyl Alcohol, Ceteareth-20, Cetyl Alcohol, Glyceryl Monostearate, Propylene Glycol, White Petrolatum, Diazolidinyl Urea, Trolamine, Edetate Disodium, Xanthan Gum, Acrylates/C 10-30 Alkyl Acrylate Crosspolymer, Vitamin E, Iodopropynyl Butylcarbamate, Fragrance, Carbomer	**Adults & Peds >6 mo:** Apply prn.
Lubriderm Intense Skin Repair Body Cream	Water, Glycerin, Petrolatum, Mineral Oil, Cetyl Alcohol, Dimethicone, Avena Sativa (Oat) Kernel Flour, Carbomer, Ceteareth-6, Methylparaben, Sodium Citrate, Sodium Hydroxide, Tetrasodium EDTA, Stearyl Alcohol, Citric Acid, Benzalkonium Chloride, Ethylparaben, Propylparaben, Hydrolyzed Milk Protein, Benzaldeyhyde, Butyrospermum Parkii (Shea Butter), Hydrolyzed Soy Protein, Glyceryl Stearate, C12-15 Alkyl Benzoate, Polysorbate 80, Glycine Soja (Soybean) Sterols	**Adults & Peds:** Apply prn.
Lubriderm Intense Skin Repair Body Lotion	Water, Glycerin, Ethylhexyl Isononanoate, Mineral Oil, Petrolatum, Cetyl Alcohol, Sorbitan Stearate, Hydrogenated Polydecene, Sodium Behenoyl Lactylate, Synthetic Wax, Trimethylpentanediol/Adipic Acid/Glycerin Crosspolymer, Butyrospermum Parkii (Shea Butter), Tri- PPG-3 Myristyl Ether Citrate, Propylene Glycol, Diazolidinyl Urea, Sorbityl Laurate, Glyceryl Stearate, Disodium EDTA, Triethanolamine, C12-15 Alkyl Benzoate, Fragrance, Polysorbate 80, Glycine Soja (Soybean) Sterols, Iodopropynyl Butylcarbamate	**Adults & Peds:** Apply prn.
Lubriderm Intense Skin Repair Calming Relief Body Lotion	Water, Glycerin, Disteraryldimonium Chloride, Petrolatum, Isopropyl Palmitate, Cetyl Alcohol, Dimethicone, Avena Sativa (Oat) Kernel Flour, Avena Sativa (Oat) Kernel Oil, Mineral Oil, Steareth-20, Methylparaben, Benzalkonium Chloride, Avena Sativa (Oat) Kernel Extract, Sodium Chloride, Panthenol, Butyrospermum Parkil (Shea Butter), Glyceryl Stearate C12-15 Alkyl Benzoate, Polysorbate 80, Glycine Soja (Soybean) Sterols, Titanium Dioxide	**Adults & Peds:** Apply prn.
Lubriderm Skin Therapy Moisturizing Lotion	Water, Butylene Glycol, Mineral Oil, Petrolatum, Glycerin, Cetyl Alcohol, Propylene Glycol Dicaprylate/Dicaprate, PEG-40 Stearate, C11-13 Isoparaffin, Glyceryl Stearate, Tri (PPG-3 Myristyl Ether) Citrate, Emulsifying Wax, Dimethicone, DMDM Hydantoin, Methylparaben, Carbomer, Ethylparaben, Propylparaben, Titanium Dioxide, Disodium EDTA, Sodium Hydroxide, Butylparaben, and Xanthan Gum	**Adults & Peds:** Apply prn.

(Continued)

BRAND	INGREDIENTS	DOSE
Lubriderm Skin Nourishing Moisturizing Lotion with Premium Oat Extract	Water, Glycerin, Caprylic/Capric Triglycerides, Glycerin, Glyceryl Stearate SE, Petrolatum, Camellia Oleifera Seed Oil, Castor Oil, Cocoa Butter, Cetyl Alcohol, Wax, Brassica Alba Seed Extract, Oat Kernel Extract, Cassia Angustifolia Seed Polysaccharide, Glyceryl Stearate, PEG 100 Stearate, Diazolidinyl Urea, Xanthan Gum Disodium EDTA, Fragrance, Iodopropynyl Butylcarbamate, and Soybean Oil	**Adults:** Apply prn.
Lubriderm Skin Nourishing Moisturizing Lotion with Shea and Cocoa Butters	Water, Glycerin, Cetyl Alcohol, Glyceryl Stearate SE, Petrolatum, Emulsifying Wax, Caprylic/Capric Triglyceride, Castor Oil, Octyldodecanol, Shea Butter, Cocoa Butter, Dimethicone, Tocopheryl Acetate, Diazolidinyl Urea, Xanthan Gum, Disodium EDTA, Fragrance, Iodopropynyl Butylcarbamate	**Adults:** Apply prn.
Lubriderm Skin Nourishing Moisturizing Lotion with Sea Kelp Extract	Water, Glycerin, Glyceryl Stearate SE, Cetyl Alcohol, Emulsifying Wax, Petrolatum, Caprylic/Capric Triglyceride, Castor Oil, Octyldodecanol, Dimethicone, Diazolidinyl Urea, Propylene Glycol, Xanthan Gum, Disodium EDTA, Fragrance, Giant Kelp Leaf Extract, Iodopropynyl Butylcarbamate	**Adults:** Apply prn.
Neutrogena Norwegian Formula Body Moisturizer	Water, Glycerin, Distearyldimonium Chloride, Petrolatum, Isopropyl Palmitate, Cetyl Alcohol, Dimethicone, Colloidal Oatmeal, Cetearyl Alcohol, Sodium Cetearyl Sulfate, Sodium Sulfate, Sodium Chloride, Benzyl Alcohol, Fragrance	**Adults & Peds:** Apply prn.
Neutrogena Norwegian Formula Hand Cream	Water Purified, Glycerin, Cetearyl Alcohol, Stearic Acid, Sodium Cetearyl Sulfate, Methylparaben, Propylparaben, Dilauryl Thiodipropionate, Sodium Sulfate, Fragrance	**Adults & Peds:** Apply prn.
Neutrogena Comforting Butter Body Cream	Water, Glycerin, Distearyldimonium Chloride, Petrolatum, Isopropyl Palmitate, Cetyl Alcohol, Dimethicone, Panthenol, Butyrospermum Parkii, Cocoa (Theobroma Cacao) Seed Butter, Mango (Mangifera Indica) Seed Butter, Benzyl Alcohol, BHT, Sodium Chloride, Yellow 5, Yellow 6, Fragrance	**Adults & Peds:** Apply prn.
Neutrogena Norwegian Formula Deep Moisture Cream	Water, Glycerin, Distearyldimonium Chloride, Petrolatum, Isopropyl Palmitate, Cetyl Alcohol, Dimethicone, Butyrospermum Parkii, Cocoa Seed Butter (Theobroma Cacao), Mango Seed Butter (Mangifera Indica), Benzyl Alcohol, BHT, Sodium Chloride, Yellow 5, Yellow 6, Fragrance	**Adults:** Apply qd.
Neutrogena Norwegian Formula Deep Moisture Hand Cream	Water, Glycerin, Distearyldimonium Chloride, Petrolatum, Isopropyl Palmitate, Cetyl Alcohol, Dimethicone, Panthenol, Butyrospermum Parkii, Cocoa Seed Butter (Theobroma Cacao), Mango Seed Butter (Mangifera Indica), Benzyl Alcohol, Phytantriol, BHT, Sodium Chloride, Yellow 5, Yellow 6, Fragrance	**Adults:** Apply prn.
Nivea Body Age Defying Moisturizer For Body	Water, Glycerin, Mineral Oil, Caprylic/Capric Triglycerides, Cetyl Alcohol, Dimethicone, Glyceryl Stearate, Cyclopentasiloxane, Cyclohexasiloxane, PEG-40 Stearate, Creatine, 1-Methylhydantoin-2-Imide, Ubiquinone, Fragrance, Carbomer, Sodium Hydroxide, Phenoxyethanol, Methylparaben, Propylparaben	**Adults:** Apply to damp skin prn.
Nivea Essentially Enriched Lotion	Water, Mineral Oil, C13-16 Isoparaffin, Glycerin, Isopropyl Palmitate, Petrolatum, PEG-40, Sorbitan Perisostearate, Polyglyceryl-3 Diisostearate, Prunus Amygdalus Dulcis (Sweet Almond) Oil, Tocopheryl Acetate, Taurine, Sea Salt, Magnesium Sulfate, Fragrance, Citric Acid, Sodium Citrate, Potassium Sorbate	Apply prn.
Nivea Body Original Moisture Daily Lotion, Dry Skin	Water, Mineral Oil, Glycerin, Isopropyl Palmitate, Glyceryl Stearate SE, Cetearyl Alcohol, Tocopheryl Acetate, Lanolin Alcohol, Isopropyl Myristate, Simethicone, Fragrance, Carbomer, Hydroxypropyl Methylcellulose, Sodium Hydroxide, Methylcellulose, Sodium Hydroxide, Methylchloroisothiazolinone, Methylisothiazolinone	**Adults:** Apply to damp skin prn.
Nivea Smooth Extra Dry Skin Body Oil	Mineral oil, Caprylic/Capric Triglycerides, Persea Gratissima Oil (Avocado), Fragrance	**Adults:** Apply to damp skin prn.

(Continued)

BRAND	INGREDIENTS	DOSE
Nivea Smooth Sensation Daily Lotion, Dry Skin	Water, Glycerin, Mineral Oil, Caprylic/Capric Triglycerides, Cetyl Alcohol, Dimethicone, Glyceryl Stearate, Cyclopentasiloxane, Cyclohexasiloxane, PEG-40 Stearate, Ginkgo Bilbo Leaf Extract, Tocopheryl Acetate, Butyrospermum Parkii (Shea Butter), Phenoxyethanol, Fragrance, Carbomer, Sodium Hydroxide, EDTA, Methylparaben, Propylparaben	**Adults:** Apply to damp skin prn.
Nivea Creme	Triple Purified Water, Mineral Oil, Petrolatum, Glycerin, Microcrystalline Wax, Lanolin Alcohol, Paraffin, Panthenol, Magnesium Sulfate, Decyl Oleate, Octyldodecanol, Aluminum Stearate, Methylchloroisothiazolinone, Methylisothiazolinone, Citric Acid, Magnesium Stearate, Fragrance	**Adults & Peds:** Apply prn.
Vaseline Intensive Care Cocoa Butter Deep Conditioning Lotion	Water, Petrolatum, Glycerin, Stearic Acid, Isopropyl Palmitate, Glycol Stearate, Dimethicone, Theobroma Cacao Seed Butter (Cocoa), Butyrospermum Parkii (Shea Butter), Helianthus Annuus Seed Oil or Glycine Soja Oil (Sunflower, Soybean), Glycine Soja Sterol (Soybean), Tocopheryl Acetate (Vitamin E Acetate), Retinyl Palmitate (Vitamin A Palmitate), Sodium Stearoyl-2-Lactylate, Collagen Amino Acids, Urea, Glyceryl Stearate, Cetyl Alcohol, Magnesium Aluminum Silicate, Carbomer, Lecithin, Mineral Water, Sodium PCA, Potassium Lactate, Lactic Acid, Fragrance, Stearamide AMP, Triethanolamine, Methylparaben, DMDM Hydantoin, Disodium EDTA, Caramel, Titanium Dioxide	**Adults & Peds:** Apply prn.
Vaseline Intensive Care Healthy Hand & Nail Lotion	Water, Potassium Lactate, Sodium Hydroxypropyl Starch Phosphate, Glycerin, Stearic Acid, Mineral Oil, Dimethicone, Lactic Acid, Glycol Stearate, PEG 100 Stearate, Keratin, Glycine Soja Sterol (Soybean), Lecithin, Tocopheryl Acetate (Vitamin E Acetate), Retinyl Palmitate (Vitamin A Palmitate), Healianthus Annuus Seed Oil (Sunflower), Sodium PCA, Sodium Stearoyl Lactate, Urea, Collagen Amino Acids, Ethylhexyl Methoxycinnamate, Petrolatum, Mineral Water, Cetyl Alcohol, Stearamide AMP, Cyclomethicone, Magnesium Aluminum Silicate, Glyceryl Stearate, Fragrance, XanthanGum,Corn Oil, BHT, Disodium EDTA, Methylparaben, DMDM Hydantoin	**Adults & Peds:** Apply prn.
Vaseline Intensive Care Aloe Cool & Fresh Moisturizing Lotion	Water, Glycerin, Stearic Acid, Glycol Stearate, Aloe Barbadensis Leaf Juice (Aloe Vera), Cucumis Sativus Extract (Cucumber), Helianthus Annuus Seed Oil (Sunflower), Glycine Soja Oil (Soybean), Glycine Soja Sterol (Soybean), Sodium Stearoyl-2 Lactylate, Tocopheryl Acetate (Vitamin E Acetate), Retinyl Palmitate (Vitamin A Palmitate), Sodium Acrylate/Acryloyldimethyl Taurate Copolymer, Dimethicone, Glyceryl Stearate, Cetyl Alcohol, Lecithin, Mineral Water, Sodium PCA, Potassium Lactate, Lactic Acid, Collagen Amino Acids, Urea, Fragrance, Triethanolamine, DMDM Hydantoin, Iodopropynyl Butylcarbamate, Disodium EDTA, Titanium Dioxide	**Adults & Peds:** Apply prn.
Vaseline Intensive Care Lotion Total Moisture	Water, Glycerin, Stearic Acid, Glycol Stearate, Petrolatum, Isopropyl Palmitate, Glycine Soja Sterol (Soybean), Helianthus Annuus Seed Oil (Sunflower), Glycine Soja Oil (Soybean), Avena Sativa Kernel Protein (Oat), Sodium Stearoyl-2 Lactylate, Tocopheryl Acetate (Vitamin E Acetate), Retinyl Palmitate (Vitamin A Palmitate), Panthenol (Provitamin B5), Carbomer, Lecithin, Keratin, Dimethicone, Glyceryl Stearate, Cetyl Alcohol, Sodium PCA, Potassium Lactate, Lactic Acid, Collagen Amino Acids, Mineral Water, Fragrance, Triethanolamine, Magnesium Aluminum Silicate, Urea, Methylparaben, DMDM Hydantoin, Iodopropynyl Butylcarbamate, Disodium EDTA, Titanium dioxide	**Adults & Peds:** Apply prn.
Vaseline Intensive Rescue Moisture Locking Lotion	Water, Glycerin, Petrolatum, Stearic Acid, Glycol Stearate, Dimethicone, Isopropyl Isostearate, Tapioca Starch, Cetyl Alcohol, Glyceryl Stearate, Magnesium Aluminum Silicate, Carbomer, Ethylene Brassylate, Triethanolamine, Disodium EDTA, Phenoxyethanol, Methylparaben, Propylparaben, Titanium Dioxide (CI 77891)	**Adults & Peds:** Apply prn.

(Continued)

BRAND	INGREDIENTS	DOSE
Vaseline Jelly	White Petrolatum	**Adults & Peds:** Apply prn.
Vaseline Intensive Rescue Clinical Therapy Lotion	Dimethicone (1.0%), Water, Glycerin, Isopropyl Palmitate, Distearlydimonium Chloride, Cetyl Alcohol, Mineral Oil, Steareth-21, Borago Officinalis Seed Oil, Glycine Soja (Soybean) Sterol, Petrolatum, Tocopheryl Acetate, Fragrance (Lightly Fragranced only), Stearic Acid, Lecithin, Tapioca Starch, Stearyl Stearate, Sodium Chloride, Linoleic Acid, Linolenic Acid, Ethylene Brassylate (Unfragranced only), Methylparaben, Propylparaben	**Adults & Peds:** Apply prn.
Vaseline Intensive Rescue Heal & Repair Balm	Water, Petrolatum, Glycerin, Cyclopentasiloxane, Caprylic/Capric Triglyceride, Isopropyl Palmitate, Stearic Acid, Glycol Stearate, Sodium Hydroxypropyl Starch Phosphate, Peg-100 Stearate, Cetyl Alcohol, Glyceryl Stearate, Ethylene Brassylate, Disodium EDTA, Potassium Hydroxide, Phenoxyethanol, Methylparaben, Propylparaben	**Adults & Peds:** Apply prn.
Vaseline Intensive Rescue Moisture Locking Body Butter	Water, Petrolatum, Glycerin, Dimethicone, Cyclopentasiloxane, Stearic Acid, Hydrogenated Polyisobutene, Ethylhexyl Cocoate, Hydrogenated Didecene, Glycol Stearate, Paraffin, Theobroma Cacao (Cocoa) Seed Butter, Butyrospermum Parkii (Shea Butter), Potato Starch Modified, PEG-90 Diisostearate, Dimethiconol, Disteareth-75 IPDI, Glyceryl Stearate, Sodium Acrylate/Sodium Acryloyldimethyl Taurate Copolymer, Microcrystalline Wax, Xanthan Gum, Triethanolamine, Polysorbate 80, Dimethicone Copolyol, Cetyl Alcohol, Isohexadecane, Phenoxyethanol, Disodium EDTA, Ethylene Brassylate, Methylparaben, Propylparaben	**Adults & Peds:** Apply prn.
Vaseline Intensive Rescue Healing Hand Cream	Water, Glycerin, Isopropyl Palmitate, Distearlydimonium Chloride, Cetyl Alcohol, Mineral Oil, Steareth-21, Dimethicone, Petrolatum, Tocopheryl Acetate (Vitamin E Acetate), Borago Officinalis Seed Oil, Tapioca Starch, Stearic Acid, Glycine Soja (Soybean) Sterol, Lecithin, Linoleic Acid, Stearyl Stearate, Sodium Chloride, DMDM Hydantoin, Ethylene Brassylate, Methylparaben, Propylparaben, Titanium Dioxide	**Adults & Peds:** Apply prn.

Psoriasis Products

BRAND	INGREDIENT/ STRENGTH	DOSE
COAL TAR		
Denorex Therapeutic Protection 2-in-1 shampoo	Coal Tar 2.5%	**Adults & Peds:** Use at least biw.
Denorex Therapeutic Protection shampoo	Coal Tar 2.5%	**Adults & Peds:** Use at least biw.
DHS Tar Shampoo	Coal Tar 0.5%	**Adults & Peds:** Use at least biw.
DHS Tar Gel Shampoo	Coal Tar 0.5%	**Adults & Peds:** Use at least biw.
Ionil-T Plus Shampoo	Coal Tar 2%	**Adults & Peds:** Use at least biw.
Ionil-T Shampoo	Coal Tar 1%	**Adults & Peds:** Use at least biw.
MG217 Medicated Tar Lotion	Coal Tar 1%	**Adults & Peds:** Apply to affected area qd-qid.
MG217 Ointment	Coal Tar 2%	**Adults & Peds:** Apply to affected area qd-qid.
MG217 Tar Shampoo	Coal Tar 3%	**Adults & Peds:** Use at least biw.
Neutrogena T/Gel Shampoo Extra Strength	Coal Tar 1%	**Adults & Peds:** Use at least biw.
Neutrogena T/Gel Shampoo Original Formula	Coal Tar 0.5%	**Adults & Peds:** Use at least biw.
Neutrogena T/Gel Stubborn Itch Shampoo	Coal Tar 0.5%	**Adults & Peds:** Use at least biw.
Psoriasin Gel	Coal Tar 1.25%	**Adults & Peds:** Apply to affected area qd-qid.
Psoriasin Liquid	Coal Tar 0.66%	**Adults & Peds:** Apply to affected area qd-qid.
Psoriasin Ointment	Coal Tar 2%	**Adults & Peds:** Apply to affected area qd-qid.
Reme-T Gel	Coal Tar 5%	**Adults & Peds:** Use at least biw.
CORTICOSTEROID		
Aveeno Hydrocortisone 1% Anti-Itch Cream	Hydrocortisone 1%	**Adults & Peds ≥2 yrs:** Apply to affected area tid-qid.
Cortaid Advanced 12-Hour Anti-Itch Cream	Hydrocortisone 1%	**Adults & Peds ≥2 yrs:** Apply to affected area tid-qid.
Cortaid Intensive Therapy Cooling Spray	Hydrocortisone 1%	**Adults & Peds ≥2 yrs:** Apply to affected area tid-qid.
Cortaid Intensive Therapy Moisturizing Cream	Hydrocortisone 1%	**Adults & Peds ≥2 yrs:** Apply to affected area tid-qid.
Cortaid Maximum Strength Cream	Hydrocortisone 1%	**Adults & Peds ≥2 yrs:** Apply to affected area tid-qid.
Cortaid Maximum Strength Ointment	Hydrocortisone 1%	**Adults & Peds ≥2 yrs:** Apply to affected area tid-qid.
Cortizone-10 Cream	Hydrocortisone 1%	**Adults & Peds ≥2 yrs:** Apply to affected area tid-qid.
Cortizone-10 Cream Plus	Hydrocortisone 1%	**Adults & Peds ≥2 yrs:** Apply to affected area tid-qid.
Cortizone-10 Ointment	Hydrocortisone 1%	**Adults & Peds ≥2 yrs:** Apply to affected area tid-qid.
Cortizone-10 Plus Intensive Healing Formula	Hydrocortisone 1%	**Adults & Peds ≥2 yrs:** Apply to affected area tid-qid.
Cortizone-10 Easy Relief Applicator	Hydrocortisone 1%	**Adults & Peds ≥2 yrs:** Apply to affected area tid-qid.
Cortizone-10 Cooling Relief Gel	Hydrocortisone 1%	**Adults & Peds ≥2 yrs:** Apply to affected area tid-qid.
SALICYLIC ACID		
Dermarest Psoriasis Overnight Treatment	Salicylic Acid 3%	**Adults & Peds:** Apply to affected area qhs. **Max:** qid.
Dermarest Psoriasis Medicated Moisturizer	Salicylic Acid 2%	**Adults & Peds:** Apply to affected area qd-qid.
Dermarest Psoriasis Medicated Scalp Treatment	Salicylic Acid 3%	**Adults & Peds:** Apply to affected area qd-qid.
Dermarest Psoriasis Medicated Shampoo/Conditioner	Salicylic Acid 3%	**Adults & Peds:** Apply to affected area at least biw.
Dermarest Psoriasis Skin Treatment	Salicylic Acid 3%	**Adults & Peds:** Apply to affected area qd-qid.
Neutrogena T/Gel Conditioner	Salicylic Acid 2%	**Adults & Peds:** Use at least biw.
Neutrogena T/Sal Shampoo	Salicylic Acid 3%	**Adults & Peds:** Use at least tiw.
Psoriasin Therapeutic Shampoo and Body Wash	Salicylic Acid 3%	**Adults & Peds:** Use biw.

WOUND CARE PRODUCTS

BRAND	INGREDIENT/STRENGTH	DOSE
NEOMYCIN/POLYMYXIN B/BACITRACIN COMBINATIONS		
Bacitracin Ointment	Bacitracin 500 U	**Adults & Peds:** Apply to affected area qd-tid.
Bactine Pain Relieving Protective Antibiotic	Neomycin/polymyxin B/bacitracin/pramoxine 3.5mg-10,000 U- 500 U- 1%	**Adults & Peds:** Apply to affected area qd-tid.
Neosporin Ointment	Neomycin/polymyxin B/bacitracin 3.5mg-5,000 U-400 U	**Adults & Peds:** Apply to affected area qd-tid.
Neosporin Plus Pain Relief Cream	Neomycin/polymyxin B/pramoxine 3.5mg-10,000 U-10mg	**Adults & Peds:** Apply to affected area qd-tid.
Neosporin Plus Pain Relief Ointment	Neomycin/polymyxin B/bacitracin/pramoxine 3.5mg-10,000 U-500 U-10mg	**Adults & Peds:** Apply to affected area qd-tid.
Neosporin To Go Ointment	Neomycin/polymyxin B/bacitracin 3.5mg-5,000 U-400 U	**Adults & Peds:** Apply to affected area qd-tid.
Polysporin Ointment	Polymyxin B/bacitracin 10,000 U-500 U	**Adults & Peds:** Apply to affected area qd-tid.
Polysporin First Aid Antibiotic Powder	Polymyxin B/bacitracin 10,000 U-500 U	**Adults & Peds:** Apply to affected area qd-tid.
BENZALKONIUM CHLORIDE COMBINATIONS		
Bactine First Aid Liquid	Lidocaine HCl/benzalkonium chloride 2.5%-0.13%	**Adults & Peds ≥2 yrs:** Apply to affected area qd-tid.
Bactine Pain Relieving Cleansing Spray	Lidocaine HCl/benzalkonium chloride 2.5%-0.13%	**Adults & Peds ≥2 yrs:** Apply to affected area qd-tid.
Neosporin Neo To Go	Benzalkonium Cl/pramoxine HCl 0.13%-1%	**Adults & Peds ≥2 yrs:** Apply to affected area qd-tid.
BENZETHONIUM CHLORIDE COMBINATIONS		
Gold Bond First Aid Quick Spray	Menthol/benzethonium chloride 1%-0.13%	**Adults & Peds ≥2 yrs:** Apply to affected area tid-qid.
Lanacane Maximum Strength Cream Anti-Itch	Benzocaine/benzethonium chloride 20%-0.2%	**Adults & Peds ≥2 yrs:** Apply to affected area tid-qid.
Lanacane Anti-Itch Crème Medication	Benzocaine/benzethonium chloride 6%-0.2%	**Adults & Peds ≥2 yrs:** Apply to affected area qd-tid.
Lanacane Maximum Strength First Aid Spray	Benzocaine/benzethonium chloride 20%-0.2%	**Adults & Peds ≥2 yrs:** Apply to affected area qd-tid.
CHLORHEXIDINE GLUCONATE		
Hibiclens	Chlorhexidine gluconate 4%	**Adults & Peds:** Apply sparingly to affected area prn.
Hibistat Hand Antiseptic	Chlorhexidine gluconate/isopropyl alcohol 0.5%-70%	**Adults:** Wipe until dry.
IODINE		
Betadine Skin Cleanser	Povidone-iodine 7.5%	**Adults & Peds:** Apply to affected area. Wash vigorously for 15 seconds and rinse.
Betadine Solution	Povidone-iodine 10%	**Adults & Peds:** Apply to affected area qd-tid.
MISCELLANEOUS		
Aquaphor Healing Ointment	Petrolatum, mineral oil, ceresin, lanolin	**Adults & Peds:** Apply to affected area prn.
Proxacol Hydrogen Peroxide	Hydrogen peroxide 3%	**Adults:** Apply to affected area qd-tid.
Wound Wash Sterile Saline Spray	Sterile sodium chloride solution 0.9%	**Adults & Peds:** Apply to affected area prn.

ANTACID AND HEARTBURN PRODUCTS

BRAND	INGREDIENT/STRENGTH	DOSE
ANTACID		
Alka-Seltzer Gold Tablets	Citric Acid/Potassium Bicarbonate/ Sodium Bicarbonate 1000mg-344mg-1050mg	**Adults ≥60 yrs:** 2 tabs q4h prn. **Max:** 6 tabs q24h. **Adults & Peds ≥12 yrs:** 2 tabs q4h prn. **Max:** 8 tabs q24h. **Peds ≤12 yrs:** 1 tab q4h prn. **Max:** 4 tabs q24h.
Alka-Seltzer Heartburn Relief Tablets	Citric Acid/Sodium Bicarbonate 1000mg-1940mg	**Adults ≥60 yrs:** 2 tabs q4h prn. **Max:** 4 tabs q24h. **Adults & Peds ≥12 yrs:** 2 tabs q4h prn. **Max:** 8 tabs q24h.
Alka-Seltzer Lemon Lime Tablets	Aspirin/Citric Acid/Sodium Bicarbonate 325mg-1000mg-1700mg	**Adults ≥60 yrs:** 2 tabs q4h prn. **Max:** 8 tabs/24h. **Adults & Peds ≥12 yrs:** 2 tabs q4h prn. **Max:** 8 tabs q24h.
Alka-Seltzer Tablets, Original	Aspirin/Citric Acid/Sodium Bicarbonate 325mg-1000mg-1916mg	**Adults ≥60 yrs:** 2 tabs q4h prn. **Max:** 4 tabs q24h. **Adults & Peds ≥12 yrs:** 2 tabs q4h prn. **Max:** 8 tabs q24h.
Alka-Seltzer Tablets, Extra-Strength	Aspirin/Citric Acid/Sodium Bicarbonate 500mg-1000mg-1985mg	**Adults ≥60 yrs:** 2 tabs q6h prn. **Max:** 3 tabs q24h. **Adults & Peds ≥12 yrs:** 2 tabs q6h prn. **Max:** 7 tabs q24h.
Brioschi Powder	Sodium Bicarbonate/Tartaric Acid 2.69g-2.43g/dose	**Adults & Peds ≥12 yrs:** 1-2 capfuls (6g) dissolved in 4-6 oz water q1h. **Max:** 6 doses q24h.
Gaviscon Extra Strength Liquid	Aluminum Hydroxide/Magnesium Carbonate 254mg-237.5mg/5mL	**Adults:** 2-4 tsp (10-20mL) qid.
Gaviscon Extra Strength Tablets	Aluminum Hydroxide/Magnesium Carbonate 160mg-105mg	**Adults:** 2-4 tabs qid. **Max:** 16 doses q24h.
Gaviscon Regular Strength Tablets	Aluminum Hydroxide/Magnesium Carbonate 80mg-14.2mg	**Adults:** 2-4 tabs qid. **Max:** 16 tabs q24h.
Gaviscon Regular Strength Liquid	Aluminum Hydroxide/Magnesium Carbonate 95mg-358mg/15mL	**Adults:** 1-2 tbl (15-30mL) qid.
Maalox Antacid Barrier Chewable Tablets	Calcium Carbonate 500mg	**Adults & Peds ≥12 yrs:** 2-4 tabs qid. **Max:** 16 tabs q24h.
Maalox Children's Relief Chewables	Calcium Carbonate 400mg	**Peds 2-5 yrs (24-47 lbs):** 1 tab prn. **Max:** 3 tabs. **Peds 6-11 yrs (48-95 lbs):** 2 tabs prn. **Max:** 6 tabs.
Maalox Regular Strength Chewable Tablets	Calcium Carbonate 600mg	**Adults:** 1-2 tabs prn. **Max:** 12 tabs q24h.
Mylanta, Children's	Calcium Carbonate 400 mg	**Peds 6-11 yrs (48-95 lbs):** Take 2 tab prn. **Max:** 6 tabs q24h. **Peds 2-5 yrs (24-47 lbs):** Take 1 tab prn **Max:** 3 tabs q24h.
Mylanta Ultimate Strength Liquid	Aluminum Hydroxide/Magnesium Hydroxide 500mg-500mg/5mL	**Adults & Peds ≥12 yrs:** 2-4 tsp (10-20mL) qid (between meals & hs). **Max:** 9 tsp (45mL) q24h for ≤2 weeks.
Mylanta Supreme Antacid Liquid	Calcium Carbonate/Magnesium Hydroxide 400mg-135mg/5mL	**Adults:** 2-4 tsp (10-20mL) qid. **Max:** 18 tsp (90mL) q24h.
Mylanta Ultimate Strength Chewable Tablets	Calcium Carbonate/Magnesium Hydroxide 700mg-300mg	**Adults:** 2-4 tabs qid. (between meals & hs). **Max:** 10 tabs q24h for ≤2 weeks.
Rolaids Extra Strength Softchews	Calcium Carbonate 1177mg	**Adults:** 2-3 chews q1h prn. **Max:** 6 chews q24h.
Rolaids Extra Strength Tablets	Calcium Carbonate/Magnesium Hydroxide 675mg-135mg	**Adults:** 2-4 tabs q1h prn. **Max:** 10 tabs q24h.
Rolaids Tablets	Calcium Carbonate/Magnesium Hydroxide 550mg-110mg	**Adults:** 2-4 tabs q1h prn. **Max:** 12 tabs q24h.

(Continued)

BRAND	INGREDIENT/STRENGTH	DOSE
ANTACID *(Continued)*		
Titralac Chewable Tablets	Calcium Carbonate 420mg	**Adults:** 2 tabs q2-3h prn. **Max:** 19 tabs q24h.
Tums Chewable Tablets	Calcium Carbonate 500mg	**Adults:** 2-4 tabs q1h prn. **Max:** 15 tabs q24h.
Tums E-X Chewable Tablets	Calcium Carbonate 750mg	**Adults:** 2-4 tabs prn. **Max:** 10 tabs q24h.
Tums E-X Sugar Free Chewable Tablets	Calcium Carbonate 750mg	**Adults:** 2-4 tabs prn. **Max:** 10 tabs q24h.
Tums Kids Chewable Tablets	Calcium Carbonate 750mg	**Peds >4 yrs (>49 lbs):** Take 1 tab tid. **Max:** 4 tabs q24h. **Peds 2-4 yrs (24-47 lbs):** Take ½ tab bid. **Max:** 2 tabs q24h.
Tums Smoothies Tablets	Calcium Carbonate 750mg	**Adults:** 2-4 tabs prn. **Max:** 10 tabs q24h.
Tums Ultra 1000 Chewable Tablets	Calcium Carbonate 1000mg	**Adults:** 2-4 tabs prn. **Max:** 7 tabs q24h for ≤2 weeks.
ANTACID/ANTIFLATULENT		
Gelusil Chewable Tablets	Aluminum Hydroxide/Magnesium Hydroxide/Simethicone 200mg-200mg-20mg	**Adults:** 2-4 tabs qid. **Max:** 12 tabs q24h.
Maalox Advanced Maximum Strength Liquid	Aluminum Hydroxide/Magnesium Hydroxide/Simethicone 400mg-400mg-40mg/5mL	**Adults & Peds ≥12 yrs:** 2-4 tsp (10-20mL) bid. **Max:** 12 tsp (60mL) q24h.
Maalox Advanced Maximum Strength Chewable Tablets	Calcium Carbonate/Simethicone 1000mg-60mg	**Adults:** 1-2 tabs prn. **Max:** 8 tabs q24h.
Maalox Junior Relief Chewables	Calcium Carbonate/Simethicone 400mg-24mg	**Peds 3–11 yrs:** 2 tabs prn. **Max:** 6 tabs q24h.
Maalox Advanced Regular Strength Liquid	Aluminum Hydroxide/Magnesium Hydroxide/Simethicone 200mg-200mg-20mg/5mL	**Adults & Peds ≥12 yrs:** 2-4 tsp (10-20mL) qid. **Max:** 12 tsp (60mL) q24h.
Mylanta Maximum Strength Liquid	Aluminum Hydroxide/Magnesium Hydroxide/Simethicone 400mg-400mg-40mg/5mL	**Adults & Peds ≥12 yrs:** 2-4 tsp (10-20mL) qid. **Max:** 12 tsp (60mL) q24h.
Mylanta Regular Strength Liquid	Aluminum Hydroxide/Magnesium Hydroxide/Simethicone 200mg-200mg-20mg/5mL	**Adults & Peds ≥12 yrs:** 2-4 tsp (10-20mL) qid. **Max:** 24 tsp (60mL) q24h.
Rolaids Multi-Symptom Chewable Tablets	Calcium Carbonate/Magnesium Hydroxide/Simethicone 675mg-135mg-60mg	**Adults:** 2-4 tabs q1h prn. **Max:** 8 tabs q24h.
Rolaids Extra Strength Plus Gas Soft Chews	Calcium Carbonate/Simethicone 1177mg-80mg	**Adults:** 2-3 chews q1h prn. **Max:** 6 chews q24h.
Titralac Plus Chewable Tablets	Calcium Carbonate/Simethicone 420mg-21mg	**Adults:** 2 tabs q2-3h prn. **Max:** 19 tabs q24h.
BISMUTH SUBSALICYLATE		
Maalox Total Relief Maximum Strength Liquid	Bismuth Subsalicylate 525mg/15mL	**Adults & Peds ≥12 yrs:** 2 tbl (30mL) q1/2-1h. **Max:** 8 tbl (120mL) q24h.
Pepto Bismol Chewable Tablets	Bismuth Subsalicylate 262mg	**Adults & Peds ≥12 yrs:** 2 tabs q1/2-1h. **Max:** 8 doses q24h.
Pepto Bismol Caplets	Bismuth Subsalicylate 262mg	**Adults & Peds ≥12 yrs:** 2 tabs q1/2-1h. **Max:** 8 doses q24h.
Pepto Bismol Liquid	Bismuth Subsalicylate 262mg/15mL	**Adults & Peds ≥12 yrs:** 2 tbl (30mL) q1/2-1h. **Max:** 8 doses (240mL) q24h.

(Continued)

BRAND	INGREDIENT/STRENGTH	DOSE
BISMUTH SUBSALICYLATE *(Continued)*		
Pepto Bismol Maximum Strength Liquid	Bismuth Subsalicylate 525mg/15mL	**Adults & Peds ≥12 yrs:** 2 tbl (30mL) q1h prn. **Max:** 4 doses (120mL) q24h.
H_2-RECEPTOR ANTAGONIST		
Pepcid AC Chewable Tablets	Famotidine 10mg	**Adults & Peds ≥12 yrs:** 1 tab qd. **Max:** 2 tabs q24h.
Pepcid AC Gelcaps	Famotidine 10mg	**Adults & Peds ≥12 yrs:** 1 cap qd. **Max:** 2 caps q24h.
Pepcid AC Maximum Strength EZ Chews	Famotidine 20mg	**Adults & Peds ≥12 yrs:** 1 tab qd. **Max:** 2 tabs q24h.
Pepcid AC Maximum Strength Tablets	Famotidine 20mg	**Adults & Peds ≥12 yrs:** 1 tab qd. **Max:** 2 tabs q24h.
Pepcid AC Tablets	Famotidine 10mg	**Adults & Peds ≥12 yrs:** 1 tab qd. **Max:** 2 tabs q24h.
Tagamet HB Tablets	Cimetidine 200mg	**Adults & Peds ≥12 yrs:** 1 tab qd. **Max:** 2 tabs q24h.
Zantac 150 Tablets	Ranitidine 150mg	**Adults & Peds ≥12 yrs:** 1 tab qd. **Max:** 2 tabs q24h.
Zantac 75 Tablets	Ranitidine 75mg	**Adults & Peds ≥12 yrs:** 1 tab qd. **Max:** 2 tabs q24h.
H_2-RECEPTOR ANTAGONIST/ANTACID		
Pepcid Complete Chewable Tablets	Famotidine/Calcium Carbonate/ Magnesium Hydroxide 10mg-800mg-165mg	**Adults & Peds ≥12 yrs:** 1 tab qd. **Max:** 2 tabs q24h.
PROTON PUMP INHIBITOR		
Prilosec OTC Tablets	Omeprazole 20mg	**Adults:** 1 tab qd x 14 days. May repeat 14 day course q 4 months.

ANTIDIARRHEAL PRODUCTS

BRAND	INGREDIENT/STRENGTH	DOSE
ABSORBENT AGENTS		
Equalactin Chewable Tablets	Calcium Polycarbophil 625mg	**Adults & Peds ≥12 yrs:** 2 tabs/dose. **Max:** 8 tabs q24h. **Peds 6-12 yrs:** 1 tab/dose. **Max:** 4 tabs q24h. **2 to ≤6 yrs:** 1 tab/dose. **Max:** 2 tabs q24h.
Fibercon Caplets	Calcium Polycarbophil 625mg	**Adults & Peds ≥12 yrs:** 2 tabs qd. **Max:** 8 tabs q24h.
Konsyl Fiber Caplets	Calcium Polycarbophil 625mg	**Adults & Peds ≥12 yrs:** 2 caps qd-qid. **Peds 6-12 yrs:** 1 cap qd-tid. **Max:** 8 caps q24h.
ANTIPERISTALTIC AGENTS		
Imodium A-D Caplets	Loperamide HCl 2mg	**Adults & Peds ≥12 yrs:** 2 caplets after first loose stool; 1 caplet after each subsequent loose stool. **Max:** 4 caplets q24h. **Peds 9-11 yrs (60-95 lbs):** 1 caplet after first loose stool; ½ caplet after each subsequent loose stool. **Max:** 3 caplets q24h. **6-8 yrs (48-59 lbs):** 1 caplet after first loose stool; ½ caplet after each subsequent loose stool. **Max:** 2 caplets q24h.
Imodium A-D E-Z Chews	Loperamide HCl 2mg	**Adults & Peds ≥12 yrs:** 2 caplets after first loose stool; 1 caplet after each subsequent loose stool. **Max:** 4 caplets q24h. **Peds 9-11 yrs (60-95 lbs):** 1 caplet after first loose stool; ½ caplet after each subsequent loose stool. **Max:** 3 caplets q24h. **6-8 yrs (48-59 lbs):** 1 caplet after first loose stool; 1/2 caplet after each subsequent loose stool. **Max:** 2 caplets q24h.
Imodium A-D Liquid	Loperamide HCl 1mg/7.5mL	**Adults & Peds ≥12 yrs:** 4 tsp (20mL) after first loose stool; 2 tsp (10mL) after each subsequent loose stool. **Max:** 8 tsp (4mL) q24h. **Peds 9-11 yrs (60-95 lbs):** 2 tsp (10mL) after the first loose stool; 1 tsp (5mL) after each subsequent loose stool. **Max:** 6 tsp (30mL) q24h. **Peds 6-8 yrs (48-59 lbs):** 2 tsp (10mL) after the first loose stool; 1 tsp (5mL) after each subsequent loose stool. **Max:** 4 tsp (20mL) q24h.
Imodium A-D Liquid For Use In Children (Mint Flavor)	Loperamide HCl 1mg/7.5mL	**Adults & Peds ≥12 yrs:** 6 tsp (30mL) after first loose stool; 3 tsp (15mL) after each subsequent loose stool. **Max:** 12 tsp (60mL) q24h. **Peds 9-11 yrs (60-95 lbs):** 3 tsp (15mL) after the first loose stool; 1½ tsp (7.5mL) after each subsequent loose stool. **Max:** 9 tsp (45mL) q24h. **Peds 6-8 yrs (48-59 lbs):** 3 tsp (15mL) after first loose stool; 1½ tsp (7.5mL) after each subsequent loose stool. **Max:** 6 tsp (30mL) q24h.

(Continued)

BRAND	INGREDIENT/STRENGTH	DOSE
ANTIPERISTALTIC/ANTIFLATULENT AGENTS		
Imodium Multi-Symptom Relief Caplets	Loperamide HCl/Simethicone 2mg-125mg	**Adults & Peds ≥12 yrs:** 2 caplets after first loose stool; 1 caplet after each subsequent loose stool. **Max:** 4 caplets q24h. **Peds 9-11 yrs (60-95 lbs):** 1 caplet after first loose stool; ½ caplet after each subsequent loose stool. **Max:** 2 caplets q24h. **6-8 yrs (48-59 lbs):** 1 caplet after first loose stool; ½ caplet after each subsequent loose stool. **Max:** 2 caplets q24h.
Imodium Multi-Symptom Relief Chewable Tablets	Loperamide HCl/Simethicone 2mg-125mg	**Adults & Peds ≥12 yrs:** 2 tabs with 4-8 oz water after first loose stool; 1 tab with 4-8 oz water after each subsequent loose stool. **Max:** 4 tabs q24h. **Peds 9-11 yrs (60-95 lbs):** 1 tab with 4-8 oz water after first loose stool; ½ tab after each subsequent loose stool. **Max:** 2 tabs q24h. **6-8 yrs (48-59 lbs):** 1 tab with 4-8 oz water after first loose stool; ½ tab with 4-8 oz water after each subsequent loose stool. **Max:** 2 tabs q24h.
BISMUTH SUBSALICYLATE		
Kaopectate Caplets	Bismuth Subsalicylate 262mg	**Adults & Peds ≥12 yrs:** 2 caplets q½-1h prn. **Max:** 8 doses q24h.
Kaopectate Extra Strength Liquid	Bismuth Subsalicylate 525mg/15mL	**Adults & Peds ≥12 yrs:** 2 tbl (30mL) q1h prn. **Max:** 4 doses (8 tbl) q24h.
Kaopectate Liquid	Bismuth Subsalicylate 262mg/15mL	**Adults & Peds ≥12 yrs:** 2 tbl (30mL) q½-1h prn. **Max:** 8 doses (16 tbl) q24h.
Maalox Total Relief Liquid	Bismuth Subsalicylate 525mg/15mL	**Adults & Peds ≥12 yrs:** 2 tbl (30mL) q1h prn. **Max:** 4 doses (8 tbl) q24h.
Pepto Bismol Caplets	Bismuth Subsalicylate 262mg	**Adults & Peds ≥12 yrs:** 2 caplets q½-1h. **Max:** 8 doses (16 caplets) q24h.
Pepto Bismol Chewable Tablets	Bismuth Subsalicylate 262mg	**Adults & Peds ≥12 yrs:** 2 tabs q½-1h. **Max:** 8 doses (16 tabs) q24h.
Pepto Bismol Liquid	Bismuth Subsalicylate 262mg/15mL	**Adults & Peds ≥12 yrs:** 2 tbl (30mL) q½-1h prn. **Max:** 8 doses (16 tbl) q24h.
Pepto Bismol Liquid Max	Bismuth Subsalicylate 525mg/15mL	**Adults & Peds ≥12 yrs:** 2 tbl (30mL) q1h prn. **Max:** 4 doses (8 tbl) q24h.

ANTIFLATULANT PRODUCTS

BRAND	INGREDIENT/STRENGTH	DOSE
ALPHA-GALACTOSIDASE		
Beano Food Enzyme Dietary Supplement Drops	Alpha-Galactosidase Enzyme 150 GalU	**Adults:** Add 5 drops to first bite of food serving.
Beano Food Enzyme Dietary Supplement Tablets	Alpha-Galactosidase Enzyme 150 GalU	**Adults:** Take 3 tabs before meals.
ANTACID/ANTIFLATULANT		
Gas-X Extra Strength with Maalox Chewable Tablets	Calcium Carbonate/Simethicone 500mg-125mg	**Adults:** 1-2 tabs prn. **Max:** 4 tabs q24h.
Gelusil Chewable Tablets	Aluminum Hydroxide/Magnesium Hydroxide/Simethicone 200mg-200mg-20mg	**Adults:** 2-4 tabs qid.
Maalox Max Liquid	Aluminum Hydroxide/Magnesium Hydroxide/Simethicone 400mg-400mg-40mg/5mL	**Adults & Peds ≥12 yrs:** 2-4 tsp (10-20mL) qid. **Max:** 8 tsp (60mL) q24h.
Maalox Max Chewable Tablets	Calcium Carbonate/Simethicone 1000mg-60mg	**Adults:** 1-2 tabs prn. **Max:** 8 tabs q24h.
Maalox Regular Strength Liquid	Aluminum Hydroxide/Magnesium Hydroxide/Simethicone 200mg-200mg-20mg/5mL	**Adults & Peds ≥12 yrs:** 2-4 tsp (10-20mL) qid. **Max:** 16 tsp (60mL) q24h.
Mylanta Maximum Strength Liquid	Aluminum Hydroxide/Magnesium Hydroxide/Simethicone 400mg-400mg-40mg/5mL	**Adults & Peds ≥12 yrs:** 2-4 tsp (10-20mL) qid. **Max:** 12 tsp (60mL) q24h.
Mylanta Regular Strength Liquid	Aluminum Hydroxide/Magnesium Hydroxide/Simethicone 200mg-200mg-20mg/5mL	**Adults & Peds ≥12 yrs:** 2-4 tsp (10-20mL) qid. **Max:** 24 tsp (120mL) q24h.
Rolaids Antacid & Antigas Soft Chews	Calcium Carbonate/Simethicone 1177mg-80mg	**Adults:** 2-3 chews hourly prn.
Titralac Plus Chewable Tablets	Calcium Carbonate/Simethicone 420mg-21mg	**Adults:** 2 tabs q2-3h prn. **Max:** 19 tabs q24h.
SIMETHICONE		
GasAid Maximum Strength Anti-Gas Softgels	Simethicone 125mg	**Adults:** Take 1-2 caps prn and qhs. **Max:** 4 caps q24h.
Baby Gas-X Infant Drops	Simethicone 20mg/0.3mL	**Peds ≥2 yrs (≥24 lbs):** 0.6mL prn. **Peds <2 yrs (<24 lbs):** 0.3mL prn. **Max:** 6 doses q24h.
Gas-X Children's Thin Strips	Simethicone 40mg	**Peds 2-12 yrs:** 1 strip prn and hs. **Max:** 6 strips q24h.
Gas-X Thin Strips	Simethicone 62.5mg	**Adults:** Allow 2-4 strips to dissolve prn after meals and hs. **Max:** 8 strips q24h.
Gas-X Antigas Chewable Tablets	Simethicone 80mg	**Adults:** Take 1-2 tabs prn and qhs. **Max:** 6 tabs q24h.
Gas-X Extra Strength Antigas Softgels	Simethicone 125mg	**Adults:** Take 1-2 caps prn and qhs. **Max:** 4 caps q24h.
Gas-X Maximum Strength Antigas Softgels	Simethicone 166mg	**Adults:** Take 1-2 caps prn and qhs. **Max:** 3 caps q24h.
Gas-X Ultra Strength Softgels	Simethicone 180mg	**Adults:** Take 1-2 caps prn after meals and qhs. **Max:** 2 caps q24h.
Little Tummys Gas Relief Drops	Simethicone 20mg/0.3mL	**Peds ≥2 yrs (≥24 lbs):** 0.6mL prn (after meals & hs). **Peds <2 yrs (<24 lbs):** 0.3mL prn (after meals & hs). **Max:** 12 doses q24h.
Mylanta Gas Maximum Strength Softgels	Simethicone 125mg	**Adults:** Chew 1-2 caps (after meals & hs). **Max:** 4 caps q24h.
Mylanta Gas Maximum Strength Chewable Tablets	Simethicone 125mg	**Adults:** Chew 1-2 tabs (after meals & hs). **Max:** 4 tabs q24h.
Mylicon Infant's Gas Relief Drops	Simethicone 20mg/0.3mL	**Peds ≥2 yrs (≥24 lbs):** 0.6mL (after meals & hs). **Peds <2 yrs (<24 lbs):** 0.3mL (after meals & hs). **Max:** 12 doses q24h.

HEMORRHOIDAL PRODUCTS

BRAND	INGREDIENT/STRENGTH	DOSE
ANESTHETICS/ANESTHETIC COMBINATIONS		
Tucks Hemorrhoidal Ointment	Pramoxine HCl/Zinc Oxide/Mineral Oil 1%-12.5% - 46.6%	**Adults ≥12 yrs:** Apply to affected area prn. **Max:** 5 times q24h.
Nupercainal Ointment	Dibucaine 1%	**Adults & Peds ≥12 yrs:** Apply to affected area qid.
Preparation H Hemorrhoidal Cream, Maximum Strength Pain Relief	Glycerin/Phenylephrine HCl/ Pramoxine HCl/White Petrolatum 14.4%-0.25%-1%-15%	**Adults ≥12 yrs:** Apply to affected area prn. **Max:** 4 times q24h.
Tronolane Anesthetic Hemorrhoid Cream	Pramoxine HCl/Zinc Oxide 1%-5%	**Adults:** Apply to affected area prn. **Max:** 5 times q24h.
BULK-FORMING LAXATIVES		
Citrucel Caplets	Methylcellulose 500mg	**Adults ≥12 yrs:** 2 tabs qd prn. **Max:** 12 tabs q24h. **Peds 6-12 yrs:** 1 tab qd prn. **Max:** 6 tabs q24h.
Citrucel Powder	Methylcellulose 2g/tbl	**Adults ≥12 yrs:** 1 tbl (11.5g) qd-tid. **Peds 6-12 yrs:** ½ tbl (5.75g) qd.
Equalactin Chewable Tablet	Calcium Polycarbophil 625mg	**Adults & Peds ≥12 yrs:** 2 tabs qd. **Max:** 8 tabs qd. **Peds 6-12 yrs:** 1 tab qd. **Max:** 4 tabs qd. **2 to <6 yrs:** 1 tab qd. **Max:** 2 tabs qd.
Fibercon Caplets	Calcium Polycarbophil 625mg	**Adults & Peds ≥12 yrs:** 2 tabs qd. **Max:** 8 tabs qd. **Peds <12 yrs:** Ask doctor.
Konsyl Easy Mix Powder	Psyllium 4.3g/tsp	**Adults ≥12 yrs:** 1 tsp qd-qid. **Peds:** ½ tsp qd-tid.
Konsyl Fiber Caplets	Calcium Polycarbophil 625mg	**Adults ≥12 yrs:** 2 tabs qd-qid. **Peds 6-12 yrs:** 1 tab qd-tid. **Max:** 8 tabs q24h.
Konsyl Orange Powder	Psyllium 3.4g/tsp	**Adults & Peds ≥12 yrs:** 1tbl qd-tid. **Peds 6-11 yrs:** ½ tbl qd-tid.
Konsyl Original Powder	Psyllium 6g/tsp	**Adults ≥12 yrs:** 1 tsp qd-tid. **Peds 6-12 yrs:** ½ tsp qd-tid.
Konsyl-D Powder	Psyllium 3.4g/tsp	**Adults ≥12 yrs:** 1 tsp qd-tid. **Peds 6-12 yrs:** ½ tsp qd-tid.
Metamucil Capsules	Psyllium 0.52g	**Adults & Peds ≥12 yrs:** 5 caps qd-tid.
Metamucil Original Texture Powder	Psyllium 3.4g/tbl	**Adults ≥12 yrs:** 1 tbl tid.
Metamucil Smooth Texture Powder	Psyllium 3.4g/tbl	**Adults ≥12 yrs:** 1 tbl tid.
Metamucil Wafers	Psyllium 3.4g/dose	**Adults ≥12 yrs:** 2 wafers qd-tid. **Peds: 6-12 yrs:** 1 wafer qd-tid.
HYDROCORTISONE		
Tucks Anti-Itch Ointment	Hydrocortisone Acetate 1.12%	**Adults & Peds ≥12 yrs:** Apply to affected area ud. **Max:** Apply to affected area tid-qid q24h.
Preparation H Anti-Itch Cream	Hydrocortisone 1.0%	**Adults & Peds ≥12 yrs:** Apply to affected area tid-qid.

(Continued)

BRAND	INGREDIENT/STRENGTH	DOSE
STOOL SOFTENER		
Colace Capsules	Docusate Sodium 100mg	**Adults ≥12 yrs:** 1-3 caps qd. **Peds 2-12 yrs:** 1 cap qd.
Colace Capsules	Docusate Sodium 50mg	**Adults ≥12 yrs:** 1-6 caps qd. **Peds 2-12 yrs:** 1-3 caps qd.
Colace Liquid	Docusate Sodium 10mg/mL	**Adults ≥12 yrs:** 5-15mL qd-bid. **Peds 2-12 yrs:** 5-15mL qd.
Colace Syrup	Docusate Sodium 60mg/15mL	**Adults ≥12 yrs:** 15-90mL qd. **Peds 2-12 yrs:** 5-37.5mL qd.
Docusol Constipation Relief, Mini Enemas	Docusate Sodium 283mg	**Adults ≥12 yrs:** Take 1-3 units qd. **Peds 6-12 yrs:** Take 1 unit qd.
Dulcolax Stool Softener Capsules	Docusate Sodium 100mg	**Adults ≥12 yrs:** 1-3 caps qd. **Peds 6-12 yrs:** 1 cap qd.
Fleet Pedia-Lax Liquid Stool Softener	Docusate 50mg/tbl	**Peds 2-11 yrs:** 1-3 tbl qd. **Max:** 3 tbl.
Fleet Sof-Lax	Docusate 100mg	**Adults & Peds ≥12 yrs:** 1-3 softgels qd. **Peds 2-11 yrs:** 1 softgel qd.
Kaopectate Liqui-Gels	Docusate Calcium 240mg	**Adults & Peds ≥12 yrs:** 1 cap qd until normal bowel movement.
Phillips Stool Softener Capsules	Docusate Sodium 100mg	**Adults ≥12 yrs:** 1-3 caps qd. **Peds 6-12 yrs:** 1 cap qd.
WITCH HAZEL/WITCH HAZEL COMBINATIONS		
Hemspray Hemorrhoid Relief Spray	Witch Hazel/Glycerin/ Phenylephrine HCl/Camphor 50%-20%-0.25%-0.15%	**Adults & Peds ≥12 yrs:** Apply to affected area prn. **Max:** 5 times q24h.
Preparation H Hemorrhoidal Cooling Gel	Phenylephrine HCl/Witch Hazel 0.25%-50.0%	**Adults ≥12 yrs:** Apply to affected area prn. **Max:** 4 times q24h.
Preparation H Medicated Wipes	Witch Hazel 50%	**Adults & Peds ≥12 yrs:** Apply to affected area prn. **Max:** 6 times q24h.
T.N. Dickinson's Witch Hazel Hemorrhoidal Pads	Witch Hazel 50%	**Adults & Peds ≥12 yrs:** Apply to affected area prn. **Max:** 6 times q24h.
Tucks Medicated Pads	Witch Hazel 50%	**Adults & Peds ≥12 yrs:** Apply to affected area prn. **Max:** 6 times q24h.
Tucks Take Alongs Medicated Towelettes	Witch Hazel 50%	**Adults & Peds ≥12 yrs:** Apply to affected area prn. **Max:** 6 times q24h.
MISCELLANEOUS		
Preparation H Hemorrhoidal Ointment	Mineral Oil/Petrolatum/ Phenylephrine HCl/Shark Liver Oil 14%-71.9%-0.25%-3.0%	**Adults ≥12 yrs:** Apply to affected area prn. **Max:** 4 times q24h.
Preparation H Hemorrhoidal Suppositories	Cocoa Butter/Phenylephrine HCl/ Shark Liver Oil 85.5%-0.25%-3.0%	**Adults & Peds ≥12 yrs:** Insert 1 supp qid.
Rectal Medicone Suppositories	Hard Fat/Phenylephrine 88.7%-0.25%	**Adults & Peds ≥12 yrs:** Insert 1 supp tid-qid.
Tronolane Suppositories	Hard Fat/Phenylephrine HCl 88.7%-0.25%	**Adults & Peds ≥12 yrs:** Insert 1 supp prn. **Max:** 4 times q24h.
Tucks Topical Starch Hemorrhoidal Suppositories	Topical Starch 51%	**Adults & Peds ≥12 yrs:** Insert 1 supp prn. **Max:** 6 times q24h.

LAXATIVE PRODUCTS

BRAND	INGREDIENT/STRENGTH	DOSE
BULK-FORMING		
Citrucel Caplets	Methylcellulose 500mg	**Adults & Peds ≥12 yrs:** 2 caps qd prn. **Max:** 12 tabs q24h. **Peds 6-12yrs:** 1 cap qd prn. **Max:** 6 tabs q24h.
Citrucel Powder	Methylcellulose 2g/tbl	**Adults & Peds ≥12 yrs:** 1 tbl (11.5g) qd-tid. **Peds 6-12 yrs:** ½ tbl (5.75g) qd.
Equalactin Chewable Tablet	Calcium Polycarbophil 625mg	**Adults & Peds ≥12 yrs:** 2 tabs/dose. **Max:** 8 tabs q24h. **Peds 6-11 yrs:** 1 tab/dose **Max:** 4 tabs q24h. **Peds 2-5 yrs:** 1 tab/dose **Max:** 2 tabs q24h.
Fibercon Caplets	Calcium Polycarbophil 625mg	**Adults & Peds ≥12 yrs:** 2 caps qd-qid. **Max:** 4 doses q24h.
Konsyl Easy Mix Powder	Psyllium 4.3g/tsp	**Adults & Peds ≥12 yrs:** 1 tsp qd-tid. **Peds 6-12 yrs:** ½ tsp qd-tid.
Konsyl Fiber Caplets	Calcium Polycarbophil 625mg	**Adults & Peds ≥12 yrs:** 2 caps qd-qid. **Peds 6-12 yrs:** 1 cap qd-tid. **Max:** 8 caps q24h.
Konsyl Orange Powder	Psyllium 3.4g/tbl	**Adults & Peds ≥12 yrs:** 1 tbl qd-tid. **Peds 6-12 yrs:** ½ tbl qd-tid.
Konsyl Original Powder	Psyllium 6g/tsp	**Adults & Peds ≥12 yrs:** 1 tsp qd-tid. **Peds 6-12 yrs:** ½ tsp qd-tid.
Konsyl-D Powder	Psyllium 3.4g/tsp	**Adults & Peds ≥12 yrs:** 1 tsp qd-tid. **Peds 6-12 yrs:** ½ tsp qd-tid.
Metamucil Capsules	Psyllium 0.52g	**Adults & Peds ≥12 yrs:** 5 caps qd-tid.
Metamucil Original Texture Powder (orange)	Psyllium 3.4g/tbl	**Adults & Peds ≥12 yrs:** 1 tbl up to tid. **Peds 6-11 yrs:** ½ tbl up to tid.
Metamucil Smooth Texture Powder (orange)	Psyllium 3.4g/tbl	**Adults & Peds ≥12 yrs:** 1 tbl up to tid. **Peds 6-11 yrs:** ½ tbl up to tid.
Metamucil Wafers	Psyllium 3.4 g/dose	**Adults & Peds ≥12 yrs:** 2 wafers qd-tid. **Peds 6-12 yrs:** 1 wafer qd-tid.
HYPEROSMOTICS		
Colace Glycerin Suppositories for Adults and Children	Glycerin 2.1g	**Adults & Peds ≥6 yrs:** 1 supp. **Max:** 1 supp q24h.
Colace Glycerin Suppositories for Infants and Children	Glycerin 1.2g	**Peds 2-5 yrs:** 1 supp. **Max:** 1 supp q24h.
Fleet Mineral Oil Enema	Mineral Oil 118mL	**Adults & Peds ≥12 yrs:** 1 bottle (118mL). **Peds 2-12 yrs:** ½ bottle (59mL).
Fleet Pedia-Lax Glycerin Suppositories	Glycerin 1g	**Peds 2-6 yrs:** 1 supp. ud.
Fleet Pedia-Lax Liquid Glycerin Suppositories	Glycerin 2.3g	**Peds 2-5 yrs:** 1 supp. ud.
SALINES		
Fleet Enema	Monobasic Sodium Phosphate/Dibasic Sodium Phosphate 19g-7g/118mL	**Adults & Peds ≥12 yrs:** 1 bottle (118mL).
Fleet Enema Extra	Monobasic Sodium Phosphate/Dibasic Sodium Phosphate 19g-7g/197mL	**Adults & Peds ≥12 yrs:** 1 bottle (197mL).

(Continued)

BRAND	INGREDIENT/STRENGTH	DOSE
SALINES *(Continued)*		
Fleet Pedia-Lax Chewable Tablets	Magnesium Hydroxide 400mg	**Peds 6-11 yrs:** 3-6 tabs qd. **Max:** 6 tabs q24h. **Peds 2-5 yrs:** 1-3 tabs qd. **Max:** 3 tabs q24h.
Fleet Pedia-Lax Enema	Monobasic Sodium Phosphate/Dibasic Sodium Phosphate 9.5g-3.5g/59mL	**Peds 5-11 yrs:** 1 bottle (59mL) **Peds 2-5 yrs:** ½ bottle (29.5mL)
Magnesium Citrate Solution	Magnesium Citrate 1.75g/30mL	**Adults & Peds ≥12 yrs:** 300mL. **Peds 6-12 yrs:** 90-210mL. **Peds 2-6 yrs:** 60-90mL.
Phillips Antacid/Laxative Chewable Tablets	Magnesium Hydroxide 311mg	**Adults & Peds ≥12 yrs:** 8 tabs qd. **Peds 6-11 yrs:** 4 tabs qd. **Peds 3-5 yrs:** 2 tabs qd.
Phillips Cramp-Free Laxative Caplets	Magnesium 500 mg	**Adults & Peds ≥12 yrs:** Take 2-4 tabs qd. **Max:** 4 tabs q24h.
Phillips Milk of Magnesia Concentrated Liquid	Magnesium Hydroxide 800mg/5mL	**Adults & Peds ≥12 yrs:** 1-2 tbl qd. **Peds 6-11 yrs:** ½-1 tbl qd.
Phillips Milk of Magnesia Liquid	Magnesium Hydroxide 400mg/5mL	**Adults & Peds ≥12 yrs:** 2-4 tbl qd. **Peds 6-11 yrs:** 1-2 tbl qd.
SALINE COMBINATION		
Phillips M-O Liquid	Magnesium Hydroxide/Mineral Oil 300mg-1.25mL/5mL	**Adults & Peds ≥12 yrs:** 3-4 tbl qd. **Peds 6-11 yrs:** 4-6 tsp qd.
STIMULANTS		
Alophen Enteric Coated Stimulant Laxative Pills	Bisacodyl 5mg	**Adults & Peds ≥12 yrs:** Take 1-3 tabs qd. **Peds 6-12 yrs:** Take 1 tab qd.
Carter's Laxative, Sodium Free Pills	Bisacodyl 5mg	**Adults & Peds ≥12 yrs:** Take 1-3 tabs (usually 2 tabs) qd. **Peds 6-12 yrs:** Take 1 tab qd.
Castor Oil	Castor Oil	**Adults & Peds ≥12 yrs:** 15-60mL. **Peds 2-12 yrs:** 5-15mL.
Doxidan Capsules	Bisacodyl 5mg	**Adults & Peds ≥12 yrs:** 1-3 caps (usually 2) qd. **Peds 6-12 yrs:** 1 cap qd.
Dulcolax Suppository	Bisacodyl 10mg	**Adults & Peds ≥12 yrs:** 1 supp qd. **Peds 6-12 yrs:** ½ supp qd.
Dulcolax Tablets	Bisacodyl 5mg	**Adults & Peds ≥12 yrs:** 1-3 tabs (usually 2) qd. **Peds 6-12 yrs:** 1 tab qd.
Ex-Lax Maximum Strength Tablets	Sennosides 25mg	**Adults & Peds ≥12 yrs:** 2 tabs qd-bid. **Peds 6-12 yrs:** 1 tab qd-bid.
Ex-Lax Tablets	Sennosides 15mg	**Adults & Peds ≥12 yrs:** 2 tabs qd-bid. **Peds 6-12 yrs:** 1 tab qd-bid.
Ex-Lax Ultra Stimulant Laxative Tablets	Bisacodyl 5mg	**Adults & Peds ≥12 yrs:** 1-3 tabs qd. **Peds 6-12 yrs:** 1 tab qd-bid.
Fleet Bisacodyl Enema	Bisacodyl 10mg/30mL	**Adults & Peds ≥12 yrs:** 1 bottle (30mL)
Fleet Bisacodyl Suppositories	Bisacodyl 10mg	**Adults & Peds ≥12 yrs:** 1 supp qd. **Peds 6-12 yrs:** ½ supp qd.
Fleet Pedia-Lax Quick Dissolve Strips	Sennosides 8.6mg	**Peds 6-11 yrs:** 2 strips. **Max:** 4 strips q24h. **Peds 2-5 yrs:** 1 strip. **Max:** 2 strips q24h.
Fleet Stimulant Laxative Tablets	Bisacodyl 5mg	**Adults & Peds ≥12 yrs:** 1-3 tabs (usually 2) qd. **Peds 6-12 yrs:** 1 tab qd.
Perdiem Overnight Relief Tablets	Sennosides 15mg	**Adults & Peds ≥12 yrs:** 2 tabs qd-bid. **Peds 6-12 yrs:** 1 tab qd-bid.

(Continued)

BRAND	INGREDIENT/STRENGTH	DOSE
STIMULANTS *(Continued)*		
Senokot Tablets	Sennosides 8.6mg	**Adults & Peds ≥12 yrs:** 2 tabs qd. **Max:** 4 tabs bid. **Peds 6-12 yrs:** 1 tab qd. **Max:** 2 tabs bid. **Peds 2-6 yrs:** ½ tab qd. **Max:** 1 tab bid.
SenokotXTRA tablets	Sennosides 17.2mg	**Adults & Peds ≥12 yrs:** Starting dose 1 tab qd. **Max:** 2 tabs bid. **Peds 6-12 yrs:** Starting dose: ½ tab qd. **Max:** 1 tab bid.
STIMULANT COMBINATIONS		
Konsyl Senna Prompt	Psyllium/Sennosides 500mg-9mg	**Adults & Peds ≥12 yrs:** 1-5 caps qd-bid.
Peri-Colace Tablets	Sennosides/Docusate 8.6mg-50mg	**Adults & Peds ≥12 yrs:** 2-4 tabs qd. **Peds 6-12 yrs:** 1-2 tabs qd. **Peds 2-5 yrs:** 1 tab qd.
Senokot S Tablets	Sennosides/Docusate 8.6mg-50mg	**Adults ≥12 yrs:** 2 tabs qd. **Max:** 4 tabs bid. **Peds 6-12 yrs:** 1 tab qd. **Max:** 2 tabs bid. **Peds 2-6 yrs:** ½ tab qd. **Max:** 1 tab bid.
SURFACTANTS (STOOL SOFTENERS)		
Colace Capsules	Docusate Sodium 100mg	**Adults & Peds ≥12 yrs:** 1-3 caps qd. **Peds 2-12 yrs:** 1 cap qd.
Colace Capsules	Docusate Sodium 50mg	**Adults & Peds ≥12 yrs:** 1-6 caps qd. **Peds 2-12 yrs:** 1-3 caps qd.
Colace Liquid	Docusate Sodium 10mg/mL	**Adults & Peds ≥12 yrs:** 5-15mL qd-bid. **Peds 2-12 yrs:** 5-15mL qd.
Colace Syrup	Docusate Sodium 60mg/15mL	**Adults & Peds ≥12 yrs:** 15-90mL qd. **Peds 2-12 yrs:** 15-37.5mL qd.
Docusol Constipation Relief, Mini Enemas	Docusate Sodium 283mg	**Adults & Peds ≥12 yrs:** Take 1-3 units qd. **Peds 6-12 yrs:** Take 1 unit qd
Dulcolax Stool Softener Capsules	Docusate Sodium 100mg	**Adults & Peds ≥12 yrs:** 1-3 caps qd. **Peds 2-12 yrs:** 1 cap qd.
Fleet Pedia-Lax Liquid Stool Softener	Docusate 50mg/tbl	**Peds 2-11 yrs:** 1-3 tbl qd. **Max:** 3 tbl.
Fleet Sof-Lax	Docusate 100mg	**Adults & Peds ≥12 yrs:** 1-3 softgels qd. **Peds 2-11 yrs:** 1 softgel qd.
Kaopectate Liqui-Gels	Docusate Calcium 240mg	**Adults & Peds ≥12 yrs:** 1 cap qd until normal bowel movement.
Phillips Stool Softener Capsules	Docusate Sodium 100mg	**Adults & Peds ≥12 yrs:** 1-3 caps qd. **Peds 6-12 yrs:** 1 cap qd.

ARTIFICIAL TEAR PRODUCTS

BRAND	INGREDIENT/STRENGTH	DOSE
Akwa Tears Lubricant Eye Drops	Polyvinyl Alcohol 1.4%	**Adults:** Instill 1-2 drops to affected eye prn.
Akwa Tears Lubricant Ophthalmic Ointment	White Petrolatum/Mineral Oil/ Lanolin 83%-15%-2%	**Adults:** Place 1/4 in oint inside eyelid one or more times daily.
Allergan Optive Lubricant Eye Drops	Carboxymethylcellulose/Sodium Glycerin 0.5%-0.9%	**Adults:** Instill 1-2 drops to affected eye prn.
Allergan Lacri-Lube S.O.P. Lubricant Eye Ointment	Mineral Oil/White Petrolatum 42.5%-56.8%	**Adults:** Place 1/4 in oint inside eyelid qd.
Allergan Refresh Celluvisc Lubricant Eye Drops	Carboxymethylcellulose Sodium 1%	**Adults:** Instill 1-2 drops to affected eye prn.
Allergan Refresh Dry Eye Therapy Eye Drops	Glycerin/Polysorbate 80.1%-1%	**Adults:** Instill 1-2 drops to affected eye prn.
Allergan Refresh Liquigel Lubricant Eye Drops	Carboxymethylcellulose Sodium 1%	**Adults:** Instill 1-2 drops to affected eye prn.
Allergan Refresh Lubricant Eye Drops	Polyvinyl Alcohol/Povidone 1.4%-0.6%	**Adults:** Instill 1-2 drops to affected eye prn.
Allergan Refresh Plus Lubricant Eye Drops	Carboxymethylcellulose Sodium 0.5%	**Adults:** Instill 1-2 drops to affected eye prn.
Allergan Refresh PM Lubricant Eye Ointment	White Petrolatum/Mineral Oil 57.3%-42.5%	**Adults:** Place 1/4 in oint inside eyelid.
Allergan Refresh Tears Lubricant Eye Drops	Carboxymethylcellulose Sodium 0.5%	**Adults:** Instill 1-2 drops to affected eye prn.
AMO Blink Tears Lubricating Eye Drops for Mild-Moderate Dry Eyes	Polyethylene Glycol 400 0.25%	**Adults:** Instill 1-2 drops to affected eye prn.
Bausch & Lomb Advanced Eye Relief Dry Eye Environmental Lubricant Eye Drops	Glycerin 1%	**Adults:** Instill 1 or 2 drops in the affected eye prn.
Bausch & Lomb Advanced Eye Relief Dry Eye Rejuvenation Lubricant Eye Drops	Glycerin/Propylene Glycol 0.3%-1%	**Adults:** Instill 1 or 2 drops in the affected eye prn.
Bausch & Lomb Advanced Eye Relief Night Time Lubricant Eye Ointment (Preservative Free)	Mineral Oil/White Petrolatum 20%-80%	**Adults:** Apply a small amount (1/4 inch) of ointment to the inside of lower eyelid one or more time daily.
Bausch & Lomb Soothe Lubricant Eye Drops	Glycerin/Propylene Glycol 0.6%-0.6%	**Adults:** Instill 1 or 2 drops in the affected eye prn.
Bion Tears Lubricant Eye Drops	Dextran 70/Hydroxypropyl Methylcellulose 2910 0.1%-0.3%	**Adults:** Instill 1-2 drops to affected eye prn.
Clear Eyes Eye Drops for Dry Eyes	Carboxymethylcellulose Sodium/ Glycerine 1.0%-0.25%	**Adults:** Instill 1-2 drops to affected eye prn.
GenTeal Gel	Hypromellose 0.3%	**Adults:** Instill 1 or 2 drops in the affected eye prn.
GenTeal Mild Dry Eyes Drops	Hypromellose 0.2%	**Adults:** Instill 1-2 drops to affected eye prn.
GenTeal Moderate Dry Eyes Drops	Hypromellose 0.3%	**Adults:** Instill 1-2 drops to affected eye prn.
GenTeal PM Ointment	Mineral Oil/White Petrolatum 15%-85%	**Adults:** Apply a small amount (1/4 inch) of ointment to the inside of lower eyelid one or more time daily.
GenTeal Lubricant Eye Drops for Moderate to Severe Dry Eye Relief, Gel Drops	Carboxymethylcellulose Sodium/ Hypromellose 0.25%-0.3%	**Adults:** Instill 1-2 drops to affected eye prn.
GenTeal PF Dry Eye Drops	Hydroxypropylmethylcellulose 0.3%	**Adults:** Instill 1-2 drops to affected eye prn.
Murine Tears Lubricant Eye Drops	Polyvinyl Alcohol/Povidone 0.5%-0.6%	**Adults:** Instill 1-2 drops to affected eye prn.
Optics Laboratory Minidrops Eye Therapy	Polyvinylpyrrolidone/ Polyvinyl Alcohol 6mg-14mg	**Adults:** Instill 1-2 drops to affected eye prn.

(Continued)

BRAND	INGREDIENT/STRENGTH	DOSE
Rohto Zi For Eyes Lubricant Eye Drops	Povidone 1.8%	**Adults:** Instill 1-2 drops to affected eye prn.
Soothe XP Emollient Lubricant Eye Drops	Light Mineral Oil/Mineral Oil 1%-4.5%	**Adults:** Instill 1-2 drops in the affected eye prn, or as directed by your doctor.
Soothe Lubricant Eye Drops	Glycerin/Propylene Glycol 0.6%-0.6%	**Adults:** Instill 1-2 drops in the affected eye prn, or as directed by your doctor.
Systane Lubricant Eye Drops	Polyethylene Glycol 400/ Propylene Glycol 0.4%-0.3%	**Adults:** Instill 1-2 drops to affected eye prn.
Systane Nighttime Lubricant Eye Ointment	Mineral Oil/White Petrolatum 3%-94%	**Adults:** Place ¼ inch oint inside eyelid.
Systane Preservative Free Lubricant Eye Drops	Polyethylene Glycol 400/Propylene Glycol 0.4%-0.3%	**Adults:** Instill 1 or 2 drops in the affected eye prn.
Systane Ultra Lubricant Eye Drops	Polyethylene Glycol 400/Propylene Glycol 0.4%-0.3%	**Adults:** Instill 1 or 2 drops in the affected eye prn.
Tears Naturale Forte Lubricant Eye Drops	Dextran 70/Glycerin/Hydroxypropyl Methylcellulose 1%-0.2%-0.3%	**Adults:** Instill 1-2 drops to affected eye prn.
Tears Naturale Free Lubricant Eye Drops	Dextran 70/Hydroxypropyl Methylcellulose 2910 0.1%-0.3%	**Adults:** Instill 1-2 drops to affected eye prn.
Tears Naturale II Polyquad Lubricant Eye Drops	Dextran 70/Hydroxypropyl Methylcellulose 2910 0.1%-0.3%	**Adults:** Instill 1-2 drops to affected eye prn.
Tears Naturale P.M. Lubricant Eye Ointment	White Petrolatum/Mineral Oil 94%-3%	**Adults:** Place ¼ inch oint inside eyelid qd.
TheraTears Liquid Gel Lubricant Eye Gel	Sodium Carboxymethylcellulose 1%	**Adults:** Instill 1-2 drops to affected eye prn.
TheraTears Lubricant Eye Drops	Sodium Carboxymethylcellulose 0.25%	**Adults:** Instill 1-2 drops to affected eye prn.
Visine Pure Tears Lubricant Eye Drops	Glycerin/Hypromellose/Polyethylene Glycol 400 0.2%-0.2%-1%	**Adults and Peds: >6 yrs:** Instill 1-2 drops to affected eye prn.
Viva-Drops Lubricant Eye Drops	Polysorbate 80	**Adults:** Instill 1-2 drops to affected eye prn.

OPHTHALMIC DECONGESTANT/ANTIHISTAMINE PRODUCTS

BRAND	INGREDIENT/STRENGTH	DOSE
KETOTIFEN		
Zaditor	Ketotifen 0.025%	**Adults & Peds >3 yrs:** Instill 1 drop in affected eye(s) bid every 8-12 hrs. **Max:** 2 doses qd.
Alaway	Ketotifen 0.025%	**Adults & Peds >3 yrs:** Instill 1 drop in affected eye(s) bid every 8-12 hrs. **Max:** 2 doses qd.
NAPHAZOLINE		
Bausch & Lomb Advanced Eye Relief	Naphazoline HCl/Hypromellose 0.03%-0.5%	**Adults:** Instill 1-2 drops to affected eye(s) qid.
Clear Eyes ACR Seasonal Relief	Naphazoline HCl/Glycerin/Zinc Sulfate 0.012%-0.2%-0.25%	**Adults:** Instill 1-2 drops to affected eye(s) qid.
Clear Eyes Extra Relief Lubricant Eye Redness Reliever	Naphazoline HCl/Glycerin 0.012%-0.2%	**Adults:** Instill 1-2 drops to affected eye(s) qid.
Opcon-A Allergy Relief Drops	Naphazoline HCl/Pheniramine Maleate 0.03%-0.32%	**Adults & Peds ≥6 yrs:** Instill 1-2 drops to affected eye(s) qid.
Visine-A Allergy Relief Drops	Naphazoline HCl/ Pheniramine Maleate 0.025%-0.3%	**Adults & Peds ≥6 yrs:** Instill 1-2 drops to affected eye(s) qid.
Rohto V Cool Redness Relief Drops	Naphazoline HCl/ Polysorbate 80 0.012%-0.2%	**Adults:** Instill 1-2 drops to affected eye(s) qid.
OXYMETAZOLINE		
Visine L.R. Redness Reliever Drops	Oxymetazoline HCl 0.025%	**Adults & Peds ≥6 yrs:** Instill 1-2 drops to affected eye(s) q6h prn.
PHENYLEPHRINE		
Allergan Relief Redness Reliever & Lubricant Eye Drops	Phenylephrine HCl/ Polyvinyl Alcohol 0.12%-1.4%	**Adults:** Instill 1-2 drops to affected eye(s) qid.
TETRAHYDROZOLINE		
Visine Original Drops	Tetrahydrozoline HCl 0.05%	**Adults & Peds ≥6 yrs:** Instill 1-2 drops to affected eye(s) qid.
Visine Advanced Redness Reliever drops	Tetrahydrozoline HCl/Polyethylene Glycol 400/ Povidone/Dextran 70 0.05%-1%-1%-0.1%	**Adults:** Instill 1-2 drops to affected eye(s) qid.
Murine Tears Plus Eye Drops	Tetrahydrozoline HCl/Polyvinyl Alcohol/ Povidone 0.05%-0.5%-0.6%	**Adults:** Instill 1-2 drops to affected eye(s) qid.
Rohto V. Arctic Eyedrops	Tetrahydrozoline HCl/Hypromellose 0.05%-0.35%	**Adults:** Instill 1-2 drops to affected eye(s) qid.
Rohto V. Ice Eye Drops	Tetrahydrozoline HCl/Hypromellose/Zinc Sulfate 0.05%-0.2%-0.25%	**Adults:** Instill 1-2 drops to affected eye(s) qid.
Visine A.C. Astringent Redness Reliever Drops	Tetrahydrozoline HCl/ Zinc Sulfate 0.05%-0.25%	**Adults:** Instill 1-2 drops to affected eye(s) qid.

ALLERGIC RHINITIS PRODUCTS

BRAND	INGREDIENT/STRENGTH	DOSE
ANTIHISTAMINE		
Alavert Oral Disintegrating Tablets	Loratadine 10mg	**Adults & Peds ≥6 yrs:** 1 tab qd. **Max:** 1 tab q24h.
Alavert 24-Hour Allergy Tablets	Loratadine 10mg	**Adults & Peds ≥6 yrs:** 1 tab qd. **Max:** 1 tab q24h.
Benadryl Allergy Quick Dissolve Strips	Diphenhydramine HCl 25mg	**Adults & Peds ≥12 yrs:** Dissolve 1-2 strips on tongue q4-6h. **Max:** 6 doses q24h.
Benadryl Allergy Capsules	Diphenhydramine HCl 25mg	**Adults & Peds ≥12 yrs:** 1-2 caps q4-6h. **Peds 6-12 yrs:** 1 cap q4-6h. **Max:** 6 doses q24h.
Benadryl Allergy Liquid	Diphenhydramine HCl 12.5mg/5mL	**Adults & Peds ≥12 yrs:** 2-4 tsp (10-20mL) q4-6h. **Peds 6-12 yrs:** 1-2 tsp (5-10mL) q4-6h. **Max:** 6 doses q24h.
Benadryl Allergy Ultratab	Diphenhydramine HCl 25mg	**Adults & Peds ≥12 yrs:** 1-2 tabs q4-6h. **Peds 6-12 yrs:** 1 tab q4-6h. **Max:** 6 doses q24h.
Benadryl Liqui-Gels	Diphenhydramine 25mg	**Adults & Peds ≥12 yrs:** 1-2 softgels q4-6h. **6-11 yrs:** 1 softgel q4-6h. **Max:** 6 doses q24h.
Chlor-Trimeton 4-Hour Allergy Tablets	Chlorpheniramine Maleate 4mg	**Adults & Peds ≥12 yrs:** 1 tab q4-6h. **Max:** 6 tabs q24h. **Peds 6-12 yrs:** ½ tab q4-6h. **Max:** 3 tabs q24h.
Claritin 24 Hour Allergy Tablets	Loratadine 10mg	**Adults & Peds: ≥6 yrs:** 1 tab qd. **Max:** 1 tab q24h.
Claritin Children's Chewables	Loratadine 5mg	**Adults & Peds ≥6 yrs:** 2 tabs qd. **Max:** 2 tabs q24h. **2-5 yrs:** 1 tab qd. **Max:** 1 tab q24h.
Claritin Children's Syrup	Loratadine 5mg/5mL	**Adults & Peds ≥6 yrs:** 2 tsp qd. **Max:** 2 tsp q24h. **Peds 2-6 yrs:** 1 tsp qd. **Max:** 1 tsp q24h.
Claritin RediTabs	Loratadine 10mg	**Adults & Peds ≥6 yrs:** 1 tab qd. **Max:** 1 tab q24h.
Zyrtec Tablets	Cetirizine 10mg	**Adults 18 yrs-64 yrs & Peds ≥6 yrs:** 1 tab q24h. **Max:** 1 tab q24h.
Zyrtec Children's Syrup	Cetirizine 5mg/5mL	**Adults & Peds 6-64 yrs:** 1-2 tsp qd. **Max:** 2 tsp q24h. **Adults ≥65 yrs:** 1 tsp qd. **Max:** 1 tsp q24h. **Peds 2-5 yrs:** ½ tsp qd-bid. **Max:** 1 tsp q24h.
Zyrtec Children's Chewables 5mg	Cetirizine 5mg	**Adults & Peds ≥6 yrs-64 yrs:** 1 tab q24h. **Adults ≥65 yrs:** 1 tab q24h. **Max:** 1 tab q24h.
Zyrtec Children's Chewables 10mg	Cetirizine 10mg	**Adults & Peds ≥6 yrs:** 1 tab q24h. **Adults ≥65 yrs:** Ask doctor. **Max:** 1 tab qd.
Zyrtec Children's Hive Relief Syrup	Cetirizine 5mg/5mL	**Adults & Peds ≥6 yrs-64yrs:** 1-2 tsp (5-10ml) q24h. **Max:** 2 tsp (10ml) q24h. **Adults >65:** 1 tsp q24h. **Max:** 1 tsp (5ml) q24h.
ANTIHISTAMINE COMBINATIONS		
Advil Allergy Sinus Caplets	Chlorpheniramine Maleate/ Ibuprofen/Pseudoephedrine 2mg-200mg-30mg	**Adults & Peds ≥12 yrs:** 1 tab q4-6h. **Max:** 6 tabs q24h.
Advil Allergy Sinus Caplets	Chlorpheniramine Maleate/ Ibuprofen/Pseudoephedrine 2mg-200mg-30mg	**Adults & Peds ≥12 yrs:** 1 tab q4-6h. **Max:** 6 tabs q24h.

(Continued)

BRAND	INGREDIENT/STRENGTH	DOSE
ANTIHISTAMINE COMBINATIONS *(Continued)*		
Alavert D-12 Hour Allergy and Sinus Tablets	Loratadine/Pseudoephedrine Sulfate 5mg-120mg	**Adults & Peds ≥12 yrs:** 1 tab q12h. **Max:** 2 tabs q24h.
Benadryl Allergy & Sinus Headache Caplets	Diphenhydramine HCl/ Acetaminophen/Phenylephrine HCl/ 12.5mg-325mg-5mg	**Adults & Peds ≥12 yrs:** 2 tab q4h. **Max:** 12 caps q24h. **Peds 6-11 yrs:** 1 cap q4h. **Max:** 5 caps q24h.
Benadryl Severe Allergy & Sinus Headache Caplets	Diphenhydramine HCl/ Acetaminophen/Phenylephrine HCl 25mg-325mg-5mg	**Adults & Peds ≥12 yrs:** 2 tabs q4h. **Max:** 12 tabs q24h.
Benadryl-D Allergy & Sinus Liquid	Diphenhydramine HCl/ Phenylephrine 12.5mg-5mg/5mL	**Adults & Peds ≥12 yrs:** 2 tsp q4h. **Peds 6-12 yrs:** 1 tsp q4h. **Max:** 6 doses q24h.
Benadryl-D Allergy & Sinus Tablets	Diphenhydramine/Phenylephrine HCl 25mg-10mg	**Adults & Peds ≥12 yrs:** 1 tab q4h. **Max:** 6 doses q24h.
Claritin-D 12 Hour Allergy & Congestion Tablets	Loratadine/Pseudoephedrine Sulfate 5mg-120mg	**Adults & Peds ≥12 yrs:** 1 tab q12h. **Max:** 2 tabs q24h.
Claritin-D 24 Hour Allergy & Congestion Tablets	Loratadine/Pseudoephedrine Sulfate 10mg-240mg	**Adults & Peds ≥12 yrs:** 1 tab qd. **Max:** 1 tab q24h.
Dimetapp Elixir Cold & Allergy	Brompheniramine/Phenylephrine 1mg-2.5mg/5ml	**Adults & Peds ≥12 yrs:** 4 tsp (20mL) q4h. **Peds 6-12 yrs:** 2 tsp (10mL) q4h. **Max:** 6 doses q24h.
Dimetapp Children's Chewable Tablets	Brompheniramine/Phenylephrine 1mg-2.5mg	**Peds ≥6-12 yrs:** 2 tabs q4h. **Max:** 6 doses q24h.
Sudafed PE Sinus & Allergy Tablets	Chlorpheniramine/Phenylephrine HCl 4mg-10mg	**Adults ≥12 yrs:** 1 tab q4h. **Max:** 6 tabs q24h.
Tylenol Allergy Complete Multi-Symptom Cool Burst Caplets	Chlorpheniramine Maleate/ Acetaminophen/Phenylephrine HCl 2mg-325mg-5mg	**Adults & Peds ≥12 yrs:** 2 tabs q4h. **Max:** 12 tabs q24h.
Tylenol Allergy Complete Nighttime Cool Burst Caplets	Diphenhydramine HCl/ Acetaminophen/Phenylephrine HCl 25mg-325mg-5mg	**Adults & Peds ≥12 yrs:** 2 tabs q4h. **Max:** 12 tabs q24h.
Tylenol Severe Allergy Caplets	Diphenhydramine HCl/ Acetaminophen 12.5mg-500mg	**Adults & Peds ≥12 yrs:** 2 tabs q4-6h. **Max:** 8 tabs q24h.
Zyrtec-D	Cetirizine/Pseudoephedrine HCl 5mg-120mg	**Adults 12-65 yrs:** 1 tab q12h. **Max:** 2 tabs q24h.
TOPICAL NASAL DECONGESTANTS		
4-Way Fast Acting Nasal Decongestant Spray	Phenylephrine HCl 1%	**Adults & Peds ≥12 yrs:** Instill 2-3 sprays per nostril q4h.
4-Way Mentholated Nasal Decongestant Spray	Phenylephrine HCl 1%	**Adults & Peds ≥12 yrs:** Instill 2-3 sprays per nostril q4h.
Afrin No Drip Extra Moisturizing Nasal Spray	Oxymetazoline HCl 0.05%	**Adults & Peds ≥6 yrs:** Instill 2-3 sprays per nostril q10-12h. **Max:** 2 doses q24h.
Afrin No Drip Sinus Nasal Spray	Oxymetazoline HCl 0.05%	**Adults & Peds ≥6 yrs:** Instill 2-3 sprays per nostril q10-12h. **Max:** 2 doses q24h.
Afrin No Drip Original Pump Mist Nasal Spray	Oxymetazoline HCl 0.05%	**Adults & Peds ≥6 yrs:** Instill 2-3 sprays per nostril q10-12h. **Max:** 2 doses q24h.
Afrin No Drip All Night 12 Hour Pump Mist	Oxymetazoline HCl 0.05%	**Adults & Peds ≥6 yrs:** Instill 2-3 sprays per nostril q10-12h. **Max:** 2 doses q24h.
Afrin No-Drip Severe Congestion Nasal Spray	Oxymetazoline 0.05%	**Adults & Peds ≥6 yrs:** Instill 2-3 sprays per nostril q10-12h. **Max:** 2 doses q24h.
Benzedrex Inhaler	Propylhexedrine 250mg	**Adults & Peds ≥6 yrs:** Inhale 2 sprays per nostril q2h.

(Continued)

BRAND	INGREDIENT/STRENGTH	DOSE
TOPICAL NASAL DECONGESTANTS *(Continued)*		
Dristan 12 Hour Nasal Spray	Oxymetazoline HCl 0.05%	**Adults & Peds ≥12 yrs:** Instill 2-3 sprays per nostril q10-12h. **Max:** 2 doses q24h.
Mucinex Full Force Nasal Spray	Oxymetazoline 0.05%	**Adults & Peds ≥6 yrs:** Instill 2-3 sprays per nostril q10-12h. **Max:** 2 doses q24h.
Neo-Synephrine Nasal Spray Nighttime Spray	Oxymetazoline HCl 0.05%	**Adults & Peds ≥6 yrs:** Instill 2-3 sprays per nostril q10-12h. **Max:** 2 doses per 24 hours.
Neo-Synephrine Extra Strength Nasal Spray	Phenylephrine HCl 1%	**Adults & Peds ≥12 yrs:** Instill 2-3 sprays per nostril q4h.
Neo-Synephrine Mild Formula Nasal Spray	Phenylephrine HCl 0.25%	**Adults & Peds ≥6 yrs:** Instill 2-3 sprays per nostril q4h.
Neo-Synephrine Regular Strength Nasal Decongestant Spray	Phenylephrine HCl 0.5%	**Adults & Peds ≥12 yrs:** Instill 2-3 sprays per nostril q4h.
Nostrilla Original Fast Relief	Oxymetazoline HCl 0.05%	**Adults & Peds ≥6 yrs:** Instill 2-3 sprays per nostril q10-12h. **Max:** 2 doses q24h.
Nostrilla Complete Congestion Relief	Oxymetazoline 0.05%	**Adults & Peds ≥6 yrs:** Instill 2-3 sprays per nostril q10-12h. **Max:** 2 doses q24h.
Sudafed Sinus Congestion 12 hour Nasal Spray	Oxymetazoline 0.05%	**Adults & Peds ≥6 yrs:** Instill 2-3 sprays per nostril q10-12h. **Max:** 2 doses q24h.
Sudafed Sinus Cold 12 hour Nasal Spray	Oxymetazoline 0.05%	**Adults & Peds ≥6 yrs:** Instill 2-3 sprays per nostril q10-12h. **Max:** 2 doses q24h.
Vicks Sinex 12 Hour Ultra Fine Mist For Sinus Relief	Phenylephrine HCl 0.05%	**Adults & Peds ≥6 yrs:** Instill 2-3 sprays per nostril q10-12h. **Max:** 2 doses q24h.
Vicks Sinex 12-Hour Nasal Spray	Oxymetazoline HCl 0.05%	**Adults & Peds ≥6 yrs:** Instill 2-3 sprays per nostril q10-12h. **Max:** 2 doses per day.
Vicks Sinex Nasal Spray For Sinus Relief	Phenylephrine HCl 0.5%	**Adults & Peds ≥12 yrs:** Instill 2-3 sprays per nostril q4h.
Zicam Extreme Congestion Relief	Oxymetazoline HCl 0.05%	**Adults & Peds ≥6 yrs:** Instill 2-3 sprays per nostril q10-12h. **Max:** 2 doses q24h.
Zicam Intense Sinus Relief	Oxymetazoline HCl 0.05%	**Adults & Peds ≥12 yrs:** Instill 2-3 sprays per nostril q10-12h. **Max:** 2 doses q24h.
TOPICAL NASAL MOISTURIZERS		
4-Way Saline Moisturizing Mist	Water, Boric Acid, Glycerin, Sodium Chloride, Sodium Borate, Eucalyptol, Menthol, Polysorbate 80, Benzalkonium Chloride	**Adults & Peds ≥2 yrs:** Instill 2-3 sprays per nostril prn.
Ayr Allergy & Sinus Nasal Mist	Sodium Chloride 2.65%	**Adults & Peds:** Spray bid-tid prn.
Ayr Baby's Saline Nose Spray, Drops	Sodium Chloride 0.65%	**Peds:** Instill 2 to 6 drops in each nostril.
Ayr Saline Nasal Gel With Soothing Aloe	Water, Methyl Gluceth 10, Propylene Glycol, Glycerin, Glyceryl Polymethacrylate, Triethanolamine, Aloe Barbadensis Leaf Juice (Aloe Vera Gel), PEG/PPG 18/18 Dimethicone, Carbomer, Poloxamer 184, Sodium Chloride, Xanthan Gum, Diazolidinyl Urea, Methylparaben, Propylparaben, Glycine Soja Oil (Soybean), Geraniuim Maculatum Oil, Tocopheryl Acetate, Blue 1	**Adults & Peds ≥12 yrs:** Apply to nostril prn.

(Continued)

BRAND	INGREDIENT/STRENGTH	DOSE
TOPICAL NASAL MOISTURIZERS *(Continued)*		
Ayr Saline Nasal Gel, No-Drip Sinus Spray	Water, Sodium Carbomethyl Starch, Propylene Glycol, Glycerin, Aloe Barbadensis Leaf Juice (Aloe Vera Gel), Sodium Chloride, Cetyl Pyridinium Chloride, Citric Acid, Disodium EDTA, Glycine Soja (Soybean Oil), Tocopheryl Acetate, Benzyl Alcohol, Benzalkonium Chloride, Geranium Maculatum Oil	**Adults & Peds ≥12 yrs:** Instill 1 spray in each nostril prn.
Ayr Saline Nasal Mist	Sodium Chloride 0.65%	**Adults & Peds ≥12 yrs:** Instill 2 sprays per nostril prn.
ENTSOL Mist, Buffered Hypertonic Nasal Irrigation Mist	Purified Water, Sodium Chloride, Sodium Phosphate Dibasic Edetate Disodium, Potassium Phosphate Monobasic, Benzalkonium Chloride	**Adults & Peds ≥12 yrs:** Instill 1-2 sprays per nostril prn.
ENTSOL Single Use, Pre-Filled Nasal Wash Squeeze Bottle	Purified Water, Sodium Chloride, Sodium Phosphate Dibasic, Potassium Phosphate Monobasic	**Adults & Peds ≥12 yrs:** Use as directed.
ENTSOL Spray, Buffered Hypertonic Saline Nasal Spray	Purified Water, Sodium Chloride Phosphate Dibasic, Potassium Phosphate Monobasic	**Adults & Peds ≥12 yrs:** Instill 1 spray per nostril bid, 2-6 times daily
ENTSOL Nasal Gel with Aloe and Vitamin E	Water (Purified), Propylene Glycol, Aloe, Glycerin, Dimethicone Copolyol, Poloxamer 184, Methyl Gluceth 10, Triethanolamine, Carbomer, Sodium Chloride, Vitamin E, Disodium EDTA, Xanthan Gum, Benzalkonium Chloride	**Adults & Peds:** Use prn.
Little Noses Saline Spray/Drops, Non-Medicated	Sodium Chloride 0.65%	**Peds:** 2-6 drops or sprays per nostril as directed.
Nostrilla Conditioning Double Moisture	Benzalkonium Chloride Solution, Carboxymethylcellulose Sodium, Eucalyptol, Glycine, Hyaluronic Acid Sodium, Polyethylene Glycol, Povidone, Propylene Glycol, Sodium Chloride (as 1.9% saline solution), Spearmint Oil, Wintergreen Oil, Water	**Adults & Peds:** Spray once per nostril prn.
Ocean Premium Saline Nasal Spray	Sodium Chloride 0.65%	**Adults & Peds ≥6 yrs:** Instill 2 sprays per nostril prn.
Simply Saline Sterile Saline Nasal Mist	Sodium Chloride 0.9%	**Adults & Peds ≥12 yrs:** Use prn as directed.
SinoFresh Moisturizing Nasal & Sinus Spray	Purified water, Propylene Glycol, Monobasic Sodium Phosphate, Dibasic Sodium Phosphate, Sodium Chloride, Polysorbate 80, Sorbitol Solution, Essential Oil Blend (Wintergreen Oil, Spearmint Oil, Peppermint Oil, Eucalyptus Oil) Cetylpyridinium Chloride, Benzalkonium Chloride	**Adults & Peds ≥12 yrs:** Instill 1-3 sprays per nostril bid.
MISCELLANEOUS		
NasalCrom Nasal Allergy Symptom Prevention and Controller, Nasal Spray	Cromolyn Sodium 5.2mg	**Adults & Peds ≥2 yrs:** Instill 1 spray per nostril q4-6h. **Max:** 6 doses q24h.
Similasan Hay Fever Relief, Non-Drowsy Formula, Nasal Spray	Cardiospermum HPUS 6X, Galphimia Glauca HPUS 6X, Luffa Operculata HPUS 6X, Sabadilla HPUS 6x	**Adults & Peds:** Instill 1 to 3 sprays in each nostril prn.
Zicam Allergy Relief, Homeopathic Nasal Solution, Pump	Luffa Operculata 4x, 12x, 30x, Galphimia Glauca 12x, 30x, Histaminum Hydrochloricum 12x, 30x, 200x, Sulphur 12x, 30x, 200x	**Adults & Peds ≥6 yrs:** Instill 1 spray per nostril q4h.

IS IT A COLD, THE FLU, OR AN ALLERGY?

	COLD	FLU	AIRBORNE ALLERGY
SYMPTOMS			
Chest discomfort	Mild to moderate	Common; can become severe	Sometimes
Cough	Common (hacking cough)	Sometimes	Sometimes
Duration	3-14 days	Days to weeks	Weeks (eg, 6 weeks for ragweed or grass pollen seasons)
Extreme exhaustion	Never	Early and prominent	Never
Fatigue, weakness	Sometimes	Can last up to 2-3 weeks	Sometimes
Fever	Rare	Characteristic, high (100-102°F); lasts 3-4 days	Never
General aches, pains	Slight	Usual; often severe	Never
Headache	Rare	Common	Sometimes
Itchy eyes	Rare or never	Rare or never	Common
Runny nose	Common		Common
Sneezing	Usual	Sometimes	Usual
Sore throat	Common	Sometimes	Sometimes
Stuffy nose	Common	Sometimes	Common
TREATMENT*			
	Antihistamines	Amantadine	Antihistamines
	Decongestants	Rimantadine	Nasal steroids
	Nonsteroidal anti-inflammatories	Oseltamivir	Decongestants
		Zanamivir	
PREVENTION			
	Wash your hands often; avoid close contact with anyone with a cold	Annual vaccination Amantadine Rimantadine Oseltamivir	Avoid allergens such as pollen, house flies, dust mites, mold, pet dander, cockroaches
COMPLICATIONS			
	Sinus infection	Bronchitis	Sinus infections
	Middle ear infection	Pneumonia	Asthma
	Asthma	Can be life-threatening	

Adapted from the National Institute of Allergy and Infectious Diseases, November 2008.

*Used only for temporary relief of cold symptoms.

Cough-Cold-Flu Products

BRAND NAME	ANALGESIC	ANTIHISTAMINE	DECONGESTANT	COUGH SUPPRESSANT	EXPECTORANT	DOSE
ANTIHISTAMINE + DECONGESTANT						
Actifed Cold & Allergy Tablets		Chlorpheniramine Maleate 4mg	Phenylephrine HCl 10mg			**Adults ≥12 yrs:** 1 tab q4-6h. **Max:** 6 doses q24h. **Peds 6-12 yrs:** ½ tab q4-6h. **Max:** 2 tabs q24h.
Benadryl-D Allergy/Sinus Tablets		Diphenhydramine HCl 25mg	Phenylephrine HCl 10mg			**Adults & Peds ≥12 yrs:** 1 tab q4h. **Max:** 6 tab q24h.
Children's Benadryl-D Allergy & Sinus Liquid		Diphenhydramine HCl 12.5mg/5mL	Phenylephrine HCl 5mg/5mL			**Adults ≥12 yrs:** 2 tsp (10mL) q4h. **Peds 6-12 yrs:** 1 tsp (5mL) q4h. **Max:** 6 doses q24h.
Dimetapp Children's Cold & Allergy Elixir		Brompheniramine Maleate 1mg/5mL	Phenylephrine HCl 2.5mg/5mL			**Adults & Peds ≥12 yrs:** 4 tsp q4h. **Peds 6-11 yrs:** 2 tsp q4h. **Max:** 6 doses q24h.
Dimetapp Nighttime Cold & Congestion Liquid		Diphenhydramine HCl 6.25mg/5mL	Phenylephrine HCl 2.5mg/5mL			**Adults & Peds ≥12 yrs:** 4 tsp q4h. **Peds 6-11 yrs:** 2 tsp q4h. **Max:** 6 doses q24h.
Dimetapp Children's Cold & Allergy Chewable Tablets		Brompheniramine Maleate 1mg	Phenylephrine HCl 2.5mg			**Peds 6-12 yrs:** 2 tabs q4h. **Max:** 6 doses q24h.
Pediacare Children's Allergy & Cold		Diphenhydramine HCl 12.5mg/5mL	Phenylephrine HCl 5mg/5mL			**Peds 6-11 yrs:** 1 tsp q4h. **Max:** 6 doses q24h.
Robitussin Night Time Cough & Cold Liquid		Diphenhydramine HCl 12.5mg/5mL	Phenylephrine HCl 2.5mg/5mL			**Adults & Peds ≥12 yrs:** 4 tsp q4h. **Max:** 6 doses q24h.
Sudafed Sinus & Allergy Tablets		Chlorpheniramine Maleate 4mg	Phenylephrine HCl 10mg			**Adults & Peds ≥12 yrs:** 1 tab q4h. **Max:** 6 doses q24h.
Sudafed PE Nighttime Nasal Decongestant Tablets		Diphenhydramine HCl 25mg	Phenylephrine HCl 10mg			**Adults & Peds ≥12 yrs:** 1 tab q4h. **Max:** 6 tabs q24h.
Theraflu Nighttime Cold & Cough Thin Strips		Diphenhydramine HCl 25mg/strips	Phenylephrine HCl 10mg/strip			**Adults ≥12 yrs:** 1 strip q4h. **Max:** 6 strips q24h.
Triaminic Cold & Allergy Liquid		Chlorpheniramine Maleate 1mg/5mL	Phenylephrine HCl 2.5mg/5mL			**Peds 6-12 yrs:** 2 tsp (10mL) q4h. **Max:** 6 doses q24h.

BRAND NAME	ANALGESIC	ANTIHISTAMINE	DECONGESTANT	COUGH SUPPRESSANT	EXPECTORANT	DOSE
Triaminic Nighttime Cough & Cold Liquid		Diphenhydramine HCl 6.25mg/5mL	Phenylephrine HCl 2.5mg/5mL			**Peds 6-12 yrs:** 2 tsp (10mL) q4h **Max:** 6 doses q24h.
Triaminic Nighttime Cough & Cold Thin Strips		Diphenhydramine HCl 12.5mg/strip	Phenylephrine HCl 5mg/strip			**Peds 6-12 yrs:** 1 strip q4h. **Max:** 6 strips q24h.
ANTIHISTAMINE + DECONGESTANT + ANALGESIC						
Advil Allergy Sinus Caplets	Ibuprofen 200mg	Chlorpheniramine Maleate 2mg	Pseudoephedrine HCl 30mg			**Adults & Peds ≥12 yrs:** 1 tab q4-6h. **Max:** 6 tabs q24h.
Alka-Seltzer Plus Cold Original Effervescent Tablets	Aspirin 325mg	Chlorpheniramine Maleate 2mg	Phenylephrine Bitartrate 7.8mg			**Adults & Peds ≥12 yrs:** 2 tabs q4h. **Max:** 8 tabs q24h.
Benadryl Allergy & Cold Caplets	Acetaminophen 325mg	Diphenhydramine HCl 12.5mg	Phenylephrine HCl 5mg			**Adults & Peds ≥12 yrs:** 2 tabs q4h. **Max:** 12 tabs q24h. **Peds 6-12 yrs:** 1 tab q4h. **Max:** 5 tabs q24h.
Benadryl Allergy & Sinus Headache Caplets	Acetaminophen 325mg	Diphenhydramine HCl 12.5mg	Phenylephrine HCl 5mg			**Adults & Peds ≥12 yrs:** 2 tabs q4h. **Max:** 12 tabs q24h. **Peds 6-12 yrs:** 1 tab q4h. **Max:** 5 tabs q24h.
Benadryl Severe Allergy & Sinus Headache Caplets	Acetaminophen 325mg	Diphenhydramine HCl 25mg	Phenylephrine HCl 5mg			**Adults & Peds ≥12 yrs:** 2 tabs q4h. **Max:** 12 tabs q24h.
Comtrex Day & Night Severe Cold & Sinus Caplets	Acetaminophen 325mg	Chlorpheniramine Maleate 2mg (nighttime dose only)	Phenylephrine HCl 5mg			**Adults & Peds ≥12 yrs:** *Daytime:* 2 daytime tabs q4h. **Max:** 8 daytime tabs q24h. *Nighttime:* 2 nighttime tabs q24h. **Max:** 4 nighttime tabs q24h.
Contac Cold & Flu Maximum Strength Caplets	Acetaminophen 500mg	Chlorpheniramine Maleate 2mg	Phenylephrine HCl 5mg			**Adults & Peds ≥12 yrs:** 2 tabs q4-6h **Max:** 8 tabs q24h.
Dristan Cold Multi-Symptom Tablets	Acetaminophen 325mg	Chlorpheniramine Maleate 2mg	Phenylephrine HCl 5mg			**Adults & Peds ≥12 yrs:** 2 tabs q4h. **Max:** 12 tabs q24h.
Sudafed PE Nighttime Cold Caplets	Acetaminophen 325mg	Diphenhydramine HCl 25mg	Phenylephrine HCl 5mg			**Adults & Peds ≥12 yrs:** 2 tabs q4h. **Max:** 12 tabs q24h.
Sudafed PE Severe Cold Formula Caplets	Acetaminophen 325mg	Diphenhydramine HCl 12.5mg	Phenylephrine HCl 5mg			**Adults & Peds ≥12 yrs:** 2 tabs q4h. **Max:** 12 tabs q24h. **Peds 6-11 yrs:** 1 cap q4h. **Max:** 5 tabs q24h.
Theraflu Cold & Sore Throat Hot Liquid	Acetaminophen 325mg/packet	Pheniramine Maleate 20mg/packet	Phenylephrine HCl 10mg/packet			**Adults & Peds ≥12 yrs:** 1 packet q4h. **Max:** 6 packets q24h.

(Continued)

BRAND NAME	ANALGESIC	ANTIHISTAMINE	DECONGESTANT	COUGH SUPPRESSANT	EXPECTORANT	DOSE
ANTIHISTAMINE + DECONGESTANT + ANALGESIC *(Continued)*						
Theraflu Nighttime Severe Cold & Cough Hot Liquid	Acetaminophen 325mg/packet	Diphenhydramine HCl 25mg/packet	Phenylephrine HCl 10mg/packet			**Adults & Peds ≥12 yrs:** 1 packet q4h. **Max:** 6 packets q24h.
Theraflu Sugar-Free Nighttime Severe Cold & Cough Hot Liquid	Acetaminophen 650mg/packet	Diphenhydramine HCl 25mg/packet	Phenylephrine HCl 10mg/packet			**Adults & Peds ≥12 yrs:** 1 packet q4h. **Max:** 6 packets q24h.
Theraflu Flu & Sore Throat Liquid	Acetaminophen 650mg/packet	Pheniramine Maleate 20mg/packet	Phenylephrine HCl 10mg/packet			**Adults & Peds ≥12 yrs:** 1 packet q4h. **Max:** 6 packets q24h.
Theraflu Nighttime Warming Relief Syrup	Acetaminophen 325mg/15mL	Diphenhydramine HCl 12.5mg/15mL	Phenylephrine HCl 5mg/15mL			**Adults & Peds ≥12 yrs:** 2 tbl (30mL) q4h. **Max:** 6 doses (12 tbl) q24h.
Theraflu Flu & Sore Throat Relief Syrup	Acetaminophen 325mg/15mL	Diphenhydramine HCl 12.5mg/15mL	Phenylephrine HCl 5mg/15mL			**Adults & Peds ≥12 yrs:** 2 tbl (30mL) q4h. **Max:** 6 doses (12 tbl) q24h.
Tylenol Children's Plus Cold Liquid	Acetaminophen 160mg/5mL	Chlorpheniramine Maleate 1mg/5mL	Phenylephrine HCl 2.5mg/5mL			**Peds 6-11 yrs (48-95 lbs):** 2 tsp (10mL) q4h. **Max:** 5 doses q24h.
Tylenol Children's Plus Cold and Allergy Liquid	Acetaminophen 160mg/5mL	Diphenhydramine HCl 12.5mg/5mL	Phenylephrine HCl 2.5mg/5mL			**Peds 6-11 yrs:** 2 tsp q4h. **Max:** 5 doses q24h.
Tylenol Sinus Congestion & Pain Nighttime Caplets	Acetaminophen 325mg	Chlorpheniramine Maleate 2mg	Phenylephrine HCl 5mg			**Adults & Peds ≥12 yrs:** 2 tabs q4h. **Max:** 12 tabs q24h.
Tylenol Allergy Multi-Symptom Gelcaps/Rapid-Release Gelcaps/Cool Burst Caplets	Acetaminophen 325mg	Chlorpheniramine Maleate 2mg	Phenylephrine HCl 5mg			**Adults & Peds ≥12 yrs:** 2 tabs q4h. **Max:** 12 tabs q24h.
Tylenol Allergy Multi-Symptom Nighttime Caplets	Acetaminophen 325mg	Diphenhydramine HCl 25mg	Phenylephrine HCl 5mg			**Adults & Peds ≥12 yrs:** 2 tabs q4h. **Max:** 12 tabs q24h.
Vicks NyQuil Sinus Liquicaps	Acetaminophen 325mg	Doxylamine Succinate 6.25mg	Phenylephrine HCl 5mg			**Adults & Peds ≥12 yrs:** 2 caps q4h. **Max:** 6 doses q24h.
COUGH SUPPRESSANT						
Delsym 12 Hour Cough Relief Liquid				Dextromethorphan HBr 30mg/5mL		**Adults & Peds ≥12 yrs:** 2 tsp q12h. **Max:** 4 tsp q24h. **Peds 6-11 yrs:** 1 tsp q12h. **Max:** 2 tsp q24h. **Peds 4-5 yrs:** ½ tsp q12h. **Max:** 1 dose q24h.

BRAND NAME	ANALGESIC	ANTIHISTAMINE	DECONGESTANT	COUGH SUPPRESSANT	EXPECTORANT	DOSE
COUGH SUPPRESSANT *(Continued)*						
PediaCare Long-Acting Cough Liquid				Dextromethorphan HBr 7.5mg/5mL		**Peds 6-11 yrs:** 2 tsp q6-8h. **Peds 4-5 yrs:** 1 tsp q6-8h. **Max:** 4 doses q24h.
Robitussin Cough Long-Acting Liquid				Dextromethorphan HBr 15mg/5mL		**Adults & Peds ≥12 yrs:** 2 tsp (10mL) q6-8h. **Max:** 8 tsp (40mL) q24h.
Robitussin CoughGels Liqui-gels				Dextromethorphan HBr 15mg		**Adults & Peds ≥12 yrs:** 2 caps q6-8h. **Max:** 8 caps q24h.
Robitussin Children's Cough Long-Acting Liquid				Dextromethorphan HBr 7.5mg/5mL		**Adults & Peds ≥12 yrs:** 4 tsp q6-8h. **Peds 6-11 yrs:** 2 tsp q6-8h. **Peds 4-5 yrs:** 1 tsp q6-8h. **Max:** 4 doses q24h.
Triaminic Long-Acting Cough Liquid				Dextromethorphan HBr 7.5mg/5mL		**Peds 6-11 yrs:** 2 tsp q6-8h. **Peds 4-5 yrs:** 1 tsp q6-8h. **Max:** 4 doses q24h.
Triaminic Thin Strips Long-Acting Cough				Dextromethorphan HBr 5.5mg/strip		**Peds 6-11 yrs:** 2 strips q6-8h. **Peds 4-5 yrs:** 1 strip q6-8h. **Max:** 4 doses q24h.
Vicks DayQuil Cough Liquid				Dextromethorphan HBr 15mg/15mL		**Adults & Peds ≥12 yrs:** 2 tbl (30mL) q6-8h. **Peds 6-12 yrs:** 1 tbl (15mL) q6-8h. **Max:** 4 doses q24h.
Vicks Formula 44 Custom Care Dry Cough Suppressant				Dextromethorphan HBr 30mg		**Adults & Peds ≥12 yrs:** 1 tbl q6-8h. **Peds 6-11 yrs:** 1-½ tsp q6-8h. **Max:** 4 doses q24h.
Vicks BabyRub				Eucalyptus, petrolatum, fragrance, aloe extract, eucalyptus oil, lavender oil, rosemary oil		**Peds:** Gently massage on the chest, neck, and back to help soothe and comfort.
Vicks Formula 44 Custom Care Sore Throat Lozenges				Menthol 10mg Benzocaine 10mg		**Adults & Peds >5 yrs:** 1 lozenge q2h.
Vicks VapoRub Cream				Camphor 5.2%, Menthol 2.8%, Eucalyptus 1.2%		**Adults & Peds ≥2 yrs:** Apply q8h.
Vicks VapoRub Ointment				Camphor 4.8%, Menthol 2.6%, Eucalyptus 1.2%		**Adults & Peds ≥2 yrs:** Apply q8h.
Vicks VapoSteam				Camphor 6.2%		**Adults & Peds ≥2 yrs:** 1 tbl/quart q8h.

(Continued)

BRAND NAME	ANALGESIC	ANTIHISTAMINE	DECONGESTANT	COUGH SUPPRESSANT	EXPECTORANT	DOSE
COUGH SUPPRESSANT + ANTIHISTAMINE						
Coricidin HBP Cough & Cold Tablets		Chlorpheniramine Maleate 4mg		Dextromethorphan HBr 30mg		**Adults & Peds ≥12 yrs:** 1 tab q6h. **Max:** 4 tabs q24h.
Dimetapp Children's Long-Acting Cold Plus Cough Elixir		Chlorpheniramine Maleate 1mg/5mL		Dextromethorphan HBr 7.5mg/5mL		**Peds ≥12 yrs:** 4 tsp (20mL) q6h. **6-12 yrs:** 2 tsp (10 mL) q6h. **Max:** 4 doses q24h.
Robitussin Cough & Cold Long-Acting Liquid		Chlorpheniramine Maleate 2mg/5mL		Dextromethorphan HBr 15mg/5mL		**Adults ≥12 yrs:** 2 tsp (10mL) q6h. **Max:** 4 doses q24h.
Robitussin Children's Cough & Cold Long-Acting Liquid		Chlorpheniramine Maleate 1mg/5mL		Dextromethorphan HBr 7.5mg/5mL		**Adults & Peds ≥12 yrs:** 4 tsp (20mL) q6h. **Peds 6-12 yrs:** 2 tsp (10mL) q6h. **Max:** 4 doses q24h.
Triaminic Softchews Cough and Runny Nose		Chlorpheniramine Maleate 1mg		Dextromethorphan HBr 5mg		**Peds 6-12 yrs:** 2 tabs q4-6h. **Max:** 5 doses q24h.
Vicks Children's NyQuil Liquid		Chlorpheniramine Maleate 2mg/15mL		Dextromethorphan HBr 15mg/15mL		**Adults ≥12 yrs:** 2 tbl (30mL) q6h. **Peds 6-11 yrs:** 1 tbl (15mL) q6h. **Max:** 4 doses q24h.
Vicks NyQuil Cough Liquid		Doxylamine Succinate 6.25mg/15mL		Dextromethorphan HBr 15mg/15mL		**Adults & Peds ≥12 yrs:** 2 tbl (30mL) q6h. **Max:** 8 tbl (120mL) q24h.
COUGH SUPPRESSANT + ANALGESIC						
Triaminic Cough & Sore Throat Liquid	Acetaminophen 160mg/5mL			Dextromethorphan HBr 5mg/5mL		**Peds 6-11 yrs:** 2 tsp q4h. **Peds 4-5 yrs:** 1 tsp q4h. **Max:** 5 doses q24h.
Triaminic Softchews Cough & Sore Throat	Acetaminophen 160mg			Dextromethorphan HBr 5mg		**Peds 6-11 yrs:** 2 tabs q4h. **Peds 4-5 yrs:** 1 tab q4h. **Max:** 5 doses q24h.
Tylenol Children's Plus Cough and Sore Throat Liquid	Acetaminophen 160mg/5mL			Dextromethorphan HBr 5mg/5mL		**Peds (48-95 lbs) 6-11 yrs:** 2 tsp q4h. **Peds (36-47 lbs) 4-5 yrs:** 1 tsp q4h. **Max:** 5 doses q24h.
Tylenol Cough & Sore Throat Daytime Liquid	Acetaminophen 1000mg/30mL			Dextromethorphan HBr 30mg/30mL		**Adults & Peds ≥12 yrs:** 2 tbl (30mL) q6h. **Max:** 8 tbl q24h.

BRAND NAME	ANALGESIC	ANTIHISTAMINE	DECONGESTANT	COUGH SUPPRESSANT	EXPECTORANT	DOSE
COUGH SUPPRESSANT + ANTIHISTAMINE + ANALGESIC						
Alka-Seltzer Plus Flu Effervescent Tablets	Aspirin 500mg	Chlorpheniramine Maleate 2mg		Dextromethorphan HBr 15mg		**Adults & Peds ≥12 yrs:** 2 tabs q6h. **Max:** 8 tabs q24h.
Tylenol Children's Plus Cough & Runny Nose Liquid	Acetaminophen 160mg/5mL	Chlorpheniramine Maleate 1mg/5mL		Dextromethorphan HBr 5mg/5mL		**Peds 6-11 yrs (48-95 lbs):** 2 tsp (10mL) q4h. **Max:** 5 doses q24h.
Coricidin HBP Maximum Strength Flu Tablets	Acetaminophen 500mg	Chlorpheniramine Maleate 2mg		Dextromethorphan HBr 15mg		**Adults & Peds ≥12 yrs:** 2 tabs q6h. **Max:** 8 tabs q24h.
Coricidin HBP Nighttime Multi-Symptom Cold Liquid	Acetaminophen 500mg/15mL	Doxylamine 6.25mg/15mL		Dextromethorphan HBr 15mg/15mL		**Adults & Peds ≥12 yrs:** 2 tbl q6h. **Max:** 4 doses q24h.
Triaminic Flu Cough & Fever Liquid	Acetaminophen 160mg/5mL	Chlorpheniramine Maleate 1mg/5mL		Dextromethorphan HBr 7.5mg/5mL		**Peds 6-12 yrs:** 2 tsp (10mL) q6h. **Max:** 4 doses (20mL) q24h.
Tylenol Cough & Sore Throat Nighttime Cool Burst/Honey Lemon Warming Liquid	Acetaminophen 1000mg/30mL	Doxylamine 12.5mg/30mL		Dextromethorphan HBr 30mg/30mL		**Adults & Peds ≥12 yrs:** 2 tbl q6h. **Max:** 16 tbl q24h.
Vicks Formula 44 Custom Care Cough & Cold PM	Acetaminophen 650mg/15mL	Chlorpheniramine Maleate 4mg/15mL		Dextromethorphan HBr 30mg/15mL		**Adults & Peds ≥12 yrs:** 1 tbl q6h. **Max:** 4 doses q24h.
Vicks NyQuil Liquicaps	Acetaminophen 325mg	Doxylamine Succinate 6.25mg		Dextromethorphan HBr 15mg		**Adults & Peds ≥12 yrs:** 2 caps q6h. **Max:** 8 caps q24h.
Vicks NyQuil Liquid	Acetaminophen 500mg/15mL	Doxylamine Succinate 6.25mg/15mL		Dextromethorphan HBr 15mg/15mL		**Adults & Peds ≥12 yrs:** 2 tbl (30mL) q6h. **Max:** 8 tbl (120mL) q24h.
COUGH SUPPRESSANT + ANTIHISTAMINE + ANALGESIC + DECONGESTANT						
Alka-Seltzer Plus Cough & Cold Liquid Gels	Acetaminophen 325mg	Chlorpheniramine Maleate 2mg	Phenylephrine HCl 5mg	Dextromethorphan HBr 10mg		**Adults & Peds ≥12 yrs:** 2 caps q4h. **Max:** 12 caps q24h.
Alka-Seltzer Plus Cough and Cold Effervescent Tablets	Aspirin 325mg	Chlorpheniramine Maleate 2mg	Phenylephrine Bitartrate 7.8mg	Dextromethorphan HBr 10mg		**Adults & Peds ≥12 yrs:** 2 tabs q4h. **Max:** 8 tabs q24h.
Alka-Seltzer Plus Night Cold Formula Liquid Gels	Acetaminophen 325mg	Doxylamine 6.25mg	Phenylephrine HCl 5mg	Dextromethorphan HBr 10mg		**Adults & Peds ≥12 yrs:** 2 caps q4h. **Max:** 12 caps q24h.
Alka-Seltzer Plus Cough & Cold Liquid	Acetaminophen 162.5mg/5mL	Chlorpheniramine Maleate 1mg/5mL	Phenylephrine HCl 2.5mg/5mL	Dextromethorphan HBr 5mg/5mL		**Adults & Peds ≥12 yrs:** 4 tsp q4h. **Max:** 24 tsp q24h.
Alka-Seltzer Plus Cold & Cough Formula Effervescent Tablets	Aspirin 325mg	Chlorpheniramine Maleate 2mg	Phenylephrine Bitartrate 7.8mg	Dextromethorphan HBr 10mg		**Adults & Peds ≥12 yrs:** 2 tabs q4h. **Max:** 8 tabs q24h.
Alka-Seltzer Plus Night Cold Liquid	Acetaminophen 162.5mg/5mL	Doxylamine Succinate 3.125/5mL	Phenylephrine HCl 2.5mg/5mL	Dextromethorphan HBr 5mg/5mL		**Adults & Peds ≥12 yrs:** 4 tsp q4h. **Max:** 24 tsp q24h.

(Continued)

BRAND NAME	ANALGESIC	ANTIHISTAMINE	DECONGESTANT	COUGH SUPPRESSANT	EXPECTORANT	DOSE
COUGH SUPPRESSANT + ANTIHISTAMINE + ANALGESIC + DECONGESTANT *(Continued)*						
Alka-Seltzer Plus Night Cold Formula Effervescent Tablets	Aspirin 500mg	Doxylamine 6.25mg	Phenylephrine Bitartrate 7.8mg	Dextromethorphan HBr 10mg		**Adults & Peds ≥12 yrs:** 2 tabs q4-6h. **Max:** 8 tabs q24h.
Comtrex Nighttime Cold & Cough Caplets	Acetaminophen 325mg	Chlorpheniramine Maleate 2mg	Phenylephrine HCl 5mg	Dextromethorphan HBr 10mg		**Adults & Peds ≥12 yrs:** 2 tabs q6h. **Max:** 8 tabs q24h.
Robitussin Night Time Cough, Cold & Flu Liquid	Acetaminophen 160mg/5mL	Chlorpheniramine Maleate 1mg/5mL	Phenylephrine HCl 2.5mg/5mL	Dextromethorphan HBr 5mg/5mL		**Adults & Peds ≥12 yrs:** 4 tsp q4h. **Max:** 5 doses q24h.
Theraflu Nighttime Severe Cold & Cough Caplets	Acetaminophen 325mg	Chlorpheniramine Maleate 2mg	Phenylephrine HCl 5mg	Dextromethorphan HBr 10mg		**Adults & Peds ≥12 yrs:** 2 tabs q4h. **Max:** 12 tabs q24h.
Tylenol Children's Plus Multisymptom Cold Liquid	Acetaminophen 160mg/5mL	Chlorpheniramine Maleate 1mg/5mL	Phenylephrine HCl 2.5mg/5mL	Dextromethorphan HBr 5mg/5mL		**Peds 6-11 yrs (48-95 lbs):** 2 tsp (10mL) q4h. **Max:** 5 doses q24h.
Tylenol Children's Plus Flu Liquid	Acetaminophen 160mg/5mL	Chlorpheniramine Maleate 1mg/5mL	Phenylephrine HCl 2.5mg/5mL	Dextromethorphan HBr 5mg/5mL		**Peds 6-11 yrs (48-95 lbs):** 2 tsp (10mL) q4h. **Max:** 5 doses q24h.
Tylenol Cold Head Congestion Nighttime Caplets	Acetaminophen 325mg	Chlorpheniramine Maleate 2mg	Phenylephrine HCl 5mg	Dextromethorphan HBr 10mg		**Adults & Peds ≥12 yrs:** 2 tabs q4h. **Max:** 12 tabs q24h.
Tylenol Cold Multi-Symptom Nighttime Caplets	Acetaminophen 325mg	Chlorpheniramine Maleate 2mg	Phenylephrine HCl 5mg	Dextromethorphan HBr 10mg		**Adults & Peds ≥12 yrs:** 2 tabs q4h. **Max:** 12 tabs q24h.
Tylenol Cold Multi-Symptom Nighttime Liquid	Acetaminophen 325mg/15mL	Doxylamine 6.25mg/30mL	Phenylephrine HCl 5mg/15mL	Dextromethorphan HBr 10mg/15mL		**Adults & Peds ≥12 yrs:** 2 tbl (30mL) q4h. **Max:** 12 tbl (180mL) q24h.
Vicks NyQuil D Liquid	Acetaminophen 500mg/15mL	Doxylamine 6.25mg/15mL	Pseudoephedrine HCl 30mg/15mL	Dextromethorphan HBr 15mg/15mL		**Adults & Peds ≥12 yrs:** 2 tbl (30mL) q6h. **Max:** 4 doses q24h.
COUGH SUPPRESSANT + ANTIHISTAMINE + DECONGESTANT						
Dimetapp DM Children's Cold & Cough Elixir		Brompheniramine Maleate 1mg/5mL	Phenylephrine HCl 2.5mg/5mL	Dextromethorphan HBr 5mg/5mL		**Adults ≥12 yrs:** 4 tsp (20mL) q4h. **Peds 6–12 yrs:** 2 tsp (10mL) q4h. **Max:** 6 doses q24h.
Theraflu Cold & Cough Hot Liquid		Pheniramine Maleate 20mg/packet	Phenylephrine HCl 10mg/packet	Dextromethorphan HBr 20mg/packet		**Adults & Peds ≥12 yrs:** 1 packet q4h. **Max:** 6 packets q24h.
Triaminic-D Multi-Symptom Cold		Chlorpheniramine Maleate 1mg/5mL	Pseudoephedrine HCl 15mg/5mL	Dextromethorphan HBr 7.5mg/5mL		**Peds 6-11 yrs:** 2 tsp q6h. **Max:** 4 doses q24h.

BRAND NAME	ANALGESIC	ANTIHISTAMINE	DECONGESTANT	COUGH SUPPRESSANT	EXPECTORANT	DOSE
COUGH SUPPRESSANT + DECONGESTANT						
PediaCare Children's Multi-Symptom Cold Liquid			Phenylephrine HCl 2.5mg/5mL	Dextromethorphan HBr 5mg/5mL		**Peds 6-11 yrs:** 2 tsp q4h. **Peds 4-5 yrs:** 1 tsp q4h. **Max:** 6 doses q24h.
Sudafed PE Children's Cold & Cough Liquid			Phenylephrine HCl 2.5mg/5mL	Dextromethorphan HBr 5mg/5mL		**Peds 6-11 yrs:** 2 tsp q4h. **Peds 4-5 yrs:** 1 tsp q4h. **Max:** 6 doses q24h.
Theraflu Daytime Cold & Cough Thin Strips			Phenylephrine HCl 10mg/strip	Dextromethorphan HBr 20mg/strip		**Adults & Peds ≥12 yrs:** 1 strip q4h. **Max:** 6 strips q24h.
Triaminic Day Time Cold & Cough Liquid			Phenylephrine HCl 2.5mg/5mL	Dextromethorphan HBr 5mg/5mL		**Peds 6-11 yrs:** 2 tsp q4h. **Peds 4-5 yrs:** 1 tsp q4h. **Max:** 6 doses q24h.
Triaminic Night Time Thin Strips Cough & Congestion			Phenylephrine HCl 5mg/strip	Dextromethorphan HBr 5mg/strip		**Peds 6-11 yrs:** 1 strip q4h. **Max:** 6 doses q24h.
Vicks Formula 44 Custom Care Congestion			Phenylephrine HCl 10mg/15mL	Dextromethorphan HBr 20mg/15mL		**Adults & Peds ≥12 yrs:** 1 tbl q4h. **Peds 6-11 yrs:** 1-½ tsp q4h. **Max:** 6 doses q24h.
COUGH SUPPRESSANT + DECONGESTANT + ANALGESIC						
Alka-Seltzer Plus Day Cold Liquid Gels	Acetaminophen 325mg		Phenylephrine HCl 5mg	Dextromethorphan HBr 10mg		**Adults & Peds ≥12 yrs:** 2 caps q4h. **Max:** 12 caps q24h.
Alka-Seltzer Plus Day & Night Liquid Gels	Acetaminophen 325mg		Phenylephrine HCl 5mg	Dextromethorphan HBr 10mg		**Adults & Peds ≥12 yrs:** 2 caps q4h. **Max:** 12 caps q24h.
Alka-Seltzer Plus Day & Night Effervescent Tablets	Acetaminophen 250mg		Phenylephrine Bitartrate 7.8mg	Dextromethorphan HBr 10mg		**Adults & Peds ≥12 yrs:** 2 tabs q4h. **Max:** 8 tabs q24h.
Comtrex Non-Drowsy Cold & Cough	Acetaminophen 325mg		Phenylephrine HCl 5mg	Dextromethorphan HBr 10mg		**Adults & Peds ≥12 yrs:** 2 tabs q4h. **Max:** 12 tabs q24h.
Theraflu Daytime Severe Cold & Cough Caplets	Acetaminophen 325mg		Phenylephrine HCl 5mg	Dextromethorphan HBr 10mg		**Adults & Peds ≥12 yrs:** 2 tabs q4h. **Max:** 12 tabs q24h.
Theraflu Daytime Severe Cold & Cough Hot Liquid	Acetaminophen 650mg/packet		Phenylephrine HCl 10mg/packet	Dextromethorphan HBr 20mg/packet		**Adults & Peds ≥12 yrs:** 1 pkt q4h. **Max:** 6 pkts q24h.

(Continued)

BRAND NAME	ANALGESIC	ANTIHISTAMINE	DECONGESTANT	COUGH SUPPRESSANT	EXPECTORANT	DOSE
COUGH SUPPRESSANT + DECONGESTANT + ANALGESIC *(Continued)*						
Theraflu Daytime Severe Cold Caplets	Acetaminophen 325mg		Phenylephrine HCl 5mg	Dextromethorphan HBr 15mg		**Adults & Peds ≥12 yrs:** 2 tabs q6h. **Max:** 8 tabs q24h.
Tylenol Cold Head Congestion Daytime Capsules	Acetaminophen 325mg		Phenylephrine HCl 5mg	Dextromethorphan HBr 10mg		**Adults & Peds ≥12 yrs:** 2 caps q4h. **Max:** 12 caps q24h.
Tylenol Cold Head Congestion Day/Night Pack	Acetaminophen 325mg		Phenylephrine HCl 5mg	Dextromethorphan HBr 10mg		**Adults & Peds ≥12 yrs:** 2 caps q4h. **Max:** 12 caps q24h.
Tylenol Cold Multi-Symptom Daytime Rapid-Release Gelcaps/ Citrus Burst Liquid/Gelcaps/Cool Burst Caplets	Acetaminophen 325mg		Phenylephrine HCl 5mg	Dextromethorphan HBr 10mg		**Adults & Peds ≥12 yrs:** 2 caps q4h. **Max:** 12 caps q24h.
Tylenol Cold Multi-Symptom Daytime Citrus Burst Liquid	Acetaminophen 325mg/15mL		Phenylephrine HCl 5mg/15mL	Dextromethorphan HBr 10mg/15mL		**Adults & Peds ≥12 yrs:** 2 tbl (30mL) q4h. **Max:** 6 doses (12 tbl) q24h.
Tylenol Cold Multi-Symptom Day/Night Pack	Acetaminophen 325mg		Phenylephrine HCl 5mg	Dextromethorphan HBr 10mg		**Adults & Peds ≥12 yrs:** 2 caps q4h. **Max:** 12 caps q24h.
Vicks DayQuil Liquicaps	Acetaminophen 325mg		Phenylephrine HCl 5mg	Dextromethorphan HBr 10mg		**Adults & Peds ≥12 yrs:** 2 caps q4h. **Max:** 6 caps q24h.
Vicks DayQuil Cold & Flu Relief Liquid	Acetaminophen 325mg/15mL		Phenylephrine HCl 5mg/15mL	Dextromethorphan HBr 10mg/15mL		**Adults & Peds ≥12 yrs:** 2 tbl q4h. **Max:** 6 doses q24h. **Peds 6-11 yrs:** 1 tbl q4h. **Max:** 5 doses q24h.
COUGH SUPPRESSANT + DECONGESTANT + EXPECTORANT						
Robitussin Cold & Cough CF Liquid			Phenylephrine HCl 5mg/5mL	Dextromethorphan HBr 10mg/5mL	Guaifenesin 100mg/5mL	**Adults & Peds ≥12 yrs:** 2 tsp q4h. **Max:** 6 doses q24h.
Robitussin Cough & Cold D			Pseudoephedrine HCl 30mg/5mL	Dextromethorphan HBr 10mg/5mL	Guaifenesin 100mg/5mL	**Adults & Peds ≥12 yrs:** 2 tsp q4h. **Max:** 4 doses q24h.
COUGH SUPPRESSANT + DECONGESTANT + EXPECTORANT + ANALGESIC						
Sudafed PE Cold & Cough Caplets	Acetaminophen 325mg		Phenylephrine HCl 5mg	Dextromethorphan HBr 10mg	Guaifenesin 100mg	**Adults & Peds ≥12 yrs:** 2 tabs q4h. **Max:** 12 tabs q24h.
Tylenol Cold Multi-Symptom Severe Liquid	Acetaminophen 325mg/15mL		Phenylephrine HCl 5mg/15mL	Dextromethorphan HBr 10mg/15mL	Guaifenesin 200mg/15mL	**Adults & Peds ≥12 yrs:** 2 tbl q4h. **Max:** 12 tbl q24h.
Tylenol Cold Multi-Symptom Severe Caplets	Acetaminophen 325mg		Phenylephrine HCl 5mg	Dextromethorphan HBr 10mg	Guaifenesin 200mg	**Adults & Peds ≥12 yrs:** 2 tabs q4h. **Max:** 12 tabs q24h.
Tylenol Severe Head Congestion Caplets	Acetaminophen 325mg		Phenylephrine HCl 5mg	Dextromethorphan HBr 10mg	Guaifenesin 200mg	**Adults & Peds ≥12 yrs:** 2 tabs q4h. **Max:** 12 tabs q24h.

BRAND NAME	ANALGESIC	ANTIHISTAMINE	DECONGESTANT	COUGH SUPPRESSANT	EXPECTORANT	DOSE
COUGH SUPPRESSANT & EXPECTORANT						
Alka-Seltzer Plus Mucus & Congestion Effervescent Tablets				Dextromethorphan HBr 10mg	Guaifenesin 200mg	**Adults & Peds ≥12 yrs:** 2 tabs q4h. **Max:** 8 tabs q24h.
Coricidin HBP Chest Congestion & Cough Softgels				Dextromethorphan HBr 10mg	Guaifenesin 200mg	**Adults & Peds ≥12 yrs:** 1-2 caps q4h. **Max:** 12 caps q24h.
Mucinex Cough Mini-Melts (Orange Crème)				Dextromethorphan HBr 5mg	Guaifenesin 100mg	**Adults & Peds ≥12 yrs:** 2-4 pkts q4h. **Peds 6-11 yrs:** 1-2 pkts q4h. **Peds 4-6 yrs:** 1 pkt q4h.
Mucinex DM Extended-Release Tablets				Dextromethorphan HBr 30mg	Guaifenesin 600mg	**Adults & Peds ≥12 yrs:** 1-2 tabs q12h. **Max:** 4 tabs q24h.
Robitussin Cough & Chest Congestion DM Max Liquid				Dextromethorphan HBr 10mg/5mL	Guaifenesin 200mg/5mL	**Adults & Peds ≥12 yrs:** 2 tsp q4h. **Max:** 6 doses q24h.
Robitussin Cough & Chest Congestion DM Liquid				Dextromethorphan HBr 10mg/5mL	Guaifenesin 100mg/5mL	**Adults & Peds ≥12 yrs:** 2 tsp q4h. **Max:** 6 doses q24h.
Robitussin Cough & Chest Congestion Sugar-Free DM				Dextromethorphan HBr 10mg/5mL	Guaifenesin 100mg/5mL	**Adults & Peds ≥12 yrs:** 2 tsp q4h. **Max:** 6 doses q24h.
Vicks Formula 44 Custom Care Chesty Cough				Dextromethorphan HBr 20mg/15mL	Guaifenesin 200mg/15mL	**Adults & Peds ≥12 yrs:** 1 tbl q4h. **Peds 6-11 yrs:** 1½ tsp q4h. **Max:** 6 doses q24h.
Vicks Formula 44e Pediatric Cough & Chest Congestion Relief Liquid				Dextromethorphan HBr 10mg/15mL	Guaifenesin 100mg/15mL	**Adults & Peds ≥12 yrs:** 2 tbl q4h. **Peds 6-11 yrs:** 1 tbl q4h. **Peds 4-5 yrs:** ½ tbl q4h. **Max:** 6 doses q24h.
DECONGESTANT						
Contac-D Cold Decongestant Tablets			Phenylephrine HCl 10mg			**Adults & Peds ≥12 yrs:** 1 tabs q4h. **Max:** 6 tabs q24h.
PediaCare Children's Decongestant Liquid			Phenylephrine HCl 2.5mg/5mL			**Peds 6-11 yrs:** 2 tsp q4h. **Peds 4-5 yrs:** 1 tsp q4h. **Max:** 6 doses q24h.
Sudafed 12-Hour Tablets			Pseudoephedrine HCl 120mg			**Adults & Peds ≥12 yrs:** 1 tab q12h. **Max:** 2 tabs q24h.
Sudafed 24-Hour Tablets			Pseudoephedrine HCl 240mg			**Adults & Peds ≥12 yrs:** 1 tab q24h. **Max:** 1 tab q24h.

(Continued)

BRAND NAME	ANALGESIC	ANTIHISTAMINE	DECONGESTANT	COUGH SUPPRESSANT	EXPECTORANT	DOSE
DECONGESTANT *(Continued)*						
Sudafed Children's Nasal Decongestant Liquid			Pseudoephedrine HCl 15mg/5mL			**Peds 6-11 yrs:** 2 tsp q4-6h. **Peds 4-5 yrs:** 1 tsp q4-6h. **Max:** 4 doses q24h.
Sudafed OM Sinus Cold Nasal Spray			Oxymetazoline HCl 0.05%			**Adults & Peds ≥12 yrs:** 2-3 sprays q10-12h. **Max:** 2 doses q24h.
Sudafed OM Sinus Congestion Nasal Spray			Oxymetazoline HCl 0.05%			**Adults & Peds ≥12 yrs:** 2-3 sprays q10-12h. **Max:** 2 doses q24h.
Sudafed PE Nasal Decongestant Tablets			Phenylephrine HCl 10mg			**Adults & Peds ≥12 yrs:** 1 tab q4h. **Max:** 6 tabs q24h.
Sudafed PE Children's Nasal Decongestant Liquid			Phenylephrine HCl 2.5mg/5mL			**Peds 6-11 yrs:** 2 tsp q4h. **Peds 4-5 yrs:** 1 tsp q4h. **Max:** 6 doses q24h.
Sudafed Nasal Decongestant Tablets			Pseudoephedrine HCl 30mg			**Adults ≥12 yrs:** 2 tabs q4-6h. **Peds 6-12 yrs:** 1 tab q4-6h. **Max:** 4 doses q24h.
Triaminic Thin Strips Cold with Stuffy Nose			Phenylephrine HCl 2.5mg/strip			**Peds 6-11 yrs:** 2 strips q4h. **Peds 4-5 yrs:** 1 strip q4h. **Max:** 6 doses q24h.
Triaminic Decongestant Spray Nasal & Sinus Congestion			Xylometazoline HCl 0.05%			**Peds 2-11 yrs:** 1-2 sprays q8-10h. **Max:** 3 doses q24h.
Vicks Sinex 12-Hour Nasal Spray			Oxymetazoline HCl 0.05%			**Adults & Peds ≥6 yrs:** 2-3 sprays q10-12h. **Max:** 2 doses q24h.
Vicks Sinex Nasal Spray			Phenylephrine HCl 0.5%			**Adults & Peds ≥12 yrs:** 2-3 sprays q4h. **Max:** 18 sprays q24h.
Vicks Sinex UltraFine Mist			Phenylephrine HCl 0.5%			**Adults & Peds ≥12 yrs:** 2-3 sprays q4h. **Max:** 18 sprays q24h.
Vicks Vapor Inhaler			Levmetamfetamine 50mg			**Adults ≥12 yrs:** 2 inhalations q2h. **Max:** 24 inhalations q24h **Peds 6-12 yrs:** 1 inhalation q2h. **Max:** 12 inhalations q24h.

BRAND NAME	ANALGESIC	ANTIHISTAMINE	DECONGESTANT	COUGH SUPPRESSANT	EXPECTORANT	DOSE
DECONGESTANT + ANALGESIC						
Advil Children's Cold Liquid	Ibuprofen 100mg/5mL		Pseudoephedrine HCl 15mg/5mL			**Peds 6-11 yrs (48-95 lbs):** 2 tsp (10mL) q6h. **2-5 yrs (24-47 lbs):** 1 tsp (5mL) q6h. **Max:** 4 doses q24h
Advil Cold & Sinus Caplets/Liqui-gels	Ibuprofen 200mg		Pseudoephedrine HCl 30mg			**Adults & Peds ≥12 yrs:** 1-2 caps q4-6h. **Max:** 6 caps q24h.
Alka-Seltzer Plus Sinus Formula Effervescent Tablets	Aspirin 325mg		Phenylephrine Bitartrate 7.8mg			**Adults & Peds ≥12 yrs:** 2 tabs q4h. **Max:** 8 tab q24h.
Contac Cold & Flu Day & Night Caplets	Acetaminophen 500mg		Phenylephrine HCl 5mg			**Adults & Peds ≥12 yrs:** 2 tabs q4-6h. **Max:** 8 tabs q24h.
Contac Cold & Flu Non-Drowsy Maximum Strength Caplets	Acetaminophen 500mg		Phenylephrine HCl 5mg			**Adults & Peds ≥12 yrs:** 2 tabs q4-6h. **Max:** 8 tabs q24h.
Motrin Children's Cold Suspension	Ibuprofen 100mg/5mL		Pseudoephedrine HCl 15mg/5mL			**Peds 6-12 yrs (48-95 lbs):** 2 tsp (10mL) q6h. **2-6 yrs (24-47 lbs):** 1 tsp (5mL) q6h. **Max:** 4 doses q24h.
Sinutab Sinus Tablets	Acetaminophen 325mg		Phenylephrine HCl 5mg			**Adults & Peds ≥12 yrs:** 2 tabs q4h. **Max:** 12 tabs q24h.
Sudafed PE Sinus Headache Caplets	Acetaminophen 325mg		Phenylephrine HCl 5mg			**Adults & Peds ≥12 yrs:** 2 tabs q4h. **Max:** 12 tabs q24h.
Tylenol Sinus Congestion & Pain Daytime Rapid-Release Gelcaps/Gelcaps/Cool Burst Caplets	Acetaminophen 325mg		Phenylephrine HCl 5mg			**Adults & Peds ≥12 yrs:** 2 caps q4h. **Max:** 12 caps q24h.
Vicks DayQuil Sinus Liquicaps	Acetaminophen 325mg		Phenylephrine HCl 5mg			**Adults & Peds ≥12 yrs:** 2 caps q4h. **Max:** 6 caps q24h.
DECONGESTANT + EXPECTORANT						
Mucinex Cold Liquid (Mixed Berry)			Phenylephrine HCl 2.5mg		Guaifenesin 100mg	**Peds 6-12 yrs:** 2 tsp q4h. **Peds 4-5 yrs:** 1 tsp q4h. **Max:** 6 doses q24h.
Mucinex D Extended-Release Tablets			Pseudoephedrine HCl 60mg		Guaifenesin 600mg	**Adults & Peds ≥12 yrs:** 2 tabs q12h. **Max:** 4 tabs q24h.
Sudafed PE Non-Drying Sinus Caplets			Phenylephrine HCl 5mg		Guaifenesin 200mg	**Adults & Peds ≥12 yrs:** 2 tabs q4h. **Max:** 12 tabs q24h.

(Continued)

BRAND NAME	ANALGESIC	ANTIHISTAMINE	DECONGESTANT	COUGH SUPPRESSANT	EXPECTORANT	DOSE
DECONGESTANT + EXPECTORANT *(Continued)*						
Triaminic Chest & Nasal Congestion			Phenylephrine HCl 2.5mg/5mL		Guaifenesin 50mg/5mL	**Peds 6-11 yrs:** 2 tsp q 4h. **Peds 4-5 yrs:** 1 tsp q4h. **Max:** 6 doses q24h.
DECONGESTANT + EXPECTORANT + ANALGESIC						
Theraflu Cold & Chest Congestion Warming Relief	Acetaminophen 325mg/15mL		Phenylephrine HCl 5mg/15mL		Guaifenesin 200mg/15mL	**Adults & Peds ≥12 yrs:** 2 tbl q4h. **Max:** 6 doses q24h.
Tylenol Sinus Congestion & Severe Pain Caplets	Acetaminophen 325mg		Phenylephrine HCl 5mg		Guaifenesin 200mg	**Adults & Peds ≥12 yrs:** 2 caps q4h. **Max:** 12 caps q24h.
Tylenol Sinus Severe Congestion Daytime Cool Burst Capsules	Acetaminophen 325mg		Pseudoephedrine HCl 30mg		Guaifenesin 200mg	**Adults & Peds ≥12 yrs:** 2 caps q6h. **Max:** 8 caps q24h.
EXPECTORANT						
Mucinex Extended-Release Tablets					Guaifenesin 600mg	**Adults & Peds ≥12 yrs:** 1-2 tabs q12h. **Max:** 4 tabs q24h.
Mucinex Kids Mini-Melts (Bubble Gum and Grape)					Guaifenesin 100mg	**Adults & Peds ≥12 yrs:** 2-4 packets q4h. **Peds 6-11 yrs:** 1-2 packets q4h. **Peds 4-5 yrs:** 1 packet q4h. **Max:** 6 doses q24h.
Mucinex Maximum Strength					Guaifenesin 1200mg	**Adults & Peds ≥12 yrs:** 1 tab q12h.
Robitussin Chest Congestion					Guaifenesin 100mg/5mL	**Adults ≥12 yrs:** 2-4 tsp q4h. **Max:** 6 doses q24h.
EXPECTORANT + ANALGESIC						
Comtrex Deep Chest Cold Caplets	Acetaminophen 325mg				Guaifenesin 200mg	**Adults & Peds ≥12 yrs:** 2 tabs q4-6h. **Max:** 12 tabs q24h.
Tylenol Chest Congestion Caplets	Acetaminophen 325mg				Guaifenesin 200mg	**Adults & Peds ≥12 yrs:** 2 tabs q4-6h. **Max:** 12 tabs q24h.
Tylenol Chest Congestion Liquid	Acetaminophen 500mg/15mL				Guaifenesin 200mg/15mL	**Adults & Peds ≥12 yrs:** 2 tbl (30mL) q4-6h. **Max:** 8 tbl (120mL) q24h.
Theraflu Flu & Chest Liquid	Acetaminophen 1000mg/packet				Guaifenesin 400mg/packet	**Adults & Peds ≥12 yrs:** 1 packet q6h. **Max:** 4 packets q24h.

BRAND NAME	ANALGESIC	ANTIHISTAMINE	DECONGESTANT	COUGH SUPPRESSANT	EXPECTORANT	DOSE
EXPECTORANT + DECONGESTANT + ANALGESIC						
Robitussin Cough & Cold D			Pseudoephedrine HCl 30mg	Dextromethorphan HBr 10mg	Guaifenesin 100mg	**Adults & Peds ≥12 yrs:** 2 tsp q4h. **Max:** 4 doses q24h.
Tylenol Sinus Congestion & Severe Pain Caplets	Acetaminophen 325mg		Phenylephrine HCl 5mg		Guaifenesin 200mg	**Adults & Peds ≥12 yrs:** 2 tabs q4h. **Max:** 12 tabs q24h.
ANTIHISTAMINE + ANALGESIC						
Coricidin Cold & Flu Tablets	Acetaminophen 325mg	Chlorpheniramine Maleate 2mg				**Adults & Peds ≥12 yrs:** 2 tabs q4–6h. **Max:** 12 tabs q24h.
Tylenol Severe Allergy Caplets	Acetaminophen 500mg	Diphenhydramine HCl 12.5mg				**Adults & Peds ≥12 yrs:** 2 tabs q4–6h. **Max:** 8 tabs q24h.
Tylenol Sore Throat Nighttime Liquid	Acetaminophen 1000mg/30mL	Diphenhydramine HCl 50mg/30mL				**Adults & Peds ≥12 yrs:** 2 tbl q4-6h. **Max:** 8 tbl (120mL) q24h.

NASAL DECONGESTANT/MOISTURIZING PRODUCTS

BRAND	INGREDIENT/STRENGTH	DOSE
PSEUDOEPHEDRINE		
Sudafed 12 Hour Tablets	Pseudoephedrine HCl 120mg	**Adults & Peds ≥12 yrs:** 1 tab q12h. **Max:** 2 tabs/day.
Sudafed 24 Hour Tablets	Pseudoephedrine HCl 240mg	**Adults & Peds ≥12 yrs:** 1 tab q24h. **Max:** 1 tab/day.
Sudafed Children's Nasal Decongestant Liquid	Pseudoephedrine HCl 15mg/5mL	**Peds 6-11 yrs:** 2 tsp q4-6h. **4-5 yrs:** 1 tsp q4-6h. **Max:** 4 doses q24h.
Sudafed Nasal Decongestant Tablets	Pseudoephedrine HCl 30mg	**Adults ≥12 yrs:** 2 tabs q4-6h. **Peds 6-12 yrs:** 1 tab q4-6h. **Max:** 4 doses/day.
PHENYLEPHRINE		
Pediacare Children's Decongestant Liquid	Phenylephrine 2.5/5mL	**Peds 6-11 yrs:** 2 tsp q4h. **4-5 yrs:** 1 tsp q4h. **Max:** 6 doses q24h.
Sudafed PE	Phenylephrine 10mg	**Adults & Peds ≥12 yrs:** 1 tablet every 4 hours. **Max:** 6 tabs per day.
TOPICAL NASAL DECONGESTANTS		
4-Way Fast Acting Nasal Decongestant Spray	Phenylephrine HCl 1%	**Adults & Peds ≥12 yrs:** Instill 2-3 sprays per nostril q4h.
4-Way Mentholated Nasal Decongestant Spray	Phenylephrine HCl 1%	**Adults & Peds ≥12 yrs:** Instill 2-3 sprays per nostril q4h.
Afrin No Drip Extra Moisturizing Nasal Spray	Oxymetazoline HCl 0.05%	**Adults & Peds ≥6 yrs:** Instill 2-3 sprays per nostril q10-12h. **Max:** 2 doses q24h.
Afrin No Drip Sinus Nasal Spray	Oxymetazoline HCl 0.05%	**Adults & Peds ≥6 yrs:** Instill 2-3 sprays per nostril q10-12h. **Max:** 2 doses q24h.
Afrin No-Drip Original Pump Mist Nasal Spray	Oxymetazoline HCl 0.05%	**Adults & Peds ≥6 yrs:** Instill 2-3 sprays per nostril q10-12h. **Max:** 2 doses q24h.
Afrin No Drip Severe Congestion Nasal Spray	Oxymetazoline HCl 0.05%	**Adults & Peds ≥6 yrs:** Instill 2-3 sprays per nostril q10-12h. **Max:** 2 doses q24h.
Afrin No Drip All Night 12 Hour Pump Mist	Oxymetazoline HCl 0.05%	**Adults & Peds ≥6 yrs:** Instill 2-3 sprays per nostril q10-12h. **Max:** 2 doses q24h.
Benzedrex Inhaler	Propylhexedrine 250 mg	**Adults & Peds ≥6 yrs:** Inhale 2 sprays per nostril q2h.
Dristan 12 Hour Nasal Spray	Oxymetazoline HCl 0.05%	**Adults & Peds ≥12 yrs:** Instill 2-3 sprays per nostril q10-12h. **Max:** 2 doses q24h.
Mucinex Full Force Nasal Spray	Oxymetazoline HCl 0.05%	**Adults & Peds ≥6 yrs:** Instill 2-3 sprays per nostril q10-12h. **Max:** 2 doses q24h.
Neo-Synephrine Nighttime Nasal Spray	Oxymetazoline HCl 0.05%	**Adults & Peds ≥6 yrs:** Instill 2-3 sprays per nostril q10-12h. **Max:** 2 doses q24h.
Neo-Synephrine Extra Strength Nasal Spray	Phenylephrine HCl 1%	**Adults & Peds ≥12 yrs:** Instill 2-3 sprays per nostril q4h.
Neo-Synephrine Mild Formula Nasal Spray	Phenylephrine HCl 0.25%	**Adults & Peds ≥6 yrs:** Instill 2-3 sprays per nostril q4h.
Neo-Synephrine Regular Strength Nasal Decongestant Spray	Phenylephrine HCl 0.5%	**Adults & Peds ≥12 yrs:** Instill 2-3 sprays per nostril q4h.
Nostrilla Complete Congestion Relief	Oxymetazoline HCl 0.05%	**Adults & Peds ≥6 yrs:** Instill 2-3 sprays per nostril q10-12h. **Max:** 2 doses q24h.

(Continued)

BRAND	INGREDIENT/STRENGTH	DOSE
TOPICAL NASAL DECONGESTANTS *(Continued)*		
Nostrilla Original Fast Relief	Oxymetazoline HCl 0.05%	**Adults & Peds ≥6 yrs:** Instill 2-3 sprays per nostril q10-12h. **Max:** 2 doses q24h.
Sudafed Sinus Congestion 12 Hour Nasal Spray	Oxymetazoline 0.05%	**Adults & Peds ≥6 yrs:** Spray 2-3 sprays per nostril q10-12h. **Max:** 2 doses q24h.
Sudafed Sinus Cold 12 Hour Nasal Spray	Oxymetazoline 0.05%	**Adults & Peds ≥6 yrs:** Spray 2-3 sprays per nostril q10-12h. **Max:** 2 doses q24h.
Vicks Sinex 12 Hour Ultra Fine Mist For Sinus Relief	Phenylephrine HCl 0.05%	**Adults & Peds ≥12 yrs:** Instill 2-3 sprays per nostril q10-12h.
Vicks Sinex 12 Hour Nasal Spray	Oxymetazoline HCl 0.05%	**Adults & Peds ≥6 yrs:** Instill 2-3 sprays per nostril q10-12h. **Max:** 2 doses q24h.
Vicks Sinex Nasal Spray For Sinus Relief	Phenylephrine HCl 0.5%	**Adults & Peds ≥12 yrs:** Instill 2-3 sprays per nostril q4h.
Zicam Extreme Congestion Relief	Oxymetazoline HCl 0.05%	**Adults & Peds ≥12 yrs:** Instill 2-3 sprays per nostril q10-12h. **Max:** 2 doses q24h.
Zicam Intense Sinus Relief	Oxymetazoline HCl 0.05%	**Adults & Peds ≥12 yrs:** Instill 2-3 sprays per nostril q10-12h. **Max:** 2 doses q24h.
TOPICAL NASAL MOISTURIZERS		
4-Way Saline Moisturizing Mist	Water, Boric Acid, Glycerin, Sodium Chloride, Sodium Borate, Eucalyptol, Menthol, Polysorbate 80, Benzalkonium Chloride	**Adults & Peds ≥2 yrs:** Instill 2-3 sprays per nostril prn.
Ayr Allergy & Sinus Nasal Mist	Sodium Chloride 2.65%	**Adults & Peds:** Spray bid-tid prn.
Ayr Baby's Saline Nose Spray, Drops	Sodium Chloride 0.65%	**Peds:** Instill 2 to 6 drops in each nostril.
Ayr Saline Nasal Gel With Soothing Aloe	Water, Methyl Gluceth 10, Propylene Glycol, Glycerin, Glyceryl Polymethacrylate, Triethanolamine, Aloe Barbadensis Leaf Juice (Aloe Vera Gel), PEG/PPG 18/18 Dimethicone, Carbomer, Poloxamer 184, Sodium Chloride, Xanthan Gum, Diazolidinyl Urea, Methylparaben, Propylparaben, Glycine Soja Oil (Soybean), Geranium Maculatum Oil, Tocopheryl Acetate, Blue 1	**Adults & Peds:** Apply to nostril prn.
Ayr Saline Nasal Gel, No-Drip Sinus Spray	Water, Sodium Carbomethyl Starch, Propylene Glycol, Glycerin, Aloe Barbadensis Leaf Juice (Aloe Vera Gel), Sodium Chloride, Cetyl Pyridinium Chloride, Citric Acid, Disodium EDTA, Glycine Soja (Soybean Oil), Tocopheryl Acetate, Benzyl Alcohol, Benzalkonium Chloride, Geranium Maculatum Oil	**Adults & Peds ≥12 yrs:** Instill 1 spray in each nostril as directed.
Ayr Saline Nasal Mist	Sodium Chloride 0.65%	**Adults & Peds ≥12 yrs:** Instill 2 sprays per nostril prn.
ENTSOL Mist, Buffered Hypertonic Nasal Irrigation Mist	Purified Water, Sodium Chloride, Sodium Phosphate Dibasic Edetate Disodium, Potassium Phosphate Monobasic, Benzalkonium Chloride	**Adults & Peds:** Instill 1-2 sprays per nostril prn.
ENTSOL Single Use, Pre-Filled Nasal Wash Squeeze Bottle	Purified Water, Sodium Chloride, Sodium Phosphate Dibasic, Potassium Phosphate Monobasic	**Adults & Peds ≥12 yrs:** Use as directed.
ENTSOL Spray, Buffered Hypertonic Saline Nasal Spray	Purified Water, Sodium Chloride Phosphate Dibasic, Potassium Phosphate Monobasic	**Adults & Peds ≥12 yrs:** Instill 1 spray per nostril bid, 6 times daily.

(Continued)

BRAND	INGREDIENT/STRENGTH	DOSE
TOPICAL NASAL MOISTURIZERS *(Continued)*		
ENTSOL Nasal Gel with Aloe and Vitamin E	Water (Purified), Propylene Glycol, Aloe, Glycerin, Dimethicone Copolyol, Poloxamer 184, Methyl Gluceth 10, Triethanolamine, Carbomer, Sodium Chloride, Vitamin E, Disodium EDTA, Xanthan Gum, Benzalkonium Chloride	**Adults & Peds:** Use prn.
Little Noses Saline Spray/Drops, Non-Medicated	Sodium Chloride 0.65%	**Peds:** 2-6 drops per nostril as directed.
Nostrilla Conditioning Double Moisture	Benzalkonium Chloride Solution, Carboxymethylcellulose Sodium, Eucalyptol, Glycine, Hyaluronic Acid Sodium, Polyethylene Glycol, Povidone, Propylene Glycol, Sodium Chloride (as 1.9% saline solution), Spearmint Oil, Wintergreen Oil, Water	**Adults & Peds:** Spray once per nostril prn.
Ocean Premium Saline Nasal Spray	Sodium Chloride 0.65%	**Adults & Peds ≥6 yrs:** Instill 2 sprays per nostril prn.
Simply Saline Sterile Saline Nasal Mist	Sodium Chloride 0.9%	**Adults & Peds ≥12 yrs:** Use prn as directed.
SinoFresh Moisturizing Nasal & Sinus Spray	Purified Water, Propylene Glycol, Monobasic Sodium Phosphate, Dibasic Sodium Phosphate, Sodium Chloride, Polysorbate 80, Sorbitol Solution, Essential Oil Blend (Wintergreen Oil, Spearmint Oil, Peppermint Oil, Eucalyptus Oil) Cetylpyridinium Chloride, Benzalkonium Chloride	**Adults & Peds ≥12 yrs:** Instill 1-3 sprays per nostril bid.

ANALGESIC PRODUCTS

BRAND	INGREDIENT/STRENGTH	DOSE
ACETAMINOPHEN		
Anacin Extra Strength Aspirin Free Tablets	Acetaminophen 500mg	**Adults & Peds ≥12 yrs:** 2 tabs q6h. **Max:** 8 tabs q24h.
Feverall Childrens' Suppositories	Acetaminophen 120mg	**Peds 3-6 yrs:** 1-2 Supp. q4-6h. **Max:** 6 supp. q24h.
Feverall Infants' Suppositories	Acetaminophen 80mg	**Peds 3-11 months:** 1 supp. q6h. **12-36 months:** 1 supp. q4h. **Max:** 6 supp. q24h.
Feverall Jr. Strength Suppositories	Acetaminophen 325mg	**Peds 6-12 yrs:** 1 supp. q4-6h. **Max:** 6 supp. q24h.
Tylenol 8 Hour Caplets	Acetaminophen 650mg	**Adults & Peds ≥12 yrs:** 2 tabs q8h prn. **Max:** 6 tabs q24h.
Tylenol Arthritis Caplets	Acetaminophen 650mg	**Adults:** 2 tabs q8h prn. **Max:** 6 tabs q24h.
Tylenol Arthritis Geltabs	Acetaminophen 650mg	**Adults:** 2 tabs q8h prn. **Max:** 6 tabs q24h.
Tylenol Children's Suspension	Acetaminophen 160mg/5mL	**Peds 2-3 yrs (24-35 lbs):** 1 tsp (5mL). **4-5 yrs (36-47 lbs):** 1.5 tsp (7.5mL). **6-8 yrs (48-59 lbs):** 2 tsp (10mL). **9-10 yrs (60-71 lbs):** 2.5 tsp (12.5mL). **11 yrs (72-95 lbs):** 3 tsp (15mL). May repeat q4h. **Max:** 5 doses q24h.
Tylenol Extra Strength Caplets	Acetaminophen 500mg	**Adults & Peds ≥12 yrs:** 2 tabs q4-6h prn. **Max:** 8 tabs q24h.
Tylenol Extra Strength Cool Caplets	Acetaminophen 500mg	**Adults & Peds ≥12 yrs:** 2 tabs q4-6h prn. **Max:** 8 tabs q24h.
Tylenol Extra Strength Gelcaps	Acetaminophen 500mg	**Adults & Peds ≥ 12 yrs:** 2 caps q4-6h prn. **Max:** 8 caps q24h.
Tylenol Rapid Blast Liquid	Acetaminophen 500mg/15mL	**Adults & Peds ≥12 yrs:** 2 tbl (30mL) q4-6h prn. **Max:** 8 tbl (120mL) q24h.
Tylenol Extra Strength EZ Tablets	Acetaminophen 500mg	**Adults & Peds ≥12 yrs:** 2 tabs q4-6h prn. **Max:** 8 tabs q24h.
Tylenol Extra Strength Go Tablets	Acetaminophen 500mg	**Adults & Peds ≥12 yrs:** 2 tabs q4-6h prn. **Max:** 8 tabs q24h.
Tylenol Infants' Suspension	Acetaminophen 80mg/0.8mL	**Peds 2-3 yrs (24-35 lbs):** 1.6 mL q4h prn. **Max:** 5 doses (8mL) q24h.
Tylenol Junior Meltaways Tablets	Acetaminophen 160mg	**Peds 6-8 yrs (48-59 lbs):** 2 tabs. **9-10 yrs (60-71 lbs):** 2.5 tabs. **11 yrs (72-95 lbs):** 3 tabs. **12 yrs (≥96 lbs):** 4 tabs. May repeat q4h. **Max:** 5 doses q24h.
Tylenol Regular Strength Tablets	Acetaminophen 325mg	**Adults & Peds ≥12 yrs:** 2 tabs q4-6h prn. **Max:** 12 tabs q24h. **Peds 6-11 yrs:** 1 tab q4-6h. **Max:** 5 tabs q24h.
ACETAMINOPHEN COMBINATIONS		
Anacin Advanced Headache Tablets	Acetaminophen/Aspirin/Caffeine 250mg-250mg-65mg	**Adults & Peds ≥12 yrs:** 2 tabs q6h. Max: 8 tabs q24h.
Excedrin Back & Body Caplets	Acetaminophen/Aspirin Buffered 250mg-250mg	**Adults & Peds ≥12 yrs:** 2 tabs q6h **Max:** 8 tabs q24h.
Excedrin Extra Strength Caplets	Acetaminophen/Aspirin/Caffeine 250mg-250mg-65mg	**Adults & Peds ≥12 yrs:** 2 tabs q6h. **Max:** 8 tabs q24h.
Excedrin Extra Strength Geltabs	Acetaminophen/Aspirin/Caffeine 250mg-250mg-65mg	**Adults & Peds ≥12 yrs:** 2 tabs q6h. **Max:** 8 tabs q24h.

(Continued)

BRAND	INGREDIENT/STRENGTH	DOSE
ACETAMINOPHEN COMBINATIONS *(Continued)*		
Excedrin Extra Strength Express Gels	Acetaminophen/Aspirin/Caffeine 250mg-250mg-65mg	**Adults & Peds ≥12 yrs:** 2 tabs q6h. **Max:** 8 tabs q24h.
Excedrin Extra Strength Tablets	Acetaminophen/Aspirin/Caffeine 250mg-250mg-65mg	**Adults & Peds ≥12 yrs:** 2 tabs q6h. **Max:** 8 tabs q24h.
Excedrin Migraine Caplets	Acetaminophen/Aspirin/Caffeine 250mg-250mg-65mg	**Adults:** 2 tabs prn. **Max:** 2 tabs q24h.
Excedrin Migraine Geltabs	Acetaminophen/Aspirin/Caffeine 250mg-250mg-65mg	**Adults:** 2 tabs prn. **Max:** 2 tabs q24h.
Excedrin Migraine Tablets	Acetaminophen/Aspirin/Caffeine 250mg-250mg-65mg	**Adults:** 2 tabs prn. **Max:** 2 tabs q24h.
Excedrin Sinus Headache Caplets	Acetaminophen/Phenylephrine HCl 325mg-5mg	**Adults & Peds ≥12 yrs:** 2 tabs q4h. **Max:** 12 tabs q24h.
Excedrin Sinus Headache Tablets	Acetaminophen/Phenylephrine HCl 325mg-5mg	**Adults & Peds ≥12 yrs:** 2 tabs q4h. **Max:** 12 tabs q24h.
Excedrin Tension Headache Caplets	Acetaminophen/Caffeine 500mg-65mg	**Adults & Peds ≥12 yrs:** 2 tabs q6h. **Max:** 8 tabs q24h.
Excedrin Tension Headache Express Gels	Acetaminophen/Caffeine 500mg-65mg	**Adults & Peds ≥12 yrs:** 2 tabs q6h. **Max:** 8 tabs q24h.
Excedrin Tension Headache Geltabs	Acetaminophen/Caffeine 500mg-65mg	**Adults & Peds ≥12 yrs:** 2 tabs q6h. **Max:** 8 tabs q24h.
Excedrin Tension Headache Tablets	Acetaminophen/Caffeine 500mg-65mg	**Adults & Peds ≥12 yrs:** 2 tabs q6h. **Max:** 8 tabs q24h.
Goody's Body Pain Powder	Acetaminophen/Aspirin 325mg-500mg	**Adults & Peds ≥12 yrs:** 1 powder q4-6h. **Max:** 4 powders q24h.
Goody's Cool Orange	Acetaminophen/Aspirin/Caffeine 325mg-500mg-65mg	**Adults & Peds ≥12 yrs:** 1 powder q6h. **Max:** 4 powders q24h.
Goody's Extra Strength Headache Powders	Acetaminophen/Aspirin/Caffeine 260mg-520mg-32.5mg	**Adults & Peds ≥12 yrs:** 1 powder q4-6h. **Max:** 4 powders q24h.
Midol Menstrual Complete Caplets	Acetaminophen/Caffeine/Pyrilamine Maleate 500mg-60mg-15mg	**Adults & Peds ≥12 yrs:** 2 tabs q6h. **Max:** 8 tabs q24h.
Midol Menstrual Complete Gelcaps	Acetaminophen/Caffeine/Pyrilamine Maleate 500mg-60mg-15mg	**Adults & Peds ≥12 yrs:** 2 tabs q6h. **Max:** 8 tabs q24h.
Midol Teen Formula Caplets	Acetaminophen/Pamabrom 500mg-25mg	**Adults & Peds ≥12 yrs:** 2 tabs q6h. **Max:** 8 tabs q24h.
Pamprin Cramp	Acetaminophen/Magnesium Salicylate/ Pamabrom 250mg-250mg-25mg	**Adults & Peds ≥12 yrs:** 2 caps q4-6h. **Max:** 8 tabs q24h.
Pamprin Max	Acetaminophen/Aspirin/Caffeine 250mg-250mg-65mg	**Adults & Peds ≥12 yrs:** 2 caps q4-6h. **Max:** 8 tabs q24h.
Pamprin Multi-Symptom Caplets	Acetaminophen/Pamabrom/Pyrilamine 500mg-25mg-15mg	**Adults & Peds ≥12 yrs:** 2 tabs q4-6h. **Max:** 8 tabs q24h.
Premsyn PMS Caplets	Acetaminophen/Pamabrom/Pyrilamine 500mg-25mg-15mg	**Adults & Peds ≥12 yrs:** 2 tabs q4-6h. **Max:** 8 tabs q24h.
Tylenol Women's Menstrual Relief	Acetaminophen/Pamabrom 500mg-25mg	**Adults & Peds ≥12 yrs:** 2 tabs q4-6h. **Max:** 8 tabs q24h.
Vanquish Caplets	Acetaminophen/Aspirin/Caffeine 194mg-227mg-33mg	**Adults & Peds ≥12 yrs:** 2 tabs q6h. **Max:** 8 tabs q24h.
ACETAMINOPHEN/SLEEP AIDS		
Excedrin PM Caplets	Acetaminophen/Diphenhydramine 500mg-38mg	**Adults & Peds ≥12 yrs:** 2 tabs qhs.
Excedrin PM Geltabs	Acetaminophen/Diphenhydramine citrate 500mg-38 mg	**Adults & Peds ≥12 yrs:** 2 tabs qhs.
Excedrin PM Tablets	Acetaminophen/Diphenhydramine citrate 500mg-38 mg	**Adults & Peds ≥12 yrs:** 2 tabs qhs.
Goody's PM Powder	Acetaminophen/Diphenhydramine 1000mg-76mg/dose	**Adults & Peds ≥12 yrs:** 1 packet (2 powders) qhs.
Tylenol PM Caplets	Acetaminophen/Diphenhydramine 500mg-25mg	**Adults & Peds ≥12 yrs:** 2 tabs qhs.
Tylenol PM Rapid Release Gels	Acetaminophen/Diphenhydramine 500mg-25mg	**Adults & Peds ≥12 yrs:** 2 caps qhs.

(Continued)

BRAND	INGREDIENT/STRENGTH	DOSE
ACETAMINOPHEN/SLEEP AIDS *(Continued)*		
Tylenol PM Geltabs	Acetaminophen/Diphenhydramine 500mg-25mg	**Adults & Peds ≥12 yrs:** 2 tabs qhs.
Tylenol PM Vanilla Liquid	Acetaminophen/Diphenhydramine 1000mg-50mg/30 mL	**Adults & Peds ≥12 yrs:** 2 tbl (30mL) qhs. **Max:** 8 tbl (120mL) q24h.
NSAIDs		
Advil Caplets	Ibuprofen 200mg	**Adults & Peds ≥12 yrs:** 1-2 tabs q4-6h. **Max:** 6 tabs q24h.
Advil Children's Chewable Tablets	Ibuprofen 50mg	**Peds 2-3 yr (24-35 lb):** 2 tabs q6-8h. **4-5 yr (36-47 lb):** 3 tabs q6-8h. **6-8 yr (48-59 lb):** 4 tabs q6-8h. **9-10 yr (60-71 lb):** 5 tabs q6-8h. **11 yr (72-95 lb):** 6 tabs q6-8h. **Max:** 4 doses q24h
Advil Children's Suspension	Ibuprofen 100mg/5mL	**Peds 2-3 yrs (24-35 lbs):** 1 tsp (5mL). **4-5 yrs (36-47 lbs):** 1.5 tsp (7.5mL). **6-8 yrs (48-59 lbs):** 2 tsp (10mL). **9-10 yrs (60-71 lbs):** 2.5 tsp (12.5mL). **11 yrs (72-95 lbs):** 3 tsp (15mL). May repeat q6-8h. **Max:** 4 doses q24h.
Advil Gel Caplets	Ibuprofen 200mg	**Adults & Peds ≥12 yrs:** 1-2 caps q4-6h. **Max:** 6 caps q24h.
Advil Infants' Concentrated Drops	Ibuprofen 50mg/1.25mL	**Peds 6-11 months (12-17 lbs):** 1.25mL. **12-23 months (18-23 lbs):** 1.875mL. May repeat q6-8h. **Max:** 4 doses q24h.
Advil Junior Strength Swallow Tablets	Ibuprofen 100mg	**Peds 6-10 yrs (48-71 lbs):** 2 tabs. **11 yrs (72-95 lbs):** 3 tabs. May repeat q6-8h. **Max:** 4 doses q24h.
Advil Junior Strength Chewable Tablets	Ibuprofen 100mg	**Peds 6-8 yrs (48-59 lbs):** 2 tabs. **9-10 yrs (60-71 lbs):** 2.5 tabs. **11 yrs (72-95 lbs):** 3 tabs. May repeat q6-8h. **Max:** 4 doses q24h.
Advil Liqui-Gels	Ibuprofen 200mg	**Adults & Peds ≥12 yrs:** 1-2 caps q4-6h. **Max:** 6 caps q24h.
Advil Migraine Capsules	Ibuprofen 200mg	**Adults:** 2 caps prn. **Max:** 2 caps q24h.
Advil Tablets	Ibuprofen 200mg	**Adults & Peds ≥12 yrs:** 1-2 tabs q4-6h. **Max:** 6 tabs q24h.
Aleve Caplets	Naproxen Sodium 220mg	**Adults & Peds ≥12 yrs:** 1 cap q8-12h. May take 1 additional cap within 1h of first dose. **Max:** 3 caps q24h.
Aleve Liquid Gels	Naproxen Sodium 220mg	**Adults & Peds ≥12 yrs:** 1 cap q8-12h. May take 1 additional tab within 1 hour of first dose. **Max:** 3 caps q24h.
Aleve Smooth Gels	Naproxen Sodium 220mg	**Adults & Peds ≥12 yrs:** 1 cap q8-12h. May take 1 additional tab within 1 hour of first dose. **Max:** 3 caps q24h.
Aleve Tablets	Naproxen Sodium 220mg	**Adults & Peds ≥12 yrs:** 1 tab q8-12h. May take 1 additional tab within 1 hour of first dose. **Max:**: 3 tabs q24h.
Midol Cramps and Body	Ibuprofen 200mg	**Adults & Peds ≥12 yrs:** 1-2 tabs q4-6h. **Max:** 6 tabs q24h.
Midol Extended Relief Caplets	Naproxen Sodium 220mg	**Adults & Peds ≥12 yrs:** 1-2 tabs q8-12h. **Max:** 3 tabs q24h.

(Continued)

BRAND	INGREDIENT/STRENGTH	DOSE
NSAIDs *(Continued)*		
Motrin Children's Suspension	Ibuprofen 100mg/5mL	**Peds 2-3 yrs (24-35 lbs):** 1 tsp (5mL). **4-5 yrs (36-47 lbs):** 1.5 tsp (7.5mL). **6-8 yrs (48-59 lbs):** 2 tsp (10mL). **9-10 yrs (60-71 lbs):** 2.5 tsp (12.5mL). **11 yrs (72-95 lbs):** 3 tsp (15mL). May repeat q6-8h. **Max:** 4 doses q24h.
Motrin IB Caplets	Ibuprofen 200mg	**Adults & Peds ≥12 yrs:** 1-2 tabs q4-6h. **Max:** 6 tabs q24h.
Motrin IB Tablets	Ibuprofen 200mg	**Adults & Peds ≥12 yrs:** 1-2 tabs q4-6h. **Max:** 6 tabs q24h.
Motrin Infants' Drops	Ibuprofen 50mg/1.25mL	**Peds 6-11 months (12-17 lbs):** 1.25mL. **12-23 months (18-23 lbs):** 1.875mL. May repeat q6-8h. **Max:** 4 doses q24h.
Motrin Junior Strength Caplets	Ibuprofen 100mg	**Peds 6-8 yrs (48-59 lbs):** 2 tabs. **9-10 yrs (60-71 lbs):** 2.5 tabs. **11 yrs (72-95 lbs):** 3 tabs. May repeat q6-8h. **Max:** 4 doses q24h.
Motrin Junior Strength Chewable Tablets	Ibuprofen 100mg	**Peds 6-8 yrs (48-59 lbs):** 2 tabs. **9-10 yrs (60-71 lbs):** 2.5 tabs. **11 yrs (72-95 lbs):** 3 tabs. May repeat q6-8h. **Max:** 4 doses q24h.
Pamprin All Day Caplets	Naproxen Sodium 220mg	**Adults & Peds ≥12 yrs:** 1-2 tabs q8-12h. **Max:** 3 tabs q24h.
NSAID SLEEP AIDS		
Advil PM Caplets	Ibuprofen/Diphenhydramine citrate 200mg-38mg	**Adults & Peds ≥12 yrs:** 2 caps qhs. **Max:** 2 tabs q24h.
Advil PM Liqui-Gels	Ibuprofen/Diphenhydramine citrate 200mg-38mg	**Adults & Peds ≥12 yrs:** 2 caps qhs. **Max:** 2 tabs q24h.
SALICYLATES		
Anacin 81 Tablets	Aspirin 81mg	**Adults & Peds ≥12 yrs:** 2 tabs q6h. **Max:** 8 tabs q24h.
Bayer Aspirin Extra Strength Caplets	Aspirin 500mg	**Adults & Peds ≥12 yrs:** 1-2 tabs q4-6h. **Max:** 8 tabs q24h.
Bayer Aspirin Safety Coated Caplets	Aspirin 325mg	**Adults & Peds ≥12 yrs:** 1-2 tabs q4h. **Max:** 12 tabs q24h.
Bayer Children's Aspirin Chewable Tablets	Aspirin 81mg	**Adults & Peds ≥12 yrs:** 4-8 tabs q4h. **Max:** 48 tabs q24h.
Bayer Low Dose Aspirin Tablets	Aspirin 81mg	**Adults & Peds ≥12 yrs:** 4-8 tabs q4h. **Max:** 48 tabs q24h.
Bayer Sugar Free Low Dose Aspirin Tablets	Aspirin 81mg	**Adults & Peds ≥12 yrs:** 4-8 tabs q4h. **Max:** 48 tabs q24h.
Bayer Genuine Aspirin Tablets	Aspirin 325mg	**Adults & Peds ≥12 yrs:** 1-2 tabs q4h or 3 tabs q6h. **Max:** 12 tabs q24h.
Bayer Extra-Strength Plus Caplets	Aspirin 500mg Buffered with Calcium Carbonate 500mg	**Adults & Peds ≥12 yrs:** 1-2 tabs q4-6h. **Max:** 8 tabs q24h.
Doan's Caplets	Magnesium Salicylate Tetrahydrate 580mg	**Adults & Peds ≥12 yrs:** 2 tabs q4h. **Max:** 8 tabs q24h.
Ecotrin Low Strength Tablets	Aspirin 81mg	**Adults:** 4-8 tabs q4h. **Max:** 48 tabs q24h.
Ecotrin Regular Strength Tablets	Aspirin 325mg	**Adults & Peds ≥12 yrs:** 1-2 tabs q4h. **Max:** 12 tabs q24h.
Ecotrin Maximum Strength Tablets	Aspirin 500mg	**Adults & Peds ≥12 yrs:** 2 tabs q6h. **Max:** 8 tabs q24h.
Halfprin 162mg Tablets	Aspirin 162mg	**Adults & Peds ≥12 yrs:** 2-4 tabs q4h. **Max:** 24 tabs q24h.
Halfprin 81mg Tablets	Aspirin 81mg	**Adults & Peds ≥12 yrs:** 4-8 tabs q4h. **Max:** 48 tabs q24h.

(Continued)

BRAND	INGREDIENT/STRENGTH	DOSE
SALICYLATES *(Continued)*		
St. Joseph Chewable Aspirin Tablets	Aspirin 81mg	**Adults & Peds ≥12 yrs:** 4-8 tabs q4h. **Max:** 48 tabs q24h.
St. Joseph Enteric Safety-Coated Tablets	Aspirin 81mg	**Adults & Peds ≥12 yrs:** 4-8 tabs q4h. **Max:** 48 tabs q24h.
SALICYLATES, BUFFERED		
Alka-Seltzer Original Effervescent Tablets	Aspirin/Citric Acid/Sodium Bicarbonate 325mg-1000mg-1916mg	**Adults & Peds ≥12 yrs:** 2 tabs q4h. **Max:** 8 tabs q24h.
Alka-Seltzer Extra Strength Effervescent Tablets	Aspirin/Citric Acid/Sodium Bicarbonate 500mg-1000mg-1985mg	**Adults & Peds ≥12 yrs:** 2 tabs q6h. **Max:** 7 tabs q24h.
Ascriptin Regular Strength Tablets	Aspirin Buffered with Maalox/Calcium Carbonate 325mg	**Adults & Peds ≥12 yrs:** 2 tabs q4h. **Max:** 12 tabs q24h.
Bayer Extra Strength Plus Caplets	Aspirin Buffered with Calcium Carbonate 500mg	**Adults & Peds ≥12 yrs:** 1-2 tabs q4-6h. **Max:** 8 tabs q24h.
Bufferin Extra Strength Tablets	Aspirin Buffered with Calcium Carbonate/Magnesium Oxide/Magnesium Carbonate 500mg	**Adults & Peds ≥12 yrs:** 2 tabs q6h. **Max:** 8 tabs q24h.
Bufferin Tablets	Aspirin Buffered with Calcium Carbonate/Magnesium Oxide/Magnesium Carbonate 325mg	**Adults & Peds ≥12 yrs:** 2 tabs q4h. **Max:** 12 tabs q24h.
SALICYLATE COMBINATIONS		
Alka-Seltzer Wake-Up Call	Aspirin/Caffeine 500mg-65mg	**Adults & Peds ≥12 yrs:** 2 tabs q6h. **Max:** 8 tabs q24h. **≥60 yrs: Max:** 4 tabs q24h.
Anacin Max Strength Tablets	Aspirin/Caffeine 500mg-32mg	**Adults & Peds ≥12 yrs:** 2 tabs q6h. **Max:** 8 tabs q24h.
Anacin Tablets	Aspirin/Caffeine 400mg-32mg	**Adults & Peds ≥12 yrs:** 2 tabs q6h. **Max:** 8 tabs q24h.
Bayer Back & Body Pain Caplets	Aspirin/Caffeine 500mg-32.5mg	**Adults & Peds ≥12 yrs:** 2 tabs q6h. **Max:** 8 tabs q24h.
BC Arthritis Strength Powders	Aspirin/Caffeine/Salicylamide 742mg-38mg-222mg	**Adults & Peds ≥12 yrs:** 1 powder q3-4h. **Max:** 4 powders q24h.
BC Original Formula Powders	Aspirin/Caffeine/Salicylamide 650mg-33.3mg-195mg	**Adults & Peds ≥12 yrs:** 1 powder q3-4h. **Max:** 4 powders q24h.
SALICYLATE/SLEEP AID		
Alka-Seltzer PM Effervescent Tablets	Aspirin/Diphenhydramine Citrate 325mg-38 mg	**Adults & Peds ≥12 yrs:** 2 tabs qhs.
Bayer PM Caplets	Aspirin/Diphenhydramine 500mg-38.3mg	**Adults & Peds ≥12 yrs:** 2 tabs qhs.
Doan's Extra Strength PM Caplets	Magnesium Salicylate Tetrahydrate/Diphenhydramine 580mg-25mg	**Adults & Peds ≥12 yrs:** 2 tabs qhs.

CANKER AND COLD SORE PRODUCTS

BRAND	INGREDIENT/STRENGTH	DOSE
Abreva Cold Sore/Fever Blister Treatment	Docosanol 10%	**Adults & Peds ≥12 yrs:** Use 5 times a day until healed. **Max:** 10 days.
Abreva Pump Cold Sore/Fever Blister Treatment	Docosanol 10%	**Adults & Peds ≥12 yrs:** Use 5 times a day until healed. **Max:** 10 days.
Anbesol Cold Sore Therapy Ointment	Allantoin/Benzocaine/Camphor/ White Petrolatum 1%-20%-3%-64.9%	**Adults & Peds ≥2 yrs:** Apply to affected area up to tid-qid.
Anbesol Jr. Gel	Benzocaine 10%	**Adults & Peds ≥2 yrs:** Apply to affected area up to qid.
Anbesol Maximum Strength Gel	Benzocaine 20%	**Adults & Peds ≥2 yrs:** Apply to affected area up to qid.
Anbesol Maximum Strength Liquid	Benzocaine 20%	**Adults & Peds ≥2 yrs:** Apply to affected area up to qid.
Anbesol Regular Strength Gel	Benzocaine 10%	**Adults & Peds ≥2 yrs:** Apply to affected area up to qid.
Anbesol Regular Strength Liquid	Benzocaine 10%	**Adults & Peds ≥2 yrs:** Apply to affected area up to qid.
Baby Anbesol	Benzocaine 7.5%	**Peds ≥4 months:** Apply to affected area up to qid.
Campho-Phenique Cold Sore Gel	Camphor/Phenol 10.8%-4.7%	**Adults & Peds ≥2 yrs:** Apply to affected area qd-tid.
Campho-Phenique Cold Sore Treatment Cream	Pramoxine/White Petrolatum 1%-30%	**Adults & Peds ≥2 yrs:** Apply to affected area up to tid-qid.
ChapStick Cold Sore Therapy	Allantoin/Benzocaine/Camphor/White Petrolatum 1%-20%-3%-64.9%	**Adults & Peds ≥2 yrs:** Apply to affected area up to tid-qid.
Chloraseptic Max Sore Throat Relief	Phenol 15%/Glycerin 33%	**Peds ≥3 yrs:** Apply to affected area for 15 seconds, then spit. Use q2h.
Chloraseptic Pocket Pump Sore Throat Spray	Phenol 1.4%	**Adults & Peds ≥12 yrs:** Spray 5 times to affected area, then spit. Use q2h. **Peds 2-12 yrs:** Spray 3 times to affected area, then spit. Use q2h.
Dr. Snapz Swabplus Mouth Sore Relief Swabs	Benzocaine 20%	**Adults & Peds ≥2 yrs:** Apply to affected area up to qid.
Herpecin-L Lip Balm Stick, SPF 30	Dimethicone/Methyl Anthranilate/ Octyl Methoxycinnamate/Octyl Salicylate/ Oxybenzone 1%-5%-7.5%-5%- 6%	**Adults & Peds ≥12 yrs:** Apply prn.
Kank-A Soft Brush Tooth/Mouth Pain Gel	Benzocaine 20%	**Adults & Peds ≥2 yrs:** Apply to affected area up to qid.
Kanka-A Mouth Pain Liquid	Benzocaine 20%	**Adults & Peds ≥2 yrs:** Apply to affected area up to qid.
Novitra Cold Sore Maximum Strength Cream	Zincum Oxydatum 2X/HPUS	**Adults & Peds ≥2 yrs:** Apply to affected area q2-3h, 6 to 8 times daily.
Orabase with Benzocaine Gel	Benzocaine 20%	**Adults & Peds ≥2 yrs:** Apply to affected area up to qid.
Orabase with Benzocaine Paste	Benzocaine 20%	**Adults & Peds ≥2 yrs:** Apply to affected area up to qid.
Orajel Ultra Mouth Sore Medicine Film-Forming Gel	Benzocaine/Menthol 15%-2%	**Adults & Peds ≥2 yrs:** Apply to affected area up to qid.
Orajel Mouth Sore Medicine Gel	Benzocaine/Benzalkonium Chloride/Zinc Chloride 20%-0.02%-0.1%	**Adults & Peds ≥2 yrs:** Apply to affected area up to qid.
Orajel Antiseptic Mouth Sore Rinse	Hydrogen Peroxide 1.5%	**Adults & Peds ≥2 yrs:** Rinse with 2 tsp then spit. Use up to qid.
Orajel Medicated Mouth Sore Swabs	Benzocaine 20%	**Adults & Peds ≥2 yrs:** Apply to affected area up to qid.

(Continued)

BRAND	INGREDIENT/STRENGTH	DOSE
Orajel Medicated Cold Sore Brush	Allantoin/Benzocaine/Dimethicone/White Petrolatum 0.5%-20%-2%-65%	**Adults & Peds ≥2 yrs:** Apply to affected area up to tid-qid.
Orajel Protective Mouth Sore Discs	Benzocaine 15mg	**Adults & Peds ≥2 yrs:** Apply to affected area q2h prn.
Releev 1-Day Cold Sore Treatment	Benzalkonium Chloride 0.13%	**Adults & Peds ≥2 yrs:** Apply to clean dry affected area tid-qid.
Zilactin	Benzyl Alcohol 10%	**Adults & Peds ≥2 yrs:** Apply to affected area up to qid.
Zilactin B	Benzocaine 10%	**Adults & Peds ≥2 yrs:** Apply to affected area up to qid.
Zilactin L	Benzyl Alcohol 10%	**Adults & Peds ≥2 yrs:** Apply to affected area up to qid.
Zilactin Tooth & Gum	Benzocaine 20%	**Adults & Peds ≥2 yrs:** Apply to affected area up to qid.

ACE INHIBITORS

DRUG (BRAND)	PEAK PLASMA LEVEL	FOOD EFFECT ON AMOUNT ABSORBED	HYPERTENSION DOSING*	HEART FAILURE DOSING	RENAL DOSE ADJUSTMENT
Benazepril (Lotensin)	1-2 hrs (fasting); 2-4 hrs (non-fasting**)	None	**Initial:** 10mg qd. **Usual:** 20-40mg/day given qd-bid. **Max:** 80mg/day.	Not FDA approved.	CrCl<30mL/min/1.73m²: **Initial:** 5mg qd. **Max:** 40mg/day.
Captopril (Capoten)	1 hr	Reduced***	**Initial:** 25mg bid-tid. **Usual:** 25-150mg bid-tid. **Max:** 450mg/day.	**Initial:** 25mg tid. **Usual:** 50-100mg tid. **Max:** 450mg/day.	**Significant Renal Dysfunction:** Lower initial dose and titrate slowly.
Enalapril (Vasotec)	3-4 hrs**	None	**Initial:** 5mg qd. **Usual:** 10-40mg/day given qd-bid. **Max:** 40mg/day.†	**Initial:** 2.5mg qd. **Usual:** 2.5-20mg given bid. **Max:** 40mg/day.	**HTN:** CrCl ≤30mL/min: **Initial:** 2.5mg/day. **Max:** 40mg/day. **Dialysis:** 2.5mg/day on dialysis day. **HF:** SCr 1.6mg/dL: **Initial:** 2.5mg qd. **Max:** 40mg/day.
Fosinopril (Monopril)	3 hrs**	None	**Initial:** 10mg qd. **Usual:** 20-40mg/day. **Max:** 80mg/day.†	**Initial:** 10mg qd. **Usual:** 20-40mg qd. **Max:** 40mg/day.	**HTN:** No dosage adjustment needed. **HF:** Moderate to severe renal failure/vigorous diuresis: initial: 5mg qd.
Lisinopril (Prinivil, Zestril)	7 hrs	None	**Initial:** 10mg qd. **Usual:** 20-40mg qd. **Max:** 80mg/day.†	(Prinivil) **Initial:** 5mg qd. **Usual:** 5-20mg qd. (Zestril) **Initial:** 5mg qd. **Usual:** 5-40mg qd. **Max:** 40mg/day.	**HTN:** CrCl 10-30mL/min: **Initial:** 5mg qd. **Max:** 40mg/day. CrCl <10mL/min: **Initial:** 2.5mg qd. **Max:** 40mg/day. **HF:** CrCl ≤30mL/min: **Initial:** 2.5mg qd.
Moexipril (Univasc)	1.5 hrs**	Reduced***	**Initial:** 7.5mg qd. **Usual:** 7.5-30mg/day given qd-bid. **Max:** 60mg/day.	Not FDA approved.	CrCl ≤40mL/min/1.73m²: **Initial:** 3.75mg qd. **Max:** 15mg/day.
Perindopril (Aceon)	3-7 hrs**	None	**Initial:** 4mg qd. **Usual:** 4-8mg/day qd. **Max:** 16mg/day.	Not FDA approved.	CrCl >30mL/min: **Initial:** 2mg qd. **Max:** 8mg/day.
Quinapril (Accupril)	2 hrs**	Reduced (after high-fat meals)	**Initial:** 10-20mg qd. **Usual:** 20-80mg/day given qd-bid.	**Initial:** 5mg bid. **Usual:** 10-20mg bid.	CrCl 30-60mL/min: **Initial:** 5mg/day. CrCl 10-30mL/min: **Initial:** 2.5mg/day.
Ramipril (Altace)	2-4 hrs**	None	**Initial:** 2.5mg qd. **Usual:** 2.5-20mg/day given qd-bid.	**Post MI:** **Initial:** 2.5mg bid; 1.25mg bid if hypotensive. Titrate to 5mg bid.	**HTN:** **Initial:** 1.25mg qd. **Max:** 5mg/day. **Post MI:** **Initial:** 1.25mg/day. **Max:** 2.5mg/bid.
Trandolapril (Mavik)	4-10 hrs**	None	**Initial:** 1mg qd in non-black patients. 2mg qd in black patients. **Usual:** 2-4mg/day. **Max:** 8mg/day.	**Post MI:** **Initial:** 1mg qd. Titrate to 4mg qd if tolerated.	CrCl <30mL/min: **Initial:** 0.5mg qd.

* Note: Dosages may need to be adjusted when used in combination with other antihypertensives (ie, diuretics). Monitor patient closely. For more information, refer to monograph listings or drug's FDA-approved labeling.

** Peak effect of active metabolite.

*** Administer 1 hour before meals captopril and moexipril.

† Refer to monograph for pediatric dosing.

ANTIARRHYTHMIC AGENTS

DRUG (BRAND)	HOW SUPPLIED	INDICATION	DOSAGE	HEPATIC/RENAL DOSE ADJUSTMENT*
Class IA Antiarrhythmics				
Disopyramide (Norpace)	Cap: (Norpace) 100mg, 150mg; Cap, Extended-Release: (Norpace CR) 100mg, 150mg	Treatment of documented life-threatening ventricular arrhythmias.	**Adults:** Usual: 400-800mg/day in divided dose. Recommended: 150mg q6h immediate-release (IR) or 300mg q12h extended-release (CR). Adjust dose with anticholinergic effects. Rapid Control of Ventricular Arrhythmia: LD: 300mg IR (200mg if <110lbs). Follow with maint dose. Cardiomyopathy/Cardiac Decompensation: Initial: 100mg q6-8h IR. Adjust gradually. See labeling if no response or toxicity occurs. Elderly: Start at low end of dosing range. **Pediatrics:** <1 yr: 10-30mg/kg/day. 1-4 yrs: 10-20mg/kg/day. 4-12 yrs: 10-15mg/kg/day. 12-18 yrs: 6-15mg/kg/day. Give in equally divided doses q6h. Hospitalize patient during initial therapy. Start dose titration at lower end of range.	Weight <110lbs/Moderate Hepatic or Renal Insufficiency (CrCl >40mL/min): 100mg q6h IR or 200mg q12h CR. Severe Renal Insufficiency (with or without initial 150mg LD): CrCl 30-40mL/min: 100mg q8h IR. CrCl 30-15mL/min: 100mg q12h IR. CrCl <15mL/min: 100mg q24h IR.
Quinidine Gluconate	Tab, Extended-Release: 324mg; **Inj:** 80mg/mL	Conversion of symptomatic atrial fibrillation/flutter (A-Fib/Flutter) to normal sinus rhythm, and suppression of ventricular arrhythmias. Tab: reduction of relapse frequency into A-Fib/Flutter	**Adults:** A-Fib/Flutter Conversion: Initial: 2 tabs q8h. Titrate: Increase cautiously if no effect after 3-4 doses. Alternate Regimen: 1 tab q8h for 2 days, then 2 tabs q12h for 2 days, then 2 tabs q8h up to 4 days. A-Fib/Flutter Relapse Reduction: 1 tab q8-12h. Titrate: Increase cautiously if needed. Ventricular Arrhythmia: Dosing regimens not adequately studied. May break tab in half. Do not chew or crush. IV: A-Fib/Flutter and Ventricular Arrhythmia: 0.25mg/kg/min. Max: 5-10mg/kg. Consider alternate therapy if conversion to sinus rhythm not achieved. Elderly: Start at low end of dosing range.	Renal/Hepatic Impairment or CHF: Reduce dose.
Quinidine Sulfate	Tab: 200mg, 300mg; 300mg ER	Conversion of symptomatic A-fib/flutter to normal sinus rhythm, reduction of relapse frequency into A-fib/flutter, and suppression of ventricular arrhythmias.	**Adults:** A-Fib/Flutter Conversion: Initial: 400mg q6h. Titrate: Increase cautiously if no effect after 4-5 doses. (ER): 300mg q8-12h. Titrate: Increase dose cautiously. A-Fib/Flutter Relapse Reduction: 200mg q6h. (ER): 300mg q8-12h. Titrate: Increase cautiously if needed. Ventricular Arrhythmia: Dosing regimens not adequately studied.	Renal or hepatic impairment: Reduce dose.

DRUG (BRAND)	HOW SUPPLIED	INDICATION	DOSAGE	HEPATIC/RENAL DOSE ADJUSTMENT*
Class IB Antiarrhythmics				
Mexiletine	Cap: 150mg, 200mg, 250mg	Treatment of life-threatening ventricular arrhythmias.	**Adults:** Initial: 200mg q8h when rapid control is not essential. Titrate: Adjust by 50-100mg, not less than every 2-3 days. Usual: 200-300mg q8h. Max: 1200mg/day. If control with ≤300mg q8h, then may divide daily dose and give q12h. Max: 450mg q12h. For Rapid Control: LD: 400mg, then 200mg in 8 hrs. Transfer from Class I Oral Agents: Initial: 200mg and titrate as above, 6-12 hrs after last quinidine sulfate or disopyramide dose, 3-6 hrs after last procainamide dose, or 8-12 hrs after last tocainide dose. Take with food or antacid.	Severe Hepatic Disease: May need lower dose.
Class IC Antiarrhythmics				
Flecainide (Tambocor)	Tab: 50mg, 100mg*, 150mg* *scored	Prevention of paroxysmal supraventricular tachycardias (PSVT), paroxysmal atrial fibrillation/flutter (PAF) associated with disabling symptoms in patients without structural heart disease. Prevention of life-threatening ventricular arrhythmias (VT).	**Adults:** PSVT/PAF: Initial: 50mg q12h. Titrate: May increase by 50mg bid every 4 days. Max: 300mg/day. Sustained VT: Initial: 100mg q12h. Titrate: May increase by 50mg bid every 4 days. Max: 400mg/day. Reduce dose by 50% with amiodarone. **Pediatrics:** <6 months: Initial: 50mg/m^2/day given bid-tid. ≥6 months: Initial: 100mg/m^2/day given bid-tid. Max: 200mg/m^2/day. Reduce dose by 50% with amiodarone.	CrCl ≤35mL/min: Initial: 100mg qd or 50mg bid.
Propafenone (Rythmol, Rythmol SR)	Tab: 150mg*, 225mg*, 300mg*; *scored SR: 225mg, 325mg, 425mg	To prolong the time to recurrence of paroxysmal atrial fibrillation/flutter (PAF) and paroxysmal supraventricular tachycardia (PSVT) associated with disabling symptoms in patients without structural heart disease. Treatment of life-threatening documented ventricular arrhythmias.	**Adults:** Initial: 150mg q8h. Titrate: May increase at minimum 3-4 day intervals to 225mg q8h, then to 300mg q8h if needed. Max: 900mg/day. Elderly/Marked Myocardial Damage: Increase more gradually during initial phase. **SR: Adults:** Initial: 225mg q12h. Titrate: May increase at minimum 5 day intervals to 325mg q12h, then to 425mg q12h if needed. QRS Widening/ 2nd- or 3rd-degree AV Block: Reduce dose.	Hepatic Dysfunction: Give 20-30% of normal dosage. (SR) Hepatic Impairment: Reduce dose.
Class II Antiarrhythmics (Beta Blockers)				
Acebutolol (Sectral)	Cap: 200mg, 400mg	Management of hypertension and ventricular arrhythmias	**Adults:** Ventricular Arrhythmia: Initial: 200mg bid. Maint: Increase gradually to 600-1200mg/day. Elderly: Lower daily doses. Max: 800mg/day.	CrCl <50mL/min: Decrease daily dose by 50%. CrCl <25mL/min: Decrease daily dose by 75%.

(Continued)

DRUG (BRAND)	HOW SUPPLIED	INDICATION	DOSAGE	HEPATIC/RENAL DOSE ADJUSTMENT*
Class II Antiarrhythmics (Beta Blockers) *(Continued)*				
Esmolol (Brevibloc)	Inj: 10mg/mL [10mL, 250mL], 20mg/mL [5mL, 100mL]	For rapid control of ventricular rate in atrial fibrillation or atrial flutter in perioperative, postoperative, or other emergent circumstances. For non-compensatory sinus tachycardia.	**Adults:** Supraventricular Tachycardia: Titrate dose based on ventricular rate. Load: 0.5mg/kg over 1 min. Maint: 0.05mg/kg/min for next 4 min. May continue at 0.05mg/kg/min at intervals of 4 min or increase stepwise to max 0.2mg/kg/min. Rapid slowing of ventricular response: Repeat 0.5mg/kg load over 1 min, then 0.1mg/kg/min for 4 min. If needed, another (final) load of 0.5mg/kg over 1 min, then 0.15mg/kg/min for 4 min up to 0.2mg/kg/min. May continue infusions for 24hrs. Intraoperative/Postoperative Tachycardia: Immediate Control: Initial: 80mg bolus over 30 sec. Maint: 0.15mg/kg/min. May titrate up to 0.3mg/kg/min. Gradual Control: Initial: 0.5mg/kg over 1 min. Maint: 0.05mg/kg/min for 4 min. Then, if needed, may repeat load and increase to 0.1mg/kg/min.	
Propranolol (Inderal)	Inj: 1mg/mL; Tab: 10mg*, 20mg*, 40mg*, 60mg*, 80mg* *scored	(Inj) For cardiac arrhythmias (supraventricular, ventricular tachycardia, tachyarrhythmia of digitalis intoxication, resistant tachyarrhythmia). (Tab) To control ventricular rate in patients with atrial fibrillation and a rapid ventricular response.	**Adults:** (Inj) 1-3mg IV at 1 mg/min. May give 2nd dose after 2 min, subsequent doses q4h prn. A Fib: 10-30mg PO tid-qid ac and hs.	Hepatic insufficiency: May need to lower dose.
Sotalol (Betapace)	Tab: 80mg*, 120mg*, 160mg* *scored	Treatment of documented life threatening ventricular arrhythmias.	**Adults:** Initial: 80mg bid. Titrate: Increase to 120-160mg bid if needed. Allow 3 days between dose increments. Usual: 160-320mg/day given bid-tid. Refractory Patients: 480-640mg/day. May increase dose with renal impairment after at least 5-6 doses. **Pediatrics:** ≥2 yrs: Initial: 30mg/m² tid. Titrate: Wait at least 36 hrs between dose increases. Guide dose by response, HR, and QTc. Max: 60mg/m². <2 yrs: See dosing chart in PI. Reduce dose or d/c if QTc >550msec.	**Adults:** CrCl 30-59mL/min: Dose q24h. CrCl 10-29mL/min: Dose q36-48h. CrCl <10mL/min: Individualize dose. **Pediatrics:** Renal Impairment: Reduce dose or increase interval.

DRUG (BRAND)	HOW SUPPLIED	INDICATION	DOSAGE	HEPATIC/RENAL DOSE ADJUSTMENT*
Class II Antiarrhythmics (Beta Blockers) *(Continued)*				
Sotalol (Betapace AF)	Tab: 80mg*, 120mg*, 160mg* *scored	Maintenance of normal sinus rhythm with symptomatic atrial fibrillation/atrial flutter (AFIB/AFL) in patients who are currently in sinus rhythm.	**Adults:** Initiate with continuous ECG monitoring. Give dose qd for CrCl 40-60mL/min and bid for CrCl >60mL/min. Initial: 80mg. Monitor QT 2-4hrs after each dose. Reduce dose or d/c if QT ≥500msec. If QT <500msec after 3 days (after 5th or 6th dose if receiving qd dosing), discharge on current treatment. Alternately, may increase dose to 120mg during hospitalization, and follow for 3 days with bid dose and for 5 or 6 doses if receiving qd dose. Max: 160mg qd or bid depending on CrCl. **Pediatrics:** ≥2 yrs: Initial: 30mg/m² tid. Titrate: Wait at least 36 hrs between dose increases. Guide dose by response, heart rate and QTc. Max: 60mg/m². <2 yrs: See dosing chart in PI. Reduce dose or d/c if QTc >550msec.	Renal Impairment: Reduce dose or increase interval.
Class III Antiarrhythmics				
Amiodarone (Pacerone, Cordarone, Nexterone)	Tab: 100mg, 200mg*, 300mg*, 400mg* *scored; Inj: 50mg/mL [3mL]	Treatment of documented, life-threatening recurrent ventricular fibrillation and recurrent hemodynamically unstable ventricular tachycardia.	**Adults:** Give LD in hospital. LD: 800-1600mg/day in divided doses for 1-3 weeks. After control is achieved, then 600-800mg/day for 1 month. Maint: 400mg/day; up to 600mg/day if needed. Use lowest effective dose. Take with meals. Elderly: Start at low end of dosing range. IV: Adults: LD: 150mg over 1st 10 min (15mg/min), then 360mg over next 6 hrs (1mg/min), then 540mg over remaining 18 hrs (0.5mg/min). Maint: 0.5mg/min for 2-3 weeks. Breakthrough Ventricular Tachycardia/Ventricular Fibrillation: 150mg supplement IV over 10 min. Increase rate to achieve suppression. Elderly: Start at low end of dosing range. Administer infusions >2 hrs in a glass or polyolefin bottle containing D5W. Amiodarone leaches out plasticizers (eg, DEHP from IV tubing) especially at higher infusion concentrations, and lower flow rates.	

(Continued)

DRUG (BRAND)	HOW SUPPLIED	INDICATION	DOSAGE	HEPATIC/RENAL DOSE ADJUSTMENT*
Class III Antiarrhythmics *(Continued)*				
Dofetilide (Tikosyn)	Cap: 125mcg, 250mcg, 500mcg	Conversion to and maintenance of normal sinus rhythm in atrial fibrillation/flutter.	**Adults:** Individualize dose based on CrCl and QTc. Use QT interval if HR <60 beats/min. Initiate with continuous ECG monitoring. Determine QTc interval 2-3 hrs after 1st dose and adjust dose if QTc >500msec or if >15% increase from baseline. QTc Adjustment: Reduce 500mcg bid to 250mcg bid. Reduce 250mcg bid to 125mcgbid. Reduce 125mcg bid to 125mcg qd. D/C anytime after 2nd dose if QTc >500 msec (550msec with ventricular conduction abnormalities).	CrCl: >60mL/min: 500mcg bid. CrCl 40-60mL/min: 250mcg bid. CrCl 20 to <40mL/min: 125mcg bid. CrCl <20mL/min: do not use. Monitor ECG.
Ibutilide (Corvert)	Inj: 0.1mg/mL	For rapid conversion of atrial fibrillation or flutter (A-Fib/Flutter) of recent onset to sinus rhythm.	**Adults:** ≥60kg: 1mg over 10 min. <60 kg: 0.01mg/kg over 10 min. If arrhythmia still present within 10 min after the end of the initial infusion, repeat infusion 10 min after completion of 1st infusion. Continuous ECG monitoring for 4hrs after infusion or until QTc returns to baseline.	
Class IV Antiarrhythmics (Calcium Channel Blockers)				
Diltiazem Injection	Inj: 5mg/mL	Temporary control of rapid ventricular rate in atrial fibrillation/flutter (A-Fib/Flutter). Rapid conversion of paroxysmal supraventricular tachycardia (PSVT) to sinus rhythm.	**Adults:** Bolus: (Injection/Lyo-Ject) 0.25mg/kg IV over 2 minutes. If no response after 15 minutes, may give 2nd dose of 0.35mg/kg over 2 minutes. Continuous Infusion: (Injection/Lyo-Ject/Monovial) 0.25-0.35mg/kg IV bolus, then 10mg/hr. Titrate: Increase by 5mg/hr. Max: 15mg/hr and duration up to 24 hrs.	
Verapamil (Calan)	Tab: 40mg, 80mg*, 120mg* *scored Inj: 2.5mg/mL (available in generic)	(Tab): With digitalis, for control of ventricular rate at rest and during stress in patients with chronic atrial flutter and/or atrial fibrillation and prophylaxis of repetitive PSVT. (Inj): Rapid conversion of PSVT to sinus rhythm, including those associated with accessory bypass tracts and temporary control of rapid ventricular rate in A-fib/flutter except when associated with accessory bypass tracts.	**Adults:** A-Fib (Digitalized): Usual: 240-320mg/day PO given tid-qid. PSVT Prophylaxis (Non-Digitalized): 240-480mg/day PO given tid-qid. Max: 480mg/day. **(Inj): Adults:** Initial: 5-10mg IV bolus over 2 min. If 1st dose not adequate, repeat 10mg over 2 min 30 min after first dose. Elderly: Administer dose over at least 3 min. **Pediatrics:** Continuously monitor ECG. **<1yr:** 0.1-0.2mg/kg IV bolus over 2 min. If 1st dose not adequate, repeat 0.1-0.2mg/kg over 2 min 30 min after 1st dose. **1-15yrs:** 0.1-0.3 mg/kg IV bolus over 2 min. Max: 5mg. If 1st dose not adequate, repeat 0.1-0.3mg/kg over 2 min 30 min after 1st dose. Max: 10mg single dose.	Severe hepatic dysfunction: (Tab) Give 30% of normal dose.

DRUG (BRAND)	HOW SUPPLIED	INDICATION	DOSAGE	HEPATIC/RENAL DOSE ADJUSTMENT*
Class V Antiarrhythmics				
Adenosine (Adenocard)	Inj: 3mg/mL [2mL, 4mL]	Conversion of paroxysmal supraventricular tachycardia (including Wolff-Parkinson-White syndrome) to sinus rhythm (SR).	**Adults:** 6mg rapid IV bolus infusion over 1-2 seconds. If not converted to SR within 1-2 min, give 12mg rapid IV bolus; may give 2nd 12mg dose if needed. Max: 12mg/dose. **Pediatrics:** <50kg: 0.05-0.1mg/kg rapid IV bolus. If not converted to SR within 1-2 min, give additional bolus doses incrementally increasing amount by 0.05-0.1mg/kg. Follow each bolus with a saline flush. Continue process until SR or a maximum single dose of 0.3mg/kg is used. ≥50kg: 6mg rapid IV bolus infusion over 1-2 sec. If not converted to SR within 1-2 min, give 12mg rapid IV bolus; may give 2nd 12mg dose if needed. Max: 12mg/dose.	
Digoxin (Lanoxin)	Cap: (Lanoxicaps) 0.1mg, 0.2mg; Inj: (Pediatric Inj) 0.1mg/mL, 0.25mg/mL; Sol: (Pediatric Sol) 0.05mg/mL [60mL]; **Tab:** 0.125mg*, 0.25mg* *scored	Treatment of mild to moderate heart. failure and to control ventricular response rate with chronic atrial fibrillation.	**Adults:** Rapid Digitalization: LD: (Cap/Inj) 0.4-0.6mg PO/IV single dose or (Tab) 0.5-0.75mg PO, may give additional (Cap/Inj) 0.1-0.3mg or (Tab) 0.125-0.375mg at 6-8 hr intervals until clinical effect. Maint: (Tab) 0.125-0.5mg qd. A-Fib: Titrate to minimum effective dose for desired response. **Pediatrics:** See PI for full pediatric dosing information.	Elderly (>70 yrs)/Renal Dysfunction: Initial: 0.125mg qd. Marked Renal Dysfunction: Initial: 0.0625mg qd. Titrate: Increase every 2 weeks based on response.

ARBs* AND COMBINATIONS

DRUG	BRAND	USUAL HTN† DOSAGE RANGE	HOW SUPPLIED
ANGIOTENSIN II RECEPTOR BLOCKERS			
Candesartan	Atacand	8–32mg/day.	**Tab:** 4mg, 8mg, 16mg, 32mg
Eprosartan	Teveten	400–800mg/day.	**Tab:** 400mg, 600mg
Irbesartan	Avapro	150–300mg/day.	**Tab:** 75mg, 150mg, 300mg
Losartan	Cozaar	25–100mg/day.	**Tab:** 25mg, 50mg, 100mg
Olmesartan	Benicar	20–40mg/day.	**Tab:** 5mg, 20mg, 40mg
Telmisartan	Micardis	20–80mg/day.	**Tab:** 20mg, 40mg, 80mg
Valsartan	Diovan	80–320mg/day.	**Tab:** 40mg, 80mg, 160mg, 320mg
COMBINATIONS			
Candesartan-Hydrochlorothiazide	Atacand HCT	16/12.5–32/25mg/day.	**Tab:** 16mg-12.5mg, 32mg-12.5mg, 32mg-25mg
Eprosartan-Hydrochlorothiazide	Teveten HCT	600/12.5–600/25mg/day.	**Tab:** 600mg-12.5mg, 600mg-25mg
Irbesartan-Hydrochlorothiazide	Avalide	150/12.5–300/25mg/day.	**Tab:** 150mg-12.5mg, 300mg-12.5mg, 300mg-25mg
Losartan-Hydrochlorothiazide	Hyzaar	50/12.5–100/25mg/day.	**Tab:** 50mg-12.5mg, 100mg-12.5mg, 100mg-25mg
Olmesartan-Amlodipine	Azor	20/5-40/10mg/day.	**Tab:** 20mg-5mg, 20mg-10mg, 40mg-5mg, 40mg-10mg
Olmesartan-Hydrochlorothiazide	Benicar HCT	20/12.5–40/25mg/day.	**Tab:** 20mg-12.5mg, 40mg-12.5mg, 40mg-25mg
Telmisartan-Hydrochlorothiazide	Micardis HCT	40/12.5–160/25mg/day.	**Tab:** 40mg-12.5mg, 80mg-12.5mg, 80mg-25mg
Valsartan-Amlodipine	Exforge	160/5-320/10mg/day.	**Tab:** 160mg-5mg, 160mg-10mg, 320mg-5mg, 320mg-10mg
Valsartan-Hydrochlorothiazide	Diovan HCT	160/12.5–320/25mg/day.	**Tab:** 80mg-12.5mg, 160mg-12.5mg, 160mg-25mg, 320mg-12.5mg, 320mg-25mg

*ARBs: Angiotensin II receptor blockers.

†HTN: Hypertension.

Adopted from the Seventh Report of the Joint National Committee on Prevention, Detection, Evaluation, and Treatment of High Blood Pressure (JNC 7); http://www.nhlbi.nih.gov/guidelines/hypertension/jnc7full.htm.

BETA-BLOCKERS

DRUG	BRAND	HOW SUPPLIED	HYPERTENSION DOSING	ANGINA DOSING	POST-MI DOSING
NONSELECTIVE BETA-BLOCKERS					
Nadolol	Corgard	**Tab:** 20mg, 40mg, 80mg	**Initial:** 40mg qd. **Usual:** 40mg–80mg qd. **Max:** 320mg/day.	**Initial:** 40mg qd. **Usual:** 40mg–80mg qd. **Max:** 240mg/day.	Not FDA approved
Penbutolol sulfate	Levatol	**Tab:** 20mg	**Initial** and **Usual:** 20mg qd.	Not FDA approved	Not FDA approved
Pindolol	Visken	**Tab:** 5mg, 10mg	**Initial:** 5mg bid **Max:** 60mg/day.	Not FDA approved	Not FDA approved
Propranolol HCl	Inderal	**Tab:** 10mg, 20mg, 40mg, 60mg, 80mg	**Initial:** 40mg bid **Usual:** 120mg–240mg/day. **Max:** 640mg/day.	**Usual:** 80mg–320mg/day.	**Initial:** 40mg bid **Usual:** 180mg–240mg/day. **Max:** 240mg/day.
	Inderal LA	**Cap, LA:** 60mg, 80mg, 120mg, 160mg	**Initial:** 80mg qd **Usual:** 120mg–160mg qd. **Max:** 640mg/day.	**Initial:** 80mg qd. **Usual:** 160mg qd. **Max:** 320mg	Not FDA approved
	Innopran XL	**Cap, ER:** 80mg, 120mg	**Initial:** 80mg qhs. **Max:** 120mg qhs.	Not FDA approved	Not FDA approved
Timolol maleate	Various generics	**Tab:** 5mg, 10mg 20mg	**Initial:** 10mg, bid **Usual:** 20mg–40mg/day. **Max:** 60mg/day.	Not FDA approved	**Usual:** 10mg bid (post acute MI).
SELECTIVE BETA$_1$-BLOCKERS					
Acebutolol	Sectral	**Cap:** 200mg, 400mg	**Initial:** 400mg qd or bid. **Usual:** 400mg–800mg/day. **Max:** 1200mg/day.	Not FDA approved	Not FDA approved
Atenolol	Tenormin	**Tab:** 25mg, 50mg, 100mg	**Initial:** 50mg qd. **Max:** 100mg qd.	**Initial:** 50mg qd. **Usual:** 100mg qd. **Max:** 200mg qd.	**Usual:** 50mg bid or 100mg qd for 6–9 days post MI.
Betaxolol HCl	Kerlone	**Tab:** 10mg, 20mg	**Initial:** 10mg qd. **Max:** 40mg qd.	Not FDA approved	Not FDA approved
Bisoprolol fumarate	Zebeta	**Tab:** 5mg, 10mg	**Initial:** 2.5mg–5mg qd. **Usual:** 2.5mg–20mg qd. **Max:** 20mg qd.	Not FDA approved	Not FDA approved
Esmolol	Brevibloc	**Inj:** 10mg/mL [10mL, 250mL], 20mg/mL [5mL, 100mL], 250mg/mL concentrate	**Immediate Control: Initial:** 80mg bolus over 30 sec. **Maint:** 0.15mg/kg/min. May titrate up to 0.3mg/kg/min. **Gradual Control: Initial:** 0.5mg/kg over 1 min. **Maint:** 0.05mg/kg/min for 4 min. If needed, may repeat loading dose. **Maint:** follow and increase to 0.1mg/kg/min.**	Not FDA approved	Not FDA approved
Metoprolol succinate	Toprol-XL†	**Tab, XL:** 25mg, 50mg, 100mg, 200mg	**Initial:** 25mg–100mg qd. **Max:** 400mg/day.	**Initial:** 100mg qd. **Max:** 400mg/day.	Not FDA approved

(Continued)

DRUG	BRAND	HOW SUPPLIED	HYPERTENSION DOSING	ANGINA DOSING	POST-MI DOSING
SELECTIVE BETA$_1$-BLOCKERS *(Continued)*					
Metoprolol tartrate	Lopressor	**Tab:** 50mg, 100mg	**Initial:** 100mg qd or in divided doses **Usual:** 100mg–450mg/day. **Max:** 450mg/day.	**Initial:** 50mg bid **Usual:** 100mg–400mg/day. **Max:** 400mg/day.	**Usual:** 100mg bid for at least 3 months.
	Various generics	**Tab:** 25mg, 50mg 100mg	**Initial:** 100mg qd or in divided doses **Usual:** 100mg–450mg/day. **Max:** 450mg/day.	**Initial:** 50mg bid **Usual:** 100mg–400mg/day. **Max:** 400mg/day.	**Usual:** 100mg bid for at least 3 months.
Nebivolol	Bystolic	**Tab:** 2.5mg, 5mg 10mg, 20mg	**Initial:** 5mg qd. Titrate: May increase dose if needed at 2-week intervals. **Max:** 40mg. **Hepatic impairment/ CrCl <30mL/min:** 2.5mg qd.	Not FDA approved	Not FDA approved
MIXED ALPHA- AND BETA-BLOCKERS					
Carvedilol	Coreg†	**Tab:** 3.125mg, 6.25mg, 12.5mg, 25mg	**Initial:** 6.25mg bid **Max:** 25mg bid	Not FDA approved	Left Ventricular Dysfunction post MI: **Initial:** 6.25mg bid, then increase to 12.5mg bid after 3-10 days. **Usual Target:** 25mg bid.
	Coreg CR†	**Tab, CR:** 10mg, 20mg, 40mg, 80mg	**Initial:** 20mg qd. **Max:** 80mg/day.	Not FDA approved	Left Ventricular Dysfunction post MI: **Initial:** 10mg–20mg qd. **Usual:** 80mg qd.
Labetalol HCl	Trandate	**Tab:** 100mg, 200mg, 300mg	**Initial:** 100mg bid **Usual:** 200mg–400mg bid	Not FDA approved	Not FDA approved
COMBINATIONS					
Atenolol/ Chlorthalidone	Tenoretic	**Tab:** 50mg/25mg, 100mg/25mg	**Initial:** 50mg/25mg qd. **Max:** 100mg/ 25mg/day.	Not FDA approved	Not FDA approved
Nadolol/ Bendroflumethiazide	Corzide	**Tab:** 40mg/5mg, 80mg/5mg	**Initial:** 40mg/5mg qd. **Max:** 80mg/ 5mg/day.	Not FDA approved	Not FDA approved
Bisoprolol/ fumarate/ HCTZ*	Ziac	**Tab:** 2.5mg/ 6.25mg, 5mg/ 6.25mg, 10mg/ 6.25mg	**Initial:** 2.5mg/ 6.25mg qd. **Max:** 20mg/12.5mg/day.	Not FDA approved	Not FDA approved

(Continued)

DRUG	BRAND	HOW SUPPLIED	HYPERTENSION DOSING	ANGINA DOSING	POST-MI DOSING
COMBINATIONS *(Continued)*					
Metoprolol tartrate/ HCTZ*	Lopressor HCT	**Tab:** 50mg/25mg, 100mg/25mg, 100mg/50mg	Individualize dose. **Lopressor usual initial:** 100mg/day qd or divided. **Lopressor max:** 450mg/day. **HCTZ usual:** 12.5mg-50mg/day. HCTZ dose >50mg/day not recommended.	Not FDA approved	Not FDA approved
Propranolol/ HCTZ*	Inderide	**Tab:** 40mg/25mg 80mg/25mg	Individualize dose. **Propranolol alone initial:** 80mg/day. **Usual:** 160mg-480mg/day. **HCTZ alone usual:** 12.5-50mg/day. **Inderide max dose:** 160mg/50mg.	Not FDA approved	Not FDA approved

*Hydrochlorothiazide.

**Brevibloc is used for the treatment of tachycardia and hypertension that occur during induction and tracheal intubation, during surgery, on emergence from anesthesia, and in the postoperative period.

†For additional indications, refer to FDA-approved labeling.

Note: Sotalol (Betapace) is indicated for ventricular arrhythmias. Refer to FDA-approved labeling for dosing and additional information.

Source: FDA-approved labeling.

CALCIUM CHANNEL BLOCKERS

DRUG	BRAND	HOW SUPPLIED	HYPERTENSION DOSING*	ANGINA DOSING*
DIHYDROPYRIDINES				
Amlodipine besylate	Norvasc	**Tab:** 2.5mg, 5mg, 10mg	**Initial:** 5mg qd. **Max:** 10mg qd.	**Initial/Usual:** 10mg qd.
Felodipine	Plendil	**Tab, ER:** 2.5mg, 5mg, 10mg	**Initial:** 5mg qd. **Usual:** 2.5-10mg qd.	Not FDA approved
Isradipine	DynaCirc CR, generic	**Tab, CR:** 5mg, 10mg **Cap:** 2.5mg, 5mg	**Initial:** Cap: 2.5mg bid or (CR): 5mg qd. **Max:** 20mg/day.	Not FDA approved
Nicardipine HCl	Cardene	**Cap:** 20mg, 30mg	**Initial:** 20mg tid. **Usual:** 20-40mg tid.	**Initial:** 20mg tid. **Usual:** 20-40mg tid.
	Cardene SR	**Cap, ER:** 30mg, 45mg, 60mg	**Initial:** 30mg bid. **Usual:** 30-60mg bid.	Not FDA approved
Nifedipine	Adalat CC	**Tab, ER:** 30mg, 60mg, 90mg	**Initial:** 30mg qd. **Usual:** 30-60mg qd. **Max:** 90mg/day.	Not FDA approved
	Afeditab CR	**Tab, ER:** 30mg, 60mg	**Initial:** 30mg qd. **Usual:** 30-60mg qd. **Max:** 90mg/day.	Not FDA approved
	Procardia	**Cap:** 10mg, 20mg	Not FDA approved	**Initial:** 10mg tid. **Usual:** 10-20mg tid. **Max:** 180mg/day.
	Procardia XL	**Tab, ER:** 30mg, 60mg, 90mg	**Initial:** 30-60mg qd. **Max:** 120mg/day.	**Initial:** 30-60mg qd. **Max:** 90-120mg/day.
Nisoldipine	Generic	**Tab, ER:** 20mg, 30mg, 40mg	**Initial:** 20mg qd. **Usual:** 20-40mg qd. **Max:** 60mg/day.	Not FDA approved
	Sular	**Tab, ER:** 8.5mg, 17mg, 25.5mg, 34mg	**Initial:** 17mg qd. **Usual:** 17-34mg qd. **Max:** 34mg/day.	Not FDA approved
NON-DIHYDROPYRIDINES				
Diltiazem HCl	Cardizem	**Tab:** 30mg, 60mg, 90mg, 120mg	Not FDA approved	**Initial:** 30mg qid. **Usual:** 180-360mg/day.
	Cardizem CD, Cartia XT	**Cap, ER:** 120mg, 180mg, 240mg, 300mg, (Cardizem CD) 360mg	**Initial:** 180-240mg qd. **Usual:** 240-360mg qd. **Max:** 480mg qd.	**Initial:** 120-180mg qd. **Max:** 480mg/day.
	Cardizem LA	**Tab, ER:** 120mg, 180mg, 240mg, 300mg, 360mg, 420mg	**Initial:** 180-240mg qd. **Max:** 540mg/day.	**Initial:** 180 qd. **Max:** 360mg/day.
	Dilacor XR	**Cap, ER:** 120mg, 180mg, 240mg	**Initial:** 180-240mg qd. **Usual:** 180-480mg qd. **Max:** 540mg qd.	**Initial:** 120mg qd. **Max:** 480mg/day.
	Dilt-CD	**Cap, ER:** 120mg 180mg, 240mg, 300mg	**Initial:** 180-240mg qd. **Usual:** 240-360mg qd. **Max:** 540mg/day.	**Initial:** 120-180mg qd. **Max:** 540mg/day.
	Diltzac	**Cap, ER:** 120mg, 180mg, 240mg, 300mg, 360mg	**Initial:** 120-240mg qd. **Usual:** 120-540mg qd. **Max:** 540mg/day.	**Initial:** 120-180mg qd. **Max:** 540mg/day.
	Tiazac, Taztia XT	**Cap, ER:** 120mg, 180mg, 240mg, 300mg, 360mg, (Tiazac) 420mg	**Initial:** 120-240mg qd. **Usual:** 120-540mg qd. **Max:** 540mg qd.	**Initial:** 120-180mg qd. **Max:** 540mg/day.

(Continued)

DRUG	BRAND	HOW SUPPLIED	HYPERTENSION DOSING*	ANGINA DOSING*
NON-DIHYDROPYRIDINES *(Continued)*				
Verapamil HCl	Calan**	**Tab:** 40mg, 80mg, 120mg	**Initial:** 80mg tid. **Usual:** 360-480mg/day.	**Usual:** 80-120mg tid. **Max:** 480mg/day.
	Covera HS	**Tab, ER:** 180mg, 240mg	**Initial:** 180mg qhs. **Max:** 480mg qhs.	**Initial:** 180mg qhs. **Max:** 480mg qhs.
	Isoptin SR	**Tab, ER:** 120mg, 180mg, 240mg	**Initial:** 180mg qam. **Max:** 480mg/day.	Not FDA approved
	Verelan	**Cap, ER:** 120mg, 180mg, 240mg, 360mg	**Usual:** 240mg qam. **Max:** 480mg/day.	Not FDA approved
	Verelan PM	**Cap, ER:** 100mg, 200mg, 300mg	**Usual:** 200mg qhs. **Max:** 400mg qhs.	Not FDA approved

* NOTE: Adult dosing shown is for monotherapy. Dosage needs to be adjusted by titration to individual patient needs. Dosages may need to be reduced in the elderly, or with renal/hepatic impairment. When used in combination with other antihypertensives the dosage of the calcium channel blocker or the concomitant antihypertensives may need to be adjusted due to possible additive effect. Monitor patient closely. For more information refer to monograph listings or drug's FDA-approved labeling.
** For additional indications refer to monograph listings or drug's FDA-approved labeling.

CHOLESTEROL-LOWERING AGENTS

BRAND (GENERIC)	HOW SUPPLIED (MG)*	USUAL DOSAGE RANGE**	T-CHOL (% DECREASE)	LDL (% DECREASE)	HDL (% INCREASE)	TG (% DECREASE)
HMG-CoA REDUCTASE INHIBITORS (STATINS)						
Lipitor (Atorvastatin)	**Tabs:** 10, 20, 40 80	10-80mg/day	29 to 45	39 to 60	5 to 9	19 to 37
Lescol (Fluvastatin)	**Tabs:** 20, 40	20-80mg/day	17 to 27	22 to 36	3 to 6	12 to 18
Lescol XL (Fluvastatin)	**Tabs, ER:** 80	80mg/day	25	35	7	19
Altoprev (Lovastatin)	**Tab, ER:** 20, 40, 60	20-60mg/day	20.9 to 29.2	29.6 to 40.8	11.6 to 13.1	9.9 to 25.1
Mevacor (Lovastatin)	**Tabs:** 10, 20, 40	10-80mg/day given qd or bid	17 to 29	24 to 40	6.6 to 9.5	10 to 19
Pravachol (Pravastatin)	**Tabs:** 10, 20, 40, 80	40-80mg/day qd; renal/hepatic dysfunction: 10mg qd	16 to 27	22 to 37	2 to 12	11 to 24
Crestor (Rosuvastatin)	**Tabs:** 5, 10, 20, 40	5-40mg/day	33 to 46	45 to 63	8 to 14	10 to 35
Zocor (Simvastatin)	**Tabs:** 5, 10, 20, 40, 80	5-80mg/day	19 to 36	26 to 47	8 to 16	12 to 33
FIBRATES						
Tricor (Fenofibrate)	**Tab:** 48, 145	48-145mg/day	18.7	20.6	11	28.9
Lofibra (Fenofibrate)	**Tabs:** 54, 160; **Caps:** 67, 134, 200	54-160mg/day, 67-200mg/day	18.7	20.6	11	28.9
Antara (Fenofibrate)	**Caps:** 43, 130	43-130mg/day	18.7	20.6	11	28.9
Triglide (Fenofibrate)	**Tabs:** 50, 160	50-160mg/day	18.7	20.6	11	28.9
Lopid (Gemfibrozil)	**Tab:** 600	1200mg/day in divided doses	n/a	4.1	12.6	Not specified-but decrease
BILE-ACID SEQUESTRANTS						
Colestid (Colestipol)	**Granules:** 5g/pkt or scoop; **Tab:** 1000	**Granules:** 1-6 pkts or scoopfuls/day given qd or in divided doses; **Tab:** 2-16g/day given qd or in divided doses	Not specified	Not specified	Not specified	Not specified
Questran, Questran Light (Cholestyramine)	**Granules:** 4g/pkt or scoop	2-4 packets or scoopfuls daily (8-16 g) divided into two doses	7.2	10.4	n/a	n/a
WelChol (Colesevelam HCl)	**Tabs:** 625	3750mg/day given qd or bid	7	15	3	10
CHOLESTEROL ABSORPTION INHIBITOR						
Zetia (Ezetimibe)	**Tab:** 10	10mg qd	13	18	1	8
NICOTINIC ACID DERIVATIVE						
Niaspan (Niacin, Extended-Release)	**Tabs, ER:** 500, 750, 1000	1-2g qhs	3 to 10	5 to 14	18 to 22	13 to 28
LIPID-REGULATING AGENT						
Lovaza (Omega-3-Acid Ethyl Esters	**Cap:** 1000	4g/day given qd or bid	9.7	+44.5	9.1	44.9

(Continued)

BRAND (GENERIC)	HOW SUPPLIED (MG)*	USUAL DOSAGE RANGE**	T-CHOL (% DECREASE)	LDL (% DECREASE)	HDL (% INCREASE)	TG (% DECREASE)
COMBINATIONS						
Caduet (Amlodipine/ Atorvastatin)	**Tabs:** 2.5/10, 2.5/20, 2.5/40, 5/10, 5/20, 5/40, 5/80, 10/10, 10/20, 10/40, 10/80	5/10mg to 10/80mg	n/a	n/a	n/a	n/a
Vytorin (Ezetimibe/ Simvastatin)	**Tabs:** 10/10, 10/20, 10/40, 10/80	10/10 to 10/80mg/day	31 to 43	45 to 60	6 to 10	23 to 31
Advicor (Niacin ER/ Lovastatin)	**Tabs:** 500/20, 750/20, 1000/20, 1000/40	500/20mg to 2000mg/40mg	Not specified	30 to 42	20 to 30	32 to 44
Simcor (Niacin ER/ Simvastatin)	**Tabs:** 500/20, 750/20, 1000/20	500mg/20mg to 2000mg/40mg	8.8 to 11.1	11.9 to 14.3	20.7 to 29	26.5 to 38.0

* Unless otherwise indicated

** NOTE: Dosage shown is for adults and may need to be adjusted to individual patient needs. For pediatric dosing and additional information please refer to the individual monograph listing or the drug's FDA-approved labeling. According to NCEP-ATP III guidelines, lipid-altering agents should be used in addition to a diet restricted in saturated fat and cholesterol only when the response to diet and other nonpharmacological measures has been inadequate.

Abbreviation: ER: Extended-Release

COAGULATION MODIFIERS

DRUG (BRAND)	HOW SUPPLIED	INDICATIONS	DOSAGE	HEPATIC/RENAL IMPAIRMENT
THROMBOLYTICS				
Alteplase (Activase)	Inj: 50mg, 100mg	To improve ventricular function, reduce incidence of congestive heart failure, and reduce mortality with acute myocardial infarction (AMI). Management of acute ischemic stroke and acute massive pulmonary embolism (PE).	AMI: Accelerated Infusion: >67kg: 15mg IV bolus, then 50mg over next 30 min, and then 35mg over next 60 min. ≤67kg: 15mg IV bolus, then 0.75mg/kg (max 50mg) over next 30 min, then 0.5mg/kg (max 35mg) over next 60 min. Max: 100mg total dose. 3-Hr Infusion: ≥65kg: 60mg in 1st hr (give 6-10mg as IV bolus), then 20mg over 2nd hr, then 20mg over 3rd hr. <65kg: 1.25mg/kg over 3 hrs as described above. Stroke: 0.9mg/kg IV over 1 hr (max 90mg total dose). Administer 10% of total dose as IV bolus over 1 min. PE: 100mg IV over 2 hrs. Start heparin at end or immediately after infusion when PTT or PT ≤2× normal.	
Reteplase (Retavase)	Inj: 10.4 U	To improve ventricular function following acute myocardial infarction (AMI), reduce the incidence of congestive heart failure (CHF) and reduce the mortality associated with AMI.	10 U IV over 2 min. Repeat in 30 min.	
Tenecteplase (TNKase)	Inj: 50mg	To reduce mortality with AMI.	Administer as single IV bolus over 5 seconds. <60kg: 30mg. 60 to <70kg: 35mg. 70 to <80kg: 40mg. 80 to <90kg: 45mg. ≥90kg: 50mg. Max: 50mg/dose.	
Urokinase (Abbokinase, Kinlytic)	Inj: 250,000 IU	Lysis of acute massive pulmonary emboli (PE) and PE accompanied by unstable hemodynamics.	LD: 4400 IU/kg IV at 90mL/hr over 10 min. Maint: 4400 IU/kg/hr IV at 15mL/hr for 12 hrs. Flush line after each cycle. For IV use only.	
PLATELET AGGREGATION INHIBITOR				
Abciximab (Reopro)	Inj: 2mg/mL	Adjunct to percutaneous coronary intervention (PCI) for prevention of cardiac ischemic complications in patients undergoing PCI or with unstable angina unresponsive to conventional therapy when PCI is planned within 24 hrs. Intended for use with aspirin and heparin.	PCI: 0.25mg/kg IV bolus given 10-60 min before start PCI, followed by 0.125mcg/kg/min IV infusion (Max: 10mcg/min) for 12 hrs. Unstable Angina: 0.25mg/kg IV bolus followed by 10mcg/min infusion for 18-24 hrs, concluding 1 hr after PCI.	

(Continued)

DRUG (BRAND)	HOW SUPPLIED	INDICATIONS	DOSAGE	HEPATIC/RENAL IMPAIRMENT
Anagrelide (Agrylin)	Cap: 0.5mg	Treatment of thrombocythemia secondary to myeloproliferative disorders.	Initial: 0.5mg qid or 1mg bid for at least 1 week. Titrate: Increase by no more than 0.5mg/day per week. Max: 10mg/day or 2.5mg/dose. Adjust lowest effective dose to reduce and maintain platelets <600,000/mcL. Monitor platelets every 2 days during first week, then weekly thereafter until reach maintenance dose. **Pediatrics:** Initial: 0.5mg qd. Titrate: Increase by no more than 0.5mg/day per week. Max:10mg/day or 2.5mg/dose. Adjust to lowest effective dose to reduce and maintain platelets <600,000/mcL. Monitor platelets every 2 days during first week, then weekly thereafter until reach maintenance dose.	Moderate Hepatic Impairment: Initial: 0.5mg qd for at least 1 week. Titrate: Increase by no more than 0.5mg/day per week. Max: 10mg/day or 2.5mg/dose.
Aspirin (Halfprin)	Tab, Delayed-Release: 81mg, 162mg	To reduce the risk of vascular mortality and fatal and nonfatal cardiovascular and cerebrovascular events in patients with a suspected acute MI.	162mg as soon as MI suspected; continue qd for 30 days. May need to continue as prophylaxis for recurrent MI. Crush, chew, or suck the 1st dose.	
Cilostazol (Pletal)	Tab: 50mg, 100mg	Reduction of symptoms with intermittent claudication.	100mg bid, ½ hr before or 2 hrs after breakfast and dinner. Concomitant CYP3A4 and CYP2C19 Inhibitors: Consider 50mg bid.	
Clopidogrel (Plavix)	Tab: 75mg, 300mg	For reduction of thrombotic events in those with recent stroke or MI, established peripheral arterial disease (PAD); or with non-ST-segment elevation acute coronary syndrome (unstable angina/non-Q-wave MI); and patients with ST-segment elevation acute myocardial infarction (STEMI).	MI/Stroke/PAD: 75mg qd. Acute Coronary Syndrome: Take with 75-325mg ASA qd. LD: 300mg. Maint: 75mg qd. STEMI: 75mg, with 75-325mg ASA, qd with or without LD.	
Dipyridamole (Persantine)	Tab: 25mg, 50mg, 75mg	Adjunct to coumarin anticoagulants for prevention of postoperative thromboembolic complications of cardiac valve replacement.	75-100mg qid.	
Dipyridamole and aspirin (Aggrenox)	Cap: (Dipyridamole Extended-Release/ ASA) 200mg-25mg	Reduce risk of stroke in patients with transient brain ischemia or complete ischemic stroke due to thrombosis.	1 cap bid (am and pm).	
Eptifibatide (Integrilin)	Sol: 0.75mg/mL, 2mg/mL	Treatment of acute coronary syndrome (ACS) in patients being medically managed or undergoing percutaneous coronary intervention (PCI) including intracoronary stenting.	ACS: 180mcg/kg IV bolus, then 2mcg/kg/min IV infusion until discharge, initiation of CABG, or up to 72 hrs. If undergoing PCI, continue until discharge or 18-24 hrs post-PCI. PCI: 180mcg/kg IV bolus immediately before PCI, then 2mcg/kg/min IV infusion. Give 2nd bolus of 180mcg/kg 10 min after 1st bolus. Continue until discharge or 18-24 hrs post-PCI. See PI for concomitant ASA and heparin doses.	ACS: CrCl <50mL/min: 180mcg/kg IV bolus, then 1mcg/kg/min IV infusion. PCI: CrCl <50mL/min: 180mcg/kg IV bolus immediately before PCI, then 1mcg/kg/min IV infusion. Give 2nd bolus of 180mcg/kg 10 min after 1st bolus.

DRUG (BRAND)	HOW SUPPLIED	INDICATIONS	DOSAGE	HEPATIC/RENAL IMPAIRMENT
PLATELET AGGREGATION INHIBITOR *(Continued)*				
Ticlopidine (Ticlid)	Tab: 250mg	To reduce risk of thrombotic stroke in stroke patients or those with stroke precursors who are ASA intolerant, allergic, or failed ASA therapy. Adjunct to ASA to reduce incidence of subacute stent thrombosis in patients undergoing successful coronary artery stent implantation.	Take with food. Stroke: 250mg bid. Coronary Artery Stenting: 250mg bid with ASA for up to 30 days after stent implant.	
Tirofiban (Aggrastat)	Inj: 0.05mg/mL	In combination with heparin, for treatment of acute coronary syndrome, in patients being medically managed or undergoing PTCA or atherectomy.	Initial: 0.4mcg/kg/min IV for 30 min. Maint: 0.1mcg/kg/min IV. Continue through angiography and for 12-24 hrs after angioplasty or atherectomy.	CrCl <30mL/min: Administer half of the usual rate of infusion.
COAGULATION FACTOR INHIBITOR				
Dalteparin (Fragmin)	Inj: (Syringe) 2500 IU/0.2mL, 5000 IU/0.2mL, 7500 IU/0.3mL, 10,000 IU/0.4mL, 10,000 IU/1mL, 12,500 IU/0.5mL, 15,000 IU/0.6mL, 18,000 IU/0.72mL; (MDV) 25,000 IU/mL [3.8mL], 10,000 IU/mL [9.5mL]	Prevention of ischemic complications in unstable angina and non-Q-wave MI with concurrent ASA therapy. Prophylaxis of DVT in hip replacement surgery, abdominal surgery in patients who are at high risk for thromboembolic complications, and for those at risk for thromboembolic complications due to severely restricted mobility during acute illness. Extended treatment of symptomatic VTE (proximal DVT and/or PE), to reduce the recurrence of VTE in patients with cancer.	Administer SQ. Unstable Angina/Non-Q-Wave MI: 120 IU/kg up to 10,000 IU q12h with ASA (75-165mg/day) for 5-8 days. Hip Surgery: Pre-Op Start: Initial (if start 2 hrs pre-op): 2500 IU within 2 hrs pre-op, then 2500 IU 4-8 hrs post-op. Initial (if start 10-14 hrs pre-op): 5000 IU 10-14 hrs pre-op, then 5000 IU 4-8 hrs post-op. Maint (for either initial dose): 5000 IU SQ qd for 5-10 days post-op (up to 14 days). Post-Op Start: 2500 IU 4-8 hrs post-op. Maint: 5000 IU qd. Abdominal Surgery: 2500 IU 1-2 hrs pre-op. Maint: 2500 IU qd for 5-10 days post-op. Abdominal Surgery with High Risk: 5000 IU evening before surgery. Maint: 5000 IU qd for 5-10 days post-op. Abdominal Surgery with Malignancy: Initial: 2500 IU 1-2 hrs pre-op, then 2500 IU 12 hrs later. Maint: 5000 IU qd for 5-10 days post-op. Severely Restricted Mobility During Acute Illness: 5000 IU qd for 12-14 days. Symptomatic VTE in Cancer Patients: 200 IU/kg qd for first 30 days, then 150 IU/kg qd for months 2-6. Max: 18,000 IU/day. Platelet Count 50,000-100,000/mm^3: Reduce dose by 2500 IU until platelet count ≥100,000/mm^3. Platelet Count <50,000/mm^3: D/C therapy until platelet count >50,000/mm^3.	Renal Impairment (CrCl <30mL/min): Monitor anti-Xa levels to determine appropriate dose.

(Continued)

DRUG (BRAND)	HOW SUPPLIED	INDICATIONS	DOSAGE	HEPATIC/RENAL IMPAIRMENT
COAGULATION FACTOR INHIBITOR *(Continued)*				
Enoxaparin (Lovenox)	Inj: (MDV) 300mg/3mL; (Syringe) 30mg/0.3mL, 40mg/0.4mL, 60mg/0.6mL, 80mg/0.8mL, 100mg/mL, 120mg/0.8mL, 150mg/mL	Prevention of DVT in hip or knee replacement surgery, abdominal surgery, or with severely restricted mobility during acute illness. With concomitant warfarin, inpatient treatment of acute DVT with or without PE and outpatient treatment of DVT without PE. Prevention of ischemic complications in unstable angina and non-Q-wave MI with concurrent ASA therapy. Treatment of acute ST-segment elevation MI (STEMI) in patients receiving thrombolysis and being managed medically or with percutaneous coronary intervention (PCI).	Hip/Knee Surgery: 30mg SQ q12h, starting 12-24 hrs post-op, for 7-10 days (up to 14 days) or 40mg SQ qd, starting 12 hrs pre-op for hip surgery for 3 weeks. Abdominal Surgery: 40mg SQ qd, starting 2 hrs pre-op, for 7-10 days (up to12 days). DVT with or without PE treatment: (inpatient/outpatient) 1mg/kg SQ q12h or (inpatient) 1.5mg/kg SQ qd with warfarin (start within 72 hrs) for 7 days (up to 17 days). Acute Illness: 40mg SQ qd for 6-11 days (up to 14 days). Unstable Angina/Non-Q-Wave MI: 1mg/kg SQ q12h with 100-325mg/day of ASA for 2-8 days (up to 12.5 days). Acute STEMI (<75 yrs): 30mg single IV bolus plus a 1mg/kg SQ dose followed by 1mg/kg SQ q12h with ASA. Max: 100mg for 1st 2 doses only. Acute STEMI (≥75 yrs): 0.75mg/kg SQ q12h (no initial bolus) with ASA. Max: 75mg for 1st 2 doses only. When given with thrombolytic, give enoxaparin dose between 15 min before and 30 min after start of fibrinolytic therapy. With PCI, if last enoxaparin SQ dose was given >8 hrs before balloon inflation, an IV bolus of 0.3mg/kg of enoxaparin should be given.	CrCl <30mL/min: Surgery/Acute Illness: 30mg SQ qd. DVT with or without PE treatment (inpatient/outpatient)/Unstable Angina/Non-Q-Wave MI: 1mg/kg SQ qd. Acute STEMI: <75 yrs: 30mg single IV bolus plus a 1mg/kg SQ dose followed by 1mg/kg SQ qd. ≥75 yrs: 1mg/kg SQ qd (no initial bolus)
Fondaparinux (Arixtra)	Inj: (Syringe) 2.5mg/0.5mL, 5mg/0.4mL, 7.5mg/0.6mL, 10mg/0.8mL	Prophylaxis of DVT in patients undergoing hip fracture surgery, including extended prophylaxis; hip replacement surgery; knee replacement surgery; abdominal surgery who are at risk of thromboembolic complications. With concomitant warfarin, treatment of acute PE when initial therapy is administered in hospital and acute DVT.	DVT Prophylaxis: 2.5mg SQ qd, starting 6-8 hrs post-op for 5-9 days (up to 11 days). Hip Fracture Surgery: Extended prophylaxis up to 24 additional days is recommended. DVT/PE Treatment: <50kg: 5mg SQ qd. 50-100kg: 7.5mg SQ qd. >100kg: 10mg SQ qd. Add concomitant warfarin ASAP (usually within 72 hrs) and continue for 5-9 days (up to 26 days) until INR=2-3.	CrCl <30mL/min: Avoid use.
Heparin	Inj: 1000 U/mL, 5000 U/mL, 10,000 U/mL	Prophylaxis and treatment of venous thrombosis and its extension, PE in atrial fibrillation, and peripheral arterial embolism. Prevention of post-operative DVT and PE. Diagnosis and treatment of acute and chronic consumptive coagulopathies, for prevention of clotting in arterial and cardiac surgery.	Based on 68kg: Initial: 5000 U IV, then 10,000-20,000 U SQ. Maint: 8000-10,000 U SQ q8h or 15,000-20,000 U SQ q12h. Intermittent IV Injection: Initial: 10,000 U. Maint: 5000-10,000 U q4-6h. Continuous IV Infusion:Initial: 5000U. Maint: 20,000-40,000 U/24 hrs. Adjust to coagulation test results. See PI for details in specific disease states. Pediatrics: Initial: 50 U/kg IV drip. Maint: 100 U/kg IV drip q4h or 20,000 U/m^2/24 hrs continuously.	

DRUG (BRAND)	HOW SUPPLIED	INDICATIONS	DOSAGE	HEPATIC/RENAL IMPAIRMENT
COAGULATION FACTOR INHIBITOR *(Continued)*				
Phytonadione (Mephyton)	Tab: 5mg* *scored; Inj: 1mg/0.5 mL	For coagulation disorders caused by vitamin K deficiency or interference with vitamin K activity, including anticoagulant-induced prothrombin deficiency caused by coumarin or indanedione derivatives; and hypoprothrombinemia secondary to antibacterials, salicylates, obstructive jaundice, or biliary fistulas.	(Tab): Anticoagulant-Induced Prothrombin Deficiency: Initial: 2.5-10mg up to 25mg (rarely 50mg). May repeat if PT is still elevated 12-48 hrs after initial dose. Hypoprothrombinemia Due to Other Causes: 2.5-25mg or more (rarely up to 50mg). Give bile salts when endogenous bile supply to GIT is deficient. **Adults (IV):** Administer SQ when possible. Anticoagulant-Induced PT Deficiency: Initial: 2.5-10mg up to 25mg (rarely 50mg). May repeat if PT is still elevated 6-8 hrs after initial dose. Hypoprothrombinemia Due to Other Causes: 2.5-25mg or more (rarely up to 50mg); route depends on severity of condition and response. **Pediatrics** (IV): Prophylaxis of Hemorrhagic Disease in Newborn: 0.5-1mg IM within 1 hr of birth. Treatment of Hemorrhagic Disease in Newborn: 1mg SQ/IM (may need higher dose if mother has received oral anticoagulants).	
Tinzaprin (Innohep)	Inj: 20,000 anti-Xa IU/mL	Treatment of acute symptomatic DVT with or without PE with concomitant warfarin.	175 anti-Xa IU/kg SQ qd for at least 6 days and until anticoagulated with warfarin (INR is at least 2.0 for 2 consecutive days). Begin warfarin within 1-3 days of therapy.	
Warfarin (Coumadin, Jantoven)	Inj: (Coumadin) 5mg; Tab: (Coumadin, Jantoven) 1mg*, 2mg*, 2.5mg*, 3mg*, 4mg*, 5mg*, 6mg*, 7.5mg*, 10mg* *scored	Prophylaxis and treatment of venous thrombosis, PE, and thromboembolic disorders associated with atrial fibrillation and/or cardiac valve replacement. To reduce risk of death, recurrent MI, and thromboembolic events after MI.	≥18 yrs: Adjust dose based on PT/INR. Give IV as alternate to PO. Initial: 2-5mg qd. Usual: 2-10mg qd. Venous Thromboembolism (including pulmonary embolism): INR 2-3. Atrial Fibrillation: INR 2-3. Post-MI: Initiate 2-4 weeks post-infarct and maintain INR 2.5-3.5. Mechanical/Bioprosthetic Heart Valve: INR 2-3 for 12 weeks after valve insertion, then INR 2.5-3.5 long term.	
THROMBIN INHIBITOR				
Argatroban	Inj: 100mg/mL	Prophylaxis or treatment of thrombosis in heparin-induced thrombocytopenia (HIT). As an anticoagulant in patients with or at risk for HIT undergoing percutaneous coronary intervention (PCI).	Thrombosis: D/C heparin and obtain baseline aPTT. Initial: 2mcg/kg/min IV. Check aPTT after 2 hrs. Titrate: Increase dose until aPTT is 1.5-3× the initial baseline. Max: 10mcg/kg/min. PCI: Initial: 350mcg/kg bolus with 25mcg/kg/min IV. Check activated clotting time (ACT) 5-10 min after bolus. Proceed with PCI if ACT >300 seconds. See PI for detailed information for dose adjustment.	Thrombosis: Moderate Hepatic Impairment: Initial: 0.5mcg/kg/min

(Continued)

DRUG (BRAND)	HOW SUPPLIED	INDICATIONS	DOSAGE	HEPATIC/RENAL IMPAIRMENT
THROMBIN INHIBITOR *(Continued)*				
Bivalirudin (Angiomax)	Inj: 250mg	Adjunct to aspirin for anticoagulation in patients with unstable angina undergoing percutaneous transluminal coronary angioplasty (PTCA) or percutaneous coronary intervention (PCI). Patients with, or at risk of, HIT/HITTS undergoing PCI.	Initial: 0.75mg/kg IV bolus, then 1.75mg/kg/hr for duration of PCI procedure. Additional bolus of 0.3mg/kg can be given if needed based on ACT. Continuation of infusion for up to 4 hrs post-procedure is optional. After 4 hrs, if needed, an additional 0.2mg/kg/hr IV for up to 20 hrs may be initiated.	Renal Impairment: CrCl <30mL/min: 1mg/kg/hr infusion. Hemodialysis: 0.25mg/kg/hr infusion. Reduction in bolus dose not necessary; monitor anticoagulation.
Lepirudin (Refludan)	Inj: 50mg	Anticoagulant for heparin-induced thrombocytopenia (HIT) and associated thromboembolic disease.	LD: 0.4mg/kg (max 44mg) IV over 15-20 seconds. Initial: 0.15mg/kg/hr (max 16.5mg/hr) continuous infusion for 2-10 days. Adjust dose based on aPTT. Concomitant Thrombolytic Therapy: LD: 0.2mg/kg. Initial: 0.1mg/kg/hr. See PI for monitoring and adjusting therapy details.	Renal Impairment: LD: 0.2mg/kg. Initial: CrCl 45-60 mL/min: 0.075mg/kg/hr. CrCl 30-44mL/min: 0.045mg/kg/hr. CrCl 15-29 mL/min: 0.0225mg/kg/hr. CrCl <15mL/min/Hemodialysis: Avoid or stop infusion.
MISCELLANEOUS				
Aminocaproic Acid (Amicar)	Inj: 250mg/mL [20mL]; Syrup: 1.25g/5mL; Tab: 500mg*, 1000mg* *scored	To enhance hemostasis when fibrinolysis contributes to bleeding.	IV: 16-20mL (4-5g) in 250mL diluent during 1st hr, then 4mL/hr (1g) in 50mL of diluent. PO: 5g during 1st hr, then 5mL (syr) or 1g (tabs) per hr. Continue IV/PO therapy for 8 hrs or until bleeding is controlled.	
Pentoxifylline (Trental)	Tab, Extended-Release: 400mg	Treatment of intermittent claudication due to chronic occlusive arterial disease of the limbs.	400mg tid with meals for at least 8 weeks. Reduce to 400mg bid if digestive and CNS side effects occur; d/c if side effects persist.	
Thrombin (Recombinant) (Recothrom)	Powder: 5000 IU	Aid to hemostasis whenever oozing blood and minor bleeding from capillaries and small venules is accessible and control of bleeding by standard surgical techniques is ineffective or impractical. May be used in conjunction with an absorbable gelatin sponge, USP.	Apply directly on the surface of bleeding tissue or in conjunction with absorbable gelatin sponge. Required amount depends upon the tissue area to be treated. Reconstitute with sterile isotonic saline at a recommended concentration of 1000 IU/mL.	
Topical Thrombin (Thrombin-JMI)	Powder: 5,000 IU, 20,000 IU; Kit: Powder: 20,000 IU [Spray; Syringe Spray]	An aid to hemostasis whenever oozing blood and minor bleeding from capillaries and small venules is accessible. In various types of surgery, may be used in conjuction with an Absorbable Gelatin Sponge, USP for hemostasis.	Spray topically on surface of bleeding tissue. Reconstitute with sterile isotonic saline at a recommended concentration of 1,000-2,000 IU/mL. Profuse Bleeding: Use 1,000 IU/mL. General use (eg, plastic surgery, dental extractions, skin grafting): 100 IU/mL. Intermediate strengths may be prepared by diluting in appropriate isotonic saline volume if needed. Oozing surfaces: Use dry form. May be used with FlowSeal™ NT.	

DIURETICS

DRUG	BRAND	USUAL HYPERTENSION DOSAGE RANGE	HOW SUPPLIED
ALDOSTERONE-RECEPTOR BLOCKERS			
Eplerenone	Inspra	50mg qd or bid.	**Tab:** 25mg, 50mg
Spironolactone	Aldactone	50mg–100mg/day.	**Tab:** 25mg, 50mg, 100mg
LOOP DIURETICS			
Bumetanide	Bumex	0.5mg–2mg qd.	**Tab:** 0.5mg, 1mg, 2mg
Furosemide	Lasix	40mg bid.	**Tab:** 20mg, 40mg, 80mg
Torsemide	Demadex	5mg–10mg qd.	**Tab:** 5mg, 10mg, 20mg, 100mg
POTASSIUM-SPARING DIURETICS			
Amiloride	Various generics	5mg–10mg qd.	**Tab:** 5mg
Triamterene	Dyrenium	100mg–150mg bid.	**Cap:** 50mg, 100mg
THIAZIDE DIURETICS			
Chlorothiazide	Diuril	**Sus:** 0.5–1g/day.	**Sus:** 250mg/5mL
	Various generics	**Tab:** 0.5g–1g/day.	**Tab:** 250mg, 500mg
Chlorthalidone	Thalitone	15mg–50mg qd.	**Tab:** 15mg
	Various generics	25mg–100mg qd.	**Tab:** 25mg, 50mg
Hydrochlorothiazide	Microzide	12.5mg–50mg qd.	**Cap:** 12.5mg
	Various generics	25mg–50mg qd.	**Cap:** 12.5mg; **Tab:** 12.5mg, 25mg, 50mg
Indapamide	Various generics	1.25mg–5mg qd.	**Tab:** 1.25mg, 2.5mg
Metolazone	Zaroxolyn	2.5mg–5mg qd.	**Tab:** 2.5mg, 5mg, 10mg
COMBINATION DIURETICS*			
Amiloride-Hydrochlorothiazide	Various generics	1-2 tabs qd (5/50mg-10/100mg/day)	**Tab:** 5/50mg
Spironolactone-Hydrochlorothiazide	Aldactazide	50/50mg-100/100mg/day	**Tab:** 25/25mg, 50/50mg
Triamterene-Hydrochlorothiazide	Dyazide, Maxzide	37.5/25mg-75/50mg/day	**Cap:** 37.5/25mg, 25/50mg **Tab:** 37.5/25mg, 75/50mg

* Fixed combination drugs are indicated for the treatment of hypertension in patients who develop hypokalemia on hydrochlorothiazide alone.

LIPID MANAGEMENT

DRUG	BRAND	HOW SUPPLIED (mg)*	USUAL DOSAGE RANGE**	COMMENTS
HMG-CoA REDUCTASE INHIBITORS (STATINS)**				
Atorvastatin	Lipitor	**Tab:** 10, 20, 40, 80	10-80mg/day	CI: Active liver disease, unexplained persistent elevations of serum transaminases, pregnancy, nursing mothers. Generally LFTs should be monitored prior to therapy, at 12 weeks, with dose elevations, and periodically thereafter. Increased risk of myopathy with concomitant use of cyclosporine, fibrates, erythromycin, clarithromycin, HIV protease inhibitors, niacin, or azole antifungals. Use with fibrates and niacin should generally be avoided.
Fluvastatin	Lescol	**Cap:** 20, 40	20-80mg/day	
	Lescol XL	**Tab, ER:** 80		
Lovastatin	Altoprev	**Tab, ER:** 20, 40, 60	20-60mg/day	
	Mevacor	**Tab:** 20, 40	10-80mg/day given qd or bid	
Pravastatin	Pravachol	**Tab:** 10, 20, 40, 80	40-80mg qd. Renal/Hepatic dysfunction: 10mg qd	
Rosuvastatin	Crestor	**Tab:** 5, 10, 20, 40	5-40mg/day	
Simvastatin	Zocor	**Tab:** 5, 10, 20, 40, 80	5-80mg/day	
FIBRATES				
Fenofibrate	Antara	**Tab:** 43, 130	43-130mg/day	Use with statins should generally be avoided. CI: Pre-existing gallbladder disease, hepatic or severe renal dysfunction, unexplained hepatic dysfunction, primary biliary cirrhosis.
	Triglide	**Tab:** 50, 160	50-160mg/day	
	Tricor	**Tab:** 48, 145	48-145mg/day	
	Lofibra	**Cap:** 67,134, 200 **Tab:** 54, 160	67-200mg/day 54-160mg/day	
Gemfibrozil	Lopid	**Tab:** 600	1200mg/day in divided doses	
BILE-ACID SEQUESTRANTS				
Cholestyramine	Questran Questran Light Prevalite Locholest Locholest Lite	4g/pkt or scoop	8-16g/day, given bid	CI: Complete biliary obstruction. May bind to other drugs and delay/reduce absorption. Take other medications 1 hr before or 4-6 hrs after cholestyramine. Mix powder in fluid before taking. (Light): Contains phenylalanine.
Colesevelam HCl	WelChol	**Tab:** 625	3750mg/day given qd or bid	CI: Bowel obstruction, serum TG >500mg/dL, history of hypertriglyceridemia-induced pancreatitis. Take with a meal.
Colestipol	Colestid Flavored Colestid	**Granules:** 5g/pkt or scoop **Tab:** 1g	**Granules:** 1-6 pkts or scoopfuls/day given qd or in divided doses **Tab**: 2-16g/day given qd or in divided doses	May bind to other drugs and delay/reduce absorption. Take other medications 1 hr before or 4-6 hrs after Colestid. Mix granules in liquid or highly liquid food before taking. Flavored Colestid: Contains phenylalanine.
CHOLESTEROL ABSORPTION INHIBITOR				
Ezetimibe	Zetia	**Tab:** 10	10mg qd	CI: Pregnancy, nursing mothers, concomitant administration of statins in active liver disease or unexplained elevations in LFTs. Increased risk of myopathy when administered with statins. Monitor cyclosporine levels for concomitant administration.

(Continued)

DRUG	BRAND	HOW SUPPLIED (mg)*	USUAL DOSAGE RANGE**	COMMENTS
NICOTINIC ACID DERIVATIVE				
Niacin, extended-release	Niaspan	**Tab, ER:** 500, 750, 1000	1-2g qhs	CI: Significant or unexplained hepatic dysfunction, active peptic ulcer disease, arterial bleeding. Use with caution in renal insufficiency. May pretreat with ASA or NSAIDs 30 min prior to reduce flushing.
LIPID-REGULATING AGENT				
Omega-3-Acid Ethyl Esters	Lovaza	**Cap:** 1000	4g/day given qd or bid	Caution in patients with known sensitivity or allergy to fish.
COMBINATIONS				
Amlodipine-Atorvastatin	Caduet	**Tab:** (Amlodipine/Atorvastatin): 2.5/10, 2.5/20, 2.5/40, 5/10, 5/20, 5/40, 5/80, 10/10, 10/20, 10/40, 10/80	5mg/10mg to 10mg/80mg/day	See Statins.
Ezetimibe-Simvastatin	Vytorin	**Tab:** (Ezetimibe/Simvastatin): 10/10, 10/20, 10/40, 10/80	10/10 to 10/80mg/day	See Statins. Avoid use in moderate to severe hepatic insufficiency.
Niacin ER-Lovastatin	Advicor	**Tab:** (Niacin ER/Lovastatin) 500/20, 750/20, 1000/20, 1000/40	500mg/20mg to 2000mg/40mg/day qhs	See Statins and Niacin. Do not substitute for equivalent dose of immediate-release niacin. May pretreat with ASA or NSAIDs 30 min prior to reduce flushing.
Niacin ER-Simvastatin	Simcor	**Tab:** (Niacin ER/Simvastatin) 500/20, 750/20, 1000/20	500mg/20mg to 2000mg/40mg/day	See Statins and Niacin. Do not substitute for equivalent dose of immediate-release niacin. May pretreat with ASA or NSAIDs 30 min prior to reduce flushing.

* Unless otherwise indicated.

** **NOTE:** Dosages shown are for adults and may need to be adjusted to individual patient needs. For pediatric dosing and additional information please refer to the individual monograph listings or the drug's FDA-approved labeling. According to NCEP-ATP III guidelines, lipid-altering agents should be used in addition to a diet restricted in saturated fat and cholesterol only when the response to diet and other nonpharmacological measures has been inadequate.

Abbreviations: CI: Contraindications; ER: Extended-Release.

ACNE MANAGEMENT: SYSTEMIC THERAPIES

DRUG (BRAND)	**HOW SUPPLIED**	**DOSAGE**	**SIDE EFFECTS**
ANTIBIOTICS			
Doxycycline hyclate (Doryx, Vibramycin)	Doryx: (Tab, Delayed-Release) 75mg, 100mg, 150mg Vibramycin: (Cap) 50mg, 100mg	100mg q12h on 1st day, followed by 100mg qd.	Anorexia, nausea, vomiting, diarrhea, dysphagia, enterocolitis, rash, exfoliative dermatitis, renal toxicity, hypersensitivity reactions, blood dyscrasias, tooth discoloration, photosensitivity
Doxycycline monohydrate (Monodox)	Cap: 50mg, 75 mg, 100mg	100mg q12h or 50mg q6h for 1 day, then 100mg/day.	GI effects, photosensitivity, rash, blood dyscrasias, hypersensitivity reactions, tooth discoloration
Doxycycline, USP (Oracea)	Cap: 40mg	40mg qd am.	Anorexia, nausea, sinusitis, diarrhea, abdominal pain
Minocycline HCl (Dynacin, Minocin)	Cap: 50mg, 75mg, 100mg; Tab: 50mg, 75mg, 100mg	200mg initially, then 100mg q12h; alternative is 100-200mg initially, then 50mg qid.	Anorexia, nausea, vomiting, diarrhea, dysphagia, enterocolitis, pancreatitis, increased LFTs, hepatitis, liver failure, renal toxicity, rash, exfoliative dermatitis, Stevens-Johnson syndrome, skin and mucous membrane pigmentation, blood dyscrasias, headache, tooth discoloration, photosensitivity, intracranial HTN
Minocycline HCl (Solodyn)	Tab, Extended-Release: 45mg, 90mg, 135mg	1mg/kg qd for 12 weeks.	Headache, fatigue, dizziness, pruritus, malaise, mood alteration, Stevens-Johnson syndrome, photosensitivity, tooth discoloration
Tetracycline HCl (Sumycin)	Sus: 125mg/5mL; Tab: 250mg, 500mg	Mild-Moderate: 250mg qid or 500mg bid. Severe: 500mg qid. Severe Acne: Initial: 1g/day in divided doses. Maint: After improvement, 125-500mg/day.	GI effects, photosensitivity, increased BUN, hypersensitivity reactions, blood dyscrasias, dizziness, headache, tooth discoloration
ORAL CONTRACEPTIVES			
Ethinyl Estradiol and Drospirenone (YAZ)	Tab: (Ethinyl Estradiol-Drospirenone) 0.02mg-3mg	1 tab qd for 28 days, then repeat. Start on first Sunday of menses or begin 1st day of menses.	Nausea, vomiting, breakthrough bleeding, spotting, amenorrhea, migraine, vaginal candidiasis, edema, weight changes, depression, urticaria, angioedema, circulatory symptoms, dysmenorrhea
Ethinyl Estradiol and Norgestimate (Ortho Tri-Cyclen)	Tab: (Ethinyl Estradiol-Norgestimate) 0.035mg-0.18mg, 0.035mg-0.215mg, 0.035mg-0.25mg	1 tab qd for 28 days, then repeat. Start on first Sunday of menses or begin 1st day of menses.	Nausea, vomiting, breakthrough bleeding, spotting, amenorrhea, migraine, depression, vaginal candidiasis, edema, weight changes
Ethinyl Estradiol and Norethindrone (Estrostep Fe)	Tab: (Ethinyl Estradiol-Norethindrone) 0.035mg-1mg, 0.030mg-1mg, 0.020mg-1mg and 75mg ferrous fumarate	1 tab qd for 28 days, then repeat. Start on first Sunday of menses or begin 1st day of menses.	Nausea, vomiting, breakthrough bleeding, spotting, amenorrhea, migraine, depression, vaginal candidiasis, edema, weight changes

(Continued)

DRUG (BRAND)	**HOW SUPPLIED**	**DOSAGE**	**SIDE EFFECTS**
RETINOID			
Isotretinoin (Accutane, Amnesteem, Claravis, Sotret)	Accutane, Amnesteem, Claravis: (Cap) 10mg, 20mg, 40mg Sotret: (Cap) 10mg, 20mg, 30mg, 40mg	0.5-1mg/kg/day given bid for 15-20 weeks.	Cheilitis, dry skin and mucous membranes, conjunctivitis, blood dyscrasias, epistaxis, decreased HDL, elevated cholesterol and TG, elevated blood sugar, arthralgias, back pain, hearing/vision impairment, rash, photosensitivity reactions, psychiatric disorders

References:
FDA-Approved Product Labeling.

ACNE MANAGEMENT: TOPICAL THERAPIES

DRUG (BRAND)	**HOW SUPPLIED**	**DOSAGE**	**SIDE EFFECTS**
ANTIBACTERIAL/KERATOLYTIC AGENTS & COMBINATIONS			
Benzoyl peroxide (Benzac AC, Benzagel, Triaz)	Benzac AC: (Gel) 5%, 10% [60g], (Wash) 10% [60g]; Benzagel: (Gel) 5%, 10% [42.5g], (Wash) 10% [60g]; Triaz: (Gel) 3%, 6%, 9% [42.5g], (Cleanser) 3%, 6%, 9% [170.3g, 340.2g], (Pads) 3%, 6%, 9% [30g, 60g]	(Benzac) Apply qd-bid. (Benzagel) Apply wash qd-bid; apply gel qd initially or qhs for light skin. (Triaz) Apply gel/ wash qd-bid.	Erythema, peeling, contact dermatitis, dryness, irritation
Benzoyl peroxide/ Sulfur (Sulfoxyl Lotion Regular/Strong)	Lot: (Regular): 10%-2% [59mL]; (Strong): 10%-5% [59mL]	Apply initially once daily for the first week then twice daily, as tolerated.	Erythema, peeling, contact, dermatitis, dryness, irritation, itching, redness
Clindamycin/ Benzoyl peroxide (Benzaclin, Duac)	Benzaclin: (Gel) 1%-5% [25g, 50g]; Duac: (Gel) 1%-5% [45g]	(Benzaclin) Apply bid. (Duac) Apply once in the evening.	Dry skin, erythema, peeling, and burning
Benzoyl peroxide/ Erythromycin (Benzamycin)	Gel: 5%-3% [23.3g, 46.6g, 60^s]	Apply bid.	Dryness, urticaria, skin irritation, skin discoloration, oiliness
Benzoyl peroxide (Brevoxyl, Zoderm)	Brevoxyl: (Gel) 4%, 8% [42.5g], (Lot, Creamy Wash) 4%, 8% [170g]; Zoderm: (Cleanser) 4.5%, 6.5%, 8.5% [400mL], (Cre/Gel) 4.5%, 6.5%, 8.5% [125mL]	(Brevoxyl) Apply gel qd-bid; apply lotion qd for first week then bid as tolerated. (Zoderm) Apply qd-bid.	Erythema, peeling, contact dermatitis, dryness
ANTIBIOTICS & COMBINATIONS			
Clindamycin (Cleocin T, Clindagel, Clindets, Evoclin Foam)	Cleocin T: (Gel) 1% [30g, 60g], (Lot) 1% [60mL], (Sol) 1% [30mL, 60mL], (Swab, Pledgets) 1% [60^s]; Clindagel: 1% [42g, 77g]; Clindets: (Swab) 1% [69]; Evoclin: (Foam) 1% [50g, 100g]	(Cleocin T) Apply bid. (Clindagel) Apply qd. (Clindets) Apply bid. (Evoclin Foam) Apply qd.	Local irritation, stains clothing
Clindamycin/ Tretinoin (Ziana)	Gel: 1.2%-0.025% [2g, 30g, 60g]	Apply qd at bedtime.	Nasopharyngitis, erythema, scaling, itching, burning
Erythromycin (Erygel Erythromycin Topical Swabs)	Erygel: 2% [30g, 60g]; Erythromycin Topical Swabs: 2% [60g]	(Erygel) Apply qd-bid. Erythromycin Topical Swabs: Apply bid.	Local irritation, stains clothing, peeling, dryness, itching, erythema, oiliness
Sulfacetamide (Klaron)	Lot: 10% [118mL]	Apply bid.	Itching, erythema, edema
Sulfacetamide/ Sulfur (Plexion TS, Sulfacet-R)	Plexion TS: (Lot) 10%-5% [30g]; Sulfacet-R: (Lot) 10%-5% [25g]	Apply qd-tid.	Local irritation
Sulfacetamide/ Sulfur (Plexion SCT, Rosac)	Plexion SCT: (Cre) 10%-5% [4oz] Rosac: (Cre) 10%-5% [45g]	(Rosac) Apply qd-tid. (Plexion SCT) Apply qd.	Local irritation
Sulfacetamide/ Sulfur (Clenia, Plexion, Rosula)	Clenia: (Cleanser) 10%-5% [170g, 340g], Cre: 10%-5% [28g]; Plexion: (Cleanser) 10%-5% [170.3g, 340.2g]; Rosula: (Cleanser) 10%-5% [355mL], Gel 10%-5% [45mL]	(Clenia) Apply wash qd-bid; apply cream qd-tid. (Plexion) Apply qd-bid. (Rosula) Apply cleanser qd-bid; apply gel qd-tid.	Local irritation
Sulfacetamide/ Urea (Rosula NS Dicarboxylic Acids)	(Swab) 10%-10% [30^s]	Apply qd-bid.	Local hypersensitivity, instances of Stevens-Johnson syndrome

(Continued)

DRUG (BRAND)	**HOW SUPPLIED**	**DOSAGE**	**SIDE EFFECTS**
ANTIBIOTICS & COMBINATIONS *(Continued)*			
Azelaic acid (Azelex)	(Cre) 20% [30g, 50g]	Apply bid.	Dryness, scaling, erythema, burning, irritation, pruritus; rarely, hypopigmentation
Azelaic acid (Finacea)	(Gel) 15% [30g, 50g]	Apply bid.	Burning, stinging, tingling, pruritus, scaling, dry skin
Adapalene (Differin)	(Cre) 0.1% [45g]; (Gel) 0.1%, 0.3% [45g, 75g]	Apply hs.	Erythema, scaling, dryness, pruritus, burning, sunburn, acne flares
Tazarotene (Avage, Tazorac)	(Cre) 0.1% [15g, 30g]; 0.5% [30g, 60g]; (Gel) 0.05%, 0.1% [30g, 100g]	Apply hs.	Pruritus, burning/stinging, erythema, irritation, skin pain, desquamation, dry skin, rash
Tretinoin (Atralin, Avita, Retin-A)	(Cre) 0.025%, 0.05%, 0.1% [20g, 45g]; (Gel) 0.01%, 0.025% [15g, 45g]; (Sol) 0.05% [28mL]	Apply hs.	Local skin reactions (red, edematous, blistered, crusted), photosensitivity, temporary skin pigmentation changes
Tretinoin microsphere (Retin-A-Micro)	(Gel) 0.04%, 0.1% [20g, 45g]	Apply hs.	

Source: FDA-approved product labeling.

PSORIASIS MANAGEMENT: SYSTEMIC THERAPIES

DRUG (BRAND)	HOW SUPPLIED	DOSAGE	SIDE EFFECTS
ANTIMETABOLITE			
Methotrexate	**Inj:** 20mg, 1g, 25mg/mL; **Tab:** 2.5mg, 5mg, 7.5mg, 10mg, 15mg	**Initial:** 10-25mg weekly until response or use divided oral dose schedule, 2.5mg at 12-hr intervals for 3 doses. **Titrate:** Increase gradually until optimal response. **Maint:** Reduce to lowest effective dose. **Max:** 30mg/wk.	Ulcerative stomatitis, leukopenia, nausea, abdominal distress, malaise, fatigue, chills, fever, dizziness, decreased resistance to infection
IMMUNOSUPPRESSIVES			
Alefacept (Amevive)	**Inj:** (IV) 7.5mg, (IM) 15mg	7.5mg IV bolus or 15mg IM once wkly for 12 wks. May repeat cycle 12 wks after first cycle complete. Adjust dose, D/C, based on CD4+ T-lymphocyte counts.	Lymphopenia, injection-site reactions, influenza-like symptoms, pruritus, hypersensitivity reactions
Cyclosporine (Neoral)	**Cap:** 25mg, 100mg; **Sol:** 100mg/mL [50mL]	**Initial:** 1.25mg/kg bid for 4 wks. **Titrate:** May increase by 0.5mg/kg/day every 2 weeks. **Max:** 4mg/kg/day.	Infection, renal dysfunction, HTN, malignancy risk w/certain psoriasis therapies, hirsutism, muscle cramps, acne, tremor, headache, gingival hyperplasia, diarrhea, nausea, vomiting
MONOCLONAL ANTIBODIES/TNF BLOCKERS			
Adalimumab (Humira)	**Inj:** 20mg/0.4mL, 40mg/0.8mL	**Initial:** 80mg. **Maint:** 40mg every other week starting 1 week after initial dose.	URI, injection-site pain/reactions, headache, rash, sinusitis, nausea, UTI, flu syndrome, abdominal pain, hyperlipidemia, hypercholesterolemia, back pain, hematuria, HTN, immunogenicity
Infliximab (Remicade)	**Inj:** 100mg	5mg/kg IV infusion; repeat at 2 and 6 weeks. **Maint:** 5mg/kg every 8 weeks.	Infusion reactions, nausea, infections, URI, pruritus, headache, sore throat, potential risk of reactivating TB, hepatotoxicity
PSORALENS			
Methoxsalen* (8-Mop, Oxsoralen-Ultra)	**Cap:** 10mg	Take with food or milk. **Initial:** <30kg: 10mg. 30-50kg: 20mg. 51-65kg: 30mg. 66-80kg: 40mg. 81-90kg: 50mg. 91-115kg: 60mg. >115kg: 70mg. Take 2 hrs before UVA exposure. **Titrate:** May increase by 10mg after 15th treatment under certain conditions. **Max:** Do not treat more often than qod.	Nausea, nervousness, insomnia, depression, pruritus, erythema
RETINOID			
Acitretin (Soriatane)	**Cap:** 10mg, 25mg	**Initial:** 25-50mg qd w/food. Individualize dose based on intersubject variation in pharmacokinetics, clinical efficacy, and incidence of side effects. **Maint:** 25-50mg qd. Terminate therapy when lesions resolve. May treat relapses.	Ophthalmologic effects, cheilitis, rhinitis, dry mouth, epistaxis, alopecia, dry skin, rash, skin peeling, nail disorder, pruritus, paresthesia, paronychia, skin atrophy, sticky skin, xerophthalmia, arthralgia

(Continued)

DRUG (BRAND)	HOW SUPPLIED	DOSAGE	SIDE EFFECTS
TNF-BLOCKING AGENT			
Etanercept (Enbrel)	**Inj:** 25mg [vial], 25mg/0.5mL [syringe] 50mg/mL [syringe]	**Initial:** 50mg SQ twice weekly given 3 or 4 days apart for 3 months. May begin with 25-50mg/wk. **Maint:** 50mg/wk.	Injection site reactions, infections, headache

* Oxsoralen-Ultra and 8-MOP are not interchangeable due to significantly greater bioavailability and earlier photosensitization onset time of Oxsoralen-Ultra.

Sources: FDA-approved product labeling. Luba KM, Stulberg DL. Chronic plaque psoriasis. *Am Fam Physician.* 2006 Feb 15;73(4):636-44. Review.

PSORIASIS MANAGEMENT: TOPICAL THERAPIES

DRUG (BRAND)	HOW SUPPLIED	DOSAGE	SIDE EFFECTS
TOPICAL IMMUNOSUPPRESSANT			
Pimecrolimus (Elidel)	Cre: 1% [30g, 60g, 100g]	Apply bid.	Burning, headache, nasopharyngitis, pyrexia, influenza, pharyngitis, viral infection
TOPICAL STEROIDS			
Clobetasol (Temovate, Temovate-E, Clobex, Embeline E, Olux, Olux-E)	(Temovate) Cre, Oint: 0.05% [15g, 30g, 45g, 60g]; Gel: 0.05% [15g, 30g, 60g]; Sol: 0.05% [25mL, 50mL]; (Temovate-E) Cre: 0.05% [15g, 30g, 60g]; (Clobex) Lot: 0.05% [30mL, 59mL, 118mL]; Shampoo: 0.05% [118mL]; Spray: 0.05% [2oz]; (Embeline E) Cre: 0.05% [15g, 30g,60g]; (Olux) Foam: 0.05% [50g, 100g] (Olux-E) Foam: 0.05% [100g]	Apply bid.	Hypopigmentation, tachyphylaxis, striae, skin atrophy. Other common side effects: burning, stinging, pruritus, erythema, folliculitis, cracking/fissures of the skin, numbness in fingers, tenderness
Fluocinolone (Synalar)	Cre, Oint: 0.025% [15g, 60g]; Sol: 0.01% [20mL, 60mL]	Apply bid-qid.	Dryness, folliculitis, acne, skin atrophy, burning, itching, irritation
Fluocinonide (Lidex, Lidex-E, Vanos)	(Lidex) Cre, Gel, Oint: 0.05% [15g, 30g, 60g, 120mg]; Sol: 0.05% [20mL, 60mL]; (Lidex-E) Cre: 0.05% [15g, 30g, 60g]; (Vanos) Cre: 0.1% [30mg, 60mg, 120mg]	(Lidex, Lidex-E) Apply bid-qid. (Vanos) Apply qd-bid.	Burning, itching, irritation, dryness, folliculitis, acne, hypopigmentation, skin atrophy
Halcinonide (Halog, Halog-E)	(Halog) Cre, Oint: 0.1% [15g, 30g, 60g, 240g]; Sol: 0.1% [20mL, 60mL]; (Halog-E) Cre: 0.1% in a hydrophilic vanishing cream [30g, 60g]	(Cre, Oint, Sol) Apply bid-tid. (Cre, hydrophilic base) Apply qd-tid.	Burning, itching, irritation, dryness, folliculitis, hypopigmentation, contact dermatitis, skin maceration
Hydrocortisone (Hytone, Locoid, Pandel, Westcort)	(Hytone 1%, 2.5%) Cre: [1oz, 2oz] Lot: [2oz] (Locoid 0.1%) Lot: [2oz, 4oz] Oint: [15g, 45g] Cre: [15g, 45g, 60g] Sol: [20mL, 60mL] (Pandel) Cre: 0.1% [15g, 45g, 80g]; (Westcort) Cre, Oint: 0.2% [15g, 45g, 60g]	(Hytone) bid-qid; (Locoid) Lot: bid; Oint, Cre, Sol: bid-tid (Pandel) Apply qd-bid. (Westcort) Apply bid-tid.	Burning, stinging, moderate paresthesia, itching, dryness, folliculitis, hypopigmentation, skin atrophy
Hydrocortisone/ Pramoxine (Epifoam, Novacort, Pramosone)	(Epifoam) Foam: (Hydrocortisone-Pramoxine) 1%-1% [10g]; (Novacort) Gel: 2%-1% [29g]; (Pramosone) Cre: 1%-1%, 1%-2.5% Lot: 1%-1% [60mL, 120mL, 240mL], 1%-2.5% [60mL, 120mL]; Oint: 1%-1%, 1%-2.5% [30g]	Apply tid-qid.	Burning, itching, irritation, dryness, folliculitis, hypopigmentation, maceration, skin atrophy
Mometasone (Elocon)	Cre, Oint: 0.1% [15g, 45g]; Lot: 0.1% [30mL, 60mL]	Apply qd.	Burning, pruritus, skin atrophy, rosacea, acneiform reaction, tingling, stinging, furunculosis, folliculitis
Prednicarbate (Dermatop)	Cre, Oint: 0.1% [15g, 60g]	Apply bid.	Burning, itching, irritation, dryness, folliculitis, hypertrichosis, acneiform eruptions, hypopigmentation
Triamcinolone (Kenalog)	(Kenalog) Cre: 0.1% [15g, 60g, 80g], 0.5% [20g]; Lot: 0.025%, 0.1% [15mL, 60mL]; Oint: 0.025%: [15g, 80g, 240g] 0.1%: [15g, 60g, 80g, 240g] 0.5%: [20g]; Spray: 0.147mg/g [63g]	(Kenalog) Cre, Lot, Oint: Apply 0.025% bid-qid. Apply 0.1% or 0.5% bid-tid. Spray: Apply tid-qid.	Burning, itching, irrita-, tion, dryness, folliculitis, hypopigmentation, allergic contact dermatitis

(Continued)

DRUG (BRAND)	HOW SUPPLIED	DOSAGE	SIDE EFFECTS
TOPICAL RETINOID			
Tazarotene (Avage, Tazorac)	Cre: 0.05%, 0.1% [15g, 30g, 60g]; Gel: 0.05%, 0.1% [30g, 100g]	Apply hs.	Pruritus, erythema, irritation, dry skin, rash, skin discoloration
VITAMIN D DERIVATIVES & COMBINATIONS			
Calcipotriene (Dovonex, Dovonex Scalp)	(Dovonex) Cre, Oint: 0.005% [60g, 120g]; (Dovonex Scalp) Sol: 0.005% [60mL]	(Dovonex) Apply bid. (Dovonex Scalp) Apply bid.	Skin irritation, pruritus, burning, hypercalcemia
Calcipotriene/ betamethasone (Taclonex)	Oint: (Calcipotriene-Betamethasone) 0.005%-0.064% [15g, 30g, 60g] Scalp Sus: [60g]	Apply ud.	Pruritus, headache
MISCELLANEOUS AGENTS			
Anthralin (Anthra-Derm)	Cre: 1% [50g]	Apply qd-bid.	Skin irritation, erythema, staining (skin and clothing), odor
Coal Tar (Zetar)	Sol 10%: 2% [3.8oz]	Apply hs.	Skin irritation, folliculitis, odor, staining of clothing
Urea (Carmol 40)	Cre: 40% [28.35g, 85g, 198.6g]; Gel: 40% [15mL]; Lot: 40% [236.6 mL]	Apply bid.	Transient stinging, burning, itching, irritation

Sources:
FDA-approved drug labeling.
Luba KM, Stulberg DL. Chronic plaque psoriasis. *Am Fam Physician.* 2006 Feb 15;73(4):636-44. Review.

TOPICAL CORTICOSTEROIDS

STEROID	DOSAGE FORM(S)	STRENGTH (%)	POTENCY	FREQUENCY
Alclometasone Dipropionate (Aclovate)	Cre, Oint	0.05	Low-Med	bid/tid
Augmented Betamethasone Dipropionate (Diprolene, Diprolene AF)	Cre, Oint	0.05	Very High	qd/bid
	Cre, Lot	0.05	High	qd/bid
Betamethasone Dipropionate	Cre, Lot, Oint	0.05	High	qd/bid
Betamethasone Valerate (Luxiq)	Foam	0.12	Medium	bid
Clobetasol Propionate (Clobevate, Clobex, Cormax, Embeline E, Olux, Olux E, Temovate, Temovate-E)	Cre, Foam (Olux)	0.05	Very High	bid
	Cream (Embeline E), Foam, Gel (Clobevate), Lotion (Clobex), Oint, Shampoo (Clobex), Sol	0.05	Very High	qd (shampoo)
Clocortolone Pivalate (Cloderm)	Cre	0.1	Med	tid
Desonide (Desonate, DesOwen, Verdeso)	Cre, Foam, Gel (Desonate), Lot, Oint	0.05	Low-Med	bid/tid
Desoximetasone (Topicort, Topicort LP)	Cre	0.05	Medium	bid
	Cre, Oint	0.25	High	bid
	Gel	0.05	High	bid
Diflorasone Diacetate (Psorcon)	Oint, Cre (Psorcon)	0.05	Very High	bid
Fluocinolone Acetonide (Capex, Derma-Smoothe/FS, Synalar)	Cre, Oint	0.025	Medium	tid/qid
	Sol	0.01	Medium	bid/qid
	Oil (Derma-Smoothe/FS)	0.01	Medium	tid
	Shampoo (Capex)	0.01	Medium	qd
Fluocinonide (Lidex, Lidex-E, Vanos)	Cre, Gel, Oint, Sol	0.05	High	bid/qid
	Cre	0.1	Very High	qd/bid
Flurandrenolide (Cordran, Cordran SP)	Cre, Oint	0.025	Medium	bid/tid
	Cre, Lot, Oint	0.05	Medium	bid/tid
	Tape	4mcg/cm^2	Medium	qd/bid
Fluticasone Propionate (Cutivate)	Cre, Lot	0.05	Medium	qd/bid
	Oint	0.005	Medium	bid
Halcinonide (Halog, Halog-E)	Cre, Oint, Sol	0.1	High	bid/tid
Halobetasol Propionate (Ultravate)	Cre, Oint	0.05	Very High	qd/bid
Hydrocortisone (Anusol HC, Hytone)	Lot, Cre	1	Low	tid/qid
	Cre, Lot, Oint	2.5	Low	bid/qid
Hydrocortisone Butyrate (Locoid, Locoid Lipo Cream)	Cre, Lot, Oint, Sol	0.1	Medium	bid/tid
Hydrocortisone Probutate (Pandel)	Cre	0.1	Medium	qd/bid
Hydrocortisone Valerate (Westcort)	Cre, Oint	0.2	Medium	bid/tid
Mometasone Furoate (Elocon)	Cre, Lot, Oint	0.1	Medium	qd
Prednicarbate (Dermatop)	Cre, Oint	0.1	Medium	bid
Triamcinolone Acetonide (Kenalog, Triderm)	Cre, Lot, Oint	0.025	Medium	bid/qid
	Cre, Lot, Oint	0.1	Medium	bid/tid
	Cre, Oint	0.5	High	bid/tid
	Spray	0.147	Medium	tid/qid

INSULIN FORMULATIONS

TYPE OF INSULIN	BRAND	ONSET* (hrs)	PEAK* (hrs)	DURATION* (hrs)
Rapid-acting				
Insulin Glulisine	Apidra	–	0.5 to 1.7	1 to 3
Insulin Lispro	Humalog	<0.25	0.5 to 1.5	3 to 5
Insulin Aspart	Novolog	<0.25	0.5 to 1	3 to 5
Short-acting				
Regular Insulin	Humulin R†	0.5 to 1	2 to 4	4 to 12
	Novolin R	0.5	2.5 to 5	8
Intermediate-acting				
NPH (Isophane)	Humulin N	1 to 3	6 to 12	18 to 24
	Novolin N	1.5	4 to 12	24
Long-acting				
Insulin glargine	Lantus	1	Flat	24
Insulin detemir	Levemir	–	6 to 8	24
Combinations				
Isophane insulin suspension (70%)/ regular insulin (30%)	Humulin 70/30	0.5 to 1	4 to 6	24
	Novolin 70/30	0.5	2 to 12	24
Isophane insulin suspension (50%)/ regular insulin (50%)	Humulin 50/50	0.5 to 1	3 to 5	24
Insulin lispro protamine (75%)/ insulin lispro (25%)	Humalog Mix 75/25	≤0.25	0.5 to 4	24
Insulin aspart protamine (70%)/ insulin aspart (30%)	Novolog Mix 70/30	≤0.25	1 to 4	24

*Approximate parameters following SC injection of an average patient dose; insulin concentration: 100 U/mL.

†Also available as 500 U/mL for insulin-resistant patients (rapid onset; up to 24-hr duration).

ORAL ANTIDIABETIC AGENTS

DRUG	HOW SUPPLIED	INITIAL* & (MAX) DOSE	USUAL DOSE RANGE*
BIGUANIDES			
Metformin HCl			
Fortamet	**Tab: ER:** 500mg, 1000mg	1000mg qd with evening meal (2500mg/day).	500-2500mg qd.
Glumetza	**Tab: ER:** 500mg, 1000mg	1000mg qd with evening meal (2000mg/day).	1500mg-2000mg/day.
Glucophage, Riomet	**Tab:** 500mg, 850mg, 1000mg **Sol:** 500mg/5mL	500mg bid or 850mg qd with meals (2550mg/day).	850mg-2000mg/day qd or divided doses.
Glucophage XR	**Tab: ER:** 500mg, 750mg	500mg qd with evening meal (2550mg/day).	500-2000mg/day qd or divided doses.
BILE-ACID SEQUESTRANT			
Colesevelam HCl Welchol	**Tab:** 625mg	1875mg bid or 3750mg qd (3750mg/day).	3750mg qd.
DIPEPTIDYL PEPTIDASE-4 INHIBITOR			
Sitagliptin Januvia	**Tab:** 25mg, 50mg, 100mg	100mg qd.	100mg qd.
GLUCOSIDASE INHIBITORS			
Acarbose Precose	**Tab:** 25mg, 50mg, 100mg	25mg tid at start of each meal (≤60kg: 50mg tid, >60kg: 100mg tid).	25-100mg tid.
Miglitol Glyset	**Tab:** 25mg, 50mg, 100mg	25mg tid at start of each meal (300mg/day).	50-100mg tid.
MEGLITINIDES			
Nateglinide Starlix	**Tab:** 60mg, 120mg	120mg tid before meals (360mg/day).	120mg tid.
Repaglinide Prandin	**Tab:** 0.5mg, 1mg, 2mg	0.5-2mg with each meal (16mg/day).	0.5-4mg with each meal.
SULFONYLUREAS			
Chlorpropamide Diabinese	**Tab:** 100mg, 250mg	Initial: 250mg daily. Elderly: 100-125mg/day. (750mg/day).	<100-500mg daily. Most patients controlled with 250mg daily.
Glimepiride Amaryl	**Tab:** 1mg, 2mg, 4mg	1-2mg qd w/breakfast or first main meal (8mg/day).	1-4mg qd.
Glipizide			
Glucotrol	**Tab:** 5mg, 10mg	5mg qd before breakfast (40mg/day).	5-40mg qd or divided if >15mg/day.
Glucotrol XL	**Tab, ER:** 2.5mg, 5mg, 10mg	5mg qd w/breakfast (20mg/day).	5-10mg qd.
Glyburide Diabeta, Micronase	**Tab:** 1.25mg, 2.5mg, 5mg	2.5-5mg qd w/breakfast or first main meal (20mg/day).	1.25-20mg qd or divided doses.
Glynase PresTab	**Tab:** 1.5mg, 3mg, 6mg	1.5-3mg qd w/breakfast or first main meal (12mg/day).	0.75-12mg qd or divided doses.

(Continued)

DRUG	HOW SUPPLIED	INITIAL* & (MAX) DOSE	USUAL DOSE RANGE*
THIAZOLIDINEDIONES			
Pioglitazone HCl Actos	**Tab:** 15mg, 30mg, 45mg	15-30mg qd (45mg/day).	15-30mg qd.
Rosiglitazone maleate Avandia	**Tab:** 2mg, 4mg, 8mg	2mg bid or 4mg qd (8mg/day).	4mg bid or 8mg qd.
COMBINATIONS			
Glipizide/ Metformin HCl Metaglip	**Tab:** 2.5mg/250mg, 2.5mg/500mg, 5mg/500mg	2.5mg/250mg qd w/meals or 2.5mg/500mg bid (20mg/2g/day).	2.5mg/250mg qd-2.5mg/500mg bid.
Glyburide/ Metformin HCl Glucovance	**Tab:** 1.25mg/250mg, 2.5mg/500mg, 5mg/500mg	1.25mg/250mg qd or bid with meals (20mg/2g/day).	1.25mg/250mg qd-5mg/500mb bid.
Pioglitazone/ Glimepiride Duetact	**Tab:** 30mg/2mg, 30mg/4mg	30mg/2mg qd or 30mg/4mg qd Do not give more than once daily at any of the tablet strengths.	1 tab qd.
Pioglitazone/ Metformin HCl Actoplus Met	**Tab:** 15mg/500mg, 15mg/850mg	15mg/500mg or 15mg/850mg qd-bid (45mg/2250mg/day).	1 tab qd-bid.
Repaglinide/ Metformin HCl PrandiMet	**Tab:** 1mg/500mg, 2mg/500mg	1mg/500mg bid-tid before meals or 2mg/500mg bid-tid before meals (10mg/2500/day)	1 tab bid-tid.
Rosiglitazone/ Glimepiride Avandaryl	**Tab:** 4mg/1mg, 4mg/2mg, 4mg/4mg, 8mg/2mg, 8mg/4mg	4mg/1mg qd or 4mg/2mg qd w/first meal (8mg/4mg qd).	1 tab am.
Rosiglitazone/ Metformin HCl Avandamet	**Tab:** 1mg/500mg, 2mg/500mg, 4mg/500mg, 2mg/1g, 4mg/1g	2mg/500mg qd-bid w/meals (8mg/2g/day).	1 tab bid.
Sitagliptin/ Metformin Janumet	**Tab:** 50mg/500mg, 50mg/1000mg	50mg/500mg or 50mg/1000mg bid w/meals (100mg/2g qd).	1 tab bid.

*NOTE: Usual dose ranges are derived from the drug's FDA-approved labeling. There is no fixed dosage regimen for the management of diabetes mellitus with any hypoglycemic agent. The initial and maintenance dosing should be conservative, depending on the patient's individual needs, especially in elderly, debilitated or malnourished patients, and with impaired renal or hepatic function. Management of type 2 diabetes should include blood glucose and HbA1c monitoring, nutritional counseling, exercise, and weight reduction as needed. For more detailed information refer to the individual monograph listings or the drug's FDA-approved labeling.

ANTIEMETICS

DRUG (BRAND)	INDICATIONS	HOW SUPPLIED	ADULT DOSING	PEDIATRIC DOSING
Anticholinergic Agent				
Scopolamine (Transderm Scop)	Prevention of nausea and vomiting associated with motion sickness or recovery from anesthesia and surgery.	Patch: 0.33mg/24 hrs [4[S]]	Apply 1 patch the evening before surgery or 1 hr prior to cesarean section. Keep in place for 24 hrs. Apply patch to a hairless area behind the ear at least 4 hrs before needed. Do not cut patch in half.	
Antihistamines				
Dimenhydrinate (Dramamine Original Formula)	Prevention and treatment of nausea, vomiting, or vertigo caused by motion sickness.	Inj: 50mg/mL	(Inj) 50mg q4h, may increase to 100mg q4h if drowsiness is desirable. For IV administration, dilute each mL of solution in 10mL of 0.9% sodium chloride and inject over 2 minutes. IM injection is administered undiluted.	(IM) 1.25mg/kg or 37.5mg/m^2 body surface area qid. Max: 300mg/day.
Meclizine HCl (Antivert)	Management of nausea, vomiting and dizziness associated with motion sickness. Management of vertigo associated with diseases affecting the vestibular system.	Tab: 12.5mg, 25mg, 50mg* *scored	25-50mg 1 hr prior to trip/departure, repeat q24h prn.	**≥12 yrs:** Motion Sickness: 25-50mg 1 hr prior to trip/departure, repeat q24h prn. Vertigo: 25-100mg/day in divided doses.
Promethazine HCl (Phenergan)	Prevention and control of nausea and vomiting in surgery. Active and prophylactic treatment of motion sickness.	Liq: 6.25/5mL [473mL, 118mL]; Sup: 12.5mg, 25mg; Tab: 12.5mg, 25mg, 50mg; Inj: 25mg/mL, 50mg/mL	Nausea/Vomiting: 12.5-25mg q4h; Motion Sickness: 25mg bid 0.5-1h prior to trip/departure	**≥2 yrs:** Dose should not exceed half of adult dose. Premedication: Usual: 0.5mg/lb. Do not give IV administration >25mg/mL and at a rate >25mg/min.
Cannabinoids				
Dronabinol (Marinol)	Treatment of nausea and vomiting associated with chemotherapy when conventional treatment has failed.	Cap: 2.5mg, 5mg, 10mg	Initial: 5mg/m^2 given 1-3 hrs before chemotherapy, then q2-4h after chemotherapy, up to 4-6 doses/day. Titrate: May increase by 2.5mg/m^2 increments. Max: 15mg/m^2/dose.	
Nabilone (Cesamet)	Treatment of the nausea and vomiting associated with chemotherapy when conventional treatment has failed.	Cap: 1mg	Initial: 1 or 2mg bid; given 1-3 hrs before chemotherapy. A dose of 1 or 2mg the night before may be useful. Max: 6mg/day given in divided doses tid.	

(Continued)

DRUG (BRAND)	INDICATIONS	HOW SUPPLIED	ADULT DOSING	PEDIATRIC DOSING
5-HT_3 Antagonists				
Dolasetron mesylate (Anzemet)	(Inj) Prevention of nausea/vomiting associated with emetogenic cancer chemotherapy including high-dose cisplatin. Prevention and treatment of post-op nausea/vomiting (PONV). (Tab) Prevention of nausea/vomiting associated with moderately emetogenic cancer chemotherapy and prevention of PONV.	Inj: 20mg/mL; Tab: 50mg, 100mg	(Inj) Prevention of Chemotherapy-Induced Nausea/Vomiting (CINV): 1.8mg/kg IV single dose or 100mg IV 30 min before chemotherapy. Prevention/Treatment of PONV: 12.5mg IV single dose 15 min before cessation of anesthesia or as soon as nausea/vomiting presents. (Tab) Prevention of CINV: 100mg PO within 1 hr before chemotherapy. Prevention of PONV: 100mg PO within 2 hrs before surgery.	**2-16 yrs:** (Inj) Prevention of CINV: 1.8mg/kg IV single dose 30 min before chemotherapy. Max: 100mg. May mix inj in apple or grape juice and take orally within 1 hr before chemotherapy. Prevention/Treatment of PONV: 0.35mg/kg IV single dose 15 min before cessation of anesthesia or as soon as nausea/vomiting presents. Max: 12.5mg single dose. May mix 1.2mg/kg inj in apple or grape juice and take orally within 2 hrs before surgery. Max: 100mg/dose. (Tab) Prevention of CINV: 1.8mg/kg PO within 1 hr before chemotherapy. Max: 100mg. Prevention of PONV: 1.2mg/kg PO within 2 hrs before surgery. Max: 100mg.
Granisetron hydrochloride (Kytril)	(Inj, Sol, Tab) Prevention of nausea and vomiting associated with chemotherapy. (Sol, Tab) Prevention of nausea and vomiting associated with radiation. (Inj) Prevention and treatment of post-op nausea and vomiting (PONV).	Inj: 0.1mg/mL, 1mg/mL; Sol: 2mg/10mL [30mL]; Tab: 1mg	(Sol/Tab) Prevention of Chemotherapy-Induced Nausea/Vomiting (CINV): 2mg qd up to 1 hr before chemotherapy or 1mg bid (up to 1 hr before chemotherapy and 12 hrs later). (Inj) 10mcg/kg within 30 min before chemotherapy. Prevention with Radiation: (Sol/Tab) 2mg within 1 hr of radiation. Prevention of PONV: (Inj) Administer 1mg over 30 sec before induction of anesthesia or immediately before anesthesia reversal. Treatment of PONV: (Inj) Administer 1mg over 30 sec.	**2-16 yrs:** Prevention of CINV: 10mcg/kg IV within 30 min before chemotherapy.

DRUG (BRAND)	INDICATIONS	HOW SUPPLIED	ADULT DOSING	PEDIATRIC DOSING
5-HT_3 Antagonists *(Continued)*				
Ondansetron hydrochloride (Zofran)	(Inj) Prevention of nausea and vomiting associated with initial and repeat courses of emetogenic cancer chemotherapy, including high-dose cisplatin. Prevention of post-op nausea and/or vomiting (PONV). (Sol/Tab) Prevention of nausea and vomiting associated with: highly emetogenic cancer chemotherapy, including cisplatin ≥50mg/m²; initial and repeat courses of moderately emetogenic cancer of moderately emetogenic cancer chemotherapy; and radiotherapy in patients receiving either total body irradiation, single high-dose fraction to the abdomen, or daily fractions to the abdomen. Prevention of PONV.	Inj: 2mg/mL; Sol: 4mg/5mL [50mL]; Tab: 4mg, 8mg, 24mg; Tab, Disintegrating: 4mg, 8mg	Prevention of Chemotherapy-Induced Nausea/Vomiting (CINV): (Inj) 32mg single dose over 15 min or three 0.15mg/kg doses, 1st dose 30 min before chemotherapy, then 4 and 8 hrs after 1st dose. Prevention of CINV, Highly Emetogenic Therapy: (Tab) 24mg single dose tab 30 min before chemotherapy. Prevention of CINV, Moderately Emetogenic Therapy: (Sol/Tab) 8mg bid, 1st dose 30 min before chemotherapy, then 8 hrs later, then bid for 1-2 days after chemotherapy. Prevention of PONV: (Inj) 4mg IM/IV immediately before anesthesia or post-op after surgery if nausea or vomiting occurs. (Sol/Tab) 16mg 1 hr before anesthesia. Prevention of Nausea/Vomiting Associated with Radiation Therapy: (Sol/Tab) Usual: 8mg tid. Total Body Irradiation: 8mg 1-2 hrs before therapy daily. Single High-Dose Therapy To Abdomen: 8mg 1-2 hrs before therapy then q8h after 1st dose for 1-2 days after completion of therapy. Daily Fractionated Therapy To Abdomen: 8mg 1-2 hrs before therapy then q8h after 1st dose. Severe Hepatic Dysfunction (Child-Pugh ≥10): Max: 8mg/day IV single dose infused over 15 min, start 30 min before chemotherapy or 8mg/day PO.	Prevention of CINV: (Inj) **6 months-18 yrs:** Three 0.15mg/kg doses, 1st dose 30 min before chemotherapy, then 4 and 8 hrs after the 1st dose. (Sol/Tab) Prevention of CINV, Moderately Emetogenic Therapy: ≥**12 yrs:** 8mg bid, 1st dose 30 min before chemotherapy, then 8mg 8 hrs later, then bid for 1-2 days. 4-11 yrs: 4mg tid, 1st dose 30 min before chemotherapy, then 4 and 8 hrs after 1st dose, then tid for 1-2 days. Prevention of PONV: (Inj) >**12 yrs:** 4mg IM/IV immediately before anesthesia or post-op after surgery if nausea or vomiting occurs. **1 month-12 yrs:** ≤40kg: 0.1mg/kg single dose. >40kg: 4mg single dose. Severe Hepatic Dysfunction: Max: 8mg/day IV single dose infused over 15 min, start 30 min before chemotherapy or 8mg/day PO.
Palonosetron hydrochloride (Aloxi)	Prevention of acute nausea and vomiting associated with initial and repeat courses of moderately and highly emetogenic cancer chemotherapy. Prevention of delayed nausea and vomiting associated with initial and repeat courses of moderately emetogenic cancer chemotherapy. Prevention of post-op nausea and vomiting (PONV) for up to 24 hrs following surgery. Prevention of acute nausea and vomiting associated with initial and repeat courses of moderately emetogenic cancer chemotherapy.	Inj: 0.25mg/5mL, 0.075mg/1.5mL Cap: 0.5mg	(Cap) Chemo-Induced N/V: 0.5mg 1 hr prior to chemotherapy. (Inj) Chemo-Induced N/V: 0.25mg IV single dose 30 min before start of chemotherapy. Repeated dosing within a 7 day interval not recommended. PONV: 0.075mg IV single dose 10 sec before induction of anesthesia.	

(Continued)

DRUG (BRAND)	INDICATIONS	HOW SUPPLIED	ADULT DOSING	PEDIATRIC DOSING
Miscellaneous				
Dextrose glucose 1.87g, Levulose Fructose 1.87g, and Phosphoric Acid 21.5 mg (Emetrol)	For relief of nausea due to upset stomach from intestinal flu, and food or drink indiscretions.	Liq: 118mL	1-2 tblsp PO every 15 min until response is achieved.	**2-12 yrs:** 1-2 tsp PO every 15 min until response is achieved.
Droperidol (Inapsine)	To reduce incidence of nausea and vomiting associated with surgical and diagnostic procedures.	Inj: 2.5mg/mL	Initial (Max): 2.5mg IM/IV. May give additional 1.25mg cautiously to achieve desired effect. Lower initial doses in elderly, debilitated, poor-risk patients.	**2-12 yrs:** Initial (Max): 0.1 mg/kg IM/IV. May give additional dose cautiously. Lower initial doses in debilitated, poor-risk patients.
Metoclopramide	(Inj) Prevention of post-op or chemo-induced nausea/vomiting.	Inj: 5mg/mL; Syr: 5mg/5mL; Tab: 5mg, 10mg* *scored	Antiemetic: (Postoperative) 10-20mg IM near end of surgery. (Chemotherapy-Induced) 1-2mg/kg 30 min before chemotherapy then q2h for two doses, then q3h for three doses. Give 2mg/kg for highly emetogenic drugs for initial 2 doses. For CrCl <40mL/min: Give approx. half the recommended dosage.	
Trimethobenzamide hydrochloride (Tigan)	Treatment of postoperative nausea and vomiting and for nausea associated with gastroenteritis.	Cap: 300mg; Inj: 100mg/mL	(Cap) 300mg tid-qid. (Inj) 200mg IM tid-qid.	
Phenothiazine Derivative				
Prochlorperazine	Control of severe nausea and vomiting.	Inj: (Edisylate) 5mg/mL; Supp: 25mg; Tab: (Maleate) 5mg, 10mg, 25mg	Nausea/Vomiting: (Tab) Usual: 5-10mg tid-qid. Max: 40mg/day. (Supp) 25mg pr bid. (IM) 5-10mg IM q3-4h prn. Max: 40mg/day. (IV) 2.5-10mg IV (not bolus). Max: 10mg single dose and 40mg/day. Nausea/Vomiting with Surgery: 5-10mg IM 1-2 hrs or 5-10mg IV 15-30 min before anesthesia, or during or after surgery; repeat once if needed.	Nausea/Vomiting: >**2 yrs** and >20 lbs: (PO/PR) 20-29 lbs: Usual: 2.5mg qd-bid. Max: 7.5mg/day. 30-39 lbs: 2.5mg bid-tid. Max: 10mg/day. 40-85 lbs: 2.5mg tid or 5mg bid. Max: 15mg/day. (IM) 0.06mg/lb, usually single dose for control.

DRUG (BRAND)	INDICATIONS	HOW SUPPLIED	ADULT DOSING	PEDIATRIC DOSING
Substance P/neurokinin 1 Receptor Antagonist				
Aprepitant (Emend)	In combination with other antiemetics for prevention of acute and delayed nausea and vomiting associated with initial and repeat courses of highly emetogenic cancer chemotherapy (eg, high-dose cisplatin) and for moderately emetogenic cancer chemotherapy. For the prevention of post-op nausea and vomiting (PONV).	Cap: 40mg, 80mg, 125mg; Tri-Pak: (one 125mg & two 80mg caps)	Prevention of Chemotherapy-Induced Nausea/Vomiting: Day 1: 125mg 1 hr prior to chemotherapy. Days 2 and 3: 80mg qam. Regimen should include a corticosteroid and a 5-HT_3 antagonist. Prevention of PONV: 40mg within 3 hrs prior to induction of anesthesia.	
Fosaprepitant Dimeglumine (Emend for injection)	In combination with other antiemetics for prevention of acute and delayed nausea and vomiting associated with initial and repeat courses of highly emetogenic cancer chemotherapy (eg, high-dose cisplatin) and for moderately emetogenic cancer chemotherapy.	Powder (Vial): 115mg/10mL [10mL]	115mg IV over 15 min or 125mg PO 30 min prior to chemotherapy on day 1, 80mg PO days 2 and 3 only of a 3-day regimen, in addition to corticosteroid and 5-HT_3 antagonist.	

H_2 ANTAGONISTS AND PPIs COMPARISON

	DRUG	HOW SUPPLIED	INDICATIONS: Heart-burn	PUD	GERD	Zollinger-Ellison	*H.pylori*	NSAID† Induced	Upper GI‡ Bleeding
H_2 ANTAGONISTS	**CIMETIDINE**								
	Tagamet	**Inj:** 300mg/50mL** **Sol:** 300mg/5mL** **Tab:** 200mg, 300mg, 400mg, 800mg		X	X	X			X
	Tagamet HB*	**Tab:** 200mg	X						
	FAMOTIDINE								
	Pepcid, Pepcid RPD	**Inj:** 0.4mg/mL, 10mg/mL **Sus:** 40mg/5mL; **Tab:** 20mg, 40mg; **Tab, Disintegrating:** (RPD); 20mg, 40mg		X	X	X			
	Pepcid AC*	**Cap:** 10mg **Tab:** 10mg, 20mg **Tab, Chewable:** 10mg	X						
	Pepcid Complete*	**Tab, Chewable:** (Famotidine-Calcium Carbonate-Magnesium Hydroxide) 10mg-800mg-165mg	X						
	NIZATIDINE								
	Axid	**Cap:** 150mg, 300mg **Sol:** 15mg/mL		X	X				
	RANITIDINE								
	Zantac	**Inj:** 1mg/mL, 25mg/mL **Syrup:** 15mg/mL **Tab:** 150mg, 300mg **Tab, Effervescent:** 25mg		X	X	X			
	Zantac OTC*	**Tab:** 75mg, 150mg	X						
PROTON PUMP INHIBITORS	**DEXLANSOPRAZOLE**								
	Kapidex	**Cap, DR:** 30mg, 60mg	X		X				
	ESOMEPRAZOLE								
	Nexium	**Cap, DR:** 20mg, 40mg; **Inj:** 20mg, 40mg **Sus, DR:** 10mg, 20mg, 40mg (granules/packet)	X	X	X	X	X	X	
	LANSOPRAZOLE								
	Prevacid	**Cap, DR:** 15mg, 30mg; **Inj:** 30mg **Sus:** 15mg/packet, 30mg/packet **Tab, Disintegrating:** 15mg, 30mg	X	X	X	X	X	X	
	Prevpac	**Cap:** (Amoxicillin) 500mg **Tab:** (Clarithromycin) 500mg **Cap, DR:** (Lansoprazole) 30mg					X		
	Prevacid NapraPAC	**Cap, DR:** (Naproxen Lansoprazole): 500mg-15mg						X	
	OMEPRAZOLE								
	Prilosec	**Cap, DR:** 10mg, 20mg, 40mg; **Sus, DR:** 2.5mg, 10mg (granules/packet)		X	X	X	X		
	Prilosec OTC*	**Tab:** 20mg	X						
	Zegerid	(Omeprazole-Sodium Bicarbonate); **Cap:** 20mg-1100mg, 40mg-1100mg; **Pow:** 20mg-1680mg/packet, 40mg-1680mg/packet	X	X	X				X
	PANTOPRAZOLE								
	Protonix	**Inj:** 40mg; **Tab, DR:** 20mg, 40mg **Sus, DR:** 40mg (granules/packet)	X		X	X			
	RABEPRAZOLE								
	Aciphex	**Tab, DR:** 20mg		X	X	X	X		

DR=Delayed-Release *OTC. **Product available generically only. †Prevention of NSAID-induced gastric ulcers.
‡Prevention of upper GI bleeding in critically ill patients.

ANTIBIOTIC SENSITIVITY – AMINOGLYCOSIDES*

ORGANISMS	Amikacin	Gentamicin	Streptomycin	Tobramycin
ANAEROBES				
Actinomyces				
Bacillus anthracis				
Bacteroides fragilis				
Clostridium difficile				
Clostridium species				
GRAM-NEGATIVE AEROBES				
Acinetobacter baumannii	✓			
Aeromonas hydrophila				
Bartonella henselae				
Bordetella species				
Burkholderia cepacia				
Campylobacter jejuni				
Citrobacter species	✓	✓		✓
Coxiella burnetti				
Enterobacter species	✓	✓		✓
Escherichia coli	✓	✓	✓	✓

*These are generalizations. There are major differences among countries, areas, and hospitals depending on antibiotic usage patterns.

Blank = no or insufficient activity, or unknown.

ORGANISMS	Amikacin	Gentamicin	Streptomycin	Tobramycin	
GRAM-NEGATIVE AEROBES *(Continued)*					
Francisella tularensis			✓		
Haemophilus influenzae			✓		
Klebsiella species	✓	✓	✓	✓	
Legionella species					
Moraxella catarrhalis					
Morganella morganii				✓	
Neisseria gonorrhoeae					
Neisseria meningitidis					
Pasturella multocida					
Proteus mirabilis	✓	✓	✓	✓	
Proteus vulgaris	✓	✓	✓	✓	
Providencia stuartii	✓	✓		✓	
Pseudomonas aeruginosa	✓	✓		✓	
Rickettsia species					
Salmonella species		✓			
Serratia species	✓	✓		✓	
Shigella species		✓			
Stenotrophomonas maltophilia					

*These are generalizations. There are major differences among countries, areas, and hospitals depending on antibiotic usage patterns.

Blank = no or insufficient activity, or unknown.

AMINOGLYCOSIDES (CONTINUED)

ORGANISMS	Amikacin	Gentamicin	Streptomycin	Tobramycin	
GRAM-NEGATIVE AEROBES *(Continued)*					
Vibrio vulnificus					
Yersinia enterocolitica					
Yersinia pestis					
GRAM-POSITIVE AEROBES					
Enterococcus faecalis			✓		
Enterococcus faecium					
Enterococcus faecium (VRE)					
Listeria monocytogenes					
Nocardia					
Staphylococcus aureus (MSSA)		✓		✓	
Staphylococcus aureus (MRSA)					
Staphylococcus epidermidis		✓			
Staphylococcus epidermidis (MRSE)					
Streptococcus pneumoniae†					
Streptococcus pneumoniae§§					

*These are generalizations. There are major differences among countries, areas, and hospitals depending on antibiotic usage patterns.

Blank = no or insufficient activity, or unknown.

† Penicillin sensitive; MIC ≤1.0 mcg/mL. §§ Penicillin resistant; MIC ≥2.0 mcg/mL.

ORGANISMS	Amikacin	Gentamicin	Streptomycin	Tobramycin	
GRAM-POSITIVE AEROBES *(Continued)*					
Streptococcus (Group A,B,C,F,G)					
Streptococcus species					
MISCELLANEOUS					
Chlamydia pneumoniae					
Chlamydia trachomatis					
Ehrlichia/Anaplasma species					
MYCOBACTERIA					
Mycobacterium avium (MAI) (non-HIV)					
Mycoplasma pneumoniae					
SPIROCHETES					
Leptospira interrogans					
Treponema pallidum (syphilis)					

*These are generalizations. There are major differences among countries, areas, and hospitals depending on antibiotic usage patterns.

Blank = no or insufficient activity, or unknown.

ANTIBIOTIC SENSITIVITY – CARBAPENEMS/MONOBACTAMS*

ORGANISMS	Aztreonam	Ertapenem	Imipenem/Cilastatin	Meropenem
ANAEROBES				
Actinomyces				
Bacillus anthracis			✓	
Bacteroides fragilis		✓	✓	✓
Clostridium difficile				✓
Clostridium species		✓	✓	✓
GRAM-NEGATIVE AEROBES				
Acinetobacter baumannii			✓	✓
Aeromonas hydrophila	✓		✓	✓
Bartonella henselae				
Bordetella species				
Burkholderia cepacia				
Campylobacter jejuni				✓
Citrobacter species	✓	✓	✓	✓
Coxiella burnetti				
Enterobacter species	✓	✓	✓	✓
Escherichia coli	✓	✓	✓	✓

*These are generalizations. There are major differences among countries, areas, and hospitals depending on antibiotic usage patterns.

Blank = no or insufficient activity, or unknown.

ORGANISMS	Aztreonam	Ertapenem	Imipenem/Cilastatin	Meropenem	
GRAM-NEGATIVE AEROBES *(Continued)*					
Francisella tularensis					
Haemophilus influenzae	✓	✓	✓	✓	
Klebsiella species	✓	✓	✓	✓	
Legionella species					
Moraxella catarrhalis		✓		✓	
Morganella morganii	✓	✓	✓	✓	
Neisseria gonorrhoeae	✓		✓		
Neisseria meningitidis	✓		✓	✓	
Pasturella multocida	✓		✓	✓	
Proteus mirabilis	✓	✓	✓	✓	
Proteus vulgaris	✓	✓	✓	✓	
Providencia stuartii	✓	✓	✓		
Pseudomonas aeruginosa	✓		✓	✓	
Rickettsia species					
Salmonella species				✓	
Serratia species	✓	✓	✓	✓	
Shigella species				✓	
Stenotrophomonas maltophilia					

*These are generalizations. There are major differences among countries, areas, and hospitals depending on antibiotic usage patterns.

Blank = no or insufficient activity, or unknown.

CARBAPENEMS/MONOBACTAMS (CONTINUED)

ORGANISMS	Aztreonam	Ertapenem	Imipenem/Cilastatin	Meropenem	
GRAM-NEGATIVE AEROBES *(Continued)*					
Vibrio vulnificus					
Yersinia enterocolitica	✓			✓	
Yersinia pestis					
GRAM-POSITIVE AEROBES					
Enterococcus faecalis			✓	✓	
Enterococcus faecium					
Enterococcus faecium (VRE)					
Listeria monocytogenes			✓	✓	
Nocardia			✓		
Staphylococcus aureus (MSSA)		✓	✓	✓	
Staphylococcus aureus (MRSA)					
Staphylococcus epidermidis		✓	✓	✓	
Staphylococcus epidermidis (MRSE)					
Streptococcus pneumoniae†		✓	✓	✓	
Streptococcus pneumoniae§§					

*These are generalizations. There are major differences among countries, areas, and hospitals depending on antibiotic usage patterns.

Blank = no or insufficient activity, or unknown.

† Penicillin sensitive; MIC ≤1.0 mcg/mL. §§ Penicillin resistant; MIC ≥2.0 mcg/mL.

ORGANISMS	Aztreonam	Ertapenem	Imipenem/Cilastatin	Meropenem	
GRAM-POSITIVE AEROBES *(Continued)*					
Streptococcus (Group A,B,C,F,G)		✓	✓	✓	
Streptococcus species		✓	✓	✓	
MISCELLANEOUS					
Chlamydia pneumoniae					
Chlamydia trachomatis					
Ehrlichia/Anaplasma species					
MYCOBACTERIA					
Mycobacterium avium (MAI) (non-HIV)					
Mycoplasma pneumoniae					
SPIROCHETES					
Leptospira interrogans					
Treponema pallidum (syphilis)					

*These are generalizations. There are major differences among countries, areas, and hospitals depending on antibiotic usage patterns.

Blank = no or insufficient activity, or unknown.

ANTIBIOTIC SENSITIVITY – CEPHALOSPORINS*

ORGANISMS	Cefaclor	Cefadroxil	Cefazolin	Cefdinir	Cefepime	Cefixime	Cefotaxime	Cefoxitin	Cefpodoxime Proxetil	Cefprozil	Ceftazidime	Ceftibuten	Ceftizoxime	Ceftriaxone	Cefuroxime Axetil	Cephalexin
ANAEROBES																
Actinomyces																
Bacillus anthracis																
Bacteroides fragilis								✓								
Clostridium difficile																
Clostridium species							✓	✓		✓	✓			✓		
GRAM-NEGATIVE AEROBES																
Acinetobacter baumannii					✓		✓				✓			✓		
Aeromonas hydrophila													✓			
Bartonella henselae																
Bordetella species																
Burkholderia cepacia																
Campylobacter jejuni																
Citrobacter species	✓			✓	✓		✓		✓	✓	✓		✓	✓	✓	
Coxiella burnetti																
Enterobacter species					✓		✓				✓		✓	✓		
Escherichia coli	✓	✓	✓	✓	✓		✓	✓	✓	✓	✓		✓	✓	✓	✓

*These are generalizations. There are major differences among countries, areas, and hospitals depending on antibiotic usage patterns.

Blank = no or insufficient activity, or unknown.

ORGANISMS	Cefaclor	Cefadroxil	Cefazolin	Cefdinir	Cefepime	Cefixime	Cefotaxime	Cefoxitin	Cefpodoxime Proxetil	Cefprozil	Ceftazidime	Ceftibuten	Ceftizoxime	Ceftriaxone	Cefuroxime Axetil	Cephalexin
GRAM-NEGATIVE AEROBES *(Continued)*																
Francisella tularensis																
Haemophilus influenzae	✓			✓	✓	✓	✓	✓	✓	✓	✓	✓	✓	✓	✓	
Klebsiella species	✓	✓		✓	✓	✓	✓	✓	✓	✓	✓		✓	✓	✓	✓
Legionella species																
Moraxella catarrhalis	✓	✓		✓	✓	✓			✓	✓		✓	✓	✓	✓	✓
Morganella morganii					✓		✓	✓			✓			✓	✓	
Neisseria gonorrhoeae	✓					✓	✓	✓	✓	✓	✓	✓	✓	✓	✓	
Neisseria meningitidis							✓				✓		✓	✓		
Pasturella multocida						✓					✓					
Proteus mirabilis	✓	✓	✓	✓	✓	✓	✓	✓	✓	✓	✓		✓	✓	✓	✓
Proteus vulgaris					✓	✓	✓	✓	✓		✓		✓	✓		
Providencia stuartii					✓	✓	✓	✓	✓		✓		✓	✓		
Pseudomonas aeruginosa					✓						✓		✓			
Rickettsia species																
Salmonella species						✓	✓			✓	✓			✓		
Serratia species					✓	✓	✓				✓	✓	✓	✓		

*These are generalizations. There are major differences among countries, areas, and hospitals depending on antibiotic usage patterns.

Blank = no or insufficient activity, or unknown.

CEPHALOSPORINS (CONTINUED)

ORGANISMS	Cefaclor	Cefadroxil	Cefazolin	Cefdinir	Cefepime	Cefixime	Cefotaxime	Cefoxitin	Cefpodoxime Proxetil	Cefprozil	Ceftazidime	Ceftibuten	Ceftizoxime	Ceftriaxone	Cefuroxime Axetil	Cephalexin
GRAM-NEGATIVE AEROBES *(Continued)*																
Shigella species						✓	✓			✓	✓			✓		
Stenotrophomonas maltophilia																
Vibrio vulnificus										✓						
Yersinia enterocolitica											✓					
Yersinia pestis																
GRAM-POSITIVE AEROBES																
Enterococcus faecalis										✓						
Enterococcus faecium																
Enterococcus faecium (VRE)																
Listeria monocytogenes										✓						
Nocardia																
Staphylococcus aureus (MSSA)	✓	✓	✓	✓	✓		✓	✓	✓	✓	✓		✓	✓	✓	✓
Staphylococcus aureus (MRSA)																

*These are generalizations. There are major differences among countries, areas, and hospitals depending on antibiotic usage patterns.

Blank = no or insufficient activity, or unknown.

ORGANISMS	Cefaclor	Cefadroxil	Cefazolin	Cefdinir	Cefepime	Cefixime	Cefotaxime	Cefoxitin	Cefpodoxime Proxetil	Cefprozil	Ceftazidime	Ceftibuten	Ceftizoxime	Ceftriaxone	Cefuroxime Axetil	Cephalexin
GRAM-POSITIVE AEROBES *(Continued)*																
Staphylococcus epidermidis		✓	✓	✓	✓		✓	✓		✓			✓	✓	✓	
Staphylococcus epidermidis (MRSE)																
Streptococcus pneumoniae†	✓	✓	✓	✓	✓		✓	✓	✓	✓	✓	✓	✓	✓	✓	✓
Streptococcus pneumoniae§§					✓		✓		✓				✓	✓		
Streptococcus (Group A,B,C,F,G)		✓	✓	✓	✓		✓	✓	✓	✓	✓	✓	✓	✓	✓	✓
Streptococcus species	✓	✓	✓	✓	✓		✓	✓	✓	✓	✓	✓	✓	✓	✓	✓
MISCELLANEOUS																
Chlamydia pneumoniae																
Chlamydia trachomatis																
Ehrlichia/Anaplasma species																
MYCOBACTERIA																
Mycobacterium avium (MAI) (non-HIV)																

*These are generalizations. There are major differences among countries, areas, and hospitals depending on antibiotic usage patterns.

Blank = no or insufficient activity, or unknown.

† Penicillin sensitive; MIC ≤1.0 mcg/mL. §§ Penicillin resistant; MIC ≥2.0 mcg/mL.

CEPHALOSPORINS (CONTINUED)

ORGANISMS	Cefaclor	Cefadroxil	Cefazolin	Cefdinir	Cefepime	Cefixime	Cefotaxime	Cefoxitin	Cefpodoxime Proxetil	Cefprozil	Ceftazidime	Ceftibuten	Ceftizoxime	Ceftriaxone	Cefuroxime axetil	Cephalexin
MYCOBACTERIA *(Continued)*																
Mycoplasma pneumoniae																
SPIROCHETES																
Leptospira interrogans																
Treponema pallidum (syphilis)																

*These are generalizations. There are major differences among countries, areas, and hospitals depending on antibiotic usage patterns.

Blank = no or insufficient activity, or unknown.

ANTIBIOTIC SENSITIVITY – FLUOROQUINOLONES*

ORGANISMS	Ciprofloxacin	Gemifloxacin	Levofloxacin	Moxifloxacin	Norfloxacin	Ofloxacin	
ANAEROBES							
Actinomyces							
Bacillus anthracis	✓						
Bacteroides fragilis				✓			
Clostridium difficile							
Clostridium species			✓	✓		✓	
GRAM-NEGATIVE AEROBES							
Acinetobacter baumannii			✓				
Aeromonas hydrophila	✓						
Bartonella henselae							
Bordetella species			✓			✓	
Burkholderia cepacia							
Campylobacter jejuni	✓						
Citrobacter species	✓		✓	✓	✓	✓	
Coxiella burnetti			✓				
Enterobacter species	✓		✓	✓	✓	✓	
Escherichia coli	✓		✓	✓	✓	✓	

*These are generalizations. There are major differences among countries, areas, and hospitals depending on antibiotic usage patterns.

Blank = no or insufficient activity, or unknown.

FLUOROQUINOLONES (CONTINUED)

ORGANISMS	Ciprofloxacin	Gemifloxacin	Levofloxacin	Moxifloxacin	Norfloxacin	Ofloxacin	
GRAM-NEGATIVE AEROBES *(Continued)*							
Francisella tularensis							
Haemophilus influenzae	✓	✓	✓	✓		✓	
Klebsiella species	✓	✓	✓	✓	✓	✓	
Legionella species	✓	✓	✓	✓		✓	
Moraxella catarrhalis	✓	✓	✓	✓		✓	
Morganella morganii	✓		✓		✓	✓	
Neisseria gonorrhoeae	✓				✓	✓	
Neisseria meningitidis							
Pasturella multocida							
Proteus mirabilis	✓		✓	✓	✓	✓	
Proteus vulgaris	✓	✓	✓		✓	✓	
Providencia stuartii	✓		✓		✓	✓	
Pseudomonas aeruginosa	✓				✓	✓	
Rickettsia species							
Salmonella species	✓						
Serratia species	✓		✓		✓	✓	
Shigella species	✓						
Stenotrophomonas maltophilia							

*These are generalizations. There are major differences among countries, areas, and hospitals depending on antibiotic usage patterns.

Blank = no or insufficient activity, or unknown.

ORGANISMS	Ciprofloxacin	Gemifloxacin	Levofloxacin	Moxifloxacin	Norfloxacin	Ofloxacin
GRAM-NEGATIVE AEROBES *(Continued)*						
Vibrio vulnificus	✓					
Yersinia enterocolitica	✓					
Yersinia pestis						
GRAM-POSITIVE AEROBES						
Enterococcus faecalis	✓		✓	✓	✓	
Enterococcus faecium						
Enterococcus faecium (VRE)						
Listeria monocytogenes						
Nocardia						
Staphylococcus aureus (MSSA)	✓	✓	✓	✓	✓	✓
Staphylococcus aureus (MRSA)						
Staphylococcus epidermidis	✓		✓	✓	✓	✓
Staphylococcus epidermidis (MRSE)						
Streptococcus pneumoniae†	✓	✓	✓	✓		✓
Streptococcus pneumoniae§§	✓	✓	✓	✓		✓

*These are generalizations. There are major differences among countries, areas, and hospitals depending on antibiotic usage patterns.

Blank = no or insufficient activity, or unknown.

† Penicillin sensitive; MIC ≤1.0 mcg/mL. §§ Penicillin resistant; MIC ≥2.0 mcg/mL.

FLUOROQUINOLONES (CONTINUED)

ORGANISMS	Ciprofloxacin	Gemifloxacin	Levofloxacin	Moxifloxacin	Norfloxacin	Ofloxacin
GRAM-POSITIVE AEROBES *(Continued)*						
Streptococcus *(Group A,B,C,F,G)*	✓	✓	✓	✓		✓
Streptococcus species	✓	✓	✓	✓	✓	✓
MISCELLANEOUS						
Chlamydia pneumoniae		✓	✓	✓		✓
Chlamydia trachomatis						✓
Ehrlichia/Anaplasma species						
MYCOBACTERIA						
Mycobacterium avium *(MAI) (non-HIV)*						
Mycoplasma pneumoniae		✓	✓	✓		✓
SPIROCHETES						
Leptospira interrogans						
Treponema pallidum (syphilis)						

*These are generalizations. There are major differences among countries, areas, and hospitals depending on antibiotic usage patterns.

Blank = no or insufficient activity, or unknown.

ANTIBIOTIC SENSITIVITY – MACROLIDES & CLINDAMYCIN*

ORGANISMS	Azithromycin	Clarithromycin	Clindamycin	Erythromycin	Telithromycin	
ANAEROBES						
Actinomyces						
Bacillus anthracis						
Bacteroides fragilis						
Clostridium difficile						
Clostridium species			✓			
GRAM-NEGATIVE AEROBES						
Acinetobacter baumannii						
Aeromonas hydrophila						
Bartonella henselae						
Bordetella species	✓	✓		✓		
Burkholderia cepacia						
Campylobacter jejuni	✓					
Citrobacter species						
Coxiella burnetti						
Enterobacter species						
Escherichia coli						

*These are generalizations. There are major differences among countries, areas, and hospitals depending on antibiotic usage patterns.

Blank = no or insufficient activity, or unknown.

MACROLIDES & CLINDAMYCIN (CONTINUED)

ORGANISMS	Azithromycin	Clarithromycin	Clindamycin	Erythromycin	Telithromycin	
GRAM-NEGATIVE AEROBES *(Continued)*						
Francisella tularensis						
Haemophilus influenzae	✓	✓			✓	
Klebsiella species						
Legionella species	✓	✓		✓	✓	
Moraxella catarrhalis	✓	✓		✓	✓	
Morganella morganii						
Neisseria gonorrhoeae				✓		
Neisseria meningitidis						
Pasturella multocida		✓				
Proteus mirabilis						
Proteus vulgaris						
Providencia stuartii						
Pseudomonas aeruginosa						
Rickettsia species						
Salmonella species						
Serratia species						
Shigella species						
Stenotrophomonas maltophilia						

*These are generalizations. There are major differences among countries, areas, and hospitals depending on antibiotic usage patterns.

Blank = no or insufficient activity, or unknown.

ORGANISMS	Azithromycin	Clarithromycin	Clindamycin	Erythromycin	Telithromycin	
GRAM-NEGATIVE AEROBES *(Continued)*						
Vibrio vulnificus						
Yersinia enterocolitica						
Yersinia pestis						
GRAM-POSITIVE AEROBES						
Enterococcus faecalis						
Enterococcus faecium						
Enterococcus faecium (VRE)						
Listeria monocytogenes				✓		
Nocardia						
Staphylococcus aureus (MSSA)	✓	✓	✓	✓		
Staphylococcus aureus (MRSA)						
Staphylococcus epidermidis			✓			
Staphylococcus epidermidis (MRSE)						
Streptococcus pneumoniae†			✓		✓	
Streptococcus pneumoniae§§	✓				✓	

*These are generalizations. There are major differences among countries, areas, and hospitals depending on antibiotic usage patterns.

Blank = no or insufficient activity, or unknown.

† Penicillin sensitive; MIC ≤1.0 mcg/mL. §§ Penicillin resistant; MIC ≥2.0 mcg/mL.

MACROLIDES & CLINDAMYCIN (CONTINUED)

ORGANISMS	Azithromycin	Clarithromycin	Clindamycin	Erythromycin	Telithromycin	
GRAM-POSITIVE AEROBES *(Continued)*						
Streptococcus (Group A,B,C,F,G)	✓	✓	✓			
Streptococcus species		✓				
MISCELLANEOUS						
Chlamydia pneumoniae		✓			✓	
Chlamydia trachomatis	✓			✓		
Ehrlichia/Anaplasma species						
MYCOBACTERIA						
Mycobacterium avium (MAI) (non-HIV)	✓	✓			✓	
Mycoplasma pneumoniae				✓	✓	
SPIROCHETES						
Leptospira interrogans						
Treponema pallidum (syphilis)	✓			✓		

*These are generalizations. There are major differences among countries, areas, and hospitals depending on antibiotic usage patterns.

Blank = no or insufficient activity, or unknown.

ANTIBIOTIC SENSITIVITY – PENICILLINS*

ORGANISMS	Amoxicillin	Amoxicillin + Clavulanate	Ampicillin	Ampicillin + Sulbactam	Dicloxacillin	Nafcillin/ Oxacillin	Penicillin	Piperacillin	Piperacillin + Tazobactam	Ticarcillin + Clavulanic Acid
ANAEROBES										
Actinomyces							✓			
Bacillus anthracis			✓				✓			
Bacteroides fragilis		✓		✓				✓	✓	✓
Clostridium difficile										✓
Clostridium species			✓	✓			✓	✓	✓	✓
GRAM-NEGATIVE AEROBES										
Acinetobacter baumannii								✓	✓	✓
Aeromonas hydrophila										
Bartonella henselae										
Bordetella species										
Burkholderia cepacia										
Campylobacter jejuni										
Citrobacter species								✓	✓	✓
Coxiella burnetti										
Enterobacter species		✓		✓				✓	✓	✓
Escherichia coli	✓	✓	✓	✓				✓	✓	✓

*These are generalizations. There are major differences among countries, areas, and hospitals depending on antibiotic usage patterns.

Blank = no or insufficient activity, or unknown.

PENICILLINS (CONTINUED)

ORGANISMS	Amoxicillin	Amoxicillin + Clavulanate	Ampicillin	Ampicillin + Sulbactam	Dicloxacillin	Nafcillin/ Oxacillin	Penicillin	Piperacillin	Piperacillin + Tazobactam	Ticarcillin + Clavulanic Acid
GRAM-NEGATIVE AEROBES *(Continued)*										
Francisella tularensis										
Haemophilus influenzae	✓	✓	✓	✓				✓	✓	✓
Klebsiella species		✓		✓				✓	✓	✓
Legionella species										
Moraxella catarrhalis		✓		✓					✓	✓
Morganella morganii								✓	✓	✓
Neisseria gonorrhoeae	✓	✓	✓	✓			✓	✓	✓	✓
Neisseria meningitidis			✓							
Pasturella multocida										✓
Proteus mirabilis	✓	✓	✓	✓				✓	✓	✓
Proteus vulgaris				✓				✓	✓	✓
Providencia stuartii				✓						✓
Pseudomonas aeruginosa								✓	✓	✓
Rickettsia species										
Salmonella species			✓						✓	
Serratia species								✓	✓	
Shigella species			✓							

*These are generalizations. There are major differences among countries, areas, and hospitals depending on antibiotic usage patterns.

Blank = no or insufficient activity, or unknown.

ORGANISMS	Amoxicillin	Amoxicillin + Clavulanate	Ampicillin	Ampicillin + Sulbactam	Dicloxacillin	Nafcillin/ Oxacillin	Penicillin	Piperacillin	Piperacillin + Tazobactam	Ticarcillin + Clavulanic Acid
GRAM-NEGATIVE AEROBES *(Continued)*										
Stenotrophomonas maltophilia								✓		✓
Vibrio vulnificus										
Yersinia enterocolitica								✓		
Yersinia pestis										
GRAM-POSITIVE AEROBES										
Enterococcus faecalis	✓	✓	✓					✓	✓	
Enterococcus faecium								✓		
Enterococcus faecium (VRE)										
Listeria monocytogenes			✓				✓			
Nocardia										
Staphylococcus aureus (MSSA)		✓	✓	✓	✓	✓	✓		✓	✓
Staphylococcus aureus (MRSA)										
Staphylococcus epidermidis		✓		✓	✓	✓			✓	✓
Staphylococcus epidermidis (MRSE)										
Streptococcus pneumoniae†	✓	✓	✓	✓	✓		✓	✓	✓	✓
Streptococcus pneumoniae§§	✓	✓	✓	✓						✓

*These are generalizations. There are major differences among countries, areas, and hospitals depending on antibiotic usage patterns.

Blank = no or insufficient activity, or unknown.

† Penicillin sensitive; MIC ≤1.0 mcg/mL. §§ Penicillin resistant; MIC ≥2.0 mcg/mL.

PENICILLINS (CONTINUED)

ORGANISMS	Amoxicillin	Amoxicillin + Clavulanate	Ampicillin	Ampicillin + Sulbactam	Dicloxacillin	Nafcillin/ Oxacillin	Penicillin	Piperacillin	Piperacillin + Tazobactam	Ticarcillin + Clavulanic Acid
GRAM-POSITIVE AEROBES *(Continued)*										
Streptococcus (Group A,B,C,F,G)	✓	✓	✓		✓		✓	✓	✓	✓
Streptococcus species	✓	✓	✓	✓	✓		✓	✓	✓	✓
MISCELLANEOUS										
Chlamydia pneumoniae										
Chlamydia trachomatis										
Ehrlichia/Anaplasma species										
MYCOBACTERIA										
Mycobacterium avium (MAI) (non-HIV)										
Mycoplasma pneumoniae										
SPIROCHETES										
Leptospira interrogans										
Treponema pallidum (syphilis)							✓			

*These are generalizations. There are major differences among countries, areas, and hospitals depending on antibiotic usage patterns.

Blank = no or insufficient activity, or unknown.

ANTIBIOTIC SENSITIVITY – SULFONAMIDES*

ORGANISMS	Trimethoprim + Sulfamethoxazole
ANAEROBES	
Actinomyces	
Bacillus anthracis	
Bacteroides fragilis	
Clostridium difficile	
Clostridium species	
GRAM-NEGATIVE AEROBES	
Acinetobacter baumannii	
Aeromonas hydrophila	
Bartonella henselae	
Bordetella species	
Burkholderia cepacia	
Campylobacter jejuni	
Citrobacter species	
Coxiella burnetti	
Enterobacter species	✓

ANTIBIOTIC SENSITIVITY – TETRACYCLINES*

ORGANISMS	Doxycycline	Minocycline	Tetracycline	
ANAEROBES				
Actinomyces	✓	✓	✓	
Bacillus anthracis	✓	✓	✓	
Bacteroides fragilis	✓		✓	
Clostridium difficile				
Clostridium species	✓	✓	✓	
GRAM-NEGATIVE AEROBES				
Acinetobacter baumannii	✓	✓	✓	
Aeromonas hydrophila				
Bartonella henselae				
Bordetella species				
Burkholderia cepacia				
Campylobacter jejuni				
Citrobacter species				
Coxiella burnetti				
Enterobacter species	✓			

*These are generalizations. There are major differences among countries, areas, and hospitals depending on antibiotic usage patterns.

Blank = no or insufficient activity, or unknown.

SULFONAMIDES (CONTINUED)

ORGANISMS	Trimethoprim + Sulfamethoxazole
GRAM-NEGATIVE AEROBES *(Continued)*	
Escherichia coli	✓
Francisella tularensis	
Haemophilus influenzae	✓
Klebsiella species	✓
Legionella species	
Moraxella catarrhalis	✓
Morganella morganii	✓
Neisseria gonorrhoeae	
Neisseria meningitidis	
Pasturella multocida	
Proteus mirabilis	✓
Proteus vulgaris	✓
Providencia stuartii	
Pseudomonas aeruginosa	
Rickettsia species	
Salmonella species	
Serratia species	

TETRACYCLINES (CONTINUED)

ORGANISMS	Doxycycline	Minocycline	Tetracycline	
GRAM-NEGATIVE AEROBES *(Continued)*				
Escherichia coli	✓	✓	✓	
Francisella tularensis	✓	✓	✓	
Haemophilus influenzae	✓	✓	✓	
Klebsiella species	✓	✓	✓	
Legionella species				
Moraxella catarrhalis				
Morganella morganii				
Neisseria gonorrhoeae	✓	✓	✓	
Neisseria meningitidis		✓		
Pasturella multocida				
Proteus mirabilis				
Proteus vulgaris				
Providencia stuartii				
Pseudomonas aeruginosa				
Rickettsia species	✓	✓	✓	
Salmonella species				
Serratia species				

*These are generalizations. There are major differences among countries, areas, and hospitals depending on antibiotic usage patterns.

Blank = no or insufficient activity, or unknown.

ORGANISMS	Trimethoprim + Sulfamethoxazole
GRAM-NEGATIVE AEROBES *(Continued)*	
Shigella species	✓
Stenotrophomonas maltophilia	
Vibrio vulnificus	
Yersinia enterocolitica	
Yersinia pestis	
GRAM-POSITIVE AEROBES	
Enterococcus faecalis	
Enterococcus faecium	
Enterococcus faecium (VRE)	
Listeria monocytogenes	
Nocardia	
Staphylococcus aureus (MSSA)	
Staphylococcus aureus (MRSA)	
Staphylococcus epidermidis	
Staphylococcus epidermidis (MRSE)	
Streptococcus pneumoniae†	✓

ORGANISMS	Doxycycline	Minocycline	Tetracycline	
GRAM-NEGATIVE AEROBES *(Continued)*				
Shigella species	✓	✓	✓	
Stenotrophomonas maltophilia				
Vibrio vulnificus				
Yersinia enterocolitica				
Yersinia pestis	✓	✓	✓	
GRAM-POSITIVE AEROBES				
Enterococcus faecalis	✓		✓	
Enterococcus faecium	✓		✓	
Enterococcus faecium (VRE)				
Listeria monocytogenes	✓	✓	✓	
Nocardia				
Staphylococcus aureus (MSSA)		✓		
Staphylococcus aureus (MRSA)				
Staphylococcus epidermidis				
Staphylococcus epidermidis (MRSE)				
Streptococcus pneumoniae†	✓	✓	✓	

*These are generalizations. There are major differences among countries, areas, and hospitals depending on antibiotic usage patterns.

Blank = no or insufficient activity, or unknown.

† Penicillin sensitive; MIC ≤1.0 mcg/mL.

SULFONAMIDES (CONTINUED)

ORGANISMS	Trimethoprim + Sulfamethoxazole
GRAM-POSITIVE AEROBES *(Continued)*	
Streptococcus pneumoniae§§	
Streptococcus (Group A,B,C,F,G)	
Streptococcus species	
MISCELLANEOUS	
Chlamydia pneumoniae	
Chlamydia trachomatis	
Ehrlichia/Anaplasma species	
MYCOBACTERIA	
Mycobacterium avium (MAI) (non-HIV)	
Mycoplasma pneumoniae	
SPIROCHETES	
Leptospira interrogans	
Treponema pallidum (syphilis)	

TETRACYCLINES (CONTINUED)

ORGANISMS	Doxycycline	Minocycline	Tetracycline	
GRAM-POSITIVE AEROBES *(Continued)*				
Streptococcus pneumoniae§§				
Streptococcus (Group A,B,C,F,G)				
Streptococcus species	✓	✓	✓	
MISCELLANEOUS				
Chlamydia pneumoniae				
Chlamydia trachomatis	✓	✓	✓	
Ehrlichia/Anaplasma species				
MYCOBACTERIA				
Mycobacterium avium (MAI) (non-HIV)				
Mycoplasma pneumoniae	✓	✓	✓	
SPIROCHETES				
Leptospira interrogans				
Treponema pallidum (syphilis)	✓	✓	✓	

*These are generalizations. There are major differences among countries, areas, and hospitals depending on antibiotic usage patterns.

Blank = no or insufficient activity, or unknown.

§§ Penicillin resistant; MIC ≥2.0 mcg/mL.

Antibiotic Sensitivity – Miscellaneous*

ORGANISMS	Chloramphenicol	Colistimethate	Daptomycin	Fosfomycin	Linezolid	Metronidazole	Nitrofurantoin	Quinupristin + Dalfopristin	Rifampin	Vancomycin
ANAEROBES										
Actinomyces								✓		✓
Bacillus anthracis										✓
Bacteroides fragilis						✓		✓		
Clostridium difficile						✓				✓
Clostridium species						✓		✓		✓
GRAM-NEGATIVE AEROBES										
Aeromonas hydrophila										
Bartonella henselae										
Bordetella species										
Burkholderia cepacia										
Campylobacter jejuni										
Citrobacter species				✓			✓			
Coxiella burnetti										
Enterobacter species		✓		✓			✓			
Escherichia coli	✓	✓		✓			✓		✓	
Francisella tularensis										

*These are generalizations. There are major differences among countries, areas, and hospitals depending on antibiotic usage patterns.

Blank = no or insufficient activity, or unknown.

MISCELLANEOUS (CONTINUED)

ORGANISMS	Chloramphenicol	Colistimethate	Daptomycin	Fosfomycin	Linezolid	Metronidazole	Nitrofurantoin	Quinupristin + Dalfopristin	Rifampin	Vancomycin
GRAM-NEGATIVE AEROBES *(Continued)*										
Haemophilus influenzae	✓								✓	
Klebsiella species	✓	✓		✓			✓			
Legionella species										
Moraxella catarrhalis										
Morganella morganii										
Neisseria gonorrhoeae										
Neisseria meningitidis									✓	
Pasturella multocida					✓					
Proteus mirabilis	✓			✓						
Proteus vulgaris	✓			✓						
Providencia stuartii										
Pseudomonas aeruginosa	✓	✓								
Rickettsia species										
Salmonella species										
Serratia species				✓						
Shigella species										
Stenotrophomonas maltophilia										

*These are generalizations. There are major differences among countries, areas, and hospitals depending on antibiotic usage patterns.

Blank = no or insufficient activity, or unknown.

ORGANISMS	Chloramphenicol	Colistimethate	Daptomycin	Fosfomycin	Linezolid	Metronidazole	Nitrofurantoin	Quinupristin + Dalfopristin	Rifampin	Vancomycin
GRAM-NEGATIVE AEROBES *(Continued)*										
Vibrio vulnificus										
Yersinia enterocolitica										
Yersinia pestis										
GRAM-POSITIVE AEROBES										
Enterococcus faecalis			✓	✓	✓		✓		✓	✓
Enterococcus faecium			✓	✓	✓		✓	✓		✓
Enterococcus faecium (VRE)			✓		✓			✓		
Listeria monocytogenes										✓
Nocardia										
Staphylococcus aureus (MSSA)	✓		✓		✓		✓	✓	✓	✓
Staphylococcus aureus (MRSA)			✓		✓			✓	✓	✓
Staphylococcus epidermidis			✓		✓		✓	✓	✓	✓
Staphylococcus epidermidis (MRSE)			✓		✓			✓		✓
Streptococcus pneumoniae†			✓		✓					✓
Streptococcus pneumoniae§§					✓					✓

*These are generalizations. There are major differences among countries, areas, and hospitals depending on antibiotic usage patterns.

Blank = no or insufficient activity, or unknown.

† Penicillin sensitive; MIC ≤1.0 mcg/mL. §§ Penicillin resistant; MIC ≥2.0 mcg/mL.

MISCELLANEOUS (CONTINUED)

ORGANISMS	Chloramphenicol	Colistimethate	Daptomycin	Fosfomycin	Linezolid	Metronidazole	Nitrofurantoin	Quinupristin + Dalfopristin	Rifampin	Vancomycin
GRAM-POSITIVE AEROBES *(Continued)*										
Streptococcus (Group A,B,C,F,G)			✓		✓			✓		✓
Streptococcus species			✓		✓			✓		✓
MISCELLANEOUS										
Chlamydia pneumoniae										
Chlamydia trachomatis										
Ehrlichia/Anaplasma species										
MYCOBACTERIA										
Mycobacterium avium (MAI) (non-HIV)										
Mycoplasma pneumoniae										
SPIROCHETES										
Leptospira interrogans										
Treponema pallidum (syphilis)										

*These are generalizations. There are major differences among countries, areas, and hospitals depending on antibiotic usage patterns.

Blank = no or insufficient activity, or unknown.

DRUG TREATMENTS FOR COMMON STDs*

DISEASE	DRUG	RECOMMENDED DOSAGE
Bacterial Vaginosis		
Nonpregnant Women	Metronidazole (Flagyl) *or* Clindamycin cream (Cleocin) *or* Metronidazole gel (MetroGel)	500mg PO bid x 7d. 2%, 1 full applicator intravaginally qhs x 7d. 0.75%, 1 full applicator intravaginally qd x 5d.
Alternative Regimens (Nonpregnant Women)	Clindamycin *or* Clindamycin ovules	300mg PO bid x 7d. 100g intravaginally qhs x 3d.
Pregnant Women	Metronidazole (CI in 1st trimester) *or* Clindamycin	250mg or 500mg PO tid x 7d (metronidazole) 300mg PO bid x 7d (clindamycin)
Chancroid	Azithromycin (Zithromax) *or* Ceftriaxone (Rocephin) *or* Ciprofloxacin (Cipro) *or* Erythromycin base	1g PO single dose. 250mg IM single dose. 500mg PO bid x 3d. 500mg PO tid x 7d.
Chlamydial Infection		
Nonpregnant Women	Azithromycin (Zithromax) *or* Doxycycline (Vibramycin)	1g PO single dose. 100mg PO bid x 7d.
Alternative Regimens (Nonpregnant/pregnant)	Erythromycin base or Erythromycin Ethylsuccinate or Ofloxacin (Floxin) *or* Levofloxacin (Levaquin)	500mg PO qid x 7d or 250mg PO qid x 14d (pregnancy) 800mg PO qid x 7d or 400mg PO qid x 14d (pregnancy) 300mg PO bid x 7d (nonpregnant) 500mg PO qd x 7d (nonpregnant)
Pregnant Women	Azithromycin (Zithromax) *or* Amoxicillin	1g PO single dose. 500mg PO tid x 7d
Epididymitis		
Gonococcal or Chlamydial Infection	Ceftriaxone (Rocephin) *plus* Doxycycline (Vibramycin)	250mg IM single dose. 100mg PO bid x 10d.
Enteric organisms, negative gonococcal culture, or nucleic acid amplification test	Ofloxacin (Floxin) *or* Levofloxacin (Levaquin)	300mg PO bid x 10d. 500mg PO qd x 10d.
Granuloma Inguinale	Doxycycline (Vibramycin)	100mg PO bid for at least 3 weeks.
Alternative Regimens	Ciprofloxacin (Cipro) *or* Erythromycin base (during pregnancy) *or* Azithromycin (Zithromax) Trimethoprim/Sulfamethoxazole (Bactrim, Septra) plus (if no improvement w/in first few days) Aminoglycoside (ie, gentamicin)	750mg PO bid for at least 3 weeks. 500mg PO qid for at least 3 weeks. 1g PO once weekly for at least 3 weeks. 1 tab (DS) PO bid for at least 3 weeks. 1mg/kg IV q8h for at least 3 weeks.
Herpes Simplex Virus (HSV)		
First Episode	Acyclovir (Zovirax) *or* Famciclovir (Famvir) *or* Valacyclovir (Valtrex)	400mg PO tid x 7-10d or 200mg PO 5x/d x 7-10d. 250mg PO tid x 7-10d. 1g PO bid x 7-10d.
Recurrent Episodes	Acyclovir *or* Famciclovir *or* Valacyclovir	400mg PO tid x 5d or 800mg PO bid x 5d or 800mg PO tid x 2d. 1g bid x 1d or 125mg PO bid x 5d or 500mg PO bid x 3d or 1g PO qd x 5d.
Daily Suppressive Therapy	Acyclovir *or* Famciclovir *or* Valacyclovir	400mg PO bid. 250mg PO bid. 500mg PO qd (<10 episodes/yr) or 1g PO qd.

(Continued)

DISEASE	DRUG	RECOMMENDED DOSAGE
Human Papillomavirus (HPV) Infection		
External Genital Area	Podofilox (Condylox) *or*	0.5% sol or gel (patient-applied) bid x 3d, wait 4d, repeat as necessary x 4 cycles. Limit application to 0.5mL/day and to <10cm^2 wart area.
	Imiquimod (Aldara)	5% cre (patient-applied) tiw at bedtime up to 16 wks.
	Cryotherapy *or*	Physician-applied every 1-2 wks.
	Podophyllum resin	10-25% (physician-applied) qwk if necessary. Limit application to 0.5mL/day and to <10cm^2 wart area. Do not apply to area with open lesions or wounds.
	Trichloroacetic acid *or*	80-90% (physician-applied) qwk if necessary.
	Bichloroacetic acid *or*	80-90% (physician-applied) qwk if necessary.
	Surgical removal	
Alternative Regimens	Intralesional interferon *or* laser surgery	
Vaginal warts	Cryotherapy *or*	With liquid nitrogen.
	Trichloroacetic acid *or*	80-90% (physician-applied) qwk if necessary.
	Bichloroacetic acid	80-90% (physician-applied) qwk if necessary.
Urethral Meatus warts	Cryotherapy *or*	With liquid nitrogen.
	Podophyllum	10-25% (physician-applied) qwk if necessary.
Anal warts	Cryotherapy	With liquid nitrogen.
	Trichloroacetic acid *or*	80-90% (physician-applied) qwk if necessary.
	Bichloroacetic acid *or*	80-90% (physician-applied) qwk if necessary.
	Surgical removal	
Lymphogranuloma Venereum	Doxycycline (Vibramycin)	100mg PO bid x 21d.
Alternative Regimen (including pregnancy)	Erythromycin base	500mg PO qid x 21d.
Nongonococcal Urethritis	Azithromycin (Zithromax) *or*	1g PO single dose.
	Doxycycline (Vibramycin)	100mg PO bid x 7d.
Alternative Regimens	Erythromycin base or	500mg PO qid x 7d.
	Erythromycin ethylsuccinate *or*	800mg PO qid x 7d.
	Ofloxacin (Floxin) *or*	300mg PO bid x 7d.
	Levofloxacin (Levaquin)	500mg PO qd x 7d.
Recurrent and Persistent Urethritis	Metronidazole *or*	2g PO single dose.
	Tinidazole *plus*	2g PO single dose.
	Azithromycin	1g PO single dose (if not used for initial episodes).
Pediculosis Pubis	Permethrin cream (NIX)	1% cre: Apply to affected area & wash off after 10 min.
	Pyrethrins with piperonyl butoxide (compounded by pharmacist)	Apply to affected area and wash off after 10 min.
Alternative Regimens	Malathion	0.5% lotion: Apply for 8-12 hours and wash off.
	Ivermectin	250µg/kg repeat in 2 weeks.
Pelvic Inflammatory Disease		
Parenteral Regimen A	Cefotetan (Cefotan) *or*	2g IV q12h.
	Cefoxitin (Mefoxin) *plus*	2g IV q6h.
	Doxycycline (Vibramycin)	100mg IV q12h.
Parenteral Regimen B	Clindamycin (Cleocin) *plus*	900mg IV q8h.
	Gentamicin	LD: 2mg/kg IM/IV. MD: 1.5mg/kg IM/IV q8h (may substitute single daily dosing).
Alternative Regimen	Ampicillin/Sulbactam *plus*	3g IV q6h.
	Doxycycline	100mg PO/IV q12h.
Oral Regimen	Ceftriaxone (Rocephin) *plus*	250mg IM single dose
	Doxycycline w/ or w/o	100mg PO bid x 14d
	Metronidazole	500mg PO bid x 14d
	or	
	Cefoxitin *plus*	2g IM single dose with probenecid 1g PO single dose
	Doxycycline w/ or w/o	100mg PO bid x 14d
	Metronidazole	500mg PO bid x 14d
	or	
	3rd Gen Cephalosporin *plus*	Given IV/IM
	Doxycycline w/ or w/o	100mg PO bid x 14d
	Metronidazole	500mg PO bid x 14d
Alternative Oral Regimen (Use only if negative NAAT test or negative gonococcal culture)	Levofloxacin *or*	500mg PO qd x 14d
	Ofloxacin w/ or w/o	400mg PO bid x 14d
	Metronidazole	500mg PO bid x 14d

(Continued)

DISEASE	DRUG	RECOMMENDED DOSAGE
Proctitis, Proctocolitis & Enteritis	Ceftriaxone (Rocephin) *plus* Doxycycline (Vibramycin)	125mg IM single dose. 100mg PO bid x 7d.
Scabies	Permethrin cream (Elimite) or Ivermectin	5% cre: Apply to body from the neck down & wash off after 8-14h; re-evaluate in 1 week. 200mcg/kg PO; repeat in 2 weeks.
Alternative Regimens	Lindane (Kwell)	1% lot or cre: Apply 1oz lotion or 30g cream to body from the neck down & wash off after 8h; re-evaluate in 1 wk (not recommended in pregnancy, lactating women or children <2 yrs).
Syphilis		
Primary & Secondary Disease	Benzathine Penicillin G	**Adults:** 2.4 MU IM single dose. **Pediatrics:** 50,000 U/kg IM single dose. **Max:** 2.4 MU/dose.
Penicillin Allergy	Doxycycline (Vibramycin) *or* Tetracycline	100mg PO bid x 14d. 500mg PO qid x 14d.
Early Latent Disease	Benzathine Penicillin G	**Adults:** 2.4 MU IM single dose. **Pediatrics:** 50,000 U/kg IM single dose. **Max:** 2.4 MU/dose.
Late Latent, Unknown Duration	Benzathine Penicillin G	**Adults:** 2.4 MU IM qwk x 3 doses. **Pediatrics:** 50,000 U/kg IM qwk x 3 doses. **Max:** 2.4 MU/dose.
Tertiary Disease	Benzathine Penicillin G	2.4 MU IM qwk x 3 doses.
Neurosyphilis	Aqueous Crystalline Penicillin G	3-4 MU IV q4h or continuous infusion x 10-14d.
Alternative Regimen	Procaine Penicillin *plus* Probenecid	2.4 MU IM qd x 10-14d. 500mg PO qid x 10-14d.
Trichomoniasis	Metronidazole (Flagyl) Tinidazole (Tindamax)	2g PO single dose. 2g PO single dose.
Alternative Regimen	Metronidazole	500mg PO bid x 7d.
Pregnant Women	Metronidazole (CI in 1st trimester)	2g PO single dose.
Uncomplicated Gonococcal Infections		
Cervix, Urethra, and Rectum *Recommended Regimens*	Ceftriaxone or Cefixime Plus *If Chlamydial infection is not ruled out:* Azithromycin (Zithromax) *or* Doxycycline (Vibramycin)	125mg IM single dose. 400mg PO single dose. or 400mg by susp 200mg/mL 1g PO single dose. 100mg PO bid x 7d.
Alternative Regimens	Spectinomycin or *Cephalosporin regimens:* Ceftizoxime *or* Cefotaxime *or* Cefoxitin plus Probenecid	2g IM single dose. 500mg IM single dose. 500mg IM single dose. 2g IM. 1g PO.
Pharynx *Recommended Regimens*	Ceftriaxone *plus* *If Chlamydial infection is not ruled out:* Azithromycin (Zithromax) or Doxycycline (Vibramycin)	125mg IM single dose. 1g PO single dose. 100mg PO bid x 7d.

(Continued)

DISEASE	DRUG	RECOMMENDED DOSAGE
Vulvovaginal Candidiasis		
Intravaginal Agents	Butoconazole *or*	2% cre, 5g intravaginally x 3d (sustained release)
	Butoconazole *or*	2% cre, 5g intravaginally single dose.
	Clotrimazole *or*	1% cre, 5g intravaginally x 7-14d.
	Clotrimazole *or*	100mg vaginal tab qd x 7 days or 2 tabs qd x 3d.
	Miconazole *or*	2% cre, 5g intravaginally qd x 7d.
	Miconazole *or*	200mg vaginal supp qd x 3d.
	Miconazole *or*	100mg vaginal supp qd x 7d.
	Miconazole	1200mg vaginal supp single dose.
	Nystatin *or*	100,000-U vaginal tab qd x 14d.
	Tioconazole *or*	6.5% oint, 5g intravaginally single dose.
	Terconazole *or*	0.4% cre, 5g intravaginally x 7d.
	Terconazole *or*	0.8% cre, 5g intravaginally x 3d.
	Terconazole	80mg vaginal supp qd x 3d.
Oral Agent	Fluconazole	150mg tab PO single dose.

*Adapted from: Centers for Disease Control and Prevention. Sexually Transmitted Diseases Treatment Guidelines 2006. MMWR 2002; 51 (No. RR-6): 1-77.

FLU VACCINES

DRUG NAME	INDICATION	HOW SUPPLIED	DOSING	SIDE EFFECTS
Afluria	Active immunization of adults ≥18 yrs against influenza disease caused by influenza virus subtypes A and B contained in the vaccine.	**Inj:** 0.5mL [10 syringes], **MDV:** 5mL [10 doses]	**Adults ≥18 yrs:** 0.5mL IM in deltoid region of upper arm.	**Local:** tenderness, pain, redness, swelling. **Systemic:** headache, malaise, muscle aches.
Fluarix	Active immunization of adults ≥18 yrs against influenza disease caused by influenza virus subtypes A and B contained in the vaccine.	**Inj:** 0.5mL prefilled	**Adults ≥18 yrs:** 0.5mL IM in deltoid muscle.	**Local:** pain, redness, swelling. **Systemic:** muscle aches, fatigue, headache, arthralgia, shivering, fever.
FluLaval	Active immunization of adults ≥18 yrs against influenza disease caused by influenza virus subtypes A and B contained in the vaccine.	**Inj:** 45mcg/0.5mL, **MDV:** [10 doses]	**Adults ≥18 yrs:** 0.5mL IM in deltoid muscle.	**Local:** pain, redness, and/or swelling at injection site. **Systemic:** headache, fatigue, myalgia, low-grade fever, malaise.
FluMist	Active immunization of individuals 2-49 yrs against influenza disease caused by influenza virus subtypes A and B contained in the vaccine.	**Nasal Spray:** 0.2mL [10s]	**Adults ≤49 yrs:** One 0.2mL (0.1mL per nostril) dose. **Pediatrics ≥9 yrs:** One 0.2mL (0.1mL per nostril) dose. **2-8 yrs:** Not Previously Vaccinated With Influenza Vaccine: 0.2mL (0.1mL per nostril) for 2 doses at least 1 month apart. Previously Vaccinated With Influenza Vaccine: One 0.2mL (0.1mL per nostril) dose.	Runny nose, congestion, cough, irritability, headache, sore throat, fever, chills, muscle aches, vomiting, fatigue/weakness.
Fluvirin	Immunization of individuals ≥4 yrs against influenza disease caused by influenza virus subtypes A and B contained in the vaccine.	**Inj:** 45mcg/0.5mL prefilled, or **MDV:** 5mL [10 doses]	**Adults:** 0.5mL IM in deltoid muscle as a single dose. **Pediatrics 4-8 yrs:** Not Previously Vaccinated: 0.5mL IM on Day 1. Repeat dose at least 1 month later. Previously Vaccinated: 0.5mL IM as 1 dose. >**9 yrs:** 0.5mL IM as 1 dose. Administer in deltoid muscle to older children and in thigh muscle in infants and young children.	**Local:** Pain, erythema, ecchymosis, induration, swelling. **Systemic:** headache, myalgia.
Fluzone	Active immunization of individuals ≥6 months against influenza disease caused by influenza virus subtypes A and B contained in the vaccine.	**Inj:** 0.25mL, 0.5mL (prefilled) **MDV:** [10 doses]	**Adults:** 0.5mL IM in deltoid muscle. **Pediatrics:** Previously Vaccinated: 6-35 months: 0.25mL IM. 3-8 yrs: 0.5mL IM. Not Previously Vaccinated: **Children <9 yrs:** 2 doses of vaccine administered ≥1 month apart. Administer in deltoid muscle for children >36 months and anterolateral aspect of thigh for children ≤36 months. **Children <9 yrs:** 0.5mL dose	**Local:** Pain, swelling. **Systemic:** fever, malaise, myalgia.

HIV/AIDS PHARMACOTHERAPY

DRUG	BRAND	HOW SUPPLIED	USUAL DOSE	FOOD EFFECT
CCR5 ANTAGONISTS				
Maraviroc (MVC)	Selzentry	**Tab:** 150mg, 300mg	**Adults >16 yrs:** Give in combination with other antiretroviral medications. With Strong CYP3A Inhibitors (with or without CYP3A inducers) Including PIs (excepts tipranavir/ritonavir), Delavirdine: 150mg bid. With NRTIs, Tipranavir/Ritonavir, Nevirapine, Other Drugs That Are Not Strong CYP3A Inhibitors/Inducers: 300mg bid. With CYP3A Inducers (without strong CYP3A inhibitor): 600mg bid.	Take without regard to meals.
HIV INTEGRASE STRAND TRANSFER INHIBITOR				
Raltegravir	Isentress	**Tab:** 400mg	**Adults:** 400mg bid.	Take without regard to meals.
NUCLEOSIDE REVERSE TRANSCRIPTASE INHIBITORS (NRTIs)				
Abacavir (ABC)	Ziagen	**Sol:** 20mg/mL [240mL]; **Tab:** 300mg	**Adults >16 yrs:** 600mg qd. **Pediatrics 3 months-16 yrs:** 8mg/kg bid. **Max:** 300mg bid.	Take without regard to meals.
Didanosine (ddI)	Videx Powder for Oral Sol; Videx EC	**Powder for Sol:** 10mg/mL [2g, 4g]; **Cap, Delayed Release:** (Videx EC) 125mg, 200mg, 250mg, 400mg	**Adults ≥60kg: (Cap)** 400mg qd; **(Sol)** 200mg bid or 400mg qd. **<60kg: (Sol)** 125mg bid. or 250mg qd. 25-60 kg: **(Cap)** 250mg qd. 20-25 kg: **(Cap)** 200mg qd. **Pediatrics 2 weeks-8 months: (Sol)** 100mg/m^2 bid. **>8 months:** 120mg/m^2 bid.	Take on empty stomach at least 30 minutes before or 2 hrs after meals. Swallow caps whole.
Emtricitabine (FTC)	Emtriva	**Cap:** 200mg; **Sol:** 10mg/mL [170mL]	**Adults ≥18 yrs: Cap:** 200 mg qd. **Sol:** 240mg (24mL) qd. **Pediatrics 0-3 mos:** 3mg/kg qd. **3 mos-17 yrs: Cap: >33kg:** 200mg qd. **Sol:** 6mg/kg qd. **Max:** 240mg (24mL).	Take without regard to meals.
Lamivudine	Epivir	**Sol:** 10mg/mL [240mL]; **Tab:** 150mg, 300mg	**Adults:** 150mg bid or 300mg qd. **Pediatrics 3 months-16 yrs:** 4mg/kg bid. **Max:** 150mg bid.	Take without regard to meals.
Stavudine (d4T)	Zerit	**Cap:** 15mg, 20mg, 30mg, 40mg; **Sol:** 1mg/mL [200mL]	**Adults ≥60kg:** 40mg q12h. **<60kg:** 30mg q12h. **Pediatrics ≥60kg:** 40mg q12h. **30-59 kg:** 30mg q12h. **≥14 days and <30kg:** 1mg/kg q12h. **Birth-13 days:** 0.5mg/kg q12h.	Take without regard to meals.
Tenofovir Disoproxil Fumarate (TDF)	Viread	**Tab:** 300mg	**Adults:** 300mg once daily.	Take without regard to meals.
Zidovudine (AZT, ZDV)	Retrovir	**Cap:** 100mg; **Inj:** 10mg/mL; **Syrup:** 50mg/5mL [240mL]; **Tab:** 300mg	**Adults: (Cap, Tab)** 600mg/day in divided doses. (Inj) 1mg/kg IV over 1 hr 5-6 times/day. **Pediatrics 6 weeks-12 yrs:** 160mg/m^2 PO q8h. **Max:** 200mg PO q8h.	Take without regard to meals.

(Continued)

DRUG	BRAND	HOW SUPPLIED	USUAL DOSE	FOOD EFFECT
NON-NUCLEOSIDE REVERSE TRANSCRIPTASE INHIBITORS (NNRTIs)				
Delavirdine (DLV)	Rescriptor	**Tab:** 100mg, 200mg	**Adults: Usual:** 400mg tid. **Pediatrics ≥16 yrs: Usual:** 400mg tid.	Take without regard to meals.
Efavirenz (EFV)	Sustiva	**Cap:** 50mg, 100mg, 200mg; **Tab:** 600mg	**Adults Initial:** 600mg qd at bedtime. **Pediatrics ≥3 yrs: 10 to <15kg:** 200mg qd. **15 to <20kg:** 250mg qd. **20 to <25kg:** 300mg qd. **25 to <32.5kg:** 350mg qd. **32.5 to <40kg:** 400mg qd. **≥40kg:** 600mg qd at bedtime.	Take on an empty stomach.
Etravirine (ETR)	Intelence	**Tab:** 100mg	**Adults:** 200mg bid.	Take with meals.
Nevirapine (NVP)	Viramune	**Sus:** 50mg/5mL [240mL]; **Tab:** 200mg* *scored	**Adults ≥16 yrs:** 200mg qd for 14 days (lead-in period), then 200mg bid. **Pediatrics >15 days:** 150mg/m^2 qd for 14 days, then 150mg/m^2 bid. **Max:** 400mg/day.	Take without regard to meals.
PROTEASE INHIBITORS (PIs)				
Atazanavir (ATV)	Reyataz	**Cap:** 100mg, 150mg, 200mg, 300mg	**Adults:** Therapy-naive: 400mg qd. Therapy Experienced: (ATV 300mg + RTV 100mg) qd.	Take with food; avoid taking with antacids.
Darunavir (DRV)	Prezista	**Tab:** 75mg, 300mg, 400mg, 600mg	**Adults:** Therapy-naïve: (DRV 800mg + RTV 100mg) qd. Therapy-experienced: (DRV 600mg + RTV 100mg) bid. **Pediatrics:** (6 to <18 yrs): ≥40kg: (DRV 600mg + RTV 100mg) bid. ≥30- <40kg: (DRV 450mg + RTV 60mg) bid. ≥20-<30kg: (DRV 375mg + RTV 50mg) bid. **Max:** (DRV 600mg + RTV 100mg) bid.	Take with food.
Fosamprenavir (fAPV)	Lexiva	**Tab:** 700mg **Sus:** 50mg/mL [225mL]	**Adults:** Therapy-naïve: fAPV 1,400mg bid OR fAPV 1400mg qd + RTV 200mg qd OR fAPV 1400mg qd + RTV 100mg qd OR fAPV 700mg bid + RTV 100mg bid. PI-experienced: fAPV 700mg bid + RTV 100mg bid. **Pediatrics:** (Sus): Therapy-naïve: (2-5 yrs) fAPV 30mg/kg bid **Max:** fAPV 1,400mg bid. (≥6 yrs): fAPV 30mg/kg bid **Max:** fAPV 1,400mg bid. OR fAPV 18mg/kg bid + RTV 3mg/kg bid **Max:** fAPV 700mg bid + RTV 100mg bid. Therapy-experienced: (≥6 yrs) fAPV 18mg/kg bid + RTV 3mg/kg bid **Max:** fAPV 700mg bid + RTV 100mg bid.	**Tab:** Take with or w/o food. **Sus: Adults:** Take w/o food. **Pediatrics:** Take with food.

(Continued)

DRUG	BRAND	HOW SUPPLIED	USUAL DOSE	FOOD EFFECT
PROTEASE INHIBITORS (PIs) *(Continued)*				
Indinavir (IDV)	Crixivan	**Cap:** 100mg, 200mg, 333mg, 400mg	**Adults:** 800mg q8h RTV Boost: (IDV 800mg + RTV 100 or 200mg) q12h.	Take 1 hr before or 2 hr after meals; may take with skim milk or low-fat meal.
Nelfinavir (NFV)	Viracept	**Sus:** (powder) 50mg/g [144g] **Tab:** 250mg, 625mg	**Adults:** 1250mg bid or 750mg tid. **Pediatrics 2-13 yrs:** 45-55mg/kg bid; 25-35mg/kg tid. **Max:** 2500mg/day	Take with meals.
Ritonavir (RTV)	Norvir	**Cap:** 100mg **Sol:** 80mg/mL [240mL]	**Adults: Initial:** 300mg bid. **Titrate:** Increase every 2-3 days by 100mg bid. **Maint:** 600mg bid. **Pediatrics >1 month: Initial:** 250mg/m^2 po bid. **Titrate:** Increase by 50mg/m^2 every 2-3 days. **Maint:** 350-400mg/m^2 po bid or highest tolerated dose. **Max:** 600mg bid.	Take with food, may improve tolerability.
Saquinavir (SQV)	Invirase	**Hard Gel Cap:** 200mg **Tab:** 500mg	**Adults/Pediatrics >16 yrs:** 1000mg bid with RTV 100mg bid OR 1000mg bid with LPV/RTV 400/100mg bid (no additional RTV).	Take within 2 hrs after a meal when taken with RTV.
Tipranavir (TPV)	Aptivus	**Cap:** 250mg **Sol:** 100mg/mL	**Adults:** (500mg + RTV 200mg) bid. **Pediatrics:** (≥2 yrs) 14mg/kg + RTV 6mg/kg (or 375mg/m^2 + RTV 150 mg/m^2) bid. **Max:** (500mg + RTV 200mg) bid.	Take with or w/o food.
FUSION INHIBITOR				
Enfuvirtide (T20)	Fuzeon	**Inj:** 90mg/mL [60^s]	**Adults:** 90mg SQ bid. **Pediatrics 6-16 yrs:** 2mg/kg SQ bid. **Max:** 90mg bid. 11-15.5kg: 27mg bid. 15.6-20.0kg: 36mg bid. 20.1-24.5kg: 45mg bid. 24.6-29.0kg: 54mg bid. 29.1-33.5kg: 63mg bid. 33.6-38.0kg: 72mg bid. 38.1-42.5kg: 81mg bid. ≥42.6kg: 90mg bid.	
COMBINATIONS				
EFV/FTC/TDF	Atripla	**Tab:** (Efavirenz-Emtricitabine-Tenofovir DF) 600mg-200mg-300mg	**Adults ≥18 yrs:** 1 tab qd, preferably at bedtime.	Take on empty stomach.
3TC/ZDV	Combivir	**Tab:** (Lamivudine-Zidovudine) 150mg-300mg	**Adults/Pediatrics:** (≥30kg) 1 tab bid. Do not give if CrCl <50mL/min or if <30kg weight.	Take without regard to meals.
ABC/3TC	Epzicom	**Tab:** (Abacavir Sulfate-Lamivudine) 600mg-300mg	**Adults ≥18 yrs:** CrCl >50 mL/min: 1 tab qd. Do not give if CrCl <50mL/min	Take without regard to meals.

(Continued)

DRUG	BRAND	HOW SUPPLIED	USUAL DOSE	FOOD EFFECT
COMBINATIONS *(Continued)*				
LPV/RTV	Kaletra	**Cap:** (LPV-RTV) 133.3mg-33.3mg **Tab:** (LPV-RTV) 200mg-50mg; 100mg-25mg; **Sol:** (LPV-RTV) 80mg-20mg/mL [160mL]	**Adults:** Therapy-naive: 400/100mg bid or 800/200mg qd. Therapy-experienced: 400/100mg bid. **Pediatrics: Sol:** (14 days-6 months) LPV/RTV 16/4 mg/kg or 300/75 mg/m^2 bid. (6 months-18 yrs) LPV/RTV 230/57.5 mg/m^2 bid or weight-based (<15kg) 12/3 mg/kg bid (≥15-40kg) 10/2.5 mg/kg bid.	**Tab:** Take without regard to meals. **Cap/Sol:** Take with meals.
ABC/ZDV/3TC	Trizivir	**Tab:** (Abacavir-Lamivudine-Zidovudine) 300mg-150mg-300mg	**Adults/Adolescents:** >40kg and CrCl >50mL/min: 1 tab bid.	Take without regard to meals.
FTC/TDF	Truvada	**Tab:** (Emtricitabine-Tenofovir Disoproxil Fumarate) 200mg-300mg	**Adults ≥18 yrs:** CrCl ≥50mL/min: 1 tab qd. CrCl 30-49mL/min: 1 tab q48h.	Take without regard to meals.
Sources: FDA Approved Labeling; Guidelines for the Use of Antiretroviral Agents in HIV-1-Infected Adults and Adolescents - October 10, 2006.				

HIV/AIDS COMPLICATIONS THERAPY

DISEASE-RELATED COMPLICATION	GENERIC (BRAND)	RECOMMENDED DOSAGE
ASPERGILLOSIS		
Prevention	Posaconazole (Noxafil)	**Adults/Pediatrics ≥13 yrs:** 200mg PO tid. Duration of treatment based on neutropenia/immunosuppression.
Recommended Treatment Regimen	Voriconazole (VFEND)*	**Adults: LD:** 6mg/kg q12h for 1st 24 hrs. **MD:** (IV) 4mg/kg q12h or (PO) ≥40kg: 200mg q12h. <40kg: 100mg q12h. Continue treatment until at least 7 days following resolution of symptoms.
Alternative Treatment Regimen	Amphotericin B (AmBisome)	**Adults/Pediatrics:** 3-5mg/kg/day IV controlled infusion over 1-2 hrs.
	Amphotericin B lipid-formulation	**Adults/Pediatrics:** 5mg/kg at 2.5mg/kg/hr.
	Caspofungin (Cancidas)	**Adults: LD:** 70mg slow IV infusion over 1 hr on Day 1. **MD:** 50mg IV qd. **Pediatrics:** (3 months-17 yrs). **LD:** 70mg/m^2 slow IV infusion over 1 hr on Day 1. **MD:** 50mg/m^2 qd. **Max:** LD and MD should not exceed 70mg.
	Itraconazole (Sporanox)	**Adults:** 200-400mg PO qd w/ meals.
CANDIDIASIS		
Prevention/Treatment	Amphotericin B (AmBisome)	**Adults/Pediatrics:** 3-5mg/kg/day IV controlled infusion over 1-2 hrs.
	Amphotericin B lipid-formulation	**Adults/Pediatrics:** 5mg/kg at 2.5mg/kg/hr.
	Caspofungin (Cancidas)	**Adults: LD:** 70mg slow IV infusion over 1 hr on Day 1. **MD:** 50mg IV qd. **Esophageal:** 50mg/day slow IV infusion over 1 hr.
	Fluconazole (Diflucan)†	**Oropharngeal: Adults:** 200mg PO Day 1, then 100mg qd q 2 weeks. **Pediatrics:** 6mg/kg Day 1, then 3mg/kg qd q 2 weeks. **Esophageal: Adults:** 200mg Day 1, then 100mg qd. Continue until 2 weeks after resolution of symptoms. Max: 400mg/day. **Pediatrics:** 6mg/kg Day 1, then 3mg/kg qd for a minimum of 3 weeks and for at least 2 weeks following resolution of symptoms. Max: 12mg/kg/day.
	Itraconazole (Sporanox)	**Oropharngeal: Adults:** Swish and swallow 200mg (20mL) oral solution qd x 1-2 weeks.
	Posaconazole (Noxafil)	**Oropharngeal: ≥13 yrs**: 100mg bid Day 1, then 100mg qd x 13d. **Refractory to fluconazole:** 400mg bid. Duration of therapy individualized.
	Voriconazole (VFEND)*	**Esophageal: Adults:** ≥40kg: 200mg PO q12h. <40kg: 100mg PO q12h. Continue treatment until at least 7 days following resolution of symptoms.
CMV RETINITIS		
Treatment	Cidofovir (Vistide)†	**Adults:** Induction: 5mg/kg IV infusion over 1 hr q week x 2 weeks. Maint: 5mg/kg IV over 1 hr q 2 weeks.
	Foscarnet (Foscavir)	**Adults:** Induction: 90mg/kg over 1.5-2 hrs IV infusion q12h or 60mg/kg 1 hr IV infusion q8h x 2-3 weeks. **Maint:** 90-120mg/kg/day IV over 2 hrs.
	Ganciclovir (Cytovene)†	**Adults:** Induction: 5mg/kg IV over 1hr q12h x 14-21days. Maint: 5mg/kg IV over 1 hr qd x 7 days/week or 6mg/kg IV qd x 5 days/week.
	Ganciclovir (Vitrasert)	**Adults/Pediatrics ≥9 yrs:** One implant q 5-8 months.
	Valganciclovir (Valcyte)	**Adults:** Induction: 900mg PO bid x 21 days w/ food. Maint: 900mg PO qd w/ food.
CRYPTOCOCCAL MENINGITIS		
Treatment	Amphotericin B (AmBisome)	**Adults:** 6mg/kg/day IV over 1-2 hrs.
	Fluconazole (Diflucan)	**Adults:** 400mg on Day 1, then 200-400mg qd x 10-12 weeks. Relapse: 200mg qd. **Pediatrics:** 12mg/kg on Day 1, then 6-12mg/kg qd x 10-12 weeks. Relapse: 6mg/kg qd.

(Continued)

DISEASE-RELATED COMPLICATION	GENERIC (BRAND)	RECOMMENDED DOSAGE
HSV		
Recommended Regimen for Daily Suppressive Therapy	Acyclovir *or* Famciclovir (Famvir) *or* Valacyclovir	400-800mg PO bid-tid. 500mg PO bid. 500mg PO bid.
Recommended Regimen for Episodic Infection	Acyclovir *or* Famiciclovir† *or* Valacyclovir	400mg PO tid x 5-10 days. 500mg PO bid x 5-10 days. 1g PO bid x 5-10 days.
KAPOSI'S SARCOMA		
Treatment	Alitretinoin (Panretin)	**0.1% gel: Adults: Initial:** Apply bid to lesions. Can increase to tid-qid based on individual lesion tolerance.
	Daunorubicin (DaunoXome)	**Adults:** 40mg/m^2 IV over 60 min q 2 weeks.
	Doxorubicin (Doxil)	**Adults:** 20mg/m^2 IV q 3 weeks. Initial rate: 1mg/min. May be increased to administer over 1 hr if tolerated.
	Interferon alfa-2b (INTRON A)	**Adults:** 30 MIU/m^2/dose SQ/IM tiw until max response achieved after 16 weeks. Must use Powder for Injection/Reconstitution only. Solution for Injection in vials or Multidose Pens should not be used.
	Paclitaxel (Taxol)	**Adults:** 135mg/m^2 IV over 3 hrs q 3 weeks or 100mg/m2 IV over 3 hrs q 2 weeks. Dose Intensity: 45-50mg/m^2/week.
MAC		
Prevention/Treatment	Azithromycin (Zithromax)	**Adults:** Prevention: 1200mg once weekly. Treatment: 600mg qd with ethambutol 15mg/kg/day.
Prevention/Treatment	Clarithromycin (Biaxin)	**Adults:** 500mg PO bid. **Pediatrics:** 7.5mg/kg bid up to 500mg bid.
Prevention	Rifabutin (Mycobutin)†	**Adults:** 300mg PO qd. N/V/GI upset: 150mg bid w/ food.
PCP		
Prevention/Treatment	Atovaquone (Mepron)	**Adults/Pediatrics ≥13 yrs**: 1500mg PO qd w/ meals. **Adults/Pediatrics ≥13 yrs (mild-moderate PCP):** 750mg PO bid w/ meals x 21 days.
	TMP/SMX (Bactrim)	**Adults/Pediatrics:** Treatment: 15-20mg/kg/day TMP and 75-100mg/kg/day SMX in divided doses q6h x 14-21days.
	TMP/SMX DS (Bactrim DS)	**Adults:** Prevention: 1 DS tab (160/800mg) qd. **Pediatrics:** Prevention: 150mg/m^2/day TMP with 750mg/m^2/day SMX PO bid in equally divided doses on 3 consecutive days/week.
VISCERAL LEISHMANIASIS		
Treatment	Amphotericin B (AmBisome)	**Adults:** Immunocompetent: 3mg/kg/day IV Days 1-5, then on Days 14 and 21. Immunocompromised: 4mg/kg/day IV Days 1-5, then on Days 10, 17, 24, 31, and 38.
WEIGHT LOSS		
Anorexia	Dronabinol (Marinol)	**Adults:** 2.5mg qhs or bid ac. **Max:** 20mg/day in divided doses.
Anorexia, cachexia, unexplained weight loss	Megesterol (Megace)	**Adults:** Initial: 800mg/d. **Usual:** 400-800mg/day.
Cachexia/Wasting	Somatropin (Serostim)	**Adults:** >55kg: 6mg SQ qhs. 45-55kg: 5mg SQ qhs. 35-45kg: 4mg SQ qhs. <35kg: 0.1mg/kg SQ qhs. **Max:** 6mg/day.

Abbreviations: CMV=cytomegalovirus; HSV=herpes simplex virus; MAC=*Mycobacterium avium* complex; PCP=*Pneumocystis carinii* pneumonia.

*Use cautiously in patients on protease inhibitors and efavirenz.

†For dosing in special populations, see the complete prescribing information.

MANAGEMENT OF HEPATITIS B AND HEPATITIS C

BRAND NAME (GENERIC)	HOW SUPPLIED	ADULTS	COMMENTS
HEPATITIS B			
Acyclic Nucleotide Analog			
Hepsera (Adefovir dipivoxil)	**Tab:** 10mg	**Adults:** 10mg QD PO without regard to food. **Pediatrics ≥12 yrs:** 10mg QD PO without regard to food.	Renal Impairment: CrCl 30-49mL/min: 10mg q48h. CrCl 10-29mL/min: 10mg q72h. Hemodialysis Patients: 10mg every 7 days following dialysis.
Biological Response Modifier			
Intron-A (Interferon alfa-2b, recombinant)	**Inj:** 10 MIU, 18 MIU, 50 MIU, 3 MIU/0.2mL, 5 MIU/0.2mL, 10 MIU/0.2mL, 3MIU/0.5mL, 5MIU/0.5mL	**Adults ≥18 yrs:** IM/SQ: 5 MIU qd or 10 MIU IM/SQ 3x/week for 16 weeks. **Pediatrics 1-17yrs:** 3 MIU/m^2 SQ 3x/week for 1 week, then 6 MIU/m^2 3x/week (max 10 MIU TIW) for total therapy of 16-24 weeks.	Adjust dose according to severe adverse reactions and laboratory abnormalities (See PI for more information). Reduce dose by 50% or stop therapy with severe reactions. Adjust based on WBC, granulocyte, and/or platelet counts.
Guanosine Nucleoside Analogue			
Baraclude (Entecavir)	**Sol:** 0.05mg/mL; **Tab:** 0.5mg, 1mg	**Adults/Pediatrics >16 yrs:** Nucleoside-Treatment-Naive: 0.5mg qd. CrCl 30 to <50mL/min: 0.25mg qd or 0.5mg q48h. CrCl 10 to <30mL/min: 0.15mg qd or 0.5mg q72h. CrCl <10mL/min: 0.05mg qd or 0.5mg q7 days. Receiving Lamivudine or Known Lamivudine Resistance Mutation: 1mg qd. CrCl 30 to <50mL/min: 0.5mg qd or 1mg q48h. CrCl 10 to <30mL/min: 0.3mg qd or 1mg q72h. CrCl <10mL/min: 0.1mg qd or 1mg q7 days.	Take on empty stomach.
Nucleoside Analogues			
Epivir-HBV (Lamivudine)	**Sol:** 5mg/mL [240mL]; **Tab:** 100mg	**Adults:** 100mg qd. CrCl 30-49mL/min: 100mg Day 1, then 50mg qd. CrCl: 15-29mL/min: 100mg Day 1, then 25mg qd. CrCl 5-14mL/min: 35mg Day 1, then 15mg qd. CrCl <5mL/min: 35mg Day 1, then 10mg qd. **Pediatrics 2-17 yrs:** 3mg/kg qd. Max: 100mg/day.	
Tyzeka (Telbivudine)	**Tab:** 600mg	**Adults/Pediatrics ≥16 yrs:** CrCl ≥50mL/min: 600mg qd. CrCl 30-49mL/min: 600mg every 48 hrs. CrCl <30mL/min (not requiring dialysis): 600mg every 72 hrs. ESRD: 600mg every 96 hrs.	Take with or without food.
Viread (Tenofovir disoproxil fumarate)	**Tab:** 300mg	**Adults:** 300mg qd without regard to food. Renal Impairment: CrCl 30-49mL/min: 300mg q48 hrs. CrCl 10-29mL/min: 300mg q72-96 hrs.	Hemodialysis: 300mg every 7 days after total of approx. 12 hrs of dialysis.

(Continued)

BRAND NAME (GENERIC)	HOW SUPPLIED	ADULTS	COMMENTS
Pegylated Virus Proliferation Inhibitor			
Pegasys (Peginterferon alfa-2a)	**Inj:** Prefilled syringe: 180mcg/0.5mL; **Single Dose Vial:** 180mcg/mL	**Monotherapy:** 180mcg SQ in abdomen or thigh once weekly for 48 wks.	Adjust dose based on hematological parameters and depression severity (see PI for dose modifications).
Vaccines			
Engerix-B (Hepatitis B vaccine [recombinant])	**Inj:** 10mcg/0.5mL, 20mcg/mL	**Adults >19 yrs:** 20mcg/1mL IM in deltoid region at 0, 1, 6 months. Hemodialysis: 40mcg/2mL IM at 0, 1, 2, 6 months. Booster: 20mcg IM. Hemodialysis Booster: 40mcg IM. May give SQ with risk of hemorrhage. **Pediatrics ≤19 yrs:** 10mcg/0.5mL IM at 0, 1, 6 months. Booster: ≤10 yrs: 10mcg IM. 11-19 yrs: 20mcg IM.	See PI for special populations. May give SQ with risk of hemorrhage.
Recombivax HB, Recombivax HB Adult, Recombivax HB Dialysis, Recombivax HB Pediatric/Adolescent (Hepatitis B vaccine [recombinant])	**Inj:** Pediatric/Adolescent Formulation Preservative-Free: 5mcg/0.5mL, Adult Formulation Preservative-Free: 10mcg/1mL, Dialysis Formulation Preservative-Free: 40mcg/1mL	**Adults:** IM into deltoid muscle. If at risk of hemorrhage with IM injection, give SQ. ≥20 years (Adult Formulation): 10mcg at 0, 1, 6 months. Predialysis/Dialysis (Dialysis Formulation): 40mcg at 0, 1, 6 months; consider booster dose or revaccination if anti-HBs level <l0mIU/mL 1 to 2 months after the 3rd dose. **Pediatrics:** IM injection into anterolateral thigh in infants and young children. Give SQ if risk of hemorrhage following IM injection. 0-19 years (Pediatric/Adolescent Formulation): 5mcg at 0, 1, 6 months. 11-15 years (Adult Formulation): 10mcg as first dose, then 10mcg 4-6 months later.	
Combination Vaccines			
Comvax (*Haemophilus* B conjugate [Meningococcal protein conjugate] and Hepatitis B [recombinant] vaccine)	**Inj:** 7.5mcg PRP polysaccaride conjugated to about 125mcg OMPC and 5 mcg HBsAg [0.5mL]	**Pediatrics ≥6 weeks:** 0.5mL IM at 2, 4, and 12-15 months of age. If schedule cannot be followed, wait at least 6 wks between 1st 2 doses. The 2nd and 3rd dose should be close to 8-11 months apart.	
Pediarix (Diphtheria and tetanus toxoids and acellular pertussis adsorbed, Hepatitis B [recombinant] and Inactivated poliovirus vaccine combined)	**Inj:** 0.5mL	**Pediatrics ≥6 weeks to <7 yrs:** 3 doses of 0.5mL IM at 6-8 wk intervals. Start at 2 months old or as early as 6 wks old if necessary.	Preferred site is anterolateral aspect of the thigh for children <1yr. In older children, deltoid muscle. May use to complete primary series in infants who have received 1 or 2 doses of Infanrix or IPV or to complete a hepatitis B vaccine (recombinant) series. Not recommended for completion of the first 3 doses of the DTaP vaccination series initiated with a DTaP vaccine from a different manufacturer.

BRAND NAME (GENERIC)	HOW SUPPLIED	ADULTS	COMMENTS
Combination Vaccines *(Continued)*			
Twinrix Hepatitis A inactivated & Hepatitis B [recombinant] vaccine)	**Inj:** (Hepatitis A-Hepatitis B) 720 ELISA U-20mcg/mL	**Adults ≥18 yrs:** 3-Dose Schedule: 1mL IM in deltoid region at 0, 1, and 6 months. Alternative 4-Dose Schedule: 1 mL IM in deltoid region on Days 0, 7, and 21-30, followed by booster dose at 12 months.	
HEPATITIS C TREATMENT			
Biological Response Modifiers			
Infergen (Interferon alfacon-1)	**Inj:** 9mcg/0.3mL, 15mcg/0.5mL	**Adults ≥18 yrs:** 9mcg 3x/week (TIW) SQ for 24 wks, wait 48 48 hrs between doses. If No Response or Relapse: 15mcg TIW SQ as a single injection for up to 48 wks.	Hold dose temporarily in presence of severe adverse effects and reduce to 7.5mcg.
Intron-A (Interferon alfa-2b, recombinant)	**Inj:** 10 MIU, 18 MIU, 50 MIU, 3 MIU/0.2mL, 5 MIU/0.2mL, 10 MIU/0.2mL, 3MIU/0.5mL, 5MIU/0.5mL	**Adults ≥18 yrs:** 3 MIU IM/SQ TIW for 18-24 months	If severe adverse reactions develop, reduce dose by 50% or temporarily stop therapy.
Roferon-A (Interferon alfa-2a, recombinant)	**Inj:** 3 MIU/0.5mL, 6 MIU/0.5mL, 9 MIU/0.5mL	**Adults ≥18 yrs:** 3 MIU TIW SQ for 12 months (48-52 weeks) OR 6 MIU TIW for 12 weeks then 3 MIU for 36 wks.	D/C treatment if no response within 3 months. Retreat if tolerated and partial or complete response to therapy but relapsed. Retreatment: 3 MIU TIW OR 6 MIU TIW for 6 to 12 months. If intolerant to prescribed dose, temporarily reduce dose by 50%. If adverse events resolve, reinitiate prescribed dose.
Biological Response Modifier/Nucleoside Analog			
Rebetron (Ribavirin and Interferon alfa-2b, recombinant Injection)	**Inj-Cap:** (Interferon alfa-2b-Ribavirin) 3 MIU/0.2mL-200mg, 3 MIU/0.5mL-200mg	**Adults ≥18 yrs:** Previously Untreated with Interferon: Treat for 24-48 wks. Relapse After Interferon Treatment: Treat for 24 wks. Usual: ≤75kg: Interferon 3 MIU SQ TIW with ribavirin 400mg PO qam and 600mg PO qpm. >75kg: Interferon 3 MIU SQ TIW with ribavirin 600mg PO qam and 600mg PO qpm.	**Dose Reduction:** If Hgb <10g/dL with no cardiac history, decrease ribavirin to 600mg PO qd. If ≥2g/dL, decrease in Hgb during a 4-wk period with cardiac history, decrease interferon to 1.5 MIU SQ TIW and ribavirin to 600mg PO qd. If WBC <1.5x10^9/L or neutrophils <0.75x10^9/L or platelets <50x10^9/L: Decrease interferon to 1.5 MIU SQ TIW. D/C interferon and ribavirin if Hgb <8.5g/dL with no cardiac history, or Hgb <12g/dL after 4 wks of dose reduction with a cardiac history, WBC <1x10^9/L, neutrophils <0.5x10^9/L, or platelets <25x10^9/L.
Nucleoside Analog			
Copegus (Ribavirin)	**Tab:** 200mg	**Adults ≥18 yrs:** Give bid in divided doses. Treat for 24-48 wks with Pegasys 180mcg. Genotypes 1 and 4: <75kg: 1000mg/day for 48 wks. ≥75kg: 1200mg/day for 48 wks. Genotypes 2 and 3: 800mg/day for 24 wks. HCV/HIV: 800mg PO QD. Treat for 48 wks with Pegasys 180mcg SQ once weekly.	**Dose Modifications:** Reduce to 600mg/day for Copegus if Hgb <10g/dL with no cardiac history, or if Hgb decreases by ≥2g/dL during a 4-week period with stable cardiac disease. D/C Copegus if Hgb <8.5g/dL with no cardiac history or if Hgb <12g/dL after 4 wks of dose reduction with stable cardiac disease. After dose modification, may restart Copegus at 600mg/day, then may increase to 800mg/day. CrCl <50mL/min: Avoid use.

(Continued)

BRAND NAME (GENERIC)	HOW SUPPLIED	ADULTS	COMMENTS
Nucleoside Analog			
Rebetol (Ribavirin)	**Cap:** 200mg; Sol: 40mg/mL [100mL]	**Adults ≥18 yrs:** With Intron A: ≤75kg: 400mg qam and 600mg qpm PO. >75kg: 600mg qam and 600mg qpm PO. Treat for 24-48 wks in interferon-naive patients; In relapsed patients, treat for 24 wks. With Peg-Intron: 400mg bid, qam and qpm with food. **Pediatrics ≥3 yrs:** 15mg/kg/day PO in divided doses qam and qpm. Use solution if ≤25kg or cannot swallow caps. With Intron A: 25-36kg: 200mg bid PO, qam and qpm. 37-49kg: 200mg PO qam and 400mg qpm. 50-61kg: 400mg bid PO, qam and qpm. >61kg: Dose as adult. Genotype 1: Treat for 48 wks. Genotype 2/3: Treat for 24 weeks. Reduce to 7.5mg/day (divided dose AM and PM) if Hgb <10g/dL with no cardiac history, or if Hgb decreases by ≥2g/dL during a 4 week-period with a cardiac history. (Intron A for ≥3 yrs: 3 MIU/m^2 3 times weekly SQ).	**Adults:** Reduce to 600mg qd if Hgb <10g/dL with no cardiac history, or if Hgb decreases by ≥2g/dL during a 4 week-period with a cardiac history. **Adults/Peds:** D/C if Hgb <8.5g/dL with no cardiac history or if Hgb <12g/dL after 4 wks of dose reduction with a cardiac history. CrCl <50mL/min: Avoid use.
Pegylated Virus Proliferation Inhibitor			
Pegasys (Peginterferon alfa-2a)	**Inj:** Prefilled syringe: 180mcg/0.5mL; **Single Dose Vial:** 180mcg/mL	**Adults ≥18 yrs:** Monotherapy: 180mcg SQ (in abdomen or thigh) once weekly for 48 weeks. Combination Therapy With Copegus: 180mcg SQ once weekly for 24 weeks with Genotypes 2 and 3 or 48 wks with Genotypes 1 and 4. HCV/HIV: Monotherapy: 180mcg SQ in abdomen or thigh once weekly for 48 weeks. Combination Therapy with Copegus: 180mcg SQ once weekly for 48 wks, regardless of genotype.	Adjust dose based on hematological parameters and depression severity (see PI for dose modifications).
PegIntron (Peginterferon alpha-2b)	**Inj:** 50mcg/0.5mL, 80mcg/0.5mL, 120mcg/0.5mL, 150mcg/0.5mL	**Adults ≥18 yrs:** Monotherapy: 1mcg/kg/wk SQ for 1 yr administered on the same day of the week. Combination Therapy With Rebetol: 1.5mcg/kg/wk plus Rebetol 800-1400mg/day PO based on patients body weight for 48 wks in Genotype 1, and 24 wks in Genotype 2 and 3 patients. CrCl <50mL/min: D/C therapy. Adjust dose based on hematological parameters and depression severity (see PI for dose modifications). **Pediatrics 3-17 yrs:** Combination Therapy With Rebetol: 60mcg/m^2/wk SQ plus Rebetol 15mg/kg/day in 2 divided doses for 48 wks in Genotype 1, and 24 weeks in Genotype 2 and 3 patients.	**Adults:** Renal Impairment: CrCl 30-50mL/min: Reduce PegIntron dose by 25%. CrCl 10-29mL/min: Reduce PegIntron dose by 50%. D/C therapy if renal function decreases, if there is not at least a 2 $\log^{10}$ drop or loss of HCV-RNA at 12 wks, or whose HCV-RNA levels remain detectable after 24 wks of therapy. CrCl <50mL/min: D/C therapy. Adjust dose based on hematological parameters and depression severity (see PI for dose modifications). **Pediatrics:** Renal Impairment: CrCl 30-50mL/min: Reduce PegIntron dose by 25%. CrCl 10-29mL/min: Reduce PegIntron dose by 50%. D/C if renal function decreases, HCV-RNA dropped <2 $\log^{10}$ at 12 wks, or HCV-RNA levels remain detectable after 24 wks.

ORAL ANTIBIOTICS

DRUG	BRAND	FORMULATIONS (mg or mg/5mL)*
CEPHALOSPORINS		
Cefaclor	Cefaclor	**Cap:** 250, 500 **Sus:** 125, 250, 375
	Cefaclor ER	**Tab, ER:** 500
Cefadroxil	Duricef	**Cap:** 500 **Sus:** 125, 250, 500 **Tab:** 1g
Cefdinir	Omnicef	**Cap:** 300 **Sus:** 125, 250
Cefditoren	Spectracef	**Tab:** 200, 400
Cefixime	Suprax	**Sus:** 100, 200 **Tab:** 400
Cefpodoxime	Vantin	**Sus:** 50, 100 **Tab:** 100, 200
Cefprozil	Cefzil	**Sus:** 125, 250 **Tab:** 250, 500
Ceftibuten	Cedax	**Cap:** 400 **Sus:** 90
Cefuroxime	Ceftin	**Sus:** 125, 250 **Tab:** 125, 250, 500
Cephalexin	Keflex	**Cap:** 250, 500, 750
	Panixine	**Tab, Dispersible:** 125, 250
FLUOROQUINOLONES		
Ciprofloxacin**	Cipro	**Sus:** 250, 500 **Tab:** 100, 250, 500, 750
	Cipro XR	**Tab, ER:** 500, 1000
	ProQuin XR	**Tab, ER:** 500
Gemifloxacin	Factive	**Tab:** 320
Levofloxacin**	Levaquin	**Sol:** 25mg/mL; **Tab:** 250, 500, 750
Moxifloxacin	Avelox	**Tab:** 400
Norfloxacin	Noroxin	**Tab:** 400
Ofloxacin	Floxin	**Tab:** 200, 300, 400
MACROLIDES		
Azithromycin**	Zithromax	**Sus:** 100, 200, 1g/pkt **Tab:** 250, 500, 600
	Zmax	**Sus, ER:** 2g
Clarithromycin	Biaxin	**Sus:** 125, 250 **Tab:** 250, 500
	Biaxin XL	**Tab, ER:** 500
Erythromycin ethylsuccinate	E.E.S.	**Sus:** 200, 400 **Tab:** 400
	EryPed	**Sus:** 100, 200, 400 **Tab, Chewable Tab:** 200
	Eryc	**Cap, DR:** 250
	Ery-Tab	**Tab, DR:** 250, 333, 500
	Erythromycin Base	**Tab:** 250, 500
	Erythromycin Delayed-Release	**Cap: Delayed-Release:** 250
	PCE	**Tab:** 333, 500
PENICILLINS		
Amoxicillin	Amoxil	**Cap:** 250, 500 **Chew, Tab:** 200, 400 **Drops:** 50mg/mL **Sus:** 125, 200, 250, 400 **Tab:** 500, 875
	DisperMox	**Tab, Dispersible:** 200, 400, 600

(Continued)

DRUG	BRAND	FORMULATIONS (mg or mg/5mL)*
PENICILLINS *(Continued)*		
Ampicillin		**Cap:** 250, 500 **Sus:** 125, 250
Carbenicillin	Geocillin	**Tab:** 382
Dicloxacillin	Dicloxacillin Sodium	**Cap:** 125, 250, 500 **Sus:** 62.5
Penicillin V	Veetids	**Sus:** 125, 250 **Tab:** 250, 500
TETRACYCLINES		
Demeclocycline	Declomycin	**Tab:** 150, 300
Doxycycline	Doryx	**Cap:** 75, 100
	Monodox	**Cap:** 50, 75, 100
	Periostat	**Tab:** 20
	Vibramycin	**Cap:** 50, 100 **Syr:** 50 **Sus:** 25
	Vibra-Tabs	**Tab:** 100
Minocycline**	Minocin	**Cap:** 50, 100
	Dynacin	**Tab:** 50, 75, 100
	Solodyn	**Tab, Extended Release:** 45, 90, 135
Tetracycline	Sumycin	**Sus:** 125 **Tab:** 250, 500
OTHER		
Clindamycin**	Cleocin	**Cap:** 75, 150, 300 **Sus:** 75
Dapsone	Dapsone	**Tab:** 25, 100
Fosfomycin	Monurol	**Powder:** 3g/packet
Linezolid**	Zyvox	**Sus:** 100 **Tab:** 400, 600
Methanamine	Hiprex	**Tab:** 1g
Metronidazole	Flagyl	**Cap:** 375 **Tab:** 250, 500
	Flagyl ER	**Tab, ER:** 750
Nitrofurantoin	Furadantin	**Sus:** 25
	Macrobid	**Cap:** 100
	Macrodantin	**Cap:** 25, 50, 100
Telithromycin	Ketek	**Tab:** 300, 400
Trimethoprim	Primsol	**Sol:** 50
Vancomycin**	Vancocin	**Cap:** 125, 250
COMBINATIONS		
Erythromycin ethylsuccinate/ Sulfisoxazole	Pediazole	**Sus:** 200/600
Amoxicillin/Clavulanate	Augmentin	**Chew, Tab:** 125/31.25, 250/62.5, 200/28.5, 400/57 **Sus:** 125/31.2, 200/28.5, 400/57, 250/62.5 **Tab:** 250/125, 500/125, 875/125
	Augmentin ES 600	**Sus:** 600/42.9
	Augmentin XR	**Tab, ER:** 1000/62.5
Sulfamethoxazole/ Trimethoprim	Bactrim, Septra**	**Tab:** 400/80 **Sus:** 200/40
	Bactrim DS, Septra DS	**Tab, DS:** 800/160

* Unless otherwise indicated. **Injection formulation available.

SYSTEMIC ANTIBIOTICS

BRAND NAME (Generic)	DOSAGE FORM/ STRENGTH	INDICATIONS	ADULT DOSE	PEDIATRIC DOSE
AMINOGLYCOSIDES				
Amikacin (amikacin sulfate)	**Inj:** 50mg/mL, 250mg/mL	Short-term treatment of serious infections caused by gram-negative bacteria such as septicemia, and respiratory tract, bone/joint, CNS (including meningitis), skin and soft tissue, and intra-abdominal infections; burns and postoperative infections; complicated and recurrent urinary tract infections (UTI); and staphylococcal disease.	(IM/IV)15mg/kg/day given q8h or q12h. Max: 15mg/kg/day. Heavier Weight Patients: Max: 1.5g/day. Recurrent Uncomplicated UTI: 250mg bid. Duration: 7-10 days. Stop therapy if no response after 3-5 days. Reduce dose or increase dosing interval if suspect renal dysfunction. Discontinue if azotemia increases or if a progressive decrease in urinary output occurs.	15mg/kg/day given bid-tid. Newborns: LD: 10mg/kg. MD: 7.5mg/kg q12h. Duration: 7-10 days.
Amikacin Pediatric (amikacin sulfate)	**Inj:** 50mg/mL	Short-term treatment of serious infections caused by gram-negative bacteria such as septicemia, and respiratory tract, bone/joint, CNS (including meningitis), skin and soft tissue, and intra-abdominal infections; burns and postoperative infections; complicated and recurrent urinary tract infections (UTI); and staphylococcal disease.		15mg/kg/day given bid-tid. Newborns: LD: 10mg/kg. MD: 7.5mg/kg q12h. Duration: 7-10 days.
Gentamicin sulfate	**Inj:** 10mg/mL, 40mg/mL	Treatment of bacterial neonatal sepsis, bacterial septicemia, and serious bacterial infections of the CNS (meningitis), urinary tract, respiratory tract, gastrointestinal tract (including peritonitis), skin, bone and soft tissue (including burns) caused by susceptible strains of microorganisms.	(IM/IV) Serious Infections: 3mg/kg/day given q8h. Life-Threatening Infections: 5mg/kg/day tid-qid; reduce to 3mg/kg/day as soon as clinically indicated. Treat for 7-10 days; may need longer course in difficult and complicated infections. Renal Impairment: Reduced dose given q8h or usual dose given at prolonged intervals based on either CrCl or serum creatinine. Dialysis: 1-1.7mg/kg, depending on severity of infection, at end of each dialysis period. Obese Patients: Calculate dose based on estimated lean body mass.	6-7.5mg/kg/day (2-2.5mg/kg given q8h). Infants and Neonates: 7.5mg/kg/day (2.5mg/kg given q8h). Premature and Full-Term Neonates 1 week: 5mg/kg/day (2.5mg/kg given q12h). Treat for 7-10 days; may need longer course in difficult and complicated infections. Renal Impairment: Reduced dose given q8h or usual dose given at prolonged intervals based on either CrCl or serum creatinine. Dialysis: 2mg/kg at end of each dialysis period. Obese Patients: Calculate dose based on estimated lean body mass.

(Continued)

BRAND NAME (Generic)	DOSAGE FORM/ STRENGTH	INDICATIONS	ADULT DOSE	PEDIATRIC DOSE
AMINOGLYCOSIDES *(Continued)*				
Tobramycin (tobramycin sulfate)	**Inj:** 10mg/mL, 40mg/mL, 1.2g	Treatment of serious lower respiratory tract, CNS (eg, meningitis), intra-abdominal, bone, skin and skin structure, and complicated/recurrent urinary tract infections; and septicemia caused by susceptible strains of microorganisms.	(IM/IV) Serious Infections: 3mg/kg/day given q8h. Life-Threatening Infections: Up to 5mg/kg/day given tid-qid. Reduce to 3mg/kg/day as soon as clinically indicated. Max: 5mg/kg/day unless serum levels monitored. Treat for 7-10 days; may need longer course in difficult and complicated infections. Severe Cystic Fibrosis: Inital: 10mg/kg/day given qid. Measure levels to determine subsequent doses. Renal Impairment: LD: 1mg/kg followed by reduced doses given q8h or normal doses given at prolonged intervals based on either CrCl or serum creatinine. Do not use either method during dialysis. Obese Patients: Calculate dose based on estimated lean body weight plus 40% of the excess as the basic weight on which to figure mg/kg. ADD-Vantage vials are not for IM use. (IV): Infusion period: 20-60 min.	>1 week: (IM/IV) 6-7.5mg/kg/day given tid-qid (eg, 2-2.5mg/kg q8h or 1.5-1.89mg/kg q6h). 1 week: Up to 2mg/kg q12h. Treat for 7-10 days; may need longer course in difficult and complicated infections. Severe Cystic Fibrosis: Initial: 10mg/kg/day given qid. Measure levels to determine subsequent doses. Renal Impairment: LD: 1mg/kg, followed by reduced doses given q8h or normal doses given at prolonged intervals based on either CrCl or serum creatinine. Do not use either method during dialysis. Obese Patients: Calculate dose based on estimated lean body weight plus 40% of the excess as the basic weight on which to figure mg/kg. ADD-Vantage vials are not for IM use. (IV): Infusion period: 20-60 min.
Streptomycin sulfate	**Inj:** 1g/ampule	Treatment of moderate to severe infections such as mycobacterium tuberculosis (TB) and non-TB infections (eg, plague, tularemia, chancroid, granuloma inguinale, *H.influenzae* and *K.pneumoniae* infections, UTI, gram-negative bacillary bacteremia, endocardial infections).	IM only. TB: 15mg/kg/day (Max: 1g), or 25-30mg/kg twice weekly (Max: 1.5g), or 25-30mg/kg three times weekly (Max: 1.5g). Do not exceed a total dose of 120g over the course of theraphy unless no other therapeutic options exist. Elderly (>60 yrs): Reduce dose. Treat for minimum of 1 year if possible. Tularemia: 1-2g/day in divided doses for 7-14 days until afebrile for 5-7 days. Plague: 1g bid for minimum of 10 days. Streptococcal Endocarditis: With PCN, 1g bid for week 1, then 500mg bid for week 2. Elderly (>60 yrs): 500mg bid for 2 weeks. Enterococcal Endocarditis: With PCN, 1g bid for 2 weeks, then 500mg bid for 4 weeks. Renal Impairment: Reduce dose. Moderate/Severe Infections: 1-2g/day in divided doses q6-12h. Max: 2g/day.	IM only. TB: 20-40mg/kg/day (Max: 1g), or 25-30 mg/kg twice weekly (Max: 1.5g), or 25-30mg/kg three times weekly (Max: 1.5g). Do not exceed a total dose of 120g over the course of therapy unless no other therapeutic options exist. Treat for minimum of 1 year if possible. Moderate/Severe Infections: 20-40mg/kg/day (8-20mg/lb/day) in divided doses q6-12h.
TOBI (tobramycin)	**Sol:** 60mg/mL (300mg/ampule)	Management of cystic fibrosis patients with *P.aeruginosa.*	Inhale via nebulizer 300mg q12h for 28 days, then stop for 28 days. Resume therapy for next 28-day on/28-day off cycle.	≥6 yrs: Inhale via nebulizer 300mg q12h for 28 days, then stop for 28 days. Resume therapy for next 28-day on/28-day off cycle.

BRAND NAME (Generic)	DOSAGE FORM/ STRENGTH	INDICATIONS	ADULT DOSE	PEDIATRIC DOSE
CARBAPENEMS				
Invanz (ertapenem sodium)	**Inj:** 1g	Treatment of complicated intra-abdominal infections; skin and skin structure infections (SSSI), including diabetic foot infections without osteomyelitits; community acquired pneumonia (CAP); complicated urinary tract infections (UTI) including pyelonephritis; acute pelvic infections including postpartum endomyometritis, septic abortion, and post surgical gynecologic infections; prophylaxis of surgical site infection following elective colorectal surgery.	Treatment: 1g IM/IV qd. Duration: Intra-Abdominal Infections: 5-14 days. SSSI: 7-14 days. CAP/UTI: 10-14 days. Pelvic Infection: 3-10 days. May administer IV for up to 14 days and IM for up to 7 days. CrCl ≤30mL/min/1.73m^2: 500mg IM/IV qd. Hemodialysis: Give 150mg IM/IV after dialysis only if 500mg dose was given within 6 hrs prior to dialysis. Prophylaxis: 1g IV as single dose given 1 hr prior to surgical incision.	≥13 yrs: 1g IM/IV qd. 3 mo-12 yrs: 15mg/kg IM/IV bid (not to exceed 1g/day). Treatment Duration: Intra-Abdominal Infections: 5-14 days. SSSI: 7-14 days. CAP/UTI: 10-14 days. Pelvic Infections: 3-10 days. May administer IV for up to 14 days and IM for up to 7 days. CrCl ≤30mL/min/1.73 m^2: 500mg IM/IV qd.
Merrem (meropenem)	**Inj:** 500mg, 1g	Treatment of intra-abdominal infections, bacterial meningitis, and complicated skin and skin structure infections (cSSSI) caused by susceptible strains of microorganisms.	Intra-Abdominal: 1g q8h. CrCl 26-50mL/min: 1 g q12h. CrCl 10-25mL/min: 500mg q12h. CrCl <10mL/min: 500mg q24h. cSSSI: 500mg q8h. CrCl 26-50mL/min: 500mg q12h. CrCl 10-25mL/min: 250mg q12h. CrCl <10mL/min: 250mg q24h.	3 months >50kg: Intra-Abdominal: 1g q8h. Meningitis: 2g q8h. cSSSI: 500mg q8h. 50kg: Intra-Abdominal: 20mg/kg q8h. Max: 1g q8h. Meningitis: 40mg/kg q8h. Max: 2g q8h. cSSSI: 10mg/kg q8h. Max: 500mg q8h.
CEPHALOSPORINS, FIRST GENERATION				
Cefazolin (cefazolin)	**Inj:** 500mg, 1g, 10g, 20g	Treatment of respiratory tract, urinary tract (UTI), skin and skin structure, biliary tract, bone and joint, and genital infections, septicemia, and endocarditis caused by susceptible strains of microorganisms. Perioperative prophylaxis for surgical procedures classified as contaminated or potentially contaminated.	Moderate-Severe Infections: 500mg-1g q6-8h. Mild Gram-Positive Cocci Infection: 250-500mg q8h. Acute, Uncomplicated UTI: 1g q12h. Pneumococcal Pneumonia: 500mg q12h. Severe Life-Threatening Infection (eg, Endocarditis, Septicemia): 1-1.5g q6h; Max: 12g/day (rare). Perioperative Prophylaxis: 1g IM/IV 0.5-1 hr before surgery. For Procedures ≥2 hrs: 500mg-1g IM/IV during surgery. Maint: 500mg-1g IM/IV q6-8h for 24 hrs post-op. Continue for 3-5 days post-op for devastating procedures (eg, open-heart surgery and prosthetic arthroplasty). Renal Impairment: CrCl 35-54 mL/min: Full dose q8h. CrCl 11-34 mL/min ½ usual dose q12h. CrCl <10mL/min: ½ usual dose q18-24h. Apply reduced dosage recommendations after initial LD is given.	Mild-Moderately Severe Infection: 25-50mg/kg/day in 3-4 equal doses. Severe Infection: 100mg/kg/day in divided doses. Renal impairment: CrCl 40-70mL/min: 60% of normal daily dose in equally divided doses q12h. CrCl 20-40mL/min: 25% of normal daily dose in equally divided doses q12h. CrCl 5-20mL/min: 10% of normal daily dose q24h. Apply reduced dosage recommendations after initial LD is given.

(Continued)

BRAND NAME (Generic)	DOSAGE FORM/ STRENGTH	INDICATIONS	ADULT DOSE	PEDIATRIC DOSE
CEPHALOSPORINS, FIRST GENERATION *(Continued)*				
Duricef (cefadroxil monohydrate)	**Cap:** 500mg; **Sus:** 250mg/5mL [50mL, 100mL], 500mg/5mL [50mL, 75mL, 100mL]; **Tab:** 1g	Skin and skin structure infections (SSSI) and urinary tract infections (UTI), pharyngitis, and tonsillitis.	Uncomplicated Lower UTI: 1-2g/day given qd or bid. Other UTI: 1gm bid. SSSI: 1g qd or 500mg bid. Group A ß-hemolytic Strep Pharyngitis/Tonsillitis: 1g qd or 500mg bid for 10 days. CrCl ≤50mL/min: Initial: 1g. Maint: CrCl 25-50mL/min: 500mg q12h; CrCl 10-25mL/min: 500mg q24h; CrCl 0-10mL/min: 500mg q36h	UTI/SSSI: 15mg/kg q12h. Pharyngitis/Tonsillitis/Impetigo: 30mg/kg qd or 15mg/kg q12h. Treat ß-hemolytic strep infections for at least 10 days.
Keflex (cephalexin)	**Cap:** 250mg, 333mg 500mg, 750mg; **Sus:** 125mg/5mL, 250mg/5mL [100mL, 200mL]; **Tab:** 250mg, 500mg	Treatment of otitis media and skin and skin structure infections (SSSI); bone, genitourinary tract, and respiratory tract infections.	Usual adult dosage range: 1-4g/day in divided doses. Usual dose: 250mg q6h. Streptococcal Pharyngitis/SSSI/Uncomplicated Cystitis (>15 yrs): 500mg q12h. Treat cystitis for 7-14 days. Max: 4g/day.	Usual: 25-50mg/kg/day in divided doses. Streptococcal Pharyngitis (>1 yr)/SSSI: May divide dose and give q12h. Otitis Media: 75-100mg/kg/day in 4 divided doses. Administer for ≥10 days in, ß-hemolytic streptococcal infections.
Panixine (cephalexin)	**Tab, Dispersible:** 125mg, 250mg	Skin and skin structure (SSSI), bone genitourinary and respiratory tract infections, otitis media, acute prostatitis.	Usual adult dosage range: 1-4g/day in divided doses. Usual dose: 250mg q6h. Streptococcal Pharyngitis/SSSI/Uncomplicated Cystitis (>15 yrs): 500mg q12h. Treat cystitis for 7-14 days. Max: 4g/day.	Usual: 25-50mg/kg/day in divided doses. Streptococcal Pharyngitis (>1 yr)/SSSI: May divide dose and give q12h. Otitis Media: 75-100mg/kg/day in 4 divided doses. Administer for ≥10 days in, ß-hemolytic streptococcal infections.
CEPHALOSPORINS, SECOND GENERATION				
Cefaclor	**Cap:** 250mg, 500mg; **Sus:** 125mg/5mL [75mL, 150mL], 187mg/5mL [50mL, 100mL], 250mg/5mL [75mL, 150mL], 375mg/5mL [50mL, 100mL]	Treatment of otitis media, pharyngitis, tonsillitis, lower respiratory tract, urinary tract, and skin and skin structure infections caused by susceptible strains of microorganisms.	Usual: 250mg q8h. Severe Infections/Pneumonia: 500mg q8h. Treat ß-hemolytic strep for 10 days.	≥1 mo: Usual: 20mg/kg/day given q8h. Otitis Media/Serious Infections: 40mg/kg/day. Max: 1g/day. May administer q12h for otitis media and pharyngitis. Treat ß-hemolytic strep for 10 days.
Cefaclor ER	**Tab, Extended-Release:** 375mg, 500mg	Acute bacterial exacerbation of chronic bronchitis (ABECB), secondary bacterial infections of acute bronchitis, pharyngitis, tonsillitis, and uncomplicated skin and skin structure infections (SSSI) caused by susceptible strains of microorganisms.	ABECB/Acute Bronchitis: 500mg q12h for 7 days. Pharyngitis/Tonsillitis: 375mg q12h for 10 days. SSSI: 375mg q12h for 7-10 days. Take with meals. Do not crush, cut or chew tab.	≥16 yrs: ABECB/Acute Bronchitis: 500mg q12h for 7 days. Pharyngitis/Tonsillitis: 375mg q12h for 10 days. SSSI: 375mg q12h for 7-10 days. Take with meals. Do not crush, cut or chew tab.

BRAND NAME (Generic)	DOSAGE FORM/ STRENGTH	INDICATIONS	ADULT DOSE	PEDIATRIC DOSE
Cefoxitin (cefoxitin sodium)	**Inj:** 1g, 1g/50mL, 2g, 2g/50mL, 10g	Treatment of lower respiratory tract, urinary tract, intra-abdominal, gynecological, skin and skin structure, and bone and joint infections, and septicemia. For surgical prophylaxis.	Usual: 1-2g IV q6-8h. Uncomplicated Infections: 1g IV q6-8h. Moderate-Severe: 1g IV q4h or 2g IV q6-8h. Gas Gangrene/Other Infections Requiring Higher Dose: 2g IV q4h or 3g IV q6h. Renal Insufficiency: LD: 1-2g IV. Maint: CrCl 30-50mL/min: 1-2g IV q8-12h. CrCl 10-29mL/min: 1-2g IV q12-24h. CrCl 5-9mL/min: 0.5-1g IV q12-24h. CrCl <5mL/min: 0.5-1g IV q24-48h. Hemodialysis: LD: 1-2g IV after dialysis. Maint: See renal insufficiency doses above. Prophylaxis: Uncontaminated GI Surgery/Hysterectomy: 2g IV 0.5-1 hr prior to surgery, then 2g IV q6h after first dose up to 24 hrs. C-Section: 2g IV single dose after umbilical cord is clamped, or 2g IV after umbilical cord is clamped followed by 2g IV 4 and 8 hrs after initial dose.	≥3 mo: 80-160mg/kg/day divided into 4-6 equal doses. Max: 12g/day. Prophylaxis: Uncontaminated GI Surgery/Hysterectomy: 30-40mg/kg IV 0.5-1 hr prior to surgery, then 30-40mg/kg IV q6h after first dose up to 24 hrs.
Ceftin (cefuroxime axetil)	**Sus:** 125mg/5mL [100mL], 250mg/5mL [50mL, 100mL]; **Tab:** 125mg, 250mg, 500mg	(Sus/Tab) Pharyngitis/tonsillitis, acute otitis media (Sus) Impetigo. (Tab) Uncomplicated skin and skin structure (SSSI), and urinary tract infection (UTI), gonorrhea, early lyme disease, acute bacterial maxillary sinusitis, acute bacterial exacerbations of chronic bronchitis (ABECB) and secondary bacterial infections of acute bronchitis.	(Tab) Pharyngitis/Tonsillitis/Sinusitis: 250mg bid for 10 days. ABECB/SSSI: 250-500mg bid for 10 days. Acute Bronchitis: 250-500mg bid for 5-10 days. UTI: 250mg bid for 7-10 days. Gonorrhea: 1000mg single dose. Lyme Disease: 500mg bid for 20 days.	≥13 yrs: (Tab) Pharyngitis/Tonsillitis/Sinusitis: 250mg bid for 10 days. ABECB/SSSI: 250-500mg bid for 10 days. Acute Bronchitis: 250-500mg bid for 5-10 days. UTI: 125-250mg bid for 7-10 days Gonorrhea: 1000mg single dose. Lyme Disease: 500mg bid for 20 days. 3 mo-12 yrs: (Sus) Pharyngitis/Tonsillitis: 10mg/kg bid for 10 days. Max: 500mg/day. Otitis Media/Sinusitis/Impetigo: 15mg/kg bid for 10 days. Max: 1000mg/day. (Tab-if can swallow whole) Otitis Media/Sinusitis: 250mg bid for 10 days.
Cefzil (cefprozil)	**Sus:** 125mg/5mL, 250mg/5mL [50mL, 75mL, 100mL]; **Tab:** 250mg, 500mg	Mild to moderate pharyngitis/tonsillitis, otitis media, acute sinusitis, secondary bacterial infection of acute bronchitis, acute bacterial exacerbation of chronic bronchitis (ABECB), and uncomplicated skin and skin structure infections (SSSI).	≥13 yrs: Pharyngitis/Tonsillitis: 500mg q24h for 10 days. Acute Sinusitis: 250-500mg q12h for 10 days. ABECB/Acute Bronchitis: 500mg q12h for 10 days. SSSI: 250-500mg q12h or 500mg q24h. CrCl <30mL/min: 50% of standard dose.	2-12 yrs: Pharyngitis/Tonsillitis: 7.5mg/kg q12h for 10 days. SSSI: 20mg/kg q24h for 10 days. 6 mos-12 yrs: Otitis Media: 15mg/kg q12h for 10 days. Acute Sinusitis: 7.5-15mg/kg q12h for 10 days. Do not exceed adult dose. CrCl <30mL/min: 50% of standard dose.

(Continued)

BRAND NAME (Generic)	DOSAGE FORM/ STRENGTH	INDICATIONS	ADULT DOSE	PEDIATRIC DOSE
CEPHALOSPORINS, SECOND GENERATION *(Continued)*				
Mefoxin (cefoxitin sodium)	**Inj:** 1g, 1g/50mL, 2g, 2g/50mL, 10g	Treatment of lower respiratory tract, urinary tract, intra-abdominal, gynecological, skin and skin structure, and bone and joint infections, and septicemia. For surgical prophylaxis.	Usual: 1-2g IV q6-8h. Uncomplicated Infections: 1g IV q6-8h. Moderate-Severe: 1g IV q4h or 2g IV q6-8h. Gas Gangrene/Other Infections Requiring Higher Dose: 2g IV q4h or 3g IV q6h. Renal Insufficiency: LD: 1-2g IV. Maint: CrCl 30-50mL/min: 1-2g IV q8-12h. CrCl 10-29mL/min: 1-2g IV q12-24h. CrCl 5-9mL/min: 0.5-1g IV q12-24h. CrCl <5mL/min: 0.5-1g IV q24-48h. Hemodialysis: LD: 1-2g IV after dialysis. Maint: See renal insufficiency doses above. Prophylaxis: Uncontaminated GI Surgery/Hysterectomy: 2g IV 0.5-1 hr prior to surgery, then 2g IV q6h after first dose up to 24 hrs. C-Section: 2g IV single dose after umbilical cord is clamped, or 2g IV after umbilical cord is clamped followed by 2g IV 4 and 8 hrs after initial dose.	≥3 mos: 80-160mg/kg/day divided into 4-6 equal doses. Max: 12g/day. Prophylaxis: Uncontaminated GI Surgery/Hysterectomy: 30-40mg/kg IV 0.5-1 hr prior to surgery, then 30- 40mg/kg IV q6h after first dose up to 24 hrs.
Zinacef (cefuroxime)	**Inj:** 750mg, 1.5g, 7.5g, 750mg/50mL, 1.5g/50mL	Treatment of septicemia; meningitis; gonorrhea; lower respiratory tract, urinary tract, skin and skin structure (SSSI), and bone and joint infections caused by susceptible strains of microorganisms. For preoperative and perioperative surgical prophylaxis.	Usual: 750mg-1.5g q8h for 5-10 days. Uncomplicated Pneumonia and UTI/SSSI/Disseminated Gonococcal Infections: 750mg q8h. Severe/Complicated Infections: 1.5g q8h. Bone and Joint Infections: 1.5g q8h. Life-Threatening Infections/Infections With Susceptible Organisms: 1.5g q6h. Meningitis: Max: 3g q8h. Uncomplicated Gonococcal Infection: 1.5g IM single dose at 2 different sites with 1g PO probenecid. Surgical Prophylaxis: 1.5g IV 0.5-1 hr before incision, then 750mg IM/IV q8h with prolonged procedure. Open Heart Surgery (Perioperative): 1.5g IV at induction of anesthesia and q12h thereafter, for total of 6g. Renal impairment: CrCl 10-20mL/min: 750mg q12h. CrCl <10mL/min: 750mg q24h. Hemodialysis: Give further dose at end of dialysis.	>3 months: Usual: 50-100 mg/kg/day in divided doses q6-8h. Severe infections: 100mg/kg/day (not to exceed max adult dose). Bone and Joint Infections: 150mg/kg/day in divided doses q8h (not to exceed max adult dose). Meningitis: 200-240mg/kg/day IV in divided doses q6-8h. Renal Dysfunction: Modify dosing frequency consistent with adult recommendations.

BRAND NAME (Generic)	DOSAGE FORM/ STRENGTH	INDICATIONS	ADULT DOSE	PEDIATRIC DOSE
CEPHALOSPORINS, THIRD GENERATION				
Cedax (ceftibuten)	**Cap:** 400mg; **Sus:** 90mg/5mL [30mL, 60mL, 90mL, 120mL]	Acute bacterial exacerbations of chronic bronchitis (ABECB), acute bacterial otitis media, pharyngitis and tonsillitis.	ABECB/Otitis Media/Pharyngitis/Tonsillitis: 400mg qd for 10 days. Max: 400mg/day. CrCl 30-49mL/min: 4.5mg/kg or 200mg qd. CrCl 5-29mL/min: 2.25mg/kg or 100mg qd. Take 2 hrs before or at least 1 hr after a meal.	≥6 mo: Pharyngitis/Tonsillitis/Otitis Media: 9mg/kg qd for 10 days. Max: 400mg. ABECB/Otitis Media/Pharyngitis/Tonsillitis: ≥12 yrs: 400mg qd for 10 days Max: 400mg/day. CrCl 30-49mL/min: 4.5mg/kg or 200mg qd. CrCl 5-29mL/min: 2.25mg/kg or 100mg qd. Take 2 hrs before or at least 1 hr after a meal.
Fortaz (ceftazidime)	**Inj:** 500mg, 1g, 1g/50mL, 2g, 2g/50mL, 6g	Treatment of lower respiratory tract (eg, pneumonia), skin and skin structure (SSSI), bone and joint, gynecologic, CNS (eg, meningitis), intra-abdominal, and urinary tract infections (UTI), and septicemia. For use in sepsis.	Usual: 1g IM/IV q8-12h. Uncomplicated UTI: 250 mg IM/IV q12h. Complicated UTI: 500mg IM/IV q8-12h. Bone and Joint Infection: 2g IV q 12h. Uncomplicated Pneumonia/SSSI: 500mg-1g IM/IV q8h. Gynecological/Intra-Abdominal/Meningitis/Severe Life-Threatening Infection: 2g IV q8h. Lung Infection caused by Pseudomonas spp. in Cystic Fibrosis (normal renal function): 30-50mg/kg IV q8h. Max: 6g/day. CrCl 31-50mL/min; 1g q12h. CrCl 16-30mL/min: 1g q24h. CrCl 6-15mL/min: 500mg q24h. CrCl <5mL/min: 500mg q48h. For severe infections (6g/day), increase renal impairment dose by 50% or increase dosing interval. Apply reduced dosage recommendations after initial 1g LD is given. Hemodialysis: Give 1g before then 1g after each hemodialysis. Intra-Peritoneal Dialysis/Continuous Peritoneal Dialysis: Ambulatory Peritoneal Dialysis: Give 1g followed by 500mg q24h or add to fluid at 250mg/2mL.	≥12 yrs: Usual: 1g IM/IV q8-12h. Uncomplicated UTI: 250mg IM/IV q12h. Complicated UTI: 500mg IM/IV q8-12h. Bone and Joint Infection: 2g IV q12h. Uncomplicated Pneumonia/SSSI: 500mg-1g IM/IV q8h. Gynecological/Intra-Abdominal/Meningitis/Severe Life-Threatening Infection: 2g IV q8h. Lung Infection caused by Pseudomonas spp. in Cystic Fibrosis (normal renal function): 30-50mg/kg IV q8h Max: 6g/day. CrCl 31-50mL/min: 1g q12h. CrCl 16-30mL/min: 1g q24h. CrCl 6-15mL/min: 500mg q24h. CrCl <5mL/min: 500mg q48h. For severe infections (6g/day), increase renal impairment dose by 50% or increase dosing interval. Apply reduced dosage recommendations after initial 1g LD is given. Hemodialysis: Give 1g before then 1g after each hemodialysis. Intra-Peritoneal Dialysis/Continuous Ambulatory Peritoneal Dialysis: Give 1g followed by 500mg q24h or add to fluid at 250mg/2mL. 1 month-12 yrs: 30-50mg/kg IV, q8h. Max: 6mg/day. Neonates: (0-4 weeks): 30mg/kg IV, q12h. Higher doses for cystic fibrosis, meningitis, or immunocompromised patients.

(Continued)

BRAND NAME (Generic)	DOSAGE FORM/ STRENGTH	INDICATIONS	ADULT DOSE	PEDIATRIC DOSE
CEPHALOSPORINS, THIRD GENERATION *(Continued)*				
Claforan (cefotaxime sodium)	**Inj:** 500mg, 1g, 2g, 10g	Treatment of lower respiratory tract, genitourinary, gynecologic, intra-abdominal, skin and skin structure, bone and joint, and CNS infections (eg, meningitis), bacteremia, and septicemia. For surgical prophylaxis.	Gonococcal Urethritis/Cervicitis (Males/Females): 500mg single dose IM. Rectal Gonorrhea: 0.5g (females) or 1g (males) single dose IM. Uncomplicated Infections: 1g IM/IV q12h. Moderate-Severe Infections: 1-2g IM/IV q8h. Septicemia: 2g IV q6-8h. Life-Threatening Infections: 2g IV q4h. Max: 12g/day. Surgical Prophylaxis: 1g IM/IV 30-90 min before surgery. Cesarean Section: 1g IV when umbilical cord is clamped, then 1g IV/IM at 6 and 12 hrs after 1st dose. CrCl <20mL/min/1.73 m^2: Give ½ of usual dose.	≥50kg: Use adult dose. Max: 12g/day. 1mo-12 yrs and ≤50kg: 50-180mg/kg/day IM/IV divided in 4-6 doses. 1-4 weeks: 50mg/kg IV q8h. 0-1 week: 50mg/kg IV q12h. CrCl <20mL/min/1.73 m^2: Give ½ of usual dose.
Omnicef (cefdinir)	**Cap:** 300mg; **Sus:** 125mg/5mL, 250mg/5mL [60mL, 100mL]	Community acquired pneumonia (CAP), acute exacerbations of chronic bronchitis (AECB), acute maxillary sinusitis, pharyngitis/tonsillitis, uncomplicated skin and structure infections (SSSI), and acute bacterial otitis media.	(Cap) SSSI/Cap: 300mg q12h for 10 days. AECB/Pharyngitis/Tonsillitis: 300mg q12h for 5-10 days or 600mg q24h for 10 days. Sinusitis: 300mg q12h or 600mg q24h for 10 days. CrCl <30mL/min: 300mg qd. Hemodialysis: Initial: 300mg or 7mg/kg after dialysis, then 300mg or 7mg/kg every other day.	(Sus) 6 mo-12 yrs: OtitisMedia/Pharyngitis/Tonsillitis: 7mg/kg q12h for 5-10 days or 14mg/kg q24h for 10 days. Sinusitis: 7mg/kg q12h or 14mg/kg q24h for 10 days. SSSI: 7mg/kg q12h for 10 days. (Cap) ≥13 yrs: CAP/SSSI: 300mg q12h for 10 days. AECB/ Pharyngitis/Tonsillitis: 300mg q12h for 5-10 days or 600mg q24h for 10 days. Sinusitis: 300mg q12h or 600mg q24h for 10 days. CrCl <30mL/min/1.73m^2: 7mg/kg qd. Max: 300mg qd.
Rocephin (ceftriaxone sodium)	**Inj:** 250mg, 500mg, 1g	Treatment of lower respiratory tract infections, skin and skin structure infections, bone and joint infections, intra-abdominal infections, acute otitis media, uncomplicated gonorrhea, pelvic inflammatory disease, UTI, septicemia, and meningitis. For surgical prophylaxis.	Usual: 1-2g/day IV/IM given qd-bid. Max: 4g/day. Gonorrhea: 250mg IM single dose. Surgical Prophylaxis: 1g IV ½-2 hrs before surgery.	Skin Infections: 50-75mg/kg/day IV/IM given qd-bid. Max: 2g/day. Otitis Media: 50mg/kg (up to 1g) IM single dose. Serious Infections: 50-75mg/kg/day IM/IV given q12h. Max: 2g/day. Meningitis: Initial: 100mg/kg (up to 4g), then 100mg/kg/day given qd-bid for 7-14 days. Max: 4g/day.
Spectracef (cefditoren pivoxil)	**Tab:** 200mg, 400mg	Treatment of acute bacterial exacerbations of chronic bronchitis (ABECB), pharyngitis/tonsillitis, community acquired pneumonia (CAP), and uncomplicated skin and skin-structure infections (SSSI).	ABECB: 400mg bid for 10 days. Pharyngitis/ Tonsillitis/SSSI: 200mg bid for 10 days. Cap: 400mg bid for 14 days. CrCl 30-49mL/min: 200mg bid. CrCl<30mL/min: 200mg qd. Take with meals.	≥12 yrs: ABECB: 400mg bid for 10 days. Pharyngitis/ Tonsillitis/SSSI: 200mg bid for 10 days. Cap: 400mg bid for 14 days. CrCl 30-49mL/min: 200mg bid. CrCl<30mL/min: 200mg qd. Take with meals.

BRAND NAME (Generic)	DOSAGE FORM/ STRENGTH	INDICATIONS	ADULT DOSE	PEDIATRIC DOSE
Suprax (cefixime)	**Sus:** 100mg/5mL [50mL, 75mL, 100mL], 200mg/5mL; **Tab:** 400mg	(Sus/Tab)Pharyngitis, tonsillitis, acute bronchitis, acute exacerbation of chronic bronchitis, uncomplicated UTIs, and cervical/urethral gonorrhea caused by susceptible strains. (Sus) Otitis media.	Usual: 400mg qd. Gonorrhea: 400mg single dose. CrCl 21-60mL/min/Hemodialysis: Give 75% of standard dose. CrCl <20mL/min/CAPD: Give 50% of standard dose.	>12 yrs or >50kg: (Tab/Sus) Usual: 400mg qd. ≥6 mos: (Sus) 8mg/kg qd or 4mg/kg bid. Treat for at least 10 days with *S. pyogenes*. CrCl 21-60mL/min/ Hemodialysis: Give 75% of standard dose. CrCl <20mL/min/CAPD: Give 50% of standard dose.
Tazicef (ceftazidime)	**Inj:** 500mg, 1g, 2g, 6g	Treatment of lower respiratory tract (eg, pneumonia), skin and skin structure (SSSI), bone and joint, gynecologic, CNS (eg, meningitis), intra-abdominal, and urinary tract infections (UTI), and septicemia. For use in sepsis.	Usual: 1g IV q8-12h. Uncomplicated UTI: 250mg IM/IV q12h. Complicated UTI: 500mg IV q8-12h. Bone and Joint Infection: 2g IV q12h. Uncomplicated Pneumonia/SSSI: 500mg-1g IV q8h. Gynecological/Intra-Abdominal/Meningitis/Severe Life-Threatening Infection: 2g IV q8h. Lung Infection caused by Pseudomonas in Cystic Fibrosis (normal renal function): 30-50mg/kg IV q8h. Max: 6g/day. Renal Impairment: CrCl 31-50mL/min: 1g q12h CrCl 16-30mL/min: 1g q24h. CrCl 6-15mL/min: 500mg q24h. CrCl <5mL/min: 500mg q48h. For severe infections (6g/day), increase renal impairment dose by 50% or increase dosing interval. Apply reduced dosage recommendations after initial 1g LD is given. Hemodialysis: Give 1g before and 1g after each hemodialysis. Intra-Peritoneal Dialysis/Continuous Ambulatory Peritoneal Dialysis: Give 1g followed by 500mg q24h, or add to fluid at 250mg/2L.	Neonates (0-4 weeks): 30mg/kg IV q12h. 1 mo-12 yrs: 30-50mg/kg IV q8h. Max: 6g/day. Higher doses for patients with cystic fibrosis or when treating meningitis. Renal Impairment: Reduce dosing frequency.
Vantin (cefpodoxime proxetil)	**Sus:** 50mg/mL [50mL, 100mL], 100mg/5mL [50mL, 75mL, 100mL]; **Tab:** 100mg, 200mg	Acute otitis media, pharyngitis/tonsillitis, community acquired pneumonia (CAP), acute bacterial exacerbation of chronic bronchitis (ABECB), acute uncomplicated urethral and cervical gonorrhea, acute uncomplicated ano-rectal infections in women, uncomplicated skin and skin structure infections (SSSI), acute maxillary sinusitis, uncomplicated urinary tract infections (UTI).	Take tabs with food. Pharyngitis/Tonsillitis: 100mg q12h for 5-10 days. Cap: 200mg q12h for 14 days. ABECB: 200mg q12h for 10 days. Uncomplicated Gonorrhea (Men and Women)/Rectal Gonococcal Infections (women): 200mg single dose. SSSI: 400mg q12h for 7-14 days. Sinusitis: 200mg q12h for 10 days. UTI: 100mg q12h for 7 days. CrCl<30mL/min: Increase interval to q24h. Hemodialysis: Dose 3 times weekly after dialysis.	≥12 yrs: Take tabs with food. Pharyngitis/Tonsillitis: 100mg q12h for 5-10 days. Cap: 200mg q12h for 14 days. ABECB: 200mg q12h for 10 days. Uncomplicated Gonorrhea (men and women)/Rectal Gonococcal Infections (women): 200mg single dose. SSSI: 400mg q12h for 7-14 days. Sinusitis: 200mg q12h for 10 days. UTI: 100mg q12h for 7 days. 2 mos-11 yrs: Otitis Media: 5mg/kg q12h for 5 days. Max: 200mg/dose. Pharyngitis/Tonsillitis: 5mg/kg q12h for 5-10 days. Max: 100mg/dose. Sinusitis: 5mg/kg q12h for 10 days. Max:200mg/dose. CrCl<30mL/min: Increase interval to q24h. Hemodialysis: Dose 3 times weekly after dialysis.

(Continued)

BRAND NAME (Generic)	DOSAGE FORM/ STRENGTH	INDICATIONS	ADULT DOSE	PEDIATRIC DOSE
CEPHALOSPORIN, FOURTH GENERATION				
Maxipime (cefepime HCl)	**Inj:** 500mg, 1g, 2g	Treatment of uncomplicated/complicated urinary tract (UTI), uncomplicated skin and skin structure (SSSI), and complicated intra-abdominal infections, and pneumonia. Emperic therapy for febrile neutropenia.	Moderate-Severe Pneumonia: 1-2g IV q12h for 10 days. Febrile Neutropenia Emperic Therapy: 2g IV q8h for 7 days or until neutropenia resolved. Mild-Moderate UTI: 0.5-1g IM/IV q12h for 7-10 days. Severe UTI/Moderate-Severe SSSI: 2g IV q12h for 10 days. Complicated Intra-Abdominal Infections: 2g IV q12h for 7-10 days. CrCl<60mL/min: Initial: Same dose as normal renal function. Maint: Refer to prescribing information for dose-adjustment. Hemodialysis patients: 1g on Day 1, then 500mg q24h, except for neutropenia: 1g q24h. Ambulatory peritoneal dialysis: Normal recommended dose at dosing interval of q48h.	2 months-16 yrs: ≤40kg: UTI/SSSI/Pneumonia: 50mg/kg IV q12h. Febrile Neutropenia: 50mg/kg IV q8h. Max: Do not exceed adult dose. CrCl ≤60mL/min: Initial: Same dose as normal renal function. Maint: Refer to prescribing information for dose adjustment.
FLUOROQUINOLONES				
Avelox (moxifloxacin HCl)	**Inj:** 400mg/250mL; **Tab:** 400mg [ABC pack, 5 tabs]	Acute bacterial sinusitis, acute bacterial exacerbation of chronic bronchitis (ABECB), uncomplicated skin and skin structure infections (SSSI), complicated skin and skin structure infections (cSSSI), complicated intra-abdominal infections (cIAI), and community acquired pneumonia (CAP), including multi-drug resistant *S.pneumoniae.*	≥18 yrs: Sinusitis: 400mg PO/IV q24h for 10 days. ABECB: 400mg PO/IV q24h for 5 days. SSSI: 400mg PO/IV q24h for 7 days. cSSSI: 400mg PO/IV q24h for 7-21 days. cIAI: 400mg PO/IV q24h for 5-14 days. CAP: 400mg PO/IV q24h for 7-14 days.	

BRAND NAME (Generic)	DOSAGE FORM/ STRENGTH	INDICATIONS	ADULT DOSE	PEDIATRIC DOSE
Cipro (ciprofloxacin HCl)	**Sus:** 250mg/5mL, 500mg/5mL [100mL]; **Tab:** 100mg, 250mg, 500mg, 750mg	Adults: Treatment of lower respiratory tract (LRTI), complicated intra-abdominal, skin and skin structure (SSSI), bone and joint, and urinary tract infections (UTI), acute exacerbations of chronic bronchitis, acute sinusitis, acute uncomplicated cystitis in females, chronic bacterial prostatitis, infectious diarrhea, typhoid fever, uncomplicated cervical and urethral gonorrhea. Adults/Pediatrics: Post-exposure inhalation anthrax. Pediatrics: Complicated urinary tract infections and pyelonephritis.	≥18 yrs: Acute Sinusitis/Typhoid Fever: 500mg q12h for 10 days. LRTI/SSSI: Mild-Moderate: 500mg q12h for 7-14 days. Severe/Complicated: 750mg q12h for 7-14 days. Cystitis/Acute Uncompilcated UTI: 250mg q12h for 3 days. Mild-Moderate UTI: 250mg q12h for 7-14 days. Severe/Complicated UTI: 500mg q12h for 7-14 days. Chronic Bacterial Prostatitis: 500mg q12h for 28 days. Intra-Abdominal: 500mg q12h (w/ metronidazole) for 7-14 days. Bone and Joint: Mild-Moderate: 500mg q12h for ≥4-6 weeks. Severe/Complicated: 750mg q12h for ≥4-6 weeks. Infectious Diarrhea: 500mg q12h for 5-7 days. Uncomplicated Urethral/Cervical Gonococcal: 250mg single dose. Inhalational Anthrax: 500mg q12h for 60 days. CrCl 30-50mL/min: 250-500mg q12h. CrCl 5-29mL/min: 250-500mg q18h. Hemodialysis/Peritoneal Dialysis: 250-500mg q24h (after dialysis). Administer at least 2 hrs before or 6 hrs after magnesium or aluminum containing antacids, sucralfate, Videx (didanosine) chewable/buffered tablets or pediatric powder, or other products containing calcium, iron or zinc.	<18 yrs: Inhalational Anthrax: 15mg/kg q12h for 60 days. Max: 500mg/dose. 1-17 yrs: Complicated UTI/Pyelonephritis: 10-20mg/kg q12h for 10-21 days. Max: 750mg/dose.

(Continued)

BRAND NAME (Generic)	DOSAGE FORM/ STRENGTH	INDICATIONS	ADULT DOSE	PEDIATRIC DOSE
FLUOROQUINOLONES *(Continued)*				
Cipro IV (ciprofloxacin)	**Inj:** 10mg/mL, 200mg/100mL, 400mg/200mL	Adults: Treatment of skin and skin structure (SSSI), bone and joint, complicated intra-abdominal infections, lower respiratory (LRTI), and urinary tract infections(UTI), nosocomial pneumonia, acute sinusitis, chronic bacterial prostatitis, empirical therapy for febrile neutropenia. Adults/Pediatrics: Post-exposure inhalation anthrax. Pediatrics: Complicated urinary tract infections and pyelonephritis.	≥18 yrs: IV: UTI: Mild-Moderate: 200mg q12h for 7-14 days. Complicated/Severe: 400mg q12h for 7-14 days. LRTI/SSSI: Mild-Moderate: 400mg q12h for 7-14 days. Complicated/Severe: 400mg q8h for 7-14 days. Bone and Joint: Mild-Moderate: 400mg q12h for ≥4-6 weeks. Complicated/Severe: 400mg q8h for ≥4-6 weeks. Nosocomial Pneumonia: 400mg q8h for 10-14 days. Complicated Intra-Abdominal: 400mg q12h (w/metronidazole) for 7-14 days. Acute Sinusitis: 400mg q12h for 10 days. Chronic Bacterial Prostatitis: 400mg q12h for 28 days. Febrile Neutropenia: 400mg q8h (w/piperacillin 50mg/kg q4h) for 7-14 days. Max piperacillin: 24g/day. Inhalational Anthrax: 400mg q12h for 60 days. Administer over 60 min. CrCl 5-29mL/min: 200-400mg q18-24h.	<18 yrs: Inhalational Anthrax: 10mg/kg q12h for 60 days. Max: 400mg/dose; 800mg/day. 1-17 yrs: Complicated UTI/Pyleonephritis: 6-10mg/kg q8h for 10-21 days. Max: 400mg/dose.
Cipro XR (ciprofloxacin)	**Tab, Extended-Release:** 500mg, 1000mg	Uncomplicated (acute cystitis) and complicated urinary tract infections (UTI), and acute uncomplicated pyelonephritis due to *E.coli.*	≥18 yrs: Uncomplicated UTI: 500mg qd for 3 days. Complicated UTI: 1000mg qd for 7-14 days. CrCl <30mL/min: 500 mg qd. Acute Uncomplicated Pyelonephritis: 1000mg qd for 7-14 days. CrCl <30mL/min: 500mg qd. Take with fluids. Administer at least 2 hrs before or 6 hrs after magnesium or aluminum containing antacids, sucralfate, Videx (didanosine) chewable/buffered tablets or pediatric powder, metal cations (eg, iron), multivitamins with zinc. Avoid concomitant administration with dairy products alone, or with calcium-fortified products. Space concomitant calcium intake (>800mg) by at least 2 hrs. Do not split, crush, or chew. Swallow tab whole. Dialysis: Give after procedure is completed.	
Factive (gemifloxacin mesylate)	**Tab:** 320mg	Treatment of community-acquired pneumonia (CAP), including multi-drug resistant *Streptococcus pneumoniae* (MDRSP), and acute bacterial exacerbation of chronic bronchitis (ABECB).	≥18 yrs: ABECB: 320mg qd for 5 days. CAP: 320mg qd for 5 days *S.pneumoniae, H.influenzae, M. pneumoniae*, or *C.pneumoniae* or 7 days (MDRSP, *K.pneumoniae*, or *M.catarrhalis*). Renal Impairment: CrCl ≤40mL/min or Dialysis: 160mg qd. Take with fluids.	

BRAND NAME (Generic)	DOSAGE FORM/ STRENGTH	INDICATIONS	ADULT DOSE	PEDIATRIC DOSE
Floxin (ofloxacin)	**Tab:** 200mg, 300mg, 400mg	Treatment of complicated urinary tract (UTI) and uncomplicated skin and skin structure infection (SSSI), acute bacterial exacerbation of chronic bronchitis (ABECB), community acquired pneumonia (CAP), acute uncomplicated urethral and cervical gonorrhea, nongonococcal urethritis and cervicitis, mixed infections of the urethra and cervix, acute pelvic inflammatory disease (PID), uncomplicated cystitis, prostatitis.	≥18 yrs: ABECB/CAP/SSSI: 400mg q12h for 10 days. Cervicitis/Urethritis: 300mg q12h for 7 days. Gonorrhea: 400mg single dose. PID: 400mg q12h for 10-14 days. Uncomplicated Cystitis: 200mg q12h for 3 days (*E.coli* or *K.pneumoniae*) or 7 days (other pathogens). Complicated UTI: 200mg q12h for 10 days. Prostatitis: (*E.coli*) 300mg q12h for 6 weeks. CrCl 20-50mL/min: Dose q24h. CrCl <20mL/min: After regular initial dose, give 50% of normal dose q24h. Severe Hepatic Impairment: Max: 400mg/day.	
Levaquin (levofloxacin)	**Inj:** 5mg/mL, 25mg/mL; Sol: 25mg/mL; **Tab:** 250mg, 500mg, 750mg [Leva-pak, 5[s]]	Uncomplicated and complicated skin and skin structure (SSSI), and urinary tract infections (UTI), acute bacterial sinusitis, acute bacterial exacerbation of chronic bronchitis (ABECB), community acquired pneumonia (CAP), including multi-drug resistant *Streptococcus pneumoniae*, nosocomial pneumonia, chronic bacterial prostatitis (CBP), and acute pyelonephritis caused by susceptible strains of microorganisms. Prevention of inhalational anthrax following exposure to *Bacillus anthracis*.	≥18 yrs: IV/PO: ABECB: 500mg qd for 7 days. CAP: 500mg qd for 7-14 days or 750mg qd for 5 days. Sinusitis: 500mg qd for 10-14 days or 750mg qd for 5 days. CBP: 500mg qd for 28 days. Uncomplicated SSSI: 500mg qd for 7-10 days. Complicated SSSI/Nosocomial Pneumonia: 750mg qd for 7-14 days. Complicated UTI or acute pyelonephritis: 750mg qd for 5 days or 250mg qd for 10 days. Uncomplicated UTI: 250mg qd for 3 days. Inhalational Anthrax: 500mg qd for 60 days. Complicated SSSI/Nosocomial Pneumonia/CAP/Sinusitis/Complicated UTI: CrCl 20-49mL/min: 750mg, then 750mg q48h. CrCl 10-19mL/min/Hemodialysis/CAPD: 750mg, then 500mg q48h. ABECB/CAP/Sinusitis/Uncomplicated SSSI/CBP/Inhalational Anthrax: CrCl 20-49mL/min: 500mg, then 250mg q24h. CrCl 10-19mL/min/ Hemodialysis/CAPD: 500mg, then 250mg q48h. Take oral solution 1 hr before or 2 hrs after eating.	Inhalational Anthrax: 750kg and ≥6 months, 500mg q24h for 60 days. <50kg and ≥6 months: 8mg/kg q12h for 60 days. Max: 250mg/dose.

(Continued)

BRAND NAME (Generic)	DOSAGE FORM/ STRENGTH	INDICATIONS	ADULT DOSE	PEDIATRIC DOSE
FLUOROQUINOLONES *(Continued)*				
Proquin XR (ciprofloxacin HCl)	**Tab, Extended-Release:** 500mg	Treatment of uncomplicated urinary tract infections (acute cystitis) caused by *E.coli* and *K.pneumoniae.*	500mg qd with pm meal for 3 days. Administer at least 4 hrs before or 2 hrs after magnesium or aluminum containing antacids, sucralfate, Videx (didanosine) chewable/buffered tablets of pediatric powder, metal cations (eg, iron), multivitamins with zinc. Do not split, crush, or chew. Swallow tab whole.	
MACROLIDES				
Biaxin (clarithromycin)	**Sus:** 125mg/5mL, 250mg/5mL [50mL, 100mL]; **Tab:** 250mg, 500mg	Adults: Pharyngitis/tonsillitis, acute maxillary sinusitis, acute bacterial exacerbation of chronic bronchitis (ABECB), community acquired pneumonia (CAP), uncomplicated skin and skin structure infections (SSSI), disseminated mycobacterial infections, combination therapy for *H.pylori* infection with duodenal ulcers. MAC prophylaxis in advanced HIV. Pediatrics: Pharyngitis/tonsillitis, CAP, acute maxillary sinusitis, acute otitis media, uncomplicated SSSI, disseminated mycobacterial infections. MAC prophylaxis in advanced HIV.	Pharyngitis/Tonsillitis: 250mg q12h for 10 days. Sinusitis: 500mg q12h for 14 days. ABECB: 250-500mg q12h for 7-14 days. SSSI/CAP: 250mg q12h for 7-14 days. MAC Prophylaxis/Treatment: 500mg bid. *H.pylori*: Triple Therapy: 500mg + amoxicillin 1g + omeprazole 20mg, all q12h for 10 days; or 500mg + amoxicillin 1g + lansoprazole 30mg, all q12h for 10-14 days. Give additional omeprazole 20mg qd for 18 days with active ulcer. Dual Therapy: 500mg q8h + omeprazole 40mg qd for 14 days (give additional omeprazole 20mg qd for 14 days with active ulcer); or 500mg q8h or q12h + ranitidine bismuth citrate 400mg q12h for 14 days (give additional ranitidine bismuth citrate 400mg bid for 14 days with active ulcer). Avoid Biaxin and ranitidine bismuth citrate combination with CrCl<25mL/min. CrCl <30mL/min: Give 50% dose or double interval.	≥6 mo: Usual: 7.5mg/kg q12h for 10 days. MAC Prophylaxis/Treatment: ≥20 mo: 7.5mg/kg bid, up to 500mg bid. CrCl <30mL/min: Give 50% dose or double interval.
Biaxin XL (clarithromycin)	**Tab, Extended-Release:** 500mg [PAC 14 tabs]	Treatment of acute maxillary sinusitis, community acquired pneumonia (CAP), and acute bacterial exacerbation of chronic bronchitis (ABECB).	Sinusitis: 1000mg qd for 14 days. ABECB/Cap: 1000mg qd for 7 days. CrCl <30mL/min: Give 50% dose or double interval. Take with food.	

BRAND NAME (Generic)	DOSAGE FORM/ STRENGTH	INDICATIONS	ADULT DOSE	PEDIATRIC , DOSE
E.E.S. (erythromycin ethylsuccinate)	**Sus:** 200mg/5mL, 400mg/5mL (100mL, 480mL); **Tab:** 400mg	Mild to moderate upper and lower respiratory tract and skin and skin structure infections, listeriosis, pertussis, diphtheria, erythrasma, intestinal amebiasis, acute pelvic inflammatory disease (PID) *N.gonorrhoeae,* primary syphilis in PCN allergy, Legionnaires' disease, chlamydial infections (eg, newborn conjunctivitis urethral, endocervical, or rectal, etc), and nongonococcal urethritis. Prophylaxis of strep pharyngitis with history of rheumatic fever.	Usual: 1600mg/day given q6h, q8h or q12h. Max: 4g/day. Treat strep infections for 10 days. Streptococcal Infection Prophylaxis with Rheumatic Heart Disease: 400mg bid. Urethritis *C.trachomatis* or *U. urealyticum*: 800mg tid for 7 days. Primary Syphilis: 48-64g in divided doses over 10-15 days. Intestinal Amebiasis: 400mg qid for 10-14 days. Pertussis: 40-50mg/kg/day in divided doses for 5-14 days. Legionnaires' Disease: 1.6-4g/day in divided doses.	Usual: 30-50mg/kg/day in divided doses q6h, q8h or q12h. Double dose for more severe infections. Treat strep infections for 10 days. Intestinal Amebiasis: 30-50mg/kg/day in divided doses for 10-14 days. Pertussis: 40-50mg/kg/day in divided doses for 5-14 days.
ERYC (erythromycin)	**Cap, Delayed-Release:** 250mg	Mild to moderate upper and lower respiratory tract and skin and soft tissue infections, pertussis, diphtheria, erythrasma, intestinal amebiasis, acute pelvic inflammatory disease (PID) (*N.gonorrhoeae*), *Listeria monocytogenes* infections, primary syphilis in PCN allergy, Legionnaires' disease, chlamydial infections (eg, newborn conjunctivitis, urethral, endocervical, or rectal, etc), and nongonococcal urethritis. Prophylaxis of strep pharyngitis with history of rheumatic fever in PCN allergy.	Usual: 250mg q6h or 500mg q12h. Max: 4g/day. Treat strep infections for 10 days. Chlamydial Urogenital Infection During Pregnancy: 500mg qid for at least 7 days or 250mg qid for 14 days. Urethral/Endocervical/Rectal Chlamydial Infections: 500mg qid for at least 7 days. Primary Syphilis: 30-40g in divided doses for 10-15 days. Acute PID: 500mg (erythromycin lactobionate) IV q6h for 3 days, then 250mg PO q6h for 7 days. Streptococcal Infection Long-Term Prophylaxis of Rheumatic Fever: 250mg bid. Intestinal Amebiasis: 250mg qid for 10-14 days. Pertussis: 40-50mg/kg/day in divided doses for 5-14 days. Legionnaires' Disease: 1-4g/day in divided doses	Usual: 30-50mg/kg/day in divided doses without food. Max: 4g/day. Severe Infections: Double dose up to 4g/day. Treat strep infections for 10 days. Intestinal Amebiasis: 30-50mg/kg/day in divided doses for 10-14 days.
EryPed (erythromycin ethylsuccinate)	**Sus:** 200mg/5mL, 400mg/5mL [5mL, 100mL, 200mL]	Treatment of mild to moderate upper and lower respiratory tract and skin and skin structure infections, listeriosis, pertussis, diphtheria, erythrasma, intestinal amebiasis, acute pelvic inflammatory disease (PID) *N.gonorrhoeae,* primary syphilis in PCN allergy, Legionnaires' disease, chlamydial infections (eg, newborn conjunctivitis, urethral, endocervical, or rectal, etc), and nongonococcal urethritis. Prophylaxis of strep pharyngitis with history of rheumatic fever.	Usual: 1600mg/day given q6h, q8h or q12h. Max: 4g/day. Treat strep infections for 10 days. Streptococcal Infection Prophylaxis with Rheumatic Heart Disease: 400mg bid. Urethritis *C.trachomatis* or *U. urealyticum*: 800mg tid for 7 days. Primary Syphilis:48-64g in divided doses over 10-15 days. Intestinal Amebiasis: 400mg qid for 10-14 days. Pertussis:40-50mg/kg/day in divided doses for 5-14 days. Legionnaires' Disease: 1.6-4g/day in divided doses.	Usual: 30-50mg/kg/day in divided doses q6h, q8h or q12h. Double dose for more severe infections. Treat strep infections for 10 days. Intestinal Amebiasis: 30-50mg/kg/day in divided doses for 10-14 days. Pertussis: 40-50mg/kg/day in divided doses for 5-14 days.

(Continued)

BRAND NAME (Generic)	DOSAGE FORM/ STRENGTH	INDICATIONS	ADULT DOSE	PEDIATRIC DOSE
MACROLIDES *(Continued)*				
Ery-Tab (erythromycin)	**Tab, Delayed-Release:** 250mg, 333mg, 500mg	Mild to moderate upper and lower respiratory tract and skin and skin structure infections, listeriosis, pertussis, diphtheria, erythrasma, intestinal amebiasis, acute pelvic inflammatory disease (PID) *(N.gonorrhoeae)*, primary syphilis in PCN allergy, Legionnaires' disease, chlamydial infections (eg, newborn conjunctivitis urethral, endocervical, rectal, etc), and nongonococcal urethritis. Prophylaxis of rheumatic fever.	Usual: 250mg qid, 333mg q8h or 500mg q12h without food. Max: 4g/day. Do not take bid when dose is ≥1g/day. Treat strep infections for 10 days. Chlamydial Urogenital Infection During Pregnancy: 500mg qid or 666mg q8h for at least 7 days, or 500mg q12h, 333mg q8h or 250mg qid for at least 14 days. Urethral/Endocervical/Rectal Chlamydial Infections and Nongonococcal Urethritis: 500mg qid or 666mg q8h for at least 7 days. Primary Syphilis: 30-40g in divided doses for 10-15 days. Acute PID: 500mg (erythromycin lactobionate) IV q6h for 3 days, then 500mg PO q12h or 333mg q8h for 7 days. Streptococcal Infection Long-Term Prophylaxis of Rheumatic Fever: 250mg bid. Intestinal Amebiasis: 500mg q12h, 333mg q8h or 250mg q6h for 10-14 days. Pertussis: 40-50mg/kg/day in divided doses for 5-14 days. Legionnaires' Disease: 1-4g/day in divided doses.	Usual: 30-50mg/kg/day in divided doses without food. Max: 4g/day. Severe Infections: Double dose up to 4g/day. Treat strep infections for 10 days. Chlamydial Conjunctivitis of Newborns and Chlamydial Pneumonia in Infancy: 12.5mg/kg qid for 2 weeks and 3 weeks, respectively. Intestinal Amebiasis: 30-50mg/kg/day in divided doses for 10-14 days. Long-Term Prophylaxis of Rheumatic Fever: 250mg bid. Intestinal Amebiasis: 30-50mg/kg/day in divided doses for 10-14 days. Pertussis: 40-50mg/kg/day in divided doses for 5-14 days. Legionnaire's Disease: 1-4g/day in divided doses.
Erythrocin (erythromycin stearate)	**Tab:** 250mg, 500mg	Mild to moderate upper and lower respiratory tract, and skin and skin structure infections, listeriosis, pertussis, diphtheria, erythrasma, intestinal amebiasis, acute pelvic inflammatory disease (PID) (gonorrhea), primary syphilis in PCN allergy, Legionnaires' disease, chlamydial infections (eg, newborn conjunctivitis urethral, endocervical, or rectal, etc), and nongonococcal urethritis. Prophylaxis of rheumatic fever.	Usual: 250mg q6h or 500mg q12h without food. Max: 4g/day. Treat strep infections for 10 days. Streptococcal Infection Prophylaxis of Rheumatic Fever: 250mg bid. Chlamydial Urogenital Infection During Pregnancy: 500mg qid for 7 days or 250mg qid for 14 days. Urethral/Endocervical/Rectal Chlamydial Infections and Nongonococcal Urethritis: 500mg qid for at least 7 days. Primary Syphilis: 30-40g in divided doses over 10-15 days. Acute PID: 500mg (erythromycin lactobionate) IV q6h for 3 days, then 500mg PO q12h for 7 days. Intestinal Amebiasis: 250mg qid for 10-14 days. Pertussis: 40-50mg/kg/day in divided doses for 5-14 days. Legionnaires' Disease: 1-4g/day in divided doses.	Usual: 30-50mg/kg/day in divided doses without food. Severe Infections: Double dose up to 4g/day. Treat strep infections for 10 days. Streptococcal Infection Prophylaxis of Rheumatic Fever: 250mg bid. Chlamydial Conjunctivitis of Newborns/Chlamydial Pneumonia in Infancy: 12.5mg/kg qid for 2 weeks and 3 weeks, respectively. Intestinal Amebiasis: 30-50mg/kg/day in divided doses for 10-14 days. Pertussis: 40-50mg/kg/day in divided doses for 5-14 days.

BRAND NAME (Generic)	DOSAGE FORM/ STRENGTH	INDICATIONS	ADULT DOSE	PEDIATRIC DOSE
Erythromycin	**Cap, Delayed-Release:** 250mg	Mild to moderate upper and lower respiratory tract and skin and skin structure infections, listeriosis, pertussis, diphtheria, erythrasma, intestinal amebiasis, primary syphilis in PCN allergy, Legionnaires' disease, chlamydial infections (eg, newborn conjunctivitis urethral, endocervical, rectal, etc), and nongonococcal urethritis. Prophylaxis of strep infection with history of rheumatic fever.	Usual: 250mg q6h or 500mg q12h without food. Max: 4g/day. Treat strep infections for 10 days. Streptococcal Infection Prophylaxis of Rheumatic Fever: 250mg bid. Chlamydial Urogenital Infection During Pregnancy: 500mg qid for at least 7 days or 250mg qid for at least 14 days. Urethral/ Endocervical/Rectal Chlamydial Infections: 500mg qid for at least 7days. Primary Syphilis: 30-40g in divided doses over 10-15 days. Intestinal Amebiasis: 250mg q6h for 10-14 days. Pertussis: 40-50mg/ kg/day in divided doses for 5-14 days. Legionnaires' Disease: 1-4g/day in divided doses.	Usual: 30-50mg/kg/day in divided doses without food. Severe Infections: Double dose up to 4g/day. Treat strep infections for 10 days. Streptococcal Infection Prophylaxis of Rheumatic Fever: 250mg bid. Intestinal Amebiasis: 30-50mg/kg/day in divided doses for 10-14 days. Pertussis: 40-50mg/kg/day in divided doses for 5-14 days.
Erythromycin Base	**Tab:** 250mg	Mild to moderate upper and lower respiratory tract and skin and skin structure infections, listeriosis, pertussis, diphtheria, erythrasma, intestinal amebiasis, acute pelvic inflammatory disease (PID) *(N.gonorrhoeae)*, primary syphilis in PCN allergy, Legionnaires' disease, chlamydial infections (eg, newborn conjunctivitis urethral, endocervical, rectal, etc), and nongonococcal urethritis. Prophylaxis of rheumatic fever.	Usual: 250mg q6h or 500mg q12h without food. Max: 4g/day. Treat strep infections for 10 days. Streptococcal Infection Prophylaxis of Rheumatic Fever: 250mg bid. Chlamydial Urogenital Infection During Pregnancy: 500mg qid for 7 days or 250mg qid for 14 days. Urethral/Endocervical/Rectal Chlamydial Infections and Nongonococcal Urethritis: 500mg qid for at least 7 days. Primary Syphilis: 30-40g in divided doses over 10-15 days. Acute PID: 500mg (erythromycin lactobionate) IV q6h for 3 days, then 500mg PO q12h for 7 days. Intestinal Amebiasis: 250mg qid for 10-14 days. Pertussis: 40-50mg/kg/day in divided doses for 5-14 days. Legionnaires' Disease: 1-4g/day in divided doses.	Usual: 30-50mg/kg/day in divided doses without food. Severe Infections: Double dose up to 4g/day. Treat strep infections for 10 days. Streptococcal Infection Prophylaxis of Rheumatic Fever: 250mg bid. Chlamydial Conjunctivitis of Newborns and Chlamydial Pneumonia in Infancy: 12.5mg/kg qid for 2 weeks and 3 weeks, respectively. Intestinal Amebiasis: 30-50mg/kg/day in divided doses for 10-14 days. Pertussis: 40-50mg/kg/day in divided doses for 5-14 days.

(Continued)

BRAND NAME (Generic)	DOSAGE FORM/ STRENGTH	INDICATIONS	ADULT DOSE	PEDIATRIC DOSE
MACROLIDES *(Continued)*				
PCE (erythromycin)	**Tab, Delayed-Release:** 333mg, 500mg	Mild to moderate upper and lower respiratory tract and skin and skin structure infections, listeriosis, pertussis, diphtheria, erythrasma, intestinal amebiasis, acute pelvic inflammatory disease (PID) *(N.gonorrhoeae)*, primary syphilis in PCN allergy, Legionnaires' disease, chlamydial infections (eg, newborn conjunctivitis urethral, endocervical, or rectal, etc), and nongonococcal urethritis. Prophylaxis of rheumatic fever.	Usual: 333mg q8h or 500mg q12h without food. Max: 4g/day. Do not take bid when dose is ≥1g/day. Treat strep infections for 10 days. Chlamydial Urogenital Infection During Pregnancy: 500mg qid or 666mg q8h for at least 7 days, or 500mg q12h, 333mg q8h or 250mg qid for at least 14 days. Urethral/Endocervical/Rectal Chlamydial Infections and Nongonococcal Urethritis: 500mg qid or 666mg q8h for at least 7 days. Primary Syphilis: 30-40g in divided doses for 10-15 days. Acute PID: 500mg (erythromycin lactobionate) IV q6h for 3 days, then 500mg PO q12h or 333mg q8h for 7 days. Streptococcal Infection Long-Term Prophylaxis of Rheumatic Fever: 250mg bid. Intestinal Amebiasis: 500mg q12h, or 333mg q8h or 250mg q6h for 10-14 days. Pertussis: 40-50mg/kg/day in divided doses for 5-14 days. Legionnaires' Disease: 1-4g/day in divided doses.	Usual: 30-50mg/kg/day in divided doses without food. Max: 4g/day. Severe Infections: Double dose up to 4g/day. Treat strep infections for 10 days. Chlamydial Conjunctivitis of Newborns and Chlamydial Pneumonia in Infancy: 12.5mg/kg qid for 2 weeks and 3 weeks, respectively. Intestinal Amebiasis: 30-50mg/kg/day in divided doses for 10-14 days. Long-Term Prophylaxis of Rheumatic Fever: 250mg bid. Pertussis: 40-50mg/kg/day in divided doses for 5-14 days. Legionnaires' Disease: 1-4g/day in divided doses.
Zithromax (azithromycin)	**Inj:** 500mg; **Sus:** 100mg/5mL [15mL], 200mg/5mL [15mL, 22.5mL, 30mL], 1g/pkt [3^S^ 10^S^]; **Tab:** 250mg [Z-Pak, 6 tabs], 500mg [Tri-Pak, 3 tabs], 600mg	(PO) Treatment of acute bacterial exacerbations of COPD, acute bacterial sinusitis (ABS), community acquired pneumonia (CAP), pharyngitis/tonsillitis, uncomplicated skin and skin structure, urethritis/cervicitis, genital ulcer disease (men), acute otitis media, prevention of disseminated *Mycobacterium avium* complex (MAC) disease in advanced HIV infection. (IV) Treatment of CAP and pelvic inflammatory disease (PID).	(PO) COPD/CAP/Pharyngitis/Tonsillitis (second line therapy)/SSSI: ≥16 yrs: 500mg on day 1, then 250 mg qd on days 2-5. COPD: 500mg qd for 3 days. ABS: 500mg qd for 3 days. Genital Ulcer Disease and Non-Gonococcal Urethritis/Cervicitis: 1g single dose. Urethritis/Cervicitis due to gonorrhea: 2g single dose. MAC Prophylaxis: 1200mg once weekly. MAC Treatment: 600mg qd with ethambutol 15mg/kg/day. (IV) ≥16 yrs: Cap: 500mg qd for at least 2 days, then 500mg PO to complete 7-10 day course. PID: 500mg qd for 1-2 days, then 250mg PO to complete 7-day course.	(Sus) Otitis Media: ≥6 mo: 30mg/kg single dose; 10mg/kg qd for 3 days; or 10mg/kg qd on day 1, then 5mg/kg qd on days 2-5. ABS: ≥6 mo: 10mg/kg qd for 3 days. Cap: ≥6 mo: 10mg/kg qd on day 1, then 5mg/kg qd on days 2-5. (Sus, Tab) Pharyngitis/Tonsillitis: ≥2 yrs: 12mg/kg qd for 5 days. 1g suspension is not for pediatric use.

BRAND NAME (Generic)	DOSAGE FORM/ STRENGTH	INDICATIONS	ADULT DOSE	PEDIATRIC DOSE
Zmax (azithromycin)	**Sus, Extended-Release:** 2g	Treatment of mild to moderate acute bacterial sinusitis due to *Haemophilus influenzae, Moraxella catarrhalis,* or *Streptococcus pneumoniae.* Treatment of community-acquired pneumonia due to *Chlamydophila pneumoniae, Haemophilus influenzae,* Mycoplasma pneumoniae, or Streptococcus pneumoniae in patients appropriate for oral therapy.	2g single dose. Take on an empty stomach (1 hr before or 2 hrs after a meal).	≥6 months/<75lb: 60 mg/kg, single dose; >75lb: adult dose.
PENICILLINS				
Amoxil (amoxicillin)	**Cap:** 250mg, 500mg; **Sus:** 50mg/mL [15mL, 30mL], 125mg/5mL [80mL, 100mL, 150mL], 200mg/5mL [50mL, 75mL, 100mL], 250mg/5mL [80mL, 100mL, 150mL], 400mg/5mL [50mL, 75mL, 100mL]; **Tab:** 500mg, 875mg; **Tab, Chewable:** 200mg, 400mg	Infections of the ear, nose, throat, genitourinary tract, skin and skin structure, lower respiratory tract due to susceptible (beta lactamase negative) organisms; gonorrhea (acute uncomplicated). *H.pylori* eradication to reduce the risk of duodenal ulcer recurrence.	Ear/Nose/Throat/SSSI/GU: (Mild/Moderate): 500mg q12h or 250mg q8h. (Severe): 875mg q12h or 500 mg q8h. LRTI: 875mg q12h or 500mg q8h. Gonorrhea: 3g as single dose. *H.pylori:* (Dual Therapy) 1g + 30mg lansoprazole, both tid for 14 days. (Triple Therapy) 1g + 30mg lansoprazole + 500mg clarithromycin, all q12h X 14 days. CrCl <30mL/min: Do not give 875mg tab. CrCl 10-30mL/min: 250-500mg q12h. <10mL/min: 250-500mg q24h. Hemodialysis: 250-500mg q24h, additional dose during and at the end.	**Neonates:** ≤12 weeks: Max: 30mg/kg/day divided q12h. >3 mo: Ear/Nose/Throat/SSSI/GU: (Mild/Moderate): 25mg/kg/day given q12h or 20mg/kg/day given q8h. (Severe): 45mg/kg/day given q12h or 40 mg/kg/day given q8h. LRTI: 45mg/kg/day given q12h or 40mg/kg/day given q8h. Gonorrhea: (Prepubertal) 50mg/kg with 25mg/kg probenecid as single dose. (Not for <2 yrs). >40kg: Dose as adult.
Ampicillin (ampicillin sodium)	**Inj:** 125mg, 250mg, 500mg, 1g, 2g, 10g	Treatment of respiratory tract, urinary tract, and GI infections, bacterial meningitis, septicemia, endocarditis.	IM/IV: Respiratory Tract: ≥40kg: 250-500mg q6h. <40kg: 25-50mg/kg/day given q6-8h. GI/GU Caused by *N.gonorrhea* (Females): ≥40kg: 500mg q6h. <40kg: 50mg/kg/day given q6-8h. Urethritis Caused by *N.gonorrhea* (Males): 500mg q8-12h for 2 doses; may retreat if needed. Bacterial Meningitis: 150-200mg/kg/day given q3-4h. Septicemia: 150-200mg/kg/day IV for 3 days, continue with IM q3-4h. Treat for minimum of 10 days and 48-72 hrs after being asymptomatic.	Bacterial Meningitis: 150-200mg/kg/day given q3-4h. Septicemia: 150-200mg/kg/day IV given q3-4h for 3 days, continue with IM q3-4h. Treat for minimum of 10 days and 48-72 hrs after being asymptomatic.

(Continued)

BRAND NAME (Generic)	DOSAGE FORM/ STRENGTH	INDICATIONS	ADULT DOSE	PEDIATRIC DOSE
PENICILLINS *(Continued)*				
Augmentin (amoxicillin-clavulanate potassium)	(Amoxicillin-Clavulanate) **Sus:** 125-31.25mg/5mL [75mL, 100mL, 150mL] 200-28.5mg/5mL [50mL, 75mL, 100mL], 250-62.5mg/5mL [75mL, 100mL, 150mL], 400-57mg/5mL [50mL, 75mL, 100mL]; **Tab:** 250-125mg, 500-125mg, 875-125mg; Tab, Chewable: 125-31.25mg, 200-28.5mg, 250-62.5mg, 400-57mg	Treatment of lower respiratory tract (LRTI), skin and skin structure (SSSI), and urinary tract infections (UTI), otitis media (OM), sinusitis.	(Dose based on amoxicillin) 500mg q12h or 250mg q8h. Severe Infections/RTI: 875mg q12h or 500mg q8h. May use 125mg/5mL or 250mg/5mL sus in place of 500mg tab and 200mg/5mL sus or 400mg/5mL sus in place of 875mg tab. CrCl <30mL/min: Do not give 875mg tab. CrCl 10-30mL/min: 250-500mg q12h. CrCl <10mL/min: 250-500mg q24h. Hemodialysis: 250-500mg q24h, give additional dose during and at the end of dialysis.	(Dose based on amoxicillin) ≥40kg: Use adult dose. ≥12 weeks: Sinusitis/OM/LRTI/Severe Infections: (Sus/Tab, Chewable) 45mg/kg/day given q12h or 40mg/kg/day given q8h. Less Severe Infections: 25mg/kg/day given q12h or 20mg/kg/day given q8h. <12 weeks:15mg/kg q12h (use 125mg/5mL sus).
Augmentin ES-600 (amoxicillin-clavulanate potassium)	**Sus:** (Amoxicillin-Clavulanate) 600mg-42.9mg/5mL [75mL, 125mL, 200mL]	Treatment of recurrent or persistent acute otitis media.		(Dose based on amoxicillin) 3 mo-12 yrs: <40kg: 45mg/kg q12h for 10 days.
Augmentin XR (amoxicillin-clavulanate potassium)	**Tab, Extended-Release:** (Amoxicillin-Clavulanate) 1000 mg-62.5mg	Treatment of community acquired pneumonia (CAP) or acute bacterial sinusitis due to confirmed or suspected ß-lactamase producing pathogens.	Sinusitis: 2 tabs q12h for 10 days. CAP: 2 tabs q12h for 7-10 days. Take at the start of a meal.	≥16 yrs: Sinusitis: 2 tabs q12h for 10 days. CAP: 2 tabs q12h for 7-10 days. Take at the start of a meal.
Bicillin C-R (penicillin G benzathine-penicillin G procaine)	**Inj:** (Penicillin G Benzathine-Penicillin G Procaine) 300,000-300,000 U/mL	Treatment of moderately severe to severe upper-respiratory tract (URTI) and skin and soft-tissue infections (SSTI), scarlet fever and erysipelas due to streptococci. Treatment of moderately severe pneumonia and otitis media due to pneumococci.	Group A Strep: URTI/SSTI/Scarlet Fever/Erysipelas: 2.4 MU IM. Treat at a single session using multiple IM sites, or use an alternative schedule and give ½ of the total dose on Day 1 and ½ on Day 3. Pneumococcal Infections (Except Meningitis): 1.2 MU IM, repeat every 2-3 days until temperature is normal for 48 hrs. Administer IM into upper, outer quadrant of buttock.	Group A Strep: URTI/SSTI/Scarlet Fever/Erysipelas: >60 lbs: 2.4 MU IM. 30-60 lbs: 900,000 U-1.2 MU IM. <30 lbs: 600,000 U IM. Treat at a single session using multiple IM sites, or use an alternative schedule and give ½ of the total dose on Day 1 and ½ on Day 3. Pneumococcal Infections (Except Meningitis): 600,000 U IM, repeat every 2-3 days until temperature is normal for 48 hrs. Administer IM into upper, outer quadrant of buttock. Use the midlateral aspect of thigh in neonates, infants, and small children.

BRAND NAME (Generic)	DOSAGE FORM/ STRENGTH	INDICATIONS	ADULT DOSE	PEDIATRIC DOSE
Bicillin C-R 900/300 (penicillin G benzathine-penicillin G procaine)	**Inj:** (Penicillin G Benzathine-Penicillin G Procaine) 900,000-300,000 U/2mL	Treatment of moderately severe to severe upper-respiratory tract (URTI) and skin and soft-tissue infections (SSTI), scarlet fever and erysipelas due to streptococci. Treatment of moderately severe pneumonia and otitis media due to pneumococci.		Group A Strep: URTI/SSTI/Scarlet Fever/Erysipelas: 1.2 MU IM single dose. Pneumococcal Infections (Except Meningitis): 1.2 MU IM every 2-3 days until temperature is normal for 48 hrs. Administer IM into upper, outer quadrant of buttock. Use midlateral aspect of thigh in neonates, infants, and small children.
Bicillin L-A (penicillin G benzathine)	**Inj:** 300,000 U/mL, 600,000 U/mL	Treatment of mild to moderate upper respiratory tract infections (URTI) due to streptococci and venereal infections (eg, syphilis, yaws, bejel, pinta). Prophylaxis to prevent recurrence of rheumatic fever or chorea.	Group A Strep: URTI: 1.2 MU IM single dose. Primary/Secondary/Latent Syphilis: 2.4 MU IM single dose. Late Syphilis (Tertiary/Neurosyphilis): 2.4 MU IM every 7 days for 3 doses. Yaws/Bejel/Pinta: 1.2 MU IM single dose. Rheumatic Fever/Glomerulonephritis Prophylaxis: 1.2 MU IM once a mo or 600,000 U IM every 2 weeks. Administer IM into upper, outer quadrant of buttock.	Group A Strep: URTI: Older Pediatrics: 900,000 U IM single dose. <60lbs: 300,000-600,000 U IM single dose. Congenital Syphilis: 2-12 yrs: Adjust dose based on adult schedule. <2 yrs: 50,000 U/kg IM single dose. Rheumatic Fever/Glomerulonephritis Prophylaxis: 1.2 MU IM once a mo or 600,000 U every 2 weeks. Administer IM into upper, outer quadrant of buttock. Use the midlateral aspect of thigh in neonates, infants, and small children.
Dicloxacillin (dicloxacillin sodium)	**Cap:** 125mg, 250mg, 500mg	Infections caused by penicillinase-producing staphylococci.	Mild-Moderate Infection: 125mg q6h. Severe Infection: 250mg q6h for at least 14 days.	<40kg: Mild-Moderate Infection: 12.5mg/kg/day in divided doses q6h. Severe Infection: 25mg/kg/day in divided doses q6h for at least 14 days.
Geocillin (carbenicillin disodium)	**Tab:** 382mg	Treatment of acute and chronic infections of the upper and lower urinary tract (UTI) and asymptomatic bacteriuria.	UTI: *E.coli, Proteus,* and *Enterobacter:* 1-2 tabs qid. *Pseudomonas, Enterococcus:* 2 tabs qid. Prostatitis: *E.coli, Proteus, Enterococcus* and *Enterobacter:* 2 tabs qid. CrCl 10-20mL/min: Adjust dose.	
Penicillin VK, Veetids (penicillin V potassium)	**Sus:** 125mg/5mL, 250mg/5mL [100mL, 200mL]; **Tab:** 250mg, 500mg	Mild to moderately severe bacterial infections including scarlet fever, mild erysipelas, and conditions of the respiratory tract, oropharynx, skin and soft tissue. Prevention of recurrence following rheumatic fever and/or chorea.	Usual: Streptococcal Infections (Scarlet Fever, Erysipelas, Upper Respiratory Tract): 125-250mg q6-8h for 10 days. Pneumococcal Infections (Otitis Media, Respiratory Tract): 250-500mg q6h until afebrile for at least 2 days. Staphylococcus Infections (Skin/Soft Tissue): 250-500mg q6-8h. Fusospirochetosis Infections (Oropharnyx): 250-500mg. Rheumatic Fever/Chorea Prevention: 125-250mg bid. Bacterial endocarditis prophylaxis in patients with rheumatic or valvular heart disease during dental or surgical procedures of upper respiratory tract: 2g 1 hr before procedure, then 1g 6 hr later.	≥12 yrs: Usual: Streptococcal Infections (Scarlet fever, Erysipelas, Upper Respiratory Tract): 125-250mg q6-8h for 10 days. Pneumococcal Infections (Otitis media, Respiratory Tract): 250-500mg q6h until afebrile for at least 2 days. Staphylococcus Infections (Skin/Soft Tissue): 250-500mg q6-8h. Fusospirochetosis Infections (Oropharnyx): 250-500mg q6-8h. Rheumatic Fever/Chorea Prevention: 125-250mg bid. Bacterial endocarditis prophylaxis in patients with rheumatic or valvular heart disease during dental or surgical procedures of upper respiratory tract: <60lbs: 1g 1 hr before procedure, then 500mg 6 hr later.

(Continued)

BRAND NAME (Generic)	DOSAGE FORM/ STRENGTH	INDICATIONS	ADULT DOSE	PEDIATRIC DOSE
PENICILLINS *(Continued)*				
Pfizerpen (penicillin G potassium)	**Inj:** 5 MU, 20 MU	For therapy of severe infections when rapid and high blood levels of penicillin required. Management of streptococcal, pneumococcal, staphylococcal, clostridial, fusospirochetal, listeria, and gram negative bacillary, and pasteurella infections. For anthrax, actinomycosis, diphtheria, erysipeloid, meningitis (including meningococci), endocarditis, bacteremia, rat-bite fever, syphilis, and gonorrheal endocarditis and arthritis. With combined oral therapy, prophylaxis against endocarditis in patients with congenital heart disease, rheumatic, or other acquired valvular heart disease undergoing dental procedures or surgical procedures of upper respiratory tract.	Anthrax: Minimum of 5 MU/day in divided doses. Gonorrheal Endocarditis/Severe Infections (Streptococci, Pneumococci, Staphylococci): Minimum of 5 MU/day. Syphilis: Administer in hospital. Determine dose and duration based on age and weight. Meningococcic Meningitis: 1-2 MU IM q2h or 20-30 MU/day continuous IV. Actinomycosis: 1-6 MU/day for cervicofacial cases; 10-20 MU/day for thoracic and abdominal disease. Clostridial Infections: 20 MU/day (adjunct to anti-toxin). Fusospirochetal Severe Infections: 5-10 MU/day for oropharynx, lower respiratory tract, and genital area infection. Rat-bite Fever: 12-15 MU/day for 3-4 weeks. Listeria Endocarditis: 15-20 MU/day for 4 weeks. Listeria meningitis: 15-20 MU/day for 2 weeks. Pasteurella Bacteremia/Meningitis: 4-6 MU/day for 2 weeks. Erysipeloid Endocarditis: 2-20 MU/day for 4-6 weeks. Gram Negative Bacillary Bacteremia: 20-80 MU/day. Diphtheria (carrier state): 0.3-0.4 MU/day in divided doses for 10-12 days. Endocarditis Prophylaxis: 1 MU IM mixed with 0.6 MU procaine penicillin G 0.5-1 hr before procedure. Renal/Cardiac/Vascular Dysfunction: Consider dose reduction. For streptococcal infection, treat for minimum 10 days.	Listeria Infections: Neonates: 0.5-1 MU/day. Congenital Syphilis: Administer in hospital. Determine dose and duration based on age and weight. Endocarditis Prophylaxis: 30,000 U/kg IM mixed with 0.6 MU procaine penicillin G 0.5-1 hr before procedure. For streptococcal infection, treat for minimum 10 days.
Permapen (penicillin G benzathine)	**Inj:** 600,000 U/mL	Treatment of microorganisms susceptible to low and very prolonged serum levels in upper respiratory tract infections (streptococci group A—without bacteremia), syphilis, yaws, bejel, and pinta. Prophylaxis for rheumatic fever and/or chorea. Follow-up prophylactic therapy for rheumatic heart disease and acute glomerulonephritis.	Streptococcal Infection: 1.2 MU IM single dose. Primary/Secondary/Latent Syphilis: 2.4 MU IM single dose. Late (Tertiary/Neurosyphilis) Syphilis: 3 MU IM every 7 days for total of 6-9 MU. Yaws/Bejel/Pinta: 1.2 MU IM single dose. Rheumatic Fever/Glomerulonephritis Prophylaxis: 1.2 MU IM once a month or 600,000 U IM q 2 weeks. Use upper outer quadrant of buttock. Rotate injection site.	≤12 yrs: Adjust dose according to age and weight and severity of infection. Streptococcal Infection: 900,000 U IM single dose in older children. Congenital Syphilis: <2 yrs: 50,000 U/kg IM single dose. 2-12 yrs: Adjust dose based on adult schedule. Use midlateral aspect of thigh in infants and small children. May divide dose between 2 buttocks in peds <2 yrs. Rotate injection site.

BRAND NAME (Generic)	DOSAGE FORM/ STRENGTH	INDICATIONS	ADULT DOSE	PEDIATRIC DOSE
Piperacillin	**Inj:** 2g, 3g, 4g	Treatment of serious intra-abdominal, urinary tract, gynecologic, lower respiratory tract, skin and skin structure, bone and joint, and gonococcal infections, septicemia, and perioperative surgical prophylaxis.	Usual: 3-4g IM/IV q4-6h. Max: 24g/day; IM: 2g/site. Serious Infections: 200-300mg/kg/day IV divided q4-6h. Complicated UTI: 125-200mg/kg/day IV divided q6-8h. Uncomplicated UTI/Community Acquired Pneumonia: 100-125mg/kg/day IM/IV divided q6-12h. Uncomplicated Gonorrhea: 2g IM single dose with 1g PO probenecid 1/2 hr before injection. Surgical Prophylaxis: 2g IV 20-30 min just prior to anesthesia (See labeling for follow-up dosing). C-Section: 2g IV after cord is clamped, then 2g 4 hrs and 8 hrs after 1st dose. Renal Impairment: Uncomplicated/Complicated UTI: CrCl<20mL/min: 3g q12h. Complicated UTI: CrCl 20-40mL/min: 3g q8h. Serious Infection: CrCl 20-40mL/min: 4g q8h. CrCl<20mL/min: 4g q12h. Hemodialysis: Give 1g additional dose after each dialysis. Max: 2g q8h. Usual treatment is for 7-10 days; treat gynecologic infections for 3-10 days; treat *S.pyogenes* infections for at least 10 days.	≥12 yrs: Usual: 3-4g IM/IV q4-6h. Max: 24g/day; IM: 2g/site. Serious Infections: 200-300mg/kg/day IV divided q4-6h. Complicated UTI: 125-200mg/kg/day IV divided q6-8h. Uncomplicated UTI/Community Acquired Pneumonia: 100-125mg/kg/day IM/IV divided q6-12h. Uncomplicated Gonorrhea: 2g IM single dose with 1g PO probenecid 1/2 hr before injection. Surgical Prophylaxis: 2g IV 20-30 minute just prior toanesthesia (See labeling for follow-up dosing). C-section: 2g IV after cord is clamped, then 2g 4 hrs and 8 hrs after 1st dose. Renal Impairment: Uncomplicated/Complicated UTI: CrCl <20mL/min: 3g q12h. Complicated UTI: CrCl 20-40mL/min: 3g q8h. Serious Infection: CrCl 20-40mL/min: 4g q8h. CrCl <20mL/min: 4g q12h. Hemodialysis: Give 1g additional dose after each dialysis. Max: 2g q8h. Usual treatment is for 7-10 days; treat gynecologic infections for 3-10 days; treat *S.pyogenes* infections for at least 10 days.
Timentin (ticarcillin-clavulanate potassium)	**Inj:** (Ticarcillin-Clavulanate) 3g-100mg, 3g-200mg, 3g-100mg/100mL, 30g-1g	Treatment of lower respiratory tract, bone and joint, skin and skin structure, urinary tract (UTI), gynecologic, and intra-abdominal infections, and septicemia.	≥60kg: UTI/Systemic Infection: 3g-100mg (3.1g vial) IV q4-6h. Gynecologic Infections: Moderate: 200mg/kg/day ticarcillin IV given q6h. Severe: 300mg/kg/day ticarcillin IV given q4h.<60kg: Usual: 200-300mg/kg/day ticarcillin IV given q4-6h. UTI: 3g-200mg (3.2g vial) q8h. Renal Impairment (based on ticarcillin): CrCl 60-30mL/min: 2g IV q4h. CrCl 30-10mL/min: 2g IV q8h. CrCl<10mL/min: 2g IV q12h (2g IV q24h with hepatic dysfunction). Peritoneal Dialysis: 3.1g IV q12h. Hemodialysis: 2g IV q12h, and 3.1g after each dialysis. Apply reduced dosage after initial 3.1g LD is given.	≥3 mo: >60kg: Mild to Moderate: 3g-100mg (3.1g vial) IV q6h. Severe: 3g-100mg (3.1g vial) IV q4h. <60kg: Mild to Moderate: 50mg/kg ticarcillin IV q6h. Severe: 50mg/kg ticarcillin IV q4h.

(Continued)

BRAND NAME (Generic)	DOSAGE FORM/ STRENGTH	INDICATIONS	ADULT DOSE	PEDIATRIC DOSE
PENICILLINS *(Continued)*				
Unasyn (ampicillin sodium/ sulbactam sodium)	**Inj:** (Ampicillin-Sulbactam) 1g-0.5g, 2g-1g, 10g-5g	Treatment of skin and skin structure (SSSI), intra-abdominal, and gynecological infections caused by susceptible microorganisms.	1.5-3g (ampicillin + sulbactam) IM/IV q6h. Max: 4g/day sulbactam. Renal Impairment: CrCl ≥30mL/min: 1.5-3g q6-8h. CrCl 15-29mL/min: 1.5-3g q12h. CrCl 5-14mL/min: 1.5-3g q24h.	≥40kg: Dose according to adult recommendations. Max: 4g/day sulbactam. <40kg: 300mg/kg IV in divided doses q6h.
Zosyn	**Inj:** (Piperacillin-Tazobactam) 40mg-5mg/mL, 60mg-7.5mg/mL, 2g-0.25g, 3g-0.375g, 4g-0.5g, 4g-0.5g/100mL, 36g-4.5g	Treatment of appendicitis, peritonitis, uncomplicated/complicated skin and skin structure infections, postpartum endometritis, pelvic inflammatory disease, moderate severity of community acquired pneumonia, and moderate to severe nosocomial pneumonia.	Usual: 3.375g q6h for 7-10 days. Nosocomial Pneumonia: 4.5g q6h for 7-14 days plus aminoglycoside. Renal Impairment (all indications except Nosocomial Pneumonia): CrCl 20-40mL/min: 2.25g q6h, CrCl <29mL/min: 2.25g q8h. Hemodialysis: 2.25g q12h. Give 1 additional 0.75g dose after each dialysis period. Nosocomial Pneumonia: CrCl 20-40 mL/min: 3.375g q6h, CrCl <20 mL/min: 2.25g q6h. Hemodialysis: 2.25g q8h. Give 1 addtional 0.75g dose after each dialysis period.	Appendicitis/peritonitis: ≥9 months (≤40kg) normal renal function: 100mg piperacillin/12.5mg tazobactam per kg q8h. 2-9 months: 80mg piperacillin/10mg tazobactam per kg q8h. (>40kg): Give adult dose.
STREPTOMYCES DERIVATIVES				
Sumycin (tetracycline HCl)	**Sus:** 125mg/5mL; **Tab:** 250mg, 500mg	Treatment of respiratory tract, urinary tract, and skin and skin structure infections, lymphogranuloma, psittacosis, trachoma, uncomplicated urethral/endocervical/rectal infection caused by *Chlamydia,* nongonococcal urethritis, chancroid, plague, cholera, brucellosis, and others. When PCN is contraindicated, treatment of uncomplicated gonorrhea, syphilis, listeriosis, anthrax, *Clostridium* species, and others. Adjunct therapy for amebicides and severe acne.	Mild-Moderate: 250mg qid or 500mg bid. Severe: 500mg qid. Continue for 24-48 hrs after symptoms subside (minimum 10 days with streptococci infections). Severe Acne: Initial: 1g/day in divided doses. Maint: After improvement, 125-500mg/day. Brucellosis: 500mg qid for 3 weeks plus streptomycin 1g IM bid for 1 week, then qd for 1 week. Syphilis: 30-40g equally divided over 10-15 days. Gonorrhea: 500mg q6h for 7 days. Chlamydia: 500mg qid for at least 7 days. Renal Dysfunction: Reduce dose or extend dose interval.	Usual: >8 yrs: 25-50mg/kg divided qid. Continue for 24-48 hrs after symptoms subside (minimum 10 days with streptococci infections). Severe Acne: Initial: 1g/day in divided doses. Maint: After improvement, 125-500mg/day. Renal Dysfunction: Reduce dose or extend dose interval.
Lincocin (lincomycin HCl)	**Inj:** 300mg/mL	Treatment of serious infections due to streptococci, pneumococci, and staphylococci. Reserve for PCN allergy or if PCN is inappropriate.	IM: Serious Infection: 600mg q24h. More Severe Infection: 600mg q12h or more often. IV: Dose depends on severity. Serious Infection: 600mg-1g q8-12h. More Severe Infection: Increase dose. Infuse over ≥1 hr. Life-Threatening Situation: Up to 8g/day has been given. Max: 8g/day. Severe Renal Dysfunction: 25-30% of normal dose.	>1 mo: IM: Serious Infection: 10mg/kg q24h. More Severe Infection: 10mg/kg q12h or more often. IV: 10-20mg/kg/day, depending on severity infused in divided doses as described for adults. Severe Renal Dysfunction: 25-30% of normal dose.

BRAND NAME (Generic)	DOSAGE FORM/ STRENGTH	INDICATIONS	ADULT DOSE	PEDIATRIC DOSE
TETRACYCLINE DERIVATIVES				
Declomycin (demeclocycline HCl)	**Tab:** 150mg, 300mg	Treatment of infections due to *rickettsiae, Mycoplasma pneumoniae, B.recurrentis,* agents of psittacosis, ornithosis, lymphomagranuloma venereum or granuloma inguinale. Treatment of gram-negative infections (eg, respiratory, urinary tract), gram-positive infections (eg, respiratory tract, skin and soft tissue), trachoma, inclusion conjunctivitis. When PCN is contraindicated, treatment of gonorrhea, syphilis, listeriosis, anthrax, *Clostridium* species, and others. Adjunct therapy for amebicides.	Usual: 150mg qid or 300mg bid. Gonorrhea: 600mg followed by 300mg q12h for 4 days to a total of 3g. Renal/Hepatic Impairment: Reduce dose and/or extend dose intervals. Continue therapy for at least 24-48 hrs after symptoms subside. Take at least 1 hr before or 2 hrs after meals with plenty of fluids.	>8 yrs: 7-13mg/kg/day, depending upon severity of the disease, divided into bid to qid. Max: 600mg/day. Gonorrhea: 600mg followed by 300mg q12h for 4 days to a total of 3g. Renal/Hepatic Impairmenrt: Reduce dose and/or extend dose intervals. Continue therapy for at least 24-48 hrs after symptoms subside. Take at least 1 hr before or 2 hrs after meals with plenty of fluids.
Doryx (doxycycline hyclate)	**Tab:** 75mg, 100mg, 150mg	Treatment of susceptible infections including respiratory, urinary, lymphogranuloma, psittacosis, trachoma, uncomplicated urethral/endocervical/rectal, nongonococcal urethritis, rickettsiae, chancroid, plague, cholera, brucellosis, anthrax. When penicillin is contraindicated, treatment of syphilis, listeriosis, *Clostridium* species, and others. Adjunct therapy for amebiasis and severe acne.	Usual: 100mg q12h on 1st day, followed by 100mg qd. Severe Infections/Chronic UTI: 100mg q12h. Uncomplicated Gonococcal Infections (except anorectal infections in men): 100mg bid for 7 days, or 300mg followed in 1 hr by another 300mg dose. Acute Epididymo-Orchitis: 100mg bid for at least 10 days. Syphilis, early: Patients who are allergic to penicillin: 100mg bid for 2 weeks. Duration of more than 1 year: 100 bid for 4 weeks. Nongonococcal Urethritis, Uncomplicated Urethral/Endocervical/Rectal Infection: 100mg bid for at least 7 days. Inhalational Anthrax (post-exposure): 100mg bid for 60 days. Treat Strep infections for 10 days.	>8 yrs: >100 lbs: 100mg q12h on 1st day, followed by 100mg qd. Severe Infections/Chronic UTI: 100mg q12h. ≤100 lbs: 2mg/lb/day given bid on Day 1, followed by 1mg/lb/day given qd-bid thereafter. Severe Infections: Up to 2mg/lb. Inhalational Anthrax (post-exposure): <100 lbs: 1mg/lb bid for 60 days. >100 lbs: Give adult dose.

(Continued)

BRAND NAME (Generic)	DOSAGE FORM/ STRENGTH	INDICATIONS	ADULT DOSE	PEDIATRIC DOSE
TETRACYCLINE DERIVATIVES *(Continued)*				
Dynacin (minocycline HCl)	**Tab:** 50mg, 75mg, 100mg	Treatment of inclusion conjunctivitis, nongonococcal urethritis, and other infections (eg, respiratory tract, endocervical, rectal, urinary tract, skin and skin structure) caused by susceptible strains of microorganisms. Alternative treatment in certain other infections (eg, urethritis, gonococcal, syphilis, anthrax). Adjunctive therapy in acute intestinal amebiasis and severe acne. Treatment of *Mycobacterium marinum* and asymptomatic carriers of *Neisseria meningitidis.*	Usual: 200mg initially, then 100mg q12h; alternative is 100-200mg initially, then 50mg qid. Uncomplicated Gonococcal Infection (Men, Other Than Urethritis and Anorectal Infections): 200mg initially, then 100mg q12h for minimum 4 days. Uncomplicated Gonococcal Urethritis (Men): 100mg q12h for 5 days. Syphilis: Administer usual dose for 10-15 days. Meningococcal Carrier State: 100mg q12h for 5 days. *Mycobacterium marinum:* 100mg q12h for 6-8 weeks. Uncomplicated urethral, endocervical, or rectal infection: 100mg q12h for at least 7 days. Renal Dysfunction: Reduce dose and/or extend dose intervals.	>8 yrs: 4mg/kg initially followed by 2mg/kg q12h. Take with plenty of fluids.
Minocin (minocycline HCl)	**Cap:** 50mg, 100mg;	Treatment of inclusion conjunctivitis, nongonococcal urethritis, and other infections (eg, respiratory tract, endocervical, rectal, urinary tract, skin and skin structure) caused by susceptible strains of microorganisms. Alternative treatment in certain other infections (eg, urethritis, gonococcal, syphilis, anthrax). Adjunctive therapy in acute intestinal amebiasis and severe acne. Treatment of *Mycobacterium marinum* and asymptomatic carriers of *Neisseria meningitidis.*	Usual: 200mg initially, then 100mg q12h; alternative is 100-200mg initially, then 50mg qid. Uncomplicated Gonococcal Infection (other than urethritis and anorectal infections in men): 200mg initially, then 100mg q12h for minimum 4 days. Uncomplicated Gonococcal Urethritis (Men): 100mg q12h for 5 days. Syphilis: Administer usual dose for 10-15 days. Meningococcal Carrier State: 100mg q12h for 5 days. *Mycobacterium marinum:* 100mg q12h for 6-8 weeks. Uncomplicated Urethral, Endocervical, or Rectal Infection Caused by *Chlamydia trachomatis* or *Ureaplasma urealyticum:* 100mg q12h for at least 7 days. Gonorrhea in Patients Sensitive to PCN: 200mg initially, then 100mg q12h for at least 4 days, with post-therapy cultures within 2-3 days. Take with plenty of fluids. Renal Dysfunction: Max: 200mg/24hrs.	>8 yrs: 4mg/kg initially followed by 2mg/kg q12h. Take with plenty of fluids. Renal Dysfunction: Max: 200mg/24 hrs.

BRAND NAME (Generic)	DOSAGE FORM/ STRENGTH	INDICATIONS	ADULT DOSE	PEDIATRIC DOSE
Monodox (doxycycline monohydrate)	**Cap:** 50mg, 75mg, 100mg	Treatment of respiratory tract, urinary tract, skin and skin structure, uncomplicated urethral/endocervical/rectal infection caused by *C.trachomatis,* nongonococcal urethritis caused by *C.trachomatis* and *U.urealyticum,* lymphogranuloma, psittacosis, trachoma, chancroid, plague, cholera, brucellosis. Treatment of uncomplicated gonorrhea, syphilis, listeriosis, anthrax, *Clostridium* species when PCN is contraindicated. Adjunct therapy for amebicides and severe acne.	Usual: 100mg q12h or 50mg q6h for 1 day, then 100 mg/day. Severe Infection: 100mg q12h. Uncomplicated Gonococcal Infections (except anorectal infections in men): 100mg bid for 7 days or 300mg stat, then repeat in 1 hr. Acute Epididymo-Orchitis caused by *N.gonorrhea* or *C.trachomatis:* 100mg bid for at least 10 days. Primary/Secondary Syphilis: 300mg/day in divided dose for at least 10 days. Uncomplicated Urethral/ Endocervical/Rectal Infection caused by *C.trachomatis:* 100mg bid for at least 7 days. Nongonococcal Urethritis caused by *C.trachomatis* and *U.urealyticum:* 100mg bid for at least 7 days. Take with full glass of water. Take with food if GI upset occurs.	>8 yrs: ≤100 lbs: 2mg/lb divided in 2 doses for 1 day, then 1mg/lb daily in single or 2 divided doses. Severe Infection: May use up to 2mg/lb/day. >100 lbs; 100mg q12h or 50mg q6h for 1 day, then 100mg/day. Severe Infection: 100mg q12h. Take with a full glass of water. Take with food if GI upset occurs.
Oracea (doxycycline)	**Cap:** 40mg	Treatment of only inflammatory lesions (papules and pustules) of rosacea.	40mg qd in am. Take on empty stomach.	
Periostat (doxycycline hyclate)	**Tab:** 20mg	Adjunct to scaling and root planing to promote attachment level gain and reduces pocket depth in patients with adult periodontitis.	Following scaling and root planing, 20mg bid, 1 hour prior to or 2hr after morning and evening meals for up to 9 months. Maintain adequate fluid intake with caps to reduce risk of esophageal irritation and ulceration.	
Solodyn (minocycline HCl)	**Tab, Extended-Release:** 45mg, 90mg, 135mg.	Treatment of inflammatory lesions of non-nodular moderate to severe acne vulgaris in patients ≥12 yrs.	1mg/kg qd for 12 weeks. Reduce dose or extend interval with renal impairment.	≥12 yrs: 1mg/kg qd for 12 weeks. Reduce dose or extend interval with renal impairment.
Vibra-tabs (doxycycline hyclate)	**Tab:** 100mg	Treatment of susceptible infections including respiratory, urinary, skin and skin structure, lymphogranuloma, psittacosis, trachoma, uncomplicated urethral/endocervical/rectal, nongonococcal urethritis, rickettsiae, chancroid, plague, cholera, brucellosis, anthrax. When penicillin is contraindicated, treatment of uncomplicated gonorrhea, syphilis, listeriosis, *Clostridium species,* and others. Adjunct therapy for amebiasis and severe acne. Prophylaxis of malaria.	Usual: 100mg q12h on day 1, then 100mg qd or 50mg q12h. Severe Infection: 100mg q12h. Treat for 10 days with strep infection. Uncomplicated Gonococcal Infection (Except Anorectal in Men): 100mg bid for 7 days or 300mg followed by 300mg in 1 hr. Uncomplicated Urethral/Endocervical/Rectal Infection and Nongonococcal Urethritis: 100mg bid for 7 days. Syphilis: 100mg bid for 2 weeks. Syphilis for >1 yr: 100mg bid for 4 weeks. Acute Epididymo-orchitis: 100mg bid for at least 10 days. Inhalation Anthrax (Post-Exposure): 100mg bid for 60 days. Malaria Prophylaxis: 100mg qd. Begin 1-2 days before travel and continue for 4 weeks after leaving malarious area.	>8 yrs: >100 lbs: 100mg q12h on Day 1, then 100mg qd or 50mg q12h. For severe infections, 100mg q12h. ≤100 lbs: 2mg/lb divided bid on Day 1, then 1mg/lb qd or bid. For severe infections, up to 2mg/lb. Inhalation Anthrax (post-exposure): <100 lbs: 1mg/lb bid for 60 days. ≥100 lbs: 100mg bid for 60 days. Malaria Prophylaxis: >8 yrs: 2mg/kg qd, up to 100mg qd. Begin 1-2 days before travel and continue for 4 weeks after leaving malarious area.

(Continued)

BRAND NAME (Generic)	DOSAGE FORM/ STRENGTH	INDICATIONS	ADULT DOSE	PEDIATRIC DOSE
TETRACYCLINE DERIVATIVES *(Continued)*				
Vibramycin (doxycycline)	**Cap:** (Doxycycline Hyclate) 50mg, 100mg; **Syrup:** (Doxycycline Calcium) 50mg/5mL; **Sus:** (Doxycycline Monohydrate) 25mg/5mL [60mL]	Treatment of susceptible infections including respiratory, urinary, lymphogranuloma, psittacosis, trachoma, uncomplicated urethral/endocervical/rectal, nongonococcal urethritis, rickettsiae, chancroid, plague, cholera, brucellosis, anthrax. When penicillin is contraindicated, treatment of uncomplicated gonorrhea, syphilis, listeriosis, *Clostridium species,* and others. Adjunct therapy for amebiasis and severe acne. Prophylaxis of malaria.	Usual: 100mg q12h on day 1, then 100mg qd or 50mg q12h. Severe Infection: 100mg q12h. Treat for 10 days with strep infection. Uncomplicated Gonococcal Infection (Except Anorectal in Men): 100mg bid for 7 days or 300mg followed by 300mg in 1 hr. Uncomplicated Urethral/Endocervical/Rectal Infection and Nongonococcal Urethritis: 100mg bid for 7 days. Syphilis: 100mg bid for 2 weeks. Syphilis for >1 yr: 100mg bid for 4 weeks. Acute Epididymo-orchitis: 100mg bid for at least 10 days. Inhalation Anthrax (Post-Exposure): 100mg bid for 60 days. Malaria Prophylaxis: 100mg qd. Begin 1-2 days before travel and continue for 4 weeks after leaving malarious area.	>8 yrs: ≤100 lbs: 1mg/lb bid on day 1, then 1mg/lb qd or 0.5mg/lb bid. Severe Infections: Maint: 2mg/lb. >100 lbs: Usual: 100mg q12h on day 1, then 100mg qd or 50mg q12h. Severe Infection: 100mg q12h. Treat for 10 days with strep infection. Inhalation Anthrax (Post-Exposure): <100 lbs: 1mg/lb bid for 60 days. ≥100 lbs: 100mg bid for 60 days. Malaria Prophylaxis: 2mg/kg qd. Max: 100mg/day. Begin 1-2 days before travel and continue for 4 weeks after leaving malarious area.
MISCELLANEOUS				
Bactrim (trimethoprim-sulfamethoxazole)	(Sulfamethoxazole [SMX]-Trimethoprim [TMP]) **Tab:** 400mg-80mg; **Tab, DS:** 800mg-160mg	Treatment of urinary tract infection (UTI), acute otitis media, acute exacerbation of chronic bronchitis (AECB), travelers' diarrhea, Shigellosis, and pneumocystitis carinii pneumonia (PCP).	UTI: 800mg SMX-160mg TMP q12h for 10-14 days. Shigellosis: 800mg SMX-160mg TMP q12h for 5 days. AECB: 800mg SMX-160mg TMP q12h for 14 days. PCP Treatment: 15-20mg/kg TMP and 75-100 mg/kg SMX per 24 hrs given q6h for 14-21 days. PCP Prophylaxis: 800mg SMX-160mg TMP qd. Traveler's Diarrhea: 800mg SMX-160mg TMP q12h for 5 days. CrCl: 15-30mL/min: 50% usual dose. CrCl: <15mL/min: Not recommended.	≥2 mo: UTI/Otitis Media: 4mg/kg TMP and 20mg/kg SMX q12h for 10 days. Shigellosis: 8mg/kg TMP and 40mg/kg SMX per 24 hrs given q12h for 5 days. PCP Treatment: 15-20mg/kg TMP and 75-100mg/kg SMX per 24 hrs given q6h for 14-21 days. PCP Prophylaxis: 150mg/m2/day TMP with 750mg/m2/day SMX given bid, on 3 consecutive days/week. Max: 320mg TMP/1600mg SMX/day. CrCl: 15-30mL/min: 50% usual dose. CrCl: <15mL/min: Not recommended.
Cleocin (clindamycin)	**Cap:** (HCl) 75mg, 150mg, 300mg; **Inj:** (Phosphate) 150mg/mL, 300mg/50mL, 600mg/50mL, 900mg/50mL; **Sus:** (HCl) 75mg/5mL [100mL]	Serious infections caused by anaerobes, *streptococci, pneumococci* and *staphylococci.*	Serious Infection: 150-300mg PO q6h or 600-1200 mg/day IM/IV given bid-qid. More Severe Infection: 300-450mg PO q6h or 1200-2700mg/day IM/IV given bid-qid. Life-threatening Infections: Up to 4800mg/day IV. Max: 600mg per IM injection. Take oral form with full glass of water. Treat ß-hemolytic strep for at least 10 days.	Birth-16 yrs: Serious Infection: 8-16mg/kg/day tid-qid. More Severe Infection: 16-20mg/kg/day tid-qid. 1 mo-16 yrs: 20-40mg/kg/day IM/IV given tid-qid; use higher dose for more severe infection. <1 mo: 15-20mg/kg/day IM/IV given tid-qid. Take oral form with full glass of water. Treat ß-hemolytic strep for at least 10 days.

BRAND NAME (Generic)	DOSAGE FORM/ STRENGTH	INDICATIONS	ADULT DOSE	PEDIATRIC DOSE
Coly-Mycin M (colistimethate sodium)	**Inj:** 150mg	Treatment of acute or chronic infections due to certain gram-negative bacilli (eg, *Pseudomonas aeruginosa, Enterobacter aerogenes, E.coli, Klebsiella pneumoniae).*	Usual: 2.5-5mg/kg/day IV/IM in 2-4 divided doses. Max: 5mg/kg/day. SCr 1.3-1.5mg/dL: 2.5-3.8mg/kg/day IV/IM in 2 divided doses. SCr 1.6-2.5mg/dL: 2.5mg/kg/day IV/IM in 1-2 divided doses. SCr 2.6-4mg/dL: 1.5mg/kg/day IV/IM q36h. Obesity: Base dose on IBW.	Usual: 2.5-5mg/kg/day IV/IM in 2-4 divided doses. Max: 5mg/kg/day. SCr 1.3-1.5mg/dL: 2.5-3.8mg/kg/day IV/IM in 2 divided doses. SCr 1.6-2.5mg/dL: 2.5mg/kg/day IV/IM in 1-2 divided doses. SCr 2.6-4mg/dL: 1.5mg/kg/day IV/IM q36h. Obesity: Base dose on IBW.
Cubicin (daptomycin)	**Inj:** 500mg/vial	Susceptible complicated skin and skin structure infections (cSSSI). *Staphylococcus aureus* blood stream infections (bacteremia).	≥18 yrs: Administer as IV infusion over 30 minutes. cSSSI: 4mg/kg once every 24 hrs for 7-14 days. *S.aureus* Bacteremia: 6mg/kg once every 24 hrs for minimum 2-6 weeks. Renal impairment: CrCl <30 mL/min, Hemodialysis or CAPD: (cSSSI) 4mg/kg or *(S.aureus bacteremia)* 6mg/kg once every 48 hrs.	
Flagyl IV (metronidazole HCl)	**Inj:** 500mg (RTU)	Treatment of anaerobic intra-abdominal, skin and skin structure, gynecologic, bone and joint, CNS, lower respiratory tract infections, endocarditis, and septicemia. Prophylaxis for colorectal surgery.	LD: 15mg/kg IV. Maint: 6 hrs later, 7.5mg/kg IV q6h for 7-10 days or more. Max: 4g/24 hrs. Infuse over 1 hr. Colorectal surgery prophylaxis: 15mg/kg IV over 30-60 min. Complete infusion 1 hr before surgery, then 7.5mg/kg IV over 30-60 min at 6 hrs and 12 hrs after initial dose.	
Hiprex (methenamine hippurate)	**Tab:** 1g	Prophylaxis or suppression of recurrent urinary tract infections when long-term therapy is necessary. For use only after infection is eradicated by other appropriate antimicrobials.	1g bid. Contraindicated in renal or severe hepatic insufficiency.	>12 yrs: 1g bid. 6 to 12 yrs: 0.5g-1g bid. Contraindicated in renal or severe hepatic insufficiency.
Ketek (telithromycin)	**Tab:** 300mg [20[S]], 400mg [60[S], Ketek Pak, 100[S]]	Treatment of mild to moderate community-acquired pneumonia (CAP) due to *S.pneumoniae* (including MDRSP), *H.influenzae, M.catarrhalis, C.pneumoniae*, or *M.pneumoniae.*	800mg qd for 7-10 days. Severe Renal Impairment (CrCl <30mL/min): 600mg qd. Hemodialysis: Give after dialysis session on dialysis days. Severe Renal Impairment (CrCl <30mL/min) with Hepatic Impairment: 400mg qd.	
Macrobid (nitrofurantoin monohydrate)	**Cap:** 100mg	Treatment of acute uncomplicated urinary tract infections (acute cystitis).	100mg every 12 hrs for 7 days. Take with food.	>12 yrs: 100mg every 12 hrs for 7 days. Take with food.
Macrodantin (nitrofurantoin macrocrystals)	**Cap:** 25mg, 50mg, 100mg	Treatment of urinary tract infection.	50-100mg qid for at least 7 days. Take with food. Long-term Suppressive Use: 50-100mg at bedtime.	≥1 mo: 5-7mg/kg/day given qid for at least 7 days. Take with food. Long-term Suppressive Use: 1mg/kg/day given qd-bid.

(Continued)

BRAND NAME (Generic)	DOSAGE FORM/ STRENGTH	INDICATIONS	ADULT DOSE	PEDIATRIC DOSE
MISCELLANEOUS *(Continued)*				
Monurol (fosfomycin tromethamine)	**Pow:** 3g/sachet	Uncomplicated urinary tract infection (acute cystitis) in women.	≥18 yrs: 1 single-dose sachet. Mix with 3-4oz of water before ingesting.	
Primsol (trimethoprim HCl)	**Sol:** 50mg/5mL	Treatment of acute otitis media in pediatrics and urinary tract infection (UTI) in adults.	UTI: Usual: 100mg q12h or 200mg q24h for 10 days. CrCl: 15-30mL/min: Give 50% of usual dose. CrCl <15mL/min: Use not recommended.	Otitis Media: ≥6 mos: 5mg/kg q12h for 10 days. CrCl: 15-30mL/min: Give 50% of usual dose.
Rifadin (rifampin)	**Cap:** 150mg, 300mg; **Inj:** 600mg	Treatment of all forms of tuberculosis (TB). Treatment of asymptomatic carriers of *Neisseria meningitidis* to eliminate meningococci from the nasopharynx.	TB: 10mg/kg PO/IV qd. Max: 600mg/day. Meningococcal Carriers: 600mg bid for 2 days. Take 1 hr before or 2 hrs after a meal with a full glass of water.	TB: 10-20mg/kg PO/IV qd. Max: 600mg/day. Meningococcal Carriers: ≥1 mo: 10mg/kg q12h for 2 days. Max: 600mg/dose. <1 mo: 5mg/kg q12h for 2 days. Take 1 hr before or 2 hrs after a meal with a full glass of water.
Rifamate (isoniazid-rifampin)	**Cap:** (Isoniazid-Rifampin) 150mg-300mg	For pulmonary tuberculosis (TB). Not for initial therapy or prevention of TB.	2 caps qd. Take 1 hr before or 2 hrs after meals. Give with pyridoxine in the malnourished, those predisposed to neuropathy (eg, alcoholics, diabetics), and adolescents.	
Rifater (isoniazid-rifampin-pyrazinamide)	**Tab:** (Isoniazid-Pyrazinamide-Rifampin) 50mg-300mg-120mg	For initial phase of the short-course treatment of pulmonary tuberculosis.	≤44kg: 4 tabs single dose qd. 45-54kg: 5 tabs single dose. ≥55kg: 6 tabs single dose. Give pyridoxine in malnourished, if predisposed to neuropathy (eg, alcoholics, diabetics), and adolescents. Take 1 hr before or 2 hrs after meals with full glass of water. Treatment usually lasts 2 months.	≥15 yrs: ≤44kg: 4 tabs single dose qd. 45-54kg: 5 tabs qd single dose. ≥55kg: 6 tabs qd single dose. Give pyridoxine in malnourished, if predisposed to neuropathy (eg, alcoholics, diabetics), and adolescents. Take 1 hr before or 2 hrs after meals with full glass of water. Treatment usually lasts 2 months.
Septra (sulfamethoxazole-trimethoprim)	(Sulfamethoxazole [SMX]-Trimethoprim [TMP]) **Inj:** 80mg-16mg/mL; **Sus:** 200mg-40mg/5mL [100mL, 473mL]; **Tab:** 400mg-80mg; **Tab, DS:** 800mg-160mg	(Inj, Sus, Tab) Treatment of urinary tract infection (UTI), pneumocystitis carinii pneumonia (PCP) and enteritis caused by *Shigella.* (Sus, Tab). Treatment of acute exacerbation of chronic bronchitis (AECB), travelers' diarrhea, and acute otitis media.	(Sus, Tab) UTI: 800mg-160mg PO q12h for 10-14 days. Shigellosis/Traveler's Diarrhea: 800mg-160mg PO q12h for 5 days. AECB: 800mg-160mg PO q 12h for 14 days. PCP Treatment: 15-20mg/kg TMP and 75-100mg/kg SMX per 24 hrs given PO q6h for 14-21 days PCP Prophylaxis: 800mg-160mg PO qd. (Inj) Severe UTI: 8-10mg/kg TMP IV given in divided doses q6, 8 or 12h for up to 14 days. PCP Treatment: 15-20mg/kg TMP IV given in divided doses q6-8h for up to 14 days. Shigellosis: 8-10mg/kg TMP IV given in divided doses q6, 8 or 12h for 5 days. (Inj, Sus, Tab) Renal Impairment: CrCl 15-30 mL/min: 50% usual dose. CrCl <15mL/min: Not recommended.	(Sus, Tab) ≥2 mo: UTI/Otitis Media: 4mg/kg TMP and 20mg/kg SMX q12h for 10 days. Shigellosis: 4mg/kg TMP and 20mg/kg SMX q12h for 5 days. PCP Treatment: 15-20mg/kg TMP and 75-100mg/kg SMX/24 hrs given q6h for 14-21 days. PCP Prophylaxis: 150mg/m2/day TMP and 750mg/m2/ day SMX PO given bid, on 3 consecutive days per week. Max: 320mg TMP and 1600mg SMX per day. (Inj) Severe UTI: 8-10mg/kg TMP IV given in divided doses q6, 8 or 12h for up to 14 days. PCP Treatment: 15-20mg/kg TMP IV given in divided doses q6-8h for up to 14 days. Shigellosis: 8-10mg/kg TMP given in divided doses q6, 8 or 12h for 5 days. (Inj, Sus, Tab) Renal Impairment: CrCl 15-30mL/mL/min: 50% usual dose. CrCl <15mL/min: Not recommended.

BRAND NAME (Generic)	DOSAGE FORM/ STRENGTH	INDICATIONS	ADULT DOSE	PEDIATRIC DOSE
Synercid (dalfopristin-quinupristin)	**Inj:** (Dalfopristin-Quinupristin) 350mg-150mg per 500mg vial	Treatment of serious or life-threatening infections associated with vancomycin-resistant *Enterococcus faecium* (VREF) bacteremia and complicated skin and skin structure infections (SSSI) caused by *Staphylococcus aureus* (methicillin susceptible) or *Streptococcus pyogenes.*	VREF: 7.5mg/kg IV q8h. Duration depends on site and severity of infection. Complicated SSSI: 7.5mg/kg IV q12h for at least 7 days. Hepatic Cirrhosis (Child Pugh A or B): May need dose reduction.	≥16 yrs: VREF: 7.5mg/kg IV q8h. Duration depends on site and severity of infection. Complicated SSSI: 7.5mg/kg IV q12h for at least 7 days. Hepatic Cirrhosis (Child Pugh A or B): May need dose reduction.
Vancocin (vancomycin HCl)	**Inj:** 500mg/100mL, 500mg/vial, 1g/vial, 5g/vial, 10g/vial	Treatment of severe infections caused by susceptible strains of methicillin-resistant staphylococci. Indicated for penicillin-allergic patients, those who cannot receive or have failed to respond to other drugs, and for vancomycin-susceptible organisms that are resistant to other antimicrobials.	Usual: 500mg IV q6h or 1g IV q12h. Mild to Moderate Renal Impairment: Initial: ≥15mg/kg/day. Maint: 1.9mg/kg/d. Administer 10mg/min or over at least 60 min, whichever is longer. Renal Dysfunction: Initial: 15mg/kg. Dose is about 15x the GFR in mL/min (refer to table in labeling). Elderly: Require greater dose reduction. Functionally Anephric: Initial: 15mg/kg, then 1.9mg/kg/24hrs. Marked Renal Dysfunction: 250-1000mg once every several days. Anuria: 1000mg every 7-10 days.	Usual: 10mg/kg IV q6h. Infants/Neonates: Initial: 15mg/kg, then 10mg/kg q12h for neonates in the 1st week of life and q8h thereafter until 1 mo of age. Administer over at least 60 min. Renal Dysfunction: Initial: 15mg/kg. Dose is about 15x the GFR in mL/min (refer to table in labeling). Premature Infants: May need to increase dosing intervals.
Vancocin Oral (vancomycin HCl)	**Cap:** 125mg, 250mg	Staphylococcal enterocolitis and antibiotic-associated pseudomembranous colitis caused by *C.difficile.*	500mg-2g/day given tid-qid for 7-10 days.	40mg/kg/day given tid-qid for 7-10 days. Max: 2g/day.
Zyvox (linezolid)	**Inj:** 2mg/mL [100mL, 200mL, 300mL]; **Sus:** 100mg/5mL; **Tab:** 600mg	Vancomycin resistant *Enterococcus faecium* (VRE) infections, nosocomial pneumonia caused by *Staphylococcus aureus* (methicillin-susceptible and-resistant strains) or *Streptococcus pneumoniae* (including multi-drug resistant strains [MDRSP]), complicated skin and skin structure infections (SSSI) including diabetic foot infections without concomitant osteomyelitis caused by *Staphylococcus aureus* (methicillin-susceptible and -resistant strains), *Streptococcus pyogenes,* or *Streptococcus agalactiae,* uncomplicated SSSI caused by *Staphylococcus aureus* (methicillin-susceptible only) or *Streptococcus pyogenes,* community-acquired pneumonia (CAP) caused by *Streptococcus pneumoniae* (MDRSP), including concurrent bacteremia, or *Staphylococcus aureus* (methicillin-susceptible strains only).	Complicated SSSI/CAP/Nosocomial Pneumonia: 600mg IV/PO q12h for 10-14 days. VRE: 600mg IV/PO q12h for 14-28 days. Uncomplicated SSSI: 400mg PO q12h for 10-14 days.	Complicated SSSI/CAP/Nosocomial Pneumonia: Treat for 10-14 days. ≥12 yrs: 600mg IV/PO q12h. Birth-11 yrs: 10mg/kg IV/PO q8h. VRE: Treat for 14-28 days: 10mg/kg IV/PO q8h. Uncomplicated SSSI: Treat for 10-14 days: ≥12 yrs: 600mg PO q12h. 5-11 yrs: 10mg/kg PO q12h. <5 yrs: 10mg/kg PO q8h. Neonates <7 days should be initiated with dosing regimen of 10mg/kg q12h; may increase to 10mg/kg q8h if suboptimal response. All neonatal patients should receive 10mg/kg q8h by 7 days of life.

SYSTEMIC ANTIFUNGALS

GENERIC	BRAND	INDICATION	DOSAGE FORM	DOSAGE
Amphotericin B	Amphocin	Progressive, potentially life-threatening fungal infections: Aspergillosis, cryptococcosis, North American blastomycosis, systemic candidiasis, coccidioidomycosis, histoplasmosis, zygomycosis, sporotrichosis, and infections due to *Conidiobolus* and *Basidiobolus* species.	**Inj:** 50mg	Initial: 0.25mg/kg. Titrate: Increase by 5-10mg/day, depending on cardio-renal status, up to 0.5-0.7mg/kg/day.
Amphotericin B cholesteryl sulfate	Amphotec	Treatment of invasive aspergillosis in patients with renal impairment, unacceptable toxicity, or previous failure to amphotericin deoxycholate.	**Inj:** 50mg, 100mg	3-4mg/kg/day IV at 1mg/kg/hr.
Amphotericin B lipid complex injection	Abelcet	Invasive fungal infections in patients who are refractory to or intolerant of conventional amphotericin B therapy.	**Inj:** 5mg/mL	Single infusion 5mg/kg.
Amphotericin B liposome injection	AmBisome	Treatment of patients with *Aspergillus* species, *Candida* species, and/or *Cryptococcus* species infections refractory to amphotericin B deoxycholate, cryptococcal meningitis in HIV patients, fungal infection in febrile, neutropenic patients, and treatment of visceral leishmaniasis. Empirical therapy for presumed fungal infections in febrile neutropenic patients. Treatment of cryptococcal meningitis in HIV-infected patients.	**Inj:** 50mg	3-6mg/kg/day. Empiric therapy = 3mg/kg/day IV. Systemic infections (*Aspergillus, Candida, Cryptococcus*): 3-5mg/kg/day IV. Cryptococcal Meningitis in HIV: 6mg/kg/day IV. Visceral Leishmaniasis for Immunocompetent patients: 3mg/kg/day on Days 1-5 and 3mg/kg/day on Days 14, 21. Visceral Leishmaniasis in Immunocompromised patients: 4mg/kg/day on Days 1-5 and 4mg/kg/day on Days 10, 17, 24, 31, 38.
Anidulafungin	Eraxis	Treatment of candidemia and other forms of *Candida* infections, esophageal candidiasis.	**Inj:** 50mg, 100mg	Candidemia: LD 200mg on Day 1, MD 100mg x 14d. Esophageal Candidiasis: 100mg qd x 1 day then 50mg qd x 14 days.
Caspofungin Acetate	Cancidas	Treatment of candidemia, esophageal candidiasis, fungal infections in febrile, neutropenic patients, invasive aspergillosis in patients who are refractory to or intolerant of other therapies.	**Inj:** 50mg, 70mg	70mg LD on Day 1 and then 50mg qd. Esophageal candidasis: 50mg qd.
Clotrimazole	Mycelex Troche	Oropharyngeal candidiasis. To prevent oropharyngeal candidiasis in immuno-compromised conditions.	**Loz/Troche:** 10mg	1 troche in mouth 5 times/day for 14 days. Prophylaxis: 1 troche tid.
Fluconazole	Diflucan	Treatment of vaginal, oropharyngeal, esophageal, and systemic candidiasis. Treatment of peritonitis and UTI caused by *Candida*. Treatment of cryptococcal meningitis. Prophylaxis in patients undergoing BMT.	**Inj:** 200mg/100mL, 400mg/200mL; **Sus:** 50mg/5mL, 200mg/5mL [35mL]; **Tab:** 50mg, 100mg, 150mg, 200mg	Vaginal *Candida*: 150mg po x 1 day. All other: 100-200mg/day. Max: 400mg/day.

(Continued)

GENERIC	BRAND	INDICATION	DOSAGE FORM	DOSAGE
Flucytosine	Ancobon	Treatment of septicemia, endocarditis, and urinary tract infections caused by *Candida*. Treatment of meningitis and pulmonary infection caused by *Cryptococcus*.	**Cap:** 250mg, 500mg	50-150mg/kg/day given q6h.
Griseofulvin	Grifulvin V	Treatment of ringworm.	**Sus:** 125mg/5mL [120mL]; **Tab:** 500mg, 250mg	0.5-1g qd.
Griseofulvin	Gris-PEG	Treatment of ringworm.	**Tab (ultramicrosize):** 125mg, 250mg	375mg as a single dose or in divided doses.
Itraconazole	Sporanox	Onychomycosis of the toenail and fingernail, blastomycosis and histoplasmosis. Treatment of aspergillosis if refractory to or intolerant of amphotericin B. (Sol) Treatment of oropharyngeal and esophageal candidiasis.	**Cap:** 100mg; **Inj:** 10mg/mL; **Sol:** 10mg/mL [150mL]	(Cap) Blastomycosis: 200mg once daily (2 capsules). Aspergillosis: 200-400mg. Max: 400mg/day. (Inj): 200mg bid for four doses, followed by 200mg once daily for up to 14 days. (Sol): Swish (10mL at a time) for several seconds and swallow.
Ketoconazole	Nizoral	Candidiasis, chronic mucocutaneous candidiasis, oral thrush, candiduria, blastomycosis, coccidioidomycosis, histoplasmosis, chromomycosis, and paracoccidioidomycosis. Treatment of patients with severe recalcitrant cutaneous dermatophyte infections not responsive to topical therapy or oral griseofulvin. Not for treatment of fungal meningitis.	**Tab:** 200mg	200mg qd. Max: 400mg qd.
Micafungin sodium	Mycamine	Esophageal candidiasis and prophylaxis of *Candida* infection in HSCT patients. Treatment of candidemia, acute disseminated candidiasis, *Candida* peritonitis, and abscesses.	**Inj:** 50mg, 100mg	Treatment of Candidemia, Acute Disseminated Candidiasis, *Candida* Peritonitis and Abscesses: 100mg IV qd (usual range 10-47 days). Treatment of Esophageal Candidiasis: 150mg/day (usual range 10-30 days); Prophylaxis (HSCT): 50mg IV qd (usual range 6-51 days).
Nystatin	Mycostatin	(Cream, Powder) Treatment of cutaneous or mucocutaneous mycotic infections caused by *Candida*.	**Cream:** 100,000 U/g; **Powder:** 100,000 U/g	Powder: Apply to affected area twice daily or as indicated until healing is complete. Cream: Apply to candidal lesions two or three times daily until healing is complete.
Posaconazole	Noxafil	Prophylaxis of invasive *Aspergillus* and *Candida*, oropharyngeal candidiasis, including oropharyngeal candidiasis refractory to itraconazole and/or fluconazole.	**Sus:** 40mg/mL [105mL]	Prophylaxis: 200mg tid. Oropharyngeal Candidiasis: 100mg bid x 1 day, 100mg qd x 13 days. Oropharyngeal Candidiasis refractory to itraconazole and/or fluconazole = 400mg bid.

(Continued)

GENERIC	BRAND	INDICATION	DOSAGE FORM	DOSAGE
Terbinafine HCl	Lamisil	(Tab): Onychomycosis of the toenail or fingernail. (Granules): Tinea capitis in patients ≥4 years old.	**Tab:** 250mg; **Granules:** 125mg/packet and 187.5mg/packet	(Tab) 250mg po qd for 6 weeks for fingernail and 12 weeks for toenail. (Gran) ≤25kg: 125mg/day, 25-35kg: 187.5mg/day, >35kg: 250mg/day. Take for 6 weeks.
Voriconazole	Vfend	Invasive aspergillosis, esophageal candidiasis, serious fungal infections caused by *Scedosporium apiospermum* and *Fusarium* spp. including *Fusarium solani*, candidemia in nonneutropenic patients.	**Inj:** 200mg; **Sus:** 40mg/mL [100mL]; **Tab:** 50mg, 200mg	200mg po q12h. IV LD: 6mg/kg q12h for first 24h. IV MD: 3-4mg/kg q12h.

ANKYLOSING SPONDYLITIS AGENTS

DRUG (BRAND)	HOW SUPPLIED	USUAL DOSE RANGE	MAX DOSE
COX-2 INHIBITOR			
Celecoxib (Celebrex)	**Cap:** 50mg, 100mg, 200mg, 400mg	200mg qd or 100mg bid.	400mg/day with food.
MONOCLONAL ANTIBODIES/TNF-RECEPTOR BLOCKERS			
Infliximab (Remicade)	**Inj:** 100mg [20 mL]	5mg/kg as IV infusion repeat at 2 and 6 wks then every 6 wks thereafter.	20mg/kg.
Adalimumab (Humira)	**Inj:** 40mg/0.8mL	40mg SQ every other wk.	n/a
NSAIDs			
Sulindac (Clinoril)	**Tab:** 150mg, 200mg*	150mg bid with food.	400mg/day with food.
Diclofenac Sodium (Voltaren)	**Tab, Delayed-Release:** 25mg, 50mg, 75mg **Tab, Extended-Release:** 100mg	25mg qid and 25mg qhs prn.	125mg/day.
Indomethacin (Indocin, Indocin SR)	**Cap:** 25mg, 50mg; **Sus:** 25mg/5mL [237]; **Cap, Extended-Release:** 75mg	Take with food. **Cap/Sus:** 25mg PO bid-tid; **ER:** 75mg qd.	**Cap/Sus:** 200mg/day. **ER:** 75mg bid.
Naproxen (EC-Naprosyn, Naprosyn)	**Sus:** 25mg/mL; **Tab:** 250mg, 375mg, 500mg; **Tab, Delayed-Release:** 375mg, 500mg	250mg, 375mg, or 500mg bid; 375mg or 500mg bid.	1500mg/day.
Naproxen sodium (Anaprox)	**Tab:** 275mg	275mg bid or 550mg bid.	1650mg/day.
(Anaprox DS)	**Tab:** 550mg*	275mg bid or 550mg bid.	1650mg/day.
(Naprelan)	**Tab, Extended-Release:** 375mg, 500mg, 750mg	750mg-1g qd.	1500mg/day.
SALICYLATE			
Aspirin (Genuine Bayer Aspirin, Bayer Extra Strength)	**Tab:** 325mg; **Tab, Extra-Strength:** 500mg	Up to 4g/day in divided doses.	4g/day.
(Ecotrin)	**Tab, Delayed-Release:** 81mg, 325mg, 500mg	Up to 4g/day in divided doses.	4g/day.
TNF-RECEPTOR BLOCKER			
Etanercept (Enbrel)	**Inj:** 25mg [vial], 50mg/mL [syringe]	50mg SQ per wk, given as one SQ injection.	50mg/wk.

*Scored.

BONE MINERAL DENSITY CLASSIFICATION/TESTS

World Health Organization (WHO) Definition of Osteoporosis	
Normal	Bone mineral density within 1 standard deviation (SD) of the young adult mean (T-score ≥ -1.0)
Osteopenia (low bone mass)	Bone mineral density between 1.0 and 2.5 SD below the young adult mean ($-2.5 <$ T-score < -1.0)
Osteoporosis	Bone mineral density 2.5 SD or more below the young adult mean (T-score ≤ -2.5)
Note: The definitions above should not be applied to premenopausal women, men <50 years of age, and children.	

Bone mineral density (BMD) tests

- BMD tests provide a measurement of T-score for bone density at hip and spine to:
  - —Establish and confirm a diagnosis of osteoporosis
  - —Predict future fracture risk
  - —Measure response to osteoporosis treatment
- BMD is measured in grams of mineral per square centimeter scanned (g/cm^2) and compared to the expected BMD for the patient's age and sex (Z-score) or compared with "normal adults" of the same sex (T-score).
- The difference between the patient's score and the optimal BMD is expressed in standard deviations (SD) above and below the mean. Usually 1 SD equals about 10-15% of the bone density value in g/cm^2.
- Negative values for T-score, such as -1.5, -2, or -2.5, indicate low bone mass.
- The greater the negative score, the greater the risk of fracture.

DIETARY CALCIUM INTAKE

Recommended Calcium Intakes*

Age	Daily Intake (mg)
Birth-6 months	210
6 months-1 year	270
1-3 years	500
4-8 years	800
9-13 years	1300
14-18 years	1300
19-30 years	1000
31-50 years	1000
51-70 years	1200
70 years or older	1200
Pregnant or Lactating	
14-18 years	1300
19-50 years	1000

*Source: National Institute of Arthritis and Musculoskeletal and Skin Diseases (NIAMS); National Institutes of Health

Estimating Daily Dietary Calcium Intake

Step 1: Estimate calcium intake from calcium-rich foods.*

Product	Servings/Day	Calcium/Serving (mg)		Calcium (mg)
Milk (8 oz)	______	× 300	=	______
Yogurt (8 oz)	______	× 400	=	______
Cheese (1 oz, or 1 cubic inch)	______	× 200	=	______
Fortified foods or juices	______	× 80-1000**	=	______

Step 2: Total from above + 250 mg for nondairy sources = total dietary calcium.

* About 75-80% of the calcium consumed in American diets is from dairy products.
** Calcium content of fortified foods varies.

Factors related to vitamin D that may affect calcium absorption:

- National Osteoporosis Foundation recommends an intake of 800 to 1000 International Units (IU) of vitamin D_3 per day for adults over age 50
- Desired level for the average adult's serum 25(OH)D concentration is 30 ng/mL (75 nmol/L) or higher
- Safe upper limit for vitamin D intake for normal adult population was set at 2000 IU per day in 1997
- Patients with malabsorption (eg, celiac disease) or chronic renal insufficiency, or those who are housebound, chronically ill, or have limited sun exposure, may need vitamin D supplements

Source: National Institute of Arthritis and Musculoskeletal and Skin Diseases (NIAMS), National Institutes of Health.

GOUT AGENTS

DRUG (BRAND)	HOW SUPPLIED	USUAL DOSE RANGE	MAX DOSE
ALKALINIZING AGENT			
Citric acid/ Potassium citrate (Polycitra)	**Packet:** 1002mg-3300mg/pack [100[S]]; **Sol:** (Citric Acid-Potassium Citrate) 334mg-550mg/5mL [480mL]	15mL or 1 packet qid, pc and hs. Dilute in 6 oz of water or juice.	
CORTICOSTEROIDS			
Hydrocortisone sodium succinate (A-Hydrocort)	**Inj:** 100mg/2mL	**Acute Gout:** Individualized dosing. May repeat dose at intervals of 2,4, or 6 hours based on patient response.	
Hydrocortisone (Cortef)	**Tab:** 5mg, 10mg, 20mg	**Acute Gout:** Individualized dosing.	
Methylpredni-solone (Medrol)	**Tab:** 4mg, 8mg, 16mg, 24mg, 32mg	**Acute Gout:** Individualized dosing.	
Prednisone	**Tab:** 1mg, 2.5mg, 5mg, 10mg, 20mg, 25mg, 50mg	**Acute Gout:** Individualized dosing.	
NSAIDs			
Indomethacin (Indocin)	**Cap:** 25mg, 50mg; **Sus:** 25mg/5mL [237mL]	**Acute Gout:** 50mg PO tid until pain is tolerable, then d/c.	
Naproxen (Anaprox)	**Tab:** 275mg	**Acute Gout:** 825mg followed by 275mg q8h.	
(Anaprox DS)	550mg*	**Acute Gout:** 825mg followed by 275mg q8h.	
(Naprelan)	**Tab, Controlled-Release:** 375mg, 500mg, 750mg	**Acute Gout:** 1-1.5g qd x 1 day, then 1g qd until attack subsides.	1.5g/day.
(Naprosyn)	**Sus:** 25mg/mL; Tab: 250mg*, 375mg, 500mg*	**Acute Gout:** 750mg followed by 250mg q8h until attack subsides.	1500mg/day.
Sulindac (Clinoril)	**Tab:** 150mg, 200mg*	**Acute Gout:** 200mg bid, usually for 7 days.	400mg/day
PHENANTHRENE DERIVATIVE			
Colchicine	**Tab:** 0.6mg	**Acute Gout:** 0.6-1.2mg, then 0.6mg/hr or 1.2mg q2h until pain relieved or diarrhea ensues (wait 3 days between courses). **Prophylaxis:** <1attack/yr: 0.6mg/day given 3-4x/wk; >1 attack/year, 0.6mg qd.	4-8mg/acute
URICOSURIC AGENTS			
Probenecid	**Tab:** 500mg	**Initial:** 250mg bid x 1 wk **Maint:** 500mg bid. **Titrate:** May increase by 500mg every 4 wks.	2g/day.
Sulfinpyrazone	**Tab:** 100mg, 200mg	**Initial:** 100-200mg bid x 1 wk. **Maint:** 200mg bid.	800mg/day.
XANTHINE OXIDASE INHIBITORS			
Allopurinol (Zyloprim)	**Tab:** 100mg*, 300mg*	**Mild Gout: Usual:** 200-300mg/day. **Moderately-Severe Gout: Usual:** 400-600mg/day.	800mg/day.
Febuxostat (Uloric)	**Tab:** 40mg, 80mg	**Initial:** 40mg qd. Increase to 80mg qd if serum uric acid >6mg/dL after 2 weeks.	80mg/day.
COMBINATION			
Colchicine/ Probenecid	**Tab:** (Colchicine-Probenecid) 0.5mg-500mg	1 tab qd x 1 wk, then 1 tab bid. **Titrate:** May increase by 1 tab/day every 4 wks.	4 tabs/day.

*Scored.

OSTEOARTHRITIS AGENTS

DRUG (BRAND)	HOW SUPPLIED	USUAL DOSE RANGE	MAX DOSE
COX-2 INHIBITOR			
Celecoxib (Celebrex)	**Cap:** 50mg, 100mg, 200mg, 400mg	200mg qd or 100mg bid.	
NSAIDs			
Diclofenac Epolamine (Flector)	**Patch:** 180mg [5[s]]	Apply 1 patch to most painful area bid.	1 patch bid.
Diclofenac sodium (Voltaren)	**Tab, Delayed-Release:** 25mg, 50mg, 75mg	50mg bid-tid or 75mg bid.	150mg/day.
(Voltaren-XR)	**Tab, Extended-Release:** 100mg	100mg qd.	100mg/day.
(Voltaren Gel)	**Gel:** 1%	Measure onto enclosed dosing card to appropriate 2g or 4g line. Lower Extremities: Apply 4g to affected foot, knee, or ankle qid. Upper Extremities: Apply 2g to affected hand, elbow, or wrist qid.	Lower Extremities: 16g/day to any single joint. Upper Extremities: 8g/day to any single joint. 32g/day over all affected joints.
Diflunisal (Dolobid)	**Tab:** 500mg	250-500mg bid.	1500mg/day.
Etodolac	**Cap:** 200mg, 300mg; **Tab:** 400mg, 500mg	300mg bid-tid or 400-500mg bid.	1200mg/day.
(Etodolac XR)	**Tab, Delayed-Release:** 400mg, 500mg, 600mg	400-1000mg qd.	1200mg/day.
Fenoprofen (Nalfon)	**Cap:** 200mg; **Tab:** 600mg	300-600mg tid-qid.	3200mg/day.
Flurbiprofen (Ansaid)	**Tab:** 50mg, 100mg	200-300mg/day given bid, tid or qid.	300mg/day or 100mg/dose.
Ketoprofen	**Cap:** 25mg, 50mg, 75mg; **Cap, Extended-Release:** 100mg, 150mg, 200mg	75mg tid or 50mg qid. ER: 200mg qd.	300mg/day. ER: 200mg/day.
Ibuprofen (Motrin, Motrin IB)	**Sus:** 100mg/5mL [120mL, 480mL]; **Tab:** 300mg, 400mg, 600mg, 800mg **Tab:** 200mg	300mg qid or 400mg, 600mg or 800mg tid-qid. (Motrin IB) 200mg q4-6h. 400mg with meals/milk.	3200mg/day. 1200mg/day. (Motrin IB)
Meclofenamate	**Cap:**50mg, 100mg	200-400mg/day in 3-4 divided doses.	400mg/day.
Meloxicam (Mobic)	**Sus:** 7.5mg/5mL **Tab:** 7.5mg, 15mg	7.5mg qd.	15mg/day.
Nabumetone	**Tab:** 500mg, 750mg	1000mg qd.	2000mg/day.
Naproxen (Naprosyn, EC-Naprosyn)	**Sus:** 25mg/mL **Tab:** 250mg, 375mg, 500mg; **Tab, Delayed-Release:** 375mg, 500mg	250, 375, or 500mg bid.	1500mg/day.
Naproxen sodium (Anaprox)	**Tab:** 275mg	275mg bid.	1650mg/day.
(Anaprox DS)	**Tab:** 550mg*	550mg bid.	1650mg/day.
(Naprelan)	**Tab, Extended-Release:** 375mg, 500mg, 750mg	750mg-1g qd.	1.5g/day.
Oxaprozin (Daypro)	**Tab:** 600mg*	1200mg qd.	1800mg/day in divided doses (not to exceed 26mg/kg/day).
Piroxicam (Feldene)	**Cap:** 10mg, 20mg	20mg qd or 10mg bid.	
Sulindac (Clinoril)	**Tab:** 150mg, 200mg	150mg bid with food.	400mg/day with food.
Tolmetin (Tolectin)	**Cap:** (DS) 400mg; **Tab:** 200mg*, 600mg	400mg tid.	1800mg/day.

(Continued)

DRUG (BRAND)	HOW SUPPLIED	USUAL DOSE RANGE	MAX DOSE
NON-SALICYLATE ANALGESIC			
Acetaminophen (Tylenol Arthritis Pain)	**Tab, Extended-Release:** 650mg	1300mg q8h.	4g/day (6 tabs/day)
SALICYLATE			
Aspirin (Genuine Bayer Aspirin, Bayer Extra Strength, Ecotrin)	**Tab:** 325mg Tab, Extra Strength: **Tab, Delayed-Release:** 81mg, 325mg, 500mg	Up to 3g/day in divided doses.	4g/day.
Salsalate (Salflex)	**Tab:** 500mg, 750mg*	1000mg tid or 1500mg bid.	
Choline Magnesium Trisalicylate (Trilisate)	**Liq:** 500mg/5mL; **Tab:** 500mg*, 750mg*, 1000mg*	1500mg bid.	3g/d.
NSAID COMBINATION			
Diclofenac sodium/Misoprostol (Arthrotec)	**Tab:** 50mg-0.2mg, 75mg-0.2mg	50mg tid. Do not crush, chew or divide.	150mg/day.
MISCELLANEOUS			
Botanical/Mineral substances (Traumeel Inj)	**Inj:** 2.2mL amps [10s]	1 amp qd for acute disorders or 1-2 amps 1-3 times weekly. May administer IV, IM, SQ, or intradermally.	NA
Flavocoxid (Limbrel)	**Cap:** 250mg, 500mg	250-500mg q12h.	500-1000mg/day.
Hyaluronan (Euflexxa)	**Inj:** 1% [2mL]	Inject 2mL intra-articularly into the knee weekly for 3 wks. Total 3 injections.	3 injections.
(Hyalgan)	**Inj:** 2mL	2mL by intra-articular injection once a wk. Some patients may experience benefit with 3 injections given at weekly intervals.	5 injections.
(Orthovisc)	**Inj:** 30mg/2mL	30mg intra-articularly once a wk. Total 3-4 injections.	3-4 injections.
(Supartz)	**Inj:** 2.5mL	2.5mL by intra-articular injection once a wk. Total 5 injections. Some patients may experience benefit with 3 injections given at weekly intervals.	5 injections.
Hylan G-F 20 (Synvisc)	**Inj:** 8mg/mL	Intra-articular injection once weekly (one wk apart). Total 3 injections.	3 injections.

*Scored

Osteoporosis Agents

DRUG (BRAND)	INDICATIONS	HOW SUPPLIED	DOSAGE
BISPHOSPHONATES & COMBINATIONS			
Alendronate Sodium (Fosamax)	Treatment and prevention of osteoporosis in postmenopausal women. Treatment to increase bone mass in men with osteoporosis. Treatment of glucocorticoid-induced osteoporosis.	Sol: 70mg [75mL]; Tab: 5mg, 10mg, 35mg, 40mg, 70mg	Osteoporosis: Treatment: 70mg once weekly or 10mg qd. Prevention: 35mg once weekly or 5mg qd. Increase bone mass in men with osteoporosis: 70mg once weekly or 10mg qd. Glucocorticoid-Induced: 5mg qd; 10mg qd for post-menopausal women not on estrogen.Take at least 30 min before the first food, beverage (other than plain water), or medication (Take tabs with 6-8 oz plain water or 2oz with oral sol). Do not lie down for at least 30 min and until after 1st food of day.
Alendronate Sodium/ Cholecalciferol (Fosamax Plus D)	Treatment of osteoporosis in postmenopausal women. Treatment to increase bone mass in men with osteoporosis.	Tab: (Alendronate Sodium-Cholecalciferol) 70mg-2800 IU, 70mg-5600 IU	Adults: 1 tab (70mg/5600 IU or 70mg/2800 IU) once weekly. Take at least 30 min before 1st food, beverage (other than plain water), or medication. Do not lie down for at least 30 min and until after 1st food of day.
Ibandronate Sodium (Boniva)	(Inj) Treatment of osteoporosis in postmenopausal women. (PO) Treatment and prevention of postmenopausal osteoporosis.	Inj: 3mg/3mL; Tab: 2.5mg, 150mg	Inj: 3mg IV over 15-30 sec every 3 months. PO: 2.5mg qd or 150mg once monthly. Swallow whole with 6-8 oz plain water. Do not lie down for 60 min after dose. Take at least 60 min before 1st food, drink (other than plain water), medication, or supplementation.
Risedronate Sodium (Actonel)	Prevention and treatment of osteoporosis in postmenopausal women, glucocorticoid-induced osteoporosis in men and women. Increase bone mass in men with osteoporosis.	Tab: 5mg, 30mg, 35mg, 75mg, 150mg	Postmenopausal Osteoporosis Prevention/Treatment: 5mg qd or 35mg once weekly or 75mg on 2 consecutive days each month or 150mg once a month. Glucocorticoid-Induced Osteoporosis: 5mg qd. Increase Bone Mass in Men with Osteoporosis: 35mg once weekly. Take at least 30 min before the first food or drink of the day other than water. Swallow tab in upright position with 6-8 oz of plain water. Do not lie down for 30 min after dose.
Risedronate Sodium/ Calcium Carbonate (Actonel with Calcium)	Treatment and prevention of postmenopausal osteoporosis.	Tab: (Risedronate Sodium) 35mg; Tab: (Calcium Carbonate) 1250mg	Risedronate: 35mg once weekly (Day 1 of 7-day treatment cycle). Take at least 30 min before 1st food or drink of day other than water. Swallow tab in upright position with 6-8oz of plain water. Do not lie down for 30 min after dose. Calcium: 1250mg qd with food on each of remaining 6 days (Days 2-7 of the 7-day treatment cycle).
Zoledronic Acid (Reclast)	Treatment of osteoporosis in postmenopausal women and to reduce incidence of new clinical fractures in patients at high risk of fractures. Treatment to increase bone mass in men with osteoporosis. Treatment and prevention of glucocorticoid-induced osteoporosis in men and women.	Sol: 5mg/100mL [100mL]	5mg IV once a year. Infuse for >15 min at constant rate. Hydrate prior to administration.

DRUG (BRAND)	INDICATIONS	HOW SUPPLIED	DOSAGE
HORMONE THERAPY			
Conjugated Estrogens (Premarin Tabs)	Prevention of postmenopausal osteoporosis.	Tab: 0.3mg, 0.45mg, 0.625mg, 0.9mg, 1.25mg	0.3mg qd continuous or cyclically (eg, 25 days on, 5 days off).
Conjugated Estrogens/ Medroxyprogesterone Acetate (Premphase)	For prevention of osteoporosis in women with intact uterus.	Tab: 0.625mg (Estrogens, Conjugated) and 0.625mg-5mg (Estrogens, Conjugated-Medroxyprogesterone)	0.625mg tab qd on Days 1-14 and 0.625mg-5mg tab qd on Days 15-28. Re-evaluate after 3-6 months.
Conjugated Estrogens/ Medroxyprogesterone Acetate (Prempro)	Prevention of postmenopausal osteoporosis in women with intact uterus.	Tab: (Estrogens, Conjugated-Medroxyprogesterone) 0.3mg-1.5mg, 0.45mg-1.5mg, 0.625mg-2.5mg, 0.625mg-5mg	Initial: 0.3mg-1.5mg qd. Adjust dose based on response. Re-evaluate after 3-6 months.
Estradiol (Alora)	Prevention of postmenopausal osteoporosis.	Patch: 0.025mg/24 hrs, 0.05mg/24 hrs [8s 24s], 0.075mg/24 hrs, 0.1mg/24 hrs [8s]	Apply to lower abdomen, upper quadrant of the buttocks or the hip; avoid breasts and waistline. Rotate application sites. Osteoporosis: Apply 0.025mg/day twice weekly. Titrate: May increase depending on bone mineral density and adverse events.
Estradiol (Climara)	Prevention of postmenopausal osteoporosis.	Patch: 0.025mg/day, 0.0375mg/day, 0.05mg/day, 0.06mg/day, 0.075mg/day, 0.1mg/day [4s]	Apply 1 patch weekly to lower abdomen or upper area of buttocks (avoid breasts and waistline). Rotate application sites. Minimum Effective Dose: 0.025mg/day once weekly. Re-evaluate after 3-6 months.
Estradiol (Estrace)	Prevention of osteoporosis.	Tab: 0.5mg*, 1mg*, 2mg* *scored	0.5mg qd cyclically (23 days on and 5 days off).
Estradiol (Estraderm)	Prevention of postmenopausal osteoporosis.	Patch: 0.05mg/24 hrs, 0.1mg/24 hrs [1s, 8s, 48s]	Initial: 0.05mg/day. May give continuously without intact uterus. May give cyclically (3 weeks on, 1 week off) with intact uterus. Apply to clean, dry area on trunk of body. Do not apply to breast or waistline. Replace twice weekly. Rotate application site.
Estradiol (Menostar)	Prevention of postmenopausal osteoporosis.	Patch: 14mcg/day [4s]	Apply 1 patch weekly to lower abdomen (avoid breasts, waistline, and areas where sitting would dislodge the patch). Rotate application sites.
Estradiol (Vivelle, Vivelle-Dot)	Prevention of postmenopausal osteoporosis.	Patch: (Vivelle) 0.05mg/day, 0.1mg/day [8s, 48s]; (Vivelle-Dot) 0.025mg/day, 0.0375mg/day, 0.05mg/day, 0.075mg/day, 0.1mg/day [8s, 24s]	Minimum Effective Dose: 0.025mg/day twice weekly. Apply to clean, dry area of the trunk; avoid breasts and waistline. Rotate sites; allow 1 week between same site. Without intact uterus, may give continuously; with intact uterus, may give cyclically (3 weeks on, 1 week off) with a progestin.
Estradiol/Levonorgestrel (Climara Pro)	Prevention of postmenopausal osteoporosis.	Patch: (Estradiol-Levonorgestrel): 0.045mg-0.015mg/day [4s]	Apply 1 patch weekly to lower abdomen (avoid breasts and waistline). Rotate application site; allow 1 week between same site. Re-evaluate periodically (3-6 month intervals).
Estradiol/Norethindrone (Activella)	Prevention of postmenopausal osteoporosis in women with intact uterus.	Tab: (Estradiol-Norethindrone) 1mg-0.5mg, 0.5mg-0.1mg	1 tab qd.

DRUG (BRAND)	**INDICATIONS**	**HOW SUPPLIED**	**DOSAGE**
HORMONE THERAPY *(Continued)*			
Estradiol/Norgestimate (Prefest)	Prevention of postmenopausal osteoporosis in women with intact uterus.	Tab: (Estradiol) 1mg and (Estradiol-Norgestimate) 1mg-0.09mg	1 estradiol (pink color) tab for three days followed by 1 estradiol-norgestimate (white color) tab for three days. Repeat regimen continuously.
Estropipate (Ogen)	Prevention of postmenopausal osteoporosis.	Tab: 0.625mg* (0.75mg estropipate), 1.25mg* (1.5mg estropipate), 2.5mg* (3mg estropipate), 5mg (6mg estropipate) *scored	0.75mg (as estropipate) qd for 25 days of 31-day cycle.
Estropipate (Ortho-Est)	Prevention of osteoporosis.	Tab: 0.625mg* (0.75mg estropipate), 1.25mg* (1.5mg estropipate) *scored	0.75mg (as estropipate) qd for 25 days of a 31-day cycle.
Ethinyl Estradiol/ Norethindrone (Femhrt)	Prevention of postmenopausal osteoporosis in women with intact uterus.	Tab: (Ethinyl Estradiol-Norethindrone) 2.5mcg-0.5mg, 5mcg-1mg	1 tab qd. Assess response by measuring bone mineral density.
MISCELLANEOUS			
Calcitonin-Salmon (Miacalcin)	Treatment of postmenopausal osteoporosis in females >5 yrs postmenopause.	Inj: 200 IU/mL; Nasal Spray: 200 IU/inh [2mL 2s]	(Inj) 100 IU IM/SQ every other day. If >2mL, use IM injection. (Spray) 200 IU qd intranasally. Alternate nostrils daily. Take with supplemental calcium and vitamin D for postmenopausal osteoporosis.
Calcitonin-Salmon (Fortical)	Treatment of postmenopausal osteoporosis in females >5 yrs postmenopause in conjunction with an adequate calcium and vitamin D intake.	Nasal Spray: 200 IU/inh	200 IU qd intranasally. Alternate nostrils daily.
Raloxifene (Evista)	Treatment and prevention of osteoporosis in postmenopausal women.	Tab: 60mg	60mg qd.
Teriparatide (Forteo)	Treatment of postmenopausal women with osteoporosis who are at high risk for fracture. To increase bone mass in men with primary or hypogonadal osteoporosis who are at high risk for fracture.	Inj: 250mcg/mL [2.4mL, 3mL pen]	20mcg qd SQ into thigh or abdominal wall. Administer initially under circumstances where patient can sit or lie down if symptoms of orthostatic hypotension occur. Discard pen after 28 days. Use for >2 yrs is not recommended.

RHEUMATOID ARTHRITIS AGENTS

DRUG (Brand)	**HOW SUPPLIED**	**USUAL DOSE RANGE**	**MAX DOSE**
5-AMINOSALICYLIC ACID DERIVATIVE			
Sulfasalazine (Azulfidine EN)	**Tab, Delayed-Release:** 500mg	1g bid.	3g/day.
COPPER CHELATING AGENT			
Penicillamine (Cuprimine, Depen)	**Cap:** (Cuprimine) 250mg; **Tab:** (Depen) 250mg*	500-750mg/day.	1.5g/day.
COX-2 INHIBITOR			
Celecoxib (Celebrex)	**Cap:** 50, 100mg, 200mg, 400mg	100-200mg bid.	
DIHYDROFOLIC ACID REDUCTASE INHIBITOR			
Methotrexate sodium (Trexall)	**Inj:** 25mg/mL; **Tab:** 2.5mg, 5mg, 7.5mg, 10mg, 15mg	7.5mg once weekly.	20mg/wk.
GOLD AGENT			
Auranofin (Ridaura)	**Cap:** 3mg	6mg qd or 3mg bid.	9mg/day.
IMMUNOSUPPRESSANTS			
Azathioprine (Imuran)	**Tab:** 50mg*; **Inj:** 100mg/20mL	**Initial:** 1mg/kg/day given qd-bid. **Titrate:** Increase by 0.5mg/kg/day after 6-8 wks, then at 4 wk intervals.	2.5mg/kg/day.
Cyclosporine (Neoral)	**Cap:** 25mg, 100mg; **Sol:** 100mg/mL [50mL]	**Initial:** 1.25mg/kg bid. **Titrate:** Increase by 0.5-0.75mg/kg/day after 8 wks, again after 12 wks. D/C if no benefit by wk 16.	4mg/kg/day.
INTERLEUKIN-1 RECEPTOR ANTAGONIST			
Anakinra (Kineret)	**Inj:** 100mg/0.67mL	100mg SQ qd.	
MONOCLONAL ANTIBODIES/CD20-BLOCKER			
Rituximab (Rituxan)	**Inj:** 10mg/mL	Two-1000mg IV infusions separated by 2 wks, with MTX.	400mg/hr infusion rate
MONOCLONAL ANTIBODIES/TNF-BLOCKERS			
Adalimumab (Humira)	**Inj:** 40mg/0.8mL	40mg SQ every other wk.	40mg every week w/o MTX.
Infliximab (Remicade)	**Inj:** 100mg/20mL	3mg/kg IV infusion repeat at 2 and 6 wks. **Maint:** 3mg/kg every 8 wks.	10mg/kg or every 4 wks.
NONSTEROIDAL ANTI-INFLAMMATORY DRUGS (NSAIDs)			
Diclofenac (Voltaren XR)	**Tab, Delayed-Release:** (Voltaren) 25mg, 50mg, 75mg; **Tab, Extended-Release:** (Voltaren-XR) 100mg	50mg tid-qid or 75mg bid. **ER:** 100mg qd.	225mg/day. **ER:** 200mg/day.
Diflunisal (Dolobid)	**Tab:** 500mg	250-500mg bid.	1500mg/day.
Etodolac	**Cap:** 200mg, 300mg **Tab:** 400mg, 500mg	300mg bid-tid or 400-500mg bid.	1000mg/day.
(Etodolac XR)	**Tab, Extended-Release:** 400mg, 500mg, 600mg	400-1000mg qd.	1200mg/day.
Fenoprofen (Nalfon)	**Cap:** 200mg; **Tab:** 600mg	300-600mg tid-qid.	3200mg/day.
Flurbiprofen (Ansaid)	**Tab:** 50mg, 100mg	200-300mg/day bid, tid or qid.	300mg/day 100mg/dose.

(Continued)

DRUG (Brand)	HOW SUPPLIED	USUAL DOSE RANGE	MAX DOSE
NONSTEROIDAL ANTI-INFLAMMATORY DRUGS (NSAIDs) *(Continued)*			
Ibuprofen (Motrin)	**Sus:** 100mg/5mL; **Tab:** 300mg, 400mg, 600mg, 800mg	300mg qid or 400mg, 600mg or 800mg tid-qid.	3200mg/day.
(Motrin IB)	**Tab:** 200mg	200mg q4-6h. 400mg if no response.	1200mg/day.
Ketoprofen	**Cap:** 25mg, 50mg, 75mg; **Cap, Extended-Release:** 100mg, 150mg, 200mg	75mg tid or 50mg qid. **ER:** 200mg qd	300mg/day. **ER:** 200mg/day
Meclofenamate	**Cap:** 50mg, 100mg	200-400mg/day in 3-4 divided doses.	400mg/day.
Meloxicam (Mobic)	**Sus:** 7.5mg/5mL; **Tab:** 7.5mg, 15mg	7.5mg qd.	15mg/day.
Nabumetone (Relafen)	**Tab:** 500mg, 750mg	1000mg qd.	2000mg/day.
Naproxen (Anaprox DS)	**Tab:** 275mg, 550mg*	275mg bid or 550mg bid.	1650mg/day.
(Naprelan)	**Tab, Extended-Release:** 375mg, 500mg, 750mg	750mg-1g qd.	1.5g/day.
(Naprosyn)	**Sus:** 25mg/mL; **Tab:** 250mg*, 375mg, 500mg*; **Tab, Delayed-Release:** (EC-Naprosyn) 375mg, 500mg	250, 375, or 500mg bid (EC-Naprosyn) 375 or 500mg bid.	1500mg/day.
Oxaprozin (Daypro)	**Tab:** 600mg*	1200mg qd.	1800mg/day.
Piroxicam (Feldene)	**Cap:** 10mg, 20mg	20mg qd or 10mg bid.	20mg/day.
Sulindac (Clinoril)	**Tab:** 150mg, 200mg*	150mg bid.	400mg/day.
Tolmetin (Tolectin)	**Cap:** (DS) 400mg; **Tab:** 200mg*, 600mg	200-600mg tid.	1800mg/day.
NSAID/PROSTAGLANDIN E_1 ANALOGUE			
Diclofenac/Misoprostol (Arthrotec)	**Tab:** (Diclofenac-Misoprostol) 50mg-0.2mg, 75mg-0.2mg	50mg tid-qid.	**Diclofenac:** 225mg/day **Misoprostol:** 800mcg/day 200mcg/dose
PYRIMIDINE SYNTHESIS INHIBITOR			
Leflunomide (Arava)	**Tab:** 10mg, 20mg, 100mg	**Load:** 100mg qd for 3 days. **Maint:** 20mg/day.	20mg/day
SALICYLATE			
Aspirin (Bayer Aspirin)	**Tab:** (Genuine Bayer Aspirin) 325mg **Tab:** (Bayer Extra Strength) 500mg	**Initial:** 3g/day in divided doses.	4g/day.
(Ecotrin)	**Tab, Delayed-Release:** 81mg, 325mg, 500mg	3g qd in divided doses.	4g/day.
Choline Magnesium Trisalicylate	500mg,* 750mg,* 1000mg*	1500mg bid.	3g/d.
SELECTIVE COSTIMULATION MODULATOR			
Abatacept (Orencia)	**Inj:** 250mg	**Initial:** <60kg: 500mg; 60-100kg: 750mg; >100kg: 1g. **Maint:** Give at 2 and 4 wks after initial infusion, then q 4 wks thereafter.	
TNF-RECEPTOR BLOCKER			
Etanercept (Enbrel)	**Inj:** 25mg [vial], 50mg/mL [syringe]	50mg SQ per wk.	50mg/week.
MISCELLANEOUS			
Hydroxychloroquine (Plaquenil)	**Tab:** 200mg	**Initial:** 400-600mg qd. **Maint:** After 4-12 wks, 200-400mg qd with food or milk.	

*scored

GYNECOLOGICAL ANTI-INFECTIVES

DRUG	CLASS	FORMULATION	ROUTE	RECOMMENDED DOSAGE
ANTIBACTERIALS				
Clindamycin				
Cleocin Vaginal, Clindamax	RX	**Cream:** 2%	Vaginal	**Bacterial Vaginosis: Adults:** 1 applicatorful qhs x 3-7 days (non-pregnant) or x 7 days (2nd or 3rd trimester).
Cleocin Vaginal Ovules	RX	**Sup:** 100mg	Vaginal	**Bacterial Vaginosis: Adults:** 1 sup qhs x 3 days (non-pregnant).
Clindesse	RX	**Cream:** 2%	Vaginal	**Bacterial Vaginosis: Adults:** 1 applicatorful once (non-pregnant).
Metronidazole				
Flagyl	RX	**Cap:** 375mg **Tab:** 250mg, 500mg	Oral	**Trichomoniasis: Adults:** 375mg bid or 250mg tid x 7 days. **Alternate Regimen (Tab):** If non-pregnant, 2g as single or divided dose. Contraindicated in 1st trimester.
Flagyl ER	RX	**Tab, ER:** 750mg	Oral	**Bacterial Vaginosis: Adults:** 750mg qd x 7 days. Contraindicated in 1st trimester.
MetroGel Vaginal	RX	**Gel:** 0.75%	Vaginal	**Bacterial Vaginosis: Adults:** 1 applicatorful qd-bid x 5 days (non-pregnant).
Vandazole	RX	**Gel:** 0.75%	Vaginal	**Bacterial Vaginosis: Adults:** 1 applicatorful qd-bid x 5 days (non-pregnant).
ANTIFUNGALS: CANDIDIASIS TREATMENT				
Butoconazole				
Gynazole-1	RX	**Cream:** 2%	Vaginal	**Adults:** 1 applicatorful single dose.
Clotrimazole				
Mycelex-3	OTC	**Cream:** 2%	Vaginal	**Adults/Pediatrics ≥12 yrs:** 1 applicatorful qhs x 3 days.
Mycelex-7	OTC	**Cream:** 1%	Vaginal	**Adults/Pediatrics ≥12 yrs:** 1 applicatorful qhs x 7 days.
Mycelex-7 Combination Pack	OTC	**Cream:** 1% + **Sup:** 100mg	Vaginal	**Adults/Pediatrics ≥12 yrs:** 1 sup qhs x 7 days. Apply cream externally qd-bid up to 7 days prn.
Gyne-Lotrimin 3	OTC	**Cream:** 2% **Sup:** 200mg	Vaginal	**Adults/Pediatrics ≥12 yrs:** 1 applicatorful or 1 sup qhs x 3 days.
Gyne-Lotrimin 3 Combination Pack	OTC	**Cream:** 1% + **Sup:** 200mg	Vaginal	**Adults/Pediatrics ≥12 yrs:** 1 sup qhs x 3 days. Apply cream externally qd-bid prn.
Gyne-Lotrimin	OTC	**Cream:** 1% + **Sup:** 100mg	Vaginal	**Adults/Pediatrics ≥12 yrs:** 1 applicatorful or 1 sup qhs x 7 days.
Gyne-Lotrimin Combination Pack	OTC	**Cream:** 1% + **Sup:** 100mg	Vaginal	**Adults/Pediatrics ≥12 yrs:** 1 sup qhs x 7 days. Apply cream externally qd-bid prn.
Fluconazole				
Diflucan	RX	**Tab:** 150mg	Oral	**Adults:** 150mg single dose.
Miconazole				
Monistat 1 Combination Pack	OTC	**Cream:** 2% + **Sup:** 1200mg	Vaginal	**Adults/Pediatrics ≥12 yrs:** 1 sup single dose. Apply cream externally bid up to 7 days prn.
Monistat 3	OTC	**Cream:** 4%	Vaginal	**Adults/Pediatrics ≥12 yrs:** 1 applicatorful qhs x 3 days.
Monistat 3 Combination Pack	OTC	**Cream:** 2% + **Sup:** 200mg, **Cream:** 4% + **(External) Cream:** 2%	Vaginal	**Adults/Pediatrics ≥12 yrs:** 1 sup or applicatorful qhs x 3 days. Apply cream bid externally prn x 7 days.

(Continued)

DRUG	CLASS	FORMULATION	ROUTE	RECOMMENDED DOSAGE
ANTIFUNGALS: CANDIDIASIS TREATMENT *(Continued)*				
Monistat 7	OTC	**Cream:** 2%	Vaginal	**Adults/Pediatrics ≥12 yrs:** 1 applicatorful qhs x 7 days.
Monistat 7 Combination Pack	OTC	**Cream:** 2% + **Sup:** 100mg, **Cream:** 2% + **(External) Cream:** 2%	Vaginal	**Adults/Pediatrics ≥12 yrs:** 1 sup or applicatorful qhs x 7 days. Apply cream bid externally x 7 days.
Nystatin	RX	**Tab, Vaginal:** 100,000U	Vaginal	**Adults:** 1 tablet daily x 14 days.
Sulfanilamide				
AVC	RX	**Cream:** 15%	Vaginal	**Candidiasis: Adults:** 1 applicatorful qd-bid x 30 days.
Terconazole				
Terazol 3	RX	**Cream:** 0.8% **Sup:** 80mg	Vaginal	**Adults:** 1 applicatorful or 1 sup qhs x 3 days.
Terazol 7	RX	**Cream:** 0.4%	Vaginal	**Adults:** 1 applicatorful qhs x 7 days.
Tioconazole				
Monistat 1, Vagistat 1	OTC	**Oint:** 6.5%	Vaginal	**Adults/Pediatrics ≥12 yrs:** 1 applicatorful single dose hs.

HORMONE THERAPY

DRUG	BRAND	DOSAGE (mg)
INTRAMUSCULAR ESTROGEN PRODUCTS		
Estradiol valerate	Delestrogen	**(mg/mL)** 10mg/mL, 20mg/mL, 40mg/mL
Estradiol cypionate	Depo-Estradiol	5mg/mL
ORAL ESTROGEN PRODUCTS		
Conjugated equine estrogens	Premarin	0.3, 0.45, 0.625, 0.9, 1.25
	Enjuvia	0.3, 0.45, 0.625, 0.9, 1.25
SYNTHETIC CONJUGATED ESTROGEN PRODUCTS		
Estradiol acetate	Femtrace	0.45, 0.9, 1.8
Synthetic conjugated estrogens	Cenestin	0.3, 0.45, 0.625, 0.9, 1.25
Esterified estrogens	Menest	0.3, 0.625, 1.25, 2.5
Micronized 17ß-estradiol	Estrace, Innofem	0.5, 1, 2
Estropipate (piperazine estrone sulfate)	Ortho-Est	0.75, 1.5
	Ogen	0.75 (0.625), 1.5 (1.25), 3 (2.5), 6 (5)
TRANSDERMAL ESTROGEN PRODUCTS		
17ß-estradiol matrix patch	Alora	**RELEASE RATE (mg/day)** 0.025, 0.05, 0.075, 0.1
	Climara	0.025, 0.0375, 0.05, 0.06, 0.075, 0.1
	Vivelle, Vivelle-Dot	0.025, 0.0375, 0.05, 0.075, 0.1
17ß-estradiol reservoir patch	Estraderm	0.05, 0.1
17ß-estradiol	Elestrin	(0.06% gel): 1 metered pump actuation/day applied to upper arm. Adjust dosage as necessary.
17ß-estradiol	Estrogel	(0.06% gel): 1 metered pump actuation/day applied to arm (from wrist to shoulder).
Estradiol hemihydrate	Estrasorb	(emulsion): 3.48g/day (two 1.74g pouches) applied qam to each leg from thigh to calf. Rub for 3 minutes until absorbed.
17ß-estradiol	Evamist	(spray): Initial: 1 metered spray/day qam. Usual: 1-3 sprays/day qam to adjacent, non-overlapping areas on inner forearm, start near elbow.
VAGINAL ESTROGEN PRODUCTS		
Vaginal Creams 17ß-estradiol	Estrace Vaginal Cream	2-4g/day x 1-2 wks, reduce to 1-2g/day x 1-2 wks, then 1g/day x 1-3x/wk
Conjugated equine estrogens	Premarin Vaginal Cream	0.5-2g/day x 3 wks on 1 wk off
Estropipate USP	Ogen Vaginal Cream	2-4g/day. Discontinue/taper at 3-6 month intervals.
Vaginal Ring 17ß-estradiol	Estring	Releases 0.0075mg/day x 90 days
	Femring	Releases 0.05 or 0.1mg/day x 90 days
Vaginal Tablet Estradiol hemihydrate	Vagifem	25mcg/day x 2 wks then 25mcg BIW
PROGESTOGEN ONLY PRODUCTS		
Medroxyprogesterone acetate	Provera	2.5, 5, 10
Norethindrone acetate	Aygestin	5
Progesterone USP (in peanut oil)	Prometrium	100, 200

(Continued)

DRUG	BRAND	DOSAGE (mg)		
ESTROGEN + PROGESTOGEN COMBINATIONS				
Oral continuous-cyclic regimen Conjugated equine estrogens (E) + Medroxyprogesterone acetate (P)	Premphase	0.625mg (E), 5mg (P) [E alone for days 1-14, followed by E+P on days 15-28]		
17ß-estradiol (E) + Norgestimate (P)	Prefest	1mg (E), 0.09mg (P) [E alone for days 1-3, followed by E+P on days 4-6, repeat continuously]		
Oral continuous-combined regimen Conjugated equine estrogens (E) + Medroxyprogesterone (P)	Prempro	0.3mg (E) + 1.5mg (P)	0.45mg + 1.5mg	0.625mg + 2.5 or 5mg
Ethinyl estradiol (E) + Norethindrone acetate (P)	femhrt	2.5mcg (E) + 0.5mg (P); 5mcg (E) + 1mg (P)		
17ß-estradiol (E) + Norethindrone acetate (P)	Activella	1mg (E) + 0.5mg (P); 0.5mg (E) + 0.1mg (P)		
Transdermal continuous-cyclic or continuous-combined regimen 17ß-estradiol (E) + Norethindrone acetate (P)	CombiPatch	0.05mg/day (E) + 0.14 or 0.25mg/day (P)		
Estradiol (E) + Levonorgestrel (P)	Climara Pro	0.045mg/day (E) + 0.015mg/day (P)		
ESTROGEN + ANDROGEN COMBINATIONS				
Oral cyclic regimen Esterified estrogens (E) +	Estratest*	1.25 (E) + 2.5 (A)		
Methyltestosterone (A)	Estratest H.S.*	0.625 (E) + 1.25 (A)		

NOTE: This list is not inclusive of all estrogen and progestogen products available. Indications vary among the different products. For more detailed information please refer to the individual monograph listings or the drug's FDA-approved labeling. Unopposed estrogen replacement therapy (ERT) is for use in women without an intact uterus. For women with an intact uterus, progestin must be added to the estrogen (HRT) for protection against estrogen-induced endometrial cancer. As with any therapy, the lowest possible effective dosage should be used. Re-evaluate periodically.

* This product has not obtained FDA premarket approval applicable for new drugs.

ORAL CONTRACEPTIVES

DRUG	ESTROGEN	PROGESTIN	STRENGTH (ESTROGEN/PROGESTIN)
MONOPHASIC			
Levlite	Ethinyl Estradiol	Levonorgestrel	20mcg/0.1mg
Brevicon, Modicon	Ethinyl Estradiol	Norethindrone	35mcg/0.5mg
Demulen 1/35	Ethinyl Estradiol	Ethynodiol Diacetate	35mcg/1mg
Demulen 1/50	Ethinyl Estradiol	Ethynodiol Diacetate	50mcg/1mg
Desogen, Ortho-Cept	Ethinyl Estradiol	Desogestrel	30mcg/0.15mg
Nordette-28	Ethinyl Estradiol	Levonorgestrel	30mcg/0.15mg
Loestrin 21 1/20, Loestrin Fe 1/20 Loestrin 24 Fe	Ethinyl Estradiol	Norethindrone Acetate	20mcg/1mg
Loestrin 21 1.5/30, Loestrin Fe 1.5/30	Ethinyl Estradiol	Norethindrone Acetate	30mcg/1.5mg
Lo/Ovral	Ethinyl Estradiol	Norgestrel	30mcg/0.3mg
Lybrel*	Ethinyl Estradiol	Levonorgestrel	20mcg/0.09mg
Norinyl 1/35, Ortho-Novum 1/35	Ethinyl Estradiol	Norethindrone	35mcg/1mg
Norinyl 1/50, Ortho-Novum 1/50	Mestranol	Norethindrone	50mcg/1mg
Ortho-Cyclen	Ethinyl Estradiol	Norgestimate	35mcg/0.25mg
Ovcon 35	Ethinyl Estradiol	Norethindrone	35mcg/0.4mg
Ovcon 50*	Ethinyl Estradiol	Norethindrone	50mcg/1mg
Seasonale	Ethinyl Estradiol	Levonorgestrel	30mcg/0.15mg
Yasmin	Ethinyl Estradiol	Drospirenone	30mcg/3mg
YAZ*	Ethinyl Estradiol	Drospirenone	20mcg/3mg
BIPHASIC			
Ortho-Novum 10/11	Ethinyl Estradiol	Norethindrone	**Phase 1:** 35mcg/0.5mg **Phase 2:** 35mcg/1mg
Mircette	Ethinyl Estradiol	Desogestrel	**Phase 1:** 20mcg/0.15mg **Phase 2:** 10mcg/NONE
Loseasonique*	Ethinyl Estradiol	Levonorgestrel	0.1mg, 0.02mg, 0.01mg
Seasonique*	Ethinyl Estradiol	Levonorgestrel	0.01mg, 30mcg/0.15mg
TRIPHASIC			
Cyclessa	Ethinyl Estradiol	Desogestrel	**Phase 1:** 25mcg/0.1mg **Phase 2:** 25mcg/0.125mg **Phase 3:** 25mcg/0.15mg
Estrostep Fe	Ethinyl Estradiol	Norethindrone Acetate	**Phase 1:** 20mcg/1mg **Phase 2:** 30mcg/1mg **Phase 3:** 35mcg/1mg
Ortho-Novum 7/7/7	Ethinyl Estradiol	Norethindrone	**Phase 1:** 35mcg/0.5mg **Phase 2:** 35mcg/0.75mg **Phase 3:** 35mcg/1mg
Ortho Tri-Cyclen	Ethinyl Estradiol	Norgestimate	**Phase 1:** 35mcg/0.18mg **Phase 2:** 35mcg/0.215mg **Phase 3:** 35mcg/0.25mg
Ortho Tri-Cyclen Lo*	Ethinyl Estradiol	Norgestimate	**Phase 1:** 25mcg/0.18mg **Phase 2:** 25mcg/0.215mg **Phase 3:** 25mcg/0.25mg

(Continued)

DRUG	ESTROGEN	PROGESTIN	STRENGTH (ESTROGEN/PROGESTIN)
TRIPHASIC *(Continued)*			
Tri-Levlen, Triphasil, Trivora 28	Ethinyl Estradiol	Levonorgestrel	**Phase 1:** 30mcg/0.05mg **Phase 2:** 40mcg/0.075mg **Phase 3:** 30mcg/0.125mg
Tri-Norinyl	Ethinyl Estradiol	Norethindrone	**Phase 1:** 35mcg/0.5mg **Phase 2:** 35mcg/1mg **Phase 3:** 35mcg/0.5mg
PROGESTIN ONLY			
Nor-Q.D., Ortho-Micronor		Norethindrone	0.35mg
*Currently NO generics available.			

BREAST CANCER TREATMENT OPTIONS

DRUG (BRAND)	INDICATIONS	HOW SUPPLIED	DOSAGE
ANDROGEN			
Fluoxymesterone (Halotestin)	Palliation of androgen-responsive recurrent mammary cancer in females who are >1 to <5 yrs post-menopausal or who have a hormone-dependent tumor as shown by previous beneficial response to castration.	Tab: 2mg*, 5mg*, 10mg* *scored	10-40mg/day in divided doses tid-qid. Continue therapy for at least 1 month for satisfactory subjective response, and for 2-3 months for objective response.
Methyltestosterone (Testred)	Secondary treatment of advancing inoperable metastatic (skeletal) breast cancer in females 1-5 yrs postmenopausal.	Cap: 10mg	50-200mg/day.
Testosterone (Delatestryl)	May also be used secondarily in females with advancing inoperable metastatic (skeletal) mammary cancer who are 1-5 years postmenopausal.	Inj: 200mg/mL	200-400mg every 2-4 weeks.
ANTIESTROGEN			
Faslodex (Fulvestrant)	Treatment of hormone receptor positive metastatic breast cancer in postmenopausal women with disease progression following anti-estrogen therapy.	Inj: 50mg/mL [2.5mL, 5mL]	250mg IM into buttock once monthly as either a single 5mL injection or two concurrent 2.5mL injections. Administer slowly.
ESTROGEN			
Estrace (Estradiol)	Palliative treatment of metastatic breast cancer.	Tab: 0.5mg*, 1mg*, 2mg* *scored	10mg tid for at least 3 months.
Menest (Esterified estrogens)	Palliative therapy for metastatic breast cancer in selected men and women.	Tab: 0.3mg, 0.625mg, 1.25mg, 2.5mg	10mg tid for at least 3 months.
Premarin Tablets (Conjugated estrogens)	Palliative treatment of breast cancer in patients with metastatic disease.	Tab: 0.3mg, 0.45mg, 0.625mg, 0.9mg, 1.25mg	10mg tid for minimum 3 months.
LHRH AGONIST			
Zoladex 1-Month (Goserelin)	Palliative treatment of advanced breast cancer in pre-and perimenopausal women.	Implant: 3.6mg	Inject SQ into anterior abdominal wall below navel line. 3.6mg every 28 days.
PROGESTIN			
Megestrol (Megestrol)	Palliative treatment of advanced breast carcinoma (eg, recurrent, inoperable or metastatic disease).	Tab: 20mg*, 40mg* *scored Susp: 40mg/mL	40mg qid for a minimum of 2 months. Elderly: Start at lower end of dosing range.
SELECTIVE ESTROGEN RECEPTOR MODULATORS			
Raloxifene (Evista)	Reduction in risk of invasive breast cancer in post-menopausal women with osteoporosis or at high risk for invasive breast cancer.	Tab: 60mg	60mg qd.

DRUG (BRAND)	INDICATIONS	HOW SUPPLIED	DOSAGE
SELECTIVE ESTROGEN RECEPTOR MODULATORS *(continued)*			
Tamoxifen (Soltamox)	Treatment of metastatic breast cancer in women and men. Treatment of node-positive and axillary node-negative breast cancer in women following mastectomy, axillary dissection and breast irradiation. To reduce risk of invasive breast cancer in women with DCIS. Reduction of breast cancer incidence in high risk women. Use for up to 5 yrs.	Sol: 10mg/5mL	Treatment: 20-40mg qd. Divide dosages >20mg into AM and PM doses. Risk Reduction/DCIS: 20mg qd for 5 yrs.
Tamoxifen (Tamoxifen)	Treatment of metastatic breast cancer in women and men. Treatment of node-positive and axillary node-negative breast cancer in women following mastectomy, axillary dissection and breast irradiation. To reduce risk of invasive breast cancer in women with DCIS. Reduction of breast cancer incidence in high risk women. Use for up to 5 yrs.	Tab: 10mg, 20mg	Treatment: 20-40mg qd. Divide dosages >20mg into AM and PM doses. Risk Reduction/DCIS: 20mg qd for 5 yrs.
Toremifene (Fareston)	Treatment of metastatic breast cancer in post-menopausal women with estrogen-receptor positive or unknown tumors.	Tab: 60mg	60mg qd. Treat until disease progression is evident.
SELECTIVE NONSTEROIDAL AROMATASE INHIBITORS (POSTMENOPAUSAL WOMEN ONLY)			
Anastrozole (Arimidex)	Adjuvant treatment of post-menopausal women with hormone-receptor positive early breast cancer. First-line treatment of post-menopausal women with hormone-receptor positive or hormone-receptor unknown locally advanced or metastatic breast cancer. Treatment of advanced breast cancer in post-menopausal women with disease progression following tamoxifen therapy. Patients with ER-negative disease and patients who did not respond to previous tamoxifen therapy rarely respond.	Tab: 1mg	1mg qd. Continue until tumor progression with advanced breast cancer.
Letrozole (Femara)	First-line treatment of hormone-receptor positive or hormone-receptor unknown locally advanced or metastatic breast cancer in postmenopausal women. Treatment of advanced breast cancer with disease progression following antiestrogen therapy in postmenopausal women.	Tab: 2.5mg	2.5mg qd. Continue until tumor progression is evident. Cirrhosis/ Severe Liver Dysfunction: 2.5mg every other day.

DRUG (BRAND)	INDICATIONS	HOW SUPPLIED	DOSAGE
CHEMOTHERAPY AGENTS			
ANTHRACYCLINES			
Epirubicin (Ellence)	Adjuvant treatment of primary breast cancer with axillary node tumor involvement following resection of primary breast cancer.	Inj: 2mg/mL [25mL, 100mL]	Initial: 100-120mg/m² IV infusion, repeat at 3-4 week cycles. May give total dose on Day 1 of each cycle or divide equally on Days 1 and 8. Bone Marrow Dysfunction: Initial: 75-90mg/m². Hepatic Dysfunction: Bilirubin 1.2-3mg/dL or AST 2-4X ULN: Give 1/2 of initial dose. Bilirubin >3mg/dL or AST 4X ULN: Give 1/4 of initial dose. Severe Renal Dysfunction: Serum Creatinine >5mg/dL: Lower dose. Give prophylactic therapy with SMZ-TMP or fluoroquinolone with 120mg/m² regimen. Consider pretreatment with antiemetics. Adjust dose after 1st treatment cycle based on hematologic and nonhematologic toxicities (see PI).
Doxorubicin	To produce regression in disseminated neoplastic conditions such as breast carcinoma. Adjuvant therapy in women with evidence of axillary lymph node involvement following resection of primary breast cancer.	Inj: (2mg/mL) 10mg, 20mg, 50mg	Monotherapy: 60-75mg/m² IV every 21 days. Use the lower dose with inadequate bone marrow reserves due to old age, prior therapy, or neoplastic marrow infiltration. Concomitant Chemotherapy: 40-60mg/m² IV every 21-28 days. Hyperbilirubinemia: Reduce dose by 50% if 1.2-3mg/dL; reduce dose by 75% if 3.1-5mg/dL. See PI for pediatric dosing.
ANTIMICROTUBULE AGENT			
Ixempra (Ixabepilone)	In combination with capecitabine for treatment of patients with metastatic or locally advanced breast cancer resistant to treatment with an anthracycline and a taxane, or whose cancer is taxane resistant and for whom further anthracycline therapy is contraindicated. As monotherapy for treatment of metastatic or locally advanced breast cancer in patients whose tumors are resistant or refractory to anthracyclines, taxanes, and capecitabine.	Inj: 15mg, 45mg	40mg/m² IV infusion over 3 hrs every 3 weeks. Adjust dose based on toxicities (see PI). Premedicate with H1-antagonist (eg, diphenhydramine 50mg PO) and H2-antagonist (eg, ranitidine 150-300mg PO) approximately 1hr before infusion. Also premedicate with corticosteroid (eg, dexamethasone 20mg, IV 30 min before infusion or PO 60 min before infusion) if prior hypersensitivity reaction to ixabepilone. Hepatic Impairment: Monotherapy: Mild: AST and ALT ≤2.5x ULN and Bilirubin ≤1x ULN: 40mg/m². AST or ALT ≤10x ULN and Bilirubin ≤1.5x ULN: 32mg/m². Moderate (AST and ALT ≤10x ULN and Bilirubin >1.5 to ≤3x ULN): 20-30mg/m². Strong CYP3A4 Inhibitors: Avoid or reduce dose to 20mg/m².
KINASE INHIBITOR			
Tykerb (Lapatinib)	Treatment of patients with advanced or metastatic breast cancer, in combination with capecitabine, whose tumors overexpress HER2 and received prior therapy including an anthracycline, a taxane, and trastuzumab.	Tab: 250mg	Usual: 1250mg qd on Days 1-21 continuously with capecitabine 2000mg/m²/day (administered orally in 2 doses 12 hrs apart) on Days 1-14 in a repeating 21-day cycle. Give at least 1 hr before or after a meal (however, give capecitabine with food). ≥ Grade 2 LVEF: D/C dose. If LVEF recovers and asymptomatic after 2 weeks,

DRUG (BRAND)	INDICATIONS	HOW SUPPLIED	DOSAGE
KINASE INHIBITOR *(continued)*			
			restart at 1000mg/day. Hepatic Impairment (Child-Pugh Class C): Consider dose reduction to 750mg/day. Concomitant Strong CYP3A4 Inhibitors: Avoid use. Concomitant Strong CYP3A4 Inducers: Avoid use and if must coadminister titrate gradually from 1250mg/day up to 4500mg/day based on tolerability. ≥ Grade 2 NCI CTC Toxicity: D/C or interrupt dose and restart with 1250mg/day when toxicity <Grade 1. Restart at 1000mg/day if toxicity recurs.
MISCELLANEOUS			
Capecitabine (Xeloda)	Treatment of metastatic breast cancer in combination with docetaxel after failure of prior anthracycline-containing chemotherapy. Treatment of metastatic breast cancer in patients resistant to paclitaxel and anthracycline-containing chemotherapy or resistant to paclitaxel and for whom further anthracycline therapy is not indicated.	Tab: 150mg, 500mg	Take with water within 30 min after meals. Usual/Concomitantly w/ docetoxel: 1250mg/m^2 bid for 2 weeks, then 1 week off. Give as 3-week cycles. CrCl 30-50mL/min: Reduce to 75% of starting dose. Interrupt and/or reduce dose if toxicity occurs. Readjust according to adverse effects (see PI for details).
Cytoxan (Cyclophosphamide)	Treatment of breast carcinoma.	Inj (Lyophilized): 500mg, 1g, 2g; Tab: 25mg, 50mg	Malignant Diseases (Without Hematologic Deficiency): Monotherapy: Initial: 40-50mg/kg IV in divided doses over 2-5 days, or 10-15mg/kg IV given every 7-10 days, or 3-5mg/kg twice weekly. Oral Dosing: Initial/Maint: 1-5mg/kg/day PO. Adjust dose according to antitumor activity and/or leukopenia. May need to reduce dose when combined with other cytotoxic drugs. See PI for pediatric dosing.
Dexrazoxane (Zinecard)	To reduce the incidence and severity of cardiomyopathy associated with doxorubicin in women with metastatic breast cancer who received a cumulative doxorubicin dose of 300mg/m^2 and who will continue doxorubicin therapy.	Inj: 250mg, 500mg	IV: 10:1 ratio of dexrazoxane: doxorubicin (eg, 500mg/m^2 dexrazoxane: 50mg/m^2 doxorubicin). Hepatic Impairment: Reduce dose proportionally. Give by slow IV push or rapid IV infusion. Give doxorubicin within 30 min after start of infusion. If CrCl <40 mL/min, the recommended dosage ratio is 5:1 (dexrazoxane: doxorubicin)
Fluorouracil	Palliative management of colon, rectum, breast, stomach, and pancreatic carcinomas.	Inj: 50mg/mL, [10mL, 20mL, 50mL, 100mL]	12mg/kg IV qd for 4 days. Max: 800mg/day. If no toxicity, give 6mg/kg IV on 6th, 8th, 10th, and 12th days. Skip Days 5, 7, 9, and 11. Inadequate Nutritional State: 6mg/kg IV for 3 days. If no toxicity, give 3mg/kg IV on 5th, 7th, and 9th days. Max: 400mg/day. Skip Days 4, 6, and 8. Maint (Use Schedule 1 or Schedule 2): Schedule 1: If no toxicity, repeat 1st course every 30 days after last day of previous course. Schedule 2: When toxic signs from initial course subside, give 10-15mg/kg/week IV single dose; do not exceed 1g/week.

DRUG (BRAND)	INDICATIONS	HOW SUPPLIED	DOSAGE
MISCELLANEOUS *(continued)*			
Methotrexate (Methotrexate)	(Inj/PO) Treatment of neoplastic diseases, eg, acute lymphocytic leukemia, gestational choriocarcinoma, chorioadenoma destruens, hydatidiform mole, breast cancer, epidermoid cancer of the head and neck, advanced mycosis fungoides, lung cancer, advanced stage non-Hodgkin's lymphoma.	Inj: (Generic) (Methotrexate Sodium) 25mg/mL, 1g; Tab: (Generic) (Methotrexate) 2.5mg*; Tab: (Rheumatrex) (Methotrexate) 2.5mg* [Dose Pack 15mg, 4 x 6 tabs; 12.5mg, 4 x 5 tabs; 10mg, 4 x 4 tabs; 7.5mg, 4 x 3 tabs; 5mg, 4 x 2 tabs] *scored	Choriocarcinoma/Trophoblastic Disease: 15-30mg qd PO/IM for 5 days. May repeat 3-5 times as required with rest period of ≥ 1 week. Leukemia: Induction: 3.3mg/m² with prednisone 60mg/m² qd. Remission Maintenance: 15mg/m² PO/IM twice weekly or 2.5mg/kg IV every 14 days. Burkitt's Tumor: Stages I-II: 10-25mg/day PO for 4-8 days. Administer several courses with rest periods of 7-10 days in between. Lymphosarcoma: Stage III: 0.625-2.5mg/kg/day with other antitumor agents.
MONOCLONAL ANTIBODY/HER2 BLOCKER			
Transtuzumab (Herceptin)	Part of treatment regimen containing doxorubicin, cyclophosphamide, and either paclitaxel or docetaxel or with docetaxel and carboplatin for adjuvant treatment of HER2-over-expressing breast cancer. Single agent for adjuvant treatment of HER2-over-expressing breast cancer in patients who received 1 or more chemotherapy regimens for metastatic disease.	Inj: 440mg	Adjuvant Treatment: Following Anthracycline/Concurrently With Paclitaxel for First 12 Weeks: IV infusion: Initial: 4mg/kg over 90 min. Maint: 2mg/kg/week over 30 min for total 52 doses. Following Completion of All Chemotherapy: IV Infusion: Initial: 8mg/kg. Maint: 6mg/kg every 3 weeks for total of 17 doses; give doses ≥4mg/kg over 90 min. Metastatic Breast Cancer: IV Infusion: Alone or With Paclitaxel: Initial: 4mg/kg over 90 min. Maint: 2mg/kg/week over 30 min until disease progression.
NUCLEOSIDE ANALOGUE/ANTIMETABOLITE			
Gemcitabine (Gemzar)	Adjunct with paclitaxel for 1st-line treatment of metastatic breast cancer after failure of prior anthracycline-containing adjuvant chemotherapy, unless anthracyclines were clinically contraindicated.	Inj: 200mg, 1g	1250mg/m² IV on Days 1 and 8 of each 21-day cycle. Give paclitaxel 175mg/m² IV on Day 1 before gemcitabine. All IV infusions given over 30 min. Adjust dose based on hematologic toxicity.
TAXANES			
Docetaxel (Taxotere)	Treatment of locally advanced or metastatic breast cancer after failure of prior chemotherapy. In combination with doxorubicin and cyclophosphamide for the adjuvant treatment of operable, node-positive breast cancer.	Inj: 20mg/0.5mL, 80mg/2mL	Premedicate with oral corticosteroids. Adjust dose based on febrile neutropenia, neutrophil count, cutaneous reactions, peripheral neuropathy, neurosensory signs/ symptoms, or GI toxicities (see PI). Breast Cancer: 60-100mg/m² IV over 1 hr every 3 weeks. Adjuvant Treatment Operable Node-Positive Breast CA: 75mg/m² 1 hr after doxorubicin 50mg/m² and cyclophosphamide 500mg/m² every 3 weeks for 6 courses. Administer every 3 weeks for 3 cycles.
Paclitaxel (Taxol)	Treatment of breast cancer after failure with combination chemotherapy for metastatic disease or relapse within 6 months of adjuvant chemotherapy. Adjuvant treatment of node-positive breast cancer administered sequentially to doxorubicin-containing chemotherapy.	Inj: 6mg/mL	IV: Breast Cancer: 175mg/m² over 3 hrs every 3 weeks for 4 courses. Non-Small Cell Lung Cancer: 135mg/m² over 24 hrs every 3 weeks followed by cisplatin. Reduce dose of subsequent courses by 20% if neutrophils <500 cells/mm³ for ≥1 week or severe peripheral neuropathy occurs. Premedicate prior to administration with appropriate medications; see PI for additional information.

DRUG (BRAND)	INDICATIONS	HOW SUPPLIED	DOSAGE
TAXANES *(continued)*			
Paclitaxel protein-bound particle for injectable suspension (Abraxane)	Treatment of breast cancer after failure of combination chemotherapy for metastatic disease or relapse within 6 months of adjuvant chemotherapy. Prior therapy should have included an anthracyline unless clinically contraindicated.	Inj: 100mg	260mg/m² IV over 30 min every 3 weeks. Severe neutropenia (neutrophil <500 cells/mm³ for week or longer) or severe sensory neuropathy (Grade 3 or 4): Hold dose until neutrophil >1500 cells/mm³ or sensory neuropathy resolves to Grade 1 or 2. Reduce subsequent courses to 220mg/m², if recurrence reduce subsequent courses to 180mg/m².
VASCULAR ENDOTHELIAL GROWTH INHIBITOR			
Bevacizumab (Avastin)	Treatment of patients who have not received chemotherapy for metastatic HER2 negative breast cancer, in combination with paclitaxel.	Inj: 25mg/mL [4mL, 16mL]	10mg/kg every 2 weeks. Give as IV infusion over 90 min, if 1st infusion is well tolerated, give 2nd infusion over 60 min and subsequent doses over 30 min.
VINCA ALKALOID			
Vinblastine	Palliative treatment of breast carcinoma unresponsive to appropriate endocrine surgery and hormonal therapy.	Inj: 1mg/mL [10mL]	Dose at intervals of ≤7 days. 1st Dose: 3.7mg/m². 2nd Dose: 5.5mg/m². 3rd Dose: 7.4mg/m². 4th Dose: 9.25mg/m². 5th Dose: 11.1mg/m². Max: 18.5mg/m². Do not increase dose after that dose which reduces WBC to 3000 cells/mm³. Maint: Use dose of 1 increment smaller than this dose at weekly intervals. Reduce to 50% dose if direct serum bilirubin >3mg/100mL. Only dose if WBC ≥4000 cells/mm³.

Breast Cancer Risk Factors

Unmodifiable risk factors	
Gender	Women > men
Age	1 out of 8 breast cancer diagnoses are among women <45 yrs, while about 2 out of 3 occur in women >55 yrs
Genetic	BRCA1 and BRCA2, ATM gene, CHEK2 gene, p53 tumor suppressor gene, PTEN gene mutations
Race	Whites > African Americans
Family history	Having a first-degree relative with breast cancer doubles risk; having 2 first-degree relatives increases risk about 5-fold
Personal history of breast cancer	Women with cancer in one breast have 3- to 4-fold increased risk of developing a new cancer in another area of the same breast or in the opposite breast
Abnormal breast biopsy	Nonproliferative lesions, proliferative lesions with or without atypia
Early menarche	Women who started menstruating at an early age (<12 yrs)
Age at menopause	Women who went through menopause at a late age (>55 yrs)
Personal history of breast abnormalities	Two breast tissue abnormalities–ductal carcinoma in situ (DCIS) and lobular carcinoma in situ (LCIS)–are associated with increased risk for developing invasive breast cancer
Earlier breast radiation exposure	Women who had radiation therapy to the chest area as treatment for another cancer
Breast density	Women with a higher proportion of dense breast tissue (eg, connective and milk duct tissue)

Lifestyle factors associated with increased risk of breast cancer

- Alcohol (2 drinks/day)
- High body mass index
- Not having children or having them when >30 yrs
- Lack of physical activity
- Not breastfeeding

Drugs associated with increased risk of breast cancer

- Birth control pills
- DES (diethylstilbestrol)
- Postmenopausal hormone therapy or hormone replacement therapy

Uncertain risk factors

- Antiperspirants
- Bras
- Breast implants
- High-fat diets
- Induced abortion
- Miscarriages
- Night work
- Pollution (chemicals)
- Smoking (active or passive)

Sources: American Cancer Society and National Cancer Institute.

Chemotherapy Regimens*†

CANCER TYPE	DRUGS OF CHOICE	ALTERNATIVE THERAPIES
Bladder	*Non-muscle invasive:* Bacillus Calmette-Guerin (BCG) *Neoadjuvant, adjuvant, and metastatic:* Gemcitabine/cisplatin	*Non-muscle invasive:* Mitomycin C (MMC) *Neoadjuvant, adjuvant, and metastatic:* Methotrexate/vinblastine/doxorubicin/cisplatin (MVAC)
Breast		
Risk reduction	Tamoxifen (premenopausal); tamoxifen or raloxifene (postmenopausal)	
Adjuvant (trastuzumab containing)	Doxorubicin/cyclophosphamide followed by paclitaxel + trastuzumab (Ac → T + trastuzumab)	Cyclophosphamide/epirubicin/5-FU (Docetaxel/trastuzumab → FEC) Docetaxel/carboplatin/trastuzumab (TCH) Doxorubicin/cyclophosphamide → docetaxel/trastuzumab (AC)
Adjuvant (nontrastuzumab containing)	Fluorouracil/doxorubicin/cyclophosphamide (FAC/CAF) Cyclophosphamide/epirubicin/fluorouracil (FEC/CEF) (Doxorubicin/cyclophosphamide) ± sequential paclitaxel (AC) Epirubicin/cyclophosphamide (EC) Docetaxel/doxorubicin/cyclophosphamide with filgrastim support (TAC) Doxorubicin followed by cyclophosphamide/methotrexate/fluorouracil (A→CMF) Epirubicin followed by cyclophosphamide/methotrexate/fluorouracil (E→CMF) Cyclophosphamide/methotrexate/fluorouracil (CMF) Doxorubicin/cyclophosphamide + sequential paclitaxel x4 with filgrastim support (ACx4) Doxorubicin followed by paclitaxel followed by cyclophosphamide with filgrastim support (A → T → C) Fluorouracil/epirubicin/cyclophosphamide followed by docetaxel (FEC → T) Docetaxel/cyclophosphamide (TC)	
Neoadjuvant	Paclitaxel + trastuzumab followed by cyclophosphamide/epirubicin/fluorouracil + trastuzumab (T + trastuzumab → CEF + trastuzumab)	
Recurrent or metastatic	*Single agents:* Doxorubicin, epirubicin, paclitaxel, docetaxel, capecitabine, vinorelbine, gemcitabine *Combinations:* Cyclophosphamide/doxorubicin/fluorouracil (CAF/FAC); fluorouracil/epirubicin/cyclophosphamide (FEC); epirubicin/cyclophosphamide (EC); doxorubicin/docetaxel (AT); doxorubicin/paclitaxel; cyclophosphamide/methotrexate/fluorouracil (CMF); docetaxel/capecitabine; gemcitabine/paclitaxel (GT)	
HER2-positive metastatic disease	1) Trastuzumab + (paclitaxel ± carboplatin) or (docetaxel) or (vinorelbine) 2) Lapatnib + capecitabine	
Colorectal	*Adjuvant Stage III:* 5-FU + oxaliplatin + leucovorin (FOLFOX) *Metastatic:* Bevacizumab + 1) 5-FU + oxaliplatin + leucovorin (FOLFOX) or 2) irinotecan + leucovorin (FOLFIRI) + 5-FU or 3) oxaliplatin + capecitabine (CapeOX) or 4) 5-FU/LV	*Adjuvant Stage III:* 5-FU/LV or capecitabine

(Continued)

CANCER TYPE	DRUGS OF CHOICE	ALTERNATIVE THERAPIES
Esophageal		
Chemoradiation	Cisplatin + 5-FU	Cisplatin + 1) irinotecan or 2) paclitaxel or 3) docetaxel Docetaxel or paclitaxel + 5-FU or capecitabine Oxaliplatin + fluoropyrimidine (5-FU or capecitabine)
Recurrent or metastatic	Docetaxel/cisplatin/5-FU (DCF) Epirubicin/cisplatin/5-FU (ECF)	Irinotecan + cisplatin or fluoropyrimidine (5-FU or capecitabine)
Leukemia		
Acute lymphocytic leukemia (ALL)	*Induction:* Vincristine/L-asparaginase/dexamethasone ± daunorubicin *CNS prophalaxis:* Intrathecal methotrexate ± hydrocortisone ± cytarabine *Consolidation:* L-asparaginase/doxorubicin/etoposide/cyclophosphamide/cytarabine *Maintenance:* Methotrexate/6-MP/vincristine/dexamethasone *Recurrent:* Vincristine/L-asparaginase/doxorubicin or daunorubicin/cyclophosphamide/cytarabine/etoposide or tenoposide	*Induction:* Addition of methotrexate ± 6-MP
Acute myelogenous leukemia (AML)	*Induction:* (pt <60) cytarabine + 1) daunorubicin or 2) idarubicin *Induction:* (pt >60) subQ cytarabine or hydroxyurea *Post-induction:* High-dose cytarabine	
Acute promyelocyctic leukemia (APL)	*Induction:* All-trans retinoic acid (ATRA) *Relapse:* Arsenic trioxide ± gemtuzumab	*Induction:* Arsenic trioxide
Chronic lymphocyctic leukemia (CLL)	Bendamustine (Fludarabine/cyclophosphamide) ± rituximab (FC) Fludarabine ± rituximab Pentostatin/cyclophosphamide/rituximab (PCR) Cyclophosphamide/doxorubicin/vincristine/prednisone (CHOP) + rituximab Chlorambucil ± prednisone ± rituximab	Alemtuzumab
Chronic myelogenous leukemia (CML)	High-dose imatinib	Dasatinib Nilotinib Interferon therapy
Hairy cell leukemia	Cladribine	Pentostatin Interferon alpha 2a or 2b Rituximab
Liver	5-FU ± mitomycin or gemcitabine	
Lung		
Non-small cell	Carboplatin or cisplatin/paclitaxel Cisplatin/vinorelbine Gemcitabine/cisplatin Docetaxel/cisplatin	Gemcitabine/carboplatin Docetaxel/carboplatin Gemcitabine/docetaxel
Small cell	Cisplatin or carboplatin + etoposide	Cisplatin/irinotecan Carboplatin/irinotecan Cyclophosphamide/doxorubicin/vincristine
Lymphoma		
Hodgkin's disease/lymphoma	Doxorubicin/bleomycin/vinblastine/dacarbazine (ABVD) Doxorubicin/vinblastine/mechlorethamine/etoposide/vincristine/bleomycin/prednisone (Stanford V)	Bleomycin/etoposide/doxorubicin/cyclophosphamide/vincristine/procarbazine/prednisone (BEACOPP)

(Continued)

CANCER TYPE	DRUGS OF CHOICE	ALTERNATIVE THERAPIES
Non-Hodgkin's lymphoma		
Follicular lymphoma	Cyclophosphamide/doxorubicin/vincristine/prednisone (CHOP) + rituximab Cyclophosphamide/vincristine/prednisone (CVP) + rituximab Fludarabine/mitoxantrone/dexamethasone (FND) + rituximab Rituximab	Bendamustine ± rituximab
Mantle cell lymphoma	Cyclophosphamide/doxorubicin/vincristine/prednisone (CHOP) ± rituximab	Bendamustine
	Rituximab + etoposide/prednisone/vincristine/cyclophosphamide/doxorubicin (R-EPOCH)	Bortezomib
	Rituximab and cyclophosphamide/vincristine/doxorubicin/dexamethasone (R-hyper CVAD) alternating with methotrexate and cytarabine	Cladribine
Diffuse large B-cell	Rituximab + Cyclophosphamide/doxorubicin/vincristine/prednisone (CHOP)	Dexamethasone/cisplatin/cytarabine (DHAP) ± rituximab Etoposide/methylprednisone/cytarabine/cisplatin (ESHAP) ± rituximab Gemcitabine/dexamethasone/cisplatin (GDP) ± rituximab Ifosfamide/carboplatin/etoposide (ICE) ± rituximab Carmustine/etoposide/cytarabine/melphalan (miniBEAM) ± rituximab Mesna/ifosfamide/mitoxantrone/etoposide (MINE) ± rituximab
Burkitt's	*Low risk-combination:* Cyclophosphamide/vincristine/doxorubicin/high-dose methotrexate ± rituximab (CODOX-M) *Low risk-combination:* Cyclophosphamide/vincristine/doxorubicin/dexamethasone (HyperCVAD) alternating with methotrexate + cytarabine ± rituximab *High risk-combination:* Cyclophosphamide/vincristine/doxorubicin/high-dose methotrexate (CODOX-M) alternating with ifosfamide/etoposide/and high-dose cytarabine (IVAC) ± rituximab *High risk-combination:* Cyclophosphamide/vincristine/doxorubicin/dexamethasone (Hyper CVAD) alternating with methotrexate and cytarabine ± rituximab	
Lymphoblastic	Cyclophosphamide/anthracycline/vincristine/asparaginase High-dose cytarabine + rituximab or high-dose methotrexate + rituximab Cyclophosphamide/vincristine/doxorubicin/dexamethasone (Hyper CVAD) alternating with methotrexate + cytarabine ± rituximab Vincristine/prednisone	
Peripheral T-cell	Cyclophosphamide/doxorubicin/vincristine/prednisone (CHOP) Etoposide/prednisone/vincristine/cyclophosphamide/doxorubicin (EPOCH) Cyclophosphamide/vincristine/doxorubicin/dexamethasone (Hyper CVAD) alternating with methotrexate + cytarabine ± rituximab	Dexamethasone/cisplatin/cytarabine (DHAP) Etoposide/methylprednisolone/cytarabine/cisplatin (ESHAP) Gemcitabine/dexamethasone/cisplatin (GDP) Ifosfamide/carboplatin/etoposide (ICE) Carmustine/etoposide/cytarabin/melphalan (miniBEAM) Mesna/ifosfamide/mitoxantrone/etoposide (MINE)

(Continued)

CANCER TYPE	DRUGS OF CHOICE	ALTERNATIVE THERAPIES
Ovarian	Paclitaxel/carboplatin	Docetaxel/carboplatin Paclitaxel/cisplatin
Germ cell tumor	Bleomycin/etoposide/platinum (BEP)	Paclitaxel/ifosfamide/cisplatin (TIP)
Pancreatic	Locally advanced or metastatic: Gemcitabine	Gemcitabine/cisplatin or fluoropyrimidines Capecitabine ± oxaliplatin 5-FU + oxaliplatin
Prostate	Docetaxel/prednisone Androgen deprivation therapy: Finasteride or dutasteride	Docetaxel/estramustine, docetaxel/prednisone, mitoxantrone/prednisone

Abbreviations: MTX: methotrexate; 5-FU: 5-fluorouracil; LV: leucovorin.

* Selected cancers. For more detailed information, refer to the individual monograph listings or the drug's FDA-approved labeling.

† Source: National Comprehensive Cancer Network Clinical Practice Guidelines in Oncology, 2008-2009.

COLORECTAL CANCER TREATMENT OPTIONS

DRUG (BRAND)	INDICATIONS	HOW SUPPLIED	DOSAGE
Bevacizumab (Avastin)	First- or second-line treatment of metastatic carcinoma of the colon or rectum, in combination with 5-fluorouracil-based chemotherapy.	Inj: 25mg/mL [4mL, 16mL]	Colon/Rectum Metastatic Carcinoma: 5mg/kg (in combination with bolus IFL) or 10 mg/kg (in combination with FOLFOX4) given once every 14 days. Give as IV infusion over 90 min; if 1st infusion is well tolerated, give 2nd infusion over 60 min and subsequent doses over 30 min.
Capecitabine (Xeloda)	First-line treatment of metastatic colorectal carcinoma when fluoropyrimidine therapy alone is preferred. Adjuvant treatment in patients with Dukes' C colon cancer who have undergone complete resection of the primary tumor when treatment with fluoropyrimidine therapy alone is preferred.	Tab: 150mg, 500mg	1250mg/m^2 bid for 2 weeks followed by 1-week rest period given as 3-week cycles. Take with water within 30 min after meals. Give as 3-week cycles for a total of 8 cycles (24 weeks). CrCl 30-50mL/min: Reduce to 75% of starting dose. Interrupt and/or reduce dose if toxicity occurs. Readjust according to adverse effects (see PI for details).
Cetuximab (Erbitux)	In combination with irinotecan for the treatment of epidermal growth factor receptor (EGFR)-expressing, metastatic colorectal carcinoma in patients who are refractory to irinotecan-based chemotherapy. As monotherapy, for the treatment of EGFR-expressing, metastatic colorectal carcinoma after failure of both irinotecan- and oxaliplatin-based regimens.	Inj: 2mg/mL [50mL, 100mL]	Premedication with H_1 antagonist (eg, diphenhydramine 50mg) IV 30-60 min prior to 1st dose is recommended. Colorectal Cancer: LD: 400mg/m^2 IV infusion over 120 min. Maint: 250mg/m^2 IV infusion over 60 min once weekly. Max Infusion Rate: 10mg/min. See PI for dose modifications for infusion reactions and severe acneform rash.
Fluorouracil	Palliative management of colon, rectum, breast, stomach, and pancreatic carcinomas.	Inj: 50mg/mL [10mL, 20mL]	12mg/kg IV qd for 4 days. Max: 800mg/day. If no toxicity, give 6mg/kg IV on 6th, 8th, 10th, and 12th days. Skip Days 5, 7, 9, and 11. Inadequate Nutritional State: 6mg/kg IV for 3 days. If no toxicity, give 3mg/kg IV on 5th, 7th, and 9th days. Max: 400mg/day. Skip Days 4, 6, and 8. Maint (Use Schedule 1 or Schedule 2): Schedule 1: If no toxicity, repeat 1st course every 30 days after last day of previous course. Schedule 2: When toxic signs from initial course subside, give 10-15mg/kg/ week IV single dose; do not exceed 1g/week.
Irinotecan hydrochloride (Camptosar)	First-line therapy in combination with 5-fluorouracil (5-FU) and leucovorin (LV) for metastatic colon or rectal carcinomas, and for disease that has progressed or recurred following initial 5-FU therapy.	Inj: 20mg/mL [2mL, 5mL]	Combination Therapy (5-FU/LV, see PI for dosage): 125mg/m^2 IV over 90 min on days 1, 8, 15, 22 for 6 weeks; or 180mg/m^2 IV over 90 min on days 1, 15, and 29 for 6 weeks. Both regimens: Begin next cycle on Day 43. Single Therapy: 125mg/m^2 IV over 90 min on days 1, 8, 15, 22, followed by a 2-week rest; or 350mg/m^2 IV over 90 min once every 3 weeks. Premedicate with antiemetics at least 30 min prior to therapy. Dose modifications for reduced UGT1A1 activity, neutropenia, diarrhea, and other toxicities: See PI. All dose modifications should be based on worst preceding toxicity.

(Continued)

DRUG (BRAND)	INDICATIONS	HOW SUPPLIED	DOSAGE
Leucovorin Calcium	Adjunct to 5-fluorouracil (5-FU) for palliative treatment of advanced colorectal cancer.	Inj: 50mg, 100mg, 200mg, 350mg, 500mg Tab: 5mg, 10mg, 15mg, 25mg	Colorectal Cancer: 200mg/m^2 slow IV push over 3 min followed by 5-FU 370mg/m^2 IV qd for 5 days, or 20mg/m^2 IV qd followed by 5-FU 425mg/m^2 IV qd for 5 days. May repeat at 4-week intervals for 2 courses, then at 4-5 week intervals. May increase 5-FU dose by 10% if no toxicity. Reduce 5-FU dose by 20% with moderate GI/hematologic toxicity and by 30% with severe toxicity.
Oxaliplatin (Eloxatin)	In combination with infusional 5-fluorouracil (5-FU) and leucovorin (LV) for treatment of advanced metastatic carcinoma of colon or rectum and adjuvant treatment of Stage III colon cancer patients who have undergone complete resection of the primary tumor.	Inj: 50mg, 100mg	Advanced colorectal cancer: Day 1: 85mg/m^2 IV with LV 200mg/m^2; give over 120 min in separate bags using a Y-line; followed by 5-FU 400mg/m^2 bolus over 2-4 min, then 5-FU 600mg/m^2 as a 22 hr-infusion. Day 2: LV 200mg/m^2 over 120 min; followed by 5-FU 400mg/m^2 bolus over 2-4 min, then 5-FU 600mg/m^2 as a 22 hr-infusion. Repeat cycle every 2 weeks. See PI for dose modifications for persistent grade 2 neurosensory events, grade 3 or 4 GI or grade 4 hematologic toxicity. Adjuvant Therapy Stage III Colon Cancer: Recommended cycle every 2 weeks for 6 months.
Panitumumab (Vectibix)	Treatment of EGFR-expressing, metastatic colorectal carcinoma with disease progression on or following fluoropyrimidine-, oxaliplatin-, and irinotecan-containing chemotherapy regimens.	Inj: 20mg/mL [5mL, 10mL, 20mL]	6mg/kg IV infusion over 60 min every 14 days. Infuse doses >1000mg over 90 min. See PI for dose modifications.

ADMINISTRATION GUIDELINES FOR EYE DROPS & OINTMENT

Administration guidelines for eye drops:

1. Wash hands thoroughly.
2. Tilt head back.
3. Gently pull the lower eyelid away from the eye to create a pocket.
4. Hold the bottle upside down and look up just before applying a single drop. **NOTE:** To prevent contamination, do not let the tip of the eye drop applicator touch any surface (including the eye or eyelid). When not in use, keep the container tightly closed.
5. After applying the drop, look down for several seconds (still holding the eyelid away from the eye).
6. Slowly release the eyelid and close the eyes for 1 to 2 minutes. Do not blink.
7. Gently press on the inside corner of the eye (where the eyelid meets the nose) with a finger.
8. Blot excessive solution from around the eye with a tissue.

Administration guidelines for eye ointment:

1. Wash hands thoroughly.
2. Tilt head back.
3. Gently grasp lower outer eyelid below lashes, and pull eyelid away from the eye.
4. Place ointment tube over eye by directly looking at it. With a sweeping motion, place ¼ to ½-inch of ointment inside the lower eyelid by gently squeezing the tube. **NOTE:** To prevent contamination, do not let the tip of the tube touch any surface (including the eye or eyelid). When not in use, keep the tube tightly closed.
5. Slowly release eyelid and close eyes for 1 to 2 minutes.
6. Blot excessive ointment from around the eye with a tissue.
7. Vision may be temporarily blurred. Until vision clears, avoid activities requiring good visual ability.

Counseling tips:

- If having difficulty determining whether an eye dropper has touched the eye surface, keep the dropper in a refrigerator (not in a freezer).
- If more than one drop is needed, wait at least 5 minutes before instilling the next drop to prevent flushing away or diluting the first drop.
- If both eye drop and ointment therapy are needed, instill the eye drop at least 10 minutes before the ointment.

GLAUCOMA AGENTS

BRAND (generic)	INGREDIENT/STRENGTH	DOSE
BETA-BLOCKER, NONSELECTIVE		
Betagan (levobunolol HCl)	**Sol:** 0.25% [10mL], 0.5% [2mL, 10mL, 15mL]	**Adults:** (0.5%): 1-2 drops in affected eye(s) qd; bid for more severe or uncontrolled glaucoma. (0.25%): 1-2 drops bid.
Betimol (timolol)	**Sol:** 0.25%, 0.5% [5mL, 10mL, 15mL]	**Adults: Initial:** 1 drop in affected eye(s) 0.25% bid. May increase to max of 1 drop 0.5% bid. **Maint:** if adequate control, may try 1 drop of 0.25%-0.5% qd.
Carteolol (carteolol HCl)	**Sol:** 1% [5mL, 10mL, 15mL]	**Adults:** 1 drop in affected eye(s) bid.
Istalol (timolol maleate)	**Sol:** 0.5% [2.5mL, 5mL]	**Adults:** 1 drop in affected eye(s) qam.
Ocupress (carteolol HCl)	**Sol:** 1% [5mL, 10mL, 15mL]	**Adults:** 1 drop in affected eye(s) bid.
OptiPranolol (metipranolol)	**Sol:** 0.3% [5mL, 10mL]	**Adults:** 1 drop in affected eye(s) bid.
Timolol GFS (timolol maleate)	**Sol, Gel Forming:** 0.25%, 0.5% [2.5mL, 5mL]	**Adults: Initial:** 1 drop in affected eye(s) 0.25%-0.5% qd. Evaluate IOP 4 weeks after starting treatment. **Max:** 1 drop 0.5% qd. Dose other ophthalmic drugs 10 min prior to gel forming drops.
Timoptic (timolol maleate)	**Sol:** (Timoptic) 0.25% (5mL), 0.5% [5mL, 10mL]	**Adults:** Initial: 1 drop in affected eye(s) 0.25% bid. May increase to max of 1 drop 0.5% bid. **Maint:** if adequate control, may try 1 drop of 0.25%-0.5% qd.
BETA-BLOCKER, SELECTIVE		
Betaxolol Ophthalmic (betaxolol HCl)	**Sol:** 5mL, 10mL, 15mL	**Adults:** 1-2 drops in the affected eye(s) bid.
Betoptic S (betaxolol HCl)	**Sus:** 0.25% [2.5mL, 5mL, 10mL, 15mL]	**Adults:** 1 drop in the affected eye(s) bid.
CARBONIC ANHYDRASE INHIBITORS		
Acetazolamide	**Cap, Extended-Release:** 500mg; **Inj:** 500mg	**Adults:** (Cap, ER) Glaucoma: 500mg bid. Inj: Open-Angle Glaucoma: Usual: 250mg-1g IV/PO qd in divided doses. Secondary Glaucoma/Pre-op Treatment of Closed-Angle Glaucoma: (IV/PO) 250mg q4h or 250 mg bid if on short-term therapy or 500mg followed by 125 mg or 250mg q4h in severe cases.
Azopt (brinzolamide)	**Sus:** 1% [5mL, 10mL, 15mL]	**Adults:** 1 drop in affected eye(s) tid. Space dosing of other ophthalmic drugs by 10 min.
Methazolamide	**Tab:** 25mg, 50mg	**Adults:** 50-100mg bid-tid. May use with miotic or osmotic agents.
Trusopt (dorzolamide HCl)	**Sol:** 2% [10mL]	**Adults:** 1 drop in affected eye(s) tid. Space dosing of other ophthalmic drugs by 10 min.
CHOLINERGIC AGENTS		
Isopto carbachol	**Sol:** 1.5% [15mL], 3% [15mL, 30mL]	**Adults:** 2 drops in eye up to tid.
Phospholine Iodide (echothiophate iodide)	**Sol:** 0.03%, 0.06%, 0.125%, 0.25% [5mL]	**Adults:** Early Chronic Simple Glaucoma: (0.3%): 1 drop in affected eye(s) bid, am and hs. Advanced Chronic Simple Glaucoma/Glaucoma Secondary to Cataract Surgery: **Initial:** (0.3%): 1 drop bid, am and hs. **Titrate:** May increase to higher strengths prn.
Pilocarpine	**Sol:** 0.5%, 1%, 2%, 3%, 4%, 6% [15mL]	**Adults:** 2 drops tid-qid or more if needed. Heavily pigmented irises may require higher strengths.

(Continued)

BRAND	INGREDIENT/STRENGTH	DOSE
PROSTAGLANDIN ANALOGS		
Lumigan (bimatoprost)	**Sol:** 0.03% [2.5mL, 5mL, 7.5 mL]	**Adults:** 1 drop qd in affected eye(s) pm. **Max:** Once-daily dosing. Space dosing of other ophthalmic drugs by 5 min.
Travatan (travoprost)	**Sol:** 0.004% [2.5mL, 5mL]	**Adults:** 1 drop qd in affected eye(s) pm. **Max:** Once-daily dosing. Space dosing of other ophthalmic drugs by 5 min.
Xalatan (latanoprost)	**Sol:** 0.005% [2.5mL, 2.5mL x 3]	**Adults:** 1 drop qd in affected eye(s) pm. **Max:** Once-daily dosing. Space dosing of other ophthalmic drugs by 5 min.
COMBINATION DRUGS		
Combigan (brimonidine tartrate-timolol maleate)	**Sol:** (Brimonidine-Timolol) 2mg-5mg/mL	**Adults:** 1 drop in affected eye(s) bid approximately 12 hrs apart. Space dosing of other ophthalmic products at least 5 min apart.
Cosopt (dorzolamide HCl-timolol maleate)	**Sol:** (Dorzolamide-Timolol) 2%-5% [10mL]	**Adults:** 1 drop in affected eye(s) bid. Space dosing of other ophthalmic drugs by 10 min.
MISCELLANEOUS		
Alphagan P (brimonidine tartrate)	**Sol:** 0.1% [5mL, 10mL, 15mL], 0.15% [5mL, 10mL, 15mL] (contains Purite)	**Adults:** 1 drop in affected eye(s) tid, give q8h. Space dosing of other ophthalmic products that lower IOP by 5 min.
Iopidine (apraclonidine HCl)	**Sol:** 0.5% [5mL, 10mL], 1% [0.1mL, 24s]	**Adults:** (0.5%): 1-2 drops in affected eye(s) tid. Space dosing of other ophthalmic drugs by 5 min. (1%): 1 drop 1 hr pre-op, then 1 drop immediately post-op.
Pilopine HS (pilocarpine HCl)	**Gel:** 4% [4g]	**Adults:** Apply ½ inch into conjunctival sac hs.
Propine (dipivefrin HCl)	**Sol:** 0.1% [10mL, 15mL]	**Adults:** Usual: 1 drop in affected eye(s) q12h.

ADHD AGENTS

BRAND (GENERIC)	HOW SUPPLIED	ADULT DOSE	PEDIATRIC DOSE
Adderall (Amphetamine plus dextroamphetamine)	Tab: 5mg*, 7.5mg*, 10mg*, 12.5mg*, 15mg*, 20mg*, 30mg* *scored		**3-5 yrs:** Initial: 2.5mg qd. Titrate: May increase by 2.5mg weekly. **≥6 yrs:** 5mg qd-bid. May increase by 5mg weekly. Give 1st dose upon awakening and add'l doses q4-6h. Max (usual): 40mg/day.
Adderall XR* (Amphetamine salt combo)	Cap: 5mg, 10mg, 15mg, 20mg, 25mg, 30mg	Initial: 20mg qam. Currently Using Adderall: Switch to Adderall XR at the same total daily dose, taken once daily. Titrate at weekly intervals as needed.	**≥6 yrs:** Initial: 10mg qam. Titrate: May increase weekly by 5-10mg/day. Max: 30mg/day. **13-17 yrs:** Initial: 10mg/day. Titrate: May increase to 20mg/day after one week. Currently Using Adderall: Switch to Adderall XR at the same total daily dose, taken once daily. Titrate at weekly intervals as needed.
Concerta** (Methylphenidate HCl)	Tab, Extended-Release: 18mg, 27mg, 36mg, 54mg	Methylphenidate-Naive or Receiving Other Stimulant: Initial: 18 or 36mg qam. Titrate: Adjust dose at weekly intervals. Previous Methylphenidate Use: Initial: 18mg qam if previous dose 10-15mg/day; 36mg qam if previous dose 20-30mg/day; 54mg qam if previous dose 30-45mg/day; 72mg qam if previous dose 40-60mg/day. Initial conversion should not exceed 72mg/day. Titrate: Adjust dose at weekly intervals. Max: 72mg/day. Reduce dose or d/c if paradoxical aggravation of symptoms occurs. D/C if no improvement after appropriate dosage adjustments over 1 month.	**≥6 yrs:** Methylphenidate-Naive or Receiving Other Stimulant: Initial: 18mg qam. Titrate: Adjust dose at weekly intervals. Max: **6-12 yrs:** 54mg/day; **13-17 yrs:** 18-72mg/day not to exceed 2mg/kg/day. Previous Methylphenidate Use: Initial: 18mg qam if previous dose 10-15mg/day; 36mg qam if previous dose 20-30mg/day; 54mg qam if previous dose 30-45mg/day; 72mg qam if previous dose 40-60mg/day. Initial conversion should not exceed 72mg/day. Titrate: Adjust dose at weekly intervals. Max: 72mg/day. Reduce dose or d/c if paradoxical aggravation of symptoms occurs. D/C if no improvement after appropriate dosage adjustments over 1 month.
Daytrana (Methylphenidate transdermal system)	Patch: 10mg/9 hrs, 15mg/9 hrs, 20mg/9 hrs, 30mg/9 hrs [10[S], 30[S]]	Individualize dose. Apply to hip area 2 hrs before effect is needed and remove 9 hrs after application. Recommended Titration Schedule: Week 1: 10mg/9 hrs. Week 2: 15mg/9 hrs. Week 3: 20mg/9 hrs. Week 4: 30mg/9 hrs.	**≥6 yrs:** Individualize dose. Apply to hip area 2 hrs before effect is needed and remove 9 hrs after application. Recommended Titration Schedule: Week 1: 10mg/9 hrs. Week 2: 15mg/9 hrs. Week 3: 20mg/9 hrs. Week 4: 30mg/9 hrs.
Desoxyn (Methamphetamine HCl)	Tab: 5mg		**≥6 yrs:** Initial: 5mg qd-bid. Titrate: Increase weekly by 5mg/day until optimum response. Usual: 20-25mg/day; may be given in 2 divided doses.
Dexedrine (Dextroamphetamine sulfate)	Cap, Extended-Release: (Spansules) 5mg, 10mg, 15mg		**3-5 yrs:** Initial: 2.5mg qd. Titrate: Increase weekly by 2.5mg/day. **≥6 yrs:** 5mg qd-bid. Titrate: Increase weekly by 5mg/day. Max: 40mg/day.

(Continued)

BRAND (GENERIC)	HOW SUPPLIED	ADULT DOSE	PEDIATRIC DOSE
DextroStat (Dextroamphetamine sulfate)	Tab: 5mg*, 10mg* *scored		**3-5 yrs:** Initial: 2.5mg/day. Titrate: Increase weekly by 2.5mg/day until optimum response. **≥6 yrs:** Initial 5mg qd-bid. Titrate: Increase weekly by 5mg/day until optimum response. Give 1st dose upon awakening, and additional doses q4-6h.
Focalin (Dexmethylphenidate HCl)	Tab: 2.5mg, 5mg, 10mg	Take bid at least 4 hrs apart. Methylphenidate Naive: Initial: 2.5mg bid. Titrate: Increase weekly by 2.5-5mg/day. Max: 20mg/day. Currently on Methylphenidate: Initial: Take ½ of methylphenidate dose. Max: 20mg/day. Reduce or d/c if paradoxical aggravation of symptoms. D/C if no improvement after appropriate dosage adjustments over 1 month.	**≥6 yrs:** Take bid at least 4 hrs apart. Methylphenidate Naive: Initial: 2.5mg bid. Titrate: Increase weekly by 2.5-5mg/day. Max: 20mg/day. Currently on Methylphenidate: Initial: Take ½ of methylphenidate dose. Max: 20mg/day. Reduce or d/c if paradoxical aggravation of symptoms. D/C if no improvement after appropriate dosage adjustments over 1 month.
Focalin XR* (Dexmethylphenidate HCl)	Cap, Extended-Release: 5mg, 10mg, 15mg, 20mg	Methylphenidate Naive: Initial: 10mg/day. Titrate: May adjust weekly by 10mg/day. Max: 20mg/day. Currently on Methylphenidate: Initial: Take ½ of methylphenidate dose. Max: 20mg/day. Currently on Focalin: May switch to same daily dose of Focalin XR. Reduce or d/c if paradoxical aggravation of symptoms. D/C if no improvement after appropriate dosage adjustments over 1 month.	**≥6 yrs:** Methylphenidate Naive: Initial: 5mg/day. Titrate: May adjust weekly by 5mg/day. Max: 20mg/day. Currently on Methylphenidate: Initial: Take ½ of methylphenidate dose. Max: 20mg/day. Currently on Focalin: May switch to same daily dose of Focalin XR. Reduce or d/c if paradoxical aggravation of symptoms. D/C if no improvement after appropriate dosage adjustments over 1 month.
Metadate CD* (Methylphenidate HCl)	Cap, Extended-Release: 10mg, 20mg, 30mg, 40mg, 50mg, 60mg	Usual: 20mg qam before breakfast. Titrate: Increase weekly by 10-20mg depending on tolerability/efficacy. Max: 60mg/day. Reduce dose or d/c if paradoxical aggravation of symptoms occur. D/C if no improvement after appropriate dose adjustments over 1 month.	**≥6 yrs:** Usual: 20mg qam before breakfast. Titrate: Increase weekly by 10-20mg depending on tolerability/efficacy. Max: 60mg/day. Reduce dose or d/c if paradoxical aggravation of symptoms occur. D/C if no improvement after appropriate dose adjustments over 1 month.
Metadate ER** (Methylphenidate HCl)	Tab, Extended-Release: 10mg, 20mg	(Immediate-Release Methylphenidate) 10-60mg/day given bid-tid 30-45 min ac. If insomnia occurs, take last dose before 6 pm.†	**≥6 yrs:** (Immediate-Release Methylphenidate) Initial: 5mg bid before breakfast and lunch. Titrate: Increase gradually by 5-10mg weekly. Max: 60mg/day. Reduce dose or d/c if paradoxical aggravation of symptoms occur. D/C if no improvement after appropriate dose adjustment over 1 month.†
Methylin** (Methylphenidate HCl)	Sol: 5mg/5mL [500mL], 10mg/5mL [500mL]; Tab: 5mg, 10mg, 20mg; Tab, Chewable: 2.5mg, 5mg, 10mg; Tab, Extended-Release: 10mg, 20mg	(Sol/Tab/Tab, Chewable) 10-60mg/day given bid-tid 30-45 min ac. If insomnia occurs, take last dose before 6 pm.†	**≥6 yrs:** (Sol/Tab/Tab, Chewable) Initial: 5mg bid before breakfast and lunch. Titrate: Increase gradually by 5-10mg weekly. Max: 60mg/day. Reduce dose or d/c if paradoxical aggravation of symptoms occur. D/C if no improvement after appropriate dose adjustment over 1 month.†

BRAND (GENERIC)	HOW SUPPLIED	ADULT DOSE	PEDIATRIC DOSE
Ritalin, Ritalin LA*, Ritalin SR** (Methylphenidate HCl)	Cap, Extended-Release (Ritalin LA): 10mg, 20mg, 30mg, 40mg; Tab (Ritalin): 5mg, 10mg*, 20mg*; Tab, Extended-Release (Ritalin SR): 20mg **scored*	(Tab) 10-60mg/day given bid-tid 30-45 min ac. Take last dose before 6 pm if insomnia occurs. (Cap, ER) Initial: 20mg qam. Titrate: Adjust weekly by 10mg. Max: 60mg qam.† Previous Methylphenidate Use: May use as qd in place of IR dosed bid or daily dose of methylphenidate-SR. Reduce dose or d/c if paradoxical aggravation of symptoms occurs. D/C if no improvement after appropriate dose adjustment over 1 month.†	**≥6 yrs:** (Tab) Initial: 5mg bid before breakfast and lunch. Titrate: Increase gradually by 5-10mg weekly. Max: 60mg/day. (Cap, ER) Initial: 20mg qam. Titrate: Adjust weekly by 10mg. Max: 60mg qam. Previous Methylphenidate Use: May use as qd in place of IR dosed bid or daily dose of methylphenidate-SR. Reduce dose or d/c if paradoxical aggravation of symptoms occurs. D/C if no improvement after appropriate dose adjustment over 1 month.†
Strattera (Atomoxetine HCl)	Cap: 10mg, 18mg, 25mg, 40mg, 60mg, 80mg, 100mg	Initial: 40mg/day given qam or evenly divided doses in the am and late afternoon/early evening. Titrate: Increase after minimum of 3 days to target dose of about 80mg/day. After 2-4 weeks, may increase to max of 100mg/day. Max: 100mg/day. Dose adjust in hepatic insufficiency and when used with concomitant CYP450 2D6 inhibitors. See PI for detailed dosing information	**≥6 yrs:** ≤70kg: Initial: 0.5mg/kg/day given qam or evenly divided doses in the am and late afternoon or early evening. Titrate: Increase after minimum of 3 days to target dose of about 1.2mg/kg/day. Max: 1.4mg/kg/day or 100mg, whichever is less. >70kg: Initial: 40mg/day given qam or evenly divided doses in the am and late afternoon/early evening. Titrate: Increase after minimum of 3 days to target dose of about 80mg/day. After 2-4 weeks, may increase to max of 100mg/day. Max: 100mg/day. Dose adjust in hepatic insufficiency and when used with concomitant CYP450 2D6 inhibitors. See PI for detailed dosing information.
Vyvanse (Lisdexamfetamine dimesylate)	Cap: 20mg, 30mg, 40mg, 50mg, 60mg, 70mg	Individualize dose. Usual: 30mg qam. Titrate: If needed, may increase in increments of 10mg or 20mg at weekly intervals. Max: 70mg/day. Swallow caps or dissolve contents in glass of water; do not store once dissolved. Re-evaluate periodically.	Individualize dose. **6-12 yrs:** Usual: 30mg qam. Titrate: If needed, may increase in increments of 10mg or 20mg at weekly intervals. Max: 70mg/day. Swallow caps or dissolve contents in glass of water; do not store once dissolved. Re-evaluate periodically.

ADHD = attention-deficit/hyperactivity disorder.
*Swallow cap whole or open cap and sprinkle contents on applesauce; do not chew beads.
**Swallow whole; do not chew, crush, or divide.
†Tab, Extended-Release: May use in place of immediate-release tabs when the 8-hr dose corresponds to the titrated 8-hr immediate-release dose.

ALZHEIMER'S DISEASE AGENTS

DRUG (BRAND)	INDICATIONS	HOW SUPPLIED	DOSAGE	SIDE EFFECTS
Donepezil HCl (Aricept)	Treatment of dementia of the Alzheimer's type.	Tab: 5mg, 10mg; Tab, Disintegrating: 5mg, 10mg	Mild to Moderate Alzheimer's Disease: Initial: 5mg qd. Titrate: May increase to 10mg after 4-6 weeks. Severe Alzheimer's Disease: 10mg qd. Start with 5mg qd and increase to 10mg after 4-6 weeks.	Nausea, diarrhea, insomnia, vomiting, muscle cramps, fatigue, anorexia, dizziness, depression, weight decrease, infection, HTN, back pain, abnormal dreams, ecchymosis
Ergoloid Mesylates (Ergoloid mesylates)	Treatment of symptomatic decline in mental capacity of unknown etiology (eg, Alzheimer's dementia, multi-infarct dementia).	Tab: 1mg; Tab, Sublingual: 1mg, 0.5mg	Usual: 1mg tid.	Transient nausea, gastric disturbances
Galantamine HBr (Razadyne, Razadyne ER)	Treatment of mild to moderate dementia of the Alzheimer's type.	Sol: (Razadyne) 4mg/mL [100mL]; Tab: (Razadyne) 4mg, 8mg, 12mg. Cap, Extended-Release; (Razadyne ER) 8mg, 16mg, 24mg	(Sol, Tab) Initial: 4mg bid with am and pm meals. Titrate: Increase to 8mg bid after 4 weeks if tolerated, then increase to 12mg bid after 4 weeks if tolerated. Usual: 16-24mg/day. Max: 24mg/day. (Cap, ER) Initial: 8mg qd with am meal. Titrate: Increase to 16mg qd after 4 weeks, then increase to 24mg qd after 4 weeks if tolerated. Usual: 16-24mg/day. Max: 24mg/day. If therapy is interrupted, restart at lowest dose and increase to current dose. See PI for dose modification in moderate renal/hepatic impairment.	Nausea, vomiting, diarrhea, anorexia, weight loss, fatigue, dizziness, headache, depression, insomnia, abdominal pain, dyspepsia
Memantine HCl (Namenda)	Treatment of moderate to severe dementia of the Alzheimer's type.	Sol: 2mg/mL [360mL]; Tab: 5mg, 10mg; Titration-Pak: 5mg [28^S], 10mg [21^S]	Initial: 5mg qd. Titrate: Increase at intervals of at least one week to 5mg bid, then 5mg and 10mg as separate doses, then to 10mg bid. Severe Renal Impairment: Reduce dose.	Dizziness, confusion, headache, constipation, coughing, HTN, pain, vomiting, somnolence, hallucinations
Rivastigmine tartrate (Exelon)	Treatment of mild to moderate dementia of the Alzheimer's type.	Cap: 1.5mg, 3mg, 4.5mg, 6mg; Sol: 2mg/mL [120mL]; Patch: 4.6mg/24hrs, 9.5 mg/24 hrs [30^S]	Initial: 1.5mg bid. Titrate: May increase by 1.5mg bid every 2 weeks. Max: 12mg/day. If not tolerating, suspend therapy for several doses and restart at same or next lower dose. If interrupted longer than several days, reinitiate with lowest daily dose and titrate as above. (Patch) Initial: Apply 4.6mg/24 hrs patch qd to clean, dry, hairless intact skin. Maint: Increase dose after 4 weeks. Max: 9.5mg/24 hrs if well tolerated. Switching from Capsules/Oral Sol: Total Oral Daily Dose <6mg: Switch to 4.6mg/24 hrs patch. Total Oral Daily Dose 6-12mg: Switch to 9.5mg/24 hrs patch. Apply 1st patch on day following last oral dose.	Nausea, vomiting, abdominal pain, dyspepsia, constipation, somnolence, anorexia, asthenia, headache, dizziness, fatigue, diarrhea, tremor, depression
Tacrine HCl (Cognex)	Treatment of mild to moderate dementia of the Alzheimer's type.	Cap: 10mg, 20mg, 30mg, 40mg	Initial: 10mg qid. Titrate: Increase to 20mg qid after 4 weeks, then increase at 4-week intervals to 30mg qid then to 40mg qid. See PI for dose modification in case of elevated AST/SGPT elevations.	Elevated LFTs, nausea, vomiting, diarrhea, dyspepsia, myalgia, anorexia, ataxia, dizziness

ANTIPARKINSON'S AGENTS

DRUG (BRAND)	INDICATIONS	HOW SUPPLIED	DOSAGE	SIDE EFFECTS
Bromocriptine mesylate (Parlodel)	Treatment of symptoms of Parkinson's disease; adjunctive treatment to levodopa.	Tab, Snap: 2.5mg*; Cap: 5mg *scored	Initial: 1.25mg bid. Titrate: If needed, increase by 2.5mg/day every 2-4 weeks. Max: 100mg/day. Take with food. See PI for detailed dosing information with levodopa.	Headache, dizziness, GI effects, orthostatic hypotension, fatigue, arrhythmia, insomnia, hallucinations, abnormal involuntary movements, depression, syncope
Carbidopa (Lodosyn)	For use with Sinemet or levodopa in treatment of symptoms of idiopathic Parkinson's disease, postencephalitic parkinsonism, and symptomatic parkinsonism. For use in patients for whom the dosage of Sinemet provides less than adequate daily dosage (usually 70mg daily) of carbidopa.	Tab: 25mg* *scored	With Sinemet or Levodopa: Determine dose by careful titration. Most patients respond to a 1:10 proportion of carbidopa: levodopa provided carbidopa dose is ≥70mg/day. Max: 200mg/day. Consider amount of carbidopa in Sinemet when calculating dose. See PI for detailed dosing information.	Dyskinesia, psychotic episodes, delusions, hallucinations, paranoid ideation, depression with or without suicidal tendencies, dementia
Carbidopa/levodopa (Sinemet, Sinemet CR)	Treatment of symptoms of idiopathic Parkinson's disease, postencephalitic parkinsonism, and symptomatic parkinsonism.	Tab: (Carbidopa-Levodopa) 10mg-100mg*, 25mg-100mg*, 25mg-250mg*; Tab, Extended Release: (Carbidopa-Levodopa) 25mg-100mg, 50mg-200mg* *scored	(Tab) 25mg-100mg tab: Initial: 1 tab tid. Titrate: Increase by 1 tab qd or every other day up to 8 tabs/day. 10mg-100mg tab: Initial: 1 tab tid-qid. Titrate: Increase by 1 tab qd or every other day up to 2 tabs qid. 70-100mg/day carbidopa required. Max: 200mg/day carbidopa. (Tab, Extended-Release) No Prior Levodopa Use: Initial: 1 50mg-200mg tab bid at intervals >6 hrs. Titrate: Increase or decrease dose or interval accordingly. Adjust dose every 3 days. Usual: 400-1600mg/day levodopa, given in 4-8 hr intervals while awake. Conversion to Extended-Release Tabs: See PI.	Dyskinesia, nausea, cardiac irregularities, hypotension, dark saliva, GI bleeding, psychotic episodes, NMS, confusion, agitation, dizziness, somnolence, dream abnormalities
Carbidopa/levodopa (Parcopa)	Treatment of symptoms of idiopathic Parkinson's disease, postencephalitic parkinsonism, and symptomatic parkinsonism.	Tab, Disintegrating: (Carbidopa-Levodopa) 10mg-100mg*, 25mg-100mg*, 25mg-250mg* *scored	25mg-100mg tab: Initial: 1 tab tid. Titrate: Increase by 1 tab qd or qod up to 8 tabs/day. 10mg-100mg tab: Initial: 1 tab tid-qid. Titrate: Increase by 1 tab qd or qod up to 2 tabs qid. 70-100mg/day carbidopa required. Max: 200mg/day carbidopa.	Dyskinesia, choreiform, dystonic and other involuntary movements, nausea

DRUG (BRAND)	INDICATIONS	HOW SUPPLIED	DOSAGE	SIDE EFFECTS
Carbidopa/levodopa/entacapone (Stalevo)	Treatment of idiopathic Parkinson's disease to substitute for equivalent doses of previously administered carbidopa/levodopa and entacapone, or for those experiencing signs and symptoms of end-of-dose "wearing off" and taking up to 600mg/day levodopa without experiencing dyskinesias.	Tab: (Carbidopa/Levodopa/Entacapone): Stalevo 50: 12.5mg/50mg/200mg; Stalevo 75: 18.75mg/75mg/200 mg; Stalevo 100: 25mg/100mg/200mg; Stalevo 125: 31.25mg/125mg/200mg; Stalevo 150: 37.5mg/150mg/200mg; Stalevo 200: 50mg/200mg/200mg	Currently Taking Carbidopa/Levodopa and Entacapone: May switch directly to corresponding strength of levodopa/carbidopa/entacapone. Currently Taking Carbidopa/Levodopa, but not Entacapone: First, titrate individually with carbidopa/levodopa product and entacapone product, then transfer to corresponding dose. Max dose: 8 tabs/day except Stalevo 200. Max: 6 tabs/day.	Dyskinesia, hyperkinesia, hypokinesia, dizziness, nausea, diarrhea, abdominal pain, constipation, vomiting, urine discoloration, back pain, fatigue
Diphenhydramine HCl Injection	For parkinsonism when oral therapy is not possible or contraindicated.	Inj: 50mg/mL	Usual: 10-50mg IV at ≤25 mg/min or up to 100mg IM if needed. Max: 400mg/day.	Sedation, drowsiness, dizziness, disturbed coordination, epigastric distress, thickening of bronchial secretions
Pramipexole dihydrochloride (Mirapex)	Treatment of signs and symptoms of idiopathic Parkinson's disease.	Tab: 0.125mg, 0.25mg*, 0.5mg*, 0.75mg, 1mg*, 1.5mg* *scored	Initial: 0.125mg tid. Titrate: May increase every 5-7 days (eg, Week 2: 0.25mg tid; Week 3: 0.5mg tid; Week 4: 0.75mg tid; Week 5: 1mg tid; Week 6: 1.25mg tid; Week 7: 1.5mg tid). Maint: 0.5-1.5mg tid. Max: 1.5mg tid.†	Nausea, dizziness, somnolence, insomnia, constipation, asthenia, hallucinations, vision abnormalities, peripheral edema, arthritis, dry mouth, postural hypotension, chest pain, malaise
Rasagiline mesylate (Azilect)	Treatment of signs and symptoms of idiopathic Parkinson's disease as initial monotherapy and adjunct therapy to levodopa.	Tab: 0.5mg, 1mg	Monotherapy: 1mg qd. Adjunctive Therapy: Initial: 0.5mg qd. Titrate: May increase to 1mg qd. Adjust dose of levodopa with concomitant use. Concomitant Ciprofloxacin or Other CYP1A2 Inhibitors/Hepatic Impairment: 0.5mg qd.	Headache, arthralgia, depression, fall, flu syndrome, dyskinesia, accidental injury, nausea, weight loss, constipation, postural hypotension, vomiting, dry mouth, rash, somnolence
Rivastigmine (Exelon)	Treatment of mild to moderate dementia associated with Parkinson's disease.	Cap: 1.5mg, 3mg, 4.5mg, 6mg; Patch: 4.6mg/24h, 9.5mg/24h; Sol: 2mg/mL (120mL)	(Cap, Sol): Initial: 1.5mg bid with meals in am and pm. Titrate: May increase at 4-week intervals to 3mg bid, then 4.5mg bid, and 6mg bid if tolerable. Usual: 1.5-6mg bid. Patch: Initial: 4.6mg/24h. Titrate: After 4 weeks, may increase to 9.5mg/24h if tolerated. Recommended: 9.5mg/24h.	Nausea, vomiting, anorexia, tremor, chest pain, dyskinesia, dyspepsia, back pain

(Continued)

DRUG (BRAND)	INDICATIONS	HOW SUPPLIED	DOSAGE	SIDE EFFECTS
Ropinirole HCl (Requip) (Requip XL)	Treatment of symptoms of idiopathic Parkinson's disease.	Tab: 0.25mg, 0.5mg, 1mg, 2mg, 3mg, 4mg, 5mg Tab, Extended-Release: 2mg, 4mg, 8mg, 12mg	Initial: 0.25mg tid. Titrate: May increase weekly by 0.25mg tid (0.75mg/day) for 4 weeks. After Week 4, may increase weekly by 1.5mg/day up to 9mg/day, then by 3mg/day weekly to 24mg/day. Max: 24mg/day. Withdrawal: Decrease dose to bid for 4 days, then qd for 3 days. (Requip XL) Tab, Extended-Release: Initial: 2mg qd for 1-2 weeks. Swallow whole. Titrate: May increase at ≥1 week intervals by 2mg/day. Max: 24mg/day. Levodopa dose may be gradually decreased as tolerated. Switching from IR to ER: Closely match total daily IR dose with initial extended-release dose. See PI for detailed information.	Neuralgia, increased BUN, hallucinations, somnolence, vomiting, headache, sweating, asthenia, edema, fatigue, syncope, orthostatic symptoms
ADJUNCT THERAPY				
Amantadine HCl (Symmetrel)	Treatment of parkinsonism and drug-induced extrapyramidal reactions.	Tab: 100mg	Parkinsonism: Initial: 100mg bid. Serious Associated Illness/Concomitant High-Dose Antiparkinson Agent: Initial: 100mg qd. Titrate: May increase to 100mg bid.	Nausea, dizziness, insomnia, depression, anxiety, hallucinations, confusion, anorexia, dry mouth, constipation, ataxia
Apomorphine HCl (Apokyn)	Acute, intermittent treatment of hypomobility, "off" episodes (end-of-dose "wearing off" and unpredictable "on/off" episodes) associated with advanced Parkinson's disease.	Inj: 10mg/mL [3mL]	Initial: Test Dose: 2mg SC; monitor BP closely. Titrate: Increase by 1mg every few days; assess efficacy/tolerability. Max: 6mg/day. Renal Impairment: Initial: 1mg SC.	Yawning, dyskinesia, nausea, vomiting, somnolence, dizziness, rhinorrhea, edema, chest pain, increased sweating, flushing, pallor
Benztropine mesylate (Cogentin)	Adjunct in all forms of parkinsonism. Control of drug-induced extrapyramidal disorders.	Inj: 1mg/mL; Tab: 0.5mg, 1mg, 2mg	Parkinsonism: Initial: 0.5-1mg PO/IV/IM qhs. Titrate: May increase every 5-6 days by 0.5mg. Usual: 1-2mg PO/IV/IM qhs. Max: 6mg/day. Extrapyramidal Disorders: 1-4mg PO/IV/IM qd-bid. Acute Dystonic Reactions: 1-2mg IM/IV, then 1-2mg PO bid.	Tachycardia, paralytic ileus, constipation, vomiting, nausea, dry mouth, confusion, blurred vision, urinary retention, heat stroke, hyperthermia, fever
Entacapone (Comtan)	Adjunct to levodopa/carbidopa for treatment of idiopathic Parkinson's disease if experience signs of end-of-dose "wearing-off."	Tab: 200mg	200mg with each levodopa/carbidopa dose. Max: 1600mg/day. Withdraw slowly for discontinuation.	Sweating, back pain, dyskinesia, hyperkinesia, hypokinesia, nausea, diarrhea, abdominal pain, urine discoloration

DRUG (BRAND)	INDICATIONS	HOW SUPPLIED	DOSAGE	SIDE EFFECTS
Hyoscyamine sulfate (Levsin, Levbid, Levsinex)	To reduce rigidity and tremors of Parkinson's disease.	(Levbid) Tab, Extended-Release: 0.375mg. (Levsin) Drops: 0.125mg/mL [15mL]; Elixir: 0.125mg/5mL [473mL]; Inj: 0.5mg/mL; Tab: 0.125mg*; Tab, Sublingual: 0.125mg*. (Levsinex) Cap, Extended-Release: 0.375mg *scored	May also chew or swallow SL tab. (Drops; Elixir; Tab; and Tab, SL) 0.125-0.25mg q4h or prn. Max: 1.5mg/24 hrs. (Cap and Tab, Extended-Release) 0.375-0.75mg q12h; or 1 cap q8h. Max: 1.5mg/24 hrs. Do not crush or chew.	Anticholinergic effects, drowsiness, headache, nervousness
Selegiline HCl (Eldepryl)	Adjunct to levodopa/carbidopa for management of Parkinson's disease.	Cap: 5mg	5mg bid, at breakfast and lunch. Max: 10mg/day. May reduce levodopa/carbidopa by 10-30% after 2-3 days of therapy. May reduce further with continued therapy.	Nausea, dizziness, lightheadedness, fainting, abdominal pain, confusion, hallucinations, dry mouth
Selegiline HCl (Zelapar)	Adjunct in the management of Parkinson's disease in patients exhibiting a deteriorated response to levodopa/carbidopa therapy.	Tab, Orally Disintegrating: 1.25mg	1.25mg qd for 6 weeks. Titrate: After 6 weeks, may increase to 2.5mg qd if desired benefit not achieved. Max: 2.5mg/day.	Nausea, dizziness, pain, headache, insomnia, rhinitis, skin disorders, dyskinesia, backache, dyspepsia, stomatitis, constipation, hallucinations, pharyngitis, rash
Tolcapone (Tasmar)	Adjunct to levodopa/carbidopa for the treatment of symptoms of idiopathic Parkinson's disease.	Tab: 100mg, 200mg	Initial: 100mg tid. Use 200mg tid only if clinical benefit is justified. May need to decrease levodopa dose.	Dyskinesia, nausea, dystonia, excessive dreaming, anorexia, muscle cramps, orthostatic complaints, diarrhea, dizziness, headache
Trihexyphenidyl HCl	Adjunct treatment for all forms of parkinsonism (postencephalitic, arteriosclerotic, and idiopathic). For control of extrapyramidal disorders caused by CNS drugs.	Sol: 2mg/5mL [473mL]; Tab: 2mg*, 5mg* *scored	Idiopathic Parkinsonism: 1mg on Day 1. Titrate: Increase by 2mg every 3-5 days. Usual: 6-10mg/day. Max: 15mg/day. Drug-Induced Parkinsonism: Initial: 1mg. If extrapyramidal manifestations not controlled in a few hrs, increase dose until achieve control. Usual: 5-15mg/day.	Dry mouth, blurred vision, dizziness, nausea, nervousness, constipation, drowsiness, urinary hesitancy/retention, tachycardia, pupil dilation, increased intraocular tension, vomiting, weakness, headache

†For specific dosing information on different creatinine clearance values, see full Prescribing Information.

Opioid Products

GENERIC	BRAND	DOSAGE FORMS	ORAL EQUI-ANALGESIC DOSE	EQUI-ANALGESIC DOSE	USUAL ADULT DOSE	MAX DOSE	INDICATION	DEA SCHEDULE
Codeine		**Inj, Oral Sol:** (15mg/5mL); **Tab:** 15mg, 30mg, 60mg	200mg.	130mg.	PO, IM, SC, IV 15-60mg q4-6h.	360mg/24 hrs.	Relief of mild to moderate pain; cough suppression.	Schedule II
Codeine phosphate/ Acetaminophen	Tylenol w/Codeine	**Elixir:** 12mg-120mg/5mL			15mL q4h prn. 15-60mg codeine/dose and 300-1000mg APAP.	Codeine: 360mg/day. APAP: 4g/day.	Relief of mild to moderately severe pain.	Schedule V
	Tylenol #2	**Tab:** 15mg/300mg						Schedule III
	Tylenol #3	**Tab:** 30mg/300mg						Schedule III
	Tylenol #4	**Tab:** 60mg/300mg						Schedule III
Hydrocodone bitartrate/ Acetaminophen	Anexsia	**Tab:** 5mg-325mg, 7.5mg-325mg, 5mg-500mg, 7.5mg-650mg			1-2 tabs q4-6h (5/325, 5/500). 1 tab q4-6h (7.5/325, 7.5/650).	(5/325): 12 tabs/day. (5/500, 7.5/325): 8 tabs/day. (7.5/650): 6 tabs/day.	Relief of moderate to moderately severe pain.	Schedule III
	Lorcet, Lorcet-HD Lorcet Plus	**Cap:** (HD) 5mg-500mg; **Tab:** (Plus) 7.5mg-650mg, (10/650) 10mg-650mg			(Plus)1 tab q4-6h prn pain. (HD) 1-2 caps q4-6h prn pain.	(Plus) Max: 6 tabs/day. (HD) 8 caps/day.		
	Lortab Elixir Lortab	**Sol:** 7.5mg-500mg/15mL **Tab:** 2.5mg/500mg, 5mg/500mg, 7.5mg/500mg, 10mg/500mg			1 tbs q4-6h prn. (2.5/500, 5/500): 1-2 tabs q4-6h prn. (7.5/500,10/500): 1 tab q4-6h prn.	6 tbs. (2.5/500, 5/500): 8 tabs/day. (7.5/500, 10/500): 6 tabs/day.		
	Norco	**Tab:** 5mg/325mg, 7.5mg/325mg, 10mg/325mg			(5/325): 1-2 tabs q4-6h prn. (7.5/325, 10/325): 1 tab q4-6h prn.	(7.5/325,10/325): 6 tabs/day.		
	Vicodin	**Tab:** 5mg/500mg			1-2 tabs q4-6h prn.	8 tabs/day.		
	Vicodin ES	**Tab:** 7.5mg/750mg			1 tab q4-6h prn.	5 tabs/day.		
	Vicodin HP	**Tab:** 10mg/660mg			1 tab q4-6h prn.	6 tabs/day.		
	Zydone	**Tab:** 5mg/400mg, 7.5mg/400mg, 10mg/400mg			(5/400): 1-2 tabs q4-6h prn. (7.5/400, 10/400): 1 tab q4-6h prn.	(5/400): 8 tabs/day. (7.5/400, 10/400): 6 tabs/day.		
Hydrocodone bitartrate/Ibuprofen	Vicoprofen	**Tab:** 7.5/200mg			1 tab q4-6h prn.	5 tabs/day.	Short-term (generally <10 days) management of acute pain.	Schedule III

GENERIC	BRAND	DOSAGE FORMS	ORAL EQUI-ANALGESIC DOSE	EQUI-ANALGESIC DOSE	USUAL ADULT DOSE	MAX DOSE	INDICATION	DEA SCHEDULE
Oxycodone HCl	OxyContin	**Tab, ER:** 10mg, 20mg, 40mg, 80mg, 160mg			10mg q12h. Titrate: May increase the q12h dose (not the dosing frequency). May increase the total daily dose by 25-50% of the current dose.		Management of moderate to severe pain when a continuous around the clock analgesic is needed for an extended period. Only for postoperative use in patients already receiving the drug before surgery or those expected to have moderate-severe postoperative pain for an extended period of time.	Schedule II
	OxyFast	**Sol:** 20mg/mL			5mg q6h prn for pain.		Relief of moderate to moderately severe pain.	
	OxyIR	**Cap, IR:** 5mg			5mg q6h prn.			
	Roxicodone	**Sol:** 5mg/5mL; **Liq:** 20mg/mL; **Tab:** 5mg,15mg, 30mg			Tab: 15mg q4-6h prn; Sol/Liq: 10-30mg q4h prn.			
Oxycodone/Acetaminophen	Percocet	**Tab:** 2.5mg/325mg, 5mg/325mg, 7.5mg/325mg 7.5mg/500mg, 10mg/325mg,10mg/650mg			(2.5/325): 1-2 tabs q6h. (5/325): 1 tab q6h prn. (7.5/500): 1 tab q6h prn. (10-650) 1 tab q6h prn. (7.5/325): 1 tab q6h prn. (10/325): 1 tab q6h prn.	(2.5/325): 12 tabs/day. (5/325):12 tabs/day. (7.5/500): 8 tabs/day. (10-650) 6 tabs/day. (7.5/325):8 tabs/day. (10/325): 6 tabs/day.	Relief of moderate to moderately severe pain.	Schedule II
	Tylox	**Cap:** 5mg/500mg			1 cap q6h prn.	APAP: 4g/day.		
Oxycodone/Ibuprofen	Combunox	**Tab:** 5mg/400mg			1 tab/dose.	4 tabs/day for 7 days.	Short term (<7 days) management of acute, moderate to severe pain.	Schedule II
Oxycodone HCl/Aspirin	Percodan	**Tab:** 4.8355mg/325mg			1 tab q6h prn.	12 tabs/day or ASA 4g/day.	Relief of moderate to moderately severe pain.	Schedule II
Oxymorphone HCl	Opana	**Inj:** 1mg/1mL **Tab:** 5mg, 10mg			Inj: SQ/IM: 1-1.5mg q4-6h, IV: 0.5mg initial. Tab: 10-20mg q4-6h.		Relief of moderate to severe acute pain. (Tab, ER) Relief of moderate to severe pain in patients requiring continuous, around-the-clock opioid treatment for extended period of time.	Schedule II
	Opana ER	**Tab:** 5mg, 7.5mg, 10mg, 15mg, 20mg, 30mg, 40mg			5mg q12h. Titrate individually at increments of 5-10mg q12h every 3-7 days.			

(Continued)

GENERIC	BRAND	DOSAGE FORMS	ORAL EQUI-ANALGESIC DOSE	EQUI-ANALGESIC DOSE	USUAL ADULT DOSE	MAX DOSE	INDICATION	DEA SCHEDULE
Meperidine HCl	Demerol	**Syr:** 50mg/5mL; **Tab:** 50mg, 100mg; **Inj:** 25mg/mL, 50mg/mL, 75mg/mL, 100mg/mL	300mg.	75mg.	Tab: 50-150mg q3-4h prn. Inj: 50-150mg IM/SC q3-4h prn.		Moderate to severe pain. Inj: also for preoperative medication, anesthesia support, and obstetrical analgesia.	Schedule II
Propoxyphene HCl	Darvon	**Cap:** 65mg			65mg q4h prn.	390mg/day.	Relief of mild to moderate pain.	Schedule IV
Propoxyphene napsylate	Darvon-N	**Tab:** 100mg			100mg q4h prn.	600mg/day.	Relief of mild to moderate pain.	Schedule IV
Propoxyphene napsylate/ Acetaminophen	Darvocet-N 50	**Tab:** 50mg/325mg			100mg propoxyphene napsylate/650mg APAP q4h prn.	600mg propoxyphene napsylate/day. APAP: 4g/day.	Relief of mild to moderate pain.	Schedule IV
	Darvocet-N 100	**Tab:** 100mg/650mg						
	Darvocet-A 500	**Tab:** 100mg/500mg			100mg propoxyphene napsylate/500 mg APAP q4h prn.	6 tabs q24h.		
Tramadol	Ultram	**Tab:** 50mg; **Tab, ER:** 100mg, 200mg, 300mg			Tab: 50-100mg q4-6h prn. Tab, ER: 100mg/day. Titrate: 100mg q 5 days.	Tab: 400mg/day. Tab, ER: 300mg/day.	Management of moderate to moderately severe pain.	Rx only
Morphine sulfate	Astramorph PF	**Inj:** 0.5mg/mL, 1mg/mL	40-60mg.	10mg.	IV: 2-10mg/70kg of body weight. Epidural: 2-4mg/ 24 hrs. IT: 0.2-1mg/24 hrs.	Epidural: 10mg q24h.	Management of pain not responsive to non-narcotic analgesics.	Schedule II
	Duramorph	**Inj:** 0.5mg/mL, 1mg/mL			IV: 2-10mg/70kg of body weight. Epidural: 2-4mg/ 24 hrs. IT: 0.2-1mg/24 hrs.	Epidural: 10mg q24h.	Management of pain not responsive to non-narcotic analgesics.	
	Avinza	**Cap, ER:** 30mg, 60mg, 90mg, 120mg			30mg q24h.	1600mg/day.	Relief of moderate to severe pain requiring continuous opioid therapy for an extended period of time.	
	Infumorph	**Inj:** 0.5mg/mL (5mg), 1mg/mL (10mg), 10mg/mL (200mg), 25mg/mL (500mg)			1-10mg/day		Treatment of intractable chronic pain in microinfusion devices.	

GENERIC	BRAND	DOSAGE FORMS	ORAL EQUI-ANALGESIC DOSE	EQUI-ANALGESIC DOSE	USUAL ADULT DOSE	MAX DOSE	INDICATION	DEA SCHEDULE
	Kadian	**Cap, ER:** 10mg, 20mg, 30mg, 50mg, 60mg, 80mg, 100mg, 200mg			Give 50% of daily oral morphine dose q12h or give 100% oral morphine dose q24h.	Do not give more frequently than q12h.	Management of moderate to severe pain.	
	MS Contin	**Tab, ER:** 15mg, 30mg, 60mg, 100mg, 200mg			Give 50% of pts 24-hr requirement q12h or $^1/_3$ of pts 24-hr requirement q8h.		Relief of moderate to severe pain for patients who require repeated dosing with potent opioid analgesics over periods of more than a few days.	
	Oramorph SR	**Tab, ER:** 15mg, 30mg, 60mg, 100mg			Single dose is 1/2 of daily morphine requirement q12h.		Relief of pain in patients who require opioid analgesics for more than a few days.	
Hydromorphone HCl	Dilaudid, Dilaudid-HP	**Tab:** 2mg, 4mg, 8mg; **Sol:** 5mg/5mL; **HP:** 10mg/mL, 50mg/5mL, 500mg/50mL; **Pow:** 250mg	6.5-7.5mg.	1.3-2mg.	Tab: 2-4mg, PO every 4 to 6 hours. Sol: 2.5-10mL q3-6h as directed. HP: Individualized for each patient.		Management of pain. (HP) Relief of moderate to severe pain in opioid-tolerant patients who require larger than usual doses of opioids to provide adequate pain relief.	Schedule II
Methadone HCl	Dolophine	**Tab:** 5mg, 10mg; **Inj:** 10mg/mL	10-20mg.	10mg.	Dolophine: 2.5mg to 10mg every 8 to 12 hrs, slowly titrated to effect. Detox: Titrate to a total daily dose of about 40mg in divided doses. Inj: 2.5-10mg q8-12h.		To treat moderate to severe pain not responsive to non-narcotic analgesics. For detoxification treatment of opioid addiction. For maintenance treatment of opioid addiction.	Schedule II
	Methadose	**Concentrate:** 10mg/mL; **Tab:** 5mg, 10mg; **Tab, Dispersible:** 40mg			Detox: Initiate at 20-30mg and re-evaluate after 2-4hrs. Give additional 5-10mg if needed. Maintenance: Titrate to symptoms.			

(Continued)

GENERIC	BRAND	DOSAGE FORMS	ORAL EQUI-ANALGESIC DOSE	EQUI-ANALGESIC DOSE	USUAL ADULT DOSE	MAX DOSE	INDICATION	DEA SCHEDULE
Fentanyl	Duragesic	**Patch:** 12.5mcg/hr, 25mcg/hr, 50mcg/hr, 75mcg/hr, 100mcg/hr			Initial: 25mcg/hr for 72 hrs. Individualize dose.		Management of moderate to severe chronic pain when continuous opioid analgesia is required and cannot be managed by lesser means.	Schedule II
Fentanyl citrate	Actiq	**Loz:** 200mcg, 400mcg, 600mcg, 800mcg, 1200mcg, 1600mcg			200mcg. Dispense no more than 6 units. Individually titrate.	4 units/day.	Management of breakthrough cancer pain in patients with malignancies who are already receiving and are tolerant to opioid therapy for their underlying persistent cancer pain.	Schedule II
	Fentora	**Tab, Buccal:** 100mcg, 200mcg, 300mcg, 400mcg, 600mcg, 800mcg			Initial:100mcg.	Not more than 4 tabs simultaneously.	Management of breakthrough pain in patients with cancer who are already receiving and who are tolerant to opioid therapy for their underlying persistent cancer pain.	

ORAL ANTICONVULSANTS

DRUG (BRAND)	INDICATIONS	USUAL ADULT DOSE*	THERAPEUTIC SERUM LEVELS
BARBITURATES			
Mephobarbital (Mebaral)	Grand mal and petit mal epilepsy	400-600mg/day	NA
Phenobarbital	Generalized and partial	60-200mg/day	10-40mcg/mL
Primidone (Mysoline)	Tonic-clonic, psychomotor, focal	750-2000mg/day	5-12mcg/mL
BENZODIAZEPINES			
Clonazepam (Klonopin, Klonopin Wafers)	Myoclonic, akinetic, Lennox-Gastaut syndrome, absence seizures (if failed succinimides)	1.5-20mg/day	NA
Clorazepate dipotassium (Tranxene, Tranxene-SD)	Adjunct therapy in partial seizures, partial	22.5-90mg/day	NA
Diazepam (Valium)	Adjunct in convulsive disorders	4-40mg/day	NA
Diazepam (Diastat)	Refractory patients with epilepsy who require intermittent use to control bouts of increased seizure activity.	0.2mg/kg rectally	NA
HYDANTOIN			
Phenytoin (Dilantin, Phenytek)	Tonic-clonic partial (psychomotor, temporal lobe), prevent/treat seizures during/following neurosurgery.	300-600mg/day	10-20mcg/mL
SUCCINIMIDES			
Ethosuximide (Zarontin)	Absence	(Pediatrics): 20mg/kg/day	40-100mcg/mL
Methsuximide (Celontin)	Absence	300-1200mg/day	Toxic level: >40mcg/mL
MISCELLANEOUS			
Carbamazepine (Carbatrol, Tegretol)	Tonic-clonic, mixed, partial (psychomotor, temporal lobe)	800-1200mg/day	4-12mcg/mL
Divalproex sodium (Depakote, Depakote ER) **Valproic acid** (Depakene, Stavzor)	Absence, partial	10-60mg/kg/day	50-100mcg/mL
Felbamate** (Felbatol)	Partial with or w/o generalization (adults), partial/generalized with Lennox-Gastaut syndrome (pediatrics)	3600mg/day	NA
Gabapentin (Neurontin)	Partial with and without secondary generalization (>12 yrs), partial (pediatrics)	900-1800mg/day	NA
Lacosamide (Vimpat)	Partial	400mg/day	NA
Lamotrigine (Lamictal, Lamictal CD)	Partial, generalized seizures of Lennox-Gastaut syndrome, tonic-clonic (≥2 yrs)	100-400mg/day	NA
Levetiracetam (Keppra, Keppra XR)	Partial (Keppra): myoclonic, tonic-clonic	1000-3000mg/day	NA

(Continued)

DRUG (BRAND)	INDICATIONS	USUAL ADULT DOSE*	THERAPEUTIC SERUM LEVELS
MISCELLANEOUS (*Continued*)			
Oxcarbazepine (Trileptal)	Partial	600-2400mg/day	NA
Pregabalin (Lyrica)	Partial	150-600mg/day	NA
Rufinamide (Banzel)	Lennox-Gastaut syndrome	3200mg/day	NA
Tiagabine (Gabitril)	Partial	32-56mg/day	NA
Topiramate (Topamax)	Partial, tonic-clonic, Lennox-Gastaut syndrome (≥2 yrs)	200-400mg/day	NA
Zonisamide (Zonegran)	Partial	100-400mg/day	NA

*Please refer to complete monograph for pediatric dosing.
**For severe epilepsy refractory to other treatment where the risk of aplastic anemia and/or liver failure is deemed acceptable. Fully advise patient and obtain written, informed consent before treatment. Closely monitor patient.
NA = Not Available.

ORAL NARCOTIC ANALGESICS

DRUG	BRAND	FORMULATION	STRENGTH	FREQUENCY*
SINGLE-SOURCE PRODUCTS				
Butorphanol tartrate	Stadol NS	Nasal Spray	10mg/mL	3 to 4 hours
Codeine sulfate		Tablet	15mg, 30mg, 60mg	4 to 6 hours
Fentanyl	Duragesic	Patch	12.5mcg/hr, 25mcg/hr, 50mcg/hr, 75mcg/hr, 100mcg/hr	72 hours
Fentanyl citrate	Actiq	Lozenge	0.2mg, 0.4mg, 0.6mg, 0.8mg, 1.2mg, 1.6mg	15 minutes (Max: 2 doses)
	Fentora	Tablet, Buccal	100mcg, 200mcg, 300mcg, 400mcg, 600mcg, 800mcg	30 minutes (Max: 4 tabs/dose)
Hydromorphone HCl**	Dilaudid	Solution	1mg/mL	3 to 6 hours
		Suppository	3mg	6 to 8 hours
		Tablet	2mg, 4mg, 8mg	4 to 6 hours
Meperidine HCl**	Demerol	Syrup	50mg/5mL	3 to 4 hours
		Tablet	50mg, 100mg	3 to 4 hours
Methadone HCl	Dolophine	Tablet	5mg, 10mg	8 to 12 hours
	Methadose	Tablet	5mg, 10mg, 40mg (Dispersible)	8 to 12 hours
		Concentrate	10mg/mL	
Morphine sulfate**	Avinza	Capsule, Extended-Release	30mg, 45 mg, 60mg, 75mg, 90mg, 120mg	24 hours
	Kadian	Capsule, Extended-Release	10mg, 20mg, 30mg, 50mg, 60mg, 80mg, 100mg, 200mg	12 or 24 hours
	MS Contin	Tablet, Extended-Release	15mg, 30mg, 60mg, 100mg, 200mg	8 or 12 hours
	MSIR	Capsule, Tablet	15mg, 30mg	4 hours
		Solution	10mg/5mL	4 hours
		Solution	20mg/5mL	4 hours
	Oramorph SR	Tablet, Extended-Release	15mg, 30mg, 60mg, 100mg	12 hours
	Roxanol	Sol, Concentrate	20mg/mL	4 hours
	Roxanol-T	Sol, Concentrate	20mg/mL	4 hours
Oxycodone HCl	OxyContin	Tablet, Extended-Release	10mg, 15mg, 20mg, 30mg, 40mg, 60mg, 80mg, 160mg	12 hours
	OxyFast	Solution	20mg/mL	6 hours
	OxyIR	Capsule	5mg	6 hours
	Percolone	Tablet	5mg	4 hours
	Roxicodone	Solution	5mg/5mL	4 to 6 hours
		Solution (Intensol)	20mg/mL	4 to 6 hours
		Tablet	5mg, 15mg, 30mg	4 to 6 hours
Oxymorphone HCl	Opana	Tablet	5mg, 10mg	4 to 6 hours
	Opana ER	Tablet, Extended-Release	5mg, 7.5mg, 10mg, 15mg, 20mg, 30mg, 40mg	12 hours
Propoxyphene HCl	Darvon	Capsule	65mg	4 hours
Propoxyphene napsylate	Darvon-N	Tablet	100mg	4 hours
MULTI-SOURCE PRODUCTS				
Aspirin/Codeine		Tablet	325mg/30mg, 325mg/60mg	4 hours
Codeine phosphate/Acetaminophen	Tylenol w/Codeine	Elixir	12mg-120mg/5mL	4 hours
	Tylenol #2	Tablet	15mg/300mg	4 hours
	Tylenol #3	Tablet	30mg/300mg	4 hours
	Tylenol #4	Tablet	60mg/300mg	4 hours

(Continued)

DRUG	BRAND	FORMULATION	STRENGTH	FREQUENCY*
MULTI-SOURCE PRODUCTS *(Continued)*				
Dihydrocodeine/Aspirin/ Caffeine	Synalgos DC	Capsule	16mg/356.4mg/30mg	4 hours
Hydrocodone bitartrate/ Acetaminophen	Anexsia	Tablet	5mg/325mg, 7.5mg/325mg, 5mg/500mg, 7.5mg/650mg	4 to 6 hours
	Lorcet-HD	Capsule	5mg/500mg	4 to 6 hours
	Lorcet Plus	Tablet	7.5mg/650mg	4 to 6 hours
	Lorcet 10/650	Tablet	10mg/650mg	4 to 6 hours
	Lortab Elixir	Solution	7.5mg-500mg/15mL	4 to 6 hours
	Lortab 2.5/500	Tablet	2.5mg/500mg	4 to 6 hours
	Lortab 5/500	Tablet	5mg/500mg	4 to 6 hours
	Lortab 7.5/500	Tablet	7.5mg/500mg	4 to 6 hours
	Lortab 10/500	Tablet	10mg/500mg	4 to 6 hours
	Norco 5/325	Tablet	5mg/325mg	4 to 6 hours
	Norco 7.5/325	Tablet	7.5mg/325mg	4 to 6 hours
	Norco 10/325	Tablet	10mg/325mg	4 to 6 hours
	Vicodin	Tablet	5mg/500mg	4 to 6 hours
	Vicodin ES	Tablet	7.5mg/500mg	4 to 6 hours
	Vicodin HP	Tablet	10mg/660mg	4 to 6 hours
	Zydone 5/400	Tablet	5mg/400mg	4 to 6 hours
	Zydone 7.5/400	Tablet	7.5mg/400mg	4 to 6 hours
	Zydone 10/400	Tablet	10mg/400mg	4 to 6 hours
Hydrocodone bitartrate/ Ibuprofen	Vicoprofen	Tablet	7.5mg/200mg	4 to 6 hours
Oxycodone/ Acetaminophen	Percocet 2.5/325	Tablet	2.5mg/325mg	6 hours
	Percocet 5/325	Tablet	5mg/325mg	6 hours
	Percocet 7.5/325	Tablet	7.5mg/325mg	6 hours
	Percocet 7.5/500	Tablet	7.5mg/500mg	6 hours
	Percocet 10/325	Tablet	10mg/325mg	6 hours
	Percocet 10/650	Tablet	10mg/650mg	6 hours
	Roxicet	Tablet	5mg/325mg	6 hours
	Roxicet	Solution	5mg-325mg/5mL	6 hours
	Roxicet	Tablet	5mg/500mg	6 hours
	Tylox	Capsule	5mg/500mg	6 hours
Oxycodone/Ibuprofen	Combunox	Tablet	5mg/400mg	24 hours (Max: 4 tabs/day)
Oxycodone (HCl/ Terephthalate)/Aspirin	Percodan	Tablet	4.5mg/0.38mg/325mg	6 hours
Pentazocine/ Acetaminophen	Talacen	Tablet	25mg/650mg	4 hours
Pentazocine HCl/ Naloxone	Talwin NX	Tablet	50mg/0.5mg	3 to 4 hours
Propoxyphene napsylate/ Acetaminophen	Darvocet A500	Tablet	100mg/500mg	4 hours
	Darvocet-N 50	Tablet	50mg/325mg	4 hours
	Darvocet-N 100	Tablet	100mg/650mg	4 hours

*Usual dosage interval.
**Injection formulation available.

TRIPTANS FOR ACUTE MIGRAINE

DRUG	BRAND	HOW SUPPLIED	INITIAL & (MAX) DOSE*	HEPATIC/RENAL DOSE ADJUSTMENT*
Almotriptan malate	Axert	Tab: 6.25mg, 12.5mg	6.25-12.5mg. May repeat after 2 hours. (2 doses/24 hours)	Initial: 6.25mg. Max: 12.5mg/24 hours.
Eletriptan hydrobromide	Relpax	Tab: 20mg, 40mg	20-40mg. May repeat after 2 hours. (40mg/dose or 80mg/day)	Severe Hepatic Impairment: Avoid use.
Frovatriptan succinate	Frova	Tab: 2.5mg	2.5mg. May repeat after 2 hours. (7.5mg/day)	No adjustment.
Naratriptan hydrochloride	Amerge	Tab: 1mg, 2.5mg	1-2.5mg. May repeat after 4 hours. (5mg/24 hours)	Severe Renal/Hepatic Impairment: Avoid use. Mild-Moderate Renal/Hepatic Impairment: Use lower dose. Max: 2.5mg/24 hours.
Rizatriptan benzoate	Maxalt	Tab: 5mg, 10mg	5-10mg. May repeat after 2 hours. (30mg/24 hours)	No adjustment.
	Maxalt-MLT	Tab, Disintegrating: 5mg, 10mg	5-10mg. May repeat after 2 hours. (30mg/24 hours)	No adjustment.
Sumatriptan	Imitrex	Inj**: 6mg/0.5mL, inj**, stat dose system: 4mg, 6mg	6mg SQ. May repeat after 1 hour. (12mg/24 hours)	Severe Hepatic Impairment: Avoid use.
		Nasal Spray: 5mg, 20mg	5mg, 10mg, or 20mg single dose. May repeat after 2 hours. (40mg/24 hours)	Severe Hepatic Impairment: Avoid use.
		Tab: 25mg, 50mg, 100mg	25-100mg. May repeat after 2 hours. (200mg/24 hours)	Severe Hepatic Impairment: Avoid use. Hepatic Disease: Max: 50mg/single dose.
Zolmitriptan	Zomig	Nasal Spray: 5mg	5mg. May repeat after 2 hours. (10mg/24 hours)	Hepatic Impairment: Use lower dose.
		Tab: 2.5mg, 5mg	2.5mg or lower. May repeat after 2 hours. (10mg/24 hours)	Hepatic Impairment: Use lower dose.
	Zomig-ZMT	Tab, Disintegrating: 2.5mg, 5mg	2.5mg or lower. May repeat after 2 hours. (10mg/24 hours)	Hepatic Impairment: Use lower dose.
COMBINATION DRUG				
Naproxen-Sumatriptan	Treximet	Tab: (Naproxen-Sumatriptan): 500mg/85mg [9[s]]	1 tab; may repeat after 2 hrs. (2 tabs/24 hrs) Do not split, crush, or chew.	Advanced renal disease: Avoid use.

***NOTE:** Dosages shown are for adults ≥18 yrs. For more detailed information, refer to the individual monograph or the drug's FDA-approved labeling.

**Also indicated for acute treatment of cluster headaches.

ANTIDEPRESSANTS

DRUG (BRAND)	HOW SUPPLIED	DAILY DOSE Initial (I), Usual (U), Max (M)	TITRATE
AMINOKETONE			
Bupropion (Wellbutrin)	**Tab:** 75mg, 100mg	**(I)**200mg **(U)**300mg **(M)**450mg	Increase by 100mg/d q3d.
(Wellbutrin SR)	**Tab, SR:** 100mg, 150mg, 200mg	**(I)**150mg **(U)**300mg **(M)**400mg	Increase by 150mg/d q4d.
(Wellbutrin XL)	**Tab, ER:** 150mg, 300mg	**(I)**150mg **(U)**300mg **(M)**450mg	Increase by 150mg/d q4d.
Bupropion HBr (Aplenzin)	**Tab, Extended-Release:** 174mg, 348mg, 522mg	**(I)**174mg **(U)**348mg **(M)**522mg	Increase by 174mg/d q4d.
MONOAMINE OXIDASE INHIBITORS			
Phenelzine (Nardil)	**Tab:** 15mg	**(I)**45mg **(U)**15mg qd or qod	Increase rapidly to 60-90mg/d then decrease to maintenance dose.
Tranylcypromine (Parnate)	**Tab:** 10mg	**(I,U)**30mg **(M)**60mg	Increase by 10mg/d q1-3 weeks.
PHENYLETHYLAMINE			
Venlafaxine (Effexor)	**Tab:** 25mg*, 37.5mg*, 50mg*, 75mg*, 100mg*	**(I)**75mg **(U)**150-225mg **(M)**375mg	Increase by 75mg/d q4d.
(Effexor XR)	**Cap, ER:** 37.5mg, 75mg, 150mg	**(I)**37.5-75mg **(U)**75-225mg **(M)**225mg	Increase by 75mg/d q4d.
Selegeline (Emsam)	**Patch:** 6mg/24hrs, 9mg/24hrs, 12mg/24hrs	**(I)**6mg/24hrs **(U)**6mg/24hrs **(M)**12mg/24hrs	Increase by 3mg/24hrs q2wk.
PHENYLPIPERAZINE			
Nefazodone	**Tab:** 50mg, 100mg*, 150mg*, 200mg, 250mg	**(I)**200mg **(U)**300-600mg **(M)**600mg	Increase by 100-200mg/d in no less than 1 week.
SELECTIVE SEROTONIN NOREPINEPHRINE REUPTAKE INHIBITOR			
Duloxetine (Cymbalta)	**Cap:** 20mg, 30mg, 60mg	**(I,U)**40-60mg **(M)**60mg	N/A
Desvenlafaxine (Pristiq)	**Tab, Extended-Release:** 50mg, 100mg	**(I)**50mg **(M)**400mg	N/A
SELECTIVE SEROTONIN REUPTAKE INHIBITORS			
Citalopram (Celexa)	**Sol:** 10mg/5mL; **Tab:** 10mg, 20mg*, 40mg*	**(I)**20mg **(U)**40mg **(M)**60mg	Increase by 20mg/d qwk.
Escitalopram (Lexapro)	**Sol:** 5mg/5mL; **Tab:** 5mg, 10mg*, 20mg*	**(I)**10mg **(U)**10-20mg	Increase to 20mg/d after 1 week.
Fluoxetine (Prozac)	**Cap:** 10mg, 20mg, 40mg; **Sol:** 20mg/5mL; **Tab:** 10mg*	**(I)**20mg **(M)**80mg	Consider after several weeks of therapy.
Paroxetine (Paxil)	**Sus:** 10mg/5mL; **Tab:** 10mg*, 20mg*, 30mg, 40mg	**(I)**20mg **(M)**50mg	Increase by 10mg/d qwk.
(Paxil CR)	**Tab, CR:** 12.5mg, 25mg, 37.5mg	**(I)**25mg **(M)**62.5mg	Increase by 12.5mg/d qwk.
(Pexeva)	**Tab:** 10mg, 20mg, 30mg, 40mg	**(I)**20mg **(M)**50mg	Increase by 10mg/d qwk.
Sertraline (Zoloft)	**Sol:** 20mg/mL; **Tab:** 25mg*, 50mg*, 100mg*	**(I)**50mg **(M)**200mg	Increase at 1-week intervals.

(Continued)

DRUG (BRAND)	HOW SUPPLIED	DAILY DOSE Initial (I), Usual (U), Max (M)	TITRATE
TETRACYCLIC			
Mirtazapine (Remeron)	**Tab:** 15mg*, 30mg*, 45mg; **Tab, Disintegrating:** 15mg, 30mg, 45mg	**(I)**15mg **(M)**45mg	Increase q1-2 wk.
TRIAZOLOPYRIDINE			
Trazodone (Desyrel)	**Tab:** 50mg*, 100mg*, 150mg*, 300mg*	**(I)**150mg **(M)**400-600mg	Increase by 50mg/d q3-4d.
TRICYCLICS			
Amitriptyline	**Tab:** 10mg, 25mg, 50mg, 75mg, 100mg, 150mg	**(I)**OP: 50-100mg, IP: 100mg **(U)**50-100mg **(M)**OP: 150mg, IP: 300mg	OP: Increase by 25-50mg/d. IP: Increase to 200mg/d.
Amoxapine	**Tab:** 25mg*, 50mg*, 100mg*, 150mg*	**(I)**100-150mg **(U)**200-300mg **(M)**OP: 400mg IP: 600mg	Increase to 100mg bid-tid by end of first week.
Clomipramine (Anafranil)	**Cap:** 25mg, 50mg, 75mg	**(I)**25mg **(U)**100-250mg **(M)**250mg	Increase to 100mg/d in 2 weeks, then increase gradually.
Desipramine (Norpramin)	**Tab:** 10mg, 25mg, 50mg, 75mg, 100mg, 150mg	**(I,U)**100-200mg **(M)**300mg	N/A
Doxepin (Sinequan)	**Cap:** 10mg, 25mg, 50mg, 75mg, 100mg, 150mg; **Sol:** 10mg/mL	**(I)**75mg **(U)**75-150mg **(M)**300mg	Increase gradually.
Imipramine (Tofranil PM)	**Cap:** 75mg, 100mg, 125mg, 150mg	**(I)**OP: 75mg, IP: 100mg **(U)**75-150mg **(M)**OP: 200mg, IP: 250-300mg	OP: Increase to 150mg/d. IP: Increase to 200mg/d.
(Tofranil)	**Tab:** 10mg, 25mg, 50mg	**(I)**OP: 75mg, IP: 100mg **(U)**50-150mg **(M)**OP: 200mg, IP: 250-300mg	OP: Increase to 150mg/d. IP: Increase to 200mg/d.
Nortriptyline (Pamelor, Aventyl)	**Cap:** 10mg, 25mg, 50mg, 75mg; **Sol:**10mg/5mL	**(I,U)**75-100mg **(M)**150mg	N/A
Protriptyline (Vivactil)	**Tab:** 5mg, 10mg	**(U)**15-40mg **(M)**60mg	Titrate morning dose.
Trimipramine (Surmontil)	**Cap:** 25mg, 50mg, 100mg	**(I)**OP: 75mg, IP: 100mg **(U)**OP: 50-150mg, IP: 200mg **(M)**OP: 200mg, IP: 250-300mg	OP: Increase to 150mg/d. IP: Increase to 200mg/d.

Abbreviations: IP=Inpatient; OP=Outpatient *Scored.

ANTIPSYCHOTIC AGENTS

DRUG (BRAND)	HOW SUPPLIED (mg)*	INITIAL & (MAX) DOSE**	USUAL DOSE RANGE**
ATYPICAL			
Aripiprazole (Abilify)	**Tab:** 2, 5, 10, 15, 20, 30 **Sol:** 1mg/mL; **Inj:** 7.5mg/mL	10-15mg qd (30mg/day)	10-15mg qd
(Abilify Discmelt)	**Tab, Orally Disintegrating:** (Discmelt) 10, 15	10-15mg qd (30mg/day)	10-15mg qd
Clozapine (Clozaril)	**Tab:** 12.5†, 25, 50, 100, 200mg	12.5mg qd-bid (900mg/day)	100-900mg/day given tid
(Fazaclo)	**Tab, Orally Disintegrating:** 12.5, 25*, 100**scored	12.5mg qd-bid (900mg/day)	100-900mg/day given tid
Olanzapine (Zyprexa, Zyprexa Zydis)	**Tab:** 2.5, 5, 7.5, 10, 15, 20 **Tab, Orally Disintegrating:** 5, 10, 15, 20	Schizophrenia: 5-10mg qd Bipolar Mania: 10-15mg qd (20mg/day for both)	Schizophrenia: 10-15mg qd Bipolar Mania: 5-20mg qd
(Zyprexa IntraMuscular)	**Inj:** 10mg	Agitation: 10mg IM (3 doses)	Agitation: 2.5-10mg IM
Paliperidone (Invega)	**Tab, Extended-Release:** 3, 6, 9	6mg qd (12mg/day)	3-12mg/day
Quetiapine fumarate (Seroquel)	**Tab:** 25, 50, 100, 200, 300, 400mg	Schizophrenia: 25mg bid Bipolar Mania: 50mg bid (800mg/day for both)	Schizophrenia: 150-750mg/day Bipolar Mania: 400-800mg/day
(Seroquel XR)	**Tab, Extended-Release:** 50, 150, 200, 300, 400	Initial: 300mg/day (800mg/day)	400-800mg/day
Risperidone (Risperdal)	**Sol:** 1mg/mL **Tab:** 0.25, 0.5, 1, 2, 3, 4	Schizophrenia: 1mg bid (16mg/day)	Schizophrenia: 4-8mg/day Bipolar Mania: 1-6mg/day
(Risperdal M-Tab)	**Tab, Orally Disintegrating:** 0.5, 1, 2 (6mg/day) 3mg, 4mg	Bipolar Mania: 2-3mg qd	
(Risperdal Consta)	**Inj:** 12.5, 25, 37.5, 50mg	Schizophrenia: 25mg IM (50mg IM q2wk)	Schizophrenia: 25-50mg IM q2wks
Ziprasidone HCl (Geodon)	**Cap:** 20, 40, 60, 80	20mg bid (160mg/day)	20-80mg bid
Ziprasidone mesylate (Geodon) for Injection)	**Inj:** 20mg/mL	10mg IM q2h or 20mg IM q4h (40mg/day)	Switch to oral for long-term therapy
CONVENTIONAL			
Chlorpromazine	**Cap, Extended-Release:** 30, 75, 150; **Inj:** 25mg/mL; **Sup:** 25, 100; **Syrup:** 10mg/5mL; **Tab:** 10, 25,50, 100, 200	10-25mg PO bid-qid or 25mg IM (1000mg/day PO)	PO: 10-800mg/day IM: 25-50mg IM q4-6h‡ Switch to PO when controlled
Fluphenazine HCl (Prolixin)	**Elixir:** 2.5mg/5mL **Sol, Conc:** 5mg/mL **Tab:** 1†, 2.5, 5, 10 **Inj:** 2.5mg/mL	2.5mg-10mg/day in divided doses (40mg/day) 1.25mg IM q6-8h (10mg/day)	1-5mg qd
Fluphenazine decanoate (Prolixin Decanoate)	**Inj:** 25mg/mL	12.5-25mg IM/SQ q4-6 wks (100mg/dose)	Individualize to patient.

(Continued)

DRUG (BRAND)	**HOW SUPPLIED (mg)***	**INITIAL & (MAX) DOSE****	**USUAL DOSE RANGE****
CONVENTIONAL *(Continued)*			
Haloperidol	**Sol, Conc:** 2mg/mL **Tab:** 0.5, 1, 2, 5, 10, 20	Moderate: 0.5-2mg bid-tid Sev/Resist: 3-5mg bid-tid (100mg/day)	2-20mg/day
Haloperidol lactate (Haldol)	**Inj:** 5mg/mL	2-5mg IM q4-8h or hourly if needed (100mg/day)	Individualize to patient.
Haloperidol decanoate (Haldol Decanoate)	**Inj:** 50mg/mL, 100mg/mL	10-20x daily oral dose up to 100mg/dose (450mg/month)	10-15x daily oral dose
Loxapine succinate (Loxitane)	**Cap:** 5, 10, 25, 50	10mg bid, up to 50mg/day (250mg/day)	60-100mg/day
Molindone (Moban)	**Tab:** 5, 10, 25, 50	50-75mg/day (225mg/day)	5-25mg tid/qid
Perphenazine	**Tab:** 2, 4, 8, 16	Non-hospitalized: 4-8mg tid Hospitalized: 8-16mg (64mg/day)	Reduce dose as soon as possible to minimum effective dose.
Prochlorperazine maleate	**Tab:** 5, 10	5-10mg tid-qid	Moderate/Severe: 50-75mg/day Severe: 100-150mg/day
Thioridazine HCl (Mellaril)	**Sol, Conc:** 100mg/mL **Tab:** 10†, 15, 25†, 50†, 100	50-100mg tid (800mg/day)	200-800mg/day given bid-qid
Thiothixene (Navane)	**Cap:** 1, 2, 5, 10, 20	Mild: 2mg tid Severe: 5mg bid (60mg/day)	20-30mg/day
Trifluoperazine HCl	**Tab:** 1, 2, 5, 10	2-5mg bid (40mg/day or higher if needed)	15-20mg/day

Note: This list is not inclusive of all antipsychotic agents. Indications may vary among the different products.

* Unless otherwise indicated.

** Doses shown are for adults. For pediatric dosing and additional information please refer to the individual monograph listings or the drug's FDA-approved labeling. Dosages need to be adjusted by titration to individual patient needs and may need to be reduced in the elderly, debilitated, or with renal/hepatic impairment. Periodically reassess to determine the need for maintenance treatment.

† Available only in generic forms.

‡ Severe cases may require up to 2g/day or 400mg/dose IM.

BIPOLAR DISORDER PHARMACOTHERAPY

DRUG	BRAND	HOW SUPPLIED	USUAL DOSE	COMMENTS
MOOD STABILIZER				
Lithium	Various	**Cap:** 150mg, 300mg, 600mg; **Tab:** 300mg; **Tab, Extended-Release:** 450mg	**Adults/Pediatrics:** ≥**12 yrs:** Acute Mania: 600mg tid to achieve effective serum levels of 1-1.5mEq/L; monitor levels twice a week until stabilized. Maintenance Therapy: 300mg tid-qid or (ER) 450mg bid to maintain serum levels of 0.6-1.2 mEq/L; monitor levels every 2 months.	Treatment of manic episodes of bipolar disorder and maintenance treatment of bipolar disorder.
ANTICONVULSANTS				
Carbamazepine	Equetro	**Cap, Extended-Release:** 100mg, 200mg, 300mg	**Adults:** Initial: 400mg/day, given in divided doses, bid. Titrate: 200mg qd. **Max:** 1600mg/day. Do not crush or chew.	Treatment of acute manic and mixed episodes associated with bipolar I disorder.
Divalproex sodium	Depakote ER	**Tab, Extended-Release:** 250mg, 500mg	**Adults:** Mania: Initial: 25mg/kg/day given once daily. Titrate: Increase dose rapidly to clinical effect. **Max:** 60mg/kg/day. Conversion from Depakote: Administer Depakote ER qd using a dose 8-20% higher than the total daily dose of Depakote. If cannot directly convert to Depakote ER, consider increasing to next higher Depakote total daily dose before converting to appropriate total daily Depakote ER dose. Elderly: Give lower initial dose and titrate slowly. Decrease dose or discontinue if decreased food or fluid intake or if excessive somnolence occurs. Swallow whole; do not crush or chew.	Acute manic or mixed episodes associated with bipolar disorder.
	Depakote	**Tab, Delayed-Release:** 125mg, 250mg, 500mg	**Adults:** Mania: 750mg daily in divided doses. Titrate: Increase dose rapidly to clinical effect. **Max:** 60mg/kg/day. Decrease dose or discontinue if decreased food or fluid intake or if excessive somnolence occurs.	Treatment of mania associated with bipolar disorder.
Lamotrigine	Lamictal	**Tab:** 25mg*, 100mg*, 150mg*, 200mg*; **Tab, Chewable:** (Lamictal CD) 2mg, 5mg, 25mg *scored	**Adults:** Bipolar Disorder: Patients not taking carbamazepine, other enzyme-inducing drugs (EIDs) or VPA: **Weeks 1 and 2:** 25mg qd. **Weeks 3 and 4:** 50mg qd. **Week 5:** 100mg qd. **Weeks 6 and 7:** 200mg qd. Patients taking VPA: **Weeks 1 and 2:** 25mg every other day. **Weeks 3 and 4:** 25mg qd. **Week 5:** 50mg qd. **Weeks 6 and 7:** 100mg qd. Patients taking carbamazepine (or other EIDs) and not taking VPA: **Weeks 1 and 2:** 50mg qd. **Weeks 3 and 4:** 100mg qd (divided doses). **Week 5:** 200mg qd (divided doses). **Week 6:** 300mg qd (divided doses). **Week 7:** Up to 400mg qd (divided doses). After discontinuation of psychotropic drugs excluding VPA, carbamazepine, or other EIDs: Maintain current dose. After discontinuation of VPA and current lamotrigine dose of 100mg qd: **Week 1:** 150mg qd. Week 2 and onward: 200mg qd. After discontinuation of carbamazepine or other EIDs and current lamotrigine dose of 400mg qd: **Week 1:** 400mg qd. **Week 2:** 300mg qd. **Week 3 and onward:** 200mg	Maintenance treatment of bipolar I disorder to delay the time to occurrence of mood episodes (depression, mania, hypomania, mixed episodes) in patients treated for mood episodes with standard therapy.

(Continued)

DRUG	BRAND	HOW SUPPLIED	USUAL DOSE	COMMENTS
ANTICONVULSANTS *(Continued)*				
Valproic Acid	**Stavzor**	**Cap, Delayed Release:** 125mg, 250mg, 500mg	**Adults:** Mania: Initial: 750mg daily in divided doses. Titrate: Increase rapidly to produce the desired clinical effect or plasma level (50-125mcg/mL). **Max:** 60mg/kg/day.	Acute treatment of manic episodes associated with bipolar disorder.
CONVENTIONAL ANTIPSYCHOTIC				
Chlorpromazine HCl	**Thorazine**	**Cap, Extended-Release:** 30mg, 75mg, 150mg, **Inj:** 25mg/mL; **Sup:** 25mg, 100mg; **Syrup:** 10mg/5mL; **Tab:** 10mg, 25mg, , 50mg, 100mg, 200mg	**Adults:** Inpatient: Acute Schizophrenic/Manic State: 25mg IM, then 25-50mg IM in 1 hr if needed. Titrate: Increase over several days up to 400mg q4-6h until controlled then switch to PO. Usual: 500mg/day PO. **Max:** 1000mg/day PO. Less acutely disturbed: 25mg PO tid. Titrate: Increase gradually to 400mg/day. Outpatient: 10mg PO tid-qid or 25mg PO bid-tid. More Severe: 25mg PO tid. Titrate: After 1-2 days, increase by 20-50mg twice weekly until calm. Prompt control of severe symptoms: 25mg IM, may repeat in 1 hr then 25-50mg PO tid.	Control manifestations of manic type of manic-depressive illness.
ATYPICAL ANTIPSYCHOTICS				
Aripiprazole	**Abilify**	**Tab:** 2mg, 5mg, 10mg, 15mg, 20mg, 30mg; **Tab, Disintegrating:** 10mg, 15mg, (Discmelt) **Sol:** 1mg/mL [50mL, 150mL, 480mL]. **Inj:** 7.5mg/mL	**Adults:** (PO) Bipolar Disorder (Monotherapy or Adjunct): Initial/Target: 15mg/day. Max: 30mg/day. (Inj) Agitation: 9.75mg IM. Range: 5.25-15mg IM. Max: 30mg/day; initiate PO therapy as soon as possible. **Pediatrics:** Bipolar Disorder (Monotherapy or Adjunct) (10-17 yrs): Initial: 2mg/day. Titrate: 5mg after 2 days. May adjust dose in 5mg/day increments. Recommended: 10mg/day. Max: 30mg/day. Periodically reassess need for maintenance therapy. Oral sol can be given on mg-per-mg basis up to 25mg. Patients receiving 30mg tabs should receive 25mg of oral sol. Concomitant Strong CYP3A4 Inhibitors (eg, ketoconazole, clarithromycin): Reduce usual aripiprazole dose by 50%. Concomitant CYP2D6 Inhibitors (eg, quinidine, fluoxetine, paroxetine): Reduce usual aripiprazole dose by 50%. Concomitant CYP3A4 Inducers (eg, carbamazepine): Double aripiprazole dose.	(PO) Acute and maintenance treatment of manic and mixed episodes associated with bipolar I disorder with or without psychotic features in adults and pediatrics aged 10-17 yrs. Adjunctive therapy to either lithium or valproate for the acute treatment of manic and mixed episodes associated with bipolar I disorder with or without psychotic features in adults and pediatrics aged 10-17 yrs. (Inj) Acute treatment of agitation associated with schizophrenia or bipolar disorder, manic or mixed, in adults.
Olanzapine	**Zyprexa, Zyprexa Zydis**	**Inj:** 10mg; **Tab:** 2.5mg, 5mg, 7.5mg, 10mg, 15mg, 20mg; **Tab, Disintegrating:** (Zydis) 5mg, 10mg, 15mg, 20mg	**Adults:** Bipolar Mania: Initial: 10-15mg qd. Titrate: Increase/decrease by 5mg daily. **Max:** 20mg/day. With Lithium or Valproate: Initial/Usual: 10mg qd. Max: 20mg/day. Debilitated/Hypotension risk/slow metabolizers/sensitivity to olanzapine effects: Initial: 5mg qd. Titrate: Increase cautiously. (IM) Agitation: Initial: 10mg IM. Usual: 2.5-10mg IM. **Max:** 3 doses of 10mg q 2-4h. Elderly: 5mg IM. Debilitated/Hypotension risk/sensitivity to olanzapine effects: 2.5mg IM. May initiate PO therapy when clinically appropriate.	(PO) Treatment of acute mixed or manic episodes in bipolar I disorder. Short-term treatment of acute manic episodes associated with bipolar I disorder in combination with lithium or valproate. (Inj) Agitation associated with schizophrenia, bipolar I mania.

(Continued)

DRUG	BRAND	HOW SUPPLIED	USUAL DOSE	COMMENTS
ATYPICAL ANTIPSYCHOTICS *(Continued)*				
Olanzapine-fluoxetine	**Symbyax**	**Cap:** (Olanzapine-Fluoxetine): 3-25mg, 6-25mg, 6-50mg, 12-25mg, 12-50mg	**Adults:** ≥18 yrs: Initial: 6-25mg cap qpm. Titrate: Adjust dose based on efficacy and tolerability. **Max:** 18mg/75mg. Hypotension risk/hepatic impairment/metabolizers: Initial: 3/25mg-6/25mg qpm. Titrate: Increase cautiously. Re-evaluate periodically.	Treatment of depressive episodes associated with bipolar disorder.
Quetiapine	**Seroquel**	**Tab:** 25mg, 50mg, 100mg, 200mg, 300mg, 400mg	**Adults:** Bipolar Depressive Episodes: Give once daily hs. Day 1: 50mg/day. Day 2: 100mg/day. Day 3: 200mg/day. Day 4: 300mg/day. Bipolar Mania: Monotherapy/Adjunctive: Give bid. Initial: 100mg/day on Day 1. Titrate: Increase to 400mg/day on Day 4 in increments of up to 100mg/day in bid divided doses. Adjust doses up to 800mg/day by Day 6 in increments ≤200mg/day. Max: 800mg/day. Maintenance for Bipolar I Disorder: Give bid. 400-800mg/day. Hepatic Impairment: Initial: 25mg/day. Titrate: Increase by 25-50mg/day to effective dose. Elderly/Debilitated/Predisposition to Hypotension: Consider slower rate of dose titration and lower target dose.	Treatment of depressive episodes associated with bipolar disorder. Treatment of acute manic episodes associated with bipolar I disorder, as monotherapy or adjunct therapy to lithium or divalproex. Maintenance treatment of bipolar I disorder as adjunct therapy to lithium or divalproex.
Quetiapine	**Seroquel XR**	**Tab, Extended Release:** 50mg, 150mg, 200mg, 300mg, 400mg	**Adults:** Bipolar Disorder: Depressive Episodes: Give once daily in evening. Day 1: 50mg/day. Day 2: 100mg/day. Day 3: 200mg/day. Day 4: 300mg/day. Bipolar Mania: Monotherapy/Adjunct: Give once daily in evening. Day 1: 300mg. Day 2: 600mg. Titrate: May adjust dose between 400-800mg beginning on Day 3 depending on response and tolerance. Maintenance of Bipolar I Disorder: 400-800mg/day given bid. Re-evaluate periodically.	Treatment of acute depressive episodes associated with bipolar disorder. Treatment of acute manic or mixed episodes associated with bipolar I disorder, as monotherapy and as adjunct to lithium or divalproex. Maintenance treatment of bipolar I disorder as adjunct therapy to lithium or divalproex.
Risperidone	**Risperdal**	**Sol:** 1mg/mL [30mL]; **Tab:** 0.25mg, 0.5mg, 1mg, 2mg, 3mg, 4mg; **Tab, Disintegrating:** (M-Tab) 0.5mg, 1mg, 2mg, 3mg, 4mg	**Adults:** Bipolar Mania: Initial: 2-3mg qd. Titrate: Adjust dose at intervals no <24hrs and in increments/decrements of 1mg/day. Range: 1-6mg/day. **Max:** 6mg/day. **Pediatrics:** 10-17 yrs: Bipolar Mania: Initial: 0.5mg qd in morning or evening. Titrate: Adjust dose, if needed, in increments of 0.5 or 1mg/day and at intervals not <24hrs, as tolerated, to recommended dose of 2.5mg/day. **Max:** 6mg/day. Elderly/Debilitated/Hypotension/Severe Renal or Hepatic Impairment: Initial: 0.5mg bid. Titrate: Adjust dose in increments not >0.5mg bid. Increases to doses >1.5mg bid should occur at intervals of ≥1 week. Periodically reassess to determine maintenance treatment.	Short-term treatment of acute manic or mixed episodes associated with bipolar I disorder as monotherapy (Adults and Adolescents 10-17 yrs) or in combination with lithium or valproate (Adults).
Ziprasidone	**Geodon**	**Cap:** (HCl) 20mg, 40mg, 60mg, 80mg **Inj:** 20mg/mL	**Adults:** Bipolar Mania: Initial: 40mg bid with food. Titrate: Increase to 60-80mg bid on 2nd day of treatment. Maint: 40-80mg bid.	Treatment of acute manic or mixed episodes associated with bipolar disorder, with or without psychotic features.

Source: FDA approved labeling.

ADMINISTRATION GUIDELINES FOR DRY POWDER INHALERS

Guidelines for Specific Products

Spiriva HandiHaler Administration

1. Open the dust cap of the HandiHaler by pressing the green button. Pull the dust cap upward.
2. Open the mouthpiece by pulling it upward and away from the base.
3. Insert one Spiriva capsule in the center chamber of the HandiHaler device. Close the mouthpiece firmly until you hear a click. Leave the dust cap open.
4. Hold the HandiHaler device with the mouthpiece upward and press the green button until it is flush against the base, then release. Only press the green button once. **Note:** Do not block the air intake vents.
5. Exhale completely. **Note:** Do not exhale into the HandiHaler mouthpiece.
6. Raise the HandiHaler device to your mouth and close your lips tightly around the mouthpiece.
7. Keep your head upright and breathe in slowly and deeply until your lungs are full. You should hear or feel the Spiriva capsule vibrate.
8. Hold your breath as long as is comfortable and remove the HandiHaler from your mouth. Breathe normally again.
9. To get the full dose of Spiriva, exhale completely and inhale medication again as in steps 6-8.
10. Remove and discard empty capsule. Close mouthpiece and replace dust cap for storage.

Counseling Tips:

- Spiriva capsules should not be removed from the package until ready to use. Do not store the capsules in the HandiHaler device. Discard any unused capsules that are exposed to the air.
- Do not swallow Spiriva capsules.
- If you do not hear or feel the capsule vibrate, hold the HandiHaler upright and tap the device gently on a hard surface. Check to see that the mouthpiece is completely closed and continue steps.
- Clean the HandiHaler device at least once a month. Rinse with warm water and allow to air dry completely for 24 hours. **Note:** Do not use cleaning agents.
- Keep the HandiHaler device and Spiriva capsules in a dry place.

Source: Spiriva HandiHaler Prescribing Information.

Guidelines for Specific Products

Foradil Aerolizer Administration

1. Remove Aerolizer inhaler cover. Hold the base of Aerolizer and twist the mouthpiece in direction of arrow to open.
2. Place the Foradil capsule in capsule chamber. **Note:** Do not place capsule directly in mouthpiece.
3. Hold the mouthpiece upright and press both buttons at the same time once, then release. You should hear a click as the capsule is pierced. **Note:** If the buttons stay depressed, grasp the wings on the buttons and pull them out. Do not push the buttons a second time.
4. Exhale fully. **Note:** Do not exhale into Aerolizer mouthpiece.
5. Tilt head back slightly and keep inhaler level with blue buttons to left and right (not up and down).
6. Raise the inhaler to your mouth and close your lips tightly around the mouthpiece. Inhale quickly and deeply. **Note:** You will hear a whirring noise and experience a sweet taste.
7. Remove inhaler from the mouth. Continue to hold your breathe as long as you can then exhale.
8. Open the inhaler and check that the capsule is empty. If not, close inhaler and repeat steps 4-7.
9. Remove and discard the empty capsule. Close mouthpiece and replace cover for storage.

Counseling Tips:

- Never take the Aerolizer apart.
- Use Aerolizer in a level position.
- If you do not hear whirring noise, the capsule may be stuck. Open inhaler and loosen the capsule. **Note:** Do not press the buttons again.
- Do not wash Aerolizer inhaler. Keep inhaler and Foradil capsules in a dry place.
- Do not store the capsules in the Aerolizer inhaler.
- Use new Aerolizer inhaler with each refill.

Source: Foradil Aerolizer Prescribing Information, http://www.spfiles.com/piforadil.pdf.

ADMINISTRATION GUIDELINES FOR METERED-DOSE INHALERS

General Guidelines

1. Remove dust cap and hold inhaler upright.
2. Shake canister well before each use.
3. Tilt head back slightly and breathe out slowly and completely.
4. For **closed mouth** technique: Place mouthpiece in mouth and close lips tightly around (not recommended for steroid inhaler). For **open mouth** technique: Hold inhaler 1 to 2 inches from open mouth (about the width of 2 fingers).
5. Inhale slowly and deeply, and press down on the inhaler to release the medication. (The slower the breath, the greater the likelihood that the drug will reach the smaller airways.) **NOTE:** If needed, a spacer or holding chamber can be used in children or elderly patients having difficulty with coordination of technique. If using a spacer, put the mouthpiece of the spacer between teeth, and into mouth. Then, close mouth around the spacer. With the device in place, actuate the inhaler once and inhale the medication immediately after actuating the aerosol.
6. Breathe in slowly and hold breath for about 10 seconds to allow the medication to go into lungs.
7. Breathe out slowly and wait about 30 seconds to 1 minute before administering second inhalation. **NOTE:** Expect relief of symptoms within 5 to 15 minutes. Seek medical attention if symptomatic relief takes longer than 20 minutes (this should occur with short-acting medications like albuterol).
8. If using a steroid inhaler, rinse mouth with water after use. **NOTE:** Spit out the water after last puff; do not swallow.

Counseling Tips:

- Rinse only the inhaler mouthpiece and cap with warm running water and air dry. Do not wash the canister or immerse in water.
- Keep the dust cap over the mouthpiece of the inhaler when not in use.
- Do not puncture the canister. The contents are under pressure.
- Store the canister at room temperature (15°C to 30°C), away from heat (>48.9°F) or open flames.

Guidelines for Specific Products

Advair Diskus Administration

1. Hold the Diskus in one hand. Then, push the thumbgrip back as far as it will go, until the mouthpiece appears and snaps into position.
2. Hold the Diskus in a level, flat position with the mouthpiece towards you.
3. Slide the lever away as far as it will go until it clicks.
4. Breathe out completely while holding the Diskus level and away from your mouth.
5. Put the mouthpiece between the lips. Breathe in quickly and deeply through the Diskus. **NOTE:** Do not breathe in through the nose.
6. Remove the Diskus from the mouth.
7. Hold breathe for about 10 seconds. Then, breathe out slowly.
8. Close the Diskus by sliding the thumbgrip back as far as it will go.
9. Rinse the mouth with water after each use and spit out. Without swallowing.

Counseling Tips:

- Never breathe into the Diskus.
- Never take the Diskus apart.
- Use the Diskus in a level, flat position.
- Do not use with a spacer device.
- Rinse mouth with water after use. **NOTE:** Spit out the water after last puff and do not swallow the water.
- Never wash the mouthpiece or any part of the Diskus.
- Keep the Diskus in a dry place, away from heat.

Source: Advair Diskus Prescribing Information, http://us.gsk.com/products/assets/us_advair.pdf.

(Continued)

Pulmicort Flexhaler Administration

Loading a dose:

1. Turn the cover and lift it off.
2. Hold the Flexhaler upright, with mouthpiece up.
3. Twist the brown grip fully in one direction as far as it will go and twist back again in the opposite direction as far as it will go.

Inhaling the dose:

1. Twist the cover and lift it off. Hold the Flexhaler upright (mouthpiece up).
2. Twist the brown grip to the right as far as it will go, then back to the left until it clicks.
3. Turn your head away from the Flexhaler and breathe out completely. **NOTE:** Do not shake the inhaler after loading it.
4. Place the mouthpiece in your mouth, close your lips around the mouthpiece, and inhale deeply and forcefully.
5. Remove the Flexhaler from the mouth and breathe out. **NOTE:** Do not blow into the mouthpiece.
6. Replace the cover and twist shut when finished.
7. Rinse mouth with water after each use. Spit out the water after last puff and do not swallow the water.

Counseling Tips:

- A new Flexhaler needs to be primed once before its first use. No further priming is indicated, even if it has been put aside for a long time.
- Flexhaler will deliver only one dose at a time, regardless of number of times you click the brown grip. **NOTE:** The dose indicator will continue to advance.
- Do not repeat inhalations even if you do not feel the sensation of medication when inhaling.
- Do not use with a spacer device.
- Do not chew or bite on the mouthpiece.
- Do not use Flexhaler if it has been damaged or if the mouthpiece has become detached.
- Wipe the outside of the mouthpiece once a week with a tissue.
- Keep the Flexhaler in a dry place, away from heat.

Source: Pulmicort Prescribing Information.

ASTHMA MANAGEMENT

DRUG (BRAND)	DOSAGE FORM	ADULT DOSE	CHILD DOSE*
ANTICHOLINERGIC			
Ipratropium (Atrovent HFA)	**MDI:** 0.017mg/inh [12.9g]	2 inh qid	
Tiotropium (Spiriva)	**Cap, Inhalation:** 18mcg	1 cap qd	
SYSTEMIC CORTICOSTEROIDS			
Methylprednisolone	**Tab:** 2, 4, 8, 16, 32mg	7.5-60mg qd in a single dose or qod prn for control. Short course "burst": 40-60 mg/day as single dose or 2 divided doses for 3-10 days.	0.25-2mg/kg qd in a single dose or qod prn for control. Short course "burst": 1-2mg/kg/day. **Max:** 60mg/day for 3-10 days.
Prednisolone	**Tab:** 5mg; **Liq:** 5mg/5mL, 15mg/5mL		
Prednisone	**Tab:** 1, 2.5, 5, 10, 20, 50mg **Liq:** 5mg/mL, 5mg/5mL		
CROMOLYN & NEDOCROMIL			
Cromolyn (Intal)	**MDI:** 800mcg/puff	2 puffs qid	1-2 puffs tid-qid
Nedocromil (Tilade)	**MDI:** 1.75mg/puff	2 puffs bid-qid	1-2 puffs bid-qid
SHORT-ACTING β_2-AGONISTS			
Albuterol	**MDI:** 0.09mg/inh; **Sol (neb):** 0.083%, 0.5%; **Syrup:** 2mg/5mL; **Tab:** 2mg*, 4mg*; **Tab, Extended-Release (Repetabs):** 4mg, 8mg *scored	2 inh q4-6h or 1 inh q4h. **(Repetabs) Initial:** 4-8mg q12h. **Max:** 32mg/day. **(Sol)** 2.5mg tid-qid by nebulizer. **(Syrup, Tabs)** 2-4mg tid qid. **Max:** 32mg/day (8mg qid).	**(Syrup) Initial:** 2-4mg tid-qid. **Max:** 8mg (Aerosol) 2 inh q4-6h or 1 inh q4h. **(Sol)** 2.5mg tid-qid by nebulizer. **(Tabs) Initial:** 2-4mg tid-qid.
Albuterol Sulfate (ProAir HFA, Proventil HFA, Ventolin HFA)	**MDI:** 90mcg/inh	2 inh q4-6h or 1 inh q4h	2 inh q4-6h or 1 inh q4h
Aformoterol (Brovana)	**Sol, Inhalation:** 15mcg/2mL	15mcg bid	
Levalbuterol (Xopenex, Xopenex HFA)	**Sol:** 0.31mg/3mL, 0.63mg/3mL, 1.25mg/3mL (HFA) 45mcg/inh	0.63mg tid, q6-8h (HFA) 2 inh (90mcg) q4-6h or 1 inh (45mcg) q4h	0.31mg/tid (max: 0.63mg tid) q6-8h (HFA) 2 inh (90mcg) q4-6h or 1 inh (45mcg) q4h
Pirbuterol (Maxair)	**Autohaler:** 0.2mg/inh; **MDI:** 0.2mg/inh [14g]	1-2 inh q4-6h	1-2 inh q4-6h
LONG-ACTING β_2-AGONISTS			
Salmeterol (Serevent)	**DPI:** 50mcg/blister	1 blister q 12 hours	1 blister q 12 hours
Formoterol (Foradil)	**DPI:** 12mcg	1 cap q 12 hours	1 cap q 12 hours
COMBINATION AGENTS			
Ipratropium/Albuterol (Combivent)	**MDI:** (Albuterol-Ipratropium) 0.09mg-0.018mg/inh [14.7g]	2 inh qid.	
Ipratropium/Albuterol (Duoneb)	**Sol, Inhalation:** (Albuterol-Ipratropium) 3mg-0.5mg/3mL	3mL qid via nebulizer	
Fluticasone/ Salmeterol (Advair)	**DPI:** 100, 250, 500mcg/50mcg	1 puff bid	(100mcg/50mcg) 1 puff bid
Fluticasone/ Salmeterol (Advair HFA)	**MDI:** (45/21) 0.045mg-0.021mg/inh, (115/21) 0.115mg-0.021mg/inh, (230/21) 0.230mg-0.021mg/inh	Initial: 2 inh of 45/21 bid or 1 inh of 115/21 bid. **Max:** 2 inh of 230/21 bid.	
Budesonide/Formoterol (Symbicort)	**MDI:** (Budesonide-Formoterol) 80mcg-4.5mcg/inh, 160mcg-4.5mcg/inh [10.2g]	2 puff bid of 80/4.5 or 160/4.5 depending on asthma severity. **Max:** 640mcg/18mcg (2 puff bid of 160/4.5).	2 inh bid of 80/4.5 or 160/4.5 depending on asthma severity. **Max:** 640mcg/18mcg (2 inh of 160/4.5).

(Continued)

DRUG (BRAND)	DOSAGE FORM	ADULT DOSE	CHILD DOSE*
METHYLXANTHINE			
Theophylline	**Elixir; Caps & Tabs, Extended-Release**	**Initial:** 300mg/day divided q6-8h; 300mg max. **Usual Max:** 800mg/day.	**Initial:** 10mg/kg/day. **Usual Max:** <1 yr: 0.2 x age in weeks + 5 = mg/kg/day. 1 yr: 16mg/kg/day.
LEUKOTRIENE MODIFIERS			
Montelukast (Singulair)	**Tab:** 10mg; **Tab, Chewable:** 4mg, 5mg, **Granules:** 4mg	10mg qhs	6-23 mo: 4mg granules qhs. 2-5 yrs: 4mg qhs. 6-14 yrs: 5mg qhs. 15 yrs: 10mg qhs.
Zafirlukast (Accolate)	**Tab:** 10mg, 20mg	20mg bid	≥12 yrs: 20mg bid. 5-11 yrs: 10mg bid.
Zileuton (Zyflo)	**Tab:** 600mg	600mg qid	≥12 yr: 600mg qid

ESTIMATED COMPARATIVE DAILY DOSAGES FOR INHALED CORTICOSTEROIDS

	LOW DAILY DOSE		MEDIUM DAILY DOSE		HIGH DAILY DOSE	
DRUG	**ADULT**	**CHILD***	**ADULT**	**CHILD***	**ADULT**	**CHILD***
Beclomethasone HFA 40, 80mcg/inh (QVAR)	80-240mcg	80-160mcg	240-480mcg	160-320mcg	>480mcg	>320mcg
Budesonide DPI 90mcg, 180mcg, 200mcg/inh (Pulmicort Turbuhaler)	180-600mcg	180-400mcg	600-1200mcg	400-800mcg	>1200mcg	>800mcg
Budesonide Neb Sol: 0.25, 0.5mg/2mL (Pulmicort Respules)	N/A	0.5mg	N/A	1.0mg	N/A	2mg
Ciclesonide 80 mcg, 160mcg (Alvesco)	80-160mcg	80-160mcg	160-320mcg	160-320mcg	>320mcg	>320mcg
Flunisolide 250mcg/inh (Aerobid)	500-1000mcg	500-750mcg	1000-2000mcg	1000-1250mcg	>2000mcg	>1250mcg
Fluticasone DPI (Flonase)	100-300mcg	100-200mcg	300-500mcg	200-400mcg	500mcg	400mcg
Fluticasone MDI 44, 110, or 220mcg/inh (Flovent HFA)	88-264mcg	88-176mcg	264-440mcg	176-352mcg	440mcg	352mcg
Mometasone Twisthaler 110mcg/inh, 200mcg/inh 220mcg/inh (Asmanex)	200mcg	N/A	400mcg	N/A	400mcg	N/A
Triamcinolone acetonide 75mcg/inh 100mcg/inh (Azmacort)	300-750mcg	300-600mcg	750-1500mcg	600-900mcg	1500mcg	900mcg

*Children 5-11 yrs unless otherwise noted. MDI: metered-dose inhaler; DPI: dry powder inhaler.
Adopted from: The NAEPP Expert Panel Report: Guidelines for the Diagnosis and Management of Asthma–Update on Selected Topics 2007. http://www.nhlbi.nih.gov/guidelines/asthma/asthsumm.htm

ASTHMA TREATMENT PLAN

CLASSIFICATION	LUNG FUNCTION	STEPWISE APPROACH TO THERAPY IN PATIENTS >12 YEARS OF AGE
Intermittent • Symptoms $\leq$2 days a week • Short-acting β_2-agonist use for symptom control $\leq$2 days a week • Nighttime awakenings $\leq$2 times/month • Interference with normal activity - none	• Normal FEV_1 b/w exacerbations • FEV_1 $\geq$80% predicted • FEV_1/FVC - normal	**Step 1** • **Short-acting inhaled β_2-agonists as needed (2-4 puffs prn).** • Severe exacerbations may occur, separated by long periods of normal lung function and no symptoms; a course of systemic corticosteroids is recommended.
Mild persistent • Symptoms >2 days/week but not daily • Short-acting β_2-agonist use for symptom control >2days/wk but not daily, and not more than 1x on any day • Nighttime awakenings 3-4x/month • Interference with normal activity - minor limitation	• FEV_1 $\geq$80% predicted • FEV_1/FVC - normal	**Step 2** • **Low-dose inhaled corticosteroids.** • **Short-acting inhaled β_2-agonists as needed (2-4 puffs prn).** ALTERNATIVE TREATMENT: • Cromolyn, leukotriene modifier, nedocromil OR theophylline
Moderate persistent • Daily symptoms • Short-acting β_2-agonist use for symptom control daily • Nighttime awakenings >1x/wk but not nightly • Interference with normal activity - some limitation	• FEV_1 >60% but <80% predicted • FEV_1/FVC reduced 5%	**Step 3** • **Low- to medium-dose inhaled corticosteroids** AND • **Long-acting inhaled β_2-agonists.** • **Short-acting inhaled β_2-agonists as needed (2-4 puffs prn).** ALTERNATIVE TREATMENT: • Low-dose ICS + either LTRA, theophylline, OR Zileuton
Severe persistent • Symptoms throughout the day • Short-acting β_2-agonist use for symptom several times per day • Nighttime awakenings often >7x/week • Interference with normal activity - extreme limitation	• FEV_1 $\leq$60% predicted • FEV_1/FVC reduced >5%	**Step 4 or Step 5** • **Medium-dose ICS + LABA OR** • **High-dose ICS + LABA** AND • Consider Omalizumab for patients who have allergies • **Short-acting inhaled β_2-agonists as needed (2-4 puffs prn).** ALTERNATIVE TREATMENT: • Medium-dose ICS + either LTRA, Theophylline, OR Zileuton

Note: Preferred treatments are in bold.

Key Points:

- Stepwise approach presents general guidelines. Review treatment every 1 to 6 months; a gradual stepwise reduction in treatment may be possible. If control is not maintained, consider step up.
- The presence of one of the features of severity is sufficient to place a patient in that category. An individual should be assigned to the most severe grade in which any feature occurs (PEF is % of personal best; FEV is % predicted).
- Intensity of treatment will depend on severity of exacerbation; up to 3 treatments at 20-minute intervals or a single nebulizer treatment as needed. Course of systemic corticosteroids may be needed.
- Use of short-acting beta$_2$-agonists >2 days/week for a symptom relief generally indicates inadequate control and the need to step up treatment
- Airflow obstruction is indicated by reduced FEV_1 and FEV_1/FVC values relative to reference or predicted values.
- Abnormalities of lung function are categorized as restrictive and obstructive defects. A reduced ratio of FEV_1/FVC (eg, <65%) indicates obstruction to the flow of air from the lungs, whereas a reduced FVC with a normal FEV_1/FVC ratio suggests a restrictive pattern.

Abbreviations: FEV_1: Forced expiratory volume in one second. FVC: Forced vital capacity.

*Adapted from the Full Report 2007 *Guidelines for the Diagnosis and Management of Asthma.* NAEPP Expert Panel Report III.

UROLOGICAL THERAPIES

OVERACTIVE BLADDER AGENTS

DRUG	BRAND	HOW SUPPLIED	DOSING	COMMENTS
Darifenacin	Enablex	**Tab, ER:** 7.5mg, 15mg	**Initial:** 7.5mg qd. **Max:** 15mg qd.	Swallow whole. Moderate Hepatic Impairment/ Concomitant Potent CYP3A4 Inhibitors: Do not exceed 7.5mg/day. Severe Hepatic Impairment: Avoid use.
Fesoterodine	Toviaz	**Tab, ER:** 4mg, 8mg	**Initial:** 4mg qd. **Max:** 8mg/day	Swallow whole. CrCl <30mL/min. Concomitant Potent CYP3A4 Inhibitors: Do not exceed 4mg/day. Severe Hepatic Impaiment: Avoid use.
Oxybutynin	Ditropan	**Syrup:** 5mg/5mL **Tab:** 5mg	**Usual:** 5mg bid-tid. **Max:** 5mg qid.	A lower starting dose of 2.5mg bid-tid is recommended for elderly patients.
	Ditropan XL	**Tab, ER:** 5mg, 10mg, 15mg	**Initial:** 5mg or 10mg qd. **Max:** 30mg/day.	Swallow whole. Increase dose by 5mg weekly if needed.
	Gelnique	**Gel:** 10% (1g/pkt)	Apply contents of 1 pkt qd to skin on abdomen, upper arms/shoulders, or thighs.	Rotate application sites.
	Oxytrol	**Patch:** 3.9mg/day	**Usual:** Apply 1 patch twice weekly (every 3-4 days).	Rotate application sites.
Solifenacin	VESIcare	**Tab:** 5mg, 10mg	**Usual:** 5mg qd. **Max:** 10mg qd.	Swallow whole. Renal (CrCl <30mL/min)/Hepatic (Child Pugh B)/Concomitant Potent CYP3A4 Inhibitors: Do not exceed 5mg/day. Hepatic (Child Pugh C): Avoid use.
Tolterodine	Detrol	**Tab:** 1mg, 2mg	**Initial:** 2mg bid.	Decrease dose to 1mg bid if needed. Significant Hepatic/Renal Dysfunction/Concomitant CYP3A4 Inhibitors: 1mg bid.
	Detrol LA	**Cap, ER:** 2mg, 4mg	**Initial:** 4mg qd.	Swallow whole. Decrease dose to 2mg qd if needed. Significant Hepatic/ Renal Dysfunction/ Concomitant CYP3A4 Inhibitors: 2mg qd.
Trospium	Sanctura	**Tab:** 20mg	**Usual:** 20mg bid.	Take 1 hr before meals or on empty stomach. CrCl <30mL/min: 20mg qhs. Elderly ≥75 yrs: May titrate to 20mg qd based upon tolerability.
	Sanctura XR	**Cap, ER:** 60mg	**Usual:** 60mg qam	Take on empty stomach, 1 hr before meal. CrCl <30mL/min: Avoid use.

BENIGN PROSTATIC HYPERTROPHY AGENTS

DRUG	BRAND	HOW SUPPLIED	DOSING	COMMENTS
ALPHA-BLOCKERS				
Alfuzosin	Uroxatral	**Tab, ER:** 10mg	**Usual:** 10mg qd.	Take dose immediately after the same meal each day. Swallow whole.
Doxazosin	Cardura	**Tab:** 1mg, 2mg, 4mg, 8mg	**Initial:** 1mg qd. **Max:** 8mg/day.	Stepwise titration every 1-2 weeks if needed.
	Cardura XL	**Tab, ER:** 4mg, 8mg	**Initial:** 4mg qd. **Max:** 8mg qd.	Take with breakfast. Swallow whole. Titrate after 3-4 weeks if needed.
Silodosin	Rapaflo	**Cap:** 4mg, 8mg	**Usual:** 8mg qd.	Take with food. CrCl 30-50mL/min: 4mg qd.
Tamsulosin	Flomax	**Cap:** 0.4mg	**Initial:** 0.4mg qd. **Max:** 0.8mg qd.	Take dose ½ hour after the same meal each day. Titrate after 2-4 weeks if needed. Restart at initial dose if therapy is interrupted.
Terazosin	Hytrin	**Tab/cap:** 1mg, 2mg, 5mg, 10mg	**Initial:** 1mg qhs. **Usual:** 10mg/day. **Max:** 20mg/day.	Increase stepwise as needed. Restart at initial dose if therapy is interrupted.
5-ALPHA-REDUCTASE INHIBITORS				
Dutasteride	Avodart	**Cap:** 0.5mg	**Usual:** 0.5mg qd.	Swallow whole.
Finasteride	Proscar	**Tab:** 5mg	**Usual:** 5mg qd.	May be administered with doxazosin.

RECOMMENDED IMMUNIZATION SCHEDULE FOR PERSONS AGED 0-6 YEARS

Vaccine ▼ Age ▶	Birth	1 month	2 months	4 months	6 months	12 months	15 months	18 months	19–23 months	2–3 years	4–6 years
Hepatitis B[1]	HepB	HepB		see footnote 1			HepB				
Rotavirus[2]			RV	RV	*RV*[2]						
Diphtheria, Tetanus, Pertussis[3]			DTaP	DTaP	DTaP	see footnote 3	DTaP				DTaP
Haemophilus influenzae type b[4]			Hib	Hib	*Hib*[4]	Hib					
Pneumococcal[5]			PCV	PCV	PCV	PCV				PPSV	
Inactivated Poliovirus			IPV	IPV		IPV					IPV
Influenza[6]								Influenza (Yearly)			
Measles, Mumps, Rubella[7]						MMR			see footnote 7		MMR
Varicella[8]						Varicella			see footnote 8		Varicella
Hepatitis A[9]								HepA (2 doses)		HepA Series	
Meningococcal[10]										MCV	

Range of recommended ages

Certain high-risk groups

This schedule indicates the recommended ages for routine administration of currently licensed vaccines, as of December 1, 2008, for children aged 0 through 6 years. Any dose not administered at the recommended age should be administered at any subsequent visit, when indicated and feasible. Licensed combination vaccines may be used whenever any component of the combination is indicated and other components are not contraindicated and if approved by the Food and Drug Administration for that dose of the series. Providers should consult the relevant Advisory Committee on Immunization Practices statement for detailed recommendations, including high-risk conditions: **http://www.cdc.gov/vaccines/pubs/acip-list.htm**. Clinically significant adverse events that follow immunization should be reported to the Vaccine Adverse Event Reporting System (VAERS). Guidance about how to obtain and complete a VAERS form is available at **http://www.vaers.hhs.gov** or by telephone, **800-822-7967**.

1. **Hepatitis B vaccine (HepB). (Minimum age: birth)**
   At birth:
   - Administer monovalent HepB to all newborns prior to hospital discharge.
   - If mother is hepatitis B surface antigen (HBsAg)-positive, administer HepB and 0.5 mL of hepatitis B immune globulin (HBIG) within 12 hours of birth.
   - If mother's HBsAg status is unknown, administer HepB within 12 hours of birth. Determine mother's HBsAg status as soon as possible and if HBsAg-positive, administer HBIG (no later than age 1 week).

   After the birth dose:
   - The HepB series should be completed with either monovalent HepB or a combination vaccine containing HepB. The second dose should be administered at age 1 or 2 months. The final dose should be administered no earlier than age 24 weeks.
   - Infants born to HBsAg-positive mothers should be tested for HBsAg and antibody to HBsAg (anti-HBs) after completion of at least 3 doses of the HepB series, at age 9 through 18 months (generally at the next well-child visit).

   4-month dose:
   - Administration of 4 doses of HepB to infants is permissible when combination vaccines containing HepB are administered after the birth dose.
2. **Rotavirus vaccine (RV). (Minimum age: 6 weeks)**
   - Administer the first dose at age 6 through 14 weeks (maximum age: 14 weeks 6 days). Vaccination should not be initiated for infants aged 15 weeks or older (i.e., 15 weeks 0 days or older).
   - Administer the final dose in the series by age 8 months 0 days.
   - If Rotarix® is administered at ages 2 and 4 months, a dose at 6 months is not indicated.
3. **Diphtheria and tetanus toxoids and acellular pertussis vaccine (DTaP). (Minimum age: 6 weeks)**
   - The fourth dose may be administered as early as age 12 months, provided at least 6 months have elapsed since the third dose.
   - Administer the final dose in the series at age 4 through 6 years.
4. ***Haemophilus influenzae* type b conjugate vaccine (Hib). (Minimum age: 6 weeks)**
   - If PRP-OMP (PedvaxHIB® or Comvax® [HepB-Hib]) is administered at ages 2 and 4 months, a dose at age 6 months is not indicated.
   - TriHiBit® (DTaP/Hib) should not be used for dosages at 2, 4, or 6 months but can be used as the final dose in children age 12 months or older.
5. **Pneumococcal vaccine. (Minimum age: 6 weeks for pneumococcal conjugate vaccine [PCV]; 2 years for pneumococcal polysaccharide vaccine [PPSV])**
   - PCV is recommended for all children aged younger than 5 years. Administer one dose of PCV to all healthy children aged 24 through 59 months who are not completely vaccinated for their age.
   - Administer PPSV to children aged 2 years or older with certain underlying medical conditions. (See *MMWR* 2000;49[No. RR-9]), including a cochlear implant.

(Continued)

6. Influenza vaccine. (Minimum age: 6 months for trivalent inactivated influenza vaccine [TIV]; 2 years for live, attenuated influenza vaccine [LAIV])

- Administer annually to children aged 6 through 18 years.
- For healthy nonpregnant persons (i.e., those who do not have underlying medical conditions that predispose them to influenza complications) ages 2 through 49 years, either LAIV or TIV may be used.
- Children receiving TIV should receive 0.25 mL if aged 6 through 35 months or 0.5 mL if age 3 years or older.
- Administer 2 doses (separated by at least 4 weeks) to children aged younger than 9 years who are receiving influenza vaccine for the first time or who were vaccinated for the first time during previous influenza season but only received one dose.

7. Measles, mumps, and rubella vaccine (MMR). (Minimum age: 12 months)

- Administer the second dose at age 4 through 6 years. However, the second dose may be administered before age 4 years, provided at least 28 days have elapsed since the first dose.

8. Varicella vaccine. (Minimum age: 12 months)

- Administer second dose at age 4 through 6 years. However, the second dose may be administered before age 4, provided at least 3 months have elapsed since the first dose.
- For children aged 12 months through 12 years the minimum interval between doses is 3 months. However, if the second dose was administered at least 28 days after the first dose, it can be accepted as valid.

9. Hepatitis A vaccine (HepA). (Minimum age: 12 months)

- Administer to all children aged 1 year (i.e., aged 12 through 23 months). Administer the 2 doses at least 6 months apart.
- Children not fully vaccinated by age 2 years can be vaccinated at subsequent visits.
- HepA is also recommended for children older than 1 year who live in areas where vaccination programs target older children or who are at increased risk of infection. See *MMWR* 2006;55(No. RR-7).

10. Meningococcal vaccine. (Minimum age: 2 years for meningococcal conjugate vaccine [MCV] and for meningococcal polysaccharide vaccine [MPSV])

- Administer MCV to children aged 2 through 10 years with terminal complement component deficiency, anatomic or functional asplenia, and certain other high-risk groups. See *MMWR* 2005;54(No. RR-7).
- Persons who received MPSV 3 or more years previously and who remain at increased risk for meningococcal disease should be revaccinated with MCV.

The Recommended Immunization Schedules for Persons Aged 0–18 Years are approved by the Advisory Committee on Immunization Practices (**http://www.cdc.gov/vaccines/recs/acip**), the American Academy of Pediatrics (**http://www.aap.org**), and the American Academy of Family Physicians (**http://www.aafp.org**).

RECOMMENDED IMMUNIZATION SCHEDULE FOR PERSONS AGED 7-18 YEARS

Vaccine ▼ Age ▶	7–10 years	11–12 years	13–18 years
Tetanus, Diphtheria, Pertussis[1]	*see footnote 1*	Tdap	Tdap
Human Papillomavirus[2]	*see footnote 2*	HPV (3 doses)	HPV Series
Meningococcal[3]	MCV	MCV	MCV
Influenza[4]		Influenza (Yearly)	
Pneumococcal[5]		PPSV	
Hepatitis A[6]		HepA Series	
Hepatitis B[7]		HepB Series	
Inactivated Poliovirus[8]		IPV Series	
Measles, Mumps, Rubella[9]		MMR Series	
Varicella[10]		Varicella Series	

Range of recommended ages

Catch-up immunization

Certain high-risk groups

This schedule indicates the recommended ages for routine administration of currently licensed vaccines, as of December 1, 2008, for children aged 7 through 18 years. Any dose not administered at the recommended age should be administered at a subsequent visit, when indicated and feasible. Licensed combination vaccines may be used whenever any component of the combination is indicated and other components are not contraindicated and if approved by the Food and Drug Administration for that dose of the series. Providers should consult the relevant Advisory Committee on Immunization Practices statement for detailed recommendations, including high risk conditions: **http://www.cdc.gov/vaccines/pubs/acip-list.htm**. Clinically significant adverse events that follow immunization should be reported to the Vaccine Adverse Event Reporting System (VAERS). Guidance about how to obtain and complete a VAERS form is available at **http://www.vaers.hhs.gov** or by telephone, **800-822-7967**.

1. Tetanus and diphtheria toxoids and acellular pertussis vaccine (Tdap). (Minimum age: 10 years for BOOSTRIX® and 11 years for ADACEL®)

- Administer at age 11 or 12 years for those who have completed the recommended childhood DTP/DTaP vaccination series and have not received a tetanus and diphtheria toxoid (Td) booster dose.
- Persons aged 13 through 18 years who have not received Tdap should receive a dose.
- A 5-year interval from the last Td dose is encouraged when Tdap is used as a booster dose; however, a shorter interval may be used if pertussis immunity is needed.

2. Human papillomavirus vaccine (HPV). (Minimum age: 9 years)

- Administer the first dose to females at age 11 or 12 years.
- Administer the second dose 2 months after the first dose and the third dose 6 months after the first dose (at least 24 weeks after the first dose).
- Administer the series to females at age 13 through 18 years if not previously vaccinated.

3. Meningococcal conjugate vaccine (MCV).

- Administer at age 11 or 12 years, or at age 13 through 18 years if not previously vaccinated.
- Administer to previously unvaccinated college freshmen living in a dormitory.
- MCV is recommended for children aged 2 through 10 years with terminal complement deficiency, anatomic or functional asplenia, and certain other groups at high risk. See *MMWR* 2005;54 (No. RR-7).
- Persons who received MPSV 5 or more years previously and remain at increased risk for meningococcal disease should be revaccinated with MCV.

4. Influenza vaccine.

- Administer annually to children aged 6 months through 18 years.
- For healthy nonpregnant persons (i.e., those who do not have underlying medical conditions that predispose them to influenza complications) ages 2–49 years, either LAIV or TIV may be used.
- Administer 2 doses (separated by at least 4 weeks) to children younger than 9 years who are receiving influenza vaccine for the first time or who were vaccinated for the first time during the previous influenza season but only received one dose.

5. Pneumococcal polysaccharide vaccine (PPV).

- Administer to children with certain underlying medical conditions (see *MMWR* 1997;46[No. RR-8]), including a cochlear implant. A single revaccination should be administered to children with functional or anatomic asplenia or other immunocompromising condition after 5 years.

6. Hepatitis A vaccine (HepA).

- Administer the 2 doses at least 6 months apart.
- HepA is recommended for children older than 1 year who live in areas where vaccination programs target older children or who are at increased risk of infection. See *MMWR* 2006;55(No. RR-7).

(Continued)

7. Hepatitis B vaccine (HepB).

- Administer the 3-dose series to those not previously vaccinated.
- A 2-dose series (separated by at least 4 months) of adult formulation Recombivax HB® is licensed for children aged 11 through 15 years.

8. Inactivated poliovirus vaccine (IPV).

- For children who received an all-IPV or all-oral poliovirus (OPV) series, a fourth dose is not necessary if the third dose was administered at age 4 years or older.
- If both OPV and IPV were administered as part of a series, a total of 4 doses should be administered, regardless of the child's current age.

9. Measles, mumps, and rubella vaccine (MMR).

- If not previously vaccinated, administer 2 doses or the second dose for those who have received only 1 dose, with at least 28 days between doses.

10. Varicella vaccine.

- For persons aged 7 through 18 years without evidence of immunity (see *MMWR* 2007;56 [No. RR-4]), administer 2 doses if not previously vaccinated or the second dose if they have received only 1 dose.
- For persons aged 7 through 12 years, the minimum interval between doses is 3 months. However, if the second dose was administered at least 28 days after the first dose, it can be accepted as valid.
- For persons aged 13 years and older, the minimum interval between doses is 28 days.

The Recommended Immunization Schedules for Persons Aged 0–18 Years are approved by the Advisory Committee on Immunization Practices **(http://www.cdc.gov/vaccines/recs/acip)**, the American Academy of Pediatrics **(http://www.aap.org)**, and the American Academy of Family Physicians **(http://www.aafp.org)**.

CATCH-UP IMMUNIZATION SCHEDULE FOR PERSONS AGED 4 MONTHS-18 YEARS WHO START LATE OR WHO ARE MORE THAN 1 MONTH BEHIND

CATCH-UP SCHEDULE FOR PERSONS AGED 4 MONTHS THROUGH 6 YEARS					
Vaccine	Minimum Age for Dose 1	Minimum Interval Between Doses			
		Dose 1 to Dose 2	Dose 2 to Dose 3	Dose 3 to Dose 4	Dose 4 to Dose 5
Hepatitis B[1]	Birth	4 weeks	8 weeks (and at least 16 weeks after first dose)		
Rotavirus[2]	6 wks	4 weeks	4 weeks[2]		
Diphtheria, Tetanus, Pertussis[3]	6 wks	4 weeks	4 weeks	6 months	6 months[3]
Haemophilus influenzae type b[4]	6 wks	**4 weeks** if first dose administered at younger than age 12 months **8 weeks (as final dose)** if first dose administered at age 12-14 months **No further doses needed** if first dose administered at age 15 months or older	**4 weeks**[4] if current age is younger than 12 months **8 weeks (as final dose)**[4] if current age is 12 months or older and second dose administered at younger than age 15 months **No further doses needed** if previous dose administered at age 15 months or older	**8 weeks (as final dose)** This dose only necessary for children aged 12 months through 59 months who received 3 doses before age 12 months	
Pneumococcal[5]	6 wks	**4 weeks** if first dose administered at younger than age 12 months **8 weeks** (as final dose for healthy children) if first dose administered at age 12 months or older or current age 24 through 59 months **No further doses needed** for healthy children if first dose administered at age 24 months or older	**4 weeks** if current age is younger than 12 months **8 weeks** (as final dose for healthy children) if current age is 12 months or older **No further doses needed** for healthy children if previous dose administered at age 24 months or older	**8 weeks (as final dose)** This dose only necessary for children aged 12 months through 59 months who received 3 doses before age 12 months or for high-risk children who received 3 doses at any age	
Inactivated Poliovirus[6]	6 wks	4 weeks	4 weeks	4 weeks[6]	
Measles, Mumps, Rubella[7]	12 mos	4 weeks			
Varicella[8]	12 mos	3 months			
Hepatitis A[9]	12 mos	6 months			
CATCH-UP SCHEDULE FOR PERSONS AGED 7 THROUGH 18 YEARS					
Tetanus, Diphtheria/ Tetanus, Diphtheria, Pertussis[10]	7 yrs[10]	4 weeks	**4 weeks** if first dose administered at younger than age 12 months **6 months** if first dose administered at age 12 months or older	**6 months** if first dose administered at younger than age 12 months	
Human Papillomavirus[11]	9 yrs	Routine dosing intervals are recommended[11]			
Hepatitis A[9]	12 mos	6 months			
Hepatitis B[1]	Birth	4 weeks	8 weeks (and at least 16 weeks after first dose)		
Inactivated Poliovirus[6]	6 wks	4 weeks	4 weeks	4 weeks[6]	
Measles, Mumps, Rubella[7]	12 mos	4 weeks			
Varicella[8]	12 mos	**3 months** if the person is younger than age 13 years **4 weeks** if the person is aged 13 years or older			

The table above provides catch-up schedules and minimum intervals between doses for children whose vaccinations have been delayed. A vaccine series does not need to be restarted, regardless of the time that has elapsed between doses. Use the section appropriate for the child's age.

1. **Hepatitis B vaccine (HepB).**
   - Administer the 3-dose series to those not previously vaccinated.
   - A 2-dose series (separated by at least 4 months) of adult formulation Recombivax HB® is licensed for children aged 11 through 15 years.
2. **Rotavirus vaccine (RV).**
   - The maximum age for the first dose is 14 weeks 6 days. Vaccination should not be initiated for infants aged 15 weeks or older (i.e., 15 weeks, 0 days or older).
   - Administer the final dose in the series by age 8 months 0 days.
   - If Rotarix® was administered for the first and second doses, a third dose is not indicated.
3. **Diphtheria and tetanus toxoids and acellular pertussis vaccine (DTaP).**
   - The fifth dose is not necessary if the fourth dose was administered at age 4 years or older.
4. ***Haemophilus influenzae* type b conjugate vaccine (Hib).**
   - Hib vaccine is not generally recommended for persons aged 5 years or older. No efficacy data are available on which to base a recommendation concerning use of Hib vaccine for older children and adults. However, studies suggest good immunogenicity in persons who have sickle cell disease, leukemia, or HIV infection, or who have had a splenectomy; administering 1 dose of Hib vaccine to these persons is not contraindicated.
   - If the first 2 doses were PRP-OMP (PedvaxHIB® or Comvax®), and administered at age 11 months or younger, the third (and final) dose should be administered at age 12 through 15 months and at least 8 weeks after the second dose.
   - If first dose was administered at age 7 through 11 months, administer 2 doses separated by 4 weeks and a final dose at age 12 through 15 months.

(Continued)

5. Pneumococcal vaccine.

- Administer one dose of pneumococcal conjugate vaccine (PCV) to all healthy children aged 24 through 59 months who have not received at least 1 dose of PCV on or after age 12 months.
- For children aged 24 through 59 months with underlying medical conditions, administer 1 dose of PVC if 3 doses were received previously or administer 2 doses of PCV at least 8 weeks apart if fewer than 3 doses were received previously.
- Administer pneumococcal polysaccharide vaccine (PPSV) to children aged 2 years or older with certain underlying medical conditions (see *MMWR* 2000;49[No. RR-9]), including a cochlear implant, at least 8 weeks after the last dose of PCV.

6. Inactivated poliovirus vaccine (IPV).

- For children who received an all-IPV or all-oral poliovirus (OPV) series, a fourth dose is not necessary if third dose was administered at age 4 years or older.
- If both OPV and IPV were administered as part of a series, a total of 4 doses should be administered, regardless of the child's current age.

7. Measles, mumps, and rubella vaccine (MMR).

- Administer the second dose at age 4 through 6 years. However, the second dose may be administered before age 4, provided at least 28 days have elapsed since the first dose.
- If not previously vaccinated, administer 2 doses with at least 28 days between doses.

8. Varicella vaccine.

- Administer the second dose at age 4 through 6 years. However, the second dose may be administered before age 4, provided at least 3 months have elapsed since the first dose.
- For persons aged 12 months through 12 years, the minimum interval between doses is 3 months. However, if the second dose was administered at least 28 days after the first dose, it can be accepted as valid.
- For persons aged 13 years and older, the minimum interval between doses is 28 days.

9. Hepatitis A vaccine (HepA).

- HepA is recommended for children older than 1 year who live in areas where vaccination programs target older children or who are at increased risk of infection. See *MMWR* 2006;55 (No. RR-7).

10. Tetanus and diphtheria toxoids vaccine (Td) and tetanus and diphtheria toxoids and acellular pertussis vaccine (Tdap).

- Doses of DTaP are counted as part of the Td/Tdap series
- Tdap should be substituted for a single dose of Td in the catch-up series or as a booster for children aged 10 through 18 years; use Td for other doses.

11. Human papillomavirus vaccine (HPV).

- Administer the series to females at age 13 through 18 years if not previously vaccinated.
- Use recommended routine dosing intervals for series catch-up (i.e., the second and third doses should be administered at 2 and 6 months after the first dose). However, the minimum interval between the first and second doses is 4 weeks. The minimum interval between the second and third doses is 12 weeks, and the third dose should be given at least 24 weeks after the first dose.

Information about reporting reactions after immunization is available online at **http://www.vaers.hhs.gov** or by telephone, 800-822-7967. Suspected cases of vaccine-preventable diseases should be reported to the state or local health department. Additional information, including precautions and contraindications for immunization, is available from the National Center for Immunization and Respiratory Diseases at **http://www.cdc.gov/vaccines** or telephone, **800-CDC-INFO (800-232-4636)**.

RECOMMENDED ADULT IMMUNIZATION SCHEDULE, BY VACCINE AND AGE GROUP

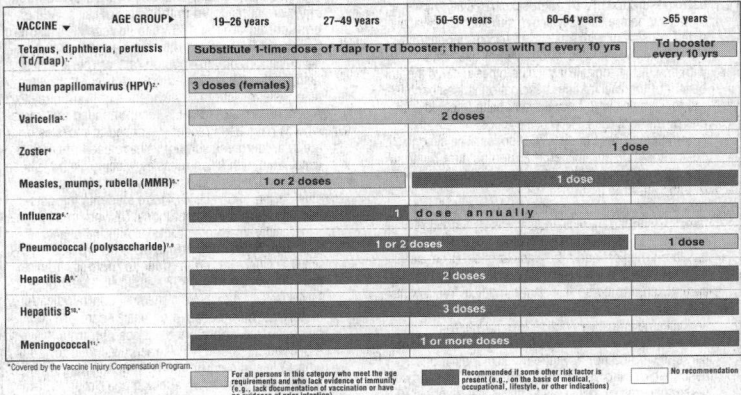

<table>
<tr><th>VACCINE ▼ / AGE GROUP ▶</th><th>19–26 years</th><th>27–49 years</th><th>50–59 years</th><th>60–64 years</th><th>≥65 years</th></tr>
<tr><td>Tetanus, diphtheria, pertussis (Td/Tdap)[1,*]</td><td colspan="4">Substitute 1-time dose of Tdap for Td booster; then boost with Td every 10 yrs</td><td>Td booster every 10 yrs</td></tr>
<tr><td>Human papillomavirus (HPV)[2,*]</td><td>3 doses (females)</td><td></td><td></td><td></td><td></td></tr>
<tr><td>Varicella[3,*]</td><td colspan="5">2 doses</td></tr>
<tr><td>Zoster[4]</td><td></td><td></td><td></td><td colspan="2">1 dose</td></tr>
<tr><td>Measles, mumps, rubella (MMR)[5,*]</td><td colspan="2">1 or 2 doses</td><td colspan="3">1 dose</td></tr>
<tr><td>Influenza[6,*]</td><td colspan="5">1 dose annually</td></tr>
<tr><td>Pneumococcal (polysaccharide)[7,8]</td><td colspan="4">1 or 2 doses</td><td>1 dose</td></tr>
<tr><td>Hepatitis A[9,*]</td><td colspan="5">2 doses</td></tr>
<tr><td>Hepatitis B[10,*]</td><td colspan="5">3 doses</td></tr>
<tr><td>Meningococcal[11,*]</td><td colspan="5">1 or more doses</td></tr>
</table>

*Covered by the Vaccine Injury Compensation Program.

Light shading: For all persons in this category who meet the age requirements and who lack evidence of immunity (e.g., lack documentation of vaccination or have no evidence of prior infection)

Dark shading: Recommended if some other risk factor is present (e.g., on the basis of medical, occupational, lifestyle, or other indications)

Unshaded: No recommendation

Report all clinically significant postvaccination reactions to the Vaccine Adverse Event Reporting System (VAERS). Reporting forms and instructions on filing a VAERS report are available at **www.vaers.hhs.gov** or by telephone, 800-822-7967.

Information on how to file a Vaccine Injury Compensation Program claim is available at **www.hrsa.gov/vaccine compensation** or by telephone, 800-338-2382. To file a claim for vaccine injury, contact the U.S. Court of Federal Claims, 717 Madison Place, N.W., Washington, D.C. 20005; telephone, 202-357-6400.

Additional information about the vaccines in this schedule, extent of available data, and contraindications for vaccination is also available at **www.cdc.gov/vaccines** or from the CDC-INFO Contact Center at 800-CDC-INFO (800-232-4636) in English and Spanish, 24 hours a day, 7 days a week.

Use of trade names and commercial sources is for identification only and does not imply endorsement by the U.S. Department of Health and Human Services.

This schedule indicates the recommended age groups for which administration of currently licensed vaccines is commonly indicated for adults ages 19 years and older, as of January 1, 2009. Licensed combination vaccines may be used whenever any components of the combination are indicated and when the vaccine's other components are not contraindicated. For detailed recommendations on all vaccines, including those used primarily for travelers or that are issued during the year, consult the manufacturers' package inserts and the complete statements from the Advisory Committee on Immunization Practices **(www.cdc.gov/vaccines/pubs/acip-list.htm)**.

1. **Tetanus, diphtheria, and acellular pertussis (Td/Tdap) vaccination.** Tdap should replace a single dose of Td for adults aged 19 through 64 years who have not received a dose of Tdap previously. Adults with uncertain or incomplete history of primary vaccination series with tetanus and diphtheria toxoid–containing vaccines should begin or complete a primary vaccination series. A primary series for adults is 3 doses of tetanus and diphtheria toxoid–containing vaccines; administer the first 2 doses at least 4 weeks apart and the third dose 6–12 months after the second. However, Tdap can substitute for any one of the doses of Td in the 3-dose primary series. The booster dose of tetanus and diphtheria toxoid–containing vaccine should be administered to adults who have completed a primary series and if the last vaccination was received 10 or more years previously. Tdap or Td vaccine may be used, as indicated.
   If a woman is pregnant and received the last Td vaccination 10 or more years previously, administer Td during the second or third trimester. If the woman received the last Td vaccination less than 10 years previously, administer Tdap during the immediate postpartum period. A dose of Tdap is recommended for postpartum women, close contacts of infants aged less than 12 months, and all health-care personnel with direct patient contact if they have not previously received Tdap. An interval as short as 2 years from the last Td is suggested; shorter intervals can be used. Td may be deferred during pregnancy and Tdap substituted in the immediate postpartum period, or Tdap may be administered instead of Td to a pregnant woman after an informed discussion with the woman. Consult the ACIP statement for recommendations for administering Td as prophylaxis in wound management.
2. **Human papillomavirus (HPV) vaccination.** HPV vaccination is recommended for all females aged 11 through 26 years (and may begin at 9 years) who have not completed the vaccine series. History of genital warts, abnormal Papanicolaou test, or posi-

(Continued)

tive HPV DNA test is not evidence of prior infection with all vaccine HPV types; HPV vaccination is recommended for persons with such histories.
Ideally, vaccine should be administered before potential exposure to HPV through sexual activity; however, females who are sexually active should still be vaccinated consistent with age-based recommendations. Sexually active females who have not been infected with any of the four HPV vaccine types receive the full benefit of the vaccination. Vaccination is less beneficial for females who have already been infected with one or more of the HPV vaccine types.
A complete series consists of 3 doses. The second dose should be administered 2 months after the first dose; the third dose should be administered 6 months after the first dose.
HPV vaccination is not specifically recommended for females with the medical indications described in Figure 2, "Vaccines that might be indicated for adults based on medical and other indications." Because HPV vaccine is not a live-virus vaccine it may be administered to persons with the medical indications described in Figure 2. However, immune response and vaccine efficacy might be less for persons with the medical indications described in Figure 2 than in persons who do not have the medical indications described or who are immunocompetent. Healthcare personnel are not at increased risk because of occupational exposure, and should be vaccinated consistent with age-based recommendations.

3. **Varicella vaccination.** All adults without evidence of immunity to varicella should receive 2 doses of single-antigen varicella vaccine if not previously vaccinated or the second dose if they have only received one dose unless they have a medical contraindication. Special consideration should be given to those who 1) have close contact with persons at high risk for severe disease (e.g., health-care personnel and family contacts of persons with immunocompromising conditions) or 2) are at high risk for exposure or transmission (e.g., teachers; child care employees; residents and staff members of institutional settings, including correctional institutions; college students; military personnel; adolescents and adults living in households with children; nonpregnant women of childbearing age; and international travelers).
Evidence of immunity to varicella in adults includes any of the following: 1) documentation of 2 doses of varicella vaccine at least 4 weeks apart; 2) U.S.-born before 1980 (although for health-care personnel and pregnant women, birth before 1980 should not be considered evidence of immunity); 3) history of varicella based on diagnosis or verification of varicella by a health-care provider (for a patient reporting a history of or presenting with an atypical case, a mild case, or both, health-care providers should seek either an epidemiologic link with a typical varicella case or to a laboratory-confirmed case or evidence of laboratory confirmation, if it was performed at the time of acute disease); 4) history of herpes zoster based on health-care provider diagnosis or verification of herpes zoster by a healthcare provider; or 5) laboratory evidence of immunity or laboratory confirmation of disease.
Pregnant women should be assessed for evidence of varicella immunity. Women who do not have evidence of immunity should receive the first dose of varicella vaccine upon completion or termination of pregnancy and before discharge from the health-care facility. The second dose should be administered 4–8 weeks after the first dose.

4. **Herpes zoster vaccination.** A single dose of zoster vaccine is recommended for adults aged 60 years and older regardless of whether they report a prior episode of herpes zoster. Persons with chronic medical conditions may be vaccinated unless their condition constitutes a contraindication.

5. **Measles, mumps, rubella (MMR) vaccination.**
Measles component: Adults born before 1957 generally are considered immune to measles. Adults born during or after 1957 should receive 1 or more doses of MMR unless they have a medical contraindication, documentation of 1 or more doses, history of measles based on health-care provider diagnosis, or laboratory evidence of immunity.
A second dose of MMR is recommended for adults who 1) have been recently exposed to measles or are in an outbreak setting; 2) have been previously vaccinated with killed measles vaccine; 3) have been vaccinated with an unknown type of measles vaccine during 1963–1967; 4) are students in postsecondary educational institutions; 5) work in a health-care facility; or 6) plan to travel internationally.
Mumps component: Adults born before 1957 generally are considered immune to mumps. Adults born during or after 1957 should receive 1 dose of MMR unless they have a medical contraindication, history of mumps based on health-care provider diagnosis, or laboratory evidence of immunity.
A second dose of MMR is recommended for adults who 1) live in a community experiencing a mumps outbreak and are in an affected age group; 2) are students in postsecondary educational institutions; 3) work in a health-care facility; or 4) plan to travel internationally. For unvaccinated health-care personnel born before 1957 who do not have other evidence of mumps immunity, administering 1 dose on a routine basis should be considered and administering a second dose during an outbreak should be strongly considered.
Rubella component: 1 dose of MMR vaccine is recommended for women whose rubella vaccination history is unreliable or who lack laboratory evidence of immunity. For women of childbearing age, regardless of birth year, routinely determine rubella immunity and counsel women regarding congenital rubella syndrome. Women who do not have evidence of immunity should receive MMR upon completion or termination of pregnancy and before discharge from the health-care facility.

6. **Influenza vaccination.** *Medical indications:* Chronic disorders of the cardiovascular or pulmonary systems, including asthma; chronic metabolic diseases, including diabetes mellitus, renal or hepatic dysfunction, hemoglobinopathies, or immunocompromising conditions (including immunocompromising conditions caused by medications or human immunodeficiency virus [HIV]); any condition that compromises respiratory function or the handling of respiratory secretions or that can increase the risk of aspiration (e.g., cognitive dysfunction, spinal cord injury, or seizure disorder or other neuromuscular disorder); and pregnancy during the influenza season. No data exist on the risk for severe or complicated influenza disease among persons with asplenia; however, influenza is a risk factor for secondary bacterial infections that can cause severe disease among persons with asplenia.
Occupational indications: All health-care personnel, including those employed by long-term care and assisted-living facilities, and caregivers of children less than 5 years old.
Other indications: Residents of nursing homes and other long-term care and assisted-living facilities; persons likely to transmit influenza to persons at high risk (e.g., in-home household contacts and caregivers of children aged less than 5 years old, persons 65 years old and older and persons of all ages with high-risk conditions); and anyone who would like to decrease their risk of getting influ-

(Continued)

enza. Healthy, nonpregnant adults aged less than 50 years without high-risk medical conditions who are not contacts of severely immunocompromised persons in special care units can receive either intranasally administered live, attenuated influenza vaccine (FluMist®) or inactivated vaccine. Other persons should receive the inactivated vaccine.

7. **Pneumococcal polysaccharide (PPSV) vaccination.** *Medical indications:* Chronic lung disease (including asthma); chronic cardiovascular diseases; diabetes mellitus; chronic liver diseases, cirrhosis; chronic alcoholism, chronic renal failure or nephritic syndrome; functional or anatomic asplenia (e.g., sickle cell disease or splenectomy [if elective splenectomy is planned, vaccinate at least 2 weeks before surgery]); immunocompromising conditions; and cochlear implants and cerebrospinal fluid leaks. Vaccinate as close to HIV diagnosis as possible.
Other indications: Residents of nursing homes or long-term care facilities and persons who smoke cigarettes. Routine use of PPSV is not recommended for Alaska Native or American Indian persons younger than 65 years unless they have underlying medical conditions that are PPSV indications. However, public health authorities may consider recommending PPSV for Alaska Natives and American Indians aged 50 through 64 years who are living in areas in which the risk of invasive pneumococcal disease is increased.

8. **Revaccination with PPSV.** One-time revaccination after 5 years for persons with chronic renal failure or nephritic syndrome; functional or anatomic asplenia (e.g., sickle cell disease or splenectomy); and for persons with immunocompromising conditions. For persons aged 65 years and older, one-time revaccination if they were vaccinated 5 or more years previously and were aged less than 65 years at the time of primary vaccination.

9. **Hepatitis A vaccination.** *Medical indications:* Persons with chronic liver disease and persons who receive clotting factor concentrates.
Behavioral indications: Men who have sex with men and persons who use illegal drugs.
Occupational indications: Persons working with hepatitis A virus (HAV)–infected primates or with HAV in a research laboratory setting.
Other indications: Persons traveling to or working in countries that have high or intermediate endemicity of hepatitis A (a list of countries is available at wwwn.cdc.gov/travel/contentdiseases.aspx) and any person seeking protection from HAV infection.
Single-antigen vaccine formulations should be administered in a 2-dose schedule at either 0 and 6–12 months (Havrix®), or 0 and 6–18 months (Vaqta®). If the combined hepatitis A and hepatitis B vaccine (Twinrix®) is used, administer 3 doses at 0, 1, and 6 months; alternatively, a 4-dose schedule, administered on days 0, 7 and 21 to 30 followed by a booster dose at month 12 may be used.

10. **Hepatitis B vaccination.** *Medical indications:* Persons with end-stage renal disease, including patients receiving hemodialysis; persons with HIV infection; and persons with chronic liver disease.
Occupational indications: Health-care personnel and public-safety workers who are exposed to blood or other potentially infectious body fluids.
Behavioral indications: Sexually active persons who are not in a long-term, mutually monogamous relationship (e.g., persons with more than 1 sex partner during the previous 6 months); persons seeking evaluation or treatment for a sexually transmitted disease (STD); current or recent injection-drug users; and men who have sex with men.
Other indications: Household contacts and sex partners of persons with chronic hepatitis B virus (HBV) infection; clients and staff members of institutions for persons with developmental disabilities; international travelers to countries with high or intermediate prevalence of chronic HBV infection (a list of countries is available at **wwwn.cdc.gov/travel/contentdiseases.aspx**); and any adult seeking protection from HBV infection.
Hepatitis B vaccination is recommended for all adults in the following settings: STD treatment facilities; HIV testing and treatment facilities; facilities providing drug-abuse treatment and prevention services; health-care settings targeting services to injection-drug users or men who have sex with men; correctional facilities; end-stage renal disease programs and facilities for chronic hemodialysis patients; and institutions and nonresidential daycare facilities for persons with developmental disabilities.
If the combined hepatitis A and hepatitis B vaccine (Twinrix®) is used, administer 3 doses at 0, 1, and 6 months; alternatively, a 4-dose schedule, administered on days 0, 7 and 21 to 30 followed by a booster dose at month 12 may be used.
Special formulation indications: For adult patients receiving hemodialysis or with other immunocompromising conditions, 1 dose of 40 μg/mL (Recombivax HB®), administed on a 3-dose schedule or 2 doses of 20 μg/mL (Engerix-B®) administered simultaneously on a 4-dose schedule at 0, 1, 2 and 6 months.

11. **Meningococcal vaccination.** *Medical indications:* Adults with anatomic or functional asplenia, or terminal complement component deficiencies.
Other indications: First-year college students living in dormitories; microbiologists who are routinely exposed to isolates of *Neisseria meningitidis*; military recruits; and persons who travel to or live in countries in which meningococcal disease is hyperendemic or epidemic (e.g., the "meningitis belt" of sub-Saharan Africa during the dry season [December–June]), particularly if their contact with local populations will be prolonged. Vaccination is required by the government of Saudi Arabia for all travelers to Mecca during the annual Hajj.
Meningococcal conjugate (MCV) vaccine is preferred for adults with any of the preceding indications who are aged 55 years or younger, although meningococcal polysaccharide vaccine (MPSV) is an acceptable alternative. Revaccination with MCV after 5 years might be indicated for adults previously vaccinated with MPSV who remain at increased risk for infection (e.g., persons residing in areas in which disease is epidemic).

12. **Selected conditions for which *Haemophilus influenzae* type b (Hib) vaccine may be used.** Hib vaccine generally is not recommended for persons 5 years and older. No efficacy data are available on which to base a recommendation concerning use of Hib vaccine for older children and adults. However, studies suggest good immunogenicity in persons who have sickle cell disease, leukemia, or HIV infection or who have had a splenectomy; administering 1 dose of vaccine to these persons is not contraindicated.

13. **Immunocompromising conditions.** Inactivated vaccines are generally acceptable (e.g., pneumococcal, meningococcal, and influenza [trivalent inactivated influenza vaccine]), and live vaccines generally are avoided in persons with immune deficiencies or immunocompromising conditions. Information on specific conditions is available at **www.cdc.gov/vaccines/pubs/acip-list.htm**.

Vaccines That Might Be Indicated for Adults Based on Medical and Other Indications

INDICATION ▶ / VACCINE ▼	Pregnancy	Immunocompromising conditions (excluding human immunodeficiency virus [HIV])[13]	HIV infection[3,12,13] CD4+ T lymphocyte count <200 cells/μL	HIV infection[3,12,13] CD4+ T lymphocyte count ≥200 cells/μL	Diabetes, heart disease, chronic lung disease, chronic alcoholism	Asplenia[12] (including elective splenectomy and terminal complement component deficiencies)	Chronic liver disease	Kidney failure, end-stage renal disease, receipt of hemodialysis	Health-care personnel
Tetanus, diphtheria, pertussis (Td/Tdap)[1,*]	Td	Substitute 1-time dose of Tdap for Td booster; then boost with Td every 10 yrs							
Human papillomavirus (HPV)[2,*]		3 doses for females through age 26 yrs							
Varicella[3,*]	Contraindicated			2 doses					
Zoster[4]	Contraindicated				1 dose				
Measles, mumps, rubella (MMR)[5,*]	Contraindicated			1 or 2 doses					
Influenza[6,*]	1 dose TIV annually								1 dose TIV or LAIV annually
Pneumococcal (polysaccharide)[7,8]		1 or 2 doses							
Hepatitis A[9,*]	2 doses								
Hepatitis B[10,*]	3 doses								
Meningococcal[11,*]	1 or more doses								

*Covered by the Vaccine Injury Compensation Program.

- For all persons in this category who meet the age requirements and who lack evidence of immunity (e.g., lack documentation of vaccination or have no evidence of prior infection)
- Recommended if some other risk factor is present (e.g., on the basis of medical, occupational, lifestyle, or other indications)
- No recommendation

Report all clinically significant postvaccination reactions to the Vaccine Adverse Event Reporting System (VAERS). Reporting forms and instructions on filing a VAERS report are available at **www.vaers.hhs.gov** or by telephone, 800-822-7967.

Information on how to file a Vaccine Injury Compensation Program claim is available at **www.hrsa.gov/vaccinecompensation** or by telephone, 800-338-2382. To file a claim for vaccine injury, contact the U.S. Court of Federal Claims, 717 Madison Place, N.W., Washington, D.C. 20005; telephone, 202-357-6400.

Additional information about the vaccines in this schedule, extent of available data, and contraindications for vaccination is also available at **www.cdc.gov/vaccines** or from the CDC-INFO Contact Center at 800-CDC-INFO (800-232-4636) in English and Spanish, 24 hours a day, 7 days a week.

Use of trade names and commercial sources is for identification only and does not imply endorsement by the U.S. Department of Health and Human Services.

This schedule indicates the recommended medical indications for which administration of currently licensed vaccines is commonly indicated for adults ages 19 years and older, as of January 1, 2009. Licensed combination vaccines may be used whenever any components of the combination are indicated and when the vaccine's other components are not contraindicated. For detailed recommendations on all vaccines, including those used primarily for travelers or that are issued during the year, consult the manufacturers' package inserts and the complete statements from the Advisory Committee on Immunization Practices **(www.cdc.gov/vaccines/pubs/acip-list.htm)**.

1. **Tetanus, diphtheria, and acellular pertussis (Td/Tdap) vaccination.** Tdap should replace a single dose of Td for adults aged 19 through 64 years who have not received a dose of Tdap previously. Adults with uncertain or incomplete history of primary vaccination series with tetanus and diphtheria toxoid–containing vaccines should begin or complete a primary vaccination series. A primary series for adults is 3 doses of tetanus and diphtheria toxoid–containing vaccines; administer the first 2 doses at least 4 weeks apart and the third dose 6–12 months after the second. However, Tdap can substitute for any one of the doses of Td in the 3-dose primary series. The booster dose of tetanus and diphtheria toxoid–containing vaccine should be administered to adults who have completed a primary series and if the last vaccination was received 10 or more years previously. Tdap or Td vaccine may be used, as indicated.

   If a woman is pregnant and received the last Td vaccination 10 or more years previously, administer Td during the second or third trimester. If the woman received the last Td vaccination less than 10 years previously, administer Tdap during the immediate postpartum period. A dose of Tdap is recommended for postpartum women, close contacts of infants aged less than 12 months, and all health-care personnel with direct patient contact if they have not previously received Tdap. An interval as short as 2 years from the last Td is suggested; shorter intervals can be used. Td may be deferred during pregnancy and Tdap substituted in the immediate postpartum period, or Tdap may be administered instead of Td to a pregnant woman after an informed discussion with the woman. Consult the ACIP statement for recommendations for administering Td as prophylaxis in wound management.

(Continued)

2. **Human papillomavirus (HPV) vaccination.** HPV vaccination is recommended for all females aged 11 through 26 years (and may begin at 9 years) who have not completed the vaccine series. History of genital warts, abnormal Papanicolaou test, or positive HPV DNA test is not evidence of prior infection with all vaccine HPV types; HPV vaccination is recommended for persons with such histories.
   Ideally, vaccine should be administered before potential exposure to HPV through sexual activity; however, females who are sexually active should still be vaccinated consistent with age-based recommendations. Sexually active females who have not been infected with any of the four HPV vaccine types receive the full benefit of the vaccination. Vaccination is less beneficial for females who have already been infected with one or more of the HPV vaccine types.
   A complete series consists of 3 doses. The second dose should be administered 2 months after the first dose; the third dose should be administered 6 months after the first dose.
   HPV vaccination is not specifically recommended for females with the medical indications described in Figure 2, "Vaccines that might be indicated for adults based on medical and other indications." Because HPV vaccine is not a live-virus vaccine it may be administered to persons with the medical indications described in Figure 2. However, immune response and vaccine efficacy might be less for persons with the medical indications described in Figure 2 than in persons who do not have the medical indications described or who are immunocompetent. Healthcare personnel are not at increased risk because of occupational exposure, and should be vaccinated consistent with age-based recommendations.
3. **Varicella vaccination.** All adults without evidence of immunity to varicella should receive 2 doses of single-antigen varicella vaccine if not previously vaccinated or the second dose if they have only received one dose unless they have a medical contraindication. Special consideration should be given to those who 1) have close contact with persons at high risk for severe disease (e.g., health-care personnel and family contacts of persons with immunocompromising conditions) or 2) are at high risk for exposure or transmission (e.g., teachers; child care employees; residents and staff members of institutional settings, including correctional institutions; college students; military personnel; adolescents and adults living in households with children; nonpregnant women of childbearing age; and international travelers).
   Evidence of immunity to varicella in adults includes any of the following: 1) documentation of 2 doses of varicella vaccine at least 4 weeks apart; 2) U.S.-born before 1980 (although for health-care personnel and pregnant women, birth before 1980 should not be considered evidence of immunity); 3) history of varicella based on diagnosis or verification of varicella by a health-care provider (for a patient reporting a history of or presenting with an atypical case, a mild case, or both, health-care providers should seek either an epidemiologic link with a typical varicella case or to a laboratory-confirmed case or evidence of laboratory confirmation, if it was performed at the time of acute disease); 4) history of herpes zoster based on health-care provider diagnosis or verification of herpes zoster by a healthcare provider; or 5) laboratory evidence of immunity or laboratory confirmation of disease.
   Pregnant women should be assessed for evidence of varicella immunity. Women who do not have evidence of immunity should receive the first dose of varicella vaccine upon completion or termination of pregnancy and before discharge from the health-care facility. The second dose should be administered 4–8 weeks after the first dose.
4. **Herpes zoster vaccination.** A single dose of zoster vaccine is recommended for adults aged 60 years and older regardless of whether they report a prior episode of herpes zoster. Persons with chronic medical conditions may be vaccinated unless their condition constitutes a contraindication.
5. **Measles, mumps, rubella (MMR) vaccination.** *Measles component:* Adults born before 1957 generally are considered immune to measles. Adults born during or after 1957 should receive 1 or more doses of MMR unless they have a medical contraindication, documentation of 1 or more doses, history of measles based on health-care provider diagnosis, or laboratory evidence of immunity.
   A second dose of MMR is recommended for adults who 1) have been recently exposed to measles or are in an outbreak setting; 2) have been previously vaccinated with killed measles vaccine; 3) have been vaccinated with an unknown type of measles vaccine during 1963–1967; 4) are students in postsecondary educational institutions; 5) work in a health-care facility; or 6) plan to travel internationally.
   Mumps component: Adults born before 1957 generally are considered immune to mumps. Adults born during or after 1957 should receive 1 dose of MMR unless they have a medical contraindication, history of mumps based on health-care provider diagnosis, or laboratory evidence of immunity.
   A second dose of MMR is recommended for adults who 1) live in a community experiencing a mumps outbreak and are in an affected age group; 2) are students in postsecondary educational institutions; 3) work in a health-care facility; or 4) plan to travel internationally. For unvaccinated health-care personnel born before 1957 who do not have other evidence of mumps immunity, administering 1 dose on a routine basis should be considered and administering a second dose during an outbreak should be strongly considered.
   Rubella component: 1 dose of MMR vaccine is recommended for women whose rubella vaccination history is unreliable or who lack laboratory evidence of immunity. For women of childbearing age, regardless of birth year, routinely determine rubella immunity and counsel women regarding congenital rubella syndrome. Women who do not have evidence of immunity should receive MMR upon completion or termination of pregnancy and before discharge from the health-care facility.
6. **Influenza vaccination.** *Medical indications:* Chronic disorders of the cardiovascular or pulmonary systems, including asthma; chronic metabolic diseases, including diabetes mellitus, renal or hepatic dysfunction, hemoglobinopathies, or immunocompromising conditions (including immunocompromising conditions caused by medications or human immunodeficiency virus [HIV]); any condition that compromises respiratory function or the handling of respiratory secretions or that can increase the risk of aspiration (e.g., cognitive dysfunction, spinal cord injury, or seizure disorder or other neuromuscular disorder); and pregnancy during the influenza season. No data exist on the risk for severe or complicated influenza disease among persons with asplenia; however, influenza is a risk factor for secondary bacterial infections that can cause severe disease among persons with asplenia.
   Occupational indications: All health-care personnel, including those employed by long-term care and assisted-living facilities, and caregivers of children less than 5 years old.
   Other indications: Residents of nursing homes and other long-term care and assisted-living facilities; persons likely to transmit influenza to persons at high risk (e.g., in-home household contacts and caregivers of children aged less than 5 years old,

(Continued)

persons 65 years old and older and persons of all ages with high-risk conditions); and anyone who would like to decrease their risk of getting influenza. Healthy, nonpregnant adults aged less than 50 years without high-risk medical conditions who are not contacts of severely immunocompromised persons in special care units can receive either intranasally administered live, attenuated influenza vaccine (FluMist®) or inactivated vaccine. Other persons should receive the inactivated vaccine.

7. **Pneumococcal polysaccharide (PPSV) vaccination.** *Medical indications:* Chronic lung disease (including asthma); chronic cardiovascular diseases; diabetes mellitus; chronic liver diseases, cirrhosis; chronic alcoholism, chronic renal failure or nephritic syndrome; functional or anatomic asplenia (e.g., sickle cell disease or splenectomy [if elective splenectomy is planned, vaccinate at least 2 weeks before surgery]); immunocompromising conditions; and cochlear implants and cerebrospinal fluid leaks. Vaccinate as close to HIV diagnosis as possible. *Other indications:* Residents of nursing homes or long-term care facilities and persons who smoke cigarettes. Routine use of PPSV is not recommended for Alaska Native or American Indian persons younger than 65 years unless they have underlying medical conditions that are PPSV indications. However, public health authorities may consider recommending PPSV for Alaska Natives and American Indians aged 50 through 64 years who are living in areas in which the risk of invasive pneumococcal disease is increased.

8. **Revaccination with PPSV.** One-time revaccination after 5 years for persons with chronic renal failure or nephritic syndrome; functional or anatomic asplenia (e.g., sickle cell disease or splenectomy); and for persons with immunocompromising conditions. For persons aged 65 years and older, one-time revaccination if they were vaccinated 5 or more years previously and were aged less than 65 years at the time of primary vaccination.

9. **Hepatitis A vaccination.** *Medical indications:* Persons with chronic liver disease and persons who receive clotting factor concentrates.
Behavioral indications: Men who have sex with men and persons who use illegal drugs.
Occupational indications: Persons working with hepatitis A virus (HAV)–infected primates or with HAV in a research laboratory setting.
Other indications: Persons traveling to or working in countries that have high or intermediate endemicity of hepatitis A (a list of countries is available at wwwn.cdc.gov/travel/contentdiseases.aspx) and any person seeking protection from HAV infection. Single-antigen vaccine formulations should be administered in a 2-dose schedule at either 0 and 6–12 months (Havrix®), or 0 and 6–18 months (Vaqta®). If the combined hepatitis A and hepatitis B vaccine (Twinrix®) is used, administer 3 doses at 0, 1, and 6 months; alternatively, a 4-dose schedule, administered on days 0, 7 and 21 to 30 followed by a booster dose at month 12 may be used.

10. **Hepatitis B vaccination.** *Medical indications:* Persons with end-stage renal disease, including patients receiving hemodialysis; persons with HIV infection; and persons with chronic liver disease.
Occupational indications: Health-care personnel and public-safety workers who are exposed to blood or other potentially infectious body fluids.
Behavioral indications: Sexually active persons who are not in a long-term, mutually monogamous relationship (e.g., persons with more than 1 sex partner during the previous 6 months); persons seeking evaluation or treatment for a sexually transmitted disease (STD); current or recent injection-drug users; and men who have sex with men.
Other indications: Household contacts and sex partners of persons with chronic hepatitis B virus (HBV) infection; clients and staff members of institutions for persons with developmental disabilities; international travelers to countries with high or intermediate prevalence of chronic HBV infection (a list of countries is available at **wwwn.cdc.gov/travel/contentdiseases.aspx**); and any adult seeking protection from HBV infection. Hepatitis B vaccination is recommended for all adults in the following settings: STD treatment facilities; HIV testing and treatment facilities; facilities providing drug-abuse treatment and prevention services; health-care settings targeting services to injection-drug users or men who have sex with men; correctional facilities; end-stage renal disease programs and facilities for chronic hemodialysis patients; and institutions and nonresidential daycare facilities for persons with developmental disabilities.
If the combined hepatitis A and hepatitis B vaccine (Twinrix®) is used, administer 3 doses at 0, 1, and 6 months; alternatively, a 4-dose schedule, administered on days 0, 7 and 21 to 30 followed by a booster dose at month 12 may be used.
Special formulation indications: For adult patients receiving hemodialysis or with other immunocompromising conditions, 1 dose of 40 μg/mL (Recombivax HB®), administed on a 3-dose schedule or 2 doses of 20 μg/mL (Engerix-B®) administered simultaneously on a 4-dose schedule at 0, 1, 2 and 6 months.

11. **Meningococcal vaccination.** *Medical indications:* Adults with anatomic or functional asplenia, or terminal complement component deficiencies.
Other indications: First-year college students living in dormitories; microbiologists who are routinely exposed to isolates of *Neisseria meningitidis*; military recruits; and persons who travel to or live in countries in which meningococcal disease is hyperendemic or epidemic (e.g., the "meningitis belt" of sub-Saharan Africa during the dry season [December–June]), particularly if their contact with local populations will be prolonged. Vaccination is required by the government of Saudi Arabia for all travelers to Mecca during the annual Hajj. Meningococcal conjugate (MCV) vaccine is preferred for adults with any of the preceding indications who are aged 55 years or younger, although meningococcal polysaccharide vaccine (MPSV) is an acceptable alternative. Revaccination with MCV after 5 years might be indicated for adults previously vaccinated with MPSV who remain at increased risk for infection (e.g., persons residing in areas in which disease is epidemic).

12. **Selected conditions for which *Haemophilus influenzae* type b (Hib) vaccine may be used.** Hib vaccine generally is not recommended for persons 5 years and older. No efficacy data are available on which to base a recommendation concerning use of Hib vaccine for older children and adults. However, studies suggest good immunogenicity in persons who have sickle cell disease, leukemia, or HIV infection or who have had a splenectomy; administering 1 dose of vaccine to these persons is not contraindicated.

13. **Immunocompromising conditions.** Inactivated vaccines are generally acceptable (e.g., pneumococcal, meningococcal, and influenza [trivalent inactivated influenza vaccine]), and live vaccines generally are avoided in persons with immune deficiencies or immunocompromising conditions. Information on specific conditions is available at **www.cdc.gov/vaccines/pubs/acip-list.htm**.

ALCOHOL-FREE PRODUCTS

The following is a selection of alcohol-free products grouped by therapeutic category. This list is not comprehensive. Generic and alternate brands may exist. Always check product labeling for definitive information on specific ingredients.

Analgesics

Advil Children's Suspension	Wyeth Consumer
APAP Elixir	Bio-Pharm
Genapap Children's Elixir	Teva
Motrin Children's Suspension	McNeil Consumer
Motrin Infants' Suspension	McNeil Consumer
Silapap Infant's Drops	Silarx
Tylenol Children's Suspension	McNeil Consumer
Tylenol Extra Strength Solution	McNeil Consumer
Tylenol Infant's Suspension	McNeil Consumer

Antiasthmatic Agents

Dy-G Liquid	Cypress
Jay-Phyl Syrup	Pharmakon

Anticonvulsant

Zarontin Syrup	Pfizer

Antiviral Agent

Epivir Oral Solution	GlaxoSmithKline

Cough/Cold/Allergy Preparations

Accuhist PDX Drops Solution	Pediamed
Accuhist PDX Syrup	Pediamed
Alacol Solution	Ballay
Alacol DM Syrup	Ballay
Allanhist PDX Syrup	Allan
Anaplex DM Syrup	ECR
Anaplex DMX Suspension	ECR
Andehist DM NR Syrup	Cypress
Andehist NR Syrup	Cypress
Aridex Solution	Gentex
Aridex-D Solution	Gentex
Atuss G Syrup	Atley
Baltussin Solution	Ballay
Banophen Elixir	Major
Benadryl Allergy Solution	Pfizer Consumer
Benadryl-D Allergy & Sinus Children's Solution	Johnson & Johnson Consumer
Bromaline Syrup	Rugby
Bromaline DM Elixir	Rugby
Bromhist PDX Solution	Cypress
Bromhist Pediatric Solution	Cypress
Bromhist-DM Pediatric Syrup	Cypress
Bromhist-DM Solution	Cypress
Bromhist-NR Solution	Cypress
Bromhist-PDX Syrup	Cypress
Bromphenex DM Solution	Breckenridge
Bromphenex HD Solution	Breckenridge
Bromplex DM Solution	Prasco
Bromplex HD Solution	Prasco
Bromtuss DM Solution	Breckenridge
Broncotron Liquid	Seyer Pharmatec
Broncotron-D Suspension	Seyer Pharmatec
B-Tuss Liquid	Blansett
Carbaphen 12 Ped Suspension	Gil
Carbaphen 12 Suspension	Gil
Carbatuss Liquid	GM
Carbatuss-12 Suspension	GM
Carbatuss-CL Solution	GM
Carbetaplex Solution	Breckenridge
Carbetaplex TS Suspension	Breckenridge
Carbofed DM Syrup	Hi-Tech Pharmacal
Cardec Solution	Qualitest
Cardec DM Solution	Qualitest
Children's Dimetapp Cold & Allergy Solution	Wyeth Consumer
Children's Dimetapp Long Acting Cough Plus Cold Solution	Wyeth Consumer
Children's Dimetapp Nighttime Flu Syrup	Wyeth Consumer
Children's Dimetapp DM Cold & Cough Solution	Wyeth Consumer
Children's Mucinex Cold Solution	Adams
Children's Mucinex Cough Syrup	Adams
Children's Mucinex Syrup	Adams
Chlordex GP Syrup	Cypress
Chlor-Mes D Solution	Cypress
Codal-DM Syrup	Cypress
Complete Allergy Elixir	Cardinal Health
Corfen DM Solution	Cypress
Coughtuss Solution	Breckenridge
Crantex HC Syrup	Breckenridge
Crantex Syrup	Breckenridge
Creomulsion Cough Syrup	Summit Industries
Creomulsion for Children Syrup	Summit Industries
Dacex-DM Solution	Cypress
Dallergy Solution	Laser
De-Chlor DM Solution	Cypress
De-Chlor DR Solution	Cypress
Dehistine Syrup	Cypress
Despec Liquid	International Ethical
Dex PC Syrup	Boca Pharmacal
Diabetic Tussin Allergy Relief Liquid	Health Care Products
Diabetic Tussin Cough Lozenges	Health Care Products
Diabetic Tussin Night Time Formula Solution	Health Care Products
Diabetic Tussin Solution	Health Care Products

Cough/Cold/Allergy Preparations (Continued)

Diabetic Tussin DM Solution	Health Care Products
Diabetic Tussin DM Maximum Strength Liquid	Health Care Products
Diabetic Tussin EX Liquid	Health Care Products
Dimetapp Decongestant Pediatric Drops	Wyeth Consumer
Donatussin Solution	Laser
Donatussin DC Syrup	Laser
Donatussin DM Solution	Laser
Donatussin DM Suspension	Laser
Donatussin DM Syrup	Laser
Double-Tussin DM Liquid	Reese
Duratuss AC12 Suspension	Victory
Duratuss DM Solution	Victory
Duratuss DM12 Suspension	Victory
Dynatuss EX Syrup	Breckenridge
Dynatuss HC Solution	Breckenridge
Endacof DM Solution	Larken
Endal HD Plus Liquid	Pediamed
Father John's Medicine Plus Drops	Oakhurst
Ganidin NR Liquid	Cypress
Gani-Tuss NR Liquid	Cypress
Gani-Tuss-DM NR Liquid	Cypress
Genebronco-D Liquid	PGD
Genecof-HC Liquid	PGD
Genecof-XP Liquid	PGD
Genecof-XP Syrup	PGD
Genedel Syrup	PGD
Genedotuss-DM Liquid	PGD
Genepatuss Liquid	PGD
Genetuss-2 Liquid	PGD
Genexpect-DM Liquid	PGD
Genexpect-PE Liquid	PGD
Genexpect-SF Liquid	PGD
Giltuss Liquid	Gil
Giltuss Pediatric Liquid	Gil
Giltuss Ped-C Solution	Gil
H-C Tussive Syrup	Vintage
Histacol DM Pediatric Syrup	Breckenridge
Histinex HC Syrup	Ethex
Histinex PV Syrup	Ethex
Hydramine Elixir	Teva
Hydro-Tussin HC Syrup	Ethex
Hydro-Tussin HD Liquid	Ethex
Hydro-Tussin XP Syrup	Ethex
Jaycof Expectorant Syrup	Pharmakon
Jaycof-HC Liquid	Pharmakon
Jaycof-XP Syrup	Pharmakon
Levall Solution	Auriga
Lodrane D Suspension	ECR
Lohist D Syrup	Larken
Lohist DM Syrup	Larken
Marcof Expectorant Syrup	Marnel
M-Clear Jr Solution	McNeil, R.A.
M-Clear Solution	McNeil, R.A.
Medi-Brom Elixir	Medicine Shoppe
Mintuss G Syrup	Breckenridge
Mintuss MR Syrup	Breckenridge
Mintuss MS Syrup	Breckenridge
Mintuss NX Solution	Breckenridge
Motrin Cold Children's Suspension	McNeil Consumer
Myhist-DM Solution	Larken
Myhist-PD Solution	Larken
Nalex DH Liquid	Blansett Pharmacal
Nalex-A Liquid	Blansett Pharmacal
Nasop Suspension	Hawthorn
Neotuss S/F Liquid	A.G. Marin
Neotuss-D Liquid	A.G. Marin
Norel DM Liquid	U.S.Pharmaceutical
Organidin NR Liquid	Meda
PediaCare Cough + Cold Children's Liquid	Johnson & Johnson Consumer
PediaCare Decongestant & Cough Liquid	Johnson & Johnson Consumer
PediaCare Long-Acting Cough Solution	Johnson & Johnson Consumer
PediaCare Multi-Symptom Cold Liquid	Johnson & Johnson Consumer
PediaCare Nightrest Liquid	Johnson & Johnson Consumer
Pediahist DM Syrup	Boca Pharmacal
Pedia-Relief Liquid	Major
Phanasin Diabetic Choice Syrup	Pharmakon
Phanasin Syrup	Pharmakon
Phanatuss Syrup	Pharmakon
Phanatuss DM Diabetic Choice Syrup	Pharmakon
Phanatuss-HC Diabetic Choice Solution	Pharmakon
Phena-HC Solution	GM
Phena-S Liquid	GM
Phena-S 12 Suspension	GM
Poly Hist DM Solution	Poly
Poly Hist HC Solution	Poly
Poly Hist PD Solution	Poly
Poly-Tussin Solution	Poly
Poly-Tussin DM Syrup	Poly
Poly-Tussin HD Syrup	Poly
Poly-Tussin XP Solution	Poly

Pro-Clear Solution	Pro-Pharma
Prolex DM Liquid	Blansett Pharmacal
Pro-Red Solution	Pro-Pharma
Q-Tussin Liquid	Qualitest
Q-Tussin PE Liquid	Qualitest
Rescon-DM Liquid	Capellon
Rescon-GG Liquid	Capellon
Rindal HD Liquid	Breckenridge
Rindal HD Plus Solution	Breckenridge
Robitussin Chest Congestion Syrup	Wyeth Consumer
Robitussin Cough & Allergy Solution	Wyeth Consumer
Robitussin Cough & Cold CF Syrup	Wyeth Consumer
Robitussin Cough, Cold & Flu Nighttime Solution	Wyeth Consumer
Robitussin Cough & Congestion Liquid	Wyeth Consumer
Robitussin Cough DM Syrup	Wyeth Consumer
Robitussin Head & Chest Congestion PE Syrup	Wyeth Consumer
Robitussin Pediatric Cough & Cold CF Solution	Wyeth Consumer
Robitussin Pediatric Cough & Cold Long-Acting Solution	Wyeth Consumer
Robitussin Pediatric Night Relief Liquid	Wyeth Consumer
Rondec Solution	Sciele
Rondec DM Drops	Sciele
Rondec DM Solution	Sciele
Ru-Tuss DM Solution	Carwin
Scot-Tussin Diabetes CF Liquid	Scot-Tussin
Scot-Tussin DM Solution	Scot-Tussin
Scot-Tussin Expectorant Solution	Scot-Tussin
Scot-Tussin Original Solution	Scot-Tussin
Scot-Tussin Senior Solution	Scot-Tussin
Siladryl Allergy Solution	Silarx
Sildec Syrup	Silarx
Sildec-DM Syrup	Silarx
Sildec-PE Solution	Silarx
Sildec PE-DM Solution	Silarx
Siltussin DAS Liquid	Silarx
Siltussin DM DAS Cough Formula Syrup	Silarx
Siltussin SA Syrup	Silarx
Simply Cough Liquid	McNeil Consumer
Sudafed Children's Cold & Cough Solution	Johnson & Johnson
Sudafed Children's Solution	Johnson & Johnson
Sudatuss DM Syrup	PGD
Sudatuss-2 Liquid	PGD
Sudatuss-SF Liquid	PGD
Triant-HC Solution	Hawthorn
TriTuss Solution	Everett
Tusdec-DM Solution	Cypress
Tusnel Pediatric Solution	Llorens
Tusnel Solution	Llorens
Tussafed-EX Syrup	Everett
Tussafed-EX Pediatric Drops	Everett
Tussafed-HC Syrup	Everett
Tussafed-HCG Solution	Everett
Tussall Solution	Everett
Tussinate Syrup	Pediamed
Tussi-Organidin DM NR Solution	Victory
Tussi-Organidin DM-S NR Solution	Victory
Tussi-Organidin NR Solution	Victory
Tussi-Organidin-S NR Solution	Victory
Tussi-Pres Liquid	Kramer-Novis
Tussi-Pres Pediatric Solution	Kramer-Novis
Tylenol Cold Children's Suspension	McNeil Consumer
Tylenol Cold Infants' Drops	McNeil Consumer
Tylenol Cold Plus Cough Children's Suspension	McNeil Consumer
Tylenol Cold Plus Cough Infants' Suspension	McNeil Consumer
Tylenol Flu Children's Suspension	McNeil Consumer
Tylenol Flu Night Time Max Strength Liquid	McNeil Consumer
Tylenol Sinus Children's Suspension	McNeil Consumer
Vazol Solution	Wraser Pharm
Vicks 44E Pediatric Liquid	Procter & Gamble
Vicks 44M Pediatric Liquid	Procter & Gamble
Vicks Dayquil Multi-Symptom Liquid	Procter & Gamble
Vicks Nyquil Children's Liquid	Procter & Gamble
V-Tann Suspension	Breckenridge
Welltuss EXP Solution	Prasco
Z-Cof 12 DM Suspension	Zyber
Z-Cof 8 DM Suspension	Zyber
Z-Cof DM Solution	Zyber
Z-Cof DMX Solution	Zyber
Z-Cof HC Solution	Zyber
Z-Cof HCX Solution	Zyber
Z-Tuss DM Syrup	Magna

Ear/Nose/Throat Products

4-Way Saline Moisturizing Mist Spray	Bristol-Myers
Ayr Baby Saline Spray	Ascher
Bucalcide Spray	Seyer Pharmatec

Ear/Nose/Throat Products (Continued)

Bucalsep Solution	Gil
Bucalsep Spray	Gil
Cheracol Sore Throat Spray	Lee
Fresh N Free Solution	Geritrex
Gly-Oxide Solution	GlaxoSmithKline
Larynex Lozenges	Dover
Listermint Solution	Johnson & Johnson Consumer
Nasal Moist Gel	Blairex
Orajel Baby Day & Night Gel	Del
Orajel Baby Nighttime Teething Pain Medicine Gel	Del
OraMagic Plus Powder	MPM Medical
OraMagicRx Powder	MPM Medical
Orasept Mouthwash/ Gargle Liquid	Pharmakon
Tanac Liquid	Del
Throto-Ceptic Spray	S.S.S.
Triaminic Sore Throat Spray	Novartis Consumer
Vicks Sinex Spray	P&G Company
Vicks Sinex 12 Hour Spray	P&G Company
Zilactin Baby Extra Strength Gel	Zila

Gastrointestinal Agents

Axid Solution	Braintree
Colidrops Pediatric Drops	A.G. Marin
Colace Solution	Purdue
Gas Relief Solution	Perrigo
Imogen Liquid	PGD
Kaodene NN Suspension	Pfeiffer
Kaopectate Advanced Formula Suspension	Pharmacia Consumer
Liqui-Doss Liquid	Ferndale
Mylicon Infants' Drops	Johnson & Johnson/ Merck

Topical Products

Aloe Vesta 2-N-1 Antifungal Ointment	Convatec
Dermatone Lips N Face Protector Ointment	Dermatone
Dermatone Moisturizing Sunblock Cream	Dermatone
Dermatone Skin Protector Cream	Dermatone
Fleet Pain Relief Pads	Fleet
Fresh & Pure Douche Solution	Unico
Handclens Solution	Woodward
Joint-Ritis Maximum Strength Ointment	Naturopathic
Neutrogena Acne Wash Liquid	Neutrogena
Neutrogena Antiseptic Solution	Neutrogena
Neutrogena Clear Pore Gel	Neutrogena
Neutrogena T/Derm Liquid	Neutrogena
Neutrogena Toner Solution	Neutrogena
Podiclens Spray	Woodward
Sea Breeze Foaming Face Wash Gel	Clairol
Sportz Bloc Cream	Med-Derm
Therasoft Anti-Acne Cream	SFC
Therasoft Skin Protectant Cream	SFC
Tiger Balm Arthritis Rub Lotion	Prince of Peace

Vitamins/Minerals/Supplements

Adaptosode For Stress Liquid	HVS
Adaptosode R+R For Acute Stress Liquid	HVS
Apetigen Elixir	Kramer-Novis
Biosode Liquid	HVS
Detoxosode Products Liquid	HVS
Genesupp-500 Liquid	PGD
Genetect Plus Liquid	PGD
Multi-Delyn Liquid	Silarx
Multi-Delyn w/Iron Liquid	Silarx
Nutrivit Solution	Llorens
Poly-Vi-Sol Drops	Mead Johnson
Poly-Vi-Sol w/Iron Drops	Mead Johnson
Protect Plus Liquid	Gil
Strovite Forte Syrup	Everett
Supervite Liquid	Seyer Pharmatec
Suplevit Liquid	Gil
Tri-Vi-Sol w/Iron Drops	Mead Johnson
Vitafol Syrup	Everett

Miscellaneous

Cytra-2 Solution	Cypress
Cytra-K Solution	Cypress
Fluorinse Solution	Oral B
Namenda Solution	Forest
Primsol Solution	FSC

COMMON LABORATORY TEST VALUES

Listed below are generally accepted normal values for a selection of common laboratory assays conducted on serum, plasma, and blood. Remember that norms may vary from laboratory to laboratory in accordance with the methodology and quality control measures employed by the facility. When in doubt, check with the laboratory that performed the analysis.

"SI range" refers to Système International d'Unités, a uniform system of reporting numerical values that permits interchangeability of information among nations and disciplines.

TEST	US RANGE	SI RANGE
Acid phosphatase	≤2.5 ng/mL	≤2.5 μg/L
Prostatic Total	≤5.8 U/L	<97 nkat/L
Alanine aminotransferase [ALT] (SGPT)	≤48 U/L	≤0.8 μkat/L
Albumin, serum	3.5-5.5 g/dL	35-55 g/L
Alkaline phosphatase	20-125 U/L	0.33-2.08 μkat/L
Ammonia [NH_3^+]	10-80 μg/dL	6-47 μmol/L
Amylase, serum	60-180 U/L	0.8-3.2 μkat/L
Antinuclear antibodies (ANA)	Negative at 1:40 dilution	
Aspartate aminotransferase (AST) (SGOT)	≤42 U/L	<0.7 μkat/L
Bilirubin		
Total	0.3-1.0 mg/dL	5.1-17 μmol/L
Direct	0.1-0.3 mg/dL	1.7-5.1 μmol/L
Indirect	0.2-0.7 mg/dL	3.4-12 μmol/L
Blood urea nitrogen/ creatinine ratio	10:1-20:1	Average 15:1
Calcium, plasma	9-10.5 mg/dL	2.2-2.6 mmol/L
Calcium, ionized	4.5-5.6 mg/dL	1.1-1.4 mmol/L
Chloride, serum	95-108 mEq/L	95-108 mmol/L
Cholesterol (total plasma)		
Desirable level	<200 mg/dL	<5.20 mmol/L
Moderate risk	200-240 mg/dL	5.2-6.3 mmol/L
High risk	>240 mg/dL	>6.3 mmol/L
Copper	70-140 μg/dL	11-22 μmol/L
Cortisol, serum		
0800 hours	5-25 μg/dL	140-690 nmol/L
1600 hours	3-12 μg/dL	80-330 nmol/L
Creatinine kinase (CK)		
Isoenzymes	CK-MM: 97-100% of total CK-MB: <3% of total CK-BB: 0% of total	CK-MM: 0.97-1.00 of total CK-MB: <0.03 of total CK-BB: 0 of total
Total	Male: ≤235 U/L Female: ≤190 U/L	Male: ≤3.92 μkat/L Female: ≤3.17 μkat/L
Creatinine, serum	<1.5 mg/dL	<133 μmol/L
Creatinine clearance	75-125 mL/min	1.24-2.08 mL/sec
Digoxin		
Therapeutic	0.8-2.0 ng/mL	1.0-2.6 nmol/L
Toxic	>2.5 ng/mL	>3.2 nmol/L
Erythrocyte count (RBC)	4.15-4.90 $\times 10^6/mm^3$	4.15-4.90 $\times 10^{12}/L$
Erythrocyte sedimentation rate (ESR)		
Male	0-20 mm/hr	0-20 mm/hr
Female	0-30 mm/hr	0-30 mm/hr
Ferritin		
Male	15-400 ng/mL	15-400 μg/L
Female	10-200 ng/mL	10-200 μg/L
Folic acid	3-16 ng/mL	7-36 nmol/L

COMMON LABORATORY TEST VALUES

TEST	US RANGE	SI RANGE
Follicle-stimulating hormone (FSH)		
Female	1.4-9.6 mIU/mL	1.4-9.6 IU/L
Ovulation	2.3-21 mIU/mL	2.3-21 IU/L
Postmenopausal	34-96 mIU/mL	34-96 IU/L
Male	0.9-15 mIU/mL	0.9-15 IU/L
Gamma-glutamyl transferase (GGT)		
Male	≤65 U/L	≤1.08 µkat/L
Female	≤45 U/L	≤0.75 µkat/L
Gases, arterial blood		
pO_2	80-100 mmHg	11-13 kPa
pCO_2	35-45 mmHg	4.7-6 kPa
Glucose, plasma		
Fasting	75-115 mg/dL	4.2-6.4 mmol/L
Postprandial (2 h)	<140 mg/dL	<7.8 mmol/L
Immunoglobulins (Ig)		
IgG	800-1500 mg/dL	8.0-15.0 g/L
IgA	90-325 mg/dL	0.9-3.2 g/L
IgM	45-150 mg/dL	0.45-1.5 g/L
IgD	0-8 mg/dL	0-0.08 g/L
IgE	<0.025 mg/dL	<0.00025 g/L
Iron, serum	50-150 µg/dL	9-27 µmol/L
Iron binding capacity	250-370 µg/dL	45-66 µmol/L
Iron saturation	20-45%	
Lactic acid (plasma, venous)	9-16 mg/dL	1.0-1.8 mmol/L
Lactic dehydrogenase (LDH)	100-190 U/L	1.7-3.2 µkat/L
Lead	<20 µg/dL	1.0 µmol/L
Leukocyte count (WBC)	$4.3\text{-}10.8 \times 10^3$	$4.3\text{-}10.8 \times 10^9$/L
Lipase	0-160 U/L	0-2.66 µkat/L
Lipoproteins (desirable levels)		
Low density (LDL)	<130 mg/dL	<3.36 mmol/L
High density (HDL)	>60 mg/dL	>1.55 mmol/L
Lithium ion (therapeutic)	0.6-1.2 mEq/L	0.6-1.2 mmol/L
Luteinizing hormone		
Female	0.8-26 mIU/mL	0.8-26 IU/L
Ovulation	25-57 mIU/mL	25-57 IU/L
Postmenopausal	40-104 mIU/mL	40-104 IU/L
Male	1.3-13 mIU/mL	1.3-13 IU/L
Osmolality, plasma	285-295 mOsm/kg	285-295 mmol/kg
Phenytoin		
Therapeutic	10-20 mg/L	40-80 µmol/L
Toxic	>30 mg/L	>120 µmol/L
Phosphorus, serum	2.5-4.5 mg/dL	0.8-1.45 mmol/L
Potassium, serum	3.5-5 mEq/L	3.5-5 mmol/L
Prolactin	2-15 ng/mL	2-15 µg/L
Prostate-specific antigen (PSA)	≤4 ng/mL	≤4 µg/L
Protein		
Total	5.5-8.0 g/dL	55-80 g/L
Albumin	3.5-5.5 g/dL	35-55 g/L
Globulin	2.0-3.5 g/dL	20-35 g/L
Reticulocyte count	0.5-2.3% of RBCs	0.005-0.023 of RBCs
Rheumatoid factor	<40 IU/mL	<40 kIU/L
Sodium, serum	136-145 mEq/L	136-145 mmol/L
Theophylline (therapeutic)	10-20 mg/L	55-110 µmol/L
Thyroxine-binding globulin (TBG)	16-34 mg/L	16-34 mg/L

TEST	US RANGE	SI RANGE
Thyroid-stimulating hormone (TSH)	0.4-5 μU/mL	0.4-5 mU/L
Thyroxine (T_4)		
Free	0.8-1.8 ng/dL	10-23 pmol/L
Total	4.5-12.5 μg/dL	58-161 nmol/L
Transferrin	230-390 μg/dL	2.3-3.9 mg/L
Triglycerides	<160 μg/dL	<1.8 mmol/L
Triiodothyronine (T_3)	70-190 ng/dL	1.1-2.9 nmol/L
T_3 uptake	25-35%	0.25-0.35 (proportion of 1.0)
Urea nitrogen, blood (BUN)	7-30 mg/dL	2.5-10.7 mmol/L
Uric acid		
Male	4.0-8.5 mg/dL	238-506 μmol/L
Female	2.5-7.5 mg/dL	149-446 μmol/L
Vitamin B_{12}	200-600 pg/mL	148-443 pmol/L

SOURCES:

Beers MH, Porter RS, Jones TV, et al. *Merck Manual of Diagnosis and Therapy,* ed 18. Whitehouse Station, NJ: Merck Research Laboratories; 2006.

Cahill M. *Illustrated Guide to Diagnostic Tests,* ed 2. Springhouse, PA: Springhouse Corporation; 1998.

Fauci AS, Braunwald E, Kasper DL, et al. *Harrison's Principles of Internal Medicine,* ed 17. New York, NY: McGraw Hill; 2008.

Goldman L, Ausiello D. *Cecil Medicine,* ed 23. Philadelphia, PA: Saunders Elsevier; 2008.

Sacher RA, McPherson RA, Campos JM. *Wildmann's Clinical Interpretation of Laboratory Tests.* Philadelphia, PA: FA Davis Company; 2000.

CYTOCHROME P450 ENZYMES: SUBSTRATES, INDUCERS, AND INHIBITORS

SUBSTRATES	INDUCERS	INHIBITORS
CYP1A2		
Acetaminophen	Broccoli	Amiodarone HCl
Aminophylline	Brussels Sprouts	Anastrozole
Amiodarone HCl	Carbamazepine	Cimetidine
Amitriptyline HCl	Charbroiled Food	Ciprofloxacin
Amoxapine	Citalopram Hydrobromide	Clarithromycin
Anagrelide HCl	Diltiazem HCl	Desogestrel
Caffeine	Erythromycin	Esomeprazole Sodium
Chlordiazepoxide	Escitalopram Oxalate	Ethinyl Estradiol
Cimetidine HCl	Esomeprazole Sodium	Fluvoxamine
Ciprofloxacin	Fluvoxamine	Gatifloxacin
Clomipramine HCl	Hypericum	Gemifloxacin Mesylate
Clopidogrel Bisulfate	Insulin	Grapefruit
Clozapine	Lansoprazole	Isoniazid
Cyclobenzaprine	Nafcillin Sodium	Ketoconazole
Desipramine HCl	Nicotine	Levofloxacin
Diazepam	Omeprazole	Levonorgestrel
Diltiazem HCl	Phenobarbital	Mestranol
Doxepin HCl	Phenytoin	Methoxsalen
Erythromycin	Primidone	Mexiletine HCl
Estradiol	Rifampicin	Moxifloxacin HCl
Flutamide	Rifampin	Nalidixic Acid
Fluticasone Propionate	Ritonavir	Norethindrone
Fluvoxamine Maleate	Tobacco	Norfloxacin
Haloperidol		Norgestrel
Imipramine HCl		Ofloxacin
Levobupivacaine HCl		Omeprazole
Maprotiline HCl		Paroxetine
Methadone HCl		Ranitidine HCl
Mexiletine HCl		Ritonavir
Mirtazapine		Sildenafil Citrate
Moxifloxacin HCl		Tacrine HCl
Nafcillin Sodium		Ticlopidine HCl
Naproxen		Trovafloxacin Mesylate
Nicotine		Vardenafil HCl
Norethindrone Acetate		Zileuton
Norfloxacin		
Nortriptyline HCl		
Ofloxacin		
Olanzapine		
Ondansetron		
Phenobarbital		
Phenytoin		
Propafenone HCl		
Propranolol HCl		
Protriptyline HCl		
Riluzole		
Ritonavir		
Ropinirole HCl		
Ropivacaine HCl		
Tacrine HCl		

(Continued)

SUBSTRATES	INDUCERS	INHIBITORS
CYP1A2 *(Continued)*		
Tamoxifen Citrate		
Theobromine		
Theophylline		
Tizanidine		
Trimethaphan Camsylate		
Trimipramine Maleate		
Trovafloxacin Mesylate		
Verapamil HCl		
Warfarin Sodium		
Zileuton		
Zolmitriptan		
CYP2C18		
Naproxen		Cimetidine
Omeprazole		
Piroxicam		
Propranolol HCl		
Tretinoin		
Warfarin Sodium		
CYP2C19		
Amitriptyline HCl	Carbamazepine	Cimetidine
Amoxapine	Norethindrone	Citalopram Hydrobromide
Carisoprodol	Phenobarbital	Delavirdine Mesylate
Cilostazol	Phenytoin	Desogestrel
Citalopram Hydrobromide	Prednisone	Efavirenz
Clomipramine HCl	Rifampin	Ethinyl Estradiol
Cyclophosphamide		Ethynodiol Diacetate
Desipramine HCl		Felbamate
Dextromethorphan		Fluoxetine
Diazepam		Fluvastatin Sodium
Divalproex Sodium		Fluvoxamine
Doxepin HCl		Indomethacin
Esomeprazole Magnesium		Isoniazid
Ethosuximide		Ketoconazole
Ethotoin		Lansoprazole
Felbamate		Letrozole
Formoterol Fumarate		Levonorgestrel
Fosphenytoin		Mestranol
Gabapentin		Modafinil
Imipramine HCl		Norethindrone
Indomethacin		Norethynodrel
Lamotrigine		Norgestimate
Lansoprazole		Norgestrel
Levetiracetam		Omeprazole
Maprotiline HCl		Oxcarbazepine
Mephenytoin		Paroxetine HCl
Mephobarbital		Ritonavir
Meprobamate		Sertraline HCl
Methsuximide		Sildenafil Citrate
Midazolam HCl		Sulfaphenazole
Nelfinavir Mesylate		Telmisartan
Nilutamide		Ticlopidine HCl

(Continued)

SUBSTRATES	INDUCERS	INHIBITORS
CYP2C19 *(Continued)*		
Nortriptyline HCl		Tolbutamide
Omeprazole		Topiramate
Oxcarbazepine		Vardenafil HCl
Pantoprazole Sodium		Voriconazole
Pentamidine Isethionate		
Phenacemide		
Phenobarbital		
Phenytoin		
Primidone		
Progesterone		
Proguanil HCl		
Propranolol HCl		
Protriptyline HCl		
Rabeprazole Sodium		
Sertraline HCl		
Teniposide		
Thioridazine		
Tiagabine HCl		
Tolbutamide		
Topiramate		
Trimethadione		
Trimipramine Maleate		
Valproate Sodium		
Valproic Acid		
Voriconazole		
Warfarin Sodium		
Zonisamide		
CYP2C8		
Amiodarone HCl	Carbamazepine	Anastrozole
Amitriptyline HCl	Phenobarbital	Cimetidine
Amoxapine	Primidone	Gemfibrozil
Benzphetamine HCl	Rifabutin	Nicardipine
Carbamazepine	Rifampin	Omeprazole
Clomipramine HCl		Sulfaphenazole
Desipramine HCl		Sulfinpyrazone
Diazepam		Trimethoprim
Diclofenac Sodium		
Docetaxel		
Doxepin HCl		
Fluvastatin Sodium		
Imipramine HCl		
Isotretinoin		
Maprotiline HCl		
Mephobarbital		
Nortriptyline HCl		
Omeprazole		
Paclitaxel		
Phenytoin		
Pioglitazone HCl		
Protriptyline HCl		
Repaglinide		
Rosiglitazone Maleate		

(Continued)

SUBSTRATES	INDUCERS	INHIBITORS
CYP2C8 *(Continued)*		
Rosiglitazone/Metformin		
Tolbutamide		
Tretinoin		
Trimipramine Maleate		
Verapamil HCl		
Vitamin A		
Warfarin Sodium		
CYP2C9		
Acarbose	Aprepitant	Amiodarone HCl
Amitriptyline HCl	Carbamazepine	Anastrozole
Candesartan Cilexetil	Dexamethasone	Bendroflumethiazide
Carbamazepine	Phenobarbital	Chloramphenicol
Carvedilol	Phenytoin	Chlorothiazide
Celecoxib	Primidone	Chlorpropamide
Chlorpropamide	Rifampin	Cimetidine
Clomipramine HCl	Rifapentine	Clopidogrel Bisulfate
Desogestrel	Secobarbital Sodium	Clotrimazole
Dextromethorphan		Diclofenac Epolamine
Diazepam		Disulfiram
Diclofenac Potassium		Efavirenz
Dronabinol		Fenofibrate
Eprosartan Mesylate		Fluconazole
Etodolac		Fluorouracil
Fenoprofen Calcium		Fluoxetine HCl
Fluoxetine HCl		Flurbiprofen
Flurbiprofen		Fluvastatin Sodium
Fluvastatin Sodium		Fluvoxamine Maleate
Glimepiride		Gemfibrozil
Glipizide		Glipizide
Ibuprofen		Glyburide
Imipramine HCl		Hydrochlorothiazide
Indomethacin		Hydroflumethiazide
Irbesartan		Imatinib Mesylate
Ketoprofen		Isoniazid
Ketorolac Tromethamine		Itraconazole
Lansoprazole		Ketoconazole
Losartan Potassium		Ketoprofen
Meclofenamate Sodium		Leflunomide
Mefenamic Acid		Lovastatin
Meloxicam		Methyclothiazide
Metformin HCl		Metronidazole
Miglitol		Miconazole
Mirtazapine		Modafinil
Montelukast Sodium		Nifedipine
Nabumetone		Omeprazole
Naproxen		Oxiconazole Nitrate
Nateglinide		Paroxetine HCl
Nifedipine		Phenylbutazone
Omeprazole		Polythiazide
Oxaprozin		Ritonavir
Phenylbutazone		Sertraline HCl
Phenytoin		Sildenafil Citrate

(Continued)

SUBSTRATES	INDUCERS	INHIBITORS
CYP2C9 *(Continued)*		
Pioglitazone HCl		Sulfacytine
Piroxicam		Sulfamethizole
Repaglinide		Sulfamethoxazole
Rofecoxib		Sulfasalazine
Rosiglitazone Maleate		Sulfinpyrazone
Sildenafil Citrate		Sulfisoxazole Acetyl
Sulfamethoxazole		Terconazole
Sulindac		Ticlopidine HCl
Suprofen		Tolazamide
Tamoxifen Citrate		Tolbutamide
Telmisartan		Vardenafil HCl
Tolazamide		Voriconazole
Tolbutamide		Zafirlukast
Tolmetin Sodium		
Torsemide		
Valsartan		
Vardenafil HCl		
Verapamil HCl		
Voriconazole		
Warfarin Sodium		
Zafirlukast		
Zileuton		
CYP2D6		
Amitriptyline HCl	Carbamazepine	Amiodarone HCl
Amphetamine Aspartate	Ethanol	Amitriptyline HCl
Atomoxetine HCl	Hypericum	Amoxapine
Bisoprolol Fumarate	Phenobarbital	Bupropion HCl
Captopril	Phenytoin	Celecoxib
Carvedilol	Primidone	Chloroquine
Cevimeline HCl	Rifampin	Chlorpheniramine
Chlorpromazine	Ritonavir	Cimetidine
Chlorpropamide		Citalopram Hydrobromide
Clomipramine HCl		Clomipramine HCl
Clozapine		Cocaine HCl
Codeine Phosphate		Desipramine HCl
Cyclobenzaprine HCl		Diphenhydramine
Desipramine HCl		Doxepin HCl
Dexfenfluramine HCl		Escitalopram Oxalate
Dextromethorphan Hydrobromide		Fluoxetine
Dolasetron Mesylate		Fluphenazine Decanoate
Donepezil HCl		Fluvoxamine Maleate
Doxepin HCl		Haloperidol
Fentanyl		Hydroxychloroquine Sulfate
Flecainide Acetate		Imatinib Mesylate
Fluoxetine		Imipramine HCl
Fluphenazine Decanoate		Maprotiline HCl
Fluvoxamine Maleate		Methadone HCl
Formoterol Fumarate		Nortriptyline HCl
Galantamine Hydrobromide		Paroxetine HCl
Haloperidol		Perphenazine
Hydrocodone Bitartrate		Propafenone HCl
Imipramine HCl		Propoxyphene HCl

(Continued)

SUBSTRATES	INDUCERS	INHIBITORS
CYP2D6 *(Continued)*		
Labetalol HCl		Protriptyline HCl
Lidocaine		Quinacrine HCl
Maprotiline HCl		Quinidine
Meperidine HCl		Ranitidine Bismuth Citrate
Methadone HCl		Ritonavir
Methamphetamine HCl		Sertraline HCl
Metoprolol Succinate		Sildenafil Citrate
Mexiletine HCl		Terbinafine HCl
Mirtazapine		Thioridazine HCl
Morphine Sulfate		Trimipramine Maleate
Nelfinavir Mesylate		Vardenafil HCl
Nortriptyline HCl		
Olanzapine		
Omeprazole		
Ondansetron		
Oxycodone HCl		
Paclitaxel		
Paroxetine HCl		
Pindolol		
Propafenone HCl		
Propoxyphene HCl		
Propranolol HCl		
Quetiapine Fumarate		
Quinidine Gluconate		
Risperidone		
Ritonavir		
Tamoxifen Citrate		
Teniposide		
Testosterone		
Thioridazine		
Timolol Maleate		
Tolterodine Tartrate		
Tramadol HCl		
Trazodone HCl		
Triazolam		
Trimipramine Maleate		
Venlafaxine HCl		
Vinblastine Sulfate		
Zonisamide		
CYP3A4		
		Potent inhibitors
Alfentanil HCl	Allium sativum	Amprenavir
Alprazolam	Aminoglutethimide	Atazanavir
Amiodarone HCl	Aprepitant	Clarithromycin
Amitriptyline HCl	Betamethasone	Delaviridine
Amlodipine Besylate	Bosentan	Delavirine
Aprepitant	Carbamazepine	Fosamprenavir Calcium
Astemizole	Ciprofloxacin	Indinavir Sulfate
Atorvastatin Calcium	Cisplatin	Itraconazole
Belladonna Ergotamine	Cortisone Acetate	Ketoconazole
Buspirone HCl	Dexamethasone	Lopinavir
Busulfan	Doxorubicin HCl	Nefazodone HCl

(Continued)

SUBSTRATES	INDUCERS	INHIBITORS
CYP3A4 *(Continued)*		
		Potent inhibitors, cont.
Carbamazepine	Efavirenz	Nelfinavir Mesylate
Chlorpheniramine	Ethosuximide	Ritonavir
Cisapride	Felbamate	Saquinavir
Clarithromycin	Fludrocortisone Acetate	Telithromycin
Cyclosporine	Fosphenytoin Sodium	Voriconazole
Desogestrel	Garlic Extract	
Diazepam	Hydrocortisone	**Inhibitors (potency not specified)**
Dihydroergotamine Mesylate	Hypericum	Acetazolamide
Diltiazem HCl	Mephenytoin	Amiodarone HCl
Disopyramide	Methsuximide	Amprenavir
Disulfiram	Methylprednisolone	Anastrozole
Doxorubicin HCl	Modafinil	Aprepitant
Dronabinol	Nafcillin Sodium	Atazanavir
Ergotamine Tartrate	Nevirapine	Cimetidine
Erythromycin	Oxcarbazepine	Ciprofloxacin
Estradiol	Phenobarbital	Clarithromycin
Ethinyl Estradiol	Phenytoin	Clotrimazole
Ethosuximide	Prednisolone	Conivaptan HCl
Ethynodiol Diacetate	Prednisone	Cyclosporine
Etoposide	Primidone	Dalfopristin
Felodipine	Rifabutin	Danazol
Fentanyl	Rifampicin	Darunavir
Haloperidol	Rifampin	Dasatinib Monohydrate
Indinavir Sulfate	Rifapentine	Delavirdine Mesylate
Isradipine	Sulfinpyrazone	Delaviridine
Itraconazole	Theophyllinate	Delavirine
Ixabepilone	Theophylline	Desloratadine
Ketoconazole	Triamcinolone	Diltiazem HCl
Levonorgestrel		Efavirenz
Lidocaine		Erythromycin
Lovastatin		Esomeprazole Magnesium
Mestranol		Fluconazole
Methadone HCl		Fluoxetine
Midazolam HCl		Fluvoxamine Maleate
Nefazodone HCl		Fosamprenavir Calcium
Nelfinavir Mesylate		Grapefruit
Nicardipine HCl		Imatinib Mesylate
Nifedipine		Indinavir Sulfate
Nimodipine		Isoniazid
Nisoldipine		Itraconazole
Nitrendipine		Ketoconazole
Norethindrone		Lapatinib
Norgestrel		Lopinavir
Ondansetron		Loratadine
Paclitaxel		Metronidazole
Pimozide		Miconazole
Polyestradiol Phosphate		Mifepristone
Quinidine Gluconate		Nefazodone HCl
Rifabutin		Nelfinavir Mesylate
Ritonavir		Nevirapine
Saquinavir		Niacin

(Continued)

SUBSTRATES	INDUCERS	INHIBITORS
CYP3A4 *(Continued)*		
Sertraline HCl Sildenafil Citrate Simvastatin Sirolimus Tacrolimus Tadalafil Tamoxifen Citrate Tiagabine HCl Tolterodine Tartrate Trazodone HCl Triazolam Vardenafil HCl Verapamil HCl Vinblastine Sulfate Vincristine Sulfate Warfarin Sodium		**Inhibitors (potency not specified, cont.)** Niacinamide Nicotinamide Nifedipine Norfloxacin Omeprazole Paroxetine HCl Posaconazole Propoxyphene HCl Quinidine Quinine Quinupristin Ranitidine HCl Ritonavir Saquinavir Sertraline HCl Sildenafil Citrate Telithromycin Troglitazone Valproate Sodium Vardenafil HCl Verapamil HCl Voriconazole Zafirlukast Zileuton
CYP3A		
Alfentanil HCl Alprazolam Aminophylline Amitriptyline HCl Amlodipine Besylate Aprepitant Astemizole Atorvastatin Calcium Buspirone HCl Busulfan Carbamazepine Chlorpheniramine Cisapride Clarithromycin Cyclosporine Desogestrel Dexamethasone Diazepam Dihydroergotamine Mesylate Diltiazem HCl Disopyramide Phosphate Doxorubicin HCl Dronabinol Dyphylline Ergotamine Tartrate	Allium sativum Aprepitant Carbamazepine Dexamethasone Efavirenz Ethosuximide Modafinil Nevirapine Phenobarbital Phenytoin Rifabutin Rifampicin Rifampin Rifapentine	Amiodarone HCl Amprenavir Aprepitant Cimetidine Ciprofloxacin Clarithromycin Cyclosporine Delavirdine Mesylate Diltiazem HCl Efavirenz Erythromycin Fluconazole Fluoxetine Fluvoxamine Maleate Grapefruit Indinavir Sulfate Isoniazid Itraconazole Ketoconazole Lopinavir Metronidazole Miconazole Nefazodone HCl Nelfinavir Mesylate Nifedipine

(Continued)

SUBSTRATES	INDUCERS	INHIBITORS
CYP3A *(Continued)*		
Erythromycin		Norfloxacin
Estrogen		Paroxetine HCl
Ethinyl Estradiol		Quinine
Ethosuximide		Ritonavir
Ethynodiol Diacetate		Saquinavir
Etoposide		Sertraline HCl
Felodipine		Venlafaxine HCl
Fentanyl		Verapamil HCl
Glyburide		Voriconazole
Haloperidol		Zafirlukast
Imipramine HCl		Zileuton
Indinavir Sulfate		
Isradipine		
Itraconazole		
Ketoconazole		
Levonorgestrel		
Lidocaine		
Lovastatin		
Mestranol		
Methadone HCl		
Midazolam HCl		
Nefazodone HCl		
Nelfinavir Mesylate		
Nicardipine		
Nifedipine		
Nimodipine		
Nisoldipine		
Norethindrone		
Norgestrel		
Ondansetron HCl		
Paclitaxel		
Pimozide		
Quinidine Gluconate		
Quinine		
Rifabutin		
Ritonavir		
Saquinavir		
Sertraline HCl		
Sildenafil Citrate		
Simvastatin		
Sirolimus		
Tacrolimus		
Tamoxifen Citrate		
Testosterone		
Theophylline		
Tiagabine HCl		
Tolterodine Tartrate		
Trazodone HCl		
Triazolam		
Venlafaxine HCl		
Verapamil HCl		
Vinblastine Sulfate		
Vincristine Sulfate		
Warfarin Sodium		

Note: This list is not comprehensive. For more information, refer to the specific product's full Prescribing Information.

DRUGS EXCRETED IN BREAST MILK

The following list is not comprehensive; generic forms and alternate brands of some products may be available. When recommending drugs to pregnant or nursing patients, always check product labeling for specific precautions.

Accolate
Accuretic
Aciphex
Actiq
Activella
Actonel
Actonel with Calcium
ActoPlus Met
Adalat
Adderall
Advicor
Aggrenox
Aldactazide
Aldactone
Aldomet
Aldoril
Alesse
Alfenta
Allegra-D
Aloprim
Altace
Ambien
Amerge
Anafranil
Anaprox
Androderm
Aplenzin
Apresoline
Aralen
Arthrotec
Asacol
Ativan
Augmentin
Avalide
Avandamet
Axid
Axocet
Azactam
Azasan
Azathioprine
Azulfidine
Bactrim
Baraclude
Benadryl
Bentyl
Betapace
Bextra
Bexxar
Bicillin
Blocadren
Boniva
Brethine
Brevicon
Brontex
Byetta
Caduet
Cafergot
Calan
Campral
Capoten
Capozide
Captopril
Carbatrol
Cardizem
Cataflam
Catapres
Ceclor
Cefizox
Cefobid
Cefotan
Ceftin
Celebrex
Celexa
Cerebyx
Ceredase
Cipro
Ciprodex
Claforan
Clarinex
Claritin
Claritin-D
Cleocin
Climara
Clozaril
Codeine
Combigan
CombiPatch
Combipres
Combivir
Combunox
Compazine
Cordarone
Corgard
Cortisporin
Corzide
Cosopt
Coumadin
Covera-HS
Cozaar
Crestor
Crinone
Cyclessa
Cymbalta
Cystospaz
Cytomel
Cytotec
Cytoxan
Dapsone
Daraprim
Darvon
Darvon-N
Decadron
Deconsal II
Demerol
Demulen
Depacon
Depakene
Depakote
DepoDur
Depo-Provera
Desogen
Desoxyn
Desyrel
Dexedrine
DextroStat
D.H.E. 45
Diabinese
Diastat
Diflucan
Digitek
Dilacor
Dilantin
Dilaudid
Diovan
Diprivan
Diuril
Dolobid
Dolophine
Doral
Doryx
Droxia
Duraclon
Duragesic
Duramorph
Duratuss
Duricef
Dyazide
Dyrenium
E.E.S.
EC-Naprosyn
Ecotrin
Effexor
Elavil
EMLA
Enduron
Epzicom
Equetro
ERYC
EryPed
Ery-Tab
Erythrocin
Erythromycin
Esgic-plus
Eskalith
Estrogel
Estrostep
Evista
Factive
FazaClo
Felbatol
Feldene
femhrt
Fiorinal
Flagyl
Floxin
Foradil
Fortamet
Fortaz
Fosamax
Furosemide
Gabitril
Galzin
Garamycin
Glucophage
Glucovance
Glumetza
Glyset
Guaifed
Halcion
Haldol
Helidac
Hycamtin
Hydrocet
Hydrocortone
Iberet-Folic
Ifex
Imitrex
Imuran
Inderal
Indocin
INFeD
Inspra
Invanz
Invega
Inversine
Ionsys
Isoptin
Janumet
Kadian
Kaletra
Keflex
Keppra
Kerlone
Ketek
Klonopin
Kronofed-A
Lamictal
Lamisil
Lamprene
Lanoxicaps
Lanoxin
Lariam
Lescol
Letairis
Levbid
Levitra
Levlen
Levlite
Levora
Levothroid
Levoxyl
Levsin
Levsinex
Lexapro
Lexiva
Lialda
Lindane
Lioresal
Lithium
Lithobid
Lo/Ovral
Loestrin
Lomotil
Loniten

(Continued)

Lopressor
Lortab
Lotensin
Lotrel
Luminal
Luvox
Lyrica
Macrobid
Macrodantin
Marinol
Maxipime
Maxzide
Menostar
Metaglip
Methergine
Methotrexate
MetroCream/Gel/Lotion
Mexitil
Micronor
Microzide
Migranal
Miltown
Minizide
Minocin
Mirapex
Mircette
M-M-R II
Mobic
Modicon
Moduretic
Monodox
Monopril
Morphine
MS Contin
MSIR
Myambutol
Mycamine
Mysoline
Namenda
Naprelan
Naprosyn
Nascobal
Naturethroid
Necon
Nembutal
Neoral
Neurontin
Niaspan
Nicotrol
Niravam
Nizoral
Norco
Nor-QD
Nordette
Norinyl
Noritate
Normodyne
Norpace
Norplant
Norpramin
Novantrone
Nubain
Nucofed
Nydrazid
Oramorph
Ortho-Cept
Ortho-Cyclen
Ortho-Novum
Ortho Tri-Cyclen
Orudis
Ovcon
Oxistat
OxyContin
OxyFast
OxyIR
Pacerone
Pamelor
Pancrease
Paxil
PCE
Pediapred
Pediazole
Pediotic
Pentasa
Pepcid
Periostat
Persantine
Pfizerpen
Phenergan
Phenobarbital
Phenytek
Phrenilin
Plan B
Ponstel
Prandimet
Pravachol
Premphase
Prempro
Prevacid
Prevacid NapraPAC
PREVPAC
Prinzide
Pristiq
Prograf
Proloprim
Prometrium
Pronestyl
Propofol
Prosed/DS
Protonix
Provera
Prozac
Pseudoephedrine
Pulmicort
Pyrazinamide
Quinidex
Quinine
Raptiva
Reglan
Relpax
Renese
Requip
Reserpine
Restoril
Retrovir
Rifadin
Rifamate
Rifater
Risperdal
Rocaltrol
Rocephin
Roxanol
Rozerem
Sanctura
Sanctura XR
Sandimmune
Sarafem
Seconal
Sectral
Semprex-D
Septra
Seroquel
Seroquel XR
Sinequan
Slo-bid
Soma
Sonata
Soriatane
Spiriva
Sprycel
Stadol
Stavzor
Streptomycin
Stromectol
Symbyax
Symmetrel
Synthroid
Tagamet
Tambocor
Tapazole
Tarka
Tasigna
Tavist
Tazicef
Tegretol
Tenoretic
Tenormin
Tenuate
Testoderm
Thalitone
Theo-24
Theo-Dur
Thorazine
Tiazac
Timoptic
Tindamax
Tobi
Tofranil
Toprol-XL
Toradol
Trandate
Tranxene
Trental
Tricor
Triglide
Trilafon
Trileptal
Tri-Levlen
Tri-Norinyl
Triostat
Triphasil
Trisenox
Trivora
Trizivir
Truvada
Tygacil
Tylenol
Tylenol with Codeine
Ultane
Ultram
Unasyn
Uniphyl
Uniretic
Unithroid
Urimax
Valium
Valtrex
Vanceril
Vancocin
Vantin
Vaseretic
Vasotec
Ventavis
Verelan
Vermox
Versed
Vibramycin
Vibra-Tabs
Vicodin
Vigamox
Viramune
Voltaren
Vytorin
Vyvanse
Wellbutrin
Xanax
Xolair
Zantac
Zarontin
Zaroxolyn
Zegerid
Zemplar
Zestoretic
Zetia
Ziac
Zinacef
Zithromax
Zoloft
Zomig
Zonalon
Zonegran
Zosyn
Zovia
Zovirax
Zyban
Zydone
Zyloprim
Zyprexa
Zyrtec

Drugs That May Cause Photosensitivity

The drugs in this table are known to cause photosensitivity in some individuals. Effects can range from itching, scaling, rash, and swelling to skin cancer, premature skin aging, skin and eye burns, cataracts, reduced immunity, blood vessel damage, and allergic reactions. The list is not all-inclusive, and shows only representative brands of each generic. When in doubt, always check specific product labeling. Individuals should be advised to wear protective clothing and to apply sunscreens while taking the medications listed below.

GENERIC	BRAND
Acamprosate	Campral
Acetazolamide	Diamox
Acitretin	Soriatane
Acyclovir	Zovirax
Alendronate	Fosamax
Aliskiren/hydrochlorothiazide	Tekturna HCT
Alitretinoin	Panretin
Almotriptan	Axert
Amiloride/hydrochlorothiazide	Amiloride/HCT
Aminolevulinic acid	Levulan Kerastick
Amiodarone	Cordarone, Pacerone
Amitriptyline	Elavil
Amitriptyline/chlordiazepoxide	Etrafon, Limbitrol
Amitriptyline/perphenazine	
Amlodipine/atorvastatin	Caduet
Amoxapine	
Amphetamine aspartate/amphetamine sulfate/dextroamphetamine saccharate/dextroamphetamine sulfate	Adderall XR
Anagrelide	Agrylin
Aripiprazole	Abilify
Atazanavir	Reyataz
Atenolol/chlorthalidone	Tenoretic
Atorvastatin	Lipitor
Atovaquone/proguanil	Malarone
Azithromycin	Zithromax
Benazepril	Lotensin
Benazepril/hydrochlorothiazide	Lotensin HCT
Bendroflumethiazide/nadolol	Corzide
Bexarotene	Targretin
Bismuth/metronidazole/tetracycline	Helidac
Bismuth subcitrate potassium/metronidazole/tetracycline	Pylera
Bisoprolol/hydrochlorothiazide	Ziac
Brompheniramine/dextromethorphan/phenylephrine	Alacol DM
Brompheniramine/dextromethorphan/pseudoephedrine	Bromfed-DM
Bupropion	Wellbutrin, Wellbutrin SR, Wellbutrin XL, Zyban
Candesartan/hydrochlorothiazide	Atacand HCT
Capecitabine	Xeloda
Captopril	Capoten
Captopril/hydrochlorothiazide	Capozide
Carbamazepine	Carbatrol, Equetro, Tegretol, Tegretol-XR
Carvedilol	Coreg
Carvedilol phosphate	Coreg CR
Celecoxib	Celebrex
Cetirizine	Zyrtec
Cetirizine/pseudoephedrine	Zyrtec-D
Cevimeline	Evoxac
Chlorhexidine gluconate	Hibistat
Chloroquine	Aralen
Chlorothiazide	Diuril
Chlorpheniramine/phenylephrine	Rynatan
Chlorpromazine	Thorazine
Chlorpropamide	
Chlorthalidone	Thalitone
Cidofovir	Vistide
Ciprofloxacin	Cipro, Cipro XR
Citalopram	Celexa
Clemastine	Tavist
Clindamycin phosphate	Clindagel
Clozapine	Clozaril, Fazaclo
Coagulation Factor IX (recombinant)	BeneFIX
Cromolyn sodium	Gastrocrom
Cyclobenzaprine	Flexeril
Cyproheptadine	Cyproheptadine
Dacarbazine	DTIC-Dome
Dantrolene	Dantrium
Demeclocycline	Declomycin
Desipramine	Norpramin
Diclofenac potassium	Cataflam
Diclofenac sodium	Voltaren
Diclofenac sodium/misoprostol	Arthrotec
Diflunisal	Dolobid
Dihydroergotamine	D.H.E. 45
Diltiazem	Cardizem, Tiazac
Diphenhydramine	Benadryl
Divalproex	Depakote
Doxepin	Sinequan
Doxycycline hyclate	Doryx, Periostat, Vibra-Tabs, Vibramycin
Doxycycline monohydrate	Monodox
Duloxetine	Cymbalta
Efalizumab	Raptiva
Enalapril	Vasotec
Enalapril/hydrochlorothiazide	Vaseretic
Enalaprilat (injection)	Enalaprilat
Epirubicin	Ellence
Eprosartan mesylate/hydrochlorothiazide	Teveten HCT
Erythromycin/sulfisoxazole	Pediazole
Escitalopram oxalate	Lexapro
Esomeprazole	Nexium
Estazolam	
Estradiol	Gynodiol, Estrogel
Eszopiclone	Lunesta
Ethionamide	Trecator-SC
Etodolac	Lodine

(Continued)

GENERIC	BRAND
Felbamate	Felbatol
Fenofibrate	Lofibra, Tricor, Triglide
Floxuridine	Sterile FUDR
Flucytosine	Ancobon
Fluorouracil	Efudex
Fluoxetine	Prozac, Sarafem
Fluoxetine/olanzapine	Symbyax
Fluphenazine	Prolixin
Flutamide	Flutamide
Fluvastatin	Lescol, Lescol XL
Fluvoxamine	Luvox, Luvox CR
Fosinopril	Monopril
Fosphenytoin	Cerebyx
Furosemide	Lasix
Gabapentin	Neurontin
Gemfibrozil	Lopid
Gemifloxacin mesylate	Factive
Gentamicin	Gentamicin
Glatiramer acetate	Copaxone
Glimepiride	Amaryl
Glimepiride/pioglitazone hydrochloride	Duetact
Glimepiride/rosiglitazone maleate	Avandaryl
Glipizide	Glucotrol
Glyburide	DiaBeta, Glynase, Micronase
Glyburide/metformin HCl	Glucovance
Griseofulvin	Grifulvin, Gris-PEG
Haloperidol	Haldol
Hexachlorophene	pHisoHex
Hydralazine/hydrochlorothiazide	Hydra-zide
Hydrochlorothiazide	Microzide
Hydrochlorothiazide/fosinopril	Monopril HCT
Hydrochlorothiazide/irbesartan	Avalide
Hydrochlorothiazide/lisinopril	Prinzide, Zestoretic
Hydrochlorothiazide/losartan potassium	Hyzaar
Hydrochlorothiazide/methyldopa	Aldoril
Hydroclorothiazide/metoprolol tartrate	Lopressor HCT
Hydrochlorothiazide/moexipril	Uniretic
Hydrochlorothiazide/quinapril	Accuretic
Hydrochlorothiazide/spironolactone	Aldactazide
Hydrochlorothiazide/telmisartan	Micardis HCT
Hydrochlorothiazide/triamterene	Dyazide, Maxzide
Hydrochlorothiazide/valsartan	Diovan HCT
Hydroxocobalamin	Cyanokit Antidote
Hydroxychloroquine	Plaquenil
Hypericum	St. John's wort
Ibuprofen	Motrin
Imatinib Mesylate	Gleevec
Imipramine	Tofranil
Imiquimod	Aldara
Indapamide	Lozol
Interferon alfa-2b, recombinant	Intron A
Interferon alfa-n3 (human leukocyte derived)	Alferon-N
Interferon beta-1a	Avonex
Interferon beta-1b	Betaseron
Irbesartan/hydrochlorothiazide	Avalide
Isocarboxazid	Marplan
Isoniazid/pyrazinamide/rifampin	Rifater
Isotretinoin	Accutane, Amnesteem
Itraconazole	Sporanox
Ketoprofen	Orudis, Oruvail
Lamotrigine	Lamictal
Leuprolide acetate	Lupron, Lupron Depot
Levamisole	Levamisole
Levofloxacin	Levaquin
Levofloxacin/5% dextrose	Levaquin Injection
Lisinopril	Prinivil, Zestril
Lisinopril/hydrochlorothiazide	Prinzide, Zestoretic
Lomefloxacin	Maxaquin
Loratadine	Claritin
Loratadine/pseudoephedrine	Claritin-D
Losartan	Cozaar
Losartan/hydrochlorothiazide	Hyzaar
Lovastatin	Altoprev, Mevacor
Lovastatin/niacin	Advicor
Maprotiline	Maprotiline
Mefenamic acid	Ponstel
Meloxicam	Mobic
Mesalamine	Pentasa
Methazolamide	
Methotrexate	Trexall
Methoxsalen	Uvadex, Oxsoralen, 8-MOP
Methyclothiazide	Enduron
Methyldopa/hydrochlorothiazide	Aldoril
Metolazone	Mykrox, Zaroxolyn
Metoprolol succinate	Toprol-XL
Metoprolol tartrate	Lopressor
Minocycline	Dynacin, Minocin, Solodyn
Mirtazapine	Remeron
Moexipril	Univasc
Moexipril/hydrochlorothiazide	Uniretic
Moxifloxacin	Avelox
Nabilone	Cesamet
Nabumetone	Relafen
Nadolol/bendroflumethiazide	Corzide
Nalidixic acid	Nalidixic acid
Naproxen	Naprosyn, EC-Naprosyn
Naproxen sodium	Anaprox, Anaprox DS, Naprelan
Naratriptan	Amerge
Nefazodone	Serzone
Nifedipine	Adalat CC, Procardia
Nisoldipine	Sular
Norfloxacin	Noroxin
Nortriptyline	Pamelor
Ofloxacin	Floxin
Olanzapine	Zyprexa
Olanzapine/fluoxetine	Symbyax

GENERIC	BRAND
Olmesartan medoxomil/ hydrochlorothiazide	Benicar HCT
Olsalazine	Dipentum
Omeprazole/ sodium bicarbonate	Zegerid
Oxaprozin	Daypro
Oxcarbazepine	Trileptal
Oxycodone	Roxicodone
Panitumumab	Vectibix
Pantoprazole	Protonix
Paroxetine hydrochloride	Paxil
Paroxetine mesylate	Pexeva
Pentosan polysulfate	Elmiron
Pentostatin	Nipent
Perphenazine	Perphenazine
Pilocarpine	Salagen
Piroxicam	Feldene
Polymyxin B sulfate/ trimethopim sulfate	Polytrim
Polythiazide	Renese
Porfimer sodium	Photofrin
Pramipexole dihydrochloride	Mirapex
Pravastatin	Pravachol
Pregabalin	Lyrica
Prochlorperazine	Compro
Promethazine	Phenergan
Protriptyline	Vivactil
Pyrimethamine/sulfadoxine	Fansidar
Pyrazinamide	Pyrazinamide
Quetiapine	Seroquel
Quinapril	Accupril
Quinapril/ hydrochlorothiazide	Accuretic
Quinidine gluconate	Quinidine
Quinidine sulfate	Quinidex
Quinine sulfate	Quinine sulfate
Rabeprazole sodium	Aciphex
Ramipril	Altace
Rasagiline mesylate	Azilect
Riluzole	Rilutek
Risperidone	Risperdal, Risperdal Consta
Ritonavir	Norvir
Rizatriptan	Maxalt, Maxalt-MLT
Ropinirole	Requip
Rosuvastatin	Crestor
Ruta graveolens	Rue
Saquinavir mesylate	Invirase
Selegiline	Eldepryl, Emsam
Sertraline	Zoloft
Sibutramine	Meridia
Sildenafil	Viagra
Simvastatin	Zocor
Simvastatin/ezetimibe	Vytorin
Sirolimus	Rapamune
Somatropin	Serostim
Sotalol	Betapace, Betapace AF
Sulfamethoxazole/ trimethoprim	Bactrim, Septra
Sulfasalazine	Azulfidine
Sulfisoxazole acetyl	Gantrisin Pediatric
Sulindac	Clinoril
Sumatriptan	Imitrex
Tacrolimus	Prograf, Protopic
Tazarotene	Tazorac
Telmisartan/ hydrochlorothiazide	Micardis HCT
Tetracycline	Sumycin
Thalidomide	Thalomid
Thioridazine hydrochloride	Thioridazine HCl
Thiothixene	Navane
Tiagabine	Gabitril
Tigecycline	Tygacil
Tolazamide	Tolazamide
Tolbutamide	Tolbutamide
Topiramate	Topamax
Tretinoin	Avita, Retin-A
Triamcinolone acetonide	Azmacort Inhalation
Triamterene	Dyrenium
Triamterene/ hydrochlorothiazide	Dyazide, Maxzide
Trifluoperazine	Trifluoperazine
Trimipramine	Surmontil
Valacyclovir	Valtrex
Valproate	Depacon
Valproic acid	Depakene
Valsartan/ hydrochlorothiazide	Diovan HCT
Vardenafil	Levitra
Varenicline tartrate	Chantix
Venlafaxine	Effexor, Effexor XR
Verteporfin	Visudyne
Vinblastine	Vinblastine
Voriconazole	Vfend
Zalcitabine	Hivid
Zaleplon	Sonata
Ziprasidone	Geodon
Zolmitriptan	Zomig
Zolpidem	Ambien, Ambien CR

DRUGS THAT MAY CAUSE QT PROLONGATION

BRAND NAME	GENERIC NAME
Abilify	Aripiprazole
AcipHex	Rabeprazole sodium
Advair	Fluticasone propionate/ salmeterol xinafoate
Advair HFA	Fluticasone propionate/ salmeterol xinafoate
Aloxi Injection	Palonosetron HCl
Amerge	Naratriptan HCl
Amitriptyline	Amitriptyline
Anzemet	Dolasetron mesylate
Apokyn	Apomorphine HCl
Avelox	Moxifloxacin HCl
Betapace	Sotalol HCl
Betapace AF	Sotalol HCl
Biaxin	Clarithromycin
Brovana	Arformoterol tartrate
Celexa	Citalopram HBr
Cipro	Ciprofloxacin
Cipro XR	Ciprofloxacin
Cordarone	Amiodarone HCl
Corvert	Ibutilide fumarate
Detrol LA	Tolterodine tartrate
Dolophine	Methadone HCl
Doxepin	Doxepin
E.E.S.	Erythromycin ethylsuccinate
Effexor XR	Venlafaxine HCl
Eraxis	Anidulafungin
ERYC	Erythromycin
EryPed	Erythromycin ethylsuccinate
Erythrocin stearate	Erythromycin stearate
Erythromycin Base Filmtab	Erythromycin
Erythromycin Delayed-Release	Erythromycin
Exelon Patch	Rivastigmine
Factive	Gemifloxacin mesylate
Fleet Enema/Enema Extra/ Enema for Children	Monobasic sodium phosphate/dibasic sodium phosphate
Foradil	Formoterol
Geodon	Ziprasidone HCl
Haldol	Haloperidol
Halfan*	Halofantrine HCl
Imitrex Injection	Sumatriptan succinate
Inapsine	Droperidol
Invega	Paliperidone
Ketek	Telithromycin
Levaquin	Levofloxacin
Levitra	Vardenafil HCl
Lexapro	Escitalopram oxalate
Maxaquin	Lomefloxacin HCl
Methadose	Methadone HCl
Namenda	Memantine HCl
Nizoral	Ketoconazole
Noroxin	Norfloxacin
Norpace	Disopyramide phosphate
Norpramin	Desipramine
Noxafil	Posaconazole
Orap	Pimozide
OsmoPrep	Sodium phosphate monobasic monohydrate/ sodium phosphate dibasic anhydrous
Pacerone	Amiodarone HCl
PCE	Erythromycin particles
Perforomist	Formoterol fumarate
Plenaxis*	Abarelix
Pletal	Cilostazol
PREVPAC	Lansoprazole/amoxicillin/ clarithromycin
Procainamide	Procainamide
Prograf	Tacrolimus
Prozac	Fluoxetine
Quinidine gluconate	Quinidine gluconate
Quinidine sulfate	Quinidine sulfate
Ranexa	Ranolazine
Raxar*	Grepafloxacin
Razadyne	Galantamine HBr
Risperdal Consta	Risperidone
Rythmol SR	Propafenone HCl
Serentil*	Mesoridazine besylate
Serevent	Salmeterol
Seroquel	Quetiapine fumarate
Sporanox	Itraconazole
Sprycel	Dasatinib
Strattera	Atomoxetine HCl
Sutent	Sunitinib malate
Symbicort	Budesonide/formoterol fumarate dihydrate
Symbyax	Olanzapine/fluoxetine HCl
Tambocor	Flecainide acetate
Tasigna	Nilotinib
Tequin*	Gatifloxacin
Thioridazine HCl	Thioridazine HCl
Tikosyn	Dofetilide
Tofranil, Tofranil-PM	Imipramine
Trisenox Injection	Arsenic trioxide
Tykerb	Lapatinib
Uroxatral	Alfuzosin HCl
Vascor*	Bepridil HCl
VFEND	Voriconazole
Viracept	Nelfinavir mesylate
Visicol	Sodium phosphate
Zagam*	Sparfloxacin
Zanaflex	Tizanidine
Zmax	Azithromycin
Zofran	Ondansetron HCl
Zolinza	Vorinostat
Zoloft	Sertraline HCl
Zomig	Zolmitriptan
Zomig-ZMT	Zolmitriptan

* Drug no longer available in the U.S.

NOTE: This list does not include all of the drugs that may cause QT disturbance. For more information, please refer to the specific product's full Prescribing Information.

DRUGS THAT MAY CAUSE STEVENS-JOHNSON SYNDROME AND TOXIC EPIDERMAL NECROLYSIS (TEN)

BRAND NAME	GENERIC NAME
ACAM2000	Smallpox vaccine, live
AcipHex	Rabeprazole sodium
Adderall XR	Dextroamphetamine sulfate/dextroamphetamine saccharate/amphetamine sulfate/amphetamine aspartate
Advicor	Niacin/lovastatin
Agenerase	Amprenavir
Aggrenox	Aspirin/dipyridamole
Albenza	Albendazole
Aldoril	Methyldopa/ hydrochlorothiazide
Aloprim	Allopurinol sodium
Altace	Ramipril
Amoxil	Amoxicillin
Anaprox	Naproxen
Ancobon	Flucytosine
Ansaid	Flurbiprofen
Arava	Leflunomide
Arimidex	Anastrozole
Arthrotec	Diclofenac sodium/ misoprostol
Atacand HCT	Candesartan cilexetil/ hydrochlorothiazide
Atripla	Efavirenz/emtricitabine/ tenofovir disoproxil fumarate
Attenuvax	Measles virus vaccine, live
Augmentin	Amoxicillin/clavulanate potassium
Avalide	Irbesartan/ hydrochlorothiazide
Avandamet	Rosiglitazone maleate/ metformin HCl
Avandia	Rosiglitazone maleate
Avelox	Moxifloxacin HCl
Azulfidine	Sulfasalazine
Bactrim	Sulfamethoxazole/ trimethoprim
Betagan	Levobunolol HCl
Betoptic S	Betaxolol HCl
Biaxin	Clarithromycin
Bleph-10	Sulfacetamide sodium
Blephamide	Sulfacetamide sodium/ prednisolone acetate
Caduet	Amlodipine besylate/ atorvastatin calcium
Capoten	Captopril
Carbatrol	Carbamazepine
Cataflam	Diclofenac potassium
Ceftin	Cefuroxime axetil
Celebrex	Celecoxib
Cialis	Tadalafil
Cimzia	Certolizumab pegol
Cipro	Ciprofloxacin
Cleocin vaginal ovules	Clindamycin phosphate vaginal suppositories
Clinoril	Sulindac
Clorpres	Clonidine HCl/chlorthalidone
Clozaril	Clozapine
Combivir	Lamivudine/zidovudine
Combunox	Oxycodone HCl/ibuprofen
Comvax	*Haemophilus* b conjugate (meningococcal protein conjugate)/ hepatitis B (recombinant) vaccine

BRAND NAME	GENERIC NAME
Covera-HS	Verapamil HCl
Crixivan	Indinavir sulfate
Cymbalta	Duloxetine HCl
Daraprim	Pyrimethamine
Daypro	Oxaprozin
Depakote ER	Divalproex sodium
Diamox	Acetazolamide
Didronel	Etidronate disodium
Dilantin	Phenytoin sodium
Diovan HCT	Valsartan/ hydrochlorothiazide
Diuril	Chlorothiazide
Dolobid	Diflunisal
Donnatal Extentabs	Phenobarbital
Duac Topical Gel	Clindamycin, 1%/benzoyl peroxide, 5%
Dynacin	Minocycline HCl
EC-Naprosyn	Naproxen
E.E.S.	Erythromycin ethylsuccinate
Effexor XR	Venlafaxine HCl
Emend	Aprepitant
Engerix-B Vaccine	Hepatitis B vaccine (recombinant)
Epzicom	Abacavir sulfate/lamivudine
Equetro	Carbamazepine
EryPed	Erythromycin ethylsuccinate
Ethyol	Amifostine
Etodolac	Etodolac
Exelon	Rivastigmine tartrate
Fansidar	Sulfadoxine/pyrimethamine
Feldene	Piroxicam
Flebogamma 5%	Immune globulin intravenous (human)
Flector	Diclofenac epolamine topical patch
Fluarix	Influenza virus vaccine
Fortaz	Ceftazidime for injection
Fosamax	Alendronate sodium
Fosamax Plus D	Alendronate sodium/ cholecalciferol
Furadantin	Nitrofurantoin
Gammagard	Immune globulin intravenous (human)
Gamunex	Immune globulin intravenous (human), 10% caprylate/ chromatography purified
Gantrisin	Acetyl sulfisoxazole
Gleevec	Imatinib mesylate
Hyzaar	Losartan potassium/ hydrochlorothiazide
Inderal LA	Propranolol HCl
Intelence	Etravirine
Intron A	Interferon alfa-2b
Lozol	Indapamide
Indocin	Indomethacin
Lamictal	Lamotrigine
Lamisil	Terbinafine HCl
Lariam	Mefloquine HCl
Lescol	Fluvastatin sodium
Leukeran	Chlorambucil
Leustatin	Cladribine
Levaquin	Levofloxacin
Lexapro	Escitalopram oxalate
Lexiva	Fosamprenavir calcium
Lipitor	Atorvastatin calcium
Lyrica	Pregabalin

BRAND NAME	GENERIC NAME
Malarone	Atovaquone/proguanil HCl
Maxalt	Rizatriptan benzoate
Mefoxin	Cefoxitin injection
Merrem	Meropenem for injection
Meruvax II	Rubella virus vaccine, live
Mevacor	Lovastatin
Micardis HCT	Telmisartan/ hydrochlorothiazide
Minocin	Minocycline HCl
Mintezol	Thiabendazole
M-M-R II	Measles, mumps, and rubella virus vaccine, live
Mobic	Meloxicam
Moduretic	Amiloride HCl/ hydrochlorothiazide
Motrin	Ibuprofen
Mumpsvax	Mumps virus vaccine, live
Nalfon	Fenoprofen calcium
Namenda	Memantine HCl
Naprelan	Naproxen sodium
Naprosyn	Naproxen
Neurontin	Gabapentin
Nexium	Esomeprazole magnesium
Niravam	Alprazolam orally disintegrating
Noroxin	Norfloxacin
Norvir	Ritonavir
Nuvigil	Armodafinil
Nystatin Oral	Nystatin
Omnicef	Cefdinir
Orthoclone OKT3 Sterile Solution	Muromonab-CD3
Ovace	Sodium sulfacetamide
Paxil	Paroxetine HCl
PCE	Erythromycin particles in tablets
PegIntron	Peginterferon alfa-2b
Pepcid	Famotidine
Phenytek	Phenytoin sodium
Plavix	Clopidogrel bisulfate
Pletal	Cilostazol
Ponstel	Mefenamic acid
Prevacid NapraPAC	Lansoprazole/naproxen
PREVPAC	Lansoprazole/ amoxicillin/clarithromycin
Prezista	Darunavir
Primaxin I.M./I.V.	Imipenem/cilastatin
Prinivil	Lisinopril
Prinzide	Lisinopril/ hydrochlorothiazide
Prograf	Tacrolimus
Proleukin	Aldesleukin
ProQuad	Measles, mumps, rubella and varicella virus vaccine, live
Protonix	Pantoprazole sodium
Provigil	Modafinil
Prozac	Fluoxetine
Raniclor	Cefaclor
Recombivax HB	Hepatitis B vaccine (recombinant)
Relafen	Nabumetone
Remicade for IV Injection	Infliximab
Rescriptor	Delavirdine mesylate
Retrovir	Zidovudine
Reyataz	Atazanavir sulfate
Rituxan	Rituximab
Rosula NS	Sodium sulfacetamide
Septra	Trimethoprim/ sulfamethoxazole
Seroquel	Quetiapine fumarate
Solodyn	Minocycline HCl
Stromectol	Ivermectin
Suprax	Cefixime for oral suspension
Sustiva	Efavirenz
Tamiflu	Oseltamivir phosphate
Tarka	Trandolapril/verapamil HCl
Taxotere	Docetaxel
Tegretol	Carbamazepine
Teveten HCT	Eprosartan mesylate/ hydrochlorothiazide
Thalomid	Thalidomide
Tiazac	Diltiazem HCl
Ticlid	Ticlopidine HCl
Timentin	Ticarcillin disodium/ clavulanate potassium
Timolide	Timolol maleate/ hydrochlorothiazide
Tindamax	Tinidazole
Topamax	Topiramate
Tricor	Fenofibrate
Trileptal	Oxcarbazepine
Trizivir	Abacavir sulfate/ lamivudine/zidovudine
Trusopt	Dorzolamide HCl
Twinrix	Hepatitis A inactivated/ hepatitis B (recombinant) vaccine
Vancocin	Vancomycin HCl
Varivax	Varicella virus vaccine, live
VFEND	Voriconazole
Viramune	Nevirapine
Voltaren	Diclofenac sodium
VoSpire ER	Albuterol sulfate
Vytorin	Ezetimibe/simvastatin
Vyvanse	Lisdexamfetamine dimesylate
Wellbutrin	Bupropion HCl
Zegerid	Omeprazole/sodium bicarbonate
Ziagen	Abacavir sulfate
Zinacef	Cefuroxime for injection
Zmax	Azithromycin extended release for oral suspension
Zocor	Simvastatin
Zoloft	Sertraline HCl
Zonegran	Zonisamide
Zosyn	Piperacillin/tazobactam
Zovirax	Acyclovir
Zyban	Bupropion HCl
Zyvox	Linezolid

Note: This list is not comprehensive. For more information, refer to the specific product's full Prescribing Information.

DRUGS THAT SHOULD NOT BE CRUSHED

Listed below are various slow-release as well as enteric-coated products that should not be crushed or chewed. Slow-release (sr) represents products that are controlled-release, extended-release, long-acting, or timed-release. Enteric-coated (ec) represents products that are delayed-release.

In general, capsules containing slow-release or enteric-coated particles may be opened and their contents administered on a spoonful of soft food. Instruct patients not to chew the particles, though. (Patients should, in fact, be discouraged from chewing any medication unless it is specifically formulated for that purpose.)

This list should not be considered all-inclusive. Generic and alternate brands of some products may exist. Tablets intended for sublingual or buccal administration (not included in this list) should also be administered only as intended, in an intact form.

DRUG	MANUFACTURER	FORM
AcipHex	Eisai	ec
Adalat CC	Schering Plough	sr
Adderall XR	Shire U.S.	sr
Advicor	KOS	sr
Aerohist	Aero	sr
Aerohist Plus	Aero	sr
Afeditab CR	Watson	sr
Aggrenox	Boehringer Ingelheim	sr
Ala-Hist	Poly	sr
Ala-Hist D	Poly	sr
Aleve Cold & Sinus	Bayer Healthcare	sr
Aleve Sinus & Headache	Bayer Healthcare	sr
Allegra-D 12 Hour	sanofi-aventis	sr
Allegra-D 24 Hour	sanofi-aventis	sr
Allerx	Cornerstone	sr
Allerx-D	Cornerstone	sr
Allfen	MCR American	sr
Allfen-DM	MCR American	sr
Alophen	Numark	ec
Altoprev	First Horizon	sr
Ambien CR	sanofi-aventis	sr
Ambifed-G	MCR American	sr
Ambifed-G DM	MCR American	sr
Amdry-C	Prasco	sr
Amdry-D	Prasco	sr
Amibid LA	Amide	sr
Amrix	ECR	sr
Anextuss	Cypress	sr
Aplenzin	Biovail	sr
Arthrotec	Pfizer	ec
Asacol	Procter & Gamble	ec
Ascriptin Enteric	Novartis Consumer	ec
Atrohist Pediatric	Celltech	sr
Augmentin XR	GlaxoSmithKline	sr
Avinza	Ligand	sr
Azulfidine Entabs	Pharmacia	ec
Bayer Aspirin Regimen	Bayer Healthcare	ec
Biaxin XL	Abbott	sr
Bidex-A	SJ	sr
Bidhist	Cypress	sr
Bisac-Evac	G & W	ec
Biscolax	Global Source	ec
Blanex-A	Blansett	sr
Bontril Slow-Release	Valeant	sr
Bromfed	Victory	sr
Bromfed-PD	Victory	sr
Bromfenex	Ethex	sr
Bromfenex PD	Quality Care	sr
Bromfenex PE	Quality Care	sr
Bromfenex PE Pediatric	Ethex	sr
Budeprion SR	Teva	sr
Budeprion XL	Teva	sr
Buproban	Teva	sr
Calan SR	Pfizer	sr
Campral	Forest	ec
Carbatrol	Shire U.S.	sr
Cardene SR	Roche	sr
Cardizem CD	Biovail	sr
Cardizem LA	KOS	sr
Cardura XL	Pfizer	sr
Cartia XT	Watson	sr
Cemill 500	Miller	sr
Cemill 1000	Miller	sr
Certuss-D	Capellon	sr
Chlorex-A	Cypress	sr
Chlor-Phen	Truxton	sr
Chlor-Trimeton Allergy	Schering Plough	sr
Chlor-Trimeton Allergy Decongestant	Schering Plough	sr
Cipro XR	Schering Plough	sr
Clarinex-D 24 Hour	Schering Plough	sr
Claritin-D	Schering	sr
Claritin-D 12 Hour	Schering	sr
Claritin-D 24 Hour	Schering	sr
Coldamine	Breckenridge	sr
Concerta	McNeil Pediatrics	sr
Contac 12-Hour	GlaxoSmithKline	sr
Correctol	Schering Plough	ec
Coreg CR	GlaxoSmithKline	sr
Covera-HS	Pfizer	sr
CPM 8/PE 20/MSC 1.25	Cypress	sr
CPM-12	Brighton	sr
Creon 5	Solvay	ec
Creon 10	Solvay	ec
Creon 20	Solvay	ec
Cymbalta	Eli Lilly	ec
Dairycare	Plainview	ec
Dallergy	Laser	sr

Enteric-coated = ec **Slow-released = sr**

DRUG	MANUFACTURER	FORM
Dallergy-Jr	Laser	sr
Deconamine SR	Kenwood Therapeutics	sr
Deconsal II	Carolina	sr
Deconex	Poly	sr
Deconex DM	Poly	sr
Depakote	Abbott	ec
Depakote ER	Abbott	sr
Depakote Sprinkles	Abbott	ec
Despec SR	International Ethical	sr
Detrol LA	Pfizer	sr
Dexedrine Spansules	GlaxoSmithKline	sr
D-Feda II	Dexo	sr
D-Hist D	Midlothian	sr
Diabetes Trio	Mason Vitamins	sr
Diamox Sequels	Duramed	sr
Dilacor XR	Watson	sr
Dilantin	Pfizer	sr
Dilantin Kapseals	Pfizer	sr
Dilatrate-SR	UCB	sr
Diltia XT	Andrx	sr
Dilt-CD	Apotex	sr
Disophrol Chronotab	Schering Plough	sr
Ditropan XL	Ortho-McNeil	sr
Donnatal Extentabs	PBM	sr
Doryx	Warner Chilcott	ec
D-Phen 1000	Midlothian	sr
Drihist SR	Prasco	sr
Drixoral	Schering Plough	sr
Drixoral Plus	Schering Plough	sr
Drixoral Sinus	Schering Plough	sr
Drysec	A.G. Marin	sr
D-Tab	Palm	sr
Dulcolax	Boehringer Ingelheim	ec
Duomax	Capellon	sr
Durahist	Kowa	sr
Durahist D	Kowa	sr
Durahist PE	Kowa	sr
Duratuss	Victory	sr
Duratuss DA	Victory	sr
Dynacirc CR	GlaxoSmithKline	sr
Dynahist-ER Pediatric	Breckenridge	sr
Dynex LA	Athlon	sr
Dynex VR	Athlon	sr
Dytan-CS	Hawthorn	sr
Easprin	Rosedale	ec
EC Naprosyn	Roche	ec
Ecotrin	GlaxoSmithKline	ec
Ecotrin Adult Low Strength	GlaxoSmithKline	ec
Ecotrin Maximum Strength	GlaxoSmithKline	ec
Ecpirin	Prime Marketing	ec
Ed A-Hist	Edwards	sr
Effexor-XR	Wyeth	sr
Enablex	Novartis	sr
Entercote	Global Source	ec
Entex LA	Andrx	sr
Entex PSE	Andrx	sr
Entocort EC	Prometheus	ec
Equetro	Shire U.S.	sr
ERYC	Warner Chilcott	sr
Ery-Tab	Abbott	ec
Eskalith-CR	GlaxoSmithKline	sr
Extendryl G	Auriga	sr
Extendryl Jr	Auriga	sr
Extendryl SR	Auriga	sr
Extress-30	Key	sr
Exetuss-DM	Larken	sr
Extress-60	Key	sr
Feen-A-Mint	Schering Plough	ec
Femilax	G & W	ec
Fero-Folic-500	Abbott	sr
Fero-Grad-500	Abbott	sr
Ferro-Sequels	Inverness Medical	sr
Ferrous Fumarate DS	Vita-Rx	sr
Fetrin	Lunsco	sr
Flagyl ER	Pharmacia	sr
Fleet Bisacodyl	Fleet, C.B.	ec
Focalin XR	Novartis	sr
Folitab 500	Rising	sr
Fortamet	First Horizon	sr
Fumatinic	Laser	sr
Genacote	Teva	ec
GFN 600/ Phenylephrine 20	Cypress	sr
GFN 600/PSE 60/DM 30	Cypress	sr
GFN 1200/DM 60	Cypress	sr
GFN 1200/ Phenylephrine 40	Cypress	sr
Gilphex TR	Gil	sr
Giltuss TR	Gil	sr
Glucophage XR	Bristol-Myers Squibb	sr
Glucotrol XL	Pfizer	sr
Glumetza	Depomed	sr
Guaifenex DM	Ethex	sr
Guaifenex GP	Ethex	sr
Guaifenex PSE 60	Ethex	sr
Guaifenex PSE 80	Ethex	sr
Guaifenex PSE 85	Ethex	sr
Guaifenex PSE 120	Ethex	sr
Halfprin	Kramer	ec
Hemax	Pronova	sr
Histacol LA	Breckenridge	sr
Humavent LA	Dexo	sr
Humibid	Adams	sr
Humibid DM	Carolina	sr
Humibid LA	Carolina	sr
Iberet-500	Abbott	sr
Iberet-Folic-500	Abbott	sr
Icar-C Plus SR	Hawthorn	sr
Imdur	Schering Plough	sr
Inderal LA	Wyeth	sr

DRUG	MANUFACTURER	FORM
Indocin SR	Forte Pharma	sr
Innopran XL	GlaxoSmithKline	sr
Invega	Janssen	sr
Isochron	Forest	sr
Isopro	Rugby	sr
Isoptin SR	Ranbaxy	sr
Kadian	Alpharma	sr
Kaon-Cl 10	Savage	sr
Keppra XR	UCB	sr
Klor-Con 8	Upsher-Smith	sr
Klor-Con 10	Upsher-Smith	sr
Klor-Con M10	Upsher-Smith	sr
Klor-Con M15	Upsher-Smith	sr
Klor-Con M20	Upsher-Smith	sr
Klotrix	Bristol-Myers Squibb	sr
K-Tab	Abbott	sr
K-Tan	Prasco	sr
Lescol XL	Novartis	sr
Levall G	Auriga	sr
Levbid	Alaven	sr
Levsinex	Alaven	sr
Lialda	Shire	ec
Lipram 4500	Global	ec
Lipram-PN10	Global	ec
Lipram-PN16	Global	ec
Lipram-PN20	Global	ec
Liquibid-D	Capellon	sr
Liquibid-D 1200	Capellon	sr
Liquibid-PD	Capellon	sr
Lithobid	JDS Pharmaceuticals	sr
Lodrane-12 Hour	ECR	sr
Lodrane-12D	ECR	sr
Lodrane 24	ECR	sr
Lodrane 24D	ECR	sr
Lohist-12	Larken	sr
Lohist-12D	Larken	sr
Luvox CR	Jazz Pharmaceuticals	sr
Mag Delay	Major	ec
Mag64	Rising	ec
Mag-SR Plus Calcium	Cypress	sr
Mag-Tab SR	Niche	sr
Maxifed	MCR American	sr
Maxifed DM	MCR American	sr
Maxifed DMX	MCR American	sr
Maxifed-G	MCR American	sr
Maxiphen DM	MCR American	sr
Medent DM	SJ	sr
Medent PE	SJ	sr
Mega-C	Merit	sr
Menopause Trio	Mason Vitamins	sr
Mestinon Timespan	Valeant	sr
Metadate CD	UCB	sr
Metadate ER	UCB	sr
Methylin ER	Mallinckrodt	sr
Micro-K	Ther-Rx	sr
Micro-K 10	Ther-Rx	sr
Mild-C	Carlson, J.R.	sr
Montephen	Monte Sano	sr
MS Contin	Purdue	sr
Mucinex	Adams	sr
Mucinex D	Adams	sr
Mucinex DM	Adams	sr
Multiret Folic-500	Actavis	sr
Mydocs	Centurion	sr
Myfortic	Novartis	ec
Nalex-A	Blansett	sr
Naprelan	Victory	sr
Nasatab LA	ECR	sr
New Ami-Tex LA	Actavis	sr
Nexium	AstraZeneca	ec
Niaspan	Abbott	sr
Nicomide	Sirius	sr
Nifediac CC	Teva	sr
Nifedical XL	Teva	sr
Nitro-Time	Time-Cap	sr
Nohist	Larken	sr
Nohist-Plus	Larken	sr
Nohist-Plus Jr	Larken	sr
Norel SR	U.S. Pharmaceutical	sr
Norpace CR	Pfizer	sr
Obstetrix EC	Seyer Pharmatec	ec
Omnihist LA	Dexo	sr
Opana ER	Endo	sr
Oramorph SR	Xanodyne	sr
Oracea	Collagenex	sr
Oxycontin	Purdue	sr
Palcaps 10	Breckenridge	ec
Palcaps 20	Breckenridge	ec
Pancrease MT 10	McNeil Consumer	ec
Pancrease MT 16	McNeil Consumer	ec
Pancrease MT 20	McNeil Consumer	ec
Pancrecarb MS-4	Digestive Care	ec
Pancrecarb MS-8	Digestive Care	ec
Pancrecarb MS-16	Digestive Care	ec
Pangestyme CN-10	Ethex	ec
Pangestyme CN-20	Ethex	ec
Pangestyme EC	Ethex	ec
Pangestyme MT16	Ethex	ec
Pangestyme UL12	Ethex	ec
Pangestyme UL18	Ethex	ec
Pangestyme UL20	Ethex	ec
Panocaps	Breckenridge	ec
Panocaps MT 16	Breckenridge	ec
Panocaps MT 20	Breckenridge	ec
Para-Time SR	Time-Cap	sr
Paser	Jacobus	sr
Pavacot	Truxton	sr
Paxil CR	GlaxoSmithKline	sr
PCE Dispertab	Abbott	sr
PCM LA	Cypress	sr
Pendex	Cypress	sr
Pentasa	Shire U.S.	sr

Drugs That Should Not Be Crushed

DRUG	MANUFACTURER	FORM
Pentoxil	Upsher-Smith	sr
Phenabid	Gil	sr
Phenabid DM	Gil	sr
Phenavent D	Ethex	sr
Phendiet-105	Truxton	sr
Phenytek	Mylan Bertek	sr
Phlemex-PE	Cypress	sr
Plendil	AstraZeneca	sr
Poly Hist Forte	Poly	sr
Poly-Vent	Poly	sr
Poly-Vent Jr	Poly	sr
Prehist D	Marnel	sr
Prevacid	Tap	ec
Prilosec	AstraZeneca	ec
Prilosec OTC	Procter & Gamble	sr
Pristiq	Wyeth	sr
Procardia XL	Pfizer	sr
Prolex PD	Blansett	sr
Prolex-D	Blansett	sr
Pronestyl-SR	Bristol-Myers Squibb	sr
Proquin XR	Depomed	sr
Protid	Lunsco	sr
Protonix	Wyeth	ec
Prozac Weekly	Eli Lilly	ec
Pseudocot-C	Truxton	sr
Pseudocot-G	Truxton	sr
Pseudovent DM	Ethex	sr
Ralix	Cypress	sr
Ranexa	CV Therapeutics	sr
Razadyne ER	Ortho-McNeil	sr
Reliable Gentle Laxative	Ivax	ec
Requip XL	GlaxoSmithKline	sr
Rescon-Jr	Capellon	sr
Rescon-MX	Capellon	sr
Respa-AR	Respa	sr
Respa-BR	Respa	sr
Respahist-II	Respa	sr
Respaire-60 SR	Laser	sr
Respaire-120 SR	Laser	sr
Rhinacon A	Breckenridge	sr
Risperdal Consta	Janssen	sr
Ritalin LA	Novartis	sr
Ritalin-SR	Novartis	sr
Rodex Forte	Legere	sr
Ru-Tuss	Carwin	sr
Rythmol SR	GlaxoSmithKline	sr
SAM-e	Pharmavite	ec
Sanctura XR	Allergan	sr
Scopohist-PE	Larken	sr
Seroquel XR	AstraZeneca	sr
Simcor	Abbott	sr
Sinemet CR	Bristol-Myers Squibb	sr
Sinutuss DM	Dexo	sr
Sinuvent PE	Dexo	sr
Slo-Niacin	Upsher-Smith	sr
Slow Fe	Novartis Consumer	sr
Slow Fe With Folic Acid	Novartis Consumer	sr
Slow-Mag	Purdue	ec
Solodyn	Medicis	sr
St. Joseph Pain Reliever	McNeil Consumer	ec
Stahist	Magna	sr
Stavzor	Noven	sr
Sudafed 12 Hour	Johnson & Johnson	sr
Sudafed 24 Hour	Johnson & Johnson	sr
Sudahist	Larken	sr
Sudatrate	Larken	sr
Sudex Tab	Atley	sr
Sular	Sciele	sr
Sulfazine EC	Qualitest	ec
Symax Duotab	Capellon	sr
Symax-SR	Capellon	sr
Tarka	Abbott	sr
Taztia XT	Andrx	sr
Tegretol-XR	Novartis	sr
Theo-24	UCB	sr
Theochron	Forest	sr
Theo-Time	Major	sr
Tiazac	Forest	sr
Toprol XL	AstraZeneca	sr
Totalday	National Vitamin	sr
Touro Allergy	Dartmouth	sr
Touro CC	Dartmouth	sr
Touro CC-LD	Dartmouth	sr
Touro DM	Dartmouth	sr
Touro HC	Dartmouth	sr
Touro LA	Dartmouth	sr
Touro LA-LD	Dartmouth	sr
Tranxene-SD	Ovation	sr
Trental	sanofi-aventis	sr
Trituss-ER	Everett	sr
Tussafed-LA	Everett	sr
Tussall-ER	Everett	sr
Tussi-Bid	Capellon	sr
Tussicaps	Mallinckrodt	sr
Tusso-DM	Everett	sr
Tusso-HC	Everett	sr
Tylenol Arthritis	McNeil Consumer	sr
Ultrabrom	Dexo	sr
Ultrabrom PD	Dexo	sr
Ultracaps MT 20	Breckenridge	ec
Ultram ER	Ortho-McNeil	sr
Ultrase	Axcan Scandipharm	ec
Ultrase MT12	Axcan Scandipharm	ec
Ultrase MT18	Axcan Scandipharm	ec
Ultrase MT20	Axcan Scandipharm	ec
Uniphyl	Purdue	sr
Urocit-K 5	Mission	sr
Urocit-K 10	Mission	sr
Uroxatral	sanofi-aventis	sr
Utira	Hawthorn	sr
Veracolate	Numark	ec
Verelan	UCB	sr

DRUG	MANUFACTURER	FORM
Verelan PM	UCB	sr
Videx EC	Bristol-Myers Squibb	ec
Vivitrol	Cephalon	sr
Voltaren	Novartis	ec
Voltaren-XR	Novartis	sr
Vospire	Dava	sr
Vospire ER	Dava	sr
We Mist LA	WE Pharmaceuticals	sr
We Mist II LA	WE Pharmaceuticals	sr
Wellbid-D	Prasco	sr
Wellbid-D 1200	Prasco	sr
Wellbutrin SR	GlaxoSmithKline	sr
Wellbutrin XL	GlaxoSmithKline	sr
Wobenzym N	Marlyn	ec
Woman's Wellbeing Menopause Relief	Consumer Choice	sr
Xanax XR	Pfizer	sr
Xedec II	Cypress	sr
Xpect-AT	Hawthorn	sr
Xpect-HC	Hawthorn	sr
Xpect PE	Hawthorn	sr
Zmax	Pfizer	sr
Zorprin	Par	sr
Zotex-12D	Vertical	sr
Zyban	GlaxoSmithKline	sr
Zyflo CR	Critical Therapeutics	sr
Zyrtec-D	McNeil Consumer	sr

GENERIC AVAILABILITY GUIDE

This section allows you to quickly determine which forms and strengths of a brand-name drug are also available generically. The entries are organized alphabetically by brand name and dosage form, with strengths in ascending order. Generic availability is indicated by a mark in the "Yes" column. Included are prescription products described in *PDR*® and *PDR® for Ophthalmic Medicines* that have generic equivalents. This list does not include every drug that is available as a generic. Generic availability information is drawn from the Drug Database maintained by *Red Book*® affiliate Thomson Micromedex. **Note: Brand-name products with no generic equivalents have been omitted.**

STRENGTH	GENERIC YES	GENERIC NO
Accutane Capsules		
10 mg	■	
20 mg	■	
40 mg	■	
Accuzyme Debriding Ointment		
830000 u/gm-10%	■	
Accuzyme SE Spray Emulsion		
830000 u/gm-10%		■
Actiq		
0.2 mg	■	
0.4 mg	■	
0.6 mg	■	
0.8 mg	■	
1.2 mg	■	
1.6 mg	■	
Active Calcium Tablets		
200 mg-100 iu	■	
Activella Tablets		
0.5 mg-0.1 mg		■
1 mg-0.5 mg	■	
Adenocard IV Injection		
3 mg/ml	■	
Adenoscan		
3 mg/ml	■	
Adipex-P Capsules		
37.5 mg	■	
Adipex-P Tablets		
37.5 mg	■	
Agrylin Capsules		
0.5 mg	■	
1 mg	■	
Albutein 5%		
5%	■	
Albutein 25%		
25%	■	
Allegra Oral Solution		
30 mg/5 ml		■
Allegra Tablets		
30 mg	■	
60 mg	■	
180 mg	■	
Allegra-D 24 Hour Extended-Release Tablets		
180 mg-240 mg		■
AlphaNine SD		
150 iu/mg	■	
Ambien Tablets		
5 mg	■	
10 mg	■	
Ambien CR Tablets		
6.25 mg		■
12.5 mg		■
Amoxil Capsules		
250 mg	■	
500 mg	■	
Amoxil Chewable Tablets		
125 mg	■	
200 mg	■	
250 mg	■	
400 mg	■	
Amoxil Pediatric Drops for Oral Suspension		
50 mg/ml	■	
Amoxil Powder for Oral Suspension		
250 mg/5 ml	■	
400 mg/5 ml	■	
Amoxil Tablets		
500 mg	■	
875 mg	■	
Anaprox Tablets		
275 mg	■	
Anaprox DS Tablets		
550 mg	■	
AndroGel		
1%	■	
Anzemet Injection		
20 mg/ml	■	
Anzemet Tablets		
50 mg		■
100 mg		■
Atrovent HFA Inhalation Aerosol		
0.017 mg/actuation		■
Atrovent Nasal Spray 0.03%		
0.03%	■	
Atrovent Nasal Spray 0.06%		
0.06%	■	
Augmentin Chewable Tablets		
125 mg-31.25 mg		■
200 mg-28.5 mg	■	
250 mg-62.5 mg		■
400 mg-57 mg	■	
Augmentin Powder for Oral Suspension		
125 mg/5 ml-31.25 mg/5 ml		■
200 mg/5 ml-28.5 mg/5 ml	■	
250 mg/5 ml-62.5 mg/5 ml		■
400 mg/5 ml-57 mg/5 ml	■	
Augmentin Tablets		
250 mg-125 mg	■	
500 mg-125 mg	■	
875 mg-125 mg	■	
Augmentin XR Extended-Release Tablets		
1000 mg-62.5 mg		■
Augmentin ES-600 Powder for Oral Suspension		
600 mg/5 ml-42.9 mg/5 ml	■	
Bactroban Cream		
2%		■
Bactroban Nasal		
2%		■
Bactroban Ointment		
2%	■	
Biaxin Filmtab Tablets		
250mg	■	
500mg	■	
Biaxin Granules		
125 mg/5 ml	■	
250 mg/5 ml	■	
Biaxin XL Filmtab Tablets		
500 mg	■	
Bleph-10 Ophthalmic Solution 10%		
10%	■	

STRENGTH	GENERIC YES	GENERIC NO
Brevoxyl-4 Creamy Wash		
4%	■	
Brevoxyl-4 Gel		
4%		■
Brevoxyl-8 Creamy Wash		
8%	■	
Brevoxyl-8 Gel		
8%		■
Calcijex Injection		
1 mcg/ml	■	
2 mcg/ml	■	
Captopril Tablets		
12.5 mg	■	
25 mg	■	
50 mg	■	
100 mg	■	
Carafate Suspension		
1 gm/10 ml	■	
Carafate Tablets		
1 gm	■	
Cardene I.V.		
2.5 mg/ml	■	
Catapres Tablets		
0.1 mg	■	
0.2 mg	■	
0.3 mg	■	
Catapres-TTS		
0.1 mg/24 hr		■
0.2 mg/24 hr		■
0.3 mg/24 hr		■
Ceftin for Oral Suspension		
125 mg/5 ml	■	
250 mg/5 ml	■	
Ceftin Tablets		
125 mg	■	
250 mg	■	
500 mg	■	
Celexa Oral Solution		
10 mg/5 ml	■	
Celexa Tablets		
10 mg	■	
20 mg	■	
40 mg	■	
CellCept Capsules		
250 mg	■	
CellCept Intravenous		
500 mg		■
CellCept Oral Suspension		
200 mg/ml		■
CellCept Tablets		
500 mg		■
Cipro Oral Suspension		
250 mg/5 ml		■
500 mg/5 ml		■
Cipro Tablets		
100 mg	■	
250 mg	■	
500 mg	■	
750 mg	■	
Cipro XR Tablets		
500 mg		■
1000 mg		■
CitraNatal DHA Tablets		
120 mg-125 mg-27 mg-400 iu-30 iu-3 mg-3.4 mg-20 mg-20 mg-1 mg-0.15 mg-25 mg-2 mg-50 mg-250 mg		■
CitraNatal 90 DHA Capsules		
120 mg-200 mg-90 mg-400 iu-30 iu-3 mg-3.4 mg-20 mg-20 mg-1 mg-0.15 mg-25 mg-2 mg-50 mg-250 mg	■	
Climara Transdermal System		
0.025 mg/24 hr	■	
0.0375 mg/24 hr	■	
0.05 mg/24 hr	■	
0.06 mg/24 hr		■
0.075 mg/24 hr	■	
0.1 mg/24 hr	■	
Clinoril Tablets		
200 mg	■	
Clorpres Tablets		
15 mg-0.1 mg	■	
15 mg-0.2 mg	■	
15 mg-0.3 mg	■	
CordyMax Cs-4 Capsules		
525 mg	■	
Coreg Tablets		
3.125 mg	■	
6.25 mg	■	
12.5 mg	■	
25 mg	■	
Creon 5 Capsules		
16600 u-5000 u-18750 u		■
Creon 10 Capsules		
33200 u-10000 u-37500 u	■	
Creon 20 Capsules		
66400 u-20000 u-75000 u	■	
Dantrium Capsules		
25 mg	■	
50 mg	■	
100 mg	■	
Delatestryl Injection		
200 mg/ml	■	
Demadex Injection		
10 mg/ml		■
Demadex Tablets		
5 mg	■	
10 mg	■	
20 mg	■	
100 mg	■	
Dexedrine Spansule Sustained-Release Capsules		
5 mg	■	
10 mg	■	
15 mg	■	
Dexedrine Tablets		
5 mg	■	
Didronel Tablets		
200 mg	■	
400 mg	■	
Diprolene Lotion 0.05%		
0.05%	■	
Diprolene Ointment 0.05%		
0.05%	■	
Diprolene AF Cream 0.05%		
0.05%	■	
Duragesic Transdermal System		
12.5 mcg/hr	■	
25 mcg/hr	■	
50 mcg/hr	■	
75 mcg/hr	■	
100 mcg/hr	■	
Dyazide Capsules		
25 mg-37.5 mg	■	
25 mg-50 mg	■	
EC-Naprosyn Delayed-Release Tablets		
375 mg	■	
500 mg	■	
Edex Injection		
10 mcg	■	
20 mcg	■	
40 mcg	■	
E.E.S. 200 Liquid		
200 mg/5 ml	■	
E.E.S. 400 Liquid		
400 mg/5 ml	■	
E.E.S. 400 Filmtab Tablets		
400 mg	■	

STRENGTH	GENERIC YES	GENERIC NO
E.E.S. Granules		
200 mg/5 ml	■	
Eldepryl Capsules		
5 mg	■	
Elocon Cream 0.1%		
0.1%	■	
Elocon Lotion 0.1%		
0.1%	■	
Elocon Ointment 0.1%		
0.1%	■	
EryPed 200 & EryPed 400 Oral Suspension		
200 mg/5 ml	■	
400 mg/5 ml	■	
EryPed Drops		
100 mg/2.5 ml		■
Estratest Tablets		
1.25 mg-2.5 mg	■	
Estratest H.S. Tablets		
0.625 mg-1.25 mg	■	
Exelon Capsules		
1.5 mg	■	
3 mg	■	
4.5 mg	■	
6 mg	■	
Exelon Patch		
4.6 mg/24 hr		■
9.5 mg/24 hr		■
Flexbumin 25% I.V.		
25%	■	
Flolan for Injection		
0.5 mg	■	
1.5 mg	■	
Flonase Nasal Spray		
0.05 mg/actuation	■	
Fluarix Vaccine		
45 mcg/0.5 ml	■	
Flumadine Syrup		
50 mg/5 ml		■
Flumadine Tablets		
100 mg	■	
FML Ophthalmic Ointment		
0.1%		■
FML Ophthalmic Suspension		
0.1%	■	
FML Forte Ophthalmic Suspension		
0.25%		■
Fortaz Injection		
1 gm	■	
2 gm	■	
6 gm	■	
500 mg	■	

STRENGTH	GENERIC YES	GENERIC NO
Fortaz for Injection		
1 gm/50 ml-2.2 gm/50 ml		■
2 gm/50 ml-1.6 gm/50 ml		■
Fosamax Oral Solution		
70 mg/75 ml		■
Fosamax Tablets		
5 mg	■	
10 mg	■	
35 mg	■	
40 mg	■	
70 mg	■	
Fosamax Plus D Tablets		
70 mg-2800 iu		■
Furosemide Tablets		
20 mg	■	
40 mg	■	
80 mg	■	
Gammagard Liquid		
100 mg/ml		■
Gammagard S/D		
0.5 gm	■	
2.5 gm	■	
5 gm	■	
10 gm	■	
Gengraf Capsules		
25 mg	■	
100 mg	■	
Hyalgan Solution		
10 mg/ml	■	
Indapamide Tablets		
1.25 mg	■	
2.5 mg	■	
Indocin Capsules		
25 mg	■	
50 mg	■	
Indocin I.V.		
1 mg		■
Indocin Oral Suspension		
25 mg/5 ml		■
Indocin Suppositories		
50 mg	■	
Klonopin Tablets		
0.5 mg	■	
1 mg	■	
2 mg	■	
Klonopin Wafers		
0.125 mg	■	
0.25 mg	■	
0.5 mg	■	
1 mg	■	
2 mg	■	

STRENGTH	GENERIC YES	GENERIC NO
K-Phos Original (Sodium Free) Tablets		
500 mg		■
K-Phos Neutral Tablets		
155 mg-852 mg-130 mg	■	
Lamictal Chewable Dispersible Tablets		
2 mg		■
5 mg	■	
25 mg	■	
Lamictal Tablets		
25 mg	■	
100 mg	■	
150 mg	■	
200 mg	■	
Lamisil Oral Granules		
125 mg/packet		■
187.5 mg/packet		■
Lamisil Tablets		
250 mg	■	
Lanoxin Injection		
0.25 mg/ml	■	
Lanoxin Injection Pediatric		
0.1 mg/ml		■
Lanoxin Tablets		
0.125 mg	■	
0.25 mg	■	
Leustatin Injection		
1 mg/ml	■	
Levothroid Tablets		
0.025 mg	■	
0.05 mg	■	
0.075 mg	■	
0.088 mg	■	
0.1 mg	■	
0.112 mg	■	
0.125 mg	■	
0.137 mg	■	
0.15 mg	■	
0.175 mg	■	
0.2 mg	■	
0.3 mg	■	
Levoxyl Tablets		
0.025 mg	■	
0.05 mg	■	
0.075 mg	■	
0.088 mg	■	
0.1 mg	■	
0.112 mg	■	
0.125 mg	■	
0.137 mg	■	
0.15 mg	■	
0.175 mg	■	
0.2 mg	■	

STRENGTH	GENERIC YES	GENERIC NO
Lexapro Oral Suspension		
5 mg/5 ml		■
Lexapro Tablets		
5 mg	■	
10 mg	■	
20 mg	■	
Lortab Tablets		
500 mg-2.5 mg	■	
500 mg-5 mg	■	
500 mg-7.5 mg	■	
500 mg-10 mg	■	
Lotrisone Cream		
0.05%-1%	■	
Marinol Capsules		
2.5 mg	■	
5 mg	■	
10 mg	■	
Marlyn Formula 50 Capsules		
252 mg-1 mg-320 mg	■	
Mavik Tablets		
1 mg	■	
2 mg	■	
4 mg	■	
Mevacor Tablets		
20 mg	■	
40 mg	■	
Mobic Tablets		
7.5 mg	■	
15 mg	■	
MS Contin Tablets		
15 mg	■	
30 mg	■	
60 mg	■	
100 mg	■	
200 mg	■	
Nadolol Tablets		
20 mg	■	
40 mg	■	
80 mg	■	
160 mg	■	
Naprosyn Suspension		
25 mg/ml	■	
Naprosyn Tablets		
250 mg	■	
375 mg	■	
500 mg	■	
Neoral Oral Solution		
100 mg/ml	■	
Neoral Soft Gelatin Capsules		
25 mg	■	
100 mg	■	

STRENGTH	GENERIC YES	GENERIC NO
Nimotop Capsules		
30 mg	■	
Nitro-Dur Transdermal Infusion System		
0.1 mg/hr	■	
0.2 mg/hr	■	
0.3 mg/hr		■
0.4 mg/hr	■	
0.6 mg/hr	■	
0.8 mg/hr		■
Novantrone for Injection Concentrate		
2 mg/ml	■	
Nu-Iron 150 Capsules		
150 mg	■	
Nystop Topical Powder USP		
100000 u/gm	■	
Olux Foam		
0.05%	■	
Olux E-Foam		
0.05%		■
Omnicef Capsules		
300 mg	■	
Omnicef for Oral Suspension		
125 mg/5 ml	■	
250 mg/5 ml	■	
OptiPranolol Metipranolol Ophthalmic Solution 0.3%		
0.3%	■	
Ortho-Cyclen Tablets		
35 mcg-0.25 mg	■	
Ortho Micronor Tablets		
0.35 mg	■	
OxyContin Tablets		
10 mg	■	
15 mg		■
20 mg	■	
30 mg		■
40 mg	■	
60 mg		■
80 mg	■	
OxyIR Capsules		
5mg	■	
Panafil Ointment		
0.5%-10%-10%		■
Panafil SE Spray Emulsion		
0.5%-10%	■	
Parnate Tablets		
10 mg	■	
Paxil Oral Suspension		
10 mg/5 ml	■	

STRENGTH	GENERIC YES	GENERIC NO
Paxil Tablets		
10 mg	■	
20 mg	■	
30 mg	■	
40 mg	■	
Paxil CR Controlled-Release Tablets		
12.5 mg	■	
25 mg	■	
37.5 mg	■	
Pentacel		
0.5 ml	■	
Pepcid Tablets		
20 mg	■	
40 mg	■	
Percocet Tablets		
325 mg-2.5 mg		■
325 mg-5 mg	■	
325 mg-7.5 mg	■	
325 mg-10 mg	■	
500 mg-7.5 mg	■	
650 mg-10 mg	■	
Percodan Tablets		
325 mg-4.5 mg-0.38 mg	■	
Persantine Tablets		
25 mg	■	
50 mg	■	
75 mg	■	
Plavix Tablets		
75 mg	■	
300 mg		■
Pletal Tablets		
50mg	■	
100mg	■	
Potaba Envules		
2 gm/packet	■	
Potaba Tablets		
0.5 gm		■
Precose Tablets		
25 mg	■	
50 mg	■	
100 mg	■	
Pred Forte Ophthalmic Suspension		
1%	■	
Pred Mild Ophthalmic Suspension		
0.12%		■
Pred-G Ophthalmic Ointment		
0.12%	■	
Pred-G Ophthalmic Suspension		
0.3%-1%		■

STRENGTH	GENERIC YES	GENERIC NO
Prinivil Tablets		
5 mg	■	
10 mg	■	
20 mg	■	
Prinzide Tablets		
12.5 mg-10 mg	■	
12.5 mg-20 mg	■	
ProAmatine Tablets		
2.5 mg	■	
5 mg	■	
10 mg	■	
Profilnine SD Solvent Detergent		
1 iu	■	
Propecia Tablets		
1 mg	■	
Proscar Tablets		
5 mg	■	
Protonix Delayed-Release Tablets		
20 mg	■	
40 mg	■	
Protonix I.V.		
40 mg		■
Prozac Weekly Capsules		
90 mg		■
Prozac Pulvules and Liquid		
10 mg	■	
20 mg	■	
20 mg/5 ml	■	
40 mg	■	
Rebetol Capsules		
200 mg	■	
Remeron Tablets		
15 mg	■	
30 mg	■	
45 mg	■	
RemeronSolTab Tablets		
15 mg	■	
30 mg	■	
45 mg	■	
Requip Tablets		
0.25 mg	■	
0.5 mg	■	
1 mg	■	
2 mg	■	
3 mg	■	
4 mg	■	
5 mg	■	
Requip XL Tablets		
2 mg		■
4 mg		■
8 mg		■
12 mg		■
Retrovir Capsules		
100 mg	■	
Retrovir IV Infusion		
10 mg/ml		■
Retrovir Syrup		
50 mg/5 ml	■	
Retrovir Tablets		
300 mg	■	
Rocaltrol Capsules		
0.25 mcg	■	
0.5 mcg	■	
Rocaltrol Oral Solution		
1 mcg/ml	■	
Rocephin Injectable Vials, ADD-Vantage, Galaxy, Bulk		
1 gm	■	
1 gm/50 ml	■	
2 gm	■	
2 gm/50 ml	■	
10 gm	■	
250 mg	■	
500 mg	■	
Romazicon Injection		
0.1 mg/ml	■	
Rythmol Tablets		
150 mg	■	
225 mg	■	
300 mg	■	
Rythmol SR Capsules		
150 mg		■
225 mg		■
300 mg		■
Salagen Tablets		
5 mg	■	
7.5 mg	■	
Sandimmune Oral Solution		
100 mg/ml	■	
Sandimmune I.V. Ampules for Infusion		
50 mg/ml	■	
Sandimmune Soft Gelatin Capsules		
25 mg	■	
100 mg	■	
Sandostatin Injection		
50 mcg/ml	■	
100 mcg/ml	■	
200 mcg/ml	■	
500 mcg/ml	■	
1000 mcg/ml	■	
Sandostatin LAR Depot		
10 mg		■
20 mg		■
30 mg		■
Soma Tablets		
250 mg		■
350 mg	■	
Synthroid Tablets		
0.025 mg	■	
0.05 mg	■	
0.075 mg	■	
0.088 mg	■	
0.1 mg	■	
0.112 mg	■	
0.125 mg	■	
0.137 mg	■	
0.15 mg	■	
0.175 mg	■	
0.2 mg	■	
0.3 mg	■	
Tegreen 97 Capsules		
250 mg	■	
Tessalon Capsules		
200 mg	■	
Tessalon Perles		
100 mg	■	
Thioridazine Hydrochloride Tablets		
10 mg	■	
25 mg	■	
50 mg	■	
100 mg	■	
Thiothixene Capsules		
1 mg	■	
2 mg	■	
5 mg	■	
10 mg	■	
Timoptic Sterile Ophthalmic Solution		
0.25%	■	
0.5%	■	
Timoptic in Ocudose		
0.25%		■
0.5%		■
Timoptic-XE Sterile Ophthalmic Gel Forming Solution		
0.25%	■	
0.5%	■	

STRENGTH	GENERIC YES	GENERIC NO
Toprol-XL Tablets		
25 mg	■	
50 mg	■	
100 mg	■	
200 mg	■	
Trusopt Sterile Ophthalmic Solution		
2%	■	
Tylenol with Codeine Tablets		
300 mg-30 mg	■	
300 mg-60 mg	■	
Ultane Liquid for Inhalation		
100%	■	
Ultrase Capsules		
20000 u-4500 u-25000 u	■	
Ultrase MT Capsules		
39000 u-12000 u-39000 u	■	
58500 u-18000 u-58500 u	■	
65000 u-20000 u-65000 u	■	
Uniphyl Tablets		
400 mg	■	
600 mg	■	
Urocit-K Tablets		
5 meq	■	
10 meq	■	
Valium Tablets		
2 mg	■	
5 mg	■	
10 mg	■	
Valtrex Caplets		
500 mg	■	
1 gm	■	
Venlafaxine Hydrochloride Tablets		
25 mg	■	
37.5 mg	■	
50 mg	■	
100 mg	■	
Vesanoid Capsules		
10 mg	■	
Vicodin Tablets		
500 mg-5 mg	■	
Vicodin ES Tablets		
750 mg-7.5 mg	■	
Vicodin HP Tablets		
660 mg-10 mg	■	
Vicoprofen Tablets		
7.5 mg-200 mg	■	
Viokase Powder		
70000 u-16800 u-70000 u/0.7 gm		■
Viokase Tablets		
30000 u-8000 u-30000 u	■	
60000 u-16000 u-60000 u	■	
Viroptic Ophthalmic Solution		
1%	■	
Voltaren Ophthalmic Solution		
0.1%	■	
Voltaren Tablets		
75 mg	■	
Voltaren-XR Tablets		
100 mg	■	
Wellbutrin Tablets		
75 mg	■	
100 mg	■	
Wellbutrin SR Sustained-Release Tablets		
100 mg	■	
150 mg	■	
200 mg	■	
Wellbutrin XL Extended-Release Tablets		
150 mg	■	
300 mg	■	
Zantac 25 EFFERdose Tablets		
25 mg		■
Zantac Injection		
25 mg/ml	■	
Zantac Injection Premixed		
1 mg/ml		■
Zantac Syrup		
15 mg/ml	■	
Zantac 150 Tablets		
150 mg	■	
Zantac 300 Tablets		
300 mg	■	
Zinacef Injection		
1.5 gm	■	
1.5 gm/50 ml	■	
7.5 gm	■	
750 mg	■	
750 mg/50 ml	■	
Zinc-220 Capsules		
220 mg	■	
Zocor Tablets		
5 mg	■	
10 mg	■	
20 mg	■	
40 mg	■	
80 mg	■	
Zofran Injection		
2 mg/ml	■	
Zofran Injection Premixed		
32 mg/50 ml	■	
Zofran Oral Solution		
4 mg/5 ml	■	
Zofran Tablets		
4 mg	■	
8 mg	■	
Zofran ODT Orally Disintegrating Tablets		
4 mg	■	
8 mg	■	
Zovirax Capsules		
200 mg	■	
Zovirax Cream		
5%		■
Zovirax Ointment		
5%		■
Zovirax Suspension		
200 mg/5 ml	■	
Zovirax Tablets		
400 mg	■	
800 mg	■	
Zyban Sustained-Release Tablets		
150 mg	■	

LACTOSE- AND GALACTOSE-FREE DRUGS

The following is a selection of lactose- and galactose-free products. The list is not comprehensive. Generic and alternate brands may exist. Always check product labeling for definitive information on specific ingredients.

TRADE NAME (OTC)	FORM
Advil	Tablets, Caplets, Gel Caplets, Liquigels
Advil PM Liquigels	
Advil Cold and Sinus	Caplets
Aleve	Caplets, Gelcaps, Tablets, Gel Tablets
Aleve Smooth Gels	Gel Tablets
Align	Capsules
Alka-Mints	Tablets
Alka-Seltzer	Effervescent Tablets
Alka-Seltzer Plus Cold	Effervescent Tablets
Ascriptin	Tablets
Axid AR	Tablets
Benadryl	Liquid, Tablets
Benadryl Allergy & Cold	Caplets
Caltrate 600 PLUS	Tablets
Claritin-D 24	Tablets
Claritin-D Reditabs	Tablets
Colace	Capsules
Dramamine Chewable	Tablets
Elecare	Powder
Enfamil Poly-Vi-Sol	Drops
Enfamil Poly-Vi-Sol with Iron	Drops
Enfamil Tri-Vi-Sol	Drops
Enfamil Tri-Vi-Sol with Iron	Drops
Ensure	Liquid, Powder, Pudding
Ensure Fiber	Liquid
Ensure High Calcium	Liquid
Ensure High Protein	Liquid
Ensure Plus	Liquid
Excedrin Extra-Strength	Caplets
Ex-Lax Maximum Strength	Tablets
Ex-Lax Regular Strength	Tablets
Ex-Lax Regular Strength Chocolate	Chewable
Fergon Iron	Tablets
Gaviscon Regular Strength	Tablets
Imodium A-D	Liquid, Tablets
Imodium A-D EZ Chews	Tablets
Imodium Multi Symptom Relief Chewable	Tablets, Caplets
Jevity	Liquid
Kaopectate Cherry	Liquid
Kaopectate Peppermint	Liquid
Kaopectate Peppermint Extra Strength	Liquid
Kaopectate Stool Softener	Softgel
Kaopectate Vanilla	Liquid
Konsyl	Powder
Lactaid	Tablets
Lactaid Fast Act	Caplets, Chewables
MCT Oil	Oil
Medi-Lyte	Tablets
Metamucil	Powder, Wafers
Metamucil Heart and Digestive Health	Capsules
Metamucil Strong Bones	Capsules
Motrin Children's	Suspension
Motrin Children's Cold	Suspension
Motrin IB	Tablets
Motrin Infant's	Drops
Motrin Junior Strength	Caplets, Tablets
Mylanta Children's	Tablets
Mylanta Gas	Tablets
Mylanta Gas Maximum Strength	Softgels
Mylanta Maximum Strength	Liquid
Mylanta Regular Strength	Liquid
Mylanta Supreme	Liquid
Mylanta Ultimate Strength	Liquid, Tablets
Mylicon Infants'	Drops
Nepro	Liquid
Ocuvite Vitamin and Mineral Supplement	Tablets
One-A-Day Cholesterol Plus	Tablets
One-A-Day Energy	Tablets
One-A-Day Essential	Tablets
One-A-Day Maximum	Tablets
One-A-Day Men's	Tablets
One-A-Day Men's Health Formula	Tablets
One-A-Day Men's 50+ Advantage	Tablets
One-A-Day Weightsmart Advanced	Tablets
One-A-Day Women's	Tablets
One-A-Day Women's 50+ Advantage	Tablets
One-A-Day Women's Active Mind & Body	Tablets
One-A-Day Women's Prenatal	Tablets
Pepto-Bismol	Suspension, Tablets
Pepto-Bismol Max. Strength	Suspension
Percy Medicine	Liquid
Polycose	Liquid, Powder
Portagen	Powder
Prilosec OTC	Tablets
Promote	Liquid
Promote with Fiber	Liquid
Pulmocare	Liquid
RCF	Liquid
Simply Sleep	Caplets
St. Joseph Adult Low Strength Aspirin	Tablets
Sucrets Maximum Strength	Lozenges
Sudafed	Tablets
Sudafed Children's	Liquid
Sudafed OM Sinus Congestion Spray	Liquid
Sudafed PE Cold and Cough	Caplets
Sudafed PE Maximum Strength Sinus & Allergy	Tablets
Sudafed PE Nighttime Cold	Caplets
Sudafed PE Non-Drying Sinus	Caplets
Sudafed PE Severe Cold Formula	Caplets
Sudafed PE Sinus Headache	Caplets
Sudafed Sinus	Tablets
Titralac	Tablets
Titralac Plus	Tablets
Tums	Tablets
Tums E-X 750	Tablets
Tums E-X Sugar Free	Tablets
Tums Kids	Tablets
Tums Quik Pak	Powder
Tums Smoothies	Tablets
Tums Ultra 1000	Tablets
Tylenol	Drops, Liquid, Tablets
Tylenol Children's Plus Cold	Liquid
Tylenol Children's Plus Cold & Allergy	Liquid
Tylenol Children's Plus Cough & Runny Nose	Liquid
Tylenol Children's Plus Cough &Sore Throat	Liquid
Tylenol Children's Plus Flu	Liquid
Tylenol Children's Plus Multi-Symptom Cold	Liquid
Tylenol Meltaways Jr.	Tablets
Unisom SleepTabs	Gels, Melts, Tablets
Zantac 75	Tablets
Zantac 150 Cool Mint	Tablets
Zantac Maximum Strength 150	Tablets

TRADE NAME (OTC)	FORM
Accutane	Capsules
Actigall	Capsules
Advicor	Tablets
Aldactazide	Tablets
Aldactone	Tablets
Allegra	Solution, Tablets
Allegra-D 12 Hr, 24 Hr	Tablets
Allegra Oral	Suspension
Altace	Capsules
Amicar	Solution, Tablets
Antivert	Tablets
Aromasin	Tablets
Augmentin	Suspension, Tablets

Augmentin Chewable	Tablets
Augmentin ES 600	Powder
Augmentin XR	Tablets
Axid	Capsules, Solution
Bactrim	Tablets
Biaxin Granules	Suspension
Calan SR	Tablets
Carafate	Suspension, Tablets
Cardene	Capsules
Cardizem CD	Capsules
Ceftin	Suspension, Tablets
Cefzil	Suspension, Tablets
Cipro	Suspension, Tablets
Cipro XR	Tablets
Clinoril	Tablets
Combivir	Tablets
Comtan	Tablets
Covera-HS	Tablets
Creon	Capsules
Cytotec	Tablets
Daypro	Tablets
Demerol	Tablets
Depakene	Capsules
Depakote	Tablets
Depakote Sprinkle	Capsules
Detrol	Tablets
Detrol LA	Tablets
DiaBeta	Tablets
Diabinese	Tablets
Diovan	Tablets
Diovan HCT	Tablets
E.E.S.	Suspension, Tablets
Epivir	Tablets, Solution
Epivir-HBV	Tablets
Ery-Tab	Tablets
Esgic-Plus	Capsules, Tablets
Exelon	Capsules
Fioricet	Tablets
Fioricet with Codeine	Capsules
Flomax	Capsules
Gleevec	Tablets
Glucotrol XL	Tablets
Glucovance	Tablets
Glyset	Tablets
GoLYTELY	Powder
Grifulvin V	Suspension, Tablets
Inderal LA	Capsules
Isoptin SR	Tablets
Kaletra	Solution, Tablets
Keppra	Solution, Tablets
K-Lor	Powder
K-Phos Neutral	Tablets
K-Phos Original Formula	Tablets
K-Tab	Tablets
Lamisil	Tablets
Lescol	Capsules
Lescol XL	Tablets
Levaquin	Solution, Tablets
Levothroid	Tablets
Levoxyl	Tablets
Lexapro	Suspension, Tablets
Librium	Capsules
Lomotil	Solution, Tablets
Lopid	Tablets
Malarone	Tablets
Malarone Pediatric	Tablets
Maxzide	Tablets
Methylin ER	Tablets
Micardis	Tablets
Micro-K	Capsules
Micronase	Tablets
Minipress	Capsules
Minocin	Capsules
Niaspan	Tablets
Niferex-150	Capsules, Elixir
Niferex-150-Forte	Capsules
Norpramin	Tablets
Norvasc	Tablets
Omnicef	Capsules, Suspension
Pamelor	Capsules, Suspension
Pamine Forte	Tablets
Pancrease MT	Capsules
Paxil	Suspension, Tablets
Pepcid	Suspension, Tablets
Percocet	Tablets
Percodan	Tablets
Plaquenil	Tablets
Pletal	Tablets
Prandin	Tablets
Precare	Tablets
Precose	Tablets
Prevacid	Capsules, Suspension
Prinivil	Tablets
ProAmatine	Tablets
Procardia	Capsules
Procardia XL	Tablets
Prometrium	Capsules
Protonix	Suspension, Tablets
Prozac	Capsules, Solution
Questran	Powder
Questran Light	Powder
Remeron SolTab	Tablets
Rifadin	Capsules
Robaxin	Tablets
Sarafem	Pulvules, Tablets
Sectral	Capsules
Sinemet	Tablets
Sinemet CR	Tablets
Soma	Tablets
Stalevo	Tablets
Symmetrel	Syrup, Tablets
Tamiflu	Capsules, Suspension
Tegretol/Tegretol-XR	Tablets, Suspension
Tenoretic	Tablets
Tenormin	Tablets
Tessalon	Capsules
Tiazac	Capsules
Ticlid	Tablets
Tikosyn	Capsules
Tofranil-PM	Capsules
Toprol-XL	Tablets
Trental	Tablets
Trileptal	Suspension, Tablets
Trizivir	Tablets
Ultrase	Capsules
Ultrase MT	Capsules
Uniphyl	Tablets
Valcyte	Tablets
Valtrex	Caplets
Vibramycin Hyclate	Capsules, Suspension
Vicodin	Tablets
Vicodin ES	Tablets
Vicodin HP	Tablets
Vicoprofen	Tablets
Videx EC	Capsules, Delayed Release
Visicol	Tablets
Vistaril	Capsules, Suspension
Welchol	Tablets
Wellbutrin	Tablets
Wellbutrin SR	Tablets
Wellbutrin XL	Tablets
Xenical	Capsules
Zantac	Efferdose Tablets, Syrup, Tablets
Zarontin	Capsules, Solution
Zebeta	Tablets
Zestril	Tablets
Ziac	Tablets
Ziagen	Solution, Tablets
Zofran	Solution, Tablets (disintegrating)
Zoloft	Oral Concentrate, Tablets
Zonegran	Capsules
Zyban	Tablets
Zyvox	Suspension, Tablets

Poison Antidote Chart

WARNING: While every effort has been made to ensure the accuracy of this chart, it is not intended to serve as the sole source of information on antidotes. Guidelines may need to be adjusted based on factors such as anticipated usage in the hospital's local area, the nearest alternate sources of antidotes, and distance to tertiary care institutions. Contact your nearest regional poison control center (1-800-222-1222) for treatment information regarding any exposure, including indications for use of antidote therapy. Directions in this chart assume that all basic life support and decontamination measures have been initiated as needed.

ANTIDOTE	POISON/DRUG/TOXIN	SUGGESTED MINIMUM STOCK QUANTITY	COMMENTS
N-Acetylcysteine (Acetadote®, Mucomyst®)	Acetaminophen Carbon tetrachloride Other hepatotoxins	Oral product: 600 mL in 10 mL or 30 mL vials of 20% solution IV product: One carton of four 30 mL vials of 20% solution	Acetaminophen is the most common drug involved in intentional and unintentional poisonings. 600 mL (120 g) of the oral product provides enough antidote to treat an adult for an entire 3-day course of therapy, or enough to treat three adults for 24 h. Several vials may be stocked in the ED to provide a loading dose and the remaining vials in the pharmacy for the q 4 h maintenance doses. The IV product dose of 120 mL (24 g) will treat one adult patient for an entire 20-hour IV protocol.
Amyl nitrite, sodium nitrite, and sodium thiosulfate (Cyanide antidote kit)	Acetonitrile Acrylonitrile Bromates (thiosulfate only) Chlorates (thiosulfate only) Cyanide (e.g., HCN, KCN and NaCN) Cyanogen chloride Cyanogenic glycoside natural sources (e.g., apricot pits and peach pits) Hydrogen sulfide (nitrites only) Laetrile Mustard agents (thiosulfate only) Nitroprusside (thiosulfate only) Smoke inhalation (combustion of synthetic materials)	One to two kits Each kit contains: Twelve 0.3 mL amyl nitrite ampules Two vials 3% sodium nitrite, 10 mL each Two vials 25% sodium thiosulfate, 50 mL each	Stock one kit in the ED. Consider also stocking one kit in the pharmacy. Note: This kit has a short shelf life of 24 months. Note: Stocking this kit may be unnecessary if adequate supply of hydroxocobalamin is available.
Antivenin, *Crotalidae* Polyvalent (equine origin)	Pit viper envenomation (e.g., rattlesnakes, cottonmouths, and timber rattlers)	None	As of March 31, 2007, this product is no longer available from the manufacturer. See Antivenin, *Crotalidae* Polyvalent Immune Fab–Ovine in this chart.

(Continued)

This chart is adapted from material furnished by the Illinois Poison Center, a program of the Metropolitan Chicago Healthcare Council (MCHC).

ANTIDOTE	POISON/DRUG/TOXIN	SUGGESTED MINIMUM STOCK QUANTITY	COMMENTS
Antivenin, *Crotalidae* Polyvalent Immune Fab–Ovine (CroFab®)	Pit viper envenomation (e.g., rattlesnakes, cottonmouths, copperheads, and timber rattlers)	Four to six vials	Advised in geographic areas with endemic populations of copperhead, water moccasin, eastern massasauga, or timber rattlesnake. In low-risk areas, know nearest alternate source of antivenin. This product may have a lower risk of hypersensitivity reaction than previously marketed equine product. Average dose in premarketing trials was 12 vials, but more may be needed. Stock in pharmacy. Store in refrigerator. Equine unavailable after March 31, 2007.
Antivenin, *Latrodectus mactans* (Black widow spider)	Black widow spider envenomation	Zero to one vial	Serious *Latrodectus* envenomations are rare. This product is only used for severe envenomations. Antivenin must be given in a critical care setting since it is an equine-derived product. Know the nearest source of antidote. Note: Product must be refrigerated at all times.
Atropine sulfate	Alpha$_2$ agonists (e.g., clonidine, guanabenz, and guanfacine) Alzheimer's drugs (e.g., donepezil, galantamine, rivastigmine, tacrine) Antimyesthenic agents (e.g., pyridostigmine) Bradyarrhythmia-producing agents (e.g., beta blockers, calcium channel blockers, and digitalis glycosides) Cholinergic agonists (e.g., bethanechol) Muscarine-containing mushrooms (e.g., Clitocybe and Inocybe) Nerve agents (e.g., sarin, soman, tabun, and VX) Organophosphate and carbamate insecticides	Total 100 mg to 150 mg Available in various formulations: 0.4 mg/mL (1 mL, 0.4 mg ampules) 0.4 mg/mL (20 mL, 8 mg vials) 0.1 mg/mL (10 mL, 1 mg ampules) Atropine sulfate military-style auto-injectors: (Atropen®) 2mg/0.7 mL, 1 mg/0.7 mL, 0.5 mg/0.7 mL, 0.25 mg/0.3 mL Atropine sulfate 2.1 mg/0.7 mL with pralidoxime chloride 600 mg/2 mL (DuoDote®)	The product should be immediately available in the ED. Some may also be stored in the pharmacy or other hospital sites, but should be easily mobilized if a severely poisoned patient needs treatment. Note: Product is necessary for adequate preparedness for a weapon of mass destruction (WMD) incident; the suggested amount may not be sufficient for mass-casualty events. Auto-injectors are available from Bound Tree Medical, Inc. Drug stocked in chempack container is intended only for use in mass-casualty events.
Calcium disodium EDTA (Versenate®)	Lead Zinc salts (e.g., zinc chloride)	One 5 mL ampule (200 mg/mL)	Stock in pharmacy. One vial provides one day of therapy for a child. More may be needed in lead-endemic areas. Important note: Edetate disodium (Endrate®) is not the same as calcium disodium EDTA, and is used primarily as an IV chelator for emergent treatment of hypercalcemia, etc.
Calcium chloride and Calcium gluconate	Beta blockers Calcium channel blockers Fluoride salts (e.g., NaF) Hydrofluoric acid (HF) Hyperkalemia (not digoxin-induced) Hypermagnesemia	10% calcium chloride: fifteen 10-mL vials 10% calcium gluconate: five 10-mL vials	Stock in ED. More may be stocked in pharmacy. Many ampules of calcium chloride may be necessary in life-threatening calcium channel blocker or hydrofluoric acid poisoning.

(Continued)

ANTIDOTE	POISON/DRUG/TOXIN	SUGGESTED MINIMUM STOCK QUANTITY	COMMENTS
Deferoxamine mesylate (Desferal®)	Iron	Twelve 500-mg vials	Stock in pharmacy. Note: Per package insert, the maximum daily dose is 6 g (12 vials). However, this dose may be exceeded in serious poisonings.
Digoxin immune Fab (Digibind®, DigiFab®)	Cardiac glycoside-containing plants (e.g., foxglove and oleander) Digitoxin Digoxin	Ten vials	Stock in ED or pharmacy. This amount (ten vials) may be given to a digoxin-poisoned patient in whom the digoxin level is unknown. This amount would effectively neutralize a steady-state digoxin level of 14.2 ng/mL in a 70-kg patient. More may be necessary in severe intoxications. Know nearest source of additional supply.
Dimercaprol (BAL in oil)	Arsenic Copper Gold Lead Lewisite Mercury	Two 3mL-amps (100 mg/mL)	Stock in pharmacy. This amount provides two doses of 3 to 5 mg/kg/dose given q 4 h to treat one seriously poisoned adult or provides enough to treat a 15-kg child for 24 h.
Ethanol	Ethylene glycol Methanol	10% alcohol in D_5W was discontinued in 2004; 5% alcohol in D_5W was discontinued in 2007. However, 10% alcohol can be prepared from dehydrated alcohol and D_5W. 180 mL of 100% ethanol or equivalents. Consult regional poison control center.	Stock in pharmacy. This amount provides enough to treat two adults with a loading dose followed by a maintenance infusion for 4 hours each. More alcohol or fomepizole will be needed during dialysis or prolonged treatment. 95% or 40% alcohol diluted in juice may be given po if IV alcohol is unavailable. Note: Ethanol is unnecessary if fomepizole is stocked. See also fomepizole in this chart.
Flumazenil (Romazicon®)	Benzodiazepines Zaleplon Zolpidem	Total 1 mg: two 5 mL vials (0.1 mg/mL)	Suggested minimum is for ED stocking. Due to risk of seizures, use with extreme caution, if at all, in poisoned patients. More may be stocked in the pharmacy for use in reversal of conscious sedation.
Folic acid and Folinic acid (Leucovorin)	Formaldehyde/Formic Acid Methanol Methotrexate, trimetrexate Pyrimethamine Trimethoprim	Folic acid: three 50-mg vials Folinic acid: one 50-mg vial	Stock in pharmacy. For methanol-poisoned patients with an acidosis, give 50 mg folinic acid initially, then 50 mg of folic acid q 4 h for six doses.
Fomepizole (Antizol®)	Ethylene glycol Methanol	Two 1.5g-vials Note: Available in a kit of four 1.5g-vials	Stock in pharmacy. Know where nearest alternate supply is located. One vial will provide at least one initial adult dose. Hospitals with critical care and hemodialysis capabilities should consider stocking one kit of four vials (enough to treat one patient for up to several days). Note: Product has a 2-year shelf life; however, the manufacturer offers a credit for unused, expired product. Ethanol is unnecessary if adequate supply of fomepizole is stocked.

(Continued)

ANTIDOTE	POISON/DRUG/TOXIN	SUGGESTED MINIMUM STOCK QUANTITY	COMMENTS
Glucagon	Beta blockers Calcium channel blockers Hypoglycemia Hypoglycemic agents	Fifty 1-mg vials	Stock 20 mg in ED and remainder in pharmacy. The total amount (50 mg) provides approximately 5 to 10 hours of high-dose therapy in life-threatening beta blocker or calcium channel blocker poisoning. A protocol using high doses of insulin/dextrose also may be considered. Consult regional poison center for guidelines.
Hydroxocobalamin (Cyanokit®)	Acetonitrile Acrylonitrile Cyanide (e.g., HCN, KCN and NaCN) Cyanogen chloride Cyanogenic glycoside natural sources (e.g., apricot pits and peach pits) Laetrile Nitroprusside Smoke inhalation (combustion of synthetic materials)	Two to four kits Each kit contains two 2.5-vials Note: Diluent is not included in the kit.	Seriously poisoned cyanide patients may require 5-10 g (one to two kits). Stock two kits in ED. Consider also stocking two kits in the pharmacy. The product has a shelf-life of 30 months post-manufacture. Due to its favorable safety profile, this product may be used in a pre-hospital setting.
Hyperbaric oxygen (HBO)	Carbon monoxide Carbon tetrachloride Cyanide Hydrogen sulfide Methemoglobinemia	Post the location and phone number of nearest HBO chamber in the ED.	Consult IPC to determine if HBO treatment is indicated.
Methylene blue	Methemoglobin-inducing agents including: Aniline dyes Dapsone Dinitrophenol Local anesthetics (e.g., benzocaine) Metoclopramide Monomethylhydrazine-containing mushrooms (e.g., Gyromitra) Naphthalene Nitrates and nitrites Nitrobenzene Phenazopyridine	Three 10-mL amps (10 mg/mL)	Stock in pharmacy. This amount provides three doses of 1 to 2 mg/kg (0.1 to 0.2 mL/kg) for an adult patient.
Nalmefene (Revex®) and Naloxone (Narcan®)	ACE inhibitors $Alpha_2$ agonists (e.g., clonidine, guanabenz, and guanfacine) Coma of unknown cause Imidazoline decongestants (e.g., oxymetazoline and tetrahydrozoline) Loperamide Opioids (e.g., codeine, dextromethorphan, diphenoxylate, fentanyl, heroin, meperidine, morphine, and propoxyphene)	Nalmefene: none required Naloxone: total 40 mg, any combination of 0.4-mg, 1-mg, and 2-mg ampules	Stock 20 mg naloxone in the ED and 20 mg elsewhere in the institution. Note: Nalmefene has a longer duration of action but it offers no therapeutic advantage over a maloxone infusion.
D-Penicillamine (Cuprimine®)	Arsenic Copper Lead Mercury	None required as an antidote. Available in bottles of 100 capsules (125 mg or 250 mg/capsule)	D-penicillamine is no longer considered the drug of choice for heavy-metal poisonings. It may be stocked in the pharmacy for other indications such as Wilson's disease or rheumatoid arthritis.

(Continued)

ANTIDOTE	POISON/DRUG/TOXIN	SUGGESTED MINIMUM STOCK QUANTITY	COMMENTS
Physostigmine salicylate (Antilirium®)	Anticholinergic alkaloid-containing plants (e.g., deadly nightshade and jimson weed) Antihistamines Atropine and other anticholinergic agents Intrathecal baclofen	Two 2-mL ampules (1 mg/mL)	Stock in ED or pharmacy. Usual adult dose is 1 to 2 mg slow IV push. Note: Duration of effect is 30 to 60 min.
Phytonadione (Vitamin K_1) (AquaMEPHYTON®, Mephyton®)	Indandione derivatives Long-acting anticoagulant rodenticides (e.g., brodifacoum and bromadiolone)	Two 0.5-mL ampules (2 mg/mL) and ten 1-mL ampules (10 mg/mL) 5-mg tablets available in packages of 10, 14, 20, 30, and 100	Stock in pharmacy.
Pralidoxime chloride (2-PAM) (Protopam®)	Antimyesthenic agents (e.g., pyridostigmine) Nerve agents (e.g., sarin, soman, tabun, and VX) Organophosphate insecticides Tacrine	Six 1-g vials Pralidoxime chloride military-style auto-injectors: 600 mg/2 mL	Stock in ED or pharmacy. Note: Serious intoxications may require 500 mg/h (12 g/day). Product is necessary for adequate preparedness for a weapon of mass destruction (WMD) incident; the suggested amount may not be sufficient for mass-casualty events. Auto-injectors are available from Bound Tree Medical, Inc. Drug stocked in chempack container is intended only for use in mass-casualty events.
Protamine sulfate	Enoxaparin Heparin	Variable, consider recommendation of hospital P&T Committee Available as 5-mL ampules (10 mg/mL) and 25-mL vials (250 mg/25 mL)	Stock in pharmacy.
Pyridoxine hydrochloride (Vitamin B_6)	Acrylamide Ethylene glycol Hydrazine Isoniazid (INH) Monomethylhydrazine-containing mushrooms (e.g., Gyromitra)	100 1-mL vials (100 mg/mL vials)	Stock in ED or pharmacy. Usual dose is 1 g pyridoxine HCl for each gram of INH ingested. If amount ingested is unknown, give 5 g of pyridoxine. Repeat dose if seizures are uncontrolled. Know nearest source of additional supply. For ethylene glycol, a dose of 100 mg/day enhances the clearance of toxic metabolite.
Sodium bicarbonate	Chlorine gas Hyperkalemia Serum alkalinization: Agents producing a quinidine-like effect as noted by widened QRS complex on EKG (e.g., amantadine, carbamazepine, chloroquine, cocaine, diphenhydramine, flecainide, propafenone, propoxyphene, tricyclic antidepressants, quinidine, and related agents) Urine alkalinization: Weakly acidic agents (e.g., chlorophenoxy herbicides, chlorpropamide, phenobarbital, and salicylates)	Twenty 50-mEq vials	Stock 10 vials in the ED and 10 vials elsewhere in the hospital.
Succimer (Chemet®)	Arsenic Lead Lewisite Mercury	One bottle of 100 capsules (100 mg/capsule)	Stock in pharmacy. FDA-approved only for pediatric lead poisoning; however, it has shown efficacy for other heavy-metal poisonings.

SUGAR-FREE PRODUCTS

The following is a selection of products by therapeutic category that contain no sugar. When recommending these products to diabetic patients, keep in mind that many may contain sorbitol, alcohol, or other sources of carbohydrates. This list is not all-inclusive and generics and alternate brands may be available. Check product labeling for a current listing of inactive ingredients.

Product	Manufacturer
Analgesics	
Addaprin Tablets	Dover
Aminofen Tablets	Dover
Aminofen Max Tablets	Dover
Aspirtab Tablets	Dover
Back Pain-Off Tablets‡	Medique
Buffasal Tablets	Dover
Dyspel Tablets	Dover
I-Prin Tablets‡	Medique
Medi-Seltzer Effervescent Tablets	Medique
Methadose Sugar Free Oral Concentrate	Mallinckrodt
Ms.-Aid Tablets‡	Medique
Children's Silapap Liquid	Silarx
Antacids/Antiflatulents	
Alcalak Chewable Tablets*† ‡ §	Medique
Dimacid Chewable Tablets	Otis Clapp & Son
Diotame Chewable Tablets*† ‡ §	Medique
Neutralin Tablets	Dover
Pepto-Bismol Caplets† ‡	Procter & Gamble
Tums E-X Sugar Free Tablets* §	GlaxoSmithKline Consumer
Anti-asthmatic/Respiratory Agents	
Jay-Phyl Syrup	JayMac
Antidiarrheals	
Diarrest Tablets	Dover
Imogen Liquid	Pharm Generic
Blood Modifiers/Iron Preparations	
I.L.X. B-12 Elixir	Kenwood
Nephro-Fer Tablets‡	Rugby
Corticosteroid	
Pediapred Solution* §	UCB
Cough/Cold/Allergy Preparations	
Alacol DM Syrup	Ballay
Alacol Solution	Ballay
Anaplex DMX Syrup	ECR
Andehist DM NR Syrup	Cypress
Andehist NR Syrup	Cypress
Aquatab C Tablets	Deston
Aridex Solution	Gentex
Baltussin Solution	Ballay
Children's Benadryl-D Allergy & Sinus Liquid*† §	Johnson & Johnson
Bromhist-DM Solution	Cypress
Bromhist Pediatric Solution	Cypress
Bromphenex DM Solution*† §	Breckenridge
Bromplex DM Solution*† §	Prasco
Broncotron Liquid	Seyer Pharmatec
Broncotron-D Suspension	Seyer Pharmatec
B-Tuss Liquid	Blansett
Carbaphen 12 Ped Suspension	Gil
Carbaphen 12 Suspension	Gil
Carbatuss-12 Suspension	GM
Carbatuss-CL Solution	GM
Carbetaplex Liquid* §	Breckenridge
Carbofed DM Liquid	Hi-Tech
Carbofed DM Syrup	Hi-Tech
Cardec DM Syrup	Qualitest
Cardec Solution	Qualitest
Cetafen Cough & Cold Tablets‡	Hart Health and Safety
Cetafen Cold Tablets‡	Hart Health and Safety
Cheratussin DAC Liquid	Qualitest
Chlordex GP Syrup	Cypress
Codal-DM Syrup	Cypress
Coldcough PD Syrup* §	Breckenridge
Coldcough Syrup* §	Breckenridge
Coldonyl Tablets	Dover
Corfen DM Solution	Cypress
Crantex Syrup	Breckenridge
Dacex-DM Solution	Cypress
Dallergy Drops*† §	Laser
De-Chlor DM Solution	Cypress
De-Chlor DR Solution	Cypress
De-Chlor HD Solution	Cypress
Despec Liquid	International Ethical

* Contains sorbitol.
† May contain other sugar alcohols (eg, glycerol, isomalt, maltitol, mannitol, xylitol).
‡ May contain other sources of carbohydrates (eg, cellulose, lactose, maltodextrin, polydextrose, starch).
§ May contain natural or artificial flavors.

Despec-SF Liquid	International Ethical
Diabetic Tussin Allergy Relief Liquid§	Health Care Products
Diabetic Tussin Allergy Relief Tablets	Health Care Products
Diabetic Tussin Cold & Flu Gelcaplets†	Health Care Products
Diabetic Tussin DM Liquid§	Health Care Products
Diabetic Tussin EX Liquid§	Health Care Products
Diabetic Tussin Solution§	Health Care Products
Diphen Capsules‡	Medique
Donatussin Drops*† §	Laser
Double Tussin DM Liquid	Reese
Duratuss DM Elixir*† ‡ §	Victory
Dytan-CS Tablets	Hawthorn
Emagrin Forte Tablets	Otis Clapp & Son
Emagrin Tablets	Otis Clapp & Son
Endacof DM Solution*†	Larken Laboratories
Endacof-PD Solution† §	Larken Laboratories
Endal HD Plus Liquid	Pediamed
Ganidin NR Liquid	Cypress
Gani-Tuss NR Liquid	Cypress
Gani-Tuss-DM NR Liquid	Cypress
Genebronco-D Liquid	Pharm Generic
Genecof-HC Liquid	Pharm Generic
Genecof-XP Liquid	Pharm Generic
Genedel Syrup	Pharm Generic
Genedotuss-DM Liquid	Pharm Generic
Genelan Liquid	Pharm Generic
Genetuss-2 Liquid	Pharm Generic
Genexpect DM Liquid	Pharm Generic
Genexpect SF Liquid	Pharm Generic
Gilphex TR Tablets	Gil
Giltuss Liquid§	Gil
Giltuss Ped-C Solution§	Gil
Giltuss Pediatric Liquid§	Gil
Giltuss TR Tablets	Gil
Guiadex DM Liquid*† §	Breckenridge
Halotussin AC Liquid	Axiom
Halotussin DAC Solution	Axiom
Lodrane D Suspension	ECR
Lohist-PD Solution*† §	Larken
Marcof Expectorant Syrup	Marnel
Metanx Tablets‡	Pamlab
Nalex DH Liquid	Blansett
Nalex A Liquid	Blansett
Neo DM Drops*† §	Laser
Neo DM Syrup*† §	Laser
Neotuss-D Liquid† §	A.G. Marin
Neotuss S/F Liquid† §	A.G. Marin
Niferex Elixir* ‡ §	Ther-Rx
Norel DM Liquid*† §	U.S. Pharmaceutical
Nycoff Tablets	Dover
Organidin NR Liquid† §	Meda
Organidin NR Tablets‡	Meda
Phanasin Syrup	Pharmakon
Phanasin Diabetic Choice Syrup	Pharmakon
Phanatuss Syrup	Pharmakon
Phanatuss DM Diabetic Choice Syrup	Pharmakon
Phanatuss-HC Diabetic Choice Solution	Pharmakon
Phena-HC Solution	GM
Phenabid Tablets	Gil
Phenabid DM Tablets	Gil
Phena-S 12 Suspension	GM
Phena-S Liquid	GM
Poly Hist DM	Poly
Poly Hist PD Solution	Poly
Prolex DM Liquid	Blansett
Quintex Syrup	Qualitest
Rescon-DM Liquid* §	Capellon
Rondec Syrup*†	Sciele
Rondec DM*†	Sciele
Ru-Tuss DM Syrup*† §	Carwin
Safetussin Liquid	Kramer
Scot-Tussin Diabetes CF Liquid	Scot-Tussin
Scot-Tussin DM Cough Chasers Lozenge	Scot-Tussin
Scot-Tussin DM Maximum Strength	Scot-Tussin
Scot-Tussin Expectorant Solution	Scot-Tussin
Scot-Tussin Senior Solution	Scot-Tussin
Siladryl Allergy Solution* §	Silarx
Sildec Syrup*† §	Silarx

* Contains sorbitol.
† May contain other sugar alcohols (eg, glycerol, isomalt, maltitol, mannitol, xylitol).
‡ May contain other sources of carbohydrates (eg, cellulose, lactose, maltodextrin, polydextrose, starch).
§ May contain natural or artificial flavors.

Sildec DM Syrup*† §	Silarx
Sildec PE-DM Syrup*† §	Silarx
Sildec-PE Syrup*† §	Silarx
Silexin Syrup	Otis Clapp & Son
Silexin Tablets	Otis Clapp & Son
Siltussin DAS Liquid*† §	Silarx
Siltussin DM DAS Cough Formula Syrup*† §	Silarx
Siltussin SA Liquid*† §	Silarx
Statuss Green Liquid* §	Magna
Children's Sudafed PE Cough & Cold Liquid*† §	Pfizer
Children's Sudafed Nasal Decongestant Liquid*† §	Pfizer
Sudanyl Tablets	Dover
Sudatuss-SF Liquid	Pharm Generic Developers
Supress DX Pediatric Drops† §	Kramer-Novis
Suttar-SF Syrup	Gil
Tanacof XR Suspension*† ‡ §	Larken
Tusdec-DM Solution*† §	Cypress
Tusnel Solution	Llorens
Tussall Solution* §	Everett
Tussi-Organidin DM NR Solution*† §	Victory
Tussi-Organidin DM-S NR Solution*† §	Victory
Tussi-Organidin NR Solution*† §	Victory
Tussi-Organidin-S NR	Victory
Tussi-Pres Liquid† §	Kramer-Novis
Vazol Solution	Wraser
Vi-Q-Tuss Syrup	Qualitest
Z-Tuss DM Syrup† §	Magna
Ztuss Expectorant Solution* §	Magna

Fluoride Preparations

Fluor-A-Day Tablets*† §	Pharmascience
Fluor-A-Day Liquid	Pharmascience
Lozi-Flur Lozenge* §	Dreir
Sensodyne with Fluoride Cool Gel*† ‡ §	GlaxoSmithKline Consumer
Sensodyne Tartar Control with Whitening† ‡ §	GlaxoSmithKline Consumer
Sensodyne w/Fluoride Toothpaste Original Flavor*† ‡ §	GlaxoSmithKline Consumer

Laxatives

Benefiber Powder	Novartis
Citrucel Powder‡ §	GlaxoSmithKline Consumer
Colace Liquid 1% Solution	Purdue Products
Fiber Choice Tablets* ‡ §	GlaxoSmithKline Consumer
Fibro-XL Capsules	Key
Genfiber Powder	Teva
Konsyl Easy Mix Formula Powder‡	Konsyl
Konsyl Orange Powder‡ §	Konsyl
Konsyl Powder‡	Konsyl
Metamucil Smooth Texture Powder‡	Procter & Gamble
Reguloid Powder Regular Flavor‡	Rugby
Reguloid Powder Orange Flavor‡ §	Rugby

Mouth/Throat Preparations

Cepacol Dual Relief Sore Throat Spray† §	Combe
Cepacol Maximum Strength Spray*† §	Combe
Cepacol Sore Throat + Coating Relief Lozenge† §	Combe
Cepacol Sore Throat Lozenges† §	Combe
Cheracol Sore Throat Spray†	Lee
Chloraseptic Spray*†§	Prestige
Diabetic Tussin Cough Drops† §	Health Care Products
Fisherman's Friend Sugar Free Mint Lozenges*	Mentholatum
Fresh N Free Liquid	Geritrex
Larynex Lozenges	Dover
Listerine Pocketpaks Film‡ §	Johnson & Johnson
Luden's Sugar Free Wild Cherry Throat Drops† §	Johnson & Johnson
Medikoff Sugar Free Drops†	Medique
N'ice Lozenges* §	Heritage/Insight
Oragesic Solution* §	Parnell
Oragel Dry Mouth Moisturizing Gel*† ‡ §	Del
Orajel Dry Mouth Moisturizing Spray† ‡ §	Del
Sepasoothe Lozenges* ‡ §	Medique
Thorets Maximum Strength Lozenges	Otis Clapp & Son
Triaminic Sore Throat Spray*† §	Novartis

Vitamins/Minerals/Supplements

Action Tabs Made for Men‡	Action Labs
Adaptoside R+R For Stress Liquid	HVS

Adaptoside R+R For Acute Stress Liquid	HVS
Alamag Tablets*† ‡ §	Medique
Alcalak Tablets*† ‡	Medique
Apetigen Elixir*†	Kramer-Novis
Apptrim Capsules	Physician Therapeutics
Apptrim-D Capsules	Physician Therapeutics
Bevitamel Tablets	Westlake
Biosode Liquid	HVS
Biotect Plus Caplet	Gil
Bugs Bunny Complete	Bayer
C&M Caps-375 Capsules	Key
Cal-Cee Tablets	Key
Calcet Plus Tablets	Mission Pharmacal
Calcimin-300 Tablets	Key
Cal-Mint Chewable Tablets*† ‡	Freeda Vitamins
Cerefolin NAC Tablets	Pamlab
Chromacaps‡	Key
Delta D3 Tablets‡	Freeda Vitamins
Detoxosode Liquids	HVS
Dexfol Tablets‡	Rising
DHEA Capsules	ADH Health Products
Diatx ZN Tablets‡	Pamlab
Dimacid Tablets	Otis Clapp & Son
Diucaps Capsules	Legere
DL-Phen-500 Capsules	Key
Enterex Diabetic Liquid‡	Victus
Evening Primose Oil Capsules†	National Vitamin
Ex-L Tablets‡	Key
Extress Tablets	Key
Eyetamins Tablets‡	Rexall Consumer
Fem-Cal Citrate Tablets‡	Freeda Vitamins
Fem-Cal Tablets‡	Freeda Vitamins
Fem-Cal Plus Tablets	Freeda Vitamins
Ferrocite Plus Tablets‡	Breckenridge
Folacin-800 Tablets‡	Key
Folbee Plus Tablets‡	Breckenridge
Folbee Tablets‡	Breckenridge
Folplex 2.2 Tablets‡	Breckenridge
Foltx Tablets‡	Pamlab
Gabadone Capsules	Physician Therapeutics
Gram-O-Leci Tablets*† ‡	Freeda Vitamins
Herbal Slim Complex Capsules	ADH Health Products
Hypertensa Capsules‡	Physician Therapeutics
Lynae Calcium/Vitamin C Chewable Tablets	Boscogen
Lynae Chondroitin/ Glucosamine Capsules	Boscogen
Lynae Ginse-Cool Chewable Tablets	Boscogen
Mag-Ox 400 Tablets	Blaine
Mag-SR Tablets‡	Cypress
Mag-SR Plus Calcium Tablets‡	Cypress
Magimin Tablets‡	Key
Maginex Tablets‡	Logan
Magnacaps Capsules‡	Key
Mangimin Tablets‡	Key
Medi-Lyte Tablets‡	Medique
Metanx Tablets‡	Pamlab
Multi-Delyn with Iron Liquid†	Silarx
Natelle C Tablets	Azur
Natelle Tablets	Azur
Nephro-Fer Tablets‡	Rugby
New Life Hair Tablets‡	Rexall Consumer
Niferex Elixir* ‡ §	Ther-Rx
Nutrisure OTC Tablets	Westlake
Nutrivit Solution*† §	Llorens
Ob Complete Tablets	Vertical
O-Cal Fa Tablets‡	Pharmics
Os-Cal 500 + D Tablets‡	GlaxoSmithKline Consumer
Powervites Tablets‡	Green Turtle Bay Vitamin
Prostaplex Herbal Complex Capsules	ADH Health Products
Protect Plus Liquid	Gil
Protect Plus Liquid NR Softgels	Gil
Pulmona Capsules	Physician Therapeutics
Quintabs-M Tablets‡	Freeda Vitamins
Replace Capsules‡	Key
Replace w/o Iron Capsules‡	Key
Resource Arginaid Powder‡	Novartis Nutrition

* Contains sorbitol.
† May contain other sugar alcohols (eg, glycerol, isomalt, maltitol, mannitol, xylitol).
‡ May contain other sources of carbohydrates (eg, cellulose, lactose, maltodextrin, polydextrose, starch).
§ May contain natural or artificial flavors.

Ribo-100 T.D. Capsules	Key
Samolinic Softgels†	Key
Sea Omega 30 Softgels†	Rugby
Sea Omega 50 Softgels†	Rugby
Sentra AM Capsules	Physician Therapeutics
Sentra PM Capsules	Physician Therapeutics
Soy Care for Menopause Capsules	Inverness Medical
Span C Tablets‡	Freeda Vitamins
Strovite Forte Syrup	Everett
Sunnie Tablets	Green Turtle Bay Vitamin
Sunvite Tablets† ‡	Rexall Naturalist
Super Dec B100 Tablets‡	Freeda Vitamins
Super Quints B-50 Tablets‡	Freeda Vitamins
Supervite Liquid	Seyer Pharmatec
Suplevit Liquid	Gil
Theramine Capsules	Physician Therapeutics
Triamin Tablets	Key
Triamino Tablets* ‡	Freeda Vitamins
Ultramino Powder	Freeda Vitamins
Uro-Mag Capsules ‡	Blaine
Vitafol Tablets† ‡	Everett
Vitamin C/Rose Hips Tablets	ADH Health Products
Vitrum Jr Chewable Tablets† ‡ §	Mason Vitamins
Xtramins Tablets	Key
Yohimbe Power Max 1500 for Women Tablets‡	Action Labs
Ze Plus Softgel	Everett

Miscellaneous

Acidoll Capsules	Key
Alka-Gest Tablets	Key
Bicitra Solution† §	Ortho-McNeil
Cafergot Tablets‡	Sandoz
Cytra-2 Solution* §	Cypress
Cytra-K Solution* §	Cypress
Cytra-K Crystals	Cypress
Melatin Tablets‡	Mason Vitamins
Namenda Solution*† §	Forest
Polycitra-K Crystals	Ortho-McNeil
Prosed/DS Tablets‡	Ferring
Questran Light Powder‡ §	Par
Soltamox Solution*† ‡	Cytogen

SULFITE-CONTAINING PRODUCTS

The following is a selection of products that contain sulfites, a common allergic trigger. Please remember, however, that the list is not comprehensive. Always check product labeling for definitive information on specific ingredients.

PRODUCT	GENERIC NAME
Alphaquin HP	Hydroquinone
Amikacin Sulfate Injection	Amikacin sulfate
Amikin Injectable	Amikacin sulfate
Apokyn	Apomorphine hydrochloride
Aramine Injection	Metaraminol
Betagan Liquifilm	Levobunolol
Betagan Ophthalmic Solution, USP	Levobunolol hydrochloride
Campral (residual traces)	Acamprosate calcium
Claripel Cream	Hydroquinone
Corlopam Injection	Fenoldopam mesylate
Cortisporin Otic Solution	Hydrocortisone/neomycin sulfate/polymyxin B
Decadron Phosphate Ophthalmic Solution	Dexamethasone sodium phosphate
Decadron Phosphate Injection	Dexamethasone sodium phosphate
Dilaudid Ampules, Dilaudid Tablets, Dilaudid Non-Sterile Powder	Hydromorphone
Dilaudid-HP Injection, Dilaudid-HP Lyophilized Powder 250 mg	Hydromorphone
Dilaudid Oral Liquid; Dilaudid Tablets - 2 mg, 4 mg, 8 mg	Hydromorphone
Dobutamine Injection	Dobutamine Injection
Dopamine HCl Injection	Dopamine HCl
Eldopaque Forte 4%	Hydroquinone
Eldoquin Forte 4%	Hydroquinone
EpiPen Auto-Injector	Epinephrine
EpiPen Jr. Auto-Injector	Epinephrine
EpiQuin Micro	Hydroquinone
Gentamicin Sulfate Injection	Gentamicin sulfate
Innohep Injection	Tinzaparin sodium
Ketoconazole Cream	Ketoconazole
Klaron Lotion 10%	Sodium sulfacetamide
Levophed Injection	Norepinephrine
Lustra	Hydroquinone
Lustra-AF	Hydroquinone
Marcaine Hydrochloride/ Epinephrine 1:200,000	Bupivacaine/epinephrine bitartrate
Melpaque HP	Hydroquinone
Melquin HP	Hydroquinone
Morphine Sulfate Injection	Morphine sulfate
Nizoral A-D	Ketoconazole
Norflex Injection	Orphenadrine
Novocain Hydrochloride for Spinal Anesthesia	Procaine
Nubain Ampules/Multiple-Dose Vials	Nalbuphine
Nuquin HP	Hydroquinone
Orphenadrine Citrate Injection	Orphenadrine citrate
Perphenazine Injections/Tablets	Perphenazine
Phenergan Injection	Promethazine hydrochloride
Pred Forte Ophthalmic Solution	Prednisolone acetate
Pred Mild Ophthalmic Solution	Prednisolone acetate
Propofol Injectable Emulsion	Propofol
Rowasa Enema	Mesalamine
Sensorcaine with Epinephrine Injection	Bupivacaine/epinephrine bitartrate
Sensorcaine-MPF with Epinephrine Injection	Bupivacaine/epinephrine bitartrate
SMZ-TMP Concentrate	Trimethoprim/sulfamethoxazole
Solaquin Forte 4% Cream; 4% Gel	Hydroquinone
Soma Compound with Codeine	Carisoprodol/aspirin/ codeine
Streptomycin Sulfate Injection	Streptomycin sulfate
Sulfamylon Cream	Mafenide acetate
Sumycin Suspension	Tetracycline hydrochloride
Talacen	Pentazocine hydrochloride/ acetaminophen
Tobramycin Sulfate Injection	Tobramycin sulfate
Torecan Injection	Triethylperazine maleate
Tri-Luma	Fluocinolone acetonide/ hydroquinone/tretinoin
Twinject Injection	Epinephrine
Tylenol with Codeine Tablets	Acetaminophen/codeine
Tylox Capsules	Acetaminophen/oxycodone
Vibramycin Syrup	Doxycycline calcium
Xibrom Ophthalmic	Bromfenac
Xylocaine with Epinephrine Injection	Lidocaine/epinephrine

USE-IN-PREGNANCY RATINGS

The U.S. Food and Drug Administration's Use-in-Pregnancy rating system weighs the degree to which available information has ruled out risk to the fetus against the drug's potential benefit to the patient. Below is a listing of drugs (by generic name) for which ratings are available.

X

Contraindicated in pregnancy

Studies in animals or humans, or investigational or postmarketing reports, have demonstrated fetal risk, which clearly outweighs any possible benefit to the patient.

Acetohydroxamic Acid
Acitretin
Ambrisentan
Amlodipine Besylate/Atorvastatin Calcium
Atorvastatin Calcium
Bexarotene
Bicalutamide
Bosentan
Cetrorelix Acetate
Clomiphene Citrate
Desogestrel/Ethinyl Estradiol
Diclofenac Sodium/Misoprostol
Dihydroergotamine Mesylate
Dutasteride
Estazolam
Estradiol
Estradiol Acetate
Estradiol Cypionate/Medroxyprogesterone Acetate
Estradiol Valerate
Estradiol/Levonorgestrel
Estradiol/Norethindrone Acetate
Estrogens, Conjugated
Estrogens, Conjugated, Synthetic A
Estrogens, Conjugated/Medroxyprogesterone Acetate
Estrogens, Esterified
Estrogens, Esterified/Methyltestosterone
Estropipate
Ethinyl Estradiol/Drospirenone
Ethinyl Estradiol/Ethynodiol Diacetate
Ethinyl Estradiol/Etonogestrel
Ethinyl Estradiol/Ferrous Fumarate/Norethindrone Acetate
Ethinyl Estradiol/Levonorgestrel
Ethinyl Estradiol/Norelgestromin
Ethinyl Estradiol/Norethindrone Acetate
Ethinyl Estradiol/Norgestimate
Ethinyl Estradiol/Norgestrel
Ezetimibe/Simvastatin
Finasteride
Fluorouracil
Flurazepam Hydrochloride
Fluvastatin Sodium
Follitropin Alfa
Follitropin Beta
Ganirelix Acetate
Goserelin Acetate
Histrelin Acetate
Hydromorphone Hydrochloride
Interferon Alfa-2B, Recombinant/Ribavirin
Iodine I 131 Tositumomab/Tositumomab
Isotretinoin
Leflunomide
Leuprolide Acetate
Levonorgestrel
Lovastatin
Lovastatin/Niacin
Medroxyprogesterone Acetate
Megestrol Acetate
Menotropins
Mequinol/Tretinoin
Mestranol/Norethindrone
Methotrexate Sodium
Methyltestosterone
Miglustat
Misoprostol
Nafarelin Acetate
Niacin/Simvastatin
Norethindrone
Norethindrone Acetate
Norgestrel
Oxandrolone
Oxymetholone
Plicamycin
Pravastatin Sodium
Pravastatin Sodium/Aspirin Buffered
Raloxifene Hydrochloride
Ribavirin
Rosuvastatin Calcium
Simvastatin
Tazarotene
Testosterone
Testosterone Enanthate
Thalidomide
Tositumomab
Triptorelin Pamoate
Warfarin Sodium

D

Positive evidence of risk

Investigational or postmarketing data show risk to the fetus. Nevertheless, potential benefits may outweigh the potential risk.

Aliskiren*
Aliskiren/Hydrochlorothiazide
Alitretinoin
Alprazolam
Altretamine
Amiodarone Hydrochloride
Amlodipine Besylate/Benazepril Hydrochloride
Amlodipine Besylate/Olmesartan Medoxomil*
Amlodipine Besylate/Valsartan
Anastrozole
Arsenic Trioxide
Aspirin Buffered/Pravastatin Sodium
Aspirin/Dipyridamole
Atenolol
Azacitidine
Azathioprine
Azathioprine Sodium
Benazepril Hydrochloride
Benazepril Hydrochloride/Hydrochlorothiazide
Bendamustine Hydrochloride
Bortezomib
Busulfan
Candesartan Cilexetil*
Candesartan Cilexetil/Hydrochlorothiazide*
Capecitabine
Captopril*
Carbamazepine
Carboplatin
Carmustine (BiCNU)
Chlorambucil
Cladribine
Clofarabine
Clonazepam
Cytarabine Liposome
Dactinomycin
Dasatinib
Daunorubicin Citrate Liposome
Daunorubicin Hydrochloride
Demeclocycline Hydrochloride
Dexrazoxane
Diazepam

* Category C or D depending on the trimester the drug is given.

Divalproex Sodium
Docetaxel
Doxorubicin Hydrochloride
Doxorubicin Hydrochloride Liposome
Doxycycline
Doxycycline Calcium
Doxycycline Hyclate
Doxycycline Monohydrate
Efavirenz
Enalapril Maleate*
Enalapril Maleate/
Hydrochlorothiazide*
Epirubicin Hydrochloride
Eprosartan Mesylate
Erlotinib
Exemestane
Floxuridine
Fludarabine Phosphate
Flutamide
Fosinopril Sodium*
Fosinopril Sodium/
Hydrochlorothiazide*
Fosphenytoin Sodium
Fulvestrant
Gemcitabine Hydrochloride
Gemtuzumab Ozogamicin
Goserelin Acetate
Ibritumomab Tiuxetan
Idarubicin Hydrochloride
Ifosfamide
Imatinib Mesylate
Irbesartan*
Irbesartan/Hydrochlorothiazide*
Irinotecan Hydrochloride
Ixabepilone
Letrozole
Lisinopril*
Lisinopril/Hydrochlorothiazide*
Lithium Carbonate
Losartan Potassium*
Losartan Potassium/
Hydrochlorothiazide*
Mechlorethamine Hydrochloride
Melphalan Hydrochloride
Mephobarbital
Mercaptopurine
Methimazole
Midazolam Hydrochloride
Minocycline Hydrochloride
Mitoxantrone Hydrochloride
Moexipril Hydrochloride*
Moexipril Hydrochloride/
Hydrochlorothiazide
Mycophenolate Mofetil
Mycophenolic Acid
Nelarabine
Neomycin Sulfate/
Polymyxin B Sulfate
Nicotine
Nilotinib
Nilotinib Hydrochloride Monohydrate
Olmesartan Medoxomil
Oxaliplatin
Pamidronate Disodium
Paroxetine Hydrochloride
Paroxetine Mesylate
Pemetrexed
Penicillamine
Pentobarbital Sodium
Pentostatin
Perindopril Erbumine
Phenytoin
Procarbazine Hydrochloride
Quinapril Hydrochloride*
Quinapril Hydrochloride/
Hydrochlorothiazide*
Ramipril*
Sorafenib
Streptomycin Sulfate
Sunitinib
Tamoxifen Citrate
Telmisartan*
Telmisartan/Hydrochlorothiazide*
Temozolomide
Temsirolimus
Thioguanine
Tigecycline
Tobramycin
Topotecan Hydrochloride
Toremifene Citrate
Trandolapril*
Trandolapril/Verapamil
Hydrochloride*
Tretinoin
Valproate Sodium
Valproic Acid
Valsartan
Valsartan/Hydrochlorothiazide
Vinorelbine Tartrate
Voriconazole
Zoledronic Acid

C

Risk cannot be ruled out

Human studies are lacking, and animal studies are either positive for risk or are lacking as well. However, potential benefits may outweigh the potential risk.

Abacavir Sulfate
Abacavir Sulfate/Lamivudine
Abacavir Sulfate/
Lamivudine/Zidovudine
Abciximab
Acamprosate Calcium
Acetaminophen
Acetaminophen/
Butalbital/Caffeine
Acetaminophen/Caffeine/
Chlorpheniramine Maleate/
Hydrocodone Bitartrate/
Phenylephrine Hydrochloride
Acetazolamide
Acetazolamide Sodium
Acyclovir
Adapalene
Adefovir Dipivoxil
Adenosine
Albendazole
Albumin (Human)
Albuterol Sulfate
Albuterol Sulfate/
Ipratropium Bromide
Alclometasone Dipropionate
Aldesleukin
Alemtuzumab
Alendronate Sodium
Alendronate Sodium/Cholecalciferol
Aliskiren*
Allopurinol Sodium
Almotriptan Malate
Alpha1-Proteinase Inhibitor (Human)
Alprostadil
Alteplase
Amantadine Hydrochloride
Amifostine
Aminocaproic Acid
Aminohippurate Sodium
Aminolevulinic Acid Hydrochloride
Aminosalicylic Acid
Amlodipine Besylate
Amlodipine Besylate/
Olmesartan Medoxomil*
Amoxicillin/Clarithromycin/
Lansoprazole
Amphetamine Aspartate/
Amphetamine Sulfate/
Dextroamphetamine
Saccharate/Dextroamphetamine
Sulfate
Anagrelide Hydrochloride
Anthralin
Antihemophilic Factor (Human)
Antihemophilic Factor
(Recombinant)
Anti-Inhibitor Coagulant Complex
Anti-Thymocyte Globulin
Apomorphine Hydrochloride
Aripiprazole
Armodafinil
Arnica Montana/Herbals,
Multiple/Sulfur
Asparaginase
Atomoxetine Hydrochloride
Atovaquone
Atovaquone/Proguanil
Hydrochloride
Atropine Sulfate/Benzoic Acid/
Hyoscyamine Sulfate/
Methenamine/Methylene Blue/
Phenyl Salicylate
Atropine Sulfate/Hyoscyamine
Sulfate/Scopolamine
Hydrobromide
Azelastine Hydrochloride
Bacitracin Zinc/Neomycin
Sulfate/Polymyxin B Sulfate

Baclofen
BCG, Live (Intravesical)
Becaplermin
Beclomethasone Dipropionate
Beclomethasone Dipropionate Monohydrate
Bendroflumethiazide
Benzocaine
Benzonatate
Benzoyl Peroxide
Benzoyl Peroxide/Clindamycin
Benzoyl Peroxide/Erythromycin
Betamethasone Dipropionate
Betamethasone Dipropionate/Clotrimazole
Betamethasone Valerate
Betaxolol Hydrochloride
Bethanechol Chloride
Bevacizumab
Bimatoprost
Bisacodyl/Polyethylene Glycol/ Potassium Chloride/Sodium Bicarbonate/Sodium Chloride
Bisoprolol Fumarate
Bisoprolol Fumarate/ Hydrochlorothiazide
Black Widow Spider Antivenin (Equine)
Botulinum Toxin Type A
Botulinum Toxin Type B
Brimonidine Tartrate/ Timolol Maleate
Brinzolamide
Brompheniramine Maleate/ Dextromethorphan Hydrobromide/Phenylephrine Hydrochloride
Budesonide
Bupivacaine Hydrochloride
Bupivacaine Hydrochloride/ Epinephrine Bitartrate
Buprenorphine Hydrochloride
Buprenorphine Hydrochloride/ Naloxone Hydrochloride
Bupropion Hydrobromide
Bupropion Hydrochloride
Butabarbital/Hyoscyamine Hydrobromide/ Phenazopyridine Hydrochloride
Butalbital/Acetaminophen
Butenafine Hydrochloride
Butoconazole Nitrate
Butorphanol Tartrate
Caffeine Citrate
Calcipotriene
Calcitonin-Salmon
Calcitriol
Calcium Acetate
Candesartan Cilexetil*
Candesartan Cilexetil/ Hydrochlorothiazide*
Capreomycin Sulfate
Captopril*
Carbetapentane Tannate/ Chlorpheniramine Tannate
Carbidopa/Entacapone/ Levodopa
Carbidopa/Levodopa
Carbinoxamine Maleate/ Dextromethorphan Hydrobromide/ Pseudoephedrine Hydrochloride
Carteolol Hydrochloride
Carvedilol
Caspofungin Acetate
Celecoxib
Cetirizine Hydrochloride
Cetuximab
Cevimeline Hydrochloride
Chloramphenicol
Chloroprocaine Hydrochloride
Chlorothiazide
Chlorothiazide Sodium
Chlorpheniramine Maleate/ Pseudoephedrine Hydrochloride
Chlorpheniramine Polistirex/Hydrocodone Polistirex
Chlorpheniramine Tannate/Phenylephrine Tannate
Chlorpropamide
Chlorthalidone/ Clonidine Hydrochloride
Choline Magnesium Trisalicylate
Ciclesonide
Cidofovir
Cilostazol
Cinacalcet Hydrochloride
Ciprofloxacin Hydrochloride
Ciprofloxacin Hydrochloride/ Hydrocortisone
Ciprofloxacin/Dexamethasone
Citalopram Hydrobromide
Clarithromycin
Clobetasol Propionate
Clonidine
Clonidine Hydrochloride
Codeine Phosphate/ Acetaminophen
Colistimethate Sodium
Colistin Sulfate/Hydrocortisone Acetate/Neomycin Sulfate/ Thonzonium Bromide
Corticorelin Ovine Triflutate
Cyanocobalamin
Cycloserine
Cyclosporine
Cytomegalovirus Immune Globulin
Dacarbazine
Daclizumab
Dantrolene Sodium
Dapsone
Darbepoetin Alfa
Darifenacin
Deferoxamine Mesylate
Delavirdine Mesylate
Denileukin Diftitox
Desloratadine
Desloratadine/ Pseudoephedrine Sulfate
Desoximetasone
Desvenlafaxine
Dexamethasone
Dexamethasone Sodium Phosphate
Dexmethylphenidate Hydrochloride
Dexrazoxane
Dextroamphetamine Sulfate
Diazoxide
Diclofenac Epolamine
Diclofenac Potassium
Diclofenac Sodium
Diflorasone Diacetate
Diflunisal
Digoxin
Digoxin Immune Fab (Ovine)
Diltiazem Hydrochloride
Dimethyl Sulfoxide
Dinoprostone
Diphtheria & Tetanus Toxoids and Acellular Pertussis Vaccine Adsorbed
Diphtheria & Tetanus Toxoids and Acellular Pertussis Vaccine Adsorbed/Hepatitis B Vaccine, Recombinant/Poliovirus Vaccine Inactivated
Dofetilide
Donepezil Hydrochloride
Dorzolamide Hydrochloride
Dorzolamide Hydrochloride/ Timolol Maleate
Doxazosin Mesylate
Dronabinol
Drotrecogin Alfa (Activated)
Duloxetine Hydrochloride
Echothiophate Iodide
Econazole Nitrate
Efalizumab
Eflornithine Hydrochloride
Eletriptan Hydrobromide
Enalapril Maleate*
Enalapril Maleate/Felodipine*
Enalapril Maleate/ Hydrochlorothiazide*
Entacapone
Entecavir
Epinastine Hydrochloride
Epinephrine
Epoetin Alfa
Eprosartan Mesylate
Erythromycin Ethylsuccinate/ Sulfisoxazole Acetyl
Escitalopram Oxalate
Eszopiclone
Ethionamide
Ethotoin
Etidronate Disodium
Exenatide
Ezetimibe
Factor IX Complex
Felodipine
Fenofibrate
Fentanyl
Fentanyl Citrate

* Category C or D depending on the trimester the drug is given.

Fentanyl Hydrochloride
Ferrous Fumarate/Folic Acid/ Intrinsic Factor Concentrate/ Liver Preparations/ Vitamin B12/Vitamin C/ Vitamins with Iron
Fexofenadine Hydrochloride
Fexofenadine Hydrochloride/ Pseudoephedrine Hydrochloride
Filgrastim
Flecainide Acetate
Fluconazole
Flucytosine
Fludrocortisone Acetate
Flumazenil
Flunisolide
Fluocinolone Acetonide
Fluocinolone Acetonide/ Hydroquinone/Tretinoin
Fluocinonide
Fluorometholone
Fluorometholone/Sulfacetamide Sodium
Fluoxetine Hydrochloride
Fluoxetine Hydrochloride/ Olanzapine
Flurandrenolide
Flurbiprofen Sodium
Fluticasone Furoate
Fluticasone Propionate
Fluticasone Propionate HFA
Fluticasone Propionate/Salmeterol Xinafoate
Fluvoxamine Maleate
Formoterol Fumarate
Fosamprenavir Calcium
Foscarnet Sodium*
Fosinopril Sodium*
Fosinopril Sodium/ Hydrochlorothiazide*
Frovatriptan Succinate
Furosemide
Gabapentin
Gallium Nitrate
Ganciclovir
Ganciclovir Sodium
Gemfibrozil
Gemifloxacin Mesylate
Gentamicin Sulfate
Gentamicin Sulfate/ Prednisolone Acetate
Glimepiride
Glimepiride/Rosiglitazone Maleate
Glipizide
Glipizide/Metformin Hydrochloride
Globulin, Immune (Human)
Globulin, Immune (Human)/ Rho (D) Immune Globulin (Human)
Glyburide
Gramicidin/Neomycin Sulfate/ Polymyxin B Sulfate
Guaifenesin/Hydrocodone Bitartrate
Haemophilus B Conjugate Vaccine
Haemophilus B Conjugate Vaccine/Hepatitis B Vaccine, Recombinant
Halobetasol Propionate
Haloperidol Decanoate
Hemin
Heparin Sodium
Hepatitis A Vaccine, Inactivated
Hepatitis A Vaccine, Inactivated/ Hepatitis B Vaccine, Recombinant
Hepatitis B Immune Globulin (Human)
Hepatitis B Vaccine, Recombinant
Homatropine Methylbromide/ Hydrocodone Bitartrate
Homeopathic Formulations
Hydralazine Hydrochloride/ Isosorbide Dinitrate
Hydrochlorothiazide
Hydrocodone Bitartrate
Hydrocodone Bitartrate/ Acetaminophen
Hydrocodone Bitartrate/ Ibuprofen
Hydrocortisone
Hydrocortisone Acetate
Hydrocortisone Acetate/ Neomycin Sulfate/ Polymyxin B Sulfate
Hydrocortisone Acetate/ Pramoxine Hydrochloride
Hydrocortisone Butyrate
Hydrocortisone Probutate
Hydrocortisone/Neomycin Sulfate/Polymyxin B Sulfate
Hydromorphone Hydrochloride
Hydroquinone
Hyoscyamine Sulfate
Ibandronate Sodium
Ibutilide Fumarate
Iloprost
Imiglucerase
Imipenem/Cilastatin
Imiquimod
Immune Globulin Intravenous (Human)
Indinavir Sulfate
Indocyanine Green
Influenza Virus Vaccine
Insulin Aspart Protamine, Human/Insulin Aspart, Human
Insulin Glargine
Insulin Glulisine
Interferon Alfa-2B, Recombinant
Interferon Alfacon-1
Interferon Alfa-N3 (Human Leukocyte Derived)
Interferon Beta-1A
Interferon Beta-1B
Interferon Gamma-1B
Iodoquinol/Hydrocortisone
Irbesartan*
Irbesartan/Hydrochlorothiazide*
Iron Dextran
Isoniazid/Pyrazinamide/ Rifampin
Isosorbide Mononitrate
Isradipine
Itraconazole
Ivermectin
Ketoconazole
Ketorolac Tromethamine
Ketotifen Fumarate
Labetalol Hydrochloride
Lamivudine
Lamivudine/Zidovudine
Lamotrigine
Lanreotide Acetate
Lanthanum Carbonate
Latanoprost
Levalbuterol Hydrochloride
Levalbuterol Tartrate
Levamisole Hydrochloride
Levetiracetam
Levobunolol Hydrochloride
Levofloxacin
Linezolid
Lisdexamfetamine
Lisinopril*
Lisinopril/Hydrochlorothiazide*
Lomefloxacin
Lopinavir/Ritonavir
Losartan Potassium*
Losartan Potassium/ Hydrochlorothiazide*
Loteprednol Etabonate
Lubiprostone
Mafenide Acetate
Magnesium Salicylate Tetrahydrate
Measles Virus Vaccine, Live
Measles, Mumps & Rubella Virus Vaccine, Live
Mebendazole
Mecamylamine Hydrochloride
Mecasermin [rDNA Origin]
Medrysone
Mefenamic Acid
Mefloquine Hydrochloride
Meloxicam
Meningoccal Polysaccharide Diphtheria Toxoid Conjugate Vaccine
Meningococcal Polysaccharide Vaccine
Meperidine Hydrochloride
Mepivacaine Hydrochloride
Metaproterenol Sulfate
Metaraminol Bitartrate
Metformin Hydrochloride/ Pioglitazone Hydrochloride
Metformin Hydrochloride/ Repaglinide
Metformin Hydrochloride/ Rosiglitazone Maleate
Methamphetamine Hydrochloride
Methazolamide
Methenamine Mandelate/ Sodium Acid Phosphate

Methocarbamol
Methoxsalen
Methoxy Polyethylene Glycol/ Epoetin Beta
Methscopolamine Nitrate/ Pseudoephedrine Hydrochloride
Methyldopa/Hydrochlorothiazide
Methylphenidate Hydrochloride
Metipranolol
Metoprolol Succinate
Metoprolol Tartrate
Metoprolol Tartrate/ Hydrochlorothiazide
Metyrosine
Mexiletine Hydrochloride
Micafungin Sodium
Midodrine Hydrochloride
Modafinil
Moexipril Hydrochloride*
Moexipril Hydrochloride/ Hydrochlorothiazide*
Mometasone Furoate
Mometasone Furoate Monohydrate
Morphine Sulfate
Morphine Sulfate, Liposomal
Moxifloxacin Hydrochloride
Mumps Virus Vaccine, Live
Muromonab-CD3
Nabumetone
Nadolol
Nadolol/Bendroflumethiazide
Naloxone Hydrochloride/ Pentazocine Hydrochloride
Naltrexone Hydrochloride
Naphazoline Hydrochloride
Naproxen Sodium
Naratriptan Hydrochloride
Natamycin
Nateglinide
Nebivolol
Nefazodone Hydrochloride
Neomycin Sulfate/ Dexamethasone Sodium Phosphate
Neomycin Sulfate/Polymyxin B Sulfate/Prednisolone Acetate
Nesiritide
Nevirapine
Niacin
Nicardipine Hydrochloride
Nifedipine
Nilutamide
Nimodipine
Nisoldipine
Nitroglycerin
Norfloxacin
Ofloxacin
Olanzapine
Olmesartan Medoxomil/ Hydrochlorothiazide
Olopatadine Hydrochloride
Olsalazine Sodium
Omega-3-Acid Ethyl Esters
Omeprazole
Oprelvekin
Orphenadrine Citrate
Oseltamivir Phosphate
Oxcarbazepine
Oxycodone Hydrochloride/ Acetaminophen
Oxycodone Hydrochloride/ Ibuprofen
Oxymorphone Hydrochloride
Palifermin
Paliperidone
Palivizumab
Pancrelipase
Paricalcitol
Peg-3350/Potassium Chloride/ Sodium Bicarbonate/ Sodium Chloride
Pegademase Bovine
Pegaspargase
Pegfilgrastim
Peginterferon Alfa-2A
Peginterferon Alfa-2B
Pemirolast Potassium
Pentazocine Hydrochloride/ Acetaminophen
Pentoxifylline
Phenoxybenzamine Hydrochloride
Phentermine Hydrochloride
Pilocarpine Hydrochloride
Pimecrolimus
Pimozide
Pioglitazone Hydrochloride
Pirbuterol Acetate
Piroxicam
Plasma Fractions, Human/ Rabies Immune Globulin (Human)
Plasma Protein Fraction (Human)
Pneumococcal Vaccine, Diphtheria Conjugate
Pneumococcal Vaccine, Polyvalent
Podofilox
Polyethylene Glycol
Polyethylene Glycol/ Potassium Chloride/Sodium Bicarbonate/Sodium Chloride
Polyethylene Glycol/Potassium Chloride/Sodium Bicarbonate/ Sodium Chloride/Sodium Sulfate
Polymyxin B Sulfate/ Trimethoprim Sulfate
Polythiazide/Prazosin Hydrochloride
Porfimer Sodium
Potassium Acid Phosphate
Potassium Chloride
Potassium Citrate
Potassium Phosphate/ Sodium Phosphate
Pralidoxime Chloride
Pramipexole Dihydrochloride
Pramlintide Acetate
Pramoxine Hydrochloride/ Hydrocortisone Acetate
Prazosin Hydrochloride
Prednisolone Acetate
Prednisolone Acetate/ Sulfacetamide Sodium
Prednisolone Sodium Phosphate
Pregabalin
Promethazine Hydrochloride
Propafenone Hydrochloride
Proparacaine Hydrochloride
Propranolol Hydrochloride
Pseudoephedrine Hydrochloride
Pyrimethamine
Quetiapine Fumarate
Quinapril Hydrochloride*
Quinidine Sulfate
Rabies Vaccine
Raltegravir Potassium
Ramelteon
Ramipril*
Ranolazine
Rasburicase
Remifentanil Hydrochloride
Repaglinide
Reteplase
Rho (D) Immune Globulin (Human)
Rifampin
Rifapentine
Rifaximin
Riluzole
Rimantadine Hydrochloride
Risedronate Sodium
Risedronate Sodium/ Calcium Carbonate
Risperidone
Rituximab
Rizatriptan Benzoate
Rocuronium Bromide
Romiplostim
Ropinirole Hydrochloride
Rosiglitazone Maleate
Rubella Virus Vaccine, Live
Salmeterol Xinafoate
Sapropterin Dihydrochloride
Sargramostim
Scopolamine
Selegiline Hydrochloride
Selenium Sulfide
Sertaconazole Nitrate
Sertraline Hydrochloride
Sevelamer Carbonate
Sevelamer Hydrochloride
Sibutramine Hydrochloride Monohydrate
Sirolimus
Sodium Benzoate/ Sodium Phenylacelate
Sodium Phenylbutyrate
Sodium Polysterene Sulfonate
Sodium Sulfacetamide/Sulfur
Solifenacin Succinate
Somatropin
Somatropin (rdna Origin)
Stavudine
Streptokinase

* Category C or D depending on the trimester the drug is given.

Succimer
Sulfacetamide Sodium
Sulfamethoxazole/Trimethoprim
Sulfanilamide
Sumatriptan
Sumatriptan Succinate
Tacrine Hydrochloride
Tacrolimus
Telithromycin
Telmisartan*
Telmisartan/
  Hydrochlorothiazide*
Tenecteplase
Terazosin Hydrochloride
Teriparatide
Tetanus & Diphtheria Toxoids
  Adsorbed
Tetanus Immune Globulin (Human)
Theophylline
Theophylline Anhydrous
Thiabendazole
Thrombin
Thyrotropin Alfa
Tiagabine Hydrochloride
Tiludronate Disodium
Timolol Hemihydrate
Timolol Maleate
Timolol Maleate/
  Hydrochlorothiazide
Tinidazole
Tiotropium Bromide
Tipranavir
Tizanidine Hydrochloride
Tobramycin/Dexamethasone
Tobramycin/Loteprednol Etabonate
Tolcapone
Tolterodine Tartrate
Topiramate
Tramadol Hydrochloride
Tramadol Hydrochloride/
  Acetaminophen
Trandolapril*
Trandolapril/Verapamil
  Hydrochloride*
Travoprost
Tretinoin
Triamcinolone Acetonide
Triamterene
Triamterene/Hydrochlorothiazide
Trientine Hydrochloride
Triethanolamine Polypeptide Oleate-
  Condensate
Trifluridine
Trimethoprim Hydrochloride
Trimipramine Maleate
Tropicamide/
  Hydroxyamphetamine
  Hydrobromide
Trospium Chloride
Tuberculin Purified Protein Derivative,
  Diluted
Typhoid Vaccine Live Oral Ty21a
Urea
Valganciclovir Hydrochloride
Varenicline Tartrate
Varicella Virus Vaccine, Live
Venlafaxine Hydrochloride
Verapamil Hydrochloride
Verteporfin
Vitamin K_1
Yellow Fever Vaccine
Zaleplon
Zanamivir
Zidovudine
Ziprasidone Mesylate
Zolmitriptan
Zolpidem Tartrate
Zonisamide

B

No evidence of risk in humans

Either animal findings show risk while human findings do not, or, if no adequate human studies have been done, animal findings are negative.

Acarbose
Acrivastine
Acyclovir
Acyclovir Sodium
Adalimumab
Agalsidase Beta
Alefacept
Alfuzosin Hydrochloride
Alosetron Hydrochloride
Alvimopan
Amiloride Hydrochloride
Amiloride Hydrochloride/
  Hydrochlorothiazide
Amoxicillin
Amoxicillin/Clavulanate Potassium
Amphotericin B
Amphotericin B Lipid Complex
Amphotericin B, Liposomal
Amphotericin B/Cholesteryl Sulfate
  Complex
Ampicillin Sodium/
  Sulbactam Sodium
Anakinra
Antithrombin III
Aprepitant
Aprotinin
Argatroban
Arginine Hydrochloride
Atazanavir Sulfate
Azelaic Acid
Azithromycin
Azithromycin Dihydrate
Aztreonam
Balsalazide Disodium
Basiliximab
Bivalirudin
Brimonidine Tartrate
Budesonide
Cabergoline
Carbenicillin Indanyl Sodium
Cefaclor
Cefazolin Sodium
Cefdinir
Cefditoren Pivoxil
Cefepime Hydrochloride
Cefixime
Cefotaxime Sodium
Cefotetan Disodium
Cefoxitin Sodium
Cefpodoxime Proxetil
Cefprozil
Ceftazidime Sodium
Ceftibuten Dihydrate
Ceftizoxime Sodium
Ceftriaxone Sodium
Cefuroxime
Cefuroxime Axetil
Cephalexin
Cetirizine Hydrochloride
Certolizumab Pegol
Ciclopirox
Ciclopirox Olamine
Cimetidine Hydrochloride
Cisatracurium Besylate
Clindamycin Hydrochloride/
  Clindamycin Phosphate
Clindamycin Palmitate Hydrochloride
Clindamycin Phosphate
Clopidogrel Bisulfate
Clotrimazole
Clozapine
Colesevelam Hydrochloride
Cromolyn Sodium
Cyclobenzaprine Hydrochloride
Cyproheptadine Hydrochloride
Dalfopristin/Quinupristin
Dalteparin Sodium
Dapiprazole Hydrochloride
Daptomycin
Desflurane
Desmopressin Acetate
Dicyclomine Hydrochloride
Didanosine
Diphenhydramine Hydrochloride
Dipivefrin Hydrochloride
Dipyridamole
Dolasetron Mesylate
Doripenem
Dornase Alfa
Doxapram Hydrochloride
Doxepin Hydrochloride
Doxercalciferol
Edetate Calcium Disodium
Emtricitabine
Emtricitabine/Tenofovir Disoproxil
  Fumarate
Enfuvirtide
Enoxaparin Sodium
Eplerenone
Epoprostenol Sodium
Ertapenem
Erythromycin

Erythromycin Ethylsuccinate
Erythromycin Stearate
Esomeprazole Magnesium
Esomeprazole Sodium
Etanercept
Ethacrynate Sodium
Ethacrynic Acid
Etravirine
Famciclovir
Famotidine
Fenoldopam Mesylate
Fondaparinux Sodium
Galantamine Hydrobromide
Glatiramer Acetate
Glucagon
Glyburide/Metformin Hydrochloride
Granisetron Hydrochloride
Hydrochlorothiazide
Ibuprofen
Indapamide
Infliximab
Insulin Aspart
Insulin Lispro Protamine, Human/Insulin Lispro, Human
Insulin Lispro, Human
Ipratropium Bromide
Iron Sucrose
Isosorbide Mononitrate
Lactulose
Lansoprazole
Lansoprazole/Naproxen
Laronidase
Lepirudin
Levocarnitine
Levocetirizine Dihydrochloride
Lidocaine Hydrochloride
Lidocaine/Prilocaine
Lindane
Loperamide Hydrochloride
Loratadine
Malathion
Maraviroc
Meclizine Hydrochloride
Memantine Hydrochloride
Meropenem
Mesalamine
Metformin Hydrochloride
Metformin Hydrochloride/Sitagliptin
Methohexital Sodium
Methyldopa
Methylnaltrexone Bromide
Metolazone
Metronidazole
Miglitol
Montelukast Sodium
Mupirocin
Mupirocin Calcium
Naftifine Hydrochloride
Nalbuphine Hydrochloride
Nalmefene Hydrochloride
Naloxone Hydrochloride
Naproxen Sodium
Nedocromil Sodium
Nelfinavir Mesylate
Nitazoxanide
Nitrofurantoin Macrocrystals
Nitrofurantoin Macrocrystals/Nitrofurantoin Monohydrate
Nizatidine
Octreotide Acetate
Omalizumab
Ondansetron Hydrochloride
Orlistat
Oxiconazole Nitrate
Oxybutynin
Oxybutynin Chloride
Oxycodone Hydrochloride
Palonosetron Hydrochloride
Pancrelipase
Pantoprazole Sodium
Pegvisomant
Penciclovir
Penicillin G Benzathine
Penicillin G Benzathine/Penicillin G Procaine
Penicillin G Potassium
Pentosan Polysulfate Sodium
Permethrin
Piperacillin Sodium
Piperacillin Sodium/Tazobactam Sodium
Praziquantel
Progesterone
Propofol
Pseudoephedrine Hydrochloride
Pseudoephedrine Sulfate
Psyllium Preparations
Rabeprazole Sodium
Ranitidine Hydrochloride
Retapamulin
Rifabutin
Ritonavir
Rivastigmine Tartrate
Ropivacaine Hydrochloride
Saquinavir Mesylate
Sevoflurane
Sildenafil Citrate
Silver Sulfadiazine
Sitagliptin Phosphate
Sodium Ferric Gluconate
Somatropin
Sotalol Hydrochloride
Sucralfate
Sulfasalazine
Tadalafil
Tamsulosin Hydrochloride
Tenofovir Disoproxil Fumarate
Terbinafine Hydrochloride
Ticarcillin Disodium/Clavulanate Potassium
Ticlopidine Hydrochloride
Tirofiban Hydrochloride
Torsemide
Trastuzumab
Treprostinil Sodium
Urokinase
Ursodiol
Valacyclovir Hydrochloride
Vancomycin Hydrochloride
Vardenafil Hydrochloride
Zafirlukast

A

Controlled studies show no risk

Adequate, well-controlled studies in pregnant women have failed to demonstrate risk to the fetus.

Liothyronine Sodium
Liotrix
Nystatin

* Category C or D depending on the trimester the drug is given.

VITAMIN COMPARISON TABLE

For easy comparison, the grid below lists the contents of an assortment of widely available vitamin/mineral supplements. It includes entries for all vitamins and minerals—except sodium—assigned a Recommended Dietary Allowance (Daily Value) by the U.S. Food and Drug Administration.

The grid is divided into two parts: the first covers general multivitamin/mineral supplements for adults; the second focuses on supplements sold especially for children.

Many of the brands in the grid include other ingredients that have nutritional importance but lack an official Recommended Dietary Allowance from the government. The presence of additional ingredients is noted in the last column of the grid.

The amounts listed are drawn from the manufacturer's package labeling, primarily as published in the *PDR® for Nutritional Supplements, 2nd Edition*. For easy comparison, the figures have been converted as necessary from the unit of measure used by the manufacturer to the measurement most frequently employed in the industry. **Amounts listed are those found in the total daily dose.** Check package labeling for other usage information provided by the manufacturer.

To conserve space, units of measure are not shown in the grid; see the following key for the measurement used for a particular ingredient.

Ingredient	Measure
Vitamin A (retinol, beta-carotene)	International Units
Vitamin B1 (thiamin)	Milligrams
Vitamin B2 (riboflavin)	Milligrams
Vitamin B3 (niacin)	Milligrams
Vitamin B5 (pantothenic acid)	Milligrams
Vitamin B6 (pyridoxine)	Milligrams
Vitamin B9 (folic acid)	Micrograms
Vitamin B12 (cobalamin)	Micrograms
Vitamin C (ascorbic acid)	Milligrams
Vitamin D	International Units
Vitamin E	International Units
Biotin	Micrograms
Calcium	Milligrams
Copper	Milligrams
Iodine	Micrograms
Iron	Milligrams
Magnesium	Milligrams
Phosphorus	Milligrams
Potassium	Milligrams
Zinc	Milligrams

BRAND	A	B1	B2	B3	B5	B6	B9	B12	C	D	E	BIOTIN	CALCIUM	COPPER	IODINE	IRON	MAGNESIUM	PHOSPHORUS	POTASSIUM	ZINC	OTHER
ADULTS																					
ACES (Carlson)	5,000	—	—	—	—	—	—	—	500	—	200	—	—	—	—	—	—	—	—	—	y
Adult Chewable Multivitamin (Puritan's Pride)	5,000	15	15	—	20	15	400	15	150	400	100	20	10	0.05	100	5	0.145	—	—	0.325	y
Advanced Prenatal *per 3 tabs*	2,700	3	3.4	—	10	3	800	12	120	400	45	300	125	2	75	30	125	—	25	25	y
Centamin Liquid *per 15 ml*	2,500	1.5	1.7	20	10	2	—	6	60	400	30	300	—	—	150	9	—	—	—	3	
Centrum	3,500	1.5	1.7	—	10	2	500	6	90	400	30	300	200	0.09	150	18	50	109	80	11	y
Centrum Cardio	1,750	0.75	0.85	10	5	2.5	200	100	30	200	15	15	54	0.35	75	3	20	40	32	3.75	y
Centrum Chewable	3,500	1.5	1.7	20	10	2	400	6	60	400	30	45	108	2	150	18	40	50	—	15	y
Centrum Performance	3,500	4.5	5.1	40	12	6	400	18	120	400	60	50	100	9	150	18	40	48	80	11	y
Centrum Silver	2,500	1.5	1.7	20	10	3	500	25	90	500	50	30	220	9	150	—	50	110	80	11	y
Daily Multi (Sundown)	2,500	1.5	1.7	—	10	2	400	6	60	400	30	30	162	2	150	18	100	—	80	15	y
Duet by Stuartnatal	3,000	1.8	4	—	—	25	1,000	12	120	400	30	—	200	2	—	29	25	—	—	25	y

(Continued)

BRAND	A	B1	B2	B3	B5	B6	B9	B12	C	D	E	BIOTIN	CALCIUM	COPPER	IODINE	IRON	MAGNESIUM	PHOSPHORUS	POTASSIUM	ZINC	OTHER
Duet Chewable by Stuartnatal	3,000	1.8	4	—	—	25	—	12	120	400	30	—	100	2	—	29	25	—	—	25	y
Folgard Rx 2.2	—	—	—	—	—	25	2,200	1,000	—	—	—	—	—	—	—	—	—	—	—	—	
Formula 100 (Puritan's Pride)	10,000	100	100	—	100	100	400	100	250	400	150	100	100	0.5	150	18	50	—	10	15	y
Geritol Complete	6,100	1.5	1.7	20	13	2	380	6.7	57	400	30	44	148	1.8	120	16	86	118	36	13.5	y
Goldline Certagen	5,000	1.5	1.7	—	10	2	400	6	60	400	30	0.03	162	2	150	18	10	109	80	15	y
Goldline Prenatal S	4,000	1.84	1.7	—	—	2.6	800	4	100	400	11	—	200	—	—	27	—	—	—	25	y
Green Source *per 3 tabs*	15,000	25	25	25	25	25	400	25	1,000	400	250	50	250	0.5	150	15	125	—	50	15	y
Hair, Skin & Nails Formula (Nature's Bounty) *per 3 tabs*	5,000	5	5	—	15	5	200	8	120	100	15	3,000	834	—	150	3	100	150	—	7.5	y
Hep-Forte	1,200	1	1	10	2	0.5	60	1	10	—	10	3.3	—	—	—	—	—	—	—	2	y
Ironmin-G	4,000	4.8	2	10	1	20	800	2	100	400	—	—	57	—	—	29.5	—	—	—	—	
Mega Vita Gel Iron Free *per 2 softgels*	10,000	50	50	—	50	50	400	50	300	400	300	50	200	2	150	—	50	50	30	15	y
Mini-Multi (Carlson Laboratories)	5,000	1.5	1.7	—	10	2	400	6	120	400	60	30	20	2	75		40	—	—	15	

Mini-Prenatal (Freeda Vitamins)	2,000	2	3	—	10	3	800	10	100	400	15	100	200	2	—	27	60	—	—	15	
Multi-Day Plus Minerals (Nature's Bounty)	2,500	1.5	1.7	—	10	2	400	6	60	400	30	30	162	—	—	—	—	—	—	—	
Myadec	5,000	1.7	2	20	10	3	400	6	60	400	30	30	162	2	150	18	100	125	40	15	y
NataChew	1,000	2	3	—	—	10	1	12	120	400	11	—	—	—	—	29	—	—	—	—	y
Ocuvite	1,000	—	—	—	—	—	—	—	200	—	60	—	—	2	—	—	—	—	—	40	
One A Day Active	5,000	4.5	5.1	40	10	6	400	18	120	400	60	40	110	2	150	9	40	48	200	15	y
One A Day Men's 50+ Advantage	2,500	4.5	3.4	20	15	6	400	25	120	400	33	30	120	2	150	—	100	—	40	22.5	y
One A Day Men's	3,500	1.2	1.7	16	5	3	400	18	90	400	45	30	210	2	—	—	120	—	100	15	y
One A Day Women's	2,500	1.5	1.7	10	5	2	400	6	60	800	30	30	450	2	—	18	50	—	—	20	y
One A Day Women's 50+ Advantage	2,500	4.5	3.4	20	15	6	400	25	60	800	33	30	405	2	150	—	50	—	—	22.5	y
One A Day Women's Prenatal	4,000	1.7	2	20	10	2.5	800	8	60	400	30	300	300	2	150	28	50	—	—	15	y
Optisource Chewable	1,875	0.375	0.425	5	2.5	0.5	200	125	15	100	—	75	250	0.5	37.5	7.5	100	50	—	—	y
PreCare Chewable	—	—	2	—	—	2	1,000	—	50	6mcg	3.5	—	250	2	—	40	50	—	—	15	y
PreCare Conceive	—	3	3.4	20	—	50	1,000	12	60	—	30	—	200	2	—	30	100	—	—	15	y

(Continued)

BRAND	A	B1	B2	B3	B5	B6	B9	B12	C	D	E	BIOTIN	CALCIUM	COPPER	IODINE	IRON	MAGNESIUM	PHOSPHORUS	POTASSIUM	ZINC	OTHER
PremesisRx Tablets	—	—	—	—	—	75	1,000	12	—	—	—	—	200	—	—	—	—	—	—	—	
Prenatal Vitamins (Nature's Bounty)	4,000	1.8	1.7	—	—	2.6	800	8	120	400	30	—	200	—	—	28	—	—	—	25	
Prenatal Vitamin (Puritan's Pride)	4,000	1.84	1.7	—	—	2.6	800	4	100	400	11	—	200	—	—	27	—	—	—	25	
Puritan's Pride Complete One	10,000	25	25	—	50	50	400	50	250	400	30	50	54	2	150	54	100	23	1	15	y
Strovite Advance	3,000	20	5	25	15	25	1,000	50	300	400	100	100	—	1.5	—	—	50	—	—	25	y
Stuart Prenatal	4,000	1.8	1.7	20	—	2.6	800	8	120	400	30	—	200	—	—	28	—	—	—	25	
Viactiv Chews	2,500	1.5	1.7	15	10	2	400	6	60	400	33	30	200	—	—	—	—	—	—	—	
CHILDREN																					
Carlson for Kids Chewable	5,000	1.5	1.7	—	10	2	400	6	120	400	60	150	50	1	75	9	20	40	32	7.5	y
Centrum Kids	3,500	1.5	1.7	20	10	2	400	6	60	400	30	45	108	2	150	18	40	50	—	15	y
Enfamil Kindercal Liquid *per 8 fl oz.*	970	0.4	0.5	4.9	3.1	0.5	38	1.4	58	125	8.8	38	240	0.3	30	2.5	50	200	310	3	y
Flintstones	3,000	1.5	1.7	15	10	2	400	6	60	400	30	40	100	2	150	18	20	100	—	12	y
GNC Kid's Chewable *per 2 tabs*	5,000	5	5	—	15	5	400	10	90	400	30	100	30	0.2	100	12	15	15	—	3	y

One A Day Kids Bugs Bunny	3,000	1.5	1.7	15	10	2	400	6	60	400	30	40	100	2	150	18	20	100	—	12	y
One A Day Kids Scooby-Doo	3,000	1.5	1.7	15	10	2	400	6	60	400	30	40	100	2	150	18	20	100	—	12	y
One A Day Kids Scooby-Doo Plus Calcium	2,500	1.05	1.2	13.5	—	1.05	300	4.5	60	400	15	—	200	—	—	—	—	—	—	—	y

*USP units.

Indices

BRAND/GENERIC INDEX

Organized alphabetically, this index includes the brand and generic names of each drug in the Product Information section. Brand-name drug entries are capitalized; generic names are not. If more than one brand name is associated with a generic, each brand can be found under the generic entry.

A

Abacavir Sulfate
- Epzicom ... 369
- Trizivir ... 1049
- Ziagen ... 1160

Abatacept
- Orencia ... 725

ABBOKINASE ... 1

Abciximab
- ReoPro ... 863

ABELCET ... 2

ABILIFY ... 3

ABILIFY DISCMELT
- See Abilify ... 3

ABRAXANE ... 4

Acamprosate Calcium
- Campral ... 176

ACANYA ... 5

Acarbose
- Precose ... 787

ACCOLATE ... 6

ACCUNEB ... 7

ACCUPRIL ... 8

ACCURETIC ... 9

ACCUTANE ... 10

Acebutolol HCl
- Sectral ... 913

ACEON ... 12

Acetaminophen
- Darvocet A500 ... 276
- Darvocet-N ... 277
- Esgic ... 381
- Esgic-Plus ... 381
- Fioricet ... 412
- Fioricet with Codeine 413
- Lorcet ... 575
- Lortab ... 576
- Midrin ... 633
- Norco ... 690
- Percocet ... 764
- Roxicet ... 895
- Talacen ... 972
- Tylenol with Codeine ... 1056
- Tylox ... 1057
- Ultracet ... 1062
- Vicodin ... 1100
- Zydone ... 1184

ACETAMINOPHEN W/CODEINE ELIXIR
- See Tylenol with Codeine ... 1056

ACETAZOLAMIDE ... 13

ACETYLCYSTEINE ... 14

ACIPHEX ... 15

Acitretin
- Soriatane ... 938

ACLOVATE ... 16

ACTIGALL ... 17

ACTIQ ... 18

ACTIVASE ... 19

ACTIVELLA ... 20

ACTONEL ... 22

ACTONEL WITH CALCIUM ... 23

ACTOPLUS MET ... 24

ACTOS ... 26

ACULAR ... 27

Acyclovir
- Zovirax Cream ... 1179
- Zovirax Ointment ... 1181
- Zovirax Oral ... 1182

Acyclovir Sodium
- Zovirax Injection ... 1180

ADALAT CC ... 28

Adalimumab
- Humira ... 478

Adapalene
- Differin ... 310
- Epiduo ... 364

ADDERALL ... 28

ADDERALL XR ... 30

Adefovir Dipivoxil
- Hepsera ... 472

ADVAIR ... 31

ADVAIR HFA ... 33

ADVICOR ... 35

AEROBID ... 36

AEROBID-M
- See Aerobid ... 36

AFEDITAB CR
- See Adalat CC ... 28

AGGRASTAT ... 37

AGGRENOX ... 38

AGRYLIN ... 39

ALAMAST ... 40

Albendazole
- Albenza ... 41

ALBENZA ... 41

ALBUTEROL ... 41

Albuterol Sulfate
- AccuNeb ... 7

Albuterol ... 41
- Combivent ... 240
- Duoneb ... 337
- ProAir HFA ... 814
- Proventil HFA ... 835
- Ventolin HFA ... 1089
- VoSpire ER ... 1123

Alclometasone Dipropionate
- Aclovate ... 16

ALCORTIN ... 43

ALDACTAZIDE ... 44

ALDACTONE ... 45

ALDARA ... 45

Alefacept
- Amevive ... 64

Alemtuzumab
- Campath ... 175

Alendronate Sodium
- Fosamax ... 443
- Fosamax Plus D ... 444

ALESSE ... 47

Alfuzosin HCl
- Uroxatral ... 1071

ALIMTA ... 48

ALINIA ... 49

Aliskiren
- Tekturna ... 987
- Tekturna HCT ... 988

ALLEGRA ... 50

ALLEGRA-D ... 51

Allopurinol
- Zyloprim ... 1186

Allopurinol Sodium
- Aloprim ... 52

Almotriptan Malate
- Axert ... 129

ALOPRIM ... 52

Alosetron HCl
- Lotronex ... 582

ALOXI ... 52

ALPHAGAN P ... 53

Alprazolam
- Niravam ... 684
- Xanax ... 1131
- Xanax XR ... 1132

ALREX ... 54

ALTABAX ... 55

ALTACE ... 55

Alteplase
- Activase ... 19

ALTOPREV 56
ALVESCO 57
Amantadine HCl
  Symmetrel 965
AMARYL 59
AMBIEN 60
AMBIEN CR 61
AMBISOME 61
Ambrisentan
  Letairis 543
AMERGE 62
AMEVIVE 64
AMICAR 65
Amidrine
  See Midrin 633
AMIKACIN 66
Amikacin Sulfate
  Amikacin 66
AMILORIDE 67
Amiloride HCl
  Amiloride 67
  Amiloride/HCTZ 67
AMILORIDE/HCTZ 67
Aminocaproic Acid
  Amicar 65
Aminosalicylic Acid
  Paser 750
Amiodarone HCl
  Cordarone 248
  Cordarone IV 249
  Pacerone 744
AMITIZA 68
AMITRIPTYLINE 69
Amlodipine Besylate
  Azor 137
  Caduet 172
  Exforge 399
  Lotrel 580
  Norvasc 696
Amnesteem
  See Accutane 10
Amoxicillin
  Amoxil 70
  Augmentin 114
  Augmentin ES-600 115
  Augmentin XR 116
  Prevpac 803
AMOXIL 70
Amphetamine Salt Combo
  Adderall 28
  Adderall XR 30
AMPHOCIN 71
AMPHOTEC 73
Amphotericin B
  AmBisome 61
  Amphocin 71
Amphotericin B
  Cholesteryl Sulfate
  Amphotec 73
Amphotericin B
  Lipid Complex
  Abelcet 2
Ampicillin
  Ampicillin Oral 74
AMPICILLIN
  INJECTION 74
AMPICILLIN ORAL 74
Ampicillin Sodium
  Ampicillin Injection 74
  Unasyn 1065
AMRIX 75
Anagrelide HCl
  Agrylin 39
Anakinra
  Kineret 529
ANAPROX
  See Anaprox DS 76
ANAPROX DS 76
Anastrozole
  Arimidex 97
ANCOBON 78
ANDRODERM 78
ANDROGEL 79
ANGELIQ 80
ANGIOMAX 82
Anidulafungin
  Eraxis 372
ANSAID 83
ANTABUSE 84
ANTARA 85
ANTIVERT 86
ANZEMET 86
APIDRA 87
APLENZIN 88
Aprepitant
  Emend 355
APRI
  See Desogen 297
APRISO 90
Aprotinin
  Trasylol 1033
APTIVUS 90
ARANESP 92
ARAVA 93
AREDIA 94
Arformoterol Tartrate
  Brovana 166
ARGATROBAN 95
ARICEPT 96
ARICEPT ODT
  See Aricept 96
ARIMIDEX 97
Aripiprazole
  Abilify 3
ARIXTRA 98
Armodafinil
  Nuvigil 707
ARMOUR THYROID 99
AROMASIN 100
ARTHROTEC 101
ASACOL 102
Ascorbic Acid
  MoviPrep 649
ASMANEX 103
Aspirin
  Aggrenox 38
  Bayer Aspirin 146
  Equagesic 370
  Fiorinal 414
  Fiorinal with Codeine 415
  Percodan 765
ASTELIN 104
ASTEPRO 105
ASTRAMORPH PF 106
ATACAND 107
ATACAND HCT 107
Atazanavir Sulfate
  Reyataz 875
Atenolol
  Tenoretic 991
  Tenormin 992
ATIVAN 109
ATIVAN INJECTION 109
Atomoxetine HCl
  Strattera 946
Atorvastatin Calcium
  Caduet 172
  Lipitor 562
Atovaquone
  Malarone 598
  Mepron 608
ATRIPLA 111
Atropine Sulfate
  Donnatal 325
  Lomotil 570
ATROVENT HFA 112
ATROVENT NASAL 113
AUGMENTIN 114
AUGMENTIN ES-600 115
AUGMENTIN XR 116
AVAGE 117
AVALIDE 118
AVANDAMET 120
AVANDARYL 121
AVANDIA 122
AVAPRO 123
AVASTIN 124
AVELOX 125
Aviane
  See Alesse 47
AVINZA 127
AVODART 128

AXERT....129
AXID....130
AXID ORAL SOLUTION
See Axid....130
AYGESTIN....131
Azacitidine
Vidaza....1102
AZACTAM....132
AZASITE....133
Azathioprine
Imuran....491
Azelaic Acid
Azelex....134
Finacea....411
Azelastine HCl
Astelin....104
Astepro....105
Optivar....721
AZELEX....134
AZILECT....134
Azithromycin
Azasite....133
Zithromax....1164
Zmax....1165
AZMACORT....135
AZOPT....136
AZOR....137
Aztreonam
Azactam....132
AZULFIDINE....138
AZULFIDINE EN....139

B

Bacitracin Zinc
Neosporin Ophthalmic....672
BACLOFEN....140
Baclofen
Baclofen....140
BACTRIM....141
BACTRIM DS
See Bactrim....141
BACTROBAN....142
BACTROBAN NASAL....143
Balsalazide Disodium
Colazal....235
Balziva
See Ovcon-35....738
BANZEL....144
BARACLUDE....145
Basiliximab
Simulect....924
BAYER ASPIRIN....146
Bayer Aspirin Children's
See Bayer Aspirin....146
Bayer Aspirin Regimen
See Bayer Aspirin....146
Bayer Aspirin Regimen with Calcium
See Bayer Aspirin....146
Beclomethasone Dipropionate
Beconase AQ....147
Qvar....846
BECONASE AQ....147
Benazepril HCl
Lotensin....578
Lotensin HCT....579
Lotrel....580
BENICAR....148
BENICAR HCT....148
BENTYL....149
BENZACLIN....150
BENZAMYCIN....151
Benzonatate
Tessalon....995
Benzoyl Peroxide
Acanya....5
BenzaClin....150
Benzamycin....151
Brevoxyl....166
Duac....334
Epiduo....364
Triaz....1038
BENZTROPINE....152
Benztropine Mesylate
Benztropine....152
BETAGAN....153
Betamethasone (augmented) Dipropionate
Diprolene....320
Betamethasone Dipropionate
Betamethasone Dipropionate....153
Lotrisone....581
BETAMETHASONE DIPROPIONATE....153
Betamethasone Valerate
Luxiq....592
BETAPACE....154
BETAPACE AF....156
Betaxolol HCl
Betoptic S....158
BETIMOL....157
BETOPTIC S....158
Bevacizumab
Avastin....124
BEXXAR....159
BIAXIN....160
BIAXIN XL....161
Bicalutamide
Casodex....188
Bimatoprost
Lumigan....585
Bisacodyl
HalfLytely....467
Bismuth Subsalicylate
Helidac....470
Bisoprolol Fumarate
Zebeta....1149
Ziac....1159
Bivalirudin
Angiomax....82
BONIVA....162
BOOSTRIX....163
Bortezomib
Velcade....1087
Bosentan
Tracleer....1029
BREVIBLOC....164
Brevicon
See Ortho-Novum 1/50....734
BREVOXYL....166
Brimonidine Tartrate
Alphagan P....53
Combigan....238
Brinzolamide
Azopt....136
Bromfenac
Xibrom....1135
Bromocriptine Mesylate
Parlodel....748
BROVANA....166
Budesonide
Entocort EC....363
Pulmicort....841
Rhinocort Aqua....876
Symbicort....960
BUMETANIDE....167
BUMEX
See Bumetanide....167
BUPRENEX....168
Buprenorphine
Suboxone....951
Buprenorphine HCl
Buprenex....168
Bupropion HCl
Wellbutrin SR....1127
Wellbutrin XL....1128
Zyban....1183
Bupropion Hydrobromide
Aplenzin....88
BUSPAR....169
Buspirone HCl
BuSpar....169
Busulfan
Myleran....653
Butalbital
Esgic....381
Esgic-Plus....381
Fioricet....412
Fioricet with Codeine 413

Fiorinal....................414
Fiorinal with Codeine 415
BYETTA....................170
BYSTOLIC....................171

C

C1 inhibitor (Human)
Cinryze....................213
CADUET....................172
Caffeine
Esgic....................381
Esgic-Plus....................381
Fioricet....................412
Fioricet with Codeine 413
Fiorinal....................414
Fiorinal with Codeine 415
CALAN....................173
CALAN SR....................174
Calcipotriene
Dovonex....................329
Dovonex Scalp....................330
Calcitonin-Salmon
Miacalcin....................625
Calcitonin-Salmon (rDNA origin)
Fortical....................442
Calcium Acetate
PhosLo....................774
Calcium Carbonate
Actonel with Calcium . 23
Camila
See Micronor....................630
CAMPATH....................175
CAMPRAL....................176
CAMPTOSAR....................176
CANASA....................178
CANCIDAS....................179
Candesartan Cilexetil
Atacand....................107
Atacand HCT....................107
Capecitabine
Xeloda....................1133
CAPOTEN
See Captopril....................181
CAPOZIDE....................180
CAPTOPRIL....................181
Captopril
Capozide....................180
Captopril....................181
Carbamazepine
Carbatrol....................182
Equetro....................371
Tegretol....................985
CARBATROL....................182
Carbidopa
Parcopa....................747
Sinemet CR....................925
Stalevo....................942
CARDENE IV....................183
CARDENE SR....................184
CARDIZEM....................185
CARDIZEM CD....................186
Cardizem LA
See Cardizem CD....................186
CARDURA....................187
CARDURA XL....................187
Carisoprodol
Soma....................934
Carteolol HCl
Ocupress....................710
Cartia XT
See Cardizem CD....................186
Carvedilol
Coreg CR....................252
CASODEX....................188
Caspofungin Acetate
Cancidas....................179
CATAFLAM....................189
CATAPRES....................190
CATAPRES-TTS
See Catapres....................190
CEFACLOR....................191
Cefaclor
Cefaclor....................191
Cefaclor ER....................192
CEFACLOR ER....................192
CEFADROXIL....................193
Cefadroxil Monohydrate
Cefadroxil....................193
CEFAZOLIN....................193
Cefdinir
Omnicef....................715
Cefepime HCl
Maxipime....................603
Cefixime
Suprax....................956
CEFOXITIN....................194
Cefoxitin Sodium
Cefoxitin....................194
Cefpodoxime Proxetil
Vantin....................1080
Cefprozil
Cefzil....................198
CEFTAZIDIME....................196
Ceftazidime
Ceftazidime....................196
Fortaz....................440
Tazicef....................983
CEFTIN....................197
Ceftriaxone Sodium
Rocephin....................888
Cefuroxime
Zinacef....................1162
Cefuroxime Axetil
Ceftin....................197
CEFZIL....................198
CELEBREX....................199
Celecoxib
Celebrex....................199
CELEXA....................201
CELLCEPT....................202
CENESTIN....................203
CEPHALEXIN....................204
CEREBYX....................205
Certolizumab pegol
Cimzia....................212
CESAMET....................206
Cetuximab
Erbitux....................373
CHANTIX....................207
Chlorambucil
Leukeran....................544
Chlordiazepoxide HCl
Librax....................557
Librium....................558
Chlorophyllin Copper Complex Sodium
Panafil....................746
Chlorothiazide
Diuril....................322
Chlorpheniramine Polistirex
Tussionex Pennkinetic....................1052
CHLORPROMAZINE....208
Chlorpropamide
Diabinese....................305
Chlorthalidone
Clorpres....................231
Tenoretic....................991
Cholecalciferol
Fosamax Plus D........444
Cholestyramine
Questran....................845
CIALIS....................210
Ciclesonide
Alvesco....................57
Omnaris....................714
Ciclopirox
Loprox....................574
Penlac....................761
Cidofovir
Vistide....................1114
Cilastatin
Primaxin I.M....................808
Primaxin I.V....................809
Cilostazol
Pletal....................780
CILOXAN....................211
CIMZIA....................212
Cinacalcet HCl
Sensipar....................915
CINRYZE....................213
CIPRO HC....................213

CIPRO IV.................... 214
CIPRO ORAL.............. 215
CIPRO XR.................. 217
CIPRODEX................. 218
Ciprofloxacin
Cipro IV.................... 214
Cipro XR.................. 217
Ciprodex.................. 218
Ciprofloxacin HCl
Ciloxan..................... 211
Cipro HC.................. 213
Cipro Oral................ 215
Proquin XR 830
Citalopram Hydrobromide
Celexa..................... 201
Claravis
See Accutane............ 10
CLARINEX 219
Clarinex RediTabs
See Clarinex............. 219
Clarinex Syrup
See Clarinex............. 219
CLARINEX-D............. 220
Clarithromycin
Biaxin...................... 160
Biaxin XL 161
Prevpac................... 803
Clavulanate Potassium
Augmentin............... 114
Augmentin ES-600 115
Augmentin XR.......... 116
Timentin.................. 1011
CLEOCIN 221
CLEOCIN T............... 222
CLEOCIN VAGINAL 223
Cleocin Vaginal Ovules
See Cleocin Vaginal.. 223
Clidinium Bromide
Librax...................... 557
CLIMARA.................. 223
CLIMARA PRO 225
CLINDAGEL 226
Clindamax Vaginal
See Cleocin Vaginal.. 223
Clindamycin
BenzaClin................ 150
Duac 334
Clindamycin HCl
Cleocin..................... 221
Clindamycin Phosphate
Acanya........................ 5
Cleocin T 222
Cleocin Vaginal........ 223
Clindagel................. 226
Ziana...................... 1161
CLINORIL
See Sulindac........... 953
Clobetasol Propionate
Clobevate............... 227
Clobex..................... 228
Cormax 253
Olux 712
Olux-E 713
Temovate................ 990
CLOBEVATE.............. 227
CLOBEX................... 228
Clocortolone Pivalate
Cloderm 229
CLODERM................ 229
Clofarabine
Clolar 230
CLOLAR................... 230
Clonazepam
Klonopin................. 530
Clonidine
Catapres................. 190
Clonidine HCl
Clorpres 231
Clopidogrel Bisulfate
Plavix 779
Clorazepate Dipotassium
Tranxene-SD.......... 1032
CLORPRES............... 231
Clotrimazole
Clotrimazole Topical. 232
Lotrisone................ 581
Mycelex Troche 652
CLOTRIMAZOLE TOPICAL 232
Clozapine
Clozapine 232
Fazaclo................... 404
CLOZAPINE 232
CLOZARIL
See Clozapine......... 232
Codeine Phosphate
Fioricet with Codeine 413
Fiorinal with Codeine 415
Promethazine VC/Codeine.................. 825
Promethazine w/Codeine.................. 827
Tylenol with Codeine...................... 1056
COGENTIN
See Benztropine 152
COGNEX.................. 234
COLAZAL 235
COLCHICINE............ 235
Colchicine/Probenecid............ 236
COLCHICINE/PROBENECID 236
Colesevelam HCl
WelChol................. 1126
COLESTID................ 237
Colestipol HCl
Colestid.................. 237
Colistin Sulfate
Cortisporin-TC Otic .. 255
COMBIGAN.............. 238
COMBIPATCH........... 239
COMBIVENT............. 240
COMBIVIR................ 241
COMBUNOX............. 242
COMTAN.................. 244
CONCERTA.............. 245
Conjugated Estrogens
Cenestin.................. 203
Enjuvia 362
Premarin IV............. 793
Premarin Tablets...... 794
Premarin Vaginal...... 796
Premphase 797
Prempro 799
Constulose
See Lactulose.......... 536
COPAXONE 246
COPEGUS 247
CORDARONE............ 248
CORDARONE IV........ 249
CORDRAN 251
CORDRAN SP
See Cordran............ 251
COREG
See Coreg CR 252
COREG CR............... 252
CORGARD
See Nadolol 656
CORMAX 253
CORMAX SCALP
See Cormax 253
CORTEF................... 254
CORTISPORIN-TC OTIC....................... 255
CORVERT 256
COSOPT 257
COUMADIN.............. 258
COVERA-HS............. 259
COZAAR.................. 260
CRESTOR................. 261
CRIXIVAN 262
Cromolyn Sodium
Cromolyn Sodium Inhalation 263
CROMOLYN SODIUM INHALATION .. 263
Cryselle
See Lo/Ovral........... 565
CUBICIN 264
CUTIVATE................ 265
CYCLESSA............... 266
Cyclobenzaprine HCl
Amrix 75
Flexeril 420

Cyclophosphamide
Cytoxan....................271
Cyclosporine
Neoral 671
Restasis....................867
Sandimmune............903
CYMBALTA 267
CYTOMEL 269
CYTOVENE 270
CYTOXAN....................271

D

D.H.E. 45....................272
DACOGEN....................273
Dalfopristin
Synercid 969
DALMANE....................274
Dalteparin Sodium
Fragmin....................446
DANTRIUM....................274
DANTRIUM IV..............275
Dantrolene Sodium
Dantrium 274
Dantrium IV 275
Daptomycin
Cubicin....................264
Darbepoetin Alfa
Aranesp....................92
Darifenacin
Enablex 359
Darunavir
Prezista 805
DARVOCET A500 276
DARVOCET-N 277
DARVON....................277
DARVON-N................278
Dasatinib
Sprycel....................941
DAYTRANA..................279
DDAVP........................281
DDAVP Nasal Spray
See DDAVP..............281
DDAVP Rhinal Tube
See DDAVP..............281
DECADRON
See Dexamethasone..301
Decitabine
Dacogen....................273
Deferasirox
Exjade 400
Delavirdine Mesylate
Rescriptor..................865
DELTASONE
See Prednisone........790
DEMADEX....................282
DEMEROL
INJECTION 283
DEMEROL ORAL........284
DENAVIR....................285
DEPACON 286
DEPAKENE 287
DEPAKOTE..................288
DEPAKOTE ER............289
DEPO-ESTRADIOL.....290
DEPO-MEDROL.........292
DEPO-PROVERA........293
DEPO-PROVERA
CONTRACEPTIVE....294
DEPO-SUBQ
PROVERA 104..........295
DEPO-TESTOSTER-
ONE 296
Desloratadine
Clarinex....................219
Clarinex-D 220
Desmopressin Acetate
DDAVP 281
DESOGEN..................297
Desogestrel
Cyclessa 266
Desogen....................297
Mircette....................638
Ortho-Cept..............730
Desonide
DesOwen..................298
DESOWEN 298
Desoximetasone
Topicort....................1025
DESOXYN 299
Desvenlafaxine
Pristiq......................813
DETROL
See Detrol LA 300
DETROL LA................300
Dexamethasone
Ciprodex....................218
Dexamethasone 301
TobraDex....................1018
DEXAMETHASONE 301
DEXEDRINE 302
DEXEDRINE
SPANSULES
See Dexedrine..........302
Dexlansoprazole
Kapidex 521
Dexmethylphenidate HCl
Focalin 434
Focalin XR 435
Dexrazoxane
Zinecard....................1163
Dextroamphetamine
Sulfate
Dexedrine 302
DextroStat..................303
Dextromethorphan HBr
Promethazine DM.....823
DEXTROSTAT.............303
DIABETA....................304
DIABINESE 305
DIAMOX SEQUELS
See Acetazolamide......13
DIASTAT 306
Diazepam
Diastat......................306
Diazepam Injection ..307
Valium......................1073
DIAZEPAM
INJECTION 307
Dichloralphenazone
Midrin......................633
Diclofenac Epolamine
Flector 419
Diclofenac Potassium
Cataflam....................189
Diclofenac Sodium
Arthrotec....................101
Voltaren Gel..............1119
Voltaren Ophthalmic .1121
Voltaren-XR..............1121
DICLOXACILLIN 308
Dicloxacillin Sodium
Dicloxacillin 308
Dicyclomine HCl
Bentyl 149
Didanosine
Videx........................1103
DIDRONEL..................309
DIFFERIN....................310
Diflorasone Diacetate
Psorcon E 840
DIFLUCAN 310
DIGIBIND 312
Digitek
See Lanoxin 539
Digoxin
Lanoxin 539
Digoxin Immune Fab
(Ovine)
Digibind....................312
Dihydroergotamine
Mesylate
D.H.E. 45 272
Migranal 633
DILACOR XR..............313
DILANTIN 313
DILAUDID 315
DILAUDID-HP
See Dilaudid 315
DILTIA XT
See Dilacor XR 313
Diltiazem HCl
Cardizem....................185
Cardizem CD..............186

Dilacor XR 313
Diltiazem Injection 316
Tiazac..................... 1007

DILTIAZEM INJECTION 316

DIOVAN 317

DIOVAN HCT............... 318

Diphenhydramine HCl
Diphenhydramine HCl Injection 319

DIPHENHYDRAMINE HCL INJECTION........ 319

Diphenoxylate HCl
Lomotil.................... 570

Diphtheria Toxoid
Boostrix.................. 163
Pediarix 756
Tetanus & Diphtheria Toxoids Adsorbed 998
Tripedia 1046

DIPROLENE 320

DIPROLENE AF
See Diprolene 320

Dipyridamole
Aggrenox 38
Persantine 767

Disopyramide Phosphate
Norpace 694

Disulfiram
Antabuse.................. 84

DITROPAN
See Ditropan XL........ 321

DITROPAN XL 321

DIURIL 322

Divalproex Sodium
Depakote................ 288
Depakote ER........... 289

DOBUTAMINE 323

Docetaxel
Taxotere 982

Dofetilide
Tikosyn.................. 1010

Dolasetron Mesylate
Anzemet 86

DOLOPHINE.............. 324

Donepezil HCl
Aricept 96

DONNATAL............... 325

DONNATAL EXTENTABS
See Donnatal 325

DOPAMINE 326

DORIBAX.................. 327

Doripenem
Doribax 327

Dornase Alfa
Pulmozyme............. 843

DORYX 328

Dorzolamide HCl
Cosopt 257
Trusopt.................. 1050

DOVONEX 329

DOVONEX SCALP 330

Doxazosin Mesylate
Cardura 187
Cardura XL 187

DOXEPIN 331

Doxepin HCl
Doxepin.................. 331

DOXIL...................... 332

DOXORUBICIN HCL.... 333

Doxorubicin HCl Liposome
Doxil...................... 332

Doxycycline
Oracea 722

Doxycycline Hyclate
Doryx 328
Vibramycin 1098

Doxycycline Monohydrate
Monodox 642

Dronabinol
Marinol.................. 599

Drospirenone
Angeliq..................... 80
Yasmin 1142
YAZ....................... 1144

Drotrecogin alfa
Xigris.................... 1136

DUAC...................... 334

DUETACT................. 335

Duloxetine HCl
Cymbalta................ 267

DUONEB.................. 337

Duradrin
See Midrin.............. 633

DURAGESIC.............. 338

DURAMORPH............ 339

Dutasteride
Avodart 128

DYAZIDE.................. 340

DYNACIN.................. 341

DYNACIRC CR........... 342

DYRENIUM............... 343

E

E.E.S....................... 344

EC-NAPROSYN
See Naprosyn 660

Eculizumab
Soliris 929

Efavirenz
Atripla 111
Sustiva 958

EFFEXOR.................. 345

EFFEXOR XR............. 346

ELDEPRYL 347

ELESTAT.................. 348

Eletriptan Hydrobromide
Relpax 857

ELIDEL..................... 349

ELIGARD.................. 350

ELLENCE 350

ELMIRON 352

ELOCON 352

ELOXATIN................ 353

EMCYT.................... 354

EMEND 355

EMLA..................... 356

EMSAM 357

Emtricitabine
Atripla 111
Emtriva................... 358
Truvada 1051

EMTRIVA................. 358

ENABLEX................. 359

Enalapril Maleate
Vaseretic 1083
Vasotec 1084

Enalaprilat
Vasotec I.V............. 1085

ENBREL.................. 360

ENDOCET
See Percocet 764

ENDODAN
See Percodan.......... 765

Enfuvirtide
Fuzeon 450

ENGERIX-B 361

ENGERIX-B PEDIATRIC/ ADOLESCENT
See Engerix-B.......... 361

ENJUVIA.................. 362

Enoxaparin Sodium
Lovenox.................. 583

ENPRESSE
See Triphasil 1047
See Trivora 1048

Entacapone
Comtan 244
Stalevo 942

Entecavir
Baraclude 145

ENTOCORT EC.......... 363

Enulose
See Lactulose 536

EPIDUO 364

Epinastine HCl
Elestat.................... 348

Epinephrine
EpiPen.................... 365
Twinject................. 1053

EPIPEN 365

EPIPEN JR.
See EpiPen 365

Epirubicin HCl
Ellence ... 350
EPIVIR ... 366
EPIVIR-HBV ... 367
Eplerenone
Inspra ... 503
Epoetin Alfa
Epogen ... 368
Procrit ... 819
EPOGEN ... 368
Eprosartan Mesylate
Teveten ... 999
Teveten HCT ... 1000
Eptifibatide
Integrilin ... 504
EPZICOM ... 369
EQUAGESIC ... 370
EQUETRO ... 371
ERAXIS ... 372
ERBITUX ... 373
Erlotinib
Tarceva ... 977
Errin
See Micronor ... 630
Ertapenem Sodium
Invanz ... 508
ERYC ... 374
ERY-TAB ... 375
ERYTHROCIN ... 376
Erythromycin
Benzamycin ... 151
ERYC ... 374
Ery-Tab ... 375
Erythromycin Base ... 377
Erythromycin Delayed-Release ... 379
PCE ... 754
ERYTHROMYCIN BASE ... 377
ERYTHROMYCIN DELAYED-RELEASE 379
Erythromycin Ethylsuccinate
E.E.S. ... 344
Erythromycin Stearate
Erythrocin ... 376
Escitalopram Oxalate
Lexapro ... 554
ESCLIM ... 380
ESGIC ... 381
ESGIC-PLUS ... 381
ESKALITH ... 382
ESKALITH CR
See Eskalith ... 382
Esmolol HCl
Brevibloc ... 164
Esomeprazole Magnesium
Nexium ... 678
Esomeprazole Sodium
Nexium IV ... 680
Esterified Estrogens
Estratest ... 388
ESTRACE ... 383
ESTRADERM ... 385
Estradiol
Activella ... 20
Angeliq ... 80
Climara ... 223
Climara Pro ... 225
CombiPatch ... 239
Esclim ... 380
Estrace ... 383
Estraderm ... 385
Estrasorb ... 386
Estring ... 389
EstroGel ... 390
Prefest ... 791
Vagifem ... 1071
Vivelle ... 1117
Estradiol Cypionate
Depo-Estradiol ... 290
Estramustine Phosphate Sodium
Emcyt ... 354
ESTRASORB ... 386
ESTRATEST ... 388
ESTRATEST H.S.
See Estratest ... 388
ESTRING ... 389
ESTROGEL ... 390
Estropipate
Ogen ... 711
ESTROSTEP FE ... 392
Eszopiclone
Lunesta ... 586
Etanercept
Enbrel ... 360
Ethinyl Estradiol
Alesse ... 47
Cyclessa ... 266
Desogen ... 297
Estrostep Fe ... 392
femhrt ... 408
Lo/Ovral ... 565
Loestrin ... 568
Lybrel ... 592
Mircette ... 638
Nordette-28 ... 691
NuvaRing ... 705
Ortho Evra ... 726
Ortho Tri-Cyclen ... 727
Ortho Tri-Cyclen Lo .. 729
Ortho-Cept ... 730
Ortho-Cyclen ... 731
Ortho-Novum 1/35 ... 732
Ortho-Novum 10/11 ... 735
Ortho-Novum 7/7/7 . 736
Ovcon-35 ... 738
Ovcon-35 Fe ... 739
Seasonale ... 910
Seasonique ... 911
Tri-Levlen ... 1042
Tri-Norinyl ... 1045
Triphasil ... 1047
Trivora ... 1048
Yasmin ... 1142
YAZ ... 1144
Ethionamide
Trecator ... 1035
Ethosuximide
Zarontin ... 1147
Etidronate Disodium
Didronel ... 309
Etodolac
Etodolac ... 393
Etodolac Extended-Release ... 394
ETODOLAC ... 393
ETODOLAC EXTENDED-RELEASE .. 394
Etonogestrel
NuvaRing ... 705
ETOPOPHOS ... 395
Etravirine
Intelence ... 505
EUFLEXXA ... 396
EVISTA ... 397
EXELON ... 398
Exemestane
Aromasin ... 100
Exenatide
Byetta ... 170
EXFORGE ... 399
EXJADE ... 400
EXTINA ... 401
Ezetimibe
Vytorin ... 1123
Zetia ... 1157

F

FACTIVE ... 402
Famciclovir
Famvir ... 403
Famotidine
Pepcid ... 763
FAMVIR ... 403
FASLODEX ... 404
FAZACLO ... 404
Febuxostat
Uloric ... 1060
Felbamate
Felbatol ... 406
FELBATOL ... 406
Felodipine
Plendil ... 779
FEMARA ... 407
FEMHRT ... 408

Fenofibrate
Antara 85
Lofibra 569
Tricor 1038
Triglide 1039
Fenofibric acid
Trilipix 1043
Fentanyl
Duragesic 338
Fentanyl Citrate
Actiq 18
Fentora 409
Sublimaze 950
FENTORA 409
FERRLECIT 410
Ferrous Fumarate
Loestrin 568
Ovcon-35 Fe 739
Fesoterodine Fumarate
Toviaz 1028
Fexofenadine HCl
Allegra 50
Allegra-D 51
Filgrastim
Neupogen 675
FINACEA 411
Finasteride
Propecia 828
Proscar 831
FIORICET 412
FIORICET WITH CODEINE 413
FIORINAL 414
FIORINAL WITH CODEINE 415
FLAGYL 416
FLAGYL ER 417
FLAGYL IV 418
Flavocoxid
Limbrel 560
Flecainide Acetate
Tambocor 973
FLECTOR 419
FLEXERIL 420
FLOMAX 421
FLONASE 421
FLOVENT HFA 422
FLOXIN 424
FLOXIN OTIC 425
FLOXIN OTIC SINGLES
See Floxin Otic 425
Fluconazole
Diflucan 310
Flucytosine
Ancobon 78
FLUDROCORTISONE .. 426
FLULAVAL 427
Flumazenil
Romazicon 889
FLUMIST 427
Flunisolide
Aerobid 36
Flunisolide Nasal Spray 428
Nasarel 664
FLUNISOLIDE NASAL SPRAY 428
Fluocinolone Acetonide
Synalar 967
Tri-Luma 1044
Fluocinonide
Vanos 1078
Fluorometholone
FML 432
FML-S 433
FLUOROURACIL 429
Fluoxetine HCl
Prozac 838
Prozac Weekly 839
Sarafem 907
Symbyax 962
Flurandrenolide
Cordran 251
Flurazepam HCl
Dalmane 274
Flurbiprofen
Ansaid 83
Fluticasone Furoate
Veramyst 1090
Fluticasone Propionate
Advair 31
Advair HFA 33
Cutivate 265
Flonase 421
Flovent HFA 422
Fluvastatin Sodium
Lescol XL 542
FLUVOXAMINE 430
Fluvoxamine Maleate
Fluvoxamine 430
Luvox CR 590
FLUZONE 431
FML 432
FML FORTE
See FML 432
FML-S 433
FOCALIN 434
FOCALIN XR 435
FOLGARD RX 2.2 436
Folic Acid
Folgard RX 2.2 436
Folic Acid 436
Foltx 437
FOLIC ACID 436
FOLTX 437
Fondaparinux Sodium
Arixtra 98
FORADIL 438
Formoterol Fumarate
Foradil 438
Perforomist 766
Formoterol Fumarate dihydrate
Symbicort 960
FORTAMET 439
FORTAZ 440
FORTEO 441
FORTICAL 442
FOSAMAX 443
FOSAMAX PLUS D 444
Fosamprenavir Calcium
Lexiva 555
Fosinopril Sodium
Monopril 644
Monopril HCT 645
Fosphenytoin Sodium
Cerebyx 205
FOSRENOL 445
FRAGMIN 446
FROVA 448
Frovatriptan Succinate
Frova 448
Fulvestrant
Faslodex 404
FUROSEMIDE 449
FUZEON 450

G

Gabapentin
Neurontin 676
GABITRIL 451
Galantamine Hydrobromide
Razadyne ER 851
Ganciclovir
Cytovene 270
Vitrasert 1116
GARDASIL 452
Gatifloxacin
Zymar 1187
Gemcitabine HCl
Gemzar 452
Gemfibrozil
Lopid 571
Gemifloxacin Mesylate
Factive 402
Gemtuzumab Ozogamicin
Mylotarg 654
GEMZAR 452
Generlac
See Lactulose 536
Gentamicin Sulfate
Pred-G 789

Genuine Bayer Aspirin
See Bayer Aspirin......146
GEODON 454
GEODON FOR INJECTION
See Geodon..............454
Glatiramer Acetate
Copaxone................246
GLEEVEC...................455
Glimepiride
Amaryl 59
Avandaryl...................121
Duetact 335
GLIPIZIDE..................456
Glipizide
Glipizide..................456
Glucotrol XL 460
Metaglip 613
Glipizide ER
See Glucotrol XL......460
GLUCAGON..............457
Glucophage
See Glucophage XR..458
GLUCOPHAGE XR......458
Glucotrol
See Glucotrol XL......460
GLUCOTROL
See Glipizide...........456
GLUCOTROL XL.........460
GLUCOVANCE 461
GLUMETZA................462
Glyburide
DiaBeta 304
Glucovance..............461
Glynase PresTab.......463
Micronase................629
GLYNASE PRESTAB ... 463
GLYSET.....................464
Goserelin Acetate
Zoladex 1-Month 1168
Zoladex 3-Month......1169
Granisetron HCl
Kytril 534
GRIFULVIN V.............465
Griseofulvin
Grifulvin V 465
Gris-PEG..................466
GRIS-PEG 466

H

HALCION..................466
Haldol
See Haloperidol 468
Haldol Decanoate
See Haloperidol 468
HALFLYTELY.............467
Halobetasol Propionate
Ultravate.................1064
HALOPERIDOL..........468
HAVRIX.....................469
HELIDAC...................470
HEPARIN SODIUM.......471
Hepatitis A Vaccine (Inactivated)
Havrix......................469
Twinrix..................1054
Hepatitis B (Recombinant)
Engerix-B 361
Pediarix 756
Recombivax HB 855
Twinrix..................1054
Hepatitis B Immune Globulin
Vaqta 1081
HEPSERA..................472
HERCEPTIN...............473
Histrelin Acetate
Vantas...................1079
HUMALOG 474
HUMALOG MIX 75/25 . 475
Human Papillomavirus Recombinant Vaccine, Quadrivalent
Gardasil..................452
HUMATROPE 476
HUMIRA....................478
HUMULIN..................479
HUMULIN 50/50
See Humulin 70/30 ..480
HUMULIN 70/30.........480
Humulin N
See Humulin.............479
Humulin R
See Humulin.............479
HYALGAN..................481
HYDRALAZINE 482
Hydrochlorothiazide
Accuretic.....................9
Aldactazide 44
Amiloride/HCTZ 67
Atacand HCT 107
Avalide 118
Benicar HCT 148
Capozide 180
Diovan HCT 318
Dyazide 340
Hydrochlorothiazide. 482
Hyzaar.....................487
Inderide...................495
Lopressor HCT......... 573
Lotensin HCT 579
Maxzide...................604
Methyldopa/HCTZ 618
Micardis HCT 627
Microzide.................630
Monopril HCT...........645
Prinzide 812
Tekturna HCT...........988
Teveten HCT 1000
Uniretic 1067
Vaseretic 1083
Zestoretic 1154
Ziac........................1159
HYDROCHLOROTHIAZIDE 482
Hydrocodone Bitartrate
Lorcet..................... 575
Lortab 576
Norco 690
Vicodin...................1100
Vicoprofen..............1100
Zydone.................. 1184
Hydrocodone Polistirex
Tussionex Pennkinetic............1052
Hydrocortisone
Alcortin 43
Cipro HC..................213
Cortef......................254
Neomycin/Poly B/ Hydrocortisone Otic. 670
Hydrocortisone Acetate
Cortisporin-TC Otic .. 255
Hydrocortisone Butyrate
Locoid 567
Hydrocortisone Probutate
Pandel.....................747
Hydrocortisone Sodium Succinate
Solu-Cortef.............. 932
Hydrocortisone Valerate
Westcort 1129
Hydromorphone HCl
Dilaudid...................315
Hydroquinone
Tri-Luma.................1044
Hydroxychloroquine Sulfate
Plaquenil 778
HYDROXYZINE HCL ... 483
HYDROXYZINE PAMOATE................484
Hylan G-F 20
Synvisc....................971
Hyoscyamine Sulfate
Donnatal................. 325
Hyoscyamine Sulfate 485
Levbid 548
HYOSCYAMINE SULFATE 485
HYTRIN.....................486
HYZAAR................... 487

I

Ibandronate Sodium
Boniva.....................162
Ibritumomab Tiuxetan
Zevalin 1158
Ibuprofen
Combunox.............. 242

Motrin....................647
Vicoprofen..............1100

Ibutilide Fumarate
Corvert..................256

IFEX.....................488

IFEX/MESNEX
See Ifex.................488

Ifosfamide
Ifex.....................488

Iloprost
Ventavis................1088

Imatinib Mesylate
Gleevec..................455

IMDUR....................489

Imipenem
Primaxin I.M.............808
Primaxin I.V.............809

Imipramine HCl
Tofranil................1020

Imipramine Pamoate
Tofranil-PM.............1021

Imiquimod
Aldara....................45

IMITREX..................490

IMURAN...................491

INDAPAMIDE...............492

INDERAL..................493

INDERAL LA...............494

INDERIDE.................495

Indinavir Sulfate
Crixivan.................262

INDOCIN
See Indomethacin.........497

INDOCIN I.V..............496

INDOMETHACIN.............497

Indomethacin
Sodium Trihydrate
Indocin I.V..............496

INFERGEN.................499

Infliximab
Remicade.................859

Influenza Virus Vaccine
FluLaval.................427
Fluzone..................431

Influenza Virus
Vaccine Live
FluMist..................427

INFUMORPH................500

INNOHEP..................501

INNOPRAN XL..............502

INSPRA...................503

Insulin Aspart
Novolog..................700
Novolog Mix 70/30........701

Insulin Aspart Protamine
Novolog Mix 70/30........701

Insulin Detemir,
rDNA origin
Levemir..................549

Insulin Glargine, Human
Lantus...................541

Insulin Glulisine, rDNA
Apidra....................87

Insulin Human, rDNA
origin
Humulin..................479
Humulin 70/30............480
Novolin..................698
Novolin 70/30............699

Insulin Lispro
Humalog..................474
Humalog Mix 75/25........475

Insulin Lispro Protamine
Humalog Mix 75/25........475

Insulin, Human
(Isophane/Regular)
Humulin 70/30............480
Novolin 70/30............699

Insulin, Human Isophane
Humulin..................479
Novolin..................698

Insulin, Human Regular
Humulin..................479
Novolin..................698

INTAL
See Cromolyn
Sodium Inhalation........263

INTEGRILIN...............504

INTELENCE................505

Interferon alfa-2b
Intron A.................506

Interferon alfacon-1
Infergen.................499

Interferon beta-1a
Rebif....................853

INTRAVENOUS
SODIUM DIURIL
See Diuril...............322

INTRON A.................506

INVANZ...................508

INVEGA...................509

INVIRASE.................510

Iodine I 131 Tositumomab
Bexxar...................159

Iodoquinol
Alcortin..................43

Ipratropium Bromide
Atrovent HFA.............112
Atrovent Nasal...........113
Combivent................240
Duoneb...................337

IQUIX....................511

Irbesartan
Avalide..................118
Avapro...................123

Irinotecan HCl
Camptosar................176

ISENTRESS................512

Isometheptene Mucate
Midrin...................633

ISONIAZID................512

Isoniazid
Isoniazid................512
Rifamate.................878
Rifater..................879

ISOPTO CARPINE
See Pilocarpine..........774

Isordil
See Isosorbide
Dinitrate................513

Isordil Titradose
See Isosorbide
Dinitrate................513

ISOSORBIDE
DINITRATE................513

Isosorbide Mononitrate
Imdur....................489
Monoket..................644

Isotretinoin
Accutane..................10

Isradipine
DynaCirc CR..............342

Itraconazole
Sporanox.................940

Ivermectin
Stromectol...............949

Ixabepilone
Ixempra..................514

IXEMPRA..................514

J

JADELLE
See Norplant II..........695

JANTOVEN
See Coumadin.............258

JANUMET..................515

JANUVIA..................517

Junel 1.5/30
See Loestrin.............568

Junel 1/20
See Loestrin.............568

Junel Fe 1.5/30
See Loestrin.............568

Junel Fe 1/20
See Loestrin.............568

K

KADIAN...................518

KALETRA..................519

KAPIDEX..................521

KARIVA
See Mircette.............638

KAYEXALATE...............521

K-DUR....................522

KEFLEX
See Cephalexin...........204

KEMSTRO
See Baclofen.............140

KENALOG..................523

KEPIVANCE 524
KEPPRA 524
KEPPRA XR............... 526
KETEK 526
Ketoconazole
  Extina..................... 401
  Ketoconazole Topical 527
  Nizoral.................... 688
  Nizoral Shampoo...... 689
KETOCONAZOLE TOPICAL 527
KETOROLAC.............. 528
Ketorolac Tromethamine
  Acular 27
  Ketorolac................. 528
KINERET.................... 529
KLONOPIN................. 530
KLONOPIN WAFERS
  See Klonopin 530
K-LOR......................... 531
KLOR-CON
  See Klor-Con M........ 532
KLOR-CON M 532
KLOTRIX
  See K-Tab 533
KRISTALOSE.............. 533
K-TAB 533
KYTRIL 534

L

LABETALOL............... 535
Labetalol HCl
  Labetalol 535
  Trandate................ 1030
Lacosamide
  Vimpat 1105
LACTULOSE............... 536
Lactulose
  Kristalose 533
  Lactulose................. 536
LAMICTAL 537
LAMICTAL CD
  See Lamictal............ 537
LAMISIL..................... 539
Lamivudine
  Combivir.................. 241
  Epivir....................... 366
  Epivir-HBV............... 367
  Epzicom 369
  Trizivir 1049
Lamotrigine
  Lamictal 537
Lanoxicaps
  See Lanoxin............. 539
LANOXIN................... 539
Lanreotide
  Somatuline Depot 935
Lansoprazole
  Prevacid 800
  Prevacid NapraPAC...801
  Prevpac................... 803
Lanthanum Carbonate
  Fosrenol.................. 445
LANTUS...................... 541
Lapatinib
  Tykerb.................... 1055
LASIX
  See Furosemide....... 449
Latanoprost
  Xalatan.................. 1130
Leflunomide
  Arava 93
Lenalidomide
  Revlimid 874
Lepirudin
  Refludan.................. 855
LESCOL
  See Lescol XL 542
LESCOL XL 542
Lessina
  See Alesse 47
LETAIRIS................... 543
Letrozole
  Femara.................... 407
LEUKERAN 544
LEUKINE.................... 545
Leuprolide Acetate
  Eligard..................... 350
  Lupron 587
  Lupron Depot (GYN) 588
  Lupron Depot (Oncology) 589
  Lupron Pediatric 590
  Viadur 1096
Levalbuterol HCl
  Xopenex.................1138
Levalbuterol Tartrate
  Xopenex HFA..........1138
LEVAQUIN 546
LEVBID...................... 548
LEVEMIR................... 549
Levetiracetam
  Keppra 524
  Keppra XR 526
LEVITRA 550
Levobunolol HCl
  Betagan.................. 153
Levocetirizine Dihydrochloride
  Xyzal.....................1142
Levodopa
  Parcopa.................. 747
  Sinemet CR.............. 925
  Stalevo 942
Levofloxacin
  Iquix........................ 511
  Levaquin.................. 546
  Quixin...................... 846
Levonorgestrel
  Alesse 47
  Climara Pro.............. 225
  Lybrel...................... 592
  Mirena 639
  Nordette-28............. 691
  Norplant II 695
  Seasonale 910
  Seasonique............... 911
  Tri-Levlen 1042
  Triphasil.................1047
  Trivora.................. 1048
Levora
  See Nordette-28 691
LEVOTHROID............. 551
Levothyroxine Sodium
  Levothroid............... 551
  Levoxyl.................... 552
  Synthroid................. 970
  Unithroid 1068
LEVOXYL.................. 552
Levsin
  See Levbid............... 548
Levsinex
  See Levbid............... 548
LEXAPRO 554
LEXIVA 555
LIALDA 557
LIBRAX...................... 557
LIBRIUM.................... 558
Lidocaine
  EMLA 356
  Lidocaine Ointment.. 559
  Lidoderm Patch 560
  Synera..................... 968
Lidocaine HCl
  Xylocaine Injection...1139
  Xylocaine Jelly........ 1140
  Xylocaine Viscous 1141
LIDOCAINE OINTMENT 559
LIDODERM PATCH...... 560
LIMBREL.................... 560
LINDANE 561
Lindane
  Lindane 561
Linezolid
  Zyvox......................1189
Liothyronine Sodium
  Cytomel.................. 269
Liotrix
  Thyrolar................1006
LIPITOR 562
Lisdexamfetamine Dimesylate
  Vyvanse 1125
Lisinopril
  Prinivil 811

Prinzide 812
Zestoretic 1154
Zestril 1156
Lithium Carbonate
Eskalith 382
Lithium Carbonate 563
Lithobid 564
LITHIUM CARBONATE 563
LITHOBID 564
LO/OVRAL 565
LOCOID 567
LOESTRIN 568
Loestrin 1.5/30
See Loestrin 568
Loestrin 1/20
See Loestrin 568
Loestrin Fe 1.5/30
See Loestrin 568
Loestrin Fe 1/20
See Loestrin 568
LOFIBRA 569
Lomefloxacin HCl
Maxaquin 602
LOMOTIL 570
LONOX
See Lomotil 570
LOPID 571
Lopinavir
Kaletra 519
LOPRESSOR 572
LOPRESSOR HCT 573
LOPROX 574
LOPROX TS
See Loprox 574
Lorazepam
Ativan 109
Ativan Injection 109
LORCET 575
Lorcet 10/650
See Lorcet 575
Lorcet HD
See Lorcet 575
Lorcet Plus
See Lorcet 575
LORTAB 576
Losartan Potassium
Cozaar 260
Hyzaar 487
LOTEMAX 577
LOTENSIN 578
LOTENSIN HCT 579
Loteprednol Etabonate
Alrex 54
Lotemax 577
Zylet 1185
LOTREL 580
LOTRISONE 581
LOTRONEX 582
Lovastatin
Advicor 35
Altoprev 56
Mevacor 623
LOVAZA 583
LOVENOX 583
Low-Ogestrel
See Lo/Ovral 565
Lubiprostone
Amitiza 68
LUCENTIS 585
LUMIGAN 585
LUNESTA 586
LUPRON 587
LUPRON DEPOT (GYN) 588
LUPRON DEPOT (ONCOLOGY) 589
Lupron Depot 3.75 mg
See Lupron Depot (GYN) 588
Lupron Depot 3-Month 22.5 mg
See Lupron Depot (Oncology) 589
Lupron Depot 4-Month
See Lupron Depot (Oncology) 589
Lupron Depot 7.5mg
See Lupron Depot (Oncology) 589
Lupron Depot-3 Month 11.25mg
See Lupron Depot (GYN) 588
LUPRON DEPOT-PED
See Lupron Pediatric 590
LUPRON PEDIATRIC 590
LUVOX CR 590
LUXIQ 592
LYBREL 592
LYRICA 594

M

MACROBID 595
MACRODANTIN 596
MACUGEN 597
MALARONE 598
MALARONE PEDIATRIC
See Malarone 598
Maraviroc
Selzentry 914
MARINOL 599
MAVIK 600
MAXAIR 601
MAXAIR AUTOHALER
See Maxair 601
MAXALT 601
MAXALT-MLT
See Maxalt 601
MAXAQUIN 602
MAXIPIME 603
MAXZIDE 604
MAXZIDE-25
See Maxzide 604
Measles Vaccine Live
M-M-R II 640
ProQuad 829
Meclizine HCl
Antivert 86
MEDROL 605
MEDROL DOSE PACK
See Medrol 605
Medroxyprogesterone Acetate
Depo-Provera 293
Depo-Provera Contraceptive 294
depo-subQ provera 104 295
Premphase 797
Prempro 799
Provera 836
Mefenamic Acid
Ponstel 782
MEFOXIN
See Cefoxitin 194
MEGACE ES 606
MEGACE SUSPENSION
See Megace ES 606
Megestrol Acetate
Megace ES 606
Meloxicam
Mobic 641
Memantine HCl
Namenda 658
Meperidine HCl
Demerol Injection 283
Demerol Oral 284
Meperidine/Promethazine 607
MEPERIDINE/PROMETHAZINE 607
Meprobamate
Equagesic 370
MEPRON 608
MEPROZINE
See Meperidine/Promethazine 607
Mercaptopurine
Purinethol 843
MERIDIA 609
Meropenem
Merrem 610
MERREM 610
Mesalamine
Apriso 90
Asacol 102

Canasa 178
Lialda 557
Pentasa 762
Rowasa 893
Mestranol
Ortho-Novum 1/50 ... 734
METADATE CD 611
METADATE ER 612
METAGLIP 613
Metaxalone
Skelaxin 927
Metformin HCl
Actoplus Met 24
Avandamet 120
Fortamet 439
Glucophage XR 458
Glucovance 461
Glumetza 462
Janumet 515
Metaglip 613
Prandimet 783
METHADONE
See Dolophine 324
Methadone HCl
Dolophine 324
Methadose 614
METHADOSE 614
Methamphetamine HCl
Desoxyn 299
Methimazole
Tapazole 976
Methocarbamol
Robaxin 887
METHOTREXATE 615
Methyldopa
Methyldopa 617
Methyldopa/HCTZ 618
METHYLDOPA 617
METHYLDOPA/HCTZ .. 618
METHYLIN 619
METHYLIN ER
See Methylin 619
Methylphenidate
Daytrana 279
Methylphenidate HCl
Concerta 245
Metadate CD 611
Metadate ER 612
Methylin 619
Ritalin 884
Methylprednisolone
Medrol 605
Methylprednisolone Acetate
Depo-Medrol 292
Methylprednisolone Sodium Succinate
Solu-Medrol 933
Methyltestosterone
Estratest 388
Testred 997
Metipranolol
OptiPranolol 720
METOCLOPRAMIDE ... 620
Metoclopramide HCl
Metoclopramide 620
Metolazone
Zaroxolyn 1148
Metoprolol Succinate
Toprol-XL 1026
Metoprolol Tartrate
Lopressor 572
Lopressor HCT 573
MetroCream
See MetroGel 621
METROGEL 621
METROGEL-VAGINAL . 622
MetroLotion
See MetroGel 621
Metronidazole
Flagyl 416
Flagyl ER 417
Helidac 470
MetroGel 621
MetroGel-Vaginal 622
Noritate 693
Metronidazole HCl
Flagyl IV 418
MEVACOR 623
MEXILETINE 624
MIACALCIN 625
Micafungin Sodium
Mycamine 651
MICARDIS 626
MICARDIS HCT 627
Microgestin Fe 1.5/30
See Loestrin 568
Microgestin Fe 1/20
See Loestrin 568
MICRO-K 628
MICRONASE 629
MICRONOR 630
MICROZIDE 630
Midazolam HCl
Midazolam Injection .. 631
MIDAZOLAM INJECTION 631
Midodrine HCl
ProAmatine 815
MIDRIN 633
Miglitol
Glyset 464
Migquin
See Midrin 633
MIGRANAL 633
Migrazone
See Midrin 633
Milnacipran HCl
Savella 908
MINIPRESS 634
Minitran
See Nitro-Dur 686
MINOCIN 635
Minocycline HCl
Dynacin 341
Minocin 635
Solodyn 929
MINOXIDIL 636
MIRALAX 637
MIRAPEX 637
MIRCETTE 638
MIRENA 639
Mirtazapine
Remeron 858
Misoprostol
Arthrotec 101
M-M-R II 640
MOBIC 641
Modafinil
Provigil 837
Moexipril HCl
Uniretic 1067
Univasc 1070
Mometasone Furoate
Asmanex 103
Elocon 352
Mometasone Furoate Monohydrate
Nasonex 665
MONODOX 642
MONOKET 644
MonoNessa
See Ortho-Cyclen 731
MONOPRIL 644
MONOPRIL HCT 645
Montelukast Sodium
Singulair 926
Morphine Sulfate
Astramorph PF 106
Avinza 127
Duramorph 339
Infumorph 500
Kadian 518
Morphine Sulfate Immediate Release ... 646
MS Contin 649
Oramorph SR 723
Roxanol 894
MORPHINE SULFATE IMMEDIATE RELEASE 646
MOTRIN 647
MOVIPREP 649
Moxifloxacin HCl
Avelox 125
Vigamox 1104

MS CONTIN 649
Mumps Vaccine Live
M-M-R II 640
ProQuad 829
Mupirocin
Bactroban 142
Mupirocin Calcium
Bactroban Nasal 143
MYCAMINE 651
MYCELEX TROCHE 652
Mycophenolate Mofetil
CellCept 202
Mycophenolic Acid
Myfortic 652
MYFORTIC 652
MYLERAN 653
MYLOTARG 654

N

Nabilone
Cesamet 206
NABUMETONE 655
NADOLOL 656
Nalbuphine HCl
Nubain 703
Naloxone
Suboxone 951
NALOXONE 657
Naloxone HCl
Naloxone 657
Talwin NX 973
Naltrexone
Vivitrol 1118
Naltrexone HCl
ReVia 873
NAMENDA 658
NAPRELAN 659
NAPROSYN 660
Naproxen
Naprosyn 660
Prevacid NapraPAC 801
Naproxen Sodium
Anaprox DS 76
Naprelan 659
Naratriptan HCl
Amerge 62
NARCAN
See Naloxone 657
NARDIL 661
NAROPIN 662
NASACORT AQ 663
NASAREL 664
NASONEX 665
Natalizumab
Tysabri 1058
Nateglinide
Starlix 944
NATRECOR 666
NAVANE 667
NAVELBINE 668
Nebivolol
Bystolic 171
Necon 1/35
See Ortho-Novum 1/35 732
Necon 1/50
See Ortho-Novum 1/50 734
NECON 10/11
See Ortho-Novum 10/11 735
NEFAZODONE 669
Nefazodone HCl
Nefazodone 669
Nelfinavir Mesylate
Viracept 1108
Neomycin
Neomycin/Poly B/ Hydrocortisone Otic 670
Neomycin Sulfate
Cortisporin-TC Otic 255
Neosporin Ophthalmic 672
NEOMYCIN/POLY B/ HYDROCORTISONE OTIC 670
NEORAL 671
NEOSPORIN OPHTHALMIC 672
Nepafenac
Nevanac 677
Nesiritide
Natrecor 666
NEULASTA 673
NEUMEGA 674
NEUPOGEN 675
NEURONTIN 676
NEVANAC 677
Nevirapine
Viramune 1109
NEXAVAR 677
NEXIUM 678
NEXIUM IV 680
Niacin
Advicor 35
Niaspan 680
Simcor 923
NIASPAN 680
Nicardipine HCl
Cardene IV 183
Cardene SR 184
Nifedipine
Adalat CC 28
Nifedipine 682
Procardia XL 817
NIFEDIPINE 682
NILANDRON 682
Nilutamide
Nilandron 682
NIMODIPINE 683
NIMOTOP
See Nimodipine 683
NIRAVAM 684
Nisoldipine
Sular 952
Nitazoxanide
Alinia 49
Nitrek
See Nitro-Dur 686
NITRO-BID 685
NITRO-DUR 686
Nitrofurantoin Macrocrystals
Macrodantin 596
Nitrofurantoin Monohydrate
Macrobid 595
Nitroglycerin
Nitro-Bid 685
Nitro-Dur 686
Nitrolingual Spray 687
Nitrostat 688
NITROLINGUAL SPRAY 687
NITROMIST
See Nitrolingual Spray 687
NITROQUICK
See Nitrostat 688
NITROSTAT 688
Nizatidine
Axid 130
NIZORAL 688
NIZORAL SHAMPOO 689
NORCO 690
NORDETTE-28 691
NORDITROPIN 692
NORDITROPIN NORDIFLEX
See Norditropin 692
Norelgestromin
Ortho Evra 726
Norethindrone
Activella 20
Micronor 630
Ortho-Novum 1/35 732
Ortho-Novum 1/50 734
Ortho-Novum 10/11 735
Ortho-Novum 7/7/7 736
Ovcon-35 738
Ovcon-35 Fe 739
Tri-Norinyl 1045
Norethindrone Acetate
Aygestin 131
CombiPatch 239
Estrostep Fe 392

femhrt....................408
Loestrin....................568
Norgestimate
Ortho Tri-Cyclen...... 727
Ortho Tri-Cyclen Lo.. 729
Ortho-Cyclen............ 731
Prefest...................... 791
Norgestrel
Lo/Ovral.................. 565
Norinyl 1/35
See Ortho-Novum
1/35.......................... 732
Norinyl 1/50
See Ortho-Novum
1/50.......................... 734
NORITATE.................. 693
NORPACE.................... 694
NORPACE CR
See Norpace............ 694
NORPLANT II............. 695
Nortrel 1/35
See Ortho-Novum
1/35.......................... 732
NORTREL 7/7/7
See Ortho-Novum
7/7/7.......................... 736
Nortriptyline HCl
Pamelor.................. 745
NORVASC.................. 696
NORVIR...................... 697
NOVOLIN.................. 698
NOVOLIN 70/30......... 699
Novolin N
See Novolin 698
Novolin R
See Novolin 698
NOVOLOG 700
NOVOLOG MIX 70/30.. 701
NOXAFIL 702
NUBAIN.................... 703
NUTROPIN................ 704
NUTROPIN AQ
See Nutropin............ 704
NUVARING................ 705
NUVIGIL.................... 707
NYDRAZID
See Isoniazid............ 512
Nystatin
Nystatin Oral............ 707
Nystatin Vaginal....... 708
Nystop 709
NYSTATIN ORAL........ 707
NYSTATIN VAGINAL... 708
NYSTOP.................... 709

O

Octreotide Acetate
Sandostatin 905
Sandostatin LAR...... 906
OCUFLOX.................. 709
OCUPRESS 710
Ofloxacin
Floxin...................... 424
Floxin Otic.............. 425
Ocuflox.................... 709
OGEN 711
Olanzapine
Symbyax.................. 962
Zyprexa..................1188
Olmesartan Medoxomil
Azor 137
Benicar.................... 148
Benicar HCT 148
Olopatadine HCl
Patanol.................... 751
OLUX.......................... 712
OLUX-E...................... 713
Omalizumab
Xolair...................... 1137
Omega-3-Acid Ethyl
Esters
Lovaza.................... 583
Omeprazole
Prilosec 807
Zegerid.................. 1149
OMNARIS.................. 714
OMNICEF.................. 715
OMNITROPE 716
ONCASPAR................ 717
Ondansetron
Zofran 1167
OPANA
See Opana ER.......... 718
OPANA ER 718
Oprelvekin
Neumega................ 674
OPTIPRANOLOL 720
OPTIVAR.................... 721
ORACEA.................... 722
ORAMORPH SR.......... 723
ORAPRED.................. 724
ORAPRED ODT
See Orapred 724
ORENCIA.................. 725
Orlistat
Xenical.................... 1134
ORTHO EVRA 726
ORTHO TRI-CYCLEN .. 727
ORTHO TRI-CYCLEN LO 729
ORTHO-CEPT 730
ORTHO-CYCLEN......... 731
ORTHO-NOVUM 1/35 . 732
ORTHO-NOVUM 1/50 . 734
ORTHO-NOVUM 10/11. 735
ORTHO-NOVUM 7/7/7 736
Oseltamivir Phosphate
Tamiflu 974
OVACE...................... 737
OVCON-35................ 738
OVCON-35 FE 739
Ovcon-50
See Ovcon-35 738
Oxaliplatin
Eloxatin 353
Oxcarbazepine
Trileptal.................. 1041
Oxybutynin
Oxytrol.................... 743
Oxybutynin Chloride
Ditropan XL 321
Oxycodone HCl
Combunox.............. 242
OxyContin 741
OxyIR...................... 742
Percocet.................. 764
Percodan................ 765
Roxicet.................... 895
Roxicodone 896
Tylox 1057
OXYCONTIN................ 741
OXYIR........................ 742
Oxymorphone HCl
Opana ER 718
OXYTROL 743

P

PACERONE 744
Paclitaxel
Taxol 980
Paclitaxel Protein-
bound Particles
Abraxane.................... 4
Palifermin
Kepivance................ 524
Paliperidone
Invega 509
Palivizumab
Synagis.................... 966
Palonosetron HCl
Aloxi.......................... 52
PAMELOR 745
Pamidronate Disodium
Aredia 94
PANAFIL.................... 746
PANDEL.................... 747
Panitumumab
Vectibix................ 1086
Pantoprazole Sodium
Protonix.................. 833
Papain
Panafil 746
PARCOPA 747
Paricalcitol
Zemplar IV.............. 1151
Zemplar Oral........... 1152

PARLODEL................ 748
PARNATE.................. 749
Paroxetine HCl
  Paxil...................... 752
  Paxil CR.................. 753
Paroxetine Mesylate
  Pexeva..................... 768
PASER...................... 750
PATANOL.................. 751
PAXIL....................... 752
PAXIL CR.................. 753
PCE......................... 754
PEDIAPRED.............. 755
PEDIARIX................. 756
Pegaptanib Sodium
  Macugen................. 597
Pegaspargase
  Oncaspar................. 717
PEGASYS.................. 758
Pegfilgrastim
  Neulasta................. 673
Peginterferon alfa-2a
  Pegasys................... 758
Peginterferon alfa-2b
  PEG-Intron.............. 759
PEG-INTRON............. 759
Pegvisomant
  Somavert................ 936
Pemetrexed Disodium
  Alimta...................... 48
Pemirolast Potassium
  Alamast.................... 40
Penciclovir
  Denavir................... 285
Penicillin G Potassium
  Pfizerpen................ 769
Penicillin V Potassium
  Penicillin VK............ 761
PENICILLIN VK........... 761
PENLAC.................... 761
PENTASA.................. 762
Pentazocine HCl
  Talacen................... 972
  Talwin NX................ 973
Pentosan Sodium
  Elmiron................... 352
Pentoxifylline
  Trental.................. 1037
PEPCID.................... 763
PEPCID RPD
  See Pepcid.............. 763
PERCOCET............... 764
PERCODAN.............. 765
PERFOROMIST.......... 766
Perindopril Erbumine
  Aceon...................... 12
PERSANTINE............ 767
Pertussis Vaccine, Acellular
  Boostrix.................. 163
  Pediarix.................. 756
  Tripedia................ 1046
PEXEVA.................... 768
PFIZERPEN.............. 769
Phenelzine Sulfate
  Nardil..................... 661
Phenergan
  See Promethazine.... 822
PHENERGAN INJECTION............. 770
PHENOBARBITAL...... 772
Phenobarbital
  Donnatal................. 325
  Phenobarbital.......... 772
Phenylephrine HCl
  Promethazine VC..... 824
  Promethazine VC/Codeine.................. 825
PHENYTEK............... 773
Phenytoin
  Dilantin................... 313
Phenytoin Sodium
  Phenytek................. 773
PHOSLO................... 774
PILOCARPINE........... 774
Pilocarpine HCl
  Pilocarpine............. 774
  Pilopine HS............. 775
PILOPINE HS............ 775
Pimecrolimus
  Elidel...................... 349
PINDOLOL................ 776
Pioglitazone HCl
  Actoplus Met............ 24
  Actos....................... 26
  Duetact.................. 335
PIPERACILLIN........... 776
Piperacillin Sodium
  Piperacillin.............. 776
  Zosyn.................... 1178
Pirbuterol Acetate
  Maxair.................... 601
PLAQUENIL.............. 778
PLAVIX.................... 779
PLENDIL.................. 779
PLETAL.................... 780
Pneumococcal Vaccine
  Pneumovax 23.......... 781
Pneumococcal Vaccine, Diphtheria Conjugate
  Prevnar.................. 803
PNEUMOVAX 23......... 781
Poliovirus Vaccine, Inactivated
  Pediarix.................. 756
Polyethylene Glycol 3350
  HalfLytely............... 467
  MiraLax.................. 637
  MoviPrep................ 649
Polymyxin B Sulfate
  Neomycin/Poly B/Hydrocortisone Otic. 670
  Neosporin Ophthalmic.................. 672
  Polytrim.................. 782
POLYTRIM............... 782
PONSTEL................. 782
Portia
  See Nordette-28....... 691
Posaconazole
  Noxafil.................... 702
Potassium Chloride
  HalfLytely............... 467
  K-Dur..................... 522
  K-Lor...................... 531
  Klor-Con M............. 532
  K-Tab...................... 533
  Micro-K.................. 628
  MoviPrep................ 649
Pramipexole Dihydrochloride
  Mirapex.................. 637
Pramlintide Acetate
  Symlin.................... 964
PRANDIMET.............. 783
PRANDIN.................. 785
PRAVACHOL............. 786
Pravastatin Sodium
  Pravachol............... 786
Prazosin HCl
  Minipress................ 634
PRECOSE................. 787
PRED FORTE............ 788
PRED MILD.............. 789
PRED-G................... 789
PRED-G S.O.P.
  See Pred-G............. 789
Prednisolone Acetate
  Pred Forte.............. 788
  Pred Mild................ 789
  Pred-G................... 789
Prednisolone Sodium Phosphate
  Orapred.................. 724
  Pediapred............... 755
PREDNISONE........... 790
PREFEST................. 791
Pregabalin
  Lyrica..................... 594
PREMARIN IV........... 793
PREMARIN TABLETS.. 794

PREMARIN VAGINAL.. 796
PREMPHASE 797
PREMPRO 799
PREVACID 800
Prevacid IV
See Prevacid........... 800
PREVACID
NAPRAPAC 801
Prevacid Solutab
See Prevacid........... 800
PREVNAR 803
PREVPAC...................803
PREZISTA 805
PRIALT.......................806
Prilocaine
EMLA 356
PRILOSEC..................807
PRIMAXIN I.M............808
PRIMAXIN I.V.............809
PRIMSOL 810
PRINIVIL 811
PRINZIDE.................... 812
PRISTIQ 813
PROAIR HFA 814
PROAMATINE..............815
Probenecid
Colchicine/
Probenecid.............. 236
Probenecid..............816
PROBENECID.............816
PROCARDIA
See Nifedipine 682
PROCARDIA XL...........817
PROCHLORPERAZINE. 818
PROCRIT.....................819
PROGRAF...................820
Proguanil HCl
Malarone 598
PROMETHAZINE........822
PROMETHAZINE DM .. 823
Promethazine HCl
Meperidine/
Promethazine 607
Phenergan Injection . 770
Promethazine 822
Promethazine DM..... 823
Promethazine VC 824
Promethazine VC/
Codeine.................. 825
Promethazine w/
Codeine.................. 827
PROMETHAZINE VC... 824
PROMETHAZINE
VC/CODEINE........... 825
PROMETHAZINE W/
CODEINE................ 827
Promethegan
See Promethazine 822
Propafenone HCl
Rythmol 898
Rythmol SR..............899
PROPECIA 828
Propoxyphene HCl
Darvon 277
Propoxyphene Napsylate
Darvocet A500 276
Darvocet-N..............277
Darvon-N.................278
Propranolol HCl
Inderal.....................493
Inderal LA................494
Inderide...................495
InnoPran XL.............502
PROPYLTHIOURACIL . 828
PROQUAD 829
PROQUIN XR.............830
PROSCAR 831
PROTAMINE
SULFATE 832
PROTONIX 833
PROTONIX IV
See Protonix............833
PROTOPIC 834
PROVENTIL HFA 835
PROVERA..................836
PROVIGIL..................837
PROZAC 838
PROZAC WEEKLY 839
Pseudoephedrine HCl
Allegra-D..................51
Pseudoephedrine Sulfate
Clarinex-D 220
PSORCON E..............840
PULMICORT...............841
Pulmicort Flexhaler
See Pulmicort 841
Pulmicort Respules
See Pulmicort 841
PULMOZYME 843
PURINETHOL............843
Pyrazinamide
Rifater 879

Q

QUESTRAN...............845
QUESTRAN LIGHT
See Questran 845
Quetiapine Fumarate
Seroquel..................918
Seroquel XR.............920
Quinapril HCl
Accupril.......................8
Accuretic.....................9
Quinupristin
Synercid 969
QUIXIN 846
QVAR........................846

R

Rabeprazole Sodium
Aciphex 15
Raloxifene HCl
Evista 397
Raltegravir Potassium
Isentress.................512
Ramelteon
Rozerem..................897
Ramipril
Altace.......................55
RANEXA....................847
Ranibizumab
Lucentis..................585
Ranitidine HCl
Zantac.................. 1146
Ranolazine
Ranexa 847
RAPAFLO 848
RAPAMUNE 849
Rasagiline Mesylate
Azilect....................134
RAZADYNE
See Razadyne ER 851
RAZADYNE ER...........851
REBETOL..................852
REBIF 853
RECLAST..................854
RECOMBIVAX HB.......855
Recombivax HB Adult
See Recombivax HB . 855
Recombivax HB Dialysis
See Recombivax HB . 855
Recombivax HB
Pediatric/Adolescent
See Recombivax HB . 855
REFLUDAN 855
Reglan
See Metoclopramide 620
Reglan Injection
See Metoclopramide 620
RELENZA.................856
RELPAX 857
REMERON.................858
REMERON SOLTAB
See Remeron 858
REMICADE...............859
Remifentanil HCl
Ultiva................... 1061
REMODULIN 861
RENAGEL 862
RENOVA 862

REOPRO 863
Repaglinide
Prandimet................ 783
Prandin................... 785
REPREXAIN
See Vicoprofen 1100
REQUIP...................... 864
REQUIP XL
See Requip 864
RESCRIPTOR 865
RESERPINE............... 866
RESTASIS.................. 867
RESTORIL.................. 868
Retapamulin
Altabax...................... 55
RETAVASE 869
RETIN-A 870
RETIN-A MICRO
See Retin-A 870
RETROVIR 870
REVATIO................... 872
REVIA........................ 873
REVLIMID 874
REYATAZ.................. 875
RHEUMATREX
See Methotrexate...... 615
RHINOCORT AQUA.... 876
Ribavirin
Copegus.................. 247
Rebetol.................... 852
Virazole 1110
RIFADIN.................... 877
RIFAMATE................. 878
Rifampin
Rifadin.................... 877
Rifamate.................. 878
Rifater..................... 879
RIFATER 879
Rifaximin
Xifaxan.................... 1135
RILUTEK 881
Riluzole
Rilutek..................... 881
Riomet
See Glucophage XR.. 458
Risedronate Sodium
Actonel 22
Actonel with Calcium . 23
RISPERDAL............... 882
RISPERDAL CONSTA.. 883
RISPERDAL M-TAB
See Risperdal.......... 882
Risperidone
Risperdal 882
Risperdal Consta...... 883
RITALIN 884
Ritalin LA
See Ritalin 884
Ritalin SR
See Ritalin 884
Ritonavir
Kaletra..................... 519
Norvir....................... 697
RITUXAN 886
Rituximab
Rituxan.................... 886
Rivastigmine Tartrate
Exelon...................... 398
Rizatriptan Benzoate
Maxalt 601
ROBAXIN.................. 887
Robaxin Injection
See Robaxin............ 887
Robaxin-750
See Robaxin............ 887
ROCEPHIN................ 888
ROMAZICON............. 889
Ropinirole HCl
Requip..................... 864
Ropivacaine HCl
Naropin 662
ROSAC...................... 890
Rosiglitazone Maleate
Avandamet............... 120
Avandaryl................ 121
Avandia................... 122
ROSULA 891
ROSULA NS 892
Rosuvastatin Calcium
Crestor 261
ROTATEQ.................. 892
Rotavirus Vaccine, Live
RotaTeq................... 892
ROWASA 893
ROXANOL................. 894
ROXANOL-T
See Roxanol............ 894
ROXICET.................. 895
ROXICODONE........... 896
ROXILOX
See Tylox 1057
ROZEREM 897
Rubella Vaccine, Live
M-M-R II 640
ProQuad.................. 829
Rufinamide
Banzel...................... 144
RYTHMOL................. 898
RYTHMOL SR............ 899
RYZOLT 900

S

SAIZEN...................... 901
Salmeterol Xinafoate
Advair 31
Advair HFA 33
Serevent.................. 917
SANCTURA
See Sanctura XR 902
SANCTURA XR.......... 902
SANDIMMUNE........... 903
SANDOSTATIN.......... 905
SANDOSTATIN LAR.... 906
Saquinavir Mesylate
Invirase.................... 510
SARAFEM 907
Sargramostim
Leukine.................... 545
SAVELLA 908
Scopolamine
Transderm Scop...... 1031
Scopolamine
Hydrobromide
Donnatal.................. 325
SEASONALE.............. 910
SEASONIQUE 911
SECTRAL................... 913
Selegiline
Emsam 357
Selegiline HCl
Eldepryl................... 347
Zelapar................... 1150
SELZENTRY 914
SENSIPAR................. 915
SEPTRA 916
Septra DS
See Septra 916
SEREVENT................ 917
SEROQUEL 918
SEROQUEL XR.......... 920
SEROSTIM................ 921
Sertraline HCl
Zoloft 1171
Sevelamer HCl
RenaGel.................. 862
Sibutramine HCl
Monohydrate
Meridia 609
Sildenafil Citrate
Revatio................... 872
Viagra 1097
Silodosin
Rapaflo.................... 848
SILVADENE............... 922
Silver Sulfadiazine
Silvadene................ 922
SIMCOR 923
SIMULECT................ 924
Simvastatin
Simcor.................... 923
Vytorin................... 1123
Zocor 1166
SINEMET
See Sinemet CR 925

SINEMET CR ... 925
SINEQUAN
See Doxepin ... 331
SINGULAIR ... 926
Sirolimus
Rapamune ... 849
Sitagliptin
Janumet ... 515
Sitagliptin Phosphate
Januvia ... 517
SKELAXIN ... 927
SKELID ... 928
Sodium Ascorbate
MoviPrep ... 649
Sodium Bicarbonate
HalfLytely ... 467
Zegerid ... 1149
Sodium Chloride
HalfLytely ... 467
MoviPrep ... 649
Sodium Ferric Gluconate Complex
Ferrlecit ... 410
Sodium Hyaluronate
Euflexxa ... 396
Hyalgan ... 481
Supartz ... 956
Sodium Phosphate
Visicol ... 1113
Sodium Polystyrene Sulfonate
Kayexalate ... 521
Sodium Sulfate
MoviPrep ... 649
Solifenacin Succinate
VESIcare ... 1094
SOLIRIS ... 929
SOLODYN ... 929
SOLTAMOX ... 931
SOLU-CORTEF ... 932
SOLU-MEDROL ... 933
SOMA ... 934
Somatropin
Humatrope ... 476
Norditropin ... 692
Nutropin ... 704
Omnitrope ... 716
Saizen ... 901
Serostim ... 921
Tev-Tropin ... 1001
Valtropin ... 1075
Zorbtive ... 1177
SOMATULINE DEPOT ... 935
SOMAVERT ... 936
SONATA ... 937
Sorafenib
Nexavar ... 677
SORIATANE ... 938
Sotalol HCl
Betapace ... 154
Betapace AF ... 156
Sotret
See Accutane ... 10
SPIRIVA ... 939
Spironolactone
Aldactazide ... 44
Aldactone ... 45
SPORANOX ... 940
Sprintec
See Ortho-Cyclen ... 731
SPRYCEL ... 941
SSD
See Silvadene ... 922
STALEVO ... 942
STARLIX ... 944
Stavudine
Zerit ... 1153
STAVZOR ... 945
STRATTERA ... 946
STREPTOMYCIN ... 947
Streptomycin Sulfate
Streptomycin ... 947
STROMECTOL ... 949
SUBLIMAZE ... 950
SUBOXONE ... 951
SUBUTEX
See Suboxone ... 951
SULAR ... 952
Sulbactam Sodium
Unasyn ... 1065
Sulfacetamide Sodium
FML-S ... 433
Ovace ... 737
Rosac ... 890
Rosula ... 891
Rosula NS ... 892
Sulfamethoxazole
Bactrim ... 141
Septra ... 916
Sulfasalazine
Azulfidine ... 138
Azulfidine EN ... 139
Sulfatrim Pediatric
See Septra ... 916
Sulfur
Rosac ... 890
Rosula ... 891
SULINDAC ... 953
Sumatriptan
Imitrex ... 490
SUMYCIN ... 954
Sunitinib Malate
Sutent ... 959
SUPARTZ ... 956
SUPRAX ... 956
SURMONTIL ... 957
SUSTIVA ... 958
SUTENT ... 959
SYMBICORT ... 960
SYMBYAX ... 962
SYMLIN ... 964
SYMLINPEN
See Symlin ... 964
SYMMETREL ... 965
SYNAGIS ... 966
SYNALAR ... 967
SYNERA ... 968
SYNERCID ... 969
SYNTHROID ... 970
SYNVISC ... 971

T

Tacrine HCl
Cognex ... 234
Tacrolimus
Prograf ... 820
Protopic ... 834
Tadalafil
Cialis ... 210
TALACEN ... 972
TALWIN NX ... 973
TAMBOCOR ... 973
TAMIFLU ... 974
TAMOXIFEN ... 975
Tamoxifen Citrate
Soltamox ... 931
Tamoxifen ... 975
Tamsulosin HCl
Flomax ... 421
TAPAZOLE ... 976
TARCEVA ... 977
TARKA ... 978
TASMAR ... 980
TAXOL ... 980
TAXOTERE ... 982
Tazarotene
Avage ... 117
Tazorac ... 984
TAZICEF ... 983
Tazobactam
Zosyn ... 1178
TAZORAC ... 984
TAZTIA XT
See Tiazac ... 1007
TEGRETOL ... 985
TEGRETOL-XR
See Tegretol ... 985
TEKTURNA ... 987
TEKTURNA HCT ... 988

Telbivudine
  Tyzeka....1059
Telithromycin
  Ketek....526
Telmisartan
  Micardis....626
  Micardis HCT....627
Temazepam
  Restoril....868
TEMODAR....989
TEMOVATE....990
Temovate Scalp
  See Temovate....990
Temovate-E
  See Temovate....990
Temozolomide
  Temodar....989
Temsirolimus
  Torisel....1027
Tenecteplase
  TNKase....1016
Tenofovir Disoproxil Fumarate
  Atripla....111
  Truvada....1051
  Viread....1111
TENORETIC....991
TENORMIN....992
TERAZOL 3....993
TERAZOL 7....994
Terazosin HCl
  Hytrin....486
Terbinafine HCl
  Lamisil....539
TERBUTALINE....994
Terconazole
  Terazol 3....993
  Terazol 7....994
Teriparatide
  Forteo....441
TESSALON....995
TESTIM....996
Testosterone
  Androderm....78
  Androgel....79
  Testim....996
Testosterone Cypionate
  Depo-Testosterone....296
TESTRED....997
TETANUS & DIPHTHERIA TOXOIDS ADSORBED....998
Tetanus Toxoid
  Boostrix....163
  Pediarix....756
  Tetanus & Diphtheria Toxoids Adsorbed....998
  Tetanus Toxoid Adsorbed....999
  Tripedia....1046
TETANUS TOXOID ADSORBED....999
Tetracaine
  Synera....968
Tetracycline HCl
  Helidac....470
  Sumycin....954
TEVETEN....999
TEVETEN HCT....1000
TEV-TROPIN....1001
Thalidomide
  Thalomid....1002
THALOMID....1002
THEO-24....1004
Theophylline
  Theo-24....1004
  Uniphyl....1066
THIORIDAZINE....1005
Thiothixene
  Navane....667
Thonzonium Bromide
  Cortisporin-TC Otic....255
Thyroid
  Armour Thyroid....99
THYROLAR....1006
Tiagabine HCl
  Gabitril....451
TIAZAC....1007
Ticarcillin Disodium
  Timentin....1011
TICLID....1008
Ticlopidine HCl
  Ticlid....1008
TIGAN....1009
Tigecycline
  Tygacil....1054
TIKOSYN....1010
Tiludronate Disodium
  Skelid....928
TIMENTIN....1011
Timolol
  Betimol....157
TIMOLOL GFS....1012
TIMOLOL MALEATE....1013
Timolol Maleate
  Combigan....238
  Cosopt....257
  Timolol GFS....1012
  Timolol Maleate....1013
  Timoptic....1014
TIMOPTIC....1014
Timoptic Ocudose
  See Timoptic....1014
Timoptic-XE
  See Timoptic....1014
TINDAMAX....1015
Tinidazole
  Tindamax....1015
Tinzaparin Sodium
  Innohep....501
Tiotropium Bromide
  Spiriva....939
Tipranavir
  Aptivus....90
Tirofiban HCl
  Aggrastat....37
Tizanidine HCl
  Zanaflex....1145
TNKASE....1016
TOBI....1017
TOBRADEX....1018
TOBRAMYCIN....1018
Tobramycin
  TOBI....1017
  TobraDex....1018
  Tobrex....1020
  Zylet....1185
Tobramycin Sulfate
  Tobramycin....1018
TOBREX....1020
TOFRANIL....1020
TOFRANIL-PM....1021
Tolcapone
  Tasmar....980
TOLMETIN....1022
Tolterodine Tartrate
  Detrol LA....300
TOPAMAX....1023
TOPAMAX SPRINKLE CAPSULES
  See Topamax....1023
TOPICORT....1025
TOPICORT LP
  See Topicort....1025
Topiramate
  Topamax....1023
TOPROL-XL....1026
TORADOL
  See Ketorolac....528
TORISEL....1027
Torsemide
  Demadex....282
Tositumomab
  Bexxar....159
TOVIAZ....1028
TRACLEER....1029
Tramadol HCl
  Ryzolt....900
  Ultracet....1062
  Ultram....1063
TRANDATE....1030
Trandolapril
  Mavik....600

Tarka 978
TRANSDERM SCOP 1031
Tranxene T-Tab
See Tranxene-SD 1032
TRANXENE-SD 1032
Tranxene-SD Half Strength
See Tranxene-SD 1032
Tranylcypromine Sulfate
Parnate 749
Trastuzumab
Herceptin 473
TRASYLOL 1033
TRAVATAN 1034
TRAVATAN Z
See Travatan 1034
Travoprost
Travatan 1034
TRAZODONE 1035
TRECATOR 1035
TRELSTAR 1036
Trelstar Depot
See Trelstar 1036
Trelstar LA
See Trelstar 1036
TRENTAL 1037
Treprostinil Sodium
Remodulin 861
Tretinoin
Renova 862
Retin-A 870
Tri-Luma 1044
Vesanoid 1093
Ziana 1161
Triamcinolone Acetonide
Azmacort 135
Kenalog 523
Nasacort AQ 663
Triamterene
Dyazide 340
Dyrenium 343
Maxzide 604
TRIAZ 1038
Triazolam
Halcion 466
TRICOR 1038
Trifluridine
Viroptic 1112
TRIGLIDE 1039
TRILEPTAL 1041
TRI-LEVLEN 1042
TRILIPIX 1043
TRI-LUMA 1044
Trimethobenzamide HCl
Tigan 1009
Trimethoprim
Bactrim 141
Septra 916
Trimethoprim HCl
Primsol 810
Trimethoprim Sulfate
Polytrim 782
Trimipramine Maleate
Surmontil 957
TRI-NORINYL 1045
TRIPEDIA 1046
TRIPHASIL 1047
Tri-Previfem
See Ortho Tri-Cyclen 727
Triptorelin Pamoate
Trelstar 1036
Tri-Sprintec
See Ortho Tri-Cyclen 727
TRIVORA 1048
TRIZIVIR 1049
Trospium Chloride
Sanctura XR 902
TRUSOPT 1050
TRUVADA 1051
TUSSIONEX
PENNKINETIC 1052
TWINJECT 1053
TWINRIX 1054
TYGACIL 1054
TYKERB 1055
TYLENOL WITH
CODEINE 1056
TYLOX 1057
TYSABRI 1058
TYZEKA 1059

U

ULORIC 1060
ULTIVA 1061
ULTRACET 1062
ULTRAM 1063
ULTRAM ER
See Ultram 1063
ULTRAVATE 1064
UNASYN 1065
UNIPHYL 1066
UNIRETIC 1067
UNITHROID 1068
UNIVASC 1070
Urea
Panafil 746
Rosula NS 892
Urokinase
Abbokinase 1
UROXATRAL 1071
Ursodiol
Actigall 17

V

VAGIFEM 1071
Valacyclovir HCl
Valtrex 1074
VALCYTE 1072
Valganciclovir HCl
Valcyte 1072
VALIUM 1073
Valproate Sodium
Depacon 286
Valproic Acid
Depakene 287
Stavzor 945
Valsartan
Diovan 317
Diovan HCT 318
Exforge 399
VALTREX 1074
VALTROPIN 1075
VANCOCIN ORAL 1076
Vancomycin HCl
Vancocin Oral 1076
Vancomycin
Injection 1077
VANCOMYCIN
INJECTION 1077
VANOS 1078
VANTAS 1079
VANTIN 1080
VAQTA 1081
Vardenafil HCl
Levitra 550
Varenicline Tartrate
Chantix 207
Varicella Virus
Vaccine, Live
ProQuad 829
Varivax 1082
VARIVAX 1082
VASERETIC 1083
VASOTEC 1084
VASOTEC I.V. 1085
VECTIBIX 1086
VEETIDS
See Penicillin VK 761
VELCADE 1087
VELIVET
See Cyclessa 266
Venlafaxine HCl
Effexor 345
Effexor XR 346
VENTAVIS 1088
VENTOLIN HFA 1089
VERAMYST 1090
Verapamil HCl
Calan 173
Calan SR 174
Covera-HS 259
Tarka 978
Verelan 1091
Verelan PM 1092

VERELAN 1091
VERELAN PM 1092
Verteporfin
Visudyne 1115
VESANOID................1093
VESICARE............... 1094
VFEND......................1095
VIADUR 1096
VIAGRA 1097
VIBRAMYCIN 1098
VIBRA-TABS
See Vibramycin...... 1098
VICODIN.................. 1100
Vicodin ES
See Vicodin 1100
Vicodin HP
See Vicodin 1100
VICOPROFEN............ 1100
VIDAZA 1102
VIDEX.......................1103
VIDEX EC
See Videx 1103
VIGAMOX 1104
VIMPAT.................... 1105
VINBLASTINE 1106
VINCRISTINE 1107
Vinorelbine Tartrate
Navelbine 668
VIRACEPT................ 1108
VIRAMUNE 1109
VIRAZOLE 1110
VIREAD 1111
VIROPTIC...................1112
VISICOL......................1113
VISTARIL
See Hydroxyzine
Pamoate..................484
VISTIDE 1114
VISUDYNE 1115
Vitamin B12
Folgard RX 2.2......... 436
Foltx........................ 437
Vitamin B6
Folgard RX 2.2......... 436
Foltx........................ 437
VITRASERT............... 1116
VIVELLE 1117
VIVELLE-DOT
See Vivelle................1117
VIVITROL.................. 1118
VOLTAREN
See Voltaren-XR........1121
VOLTAREN GEL.......... 1119
VOLTAREN
OPHTHALMIC 1121
VOLTAREN-XR 1121
Voriconazole
Vfend 1095
Vorinostat
Zolinza 1170
VOSPIRE ER..............1123
VYTORIN 1123
VYVANSE 1125

W

Warfarin Sodium
Coumadin................ 258
WELCHOL.................1126
WELLBUTRIN
See Wellbutrin SR 1127
WELLBUTRIN SR........ 1127
WELLBUTRIN XL........1128
WESTCORT...............1129

X

XALATAN 1130
XANAX.......................1131
XANAX XR................1132
XELODA 1133
XENICAL...................1134
XIBROM....................1135
XIFAXAN 1135
XIGRIS......................1136
XOLAIR.....................1137
XOPENEX 1138
XOPENEX HFA...........1138
XYLOCAINE INJECTION 1139
XYLOCAINE JELLY.... 1140
XYLOCAINE VISCOUS 1141
XYLOCAINE-MPF
See Xylocaine
Injection 1139
XYZAL......................1142

Y

YASMIN 1142
YAZ 1144

Z

Zafirlukast
Accolate......................6
Zaleplon
Sonata.................... 937
ZANAFLEX 1145
Zanamivir
Relenza 856
ZANTAC....................1146
ZARONTIN............... 1147
ZAROXOLYN.............1148
ZEBETA 1149
ZEGERID...................1149
ZELAPAR..................1150
ZEMPLAR IV 1151
ZEMPLAR ORAL.........1152
ZERIT 1153
ZESTORETIC.............1154
ZESTRIL....................1156
ZETIA 1157
ZEVALIN...................1158
ZIAC 1159
ZIAGEN.................... 1160
ZIANA...................... 1161
Ziconotide Acetate
Prialt 806
Zidovudine
Combivir.................. 241
Retrovir 870
Trizivir 1049
Zileuton
Zyflo CR 1185
ZINACEF...................1162
ZINECARD 1163
Ziprasidone HCl
Geodon 454
ZITHROMAX 1164
ZMAX 1165
ZOCOR 1166
ZOFRAN 1167
ZOLADEX 1-MONTH ...1168
ZOLADEX 3-MONTH ..1169
Zoledronic Acid
Reclast 854
Zometa...................1173
ZOLINZA 1170
Zolmitriptan
Zomig......................1174
ZOLOFT.....................1171
Zolpidem Tartrate
Ambien.....................60
Ambien CR 61
Zolpimist 1173
ZOLPIMIST................1173
ZOMETA 1173
ZOMIG 1174
Zomig Nasal Spray
See Zomig 1174
Zomig-ZMT
See Zomig 1174
ZONEGRAN 1176
Zonisamide
Zonegran................1176
ZORBTIVE................1177
ZOSTAVAX................1178
Zoster Vaccine Live
Zostavax.................1178
ZOSYN......................1178

ZOVIRAX CREAM.......1179
ZOVIRAX INJECTION 1180
ZOVIRAX OINTMENT.. 1181
ZOVIRAX ORAL.........1182
ZYBAN.....................1183
ZYDONE....................1184
ZYFLO CR.................1185
ZYLET.......................1185
ZYLOPRIM.................1186
ZYMAR.....................1187
ZYPREXA.................1188
Zyprexa IntraMuscular
See Zyprexa............1188
Zyprexa Zydis
See Zyprexa............1188
ZYVOX.....................1189

THERAPEUTIC CLASS INDEX

Organized alphabetically, this index includes the therapeutic class of each drug in the Product Information section. Therapeutic class headings are based on information provided in the drug monographs. The drug entries listed under each bold therapeutic class are organized alphabetically by brand name or monograph title (shown in capitalized letters), followed by the generic name in parentheses.

A

ACE INHIBITOR

ACCUPRIL (quinapril HCl) ... 8

ACEON (perindopril erbumine) ... 12

ALTACE (ramipril) ... 55

CAPTOPRIL (captopril) ... 181

LOTENSIN (benazepril HCl) ... 578

MAVIK (trandolapril) ... 600

MONOPRIL (fosinopril sodium) ... 644

PRINIVIL (lisinopril) ... 811

UNIVASC (moexipril HCl) ... 1070

VASOTEC (enalapril maleate) ... 1084

VASOTEC I.V. (enalaprilat) ... 1085

ZESTRIL (lisinopril) ... 1156

ACE INHIBITOR/CALCIUM CHANNEL BLOCKER (NONDIHYDROPYRIDINE)

TARKA (verapamil HCl-trandolapril) ... 978

ACE INHIBITOR/THIAZIDE DIURETIC

ACCURETIC (quinapril HCl-hydrochlorothiazide) ... 9

CAPOZIDE (hydrochlorothiazide-captopril) ... 180

LOTENSIN HCT (benazepril HCl-hydrochlorothiazide) ... 579

MONOPRIL HCT (fosinopril sodium-hydrochlorothiazide) ... 645

PRINZIDE (lisinopril-hydrochlorothiazide) ... 812

UNIRETIC (moexipril HCl-hydrochlorothiazide) ... 1067

VASERETIC (enalapril maleate-hydrochlorothiazide) ... 1083

ZESTORETIC (lisinopril-hydrochlorothiazide) ... 1154

ACETAMIDE LOCAL ANESTHETIC

EMLA (prilocaine-lidocaine) ... 356

LIDOCAINE OINTMENT (lidocaine) ... 559

LIDODERM PATCH (lidocaine) ... 560

SYNERA (tetracaine-lidocaine) ... 968

XYLOCAINE JELLY (lidocaine HCl) ... 1140

XYLOCAINE VISCOUS (lidocaine HCl) ... 1141

ACETAMINOPHEN ANTIDOTE/MUCOLYTIC

ACETYLCYSTEINE (acetylcysteine) ... 14

ACETYLCHOLINESTERASE INHIBITOR

ARICEPT (donepezil HCl) ... 96

EXELON (rivastigmine tartrate) ... 398

ACTIVATED PROTEIN C

XIGRIS (drotrecogin alfa) ... 1136

ACYCLIC NUCLEOTIDE ANALOGUE

HEPSERA (adefovir dipivoxil) ... 472

AGONIST-ANTAGONIST ANALGESIC

NUBAIN (nalbuphine HCl) ... 703

ALCOHOL OXIDATION INHIBITOR

ANTABUSE (disulfiram) ... 84

ALDOSTERONE BLOCKER

INSPRA (eplerenone) ... 503

ALKYLATING AGENT

MYLERAN (busulfan) ... 653

ALKYLATING AGENT (IMIDAZOTETRAZINE DERIVATIVE)

TEMODAR (temozolomide) ... 989

ALLYLAMINE ANTIFUNGAL
LAMISIL
(terbinafine HCl) 539

ALPHA-GLUCOSIDASE INHIBITOR
GLYSET
(miglitol).. 464
PRECOSE
(acarbose) 787

ALPHA$_1$/BETA-BLOCKER
COREG CR
(carvedilol)..................................... 252

ALPHA$_{1A}$-ANTAGONIST
FLOMAX
(tamsulosin HCl) 421

ALPHA$_1$-AGONIST
PROAMATINE
(midodrine HCl) 815

ALPHA$_1$-ANTAGONIST
RAPAFLO
(silodosin)...................................... 848
UROXATRAL
(alfuzosin HCl) 1071

ALPHA$_1$-BLOCKER (QUINAZOLINE)
CARDURA
(doxazosin mesylate)...................... 187
HYTRIN
(terazosin HCl)............................... 486
MINIPRESS
(prazosin HCl)................................ 634
CARDURA XL
(doxazosin mesylate)...................... 187

ALPHA$_2$-AGONIST/BETA-BLOCKER
COMBIGAN
(timolol maleate-brimonidine
tartrate)... 238

AMINOGLYCOSIDE
AMIKACIN
(amikacin sulfate)............................ 66
STREPTOMYCIN
(streptomycin sulfate) 947
TOBI
(tobramycin).................................. 1017
TOBRAMYCIN
(tobramycin sulfate)...................... 1018
TOBREX
(tobramycin).................................. 1020

AMINOGLYCOSIDE/ CORTICOSTEROID
PRED-G
(prednisolone acetate-gentamicin
sulfate) 789
TOBRADEX
(tobramycin-dexamethasone)........ 1018
ZYLET
(loteprednol etabonate-
tobramycin) 1185

AMINOKETONE
APLENZIN
(bupropion hydrobromide).............. 88
WELLBUTRIN SR
(bupropion HCl)............................ 1127
WELLBUTRIN XL
(bupropion HCl)............................ 1128
ZYBAN
(bupropion HCl)............................ 1183

AMINOPENICILLIN/ BETA LACTAMASE INHIBITOR
AUGMENTIN
(clavulanate potassium-amoxicillin) . 114
AUGMENTIN ES-600
(clavulanate potassium-amoxicillin) . 115
AUGMENTIN XR
(clavulanate potassium-amoxicillin) . 116

ANALGESIC, URINARY
ELMIRON
(pentosan sodium).......................... 352

ANALGESIC/SEDATIVE/ SYMPATHOMIMETIC
MIDRIN
(isometheptene mucate-dichlo-
ralphenazone-acetaminophen) 633

ANDROGEN
ANDRODERM
(testosterone)..................................... 78
ANDROGEL
(testosterone)..................................... 79
DEPO-TESTOSTERONE
(testosterone cypionate) 296
TESTIM
(testosterone)................................. 996
TESTRED
(methyltestosterone)...................... 997

ANGIOTENSIN II RECEPTOR ANTAGONIST
ATACAND
(candesartan cilexetil)................... 107
AVAPRO
(irbesartan) 123
BENICAR
(olmesartan medoxomil) 148
COZAAR
(losartan potassium) 260
DIOVAN
(valsartan) 317
MICARDIS
(telmisartan)................................... 626
TEVETEN
(eprosartan mesylate) 999

ANGIOTENSIN II RECEPTOR ANTAGONIST/THIAZIDE DIURETIC
ATACAND HCT
(candesartan cilexetil-
hydrochlorothiazide)...................... 107

AVALIDE
(irbesartan-hydrochlorothiazide)..... 118
BENICAR HCT
(olmesartan medoxomil-hydro-chlorothiazide)............................... 148
DIOVAN HCT
(hydrochlorothiazide-valsartan)...... 318
HYZAAR
(losartan potassium-hydrochloro-thiazide)..487
MICARDIS HCT
(telmisartan-hydrochlorothiazide)..627
TEVETEN HCT
(eprosartan mesylate-hydrochlo-rothiazide)..................................1000

ANTHRACYCLINE

DOXIL
(doxorubicin HCl liposome)............332
DOXORUBICIN HCL
(doxorubicin HCl)...........................333
ELLENCE
(epirubicin HCl)............................ 350

ANTIBACTERIAL AGENT

BACTROBAN NASAL
(mupirocin calcium)....................... 143

ANTIBACTERIAL COMBINATION

NEOSPORIN OPHTHALMIC
(bacitracin zinc-polymyxin B sulfate-neomycin sulfate)...............672

ANTIBACTERIAL/CORTICOSTEROID COMBINATION

CIPRODEX
(dexamethasone-ciprofloxacin)...... 218
CIPRO HC
(ciprofloxacin HCl-hydrocortisone). 213
CORTISPORIN-TC OTIC
(hydrocortisone acetate-thonzo-nium bromide-neomycin sulfate-colistin sulfate)..............................255
NEOMYCIN/POLY B/ HYDROCORTISONE OTIC
(polymyxin B sulfate-hydrocortisone-neomycin).................................... 670

ANTIBACTERIAL/KERATOLYTIC

ACANYA
(clindamycin phosphate-benzoyl peroxide)... 5
BENZACLIN
(clindamycin-benzoyl peroxide)...... 150
BENZAMYCIN
(erythromycin-benzoyl peroxide)..... 151
BREVOXYL
(benzoyl peroxide)........................166
DUAC
(clindamycin-benzoyl peroxide)..... 334
EPIDUO
(benzoyl peroxide-adapalene)....... 364
TRIAZ
(benzoyl peroxide)........................1038

ANTICHOLINERGIC

TRANSDERM SCOP
(scopolamine)................................1031
BENTYL
(dicyclomine HCl)......................... 149
HYOSCYAMINE SULFATE
(hyoscyamine sulfate).................. 485
LEVBID
(hyoscyamine sulfate).................. 548
BENZTROPINE
(benztropine mesylate)................. 152
ATROVENT NASAL
(ipratropium bromide).................... 113
DITROPAN XL
(oxybutynin chloride).................... 321
OXYTROL
(oxybutynin)...................................743

ANTICHOLINERGIC BRONCHODILATOR

ATROVENT HFA
(ipratropium bromide).................... 112
SPIRIVA
(tiotropium bromide)......................939

ANTICHOLINERGIC/BARBITURATE

DONNATAL
(hyoscyamine sulfate-atropine sulfate-scopolamine hydrobromide-phenobarbital)..............................325

ANTIDOTE, DIGOXIN TOXICITY

DIGIBIND
(digoxin immune fab [ovine])......... 312

ANTIESTROGEN

SOLTAMOX
(tamoxifen citrate)........................ 931
TAMOXIFEN
(tamoxifen citrate)........................975

ANTIFOLATE

ALIMTA
(pemetrexed disodium).................. 48

ANTIHISTAMINE

DIPHENHYDRAMINE HCL INJECTION
(diphenhydramine HCl)................. 319
ANTIVERT
(meclizine HCl)............................. 86
ASTELIN
(azelastine HCl)............................104

ANTI-INFLAMMATORY AGENT

APRISO
(mesalamine)................................. 90
ASACOL
(mesalamine)................................. 102
CANASA
(mesalamine)..................................178
COLAZAL
(balsalazide disodium)...................235
LIALDA
(mesalamine)..................................557

PENTASA
(mesalamine) 762

ANTIMANIC AGENT
ESKALITH
(lithium carbonate) 382
LITHIUM CARBONATE
(lithium carbonate) 563
LITHOBID
(lithium carbonate) 564

ANTIMETABOLITE
CLOLAR
(clofarabine) 230
FLUOROURACIL
(fluorouracil) 429

ANTIMICROBIAL
HELIDAC
(tetracycline HCl-bismuth subsalicylate-metronidazole) 470

ANTIMICROTUBULE AGENT
ABRAXANE
(paclitaxel protein-bound particles) ... 4
IXEMPRA
(ixabepilone) 514
TAXOL
(paclitaxel) 980
TAXOTERE
(docetaxel) 982

ANTIPROTOZOAL AGENT
TINDAMAX
(tinidazole) 1015
ALINIA
(nitazoxanide) 49

ARB/CALCIUM CHANNEL BLOCKER (DIHYDROPYRIDINE)
AZOR
(amlodipine besylate-olmesartan medoxomil) 137
EXFORGE
(amlodipine besylate-valsartan) 399

AROMATASE INACTIVATOR
AROMASIN
(exemestane) 100

AROMATASE INHIBITOR (NON-STEROIDAL)
ARIMIDEX
(anastrozole) 97

ATYPICAL ANXIOLYTIC
BUSPAR
(buspirone HCl) 169

AVERMECTINS DERIVATIVE
STROMECTOL
(ivermectin) 949

AZOLE ANTIFUNGAL
DIFLUCAN
(fluconazole) 310
MYCELEX TROCHE
(clotrimazole) 652
NIZORAL
(ketoconazole) 688
NOXAFIL
(posaconazole) 702
SPORANOX
(itraconazole) 940
VFEND
(voriconazole) 1095
CLOTRIMAZOLE TOPICAL
(clotrimazole) 232
EXTINA
(ketoconazole) 401
KETOCONAZOLE TOPICAL
(ketoconazole) 527
NIZORAL SHAMPOO
(ketoconazole) 689
TERAZOL 3
(terconazole) 993
TERAZOL 7
(terconazole) 994

B

BACTERIAL PROTEIN SYNTHESIS INHIBITOR
BACTROBAN
(mupirocin) 142

BARBITURATE
PHENOBARBITAL
(phenobarbital) 772

BARBITURATE/ANALGESIC
ESGIC
(acetaminophen-caffeine-butalbital) 381
ESGIC-PLUS
(acetaminophen-caffeine-butalbital) 381
FIORICET
(acetaminophen-caffeine-butalbital) 412
FIORICET WITH CODEINE
(codeine phosphate-acetaminophen-caffeine-butalbital) 413
FIORINAL
(caffeine-aspirin-butalbital) 414
FIORINAL WITH CODEINE
(codeine phosphate-caffeine-aspirin-butalbital) 415

B-COMPLEX VITAMIN/HMG-COA REDUCTASE INHIBITOR
ADVICOR
(lovastatin-niacin) 35

BENZISOXAZOLE DERIVATIVE
GEODON
(ziprasidone HCl) 454
INVEGA
(paliperidone) 509
RISPERDAL
(risperidone) 882

RISPERDAL CONSTA
(risperidone)....883

BENZODIAZEPINE
ATIVAN
(lorazepam)....109
ATIVAN INJECTION
(lorazepam)....109
DALMANE
(flurazepam HCl)....274
DIAZEPAM INJECTION
(diazepam)....307
HALCION
(triazolam)....466
LIBRIUM
(chlordiazepoxide HCl)....558
MIDAZOLAM INJECTION
(midazolam HCl)....631
NIRAVAM
(alprazolam)....684
RESTORIL
(temazepam)....868
TRANXENE-SD
(clorazepate dipotassium)....1032
VALIUM
(diazepam)....1073
XANAX
(alprazolam)....1131
XANAX XR
(alprazolam)....1132
DIASTAT
(diazepam)....306
KLONOPIN
(clonazepam)....530

BENZODIAZEPINE ANTAGONIST
ROMAZICON
(flumazenil)....889

BENZODIAZEPINE/ ANTICHOLINERGIC
LIBRAX
(chlordiazepoxide HCl-clidinium bromide)....557

BENZOTHIAZOLE
RILUTEK
(riluzole)....881

BETA-BLOCKER (GROUP II/III ANTIARRHYTHMIC)
BETAPACE
(sotalol HCl)....154
BETAPACE AF
(sotalol HCl)....156

BETA$_2$-AGONIST
ACCUNEB
(albuterol sulfate)....7
ALBUTEROL
(albuterol sulfate)....41
BROVANA
(arformoterol tartrate)....166
FORADIL
(formoterol fumarate)....438
MAXAIR
(pirbuterol acetate)....601
PERFOROMIST
(formoterol fumarate)....766
PROAIR HFA
(albuterol sulfate)....814
PROVENTIL HFA
(albuterol sulfate)....835
SEREVENT
(salmeterol xinafoate)....917
TERBUTALINE
(terbutaline sulfate)....994
VENTOLIN HFA
(albuterol sulfate)....1089
VOSPIRE ER
(albuterol sulfate)....1123
XOPENEX
(levalbuterol HCl)....1138
XOPENEX HFA
(levalbuterol tartrate)....1138

BETA$_2$-AGONIST/ ANTICHOLINERGIC
COMBIVENT
(ipratropium bromide-albuterol sulfate)....240
DUONEB
(ipratropium bromide-albuterol sulfate)....337

BIGUANIDE
FORTAMET
(metformin HCl)....439
GLUCOPHAGE XR
(metformin HCl)....458
GLUMETZA
(metformin HCl)....462

BILE ACID
ACTIGALL
(ursodiol)....17

BILE ACID SEQUESTRANT
COLESTID
(colestipol HCl)....237
QUESTRAN
(cholestyramine)....845
WELCHOL
(colesevelam HCl)....1126

BIOLOGICAL RESPONSE MODIFIER
INFERGEN
(interferon alfacon-1)....499
INTRON A
(interferon alfa-2b)....506
REBIF
(interferon beta-1a)....853

BISPHOSPHONATE
ACTONEL
(risedronate sodium)....22

ACTONEL WITH CALCIUM
(risedronate sodium-calcium carbonate)....23
AREDIA
(pamidronate disodium)....94
BONIVA
(ibandronate sodium)....162
DIDRONEL
(etidronate disodium)....309
FOSAMAX
(alendronate sodium)....443
RECLAST
(zoledronic acid)....854
SKELID
(tiludronate disodium)....928
ZOMETA
(zoledronic acid)....1173

BISPHOSPHONATE/VITAMIN D ANALOGUE
FOSAMAX PLUS D
(alendronate sodium-cholecalciferol). 444

BLOOD VISCOSITY REDUCER
TRENTAL
(pentoxifylline)....1037

BOWEL CLEANSER
MOVIPREP
(ascorbic acid-sodium ascorbate-polyethylene glycol 3350-potassium chloride-sodium chloride-sodium sulfate)....649
VISICOL
(sodium phosphate)....1113

BOWEL CLEANSER/ STIMULANT LAXATIVE
HALFLYTELY
(polyethylene glycol 3350-sodium bicarbonate-potassium chloride-sodium chloride-bisacodyl)....467

BROAD-SPECTRUM ANTHELMINTIC
ALBENZA
(albendazole)....41

BROAD-SPECTRUM ANTIFUNGAL
LOPROX
(ciclopirox)....574
PENLAC
(ciclopirox)....761

BROAD-SPECTRUM PENICILLIN
PIPERACILLIN
(piperacillin sodium)....776

BROAD-SPECTRUM PENICILLIN/ BETA-LACTAMASE INHIBITOR
TIMENTIN
(ticarcillin disodium-clavulanate potassium)....1011
ZOSYN
(piperacillin sodium-tazobactam)..1178

BROAD-SPECTRUM PROTEASE INHIBITOR
TRASYLOL
(aprotinin)....1033

BUTYROPHENONE
HALOPERIDOL
(haloperidol)....468

C

CALCIMIMETIC AGENT
SENSIPAR
(cinacalcet HCl)....915

CALCIUM CHANNEL BLOCKER
NIMODIPINE
(nimodipine)....683

CALCIUM CHANNEL BLOCKER (DIHYDROPYRIDINE)
NIFEDIPINE
(nifedipine)....682
ADALAT CC
(nifedipine)....28
CARDENE IV
(nicardipine HCl)....183
CARDENE SR
(nicardipine HCl)....184
DYNACIRC CR
(isradipine)....342
NORVASC
(amlodipine besylate)....696
PLENDIL
(felodipine)....779
PROCARDIA XL
(nifedipine)....817
SULAR
(nisoldipine)....952

CALCIUM CHANNEL BLOCKER (DIHYDROPYRIDINE)/ ACE INHIBITOR
LOTREL
(benazepril HCl-amlodipine besylate)....580

CALCIUM CHANNEL BLOCKER (NONDIHYDROPYRIDINE)
CARDIZEM
(diltiazem HCl)....185
DILTIAZEM INJECTION
(diltiazem HCl)....316
CALAN
(verapamil HCl)....173
CALAN SR
(verapamil HCl)....174
CARDIZEM CD
(diltiazem HCl)....186
COVERA-HS
(verapamil HCl)....259
DILACOR XR
(diltiazem HCl)....313

TIAZAC
(diltiazem HCl)....1007
VERELAN
(verapamil HCl)....1091
VERELAN PM
(verapamil HCl)....1092

CALCIUM CHANNEL BLOCKER/ HMG-COA REDUCTASE INHIBITOR
CADUET
(atorvastatin calcium-amlodipine besylate)....172

CANNABINOID
CESAMET
(nabilone)....206
MARINOL
(dronabinol)....599

CARBAMATE DERIVATIVE/ SALICYLATE
EQUAGESIC
(meprobamate-aspirin)....370

CARBAPENEM
DORIBAX
(doripenem)....327
INVANZ
(ertapenem sodium)....508
MERREM
(meropenem)....610

CARBONIC ANHYDRASE INHIBITOR
ACETAZOLAMIDE
(acetazolamide)....13
AZOPT
(brinzolamide)....136
TRUSOPT
(dorzolamide HCl)....1050

CARBONIC ANHYDRASE INHIBITOR/ NONSELECTIVE BETA-BLOCKER
COSOPT
(dorzolamide HCl-timolol maleate)..257

CARBOXAMIDE
CARBATROL
(carbamazepine)....182
TEGRETOL
(carbamazepine)....985
EQUETRO
(carbamazepine)....371

CARBOXYLIC ACID DERIVATIVE
DEPACON
(valproate sodium)....286
DEPAKENE
(valproic acid)....287
STAVZOR
(valproic acid)....945

CARDIAC GLYCOSIDE
LANOXIN
(digoxin)....539

CATION-EXCHANGE RESIN
KAYEXALATE
(sodium polystyrene sulfonate)....521

CCR5 CO-RECEPTOR ANTAGONIST
SELZENTRY
(maraviroc)....914

CENTRALLY ACTING ANALGESIC
RYZOLT
(tramadol HCl)....900
ULTRACET
(tramadol HCl-acetaminophen)....1062
ULTRAM
(tramadol HCl)....1063

CENTRAL ALPHA-ADRENERGIC AGONIST
CATAPRES
(clonidine)....190
METHYLDOPA
(methyldopa)....617

CENTRAL ALPHA-ADRENERGIC AGONIST/THIAZIDE DIURETIC
METHYLDOPA/HCTZ
(methyldopa-hydrochlorothiazide)..618

CENTRAL ALPHA-AGONIST/ MONOSULFAMYL DIURETIC
CLORPRES
(clonidine HCl-chlorthalidone)....231

CENTRALLY ACTING ALPHA$_2$-ADRENERGIC AGONIST
ZANAFLEX
(tizanidine HCl)....1145

CEPHALOSPORIN (4TH GENERATION)
MAXIPIME
(cefepime HCl)....603

CEPHALOSPORIN (1ST GENERATION)
CEFADROXIL
(cefadroxil monohydrate)....193
CEFAZOLIN
(cefazolin)....193
CEPHALEXIN
(cephalexin)....204

CEPHALOSPORIN (3RD GENERATION)
CEFTAZIDIME
(ceftazidime)....196
FORTAZ
(ceftazidime)....440
OMNICEF
(cefdinir)....715
ROCEPHIN
(ceftriaxone sodium)....888
SUPRAX
(cefixime)....956
TAZICEF
(ceftazidime)....983
VANTIN
(cefpodoxime proxetil)....1080

CEPHALOSPORIN (2ND GENERATION)
CEFACLOR (cefaclor) ... 191
CEFACLOR ER (cefaclor) ... 192
CEFOXITIN (cefoxitin sodium) ... 194
CEFTIN (cefuroxime axetil) ... 197
CEFZIL (cefprozil) ... 198
ZINACEF (cefuroxime) ... 1162

CHLORIDE CHANNEL ACTIVATOR
AMITIZA (lubiprostone) ... 68

CHOLESTEROL ABSORPTION INHIBITOR
ZETIA (ezetimibe) ... 1157

CHOLESTEROL ABSORPTION INHIBITOR/HMG-COA REDUCTASE INHIBITOR
VYTORIN (simvastatin-ezetimibe) ... 1123

CHOLINERGIC AGENT
PILOCARPINE (pilocarpine HCl) ... 774

CLASS I ANTIARRHYTHMIC
NORPACE (disopyramide phosphate) ... 694

CLASS IB ANTIARRHYTHMIC
MEXILETINE (mexiletine HCl) ... 624

CLASS IC ANTIARRHYTHMIC
RYTHMOL (propafenone HCl) ... 898
RYTHMOL SR (propafenone HCl) ... 899
TAMBOCOR (flecainide acetate) ... 973

CLASS III ANTIARRHYTHMIC
CORDARONE (amiodarone HCl) ... 248
CORDARONE IV (amiodarone HCl) ... 249
CORVERT (ibutilide fumarate) ... 256
PACERONE (amiodarone HCl) ... 744
TIKOSYN (dofetilide) ... 1010

COMT INHIBITOR
COMTAN (entacapone) ... 244
TASMAR (tolcapone) ... 980

C1 INHIBITOR
CINRYZE (c1 inhibitor (human)) ... 213

CORTICOSTEROID
ACLOVATE (alclometasone dipropionate) ... 16
BETAMETHASONE DIPROPIONATE (betamethasone dipropionate) ... 153
CLOBEVATE (clobetasol propionate) ... 227
CLOBEX (clobetasol propionate) ... 228
CORDRAN (flurandrenolide) ... 251
CORMAX (clobetasol propionate) ... 253
CUTIVATE (fluticasone propionate) ... 265
DESOWEN (desonide) ... 298
DIPROLENE (betamethasone (augmented) dipropionate) ... 320
ELOCON (mometasone furoate) ... 352
KENALOG (triamcinolone acetonide) ... 523
LOCOID (hydrocortisone butyrate) ... 567
LUXIQ (betamethasone valerate) ... 592
OLUX (clobetasol propionate) ... 712
OLUX-E (clobetasol propionate) ... 713
PANDEL (hydrocortisone probutate) ... 747
PSORCON E (diflorasone diacetate) ... 840
SYNALAR (fluocinolone acetonide) ... 967
TEMOVATE (clobetasol propionate) ... 990
TOPICORT (desoximetasone) ... 1025
ULTRAVATE (halobetasol propionate) ... 1064
VANOS (fluocinonide) ... 1078
WESTCORT (hydrocortisone valerate) ... 1129
CORTEF (hydrocortisone) ... 254
FLUDROCORTISONE (fludrocortisone acetate) ... 426

SOLU-CORTEF
(hydrocortisone sodium succinate) . 932
ENTOCORT EC
(budesonide) 363
ALREX
(loteprednol etabonate) 54
FML
(fluorometholone) 432
LOTEMAX
(loteprednol etabonate) 577
PRED FORTE
(prednisolone acetate) 788
PRED MILD
(prednisolone acetate) 789
AEROBID
(flunisolide) 36
ASMANEX
(mometasone furoate) 103
AZMACORT
(triamcinolone acetonide) 135
FLOVENT HFA
(fluticasone propionate) 422
PULMICORT
(budesonide) 841
QVAR
(beclomethasone dipropionate) 846
BECONASE AQ
(beclomethasone dipropionate) 147
FLONASE
(fluticasone propionate) 421
FLUNISOLIDE NASAL SPRAY
(flunisolide) 428
NASACORT AQ
(triamcinolone acetonide) 663
NASAREL
(flunisolide) 664
NASONEX
(mometasone furoate monohydrate) 665
RHINOCORT AQUA
(budesonide) 876
VERAMYST
(fluticasone furoate) 1090

CORTICOSTEROID/ ANTI-INFECTIVE
ALCORTIN
(iodoquinol-hydrocortisone) 43

CORTICOSTEROID/ AZOLE ANTIFUNGAL
LOTRISONE
(betamethasone dipropionate-clotrimazole) 581

CORTICOSTEROID/BETA$_2$ AGONIST
ADVAIR
(salmeterol xinafoate-fluticasone propionate) 31
ADVAIR HFA
(salmeterol xinafoate-fluticasone propionate) 33
SYMBICORT
(formoterol fumarate dihydrate-budesonide) 960

CORTICOSTEROID/DEPIGMENTING AGENT/KERATOLYTIC
TRI-LUMA
(fluocinolone acetonide-hydroquinone-tretinoin) 1044

COX-2 INHIBITOR
CELEBREX
(celecoxib) 199

CYCLIC LIPOPEPTIDE
CUBICIN
(daptomycin) 264

CYCLIC POLYPEPTIDE IMMUNOSUPPRESSANT
NEORAL
(cyclosporine) 671
SANDIMMUNE
(cyclosporine) 903

CYCLOPHOSPHAMIDE ANALOG
IFEX
(ifosfamide) 488

D

DIBENZAPINE DERIVATIVE
CLOZAPINE
(clozapine) 232
FAZACLO
(clozapine) 404
SEROQUEL
(quetiapine fumarate) 918
SEROQUEL XR
(quetiapine fumarate) 920

DIBENZAZEPINE
TRILEPTAL
(oxcarbazepine) 1041

DICARBAMATE ANTICONVULSANT
FELBATOL
(felbamate) 406

DICARBOXYLIC ACID ANTIMICROBIAL
AZELEX
(azelaic acid) 134
FINACEA
(azelaic acid) 411

DIHYDROFOLATE REDUCTASE INHIBITOR/ANTIBIOTIC
POLYTRIM
(polymyxin B sulfate-trimethoprim sulfate) 782

DIHYDROFOLIC ACID REDUCTASE INHIBITOR
METHOTREXATE
(methotrexate) 615

DIPEPTIDYL PEPTIDASE-4 INHIBITOR
JANUVIA
(sitagliptin phosphate) 517

DIPEPTIDYL PEPTIDASE-4 INHIBITOR/BIGUANIDE
JANUMET
(metformin HCl-sitagliptin)............ 515

DIRECT ACTING PARASYMPATHOMIMETIC
PILOPINE HS
(pilocarpine HCl)...........................775

DIRECT ACTING SKELETAL MUSCLE RELAXANT
DANTRIUM
(dantrolene sodium).......................274
DANTRIUM IV
(dantrolene sodium).......................275

DIRECT THROMBIN INHIBITOR
ARGATROBAN
(argatroban) 95

DNA METHYLTRANSFERASE INHIBITOR
DACOGEN
(decitabine)...................................273

DOPA-DECARBOXYLASE INHIBITOR/ DOPAMINE PRECURSOR
PARCOPA
(levodopa-carbidopa)....................747
SINEMET CR
(levodopa-carbidopa) 925

DOPA-DECARBOXYLASE INHIBITOR/ DOPAMINE PRECURSOR/COMT INHIBITOR
STALEVO
(entacapone-levodopa-carbidopa) .942

DOPAMINE AGONIST
SYMMETREL
(amantadine HCl)............................ 965

DOPAMINE ANTAGONIST/ PROKINETIC
METOCLOPRAMIDE
(metoclopramide HCl).................. 620

DOPAMINE RECEPTOR AGONIST
PARLODEL
(bromocriptine mesylate)...............748

DOPAMINE/NOREPINEPHRINE/ SEROTONIN REUPTAKE INHIBITOR
MERIDIA
(sibutramine HCl monohydrate)..... 609

E

ECHINOCANDIN
ERAXIS
(anidulafungin) 372

ECTOPARASITICIDE/OVICIDE
LINDANE
(lindane).. 561

EDTA DERIVATIVE
ZINECARD
(dexrazoxane).............................. 1163

EMETIC RESPONSE MODIFIER
TIGAN
(trimethobenzamide HCl).............1009

ENDOTHELIN RECEPTOR ANTAGONIST
LETAIRIS
(ambrisentan) 543
TRACLEER
(bosentan)....................................1029

EPIDERMAL GROWTH FACTOR RECEPTOR (EGFR) ANTAGONIST
ERBITUX
(cetuximab) 373

EPIDERMAL GROWTH FACTOR RECEPTOR TYROSINE KINASE INHIBITOR
TARCEVA
(erlotinib) 977

ERGOT ALKALOID
D.H.E. 45
(dihydroergotamine mesylate)........ 272
MIGRANAL
(dihydroergotamine mesylate)........633

ERYTHROPOIESIS AGENT
FOLIC ACID
(folic acid) 436

ERYTHROPOIESIS STIMULATOR
ARANESP
(darbepoetin alfa) 92
EPOGEN
(epoetin alfa) 368
PROCRIT
(epoetin alfa) 819

ESTRADIOL/NORNITROGEN MUSTARD
EMCYT
(estramustine phosphate sodium).. 354

ESTROGEN
CENESTIN
(conjugated estrogens)................. 203
CLIMARA
(estradiol)......................................223
DEPO-ESTRADIOL
(estradiol cypionate)..................... 290
ENJUVIA
(conjugated estrogens) 362
ESCLIM
(estradiol)......................................380
ESTRACE
(estradiol)......................................383

ESTRADERM
(estradiol)....................................385
ESTRASORB
(estradiol)....................................386
ESTRING
(estradiol)....................................389
ESTROGEL
(estradiol)....................................390
OGEN
(estropipate)................................711
PREMARIN TABLETS
(conjugated estrogens) 794
PREMARIN VAGINAL
(conjugated estrogens) 796
VAGIFEM
(estradiol)....................................1071
VIVELLE
(estradiol)....................................1117
PREMARIN IV
(conjugated estrogens) 793

ESTROGEN RECEPTOR ANTAGONIST
FASLODEX
(fulvestrant).................................404

ESTROGEN/ANDROGEN COMBINATION
ESTRATEST
(esterified estrogens-methyltestosterone)....................................388

ESTROGEN/PROGESTOGEN COMBINATION
NUVARING
(etonogestrel-ethinyl estradiol) 705
ORTHO EVRA
(ethinyl estradiol-norelgestromin)...726
ALESSE
(ethinyl estradiol-levonorgestrel)......47
CYCLESSA
(desogestrel-ethinyl estradiol)........266
DESOGEN
(desogestrel-ethinyl estradiol)........297
ESTROSTEP FE
(norethindrone acetate-ethinyl estradiol)....................................392
LOESTRIN
(norethindrone acetate-ethinyl estradiol-ferrous fumarate)............568
LO/OVRAL
(norgestrel-ethinyl estradiol).........565
LYBREL
(ethinyl estradiol-levonorgestrel)....592
MIRCETTE
(desogestrel-ethinyl estradiol)........638
NORDETTE-28
(ethinyl estradiol-levonorgestrel).... 691
ORTHO-CEPT
(desogestrel-ethinyl estradiol)....... 730
ORTHO-CYCLEN
(ethinyl estradiol-norgestimate)...... 731
ORTHO-NOVUM 10/11
(ethinyl estradiol-norethindrone) 735
ORTHO-NOVUM 1/35
(ethinyl estradiol-norethindrone) 732
ORTHO-NOVUM 1/50
(norethindrone-mestranol)............734
ORTHO-NOVUM 7/7/7
(ethinyl estradiol-norethindrone) 736
ORTHO TRI-CYCLEN
(ethinyl estradiol-norgestimate)...... 727
ORTHO TRI-CYCLEN LO
(ethinyl estradiol-norgestimate)......729
OVCON-35
(ethinyl estradiol-norethindrone).....738
OVCON-35 FE
(ethinyl estradiol-ferrous fumarate-norethindrone)........................739
SEASONALE
(ethinyl estradiol-levonorgestrel).... 910
SEASONIQUE
(ethinyl estradiol-levonorgestrel)..... 911
TRI-LEVLEN
(ethinyl estradiol-levonorgestrel)..1042
TRI-NORINYL
(ethinyl estradiol-norethindrone) ..1045
TRIPHASIL
(ethinyl estradiol-levonorgestrel)..1047
TRIVORA
(ethinyl estradiol-levonorgestrel)..1048
YASMIN
(drospirenone-ethinyl estradiol) 1142
YAZ
(drospirenone-ethinyl estradiol) 1144
ACTIVELLA
(norethindrone-estradiol)............... 20
ANGELIQ
(drospirenone-estradiol) 80
CLIMARA PRO
(levonorgestrel-estradiol)..............225
COMBIPATCH
(norethindrone acetate-estradiol)...239
FEMHRT
(norethindrone acetate-ethinyl estradiol).................................... 408
PREFEST
(norgestimate-estradiol) 791
PREMPHASE
(medroxyprogesterone acetate-conjugated estrogens) 797
PREMPRO
(medroxyprogesterone acetate-conjugated estrogens) 799

F

FIBRIC ACID DERIVATIVE
ANTARA
(fenofibrate) 85
LOFIBRA
(fenofibrate) 569

LOPID
(gemfibrozil)........ 571
TRICOR
(fenofibrate)........ 1038
TRIGLIDE
(fenofibrate)........ 1039
TRILIPIX
(fenofibric acid)........ 1043

5-AMINOSALICYLIC ACID DERIVATIVE/SULFAPYRIDINE
AZULFIDINE
(sulfasalazine)........ 138
AZULFIDINE EN
(sulfasalazine)........ 139

5-FLUOROCYTOSINE ANTIFUNGAL
ANCOBON
(flucytosine)........ 78

5-HT_1-AGONIST
IMITREX
(sumatriptan)........ 490

5-$HT_{1B/1D}$ AGONIST
AMERGE
(naratriptan HCl)........ 62
AXERT
(almotriptan malate)........ 129
FROVA
(frovatriptan succinate)........ 448
MAXALT
(rizatriptan benzoate)........ 601
RELPAX
(eletriptan hydrobromide)........ 857
ZOMIG
(zolmitriptan)........ 1174

5-HT_3 RECEPTOR ANTAGONIST
ALOXI
(palonosetron HCl)........ 52
ANZEMET
(dolasetron mesylate)........ 86
KYTRIL
(granisetron HCl)........ 534
ZOFRAN
(ondansetron)........ 1167
LOTRONEX
(alosetron HCl)........ 582

FLAVONOID
LIMBREL
(flavocoxid)........ 560

FLUORINATED PYRIMIDINE NUCLEOSIDE ANTIVIRAL
VIROPTIC
(trifluridine)........ 1112

FLUOROPYRIMIDINE CARBAMATE
XELODA
(capecitabine)........ 1133

FLUOROQUINOLONE
AVELOX
(moxifloxacin HCl)........ 125
CIPRO IV
(ciprofloxacin)........ 214
CIPRO ORAL
(ciprofloxacin HCl)........ 215
CIPRO XR
(ciprofloxacin)........ 217
FACTIVE
(gemifloxacin mesylate)........ 402
FLOXIN
(ofloxacin)........ 424
LEVAQUIN
(levofloxacin)........ 546
MAXAQUIN
(lomefloxacin HCl)........ 602
PROQUIN XR
(ciprofloxacin HCl)........ 830
CILOXAN
(ciprofloxacin HCl)........ 211
IQUIX
(levofloxacin)........ 511
OCUFLOX
(ofloxacin)........ 709
QUIXIN
(levofloxacin)........ 846
VIGAMOX
(moxifloxacin HCl)........ 1104
ZYMAR
(gatifloxacin)........ 1187
FLOXIN OTIC
(ofloxacin)........ 425

FOLIC ACID/VITAMIN COMBINATION
FOLGARD RX 2.2
(vitamin B12-vitamin B6-folic acid). 436
FOLTX
(vitamin B12-vitamin B6-folic acid).. 437

FUSION INHIBITOR
FUZEON
(enfuvirtide)........ 450

G

GABA ANALOG
BACLOFEN
(baclofen)........ 140
LYRICA
(pregabalin)........ 594
NEURONTIN
(gabapentin)........ 676
CAMPRAL
(acamprosate calcium)........ 176

GLUCAGON
GLUCAGON
(glucagon)........ 457

GLUCAN SYNTHESIS INHIBITOR
CANCIDAS
(caspofungin acetate)........ 179
MYCAMINE
(micafungin sodium)........ 651

GLUCOCORTICOID
DEPO-MEDROL (methylprednisolone acetate) 292
DEXAMETHASONE (dexamethasone) 301
MEDROL (methylprednisolone) 605
ORAPRED (prednisolone sodium phosphate) ... 724
PEDIAPRED (prednisolone sodium phosphate) ... 755
PREDNISONE (prednisone) 790
SOLU-MEDROL (methylprednisolone sodium succinate) 933

GLYCOPROTEIN IIB/IIIA INHIBITOR
AGGRASTAT (tirofiban HCl) 37
INTEGRILIN (eptifibatide) 504
REOPRO (abciximab) 863

GLYCOSAMINOGLYCAN
HEPARIN SODIUM (heparin sodium) 471

GLYCYLCYCLINE
TYGACIL (tigecycline) 1054

GRANULOCYTE COLONY STIMULATING FACTOR
NEUPOGEN (filgrastim) 675

GRANULOCYTE-MACROPHAGE COLONY STIMULATING FACTOR
LEUKINE (sargramostim) 545

GROWTH HORMONE RECEPTOR ANTAGONIST
SOMAVERT (pegvisomant) 936

GUANOSINE NUCLEOSIDE ANALOGUE
BARACLUDE (entecavir) 145

H

***H.PYLORI* TREATMENT COMBINATION**
PREVPAC (amoxicillin-clarithromycin-lansoprazole) 803

HEMATINIC
FERRLECIT (sodium ferric gluconate complex) .. 410

HEPARIN ANTAGONIST
PROTAMINE SULFATE (protamine sulfate) 832

HISTONE DEACETYLASE INHIBITOR
ZOLINZA (vorinostat) 1170

HIV-INTEGRASE STRAND TRANSFER INHIBITOR
ISENTRESS (raltegravir potassium) 512

HMG-COA REDUCTASE INHIBITOR
ALTOPREV (lovastatin) 56
CRESTOR (rosuvastatin calcium) 261
LESCOL XL (fluvastatin sodium) 542
LIPITOR (atorvastatin calcium) 562
MEVACOR (lovastatin) 623
PRAVACHOL (pravastatin sodium) 786
ZOCOR (simvastatin) 1166

HMG-COA REDUCTASE INHIBITOR/ NICOTINIC ACID
SIMCOR (simvastatin-niacin) 923

H_1-ANTAGONIST
ALLEGRA (fexofenadine HCl) 50
CLARINEX (desloratadine) 219
XYZAL (levocetirizine dihydrochloride) 1142
ELESTAT (epinastine HCl) 348
OPTIVAR (azelastine HCl) 721
ASTEPRO (azelastine HCl) 105

H_1-ANTAGONIST AND MAST CELL STABILIZER
PATANOL (olopatadine HCl) 751

H_1-ANTAGONIST/ SYMPATHOMIMETIC AMINE
ALLEGRA-D (fexofenadine HCl-pseudoephedrine HCl) 51
CLARINEX-D (pseudoephedrine sulfate-desloratadine) 220

HORMONAL BONE RESORPTION INHIBITOR
FORTICAL
(calcitonin-salmon (rdna origin)).... 442
MIACALCIN
(calcitonin-salmon) 625

H_2-BLOCKER
AXID
(nizatidine) 130
PEPCID
(famotidine).....................................763
ZANTAC
(ranitidine HCl) 1146

HUMAN B-TYPE NATRIURETIC PEPTIDE
NATRECOR
(nesiritide)....................................... 666

HUMAN GROWTH HORMONE
HUMATROPE
(somatropin).....................................476
NORDITROPIN
(somatropin).....................................692
NUTROPIN
(somatropin)..................................... 704
OMNITROPE
(somatropin)..................................... 716
SAIZEN
(somatropin).....................................901
SEROSTIM
(somatropin)..................................... 921
TEV-TROPIN
(somatropin).....................................1001
VALTROPIN
(somatropin)..................................... 1075
ZORBTIVE
(somatropin)..................................... 1177

HYALURONAN
EUFLEXXA
(sodium hyaluronate) 396
HYALGAN
(sodium hyaluronate) 481
SUPARTZ
(sodium hyaluronate) 956

HYDANTOIN
CEREBYX
(fosphenytoin sodium) 205
DILANTIN
(phenytoin)....................................... 313
PHENYTEK
(phenytoin sodium)..........................773

HYDROXYBENZOIC ACID DERIVATIVE
PASER
(aminosalicylic acid)......................750

HYLAN POLYMER
SYNVISC
(hylan G-F 20) 971

I

IGG_4 KAPPA ANTIBODY/ CALICHEAMICIN CONJUGATE
MYLOTARG
(gemtuzumab ozogamicin)........... 654

IMIDAZOLE ANTIBACTERIAL
METROGEL-VAGINAL
(metronidazole) 622

IMIDAZOLE ANTIBIOTIC
METROGEL
(metronidazole) 621
NORITATE
(metronidazole) 693

IMIDAZOLIDINEDIONE ANTIBACTERIAL
MACROBID
(nitrofurantoin monohydrate) 595
MACRODANTIN
(nitrofurantoin macrocrystals) 596

IMIDAZOPYRIDINE HYPNOTIC
AMBIEN
(zolpidem tartrate)......................... 60
AMBIEN CR
(zolpidem tartrate)......................... 61
ZOLPIMIST
(zolpidem tartrate)....................... 1173

IMMUNE RESPONSE MODIFIER
ALDARA
(imiquimod)...................................... 45

IMMUNOMODULATORY AGENT
COPAXONE
(glatiramer acetate) 246
THALOMID
(thalidomide)...............................1002

IMMUNOSUPPRESSIVE AGENT
AMEVIVE
(alefacept).. 64

INCRETIN MIMETIC
BYETTA
(exenatide) 170

INDOLINE DIURETIC
INDAPAMIDE
(indapamide).....................................492

INOSINE MONOPHOSPHATE DEHYDROGENASE INHIBITOR
CELLCEPT
(mycophenolate mofetil) 202
MYFORTIC
(mycophenolic acid)........................652

INOTROPIC AGENT
DOBUTAMINE
(dobutamine)...................................323
DOPAMINE
(dopamine HCl)...............................326

INSULIN
APIDRA
(insulin glulisine, rdna)....................87
HUMALOG
(insulin lispro)....................474
HUMALOG MIX 75/25
(insulin lispro protamine-insulin lispro)....................475
HUMULIN
(insulin human, rdna origin-insulin, human isophane-insulin, human regular)....................479
HUMULIN 70/30
(insulin human, rdna origin-insulin, human (isophane/regular)). 480
LANTUS
(insulin glargine, human)....................541
LEVEMIR
(insulin detemir, rdna origin)....................549
NOVOLIN
(insulin human, rdna origin-insulin, human isophane-insulin, human regular)....................698
NOVOLIN 70/30
(insulin human, rdna origin-insulin, human (isophane/regular)). 699
NOVOLOG
(insulin aspart)....................700
NOVOLOG MIX 70/30
(insulin aspart protamine-insulin aspart)....................701

INTERLEUKIN-1 RECEPTOR ANTAGONIST
KINERET
(anakinra)....................529

IRON-CHELATING AGENT
EXJADE
(deferasirox)....................400

ISONICOTINIC ACID HYDRAZIDE
ISONIAZID
(isoniazid)....................512

ISONICOTINIC ACID HYDRAZIDE/ RIFAMYCIN DERIVATIVE
RIFAMATE
(rifampin-isoniazid)....................878

ISONICOTINIC ACID HYDRAZIDE/ RIFAMYCIN DERIVATIVE/ NICOTINAMIDE ANALOGUE
RIFATER
(pyrazinamide-rifampin-isoniazid)..879

K

K^+ SUPPLEMENT
K-DUR
(potassium chloride)....................522
K-LOR
(potassium chloride)....................531
KLOR-CON M
(potassium chloride)....................532
K-TAB
(potassium chloride)....................533
MICRO-K
(potassium chloride)....................628

K^+-SPARING DIURETIC
ALDACTONE
(spironolactone)....................45
AMILORIDE
(amiloride HCl)....................67
DYRENIUM
(triamterene)....................343

K^+-SPARING DIURETIC/ THIAZIDE DIURETIC
ALDACTAZIDE
(hydrochlorothiazide-spironolactone)....................44
AMILORIDE/HCTZ
(amiloride HCl-hydrochlorothiazide) .67
DYAZIDE
(triamterene-hydrochlorothiazide). 340
MAXZIDE
(triamterene-hydrochlorothiazide). 604

KERATINOCYTE GROWTH FACTOR
KEPIVANCE
(palifermin)....................524

KETOLIDE ANTIBIOTIC
KETEK
(telithromycin)....................526

KINASE INHIBITOR
TORISEL
(temsirolimus)....................1027
TYKERB
(lapatinib)....................1055

L

LEUKOTRIENE INHIBITOR
ZYFLO CR
(zileuton)....................1185

LEUKOTRIENE RECEPTOR ANTAGONIST
ACCOLATE
(zafirlukast)....................6
SINGULAIR
(montelukast sodium)....................926

LINCOMYCIN DERIVATIVE
CLEOCIN
(clindamycin HCl)....................221
CLEOCIN T
(clindamycin phosphate)....................222
CLINDAGEL
(clindamycin phosphate)....................226
CLEOCIN VAGINAL
(clindamycin phosphate)....................223

LINCOSAMIDE DERIVATIVE/ RETINOID
ZIANA
(clindamycin phosphate-tretinoin)..1161

LIPASE INHIBITOR
XENICAL
(orlistat) ... 1134

LIPID-REGULATING AGENT
LOVAZA
(omega-3-acid ethyl esters) ... 583

LOCAL ANESTHETIC
NAROPIN
(ropivacaine HCl) ... 662
XYLOCAINE INJECTION
(lidocaine HCl) ... 1139

LOOP DIURETIC
BUMETANIDE
(bumetanide) ... 167
DEMADEX
(torsemide) ... 282
FUROSEMIDE
(furosemide) ... 449

LOW MOLECULAR WEIGHT HEPARIN
FRAGMIN
(dalteparin sodium) ... 446
INNOHEP
(tinzaparin sodium) ... 501
LOVENOX
(enoxaparin sodium) ... 583

LUTEINIZING HORMONE-RELEASING HORMONE AGONIST
TRELSTAR
(triptorelin pamoate) ... 1036
VANTAS
(histrelin acetate) ... 1079

M

MACROCYCLIC LACTONE IMMUNOSUPPRESSANT
RAPAMUNE
(sirolimus) ... 849

MACROLACTAM ASCOMYCIN DERIVATIVE
ELIDEL
(pimecrolimus) ... 349

MACROLIDE
BIAXIN
(clarithromycin) ... 160
BIAXIN XL
(clarithromycin) ... 161
E.E.S.
(erythromycin ethylsuccinate) ... 344
ERYC
(erythromycin) ... 374
ERY-TAB
(erythromycin) ... 375
ERYTHROCIN
(erythromycin stearate) ... 376
ERYTHROMYCIN BASE
(erythromycin) ... 377
ERYTHROMYCIN DELAYED-RELEASE
(erythromycin) ... 379
PCE
(erythromycin) ... 754
ZITHROMAX
(azithromycin) ... 1164
ZMAX
(azithromycin) ... 1165
AZASITE
(azithromycin) ... 133

MACROLIDE IMMUNOSUPPRESSANT
PROTOPIC
(tacrolimus) ... 834
PROGRAF
(tacrolimus) ... 820

MAST CELL STABILIZER
ALAMAST
(pemirolast potassium) ... 40
CROMOLYN SODIUM INHALATION
(cromolyn sodium) ... 263

MEGLITINIDE
PRANDIN
(repaglinide) ... 785
STARLIX
(nateglinide) ... 944

MEGLITINIDE/SULFONYLUREA
PRANDIMET
(metformin HCl-repaglinide) ... 783

MELATONIN RECEPTOR AGONIST
ROZEREM
(ramelteon) ... 897

MISCELLANEOUS ANTIANGINAL
RANEXA
(ranolazine) ... 847

MISCELLANEOUS GOUT AGENT
COLCHICINE
(colchicine) ... 235

MONOAMINE OXIDASE INHIBITOR
NARDIL
(phenelzine sulfate) ... 661
PARNATE
(tranylcypromine sulfate) ... 749

MONOAMINE OXIDASE INHIBITOR (TYPE B)
EMSAM
(selegiline) ... 357
AZILECT
(rasagiline mesylate) ... 134
ELDEPRYL
(selegiline HCl) ... 347
ZELAPAR
(selegiline HCl) ... 1150

MONOAMINO CARBOXYLIC ACID ANTI-FIBRINOLYTIC
AMICAR
(aminocaproic acid) 65

MONOBACTAM
AZACTAM
(aztreonam)..................................132

MONOCLONAL ANTIBODY
ZEVALIN
(ibritumomab tiuxetan) 1158

MONOCLONAL ANTIBODY/ CD52-BLOCKER
CAMPATH
(alemtuzumab)................................175

MONOCLONAL ANTIBODY/ CD20-BLOCKER
BEXXAR
(iodine I 131 tositumomab-tositumomab) 159
RITUXAN
(rituximab).................................... 886

MONOCLONAL ANTIBODY/ EGFR-BLOCKER
VECTIBIX
(panitumumab)............................ 1086

MONOCLONAL ANTIBODY/ HER2-BLOCKER
HERCEPTIN
(trastuzumab)................................473

MONOCLONAL ANTIBODY/ IGE-BLOCKER
XOLAIR
(omalizumab)................................ 1137

MONOCLONAL ANTIBODY/ IL-2R ALPHA (CD25) BLOCKER
SIMULECT
(basiliximab)..................................924

MONOCLONAL ANTIBODY/ PROTEIN C5 BLOCKER
SOLIRIS
(eculizumab)..................................929

MONOCLONAL ANTIBODY/RSV F-PROTEIN BLOCKER
SYNAGIS
(palivizumab).................................. 966

MONOCLONAL ANTIBODY/ TNF-ALPHA RECEPTOR BLOCKER
REMICADE
(infliximab) 859

MONOCLONAL ANTIBODY/ TNF-BLOCKER
HUMIRA
(adalimumab) 478

MONOCLONAL ANTIBODY/ VCAM-1 BLOCKER
TYSABRI
(natalizumab)................................ 1058

MONOCLONAL ANTIBODY/ VEGF-A BLOCKER
LUCENTIS
(ranibizumab) 585

MULTIKINASE INHIBITOR
NEXAVAR
(sorafenib)......................................677
SUTENT
(sunitinib malate) 959

MUSCARINIC ANTAGONIST
DETROL LA
(tolterodine tartrate)...................... 300
ENABLEX
(darifenacin) 359
SANCTURA XR
(trospium chloride) 902
TOVIAZ
(fesoterodine fumarate) 1028
VESICARE
(solifenacin succinate).................1094

MUSCULAR ANALGESIC (CENTRALLY ACTING)
ROBAXIN
(methocarbamol)............................887
SKELAXIN
(metaxalone) 927

N

NAPHTHOIC ACID DERIVATIVE (RETINOID-LIKE)
DIFFERIN
(adapalene) 310

NAPTHOQUINONE ANTIPROTOZOAL
MEPRON
(atovaquone) 608

NEURAMINIDASE INHIBITOR
RELENZA
(zanamivir) 856
TAMIFLU
(oseltamivir phosphate)..................974

NICOTINIC ACETYLCHOLINE RECEPTOR AGONIST
CHANTIX
(varenicline tartrate) 207

NICOTINIC ACID
NIASPAN
(niacin).. 680

NIPECOTIC ACID DERIVATIVE
GABITRIL
(tiagabine HCl) 451

NITRATE VASODILATOR
IMDUR
(isosorbide mononitrate).............. 489
ISOSORBIDE DINITRATE
(isosorbide dinitrate)...................... 513

MONOKET
(isosorbide mononitrate)....................644
NITRO-BID
(nitroglycerin).................................685
NITRO-DUR
(nitroglycerin).................................686
NITROLINGUAL SPRAY
(nitroglycerin).................................687
NITROSTAT
(nitroglycerin).................................688

NITROGEN MUSTARD ALKYLATING AGENT
CYTOXAN
(cyclophosphamide)..........................271
LEUKERAN
(chlorambucil)................................544

NITROIMIDAZOLE
FLAGYL
(metronidazole)...............................416
FLAGYL ER
(metronidazole)...............................417
FLAGYL IV
(metronidazole HCl).........................418

NMDA RECEPTOR ANTAGONIST
NAMENDA
(memantine HCl).............................658

NONBENZODIAZEPINE HYPNOTIC AGENT
LUNESTA
(eszopiclone)...................................586

NON-ERGOLINE DOPAMINE AGONIST
REQUIP
(ropinirole HCl)..............................864

NON-ERGOT DOPAMINE AGONIST
MIRAPEX
(pramipexole dihydrochloride)........637

NON-HALOGENATED GLUCOCORTICOID
ALVESCO
(ciclesonide).....................................57
OMNARIS
(ciclesonide)...................................714

NON-NARCOTIC ANTITUSSIVE
TESSALON
(benzonatate)..................................995

NON-NUCLEOSIDE REVERSE TRANSCRIPTASE INHIBITOR
INTELENCE
(etravirine)......................................505
RESCRIPTOR
(delavirdine mesylate)....................865
SUSTIVA
(efavirenz)......................................958
VIRAMUNE
(nevirapine)...................................1109

NON-NUCLEOSIDE REVERSE TRANSCRIPTASE INHIBITOR/ NUCLEOSIDE ANALOG COMBINATION
ATRIPLA
(tenofovir disoproxil fumarate-emtricitabine-efavirenz)....................111

NONSELECTIVE BETA-BLOCKER
INDERAL
(propranolol HCl)............................493
INDERAL LA
(propranolol HCl)............................494
INNOPRAN XL
(propranolol HCl)............................502
NADOLOL
(nadolol)..656
PINDOLOL
(pindolol)..776
TIMOLOL MALEATE
(timolol maleate)............................1013
BETAGAN
(levobunolol HCl)............................153
BETIMOL
(timolol)..157
OCUPRESS
(carteolol HCl)................................710
OPTIPRANOLOL
(metipranolol)................................720
TIMOLOL GFS
(timolol maleate)............................1012
TIMOPTIC
(timolol maleate)............................1014

NONSELECTIVE BETA-BLOCKER/ ALPHA$_1$ BLOCKER
LABETALOL
(labetalol HCl)................................535
TRANDATE
(labetalol HCl)................................1030

NONSELECTIVE BETA-BLOCKER/ THIAZIDE DIURETIC
INDERIDE
(propranolol HCl-hydrochlorothiazide)....................495

NONSTEROIDAL ANTIANDROGEN
CASODEX
(bicalutamide)................................188
NILANDRON
(nilutamide)....................................682

NONSTEROIDAL AROMATASE INHIBITOR
FEMARA
(letrozole).......................................407

NSAID
ANAPROX DS
(naproxen sodium)............................76
ANSAID
(flurbiprofen)....................................83
CATAFLAM
(diclofenac potassium)..................189

ETODOLAC
(etodolac)....................................393
ETODOLAC EXTENDED-RELEASE
(etodolac).................................... 394
INDOMETHACIN
(indomethacin)..............................497
KETOROLAC
(ketorolac tromethamine)..............528
MOBIC
(meloxicam).................................. 641
MOTRIN
(ibuprofen)...................................647
NABUMETONE
(nabumetone)...............................655
NAPRELAN
(naproxen sodium)........................659
NAPROSYN
(naproxen).................................. 660
PONSTEL
(mefenamic acid)........................... 782
SULINDAC
(sulindac).....................................953
TOLMETIN
(tolmetin sodium)......................... 1022
VOLTAREN-XR
(diclofenac sodium)...................... 1121
FLECTOR
(diclofenac epolamine).................. 419
VOLTAREN GEL
(diclofenac sodium)...................... 1119
INDOCIN I.V.
(indomethacin sodium trihydrate).. 496
ACULAR
(ketorolac tromethamine)................27
NEVANAC
(nepafenac)..................................677
VOLTAREN OPHTHALMIC
(diclofenac sodium)...................... 1121
XIBROM
(bromfenac)................................ 1135

NSAID/PROSTAGLANDIN E_1 ANALOGUE

ARTHROTEC
(diclofenac sodium-misoprostol)..... 101

NSAID/PROTON PUMP INHIBITOR

PREVACID NAPRAPAC
(lansoprazole-naproxen)................ 801

N-TYPE CALCIUM CHANNEL BLOCKER

PRIALT
(ziconotide acetate)....................... 806

NUCLEOSIDE ANALOGUE COMBINATION

COMBIVIR
(zidovudine-lamivudine)................. 241
EPZICOM
(abacavir sulfate-lamivudine).......... 369
TRIZIVIR
(abacavir sulfate-zidovudine-lamivudine)................................ 1049
TRUVADA
(tenofovir disoproxil fumarate-emtricitabine)............................. 1051

NUCLEOSIDE ANALOGUE

COPEGUS
(ribavirin)......................................247
EMTRIVA
(emtricitabine).............................358
EPIVIR
(lamivudine)................................. 366
EPIVIR-HBV
(lamivudine).................................367
FAMVIR
(famciclovir)................................ 403
REBETOL
(ribavirin)......................................852
RETROVIR
(zidovudine)..................................870
TYZEKA
(telbivudine).............................. 1059
VALTREX
(valacyclovir HCl)........................ 1074
VIDEX
(didanosine)................................ 1103
VIRAZOLE
(ribavirin).....................................1110
ZOVIRAX INJECTION
(acyclovir sodium)........................ 1180
ZOVIRAX ORAL
(acyclovir).................................. 1182
DENAVIR
(penciclovir)................................285
ZOVIRAX CREAM
(acyclovir).................................. 1179
ZOVIRAX OINTMENT
(acyclovir)...................................1181
VITRASERT
(ganciclovir).................................1116

NUCLEOSIDE ANALOGUE ANTIMETABOLITE

GEMZAR
(gemcitabine HCl).........................452

NUCLEOTIDE ANALOGUE REVERSE TRANSCRIPTASE INHIBITOR

VIREAD
(tenofovir disoproxil fumarate)........1111

O

OPIOID AGONIST-ANTAGONIST ANALGESIC

TALACEN
(pentazocine HCl-acetaminophen).. 972
TALWIN NX
(pentazocine HCl-naloxone HCl)..... 973

OPIOID ANALGESIC

ACTIQ
(fentanyl citrate) 18
ASTRAMORPH PF
(morphine sulfate).......... 106
AVINZA
(morphine sulfate).......... 127
BUPRENEX
(buprenorphine HCl) 168
COMBUNOX
(oxycodone HCl-ibuprofen) 242
DARVOCET A500
(propoxyphene napsylate-acetaminophen).......... 276
DARVOCET-N
(propoxyphene napsylate-acetaminophen).......... 277
DARVON
(propoxyphene HCl) 277
DARVON-N
(propoxyphene napsylate).......... 278
DEMEROL INJECTION
(meperidine HCl).......... 283
DEMEROL ORAL
(meperidine HCl).......... 284
DILAUDID
(hydromorphone HCl) 315
DOLOPHINE
(methadone HCl).......... 324
DURAGESIC
(fentanyl) 338
DURAMORPH
(morphine sulfate).......... 339
FENTORA
(fentanyl citrate) 409
INFUMORPH
(morphine sulfate).......... 500
KADIAN
(morphine sulfate).......... 518
LORCET
(hydrocodone bitartrate-acetaminophen).......... 575
LORTAB
(hydrocodone bitartrate-acetaminophen).......... 576
METHADOSE
(methadone HCl).......... 614
MORPHINE SULFATE IMMEDIATE RELEASE
(morphine sulfate).......... 646
MS CONTIN
(morphine sulfate).......... 649
NORCO
(hydrocodone bitartrate-acetaminophen).......... 690
OPANA ER
(oxymorphone HCl).......... 718
ORAMORPH SR
(morphine sulfate).......... 723
OXYCONTIN
(oxycodone HCl).......... 741
OXYIR
(oxycodone HCl).......... 742
PERCOCET
(oxycodone HCl-acetaminophen).... 764
PERCODAN
(oxycodone HCl-aspirin).......... 765
ROXANOL
(morphine sulfate).......... 894
ROXICET
(oxycodone HCl-acetaminophen).... 895
ROXICODONE
(oxycodone HCl).......... 896
SUBLIMAZE
(fentanyl citrate) 950
TYLENOL WITH CODEINE
(codeine phosphate-acetaminophen) 1056
TYLOX
(oxycodone HCl-acetaminophen).. 1057
ULTIVA
(remifentanil HCl).......... 1061
VICODIN
(hydrocodone bitartrate-acetaminophen) 1100
VICOPROFEN
(hydrocodone bitartrate-ibuprofen) 1100
ZYDONE
(hydrocodone bitartrate-acetaminophen) 1184

OPIOID ANALGESIC/ PHENOTHIAZINE

MEPERIDINE/PROMETHAZINE
(meperidine HCl-promethazine HCl) .. 607

OPIOID ANTAGONIST

NALOXONE
(naloxone HCl).......... 657
REVIA
(naltrexone HCl).......... 873
VIVITROL
(naltrexone).......... 1118

OPIOID ANTITUSSIVE/ ANTIHISTAMINE

TUSSIONEX PENNKINETIC
(hydrocodone polistirex-chlorpheniramine polistirex) 1052

OPIOID/ANTICHOLINERGIC

LOMOTIL
(diphenoxylate HCl-atropine sulfate) 570

ORGANOPLATINUM COMPLEX

ELOXATIN
(oxaliplatin) 353

OSMOTIC LAXATIVE

KRISTALOSE
(lactulose) 533

LACTULOSE
(lactulose)....536
MIRALAX
(polyethylene glycol 3350)....637

OXAZOLIDINONE CLASS ANTIBACTERIAL
ZYVOX
(linezolid)....1189

P

PARTIAL D_2/$5HT_{1A}$ AGONIST/ $5HT_{2A}$ ANTAGONIST
ABILIFY
(aripiprazole)....3

PARTIAL OPIOID AGONIST/OPIOID ANTAGONIST
SUBOXONE
(buprenorphine-naloxone)....951

PEGYLATED GRANULOCYTE COLONY STIMULATING FACTOR
NEULASTA
(pegfilgrastim)....673

PEGYLATED VIRUS PROLIFERATION INHIBITOR
PEGASYS
(peginterferon alfa-2a)....758
PEG-INTRON
(peginterferon alfa-2b)....759

PENICILLIN
PENICILLIN VK
(penicillin V potassium)....761
PFIZERPEN
(penicillin G potassium)....769

PENICILLIN (PENICILLINASE-RESISTANT)
DICLOXACILLIN
(dicloxacillin sodium)....308

***PENICILLIUM*-DERIVED ANTIFUNGAL**
GRIFULVIN V
(griseofulvin)....465
GRIS-PEG
(griseofulvin)....466

PEPTIDE SYNTHESIS INHIBITOR
TRECATOR
(ethionamide)....1035

PERIPHERAL VASODILATOR
MINOXIDIL
(minoxidil)....636

PHENOTHIAZINE
CHLORPROMAZINE
(chlorpromazine)....208

PHENOTHIAZINE DERIVATIVE
PROMETHAZINE
(promethazine HCl)....822
PHENERGAN INJECTION
(promethazine HCl)....770
PROCHLORPERAZINE
(prochlorperazine)....818

PHENOTHIAZINE DERIVATIVE/ ANTITUSSIVE
PROMETHAZINE DM
(dextromethorphan HBr-promethazine HCl)....823
PROMETHAZINE W/CODEINE
(promethazine HCl-codeine phosphate)....827

PHENOTHIAZINE DERIVATIVE/ANTITUSSIVE/ SYMPATHOMIMETIC
PROMETHAZINE VC/CODEINE
(phenylephrine HCl-promethazine HCl-codeine phosphate)....825

PHENOTHIAZINE DERIVATIVE/ SYMPATHOMIMETIC
PROMETHAZINE VC
(phenylephrine HCl-promethazine HCl)....824

PHENYLTRIAZINE
LAMICTAL
(lamotrigine)....537

PHOSPHATE BINDER
FOSRENOL
(lanthanum carbonate)....445
PHOSLO
(calcium acetate)....774
RENAGEL
(sevelamer HCl)....862

PHOSPHODIESTERASE III INHIBITOR
PLETAL
(cilostazol)....780

PHOSPHODIESTERASE TYPE 5 INHIBITOR
REVATIO
(sildenafil citrate)....872
CIALIS
(tadalafil)....210
LEVITRA
(vardenafil HCl)....550
VIAGRA
(sildenafil citrate)....1097

PHOTOSENSITIZING AGENT
VISUDYNE
(verteporfin)....1115

PIPERAZINE ANTIHISTAMINE
HYDROXYZINE HCL
(hydroxyzine HCl)....483
HYDROXYZINE PAMOATE
(hydroxyzine pamoate)....484

PIPERAZINO-AZEPINE
REMERON
(mirtazapine)....858

PIPERIDINE PHENOTHIAZINE
THIORIDAZINE
(thioridazine HCl)....1005

PLATELET AGGREGATION INHIBITOR
AGGRENOX
(dipyridamole-aspirin).... 38
PERSANTINE
(dipyridamole)....767
PLAVIX
(clopidogrel bisulfate)....779
TICLID
(ticlopidine HCl)....1008

PLATELET-REDUCING AGENT
AGRYLIN
(anagrelide HCl).... 39

PLEUROMUTILIN ANTIBACTERIAL
ALTABAX
(retapamulin)....55

PODOPHYLLOTOXIN DERIVATIVE
ETOPOPHOS
(etoposide phosphate)....395

POLYENE ANTIFUNGAL
ABELCET
(amphotericin B lipid complex).... 2
AMBISOME
(amphotericin B).... 61
AMPHOCIN
(amphotericin B).... 71
AMPHOTEC
(amphotericin B cholesteryl sulfate)..73
NYSTATIN ORAL
(nystatin)....707
NYSTOP
(nystatin).... 709
NYSTATIN VAGINAL
(nystatin)....708

PROGESTERONE
MEGACE ES
(megestrol acetate).... 606

PROGESTOGEN
DEPO-PROVERA CONTRACEPTIVE
(medroxyprogesterone acetate) 294
DEPO-SUBQ PROVERA 104
(medroxyprogesterone acetate) 295
MIRENA
(levonorgestrel)....639
NORPLANT II
(levonorgestrel).... 695
MICRONOR
(norethindrone) 630
AYGESTIN
(norethindrone acetate).... 131
PROVERA
(medroxyprogesterone acetate) 836
DEPO-PROVERA
(medroxyprogesterone acetate) 293

PROSTAGLANDIN ANALOG
LUMIGAN
(bimatoprost) 585
TRAVATAN
(travoprost)....1034
XALATAN
(latanoprost) 1130

PROTEASE INHIBITOR
APTIVUS
(tipranavir) 90
CRIXIVAN
(indinavir sulfate)....262
INVIRASE
(saquinavir mesylate) 510
KALETRA
(ritonavir-lopinavir) 519
LEXIVA
(fosamprenavir calcium)....555
NORVIR
(ritonavir) 697
PREZISTA
(darunavir).... 805
REYATAZ
(atazanavir sulfate)....875
VIRACEPT
(nelfinavir mesylate)....1108

PROTEASOME INHIBITOR
VELCADE
(bortezomib) 1087

PROTEIN
PULMOZYME
(dornase alfa).... 843

PROTEIN SYNTHESIS INHIBITOR
ONCASPAR
(pegaspargase)....717

PROTEIN-TYROSINE KINASE INHIBITOR
GLEEVEC
(imatinib mesylate) 455

PROTEOLYTIC ENZYME (DEBRIDING/HEALING AGENT)
PANAFIL
(chlorophyllin copper complex sodium-papain-urea)....746

PROTON PUMP INHIBITOR
ACIPHEX
(rabeprazole sodium).... 15
KAPIDEX
(dexlansoprazole) 521
NEXIUM
(esomeprazole magnesium)....678
NEXIUM IV
(esomeprazole sodium).... 680
PREVACID
(lansoprazole)....800
PRILOSEC
(omeprazole) 807

PROTONIX
(pantoprazole sodium) 833
ZEGERID
(sodium bicarbonate-omeprazole). 1149

PULMONARY AND SYSTEMIC VASODILATOR
REMODULIN
(treprostinil sodium)....................... 861

PURINE ANALOG
PURINETHOL
(mercaptopurine).......................... 843

PURINE ANTAGONIST ANTIMETABOLITE
IMURAN
(azathioprine) 491

PYRAZOLOPYRIMIDINE (NON-BENZODIAZEPINE)
SONATA
(zaleplon) 937

PYRIMIDINE NUCLEOSIDE ANALOG
VIDAZA
(azacitidine).................................. 1102

PYRIMIDINE SYNTHESIS INHIBITOR
MALARONE
(proguanil HCl-atovaquone) 598
ARAVA
(leflunomide) 93

PYRROLIDINE DERIVATIVE
KEPPRA
(levetiracetam) 524
KEPPRA XR
(levetiracetam) 526

Q

QUINAZOLINE DIURETIC
ZAROXOLYN
(metolazone) 1148

QUININE DERIVATIVE
PLAQUENIL
(hydroxychloroquine sulfate).......... 778

R

RAUWOLFIA ALKALOID
RESERPINE
(reserpine).................................... 866

RECOMBINANT HUMAN PARATHYROID HORMONE
FORTEO
(teriparatide) 441

RENIN INHIBITOR
TEKTURNA
(aliskiren)..987

RENIN INHIBITOR/ THIAZIDE DIURETIC
TEKTURNA HCT
(aliskiren-hydrochlorothiazide) 988

RETINOID
ACCUTANE
(isotretinoin)..................................... 10
RETIN-A
(tretinoin) 870
TAZORAC
(tazarotene).................................. 984
SORIATANE
(acitretin)...938
AVAGE
(tazarotene).................................... 117
RENOVA
(tretinoin) 862
VESANOID
(tretinoin) 1093

REVERSIBLE CHOLINESTERASE INHIBITOR
COGNEX
(tacrine HCl) 234

RIFAMYCIN DERIVATIVE
RIFADIN
(rifampin) 877

S

SALICYLATE
BAYER ASPIRIN
(aspirin)... 146

SELECTIVE ALPHA$_2$ AGONIST
ALPHAGAN P
(brimonidine tartrate) 53

SELECTIVE BETA$_1$-BLOCKER
BREVIBLOC
(esmolol HCl) 164
BYSTOLIC
(nebivolol) 171
LOPRESSOR
(metoprolol tartrate) 572
SECTRAL
(acebutolol HCl)............................ 913
TENORMIN
(atenolol).......................................992
TOPROL-XL
(metoprolol succinate) 1026
ZEBETA
(bisoprolol fumarate) 1149
BETOPTIC S
(betaxolol HCl) 158

SELECTIVE BETA$_1$-BLOCKER/ MONOSULFAMYL DIURETIC
TENORETIC
(chlorthalidone-atenolol)............... 991

SELECTIVE BETA$_1$-BLOCKER/ THIAZIDE DIURETIC
LOPRESSOR HCT
(metoprolol tartrate-hydrochlorothiazide)..................... 573

ZIAC
(bisoprolol fumarate-hydrochlorothiazide)....1159

SELECTIVE COSTIMULATION MODULATOR
ORENCIA
(abatacept)....725

SELECTIVE ESTROGEN RECEPTOR MODULATOR
EVISTA
(raloxifene HCl)....397

SELECTIVE NOREPINEPHRINE REUPTAKE INHIBITOR
STRATTERA
(atomoxetine HCl)....946

SELECTIVE SEROTONIN REUPTAKE INHIBITOR
SARAFEM
(fluoxetine HCl)....907
CELEXA
(citalopram hydrobromide)....201
FLUVOXAMINE
(fluvoxamine maleate)....430
LEXAPRO
(escitalopram oxalate)....554
LUVOX CR
(fluvoxamine maleate)....590
PAXIL
(paroxetine HCl)....752
PAXIL CR
(paroxetine HCl)....753
PEXEVA
(paroxetine mesylate)....768
PROZAC
(fluoxetine HCl)....838
PROZAC WEEKLY
(fluoxetine HCl)....839
ZOLOFT
(sertraline HCl)....1171

SEMISYNTHETIC AMPICILLIN DERIVATIVE
AMOXIL
(amoxicillin)....70

SEMISYNTHETIC PENICILLIN DERIVATIVE
AMPICILLIN INJECTION
(ampicillin sodium)....74
AMPICILLIN ORAL
(ampicillin)....74

SEMISYNTHETIC PENICILLIN/ BETA-LACTAMASE INHIBITOR
UNASYN
(ampicillin sodium-sulbactam sodium)....1065

SEMISYNTHETIC RIFAMPIN ANALOG
XIFAXAN
(rifaximin)....1135

SEROTONIN AND NOREPINEPHRINE REUPTAKE INHIBITOR
CYMBALTA
(duloxetine HCl)....267
EFFEXOR
(venlafaxine HCl)....345
EFFEXOR XR
(venlafaxine HCl)....346
NEFAZODONE
(nefazodone HCl)....669
PRISTIQ
(desvenlafaxine)....813
SAVELLA
(milnacipran HCl)....908

SKELETAL MUSCLE RELAXANT (CENTRALLY ACTING)
AMRIX
(cyclobenzaprine HCl)....75
FLEXERIL
(cyclobenzaprine HCl)....420
SOMA
(carisoprodol)....934

SODIUM CHANNEL INACTIVATOR
VIMPAT
(lacosamide)....1105

SOMATOSTATIN ANALOGUE
SANDOSTATIN
(octreotide acetate)....905
SANDOSTATIN LAR
(octreotide acetate)....906
SOMATULINE DEPOT
(lanreotide)....935

SPECIFIC FACTOR XA INHIBITOR
ARIXTRA
(fondaparinux sodium)....98

STREPTOGRAMIN
SYNERCID
(dalfopristin-quinupristin)....969

***STREPTOMYCES* DERIVED BACTERIOSTATIC AGENT**
SUMYCIN
(tetracycline HCl)....954

SUBSTANCE P/NEUROKININ 1 RECEPTOR ANTAGONIST
EMEND
(aprepitant)....355

SUCCINIMIDE
ZARONTIN
(ethosuximide)....1147

SULFAMATE-SUBSTITUTED MONOSACCHARIDE ANTIEPILEPTIC
TOPAMAX
(topiramate)....1023

SULFONAMIDE
ROSULA NS
(sulfacetamide sodium-urea)....892

OVACE
(sulfacetamide sodium) 737
SILVADENE
(silver sulfadiazine) 922

SULFONAMIDE ANTICONVULSANT
ZONEGRAN
(zonisamide) 1176

SULFONAMIDE/CORTICOSTEROID
FML-S
(sulfacetamide sodium-fluo-
rometholone) 433

SULFONAMIDE/SULFUR COMBINATION
ROSAC
(sulfacetamide sodium-sulfur) 890
ROSULA
(sulfacetamide sodium-sulfur) 891

SULFONAMIDE/TETRAHYDROFOLIC ACID INHIBITOR
BACTRIM
(sulfamethoxazole-trimethoprim) 141
SEPTRA
(sulfamethoxazole-trimethoprim) 916

SULFONYLUREA (1ST GENERATION)
DIABINESE
(chlorpropamide) 305

SULFONYLUREA (2ND GENERATION)
AMARYL
(glimepiride) 59
DIABETA
(glyburide) 304
GLIPIZIDE
(glipizide) 456
GLUCOTROL XL
(glipizide) 460
GLYNASE PRESTAB
(glyburide) 463
MICRONASE
(glyburide) 629

SULFONYLUREA/BIGUANIDE
GLUCOVANCE
(metformin HCl-glyburide) 461
METAGLIP
(metformin HCl-glipizide) 613

SYMPATHOMIMETIC AMINE
ADDERALL
(amphetamine salt combo) 28
ADDERALL XR
(amphetamine salt combo) 30
CONCERTA
(methylphenidate HCl) 245
DAYTRANA
(methylphenidate) 279
DESOXYN
(methamphetamine HCl) 299
DEXEDRINE
(dextroamphetamine sulfate) 302
DEXTROSTAT
(dextroamphetamine sulfate) 303
FOCALIN
(dexmethylphenidate HCl) 434
FOCALIN XR
(dexmethylphenidate HCl) 435
METADATE CD
(methylphenidate HCl) 611
METADATE ER
(methylphenidate HCl) 612
METHYLIN
(methylphenidate HCl) 619
RITALIN
(methylphenidate HCl) 884
VYVANSE
(lisdexamfetamine dimesylate) 1125

SYMPATHOMIMETIC CATECHOLAMINE
EPIPEN
(epinephrine) 365
TWINJECT
(epinephrine) 1053

SYNTHETIC AMYLIN ANALOGUE
SYMLIN
(pramlintide acetate) 964

SYNTHETIC CARBOCYCLIC NUCLEOSIDE ANALOGUE
ZIAGEN
(abacavir sulfate) 1160

SYNTHETIC GONADOTROPIN RELEASING HORMONE ANALOGUE
LUPRON PEDIATRIC
(leuprolide acetate) 590
LUPRON DEPOT (GYN)
(leuprolide acetate) 588
ELIGARD
(leuprolide acetate) 350
LUPRON
(leuprolide acetate) 587
LUPRON DEPOT (Oncology)
(leuprolide acetate) 589
VIADUR
(leuprolide acetate) 1096
ZOLADEX 1-MONTH
(goserelin acetate) 1168
ZOLADEX 3-MONTH
(goserelin acetate) 1169

SYNTHETIC GUANINE DERIVATIVE
CYTOVENE
(ganciclovir) 270

SYNTHETIC GUANINE DERIVATIVE NUCLEOSIDE ANALOGUE
VALCYTE
(valganciclovir HCl) 1072

SYNTHETIC THYMIDINE NUCLEOSIDE ANALOGUE
ZERIT
(stavudine)....1153

SYNTHETIC VASOPRESSIN ANALOGUE
DDAVP
(desmopressin acetate)....281

SYSTEMIC AND PULMONARY ARTERIAL VASCULAR BED DILATOR
VENTAVIS
(iloprost)....1088

T

TETRACYCLINE DERIVATIVE
DORYX
(doxycycline hyclate)....328
DYNACIN
(minocycline HCl)....341
MINOCIN
(minocycline HCl)....635
MONODOX
(doxycycline monohydrate)....642
SOLODYN
(minocycline HCl)....929
VIBRAMYCIN
(doxycycline hyclate)....1098
ORACEA
(doxycycline)....722

TETRAHYDROFOLIC ACID INHIBITOR
PRIMSOL
(trimethoprim HCl)....810

THALIDOMIDE ANALOGUE
REVLIMID
(lenalidomide)....874

THIAZIDE DIURETIC
DIURIL
(chlorothiazide)....322
HYDROCHLOROTHIAZIDE
(hydrochlorothiazide)....482
MICROZIDE
(hydrochlorothiazide)....630

THIAZOLIDINEDIONE
ACTOS
(pioglitazone HCl)....26
AVANDIA
(rosiglitazone maleate)....122

THIAZOLIDINEDIONE/BIGUANIDE
ACTOPLUS MET
(pioglitazone HCl-metformin HCl)....24
AVANDAMET
(metformin HCl-rosiglitazone maleate)....120

THIAZOLIDINEDIONE/SULFONYLUREA
AVANDARYL
(rosiglitazone maleate-glimepiride)..121
DUETACT
(pioglitazone HCl-glimepiride)....335

THIENAMYCIN/DEHYDROPEPTIDASE I INHIBITOR
PRIMAXIN I.M.
(imipenem-cilastatin)....808
PRIMAXIN I.V.
(imipenem-cilastatin)....809

THIENOBENZODIAZEPINE
ZYPREXA
(olanzapine)....1188

THIENOBENZODIAZEPINE/SELECTIVE SEROTONIN REUPTAKE INHIBITOR
SYMBYAX
(fluoxetine HCl-olanzapine)....962

THIOUREA-DERIVATIVE ANTITHYROID AGENT
PROPYLTHIOURACIL
(propylthiouracil)....828

THIOXANTHENE
NAVANE
(thiothixene)....667

THROMBIN INHIBITOR
ANGIOMAX
(bivalirudin)....82
REFLUDAN
(lepirudin)....855

THROMBOLYTIC AGENT
ABBOKINASE
(urokinase)....1
ACTIVASE
(alteplase)....19
RETAVASE
(reteplase)....869
TNKASE
(tenecteplase)....1016

THROMBOPOIETIC AGENT
NEUMEGA
(oprelvekin)....674

THYROID HORMONE SYNTHESIS INHIBITOR
TAPAZOLE
(methimazole)....976

THYROID REPLACEMENT HORMONE
ARMOUR THYROID
(thyroid)....99
CYTOMEL
(liothyronine sodium)....269
LEVOTHROID
(levothyroxine sodium)....551
LEVOXYL
(levothyroxine sodium)....552

SYNTHROID
(levothyroxine sodium)....................970
THYROLAR
(liotrix)..1006
UNITHROID
(levothyroxine sodium)................1068

TNF-RECEPTOR BLOCKER
CIMZIA
(certolizumab pegol).......................212
ENBREL
(etanercept) 360

TOPICAL CORTICOSTEROID
CLODERM
(clocortolone pivalate) 229

TOPICAL IMMUNOMODULATOR
RESTASIS
(cyclosporine)................................867

TOPOISOMERASE I INHIBITOR
CAMPTOSAR
(irinotecan HCl) 176

TOXOID
TETANUS TOXOID ADSORBED
(tetanus toxoid) 999

TOXOID COMBINATION
TETANUS & DIPHTHERIA TOXOIDS ADSORBED
(diphtheria toxoid-tetanus toxoid) . 998

TRIAZOLE DERIVATIVE
BANZEL
(rufinamide)...................................144

TRIAZOLOPYRIDINE DERIVATIVE
TRAZODONE
(trazodone HCl).......................... 1035

TRICYCLIC ANTIDEPRESSANT
AMITRIPTYLINE
(amitriptyline HCl)..........................69
DOXEPIN
(doxepin HCl)................................ 331
PAMELOR
(nortriptyline HCl).........................745
SURMONTIL
(trimipramine maleate)...................957
TOFRANIL
(imipramine HCl).........................1020
TOFRANIL-PM
(imipramine pamoate)..................1021

TRICYCLIC GLYCOPEPTIDE ANTIBIOTIC
VANCOCIN ORAL
(vancomycin HCl)........................ 1076
VANCOMYCIN INJECTION
(vancomycin HCl)........................ 1077

TYPE I AND II 5 ALPHA-REDUCTASE INHIBITOR (2ND GENERATION)
AVODART
(dutasteride)................................. 128

TYPE II 5 ALPHA-REDUCTASE INHIBITOR
PROPECIA
(finasteride)...................................828
PROSCAR
(finasteride)................................... 831

TYROSINE KINASE INHIBITOR
SPRYCEL
(dasatinib) 941

U

URICOSURIC
COLCHICINE/PROBENECID
(probenecid-colchicine)..................236
PROBENECID
(probenecid) 816

V

VACCINE
ENGERIX-B
(hepatitis B (recombinant))............ 361
FLULAVAL
(influenza virus vaccine)................427
FLUMIST
(influenza virus vaccine live)...........427
FLUZONE
(influenza virus vaccine)................ 431
GARDASIL
(human papillomavirus recombinant vaccine, quadrivalent)...................452
HAVRIX
(hepatitis A vaccine (inactivated)) . 469
M-M-R II
(rubella vaccine live-measles vaccine live-mumps vaccine live) ... 640
PNEUMOVAX 23
(pneumococcal vaccine)................ 781
PREVNAR
(pneumococcal vaccine, diphtheria conjugate) 803
PROQUAD
(varicella virus vaccine live-rubella vaccine live-measles vaccine live-mumps vaccine live).......................829
RECOMBIVAX HB
(hepatitis B (recombinant))............855
ROTATEQ
(rotavirus vaccine, live)..................892
TWINRIX
(hepatitis A vaccine (inactivated)-hepatitis B (recombinant)) 1054
VAQTA
(hepatitis B immune globulin).......1081
VARIVAX
(varicella virus vaccine live) 1082
ZOSTAVAX
(zoster vaccine live) 1178

VACCINE/TOXOID COMBINATION
BOOSTRIX
(pertussis vaccine, acellular-diphtheria toxoid-tetanus toxoid).... 163
PEDIARIX
(pertussis vaccine, acellular-hepatitis B (recombinant)-poliovirus vaccine, inactivated-diphtheria toxoid-tetanus toxoid)....................756
TRIPEDIA
(pertussis vaccine, acellular-diphtheria toxoid-tetanus toxoid)..1046

VALPROATE COMPOUND
DEPAKOTE
(divalproex sodium) 288
DEPAKOTE ER
(divalproex sodium) 289

VASCULAR ENDOTHELIAL GROWTH FACTOR (VEGF) INHIBITOR
AVASTIN
(bevacizumab)............................... 124
MACUGEN
(pegaptanib sodium)......................597

VASODILATOR
HYDRALAZINE
(hydralazine HCl) 482

VINCA ALKALOID
NAVELBINE
(vinorelbine tartrate).................... 668
VINBLASTINE
(vinblastine sulfate)......................1106
VINCRISTINE
(vincristine sulfate)....................... 1107

VIRAL DNA SYNTHESIS INHIBITOR
VISTIDE
(cidofovir)....................................1114

VITAMIN D ANALOGUE
ZEMPLAR IV
(paricalcitol).................................. 1151
ZEMPLAR ORAL
(paricalcitol)................................. 1152

VITAMIN D_3 DERIVATIVE
DOVONEX
(calcipotriene) 329
DOVONEX SCALP
(calcipotriene) 330

VITAMIN K-DEPENDENT COAGULATION FACTOR INHIBITOR
COUMADIN
(warfarin sodium)...........................258

W

WAKEFULNESS-PROMOTING AGENT
NUVIGIL
(armodafinil).................................707
PROVIGIL
(modafinil)....................................837

X

XANTHINE BRONCHODILATOR
THEO-24
(theophylline) 1004
UNIPHYL
(theophylline) 1066

XANTHINE OXIDASE INHIBITOR
ULORIC
(febuxostat)..................................1060
ZYLOPRIM
(allopurinol)................................. 1186
ALOPRIM
(allopurinol sodium) 52

Visual Identification Guide

VISUAL IDENTIFICATION GUIDE*

ABILIFY

RX

(aripiprazole)

OTSUKA AMERICA PHARMACEUTICAL

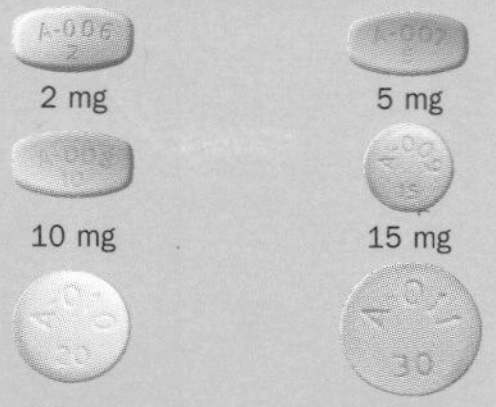

2 mg 5 mg 10 mg 15 mg 20 mg 30 mg

ABILIFY DISCMELT

RX

(aripiprazole)

OTSUKA AMERICA PHARMACEUTICAL

10 mg 15 mg

ACIPHEX

RX

(rabeprazole sodium)

EISAI/PRICARA

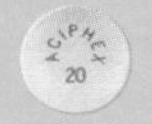

20 mg

Delayed-Release Tablets

ACTONEL

RX

(risedronate sodium)

PROCTER & GAMBLE

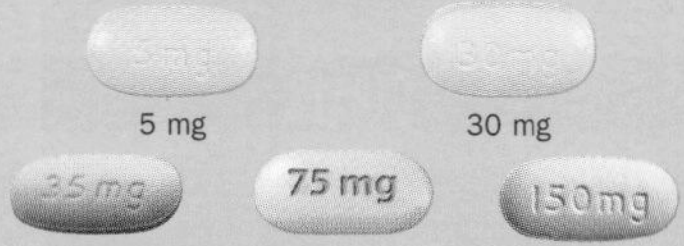

5 mg 30 mg 35 mg 75 mg 150 mg

ACTOS

RX

(pioglitazone HCl)

TAKEDA

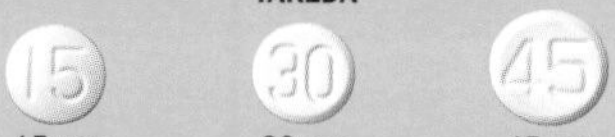

15 mg 30 mg 45 mg

ACTOPLUS MET

RX

(pioglitazone HCl/metformin HCl)

TAKEDA

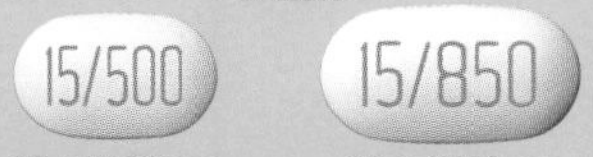

15 mg/500 mg 15 mg/850 mg

ADDERALL XR

C-II

(amphetamine salt combo)

SHIRE

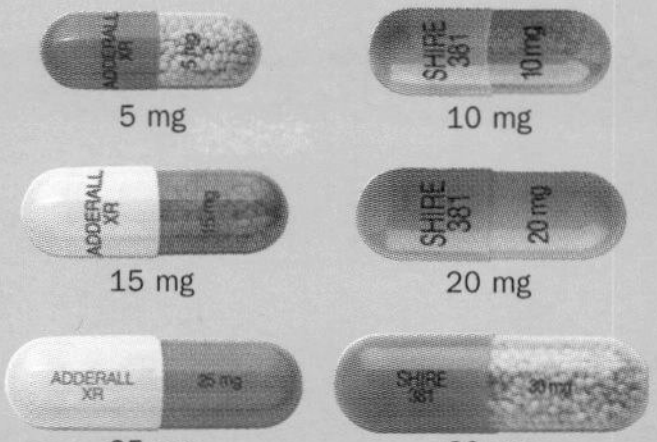

5 mg 10 mg 15 mg 20 mg 25 mg 30 mg

Extended-Release Capsules

ALLEGRA

RX

(fexofenadine HCl)

sanofi-aventis, U.S.

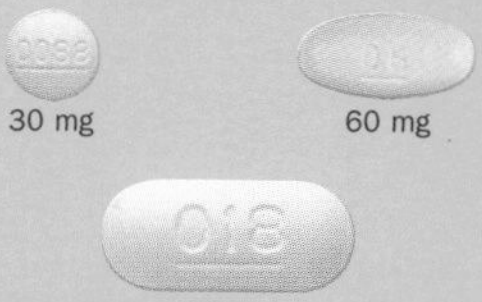

30 mg 60 mg 180 mg

ALLEGRA-D 12 HOUR

RX

(fexofenadine HCl/pseudoephedrine HCl)

sanofi-aventis, U.S.

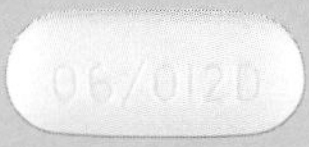

60 mg/120 mg

Extended-Release Tablets

ALLEGRA-D 24 HOUR

RX

(fexofenadine HCl/pseudoephedrine HCl)

sanofi-aventis, U.S.

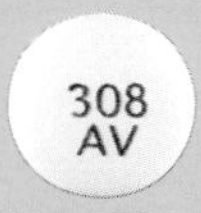

180 mg/240 mg

Extended-Release Tablets

AMBIEN

C-IV

(zolpidem tartrate)

sanofi-aventis, U.S.

5 mg 10 mg

*Other dosage forms and strengths may be available

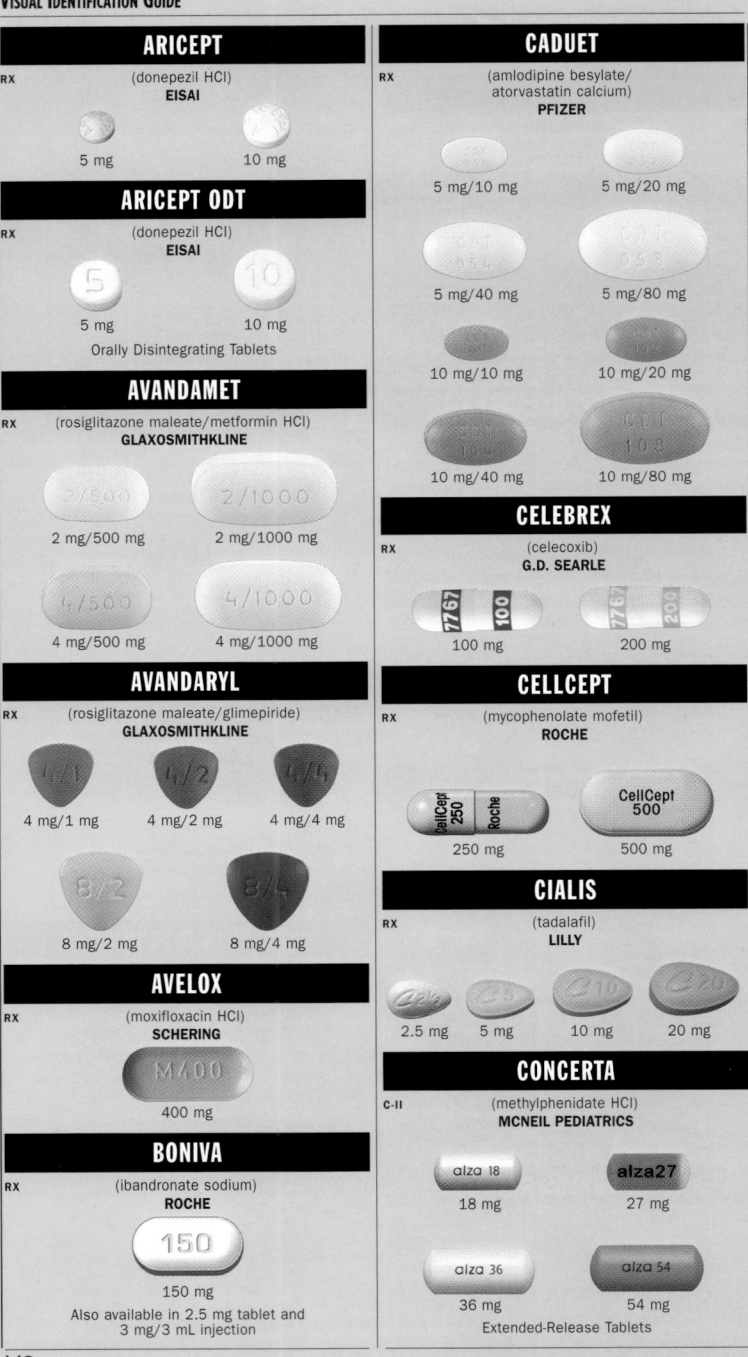

ARICEPT

RX (donepezil HCl)
EISAI

5 mg | 10 mg

ARICEPT ODT

RX (donepezil HCl)
EISAI

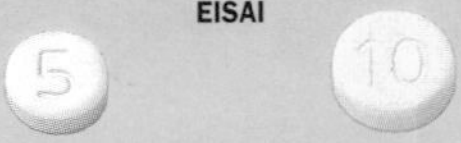

5 mg | 10 mg

Orally Disintegrating Tablets

AVANDAMET

RX (rosiglitazone maleate/metformin HCl)
GLAXOSMITHKLINE

2 mg/500 mg | 2 mg/1000 mg

4 mg/500 mg | 4 mg/1000 mg

AVANDARYL

RX (rosiglitazone maleate/glimepiride)
GLAXOSMITHKLINE

4 mg/1 mg | 4 mg/2 mg | 4 mg/4 mg

8 mg/2 mg | 8 mg/4 mg

AVELOX

RX (moxifloxacin HCl)
SCHERING

400 mg

BONIVA

RX (ibandronate sodium)
ROCHE

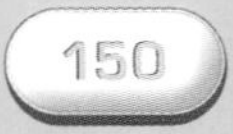

150 mg

Also available in 2.5 mg tablet and 3 mg/3 mL injection

CADUET

RX (amlodipine besylate/atorvastatin calcium)
PFIZER

5 mg/10 mg | 5 mg/20 mg

5 mg/40 mg | 5 mg/80 mg

10 mg/10 mg | 10 mg/20 mg

10 mg/40 mg | 10 mg/80 mg

CELEBREX

RX (celecoxib)
G.D. SEARLE

100 mg | 200 mg

CELLCEPT

RX (mycophenolate mofetil)
ROCHE

250 mg | 500 mg

CIALIS

RX (tadalafil)
LILLY

2.5 mg | 5 mg | 10 mg | 20 mg

CONCERTA

C-II (methylphenidate HCl)
MCNEIL PEDIATRICS

18 mg | 27 mg

36 mg | 54 mg

Extended-Release Tablets

COREG CR

RX

(carvedilol phosphate)
GLAXOSMITHKLINE

10 mg 20 mg

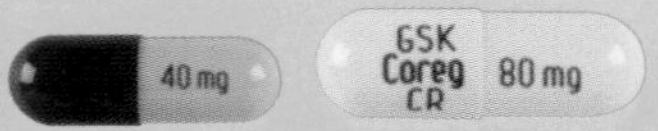

40 mg 80 mg

Extended-Release Capsules

COUMADIN

RX

(warfarin sodium)
BRISTOL-MYERS SQUIBB

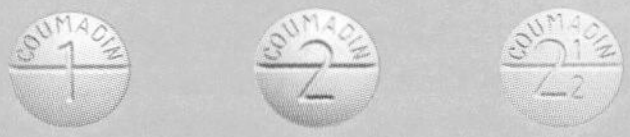

1 mg 2 mg 2.5 mg

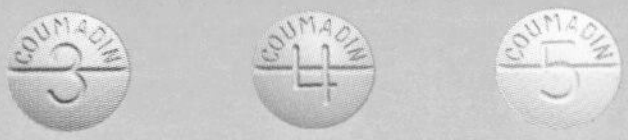

3 mg 4 mg 5 mg

6 mg 7.5 mg 10 mg

COZAAR

RX

(losartan potassium)
MERCK & CO., INC.

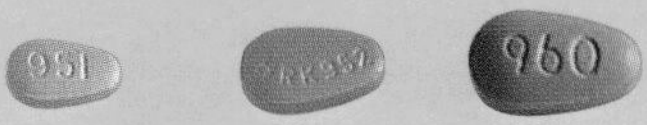

25 mg 50 mg 100 mg

Registered trademark of E.I. du Pont de Nemours and Company.

CRESTOR

RX

(rosuvastatin calcium)
ASTRAZENECA

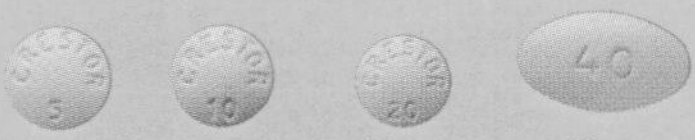

5 mg 10 mg 20 mg 40 mg

CYMBALTA

RX

(duloxetine HCl)
LILLY

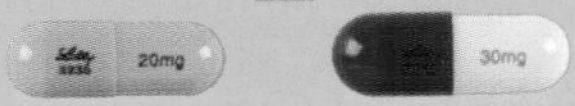

20 mg 30 mg

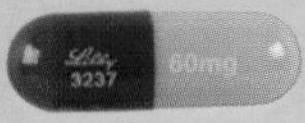

60 mg

Delayed-Release Capsules

DEPAKOTE

RX

(divalproex sodium)
ABBOTT

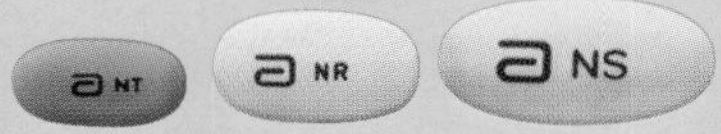

125 mg 250 mg 500 mg

Delayed-Release Tablets

DEPAKOTE ER

RX

(divalproex sodium)
ABBOTT

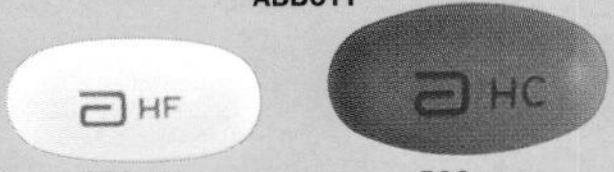

250 mg 500 mg

Extended-Release Tablets

DETROL LA

RX

(tolterodine tartrate)
PHARMACIA & UPJOHN

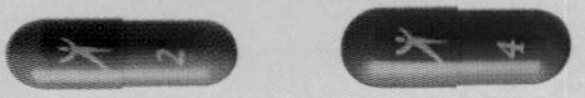

2 mg 4 mg

Extended-Release Capsules

DIOVAN

RX

(valsartan)
NOVARTIS

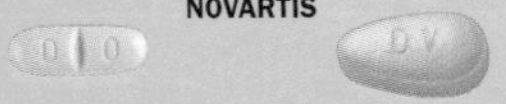

40 mg 80 mg

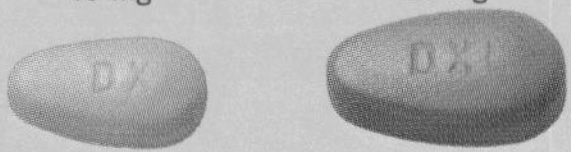

160 mg 320 mg

DIOVAN HCT

RX

(valsartan/hydrochlorothiazide)
NOVARTIS

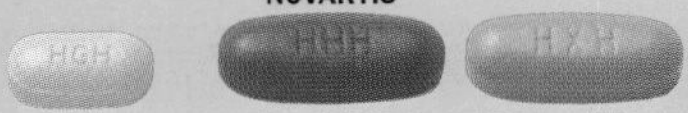

80 mg/12.5 mg 160 mg/12.5 mg 160 mg/25 mg

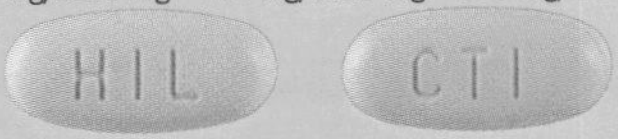

320 mg/12.5 mg 320 mg/25 mg

EFFEXOR XR

RX

(venlafaxine HCl)
WYETH

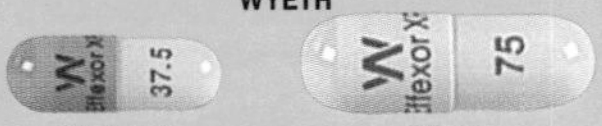

37.5 mg 75 mg

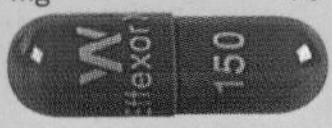

150 mg

Extended-Release Capsules

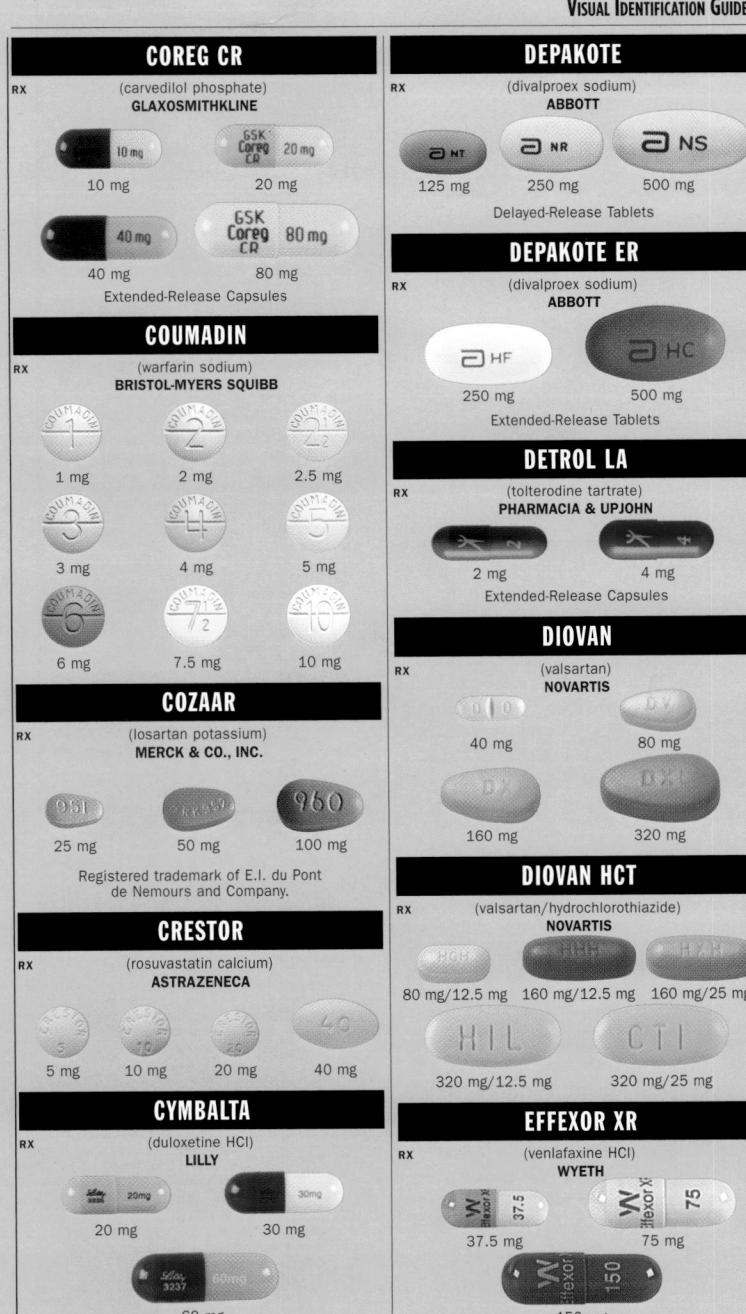

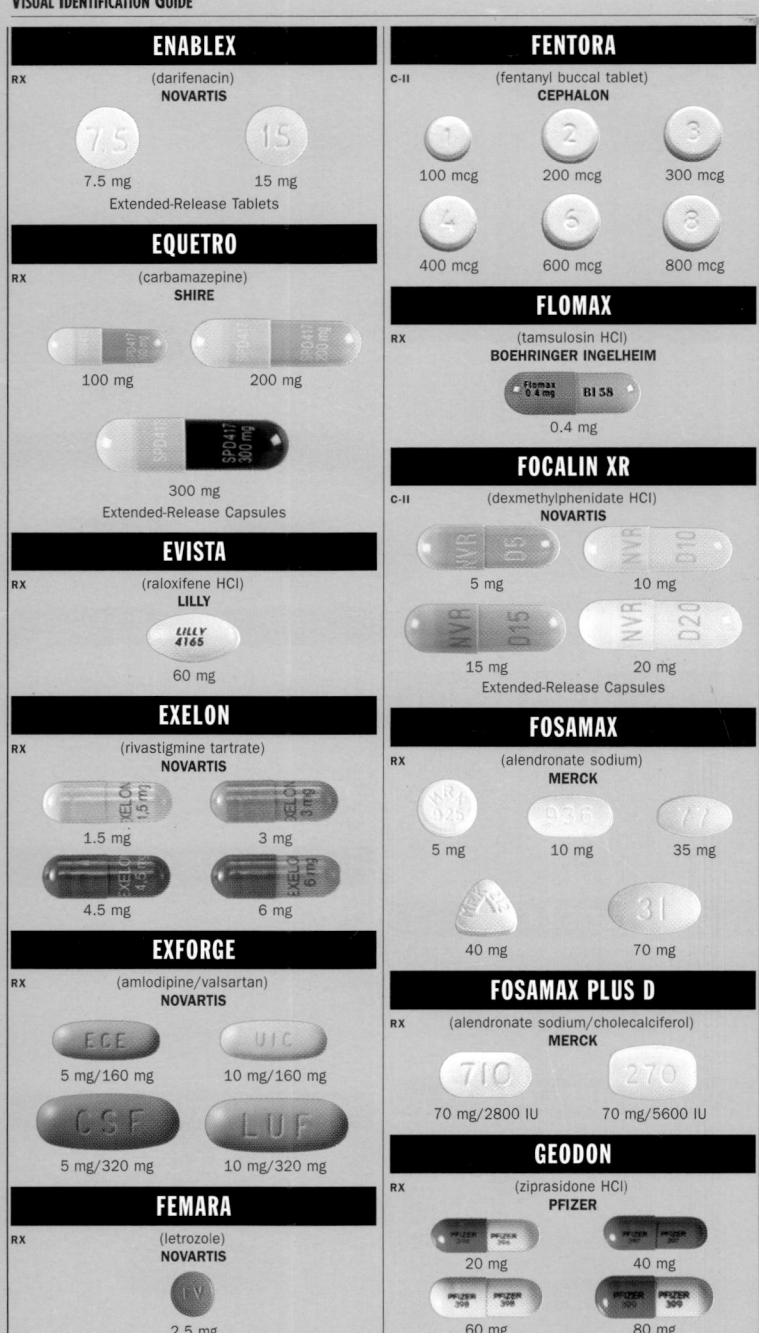

ENABLEX

RX

(darifenacin)

NOVARTIS

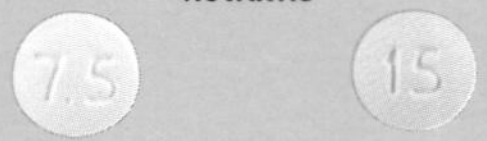

7.5 mg 15 mg

Extended-Release Tablets

EQUETRO

RX

(carbamazepine)

SHIRE

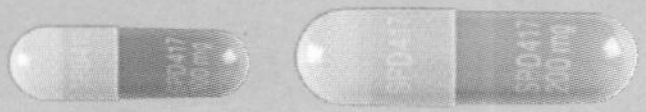

100 mg 200 mg

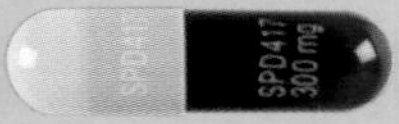

300 mg

Extended-Release Capsules

EVISTA

RX

(raloxifene HCl)

LILLY

60 mg

EXELON

RX

(rivastigmine tartrate)

NOVARTIS

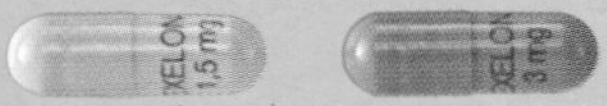

1.5 mg 3 mg

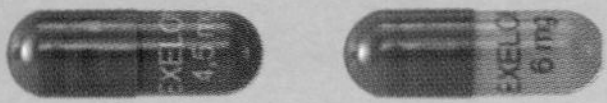

4.5 mg 6 mg

EXFORGE

RX

(amlodipine/valsartan)

NOVARTIS

5 mg/160 mg 10 mg/160 mg

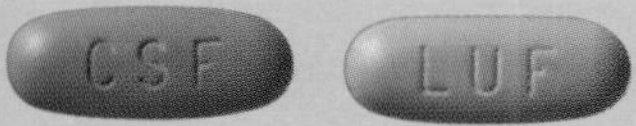

5 mg/320 mg 10 mg/320 mg

FEMARA

RX

(letrozole)

NOVARTIS

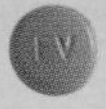

2.5 mg

FENTORA

C-II

(fentanyl buccal tablet)

CEPHALON

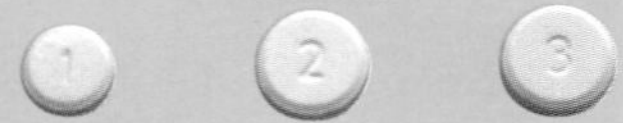

100 mcg 200 mcg 300 mcg

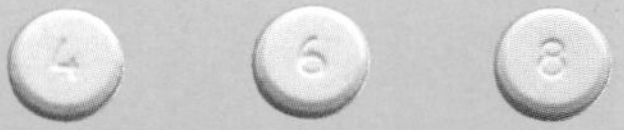

400 mcg 600 mcg 800 mcg

FLOMAX

RX

(tamsulosin HCl)

BOEHRINGER INGELHEIM

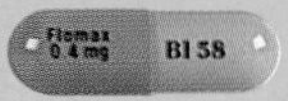

0.4 mg

FOCALIN XR

C-II

(dexmethylphenidate HCl)

NOVARTIS

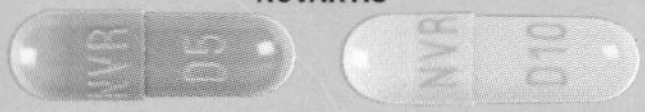

5 mg 10 mg

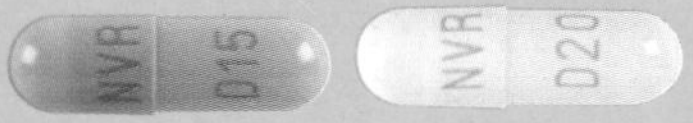

15 mg 20 mg

Extended-Release Capsules

FOSAMAX

RX

(alendronate sodium)

MERCK

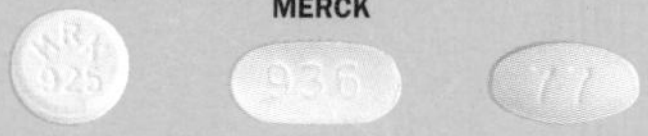

5 mg 10 mg 35 mg

40 mg 70 mg

FOSAMAX PLUS D

RX

(alendronate sodium/cholecalciferol)

MERCK

70 mg/2800 IU 70 mg/5600 IU

GEODON

RX

(ziprasidone HCl)

PFIZER

20 mg 40 mg

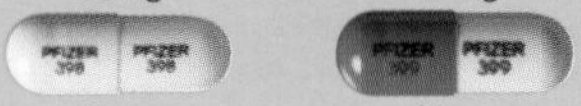

60 mg 80 mg